SYNOPSIS OF

DISEASES

of the CHEST

SYNOPSIS OF

DISEASES
of the CHEST

THIRD EDITION

Richard S. Fraser, MD, CM
Professor of Pathology
McGill University Health Centre
Montreal General Hospital
Montreal, Quebec
Canada

Neil Colman, MD
Associate Professor of Medicine
McGill University Health Centre
Montreal General Hospital
Montreal, Quebec
Canada

Nestor L. Müller, MD, PhD
Professor of Radiology
University of British Columbia and Vancouver General Hospital
Vancouver, British Columbia
Canada

P.D. Paré, MD, CM
Professor of Medicine
University of British Columbia
St. Paul's Hospital
Vancouver, British Columbia
Canada

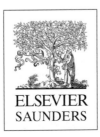

ELSEVIER
SAUNDERS

ELSEVIER
SAUNDERS

The Curtis Center
170 S Independence Mall W 300E
Philadelphia, Pennsylvania 19106

SYNOPSIS OF DISEASES OF THE CHEST   ISBN 0-7216-0445-5
Copyright © 2005, 1994, 1983, Elsevier Inc.

NOTICE

Medicine is an ever-changing field. Standard safety precautions must be followed, but as new research and clinical experience broaden our knowledge, changes in treatment and drug therapy may become necessary or appropriate. Readers are advised to check the most current product information provided by the manufacturer of each drug to be administered to verify the recommended dose, the method and duration of administration, and contraindications. It is the responsibility of the licensed prescriber, relying on experience and knowledge of the patient, to determine dosages and the best treatment for each individual patient. Neither the publisher nor the author assumes any liability for any injury and/or damage to persons or property arising from this publication.

Library of Congress Cataloging-in-Publication Data

Synopsis of diseases of the chest / [edited by] Richard S. Fraser . . . [et al.].—3rd ed.
    p.   ;   cm.
  Synopsis of: Fraser and Paré's diagnosis of diseases of the chest. 4th ed. 1999.
  Includes bibliographical references and index.
  ISBN 0-7216-0445-5
  1. Chest—Diseases.   I. Fraser, Richard S.   II. Fraser and Paré's diagnosis of diseases of the chest.
    [DNLM: 1. Thoracic Diseases.   2. Lung Diseases. WF 975 S993 2005]
RC941.P28 2005
617.5'4–dc22

Editor: Allan Ross
Developmental Editor: Denise LeMelledo
Editorial Assistant: Edward Pontee
Publishing Services Manager: Tina Rebane
Project Manager: Amy Norwitz
Designer: Gene Harris
Marketing Manager: Emily McGrath-Christie

Printed in the United States of America

Last digit is the print number: 9   8   7   6   5   4   3   2   1

This book is dedicated to our wives:

Marie-Claire

Margo

Ruth

Lisa

and children:

Emily, Nicky, Russell, Eli, Zofia, Alison,

Phillip, Peter, and Jesse

PREFACE

As in previous editions of *Diagnosis of Diseases of the Chest*, the fourth edition (1999) was so large that we thought it was likely to be used predominantly as a reference text. In an attempt to make its material more accessible, we decided to create an abbreviated version, or synopsis, aimed principally at residents in radiology (*Radiologic Diagnosis of Diseases of the Chest*, 2001). The present text, *Synopsis of Diseases of the Chest*, represents a similar effort aimed predominantly at residents and physicians in respiratory medicine or thoracic surgery and at physicians in other subspecialties seeking a relatively concise review of chest disease. Although the two synopses overlap to some extent, the text presented here has a considerably greater emphasis on clinical, pathogenetic, and pathologic features of disease and a corresponding decrease in the number of radiologic images and their description. Moreover, because there has been a 5-year period since the publication of the large book, the text has been considerably updated.

With minor exceptions, the 23 chapters in this book follow the same order and cover more or less the same material as the 79 chapters of the fourth edition of *Diagnosis of Diseases of the Chest*. The first part of the book is concerned with descriptions of the normal chest, the techniques by which chest disease can be investigated and diagnosed, and the principal radiologic abnormalities encountered during the course of investigation. The remaining chapters cover specific chest diseases organized roughly according to etiology. For ease in reading and understanding, most discussions have been subdivided into etiology and pathogenesis, pathologic characteristics, radiologic and clinical manifestations, laboratory findings, and prognosis and natural history. Because radiography and computed tomography play such important roles in diagnosis, we have retained numerous radiologic illustrations from the fourth edition; however, many have been cropped or reduced in order to restrict the length of the book to manageable proportions. A series of color figures of pathologic material has been added to better illustrate this facet of disease. Although this synopsis is not meant to be a reference text, numerous references are cited so that the interested reader can further pursue a particular subject.

As in previous editions, we invite our readers to inform us of differences of opinion they may have with the contents of this book and of areas that need improvement.

RSF

NC

NLM

PDP

ACKNOWLEDGMENTS

It is not possible to overstate our gratitude to the many individuals who helped produce this book. Donna O'Connor, Joan O'malley, Marydoolah Nundoo, and Kamillah McIntosh-Roberts of the McGill University Health Centre (MUHC) aided in the organization of the references and of the manuscript in general. Peter Thomas Paré aided in the formulation of line drawings of physiologic and pathophysiologic mechanisms. Help in production of the pathologic images was given by Larry Aubut and Leena Narsinghani, also of the MUHC. We also wish to thank the many colleagues and friends who provided us with radiologic images.

We have received considerable support and cooperation from individuals at Elsevier, particularly Denise LeMelledo, Amy Norwitz, and Allan Ross, each of whom helped to minimize the obstacles we encountered.

Finally, we would like to acknowledge the patience and understanding displayed by our wives and children throughout our work. Without their continuous encouragement this book would not have been completed, and once again we acknowledge their support with love.

RSF

NC

NLM

PDP

CONTENTS

COLOR FIGURES

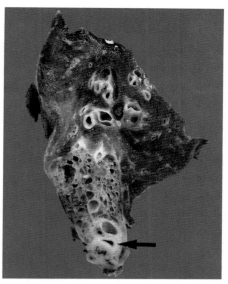

COLOR FIGURE 5–1

Intralobar sequestration. A parasagittal slice of the left lower lobe shows a well-demarcated multicystic lesion in the posterior basal aspect. A thick-walled vessel that originated in the descending aorta can be seen near the pleura (*arrow*).

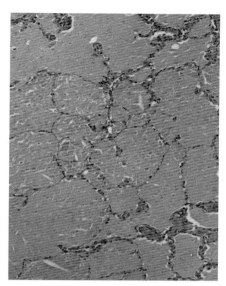

COLOR FIGURE 5–2

Pulmonary alveolar proteinosis. A section shows filling of alveolar air spaces by somewhat granular eosinophilic material. The alveolar septa are normal.

COLOR FIGURE 5–3

Pulmonary amyloidosis. A section of a pulmonary nodule (**A**) shows effacement of the parenchyma by homogeneous eosinophilic material (amyloid). Scattered multinucleated giant cells (*arrowheads*) and plasma cells (*arrow*) are present in the adjacent fibrous tissue. A section from another patient (**B**) shows mild to moderate thickening of the alveolar septa by amyloid (*large arrow*). The *small arrow* shows a normal septum.

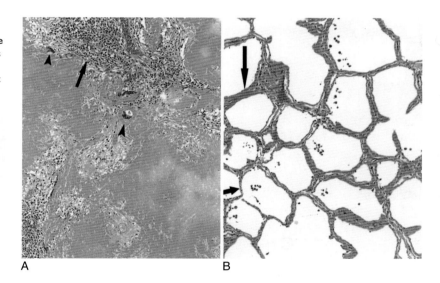

A   B

COLOR FIGURE 6–1

Acute air space pneumonia. A slice of an unfixed left lung hilum shows homogeneous consolidation of the upper lobe; histologic examination showed extensive air space filling by neutrophils (gray hepatization). Premortem blood specimens grew *Streptococcus pneumoniae*.

COLOR FIGURE 6–2

Acute bronchopneumonia. A parasagittal slice of the left lung (**A**) shows multiple foci of consolidation in the lower lobe and lingula. Confluent pneumonia associated with necrosis and hemorrhage is evident in the upper lobe and midportion of the lower lobe. A low-magnification view of a focus of very early disease (**B**) shows the patchy nature of the pneumonia to better advantage. The lumina of membranous and respiratory bronchioles and/or their accompanying pulmonary arteries can be seen in relation to the inflammatory exudate in a number of foci (*arrows*).

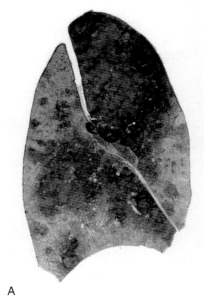

A

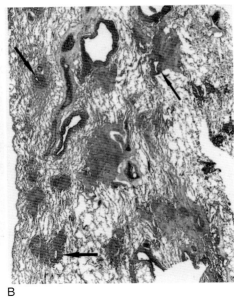

B

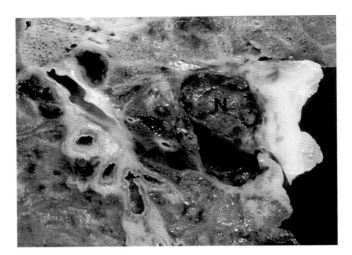

COLOR FIGURE 6–3

Chronic pulmonary abscess. A magnified view of a slice of the right lower lobe shows a well-demarcated cavity that contains necrotic tissue (N). The adjacent pleura shows marked fibrosis. The causative organism was not established.

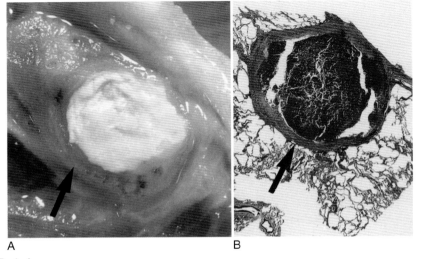

A   B

COLOR FIGURE 6–4

Tuberculosis—healed granulomas. A view of a peribronchial lymph node (**A**) shows a focus of cheese-like necrotic material completely surrounded by fibrous capsule. A low-magnification view of lung parenchyma (**B**) shows the corresponding histologic appearance of a lesion in the lung parenchyma. *Arrows* show capsule.

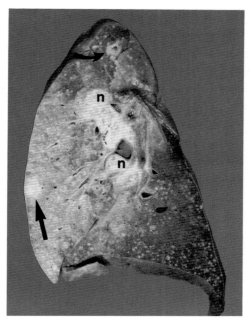

COLOR FIGURE 6–5

Progressive primary tuberculosis. A parasagittal slice of the right lung near the hilum shows a 2-cm focus of consolidation in the subpleural region of the upper lobe (*straight arrow*) (Ghon focus). The peribronchial lymph nodes (n) are enlarged and replaced by necrotic (caseous) tissue. The remaining lung parenchyma shows numerous randomly distributed nodules, 0.5 to 2 mm in diameter, that represent miliary dissemination. A single ill-defined nodular focus of consolidation approximately 1.5 cm in diameter, possibly with early cavitation, is also evident in the apical portion of the upper lobe (*curved arrow*).

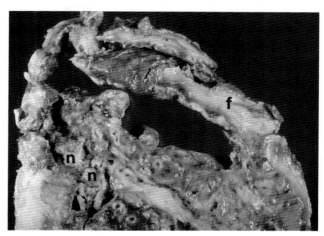

COLOR FIGURE 6–6

Tuberculosis—cavity formation. A magnified view of a slice of an upper lobe shows an irregularly shaped cavity. The adjacent lung shows fibrosis (f) and necrosis (n).

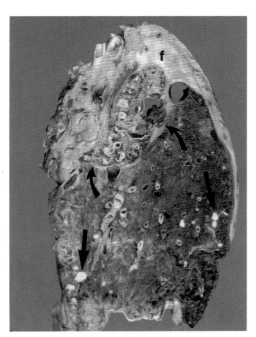

COLOR FIGURE 6–7

Tuberculosis—fibrosis and endobronchial spread. A parasagittal slice of the right lung shows marked atelectasis and fibrosis of the upper lobe (*curved arrows*) as a result of long-standing tuberculosis. A cavity is evident in its posterior aspect, and there is adjacent pleural fibrosis (f) and adherent mediastinal adipose tissue. Several foci of caseous necrosis that represent partially healed endobronchial spread of the disease can be seen in the lower and middle lobes (*long arrows*).

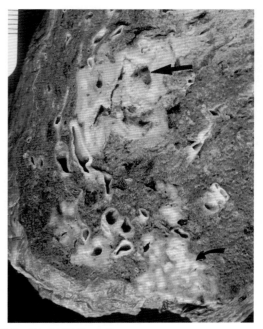

COLOR FIGURE 6–8

Tuberculosis—endobronchial spread. A magnified view of a slice of the right upper lobe shows an irregular focus of consolidation containing a small cavity (*long arrow*). A focus of bronchopneumonia confined predominantly to a single lobule in the inferior aspect (*curved arrow*) is also evident.

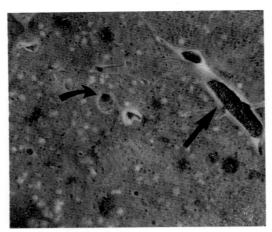

COLOR FIGURE 6–9

Miliary tuberculosis. A magnified view of lung shows a pulmonary vein (*large arrow*) and a centrilobular bronchiole (*curved arrow*). Numerous white nodules about 1 mm in diameter are scattered more or less randomly throughout the parenchyma.

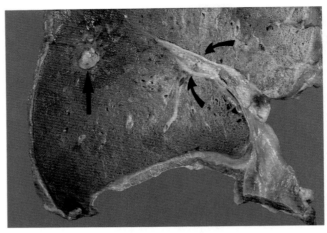

COLOR FIGURE 6–10

Histoplasmosis—chronic middle lobe collapse. A magnified view of the right lung shows a focus of white necrotic tissue surrounded by fibrous tissue in the superior segment of the lower lobe (*long arrow*). This necrotic focus represents the initial, now healed site of infection (analogous to the Ghon focus of tuberculosis). The right middle lobe (*curved arrows*) shows marked atelectasis and fibrosis as a result of obstruction of its bronchus by enlarged peribronchial lymph nodes that were replaced by similar healed granulomas (the nodes themselves are not evident on this view).

COLOR FIGURE 6–11

Histoplasmoma. A well-circumscribed subpleural nodule shows prominent laminations and a thin capsule (*arrow*). The appearance corresponds to a histoplasmoma seen on a chest radiograph.

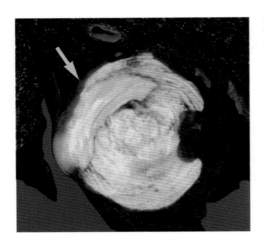

COLOR FIGURE 6–12

Pneumocystis pneumonia. A magnified view (**A**) of a transbronchial biopsy specimen from a 42-year-old man with AIDS shows mild interstitial thickening related to a mononuclear inflammatory cell infiltrate; finely vacuolated eosinophilic material is present within the alveolar air spaces. A silver stain (**B**) shows the material to contain numerous round or sickle-shaped cysts.

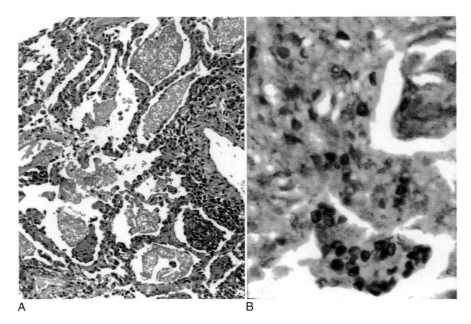

A   B

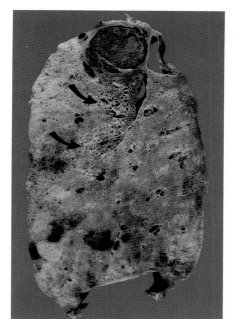

COLOR FIGURE 6–13

Aspergilloma—hemorrhage and airway obstruction. A parasagittal slice of the left lung shows a large cavity in the apex of the upper lobe that is almost completely filled by a somewhat laminated brown mass. The latter represents fungal hyphae admixed with blood from recent hemorrhage. Blood can also be seen in the airways and the parenchyma elsewhere in the lung and represents endobronchial spread. Fine fibrosis is evident in the upper lobe (*arrows*) as a result of chronic sarcoidosis. The patient was a 25-year-old woman who died as a result of the airway obstruction.

COLOR FIGURE 6–14

Aspergillus bronchopneumonia. A parasagittal slice of the right lung (**A**) shows numerous foci of necrotic white tissue distributed in a patchy fashion throughout the upper and middle lobes. A magnified view (**B**) shows these foci to be located adjacent to blood vessels (*curved arrows*) or in the centrilobular region (the *straight arrow* shows an interlobular septum), indicating an intimate association with small airways.

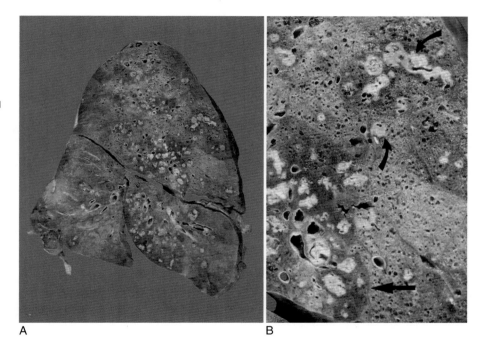

A

B

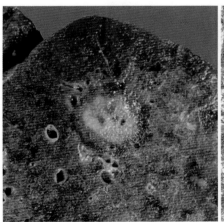

A

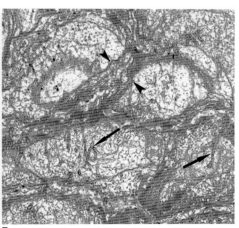

B

COLOR FIGURE 6–15

Angioinvasive aspergillosis. A magnified view of the superior segment of the right lower lobe (**A**) shows a well-circumscribed, more or less round focus of necrotic parenchyma surrounded by a hemorrhagic rim. A section of the necrotic portion (**B**) shows intact parenchymal architecture—a recognizable but edematous alveolar septum is indicated between the *arrowheads*—and alveolar air space filling by fibrin, blood, and fungal hyphae (*arrows*).

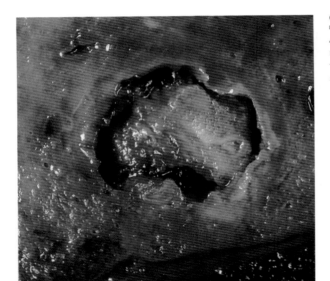

COLOR FIGURE 6-16

Angioinvasive aspergillosis. A highly magnified view of lung reveals a fragment of necrotic tissue within a thin-walled cavity. The shape of the fragment corresponds to that of the cavity, suggesting that it has developed by separation from the adjacent parenchyma.

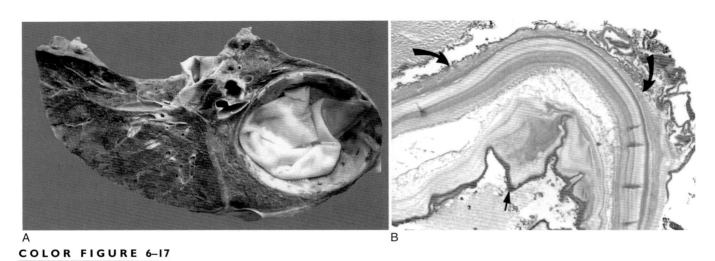

A   B

COLOR FIGURE 6-17

Hydatid cyst. A transverse slice of the right lung (**A**) shows an oval cyst in the superior segment of the lower lobe. The exo-endocyst has partially separated from the pericyst. A section (**B**) shows the laminated exocyst (*curved arrows*) and the thin, densely staining endocyst (*straight arrow*).

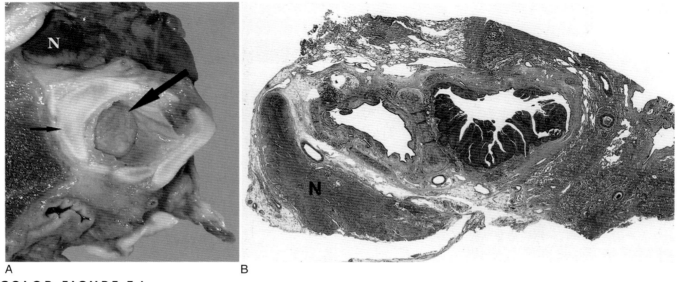

A   B

COLOR FIGURE 7-1

Squamous cell carcinoma—early lesion. A highly magnified view of lung (**A**) shows the lumen of a segmental bronchus completely occluded by a polypoid tumor (*long arrow*). A whole-mount section from another patient (**B**) demonstrates two segmental bronchi; the one on the left is normal and the other is partly occluded by a papillary tumor that shows no evidence of mucosal invasion. N, normal peribronchial lymph node; *short arrow*, bronchial cartilage.

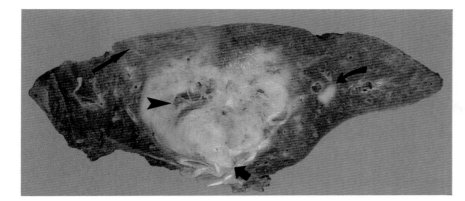

Squamous cell carcinoma. A transverse slice of the right upper lobe shows a fairly well demarcated tumor in its midportion. Some of the tumor is present in the lumen of a segmental bronchus (*short arrow*). The distal portion of lung has a granular yellow appearance indicative of obstructive pneumonitis (*long arrow*). Early cavity formation (*arrowhead*) and endobronchial spread of tumor (*curved arrow*) are also evident.

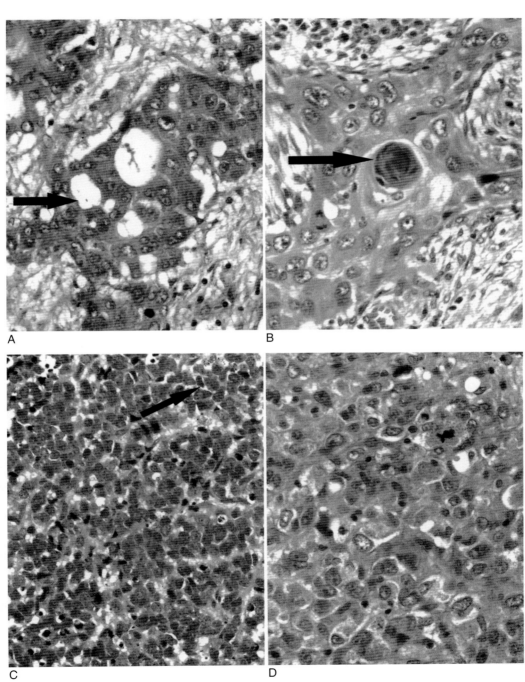

A

B

C

D

COLOR FIGURE 7–3

Pulmonary carcinoma—histologic appearance. The four main histologic types of pulmonary carcinoma are presented (all views photographed at the same magnification). **A,** adenocarcinoma (*arrow* showing glandular space); **B,** squamous cell carcinoma (*arrow* showing a keratin pearl); **C,** small cell carcinoma (*arrow* showing nuclear molding); **D,** large cell carcinoma.

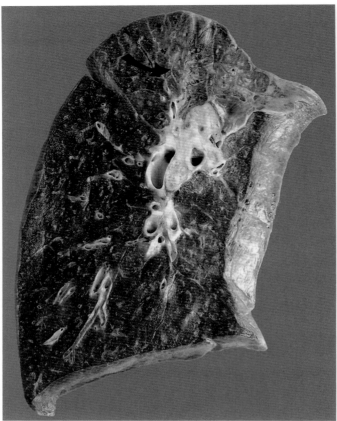

A

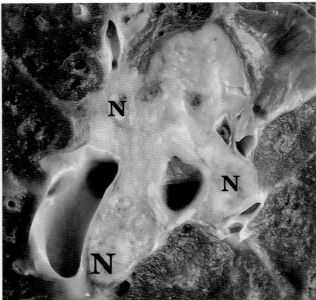

B

COLOR FIGURE 7–4

Small cell carcinoma. A parasagittal slice of the left lung near its mediastinal aspect (**A**) reveals a lobulated tumor adjacent to the upper lobe bronchus and lower lobe pulmonary artery. A magnified view (**B**) shows that the tumor occupies the interstitial space between the vessel and airway; several peribronchial lymph nodes (N) are replaced by tumor. Although the bronchus is patent on this section, extrinsic compression by carcinoma distally has resulted in partial atelectasis and obstructive pneumonitis (*curved arrow*) of the upper lobe.

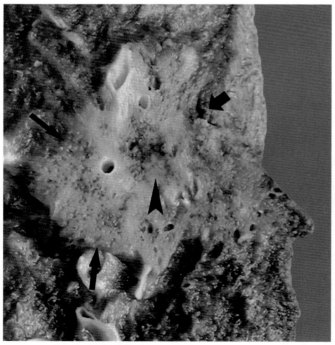

COLOR FIGURE 7–5

Adenocarcinoma—peripheral nodule. A magnified view of an upper lobe shows a well-circumscribed tumor adjacent to the pleura. Airways can be identified as small holes in the peripheral portion of the tumor (between *long arrows*), thus suggesting a bronchioloalveolar growth pattern. A focus of more solid-appearing invasive carcinoma/fibrosis is evident in the midportion (*arrowhead*). Slight pleural puckering is present (*short arrow*).

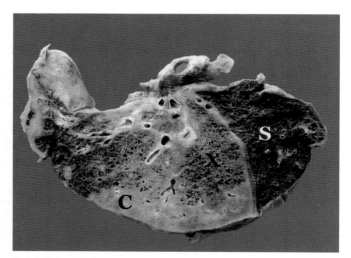

COLOR FIGURE 7–6

Bronchioloalveolar carcinoma—parenchymal consolidation. A transverse slice of the left lung shows a poorly delimited area of consolidation (C) in the upper lobe. Vessels and airways can be identified within the tumor in several places, thus suggesting a bronchioloalveolar growth pattern. Less prominent parenchymal infiltration is evident in the adjacent lung (X). S, superior segment of the lower lobe.

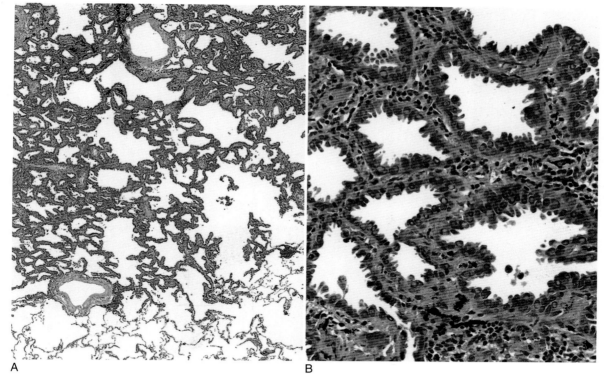

A   B

COLOR FIGURE 7–7

Bronchioloalveolar carcinoma. A low-magnification view (**A**) shows a moderate degree of parenchymal interstitial thickening by fibrous tissue and an infiltrate of lymphocytes. The underlying architecture is clearly maintained (compare with unaffected lung at the bottom). A magnified view (**B**) reveals cuboidal tumor cells lining the alveolar surface; there is no evidence of tissue invasion.

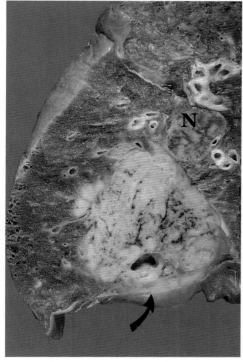

COLOR FIGURE 7–8

Large cell carcinoma. A magnified view of the left lung shows a well-circumscribed tumor occupying much of the lower lobe. Pleural invasion is evident inferiorly (*arrow*), and a peribronchial lymph node (N) is enlarged by metastatic carcinoma.

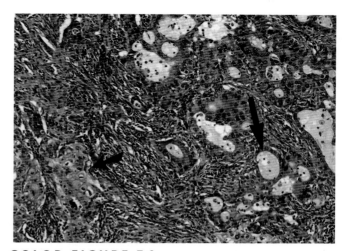

COLOR FIGURE 7–9

Adenosquamous carcinoma. A section shows a tumor with both squamous (*short arrow*) and glandular features (the latter including mucin production [*long arrow*]).

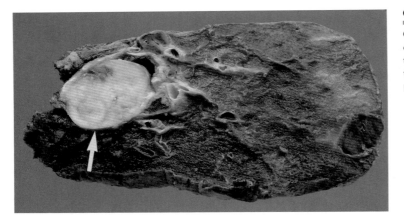

Carcinoid tumor. A transverse slice of the middle lobe shows an oval tumor almost completely occluding the lobar bronchus. The tumor does not seem to infiltrate the bronchial wall and appears to compress rather than infiltrate the lung (*arrow*). Several normal peribronchial lymph nodes are evident.

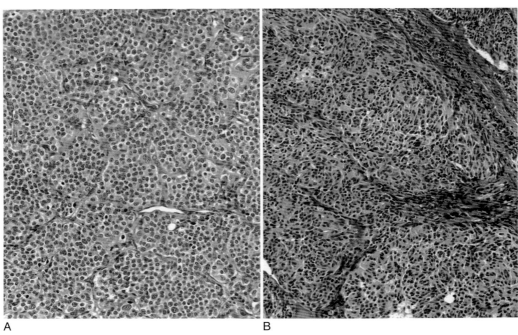

A   B

COLOR FIGURE 7–11

Carcinoid tumor—typical and atypical forms. A section of a typical carcinoid tumor (**A**) shows it to consist of uniform-sized nests of cells separated by a delicate vascular stroma. Cell nuclei are uniform in size and shape. A section of an atypical tumor (**B**) shows less well organized sheets of cells that have a greater degree of nuclear pleomorphism. Though not appreciated at this magnification, mitotic figures were easily identified.

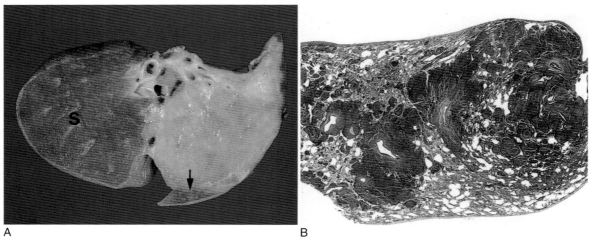

A   B

COLOR FIGURE 7–12

MALT lymphoma. A transverse slice of the right lung (**A**) shows consolidation of the middle lobe by a fleshy tan-colored tumor; the superior segment of the lower lobe (S) is unaffected. Patent airways and vessels can be seen within the tumor focally. **B**, A section from the periphery of the tumor (*arrow* in **A**) shows an infiltrate of small lymphoid cells, most prominent in the interstitial tissue around small vessels.

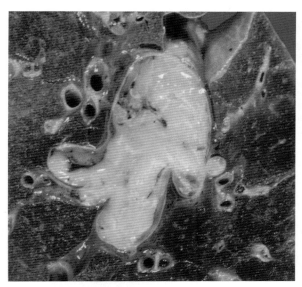

COLOR FIGURE 7–13

Pulmonary artery leiomyosarcoma. A highly magnified view of the right lung shows the interlobar artery and its segmental branches to be distended and completely occluded by a fleshy tumor that contains small foci of hemorrhage and necrosis. Histologic and immunohistochemical examination revealed the tumor to be a leiomyosarcoma.

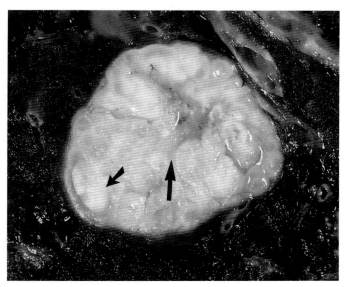

COLOR FIGURE 7–14

Chondromatous hamartoma. A magnified view of a lower lobe shows a well-circumscribed nodule composed of lobules of cartilage (*short arrow*) and fat (*long arrow*).

COLOR FIGURE 7–15

Lymphangitic carcinomatosis. A magnified view of lower lobe parenchyma (**A**) shows thickening of the interlobular septa (*straight arrow*) and perivascular interstitial tissue (*curved arrow*). The same abnormalities are apparent on a whole-mount section (**B**). A magnified view of the interlobular septa (**C**) shows tumor distending a lymphatic vessel (*arrow*) and infiltrating the connective tissue. The patient was a 48-year-old woman who had metastatic carcinoma of the breast.

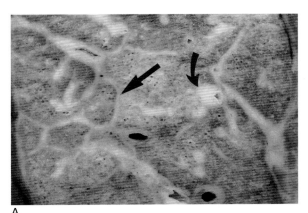

A

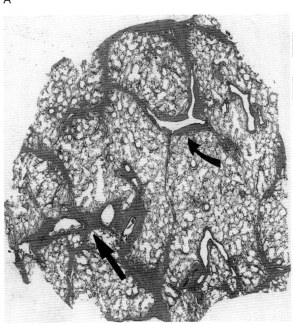

B

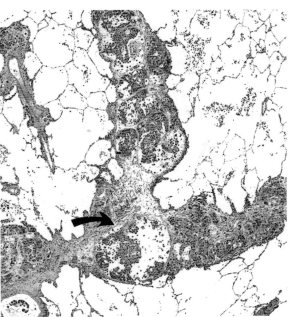

C

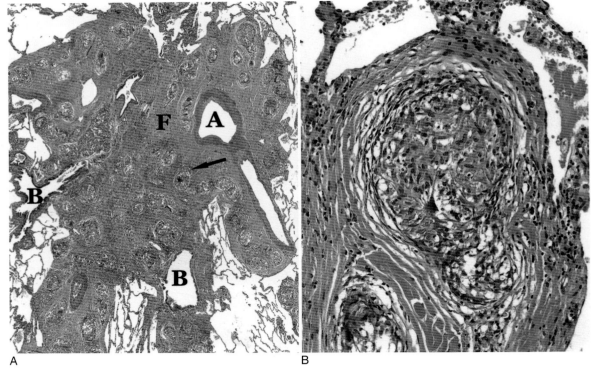

A   B

COLOR FIGURE 9–1

Sarcoidosis. A low-magnification view (**A**) shows expansion of the interstitial space surrounding several membranous bronchioles (B) and their accompanying pulmonary arteries (A) by isolated and confluent (*arrow*) non-necrotizing granulomas and mature fibrous tissue (F). A magnified view (**B**) reveals one granuloma surrounded by somewhat laminated collagen.

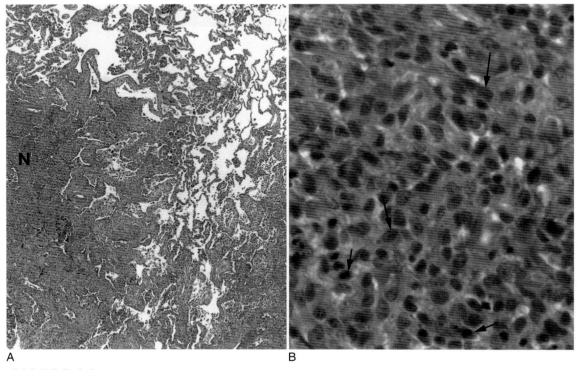

A   B

COLOR FIGURE 9–2

Langerhans cell histiocytosis. A low-magnification view of a portion of a grossly visible nodule (**A**) shows thickening of the parenchymal interstitium by a cellular infiltrate. The latter is so abundant in the central portion of the nodule (N) that the air spaces have been compressed to such a degree that they are no longer recognizable. A magnified view of the infiltrate (**B**) shows it to consist of cells that have mildly pleomorphic nuclei (*long arrows*) (Langerhans cells). Scattered eosinophils are also evident (*short arrows*).

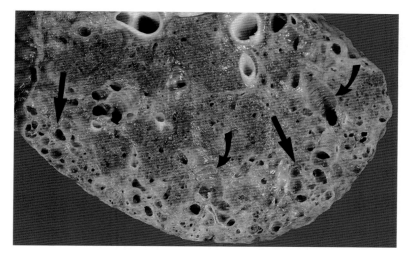

COLOR FIGURE 9–3

Usual interstitial pneumonia—gross appearance. A view of a transverse slice of a lower lobe in its basal portion shows interstitial fibrosis located predominantly in the subpleural region. Traction bronchiectasis (*curved arrows*) and a honeycomb appearance (*straight arrows*) are evident.

COLOR FIGURE 9–4

Nonspecific interstitial pneumonia. Views at low (**A**) and high (**B**) magnification show more or less uniform thickening of the parenchymal interstitium by an infiltrate of lymphocytes. There is minimal fibrosis and no evidence of active (fibroblastic) connective tissue.

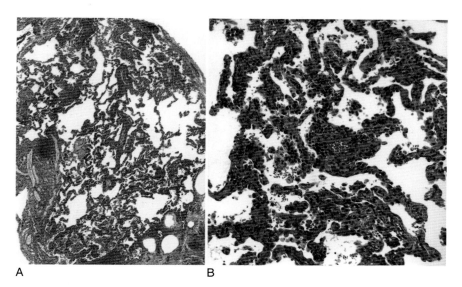

A   B

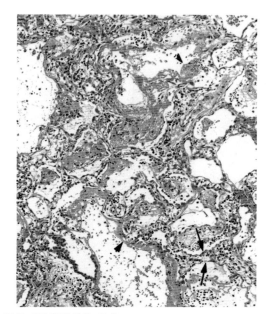

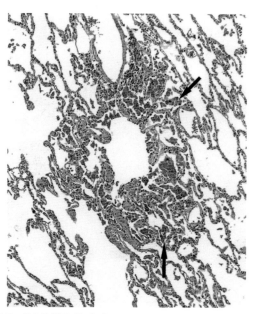

COLOR FIGURE 9–5

Acute interstitial pneumonia. A section shows mild interstitial thickening by edema fluid and neutrophils (between the *short arrows*) and filling of alveolar air spaces by fibrinous fluid. Hyaline membranes are evident in several transitional airways (*arrowheads*).

COLOR FIGURE 9–6

Respiratory bronchiolitis. A section shows the accumulation of tan-colored macrophages within alveoli in a respiratory bronchiole and the adjacent parenchyma (*arrows*). A very mild lymphocytic infiltrate is evident in the bronchiolar wall. The abnormality was an incidental finding in a lobe resected for adenocarcinoma.

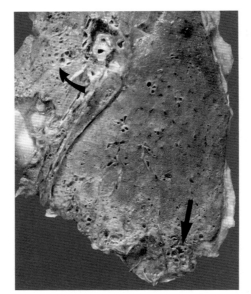

Rheumatoid disease—interstitial fibrosis. A magnified view of a slice of the right lung shows patchy interstitial thickening, predominantly in the inferior portion of the upper lobe (*curved arrow*) and basal (subpleural) portion of the lower lobe. A honeycomb appearance is evident focally (*straight arrow*).

COLOR FIGURE 10–2

Wegener's granulomatosis. A magnified view of a well-demarcated pulmonary nodule (**A**) reveals a mixed inflammatory cell infiltrate that is completely obscuring the underlying parenchyma. Scattered multinucleated giant cells (*short arrows*) and aggregates of partially necrotic neutrophils (*curved arrows*) are evident. A view of another region of the same biopsy specimen (**B**) shows a similar cellular infiltrate localized to the media of a medium-sized pulmonary artery; marked intimal proliferation is also apparent.

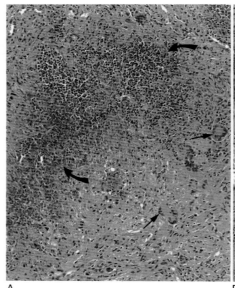

A

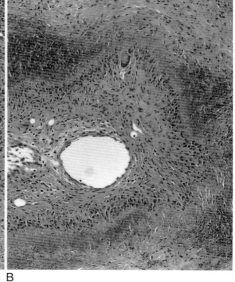

B

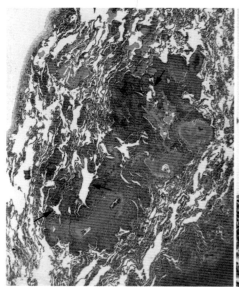

A

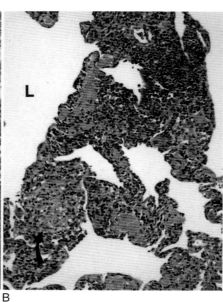

B

COLOR FIGURE 10–3

Extrinsic allergic alveolitis. A section of an open lung biopsy specimen (**A**) shows a cellular infiltrate composed predominantly of lymphocytes. The infiltrate is localized to the interstitial tissue and associated with several membranous and respiratory bronchioles and their accompanying arteries (*arrows*, bronchiolar lumen). A magnified view of one respiratory bronchiole and the adjacent parenchyma (**B**) confirms the interstitial location of the infiltrate. A poorly formed granuloma is evident (*arrow*). L, bronchiolar lumen.

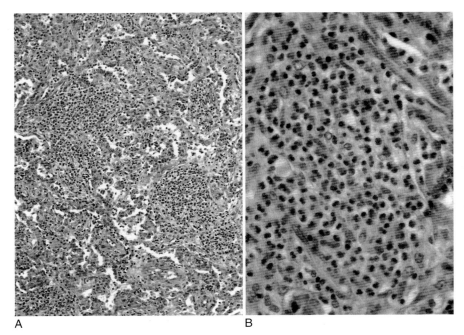

A   B

COLOR FIGURE 10-4

Chronic eosinophilic pneumonia. Views of an open lung biopsy specimen at intermediate (**A**) and high (**B**) magnification show mild parenchymal interstitial thickening and filling of alveolar air spaces by macrophages and numerous eosinophils.

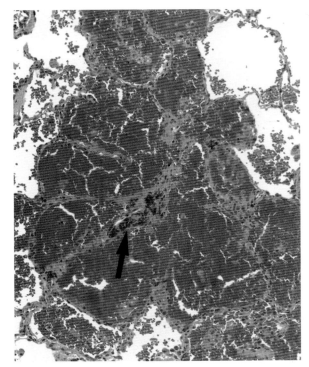

COLOR FIGURE 10-5

Goodpasture's syndrome. A section of an open lung biopsy specimen demonstrates filling of most alveolar air spaces by red blood cells. The interstitium shows a very mild mononuclear cell infiltrate and, focally (*arrow*), aggregates of hemosiderin-laden macrophages.

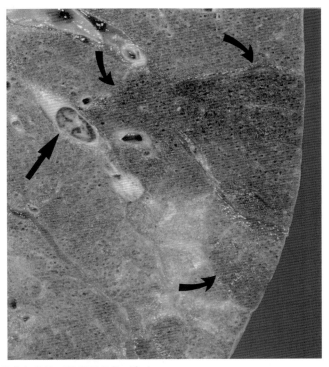

COLOR FIGURE 12-1

Pulmonary infarct. A magnified view of a slice of lower lobe reveals an early infarct (*curved arrows*). A thromboembolus is evident in the feeding artery (*straight arrow*).

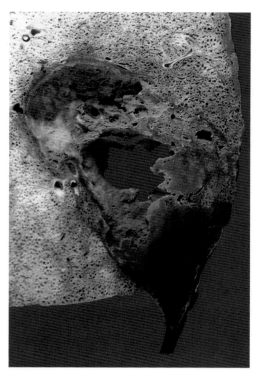

COLOR FIGURE 12-2

Pulmonary infarct—cavitation. A magnified view of a slice of lower lobe shows a well-demarcated infarct with a large cavity in its central portion. This cavity was thought to be the result of secondary bacterial infection rather than a septic embolus.

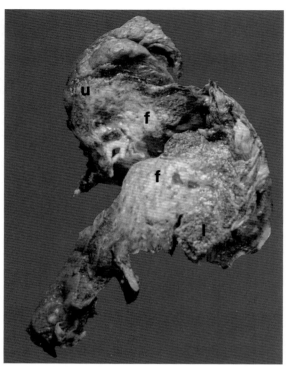

COLOR FIGURE 12-3

Intravenous talcosis—progressive massive fibrosis. A slice of a markedly distorted left lung shows foci of dense fibrosis (f) in the upper (u) and lower (l) lobes. Note the fine nodular appearance of the adjacent parenchyma, which represents foci of nonconglomerated talc granulomas.

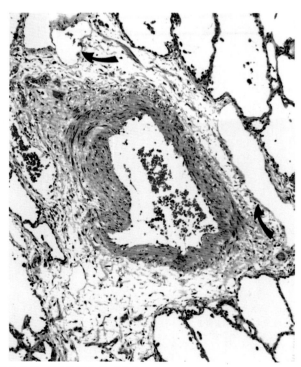

COLOR FIGURE 14-1

Acute interstitial edema. A section shows thickening of the connective tissue surrounding a pulmonary artery. The tissue has a loose appearance, characteristic of fluid accumulation. Note that the adjacent alveolar septa and air spaces are normal. Several distended lymphatics are also evident (*arrows*).

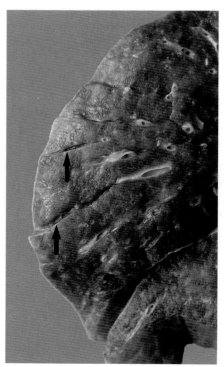

COLOR FIGURE 14-2

Acute interstitial edema—interlobular septal thickening. A magnified view of a slice of upper lobe shows the interlobular septa in the subpleural region to be thickened and to have a somewhat gelatinous appearance (*arrows*). The abnormality corresponds to Kerley B lines seen on chest radiographs.

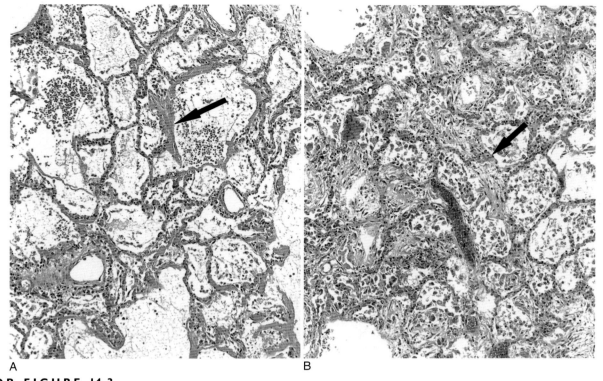

A   B

COLOR FIGURE 14–3

Diffuse alveolar damage. Sections illustrate the exudative (**A**) and proliferative (**B**) stages of the disease. In **A,** the alveolar air spaces are filled by lightly stained edema fluid and red blood cells; hyaline membranes can be seen in some transitional airways (*arrow*). In **B,** the fluid has been replaced by loose-appearing (fibroblastic) connective tissue (*arrow*) and alveolar macrophages.

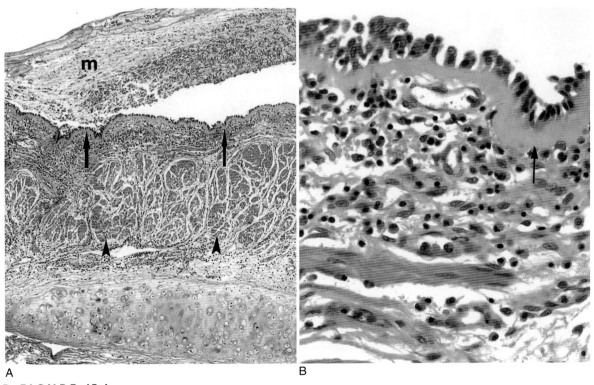

A   B

COLOR FIGURE 15–1

Asthma—histologic appearance. An autopsy section from a 30-year-old patient who died of asthma shows a marked increase in the muscularis mucosae (*arrowheads*), thickening of the basement membrane (*arrows*), and an inflammatory cellular infiltrate throughout the wall. Mucus (m) containing inflammatory and epithelial cells is evident in the airway lumen in **A**; numerous eosinophils are seen in the lamina propria in **B**.

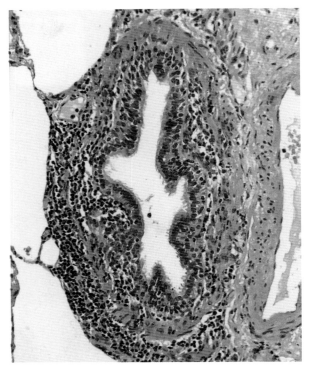

COLOR FIGURE 15–2

Cigarette smoke–associated bronchiolitis. A view of a membranous bronchiole shows a moderately severe infiltrate of lymphocytes in the mucosa and peribronchiolar interstitial tissue.

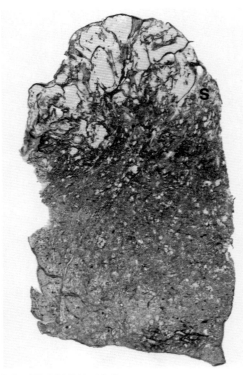

COLOR FIGURE 15–3

Centrilobular emphysema. A parasagittal paper-mounted slice of the left lung demonstrates marked emphysema with bulla formation in the apical region of the upper lobe. Less severe disease can be seen in the inferior portion of the upper lobe and superior segment (S) of the lower.

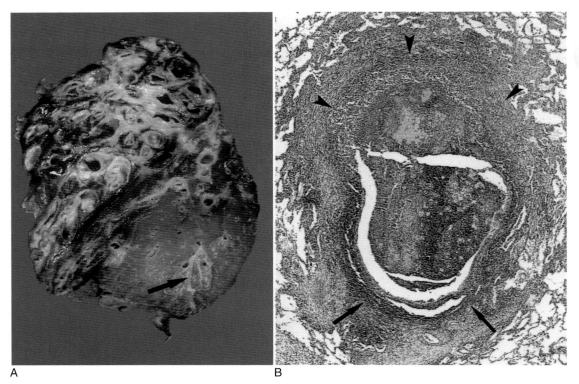

A   B

COLOR FIGURE 15–4

Cystic fibrosis. A parasagittal slice of the left lung removed at transplantation (**A**) shows extensive bronchiectasis—severe in the upper lobe, moderate in the superior segment of the lower lobe, and mild in the basal segments (*arrow*). Pus is evident in the lumina of many upper lobe airways. A section of lung between the ectatic airways (**B**) reveals a dilated membranous bronchiole whose lumen is filled by mucopurulent material. A chronic inflammatory cell infiltrate is evident in the wall at one aspect (*arrows*). The appearance at the opposite side (*arrowheads*) is that of granulation tissue secondary to epithelial ulceration.

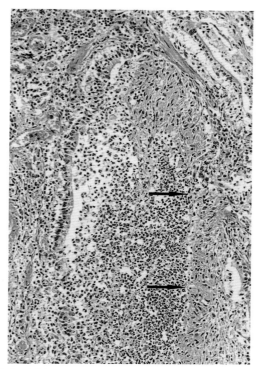

COLOR FIGURE 15–5

Acute bronchiolitis. A section shows a membranous bronchiole whose wall is focally devoid of epithelium (*arrows*). Numerous neutrophils are present in the airway lumen.

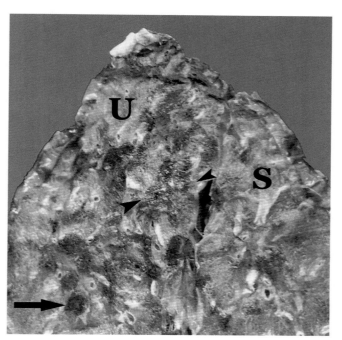

COLOR FIGURE 16–1

Simple silicosis. A magnified view of an upper lobe (U) and superior segment of lower lobe (S) demonstrates a number of sharply circumscribed gray silicotic nodules (*arrow*). Confluence of several nodules (between the *arrowheads*) indicates early progressive massive fibrosis.

COLOR FIGURE 16–2

Silicosis with progressive massive fibrosis. A slice of the left lung shows numerous gray silicotic nodules in the lower lobe (*arrows*). Confluence of nodules in the upper lobe (between the *arrowheads*) has resulted in a single masslike lesion. This lobe is much smaller than the lower one because of associated emphysema and contraction related to the fibrosis.

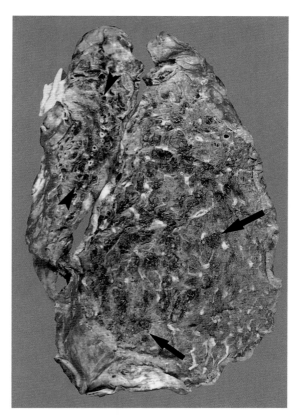

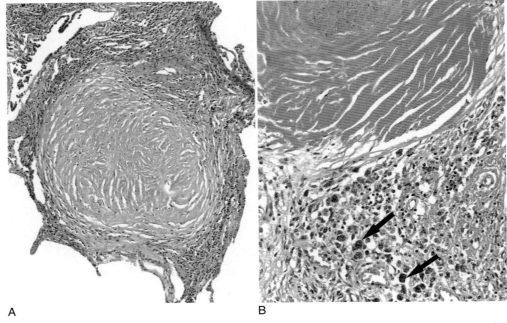

A   B

COLOR FIGURE 16–3

Silicotic nodule. Views of a parenchymal nodule at intermediate (**A**) and high (**B**) magnification reveal a focus of hypocellular collagen surrounded by an infiltrate of lymphocytes and macrophages (*arrows*), the latter containing finely granular foreign material.

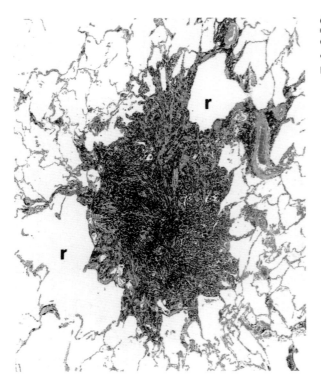

COLOR FIGURE 16–4

Coal workers' pneumoconiosis—nodular lesion. A section shows a stellate focus of connective tissue and macrophages, the later containing abundant anthracotic pigment, adjacent to two respiratory bronchioles (r).

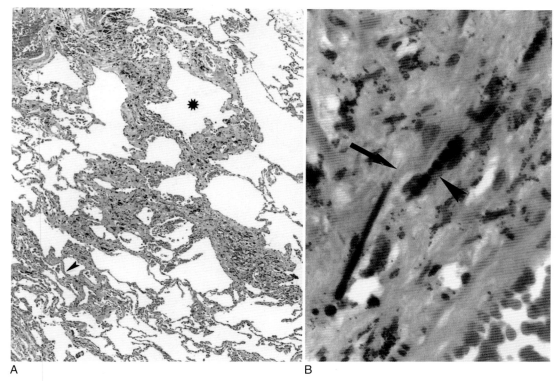

A   B

COLOR FIGURE 16–5

Peribronchiolar fibrosis associated with asbestos exposure. A section (**A**) demonstrates thickening of the wall of a respiratory bronchiole (*asterisk*) and its distal branches by fibrous tissue containing scattered lymphocytes and pigmented macrophages. Mild parenchymal interstitial fibrosis is evident (*arrowhead*). Asbestos bodies can be seen within the fibrous tissue on higher magnification (**B**). (The *arrow* indicates a fiber and the *arrowhead* a segmented iron-protein coat.) The patient was a 55-year-old man who had worked as an insulator.

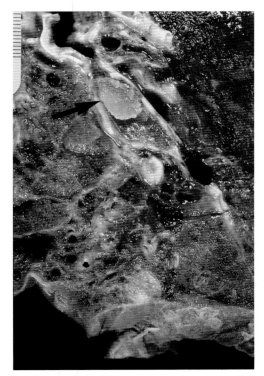

COLOR FIGURE 17–1

Aspirated foreign body. A magnified view of a slice of lower lobe shows occlusion of a basal segmental bronchus by a partially digested fragment of vegetable material (*arrow*). The adjacent mucosa is inflamed, and the distal part of the lung has mild bronchiectasis and fibrosis. The foreign body was an incidental finding at autopsy in a 78-year-old man with Alzheimer's disease.

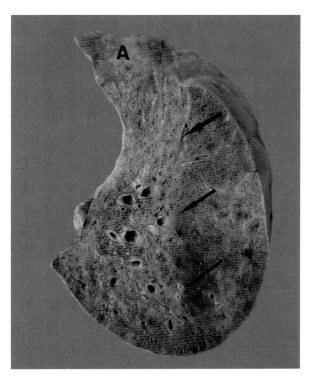

COLOR FIGURE 18–1

Radiation pneumonitis. A transverse slice of the left upper lobe (A, anterior) shows a fairly well demarcated area of parenchymal fibrosis (*arrows*) associated with mild bronchiectasis. The patient was a middle-aged woman who had been treated by mediastinal irradiation for Hodgkin's lymphoma approximately 6 months before death.

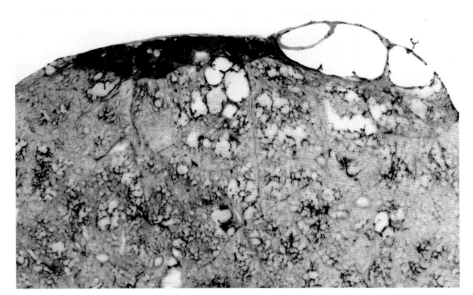

Apical cap. A magnified view of the apex of the right upper lobe shows a well-demarcated focus of subpleural fibrosis. Mild centrilobular emphysema and several blebs are also evident.

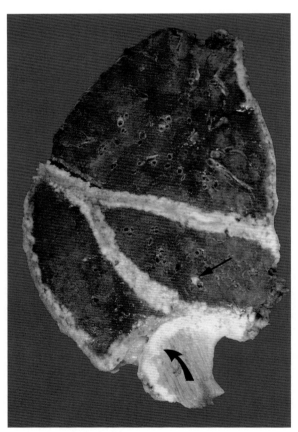

COLOR FIGURE 20–2

Mesothelioma. A parasagittal slice of the right lung shows thickening of the costal pleura and interlobar fissures by a white neoplasm. Infiltration of the hemidiaphragm is evident (*curved arrow*). The lung itself is not involved except for a small focus adjacent to one vessel (*straight arrow*) that represents lymphangitic spread.

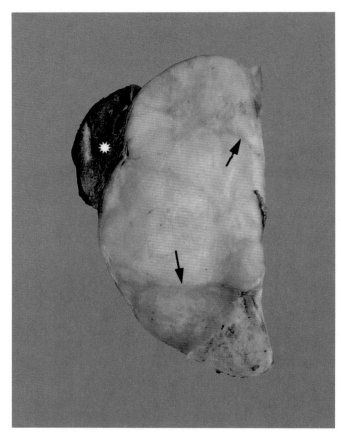

COLOR FIGURE 20–3

Pleural fibrous tumor. The cut surface of this 6-cm-diameter pleural tumor reveals it to have a uniform gray-white appearance without hemorrhage or cyst formation. Thin fibrous tissue bands (*arrows*) subdivide it into indistinct lobules. The small amount of adherent lung (*asterisk*) is not invaded.

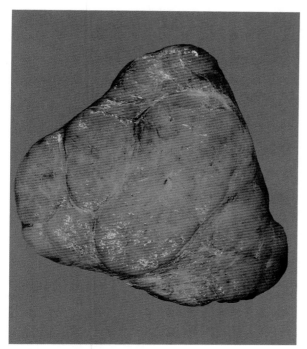

COLOR FIGURE 21–1

Thymoma. A slice of a lobulated anterior mediastinal mass shows a tan-colored tumor subdivided into variably sized lobules by thin bands of fibrous tissue.

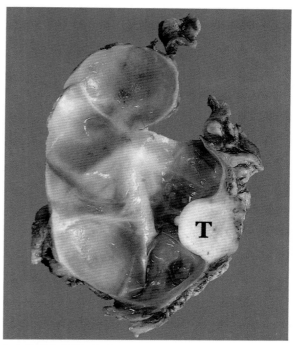

COLOR FIGURE 21–2

Cystic thymoma. A slice through the middle of an anterior mediastinal tumor shows it to consist predominantly of a thin-walled cyst; a 2-cm focus of thymoma (T) is evident at one edge.

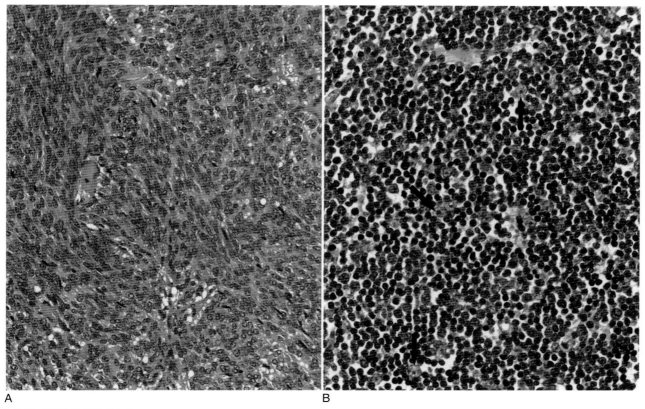

A   B

COLOR FIGURE 21–3

Thymoma—histologic appearance. A magnified view of a thymoma (**A**) shows it to consist of somewhat spindle shaped cells without an accompanying lymphocyte infiltrate (predominantly epithelial or type A thymoma). A section of another tumor (**B**) demonstrates it to be composed mostly of lymphocytes, with only occasional neoplastic epithelial cells (*arrows*) being evident (lymphocyte-predominant or type B thymoma).

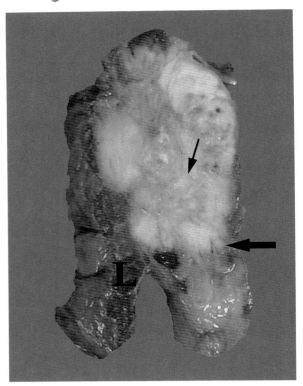

COLOR FIGURE 21–4

Thymic carcinoma. A slice of an anterior mediastinal tumor shows foci of necrosis (*thin arrow*) as well as infiltration of adipose tissue (*thick arrow*) and lung (L).

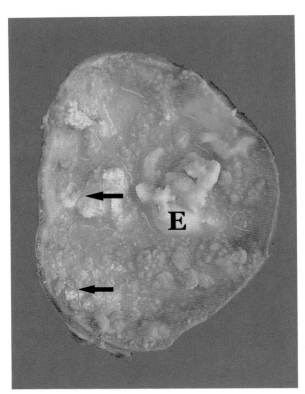

COLOR FIGURE 21–5

Mediastinal teratoma. A slice of a well-circumscribed mediastinal tumor shows foci of white tissue (E, corresponding histologically to epidermis) and scattered hairs (*arrows*). Though solid, this tumor was composed of benign (histologically mature) tissue throughout.

COLOR FIGURE 21–6

Mesothelial cyst. A thymectomy specimen—the two superior lobes of the thymus are indicated by *arrows*—shows a large thin-walled cyst in the inferior portion.

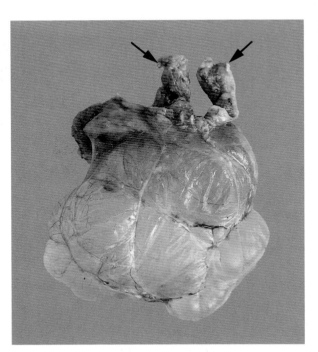

THE NORMAL CHEST

THE AIRWAYS AND PULMONARY VENTILATION

The air-containing portion of the lung can be divided into three parts, each with somewhat different but overlapping structural and functional characteristics. The *conducting airways* include the trachea, bronchi, and membranous (nonalveolated) bronchioles. Because air cannot diffuse through the walls of these airways, their primary function is to conduct air to the alveolar surface. These structures, along with the pulmonary and bronchial arteries and veins, lymphatic vessels, nerves, connective tissues of the peribronchial and perivascular spaces, and the interlobular septa, constitute the nonparenchymatous portion of the lung.

The *transitional airways* consist of respiratory bronchioles and alveolar ducts, each of which conducts air to the most peripheral alveoli. In addition to this feature, a variable number of alveoli arise from the walls of the airways of the

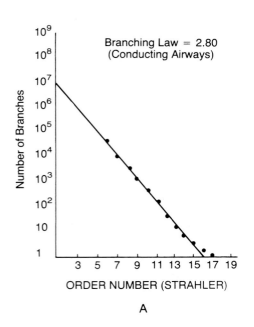

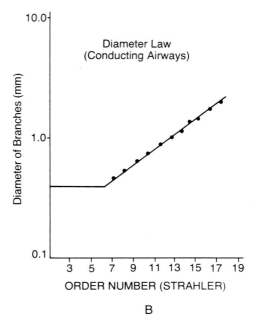

FIGURE 1–1

Number of branches (A) and their diameter (B) plotted against their order number. In **B**, note that orders 1 through 7 undergo no diameter change— diminution in caliber ceases at order 7, chiefly respiratory bronchioles. *(From Cumming G, Horsfield K, Harding LK, et al: Biological branching systems, with special reference to the lung airways. Bull Physiopathol Respir 7:31, 1971.)*

transitional zone, and thus the transitional zone has the additional function of gas exchange. The *respiratory tissue* consists of the alveolar sacs and alveoli themselves, whose primary function is exchange of gases between air and blood. Together with the transitional airways and corresponding small arteries and veins, they constitute the lung parenchyma.

Anatomy—The Conducting Airways

Geometry and Dimensions

In one study of resin casts of human lungs inflated and fixed at a volume of 5 L,[1] investigators measured the length of each branch between two points of bifurcation from an arbitrary diameter of 0.7 mm, as well as the diameter at the midpoint of every branch. One of the interesting findings was a roughly linear relationship between the order number* and the logarithm of the number, diameter, and length of the airway branches (Fig. 1–1).[1] Thus, by measuring the slope of the line relating the two, the diameter and length of any order can be predicted by dividing the diameter and length of its parent by 1.4 and 1.49, respectively. Similarly, the number of branches is linearly related to the order number, with the branching ratio of the entire conductive zone (average number of daughter branches per parent branch) being 2.8.

These "number laws" do not apply precisely at all airway levels; for example, the trachea clearly does not divide 2.8 times and, in fact, the branching pattern of the proximal conducting system is probably best described as dichotomous, with each parent dividing into two branches. However, the branching ratio of 2.8 is precise from orders 6 through 15. Similarly, the diameter law is not applicable throughout the whole airway system; at order 7 (approximately), diminution

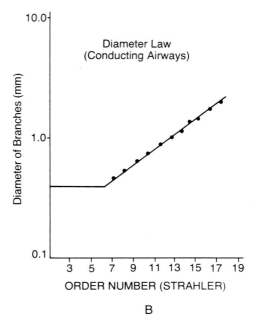

FIGURE 1–2

Frequency distribution of the number of divisions down to the lobular branches. *(From Horsfield K, Cumming G: Morphology of the bronchial tree in man. J Appl Physiol 24:373-383, 1968.)*

in airway diameter ceases, and the more distal branches (to order 1) retain the parent's diameter.

Counting distally from the trachea, the number of generations to a 0.7-mm airway ranges from 8 to 25[1]; that is, the route with the shortest path length is reached after 8 divisions and the one with the longest after 25. It is likely that local spatial constraints are most important in determining these figures. Analysis of the frequency distribution of divisions down to the lobular branches (Fig. 1–2)[2] shows a stepwise increase from division 8 to a peak at 14 and a decrease from 15 to 25.[1] The volume of airways from the carina to 0.7-mm branches has been computed to be about 70 mL[1]; when this volume is added to the volume of the upper airways from the mouth to the carina (80 mL), the sum is the total volume of the conducting airways, almost identical to the volume of anatomic dead space as determined by physiologic techniques.

Morphology and Cell Function

The basic morphology of the trachea, bronchi, and membranous bronchioles is the same and consists of a surface epithe-

---

*In this context, "order" refers to the level of airway within the conducting system. The terminal (most distal) membranous bronchiole is considered to be order 1; when two such bronchioles join, they form a single branch of order 2; when two of order 2 join, they form a branch of order 3; and so on.

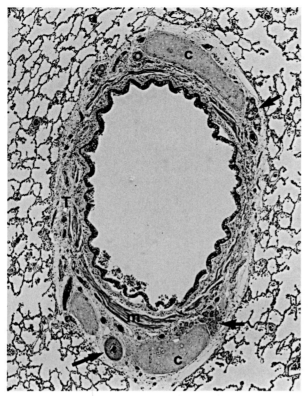

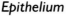

FIGURE 1–3

Normal subsegmental bronchus. C, cartilage plate; M, smooth muscle; T, interstitial connective tissue; long arrow, bronchial artery; short arrows, bronchial glands. (×30.) *(From Fraser RS, Müller NL, Colman NC, Paré PD: Fraser and Paré's Diagnosis of Diseases of the Chest, 4th ed. Philadelphia, WB Saunders, 1999.)*

lium, composed largely of ciliated and secretory cells, and subepithelial tissue containing supportive connective tissue, cells of the inflammatory and immune systems, and glands (Fig. 1–3). The proportion and type of these elements vary considerably with airway order.

Epithelium

The tracheal and proximal bronchial epithelium is composed of tall columnar cells and smaller, somewhat triangular basal cells.[2] Because not all cells reach the luminal surface and their nuclei are situated at varying levels, the epithelium possesses a pseudostratified appearance (Fig. 1–4). This appearance is gradually lost in the distal bronchi and bronchioles as the cells assume a low columnar shape. Ciliated and secretory cells, either goblet or Clara in type, constitute the bulk of the epithelium, with basal, intermediate, lymphoreticular, and neuroendocrine cells interspersed in lesser numbers.

The *ciliated cell* is the most prominent cell type in normal epithelium and is about three to five times more numerous than goblet cells in the central airways (Fig. 1–5). It extends from the luminal surface to the basement membrane, to which it is attached by a thin, tapering base. Cells are also firmly attached to one another at their apical surface by tight junctions, thus forming a barrier physically impermeable to most substances. Emanating from the surface of each cell are approximately 200 to 250 cilia, as well as numerous shorter microvilli, which have been hypothesized to function in the absorption of secretions emanating from more peripheral airways.[3] Although ciliated cells are also joined laterally to one another and to basal cells, prominent intercellular spaces containing numerous microvilli are also seen in this location, especially at the basal aspect of the cell (Fig. 1–6).[4] These spaces and the microvilli they contain are important in the transepithelial movement of fluid and electrolytes.

Each cilium is covered by a prolongation of the cell surface membrane and contains a complex structure called the *axoneme* (Fig. 1–7).[5] The axoneme consists of two central microtubules surrounded by nine peripheral doublets, which in turn are composed of two intimately related microtubules termed A and B subfibers. Two small arms composed of the protein dynein and believed to be the major focus of energy conversion into ciliary movement project from the A subfiber of one doublet to the B subfiber of the next. Also attached to each A subfiber is a radial spoke that joins it to a central sheath surrounding the inner microtubules.

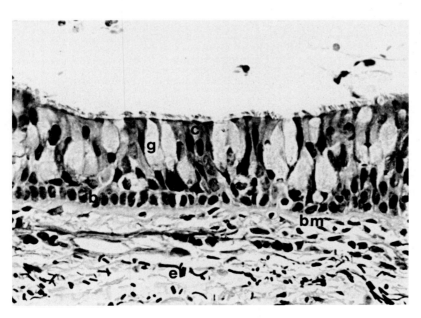

FIGURE 1–4

Normal bronchial epithelium. Ciliated (c), goblet (g), and basal (b) cells are clearly seen. Note also the thin basement membrane (bm), scattered elastic fibers (e), and inflammatory cells in the lamina propria. (Verhoeff-van Gieson, ×425.) *(From Fraser RS, Müller NL, Colman NC, Paré PD: Fraser and Paré's Diagnosis of Diseases of the Chest, 4th ed. Philadelphia, WB Saunders, 1999.)*

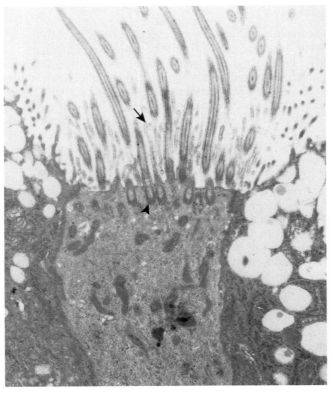

FIGURE 1–5

Ciliated cell. The luminal portion of a ciliated cell shows cilia, surface microvilli *(arrow)*, apical mitochondria, and basal bodies *(arrowhead)*. (Human bronchial epithelium, ×12,500.)

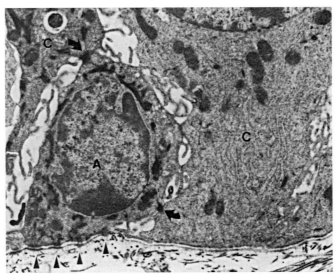

FIGURE 1–6

Tracheal epithelium—ultrastructure. A magnified view of the basal aspect of tracheal epithelium from a sheep shows a basal cell containing relatively little cytoplasm (A) and the inferior portion of several columnar cells (probably ciliated cells) (C). Intercellular spaces containing numerous microvilli are evident. Note also that the basal cell has several hemidesmosomal attachments to the underlying basement membrane *(arrowheads)* whereas the adjacent columnar cell has none. Several desmosome-like attachments are nevertheless present between the basal cell and the columnar cells *(arrows)*. (×13,200.) *(Adapted from Evans MJ, Cox RA, Shami SG, et al: The role of basal cells in the attachment of columnar cells to the basal lamina of the trachea. Am J Respir Cell Mol Biol 1:463, 1989.)*

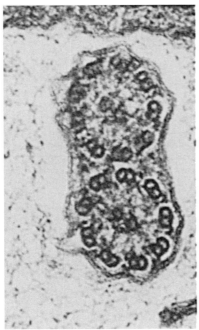

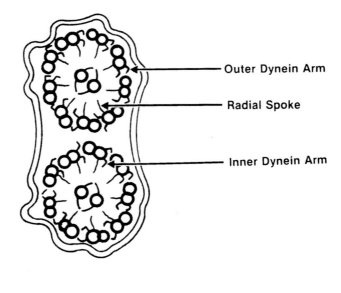

- Outer Dynein Arm
- Radial Spoke
- Inner Dynein Arm

FIGURE 1–7

Doublet cilium from a chronic smoker. Although paired within the same plasma membrane, the individual components of this cilium are normal, with nine peripheral and two central doublets and the typical arrangement of dynein arms and radial spokes. *(From Fraser RS, Müller NL, Colman NC, Paré PD: Fraser and Paré's Diagnosis of Diseases of the Chest, 4th ed. Philadelphia, WB Saunders, 1999.)*

In addition to roles in transepithelial fluid movement and mucociliary escalator function, there is evidence that ciliated cells have important effects in the control of local airway inflammation and on smooth muscle function.[6,7] The cells also express HLA-DR antigens and can therefore theoretically interact directly with intraepithelial immune cells.[8] An influence on fibroblast proliferation and production of extracellular matrix components is also likely to be important in both the normal and injured airway wall.[9]

Goblet cells (see Fig. 1–4) constitute about 20% to 30% of cells in the more proximal airways and decrease in number distally such that only occasional cells are present in normal bronchioles; in conditions of both acute and chronic airway irritation, however, they may substantially increase in number in the proximal airways and may also appear in bronchioles.[10] The apical portion of the cell is expanded by numerous membrane-bound secretory granules, whereas the basal portion has few organelles and is attenuated as it approaches the basal lamina; this combination results in the typical goblet shape from which the name of the cell is derived.

Basal cells (see Figs. 1–4 and 1–6) are relatively small, flattened, or triangular cells whose bases are adjacent to the basal lamina; their apices normally do not reach the airway lumen.[11] They are more abundant in the proximal airways, where they form a more or less continuous layer; they gradually diminish in number distally to the point that they become difficult to identify in bronchioles. Their cytoplasmic contents show little specialization, and it is believed that the cell is a reserve cell from which the epithelium is continuously repopulated.[12] It has also been speculated that these cells function as a "scaffold" for the attachment of ciliated and goblet cells to the basal lamina.[13]

Intermediate cells (see Fig. 1–4) possess somewhat more cytoplasm than basal cells do and show evidence of either ciliogenesis or mucous granule accumulation. They are generally believed to represent a stage of differentiation between the basal cell and either the goblet or the ciliated cell. It is also possible that the secretory form is important in the repair of injured airway epithelium.[14] The response to such injury is rapid; in one study in which the suprabasal epithelium of rat trachea was mechanically damaged, the epithelium was virtually reconstituted with ultrastructurally mature cells by 90 hours.[15]

The *Clara cell (nonciliated bronchiolar secretory cell)* is found primarily in bronchioles, in which it makes up the majority of the epithelium along with ciliated cells. It is columnar in shape and bulges into the airway lumen, with a slight projection above the surrounding ciliated cells (Fig. 1–8). In the apical cytoplasm are membrane-bound granules that contain several biologically active substances, including surfactant apoproteins that presumably contribute to the surface fluid layer that normally lines the bronchiolar epithelium.[16] The granules also contain a 10-kD protein known as *Clara cell–specific protein* (CC10, CC16, protein 1).[17,18] This protein has the ability to inhibit several biologic mediators, such as tumor necrosis factor-α and interleukin-1β, and has been hypothesized to have an important role in the regulation of local inflammatory and immune reactions.[19,19a] The protein can be identified in sputum, BAL fluid, and serum in a variety of conditions, including pneumonia[20] and cigarette smoking,[21] which suggests that it might be a useful marker of bronchiolar epithelial damage. It has also been implicated in the pathogenesis of several pulmonary diseases, including asthma and sarcoidosis.[19a,21a] Clara cells also function in the regeneration

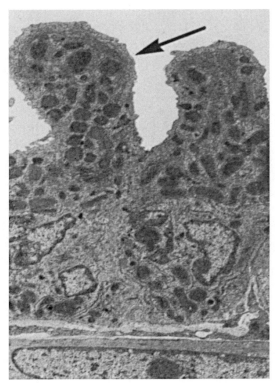

FIGURE 1–8

Clara cells. These cells possess tongue-shaped cytoplasmic processes *(arrow)* that project into the airway lumen. Nuclei are basal in position, and the apical cytoplasm contains numerous osmiophilic granules. (×4500.) *(From Wang N-S, Huang SN, Sheldon H, et al: Ultrastructural changes of Clara and type II alveolar cells in adrenalin-induced pulmonary edema in mice. Am J Pathol 62:237, 1971.)*

of damaged bronchiolar epithelium[22] and the secretion of a leukocyte protease inhibitor[23] that presumably acts to maintain the integrity of the bronchiolar epithelium.

Neuroendocrine cells have a roughly triangular shape; their bases rest on the basement membrane and their tapering apices point toward but infrequently reach the luminal surface. The cytoplasm contains numerous membrane-bound granules that have a central, electron-dense core surrounded by a thin, radiolucent halo (neurosecretory granules) (Fig. 1–9). These granules are concentrated in the basal portion of the cytoplasm and contain several biologically active peptides, including calcitonin, gastrin-releasing peptide, and 5-hydroxytryptamine (serotonin).[24] The cells are found more frequently in peripheral airways and in younger individuals, particularly fetuses and neonates, in whom they have been estimated to constitute 1% to 2% of all bronchial epithelial cells.[25]

Several potentially important functions have been hypothesized for pulmonary neuroendocrine cells.[24] Their relative prominence in fetal lungs and their fairly rapid decrease in number after birth have suggested a role in regulation of the fetal or neonatal circulation. In addition, the observation that the cells are the first to differentiate in developing airway epithelium has suggested that they may influence lung maturation. There is evidence that the cells increase in number in hypoxic conditions[26]; as a consequence, it has also been speculated that they may be mediators of the pulmonary vascular hypoxic response. Finally, a role in the regulation of epithelial growth and repair has been postulated.[27]

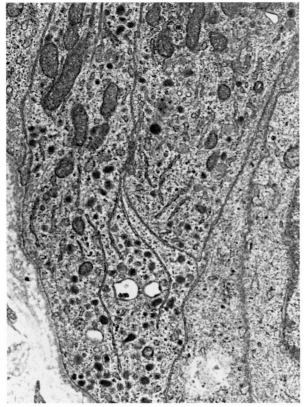

FIGURE 1–9

Neuroendocrine cell. A magnified view of the base of a neuroendocrine cell shows the lamina propria and thin basal lamina at the bottom left and numerous intracytoplasmic neurosecretory granules. (×31,000.) *(From Fraser RS, Müller NL, Colman NC, Paré PD: Fraser and Paré's Diagnosis of Diseases of the Chest, 4th ed. Philadelphia, WB Saunders, 1999.)*

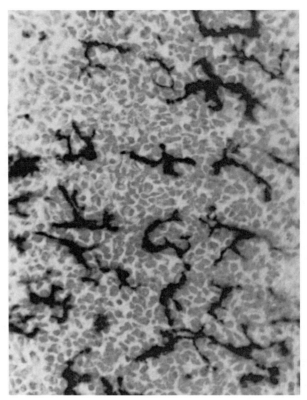

FIGURE 1–10

Airway dendritic cells. A tangential section of rat tracheal epithelium immunostained for Ia antigen shows regularly spaced dendritic cells, each with several irregular processes extending between adjacent epithelial cells. (×40.) *(From Schon-Hegrad MA, Oliver J, McMenamin PG, et al: Studies on the density, distribution, and surface phenotype of intraepithelial class II major histocompatibility complex antigen (Ia)-bearing dendritic cells (DC) in the conducting airways. J Exp Med 173:1345, 1991.)*

Clusters of neuroendocrine cells, known as *neuroepithelial bodies,* can be found throughout the tracheobronchial and bronchiolar epithelium, especially near branch points. They consist of 4 to 10 columnar cells, each of which contains neurosecretory granules that have been shown to contain serotonin and other peptides.[28] Although the individual cells of the neuroepithelial body resemble solitary neuroendocrine cells, their clustered arrangement and fairly consistent relationship to nerve fibers and possibly capillaries suggest that the two may have different functions.

Cells of the immune system can also be found within the epithelium of all conducting airways. *Dendritic* and *Langerhans cells* possess elongated cytoplasmic extensions (Fig. 1–10), highly convoluted nuclei, and an organelle-rich cytoplasm; in addition, Langerhans cells have characteristic pentalaminar cytoplasmic structures termed *Birbeck granules.*[29] Dendritic cells can be found throughout the lung, including the alveolar interstitium and peribronchiolar connective tissue[29]; Langerhans cells appear to be present only within airway epithelium, where their number is considerably greater in proximal than distal branches.[30] The cells are CD1a positive and express cell surface receptors for immunoglobulins. It is believed that they act in the initial stage of airway immunologic defense as antigen-processing and antigen-presenting cells and as stimulators of T-cell proliferation.[31]

Lymphocytes (predominantly T cells) are present throughout the conducting airway epithelium, usually singly.[32] Although they are undoubtedly involved in processing and reacting to inhaled antigens, it is also possible that they have a role in modifying airway epithelial cell function.[32] Greater numbers are occasionally seen in association with lymphoid aggregates in the lamina propria and submucosa (bronchus-associated lymphoid tissue, see page 7). *Mast cells* can also be seen within airway epithelium, possibly in increased numbers in cigarette smokers.[33]

Submucosa and Lamina Propria

The subepithelial tissue can be subdivided into a lamina propria, situated between the basement membrane and the muscularis mucosa, and a submucosa, which includes all the remaining airway tissue. The *lamina propria,* more prominent in the trachea and proximal bronchi than in the distal airways, consists principally of small blood and lymphatic vessels, a meshwork of reticulin fibers continuous with the basal lamina, and elastic tissue. The *submucosa* contains cartilage, muscle, and other supportive connective tissue elements, the major portion of the tracheobronchial glands, lymphatics, bronchial arteries and veins, and various cells related to airway function and defense mechanisms.

A primary function of the basement membrane is to provide attachment of surface epithelium to the underlying connective tissue. On the epithelial side, attachment is mediated by adhesion molecules and by hemidesmosomal junctions with basal cells[34]; on the opposite side, anchoring fibrils emanate from the basement membrane and intertwine with collagen fibers in the upper lamina propria. Ultrastructural examination shows the presence of a population of fibroblasts located immediately beneath the basement membrane ("the attenuated fibroblast sheath") that have been speculated to be capable of interaction with adjacent epithelial cells and to be involved in the regulation of local inflammatory and reparative processes.[35]

Tracheal cartilage is arranged in a series of 16 to 20 horseshoe-shaped rings oriented in a horizontal plane with their open ends directed posteriorly. This U-shaped structure is also present in the main bronchi, but in more distal branches the plates become quite irregular in size and shape. At bronchial division points, they frequently take the shape of a saddle conforming to the branching angle, thus providing extra support at sites of increased turbulence. As the airway proceeds distally, the plates become smaller and less complete until they finally disappear altogether in airways 1 to 2 mm in diameter (bronchioles). With advancing age, the plates often become ossified and may be visible on radiographs.

The bronchial cartilage plates are tethered together by dense fibroelastic tissue arranged predominantly in a longitudinal direction. At numerous points, particularly in smaller airways, elastic fibers pass obliquely from these longitudinally arranged bundles to intermingle with the elastic tissue of the lamina propria.[36] These obliquely arranged fibers are believed to help transmit to the more rigid and stronger cartilaginous-fibrous tissue the longitudinal tensions that arise in the surface epithelium and the parenchyma as a whole during respiration.

Tracheal muscle is found predominantly in the membranous (posterior) portion, where it is arranged in transverse bundles attached to the inner perichondrium. In the intrapulmonary bronchi, the muscle coat lies close to the epithelium adjacent to the lamina propria (Fig. 1–11). In the main bronchi, the orientation is mainly transverse, as in the trachea; however, in more distal airways, the fibers become obliquely oriented and arranged in branching and anastomosing bundles that form irregular spirals down the airway. There is evidence that the relative thickness of the muscle coat expressed as a proportion of airway diameter is greater in the peripheral than the proximal airways.[37]

Loose connective tissue containing collagen and reticulin fibers occupies the bulk of the remainder of the submucosa. It is continuous with adjacent periarterial connective tissue and with perivenous connective tissue near the hilum and thus, by extension, with interlobular and pleural interstitial connective tissue. This interdependence of connective tissue is important in maintaining the overall structure of the lung and providing a scaffold for the more delicate connective tissue of the parenchyma.

Tracheobronchial glands (see Fig. 1–11) are specialized extensions of the surface epithelium into the lamina propria and submucosa that are seen exclusively in the trachea and bronchi.[38] The secretory portion of the gland is connected with the airway surface by a collecting duct. Elongated secretory tubules arise from the duct and are lined proximally by mucous cells and distally by somewhat flattened serous cells. The ultrastructure of these serous cells, as well as their content of carbonic anhydrase, suggests that their principal secretion is a low-viscosity substance, possibly meant to flush out the mucus. In addition, serous cells have been shown to be a source of several substances of importance in local airway defense, including lysozyme, transferrin, and leukocyte protease inhibitor.[23,24,39] There is also evidence that the cells function both in the manufacture of secretory component and in its coupling with and ultimate secretion of dimeric immunoglobulin (IgA).[40]

Many cells concerned with airway defense and other functions are found scattered in the lamina propria and submucosa. Lymphocytes are present singly and in small clusters, the latter being variously termed lymphoid nodules, lymphoid aggregates, or *bronchus-associated lymphoid tissue* (BALT).[41,42] These clusters are not present at birth and are usually absent or rare in normal lungs[43,44]; however, they are common in association with chronic airway irritation, such as seen in association with cigarette smoke,[44] thus suggesting that the

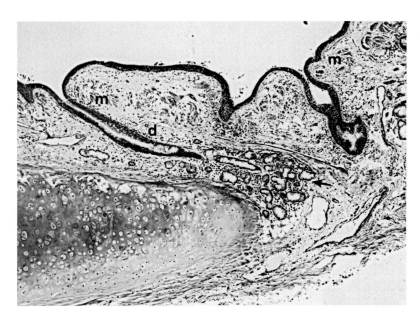

FIGURE 1–11

Normal bronchial wall with bronchial gland. A section of a lobar bronchus shows a portion of the cartilage plate, the muscularis mucosa (m), a bronchial gland duct (d), and secretory tubules (arrow). (×40.) (From Fraser RS, Müller NL, Colman NC, Paré PD: Fraser and Paré's Diagnosis of Diseases of the Chest, 4th ed. Philadelphia, WB Saunders, 1999.)

degree of BALT development is related to the presence of inhaled noxious material.

Plasma cells are commonly found in the tracheobronchial tree, particularly in relation to mucous glands and in the lamina propria close to the basal lamina.[45] Isolated *macrophages* and *mast cells* are found throughout the lamina propria and submucosa. There is evidence that macrophages in the lamina propria can modulate the activity of other lymphoreticular cells in the airway epithelium[46] and can migrate across the epithelium to the airway surface to phagocytose inhaled particulate material.[47]

Anatomy—The Transitional Zone

Geometry and Dimensions

Detailed three-dimensional studies of peripheral pulmonary tissue have shown that the geometry of the airways at this level is much more complex than usually appreciated by examining two-dimensional histologic sections.[48] Although branching can occur in a more or less symmetrical dichotomous fashion, trichotomous and even quadrivial (sometimes asymmetrical) divisions of the respiratory bronchioles are frequent. In addition, the number, overall configuration, length, and diameter of airways from the terminal bronchiole to the alveolar sac are quite variable; for example, the number of generations from the terminal bronchiole to the alveolar sac may be as many as 12 and as few as 2, although 6 to 8 is probably representative of most pathways. This geometric irregularity is probably related, at least in part, to spatial constraints imposed by pleura, interlobular septa, and larger airways and vessels.

The number of alveoli per respiratory bronchiole, alveolar duct, and alveolar sac also exhibits much variation; for example, the mean number of alveoli per alveolar sac has been calculated to range from 3.5 to 29, with most investigators having found about 10.[48] The most realistic estimate of the number of alveoli per alveolar duct is probably 15 to 20.

Morphology and Cell Function

Respiratory bronchioles have a low columnar to cuboidal epithelium (composed mostly of ciliated and Clara cells) that gradually decreases in extent as the number of alveoli increases (Fig. 1–12). In first- and second-order bronchioles, the epithelium is usually complete on one side; it overlies the lamina propria and submucosa continuous with that of the terminal bronchiole and contains a prominent pulmonary artery branch. As the number of alveoli increases, the submucosa disappears, but the muscle and elastic tissue continue in fairly prominent bundles in a spiral fashion surrounding the alveolar mouths. In the alveolar duct, bronchiolar epithelium is absent altogether, and only scanty interstitial tissue is present in the adjacent alveolar walls. Alveolar ducts terminate in a series of rounded enclosures called alveolar sacs, from each of which arise multiple alveoli.

Anatomy—The Respiratory Zone

Geometry and Dimensions

Alveoli are small, cup-shaped outpouchings of respiratory bronchioles, alveolar ducts, and alveolar sacs that are demar-

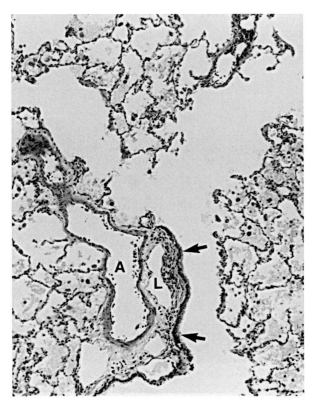

FIGURE 1–12

Respiratory bronchioles. One wall of a proximal respiratory bronchiole is completely lined by low columnar epithelium *(arrows)*. Adjacent to this is a small amount of interstitial tissue, a dilated lymphatic channel (L), and a branch of the pulmonary artery (A). The walls of the distal bronchiolar branches are almost completely alveolated. (×80.) *(From Fraser RS, Müller NL, Colman NC, Paré PD: Fraser and Paré's Diagnosis of Diseases of the Chest, 4th ed. Philadelphia, WB Saunders, 1999.)*

cated by thin septa (walls) (Fig. 1–13). In general, three septa have a common line of junction at an average angle of 120 degrees, and it is assumed that they are more or less flat if there is no pressure difference between contiguous alveoli. As a result of close packing of several alveoli of adjacent alveolar ducts and sacs, the dome of an alveolus may consist of more than three septa.

The total number of alveoli varies considerably; in one study of lungs from 32 subjects 19 to 85 years old, the computed totals ranged from 212×10^6 to 605×10^6 (mean, 375×10^6).[49] In adults, both the maximal diameter and depth of the alveolus average 250 to 300 μm.[2] Total alveolar surface area varies with body size, in one study[50] ranging from 40 to 100 m². In an average adult, it is probably between 70 and 80 m².[48]

Morphology and Cell Function

Alveolar septa are composed of a continuous, flattened epithelium overlying capillaries and a small amount of interstitial tissue. The former consists primarily of two morphologically and functionally distinct cells termed type I and type II. The interstitium itself contains a variety of cell types, as well as a small amount of connective tissue. Though not usually considered a part of the alveolar wall, the alveolar macrophage is normally present on its surface and is partly derived from

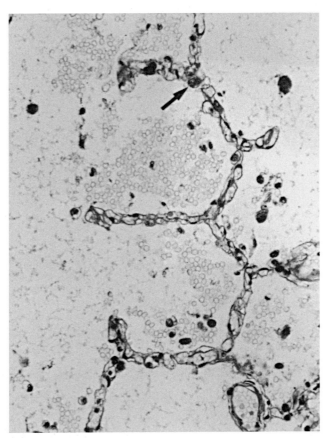

FIGURE 1–13

Normal alveoli. Note the minute amount of tissue interposed between air spaces and capillary lumina. The nucleus of a type II cell, or macrophage, is present at the junction of two septa *(arrow)*; type I cells are not clearly evident. (×350.) *(From Fraser RS, Müller NL, Colman NC, Paré PD: Fraser and Paré's Diagnosis of Diseases of the Chest, 4th ed. Philadelphia, WB Saunders, 1999.)*

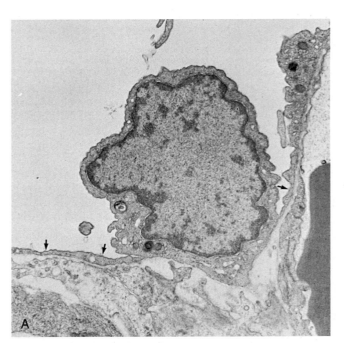

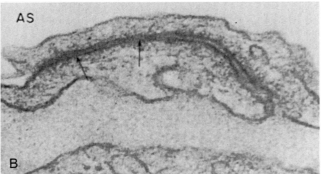

FIGURE 1–14

Type II alveolar epithelial cell. A, Low magnification showing a large nucleus and scanty cytoplasm that is attenuated on both sides over the alveolar surface *(arrows)*. **B,** High magnification of the junction between two type I cells showing a cleft extending roughly horizontally inward from the alveolar space (AS). In several areas *(arrows)* the outer leaflets of the plasma membranes appear fused. **(A,** *Courtesy of Dr. Nai-San Wang, McGill University, Montreal;* **B,** *from Schneeberger-Kelley EE, Karnovsky MJ: The ultrastructural basis of alveolar-capillary membrane permeability to peroxidase used as a tracer. J Cell Biol 37:781, 1968. Reproduced from the Journal of Cell Biology, by copyright permission of the Rockefeller University Press.)*

septal interstitial cells; thus, it is convenient to discuss its morphology and function here.

Type I Alveolar Epithelial Cell

Type I alveolar cells cover approximately 95% of the alveolar surface and have a total volume twice that of the histologically more obvious type II cells.[51] The nucleus of type I cells is small, somewhat flattened, and covered by a thin rim of cytoplasm containing few organelles (Fig. 1–14). The rest of the cytoplasm forms several broad sheets or plates that measure only 0.3 to 0.4 μm in thickness and extend for 50 μm or more over the alveolar surface, with the area covered measuring approximately 5000 μm[2].[51] The plates are joined firmly to one another and to type II cells by tight junctions that are believed to represent a more or less complete barrier to the diffusion of water-soluble substances into the alveolar lumen.[52]

The cytoplasm of type I cells contains fairly numerous pinocytotic vesicles, which have been hypothesized to transport fluid or proteins in either direction across the air-blood barrier and have been thought to be a means of resorbing neonatal or pathologic alveolar fluid.[53] The cells have also been shown to have the ability to ingest intra-alveolar particulate

material,[54] although the quantitative significance of this mechanism in relation to total lung clearance of particles is probably small when compared with alveolar macrophages.

Type II Alveolar Epithelial Cell

Type II epithelial cells are cuboidal in shape and usually located between type I cells near corners where adjacent alveoli meet. The cytoplasm contains membrane-bound granules filled with electron-dense lamellar material (Fig. 1–15) that is the source of alveolar surfactant.[55] In tissue fixed by perfusion through the vascular system, surfactant can be seen as a layer of acellular material about 4-nm thick lining the

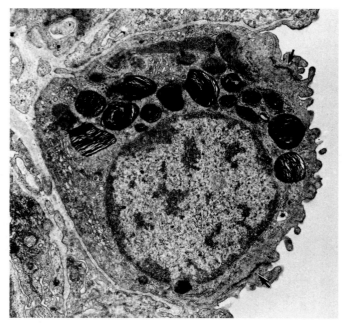

FIGURE 1–15

Type II pneumocyte. Note the short surface microvilli, junctions with type I cells *(arrows)*, and lamellated inclusion bodies. (Mouse lung, ×20,000.) *(Courtesy of Dr. Nai-San Wang, McGill University, Montreal.)*

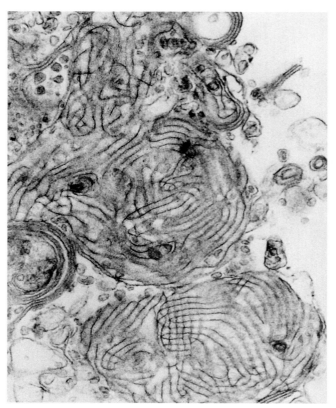

FIGURE 1–16

Surfactant. Transmission electron micrograph of free alveolar surfactant showing tubular myelin figures. *(Courtesy of Dr. David Walker, University of British Columbia, Vancouver.)*

alveolar surface.[56] It consists of two components:[57] (1) a film facing the alveolar air space that is composed of densely spaced phospholipids with a prominent tubular appearance (tubular myelin) (Fig. 1–16), and (2), deep to this film, a layer containing surface-active phospholipids in a different physicochemical configuration and representing the hypophase described by the physiologist. Components of the superficial layer are thought to be recruited from the deeper hypophase during expansion of the lung and may re-enter the hypophase layer at low lung volumes.

The type II cell has several functions in addition to that of surfactant production. In normal conditions, about 1% are mitotically active and are responsible for renewal of the alveolar surface by differentiation into type I cells.[58] This replicative ability is also important in healing after lung injury, in which the relative cytoplasmic simplicity and large surface area of type I cells makes them particularly susceptible to damage. In such circumstances, type II cells proliferate, temporarily repopulate the alveolar walls, and thereby provide epithelial integrity. As long as the air space and interstitial damage is minimal, the new type II cells can then transform into type I cells and restore the normal alveolar surface. The presence of anionic binding sites and microvilli on the type II cell surface suggests that they can act in the resorption of fluid or other substances from the alveolar lumen. There is also evidence that type II cells synthesize a variety of substances involved in alveolar structure and defense, including fibronectin and α_1-antitrypsin,[59,60] and are able to suppress lymphocyte proliferation and enhance macrophage function in the alveolar septa.[61,62]

Alveolar Septal Interstitium

A more or less continuous basement membrane underlies type I and type II cells. Over about 50% of its area, it is

intimately apposed to the underlying endothelial basement membrane; interstitial connective tissue and endothelial and epithelial cell nuclei are absent from this region of apposition, so the thickness of the air-blood barrier is determined only by the thin type I cell plate, the endothelial cell wall, and the fused basement membranes, the whole measuring about 0.5 μm (Fig. 1–17). Elsewhere, endothelial and epithelial basement membranes are separated by an interstitial space of variable width. Thus, the alveolar interstitium consists of two distinct anatomic compartments, one relatively thin, across which the major portion of gas transfer takes place, and the other thicker and functioning as mechanical support for the alveolus, a compartment for fluid transfer, and a site for various cells that contribute to alveolar function.

The septal connective tissue consists of a proteoglycan matrix into which are embedded elastic and collagen fibers that are intimately intertwined with and provide support for the capillary network. *Elastin* makes up almost 30% of dry lung weight and can stretch to about 140% of its length before breaking[63]; thus, it is of great importance in determining the mechanical properties of the lung. *Collagen* is less abundant and constitutes only about 15% of dry lung weight.[64] Both the collagen and the elastin of the alveolar septa are continuous with the fibroelastic tissue surrounding the small acinar vessels and airways and, by extension, with the connective tissue of the pleura, larger airways, and interlobular septa, thus forming a complex, three-dimensional connective tissue framework traversing and interconnecting the whole of the lung.

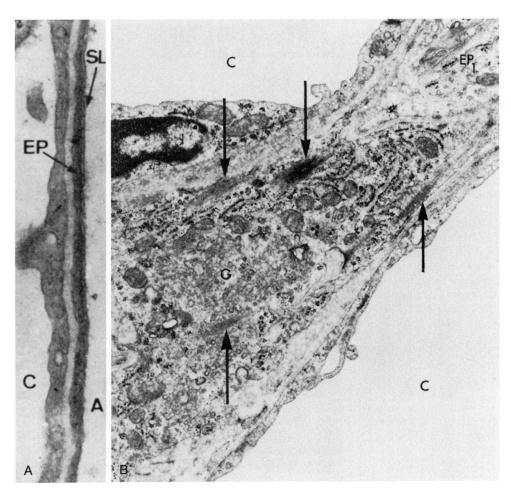

FIGURE 1–17

The air-blood barrier. A, Thin portion. A capillary (C) is present on the *left* and alveolar space (A) is on the *right*. A type I alveolar epithelial cell (EP) is covered by a clearly extracellular osmiophilic layer (SL). (Transmission electron microscopy [TEM], ×48,420.) **B,** Thick portion. Capillaries (C) and epithelial cells (EP$_1$) are separated by collagen fibers and a prominent interstitial cell containing a Golgi apparatus (G) and numerous bundles of microfilaments *(arrows)*. (Rat lung; TEM, ×24,000.) **(A,** *From Gil J, Weibel ER: Improvements in demonstration of lining layer of lung alveoli by electron microscopy. Respir Physiol 8:13-36, 1969;* **B,** *from Kapanci Y, Assimacopoulos A, Irle C, et al: "Contractile interstitial cells" in pulmonary alveolar septa: A possible regulator of ventilation-perfusion ratio? Ultrastructural, immunofluorescence, and in vitro studies. J Cell Biol 60:375-392, 1974. Copyright The Rockefeller University Press.)*

The alveolar interstitium also contains a variety of cell types. One of the more numerous, termed the *contractile interstitial cell (myofibroblast),* has ultrastructural and immunohistochemical features suggestive of both smooth muscle and fibroblast differentiation.[65] These cells appear to cross the interstitial space and attach to the basement membrane of epithelial and endothelial cells. It has been suggested that their contraction may result in a reduction in capillary blood flow and that such contraction may be the mechanism by which hypoxia causes decreased alveolar perfusion—thus, a possible means for regulation of local alveolar $\dot{V}_A/\dot{Q}$.[65] It has also been proposed that these cells may function as compliance regulators of the interstitial space by increasing resistance to interstitial expansion by edema fluid and thus propelling such fluid from the alveolar interstitium toward peribronchiolar lymphatics, where it may be effectively removed.[66] Finally, it is likely that the interstitial cells are responsible for the production of alveolar connective tissue, both in the normal state and in pathologic alveolar fibrosis.[67]

Additional cells located in the alveolar interstitium include mast cells, lymphocytes, macrophages, and dendritic cells.

The Alveolar Macrophage

Pulmonary macrophages have been considered to form several groups on the basis of differing anatomic location: (1) the *airway macrophage,* situated within the lumen or beneath the epithelial lining of conducting airways; (2) the *interstitial macrophage,* found either isolated or in relation to lymphoid tissue within interstitial connective tissue throughout the lung; (3) the *intravascular macrophage,* located adjacent to the capillary endothelial cell and possibly functioning as a reticuloendothelial cell similar to that in the liver and spleen[68]; (4) the *pleural macrophage*[69]; and (5) the *alveolar macrophage,* situated on the alveolar surface and within the air space itself.[70] Although all these cells are morphologically similar, there is evidence that the different subpopulations have different functional capabilities. However, because of its easy accessibility by BAL, the alveolar macrophage has been the most extensively studied, and the following discussion deals principally with this cell.

Numerically, the alveolar macrophage is by far the most important nonepithelial cell in the alveolar lumen. BAL of normal human air spaces yields a cell population composed of approximately 95% macrophages; dendritic cells (0.5%), lymphocytes (1% to 2%), monocyte-like cells of uncertain nature (2%), and polymorphonuclear leukocytes (less than 1%) account for the remainder.[71]

The cells range from 15 to 50 μm in diameter and are situated on the alveolar surface, with a preference for localization at the junctions between adjacent septa. Ultrastructurally, they have prominent surface microvilli and an abundance of intracytoplasmic, membrane-bound granules of variable appearance that represent primary and secondary lysosomes. They are derived from bone marrow precursors, probably via the peripheral blood monocyte.[70] In addition, there is evidence that alveolar interstitial macrophages are capable of division and thus replenishment or augmentation of the alveolar macrophage population.

The functions of the alveolar macrophage are numerous and complex,[72] and only a brief overview will be given here. These functions can be considered under three headings: (1) phagocytosis and clearance of unwanted intra-alveolar material, (2) immunologic interactions, and (3) production of inflammatory and other chemical mediators. There is evidence that different subpopulations of alveolar macrophages may have different capacities for these functions.[73]

PHAGOCYTOSIS AND CLEARANCE. Alveolar macrophages are motile and, in response to appropriate chemical stimuli, actively accumulate at the site of foreign material. Their surface possesses receptors for the Fc portion of various IgG molecules, as well as IgE, IgA, and C3; phagocytosis of foreign material occurs in association with these and other opsonins, such as fibronectin. In addition to inhaled foreign substances, alveolar macrophages ingest and eliminate endogenous pulmonary material, including dead type I and type II cells, surfactant, and the inflammatory exudate that may be produced during pneumonitis.

Although some macrophages containing foreign material enter the alveolar interstitium and either remain there or are transported via lymphatics to regional lymph nodes, there is evidence that few follow this route.[46] Instead, the majority either die within the alveoli or migrate to the terminal bronchioles, where they enter the mucociliary escalator and, along with their ingested material, are carried to the larynx and swallowed or expectorated.[74]

IMMUNOLOGIC INTERACTIONS. Alveolar macrophages have important functions in pulmonary immunologic reactions. Inhaled immunogens are phagocytosed by dendritic cells and presented to T lymphocytes, which then develop specific immunity. Subsequent antigen presentation stimulates the T cells and results in both T- and B-cell and T-cell and macrophage interactions. The latter results in activation of the macrophage and is manifested by features such as an increased number of surface receptors, increased amounts of lysosomal enzymes, and increased microbicidal activity. The importance of these interactions is illustrated by the frequency and severity of pulmonary infection in immunocompromised individuals.

PRODUCTION OF MEDIATORS. In both resting and activated conditions, alveolar macrophages synthesize and secrete a variety of substances,[72] many of which may have important effects on local pulmonary defense and structural integrity. Such substances include *fibronectin*[75]; a variety of proteases and antiproteases (*α_1-antitrypsin, α_2-macroglobulin, elastases, and collagenases*); inflammatory and immunologic mediators such as *prostaglandins, interleukins,*[76] *nitric oxide* (NO),[77] and *leukotrienes;* and antimicrobial substances such as *lysozyme and interferon.*[78]

The Lung Unit

Of the subdivisions of lung parenchyma that have been proposed as the "fundamental unit" of lung structure, the secondary lobules of Miller and the pulmonary acinus have gained the widest acceptance. The question of which most accurately represents the anatomic basis of normal and pathologic processes is controversial because each possesses

characteristics that suit one set of circumstances better than another. We believe that the subdivision most useful for descriptive and diagnostic purposes is the lobule.

The Secondary Lobule

The secondary pulmonary lobule is defined as the smallest discrete portion of lung that is surrounded by connective tissue septa. Interlobular septa are most well developed in the periphery of the lung, where they are continuous with the pleural interstitium (Fig. 1–18). They contain pulmonary veins and lymphatic vessels that drain the adjacent lobular tissue and are most numerous in the apical, anterior, and lateral aspects of the upper lobe and in the lateral and anterior regions of the right middle lobe, lingula, and lower lobe (Fig. 1–19).[79]

Each lobule contains three to five terminal bronchioles, their transitional airway branches, and the accompanying respiratory tissue. They are irregularly polyhedral in shape and generally range from 1 to 2.5 cm in diameter. A normal lobule cannot be identified on the chest radiograph. Only when the interlobular septa are rendered visible as septal lines as a result of thickening by fluid or tissue (such as edema or carcinoma) can the volume of lung between two lines be recognized as a secondary lobule. By contrast, normal interlobular septa are often identified on HRCT, most commonly in the lateral aspect of the lung as straight lines 1 to 2.5 cm in length. They can also be identified in the more central regions of both gross specimens and on HRCT when they are thickened by edema or inflammatory or neoplastic tissue (Fig. 1–20).[80-82]

From a radiologic point of view, the secondary lobule of Miller is considered the fundamental unit of lung structure for two major reasons: (1) it is the smallest anatomic unit that can be clearly identified on HRCT, and (2) assessment of the distribution of abnormalities within it can be helpful in the differential diagnosis of lung disease. For example, pathologic processes related to the terminal or respiratory bronchioles are characterized on HRCT by predominant distribution near the center of the lobule.[83] Specific abnormalities include localized areas of low attenuation in centrilobular emphysema and centrilobular nodular areas of increased attenuation in tuberculosis and hypersensitivity pneumonitis (Fig. 1–21).[84] In addition, various forms of bronchiolitis are characterized on HRCT by the presence of nodules or branching lines near the center of the lobule (Fig. 1–22) or by decreased attenuation of the lobule because of air trapping or vasoconstriction (Fig. 1–23).[83]

The Acinus

The pulmonary acinus is defined as the portion of lung distal to the terminal bronchiole. It comprises the respiratory bronchioles, alveolar ducts, alveolar sacs, alveoli, and their accompanying vessels and connective tissue (Fig. 1–24).[85] Reported measurements of acinar diameter vary between 6 and 10 mm, depending to some extent on the technique and pressure at which the lung is inflated.[86,87] In view of the size of the acinus, it is reasonable to assume that it should be visible radiologically when completely or partially filled with contrast material or inflammatory exudate.

Despite this, the concept of the acinus is of limited value in assessment of the chest radiograph or CT for several reasons. First, normal acini cannot be identified on the chest

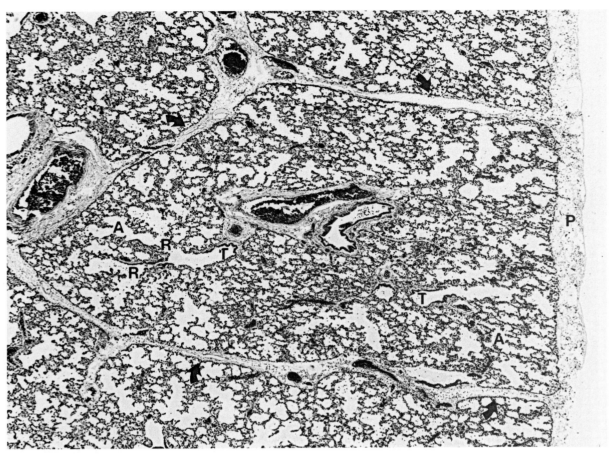

FIGURE 1–18

Secondary lobule—histologic appearance. A, alveolar duct; P, pleura; R, respiratory bronchiole; T, terminal bronchiole; *arrows,* interlobular septum. (×6.) *(From Fraser RS, Müller NL, Colman NC, Paré PD: Fraser and Paré's Diagnosis of Diseases of the Chest, 4th ed. Philadelphia, WB Saunders, 1999.)*

radiograph or with HRCT. Second, small nodular areas of consolidation cannot be assumed to represent acinar shadows radiologically. For example, in one radiologic-pathologic investigation, fluffy nodules corresponding to an acinar pattern in bronchopneumonia, "acinonodose" tuberculosis, and bronchiolitis were found to be caused predominantly by inflammation around terminal and respiratory bronchioles, with the distal air spaces usually being spared.[88] Finally, the consolidation associated with pneumonia or hemorrhage is seldom limited to the acinus but rather tends to coalesce and have a lobular, segmental, or lobar distribution.

Channels of Peripheral Airway and Acinar Communication

The first and probably the most studied of these structures are small discontinuities in the alveolar septa termed *alveolar pores (pores of Kohn)* (Fig. 1–25). They are round or oval in shape, are often situated at the junction of adjacent alveolar septa, and range in diameter from 2 to 10 μm. Because of their rarity in children, most authorities believe that they are acquired; it has been suggested that they may result from the desquamation of alveolar epithelial cells, from the action of ventilatory stress on alveolar walls, or from loss of interstitial connective tissue.[89] By transmission electron microscopy, the pore aperture is usually free of cellular or other material in airway-fixed material; in vascular-perfused tissue, however, the pore aperture is frequently occluded by a thin film of alveolar surfactant.[90] Because it is probable that vascular-perfused tissue more closely represents the normal state within the alveolar lumen, this observation casts considerable doubt on the significance of the pores in collateral ventilation.

The relationship of *alveolar fenestrae*—discontinuities measuring 20 to 100 μm in diameter—to alveolar pores is unclear. They are thought by most investigators to represent a pathologic state of the alveolar wall, some believing them to be the earliest stage of pulmonary emphysema. It has also been speculated that alveolar pores may themselves be the precursors of fenestrae.[91] Whatever their relationship, it is possible that these larger discontinuities are of greater significance than alveolar pores in providing a pathway for interacinar communication.

Direct communications between alveoli and respiratory, terminal, and preterminal bronchioles are termed *canals of Lambert;* these canals consist of epithelium-lined tubular structures that, in lungs fixed in deflation, range in diameter from "practically closed" to 30 μm.[92] It is not known whether these "airways" provide solely intra-acinar accessory communications or whether interacinar connections capable of subserving collateral ventilation occur as well.

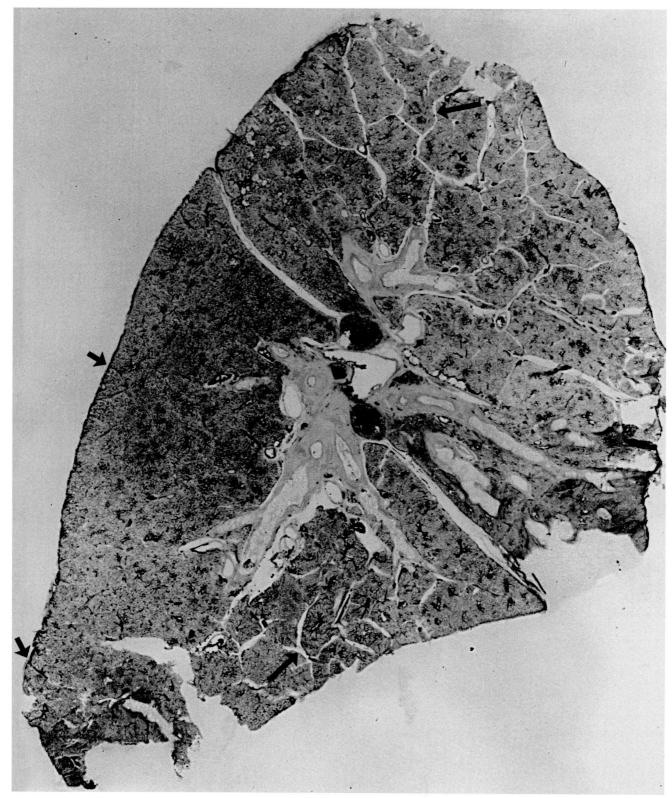

FIGURE 1–19

Interlobular septa. A paper-mounted section of a sagittal slice of the right lung shows moderately distended interlobular septa in the anterior and apical portions of the upper lobe and the basal aspect of the lower lobe *(long arrows)*. Some nondistended septa are also evident as thin black lines at the pleural surface of the lower lobe *(short arrows)*. *(From Fraser RS, Müller NL, Colman NC, Paré PD: Fraser and Paré's Diagnosis of Diseases of the Chest, 4th ed. Philadelphia, WB Saunders, 1999.)*

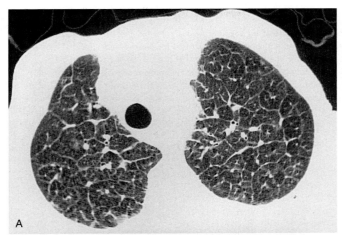

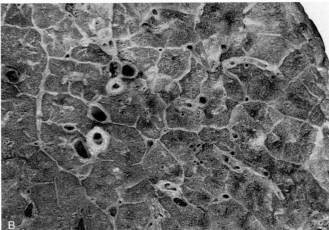

FIGURE 1–20

Interlobular septal thickening. An HRCT (1-mm collimation) scan in a patient with interstitial pulmonary edema (**A**) demonstrates thickening of the interlobular septa. Secondary pulmonary lobules are variable in size and have an irregular polyhedral shape. The patient was a 77-year-old woman with congestive heart failure. Incidental note is made of unrelated anterior mediastinal lymphadenopathy. A magnified view of a slice of upper lobe from another patient (**B**) shows mild to moderate interlobular septal thickening as a result of lymphangitic carcinomatosis. The architecture is similar to that of the HRCT image. *(From Fraser RS, Müller NL, Colman NC, Paré PD: Fraser and Paré's Diagnosis of Diseases of the Chest, 4th ed. Philadelphia, WB Saunders, 1999.)*

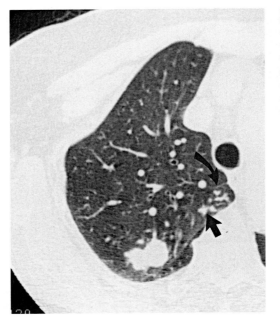

FIGURE 1–21

Centrilobular nodules in tuberculosis. An HRCT (1-mm collimation) scan at the level of the aortic arch demonstrates a lobulated, 2-cm-diameter nodule in the posterior segment of the right upper lobe. Note the centrilobular distribution of smaller nodules *(straight arrow)* and normal interlobular septum *(curved arrow)*. The patient was an 80-year-old woman with reactivation tuberculosis (large nodule) and endobronchial spread (smaller nodules). *(From Fraser RS, Müller NL, Colman NC, Paré PD: Fraser and Paré's: Diagnosis of Diseases of the Chest, 4th ed. Philadelphia, WB Saunders, 1999.)*

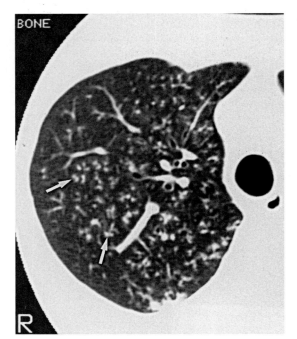

FIGURE 1–22

Centrilobular nodules caused by bronchiolitis. An HRCT (1.5-mm collimation) scan demonstrates small nodules and branching structures *(arrows)*. These abnormalities are situated approximately 5 mm away from vessels that are too large to be within the secondary pulmonary lobule and therefore represent borders of secondary pulmonary lobules. Structures and abnormalities located 5 mm away from these borders must be centrilobular in location. The patient was a 28-year-old man with bronchiolitis related to inhalation of foreign material. *(From Fraser RS, Müller NL, Colman NC, Paré PD: Fraser and Paré's Diagnosis of Diseases of the Chest, 4th ed. Philadelphia, WB Saunders, 1999.)*

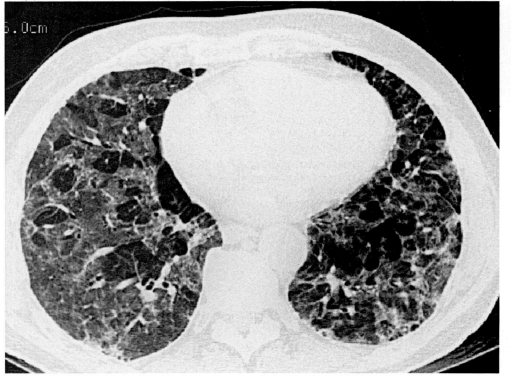

FIGURE 1–23

Decreased perfusion caused by bronchiolitis. An HRCT (1-mm collimation) scan through the lower lung zones demonstrates extensive areas of ground-glass attenuation. Note the localized polyhedral areas of decreased attenuation and small central vessels corresponding to secondary pulmonary lobules with decreased perfusion. The patient was a 74-year-old man with extrinsic allergic alveolitis and severe bronchiolitis. The areas of ground-glass attenuation correspond to alveolitis. The decreased perfusion of some of the secondary pulmonary lobules is presumably related to small-airway obstruction. *(From Fraser RS, Müller NL, Colman NC, Paré PD: Fraser and Paré's Diagnosis of Diseases of the Chest, 4th ed. Philadelphia, WB Saunders, 1999.)*

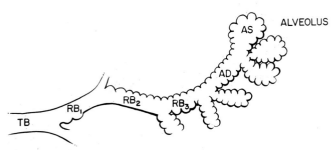

FIGURE 1–24

Component parts of the acinus. AD, alveolar duct; AS, alveolar sac; RB, respiratory bronchiole; TB, terminal bronchiole. *(From Thurlbeck WM: In Sommers SC [ed]: Pathology Annual. New York, Appleton-Century-Crofts, 1968, p 377.)*

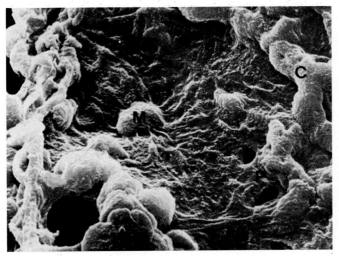

FIGURE 1–25

Surface of an alveolus. Note the capillaries (C), a macrophage (M), and alveolar pores (P). (Scanning electron microscopy, ×3650.) *(Courtesy of Dr. Nai-San Wang, McGill University, Montreal.)*

Radiology

Although several systems of bronchial nomenclature have been described, those of Boyden[93] and Jackson and Huber[94] have been the most widely adopted and remain the generally accepted terminology in North America (Table 1–1). It should be remembered, however, that the pattern of bronchial branching described, though the most common, is far from standard since there is considerable anatomic variation. The normal anatomy and common variations in the lower and upper lobe airways have also been described as viewed on HRCT.[95,96]

Trachea and Main Bronchi

For all intents and purposes, the trachea is a midline structure; a slight deviation to the right after entering the thorax is a normal finding and should not be misinterpreted as evidence of displacement. The walls of the trachea are parallel except on the left side just above the bifurcation, where the aorta commonly impresses a smooth indentation. The air columns of the

TABLE 1–1. Nomenclature of Bronchopulmonary Anatomy

Jackson-Huber	Boyden
Upper lobe	
Apical	B[1]
Anterior	B[2]
Posterior	B[3]
Right middle lobe	
Lateral	B[4]
Medial	B[5]
Right lower lobe	
Superior	B[6]
Medial basal	B[7]
Anterior basal	B[8]
Lateral basal	B[9]
Posterior basal	B[10]
Left upper lobe	
Upper division	
Apical-posterior	B[1&3]
Anterior	B[2]
Lingular division	
Superior	B[4]
Inferior	B[5]
Left lower lobe	
Superior	B[6]
Anteromedial	B[7&8]
Lateral basal	B[9]
Posterior basal	B[10]

From Fraser RS, Müller NL, Colman NC, Paré PD: Diagnosis of Diseases of the Chest, 4th ed. Philadelphia, WB Saunders, 1999.

trachea, main bronchi, and intermediate bronchus have a smoothly serrated contour created by the indentations of the cartilage rings in their walls at regular intervals.

In one CT study of 50 subjects without tracheal or mediastinal abnormalities, the length of the intrathoracic trachea ranged from 6 to 9 cm (mean, 7.5 ± 0.8 cm).[97] The most common shape was round or oval. In men 20 to 79 years old, the upper limit of normal for coronal and sagittal diameters is 25 and 27 mm, respectively[98]; in women of the same age, it is 21 and 23 mm, respectively. The lower limit of normal for both dimensions is 13 mm in men and 10 mm in women. There are only negligible differences in coronal or sagittal dimensions on radiographs exposed at full inspiration and maximal expiration.

The trachea divides into right and left main bronchi at the carina. The angle of bifurcation varies considerably; in one study of 100 normal adult subjects, the range was 35 to 90.5 degrees (mean, 60.8 ± 11.8 degrees).[99] In adults, the course of the right main bronchus distally is more direct than that of the left and is attributable, at least in part, to pressure on the left wall of the trachea by the aorta. The transverse diameter of the right main bronchus at TLC is greater than that of the left (15.3 versus 13.0 mm).[100]

Lobar Bronchi and Bronchopulmonary Segments

On this and the following pages, the anatomy of the proximal bronchi and bronchopulmonary segments is described and illustrated. Each segmental bronchus is considered separately, preceded by reproductions of a right bronchogram and corresponding drawings in anteroposterior (AP) (Fig. 1–26) and lateral (Fig. 1–27) projections and similar depictions of a left bronchogram (Figs. 1–28 and 1–29).

Text continued on page 25

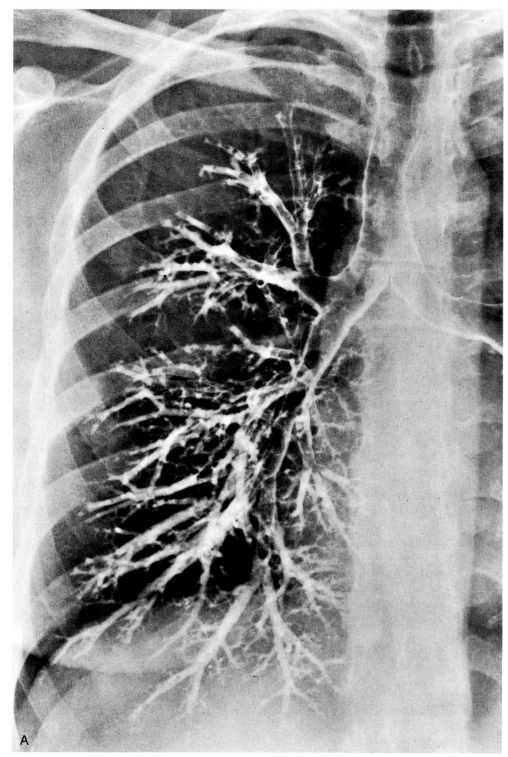

FIGURE 1–26

Right bronchial tree (frontal projection). A, Normal bronchogram of a 39-year-old woman.

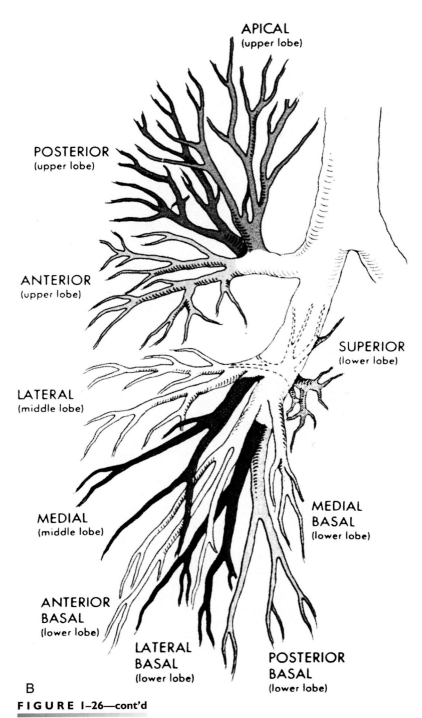

APICAL
(upper lobe)

POSTERIOR
(upper lobe)

ANTERIOR
(upper lobe)

SUPERIOR
(lower lobe)

LATERAL
(middle lobe)

MEDIAL
(middle lobe)

MEDIAL
BASAL
(lower lobe)

ANTERIOR
BASAL
(lower lobe)

LATERAL
BASAL
(lower lobe)

POSTERIOR
BASAL
(lower lobe)

B

FIGURE 1–26—cont'd

B, Normal segments of the right bronchial tree in a frontal projection. (*B from Lehman JS, Crellin JA: The normal human bronchial tree. Med Radiogr Photogr 31:81, 1955. Reprinted courtesy of Eastman Kodak Company.*)

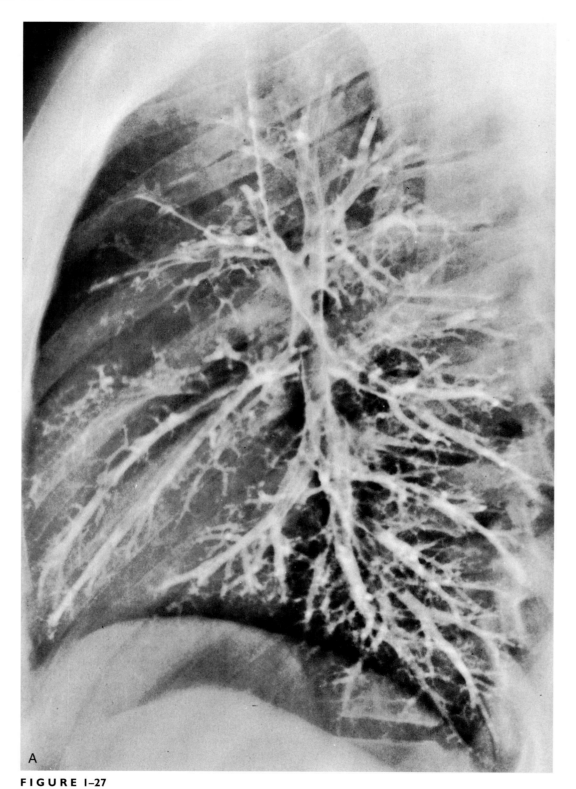

FIGURE 1–27

Right bronchial tree (lateral projection). A, Normal bronchogram of a 39-year-old woman.

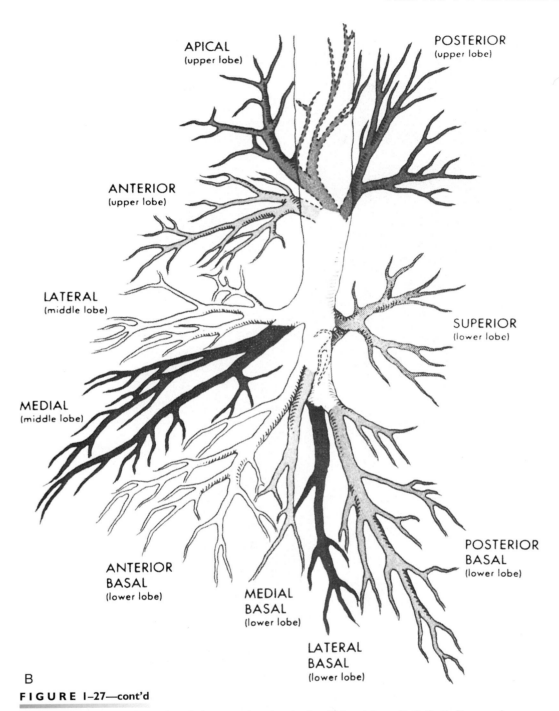

B

FIGURE 1–27—cont'd

B, Normal segments of the right bronchial tree in a lateral projection. (**B** from Lehman JS, Crellin JA: The normal human bronchial tree. Med Radiogr Photogr 31:81, 1955. Reprinted courtesy of Eastman Kodak Company.)

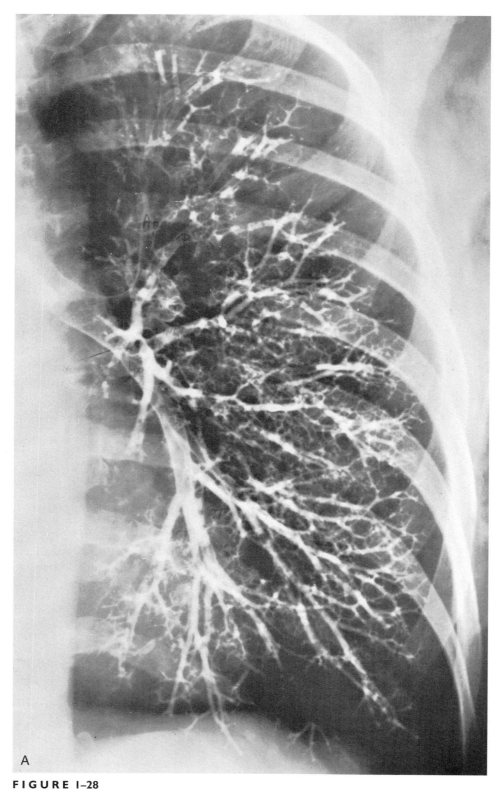

FIGURE 1–28

Left bronchial tree (frontal projection). A, Normal bronchogram of a 39-year-old woman.

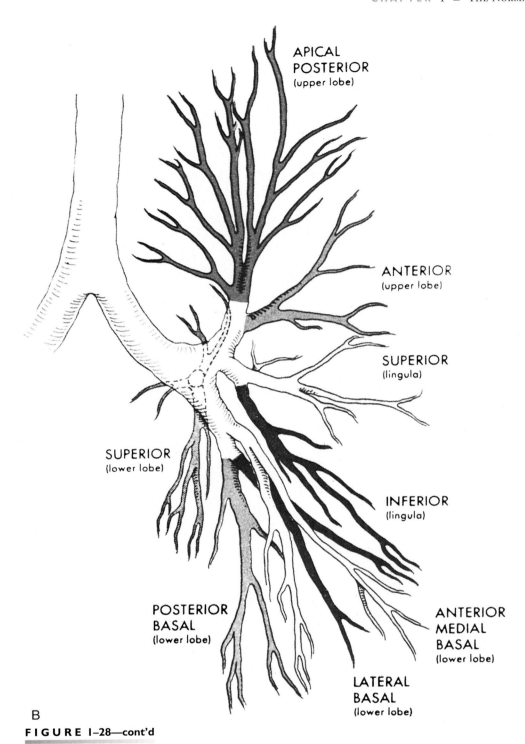

B

FIGURE 1–28—cont'd

B, Normal segments of the left bronchial tree in a frontal projection. (**B** from Lehman JS, Crellin JA: The normal human bronchial tree. Med Radiogr Photogr 31:81, 1955. Reprinted courtesy of Eastman Kodak Company.)

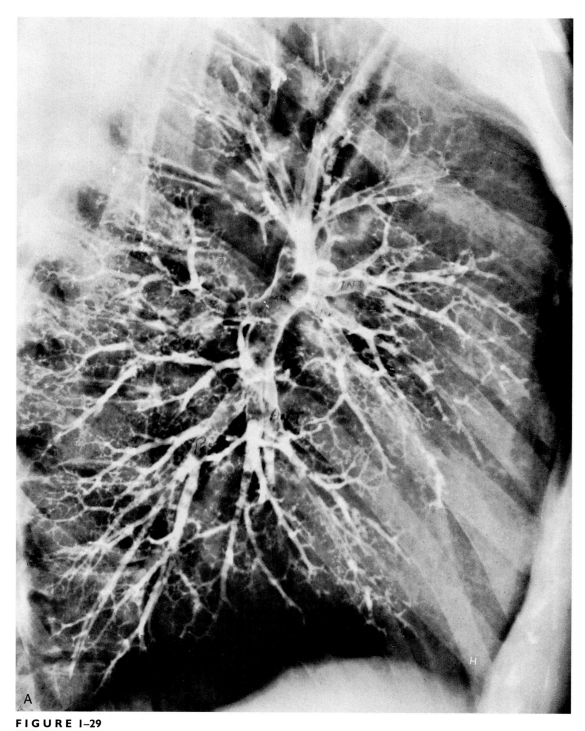

FIGURE 1–29

Left bronchial tree (lateral projection). A, Normal bronchogram of a 39-year-old woman.

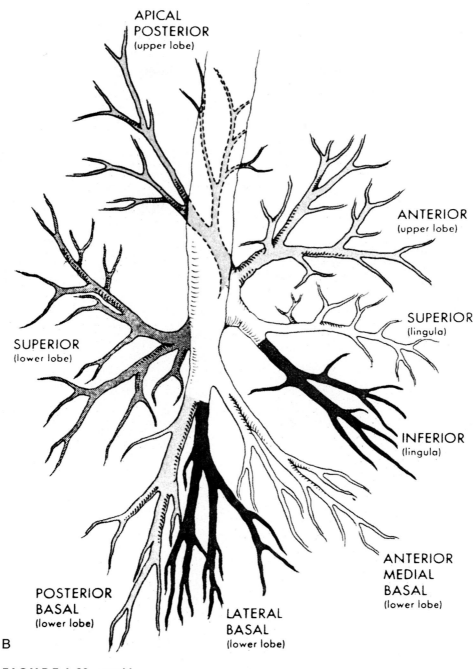

APICAL
POSTERIOR
(upper lobe)

ANTERIOR
(upper lobe)

SUPERIOR
(lingula)

INFERIOR
(lingula)

SUPERIOR
(lower lobe)

ANTERIOR
MEDIAL
BASAL
(lower lobe)

POSTERIOR
BASAL
(lower lobe)

LATERAL
BASAL
(lower lobe)

B

FIGURE 1–29—cont'd

B, Normal segments of the left bronchial tree in a lateral projection. (*B from Lehman JS, Crellin JA: The normal human bronchial tree. Med Radiogr Photogr 31:81, 1955. Reprinted courtesy of Eastman Kodak Company.*)

Right Upper Lobe. The bronchus to the right upper lobe arises from the lateral aspect of the main bronchus approximately 2.5 cm from the carina. It divides at slightly more than 1 cm from its origin, most commonly into three branches designated anterior, posterior, and apical. The branching pattern is particularly variable in relation to the axillary portion of the lobe.

Right Middle Lobe. The intermediate bronchus continues distally for 3 to 4 cm from the takeoff of the right upper lobe bronchus and then bifurcates to become the bronchi to the

middle and lower lobes. The middle lobe bronchus arises from the anterolateral wall of the intermediate bronchus, almost opposite the origin of the superior segmental bronchus of the lower lobe; 1 to 2 cm beyond its origin it bifurcates into lateral and medial segments.

Right Lower Lobe. The superior segmental bronchus arises from the posterior aspect of the lower lobe bronchus immediately beyond its origin; thus, it is almost opposite the takeoff of the middle lobe bronchus. The order of the four basal segmental bronchi of the lower lobe in the frontal projection

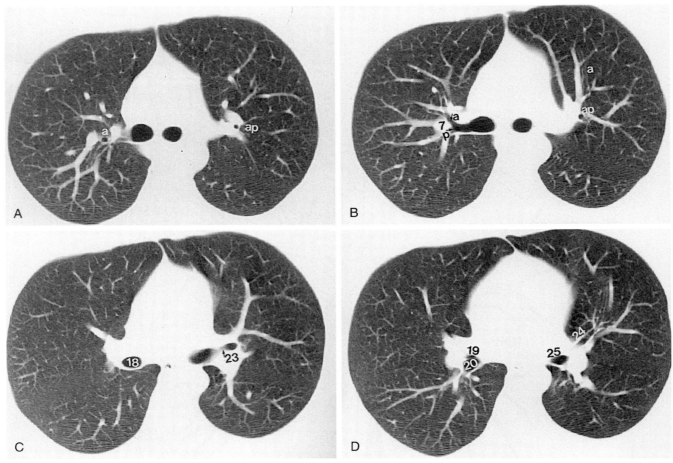

FIGURE 1–30

Bronchial anatomy on CT scan. A, A CT scan at a level immediately below the tracheal carina demonstrates the apical segmental bronchus of the right upper lobe (a) and the apical posterior segmental bronchus (ap) of the left upper lobe. **B,** CT scan at the level of the anterior (a) and posterior (p) segmental bronchi of the right upper lobe. Between them lies a branch of the right superior pulmonary vein (7). Also seen are the right and left main bronchi and the apicoposterior (ap) and anterior (a) segmental bronchi of the left upper lobe. **C,** Slightly more caudal, the apicoposterior segmental bronchus joins the left upper lobe bronchus (23). Note the local anterior and posterior indentations of the left upper lobe bronchus by the pulmonary artery. On the right, the intermediate bronchus (18) is seen in cross section. **D,** CT scan at the level of the lingular (24) and left lower lobe (25) bronchi and the carina between the right lower lobe (20) and middle lobe (19) bronchi.

from the lateral to the medial aspect of the hemithorax is *anterior-lateral-posterior-medial*. This anterior-lateral-posterior relationship is maintained in the lateral projection, hence the mnemonic "ALP."

Left Upper Lobe. About 1 cm beyond its origin from the anterolateral aspect of the main bronchus, the bronchus to the left upper lobe either bifurcates or trifurcates, usually the former. In the bifurcation pattern, the upper division almost immediately divides again into two segmental branches, the apical posterior and anterior. The lower division is the lingular bronchus, which is roughly analogous to the middle lobe bronchus of the right lung. When trifurcation of the left upper lobe bronchus occurs, the apical posterior, anterior, and lingular bronchi originate simultaneously. The lingular bronchus extends anteroinferiorly for 2 to 3 cm before bifurcating into superior and inferior divisions.

Left Lower Lobe. The divisions of the left lower lobe bronchus are similar in name and anatomic distribution to

those of the right lower lobe. The one exception lies in the absence of a separate medial basal bronchus, the anterior and medial portions of the lobe being supplied by a single anteromedial bronchus. The mnemonic ALP applies as well to the left lower lobe as to the right for identification of the order of basilar bronchi and their relationship to one another in frontal and lateral projections.

Bronchial Anatomy on Computed Tomography

Bronchi coursing horizontally within the plane of CT section are seen along their long axes (Fig. 1–30). These bronchi include the right and left upper lobe bronchi, the anterior segmental bronchi of the upper lobes, the middle lobe bronchus, and the superior segmental bronchi of the lower lobes. Bronchi coursing vertically are cut in cross section and are seen as circular lucencies. These bronchi include the apical segmental bronchus of the right upper lobe, the

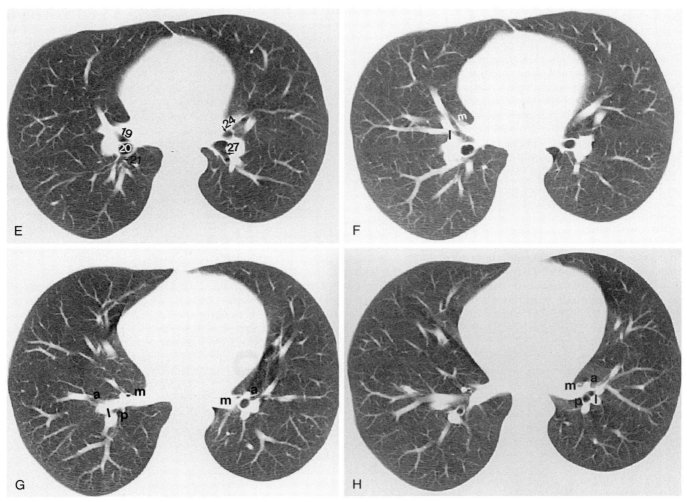

FIGURE 1–30—cont'd

E, A CT scan slightly more caudal demonstrates the superior segmental bronchus (27) of the left lower lobe, the inferior lingular bronchus (24), and the right superior segmental (21), lower lobe (20), and middle lobe bronchi (19). **F,** CT scan at the level at which the right middle lobe bronchus divides into medial (m) and lateral (l) segmental bronchi. Also seen are the lobar bronchi in cross section with the interlobar pulmonary arteries lateral to them. **G,** A CT scan at the level at which the inferior pulmonary veins join the left atrium demonstrates right medial (m) and anterior (a) segmental bronchi anterior to the right inferior pulmonary vein and posterior segmental (p) and lateral segmental (l) bronchi posterior to the vein. On the left side the medial segmental (m) and anterior segmental (a) bronchi can be seen, as well as a common trunk between the posterior and lateral segmental bronchi. More commonly, the anterior and medial bronchi originate as a common trunk to ventilate the anteromedial segmental bronchus of the left lower lobe. **H,** At a slightly lower level, the medial (m) and anterior (a) segmental bronchi of the left lower lobe can be seen anterior to the inferior pulmonary vein, whereas the lateral (l) and posterior (p) bronchi are posterior to the vein. *(From Fraser RS, Müller NL, Colman NC, Paré PD: Fraser and Paré's Diagnosis of Diseases of the Chest, 4th ed. Philadelphia, WB Saunders, 1999.)*

apicoposterior segmental bronchus of the left upper lobe, the bronchus intermedius, the lower lobe bronchi, and the basal segmental bronchi. Bronchi coursing obliquely are seen as oval lucencies and are less well visualized on CT scan. These bronchi include the lingular bronchus, the superior and inferior segmental lingular bronchi, and the medial and lateral segmental bronchi of the right middle lobe.

Function—Pulmonary Ventilation

The main purpose of breathing is to achieve and maintain alveolar and arterial blood gas homeostasis so that the oxygen demands of the organism are met and the metabolic byproduct, carbon dioxide, is exhaled. This goal is accomplished by a combination of ventilation (involving movement of gas to and from the alveoli), diffusion (involving movement of oxygen and carbon dioxide across the alveolocapillary membrane), and perfusion (involving transport of blood within the lung to and from the alveoli). The first of these three processes is discussed in this section; the remaining two are dealt with in the section on the vascular system (see page 39).

Composition of Gas in Alveoli

The composition of alveolar gas depends on the amount of oxygen removed and carbon dioxide added by capillary blood and the quantity and composition of the gas that reaches the acinus through the tracheobronchial tree.

Ventilation of the Acinus. Air contains approximately 21% oxygen and 79% nitrogen and, at sea level, has an atmospheric pressure of 760 mm Hg. The partial pressures of O_2 and N_2 are approximately 160 and 600, respectively. As air is inhaled into the tracheobronchial tree, it becomes fully saturated with water vapor at body temperature and a partial pressure of 47 mm Hg, and the partial pressure of oxygen drops to 150 mm Hg.

The quantity of gas reaching the alveoli (alveolar ventilation [$\dot{V}A$]) depends on the depth of inspiration (tidal volume [VT]), the volume of the conducting airways (the anatomic dead space [VDS]), and the number of breaths per minute (f) and can be calculated by the formula

$$\dot{V}A(L/min) = (VT - VDS) \times f$$

VDS ventilation is not considered alveolar ventilation because at the end of expiration, the dead space is filled with expired air having a composition equivalent to that in the acinus. The VA portion of each breath (ΔV) is added to the alveolar gas (Vo), and rapid diffusive mixing occurs such that gas tensions approach a uniform alveolar concentration. Failure of complete diffusive mixing within the air spaces may occur with acinar enlargement (e.g., emphysema) and with a decreased time for mixing.

Alveolar-Capillary Gas Exchange. Blood flow in the pulmonary capillaries affects the composition of alveolar gas by continuous removal of oxygen and addition of carbon dioxide. The ratio of alveolar ventilation to perfusion ($\dot{V}A/\dot{Q}$) shows regional variation within the lung, and the interaction of these two dynamic processes results in fluctuation in alveolar gas tensions not only throughout the respiratory cycle but also from breath to breath, lobe to lobe, and even acinus to acinus.

Mechanics of Acinar Ventilation. Movement of air down the conducting airways to the acinus requires force, measured as pressure, to overcome the elastic recoil of the lung parenchyma and chest wall, the frictional resistance to airflow through the tracheobronchial tree, and the inertia of the gas. Because air has very little mass, the inertial component is negligible with normal breathing frequencies; thus, elastic recoil and frictional resistance represent the major portion of the work of breathing.[101] The force necessary to inflate the lung is provided by contraction of the inspiratory muscles—mainly the diaphragm and, to a lesser extent, the external intercostal muscles. Normally, expiration is a passive phenomenon associated with relaxation of the inspiratory muscles. However, in patients who have obstructive airway disease and in normal individuals during periods of increased ventilation, expiratory muscles, especially the abdominals, may be recruited.

ELASTIC RECOIL OF LUNG PARENCHYMA AND THORACIC CAGE. At the end of a quiet breath (FRC), the chest wall recoils outward and exerts a force that is equal to and opposite the force exerted by the lung recoiling inward (Fig. 1–31). These balanced forces result in a negative pleural pressure of approximately 4 to 5 cm H_2O. On inspiration, the respiratory muscles act initially to overcome the elastic recoil of the lungs only. The chest wall actually aids inflation by its outward recoil until a volume of about 70% TLC is reached; at this point, it is inflated beyond its resting position, and the force of muscle contraction is then exerted against the recoil of both the lung and chest wall. TLC is reached when the inspiratory force

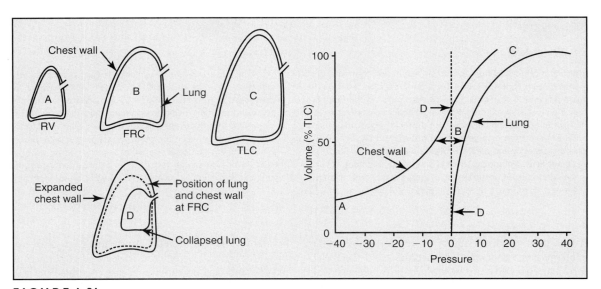

FIGURE 1–31

Static pressure-volume relationships of the lung and chest wall. In the **right panel,** lung and chest wall volumes are plotted against pressure. Transpulmonary pressure (pleural pressure – alveolar pressure) is the appropriate pressure for the lung, whereas transthoracic pressure (pleural pressure – atmospheric pressure) is the appropriate pressure for the chest wall. In the **left panel,** drawing B shows the relationship of the lung and chest wall at FRC; point B on the graph shows that at FRC, transpulmonary and transthoracic pressure is equal and opposite in sign. At RV (residual volume) (A in the **left** and **right panels**), transpulmonary pressure is near zero as the lung deflates toward the resting position, whereas transthoracic pressure is very negative because the chest wall becomes stiffer at low lung volumes. At TLC (C in the **left** and **right panels**), both the lung and the chest wall are expanded beyond their resting positions, and both exert recoil, which favors deflation. With the development of complete pneumothorax, transpulmonary and transthoracic pressure becomes zero, and the lung and chest wall assume their unstressed and relaxed positions (D).

achieved by the muscles is equaled by the combined recoil force of the lung and chest wall. It is apparent from Figure 1–31 that as lung volume increases, the elastic recoil of the lung parenchyma increases in a nonlinear fashion.

During deflation of the lung from FRC toward residual volume (RV), the expiratory muscles are aided by the elastic recoil of the lung. As RV is approached, the chest wall becomes more difficult to distort, and it is finally set at the point at which outward recoil of the chest wall equals the force exerted by the expiratory muscles. In older individuals and in patients who have obstructive lung disease, this point may not be reached because the airways may narrow and limit expiration at higher lung volumes.[102]

The relationship between changes in volume and pressure ($\Delta V/\Delta P$) is termed compliance, which can be calculated for the lung and chest wall either separately or together (respiratory system compliance). The major determinants of compliance of the lung are the quantity and anatomic arrangement of the collagen and elastic fibers in the parenchyma and airways and the surface tension at the air-fluid interface of the alveolar surface (see later). The compliance of the chest wall is determined largely by the rigidity of the rib cage. In normal individuals, the compliance of the respiratory system is the major determinant of the work of breathing; in disease, the work of breathing can increase because of decreased compliance of the lung or chest wall. It is apparent from Figure 1–31 that as lung volume increases, the compliance of the lung and chest wall decreases; therefore, hyperinflation increases the work of breathing.

SURFACE TENSION AND SURFACTANT. The surface lining of the lung has unique properties that result in a much lower surface tension than if the alveoli were lined by water or plasma and that cause a reduction in surface tension as the lung is deflated. The substance responsible for these properties is surfactant, 90% of which is composed of phospholipids; the main component of these phospholipids is dipalmitoyl phosphatidylcholine (DPPC). Surfactant is secreted as a complex of these phospholipids and protein, of which several, including apoproteins A, B, and C, have been identified.[103] Although pure phospholipid and the complex of apoprotein and phospholipids have similar capabilities for lowering surface tension, the lipoprotein complex spreads much more readily over the air-liquid interface, and the protein is probably necessary for efficient function. Surfactant proteins also have an important role in the innate immune response, where their actions contribute to microbial defense.[104]

The mechanical functions of surfactant include prevention of alveolar collapse, decrease in the work of breathing, an antisticking action that prevents adherence of alveolar walls, and an antiwetting action that may aid in keeping the alveolar surface dry. The forces that tend to decrease alveolar size are surface tension and tissue elasticity. The force generated by tissue elasticity is roughly proportional to lung volume, but it constitutes only a third of total lung elastic recoil at TLC; the other two thirds is caused by surface tension. The pressure attributable to surface factors can be calculated from the Young-Laplace relationship,

$$P = 2\gamma/r$$

where γ is the surface tension of the alveolar air-liquid interface and r is the alveolar radius. Opposed to the lung elastic recoil and surface tension forces that tend to collapse alveoli is transpulmonary pressure. Mechanical balance is achieved when transpulmonary pressure equals the pressure generated by elastic recoil and surface tension. With lung deflation, transpulmonary pressure decreases at the same time that the alveolar radius is decreasing, a situation that favors alveolar collapse. This is why a substance with the surface tension–lowering ability of surfactant is necessary to achieve alveolar stability.

The reduction in surface tension imparted by surfactant may have an important role in fluid balance in the lung distinct from its role in the mechanics of breathing. The reduced surface tension counteracts the tendency for fluid to be "sucked" into the alveolar air space from the capillary lumen.[105] Surfactant also imparts hysteresis to the lung's pressure-volume behavior; that is, at any given lung volume, surface tension and therefore lung elastic recoil are greater during inflation than during deflation. It has been suggested that in addition to an alteration in surface forces, lung hysteresis is caused partly by a different sequence of recruitment and de-recruitment of alveoli during inflation and deflation.[106]

Surfactant production and secretion are under complex neural, humoral, and chemical control.[107,108] They are stimulated by an increase in ventilation or tidal volume[109]; this effect appears to be mediated through the β-adrenergic system inasmuch as this mechanical stimulatory effect can be blocked by propranolol.[110] The ultimate metabolic fate of secreted surfactant is poorly understood. Very little passes directly up the airways; however, some is taken up by alveolar macrophages and transported in them up the mucociliary escalator. In addition, a proportion enters type I cells (via pinocytotic vesicles) and finds its way back into type II cells, where it may be reused.[111,112]

RESISTANCE OF THE AIRWAYS. Frictional resistance to airflow in the conducting airways is the second major factor in the work of breathing. The pressure necessary to produce laminar flow through a tube is described by the formula

$$\text{Pressure required} = \frac{\text{Length} \times \text{Viscosity} \times \text{Flow}}{\text{Radius}^4}$$

It is apparent from this equation that airway radius is the dominant variable in determining resistance; a doubling of airway length would only double the pressure necessary to produce a given flow (i.e., double the resistance), whereas a halving of the radius would lead to a 16-fold increase in resistance.

Under conditions of laminar flow, the flow rate is linearly related to pressure; that is, a doubling of pressure is required for a doubling of flow. However, with the development of turbulence and other nonlaminar flow states, the relationship becomes nonlinear, and a greater increase in pressure is required to produce a given increment in flow. In addition, in nonlaminar states, gas density begins to play a role, with resistance decreasing with gases of low density (e.g., a helium and oxygen mixture). In normal individuals during quiet breathing through the mouth, flow is almost totally laminar[113]; however, with breathing through the nose or through narrowed airways and during the increased flow rates of exercise, substantial turbulence may occur and result in an increasing proportion of the work of breathing devoted to overcoming resistance.

Total airway resistance represents the sum of the resistance of the various types of airway, from the larynx and large bronchi down to the respiratory bronchioles. In normal individuals, the major part of total airway resistance is provided by large airways,[114] with the relatively small component contributed by the smaller airways being related to their large cross-sectional area. However, in diseases such as asthma and chronic obstructive lung disease, the primary site of increased resistance is the small airways.

TISSUE RESISTANCE. Although the major impedance of the lungs and chest wall tissue is elastic, they do provide a small amount of frictional resistance, estimated to be between 5% and 40% of total pulmonary resistance.[115]

Collateral Ventilation

Collateral airflow between lung units can be important in preserving gas exchange capacity and in matching ventilation and perfusion in the presence of airway obstruction.[116] The resistance to airflow through collateral channels (Rcoll) can be measured by wedging a bronchoscope in a peripheral airway and measuring the pressure required to force air through that airway and the collateral channels into the surrounding lung. It varies with several parameters, including inspired gas tension, lung inflation, and the anatomic site. Increasing the partial pressure of carbon dioxide (Pco_2) in inspired gas lowers collateral resistance, whereas the response is opposite with a decrease in the partial pressure of inspired oxygen (Po_2). Collateral resistance decreases with lung inflation in a manner similar to the decrease in airway resistance that occurs with lung inflation. In normal lungs, however, collateral flow resistance at FRC is some 50 times greater than resistance to flow through the normal airways.[117]

Function—Respiratory Mucus and Mucus Rheology

The precise definitions of mucus, tracheobronchial secretions, and sputum are sometimes confused. Mucus represents the products derived from secretions of the tracheobronchial glands and epithelial goblet cells,[118] whereas tracheobronchial secretions include mucus plus other fluid and solutes derived from the alveolar and airway epithelium and the circulation; in normal individuals, the volume of these secretions has been estimated to range from 0.1 to 0.3 mL/kg of body weight, or up to about 10 mL/day.[119] Sputum consists of expectorated or swallowed mucus contaminated by saliva, transudated serum proteins, and inflammatory and desquamated epithelial cells; it is invariably associated with pulmonary disease.

Tracheobronchial secretions have three important roles:[111] (1) clearance of particulate matter deposited within the respiratory tract, (2) protection from microbial infection, and (3) humidification of inspired air and prevention of excessive fluid loss from the airway surface.

Biochemical Characteristics of Tracheobronchial Secretions. The biochemical composition of tracheobronchial secretions can be divided into two portions—a glycoprotein fraction that gives them their characteristic viscoelastic and rheologic properties, plus sol-phase proteins that are derived from both local production and transudation from serum.

The protein and nonmucous glycoprotein content in the sol phase of respiratory secretions has been characterized in sputum from patients and in bronchial lavage fluid from normal individuals.[120] It has been calculated that the quantity of IgG, IgA, transferrin, α_1-antitrypsin, and ceruloplasmin is greater than would be expected if transudation were the sole mechanism of their production, thus suggesting local production and secretion.[121] The excess immunoglobulins are synthesized by plasma cells in the airway wall; other locally produced substances, such as lysozyme and lactoferrin, are produced by airway epithelial cells.

Ninety-five percent to 98% of the weight of normal tracheobronchial secretions is water.[122] The electrolyte composition of the sol phase of the secretions is similar to that of serum; however, the relative concentration of chloride is significantly higher, and the secretions are hyperosmolar relative to plasma.

Control of Tracheobronchial Secretions. Because atropine or vagal blockade decreases the basal secretion rate of tracheobronchial secretions to approximately 60%,[123] normal secretion appears to be under a tonic cholinergic stimulation. There also appears to be both β- and α-adrenergic stimulatory influences, and β-blockade decreases basal secretions as well. α-Adrenergic stimulation increases secretion from serous cells predominantly, whereas β-adrenergic stimulation increases chiefly mucous cell secretion; cholinergic stimulation increases secretion from both cell types equally.[124] Hypoxia, stimulation of gastric mechanoreceptors, stimulation of upper airway cough receptors, and a wide variety of irritants, such as ammonia, cigarette smoke, sulfur dioxide, and organic vapors, cause an increase in mucus secretion. Inflammatory mediators such as histamine, the prostaglandins, the leukotrienes, and the neuropeptides substance P and vasoactive intestinal polypeptide are also respiratory mucus secretagogues. Neutrophil elastase is a powerful secretagogue for goblet cell mucus.[125]

Optimal mucociliary clearance by respiratory tract cilia depends on a proper balance between the volume of the mucous layer and the more fluid and less viscid sol phase through which the rapid recovery stroke of the cilia occurs.[126] Water transport—and therefore the composition of the periciliary sol phase of tracheobronchial mucus—is modulated by active ion transport across the epithelium.[127,128] A sodium-potassium adenosine triphosphatase pump located on the basolateral surface of airway epithelial cells generates an electrochemical gradient that produces a potential difference across the epithelium, the luminal fluid being approximately 30 mV negative relative to the submucosa.[129] This gradient causes a net movement of Na^+ from the lumen into the cell via an Na^+ channel in the apical (luminal) membrane.[130] The combination of the apical Na^+ channel and the basolateral pump results in transcellular Na^+ absorption. Chloride and water normally follow Na^+ passively through paracellular pathways and across a number of apical Cl^- channels, one of which is the cystic fibrosis transmembrane regulator (CFTR). Absorption of water and solutes by airway epithelium is necessary because the marked decrease in surface area between the bronchioles and the trachea would result in luminal occlusion if fluid absorption did not occur as the secretions move proximally.

Physical Characteristics of Tracheobronchial Secretions. Few data exist on the controlling mechanisms that affect the viscoelastic properties of mucus. The rate of secretion of mucous glycoprotein and periciliary fluid, as well as changes in the biochemical composition of secreted mucus and sol-phase proteins, is undoubtedly important. Vagal stimulation and methacholine inhalation tend to increase elasticity and dynamic viscosity at low stimulation frequencies and dose, whereas both viscoelastic characteristics decrease at higher frequencies and concentrations.[111] β-Adrenergic stimulation imparts a selective stimulation of mucous cells and leads to increased elasticity and dynamic viscosity; by contrast, α-adrenergic stimulation selectively stimulates serous cells and results in a more watery mucus.[111] Inhalation of prostaglandin F_2, histamine, or acetylcholine has been shown to produce alterations in the viscoelastic properties of mucus in normal subjects, but these agents also increase the transudation of serum proteins into bronchial mucus, thus suggesting altered epithelial fluid permeability.[122] Purulent sputum is more viscous, but less elastic than mucoid sputum, in part related to its DNA content.[131]

THE PULMONARY VASCULAR SYSTEM

Anatomy

Morphology and Dimensions of the Major Vessels

The conducting and transitional airways are intimately related to the pulmonary vasculature such that a branch of the pulmonary artery always accompanies the appropriate bronchial division (Fig. 1–32). In addition to these "conventional" vessels, many accessory ("supernumerary") branches of the pulmonary artery arise at points other than the corresponding bronchial divisions and directly penetrate the lung parenchyma (Fig. 1–33). These accessory branches outnumber the

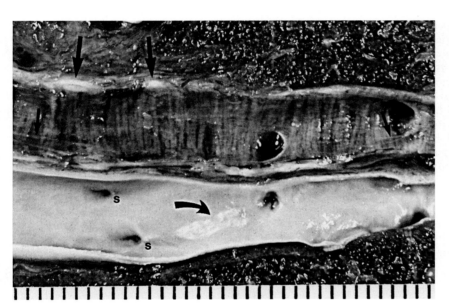

FIGURE 1–32

Normal bronchus and pulmonary artery. Longitudinal slice of a small bronchus and adjacent pulmonary artery showing cartilage plates *(long arrows)*, more or less circularly oriented smooth muscle bundles, and sparse, relatively thin, longitudinal elastic tissue bundles *(short arrows)*. Note the supernumerary artery branches (unassociated with airway branches) (S) and the small focus of mild atherosclerosis *(curved arrow)*. *(From Fraser RS, Müller NL, Colman NC, Paré PD: Fraser and Paré's Diagnosis of Diseases of the Chest, 4th ed. Philadelphia, WB Saunders, 1999.)*

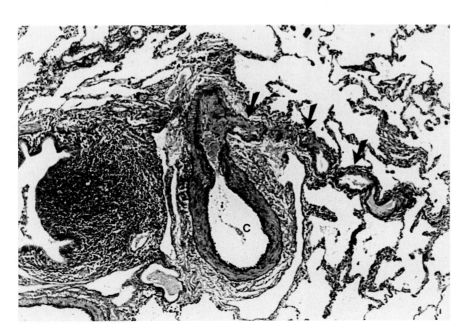

FIGURE 1–33

Pulmonary artery—conventional and supernumerary branches. The section shows a "conventional" muscular pulmonary artery (C) adjacent to a bronchiole. A small supernumerary branch *(arrows)* extends from this vessel into the adjacent lung parenchyma. *(From Fraser RS, Müller NL, Colman NC, Paré PD: Fraser and Paré's Diagnosis of Diseases of the Chest, 4th ed. Philadelphia, WB Saunders, 1999.)*

conventional ones and originate throughout the length of the arterial tree, most frequently peripherally. Thus, the branching ratio (average number of daughter branches emanating from one parent branch) increases as vessel size decreases; proximally, the ratio is about 3, a value comparable to that of the conducting airways, and distally it rises to about 3.6.[132] The precapillary pulmonary vessels can be conveniently divided into three morphologic types: elastic, muscular, and arteriolar.

Elastic arteries include the main pulmonary artery and its lobar, segmental, and subsegmental branches extending approximately to the junction of bronchi and bronchioles. Histologically, the large extrapulmonary vessels contain a multilayered latticework of elastic fibers. Within the lung the number of laminae diminishes such that at a diameter of 500 to 1000 μm, medial elastic tissue is lost altogether, with only well-developed internal and external laminae left.

Muscular arteries have an external diameter ranging from about 70 to 500 μm and possess a well-developed layer of circularly oriented smooth muscle cells between the elastic laminae. Acinar vessels with recognizable arterial features and most supernumerary arterial branches are of this type. Beyond a diameter of 70 to 80 μm, arteries gradually lose their medial smooth muscle and become arterioles composed solely of a thin intima and a single elastic lamina that is continuous with the external elastic lamina of arteries. Within the acinus, arterioles continue to divide and accompany their respective branches of the transitional airways, as well as give rise to many accessory branches. These branches and those that terminate around the alveolar sacs break up to form the capillary network of the alveoli.

The pulmonary veins arise from capillaries of the alveolar meshwork and from some of the bronchial capillaries. The larger branches are located within their own interstitial sheath separate from the bronchoarterial bundles. As in the pulmonary arterial system, numerous supernumerary vessels join the veins as they course through the lung.[133] Although their final course is somewhat variable, there are usually two large superior and two large inferior pulmonary veins, the former draining the middle and upper lobes on the right side and the upper lobe on the left and the latter draining the lower lobes.

Histologically, pulmonary veins show a variable number of elastic laminae associated with small bundles of smooth muscle cells and collagen. No valves are present; however, regularly spaced annular constrictions, possibly caused by local accumulations of smooth muscle, have been identified in animal veins and have been hypothesized to be capable of influencing blood flow.[134]

The Pulmonary Endothelium

Ultrastructurally, endothelial cells are arranged in an interlocking mosaic of platelike processes measuring as little as 0.1 μm in thickness.[135] Numerous small microvilli emanate from the cell surface; these microvilli greatly increase the cell surface area and have been shown to react immunochemically with an antibody to angiotensin-converting enzyme,[136] thus implying a role in metabolic function.

A prominent feature of the capillary endothelial cell is the presence of numerous small pits, or vesicles (*caveolae intracellulare*) (Fig. 1–34).[137] These vesicles are located in the thick, non–gas-exchanging part of the cell, either at the luminal or abluminal surface or free in the cytoplasm. Small electron-dense granules, considered to represent enzyme complexes responsible for various metabolic functions, can be seen at the bases of the vesicles. In addition to this role, it is thought that the vesicles function as a transport mechanism for fluid and proteins between blood and interstitial tissue.[138]

Endothelial cells are joined by tight junctions.[135] As seen by freeze-fracture techniques, these junctions are less complex than those of the alveolar epithelium; along with evidence

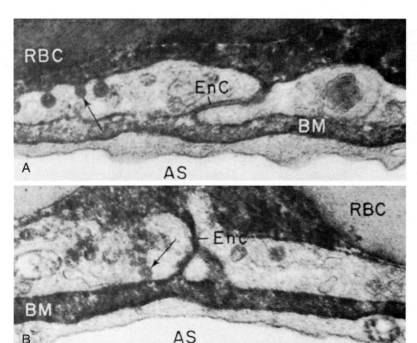

FIGURE 1–34

Endothelial intercellular cleft. Section of alveolar wall from the lung of a mouse sacrificed 90 seconds after injection of horseradish peroxidase. The reaction product in the capillary lumen (indicated by RBC) extends through the endothelial intercellular cleft (EnC) into the adjacent basement membrane (BM). In **A,** the staining of horseradish peroxidase is quite light, whereas in **B,** the basement membrane is deeply stained. Reaction product is present in endothelial invaginations (caveolae intracellulare) on both the capillary side (*arrow* in **A**) and the alveolar side (*arrow* in **B**) of the cell. (TEM; ×46,000.) (*From Schneeberger-Keeley EE, Karnovsky MJ: The ultrastructural basis of alveolar-capillary membrane permeability to peroxidase used as a tracer. J Cell Biol 37:781, 1968. Reproduced from the Journal of Cell Biology, by copyright permission of the Rockefeller University Press.*)

provided by autoradiographic tracer studies, this finding suggests that the main site of solute impermeability in the air-blood barrier is the epithelium. The complexity of the endothelial junctions is variable, being greater in arterioles (which are thought to be relatively impermeable) and less in venules (which are thought to be the major site of vascular fluid leakage). Endothelial cells produce a number of substances, such as cell adhesion molecules, antielastolytic substances, NO, and endothelin, that probably have important roles in vascular function, pulmonary defense, and even gas exchange itself.[139-141]

Geometry and Dimensions of the Alveolar Capillary Network

The pulmonary capillaries form a dense network of interconnecting vessels within the alveolar wall (Fig. 1–35). Their actual arrangement is highly complicated when one considers the three-dimensional capillary and alveolar geometry under dynamic conditions. In this situation, the shape of the alveolar septa—and the vessels that they contain—can be affected by three mechanical factors, each of which can vary in the normal respiratory cycle:[142] (1) tissue force as a result of tension on the

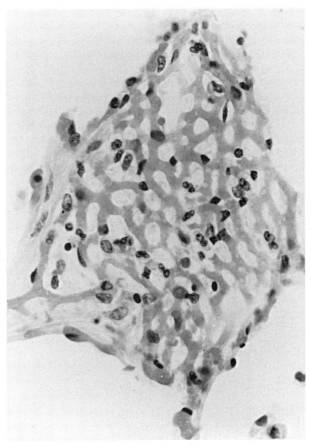

FIGURE 1–35

Alveolar capillary network. An en face section of an alveolar wall shows numerous short capillary segments interconnecting to form a complex vascular network. *(From Fraser RS, Müller NL, Colman NC, Paré PD: Fraser and Paré's Diagnosis of Diseases of the Chest, 4th ed. Philadelphia, WB Saunders, 1999.)*

interstitial connective tissue transmitted through the connective tissue of the visceral pleura, (2) capillary distending pressure, and (3) alveolar air-fluid surface forces.

The external diameter of capillary segments in fresh lung averages 8.6 μm[143]; allowing 0.3 μm for the average thickness of the capillary endothelial wall, the average internal capillary diameter is thus about 8 μm. (However, these values may vary substantially with both lung volume and capillary pressure.[144]) The axial length of capillary segments ranges from 9 to 13 μm (average, 10.3 μm). Weibel deduced that each alveolus is surrounded by about 1800 to 2000 capillary segments and that the total capillary surface of the lung is about 70 m², only slightly less than that of the alveolar surface.[143]

Intervascular Anastomoses

Because of the lungs' dual blood supply, several combinations of intervascular anastomoses are possible. Those between *bronchial arteries* and *pulmonary veins* are undoubtedly the most frequent and probably represent the normal pathway for the bulk of bronchial venous drainage. *Bronchial artery–pulmonary artery* anastomoses have been shown to occur in the normal lung; although their functional significance is unclear in normal circumstances, their number and size may increase appreciably in various disease states and potentially result in a significant *left-to-right* shunt. Though investigated extensively, the existence of *pulmonary arteriovenous anastomoses* is uncertain; some investigators have found evidence for their presence, whereas others have not.

Radiology—Vasculature

The main pulmonary artery originates in the mediastinum at the pulmonic valve and passes upward, backward, and to the left before bifurcating within the pericardium into the shorter left and longer right pulmonary arteries.

The *right pulmonary artery* courses to the right behind the ascending aorta before dividing behind the superior vena cava and in front of the right main bronchus into ascending (truncus anterior) and descending (interlobar) rami (Fig. 1–36). Though variable, the common pattern is for the ascending artery to subdivide into segmental branches that supply the right upper lobe, whereas the descending branch ultimately contributes segmental arteries to the middle and right lower lobes. The first portion of the right interlobar artery is horizontal, interposed between the superior vena cava in front and the intermediate bronchus behind. It then turns sharply downward and backward and assumes a vertical orientation within the major fissure anterolateral to the intermediate and right lower lobe bronchi before giving off segmental branches—one or two to the middle lobe and usually single branches to each of the five bronchopulmonary segments of the lower lobe.

The *left pulmonary artery*, after passing over the left main bronchus, sometimes gives off a short ascending branch that subsequently divides into segmental branches to the upper lobe; more commonly, however, it continues directly into the vertically oriented left interlobar artery, from which the segmental arteries to the upper and lower lobes arise directly. The left interlobar artery lies posterolateral to the lower lobe bronchus (see Fig. 1–36).

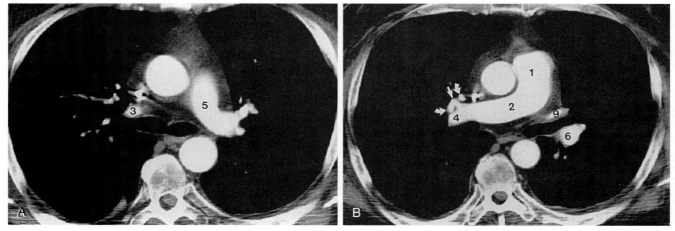

FIGURE 1–36

Anatomic features of the pulmonary artery and its main branches as seen on CT scan. A, CT at the level of the main bronchi demonstrates the ascending branch (3) of the right pulmonary artery and the main left pulmonary artery (5). **B,** CT at the level of the bronchus intermedius demonstrates the main pulmonary artery (1), right pulmonary artery (2), and right interlobar pulmonary artery (4). Also seen are the anterior segmental arteries of the right upper lobe *(straight arrow)* and right upper lobe pulmonary veins *(curved arrows)*. On the left side, the left interlobar pulmonary artery (6) can be seen behind the left upper lobe bronchus, whereas the left superior pulmonary vein (9) lies in front of the bronchus. *(From Fraser RS, Müller NL, Colman NC, Paré PD: Fraser and Paré's Diagnosis of Diseases of the Chest, 4th ed. Philadelphia, WB Saunders, 1999.)*

Measurement of arterial width can be useful in the diagnosis of pulmonary vascular disease,[145] and normal limits have been established. The upper limit of normal of the transverse diameter of the interlobar artery (measured from its lateral aspect to the air column of the intermediate bronchus) is 16 mm in men and 15 mm in women.[145] Normal ranges in size of the pulmonary arteries also have been determined by CT scan. The upper limit of normal for the diameter of the main pulmonary artery at the level of the pulmonary artery bifurcation is 29 mm, and the upper limit of normal for the diameter of the right interlobar artery measured at the level of the origin of the middle lobe bronchus is 17 mm.[146] There is no significant difference between measurements in men and women.[146]

As indicated previously, the course of the *pulmonary veins* is remote from that of the bronchoarterial bundles, so in all areas the arteries and their corresponding veins are separated by air-containing lung. Theoretically, this separation should permit distinction of artery from vein, particularly in the medial third of the lung, where the continuity of the artery with its accompanying bronchus may be more readily distinguished and where the typical course of the larger veins on their way to the mediastinum can be recognized. However, in a pulmonary angiographic study of 50 patients in AP projection, the upper lobe artery and vein were superimposed in 40% to 50% of subjects, the implication being that these vessels could not be distinguished on the chest radiograph.[147]

Segmental veins from the right upper lobe coalesce to form the *right superior pulmonary vein* (Fig. 1–37), which descends medially into the mediastinum before joining the upper posterior aspect of the left atrium (the superior venous confluence). Along its course caudad, this vessel is intimately associated with the junction of the horizontal and vertical segments of the right interlobar pulmonary artery and the anteromedial aspect of the middle lobe bronchus. The *middle lobe vein,* after passing under the middle lobe bronchus, usually joins the left atrium at the base of the superior pulmonary venous confluence, although occasionally the three veins on the right (superior, middle, and inferior) remain separate.

On the left, the segmental veins from the upper lobe join to form the *left superior pulmonary vein* (see Fig. 1–37), which after uniting with the lingular vein, courses obliquely downward and medially into the mediastinum. Along its course caudad, this vessel lies medial to the apicoposterior bronchoarterial bundle, anterolateral to the left pulmonary artery, and finally, anterior to the continuum formed by the left main and upper lobe bronchi. It thus separates these airways from the left atrium before it enters this chamber.

The horizontally oriented lower lobe segmental veins on both sides coalesce medial to the lower lobe bronchi to form the *right* and *left inferior pulmonary veins;* as they attach to the left atrium medially, they form the inferior pulmonary venous confluences (see Fig. 1–37). The left inferior pulmonary vein and venous confluence are at the same level as or slightly higher than those on the right and slightly more posterior; this vein may join with the left superior vein to form a common chamber before entering the left atrium. The normal superior and inferior venous confluences are sometimes prominent enough to simulate a mass on a lateral chest radiograph, particularly, but not exclusively, on the right.

Radiology—Hila

Posteroanterior and Lateral Radiographs

The pulmonary hila are the areas in the center of the thorax that connect the mediastinum to the lungs. The anatomic structures rendering the hila visible on radiographs are primarily the pulmonary arteries and veins, with lesser contributions from the bronchial walls, surrounding connective tissue, and lymph nodes. As viewed on a conventional posteroanterior (PA) radiograph, the hila can be divided into

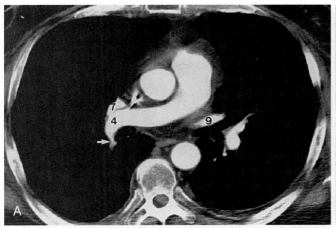

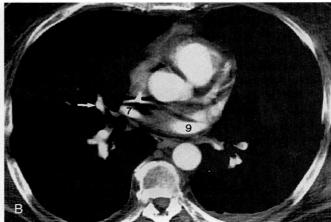

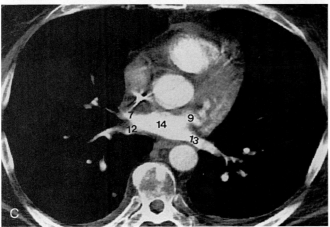

FIGURE 1–37

Pulmonary veins on CT scan. A, A CT scan at the level of the bronchus intermedius demonstrates the right superior pulmonary vein (7) immediately anterior to the descending branch of the right pulmonary artery (4). Also seen is the superior segmental artery of the right lower lobe *(straight arrow).* On the left side, the superior pulmonary vein (9) can be seen anterior to the left main and upper lobe bronchi. At this level, the left interlobar artery can be seen to be bifurcating into lingular and left lower lobe branches. **B,** A CT scan at the level of the middle lobe bronchus demonstrates right (7) and left (9) superior pulmonary veins converging toward the upper aspect of the left atrium. Also seen are the right middle lobe pulmonary artery *(arrow)* and branches of the right and left lower lobe arteries. **C,** A CT scan 5 mm more caudal demonstrates the right (7) and left (9) superior pulmonary veins and the right (12) and left (13) inferior venous confluences entering the left atrium (14). *(From Fraser RS, Müller NL, Colman NC, Paré PD: Fraser and Paré's Diagnosis of Diseases of the Chest, 4th ed. Philadelphia, WB Saunders, 1999.)*

upper and lower components by an imaginary horizontal line transecting the junction of the upper lobe and intermediate bronchi on the right and the upper and lower lobe bronchial dichotomy on the left.

The *right upper hilar opacity* is formed by the ascending pulmonary artery (truncus anterior) and the right superior pulmonary vein, including the respective branches of each (Fig. 1–38). The end-on opacity and radiolucency, respectively, of the contiguous anterior (occasionally posterior) segmental artery and bronchus can be identified in the majority of normal subjects.[148] A short segment of the upper lobe bronchus, beneath the ascending right pulmonary artery, may sometimes be observed before it trifurcates into the segmental branches serving the upper lobe.

The *lower portion of the right hilum* (Fig. 1–39) is formed by the vertically oriented interlobar artery, the right superior pulmonary vein superolaterally as it crosses the junction of the horizontal and vertical limbs of the interlobar artery, and the respective branches of these vessels. More inferiorly lies the horizontally oriented inferior pulmonary vein. The radiolucent lumen of the intermediate bronchus is invariably identified medial to the interlobar artery. Occasionally, segmental bronchi and arteries in the middle and lower lobes can be seen either in profile or end-on.

The *left superior hilum,* unlike its counterpart on the right, is often partly or completely covered by mediastinal fat and pleura between the aortic arch and the left pulmonary artery

or by a portion of the cardiac silhouette. When it is visible, the upper hilar opacity is formed by the distal left pulmonary artery, the proximal portion of the left interlobar artery, its segmental arterial branches, and the left superior pulmonary vein and its major tributaries (Fig. 1–40). Frequently, the anterior segmental or lingular bronchoarterial bundle can be identified end-on. The proximal left pulmonary artery is almost always higher than the highest point of the right interlobar artery. The reference point for the determination of this relationship is the point at which the right and left superior pulmonary veins cross their respective pulmonary arteries before entering the mediastinum.[149]

The *lower portion of the left hilum* is formed by the distal interlobar artery, the lingular artery and vein, and more caudally, the left inferior pulmonary vein (see Fig. 1–40). The air columns of the left upper lobe bronchus, its superior and inferior (lingular) divisions, and the left lower lobe bronchus may be identified.

The radiographic anatomy of the hila in *lateral projection* is complex because the right and left hilar components are to a large degree superimposed.[150,151] The most useful landmarks for the carina are the left pulmonary artery or the proximal third of the intermediate stem line, structures that bear a close approximation to the tracheal bifurcation. The air column of the normally more cephalic right upper lobe bronchus can be identified end-on in 50% of subjects, whereas that of the more caudal left upper lobe bronchus is seen in about 75%

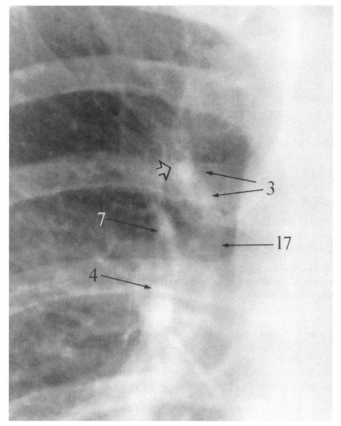

FIGURE 1–38

Right upper hilar anatomy. A detail view of the right hilum from a conventional posteroanterior radiograph demonstrates the ascending (3) and descending (4) arteries. The right superior pulmonary vein (7) crosses the hilum obliquely to form the typical V configuration. The lumen of the right upper lobe bronchus (17) and the end-on bronchus and opaque artery *(open arrow)* of the anterior segment are shown. *(From Fraser RS, Müller NL, Colman NC, Paré PD: Fraser and Paré's Diagnosis of Diseases of the Chest, 4th ed. Philadelphia, WB Saunders, 1999.)*

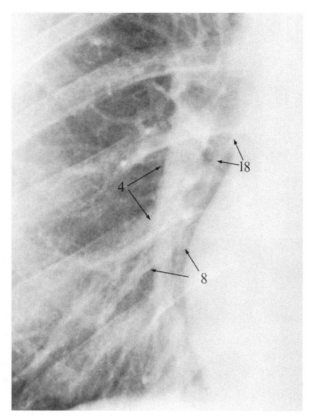

FIGURE 1–39

Right lower hilar anatomy. On this detail view from a conventional posteroanterior radiograph the interlobar (4) artery lies lateral to the intermediate bronchus (18). Note that this vessel dominates the radiographic anatomy of the lower hilum. The horizontally oriented inferior pulmonary vein (8) lies posteroinferior to the hilum. *(From Fraser RS, Müller NL, Colman NC, Paré PD: Fraser and Paré's Diagnosis of Diseases of the Chest, 4th ed. Philadelphia, WB Saunders, 1999.)*

(Fig. 1–41).[150] Occasionally, the uppermost radiolucency represents the right main bronchus, and the lowermost represents the left main bronchus.

The orifice of the right upper lobe bronchus is seldom as well circumscribed as that of the left because the latter is completely surrounded by vessels (the left pulmonary artery above, the interlobar artery behind, and the mediastinal component of the left superior pulmonary vein in front), whereas the former is devoid of vascular envelopment on its posterior aspect such that aerated upper or lower lobe parenchyma normally abuts its wall. Consequently, clear identification of the right upper lobe bronchial lumen en face constitutes highly suggestive evidence that the airway is completely surrounded by soft tissue, most likely enlarged lymph nodes.

The posterior walls of the right main and intermediate bronchi form the anatomic foundation for the *intermediate stem line* (see Fig. 1–41), a vertically oriented linear opacity measuring up to 3 mm in width[152] that is visible in 95% of individuals.[150] The posterior walls of these two bronchi are rendered visible by air in their lumina in front and aerated lung parenchyma in the azygoesophageal recess behind. On a

well-centered lateral projection, the line transects the middle or posterior third of the circular, radiolucent left upper lobe bronchus; it terminates caudally at the origin of the superior segmental bronchus of the right lower lobe, slightly proximal to or at the same level as the origin of the middle lobe bronchus anteriorly.

The physical characteristics that render the intermediate stem line visible are also operative to some extent on the left, so the posterior wall of the left main bronchus and the proximal portion of the left lower lobe bronchus may be profiled as the *left retrobronchial line* (see Fig. 1–41).[153] This short, vertical linear opacity measures 3 mm or less in width and terminates caudally at the origin of the superior segmental bronchus of the left lower lobe. Distinction between the intermediate stem line and the left retrobronchial line is not difficult if one bears in mind that the former is both longer and more anteriorly located than the latter.

There has been much confusion concerning the nomenclature of the hilar vasculature. One common misrepresentation is to depict the right hilar opacity as the "right pulmonary artery." In reality, the right pulmonary artery is a mediastinal vessel enveloped by other vessels or soft tissue elements, and it is its ascending and descending (interlobar) branches that constitute the true hilar arterial vessels. The right superior

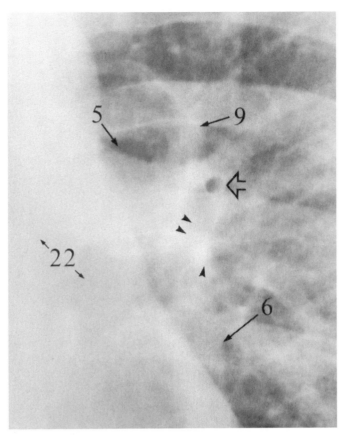

FIGURE 1–40

Left hilar anatomy. A detail view of the left hilum from a posteroanterior chest radiograph shows the left pulmonary artery (5), the interlobar artery (6), and the left superior pulmonary vein (9). The left main bronchus (22) and its superior *(two arrowheads)* and inferior *(single arrowhead)* divisions are overlapped by the hilar vessels. The end-on bronchus and opaque artery *(single open arrowhead)* of the anterior segment are seen. *(From Fraser RS, Müller NL, Colman NC, Paré PD: Fraser and Paré's Diagnosis of Diseases of the Chest, 4th ed. Philadelphia, WB Saunders, 1999.)*

pulmonary vein abuts the anterior aspect of the right interlobar artery; consequently, the right hilar complex is composed of the superior vein anteriorly, the ascending and descending arteries posteriorly, and surrounding connective tissue and lymph nodes.

The major portion of the left hilar vasculature is visible behind the intermediate stem line. The top of the left pulmonary artery is seen in 95% of subjects, usually as a sharply marginated opacity above and behind the radiolucency of the left upper lobe bronchus. Immediately posterior to this bronchus is the continuation of the left pulmonary artery, the interlobar artery. The left superior pulmonary vein, like its counterpart on the right, is closely associated with the arterial vasculature of the hilum; however, this vein is not a contour-forming vessel on lateral radiographs and thus cannot be identified.

The right and left inferior pulmonary veins are commonly imaged end-on as a result of their horizontal orientation, with a nodular opacity created below and behind the lower portion of the hila. Fortunately, vessels can usually be identified as they converge toward the opacity, thereby permitting their distinction from a true parenchymal mass.

Computed Tomography

CT is currently the imaging modality of choice for assessment of the hila. It provides a particularly detailed view that allows the diagnosis of endobronchial lesions, hilar lymph node enlargement, parahilar masses, and vascular lesions. In our opinion, non–contrast-enhanced scans suffice under most clinical circumstances; however, distinction of hilar masses or lymph node enlargement from vascular lesions and assessment of the extent of hilar tumors may require the use of an intravenous contrast agent. Anatomic features of the hila on CT can be conveniently described by examining a series of horizontal planes or levels (Fig. 1–42A). When no intravenous contrast agent is used, the anatomy is best assessed on the lung windows by relating the various structures to the bronchi.

Level I (Supracarinal Trachea) (Fig. 1–42B). On the *right*, the circular apical pulmonary artery lies medial to the radiolucent end-on apical bronchus; the apical pulmonary vein is situated lateral to this bronchoarterial bundle. On the *left*, the apicoposterior bronchus and artery are seen; the apical and anterior veins lie in front of and medial to the bronchus and artery.

Level II (Carina/Right Upper Lobe Bronchus) (Fig. 1–42C). On the *right*, the upper lobe bronchus divides into the horizontally oriented anterior and posterior segmental bronchi. In front of the main bronchus and upper lobe bronchus is the ascending branch of the right pulmonary artery; its anterior segmental branch parallels the bronchus medially or superiorly. The right superior pulmonary vein is invariably identified immediately lateral to the site at which the anterior and posterior segmental bronchi divide. In some patients, a small vein from the anterior and apical portion of the upper lobe can be seen in front of the ascending artery.

On the *left*, the circular apicoposterior bronchus and artery are located immediately lateral to the left pulmonary artery. The superior pulmonary vein is situated in front of and medial to the bronchus and artery.

Level III (Proximal Intermediate Bronchus/Left Upper Lobe Bronchus) (Fig. 1–42D). On the *right*, the intermediate bronchus is covered anteriorly by the horizontal limb of the interlobar artery and laterally by the vertical limb of the same vessel. The superior pulmonary vein abuts the junction between the horizontal and vertical components of the interlobar artery.

On the *left*, the distal main and upper lobe bronchial continuum is seen. Frequently, the end-on radiolucency of the superior division of the upper lobe can be identified. The proximal portion of the interlobar artery forms a shallow indentation on the posterior aspect of the upper lobe bronchus.

Level IV (Distal Intermediate Bronchus/Lingular Bronchus) (Fig. 1–42E). On the *right*, the anatomic features are similar to those of level III. On the *left*, the proximal portion of the lingular bronchus is separated from the end-on orifice of the lower lobe bronchus by the lingular carina. The superior segmental bronchus to the lower lobe arises posteriorly. The left interlobar artery is situated lateral to the carina separating the lingular bronchus from the lower lobe bronchus. As it enters the mediastinum, the superior pulmonary vein is joined by the lingular vein in front of and medial to the lingular bronchus.

Level V (Middle Lobe Bronchus) (Fig. 1–42F). On the *right*, the horizontal middle lobe bronchus courses obliquely into the middle lobe, where it divides after a centimeter or so into the medial and lateral segmental bronchi; posteriorly, the

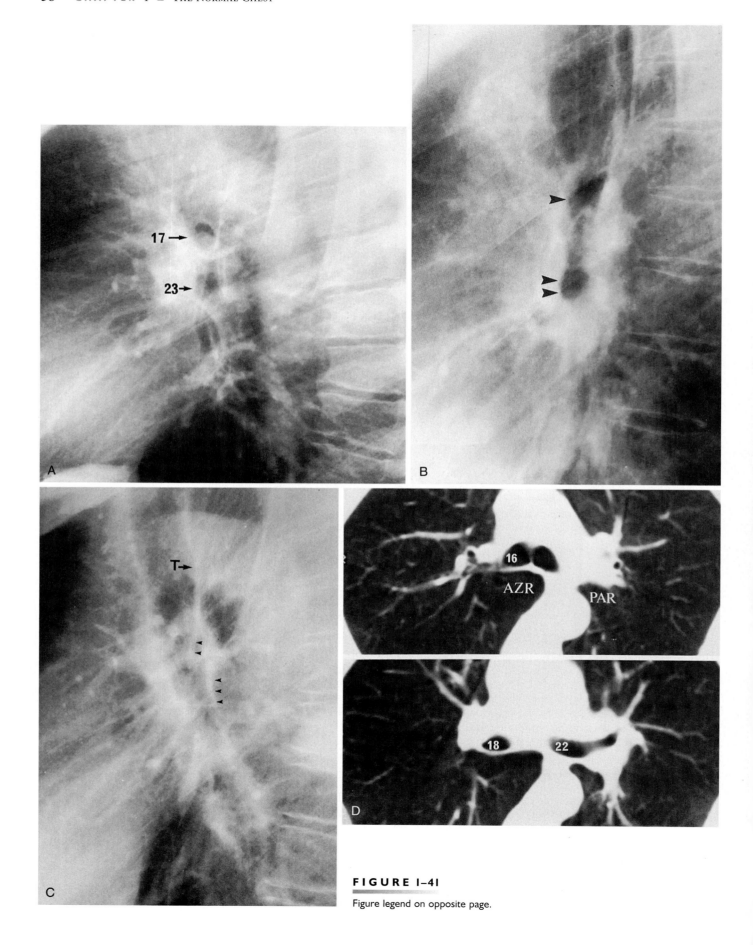

FIGURE 1–41

Figure legend on opposite page.

FIGURE 1-41

Hilar anatomy on lateral chest radiographs. A, The end-on orifices of the right (17) and left (23) upper lobe bronchi can be easily identified. Although the left hilum is normally located cephalic to the right, the right upper lobe bronchus projects cephalic to its counterpart on the left. **B,** A detail view from a conventional lateral chest radiograph reveals exceptional clarity of the right *(arrowhead)* and left *(two arrowheads)* upper lobe bronchi. This appearance should suggest an excessive quantity of soft tissue surrounding the respective bronchial lumina, the most common cause of which is hilar node enlargement, as in this patient with Hodgkin's lymphoma. **C,** In another subject, a lateral chest radiograph demonstrates the posterior tracheal stripe (T), intermediate stem line *(two arrowheads)*, and left retrobronchial line *(three arrowheads)*. On a true lateral view, the intermediate stem line may be straight or gently convex forward and characteristically bisects the orifice of the left upper lobe bronchus. **D,** CT scans through the carina *(top)* and 2 cm caudal *(bottom)* in the same patient reveal the anatomic prerequisites underlying the features described in **C.** Aerated lung in the azygoesophageal recess (AZR) and the preaortic recess (PAR) abut the posterior wall of the right main (16) and intermediate (18) bronchi and the posterior wall of the left main bronchus (22), respectively. Essentially, the intermediate stem line and the left retrobronchial line, representing the posterior wall of their respective bronchi, are rendered visible by an intrabronchial and intrapulmonary air envelope. *(From Fraser RS, Müller NL, Colman NC, Paré PD: Fraser and Paré's Diagnosis of Diseases of the Chest, 4th ed. Philadelphia, WB Saunders, 1999.)*

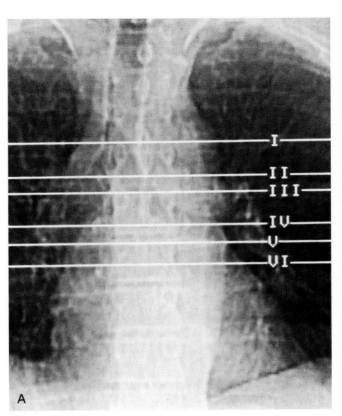

A

FIGURE 1-42

Normal CT hilar anatomy. On a scout view of the thorax (**A**), the *bars* indicate the appropriate levels for **B** through **G.** *(From Fraser RS, Müller NL, Colman NC, Paré PD: Fraser and Paré's Diagnosis of Diseases of the Chest, 4th ed. Philadelphia, WB Saunders, 1999.)*　　*Continued*

orifice of the lower lobe bronchus can be seen end-on, divided by a distinct carina or lateral spur. The superior segmental bronchus to the lower lobe arises at or slightly superior to this level and passes posterolaterally for a few millimeters before dividing into two subsegmental bronchi. The vertical part of the interlobar artery is situated posterolateral to the middle lobe bronchus and anterolateral to the lower lobe bronchus as it enters the lung parenchyma. The middle lobe artery or vein may be identified lateral to the middle lobe bronchus; the termination of the superior pulmonary vein is located anteromedial to this airway.

On the *left*, the end-on lumen of the lower lobe bronchus is seen medial to the contiguous interlobar artery. Occasionally, a portion of the inferior pulmonary vein can be identified posteromedial to this bronchus.

Level VI (Basilar Lower Lobe Bronchi/Inferior Pulmonary Veins) (Fig. 1-42G). On the *right*, the medial segmental bronchus, the first branch to be identified, is characteristically located in front of the horizontal inferior pulmonary vein. The anterior, lateral, and posterior basilar bronchi arise in succession to supply their respective segments. On the *left*, the anteromedial segmental bronchus is located anterior to the inferior pulmonary vein; the lateral and posterior segmental bronchi may be identified behind this vessel.

Function

Perfusion of the Acinar Unit

Pulmonary blood volume, comprising the volume of blood within the pulmonary arteries, pulmonary capillaries, and pulmonary veins, is about 500 mL, or 10% of total blood volume in an average adult. Capillary blood volume is about

20% to 25% of total pulmonary blood volume and can double during heavy exercise.[154]

Various pressures modify the flow of blood through the capillaries: (1) *mean intravascular pressure,* which is only 14 mm Hg in the main pulmonary artery despite the fact that it handles the same cardiac output as the systemic circulation; (2) *transmural vascular pressure,* which for extrapulmonary arteries is intravascular pressure minus intrapleural pressure, for "extra-alveolar" intraparenchymal vessels is intravascular pressure minus interstitial pressure, and for the "alveolar" vessels is intravascular pressure minus alveolar pressure; and (3) *driving pressure,* which in the pulmonary circulation in upright subjects at rest is the difference between arterial and pulmonary venous or left atrial pressure in the lower part of the lung and between arterial and alveolar pressure in the upper part of the lung.

Pulmonary vascular resistance is made up of arterial, capillary, and venous resistance arranged in series. Despite some controversy,[155] it is believed that the compliant capillary bed contributes least to total resistance and the arterioles and venules most.[156] The average capillary pressure is probably on the order of 8 to 10 cm H_2O; because colloidal osmotic pressure is between 25 and 30 mm Hg, there is a considerable force keeping fluid within the pulmonary capillaries and maintaining the alveoli dry. Even during maximal exercise when cardiac

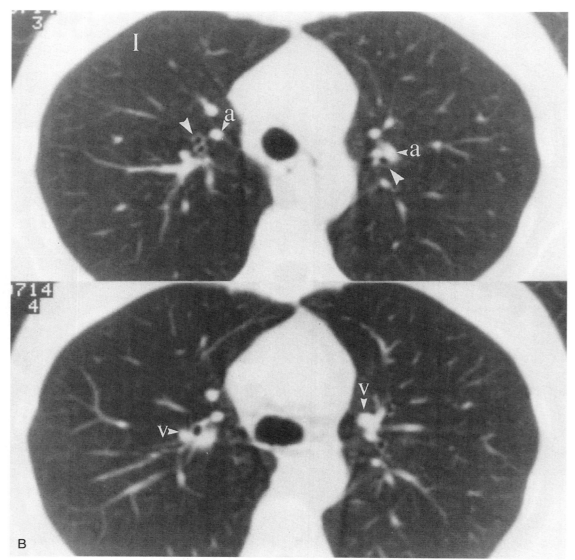

FIGURE 1–42—cont'd

In level I (supracarinal trachea) (**B**), the apical bronchus *(arrowhead)*, artery (a), and vein (v) are depicted on the right, and the apicoposterior bronchus *(arrowhead)*, artery (a), and vein (v) are on the left.

output increases to 25 to 30 L/min, hydrostatic pressure does not increase greatly because of capillary recruitment.

As with the conducting airways, doubling or halving the radius of pulmonary vessels causes a 16-fold change in resistance. When cardiac output increases, vessels widen and closed capillaries open, thereby leading to a fall in resistance. Part of this decrease may be explained by the fact that the pulmonary vascular pressure-flow curve does not have a zero pressure intercept. Put simply, this means that a critical pulmonary artery pressure must be achieved before flow begins.

Factors Influencing the Pulmonary Circulation

Gravity. By altering regional vascular transmural pressures and therefore vascular diameters, gravity has a major influence on the distribution of blood flow in the lung.[157] This distribution is governed largely by the relationship between arterial, alveolar, and venous pressure (Fig. 1–43). The lung measures approximately 30 cm from apex to base, and the hilum is positioned at about the midlevel. Because a column of blood 15 cm high is equivalent to a column of mercury 11 mm high, gravity affects intravascular pressure in an erect subject by decreasing systolic, diastolic, and mean pressures by 11 mm Hg at the apex and by increasing them 11 mm Hg at the base. If pulmonary arterial pressure in the hilar vessels is taken as 20/9 mm Hg, it follows that pressure will be 9/2 at the apex and 31/20 at the base. Since the pulmonary veins enter the left atrium at approximately the same level as the pulmonary arteries, there will also be a similar and proportional variation in venous pressure.

These gravity-dependent changes in intravascular pressure result in regional differences in capillary transmural pressure. Because extraluminal capillary pressure is 0 (atmospheric), apical vessels are virtually closed, at least during diastole; in

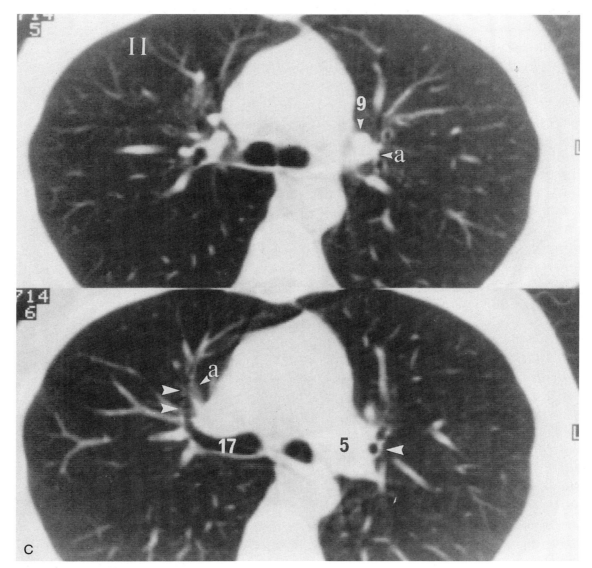

FIGURE 1–42—cont'd

In level II (carina/right upper lobe bronchus) (**C**), the upper lobe bronchus (17), anterior segmental bronchus *(two arrowheads)*, and artery (a) are shown on the right; on the left, the apicoposterior bronchus *(arrowhead)* and artery (a) are stationed immediately lateral to the left pulmonary artery (5). The left superior pulmonary vein (9) is located anteromedial to the bronchoarterial bundle.   *Continued*

this region (zone 1), the pulmonary vasculature acts as a Starling resistor in which the pertinent driving pressure is the difference between arterial and alveolar pressure (see Fig. 1–43). Farther down the lung, pulmonary artery pressure exceeds alveolar pressure throughout the cardiac cycle; however, alveolar pressure still exceeds venous pressure, and as a consequence, capillaries narrow at their downstream venous end (zone 2). Finally, as the lung base is approached, both arterial and venous pressure exceeds alveolar pressure, and the vasculature progressively dilates (zone 3). At the extreme base (zone 4), pulmonary vascular resistance increases and blood flow decreases, a phenomenon for which there is no adequate explanation.

Intrapleural Pressure and Lung Volume. Pulmonary vessels may be considered to be in extra-alveolar and alveolar compartments based on their response to changes in lung volume.[158] The former comprises arteries and veins whose extraluminal pressure is equivalent to pleural and/or interstitial pressure and that tend to dilate as lung volume increases. The alveolar compartment includes capillaries, arterioles, and venules; their extraluminal pressure is alveolar, and they tend to be compressed as the lung is inflated. Despite this compression, it is possible to perfuse the lung slowly even when alveolar pressure substantially exceeds pulmonary artery pressure. The explanation for this may be related to the presence of vessels situated at alveolar corners, which tend to be stretched and dilated rather than compressed as the lung inflates.[159]

Neurogenic and Chemical Effects. Neurogenic, humoral, blood gas, and blood chemistry changes may result in active vasomotion and modify the pulmonary circulation. Such modification may occur generally throughout the lung or, more importantly, on a regional basis, thus altering blood

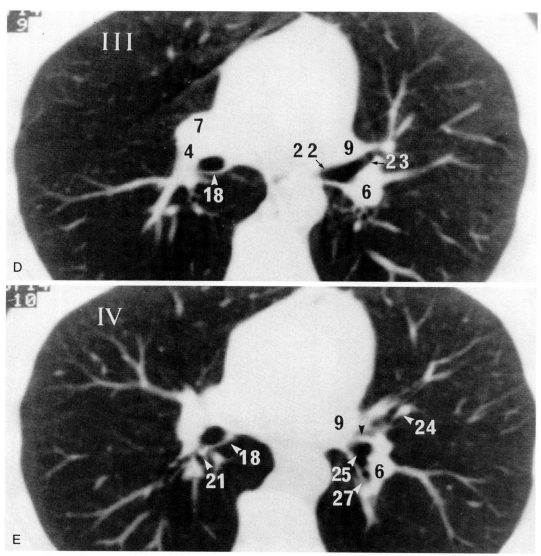

FIGURE 1–42—cont'd

In level III (proximal intermediate bronchus/left upper lobe bronchus) (**D**), on the right, the intermediate bronchus (18) is covered anteriorly and laterally by the interlobar artery (4). The close relationship of the right superior pulmonary vein (7) and the interlobar artery is creating a typical "elephant head-and-trunk" configuration. On the left, the distal main (22) and upper lobe (23) bronchial continuum is seen. Note the shallow indentation on the anterior and posterior wall of the upper lobe bronchus created by the mediastinal component of the left superior vein (9) and the proximal interlobar artery (6). In level IV (distal intermediate bronchus/lingular bronchus) (**E**), the intermediate bronchus (18) and the superior segmental bronchus (21) of the lower lobe can be identified on the right, and the lingular bronchus (24) separated by the lingular spur (arrowhead) from the end-on orifice of the lower lobe bronchus (25) is seen on the left. The superior segmental bronchus (27) lies posteriorly, the interlobar artery (6) posterolaterally, and the left superior pulmonary vein (9) anteromedially.

FIGURE 1–42—cont'd

In level V (**F**), the middle lobe bronchus (19) divides into medial (m) and lateral (l) segmental bronchi. The lower lobe bronchus (20) is separated from the middle lobe bronchus by a distinct spur or carina (arrowheads). The right superior pulmonary vein (7) lies anteromedial to the middle lobe bronchus and the interlobar artery (4) anterolateral to the lower lobe bronchus. On the left, the interlobar artery (6) lies posterolateral to the lower lobe bronchus (25). In level VI (basilar lower lobe bronchi/inferior pulmonary veins) (**G**), on the right, the medial (m), anterior (a), lateral (l), and posterior (p) segmental bronchi relate closely to the inferior pulmonary vein (8). On the left, the anteromedial (am), lateral (l), and posterior (p) segmental bronchi relate to the left inferior pulmonary vein (10). (From Fraser RS, Müller NL, Colman NC, Paré PD: Fraser and Paré's Diagnosis of Diseases of the Chest, 4th ed. Philadelphia, WB Saunders, 1999.)

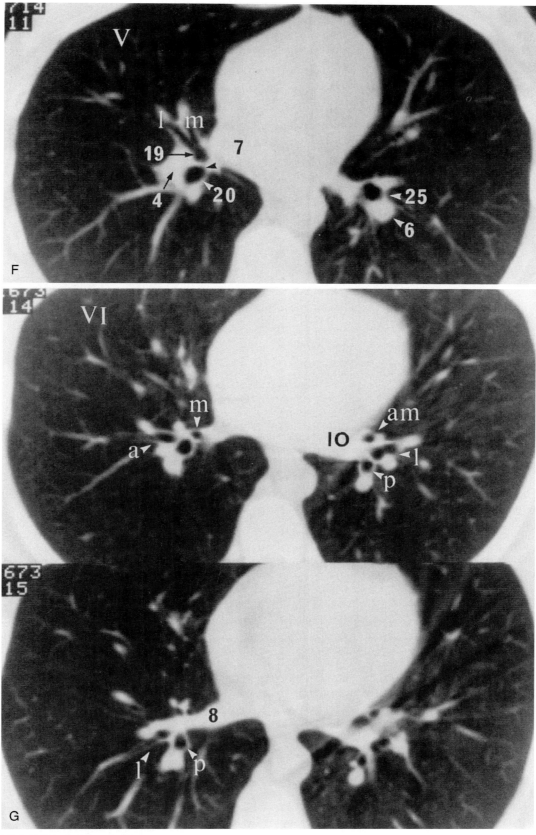

FIGURE 1–42—cont'd

Figure legend on opposite page.

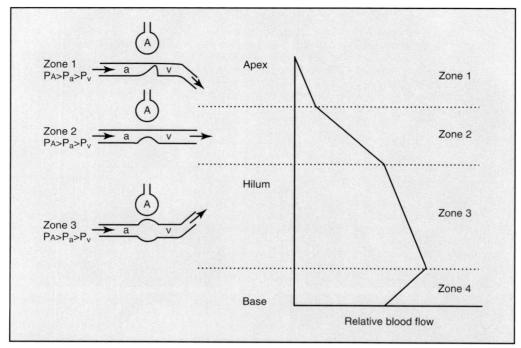

FIGURE 1–43

Regional blood flow in the lung as determined by the relationship among alveolar (A), pulmonary arterial (a), and pulmonary venous (v) pressure. At the apex, where pulmonary arterial and venous pressure may be subatmospheric, alveolar pressure will compress alveolar microvessels, increase resistance, and decrease flow (zone 1). Lower in the lung, pulmonary arterial pressure exceeds alveolar pressure, but alveolar pressure still exceeds subatmospheric venous pressure, and vessel caliber and flow depend on the differential between arterial and alveolar pressure (zone 2). Nearer the base of the lung, because arterial pressure and venous pressure exceed alveolar pressure, microvessels dilate and flow increases further (zone 3). At the lung base (zone 4), a region of decreased flow exists that cannot simply be explained by the relationship of Pa, PA, and Pv.

flow distribution and affecting local ventilation-perfusion relationships.

Hypoxia is one of the most potent stimuli of pulmonary vasoconstriction. This effect is predominantly local because the response can be demonstrated in both denervated and excised perfused lungs.[160] The mechanism of hypoxic vasoconstriction is uncertain. One currently held theory invokes a direct effect of hypoxia on the redox status of the vascular smooth muscle cell acting through potassium and calcium channels.[161] Hypoxic vasoconstriction can be modulated by endothelial release of endothelin,[162] local NO production, and red blood cell interaction with NO.[163] Most evidence suggests that it is local alveolar Po_2 that provides the major stimulus, although mixed venous Po_2 may also influence the response.[164] An increased hydrogen ion concentration, whether induced by hypercapnia or metabolic acidosis, also produces pulmonary vasoconstriction by a separate mechanism and interacts with hypoxia in increasing pulmonary arterial pressure.[165]

Although stimulation of sympathetic nerves in animals results in increased pulmonary vascular resistance and decreased compliance of large pulmonary vessels, little is known about the afferent input that could produce such reflex changes.[166] The endothelin produced by vascular endothelial cells is a powerful pulmonary vasoconstrictor. Parenterally administered epinephrine, norepinephrine, serotonin, histamine, and prostaglandin $F_{2\alpha}$ also vasoconstrict, whereas β-agonists and acetylcholine result in vasodilation.[167] The effect

of acetylcholine is mediated through the release of NO from the pulmonary vascular endothelium.

Diffusion of Gas from Acinar Units to Red Blood Cells

Diffusion in the Acinar Unit. Several factors affect diffusion of gas in the acinus. As a general rule, diffusion occurs passively from an area of higher partial pressure to one of lower partial pressure. In addition, in a gaseous medium, a light gas diffuses faster than a heavier one, whereas in a liquid or in tissue, the rate of diffusion is largely dependent on the solubility of the particular gas in that medium. Oxygen is slightly lighter than carbon dioxide and therefore diffuses more rapidly in acinar gas. In water and tissue, however, carbon dioxide is more soluble than oxygen and diffuses through these media 20 times faster than oxygen does. The alveolar ventilation portion of each tidal volume is only about 10% of the gas within the lung at FRC; however, because of the rapid diffusion of oxygen, complete mixing of this fresh air with intra-acinar gas is virtually instantaneous in normal lung.

Diffusion across the Alveolocapillary Membrane. Under resting conditions, oxygen has a driving pressure of approximately 60 mm Hg (Po_2 of alveolar gas minus the Po_2 of mixed venous blood [$100 - 40 = 60$ mm Hg]) through the alveolocapillary membrane and almost fully saturates blood in a third of the time taken by blood to traverse the pulmonary capillaries. However, the amount of *effective* alveolocapillary membrane is usually reduced because of mismatching of capillary circulation with acinar ventilation (see later).

The distance for diffusion of gas is increased in many diseases that thicken the alveolocapillary membrane. Since ventilation-perfusion mismatching is an inevitable accompaniment of such diseases, assessment of the separate contribution of diffusion impairment to arterial hypoxemia may be difficult. In these cases, arterial oxygen saturation may be normal in patients at rest despite a significant reduction in diffusing capacity; however, exercise elicits hypoxemia because the transit time through capillaries is decreased.

Measurement of the diffusing capacity of oxygen is difficult for a variety of technical reasons; therefore, that for carbon monoxide (D_{LCO}) is generally used instead. The three important variables that contribute to the overall diffusing capacity of the lung (D_L) are the alveolocapillary membrane diffusing capacity (D_m), the reaction rate of carbon monoxide with hemoglobin, and pulmonary capillary blood volume (V_c). Both the D_m and the V_c components of D_L decrease with age, the membrane component first.[168]

Matching Acinar Capillary Blood Flow with Ventilation

Ideally, alveolar ventilation and alveolar perfusion should be uniform; that is, each acinus would receive just the right amount of ventilation to oxygenate hemoglobin completely and remove all the carbon dioxide given off during gas exchange. Despite the fact that such uniformity does not occur, even in a normal lung, the concept of an "ideal" ventilation/perfusion ($\dot{V}_A/\dot{Q}$) ratio is useful as a point of reference in judging relationships between ventilation and perfusion within acini and the lung as a whole. When the $\dot{V}_A/\dot{Q}$ ratio is not ideal, it is either because perfusion is reduced relative to ventilation (high $\dot{V}_A/\dot{Q}$) or because ventilation is decreased relative to blood flow (low $\dot{V}_A/\dot{Q}$).

Figure 1–44 shows the theoretical distribution of $\dot{V}_A/\dot{Q}$ ratios in the lung in a five-compartment model. The central unit (no. 3) corresponds to the "ideal" unit with a $\dot{V}_A/\dot{Q}$ ratio of 0.9. In this acinus, ventilation is sufficient to achieve an alveolar oxygen tension (P_{AO_2}) of approximately 100 mm Hg. Unimpaired diffusion between alveolar gas and capillary blood results in a capillary oxygen tension (P_{CO_2}) of 100 mm Hg in the blood leaving this unit, a level that is sufficient to achieve 100% saturation of hemoglobin (20 mL O_2 per 100 mL of blood if the hemoglobin concentration is 15 g/dL). The resulting P_{ACO_2} and P_{CCO_2} are each 40 mm Hg, which is sufficient to lower the mixed venous carbon dioxide content from 53 to 48 mL/dL.

Unit no.1 typifies the region with the lowest possible $\dot{V}_A/\dot{Q}$ ratio—a value of 0—and represents a true intrapulmonary shunt. Capillary blood emerges from such a unit with gas partial pressures and contents identical to those of mixed venous blood (in our example, a P_{CO_2} of 40 mm Hg and a P_{CCO_2} of 46 mm Hg for a capillary O_2 content of 13 mL/dL and a capillary CO_2 content of 53 mL/dL). Unit no. 2 has a $\dot{V}_A/\dot{Q}$ ratio somewhere between 0.9 and 0, which results in alveolar and capillary gas pressures and contents that are less than "ideal" for oxygen and more than "ideal" for carbon dioxide (in our example, a P_{CO_2} of 70 mm Hg and a P_{CCO_2} of 44 mm Hg). Unit no. 5 typifies true alveolar dead space, or a

region of lung that is ventilated but not perfused ($\dot{V}_A/\dot{Q}$ = infinity); ventilation to such a unit is completely wasted ventilation because alveolar gas does not come in contact with capillary blood. Unit no. 4 has a $\dot{V}_A/\dot{Q}$ ratio between 0.9 and infinity, which results in alveolar and capillary partial pressures that are greater than "ideal" for oxygen and less than "ideal" for carbon dioxide (in our example, a P_{CO_2} of 130 mm Hg and a P_{CCO_2} of 37 mm Hg).

Because of the relationships between the oxygen and carbon dioxide content of blood and their partial pressures, $\dot{V}_A/\dot{Q}$ mismatch has quite different effects on the efficiency of the lung to take up oxygen and remove carbon dioxide. As shown in Figure 1–45, the O_2 dissociation curve is flat for values of P_{O_2} above 70 or 80 mm Hg, and therefore the overventilated unit (no. 4) cannot make up for the underventilated unit (no. 2) in terms of oxygen uptake. Although the elevated P_{O_2} in unit no. 4 results in a slight increase in the amount of dissolved oxygen in capillary blood, hemoglobin is virtually 100% saturated above a P_{O_2} of 100, and because dissolved oxygen can increase only by 0.003 mL/dL of blood per 1-mm Hg rise in P_{O_2}, little gain is achieved by overventilating units. By contrast, overventilated units can compensate for underventilated units in the removal of carbon dioxide. Since the CO_2 dissociation curve is virtually linear over the range of physiologic P_{CO_2} values, the lowered carbon dioxide content of blood from unit no. 4 can compensate for the greater than "ideal" content in unit no. 2.

When blood from units 1, 2, 3, and 4 mix in the pulmonary veins and left atrium, the resulting P_{AO_2} will be less than the mean alveolar P_{O_2} of units 2, 3, and 4, whereas P_{ACO_2} will be equal to mean alveolar P_{CO_2}. Put simply, $\dot{V}_A/\dot{Q}$ mismatch decreases the efficiency of oxygen and carbon dioxide uptake and removal; in the case of oxygen, this decreased efficiency results in a gradient between mean alveolar P_{O_2} and arterial P_{O_2} (P_{AO_2} − P_{aO_2}), whereas for carbon dioxide there is none. If a disease process leads to the development of units with low $\dot{V}_A/\dot{Q}$ ratios (no. 2) or a true shunt (no. 1), arterial hypoxemia and hypercapnia will result. Because both lowered P_{O_2} and increased P_{CO_2} stimulate increased ventilation, total alveolar ventilation will increase. Alveolar P_{O_2} in well-ventilated acinar units (no. 4) will rise while the P_{CO_2} in these units will fall. The excess carbon dioxide retained by blood circulating through the poorly ventilated units (nos. 1 and 2) will be balanced by supranormal output from the well-ventilated units, thus correcting the hypercapnia. Since increased ventilation cannot completely compensate for the hypoxemia (because of the oxygen content–partial pressure relationship), P_{O_2} will remain relatively low.

Figure 1–44 is a simplified model that spans the entire range of possible $\dot{V}_A/\dot{Q}$ ratios in five compartments. In fact, a continuous distribution of ratios is likely to exist, and even in normal lung substantial regional differences in $\dot{V}_A/\dot{Q}$ ratios have been demonstrated. This variation is caused largely by gravity.[169] As discussed previously, the effect of gravity is to increase blood flow to the dependent portions of the lung. A gravity-dependent vertical gradient in pleural pressure also results in a gravity-dependent variation in lung volume and ventilation; in erect individuals, pleural pressure at the lung apex (or anteriorly in the supine position) is more negative than at the base, and local pleural pressure (P_{pl}) increases progressively (i.e., becomes less subatmospheric) as the base of the lung is approached. This gradient is approximately

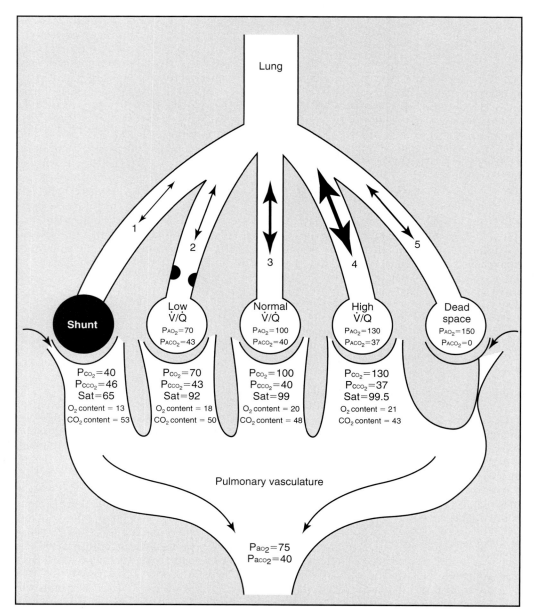

FIGURE 1–44

Theoretical distribution of $\dot{V}_A/\dot{Q}$ ratios in the lung. All possible ventilation-perfusion rations are depicted here, schematically ranging from unit 1, a shunt with a ventilation-perfusion ratio of 0, to unit 5, pure dead space with a ventilation-perfusion ratio of infinity. Blood coming from unit 1 will have gas tensions identical to that of mixed venous blood, and alveolar gas in unit 5 will have gas tensions approaching that of inspired air. Although the average alveolar PO_2 in the ventilated and perfused units (2, 3, and 4) is 100 mm Hg, the resultant arterial PO_2 after blood from all units has mixed is only 75 mm Hg. This $PA_{O_2} - Pa_{O_2}$ difference is caused by both the low oxygen content in the shunted blood and failure of the overventilated unit 4 to compensate for the underventilated unit 2 with respect to oxygen uptake.

0.25 cm H_2O per centimeter distance up and down the lung and is similar in different body positions and at different overall lung volumes. Because alveolar pressure is constant up and down the lung, this means that local transpulmonary pressure also varies in a gravity-dependent fashion. Regionally, lung parenchyma responds to the local transpulmonary pressure; therefore, at the end of a quiet expiration, acinar units in the upper lung regions are more distended and at a higher percentage of their TLC value than are the less well distended units at the base of the lung.

Despite the gradient in end-expiratory pleural and transpulmonary pressure up and down the lung, the changes in Ppl that occur during tidal breathing are similar at different vertical levels. Because of the pressure-volume characteristics of the lung (see Fig. 1–31), upper lung units are less well ventilated per unit of lung volume than are acini at the lung base, which are on a steeper portion of their pressure-volume curve. Thus, the gravity-dependent pleural pressure gradient

results in a regional variation in both lung volume (V_o) and ventilation ($\Delta V/V_o$).

If the increase in $\Delta V/V_o$ from apex to base were directly proportional to the increase in blood flow from apex to base, the $\dot{V}_A/\dot{Q}$ ratio would not vary. However, since the effect of gravity on regional perfusion is greater than its effect on regional ventilation, blood flow and ventilation are slightly mismatched even in normal lung. In the upright posture, the $\dot{V}_A/\dot{Q}$ ratio is between 2 and 3 at the lung apex and decreases to between 0.5 and 1 at the base.[170]

Although gravity-dependent variations in pulmonary artery and pleural pressure are the most important factors influencing $\dot{V}_A/\dot{Q}$ ratios, other effects may also be involved. For example, at low lung volumes, ventilation to the lung bases in the upright position or to posterior regions in the supine position may not follow the distribution suggested by regional pleural pressure because airway closure may occur in these regions.[171] The overall lung volume at which airways in

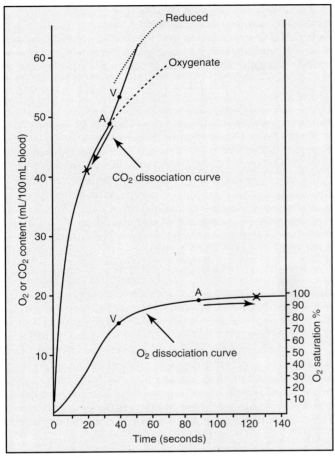

FIGURE 1–45

Carbon dioxide and oxygen dissociation curves of blood. The *arrows* (A → X) indicate the effect of doubling the ventilation on both CO_2 content and O_2 content (arterial oxygen saturation). The normal values for both arterial (A) and venous (V) oxygen and carbon dioxide are noted. It can be seen that at any given PCO_2, reduced blood can carry more carbon dioxide than oxygenated blood can.

dependent lung regions first close is termed the "closing volume." Since FRC decreases on assuming the supine posture whereas closing volume does not change, a greater number of dependent airways may close during supine tidal breathing and thereby result in a paradoxical decrease in ventilation to dependent lung regions, further $\dot{V}_A/\dot{Q}$ mismatch, and arterial hypoxemia.

Measurement of Ventilation-Perfusion Mismatch

The most commonly used and easily calculated estimate of $\dot{V}_A/\dot{Q}$ mismatch is the alveolar-arterial gradient for oxygen, $P_{AO_2} - Pa_{O_2}$. Calculation of $P_{AO_2} - Pa_{O_2}$ requires knowledge of the mean alveolar PO_2, which can be determined by using the simplified alveolar air equation:

$$1. \quad P_{AO_2} = P_{IO_2} - \frac{Pa_{CO_2}}{R}$$

in which P_{IO_2} is inspired PO_2, R is the ratio of CO_2 production to O_2 consumption (assumed to equal 0.8), and Pa_{CO_2} is the arterial PCO_2 (assumed to be equal to P_{ACO_2}).

Once P_{AO_2} is calculated, $P_{AO_2} - Pa_{O_2}$ can be obtained by comparing P_{AO_2} with the measured arterial PO_2:

$$2. \quad \text{Alveolar-arterial gradient for oxygen} = P_{AO_2} - Pa_{O_2}$$

One disadvantage of $P_{AO_2} - Pa_{O_2}$ as a measurement of gas exchange is that a given maldistribution of ventilation and perfusion or shunt will result in a different Pa_{O_2} and calculated $P_{AO_2} - Pa_{O_2}$ if there is a change in mixed venous PO_2, inspired PO_2, or the position of the O_2 dissociation curve.[172] Calculations of venous admixture and shunt provide more accurate estimates of $\dot{V}_A/\dot{Q}$ maldistribution and are less affected by mixed venous and inspired gas tensions; however, they require a sample of mixed venous blood. The same equation is used for calculation of venous admixture and shunt:

$$3. \quad \frac{\dot{Q}s}{\dot{Q}t} = \frac{Cc'_{O_2} - Ca_{O_2}}{Cc'_{O_2} - C\bar{v}_{O_2}}$$

where $\dot{Q}s/\dot{Q}t$ is the venous admixture ratio or shunt (if 100% oxygen is breathed), Cc'_{O_2} is the oxygen content of end-capillary blood, Ca_{O_2} is the oxygen content of arterial blood, and $C\bar{v}_{O_2}$ is the oxygen content of mixed venous blood; the equation assumes equilibration between alveolar and capillary PO_2. Ideal capillary PO_2 is calculated by using the alveolar air equation (see Equation 2). Content is calculated by determining the hemoglobin concentration and assuming that it is identical in venous, arterial, and capillary blood:

$$4. \quad O_2 \text{ content (mL blood/100)}$$
$$= (\text{Hgb [g/dL]} \times 1.39 \times \% \text{ saturation}) + (P_{O_2} \times 0.003)$$

where PO_2 is the PO_2 of capillary, arterial, or mixed venous blood; the first term in this equation relates to the oxygen content of hemoglobin and the second to the quantity of dissolved oxygen. When measurements for this calculation are obtained while the patient is breathing air or a gas mixture containing less than 100% oxygen, the resulting ratio is a venous admixture that is an "as if" shunt, or the amount of mixed venous blood that would have to be added to capillary blood to result in the observed arterial PO_2 and $P_{AO_2} - Pa_{O_2}$.

Although venous admixture is a more robust estimate of the lung's gas exchange ability, it is also affected by the inspired PO_2 and mixed venous PO_2.[173] Only when pure oxygen is breathed for a time sufficient to wash nitrogen out of the lung completely can a measure be obtained of gas exchange uninfluenced by inspired PO_2 and mixed venous PO_2. The calculation of shunt from Equation 3 gives an estimate of only one compartment in the $\dot{V}_A/\dot{Q}$ spectrum. Moreover, breathing pure O_2 for a prolonged period can itself increase the intrapulmonary shunt by causing alveolar collapse.[174]

A major advance in the measurement of $\dot{V}_A/\dot{Q}$ mismatch came with the development of a method to measure the "continuous" distribution of $\dot{V}_A/\dot{Q}$ ratios in normal and diseased lungs.[175] The technique involves the intravenous infusion of up to 10 inert gases dissolved in saline; the gases used have a wide range of solubility in blood, and in their passage through the lung they enter alveolar gas. The mixed expired and arterial concentration of each gas is measured by gas chromatography when a steady state is achieved; the retention and excretion of each gas can then be calculated and plotted against solubility. From the plot, the distribution of blood flow and ventilation with respect to $\dot{V}_A/\dot{Q}$ ratios can be calculated with a computer. The technique allows measurement of absolute shunt as well as alveolar dead space and also permits calculation of the proportion of perfusion and ventilation to a large number of units of varying $\dot{V}_A/\dot{Q}$ ratio.

Blood Gases and Acid-Base Balance

Blood Gases. The ability of the lung to perform its prime function—exchange of oxygen and carbon dioxide—is readily determined from analysis of a sample of arterial blood. The oxygen carried in blood is predominantly attached to hemoglobin and can be calculated by using Equation 4.

In contrast to oxygen, approximately 75% of carbon dioxide is contained in plasma. In a resting subject, mixed venous blood holds about 15 mL of oxygen per deciliter of blood at a Po_2 of 40 mm Hg and an oxygen saturation of 75%, whereas its carbon dioxide content is about 52 mL/dL of blood at a Pco_2 of 45 mm Hg. Although the red blood cell carries only 25% of the carbon dioxide, it plays an essential role in the transport of this gas to the lungs; it contains the enzyme carbonic anhydrase, which rapidly hydrates the carbon dioxide passing through the erythrocyte membrane and converts it into carbonic acid, H^+ ions, and bicarbonate ions. The bicarbonate ions (HCO_3^-) quickly permeate the cell membrane and enter plasma in exchange for chloride ions; in this manner, most of the carbon dioxide from tissues is carried by blood as bicarbonate. Because blood that contains reduced hemoglobin can carry more carbon dioxide than fully oxygenated blood can at the same Pco_2, the circumstances are ideal for uptake of carbon dioxide in tissues and for its unloading in pulmonary capillaries when the hemoglobin has been reoxygenated (see Fig. 1–45).

Arterial hypoxemia may be due to one or more of five mechanisms—diffusion defect, true shunt, ventilation-perfusion inequality, low inspired O_2, or hypoventilation. A *diffusion defect* results in hypoxemia if alveolar and capillary Po_2 fail to equilibrate in the brief transit of the red blood cell through the pulmonary capillary bed. It is probable that this mechanism contributes to the hypoxemia seen in emphysema, the increase in hypoxemia that occurs with exercise in patients who have interstitial lung disease, the hypoxemia that develops in some individuals during severe exercise, and the hypoxemia of high altitude. During exercise, the mechanism is probably a decrease in red blood cell capillary transit time, whereas at high altitudes, it is related to low alveolar Po_2. Since carbon dioxide is about 20 times more soluble than oxygen in water and tissue membranes, equilibration times are more rapid, and limitation of diffusion does not play a role in the genesis of carbon dioxide retention.

A *true shunt* is the primary cause of hypoxemia in many congenital cardiovascular abnormalities and in cardiogenic and noncardiogenic pulmonary edema and other conditions characterized by air space consolidation, such as pneumonia. The shunted blood never comes in contact with acinar gas, and for this reason the Po_2 of arterial blood cannot be raised to a normal value (approximately 600 mm Hg) during inhalation of 100% oxygen. In fact, when the shunt handles 10% or more of the cardiac output, arterial Po_2 cannot rise above 400 mm Hg. Other mechanisms that produce hypoxemia can be corrected by the inspiration of 100% oxygen, which replaces nitrogen in even the most poorly ventilated acini.

$\dot{V}_A/\dot{Q}$ *inequality* is the most common cause of the hypoxemia that accompanies pulmonary disease. As discussed earlier, $\dot{V}_A/\dot{Q}$ mismatching and shunt tend to affect oxygen transport and arterial Po_2 to a greater extent than carbon dioxide transport and Pco_2, so hypoxemia is often found in conjunction with a normal or decreased $Paco_2$. A low inspired partial pressure of oxygen causes the hypoxemia that occurs at high altitude. If overall *alveolar ventilation* decreases, carbon dioxide retention occurs as well as alveolar hypoxia and resulting hypoxemia. The hypoxemia associated with low Pio_2 and hypoventilation does not produce an increased alveolar-arterial gradient for oxygen and thus differs from the hypoxemia caused by a diffusion defect, $\dot{V}_A/\dot{Q}$ inequality, and shunt. Because hypoventilation often occurs in association with these gas exchange abnormalities, calculation of $Pao_2 - Pao_2$ aids in separating the component of hypoxemia related to hypoventilation from that caused by gas exchange problems.

Acid-Base Balance. The hydrogen ion concentration and therefore the pH of blood is dependent on at least three physicochemical systems:[176] (1) the electrochemical balance of strong ions, electrolytes that are fully dissociated at normal physiologic pH—Na^+, K^+, and Cl^- (since the law of electrical neutrality requires that the electrical charge of all dissolved strong ions equal 0, changes in the concentrations of these ions can influence the degree of dissociation of water and therefore the concentrations of hydrogen and hydroxyl ion in blood); (2) the buffering capacity of weak electrolytes such as the imidazole group of histidine molecules in tissue proteins, plasma proteins, and hemoglobin (these electrolytes can accept or donate protons and thus buffer changes in hydrogen ion concentration in blood); and (3) most important, the carbon dioxide–bicarbonate system.

The terms *alkalemia* and *acidemia* are restricted to situations in which there is a decrease or increase in the arterial hydrogen ion concentration above or below the normal range, whereas the terms *alkalosis* and *acidosis* are used to describe abnormal processes that would increase or decrease the hydrogen ion concentration of blood if there were no secondary compensatory changes. The interdependence of hydrogen ion concentration, arterial Pco_2, and bicarbonate is illustrated by the Kassirer-Bleich modification of the Henderson-Hasselbalch equation:[177]

$$[H^+] = \frac{24 \times Pco_2}{HCO_3}$$

Examination of this equation shows that the arterial concentration of hydrogen ion is dependent on the *ratio* of arterial Pco_2 to arterial bicarbonate: anything that increases the ratio will cause an increase in hydrogen ion concentration (decrease in pH), and anything that decreases the ratio will cause a decrease in hydrogen ion concentration (increase in pH).

Disturbances in acid-base balance can be divided into those that are respiratory in origin and those that are nonrespiratory or metabolic. Respiratory changes in acid-base balance are due to overventilation or underventilation with excess removal or retention of carbon dioxide. Metabolic disturbances are the result of an increase or decrease in non–carbonic acid or a loss or gain of bicarbonate in extracellular fluid. Acidosis or alkalosis may be "simple"—that is, purely respiratory or metabolic—or mixed and reflect physiologic disturbances that are both respiratory and metabolic.

RESPIRATORY ACIDOSIS. Respiratory acidosis results from alveolar hypoventilation and may be secondary to (1) a decreased central neurogenic drive to breathe, (2) an abnormality of the neural connections between the central nervous system and the respiratory muscles, (3) an abnormality in the respiratory muscles or rib cage, or (4) an abnormality of the airways or lung parenchyma that produces an inordinate increase in the work of breathing.

Respiratory acidosis may be acute or chronic. An acute increase in arterial P_{CO_2} causes a shift of the Henderson equation to the right ($H_2O + CO_2 \rightarrow H_2CO_3 \rightarrow H^+ + HCO_3^-$), thereby increasing both hydrogen and bicarbonate ion concentrations. The increase in bicarbonate tends to attenuate the increase in hydrogen ion concentration that would otherwise have occurred, thus limiting the acute change in arterial pH. As a rule of thumb, the increase in bicarbonate associated with acute CO_2 retention is approximately 1 mmol/L for each 10-mm Hg rise in P_{CO_2}. When carbon dioxide retention is prolonged, there is a renal response that consists of the formation and retention of bicarbonate. The process begins immediately, is well developed by 48 hours, and is usually complete within 5 days. During "steady-state" respiratory acidosis, an approximate 5.1-mmol/L increase in HCO_3^- occurs for each 10-mm Hg increase in P_{CO_2}. This process can return arterial pH to normal levels.[178]

RESPIRATORY ALKALOSIS. Respiratory alkalosis results from hyperventilation, the most common cause of which is an anxiety state. Traumatic, infectious, or vascular lesions of the central nervous system, hyperthyroidism, pregnancy, liver failure, and some drugs may produce prolonged respiratory alkalosis. Mild respiratory alkalosis can also be seen in pneumonia, asthma, fibrotic interstitial pulmonary diseases, and the early stages of pulmonary edema. An acute fall in serum bicarbonate occurs with hyperventilation. This change is approximately 2 mmol/L for each 10-mm Hg decrease in P_{CO_2}. With chronic respiratory alkalosis, renal excretion of bicarbonate is increased, and pH and the hydrogen ion concentration return toward normal levels. As a rule of thumb, there is a 5-mmol/L decrease in bicarbonate for each 10-mm Hg decrease in P_{CO_2}.

METABOLIC ACIDOSIS. Metabolic acidosis results from accumulation of non–carbonic acids in extracellular fluid or from loss of bicarbonate ion. It can be further subdivided on the basis of whether it results in an elevated anion gap.[144] The latter is the difference in the serum concentrations of sodium and the sum of chloride and bicarbonate [$Na^+ - (Cl^- + HCO_3^-)$] and is normally about 12 mmol/L. When an anionic acid accumulates within the body, the law of electrical neutrality requires that the sum of Cl^- and HCO_3^- plus the added anion equal the concentration of cations. Thus, with the accumulation of an unmeasured acid anion, there will be a decrease in Cl^- and HCO_3^- and an increase in the calculated difference between Na^+ and the sum of Cl^- and HCO_3^-. Although the classification of metabolic acidosis into anion gap and non–anion gap forms has proved useful, it is good to remember that certain conditions (e.g., metabolic alkalosis, methanol intoxication, or lactic acidosis) can result in an increased anion gap in the absence of acidosis or a normal anion gap despite significant acidosis.[179]

Compensation for metabolic acidosis occurs by buffering of the excess hydrogen ions by hemoglobin, plasma proteins, and phosphate and by a shift of the Henderson equation to the left as bicarbonate combines with the increased hydrogen ion to form carbonic acid ($CO_2 + H_2O \leftarrow H_2O_3 \leftarrow H^+ + HCO_3^-$). The elevated hydrogen ion concentration stimulates the central and peripheral chemoreceptors, thereby augmenting alveolar ventilation and lowering arterial P_{CO_2}. There is a time lag in the respiratory response to metabolic acidosis related to the time required for hydrogen ion and bicarbonate to equilibrate across the blood-brain barrier. In general, maximal respiratory compensation occurs by 12 hours, although the response is insufficient to return pH to normal. During steady-state metabolic acidosis, P_{CO_2} should decrease between 1 and 1.3 mm Hg for every 1-mmol/L decrease in serum bicarbonate concentration.

METABOLIC ALKALOSIS. Metabolic alkalosis results when the hydrogen ion concentration in extracellular fluid is decreased secondary to loss of acid or an increase in alkali, such as can occur with severe, protracted vomiting or after prolonged nasogastric suction. Chronic diuretic therapy, excessive exogenous administration of alkali, hyperaldosteronism, Cushing's syndrome, and excessive exogenous steroid administration are additional causes. In pulmonary practice, one of the most common causes of apparent metabolic alkalosis occurs during treatment of chronic carbon dioxide retention. If artificial ventilation is used to reduce P_{CO_2} in patients who have chronic CO_2 retention and compensated respiratory acidosis, the patient will be left with a metabolic alkalosis. The expected respiratory compensation for metabolic alkalosis is a decrease in alveolar ventilation and a rise in alveolar and arterial P_{CO_2}. Although cellular and extracellular buffers make more H^+ available to attenuate the increase in plasma HCO_3^- concentration, it is primarily an increase in P_{CO_2} that will return the P_{CO_2}-bicarbonate ratio toward normal and stabilize pH. However, the respiratory response to metabolic alkalosis is the least predictable and most variable of the compensatory mechanisms. Arterial P_{CO_2} often fails to increase or increases much less than would be expected. In some patients, "failure" to compensate may be related to concomitant respiratory or cardiovascular disorders that independently increase the drive to breathe and counteract the decreased ventilatory drive that is caused by a fall in arterial and cerebrospinal fluid hydrogen ion concentration. As a general rule, one can expect that arterial P_{CO_2} will increase by 0.4 to 0.5 mm Hg for each 1-mmol/L increase in serum bicarbonate.

THE BRONCHIAL CIRCULATION

Two to four bronchial arteries normally arise directly from the aorta or the intercostal vessels.[180] The extrapulmonary branches course to the hila, where they form an intercommunicating circular arc around the main bronchi, from which the intrapulmonary arteries radiate. The latter vessels are situated within peribronchial connective tissue and branch with the airways as far as the terminal bronchioles. Small branches penetrate into the bronchial wall and form an intercommunicating network in the mucosa. The bronchial circulation is unique in that it has dual venous drainage: a portion of bronchial flow drains into the bronchial veins to the right side of the heart via the azygos and hemiazygos systems, whereas another portion forms extensive anastomoses with the pulmonary circulation at precapillary, capillary, and postcapillary sites and drains into the left atrium via the pulmonary veins.[181]

The bronchial arteries supply the tracheal, bronchial, and bronchiolar walls; the middle third of the esophagus; the visceral pleura over the mediastinal and diaphragmatic surfaces of the lungs (the visceral pleura over the lung convexities being supplied by pulmonary arteries); the outer layers of the aortic arch, pulmonary arteries, and pulmonary veins via the vasa vasorum; the paratracheal, carinal, hilar, and intrapulmonary lymph nodes and lymphoid tissue; the vagus and bronchopulmonary nerves; and sometimes, the parietal layer of the pericardium and the thymus.[182] In addition to providing blood to all these structures, the bronchial vasculature may have other important functions, including humidification and warming of inspired air[183] and an emergency backup to maintain nutritive blood flow to the lung when the pulmonary arteries are obstructed.[184]

Because of the relative inaccessibility of the bronchial vessels, very few measurements of flow have been made in humans. Measurements of bronchopulmonary anastomotic flow have been made in patients, but the results are highly variable (ranging from 1% to almost 24% of cardiac output); flow is increased in patients who have pulmonary disease.[185]

PULMONARY DEFENSE AND OTHER NONRESPIRATORY FUNCTIONS

In addition to respiration, the lungs have several functions that are of considerable importance in the maintenance of well-being. These functions can be discussed under three headings: pulmonary defense, metabolic functions, and certain physical and related functions.

Pulmonary Defense

The entire surface of the conducting airways and lung parenchyma is normally in contact with the external environment. As a result, there is a constant risk of exposure to a variety of potentially harmful substances, including organic and inorganic particles, toxic gases and fumes, and a bewildering array of microorganisms. The defense mechanisms in response to such inhaled or aspirated substances are numerous and complex and, for convenience of discussion, can be divided into those that are specific (related to the immune system) and those that are nonspecific (including particle deposition and clearance, inflammation, and secretion of protective enzymes). The efficiency of many of these defense mechanisms may be impaired by various environmental insults and physiologic conditions, including hypoxia, hyperoxia, acidosis, cigarette smoke, and drugs (particularly corticosteroids and other suppressors of the immune or inflammatory reactions).

Particle Deposition and Clearance

The first line of defense against inhaled or aspirated noxious particles* is clearance; obviously, the faster and more efficiently the lungs can eliminate such substances, the less

---

*Strictly speaking, the term *particle* refers to a fragment of inanimate organic or inorganic matter; for purposes of this discussion, however, it includes microorganisms (such as fungal spores or conidia) and liquid droplets (on which bacteria or viruses may be adherent).

potential there is for damage. Such clearance is accomplished by several mechanisms, including transport up the mucociliary escalator, cough, phagocytosis and destruction by alveolar macrophages, and lymphatic drainage. Regional differences in these mechanisms may explain some of the variation in anatomic localization of disease in different conditions. In addition, differences in the effectiveness of clearance may partly explain differences in susceptibility to certain diseases among individual patients. For example, particles deposited on the airway mucosa are usually transported in tracheobronchial secretions to the pharynx; in healthy individuals, the time to clear the airways may be as little as several hours. However, transport is prolonged in some individuals as a result of either inherent individual variation in the mucus flow rate,[186] environmental factors such as cigarette smoke,[187] or intrinsic lung disease; such prolongation may predispose to greater particle retention and an increased risk of pulmonary disease.

A variety of physiologic mechanisms and physical factors are involved in the deposition and clearance of inhaled particles.

Size and Shape of Inhaled Particles. Four physical processes largely determine particle deposition in the lungs:

1. *Inertial impaction.* This process occurs when the momentum of a particle being carried in an air current causes it to impinge on an airway wall when the latter changes direction. This mechanism is the principal one by which large particles (from 2 to 100 μm in diameter) are deposited in the respiratory tract,[188] particularly the nose and nasopharynx. Inertial impaction also occurs within the lungs, especially at the bifurcation of proximal bronchi.
2. *Sedimentation.* Sedimentation is the mechanism by which particles are deposited on airway walls as a result of the influence of gravity; in general, the larger and denser the particle, the more rapid the settling. Sedimentation is an important mechanism of deposition of particles ranging from 0.5 to 2 μm in diameter and occurs mostly in the bronchi and membranous bronchioles.
3. *Diffusion (brownian movement).* Diffusion causes small particles (mostly less than 0.5 μm in diameter) to move randomly as a result of energy transfer from adjacent gas molecules. Although the vast majority of such particles are exhaled and therefore not retained within the lung, those that do remain are deposited in the alveoli principally by diffusion.
4. *Interception.* The first three mechanisms of deposition relate predominantly to particles that are approximately spherical in shape. When the length-to-diameter ratio of particles increases to 3:1 or greater, they are termed *fibers*, and a fourth mechanism comes into play. Such particulates, especially those with a large cross-sectional diameter such as chrysotile asbestos, are likely to come into contact with and be deposited on the airway wall. By contrast, fibers with a straight configuration and a relatively small diameter tend to travel like a javelin in the center of the airway lumen and can penetrate far into the lung periphery.[189]

Rate and Pattern of Breathing. Because the majority of large particles are trapped on the nasal mucosa, a greater concentration of such particles tends to reach the lower respiratory tract in individuals engaged in heavy exercise in whom mouth breathing is instituted. However, since the high flow rate that accompanies such exercise enhances inertial impaction, many of these particles are deposited on the proximal airways and do not reach the lung parenchyma itself. Nonetheless, increased ventilation itself results in a greater number of particles reaching the lung in a given period. Because sedimentation is a passive process related to gravity, the rate of settling and deposition of a particle by this means is dependent on the time that the particle resides within the lung. Breathing patterns that are associated with an increase in this time, such as breath-holding or quiet breathing, may result in increased deposition by this mechanism.

Distribution of Inhaled Particles. Because ventilation in the erect position is relatively greater in the lower than the upper lung regions, it might be predicted that the former would be more susceptible to lung damage from inhaled particles. That such is not always the case, however, is indicated by the predominant involvement of the upper lung zones in patients with silicosis and coal worker's pneumoconiosis. It is unclear to what extent such anatomic predilection for disease is caused by the initial distribution of particles, perhaps influenced by variations in bronchial anatomy[190] or by the phase of the respiratory cycle at which the particles are inhaled. Particle size itself may be important in this respect; in one study, investigators showed that relatively large particles (3.5 μm in diameter) were preferentially deposited in the upper lobes, as compared with particles 1.1 μm in size.[191] As might be expected, intrinsic lung disease such as emphysema can also have an appreciable effect on particle deposition.[192] In addition, particles deposited on both large and small airways can induce bronchospasm, which may influence regional particle distribution.[193]

Concentration of Inhaled Particles. The ability of the lung to cope with potentially harmful particles appears to relate to some extent to the number inhaled. For example, a concentration of less than 10 inorganic dust particles of 5 μm or less per milliliter can be completely eliminated, whereas only about 90% of a concentration of approximately 1000 such particles per milliliter is removed; the retained 10% can produce a slowly developing pneumoconiosis.

The Mucociliary Escalator. The principal function of the mucociliary escalator is to convey inhaled particles from the lung to the larynx, where they are eliminated by swallowing. Efficient functioning of this mechanism depends on the presence of a surface mucous layer of appropriate thickness and chemical composition and directed and coordinated ciliary movement sufficient to propel the mucus and entrapped particles toward the larynx.

According to the sliding microtubule hypothesis,[194] ciliary movement occurs by means of coordinated movement of the dynein arms of one ciliary doublet along an adjacent doublet, much like going up or down the rungs of a ladder. Because not all doublets move at the same time, this coordinated movement leads to a shortening of some peripheral microtubules relative to those that are either contiguous to or on the opposite side of the cilium. With the internal rigidity that is provided by the radial spokes and the basal anchoring system, the cilium bends in the direction of shortening. The ciliary beat itself can be divided into an effective (mucus-propulsive) stroke and a slower, recovery stroke. The former occurs perpendicular to the epithelial surface with the cilium almost

completely erect and its tip "grasping" the lower portion of the mucous layer with tiny clawlike structures. After a short rest at completion of the effective stroke, the cilium swings backward within the less viscous sol layer until it takes up a position compatible with the beginning of a new effective stroke (Fig. 1–46).

The surface area on which mucus lies converges about 2000-fold from small airways to the trachea; as a result, some absorption of fluid and acceleration of transport must occur to prevent plugging of the central airways.[126] A combination of an increased number of ciliated cells, increased length of cilia, and increased ciliary beat frequency also contributes to more efficient clearing of secretions.

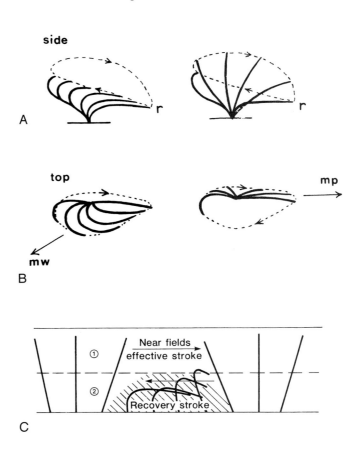

FIGURE 1–46

Beat cycle of a rabbit tracheal cilium seen from the side and from above. In the recovery stroke (**A,** *left*), the cilium starts from the rest position (r) and unrolls clockwise (**B,** *left top* view); in the effective stroke (**A,** *right*), it remains extended and bends over to reach the rest position at the right. Mucus is propelled toward the right (mp), and the recovery wave is propagated toward the lower left (mw). Cilia move in waves (**C**), with clusters in their recovery phase bordered by those undergoing their effective stroke. During the effective stroke (**D**), the ciliary tips extend into the lower portion of the mucous layer and propel it to the right. *(Adapted from Sleigh MA, Blake JR, Liron N: The propulsion of mucus by cilia. Am Rev Respir Dis 137:726, 1988.)*

A variety of pharmacologic and other factors influence normal mucociliary clearance. The mechanisms by which they act are complex and probably related to an alteration in ciliary beat frequency, the depth of the periciliary sol layer, the quantity and viscoelastic properties of the mucus, and/or the state of hydration of the secretions (for example, dehydration has been shown to decrease mucociliary clearance and rehydration to improve it).[195]

Cough. Cough is an important mechanism of respiratory defense and an adjuvant to the clearance of tracheobronchial secretions. It can be initiated voluntarily or involuntarily, the latter by stimulation of irritant receptors in the larynx, trachea, or large bronchi. The procedure begins with an inspiratory maneuver followed by glottic closure. Expiratory muscles then contract to increase pleural, abdominal, and alveolar pressure to a level of 100 mm Hg or more. The glottis is suddenly opened, and expiratory flow begins and peaks in 30 to 50 milliseconds with flows at the mouth as high as 12 L/sec. Limitation of expiratory flow within the thorax occurs as a result of airway collapse and leads to gas velocities that reach three quarters of the speed of sound (1600 to 2400 cm/sec). These high velocities produce enormous shear stress on the liquid layer lining the airways and move large amounts of mucus and any incorporated particulate debris proximally. Although cough is most effective in clearing secretions from large airways, calculations suggest that some clearance can occur down to 20th-generation airways. The greater the depth of the periciliary serous layer and the less viscous it is, the greater its effectiveness.

Clearance of the Alveolar Air Space. The majority of particles deposited in the alveoli are probably phagocytosed by alveolar macrophages, which then migrate to the mucociliary escalator, are transported to the pharynx, and are expectorated or swallowed in the same manner as free particles. When the capacity of these macrophages to clear the air spaces in this manner is overwhelmed by an abundance of particles, disease may ensue. In the case of inorganic particles, there may be penetration directly across the epithelium into alveolar or peribronchiolar interstitial tissue. Some of these particles are then transported centripetally via peribronchovascular lymphatics to bronchopulmonary and hilar lymph nodes or centrifugally via lymphatics in the interlobular septa to the pleura. Others, however, remain in the interstitial tissue (particularly peribronchiolar tissue), where they may accumulate and eventually cause significant disease.

Inflammation and Secreted Proteins

Polymorphonuclear leukocytes are normally present both in alveolar air spaces and along the conducting airways, albeit in very small numbers. Their role is presumably similar to that of alveolar macrophages, although the substances that they phagocytose and degrade may differ. In addition to these normally occurring cells, an inflammatory reaction is a common result of particle deposition, particularly if clearance mechanisms are inadequate.

Several substances secreted by airway and alveolar epithelial cells or by macrophages or derived directly from the blood also have a local nonspecific protective function. These substances include lysozyme, lactoferrin, interferon, fibronectin, surfactant, and various complement components. Surfactant apoproteins and mannose-binding lectin are members of a family of proteins called collectins that play a role in the innate immune response by binding to carbohydrate structures on the surface of pathogens and stimulating the recruitment of inflammatory cells.[196] In addition, epithelial cells produce substances, such as leukocyte antiprotease, that act to protect the lung from the deleterious side effects of the proteolytic enzymes that are probably released normally in small amounts by intrapulmonary inflammatory cells.

The reaction to irritating or noxious gases is somewhat different from that to inhaled particles. The first line of defense is cessation of ventilation; gases that do enter the conducting system are absorbed on the moist surface of the upper airways or are detoxified by dilution.

Pulmonary Immune Mechanisms

Cells of the intrapulmonary immune system are localized at a variety of sites, including lymph nodes and mucosal lymphoid nodules, and occur as isolated cells in the alveolar and bronchovascular interstitium. Numerous lymph nodes are present in the tissue adjacent to proximal bronchi. They receive lymph with admixed cells and debris from the parenchyma and conducting airways and function both as a repository for foreign particulate material and as a station for antigen processing. The precise function of mucosal lymphoid tissue is unclear; however, it has been suggested that it is a component of a common epithelial mucosal IgA system that includes the gastrointestinal tract and is involved in antigen processing and local IgA production.[197]

All immunoglobulin classes are found in tracheobronchial secretions, although the predominant forms are IgG and IgA.[198] They may be produced and secreted locally (particularly IgA and IgE) or be derived from serum by transudation (IgG). IgA is the most abundant and is present predominantly in dimeric (secretory) form. It is probably produced mostly by B cells in the connective tissue of the lamina propria and tracheobronchial glands. These antibodies have multiple functions, including opsonization and enhanced phagocytosis (particularly IgG), complement activation, toxin neutralization, and microbial agglutination.

Cell-mediated immunity is also undoubtedly important in pulmonary defense, particularly with respect to infection. BAL fluid of normal individuals yields a cellular population composed of about 80% to 85% macrophages and 10% to 15% lymphocytes, the great majority of which are T cells. Most of these cells appear to be derived from a pool of sensitized lymphocytes in the systemic circulation.[199] Such cells emigrate from pulmonary vessels at the site where an appropriate antigen is deposited and participate either in modulation and enhancement of alveolar macrophage function or in cell-mediated cytotoxicity.

Metabolic Functions

Type II alveolar cells, Clara cells, alveolar macrophages, mast cells, and pulmonary vascular endothelial cells are involved in the storage, transformation, degradation, and synthesis of a large variety of substances.[200] Surfactant production by type II alveolar cells has been discussed earlier. A variety of lipid-based mediators are synthesized by lung cells, including the products of 5-lipoxygenase (the potent contractile and vasoactive *cysteinyl-leukotrienes* LTC_4, LTD_4, and LTE_4, as well as the neutrophil chemoattractant LTB_4) and products of the cyclooxygenase enzymes that are responsible for prostaglandin metabolism.[201,202] *Prostaglandin E* causes smooth muscle relaxation and is anti-inflammatory, whereas *prostaglandin F* and *thromboxane* are contractile agonists.[203]

Mast cells are found throughout the lungs in airway, alveolar, and pleural interstitial tissue.[204] When IgE bound to their surface receptors interacts with specific antigen, they release a wide variety of mediators, including histamine, leukotrienes, prostaglandins, chemotactic factors, and proteases.

Angiotensin-converting enzyme (ACE) is produced largely by endothelial cells. ACE inactivates bradykinin, and monitoring of lung ACE content and activity has been advocated as a marker of endothelial cell function.[205] *Neutral endopeptidase,* an enzyme produced preferentially by airway epithelial cells, can inactivate inflammatory peptides, including bradykinin and the neuropeptides. The tachykinin neuropeptides *substance P* and *neurokinin A* are released from pulmonary afferent and efferent nerves and have effects on vascular and airway smooth muscle, as well as stimulate vascular leak and mucus secretion. *Vasoactive intestinal peptide* is a neurally derived peptide that acts as an endogenous bronchodilator.

NO is synthesized by the action of NO synthase (NOS) on the amino acid L-arginine and has important effects on airway and vascular function.[206,207] Two forms of the enzyme exist in the lung—a constitutively expressed form (c-NOS), which is present in the vascular endothelium, and an inducible form (i-NOS), which is expressed in the airway epithelium and lung macrophages.[77] In addition to having effects on vascular and airway smooth muscle, NO may have an immunoregulatory role by enhancing the differentiation of T_H2-type helper T cells and thereby increasing local production of the proinflammatory cytokines interleukin-4 and interleukin-5.[208]

Another group of potent, biologically active substances produced by lung cells is the *endothelins*. These are a family of small peptides that have potent vasoconstrictor and bronchoconstrictor actions, increase vascular permeability, and induce smooth muscle cell proliferation.[209] ET-1 is produced by endothelial cells; there is evidence that an increase in the production of ET-1 and a decrease in NO synthesis may contribute to pulmonary hypertension in some pulmonary vascular disorders.[210]

The lung can metabolize a number of exogenous chemicals (xenobiotics).[211] Phase 1 enzymes cause oxidation, reduction, or hydrolysis, whereas phase 2 forms usually conjugate the xenobiotic by adding an additional chemical group and thereby rendering it less toxic or more readily excretable. The phase 1 cytochrome P-450 enzymes are contained in Clara cells. Some actions of the cytochromes can be harmful, as when the P-450 breakdown products of paraquat cause pulmonary endothelial and epithelial cell damage and pulmonary edema. The lungs also contain a variety of enzymes involved in the maintenance of normal structure, such as superoxide dismutase[212] and antiproteases.[23] The vast endothelial network of the pulmonary capillaries has several metabolic functions, including modulation of blood coagulability, hydrolysis of lipids, and metabolism of biologically active substances such as serotonin and catecholamines.[203,213]

The Pulmonary Vascular Filter

The pulmonary capillary network is interposed between the systemic venous and arterial circulations and, in normal circumstances, receives the entire cardiac output. It thus has the potential to act as a sieve and protect vital organs on the systemic side of the circulation from various potentially harmful materials. Probably the most important of these materials are thrombi originating in peripheral veins. Such thrombi are not uncommon, particularly in ill individuals; although most are small and result in no significant pulmonary damage, it is clear that their potential for causing serious harm would be much greater in organs such as the heart or brain.

Normally occurring tissue elements can also be trapped within the lungs. The most common of these elements are megakaryocytes derived from the bone marrow, which are frequently seen in pulmonary capillaries, both in patients who have systemic disease and in previously healthy individuals who have died suddenly.[214] The pulmonary capillaries also serve as a storage site for blood leukocytes; a so-called marginated pool is formed in these capillaries that is two to three times larger than the number of circulating leukocytes.[215] Rather than remaining in the lung, the sequestered cells are delayed in their passage, so there is a constant turnover of cells within the pool. This sequestration is probably related in part to size. Normal leukocytes are slightly larger than most pulmonary capillaries and thus have to deform to transit the lung; because leukocytes are 1000 times less deformable than red blood cells, this process is associated with delayed passage through the capillaries. These sequestered leukocytes are presumably important in providing a ready source of cells for migration into the alveolar air spaces to combat inhaled microorganisms.[216]

DEVELOPMENT AND GROWTH OF THE LUNG

Growth and development of the lung can be divided into intrauterine and postnatal stages. Traditionally, the former itself has been divided into four periods: *embryonic, pseudoglandular, canalicular,* and *terminal sac*[217]; the addition of a fifth, or *alveolar*, phase has also been proposed.[218]

Conducting and Transitional Airways and Alveoli

The *embryonic period* of lung development begins at about 26 days of life with the formation of a ventral diverticulum of the foregut near the junction of the occipital and cervical segments. During the next 2 to 3 days, the diverticulum gives rise to right and left lung buds that progressively elongate and branch such that by days 32 to 34, the five lobar bronchi have appeared, a point marking the end of the embryonic period.

The *pseudoglandular period* extends from the end of the 5th to the 16th week of gestation and is concerned primarily with development of the bronchial tree. After the appearance of the five lobar bronchi, branching occurs quickly and more or less dichotomously. Between the 10th and 14th weeks, 65% to 75% of all bronchial branching has occurred, and by the 16th week, virtually all conducting airways are present. During this period, the airways are blind tubules lined by columnar or cuboidal epithelium—hence the term pseudoglandular (Fig. 1–47).

From the 16th to the 24th or 25th week of intrauterine life (*canalicular period*), the peripheral portion of the bronchial

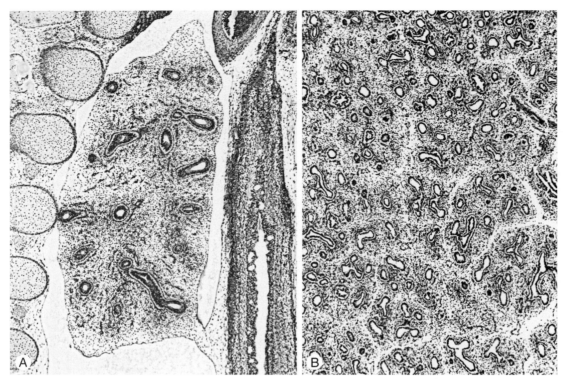

FIGURE 1–47

Developing human lung—pseudoglandular period. A, Early pseudoglandular period showing occasional tubular channels within abundant mesenchyme. Thoracic vertebrae are at the left. (×40.) **B,** Late pseudoglandular period showing more numerous branching presumptive airways. (×52.) *(From Fraser RS, Müller NL, Colman NC, Paré PD: Fraser and Paré's Diagnosis of Diseases of the Chest, 4th ed. Philadelphia, WB Saunders, 1999.)*

tree undergoes further development in the form of primitive canaliculi that represent early stages of the acinar airways (Fig. 1–48). At the same time, the mesenchyme adjacent to the canaliculi becomes vascularized through the ingrowth of capillaries.

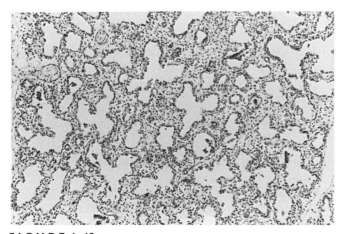

FIGURE 1–48

Developing lung—canalicular period. A section of lung during the canalicular period shows a more complex pattern, with pulmonary airways now clearly recognizable. (×120.) *(From Fraser RS, Müller NL, Colman NC, Paré PD: Fraser and Paré's Diagnosis of Diseases of the Chest, 4th ed. Philadelphia, WB Saunders, 1999.)*

By the 24th to the 25th week, terminal thin-walled spaces with flattened epithelium, termed saccules, become visible at the ends of the canaliculi. This point marks the beginning of the *terminal sac* period, which is traditionally believed to last until birth. (Nonetheless, alveolar development has been demonstrated as early as 30 weeks of gestation and, in one study, was uniformly present by 36 weeks.[218]) Acini develop rapidly, and by the 28th week, several generations of respiratory bronchioles open into so-called transitional ducts, with several generations of saccules arising from them. Further intrauterine development consists largely of saccular proliferation and a corresponding decrease in and more organized vascularization of the mesenchyme. At birth, the typical acinus consists of three generations of respiratory bronchioles, one of transitional ducts and three of saccules.[217]

Throughout the canalicular period, airway epithelium progressively decreases in height so that the entire acinar pathway is eventually lined by a cuboidal or flattened epithelium (Fig. 1–49). At about 28 weeks, differentiation into type I and type II alveolar epithelial cells has begun, and an occasional type II osmiophilic granule can be identified.[219] At this time, the blood-gas barrier is sufficiently developed to permit at least some gas exchange.

During early *postnatal* development, the acinus increases in length, and its components are remodeled, largely as a result of the appearance of alveoli. Thus, terminal bronchioles may be transformed into respiratory bronchioles and distal respiratory bronchioles into alveolar ducts. The saccules themselves

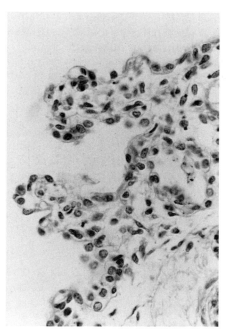

FIGURE 1–49

Developing lung—alveoli. Several presumptive alveoli are illustrated; they are still lined by cuboidal epithelium and contain a moderate amount of mesenchymal tissue in their walls. (×350.) *(From Fraser RS, Müller NL, Colman NC, Paré PD: Fraser and Paré's Diagnosis of Diseases of the Chest, 4th ed. Philadelphia, WB Saunders, 1999.)*

probably develop into both alveolar ducts and alveolar sacs. Although there is little true airway branching after birth, each terminal saccule may generate as many as four additional alveolar sacs,[217] most likely by budding. It is generally agreed that the majority of alveoli appear during early childhood, probably in the first 2 to 4 years,[220,221] and that they enlarge from childhood to adulthood. The age at which alveolar development is completed is controversial, although there is evidence that multiplication may occur until 8 years of age.[219]

The Vascular System

The pulmonary artery develops from the sixth aortic arch during the early embryonic period. On both sides, the proximal part of the arch develops into the proximal segment of the right and left pulmonary arteries; however, on the right side the distal part loses its connection with the aortic arch, whereas during intrauterine life the distal arch on the left maintains its connection with the aorta as the ductus arteriosus. Branches from both arches grow toward the developing lung buds and become incorporated with them in the future hila.

During the embryonic and pseudoglandular periods, pulmonary arteries develop at approximately the same rate and in the same manner as the airways, so the majority of preacinar branches are present by the end of the 16th week. During the latter part of fetal life, the main feature of arterial development is an increase in vessel diameter and length. In the postnatal stage, there is a small continuing increase in the development of conventional branches until about the age of 18 months; this increase in branches is related to the small increase in acinar airways that occurs during this period.[219]

By contrast, a marked increase in supernumerary branches occurs and corresponds to the prolific alveolar development of early childhood; this increase may continue, though at a decreasing rate, until about 8 years of age.[222]

In the embryonic stage, pulmonary venous blood drains via the splanchnic plexus into the primordia of the systemic venous system. Subsequently, an outpouching of the sinoatrial region of the heart (termed the common pulmonary vein) extends toward and connects with the portion of the splanchnic plexus draining the lungs. Eventually, the common pulmonary vein is incorporated into the left atrial wall and the majority of the splanchnic-pulmonary connections are obliterated, leaving four independent pulmonary veins directly entering the left atrium. Intrapulmonary development probably occurs by both vasculogenesis and angiogenesis.[223] As in the arterial system, the postacinar venous pattern is essentially complete halfway through fetal life, and the intra-acinar pattern develops during childhood.[133]

Factors Influencing Development and Growth

The factors that control lung growth and development are numerous and complex. Some evidence indicates that there is a time-dependent sequence of regulators (the "developmental program") that is responsible for such development and that this program continues into the postnatal period of alveolar development.[224] Clearly, genetic makeup has an important influence, as shown by the results of a number of experimental animal studies.[224,225] Several observations suggest that airway branching is likely to be controlled, at least partly, by signals between epithelial and mesenchymal cells. For example, if the lung buds are removed from an animal in an early stage of development and then cultured, the branching process continues, but only if the adjacent mesenchyme is included in the culture medium.[226] The precise molecular mechanisms responsible for this relationship are unclear[224]; however, it is likely that cell-cell and cell–extracellular connective tissue interactions,[227,228] as well as locally produced mediators, are involved. Regional differences in the expression of specific genes (e.g., homeobox genes)[229] and programmed death (apoptosis) of both epithelial and mesenchymal cells[230] are also likely to be important factors affecting morphogenesis.

The role of systemic hormones and locally produced peptides in growth and development, though certainly important, is for the most part poorly understood.[231] Glucocorticoids have a significant effect on the maturation of alveolar type II cells and thus on surfactant production. The precise morphologic effects of other hormones, such as thyroxine, insulin, and growth hormone, have not been well demonstrated, although such effects undoubtedly occur.[232] Pulmonary neuroendocrine cells have been hypothesized to play a role in airway development, possibly mediated by gastrin-releasing peptide.[24] An important role for hepatocyte growth factor has been hypothesized.[233]

The nature of and factors controlling postpneumonectomy compensatory lung growth are poorly understood. On the basis of animal experiments, it appears that such growth is a result of both cellular and connective tissue proliferation (as opposed to simple hypertrophy or alveolar distention) and that stretch is the initial stimulus.[234] The effects of bronchopulmonary or systemic disease acquired in childhood on lung growth are also not well understood; however, experimental evidence indicates that a variety of conditions such as viral infection[235] and starvation[236] can have an important influence. Various factors, including the amount of lung removed, age, mechanical stimulation, growth factors, retinoids, and glucocorticoids, are probably important in affecting the degree of pulmonary growth after pneumonectomy.

INNERVATION OF THE LUNG

The lung is innervated by fibers that travel in the vagus nerve and in nerves derived from the second through fifth thoracic ganglia of the sympathetic trunk (Fig. 1–50). The vagus contains preganglionic, parasympathetic efferent fibers, nonadrenergic-noncholinergic (NANC) efferent fibers, and afferent fibers from various lung receptors. The sympathetic fibers are largely postganglionic efferent in type. In addition to its obvious physiologic role, dysfunction of the pulmonary neural system has been implicated in some pulmonary inflammatory disorders.[237]

Small branches of the recurrent laryngeal nerve on the left side and the vagus itself on the right are distributed directly to the trachea, where they form several plexuses that are most prominent on the posterior wall. After giving off these branches, fibers from the vagus and sympathetic chains enter the hila, join with branches from the cardiac autonomic plexus, and form large posterior and smaller anterior plexuses in the peribronchovascular connective tissue. From these

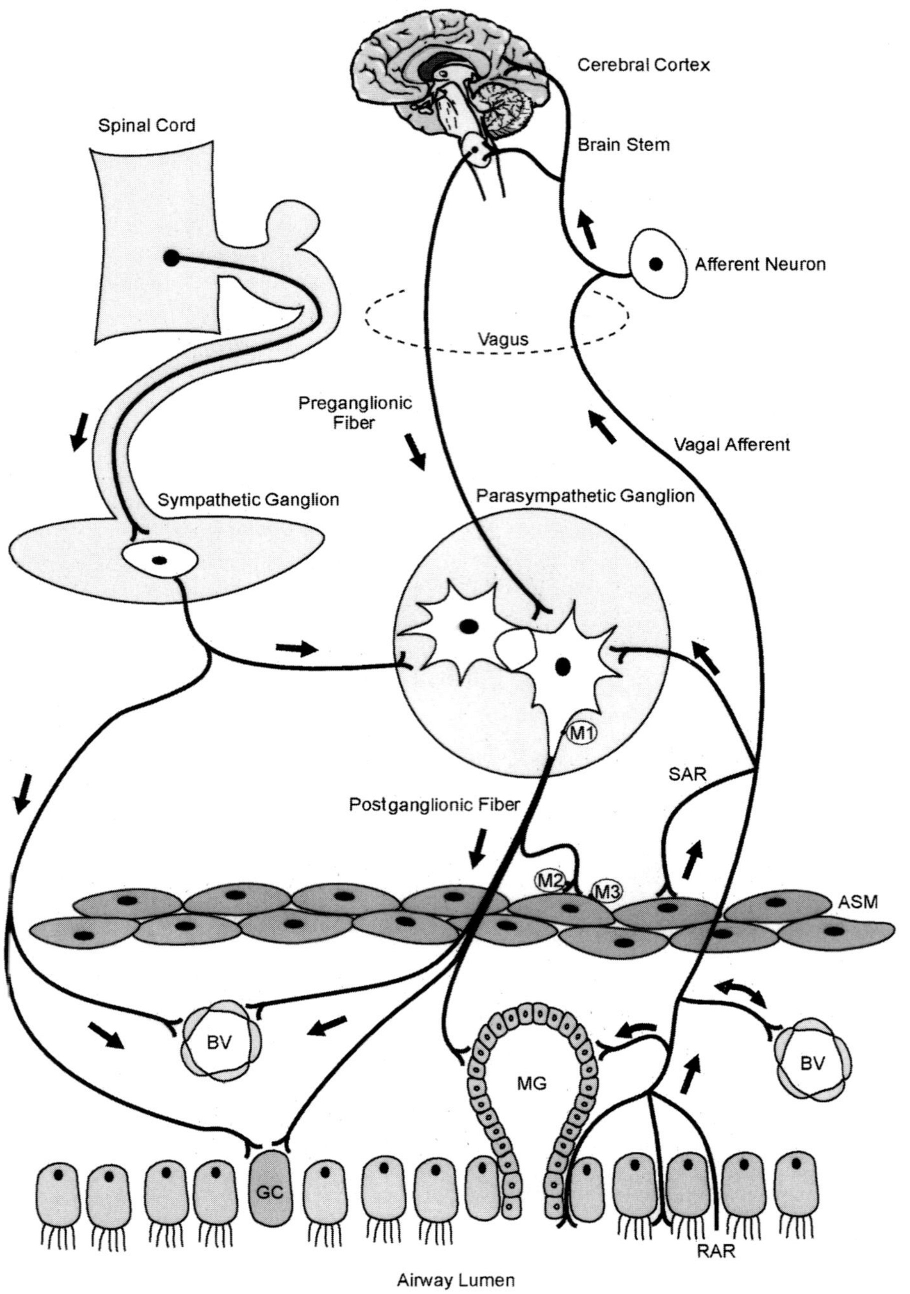

FIGURE 1–50

Innervation. Schematic diagram of the afferent and efferent innervation of the airways. Afferent nerves arise from rapidly adapting receptors (RAR), which originate as free nerve endings in the airway epithelium, and from slowly adapting receptors (SAR), which originate from nerve endings within the airway smooth muscle (ASM). Branches of the afferent nerves supply mucous glands (MG) and bronchial blood vessels (BV) and synapse with neurons within the parasympathetic airway ganglia. The afferent fibers ascend in the vagus to project to the autonomic ganglion in the brainstem, as well as the cerebral cortex. Preganglionic efferent parasympathetic nerves descend in the vagus to synapse with postganglionic neurons in the parasympathetic ganglia. Postganglionic fibers supply airway smooth muscle, mucous glands, bronchial blood vessels, and goblet cells (GC) in the airway epithelium. M_1, M_2, and M_3 represent the three subtypes of muscarinic receptor. Acetylcholine (Ach) acts on M_3 receptors to stimulate ASM contraction, on M_2 receptors to decrease further Ach release from the nerve ending, and on M_1 receptors to facilitate the transmission of preganglionic impulses through the ganglion. Sympathetic innervation originates as preganglionic fibers in the spinal cord. The preganglionic fibers synapse with postganglionic neuron fibers within the sympathetic ganglia, and the postganglionic fibers supply blood vessels and goblet cells. (From Fraser RS, Müller NL, Colman NC, Paré PD: Fraser and Paré's Diagnosis of Diseases of the Chest, 4th ed. Philadelphia, WB Saunders, 1999.)

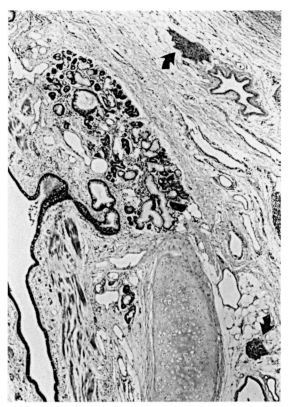

FIGURE 1–51

Bronchial wall nerves. The adventitia of the wall of a large bronchus contains two small nerves *(arrows)*. *(From Fraser RS, Müller NL, Colman NC, Paré PD: Fraser and Paré's Diagnosis of Diseases of the Chest, 4th ed. Philadelphia, WB Saunders, 1999.)*

plexuses emanate multiple peribronchial and perivascular nerve fibers that course in the same connective tissue and send branches into the adjacent airway and vessel walls (Fig. 1–51).

Afferent receptors have been divided into three functional groups on the basis of their distribution and physiologic response to various stimuli.

1. *Irritant* or *cough receptors,* located predominantly in central airways, are composed of highly arborized nets with numerous free nerve endings in the airway epithelium.[238] They respond to lung inflation or deflation and to a wide variety of chemical and mechanical stimuli. Stimulation of these receptors results in reflex bronchoconstriction, and their role is probably to inhibit inhalation of toxic material.[239]

2. *Stretch receptors* occur as tendril-like structures closely applied to the surface of individual muscle cells in the airway wall. They are responsible for sending information to the respiratory center regarding lung volume, and activation of these receptors contributes to termination of the inspiratory neural drive.

3. *Juxtacapillary (J) receptors* are situated in the lung parenchyma adjacent to alveolar septa and pulmonary capillaries.[240] They are believed to respond to stretching of these structures, such as occurs with lung congestion or interstitial edema.

Specific receptors for neurotransmitters can also be present on lung cells in the absence of innervation of the cells. An example can be seen with the response of pulmonary and bronchial endothelial cells to acetylcholine, in which the vasodilator NO is released via atropine-inhibitable receptors despite the fact that there is no direct cholinergic innervation of the endothelium.[241] Noninnervated adrenergic receptors located on airway smooth muscle respond to circulating catecholamine, which is the reason that therapeutically administered β_2-adrenergic agonists are so effective in relaxing airway smooth muscle.

Stimulation of postganglionic cholinergic efferent fibers increases secretion by the tracheobronchial glands and goblet cells, causes airway smooth muscle contraction and airway narrowing, and results in vascular smooth muscle relaxation and pulmonary vasodilation. All these effects are blocked by atropine. Postganglionic adrenergic fibers innervate pulmonary and bronchial vascular smooth muscle, and stimulation results in constriction. (Even though there is no adrenergic innervation of human airway smooth muscle, numerous β_2-adrenergic receptors are present on the muscle[242]; these receptors respond to circulating catecholamines and therapeutically administered β-agonists by relaxation.)

Although both NANC excitatory (NANCe) and inhibitory (NANCi) systems have been demonstrated in rodents, the human lung does not seem to have an excitatory pathway.[243] The most important neurotransmitter of NANCi neurons is NO.[244] Stimulation of the nerve causes release of this substance, which acts on cyclic guanylyl cyclase within smooth muscle cells to produce relaxation.

THE PLEURA

Anatomy

The pleural space is enclosed by the visceral pleura, which covers the lungs, and by the parietal pleura, which lines the chest wall, diaphragm, and mediastinum.[245] The two join at the hila. Although they may come into intimate contact locally, the left and right pleural spaces are normally separate.

The visceral pleura is a thin, but strong "membrane" that can be divided histologically into three layers (Fig. 1–52):

1. The *endopleura,* which is composed of a continuous layer of mesothelial cells and a thin underlying network of irregularly arranged collagen and elastic fibers.

2. The *external elastic lamina,* which is primarily responsible for pleural mechanical stability and consists of a thin layer of dense collagen and elastic tissue.

3. The *vascular (interstitial) layer,* which lies beneath the external elastic lamina and consists of loose connective tissue in which lymphatic channels, nerves, and bronchial vessels are situated. It is continuous with the interstitial tissue of the interlobular septa and directly overlays the *internal elastic lamina.* The latter is a thin, elastic collagen layer that is continuous with the connective tissue of the alveolar septa and surrounds almost the entire lung, thus effectively connecting the parenchyma to the pleura. The external and internal elastic laminae are only loosely attached and may be easily separated in the connective tissue plane of the vascular layer; in appropriate circumstances, liquid or gas readily accumulates in this region.

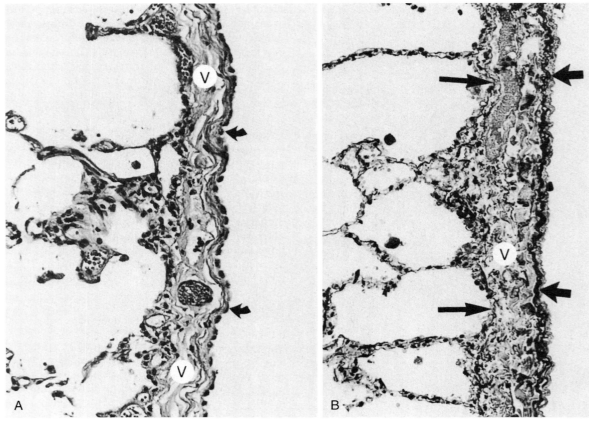

FIGURE 1–52

Normal visceral pleura. A, Mesothelial cells *(curved arrows),* vascular layer (V). **B,** Vascular layer (V), internal elastic lamina *(long arrows),* and external elastic lamina *(short arrows).* (**A,** hematoxylin-eosin; **B,** Verhoeff-van Gieson; both ×200.) *(From Fraser RS, Müller NL, Colman NC, Paré PD: Fraser and Paré's Diagnosis of Diseases of the Chest, 4th ed. Philadelphia, WB Saunders, 1999.)*

The parietal pleura consists of a layer of connective tissue deep to the endothoracic fascia of the chest wall. It is divided into two parts by a fibroelastic band, with the majority of vessels being located in the more external layer.

The blood supply to the parietal pleura is derived from the subclavian, internal mammary, and intercostal arteries.[246] The origin of the blood supply of the visceral pleura, however, is not as clear. According to some observers, the hilar, apical, mediastinal, and interlobar regions are supplied by the bronchial circulation, the remainder being nourished by the pulmonary arteries; others believe that the blood supply of the costal and diaphragmatic portions is also bronchial in origin.[246] With the exception of the hilar regions (which are drained by bronchial veins), the visceral pleural venous return is via the pulmonary veins.

The Mesothelial Cell

Mesothelial cells form a continuous layer over the whole of the visceral and parietal pleural surfaces. Their shape and size are inconstant, the diameter varying directly with transpulmonary pressure (the cells become more flattened as the lung expands).[245] When individual cells are stimulated, they enlarge, become cuboidal or columnar in shape, and develop large nuclei with prominent nucleoli; occasionally, these features are sufficient to obscure the distinction between mesothelioma and a reactive process.

Ultrastructurally, mesothelial cells are joined by tight junctions and contain pinocytotic vesicles on both the luminal and basal aspects. The cell surface is covered by numerous microvilli that are typically long and thin, about 0.1 μm in diameter and up to 3 μm in length. Presumably by means of these microvilli and the pinocytotic vesicles, mesothelial cells help regulate the composition and amount of pleural fluid. Mesothelial cells have also been shown to possess both fibrinolytic[247] and procoagulant[248] activity, features that may be important in repair and decreasing the development of fibrous adhesions after pleural injury. Surface-active phospholipids similar to alveolar surfactant, probably produced by mesothelial cells, can be found in the pleural space, where they act as lubricants to facilitate pleural surface movement.[249]

Radiology

The combined thickness of the parietal and visceral pleurae over the convexity of the lungs and over the diaphragmatic and mediastinal surfaces is normally insufficient to render them visible on the chest radiograph. By contrast, because of the presence of air-containing lung on both sides of the visceral pleura in the interlobar regions, contiguous layers of visceral pleura are visible when the x-ray beam passes tangentially along their surfaces.

Normal Fissures

Fissures form the contact surfaces between pulmonary lobes. Although they may extend to the hilum—resulting in complete lobar separation—commonly they are incomplete. For example, in one study of 100 excised lungs, an incomplete fissure was found between the right lower and upper lobes in 70% of cases, between the right lower and middle lobes in about 45%, between the left lower and upper lobes in about 40%, and between the right upper and middle lobes (minor fissure) in almost 90%.[250] Similar figures have been found in lungs examined by thin-section CT.[251] The incompleteness of interlobar fissures is important because the parenchymal "bridge" that is established provides a ready pathway for collateral air drift or for the spread of disease to another lobe, and radiographic signs may be created that can give rise to erroneous conclusions.

The *major (oblique) fissures,* which separate the upper (and on the right, the middle lobe) from the lower lobes, begin at or about the level of the fifth thoracic vertebra and extend obliquely downward and forward, roughly paralleling the sixth rib and ending at the diaphragm a few centimeters behind the anterior pleural gutter (Fig. 1–53). The *horizontal (minor) fissure* separates the anterior segment of the right

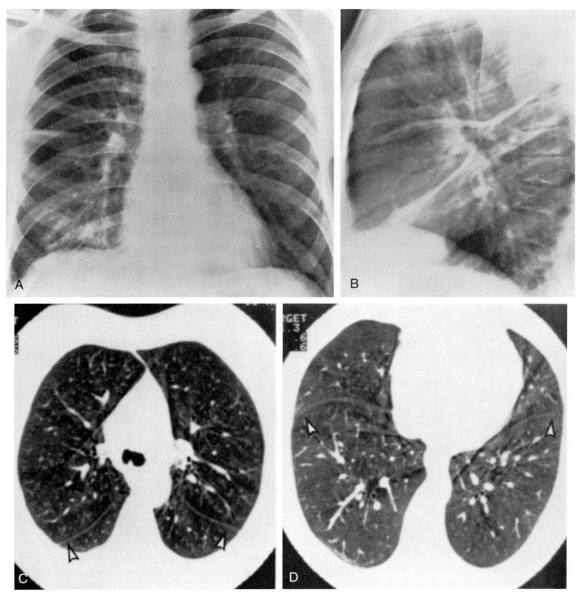

FIGURE 1–53

Interlobar fissures, right lung. The presence of minimal interlobar effusion renders the fissures clearly visible on posteroanterior (**A**) and lateral (**B**) radiographs. **C,** A CT scan through the upper part of the thorax reveals the lateral portion of the right and left major fissures *(arrowheads)* to be situated posterior to the anteromedial portion of the fissure, so-called lateral facing. **D,** A CT scan through the lower part of the thorax shows that the lateral portion of the major fissures *(arrowheads)* is located anterior to the anteromedial aspect of the major fissures, so-called medial facing. *(From Fraser RS, Müller NL, Colman NC, Paré PD: Fraser and Paré's Diagnosis of Diseases of the Chest, 4th ed. Philadelphia, WB Saunders, 1999.)*

upper lobe from the middle lobe and lies roughly horizontal at about the level of the fourth rib anteriorly. There is considerable variation in its orientation, the anterior aspect generally being lower than the posterior and the lateral part lower than the medial.[250]

The major fissures are seldom seen along their entirety on lateral chest radiographs. Such incomplete visualization is not difficult to understand in view of the underlying anatomic variability, the curved orientation of the fissures, and the fact that the major fissures are almost always oriented slightly away from the coronal plane. The minor fissure can be identified in about 55% to 80% of cases on chest radiography.[149,252] Anatomically, it rarely reaches the mediastinum and then only in its anterior portion; nonetheless, one of the more constant relationships on PA radiographs is the fissure's medial termination (or projected termination) at the lateral margin of the interlobar pulmonary artery. A fissure line or interface that projects medial to this point is almost invariably a downward-displaced major fissure and provides certain evidence of volume loss in the right lower lobe.

The appearance of the interlobar fissures on CT is influenced by section thickness. On HRCT, the major fissures are consistently visualized as continuous, smooth, thin linear opacities. On 5- to 10-mm-thick sections they may be manifested as radiolucent bands, lines, or dense bands (Fig. 1–54).[253] This variation is related to the plane of the fissure on the cross-sectional image: a perpendicular fissure (e.g., in the upper part of the thorax) is likely to produce a linear configuration, whereas a more oblique orientation causes a well-defined, dense (ground-glass) band. If the upper part of the major fissure is not quite perpendicular to the cross-sectional image, the smaller vessels at the periphery of the lobes on both sides of the fissure tend to cause the fissure to be displayed as a relatively avascular lucent band.

The minor fissure is visualized on HRCT as a curvilinear line or band of increased attenuation that forms a quarter circle or semicircle in its highest aspect (located slightly cephalic to the level of the origin of the middle lobe bronchus) (Fig. 1–55).[254] On thicker sections, the fissure is seen most commonly as a radiolucent area relatively devoid of vessels when compared with the same region in the left lung.

The Pulmonary Ligament

The pulmonary ligament consists of a double layer of pleura that drapes caudally from the lung hilum and tethers the medial aspect of the lower lobe to the mediastinum and diaphragm.[255] It is formed by the mediastinal (parietal) pleura as it reflects over the main bronchi and pulmonary arteries and veins onto the surface of the lung as the visceral pleura (Fig. 1–56). The ligament may terminate in a free falciform border anywhere between the inferior pulmonary vein and the superior aspect of the hemidiaphragm (*incomplete form*), or it may extend inferiorly and cover a portion of the medial aspect of the hemidiaphragm (*complete form*). Thus, it divides the mediastinal pleural space below the hilum into either complete or incomplete anterior and posterior compartments. The bare area of mediastinum thus created contains a network of connective tissue, small bronchial vessels, lymphatics, and lymph nodes. The left pulmonary ligament is closely related to the esophagus and is bordered posteriorly by the descending aorta; the shorter, right ligament can be situated anywhere along an arc that extends from the inferior vena cava anteriorly to the azygos vein posteriorly.

Although the pulmonary ligaments are never seen on PA or lateral chest radiographs, they can usually be identified on CT.[256] The appearance is variable, but typically consists of a small peak or pyramid on the mediastinal surface and a thin linear opacity that extends obliquely posteriorly from the apex of the peak to the lung, thus marking the intersegmental septum. It is most evident on scans obtained at or just above the level of the hemidiaphragm. Ordinarily, the right ligament is seen at a level slightly higher than the left, and both ligaments can be appreciated on only one or two slices of a series.

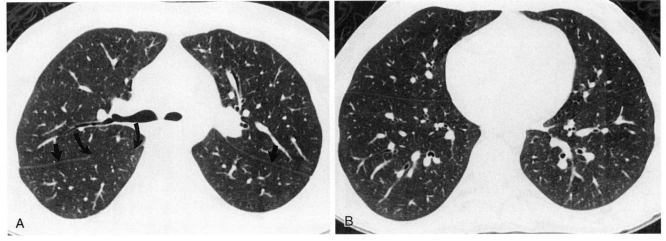

FIGURE 1–54

Normal appearance of the major fissures on HRCT scan. A, On HRCT, the major fissure is usually seen as a well-defined thin line *(straight arrows)*. Note that the medial portion of the upper aspect of the right interlobar fissure is incomplete, which has resulted in fusion of the lower and upper lobes at this level *(curved arrows)*. **B,** The lower aspect of both interlobar fissures is complete. *(From Fraser RS, Müller NL, Colman NC, Paré PD: Fraser and Paré's Diagnosis of Diseases of the Chest, 4th ed. Philadelphia, WB Saunders, 1999.)*

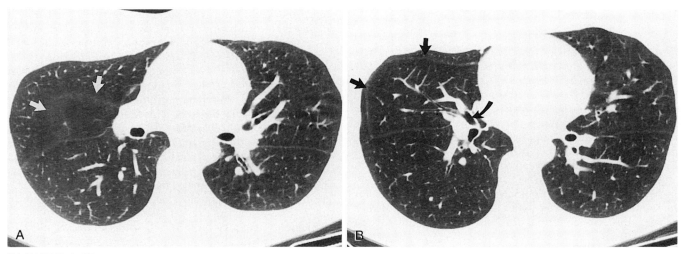

FIGURE 1–55

Normal appearance of the minor fissure on HRCT scan. A, The upper aspect of the minor fissure is seen as a curvilinear band of increased attenuation *(arrows)*. **B,** The lower and steeper portion of the minor fissure is seen as a thin line *(straight arrows)*. The right middle lobe bronchus can be seen at this level *(curved arrow)*. *(From Fraser RS, Müller NL, Colman NC, Paré PD: Fraser and Paré's Diagnosis of Diseases of the Chest, 4th ed. Philadelphia, WB Saunders, 1999.)*

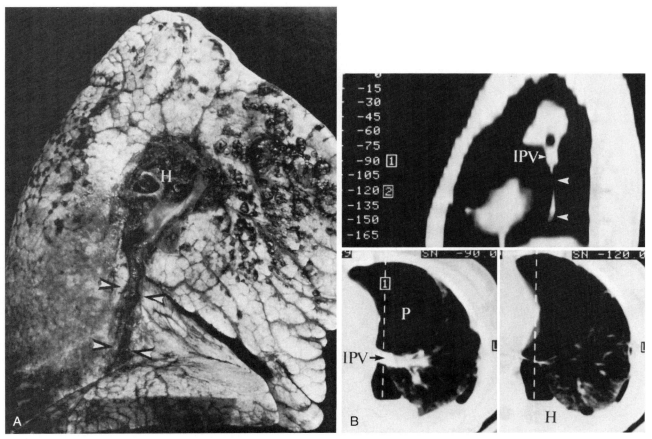

FIGURE 1–56

The pulmonary ligament. A, As seen on an inflated postmortem specimen of the left lung viewed from the medial aspect, the mediastinal (parietal) pleura reflects over the hilum superiorly, anteriorly, and posteriorly; caudally, these pleural layers are more closely apposed to compose the pulmonary ligament *(arrowheads)*. In **B** are a reformatted CT scan *(top)* and representative transverse images *(bottom)* through the plane of the left inferior pulmonary vein (IPV) and 3 cm caudally in a patient with a spontaneous hydropneumothorax (H and P). Note that the vertically oriented septum *(arrowheads)* divides the mediastinal pleural space into anterior and posterior compartments. *(From Fraser RS, Müller NL, Colman NC, Paré PD: Fraser and Paré's Diagnosis of Diseases of the Chest, 4th ed. Philadelphia, WB Saunders, 1999.)*

Accessory Fissures

Any portion of lung may be partly or completely separated from adjacent portions by an accessory pleural fissure. These fissures, which are present in about 50% of lungs, vary in their degree of development from superficial slits in the lung surface not more than 1 or 2 cm deep to complete fissures that extend all the way to the hilum. Most are of little more than academic interest radiologically. When well developed, however, recognition of such fissures is important for three reasons: (1) the lung parenchyma that they subtend may be the only site of disease whose spread is prevented by the fissure; (2) a fissure in a specific anatomic location, such as between the superior and the basal segments of the right lower lobe, can be mistaken for the minor fissure between upper and middle lobes and thus create confusion in interpretation; and (3) they are important components of linear atelectasis (see page 144).

Azygos Fissure. The azygos fissure is created by downward invagination of the azygos vein through the apical portion of the right upper lobe (Fig. 1–57).[257] The familiar curvilinear shadow extends obliquely across the upper portion of the right lung and terminates in a "teardrop" shadow caused by the vein itself at a variable distance above the right hilum.

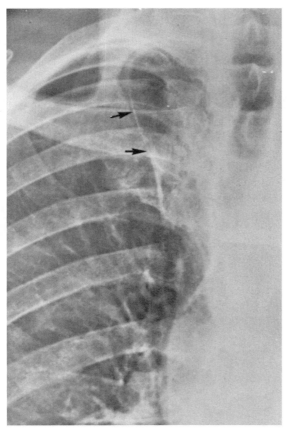

FIGURE 1–57

Accessory fissure of the azygos vein. On a posteroanterior radiograph, the fissure can be identified as a curvilinear shadow *(arrows)* extending obliquely across the upper portion of the right lung, with its lower end some distance above the right hilum. *(From Fraser RS, Müller NL, Colman NC, Paré PD: Fraser and Paré's Diagnosis of Diseases of the Chest, 4th ed. Philadelphia, WB Saunders, 1999.)*

Since the azygos vein runs outside the parietal pleura, the fissure is formed by four pleural layers (two parietal and two visceral). Although the bronchial supply of the azygos lobe is variable, either the apical bronchus or its anterior subsegmental branch is always present. The importance of the anomaly radiologically lies in failure of the apical pleural surfaces to separate when pneumothorax is present.

Inferior Accessory Fissure. This fissure is found in 30% to 45% of lungs and separates part or all of the medial basal segment from the remainder of the lower lobe. On the diaphragmatic surface of the lung, the fissure extends laterally from near the pulmonary ligament and then makes a convex arc forward to join the major fissure. On PA radiographs, the fissure line extends superiorly and slightly medially from the inner third of the right or left hemidiaphragm.

Superior Accessory Fissure. The superior accessory fissure separates part or all of the superior segment from the basal segments of the lower lobes, more often on the right. Because it commonly lies horizontally at the same level as the minor fissure, the two may be confused on a frontal radiograph, although their separate anatomic positions may be clearly established on the lateral radiograph.

Left Minor Fissure. This fissure separates the lingula from the rest of the left upper lobe; in almost all cases, the usual segmental anatomy of the left lung is preserved. In a review of 2000 consecutive PA and lateral chest radiographs it was identified in only 32 (1.6%) instances.[258] Its position is generally more cephalic than the right minor fissure, and its lateral end is usually superior to its medial end.

Function

The visceral pleura and parietal pleura form smooth membranes that facilitate movement of the lungs within the pleural space, chiefly as a result of secretion and absorption of pleural fluid.[259] The amount of fluid in normal humans ranges from less than 1 mL to 20 mL. The dynamics of transudation and absorption of fluid obeys the Starling equation and depends on a combination of hydrostatic, colloid osmotic, and tissue pressure. The tissue pressures are not known, but knowledge of the first two suggests that fluid is formed normally at the parietal pleura and absorbed at the visceral pleura (Fig. 1–58).

The net hydrostatic pressure that forces fluid out of the parietal pleura can be calculated by determining the hydrostatic pressure in systemic capillaries that supply the parietal pleura (30 cm H_2O) and the pleural pressure (−5 cm H_2O at FRC); thus, the net hydrostatic drive is 35 cm H_2O. Osmotic colloid pressure in the systemic capillaries is 34 cm H_2O, and that of the pleura is approximately 8 cm H_2O, for a net drive of 26 cm H_2O colloid osmotic pressure from the pleural space to the capillaries of the parietal pleura. The balance of these forces (35 − 26 = 9 cm H_2O) is directed from the parietal pleura to the pleural cavity.

The visceral pleura is supplied by pulmonary and bronchial vessels, and the capillary pressure is much lower than systemic capillary pressure (about 11 cm H_2O), so the net hydrostatic pressure from the visceral pleura toward the pleural cavity is 16 cm H_2O (11 + 5 cm). Osmotic colloid pressures remain constant, with a pressure of 26 cm H_2O away from the pleural cavity. Thus, the net effect of these forces is a drive of 10 cm

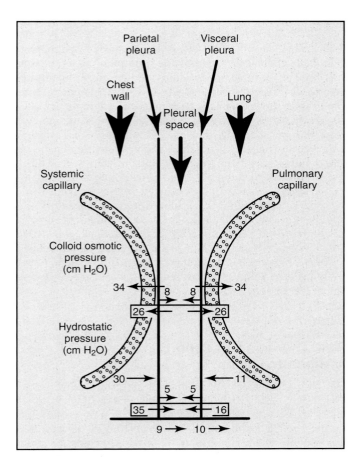

FIGURE 1–58

Diagrammatic representation of the pressures involved in the formation and absorption of pleural fluid. See text for description.

H_2O (26 − 16 cm) toward the visceral pleural capillaries. Pleural fluid is also removed by lymphatics that originate in the parietal pleura.

THE LYMPHATIC SYSTEM

Lymphatics of the Lungs and Pleura

Anatomy

Parietal pleural lymphatics are extensively distributed over the costal, mediastinal, and diaphragmatic surfaces.[260] Numerous pores (stomata) 6 to 8 μm in diameter are present between the overlying mesothelial cells (Fig. 1–59),[261] particularly on the diaphragmatic surface, where they connect with a network of lymphatics that drain to the mediastinum. These stomata and their connections are a major pathway for removal of excess fluid and cells from the pleural space.

Visceral pleural lymphatics course within the vascular layer, where they form a plexus of channels roughly following the pleural lobular boundaries. Between these channels and joining with them are smaller intercommunicating and blindly ending tributaries that ramify over the pleural surface. The entire network drains into the medial aspect of the lung near the hilum. Although lymphatic channels are present over the whole of the pleural surface, they are much better developed over the lower than the upper lobes.

Pulmonary lymphatic channels form two major pathways, one in the bronchoarterial and the other in the interlobular septal connective tissue. The bronchoarterial lymphatics originate in the region of the distal respiratory bronchioles (none are present in alveolar interstitial tissue) and run proximally (Fig. 1–60), eventually reaching the bronchial and hilar lymph nodes.[262] The interlobular lymphatics drain partly into the

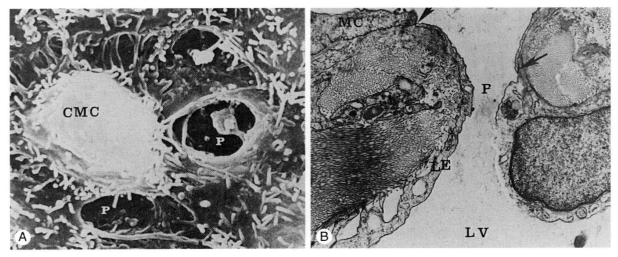

FIGURE 1–59

Diaphragmatic pores. A scanning electron micrograph of the diaphragm (**A**) shows a surface cuboidal cell (CMC) (possibly a macrophage) and numerous slender mesothelial microvilli. Two intercellular pores (P) are evident. (×8950.) A section through a pore (P) viewed by transmission electron microscopy (**B**) shows processes from two lymphatic endothelial cells (LE) extending onto the peritoneal surface to form intercellular junctions *(arrows)* with the surface mesothelial cells (MC). The close contact between the two cell types provides a direct passageway between the peritoneal cavity and the underlying lymphatic vessels (LV). (×16,200.) *(From Leak LV, Rahil K: Am Rev Respir Dis 119[Suppl]:8, 1979.)*

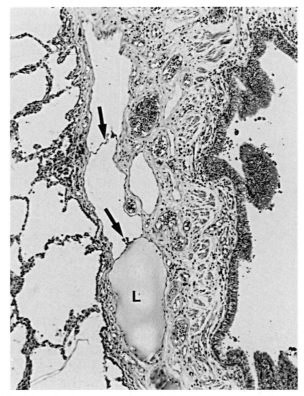

FIGURE 1–60

Peribronchial lymphatic channel. A peribronchiolar lymphatic (L) is distended by fluid (partially lost during tissue processing). Two valves are apparent *(arrows)*. (×72.) *(From Fraser RS, Müller NL, Colman NC, Paré PD: Fraser and Paré's Diagnosis of Diseases of the Chest, 4th ed. Philadelphia, WB Saunders, 1999.)*

bronchoarterial lymphatics and partly into the pleural system. Numerous funnel-shaped valves direct lymph flow in both pathways. Anastomotic channels connect the interlobular lymphatics with those in the bronchoarterial sheath; they are up to 4 cm long and are usually situated midway between the hilum and the periphery of the lung. Distension of these communicating lymphatics and edema in their surrounding connective tissue result in Kerley A lines; similar processes in the interlobular lymphatics and connective tissue result in Kerley B lines.

The lymphatic capillary endothelium rests on a discontinuous basal lamina that is entirely absent for considerable lengths.[262] In some areas, the endothelial cells are joined by intercellular junctions; in others, junctions are absent, and the vessel wall has significant gaps. The cell cytoplasm contains numerous microfilaments, some of which are thought to constitute an actin-like contractile system that possibly regulates opening or closing of the intercellular gaps. Perilymphatic collagen fibers are in close contact with the endothelial cells and their basement membrane and have been regarded as a tethering mechanism that keeps the capillaries open. These features—endothelial and basement membrane discontinuities and connective tissue anchoring system—appear to be ideal for the provision of easy and continuous access of interstitial fluid to the capillary lumen.

Function

There is evidence that the flow of lymph through pulmonary lymphatic channels is aided by the "pumping" action of ventilation. For example, in one study of 15 adult human lungs removed at autopsy,[263] ethiodized oil injected into pleural lymphatics was shown to fill the deep pulmonary lymphatics; subsequently, when a fixed inflation pressure was maintained, flow did not occur within the lymphatics. Forward flow occurred only during ventilation and appeared to depend on the lung volume at the time that the lymphatics were filled. When contrast medium was injected with lung volume maintained at FRC, forward flow occurred within the lymphatics; by contrast, when filling was achieved at a lung volume of 70% TLC, ventilation resulted in no forward movement of contrast medium within the lymphatics. The authors suggested that this difference is best explained on the basis of the smaller volume of parenchymal lymphatic segments at high rather than low lung volumes, which reduces the influence of subsequent ventilation.

The Thoracic Duct and Right Lymphatic Duct

The thoracic duct, a continuation of the cisterna chyli, enters the thorax through the aortic hiatus of the diaphragm. In most subjects it lies to the right of the aorta and follows its course cephalad; thus, in the lower portion of the thorax it lies roughly in the midline or slightly to one side. At about the level of the carina, it crosses the left main bronchus and runs cephalad in a plane parallel to the left lateral wall of the trachea and slightly posterior to it. The duct leaves the thorax between the esophagus and the left subclavian artery and runs posterior to the left innominate vein; much of the cephalic third (the cervical portion) is supraclavicular. It joins the venous system most commonly by emptying into the internal jugular vein and sometimes into the subclavian, innominate, or external jugular veins. The diameter of a normal thoracic duct ranges from 1 to 7 mm[264]; thus, this parameter cannot be used as a single determinant of obstruction. Valves are present in about 85% of vessels, primarily in the upper two thirds.

The radiologic anatomy of the right lymphatic duct has been poorly documented because this vessel cannot be suitably opacified and is inconstantly identified. The three trunks—the right jugular, right subclavian, and right mediastinal—often open separately into the jugular, subclavian, and innominate veins, respectively.

Lymph Nodes of the Mediastinum

Thoracic lymph nodes may be considered in two categories: (1) a *parietal group*, which resides outside the parietal pleura in extramediastinal tissue and drains the thoracic wall and a variety of extrathoracic structures, and (2) a *visceral group*, which is located within the mediastinum between the pleural membranes and is concerned particularly with drainage of the intrathoracic tissues.

Parietal Lymph Nodes

Parietal lymph nodes can be subdivided into three groups.

Anterior Parietal (Internal Mammary) Lymph Nodes.
Anterior parietal lymph nodes are located in the upper portion of the thorax behind the anterior intercostal spaces bilaterally, either medial or lateral to the internal mammary vessels (Fig. 1–61). They drain the anterior chest wall, medial

portion of the breasts, anterior portion of the diaphragm, and upper anterior abdominal wall.

Posterior Parietal Lymph Nodes. These nodes are found adjacent to the rib heads in the posterior intercostal spaces (*intercostal nodes*) or adjacent to the vertebrae (*juxtavertebral nodes*). Both groups drain the intercostal spaces, parietal pleura, and vertebral column. They communicate with other posterior mediastinal lymph nodes related to the descending aorta and the esophagus.

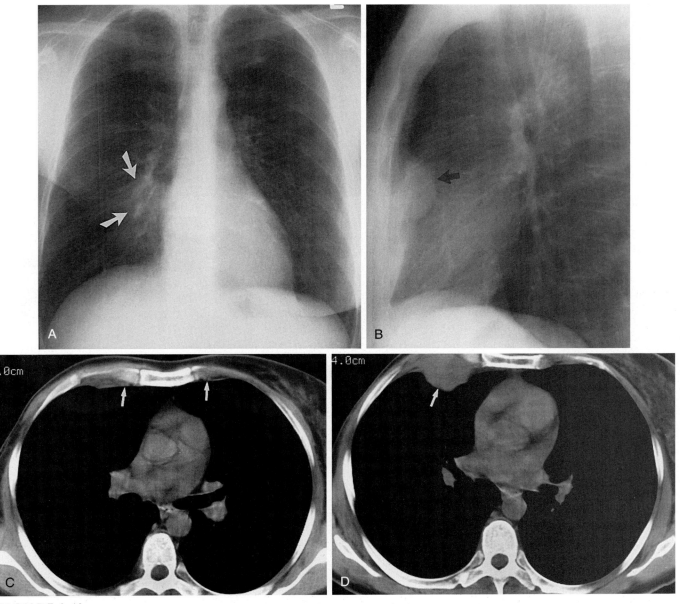

FIGURE 1–61

Enlargement of internal mammary lymph nodes. A posteroanterior radiograph (**A**) shows surgical absence of the right breast and a poorly defined, increased opacity over the right hilum *(arrows)*. A lateral chest radiograph (**B**) demonstrates a smooth, homogeneous soft tissue opacity in the retrosternal area *(arrow)* caused by enlargement of the internal mammary lymph nodes. A CT scan at the level of the bronchus intermedius (**C**) shows the right and left internal mammary artery and vein *(arrows)*; the enlarged internal mammary node is seen at a slightly lower level (**D**) *(arrow)*. The patient was a 46-year-old woman with metastatic carcinoma of the breast. *(From Fraser RS, Müller NL, Colman NC, Paré PD: Fraser and Paré's Diagnosis of Diseases of the Chest, 4th ed. Philadelphia, WB Saunders, 1999.)*

Diaphragmatic Lymph Nodes. The diaphragmatic lymph nodes are composed of the anterior (pre-pericardiac) group, located immediately behind the xiphoid and to the right and left of the pericardium anteriorly; the middle (juxtaphrenic) group, which is in proximity to the phrenic nerves as they meet the diaphragm; and the posterior (retrocrural) nodes, which reside behind the right and left crura of the diaphragm. The diaphragmatic lymph nodes drain the diaphragm and the upper part of the abdomen.

Visceral Lymph Nodes

The visceral lymph nodes can be divided into three groups.
Anterosuperior Mediastinal (Prevascular) Lymph Nodes. These lymph nodes are congregated along the anterior aspect of the superior vena cava, right and left innominate veins, and ascending aorta (Fig. 1–62). Some are situated posterior to the sternum in the lower portion of the thorax, and others reside behind the manubrium anterior to the thymus. They drain most of the structures in the anterior mediastinum, including the pericardium, thymus, diaphragmatic and mediastinal pleurae, part of the heart, and the anterior portion of the hila. Efferent channels drain into the right lymphatic or thoracic duct.

Posterior Mediastinal Lymph Nodes. These nodes are located around the esophagus (*periesophageal nodes*) and along the anterior and lateral aspects of the descending aorta (*periaortic nodes*) (Fig. 1–63); they are most numerous in the lower portion of the thorax. Their afferent channels arise from the posterior portion of the diaphragm, the pericardium, and the esophagus and directly from the lower lobes of the lungs via the right and left pulmonary ligaments. They communicate with the tracheobronchial nodes, particularly the subcarinal group, and drain chiefly via the thoracic duct.

Tracheobronchial Lymph Nodes. The tracheobronchial nodes are the most important group of visceral lymph nodes and consist in turn of several subgroups. The *paratracheal* nodes are located in front and to the right and left of the trachea (Fig. 1–64); occasionally, a retrotracheal component is present. The right paratracheal chain is usually the best developed; its lowermost member, the azygos node, is situated medial to the azygos vein arch in the pretracheal mediastinal fat. These lymph nodes receive afferent channels from

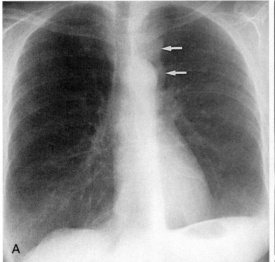
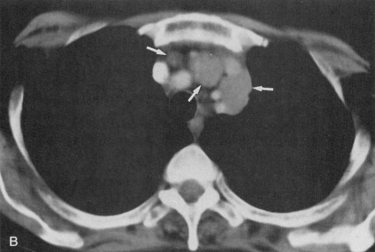
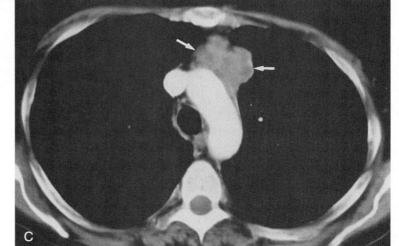

FIGURE 1–62

Enlargement of the anterior (prevascular) group of mediastinal nodes. A conventional posteroanterior radiograph (**A**) shows a widened and lobulated contour of the left upper mediastinal silhouette *(arrows)*. Intravenous contrast–enhanced CT scans through the superior mediastinum (**B** and **C**) confirm the presence of enlarged nodes *(arrows)* and reveal their intimate relationship to the great vessels. The patient was a 64-year-old woman with metastatic pulmonary carcinoma. *(From Fraser RS, Müller NL, Colman NC, Paré PD: Fraser and Paré's Diagnosis of Diseases of the Chest, 4th ed. Philadelphia, WB Saunders, 1999.)*

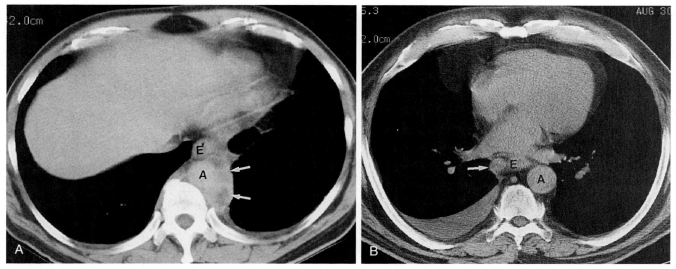

FIGURE I-63

CT scan of posterior mediastinal nodes (periesophageal and periaortic). An intravenous contrast–enhanced CT scan (**A**) demonstrates enlarged periaortic nodes *(arrows)* in a 60-year-old woman with lymphoma. A CT scan without intravenous contrast (**B**) demonstrates an enlarged periesophageal node *(arrow)* in a 63-year-old man with pulmonary carcinoma. Also noted is a small right pleural effusion. A, aorta; E, esophagus. *(From Fraser RS, Müller NL, Colman NC, Paré PD: Fraser and Paré's Diagnosis of Diseases of the Chest, 4th ed. Philadelphia, WB Saunders, 1999.)*

the bronchopulmonary and tracheal bifurcation nodes, the trachea, and the esophagus. They can also receive lymph directly from the right and left lungs without diversion through the bronchopulmonary or tracheal bifurcation nodes. Direct communication also exists with the anterior and posterior visceral mediastinal nodes. The efferent channels are the right lymphatic and thoracic ducts.

The *tracheal bifurcation (carinal)* lymph nodes are situated in the precarinal (see Fig. 1–64) and subcarinal (Fig. 1–65) fat, as well as around the circumference of the right and left main bronchi. Those in mediastinal fat between the left pulmonary artery and aortic arch are designated *aortopulmonary window* nodes (Fig. 1–66); they can be divided into medial, lateral (subpleural), and superior groups and merge above with the left prevascular nodes. Carinal lymph nodes receive afferent flow from the bronchopulmonary nodes, anterior and posterior mediastinal nodes, heart, pericardium, esophagus, and lungs. Efferent drainage is to the paratracheal group, particularly the right-sided component.

Hilar lymph nodes (Fig. 1–67) are normally too small to be detected on conventional radiographs or unenhanced CT studies. However, they are well visualized on contrast-enhanced CT (Fig. 1–68) and with MR imaging. They are located around the main bronchi and vessels and receive afferent channels from all lobes of the lungs; their efferent drainage is to the carinal and paratracheal nodes. Lymph nodes located within the right and left inferior pulmonary ligaments are often included as components of the lower hilar lymph node group.

Classification of Regional Lymph Node Stations

The mediastinal and pulmonary lymph nodes are classified according to their relationship to major anatomic structures. The preferred classification scheme is the lymph node map proposed by the American Joint Committee on Cancer and the

Union Internationale Contre le Cancer (Table 1–2, Fig. 1–69).[265] In this classification, lymph nodes are grouped according to their relationship to anatomic structures that can be identified on CT scans or MR images or at mediastinoscopy or thoracotomy. These structures include the left brachiocephalic vein, aortic arch, trachea, azygos vein, ligamentum arteriosum, left pulmonary artery, and main bronchi. Guides to this classification on CT scan have been published and are based on the demonstration of enlarged lymph nodes.[266,267]

Lymph Node Size

On CT scan or MR imaging, lymph nodes are typically ovoid. Assessment of their size is usually based on measurement of the smallest diameter (short axis) as seen on a transverse CT image because it shows much less variability than the long axis does.[268,269] The short-axis diameter above which a node should be considered enlarged depends on its location. Strictly speaking, upper paratracheal and left paraesophageal nodes should be considered enlarged when the short-axis diameter is greater than 7 mm. The threshold value is 8 mm for anterior mediastinal nodes, 10 mm for lower paratracheal and right paraesophageal nodes, and 11 mm for subcarinal nodes.[268] A more pragmatic and commonly used approach is to consider all mediastinal lymph nodes as being normal in size unless they exceed 10 mm in short-axis diameter.[266]

Lymphatic Drainage of the Lungs

According to Rouvière, the lungs can be subdivided into three main drainage areas—superior, middle, and inferior—without correspondence to pulmonary lobes.[270] In the right superior area, lymph drains directly into the paratracheal and

Text continued on page 73

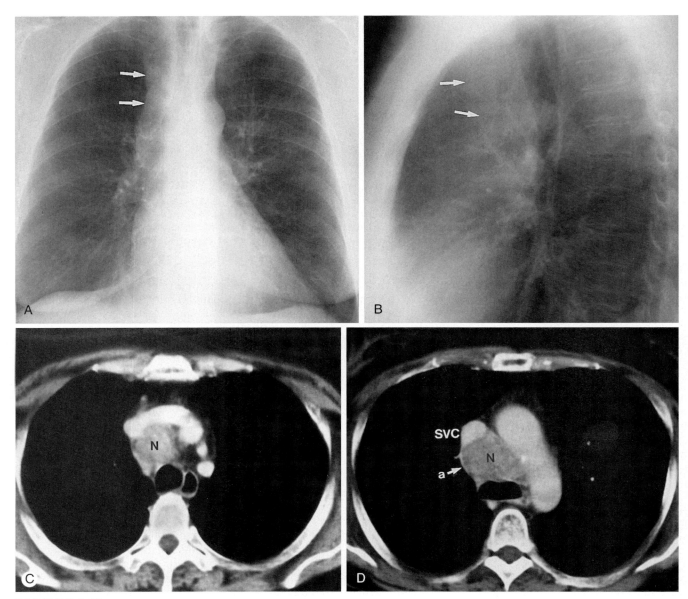

FIGURE 1–64

Enlargement of the paratracheal nodes. Posteroanterior (**A**) and lateral (**B**) chest radiographs demonstrate increased opacity to the right and anterior to the trachea *(arrows)*. An intravenous contrast–enhanced CT scan at the level of the great vessels (**C**) demonstrates enlarged paratracheal lymph nodes (N). A CT scan at the level of the tracheal carina (**D**) demonstrates anterior displacement of the superior vena cava (SVC) and lateral displacement of the azygos vein (a) by enlarged precarinal nodes (N). The patient was a 59-year-old woman with metastatic pulmonary carcinoma. *(From Fraser RS, Müller NL, Colman NC, Paré PD: Fraser and Paré's Diagnosis of Diseases of the Chest, 4th ed. Philadelphia, WB Saunders, 1999.)*

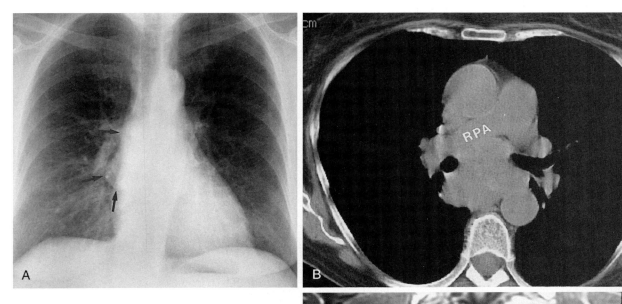

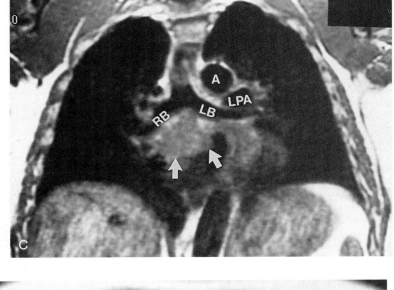

FIGURE 1–65

Enlargement of tracheal bifurcation nodes (subcarinal).
A posteroanterior chest radiograph (**A**) shows a lobulated
area of increased opacity in the subcarinal region (*arrows*). An
unenhanced CT scan 2 cm caudal to the tracheal carina
(**B**) demonstrates enlarged subcarinal nodes posterior to the
right pulmonary artery (RPA). The patient was a 61-year-old
woman with metastatic renal cell carcinoma. A coronal MR
image (**C**) in a 52-year-old man demonstrates enlarged
subcarinal nodes (*arrows*) caused by invasive thymoma. A, aorta;
LB, left main bronchus; LPA, left pulmonary artery; RB, right
main bronchus and bronchus intermedius. (*From Fraser RS,
Müller NL, Colman NC, Paré PD: Fraser and Paré's Diagnosis of
Diseases of the Chest, 4th ed. Philadelphia, WB Saunders, 1999.*)

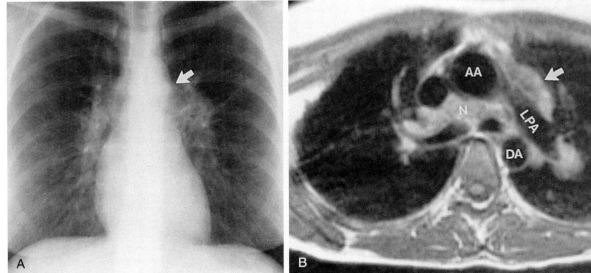

FIGURE 1–66

Enlargement of aortopulmonary window nodes. A posteroanterior chest radiograph (**A**) demonstrates a localized lateral convexity at the level of the
aortopulmonary window (*arrow*). Enlargement of the hila is also evident. A cardiac-gated MR image (**B**) demonstrates enlarged aortopulmonary window nodes
(*arrow*), as well as enlarged precarinal (N) and hilar nodes. The patient was a 31-year-old woman with sarcoidosis. AA, ascending aorta; DA, descending aorta; LPA,
left pulmonary artery. (*From Fraser RS, Müller NL, Colman NC, Paré PD: Fraser and Paré's Diagnosis of Diseases of the Chest, 4th ed. Philadelphia, WB Saunders, 1999.*)

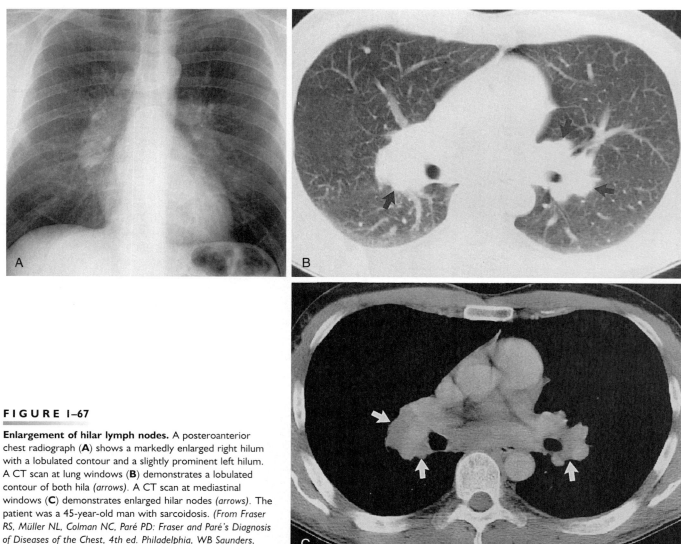

FIGURE 1–67

Enlargement of hilar lymph nodes. A posteroanterior chest radiograph (**A**) shows a markedly enlarged right hilum with a lobulated contour and a slightly prominent left hilum. A CT scan at lung windows (**B**) demonstrates a lobulated contour of both hila *(arrows)*. A CT scan at mediastinal windows (**C**) demonstrates enlarged hilar nodes *(arrows)*. The patient was a 45-year-old man with sarcoidosis. *(From Fraser RS, Müller NL, Colman NC, Paré PD: Fraser and Paré's Diagnosis of Diseases of the Chest, 4th ed. Philadelphia, WB Saunders, 1999.)*

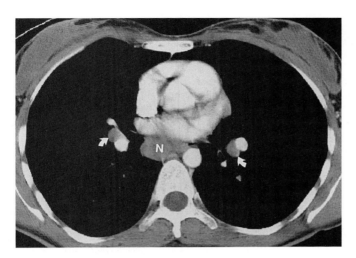

FIGURE 1–68

Enlarged hilar nodes on contrast-enhanced CT scan. A CT scan obtained after the intravenous administration of contrast material demonstrates bilateral hilar *(arrows)* and subcarinal adenopathy (N). The patient was a 22-year-old woman with sarcoidosis. *(From Fraser RS, Müller NL, Colman NC, Paré PD: Fraser and Paré's Diagnosis of Diseases of the Chest, 4th ed. Philadelphia, WB Saunders, 1999.)*

TABLE 1–2. Lymph Node Map Definitions—American Joint Committee on Cancer and the Union Internationale Contre le Cancer

Nodal Station	Anatomic Landmarks
N2 nodes—all N2 nodes lie within the mediastinal pleural envelope	
1 Highest mediastinal nodes	Nodes lying above a horizontal line at the upper rim of the brachiocephalic (left innominate) vein where it ascends to the left, crossing in front of the trachea at its midline
2 Upper paratracheal nodes	Nodes lying above a horizontal line drawn tangential to the upper margin of the aortic arch and below the inferior boundary of No. 1 nodes
3 Prevascular and retrotracheal nodes	Prevascular and retrotracheal nodes may be designated 3A and 3P; midline nodes are considered to be ipsilateral
4 Lower paratracheal nodes	The lower paratracheal nodes on the right lie to the right of the midline of the trachea between a horizontal line drawn tangential to the upper margin of the aortic arch and a line extending across the right main bronchus at the upper margin of the upper lobe bronchus and are contained within the mediastinal pleural envelope; the lower paratracheal nodes on the left lie on the left of the midline of the trachea between a horizontal line drawn tangential to the upper margin of the aortic arch and a line extending across the left main bronchus at the level of the upper margin of the left upper lobe bronchus, medial to the ligamentum arteriosum, and are contained within the mediastinal pleural envelope
Researchers may wish to designate the lower paratracheal nodes as No. 4s (superior) and No. 4i (inferior) subsets for study purposes; No. 4s nodes may be defined by a horizontal line extending across the trachea and drawn tangential to the cephalic border of the azygos vein; No. 4i nodes may be defined by the lower boundary of No. 4s and the lower boundary of No. 4, as described above
5 Subaortic (aortopulmonary window) nodes	Subaortic nodes are lateral to the ligamentum arteriosum or the aorta or left pulmonary artery and proximal to the first branch of the left pulmonary artery and lie within the mediastinal pleural envelope
6 Para-aortic (ascending aorta or phrenic) nodes	Nodes lying anterior and lateral to the ascending aorta and the aortic arch or the innominate artery, beneath a line tangential to the upper margin of the aortic arch
7 Subcarinal nodes	Nodes lying caudal to the carina of the trachea, but not associated with the lower lobe bronchi or arteries within the lung
8 Paraesophageal nodes (below the carina)	Nodes lying adjacent to the wall of the esophagus and to the right or left of the midline, excluding the subcarinal nodes
9 Pulmonary ligament nodes	Nodes lying within the pulmonary ligament, including those in the posterior wall and lower part of the inferior pulmonary vein
N1 nodes—all N1 nodes lie distal to the mediastinal pleural reflection and within the visceral pleura	
10 Hilar nodes	The proximal lobar nodes, distal to the mediastinal pleural reflection, and the nodes adjacent to the bronchus intermedius on the right; radiographically, the hilar shadow may be created by enlargement of both hilar and interlobar nodes
11 Interlobar nodes	Nodes lying between the lobar bronchi
12 Lobar nodes	Nodes adjacent to the distal lobar bronchi
13 Segmental nodes	Nodes adjacent to the segmental bronchi
14 Subsegmental nodes	Nodes around the subsegmental bronchi

From Mountain CF, Dresler CM: Regional lymph node classification for lung cancer staging. Chest 111:1718, 1997.

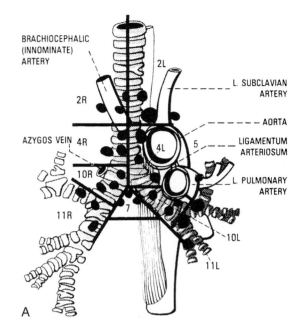

A

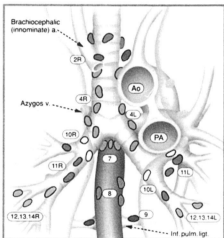

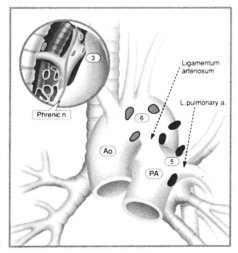

B

FIGURE 1–69

Classification of regional lymph node stations. A, 1983 American Thoracic Society scheme. **B,** 1997 American Joint Committee on Cancer and the Union Internationale Contre le Cancer scheme. *(A from Tisi GM, Friedman PJ, Peters RM, et al: Regional lymph node classification system for staging of lung cancer. Am Rev Respir Dis 127:659, 1983; B from Mountain CF, Dresler CM: Regional lymph node classification for lung cancer staging. Chest 111:1718-1723, 1997, © 1996, Mountain and Dresler. Originally adapted from Naruke T, Suemasu K, Ishikawa S: Lymph node mapping and curability of various levels of metastases in resected lung cancer. J Thorac Cardiovasc Surg 76:832-839, 1978, and American Thoracic Society: Clinical staging of primary lung cancer. Am Rev Respir Dis 127:1-6, 1983.)*

Superior Mediastinal Nodes

● **1** Highest Mediastinal

● **2** Upper Paratracheal

● **3** Pre-vascular and Retrotracheal

● **4** Lower Paratracheal (including Azygos Nodes)

N_2 = single digit, ipsilateral
N_3 = single digit, contralateral or supraclavicular

Aortic Nodes

● **5** Subaortic (A-P window)

● **6** Para-aortic (ascending aorta or phrenic)

Inferior Mediastinal Nodes

● **7** Subcarinal

● **8** Paraesophageal (below carina)

● **9** Pulmonary Ligament

N_1 Nodes

○ **10** Hilar

● **11** Interlobar

○ **12** Lobar

○ **13** Segmental

○ **14** Subsegmental

upper bronchopulmonary nodes. The middle zone drains directly into the paratracheal, the subcarinal, and the central group of bronchopulmonary nodes. The inferior zone drains into the inferior bronchopulmonary and bifurcation nodes and the posterior mediastinal chain. Thus, on the right side, all the lymph drains eventually via the right lymphatic duct.

Rouvière found that in the left superior area, lymph drains into the prevascular group of anterior mediastinal nodes and directly into the left paratracheal nodes. The middle zone drains mainly via the bifurcation and central group of bronchopulmonary nodes and partly directly into the left paratracheal group. The inferior zone drains into the bifurcation and inferior bronchopulmonary nodes and into the posterior mediastinal chain. Thus, according to Rouvière, the superior portion and part of the middle zone drain via the left paratracheal nodes into the thoracic duct, and lymph drainage from the remainder of the left lung eventually empties into the right lymphatic duct.

The "crossover" phenomenon was long thought to be of diagnostic and therapeutic importance in diseases originating in the middle or lower portion of the left lung. However, the results of some investigations have cast doubt on the validity of this concept. For example, in one study of bilateral prescalene node biopsies in 110 patients who had pulmonary carcinoma, the direction of lymphatic spread within the mediastinum was cephalad and usually ipsilateral, irrespective of the location of the primary tumor; contralateral spread was uncommon and about equally frequent from either lung.[271]

THE THORACIC INLET

The thoracic inlet represents the junction between structures at the base of the neck and those of the thorax. It parallels the first rib and is higher posteriorly than anteriorly (Fig. 1–70). On the basis of this anatomic observation, it is evident that an opacity on a PA chest radiograph that is effaced on its superior aspect and that projects at or below the level of the clavicles must be situated anteriorly, whereas one that projects above the clavicles is retrotracheal and posteriorly situated (Fig. 1–71). These characteristic findings together have been termed the *cervicothoracic sign*.[272]

From front to back, structures occupying the thoracic inlet include the right and left brachiocephalic veins (which join

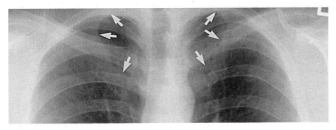

FIGURE 1–70

Normal thoracic inlet. A detail view from a posteroanterior chest radiograph in a 40-year-old man shows the normal appearance of the thoracic inlet. Because the thoracic inlet parallels the first rib (*arrows*), it is higher posteriorly than anteriorly. (*From Müller NL, Fraser RS, Colman NC, Paré PD: Radiologic Diagnosis of Diseases of the Chest. Philadelphia, WB Saunders, 2001.*)

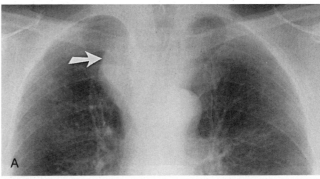

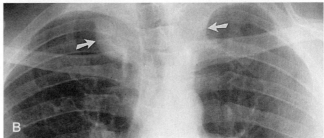

FIGURE 1–71

Cervicothoracic sign. A posteroanterior chest radiograph (**A**) from a 69-year-old man with a large thyroid goiter shows a mass (*arrow*) in the thoracic inlet displacing the trachea to the left. The mass is effaced above the level of the clavicle because it is anterior and lateral to the trachea and continuous with the soft tissues of the neck. A posteroanterior chest radiograph (**B**) in a 34-year-old patient shows bilateral paraspinal soft tissue opacities (*arrows*), well seen above the level of the clavicles. These opacities are well seen at this level because they are situated posterior to the trachea. The patient had bilateral paraspinal extension and involvement of the T3 vertebral body by hydatid disease. (*From Müller NL, Fraser RS, Colman NC, Paré PD: Radiologic Diagnosis of Diseases of the Chest. Philadelphia, WB Saunders, 2001.*)

behind the right side of the manubrium to form the superior vena cava), the common carotid arteries (lying immediately anterior to the subclavian arteries and medial to the subclavian veins), the trachea (situated immediately behind the great vessels), the esophagus (located behind the trachea and in front of the spine), and the recurrent laryngeal nerves on either side of the esophagus (Fig. 1–72).

THE MEDIASTINUM

The mediastinum separates the thorax vertically into two compartments and can be defined as the partition between the lungs (Fig. 1–73).[273] Anatomically, it can be divided into three compartments: anterior (prevascular), middle (cardiovascular), and posterior (postvascular).[273]

The *anterior compartment* is bounded anteriorly by the sternum and posteriorly by the pericardium, aorta, and brachiocephalic vessels. It merges superiorly with the anterior aspect of the thoracic inlet and extends down to the level of the diaphragm. The compartment contains the thymus, branches of the internal mammary artery and vein, lymph nodes, the inferior sternopericardial ligament, and variable amounts of fat.

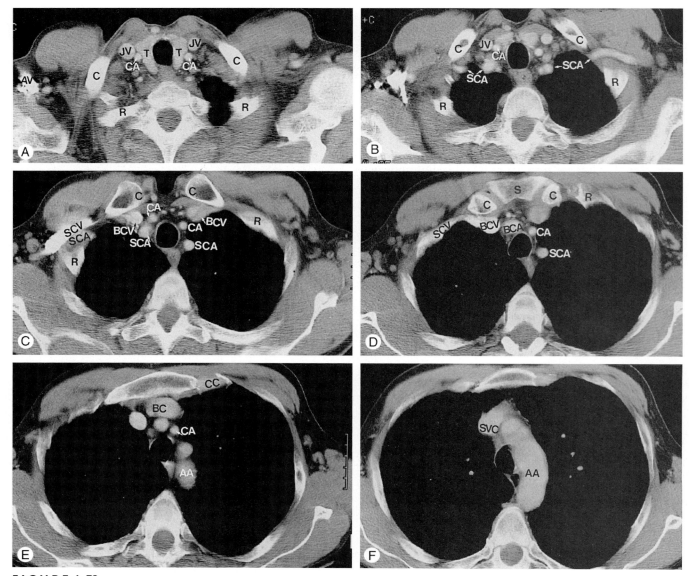

FIGURE 1–72

Normal CT scan of the thoracic inlet. A contrast-enhanced CT scan in a 51-year-old man illustrates the normal anatomy of the thoracic inlet.
A, A CT scan at the level of the posterior aspect of the first rib (R) demonstrates the left lung apex, clavicles (C), thyroid gland (T), jugular veins (JV), and carotid arteries (CA). Contrast injected into a right antecubital vein resulted in marked enhancement of the right axillary vein (AV). The thyroid gland surrounds the anterior and lateral aspects of the trachea in the lower part of the neck, whereas the esophagus lies immediately posterior to the trachea. **B,** A CT scan at the level of the lateral aspect of the first ribs demonstrates the subclavian arteries (SCA), carotid arteries, jugular veins, and inferior aspect of the thyroid gland. **C,** A CT scan at the level of the anteromedial aspect of the first ribs demonstrates the right subclavian vein (SCV) lying anterior to the subclavian artery. The proximal portions of the subclavian arteries, and the carotid arteries. The right and left brachiocephalic veins (BCV) can be seen anterior to the carotid arteries. The medial portion of the clavicle anterior to the first ribs outlines the region of the suprasternal notch. The esophagus is situated immediately posterior to the trachea. **D,** A CT scan at the level of the anterior aspect of the first ribs demonstrates the left costochondral junction, the upper aspect of the sternum (S), and the clavicles at the level of the sternoclavicular joint. At this level, the right subclavian vein (SCV) can be seen joining the brachiocephalic vein (anterolateral to the brachiocephalic artery [BCA]). The left brachiocephalic vein is seen anterolateral to the left carotid artery. At this level, as with the higher levels, the left subclavian artery and surrounding fat can be seen to form the left lateral margin of the thoracic inlet. **E,** A CT scan at the level of the first costal cartilage (CC) demonstrates the left brachiocephalic (BC) vein crossing the midline anterior to the brachiocephalic and carotid arteries. Also seen is the left subclavian artery as it originates from the uppermost aspect of the aortic arch (AA). **F,** A CT scan at the level of the aortic arch (AA) demonstrates the origin of the brachiocephalic and left carotid arteries from the aorta. At this level, the left brachiocephalic vein can be seen joining the superior vena cava (SVC).
(From Fraser RS, Müller NL, Colman NC, Paré PD: Fraser and Paré's Diagnosis of Diseases of the Chest, 4th ed. Philadelphia, WB Saunders, 1999.)

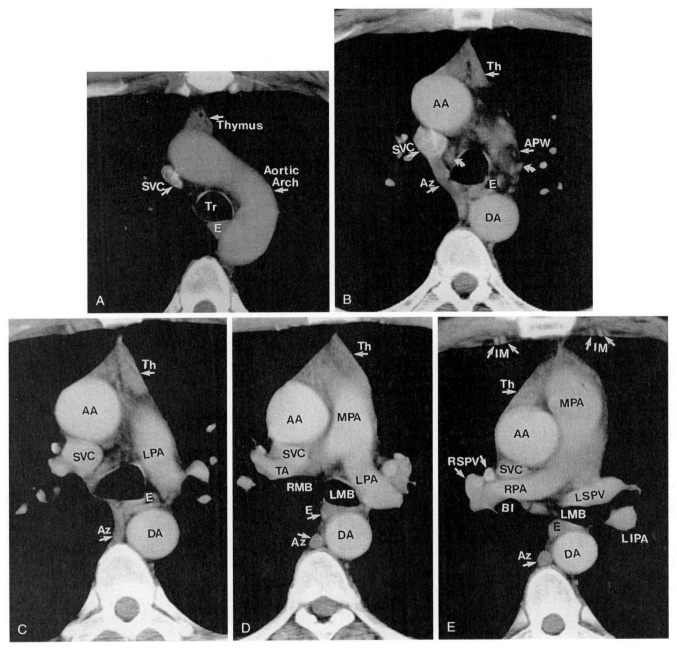

FIGURE 1–73

Normal CT anatomy of the mediastinum. An image at the level of the aortic arch (**A**) shows the thymus, superior vena cava (SVC), trachea (Tr), and esophagus (E). The paravertebral region and posterior gutters are not part of the mediastinum. An image immediately caudal to the aortic arch (**B**) shows the region of the aortopulmonary window (APW), ascending (AA) and descending aorta (DA), azygos vein (Az) draining into the superior vena cava (SVC), esophagus (E), and normal-sized mediastinal lymph nodes *(curved arrows)*. Note the triangular shape of the thymus (Th). An image at the level of the tracheal carina (**C**) shows the left pulmonary artery (LPA), superior vena cava (SVC), ascending (AA) and descending aorta (DA), thymus (Th), esophagus (E), and azygos vein (Az). An image at the level of the right (RMB) and left (LMB) main bronchi (**D**) shows the thymus (Th), ascending (AA) and descending aorta (DA), superior vena cava (SVC), truncus anterior (TA), esophagus (E), and azygos vein (Az). An image at the level of the bronchus intermedius (BI) (**E**) shows the right and left internal mammary arteries and veins (IM); thymus (Th); main (MPA), right (RPA), and left interlobular (LIPA) pulmonary arteries; superior vena cava (SVC); left superior pulmonary vein (LSPV); confluence of the right upper lobe veins to form the right superior pulmonary vein (RSPV); esophagus (E); and azygos vein (Az). *(From Müller NL, Fraser RS, Colman NC, Paré PD: Radiologic Diagnosis of Diseases of the Chest. Philadelphia, WB Saunders, 2001.)*

The *middle compartment* contains the pericardium and its contents, the ascending and transverse portions of the aorta, the superior and inferior vena cava, the brachiocephalic (innominate) arteries and veins, the phrenic nerves and cephalic portion of the vagus nerves, the trachea and main bronchi and their contiguous lymph nodes, and the main pulmonary arteries and veins.

The *posterior compartment* is bounded anteriorly by the pericardium and the vertical part of the diaphragm, laterally by the mediastinal pleura, and posteriorly by the bodies of the thoracic vertebrae. It contains the descending thoracic aorta, esophagus, thoracic duct, azygos and hemiazygos veins, autonomic nerves, fat, and lymph nodes.

The Thymus

The thymus is located in the anterosuperior portion of the mediastinum and in adults generally extends from a point above the manubrium to the fourth costal cartilage. Posteriorly, it relates to the trachea, the aortic arch and its branches, and the pericardium covering the ascending aorta and main pulmonary artery (Fig. 1–74).

On conventional radiographs, the gland is visible only in infants and young children, in whom it fills much of the anterior mediastinal space. In one CT study of 154 normal individuals, it was recognized in all those younger than 30 years, in 73% between 30 and 49, and in 17% older than 49.[274] The maximal size was observed in individuals between 12 and 19 years of age, with regression occurring between 20 and 60. Most glands have an arrowhead configuration; about a third

have separate right and left lobes.[274] The most reliable measurement of thymic size on CT scan is the thickness (short-axis or transverse dimension of a lobe). It is generally accepted that the maximum thickness of a normal thymus in individuals younger than 20 years is 1.8 cm, whereas in individuals 20 years or older, it is 1.3 cm.[275,276]

Mediastinal Lines and Interfaces

Anterior Junction Line. As the two lungs approximate anteromedially, they are separated by four layers of pleura and a variable quantity of intervening mediastinal adipose tissue to form a *septum* of variable thickness (the anterior junction line or anterior mediastinal line) (Fig. 1–75). On a PA chest radiograph, this line is typically oriented obliquely from the upper right to the lower left behind the sternum.

The Aortopulmonary Window. The aortopulmonary window consists of a space situated between the arch of the aorta and the left pulmonary artery. It is occupied largely by mediastinal fat. Its medial boundary is the ductus ligament, and its lateral boundary is the mediastinal and visceral pleura over the left lung; the latter boundary creates the aortopulmonary window interface (Fig. 1–76). Within this space are situated fat, the left recurrent laryngeal nerve, and lymph nodes. The lateral border (aortopulmonary window interface) is normally concave or straight.

Tracheal Interfaces. Normally, the trachea is bordered on its right lateral aspect by pleura covering the right upper lobe; its anterior and posterior aspects are bordered to a variable extent. Contact of the right lung in the supra-azygos area with

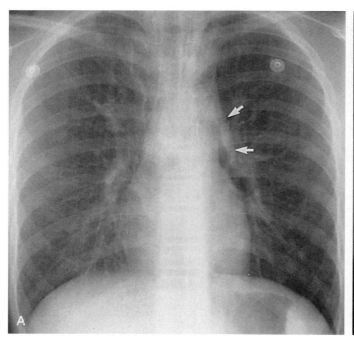
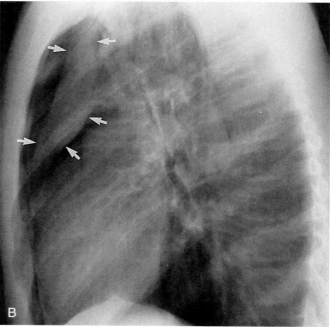

FIGURE 1–74

Normal thymus delineated by pneumomediastinum. Posteroanterior (**A**) and lateral (**B**) chest radiographs in a 10-year-old boy with pneumomediastinum demonstrate the normal location of the thymus, which is outlined by surrounding air *(arrows)*. Note that the left lobe of the thymus is larger than the right lobe. *(From Fraser RS, Müller NL, Colman NC, Paré PD: Fraser and Paré's Diagnosis of Diseases of the Chest, 4th ed. Philadelphia, WB Saunders, 1999.)*

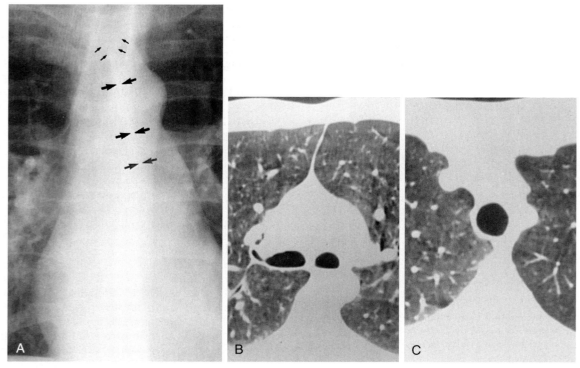

FIGURE 1–75

Anterior junction line and superior recess. A posteroanterior chest radiograph (**A**) in a 38-year-old man shows the anterior junction line *(large arrows)* extending from the right to the left caudally from the level of the aortic arch. Immediately above the arch is a V-shaped area of increased opacity *(small arrows)* representing the anterior mediastinal triangle. A CT scan at the level of the main bronchi (**B**) shows the right and left lungs to abut each other anterior to the mediastinum. The anterior junction line is formed by apposition of the visceral and mediastinal pleurae of the right and left lungs. A CT scan above the level of the aortic arch (**C**) shows that at this level the lungs are separated by the great vessels and mediastinal fat, which accounts for the anterior mediastinal triangle seen on the radiograph. *(From Müller NL, Fraser RS, Colman NC, Paré PD: Radiologic Diagnosis of Diseases of the Chest. Philadelphia, WB Saunders, 2001.)*

the right lateral wall of the trachea creates a thin stripe of soft tissue density usually visible on frontal chest radiographs that has been designated the *right paratracheal stripe.* This stripe is formed by the right wall of the trachea, contiguous parietal and visceral pleura, and a variable quantity of mediastinal fat.[277] The thickness of the stripe must be measured above the level of the azygos vein; an increase in width on serial films is a more important sign of abnormality than a single measurement.

The normal maximal width of the stripe is 4 mm.[277] Widening (greater than 5 mm) may be the result of paratracheal lymph node enlargement, mediastinal hemorrhage, or disease of the pleura or tracheal wall. It is not a particularly sensitive sign in that it is present in only approximately 30% of patients who have paratracheal lymph node enlargement shown on CT scan.[278]

The *posterior tracheal stripe* is a vertically oriented opacity formed by the posterior wall of the trachea where it comes in contact with right upper lobe parenchyma.

Posterior Junction Line. The apices of the right and left upper lobes contact the mediastinum behind the esophagus anterior to the first and second vertebral bodies. In so doing, they create a V-shaped triangular opacity that constitutes the *posterior mediastinal triangle;* margining the triangle are the *right* and *left superior recesses.* Caudally, the lungs intrude deeper into a prespinal location posterior to the esophagus

and anterior to the third through fifth vertebral bodies, where they form a pleural apposition that along with any intervening mediastinal tissue, forms the *posterior junction line.* On a PA radiograph, the posterior junction line usually projects through the air column of the trachea; it may be straight or slightly convex to the left. When intervening mediastinal tissue is abundant or a narrowed retroesophageal space precludes lung apposition, the posterior junction line can appear as a distinct stripe.[279]

Azygoesophageal Recess. The azygos vein ascends in the posterior mediastinum toward the right side or in front of the vertebral column. The esophagus is usually located slightly anterior and to the left of the vein in the prevertebral region, although they are sometimes in contact. The *azygoesophageal recess* is formed by contact of the right lower lobe with the esophagus and the ascending portion of the azygos vein (Fig. 1–77).[280,281]

The recess is frequently identified on a well-penetrated PA radiograph as an interface that extends from the diaphragm below to the level of the azygos arch above. Typically, it is seen as a continuous, shallow or deep arc concave to the right; however, in young adults, a straight or slightly dextroconvex interface may be seen.[282] A focal right-sided convexity of the azygoesophageal recess interface should raise suspicion of an underlying abnormality such as a hiatal hernia, an esophageal

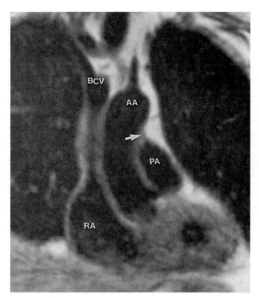

FIGURE 1–76

Aortopulmonary window. An MR image in an 83-year-old man shows the structures responsible for the left mediastinal border. Fat can be seen lateral to the aortic arch (AA) and main pulmonary artery (PA) and outlines the region of the aortopulmonary window. The ligament of the ductus arteriosus *(arrow)* can be seen to delineate the medial margin of the aortopulmonary window. Also noted are the left carotid artery, right brachiocephalic vein (BCV), superior vena cava, and right atrium (RA). *(From Müller NL, Fraser RS, Colman NC, Paré PD: Radiologic Diagnosis of Diseases of the Chest. Philadelphia, WB Saunders, 2001.)*

tumor or duplication cyst, azygos vein dilation, or subcarinal lymph node enlargement.[281]

The Heart

On a frontal radiograph of a normal chest, the position of the heart in relation to the midline of the thorax depends largely on the patient's build. Assuming radiographic exposure with the lungs fully inflated, the heart shadow is almost exactly midline in position in asthenic individuals, with only a slight projection to the left; in individuals of stockier build, it lies a little more to the left of midline.[149]

In normal individuals, the transverse diameter of the heart measured on standard PA radiographs is usually in the range of 11.5 to 15.5 cm[149]; it is less than 11.5 cm in approximately 5% and only rarely exceeds 15.5 cm (in heavy subjects of stocky build). The custom of trying to assess cardiac size by relating it to the transverse diameter of the chest (cardiothoracic ratio), though helpful, has potential pitfalls. On a PA radiograph, a cardiothoracic ratio of 50% is widely accepted as the upper limit of normal; however, the ratio exceeds 50% in at least 10% of normal individuals.[149] Measurement of the ratio is especially fallacious in individuals who have a small heart; for example, in an individual who has an 8-cm transverse cardiac diameter in a 24-cm thorax, the heart would have to enlarge 4 cm before the cardiothoracic ratio reaches 50%.[149] In our view, it is preferable to evaluate cardiac size subjectively; alternatively, it is reasonable to assume that a heart whose transverse diameter exceeds 16 cm is enlarged.

Heart size and contour are also influenced by (1) the *height of the diaphragm,* which in turn is influenced by the degree of pulmonary inflation—the lower the position of the diaphragm, the longer and narrower the cardiovascular silhouette; (2) *intrathoracic pressure,* which also influences the appearance of the pulmonary vascular pattern; (3) *body position*—assuming equality of all other factors, the heart is broader when a subject is recumbent than when erect; (4) systole and diastole—for example, in one study the change in transverse cardiac diameter between the two on PA radiographs was 0.3 cm or less in 52% of individuals, 0.4 to 0.9 cm in 41%, and 1.0 to 1.7 cm in 7%[283]; and (5) *PA versus AP radiographs*—the heart is magnified more and appears larger on radiographs taken with an AP projection of the x-ray beam.

Accumulations of fat are common in the cardiophrenic recesses bilaterally and produce an obtuse angular configuration of the inferior mediastinum at its junction with the diaphragm. The density of the fat accumulations may be

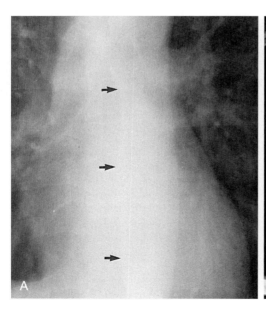

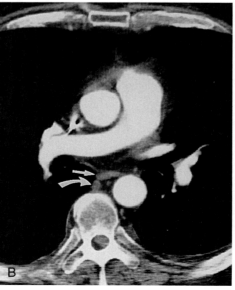

FIGURE 1–77

Azygoesophageal recess. A posteroanterior chest radiograph (**A**) in a 36-year-old man shows a normal azygoesophageal recess interface *(arrows)* extending from the level of the tracheal carina to the diaphragm to form a shallow arc convex to the right. A CT scan (**B**) shows that the interface is due to contact between the right lung and the posterior mediastinum (more specifically, between the right lung and the esophagus *[straight arrow]* and azygos vein *[curved arrow]*). *(From Müller NL, Fraser RS, Colman NC, Paré PD: Radiologic Diagnosis of Diseases of the Chest. Philadelphia, WB Saunders, 2001.)*

slightly less than that of the heart, and this contrast in density may allow identification of the approximate position of the cardiac borders. These pleuropericardial fat shadows should not be misinterpreted as cardiac enlargement or as mediastinal or diaphragmatic masses.

CONTROL OF BREATHING

The respiratory control system may be divided into four components (Fig. 1–78): (1) afferent input to a central respiratory controller, (2) the controller and its central integration, (3) output from the respiratory center, and (4) the effectors of the output—the respiratory muscles.

Input

The three major sources of input to the central regulator of respiration are (1) the peripheral and central chemoreceptors, which respond to alterations in arterial Po_2, Pco_2, and hydrogen ion concentration; (2) receptors in the respiratory tract and lungs, which are influenced by lung mechanics; and (3) muscle spindles and tendon organs in the respiratory muscles, which monitor the effectiveness of contraction of the peripheral effector system.

Peripheral Chemoreceptors. The carotid body is the major peripheral chemoreceptor.[284] It is composed in part of glomus cells that contain abundant dopamine. Because hypoxia increases dopamine release and synthesis by these cells, it is probable that they act as chemoreceptive transducers that stimulate postsynaptic afferent nerve endings contained within the carotid body. The organ has an enormous blood supply and receives as much as 2 L/min/100 g of tissue (more than 40 times the flow per gram to the brain); this massive blood supply results in a virtually unchanged Po_2 as the blood passes through the chemoreceptor tissue.

Afferent fibers from the carotid body travel in the glossopharyngeal nerve and stimulate respiration during hypoxia by release of substance P.[285] Their output is increased not only by hypoxia but also by hypercapnia and changes in pH. The hypoxic and hypercapnic responses are additive, so both stimuli together result in an enhanced response. In addition, enhanced stimulation appears to accompany rapid swings in arterial Po_2 and Pco_2, thus suggesting that the rate of change in arterial blood gas tension is as important a stimulus as the average level.[286]

In the absence of peripheral chemoreceptors, the hypoxic ventilatory response is abolished, and in fact, hypoxemia may cause ventilatory depression; however, 85% of the ventilatory response to CO_2 is preserved.

Central Chemoreceptors. The cells that function as central chemoreceptors lie 200 to 500 μm below the surface of the ventrolateral medulla oblongata. By MR imaging, these areas show increased blood flow during inhalation of hypercapnic gas mixtures.[287] Their stimulus is the hydrogen ion concentration of brain extracellular fluid. Since the blood-brain barrier is freely permeable to carbon dioxide but not to hydrogen or bicarbonate ions, hypercapnic acidosis is a more powerful stimulus to central chemoreceptors than is acute metabolic acidosis. In fact, with the increased circulating hydrogen ion concentration associated with metabolic acidosis, stimulation of the peripheral chemoreceptors occurs and results in an increase in ventilation and a decrease in Pco_2;

thus, there can actually be a paradoxical decrease in cerebrospinal fluid hydrogen ion concentration despite blood metabolic acidosis.

The higher cerebrospinal fluid pH tends to attenuate the central ventilatory response to metabolic acidosis. Similarly, the acute ventilatory response to hypoxia as a result of stimulation of peripheral chemoreceptors is partly offset by the resulting hypocapnic alkalosis. Changes in cerebrospinal fluid pH occur as hydrogen ion equilibrates across the blood-brain barrier over a period of hours. Thus, if the acidosis is prolonged, cerebrospinal pH progressively falls to more acid levels, thereby resulting in progressive stimulation of ventilation, and arterial Pco_2 continues to decrease as the metabolic acidosis is sustained.

Receptors in the Respiratory Tract and Lungs. The respiratory center receives afferent input from receptors at all levels in the respiratory tract, including the nose, the nasopharynx, and the larynx.[288,289] The tracheobronchial receptors have been the most thoroughly studied and include irritant, stretch, and J receptors. Stimulation of irritant receptors produces rapid shallow breathing and has been implicated in the altered breathing pattern seen in patients with airway disease such as asthma and COPD. Pulmonary stretch receptors are responsible for the Hering-Breuer reflex (cessation of respiratory neural drive caused by lung inflation). These receptors respond by increasing their firing frequency with lung inflation or with increases in transpulmonary pressure. Stimulation of "J" receptors causes rapid shallow breathing, laryngeal constriction, hypotension, and bradycardia. The vagus also carries afferent input from subdiaphragmatic visceral organs that can cause reflex inhibition of respiratory muscle function and a decrease in regional lung ventilation.[290]

Respiratory Muscle Afferents. The major striated muscle receptors are Golgi tendon organs and muscle spindles. The former appear to be more important in the diaphragm, muscle spindles being rare. By contrast, muscle spindles predominate in the intercostal muscles, both inspiratory and expiratory, as well as in the accessory muscles of respiration. The precise role of these receptors and their influence on the central respiratory controller is unknown, but the results of a number of studies suggest that they may be important; for example, cutting the dorsal cervical and thoracic roots can lead to temporary respiratory muscle paralysis.[291]

The Central Controller

Central control of respiratory rhythm and pattern can originate in the voluntary cortical centers or brainstem automatic centers.[292] Automatic breathing originates in a highly complex accumulation of interconnected nerve cell groups situated in the medulla and the pons. Within the former, the respiratory neurons are grouped in two distinct areas: (1) *the dorsal respiratory group* (DRG), which comprises two bilateral aggregates of neurons located near the nucleus of the tractus solitarius and consists almost exclusively of inspiratory cells, and (2) *the ventral respiratory group* (VRG), which lies close to the nucleus ambiguus and the nucleus retroambigualis and contains both inspiratory and expiratory cells.

It is thought that axons originating in the DRG project to and descend in the contralateral spinal cord and serve as the principal respiratory rhythmic drive to the anterior horn cells that innervate the diaphragm and inspiratory intercostals.

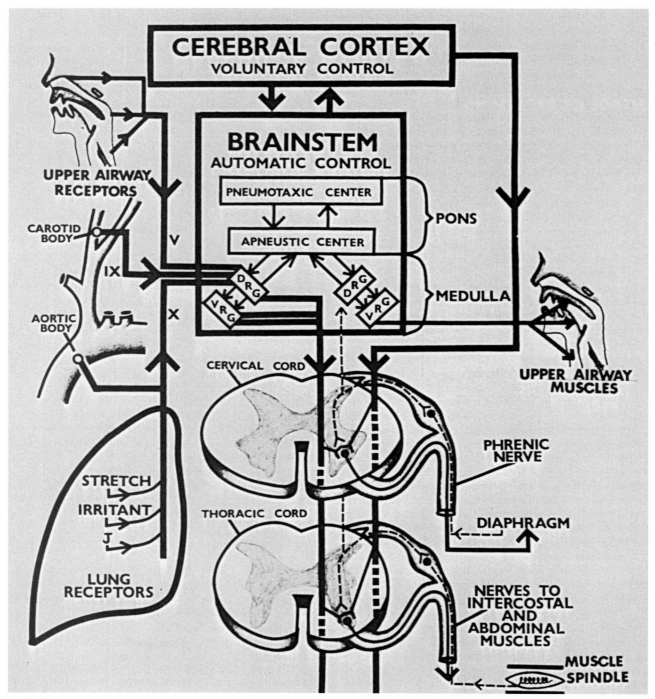

FIGURE 1–78

Respiratory control system. Central respiratory control is shared by voluntary (cerebral) and automatic (brainstem) centers. The efferent fibers from each center run in distinct spinal cord pathways, as depicted on the left side of the coronally sectioned spinal cord (right side of the drawing). A variety of interconnections exist between the cortex and the different components of the brainstem. The pontine pneumotaxic (PNC) center and the apneustic center (APC) are now termed the pontine respiratory group (PRG). Afferent fibers ascending the 5th (V), 9th (IX), and 10th (X) cranial nerves from upper airway receptors, peripheral chemoreceptors, and visceral and lung receptors connect with the ipsilateral dorsal respiratory group of neurons (DRG). In addition, afferents from Golgi tendon organs in the diaphragm and intercostal muscle spindles travel in the phrenic and intercostal nerves and reach the anterior horn cells, as well as ascend to the DRG via the dorsal columns. Respiratory neurons in the DRG are connected with those in the ventral respiratory group (VRG), from which the descending neural output originates. The efferent fibers cross in the brainstem and descend in the spinal cord to supply the diaphragm, intercostal, accessory, and expiratory muscles. Neurons in the VRG also project via the ipsilateral 9th, 10th, and 12th cranial nerves to the upper airways, where they innervate the laryngeal, genioglossal, geniohyoid, and other upper airway muscles. *(From Fraser RS, Müller NL, Colman NC, Paré PD: Fraser and Paré's Diagnosis of Diseases of the Chest, 4th ed. Philadelphia, WB Saunders, 1999.)*

Axons from the DRG also project to stimulate cells in the VRG, which does not appear to have inherent respiratory rhythmicity or sensory input from peripheral or central chemoreceptors and mechanoreceptors. Axons from the VRG cross and descend in the spinal cord to innervate anterior horn cells in the cervical and thoracic cord; these, in turn, project to the intercostal inspiratory and expiratory muscles, as well as the abdominal and accessory muscles of respiration and the muscles of the upper airway, which are important in maintaining upper airway patency.

Two additional respiratory control centers, the *pneumotaxis center* (PNC) and the *apneustic center* (APC), are located in the pons. Although their activity is not absolutely necessary for the generation of rhythmic respiratory output, they clearly influence and modulate the output of the medullary respiratory center[293]; the rhythm generated from the isolated medulla is slower and of a more gasping nature than that developed when the PNC and the APC are intact.

Inspiration is initiated by a sudden onset of inspiratory motor neuron activity in the DRG, followed by a slowly increasing ramp of activity. Inspiratory muscle activation may extend into early expiration to brake expiratory flow. Expiratory neurons are not activated during quiet breathing, but they may be recruited during increased ventilatory drive.[294]

Although most of our knowledge of central respiratory control involves the automatic brainstem controlling mechanisms, it is clear that the cerebral cortex can influence brainstem mechanisms or bypass them completely to accomplish behavior-related respiratory activity such as speech, cough, and defecation. During voluntary activity, requirements for tone or loudness may override chemical and mechanical input; for example, during speech, the response to inhaled carbon dioxide is markedly depressed and the sensation of dyspnea diminished when compared with similar carbon dioxide levels occurring without speech.[295]

Output

The basic measurements of outputs used to assess respiratory control are minute ventilation and its components tidal volume (Vt) and respiratory frequency (f). Minute ventilation itself can be divided into mean inspiratory flow (Vt/Ti) and the ratio of inspiratory time to total respiratory cycle time (Ti/Ttot). It has been proposed that Vt/Ti reflects the neural drive whereas Ti/Ttot is a measure of central timing mechanisms; these measurements have gained wide acceptance in the analysis of respiratory control.[296]

The most common inputs by which respiratory control is assessed are inhaled carbon dioxide and oxygen, administered in increasing and decreasing concentrations, respectively; the responses to added resistive and elastic loads and to exercise can also be measured. In normal individuals, progressive hypercapnia produces a linear increase in ventilation, although the slope of the curve varies widely between individuals. With progressive hypoxemia, a parabolic curve of ventilation against Po$_2$ is generated, with little increase in ventilation until Po$_2$ falls to between 50 and 60 mm Hg; however, there is also wide variability among individuals in this relationship.

Genetic or acquired alterations in ventilatory response may have profound effects on pulmonary disease. For example, it has been postulated that the genetically determined ventilatory drives to hypoxia and hypercapnia influence the pattern and course of COPD; patients with brisk or good responses to carbon dioxide and hypoxia tend to maintain blood gas tensions near normal despite significant airway obstruction (pink puffers), whereas those with depressed ventilatory responses tend to hypoventilate (blue bloaters).[297] Inherited variations in ventilatory drive may also affect the ability of normal individuals to perform various functions; for example, trained endurance athletes have a significantly reduced ventilatory drive to hypoxemia and hypercapnia when compared with normal nonathletic controls, whereas similarly fit, successful high-altitude mountain climbers have a significantly increased hypercapnic and hypoxic drive when compared with distance runners.[298]

Control of Ventilation during Exercise

The ventilatory response to exercise consists of four phases.[299] *Phase 1* is an abrupt increase in ventilation that coincides with the start of exercise. This increase occurs before any alteration in the gas tensions of mixed venous blood and is termed the "neurogenic component" of the ventilatory response, although the precise neural pathway that mediates the response is unknown. *Phase 2* begins some 10 or 15 seconds after the onset of exercise, coincident with alterations in blood gas tensions in mixed venous blood. The carotid bodies have some role in this phase because patients who do not have carotid bodies have a lag in the ventilatory response. *Phase 3* represents the steady-state response and is closely linked to carbon dioxide production. Finally, during heavy exercise *(phase 4)*, there is a further increase in ventilation coincident with the metabolic production of lactic acid. This stage is termed the anaerobic threshold, and at this point ventilation becomes uncoupled from metabolic carbon dioxide production. This final lactic acidosis–induced hyperpnea is mediated by peripheral chemoreceptors.

Compensation for Added Ventilatory Loads

The respiratory muscles act against elastic and resistive loads that may vary greatly under normal physiologic conditions and during disease. Studies in humans have shown that the decrease in tidal volume that occurs with such added loads is less than would be expected on a purely mechanical basis, thus indicating that compensatory mechanisms are brought into play to ensure adequate acinar ventilation. The first such mechanism is related to the basic mechanical properties of skeletal muscle. Since the force generated by skeletal muscle is inversely related to its velocity of shortening, an unloaded muscle will shorten rapidly and produce little force; however, with an added load, shortening is slowed and force generation increased, which results in a tendency to counteract the expected decrease in tidal volume.

The second mechanism involves reflexes initiated by mechanoreceptors in the lung and chest wall, particularly the pulmonary stretch receptors. With an added elastic or resistive load, inspiration is slowed. Because pulmonary stretch receptors adapt rapidly with time, their level of activity at any volume during inspiration is decreased; this decreased activity results in prolonged inspiration, which tends to increase tidal volume back toward control levels.[300]

Muscle spindles modulate a third mechanism by which load compensation is accomplished. These receptors contain intrafusal fibers that regulate the spindles' stretch and contract in concert with the extrafusal fibers that move the rib cage. This stimulates the gamma afferents, which through the spinal reflex enhance motor neuron output to the inspiratory muscles. A final mechanism of load compensation is initiated when central and peripheral chemoreceptors detect changes in arterial blood gas composition.[300]

Closely related to the topic of load detection and compensation are respiratory sensation and the symptom of dyspnea. Dyspnea (the unpleasant awareness of breathing or respiratory distress) should be distinguished from hyperventilation (defined as a lowered arterial P_{CO_2}) or tachypnea (rapid respiration). The balance of evidence suggests that dyspnea occurs when afferent input from respiratory muscles in some way signals an inappropriateness of the central neurogenic drive to breathe and the resulting displacement of the lung and chest wall.[301] It is not caused by alterations in arterial blood gas tensions.

Control of Breathing during Sleep

Sleep has a profound influence on the various aspects of the control of breathing (Table 1–3).[302,303] Resting ventilation is decreased during slow-wave sleep, with both tidal volume and frequency being less than during wakefulness.[304] During rapid eye movement (REM) sleep, resting ventilation varies as a result of marked irregularity of the breathing pattern, but on the whole, hyperventilation rather than hypoventilation is the rule. During stages 1 and 2 of slow-wave sleep, periodic breathing reminiscent of Cheyne-Stokes respiration may occur and change to a regular pattern during the deeper stages (3 and 4) of slow-wave sleep. The pattern of breathing during REM sleep is characterized as irregular rather than periodic.

TABLE 1–3. Effects of Sleep on Breathing

Respiratory Activity	Slow-Wave Sleep	REM Sleep
Alveolar ventilation	Decreased because of ↓ V_T and ↓ F	Variable
Arterial P_{CO_2}	↑ 4–6 mm Hg	Variable
Arterial P_{O_2}	↓ 4–8 mm Hg	Variable
Breathing pattern	Stages 1 and 2 periodic	Irregular
	Stages 3 and 4 regular	↑ F plus ↓ V_T
Diaphragmatic contraction	No change	No change
Intercostal contraction	↓	↓↓
Upper airway muscle contraction	↓	↓↓
Ventilatory response to CO_2	↓	↓↓
Ventilatory response to hypoxemia	↓	↓↓
Response to lung afferents	↓	↓↓
Response to respiratory muscle afferents	↓	↓↓

REM, rapid eye movement.
From Fraser RS, Müller NL, Colman NC, Paré PD: Diagnosis of Diseases of the Chest, 4th ed. Philadelphia, WB Saunders, 1999.

The responsiveness of the respiratory control mechanisms to afferent input is also profoundly altered during sleep; responsiveness to hypercapnia is decreased during slow-wave sleep and further decreased during REM sleep. The respiratory centers also appear to "ignore" afferent input from other sources during sleep; pulmonary stretch and irritant receptor discharge, as well as muscle spindle input, are less effective in increasing ventilation and effecting load compensation during sleep.

THE RESPIRATORY MUSCLES

The respiratory muscles can be divided into four groups that have different functions and mechanisms of action—the upper airway muscles, the diaphragm, the intercostal and accessory muscles, and the abdominal muscles.[305]

A variety of upper airway muscles are important in respiration.[306] The alae nasi are nasal dilatory muscles that are activated during increased respiratory drive. The nasal versus oral route of breathing is determined by the action of two palatal muscles, the palatoglossus and the levator palatini.[307] The genioglossal and geniohyoid muscles, as well as the muscles of the larynx and pharynx, act to stiffen the airway and prevent collapse during expiration. Receptors in the hypopharynx and larynx respond to negative pressure by reflex activation of the upper airway muscles. They contract simultaneously with the inspiratory muscles, although their electromyographic activity starts somewhat earlier and peaks during maximal inspiratory flow rather than at maximal inspired volume. The upper airway muscles are more sensitive than the other respiratory muscles to depression by sleep,[308] anesthesia, and alcohol consumption.[309]

The diaphragm is the principal muscle of inspiration. It probably acts alone during quiet breathing, with the intercostal and accessory muscles being recruited only when the demand for ventilation increases. However, there is some tonic inspiratory muscle activity in the intercostal muscles in the upright posture that prevents paradoxical inward movement of the rib cage with diaphragmatic descent. The intercostal muscles include the internal (expiratory) and external (inspiratory) intercostals. The major accessory muscles are the scalenes, the sternomastoids, and the trapezoids. The abdominal muscles include the rectus and transverse abdominis and the external and internal obliques. In healthy individuals, expiration is largely passive, with expiratory muscle activity becoming manifested only when minute ventilation exceeds about 50% of maximal voluntary ventilation.[310]

The Diaphragm

Anatomy

The central portion of the diaphragm (the central tendon) is composed of a broad sheet of decussating muscle fibers similar in shape to a boomerang, the point of the boomerang being directed toward the sternum and the concavity toward the spine (Fig. 1–79). The costal muscle fibers arise anteriorly from the xiphoid process and around the convexity of the thorax from ribs 7 to 12; posteriorly, the crural fibers arise from the lateral margins of the first, second, and third lumbar vertebrae on the right side and from the first and second

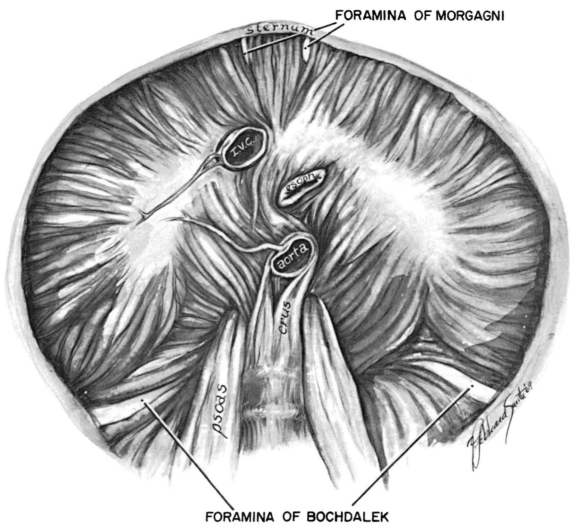

FORAMINA OF MORGAGNI

FORAMINA OF BOCHDALEK

FIGURE 1–79

Anatomy of the normal diaphragm viewed from below. See the text. I.V.C., inferior vena cava. *(From Fraser RS, Müller NL, Colman NC, Paré PD: Fraser and Paré's Diagnosis of Diseases of the Chest, 4th ed. Philadelphia, WB Saunders, 1999.)*

lumbar vertebrae on the left. These fibers converge toward the central tendon and are inserted into it nearly perpendicular to its margin.

The diaphragm can be considered as two distinct muscles that have separate nervous and vascular supplies, as well as functions.[311] The costal portion is mechanically in parallel with the intercostal and accessory muscles, and contraction of this portion results in both descent of the diaphragm and elevation of the rib cage; by contrast, the crural portion acts in parallel with the costal diaphragm and in series with the intercostal and accessory muscles, and contraction of this portion results in descent of the diaphragm without elevation of the rib cage (Fig. 1–80).

The diaphragm is composed of three types of muscle fibers: (1) slow-twitch oxidative fatigue-resistant units (type 1), (2) fast-twitch oxidative glycolytic fatigue-resistant units (type 2a), and (3) fast-twitch glycolytic fatigable units (type 2b). Each type has specific physiologic features and corresponding histochemical profiles,[312] and all fibers within individual

motor units are of the same type. Normally, type 1 fibers represent approximately 50% of muscle fibers, whereas type 2a fibers represent about 20% and type 2b about 30%; these percentages could conceivably change with atrophy or training of the respiratory muscles. It is likely that the diaphragm behaves like other skeletal muscles and that slow-twitch motor units are recruited during low-intensity contractions, such as with sustained quiet breathing, and that fast-twitch units, both fatigue resistant and fatigue susceptible, play a greater role with increasing respiratory activity.

The diaphragm receives its blood supply from the phrenic and intercostal arteries and from branches of the internal thoracic (mammary) arteries. The internal mammary and phrenic arteries anastomose to form an arterial circle around the central tendon; this circle, in turn, gives off branches that form an arcade. A second arterial circle is formed by the intercostals around the insertion of the diaphragm. This diversity of blood supply may be an important factor in the diaphragm's resistance to fatigue.[313] In contrast to limb

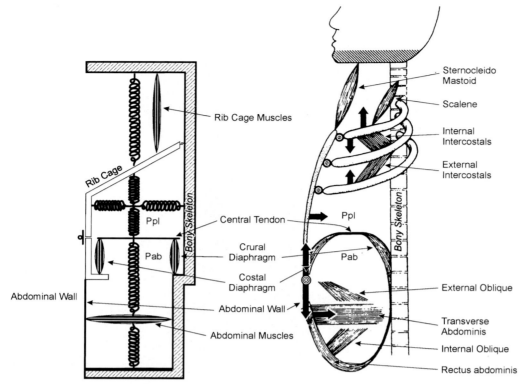

FIGURE 1–80

Mechanical model of the inspiratory musculature. The diaphragm is composed of crural and costal portions joined by the central tendon. The inverted L-shaped structure represents the rib cage; the latter is divided into a lung-apposed portion and a diaphragm-apposed portion. The *coiled springs* represent the elastic properties of the rib cage, lung, and abdomen, and the *hatched area,* the bony skeleton. The costal and crural portions of the diaphragm are arranged mechanically in parallel. In this situation, the force applied is the sum of the forces generated by the two muscles; however, the displacement (volume change) is equal to the displacement of either muscle. The costal part of the diaphragm is in series with the intercostal and accessory muscles. In this situation, the displacement of the two muscles can be added, but the forces are not summed. The *spring* linking the two portions of the rib cage indicates that the rib cage may be flexible (i.e., the lung-apposed and diaphragm-apposed portions can move independently in response to applied pressure). The drawing on the *right* represents a more anatomically realistic representation showing separation of the costal and crural parts of the diaphragm and the lung-apposed portions of the rib cage. Pab, abdominal pressure; Ppl, pleural pressure. *(Adapted from Macklem PT, Macklem DM, De Troyer A: A model of inspiratory muscle mechanics, J Appl Physiol 55:547-557, 1983; and Ward ME, Ward JW, Macklem PT: Analysis of human chest wall motion using a two-compartment rib cage model. J Appl Physiol 72:1338-1347, 1992.)*

skeletal muscle, there is no evidence in the diaphragm of blood flow limitation on contractile effort. In fact, the increasing demand for oxygen by the working diaphragm is supplied largely by augmenting blood flow rather than by increasing the extraction of oxygen from blood.[314]

The phrenic nerve is the sole motor nerve supply to the diaphragm. It arises chiefly from the fourth cervical nerve but also receives contributions from the third and fifth. At the level of the diaphragm, each phrenic nerve gives off separate branches to the anterior (sternal) region, the anterolateral region, and the crural portion. Hemidiaphragmatic and intercostal muscle innervation has a predominantly contralateral cortical representation. The conduction velocity in the phrenic nerve is high, reaching a maximum of 78 m/sec; in addition, the innervation is dense, with each nerve fiber subserving a low number of motor units—an anatomic arrangement that is usually seen in muscles performing precise movements, such as those of the eye. The intercostal

motor neurons are located between T1 and T12 in the spinal cord and reach the intercostal muscles via the intercostal nerves. Abdominal motor neurons are located between T11 and L1.

Radiology

On the chest radiograph, the upper surface of the dome-shaped diaphragm is normally visualized as it forms an interface with the lung; the soft tissues of the abdomen obscure its inferior surface. In approximately 95% of healthy adults, the level of the cupola of the right hemidiaphragm is projected in a plane ranging from the anterior end of the fifth rib to the sixth anterior interspace; in about 5%, it is projected at or below the level of the seventh rib.[315] In approximately 90% of adults, the plane of the right diaphragmatic dome is about half an interspace higher than the left; both are at the same height or the left is higher than the right in about 10% of normal

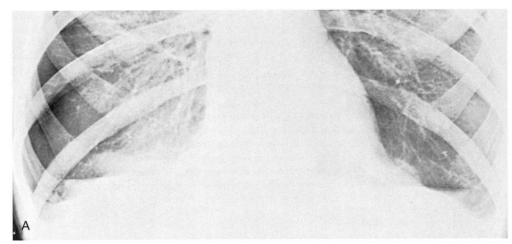

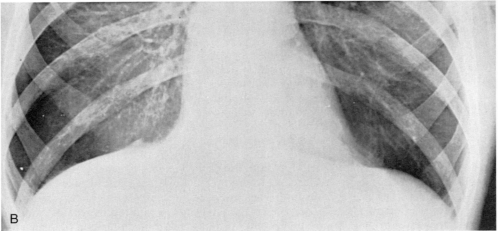

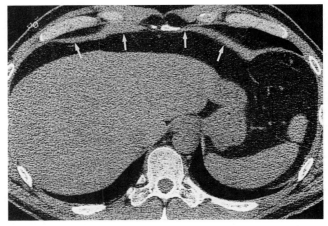

FIGURE 1–81

Diaphragmatic muscle slips.
Inspiratory (**A**) and expiratory
(**B**) radiographs of the lower half of
the thorax in a patient with severe
emphysema reveal short meniscus-
shaped shadows extending laterally
from each diaphragm. These muscle
slips are prominent during full
inspiration and disappear during
expiration. (*From Fraser RS, Müller NL,
Colman NC, Paré PD: Fraser and Paré's
Diagnosis of Diseases of the Chest, 4th
ed. Philadelphia, WB Saunders, 1999.*)

individuals.[252] The usual lower position of the left hemidiaphragm is a result of the contiguous mass of the heart on this
side rather than the presence of the liver under the right
hemidiaphragm.[316]

In some individuals, muscle slips originating from the
lateral and posterolateral aspect of the ribs can be identified
as short, meniscus-shaped shadows along the lateral half of
both hemidiaphragms; these shadows are produced by an
exceptionally low descent of the diaphragm during inspiration. In the majority of cases, the appearance is caused by
severe pulmonary overinflation (Fig. 1–81), as in asthma or
emphysema; however, it is occasionally seen in healthy young
men and should not be regarded as unequivocal evidence of
air trapping in the absence of supportive evidence.

On CT scan, the diaphragm can be visualized only where
its upper surface interfaces with the lung and the inferior
surface interfaces with intra-abdominal fat.[317] Although it is
not visualized in areas where it abuts structures of similar
soft tissue attenuation, such as the liver and spleen, its position can be inferred because at all levels, the lungs and
pleura lie adjacent and peripheral to it whereas the abdominal viscera lie central to it (Fig. 1–82).[317] The posterior or
lumbar portion of the diaphragm is well visualized at the
point where the fibers arising from the crura and arcuate
ligament arch forward to insert into the central tendon
(Fig. 1–83).

FIGURE 1–82

Anterior portion of the diaphragm. A CT scan at the level of the
xiphoid demonstrates continuity between the anterior (xiphoid) and lateral
(costal) diaphragmatic fibers *(arrows)*. The diaphragm is well visualized in
areas where it is outlined by lung and peritoneal or retroperitoneal fat.
Where it abuts structures of similar soft tissue attenuation, such as the
liver and spleen, it is not visualized; however, its position can be inferred
because of its relationship to the lungs and pleura (adjacent and peripheral
to it) and the abdominal viscera (central to it). (*From Fraser RS, Müller NL,
Colman NC, Paré PD: Fraser and Paré's Diagnosis of Diseases of the Chest,
4th ed. Philadelphia, WB Saunders, 1999.*)

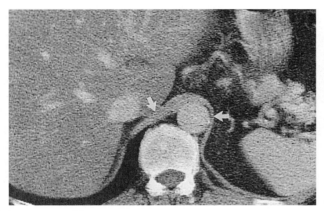

FIGURE 1–83

Lumbar portion of the diaphragm. A CT scan demonstrates the right and left crura *(arrows)* extending to the aorta. Posterolaterally, the crural fibers merge smoothly and indistinguishably with fibers arising from the medial arcuate ligaments. *(From Fraser RS, Müller NL, Colman NC, Paré PD: Fraser and Paré's Diagnosis of Diseases of the Chest, 4th ed. Philadelphia, WB Saunders, 1999.)*

The Respiratory Pump

The muscles of ventilation are striated and generally behave in the same fashion as other skeletal muscles. However, they differ in two important respects: (1) they are under voluntary as well as automatic control, and (2) in contrast to the inertial loads facing most other skeletal muscle, they must principally overcome resistive and elastic loads.[310]

The force generated by the contracting diaphragm is a function of muscle fiber length, the mechanical advantage of the muscle, the loads on the muscle, and the intensity of muscle activation. Like all skeletal muscles, respiratory muscles have a characteristic length-tension relationship. There is a specific optimal length at which maximal crossbridging between actin and myosin fibers occurs; at this length, maximal force can be generated with a given stimulation. As the fibers are lengthened or shortened beyond this point, the tension generated by a given stimulus is decreased. Thus, hyperinflation, as occurs in patients who have obstructive lung disease, decreases the efficiency of the diaphragm by shortening muscle fiber length.

When the diaphragm contracts, it not only pushes down on the abdominal viscera and displaces the abdominal wall outward but also lifts and expands the chest cage because of rib articulation and its insertion onto the lower ribs. The mechanical advantage of a dome-shaped muscle such as the diaphragm is related to its radius of curvature; the greater the curvature (the smaller the radius), the more pressure generated for a given tension (law of Laplace). The abdominal and accessory muscles can act as fixators or positioning muscles; they adjust the configuration of the diaphragm, rib cage, and abdomen in a manner that optimizes the curvature and thus the efficiency of the diaphragm.[310] This function is particularly evident in the upright position and especially during exercise when abdominal muscle contraction during expiration tends to lengthen the diaphragmatic muscle fibers.

The abdominal expiratory muscles also can aid inspiration by decreasing the end-expiratory lung volume below the relaxed volume of the rib cage and abdomen and then suddenly relaxing at the onset of inspiration; the resulting sudden descent of the diaphragm along its passive length-tension curve represents an energy-independent inspiratory contribution. This strategy is used by normal individuals in the hyperpnea of carbon dioxide rebreathing and exercise and by patients who have bilateral diaphragmatic paralysis.[318] The maneuver is effective in the upright and lateral decubitus positions but ineffective in the supine position, which probably accounts for the characteristic increase in dyspnea noted by patients with bilateral diaphragmatic paralysis when they assume the supine posture.[318]

THE CHEST WALL

Soft Tissues

The pectoral muscles form the anterior axillary fold, a structure that is normally visible on PA radiographs in both men and women; this fold curves smoothly downward and medially from the axilla to the rib cage. In men, particularly those with heavy muscular development, the inferior border of the pectoralis major may be seen as a downward extension of the anterior axillary fold that passes obliquely across the middle portion of both lungs. In women, this shadow is obscured by the breasts, whose presence and size must be taken into consideration when assessing the density of the lower lung zones.

Because of the fat planes separating the various muscle groups, CT and MR images allow identification of the majority of individual chest wall muscles. The outer anterior chest wall musculature is composed mainly of the pectoralis major (larger and more superficial) and the pectoralis minor (Fig. 1–84). The serratus anterior is located immediately superficial to the ribs on the lateral aspect of the thorax. The posterior chest wall musculature is more complex and includes superficial, intermediate, and deep muscles.[317] The first of these muscle groups controls arm motion and includes the trapezius, latissimus dorsi, levator scapulae, and rhomboid muscles. The intermediate muscles are inspiratory and include the superior and inferior serratus posterior muscles. The deep muscles lie adjacent to the vertebral column and regulate its motion.

The external and internal intercostal muscles lie between the ribs and cannot usually be distinguished from each other on CT or MR imaging. The innermost intercostal muscles together with the parietal pleura and endothoracic fascia are visualized as a 1- to 2-mm-thick line or stripe in the interspaces along the anterior and posterior costal pleural surfaces.[319] The transversus thoracis muscle is a small muscle that arises from the lower part of the sternum and attaches to the superolateral aspect of the second to the fifth costal cartilage.[317] It is seen on CT at the level of the heart as a thin line internal to the anterior costal cartilage.[319] The subcostal muscles are small muscles that extend from the angle of the rib to the internal surface of the adjacent lower rib.[317] They are seen on CT in a small number of patients as a 1- to 2-mm-thick line covering the inner surface of a posterior rib or ribs at the level of the heart.[319]

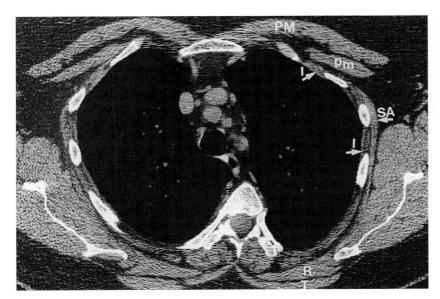

FIGURE 1–84

Chest wall muscles. A CT scan demonstrates normal chest wall muscles seen in cross section. These muscles may be divided into an anterior group (including the pectoralis major [PM] and pectoralis minor [pm]) and a posterior group (including the trapezius [T], rhomboideus [R], and the paraspinal muscles). The serratus anterior (SA) lies on the lateral aspect of the rib cage, whereas the intercostal muscles (I) lie between the ribs. *(From Fraser RS, Müller NL, Colman NC, Paré PD: Fraser and Paré's Diagnosis of Diseases of the Chest, 4th ed. Philadelphia, WB Saunders, 1999.)*

Bones

In the absence of pulmonary or pleural disease, deformity of the spine, or congenital anomalies of the ribs themselves, the rib cage should be symmetrical. Both the upper and lower borders of the ribs should be sharply defined except in the middle and lower thoracic regions; here, the thin flanges formed by the vascular sulci on the inferior aspects of the ribs posteriorly are viewed en face, thereby creating a less distinct margin.

Because of their oblique orientation, only a small portion of any given rib is seen on a single CT section.[317,320] Identification of a specific rib can be achieved by identifying the thoracic spine level adjacent to the posterior end of the rib.[317] The first rib can be identified readily because it lies adjacent to the medial end of the clavicle at the level of the sternoclavicular joint. The second, third, and fourth ribs can usually be identified at the same level by counting posteriorly along the rib cage (Fig. 1–85). By proceeding sequentially and

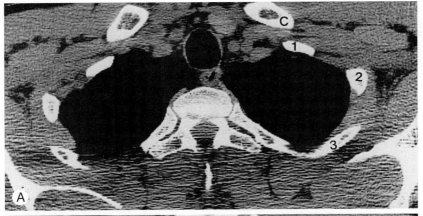
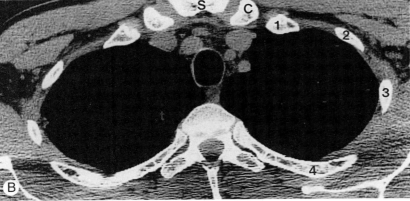

FIGURE 1–85

Ribs in cross section. An HRCT scan at the level of the thoracic inlet (**A**) demonstrates the right and left clavicles (C) and the first (1), second (2), and third (3) ribs. A second scan at the level of the sternoclavicular joint (**B**) demonstrates the upper part of the sternum (S) and the medial end of the clavicles (C). The first costal cartilage (1) and the second (2), third (3), and fourth (4) ribs can be identified by counting posteriorly along the rib cage. The fourth rib can be seen attached to the fourth thoracic vertebra. *(From Fraser RS, Müller NL, Colman NC, Paré PD: Fraser and Paré's Diagnosis of Diseases of the Chest, 4th ed. Philadelphia, WB Saunders, 1999.)*

caudad, each next vertebra and corresponding rib can be identified.

Calcification of rib cartilage is common. It usually begins with the first and is probably never of pathologic significance. The relationship between age and costal cartilage calcification differs in men and women: in the former, it is uncommon before the age of 20 years but progressively increases in frequency such that almost 90% of men 60 years and older have marginal calcification; by contrast, in women, central calcification is present in 45% of those younger than 20 years and in almost 90% older than 60 years.[321]

Thin, smooth shadows of water density that parallel the ribs and measure 1 to 2 mm in diameter project adjacent to the inferior and inferolateral margins of the first and second ribs and to the axillary portions of the lower ribs. These *"companion shadows"* (Fig. 1–86) are caused by visualization in tangential projection of parietal pleura and the soft tissues (principally fat) immediately external to the pleura and should not be interpreted as local pleural thickening. Extrapleural fat is most abundant over the fourth to eighth ribs posterolaterally and relates chiefly to the ribs rather than to the interspaces.[322]

Congenital anomalies of the ribs are relatively uncommon. *Supernumerary ribs* arising from the seventh cervical vertebra have been identified in 1% to 2% of otherwise normal individuals; nearly all are bilateral, although many are asymmetrical. Other anomalies, such as hypoplasia of the first rib, bifid or splayed anterior ribs, and rarely, local fusion of ribs, are usually important only in that they may give rise to an erroneous interpretation of abnormal lung density.

Occasionally, the inferior aspect of the clavicles has an irregular notch or indentation 2 to 3 cm from the sternal articulation; its size and shape vary from a superficial saucer-shaped defect to a deep notch 2 cm wide by 1.0 to 1.5 cm deep. These *rhomboid fossae* (Fig. 1–87) give rise to the costoclavicular, or rhomboid, ligaments that radiate downward to bind the clavicles to the first rib.[323]

The normal *thoracic spine* is straight in frontal projection and gently concave anteriorly in lateral projection. Its radiographic density in lateral projection decreases uniformly from above downward, and any deviation from this pattern should arouse suspicion of disease. The lateral and superior borders of the *manubrium* are the only portions of the sternum visible on frontal projections of the thorax, although the whole of the sternum should be clearly seen tangentially on lateral radiographs.

THE NORMAL LUNG: RADIOGRAPHY

Radiographic Density

The radiopacity of the lungs is a result of the absorptive powers of each of its component—gas, blood, and tissue. The density of bloodless collapsed lung tissue is 1.065 g/mL[324]; the density of blood is 1.052 g/mL.[325] Thus, because nonaerated lung in vivo consists of approximately half blood and half tissue,[326] the mean density of collapsed lung containing blood is approximately 1.06 g/mL.[327] By comparison, water has a density of 1.0 g/mL, and air has a density of 0. By using the average figures for total maximal tissue volume derived from anatomic and physiologic estimates and the predicted TLC of a 20-year-old man 170 cm tall (6500 mL),[328] the *average* density of lung is 740 g ÷ 7198 mL, or 0.103 g/mL. A considerable portion of lung tissue—logically, the air-containing parenchyma—must possess a density *less* than this value to compensate for the relatively high density of the visible blood vessels.

Symmetry of radiographic density of the two lungs in a normal individual depends on proper positioning for radiography. If the patient is rotated, the lung closer to the film is

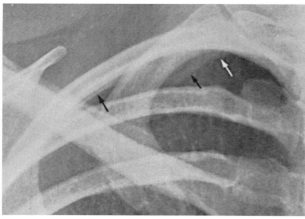

FIGURE 1–86

Companion shadows of the ribs. A magnified view of the apex of the right hemithorax reveals thin smooth shadows of water density lying roughly parallel to the inferior surfaces of the first and second ribs *(arrows)*. These companion shadows are caused by the perception in the tangential projection of a combination of parietal and visceral pleura and the soft tissues immediately external to the pleura. *(From Fraser RS, Müller NL, Colman NC, Paré PD: Fraser and Paré's Diagnosis of Diseases of the Chest, 4th ed. Philadelphia, WB Saunders, 1999.)*

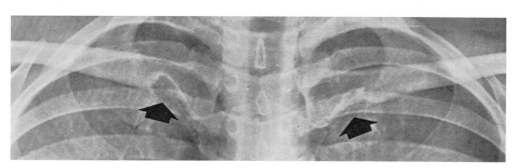

FIGURE 1–87

Rhomboid fossae. An irregular notch is present in the inferior aspect of both clavicles approximately 2 cm from their sternal end *(arrows)*. These fossae give origin to the costoclavicular or rhomboid ligaments. *(From Fraser RS, Müller NL, Colman NC, Paré PD: Fraser and Paré's Diagnosis of Diseases of the Chest, 4th ed. Philadelphia, WB Saunders, 1999.)*

more uniformly radiopaque (whiter) than the other lung (Fig. 1–88); conversely, the lung that is farthest away from the film is uniformly less radiopaque (more black), and a unilateral hyperlucent hemithorax is present that can sometimes hamper interpretation. In one investigation using phantoms, approximately 80% of this unilateral increase in radiographic

density was found to be the result of asymmetrical absorption of the primary x-ray beam, with the remaining 20% being due to scatter radiation.[329] Measurement of chest wall thickness showed that the x-ray beam traversed less tissue on the side of increased film blackening (or conversely, more tissue on the side of increased opacity), chiefly as a result of the pectoral muscles.

Provided that the patient is not rotated and the x-ray beam is centered properly, any discrepancy in the density of the two lungs must be interpreted as being abnormal. The cause varies from such benign conditions as scoliosis and congenital absence of the pectoral muscles to more significant disorders such as Swyer-James syndrome.

Pulmonary Markings

Correct interpretation of the chest radiograph requires a thorough knowledge of the pattern of linear markings throughout the normal lung. These markings are created by the pulmonary arteries, bronchi, veins, and accompanying interstitial tissue. The first two of these markings fan outward from both hila and gradually taper as they proceed distally. In the normal state, they are visible up to about 1 to 2 cm from the visceral pleural surface over the convexity of the lung, at which point it is composed predominantly of acini.

The PA chest radiograph of a normal erect individual invariably shows some discrepancy in the size of the pulmonary vessels in the upper lung zones as compared with the lower lung zones as a result of pressure-related differences in blood flow from the apex to the base (a unit volume of lung at the base of the thorax has four to eight times the blood flow of a similar volume at the apex[330]). In a recumbent individual, a decrease in the influence of gravity renders this discrepancy in vascular size minimal.

THE NORMAL LUNG: COMPUTED TOMOGRAPHY

A cross-sectional CT image of the thorax is a two-dimensional representation of a three-dimensional slice; the third dimension—slice thickness, or CT collimation—can vary from 0.5 to 10 mm. All structures within the three-dimensional unit (volume = voxel) of the slice are represented as a two-dimensional unit (area = pixel) on the image. Thicker sections (5- to 10-mm collimation) allow assessment of the entire lung volume. Such assessment can usually be made during a single breath-hold when a spiral CT technique is used. On such thick sections, vessels can be identified clearly within the lung parenchyma as they course through the slice (Fig. 1–89). Volume averaging within the plane of section results in decreased spatial resolution, however, and assessment of fine parenchymal detail requires the use of 1- to 2-mm-collimation scans. The resulting thinner sections allow assessment of airways 1.5 to 2 mm in diameter and vessels down to the level of the interlobular septal veins and centrilobular arteries.[80,331] Because of the thin section, however, vessels cut in cross section may be difficult to distinguish from small nodules.

The appearance of bronchi and vessels depends on their orientation: when imaged along their long axes, they appear as cylindrical structures that taper as they branch; when imaged at an angle to their longitudinal axes, they appear

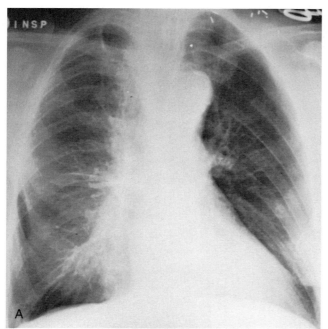

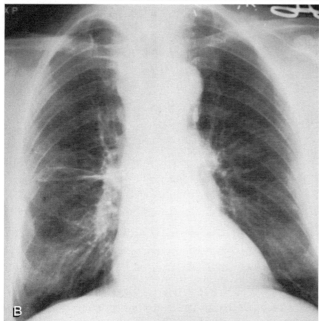

FIGURE 1–88

Alteration in lung density as a result of improper positioning. A, A radiograph of the chest in a posteroanterior projection was exposed with the patient rotated slightly into the right anterior oblique position to produce an overall increase in density of the right lung as compared with the left. In **B,** positioning has been corrected, and the asymmetry has disappeared. *(From Fraser RS, Müller NL, Colman NC, Paré PD: Fraser and Paré's Diagnosis of Diseases of the Chest, 4th ed. Philadelphia, WB Saunders, 1999.)*

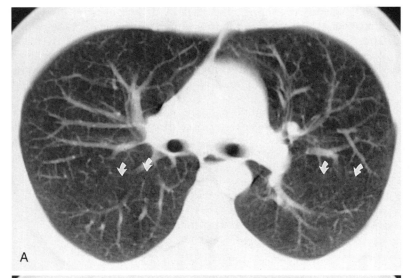

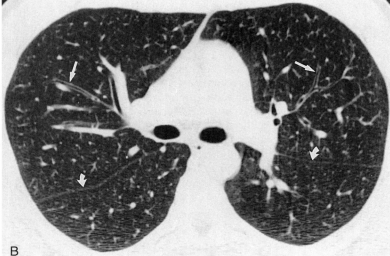

FIGURE 1-89

Comparison of conventional CT and HRCT. A 10-mm-collimation CT scan at the level of the bronchus intermedius (**A**) demonstrates normal lung parenchyma and airways as visualized on conventional CT. Pulmonary vessels can easily be identified as they course within the 10-mm thickness of the CT section. A 1-mm-collimation HRCT scan (**B**) performed at the same level reveals sharper definition between vessels and bronchi and the adjacent lung parenchyma than seen with conventional CT. Bronchi measuring approximately 2 mm in diameter *(straight arrows)* are clearly identified on the HRCT image but not on conventional CT. Interlobar fissures *(curved arrows)* appear as sharply defined lines on the HRCT image as opposed to the broad areas of slightly increased attenuation on the corresponding conventional CT image. Both images were reconstructed with a high-resolution algorithm and photographed at a window level of -700 and window width of 1500 Hounsfield units. *(From Fraser RS, Müller NL, Colman NC, Paré PD: Fraser and Paré's Diagnosis of Diseases of the Chest, 4th ed. Philadelphia, WB Saunders, 1999.)*

as rounded structures if perpendicular to the plane of the CT scan or as elliptical structures when oriented obliquely. The outer walls of pulmonary vessels form smooth, sharply defined interfaces with the surrounding lung. Central pulmonary vessels can be readily recognized as arteries by their location adjacent to bronchi. Central pulmonary veins can be identified as they course toward the left atrium. Although it is often impossible to distinguish peripheral pulmonary arteries from veins by conventional CT, differentiation can frequently be accomplished by HRCT. With this technique, veins can be identified as structures that separate secondary pulmonary lobules, extend into interlobular septa, and (sometimes) reach the pleura[332]; by contrast, pulmonary arteries lie near the center of the pulmonary lobule and do not abut the pleura.

The smallest normal airways that can be identified on CT scan are 1.5 to 2 mm in diameter[331]; smaller branches cannot be visualized because their walls are less than 0.1 mm thick and below the spatial resolution of current CT scanners. In normal individuals, no airways can be visualized within 1 cm of the costal or paravertebral pleura; however, they can be identified within 1 cm of the mediastinal pleura (but not

abutting it) in approximately 40%.[333] The smallest pulmonary artery that can be resolved by HRCT is approximately 0.2 mm in diameter and corresponds to the artery accompanying a terminal bronchiole.[331] The distance from this artery to the border of the secondary lobule or the pleural surface ranges from 3 to 5 mm.

The outer diameter of a bronchus is approximately equal to that of the adjacent pulmonary artery.[334] The *apparent* bronchial wall thickness and the diameter of bronchi and vessels are markedly influenced by the display parameters used (window level and window width). The results of studies using phantoms show that accurate assessment of the size of small parenchymal structures requires the use of a display level of -450 Hounsfield units (HU).[335,336] For clinical practice, we recommend the use of a window level of -600 to -700 HU and a window width of 1000 to 1500 HU because these settings provide the best depiction of airways and lung parenchyma. These display parameter settings result in an overestimation of the diameter of small structures and bronchial wall thickness and an underestimation of the diameter of the bronchial lumen.

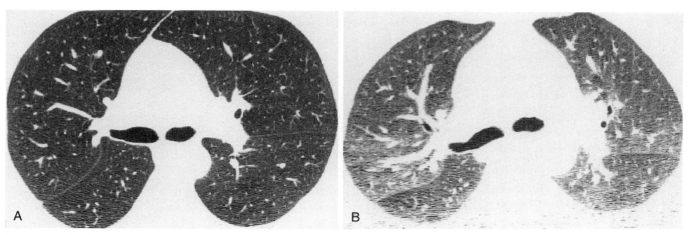

FIGURE 1–90

Increased attenuation on expiratory HRCT. Inspiratory (**A**) and expiratory (**B**) HRCT scans at the level of the main bronchi in a 35-year-old woman demonstrate the normal increase in attenuation seen at low lung volumes. The attenuation gradient from least dependent to most dependent lung regions is more readily seen on the expiratory CT scan. Note that the increase in attenuation is not homogeneous because a discontinuity is present at the level of the major fissures, with the posterior aspect of the upper lobes having greater attenuation than the superior segments of the left lower lobes. *(From Fraser RS, Müller NL, Colman NC, Paré PD: Fraser and Paré's Diagnosis of Diseases of the Chest, 4th ed. Philadelphia, WB Saunders, 1999.)*

The pulmonary artery–to–outer bronchial diameter ratio (ABR) has been assessed by many workers. In one investigation of 30 patients who did not have cardiopulmonary disease,[334] diameters were assessed at the level of subsegmental bronchi with a window level of −450 HU and a window width of 1200 to 1500 HU. The mean ABR was 0.98 ± 0.14 (range, 0.53 to 1.39)—a value comparable to that reported on chest radiographs in supine healthy individuals (1.04 ± 0.13).[145] Because an increased ratio of inner bronchial diameter to pulmonary artery diameter is one of the CT criteria for the diagnosis of bronchiectasis,[333] this ratio is another parameter that has been investigated in normal individuals. The measurement has been found to be influenced by altitude, presumably as a result of a combination of hypoxic vasoconstriction and bronchodilation.[337,338]

The attenuation of lung parenchyma is determined by its relative proportions of blood, gas, extravascular fluid, and pulmonary tissue.[339,340] Normal lung parenchyma has a fairly homogeneous attenuation that is slightly greater than that of air. A gradient is normally present, however, with attenuation being greater in dependent than nondependent regions.[340,341] This gradient is attributable primarily to the influence of gravity on blood flow and lung inflation.

CT scans of the chest are usually performed during suspended full inspiration. In selected cases, scans may be performed during or after forced expiration. As lung gas volume is reduced, lung attenuation increases, the increase being greater in the dependent than the nondependent regions (Fig. 1–90).[342,343] This increase is variable in different lung regions; for example, in one study it ranged from 84 to 372 HU.[342] Focal areas of low attenuation are frequently seen on expiratory scans, particularly in the superior segments of the lower lobes and the anterior aspects of the right middle lobe and lingula.[342] Such areas are presumably the result of focal air trapping.[342] The extent of air trapping in normal individuals is usually limited to small, localized areas involving a few secondary lobules; it can be seen on expiratory HRCT in 90% of such individuals.[344] Air trapping involving a total volume equal to or greater than that of a pulmonary segment is also seen in approximately 10% to 15% of normal individuals.[344,345] It is the extent and not simply the presence of air trapping that is important in determining the presence of airway obstruction.

Lung Density

Measurement of lung density with CT is based on the existence of an approximately linear relationship between the attenuation of an x-ray beam of 65 keV (120 kVp) and the density of materials of low atomic number (ranging from nitrogen to water).[339,346] Attenuation on a CT scan is expressed in terms of the Hounsfield unit scale, in which water is 0 HU and air is −1000 HU. The relationship between physical density—weight of tissue per unit volume—and the Hounsfield scale can be expressed by using a *scaled CT quotient,* which is obtained by adding 1000 to the Hounsfield value and then dividing by 1000. With this formulation, CT quotient values that range from air to water are approximately equal to physical density in grams per milliliter.[339,340] For example, a CT attenuation value of −880 HU (approximately the mean value for normal lung at TLC) represents a scaled CT quotient of 120 or a density equivalent of 0.12 g/mL.

Attenuation values vary considerably in different regions of the lung and are markedly influenced by pulmonary volume. Values are affected by the type of CT scanner, kilovoltage, patient size, and the particular region of lung being assessed.[347,348] As a result, measurements of lung attenuation have a limited role in the radiologic assessment of lung parenchyma. The principal exception is the use of attenuation values in determining the presence, distribution, and extent of emphysema.

REFERENCES

1. Horsfield K, Cumming G: Morphology of the bronchial tree in man. J Appl Physiol 24:373-383, 1968.
2. Gail DB, Lenfant CJ: Cells of the lung: Biology and clinical implications. Am Rev Respir Dis 127:366-387, 1983.
3. Kilburn K: A hypothesis for pulmonary clearance and its implications. Am Rev Respir Dis 98:449, 1968.
4. Nathanson I, Nadel JA: Movement of electrolytes and fluid across airways. Lung 162:125-137, 1984.
5. Kuhn C: Ciliated and Clara cells. In Bouhuys A (ed): Lung Cells in Disease. New York, Elsevier, 1976, p 91.
6. Emery N, Place GA, Dodd S, et al: Mucous and serous secretions of human bronchial epithelial cells in secondary culture. Am J Respir Cell Mol Biol 12:130-141, 1995.
7. Smith SM, Lee DK, Lacy J, et al: Rat tracheal epithelial cells produce granulocyte/macrophage colony-stimulating factor. Am J Respir Cell Mol Biol 2:59-68, 1990.
8. Rossi GA, Sacco O, Balbi B, et al: Human ciliated bronchial epithelial cells: Expression of the HLA-DR antigens and of the HLA-DR alpha gene, modulation of the HLA-DR antigens by gamma-interferon and antigen-presenting function in the mixed leukocyte reaction. Am J Respir Cell Mol Biol 3:431-439, 1990.
9. Yao PM, Delclaux C, d'Ortho MP, et al: Cell-matrix interactions modulate 92-kD gelatinase expression by human bronchial epithelial cells. Am J Respir Cell Mol Biol 18:813-822, 1998.
10. Lumsden AB, McLean A, Lamb D: Goblet and Clara cells of human distal airways: Evidence for smoking induced changes in their numbers. Thorax 39:844-849, 1984.
11. Boers JE, Ambergen AW, Thunnissen FB: Number and proliferation of basal and parabasal cells in normal human airway epithelium. Am J Respir Crit Care Med 157:2000-2006, 1998.
12. Breuer R, Zajicek G, Christensen TG, et al: Cell kinetics of normal adult hamster bronchial epithelium in the steady state. Am J Respir Cell Mol Biol 2:51-58, 1990.
13. Evans MJ, Cox RA, Shami SG, et al: The role of basal cells in attachment of columnar cells to the basal lamina of the trachea. Am J Respir Cell Mol Biol 1:463-469, 1989.
14. Shimizu T, Nishihara M, Kawaguchi S, et al: Expression of phenotypic markers during regeneration of rat tracheal epithelium following mechanical injury. Am J Respir Cell Mol Biol 11:85-94, 1994.
15. Lane BP, Gordon R: Regeneration of rat tracheal epithelium after mechanical injury. I. The relationship between mitotic activity and cellular differentiation. Proc Soc Exp Biol Med 145:1139-1144, 1974.
16. Phelps DS, Floros J: Localization of pulmonary surfactant proteins using immunohistochemistry and tissue in situ hybridization. Exp Lung Res 17:985-995, 1991.
17. Massaro GD, Singh G, Mason R, et al: Biology of the Clara cell. Am J Physiol 266:L101-L106, 1994.
18. Jorens PG, Sibille Y, Goulding NJ, et al: Potential role of Clara cell protein, an endogenous phospholipase A₂ inhibitor, in acute lung injury. Eur Respir J 8:1647-1653, 1995.
19. Stripp BR, Reynolds SD, Boe IM, et al: Clara cell secretory protein deficiency alters Clara cell secretory apparatus and the protein composition of airway lining fluid. Am J Respir Cell Mol Biol 27:170-178, 2002.
19a. Iannuzzi MC: Clara cell protein in sarcoidosis. Another job for the respiratory tract protector? Am J Respir Crit Care Med 169:143-146, 2004.
20. Nomori H, Horio H, Fuyuno G, et al: Protein 1 (Clara cell protein) serum levels in healthy subjects and patients with bacterial pneumonia. Am J Respir Crit Care Med 152:746-750, 1995.
21. Bernard AM, Roels HA, Buchet JP, et al: Serum Clara cell protein: An indicator of bronchial cell dysfunction caused by tobacco smoking. Environ Res 66:96-104, 1994.
21a. Sengler C, Heinzmann A, Jerkic SP, et al: Clara cell protein 16 (CC16) gene polymorphism influences the degree of airway responsiveness in asthmatic children. J Allergy Clin Immunol 111:515-519, 2003.
22. Evans MJ, Cabral-Anderson LJ, Freeman G: Role of the Clara cell in renewal of the bronchiolar epithelium. Lab Invest 38:648-653, 1978.
23. De Water R, Willems LN, Van Muijen GN, et al: Ultrastructural localization of bronchial antileukoprotease in central and peripheral human airways by a gold-labeling technique using monoclonal antibodies. Am Rev Respir Dis 133:882-890, 1986.
24. Johnson DE, Georgieff MK: Pulmonary neuroendocrine cells. Their secretory products and their potential roles in health and chronic lung disease in infancy. Am Rev Respir Dis 140:1807-1812, 1989.
25. Cutz E: Neuroendocrine cells of the lung. An overview of morphologic characteristics and development. Exp Lung Res 3:185-208, 1982.
26. Keith IM, Will JA: Hypoxia and the neonatal rabbit lung: Neuroendocrine cell numbers, 5-HT fluorescence intensity, and the relationship to arterial thickness. Thorax 36:767-773, 1981.
27. Sanghavi JN, Rabe KF, Kim JS, et al: Migration of human and guinea pig airway epithelial cells in response to calcitonin gene–related peptide. Am J Respir Cell Mol Biol 11:181-187, 1994.
28. Lauweryns JM, Cokelaere J, Theunynck P: Serotonin producing neuroepithelial bodies in rabbit respiratory mucosa. Science 180:410-413, 1973.
29. Hance AJ: Pulmonary immune cells in health and disease: Dendritic cells and Langerhans' cells. Eur Respir J 6:1213-1220, 1993.
30. Schon-Hegrad MA, Oliver J, McMenamin PG, et al: Studies on the density, distribution, and surface phenotype of intraepithelial class II major histocompatibility complex antigen (Ia)-bearing dendritic cells (DC) in the conducting airways. J Exp Med 173:1345-1356, 1991.
31. Toews GB: Pulmonary dendritic cells: Sentinels of lung-associated lymphoid tissues. Am J Respir Cell Mol Biol 4:204-205, 1991.
32. Erle DJ, Pabst R: Intraepithelial lymphocytes in the lung: A neglected lymphocyte population. Am J Respir Cell Mol Biol 22:398-400, 2000.
33. Lamb D, Lumsden A: Intra-epithelial mast cells in human airway epithelium: Evidence for smoking-induced changes in their frequency. Thorax 37:334-342, 1982.
34. Evans MJ, Guha SC, Cox RA, et al: Attenuated fibroblast sheath around the basement membrane zone in the trachea. Am J Respir Cell Mol Biol 8:188-192, 1993.
35. Evans MJ, Van Winkle LS, Fanucchi MV, et al: The attenuated fibroblast sheath of the respiratory tract epithelial-mesenchymal trophic unit. Am J Respir Cell Mol Biol 21:655-657, 1999.
36. Krahl V: Anatomy of the mammalian lung. In Fenn W, Rahn H (eds): Handbook of Physiology. Section 3, Respiration. Washington, DC, American Physiological Society, 1964, pp 213-284.
37. Ebina M, Yaegashi H, Takahashi T, et al: Distribution of smooth muscles along the bronchial tree. a morphometric study of ordinary autopsy lungs. Am Rev Respir Dis 141:1322-1326, 1990.
38. Whimster WF, Lord P, Biles B: Tracheobronchial gland profiles in four segmental airways. Am Rev Respir Dis 129:985-988, 1984.
39. Vogel L, Schoonbrood D, Geluk F, et al: Iron-binding proteins in sputum of chronic bronchitis patients with Haemophilus influenzae infections. Eur Respir J 10:2327-2333, 1997.
40. Brandtzaeg P: Mucosal and glandular distribution of immunoglobulin components: Differential localization of free and bound SC in secretory epithelial cells. J Immunol 112:1553-1559, 1974.
41. Bienenstock J, Clancy R, Perey D: Bronchus-associated lymphoid tissue (BALT): Its relationship to mucosal immunity. In Kirkpatrick C, Reynolds H (eds): Immunologic and Infectious Reactions in the Lung. New York, Marcel Dekker, 1976, p 29.
42. Pabst R, Gehrke I: Is the bronchus-associated lymphoid tissue (BALT) an integral structure of the lung in normal mammals, including humans? Am J Respir Cell Mol Biol 3:131-135, 1990.
43. Holt PG: Development of bronchus associated lymphoid tissue (BALT) in human lung disease: A normal host defense mechanism awaiting therapeutic exploitation? Thorax 48:1097-1098, 1993.
44. Richmond I, Pritchard GE, Ashcroft T, et al: Bronchus associated lymphoid tissue (BALT) in human lung: Its distribution in smokers and non-smokers. Thorax 48:1130-1134, 1993.
45. Soutar CA: Distribution of plasma cells and other cells containing immunoglobulin in the respiratory tract of normal man and class of immunoglobulin contained therein. Thorax 31:158-166, 1976.
46. Holt PG, Oliver J, Bilyk N, et al: Downregulation of the antigen presenting cell function(s) of pulmonary dendritic cells in vivo by resident alveolar macrophages. J Exp Med 177:397-407, 1993.
47. Geiser M, Baumann M, Cruz-Orive LM, et al: The effect of particle inhalation on macrophage number and phagocytic activity in the intrapulmonary conducting airways of hamsters. Am J Respir Cell Mol Biol 10:594-603, 1994.
48. Schreider JP, Raabe OG: Structure of the human respiratory acinus. Am J Anat 162:221-232, 1981.
49. Angus GE, Thurlbeck WM: Number of alveoli in the human lung. J Appl Physiol 32:483-485, 1972.
50. Thurlbeck WM: The internal surface area of nonemphysematous lungs. Am Rev Respir Dis 95:765-773, 1967.
51. Crapo JD, Barry BE, Gehr P, et al: Cell number and cell characteristics of the normal human lung. Am Rev Respir Dis 126:332-337, 1982.
52. Bartels H: The air-blood barrier in the human lung. A freeze-fracture study. Cell Tissue Res 198:269-285, 1979.
53. Schneeberger E: The integrity of the air-blood barrier. In Brian J, Proctor D, Reid L (eds): Respiratory Defense Mechanisms. New York, Marcel Dekker, 1977, p 687.
54. Heppleston AG, Young AE: Uptake of inert particulate matter by alveolar cells: An ultrastructural study. J Pathol 111:159-164, 1973.
55. Kikkawa Y, Smith F: Cellular and biochemical aspects of pulmonary surfactant in health and disease. Lab Invest 49:122-139, 1983.
56. Kikkawa Y: Morphology of alveolar lining layer. Anat Rec 167:389-400, 1970.
57. Gil J, Weibel ER: Improvements in demonstration of lining layer of lung alveoli by electron microscopy. Respir Physiol 8:13-36, 1969.
58. Crystal R: Biochemical processes in the normal lung. In Bouhuys A (ed): Lung Cells in Disease. New York, Elsevier, 1976, p 17.
59. Crouch EC, Moxley MA, Longmore W: Synthesis of collagenous proteins by pulmonary type II epithelial cells. Am Rev Respir Dis 135:1118-1123, 1987.
60. Boutten A, Venembre P, Seta N, et al: Oncostatin M is a potent stimulator of alpha1-antitrypsin secretion in lung epithelial cells: Modulation by transforming growth factor-beta and interferon-gamma. Am J Respir Cell Mol Biol 18:511-520, 1998.
61. Paine R 3rd, Mody CH, Chavis A, et al: Alveolar epithelial cells block lymphocyte proliferation in vitro without inhibiting activation. Am J Respir Cell Mol Biol 5:221-229, 1991.
62. van Iwaarden F, Welmers B, Verhoef J, et al: Pulmonary surfactant protein A enhances the host-defense mechanism of rat alveolar macrophages. Am J Respir Cell Mol Biol 2:91-98, 1990.
63. Starcher BC: Elastin and the lung. Thorax 41:577-585, 1986.
64. Laurent GJ: Lung collagen: More than scaffolding. Thorax 41:418-428, 1986.

65. Kapanci Y, Assimacopoulos A, Irle C, et al: "Contractile interstitial cells" in pulmonary alveolar septa: A possible regulator of ventilation-perfusion ratio? Ultrastructural, immunofluorescence, and in vitro studies. J Cell Biol 60:375-392, 1974.

66. Weibel E, Bachofen A: Structural design of the alveolar septum and fluid exchange. In Fishman A, Renkin E (eds): Pulmonary Edema. Bethesda, MD, American Physiological Society, 1979, p 1.

67. Vyalov SL, Gabbiani G, Kapanci Y: Rat alveolar myofibroblasts acquire alpha-smooth muscle actin expression during bleomycin-induced pulmonary fibrosis. Am J Pathol 143:1754-1765, 1993.

68. Dehring DJ, Wismar BL: Intravascular macrophages in pulmonary capillaries of humans. Am Rev Respir Dis 139:1027-1029, 1989.

69. Frankenberger M, Passlick B, Hofer T, et al: Immunologic characterization of normal human pleural macrophages. Am J Respir Cell Mol Biol 23:419-426, 2000.

70. Hocking WG, Golde DW: The pulmonary-alveolar macrophage (first of two parts). N Engl J Med 301:580-587, 1979.

71. van Haarst JM, Hoogsteden HC, de Wit HJ, et al: Dendritic cells and their precursors isolated from human bronchoalveolar lavage: Immunocytologic and functional properties. Am J Respir Cell Mol Biol 11:344-350, 1994.

72. Sibille Y, Reynolds HY: Macrophages and polymorphonuclear neutrophils in lung defense and injury. Am Rev Respir Dis 141:471-501, 1990.

73. Shellito J, Kaltreider HB: Heterogeneity of immunologic function among subfractions of normal rat alveolar macrophages. II. Activation as a determinant of functional activity. Am Rev Respir Dis 131:678-683, 1985.

74. Lay JC, Bennett WD, Kim CS, et al: Retention and intracellular distribution of instilled iron oxide particles in human alveolar macrophages. Am J Respir Cell Mol Biol 18:687-695, 1998.

75. Villiger B, Broekelmann T, Kelley D, et al: Bronchoalveolar fibronectin in smokers and nonsmokers. Am Rev Respir Dis 124:652-654, 1981.

76. Hancock A, Armstrong L, Gama R, et al: Production of interleukin 13 by alveolar macrophages from normal and fibrotic lung. Am J Respir Cell Mol Biol 18:60-65, 1998.

77. Fang FC, Vazquez-Torres A: Nitric oxide production by human macrophages: There's NO doubt about it. Am J Physiol Lung Cell Mol Physiol 282:L941-L943, 2002.

78. Nugent KM, Glazier J, Monick MM, et al: Stimulated human alveolar macrophages secrete interferon. Am Rev Respir Dis 131:714-718, 1985.

79. Reid L, Rubino M: The connective tissue septa in the foetal human lung. Thorax 14:3-13, 1959.

80. Webb WR, Stein MG, Finkbeiner WE, et al: Normal and diseased isolated lungs: High-resolution CT. Radiology 166:81-87, 1988.

81. Munk PL, Muller NL, Miller RR, et al: Pulmonary lymphangitic carcinomatosis: CT and pathologic findings. Radiology 166:705-709, 1988.

82. Storto ML, Kee ST, Golden JA, et al: Hydrostatic pulmonary edema: High-resolution CT findings. AJR Am J Roentgenol 165:817-820, 1995.

83. Muller NL, Miller RR: Diseases of the bronchioles: CT and histopathologic findings. Radiology 196:3-12, 1995.

84. Gruden JF, Webb WR, Warnock M: Centrilobular opacities in the lung on high-resolution CT: Diagnostic considerations and pathologic correlation. AJR Am J Roentgenol 162:569-574, 1994.

85. Raskin SP: The pulmonary acinus: Historical notes. Radiology 144:31-34, 1982.

86. Gamsu G, Thurlbeck WM, Macklem PT, et al: Roentgenographic appearance of the human pulmonary acinus. Invest Radiol 6:171-175, 1971.

87. Lui YM, Taylor JR, Zylak CJ: Roentgen-anatomical correlation of the individual human pulmonary acinus. Radiology 109:1-5, 1973.

88. Itoh H, Tokunaga S, Asamoto H, et al: Radiologic-pathologic correlations of small lung nodules with special reference to peribronchiolar nodules. AJR Am J Roentgenol 130:223-231, 1978.

89. Takaro T, Gaddy LR, Parra S: Thin alveolar epithelial partitions across connective tissue gaps in the alveolar wall of the human lung: Ultrastructural observations. Am Rev Respir Dis 126:326-331, 1982.

90. Takaro T, Price HP, Parra SC: Ultrastructural studies of apertures in the interalveolar septum of the adult human lung. Am Rev Respir Dis 119:425-434, 1979.

91. Pump KK: Fenestrae in the alveolar membrane of the human lung. Chest 65:431-436, 1974.

92. Lambert MW: Accessory bronchiole-alveolar communications. J Pathol Bacteriol 70:311-314, 1955.

93. Boyden E: Segmental Anatomy of the Lungs. New York, McGraw-Hill, 1955.

94. Jackson C, Huber J: Correlated applied anatomy of the bronchial tree and lungs with system of nomenclature. Dis Chest 9:319, 1943.

95. Naidich DP, Zinn WL, Ettenger NA, et al: Basilar segmental bronchi: Thin-section CT evaluation. Radiology 169:11-16, 1988.

96. Lee KS, Bae WK, Lee BH, et al: Bronchovascular anatomy of the upper lobes: Evaluation with thin-section CT. Radiology 181:765-772, 1991.

97. Gamsu G, Webb WR: Computed tomography of the trachea: Normal and abnormal. AJR Am J Roentgenol 139:321-326, 1982.

98. Breatnach E, Abbott GC, Fraser RG: Dimensions of the normal human trachea. AJR Am J Roentgenol 142:903-906, 1984.

99. Haskin PH, Goodman LR: Normal tracheal bifurcation angle: A reassessment. AJR Am J Roentgenol 139:879-882, 1982.

100. Fraser RG: Measurements of the calibre of human bronchi in three phases of respiration by cinebronchography. J Can Assoc Radiol 12:102-112, 1961.

101. Mead J: Mechanical properties of lungs. Physiol Rev 41:281-330, 1961.

102. Islam MS: Mechanism of controlling residual volume and emptying rate of the lung in young and elderly healthy subjects. Respiration 40:1-8, 1980.

103. Nogee LM: Abnormal expression of surfactant protein C and lung disease. Am J Respir Cell Mol Biol 26:641-644, 2002.

104. Wright JR: Pulmonary surfactant: A front line of lung host defense. J Clin Invest 111:1453-1455, 2003.

105. Albert RK, Lakshminarayan S, Hildebrandt J, et al: Increased surface tension favors pulmonary edema formation in anesthetized dogs' lungs. J Clin Invest 63:1015-1018, 1979.

106. Smaldone GC, Mitzner W, Itoh H: Role of alveolar recruitment in lung inflation: Influence on pressure-volume hysteresis. J Appl Physiol 55:1321-1332, 1983.

107. Rooney S: Regulation of surfactant associated phospholipid synthesis and secretion. In Polin R, Fox W (eds): Fetal and Neonatal Physiology. Philadelphia, WB Saunders, 1992, pp 971-985.

108. Mendelson CR, Boggaram V: Hormonal control of the surfactant system in fetal lung. Annu Rev Physiol 53:415-440, 1991.

109. Massaro GD, Massaro D: Morphologic evidence that large inflations of the lung stimulate secretion of surfactant. Am Rev Respir Dis 127:235-236, 1983.

110. Corbet A, Cregan J, Frink J, et al: Distention-produced phospholipid secretion in postmortem in situ lungs of newborn rabbits. Inhibition by specific beta-adrenergic blockade. Am Rev Respir Dis 128:695-701, 1983.

111. King M: Mucus and mucociliary clearance. Basic Respir Dis 11:1, 1982.

112. Ikegami M, Jobe AH: Surfactant metabolism. Semin Perinatol 17:233-240, 1993.

113. Lisboa C, Ross WR, Jardim J, et al: Pulmonary pressure-flow curves measured by a data-averaging circuit. J Appl Physiol 47:621-627, 1979.

114. Macklem PT, Mead J: Resistance of central and peripheral airways measured by a retrograde catheter. J Appl Physiol 22:395-401, 1967.

115. Ferris BG Jr, Mead J, Opie LH: Partitioning of respiratory flow resistance in man. J Appl Physiol 19:653-658, 1964.

116. Menkes H, Traystman R: Collateral ventilation, lung disease. In Murray J (ed): Lung Disease—State of the Art. New York, American Lung Association, 1978, p 87.

117. Inners CR, Terry PB, Traystman RJ, et al: Effects of lung volume on collateral and airways resistance in man. J Appl Physiol 46:67-73, 1979.

118. Jeffery P, Zhu J: Mucin-producing elements and inflammatory cells. Novartis Found Symp 248:51-68, discussion 68-75, 277-282, 2002.

119. Keal E: Physiological and pharmacological control of airway secretion. In Brian D, Proctor D, Reid L (eds): Respiratory Defense Mechanisms—Part 1. Lung Biology in Health and Disease. New York, Marcel Dekker, 1977.

120. Low RB, Davis GS, Giancola MS: Biochemical analyses of bronchoalveolar lavage fluids of healthy human volunteer smokers and nonsmokers. Am Rev Respir Dis 118:863-875, 1978.

121. Szabo S, Barbu Z, Lakatos L, et al: Local production of proteins in normal human bronchial secretion. Respiration 39:172-178, 1980.

122. Lopez-Vidriero MT, Das I, Smith AP, et al: Bronchial secretion from normal human airways after inhalation of prostaglandin $F_{2\alpha}$, acetylcholine, histamine, and citric acid. Thorax 32:734-739, 1977.

123. Ueki I, German VF, Nadel JA: Micropipette measurement of airway submucosal gland secretion. Autonomic effects. Am Rev Respir Dis 121:351-357, 1980.

124. Nadel JA: New approaches to regulation of fluid secretion in airways. Chest 80:849-851, 1981.

125. Nadel JA: Role of neutrophil elastase in hypersecretion during COPD exacerbations, and proposed therapies. Chest 117:386S-389S, 2000.

126. Sleigh M: The nature and action of respiratory tract cilia. In Brian J, Proctor D, Reid L (eds): Respiratory Defense Mechanisms—Part 1. Lung Biology in Health and Disease. New York, Marcel Dekker, 1977, pp 247-288.

127. Boucher RC: Human airway ion transport. Part one. Am J Respir Crit Care Med 150:271-281, 1994.

128. Boucher RC: Human airway ion transport. Part two. Am J Respir Crit Care Med 150:581-593, 1994.

129. Olver RE, Davis B, Marin MG, et al: Active transport of Na^+ and Cl^- across the canine tracheal epithelium in vitro. Am Rev Respir Dis 112:811-815, 1975.

130. Graham A, Alton EW, Geddes DM: Effects of 5-hydroxytryptamine and 5-hydroxytryptamine receptor agonists on ion transport across mammalian airway epithelia. Clin Sci (Lond) 83:331-336, 1992.

131. Fuchs HJ, Borowitz DS, Christiansen DH, et al: Effect of aerosolized recombinant human DNase on exacerbations of respiratory symptoms and on pulmonary function in patients with cystic fibrosis. The Pulmozyme Study Group. N Engl J Med 331:637-642, 1994.

132. Horsfield K: Morphometry of the small pulmonary arteries in man. Circ Res 42:593-597, 1978.

133. Hislop A, Reid L: Fetal and childhood development of the intrapulmonary veins in man—branching pattern and structure. Thorax 28:313-319, 1973.

134. Schraufnagel DE, Patel KR: Sphincters in pulmonary veins. An anatomic study in rats. Am Rev Respir Dis 141:721-726, 1990.

135. Heath D, Smith P: The pulmonary endothelial cell. Thorax 34:200-208, 1979.

136. Ryan US, Ryan JW, Whitaker C, et al: Localization of angiotensin converting enzyme (kininase II). II. Immunocytochemistry and immunofluorescence. Tissue Cell 8:125-145, 1976.

137. Smith U, Ryan J: Substructural features of pulmonary endothelial caveolae. Tissue Cell 4:49, 1972.

138. Pietra GG, Sampson P, Lanken PN, et al: Transcapillary movement of cationized ferritin in the isolated perfused rat lung. Lab Invest 49:54-61, 1983.

139. Fleming RE, Crouch EC, Ruzicka CA, et al: Pulmonary carbonic anhydrase IV: Developmental regulation and cell-specific expression in the capillary endothelium. Am J Physiol 265:L627-L635, 1993.

140. Gee MH, Albertine KH: Neutrophil–endothelial cell interactions in the lung. Annu Rev Physiol 55:227-248, 1993.
141. Kourembanas S, Bernfield M: Hypoxia and endothelial–smooth muscle cell interactions in the lung. Am J Respir Cell Mol Biol 11:373-374, 1994.
142. Assimacopoulos A, Guggenheim R, Kapanci Y: Changes in alveolar capillary configuration at different levels of lung inflation in the rat. An ultrastructural and morphometric study. Lab Invest 34:10-22, 1976.
143. Weibel E: Morphometry of the Human Lung. New York, Academic Press, 1963.
144. Glazier JB, Hughes JM, Maloney JE, et al: Measurements of capillary dimensions and blood volume in rapidly frozen lungs. J Appl Physiol 26:65-76, 1969.
145. Woodring JH: Pulmonary artery–bronchus ratios in patients with normal lungs, pulmonary vascular plethora, and congestive heart failure. Radiology 179:115-122, 1991.
146. Kuriyama K, Gamsu G, Stern RG, et al: CT-determined pulmonary artery diameters in predicting pulmonary hypertension. Invest Radiol 19:16-22, 1984.
147. Burko H, Carwell G, Newman E: Size, location, and gravitational changes of normal upper lobe pulmonary veins. AJR Am J Roentgenol 111:687-689, 1971.
148. Fraser RG, Fraser RS, Renner JW, et al: The roentgenologic diagnosis of chronic bronchitis: A reassessment with emphasis on parahilar bronchi seen end-on. Radiology 120:1-9, 1976.
149. Simon G: Principles of Chest X-ray Diagnosis, 3rd ed. London, Butterworth, 1971.
150. Proto A, Speckman J: The left lateral radiograph of the chest. 1. Med Radiogr Photogr 55:30, 1979.
151. Proto A, Speckman J: The left lateral radiograph of the chest. 2. Med Radiogr Photogr 56:38, 1980.
152. Schnur MJ, Winkler B, Austin JH: Thickening of the posterior wall of the bronchus intermedius. A sign on lateral radiographs of congestive heart failure, lymph node enlargement, and neoplastic infiltration. Radiology 139:551-559, 1981.
153. Webb WR, Gamsu G: Computed tomography of the left retrobronchial stripe. J Comput Assist Tomogr 7:65-69, 1983.
154. Newman F, Smalley BF, Thomson ML: Effect of exercise, body and lung size on CO diffusion in athletes and nonathletes. J Appl Physiol 17:649-655, 1962.
155. Cope DK, Grimbert F, Downey JM, et al: Pulmonary capillary pressure: A review. Crit Care Med 20:1043-1056, 1992.
156. Hakim TS, Michel RP, Chang HK: Partitioning of pulmonary vascular resistance in dogs by arterial and venous occlusion. J Appl Physiol 52:710-715, 1982.
157. West JB: Regional differences in the lung. Chest 74:426-437, 1978.
158. Howell JB, Permutt S, Proctor DF, et al: Effect of inflation of the lung on different parts of pulmonary vascular bed. J Appl Physiol 16:71-76, 1961.
159. Lamm WJ, Kirk KR, Hanson WL, et al: Flow through zone 1 lungs utilizes alveolar corner vessels. J Appl Physiol 157:1518-1523, 1991.
160. Isawa T, Teshima T, Hirano T, et al: Regulation of regional perfusion distribution in the lungs: Effect of regional oxygen concentration. Am Rev Respir Dis 118:55-63, 1978.
161. Michelakis ED, Archer SL, Weir EK: Acute hypoxic pulmonary vasoconstriction: A model of oxygen sensing. Physiol Res 44:361-367, 1995.
162. Shimoda LA, Sham JS, Liu Q, et al: Acute and chronic hypoxic pulmonary vasoconstriction: A central role for endothelin-1? Respir Physiol Neurobiol 132:93-106, 2002.
163. Deem S, Swenson ER, Alberts MK, et al: Red-blood-cell augmentation of hypoxic pulmonary vasoconstriction: Hematocrit dependence and the importance of nitric oxide. Am J Respir Crit Care Med 157:1181-1186, 1998.
164. Marshall C, Marshall B: Site and sensitivity for stimulation of hypoxic pulmonary vasoconstriction. J Appl Physiol 55:711-716, 1983.
165. Bergofsky EH, Lehr DE, Fishman AP: The effect of changes in hydrogen ion concentration on the pulmonary circulation. J Clin Invest 41:1492-1502, 1962.
166. Downing SE, Lee JC: Nervous control of the pulmonary circulation. Annu Rev Physiol 42:199-210, 1980.
167. Bergofsky EH: Humoral control of the pulmonary circulation. Annu Rev Physiol 42:221-233, 1980.
168. Georges R, Saumon G, Loiseau A: The relationship of age to pulmonary membrane conductance and capillary blood volume. Am Rev Respir Dis 117:1069-1078, 1978.
169. Milic-Emili J: Interregional distribution of inspired gas. Prog Respir Res 16:33, 1981.
170. West JB, Dollery CT: Distribution of blood flow and ventilation-perfusion ratio in the lung, measured with radioactive carbon dioxide. J Appl Physiol 15:405-410, 1960.
171. Engel LA, Grassino A, Anthonisen NR: Demonstration of airway closure in man. J Appl Physiol 38:1117-1125, 1975.
172. Turek Z, Kreuzer F: Effect of shifts of the O_2 dissociation curve upon alveolar-arterial O_2 gradients in computer models of the lung with ventilation-perfusion mismatching. Respir Physiol 45:133-139, 1981.
173. West JB: Ventilation-perfusion inequality and overall gas exchange in computer models of the lung. Respir Physiol 7:88-110, 1969.
174. Dantzker D, Wagner P, West J: Instability of lung units with low $\dot{V}A/\dot{Q}$ ratios during O_2 breathing. J Appl Physiol 38:886, 1975.
175. Wagner PD, Saltzman HA, West JB: Measurement of continuous distributions of ventilation-perfusion ratios: Theory. J Appl Physiol 36:588-599, 1974.
176. Jones N: Should we change our approach to acid-base physiology? Ann R Coll Phys Surg Can 23:235, 1990.
177. Narins RG, Emmett M: Simple and mixed acid-base disorders: A practical approach. Medicine (Baltimore) 59:161-187, 1980.
178. Martinu T, Menzies D, Dial S: Re-evaluation of acid-base prediction rules in patients with chronic respiratory acidosis. Can Respir J 10:311-315, 2003.
179. Salem MM, Mujais SK: Gaps in the anion gap. Arch Intern Med 152:1625-1629, 1992.
180. Cudkowicz L: Bronchial arterial circulation in man: Normal anatomy and responses to disease. In Moser K (ed): Pulmonary Vascular Diseases. New York, Marcel Dekker, 1979, p 111.
181. Murata K, Itoh H, Todo G, et al: Bronchial venous plexus and its communication with pulmonary circulation. Invest Radiol 21:24-30, 1986.
182. Botenga AS: Selective Bronchial and Intercostal Arteriography. Kroese, NV, HE Stenfert 1970.
183. McFadden ER Jr: Respiratory heat and water exchange: Physiological and clinical implications. J Appl Physiol 54:331-336, 1983.
184. Malik AB, Tracy SE: Bronchovascular adjustments after pulmonary embolism. J Appl Physiol 49:476-481, 1980.
185. Baile EM, Ling H, Heyworth JR, et al: Bronchopulmonary anastomotic and noncoronary collateral blood flow in humans during cardiopulmonary bypass. Chest 87:749-754, 1985.
186. Proctor DF, Lundqvist G: Clearance of inhaled particles from the human nose. Arch Intern Med 131:132-139, 1973.
187. Bohning DE, Atkins HL, Cohn SH: Long-term particle clearance in man: Normal and impaired. Ann Occup Hyg 26:259-271, 1982.
188. Stuart BO: Deposition of inhaled aerosols. Arch Intern Med 131:60-73, 1973.
189. Craighead JE, Mossman BT: The pathogenesis of asbestos-associated diseases. N Engl J Med 306:1446-1455, 1982.
190. Pinkerton KE, Plopper CG, Mercer RR, et al: Airway branching patterns influence asbestos fiber location and the extent of tissue injury in the pulmonary parenchyma. Lab Invest 55:688-695, 1986.
191. Pityn P, Chamberlain MJ, Fraser TM, et al: The topography of particle deposition in the human lung. Respir Physiol 78:19-29, 1989.
192. Sweeny T, Brian J, Leavitt S, et al: Emphysema alters the deposition pattern of inhaled particles in hamsters. Am J Pathol 128:19, 1987.
193. Swartenaren M, Philipson L, Linman L, et al: Regional deposition of particles in human lungs after induced bronchoconstriction. Exp Lung Res 10:223, 1986.
194. Satir P: How cilia move. Sci Am 231:45, 1974.
195. Chopra SK, Taplin GV, Simmons DH, et al: Effects of hydration and physical therapy on tracheal transport velocity. Am Rev Respir Dis 115:1009-1014, 1977.
196. Holmskov UL: Collectins and collectin receptors in innate immunity. APMIS Suppl 100:1-59, 2000.
197. Bienenstock J, Befus AD, McDermott M: Mucosal immunity. Monogr Allergy 16:1-18, 1980.
198. Burnett D: Immunoglobulins in the lung. Thorax 41:337-344, 1986.
199. Kaltreider HB, Byrd PK, Daughety TW, et al: The mechanism of appearance of specific antibody-forming cells in lungs of inbred mice after intratracheal immunization with sheep erythrocytes. Am Rev Respir Dis 127:316-321, 1983.
200. Heinemann H, Fishman A: Nonrespiratory functions of mammalian lung. Physiol Rev 49:1, 1969.
201. Holgate ST, Peters-Golden M, Panettieri RA, et al: Roles of cysteinyl leukotrienes in airway inflammation, smooth muscle function, and remodeling. J Allergy Clin Immunol 111:S18-S34, discussion S34-S36, 2003.
202. Schellenberg RR, Tsang S, Salari H: Leukotrienes mediate delayed airway effects of 15-HETE. Ann N Y Acad Sci 744:243-250, 1994.
203. Fanburg BL: Prostaglandins and the lung. Am Rev Respir Dis 108:482-489, 1973.
204. Caughey GH: The structure and airway biology of mast cell proteinases. Am J Respir Cell Mol Biol 4:387-394, 1991.
205. Muzykantov VR, Danilov SM: A new approach to the investigation of oxidative injury to the pulmonary endothelium: Use of angiotensin-converting enzyme as a marker. Biomed Sci 2:11-21, 1991.
206. Barnes PJ: Nitric oxide and airway disease. Ann Med 27:389-393, 1995.
207. Ricciardolo FL: Multiple roles of nitric oxide in the airways. Thorax 58:175-182, 2003.
208. Barnes PJ, Liew FY: Nitric oxide and asthmatic inflammation. Immunol Today 16:128-130, 1995.
209. Luscher TF, Wenzel RR: Endothelin and endothelin antagonists: Pharmacology and clinical implications. Agents Actions Suppl 45:237-253, 1995.
210. Stewart DJ: Endothelial dysfunction in pulmonary vascular disorders. Arzneimittelforschung 44:451-454, 1994.
211. Hukkanen J, Pelkonen O, Hakkola J, et al: Expression and regulation of xenobiotic-metabolizing cytochrome P450 (CYP) enzymes in human lung. Crit Rev Toxicol 32:391-411, 2002.
212. Oury TD, Chang LY, Marklund SL, et al: Immunocytochemical localization of extracellular superoxide dismutase in human lung. Lab Invest 70:889-898, 1994.
213. Becker K: The endocrine lung. In Becker K, Gazdar A (eds): The Endocrine Lung in Health and Disease. Philadelphia, WB Saunders, 1984, p 3.
214. Aabo K, Hansen KB: Megakaryocytes in pulmonary blood vessels. I. Incidence at autopsy, clinicopathological relations especially to disseminated intravascular coagulation. Acta Pathol Microbiol Scand [A] 86:285-291, 1978.
215. Hogg JC: Neutrophil kinetics and lung injury. Physiol Rev 67:1249-1295, 1987.
216. Downey GP, Worthen GS, Henson PM: Neutrophil sequestration and migration in localized pulmonary inflammation. Am Rev Respir Dis 147:168, 1993.
217. Hislop A, Reid L: Development of the acinus in the human lung. Thorax 29:90-94, 1974.
218. Langston C, Kida K, Reed M, et al: Human lung growth in late gestation and in the neonate. Am Rev Respir Dis 129:607-613, 1984.
219. Thurlbeck WM: Postnatal growth and development of the lung. Am Rev Respir Dis 111:803-844, 1975.

220. Thurlbeck WM: Postnatal human lung growth. Thorax 37:564-571, 1982.
221. Zeltner TB, Burri PH: The postnatal development and growth of the human lung. II. Morphology. Respir Physiol 67:269-282, 1987.
222. Hislop A, Reid L: Pulmonary arterial development during childhood: Branching pattern and structure. Thorax 28:129-135, 1973.
223. Hall SM, Hislop AA, Haworth SG: Origin, differentiation, and maturation of human pulmonary veins. Am J Respir Cell Mol Biol 26:333-340, 2002.
224. Cardoso WV, Williams MC: Basic mechanisms of lung development: Eighth Woods Hole Conference on Lung Cell Biology 2000. Am J Respir Cell Mol Biol 25:137-140, 2001.
225. Hackett BP, Bingle CD, Gitlin JD: Mechanisms of gene expression and cell fate determination in the developing pulmonary epithelium. Annu Rev Physiol 58:51-71, 1996.
226. Smith BT, Fletcher WA: Pulmonary epithelial-mesenchymal interactions: Beyond organogenesis. Hum Pathol 10:248-250, 1979.
227. Wendel D, Taylor D, Albertine K, et al: Impaired distal airway development in mice lacking elastin. Am J Respir Cell Mol Biol 23:320-326, 2000.
228. Kleinman HK, Schnaper HW: Basement membrane matrices in tissue development. Am J Respir Cell Mol Biol 8:238-239, 1993.
229. Bogue CW, Lou LJ, Vasavada H, et al: Expression of Hoxb genes in the developing mouse foregut and lung. Am J Respir Cell Mol Biol 15:163-171, 1996.
230. Schittny JC, Djonov V, Fine A, et al: Programmed cell death contributes to postnatal lung development. Am J Respir Cell Mol Biol 18:786-793, 1998.
231. Gross I: Regulation of fetal lung maturation. Am J Physiol 259:L337-L344, 1990.
232. Pinkerton KE, Kendall JZ, Randall GC, et al: Hypophysectomy and porcine fetal lung development. Am J Respir Cell Mol Biol 1:319-328, 1989.
233. Mason RJ: Hepatocyte growth factor: The key to alveolar septation? Am J Respir Cell Mol Biol 26:517-520, 2002.
234. Cagle PT, Thurlbeck WM: Postpneumonectomy compensatory lung growth. Am Rev Respir Dis 138:1314-1326, 1988.
235. Castleman WL: Alterations in pulmonary ultrastructure and morphometric parameters induced by parainfluenza (Sendai) virus in rats during postnatal growth. Am J Pathol 114:322-335, 1984.
236. Das RM: The effects of intermittent starvation on lung development in suckling rats. Am J Pathol 117:326-332, 1984.
237. Perez Fontan JJ: On lung nerves and neurogenic injury. Ann Med 34:226-240, 2002.
238. Laitinen A: Ultrastructural organisation of intraepithelial nerves in the human airway tract. Thorax 40:488-492, 1985.
239. Sant'Ambrogio G: Information arising from the tracheobronchial tree of mammals. Physiol Rev 62:531-569, 1982.
240. Hung KS, Hertweck MS, Hardy JD, et al: Electron microscopic observations of nerve endings in the alveolar walls of mouse lungs. Am Rev Respir Dis 108:328-333, 1973.
241. Laitenen L, Laitenen A: Neural elements in human airways. In Raeburn D, Giembycz M (eds): Airways Smooth Muscle: Structure, Innervation and Neurotransmission. Basel, Birkhäuser-Verlag, 1994, pp 309-324.
242. Nadel JA, Barnes PJ: Autonomic regulation of the airways. Annu Rev Med 35:451-467, 1984.
243. Barnes PJ: The third nervous system in the lung: Physiology and clinical perspectives. Thorax 39:561-567, 1984.
244. Belvisi M, Bai T: Inhibitory nonadrenergic, noncholinergic innervation of airway smooth muscle: Role of nitric oxide. In Raeburn D, Giembycz M (eds): Airways Smooth Muscle: Structure, Innervation and Neurotransmission. Basel, Birkhäuser-Verlag, 1994, pp 158-187.
245. Wang NS: Anatomy and physiology of the pleural space. Clin Chest Med 6:3-16, 1985.
246. Pistolesi M, Miniati M, Giuntini C: Pleural liquid and solute exchange. Am Rev Respir Dis 140:825-847, 1989.
247. Whitaker D, Papadimitriou JM, Walters M: The mesothelium: Its fibrinolytic properties. J Pathol 136:291-299, 1982.
248. Idell S, Zwieb C, Kumar A, et al: Pathways of fibrin turnover of human pleural mesothelial cells in vitro. Am J Respir Cell Mol Biol 7:414-426, 1992.
249. Hills BA: Graphite-like lubrication of mesothelium by oligolamellar pleural surfactant. J Appl Physiol 73:1034-1039, 1992.
250. Raasch BN, Carsky EW, Lane EJ, et al: Radiographic anatomy of the interlobar fissures: A study of 100 specimens. AJR Am J Roentgenol 138:1043-1049, 1982.
251. Glazer HS, Anderson DJ, DiCroce JJ, et al: Anatomy of the major fissure: Evaluation with standard and thin-section CT. Radiology 180:839-844, 1991.
252. Felson B: Chest Roentgenology. Philadelphia, WB Saunders, 1973.
253. Proto AV, Ball JB Jr: Computed tomography of the major and minor fissures. AJR Am J Roentgenol 140:439-448, 1983.
254. Berkmen YM, Auh YH, Davis SD, et al: Anatomy of the minor fissure: Evaluation with thin-section CT. Radiology 170:647-651, 1989.
255. Rabinowitz JG, Cohen BA, Mendleson DS: Symposium on Nonpulmonary Aspects in Chest Radiology. The pulmonary ligament. Radiol Clin North Am 22:659-672, 1984.
256. Rost RC Jr, Proto AV: Inferior pulmonary ligament: Computed tomographic appearance. Radiology 148:479-483, 1983.
257. Mata J, Caceres J, Alegret X, et al: Imaging of the azygos lobe: Normal anatomy and variations. AJR Am J Roentgenol 156:931-937, 1991.
258. Austin JH: The left minor fissure. Radiology 161:433-436, 1986.
259. Black LF: The pleural space and pleural fluid. Mayo Clin Proc 47:493-506, 1972.
260. Masada S, Ichikawa S, Nakamura Y, et al: Structure and distribution of the lymphatic vessels in the parietal pleura of the monkey as studied by enzyme-

261. histochemistry and by light and electron microscopy. Arch Histol Cytol 55:525-538, 1992.
261. Li J, Jiang B: A scanning electron microscopic study on three-dimensional organization of human diaphragmatic lymphatics. Funct Dev Morphol 3:129-132, 1993.
262. Lauweryns JM, Baert JH: Alveolar clearance and the role of the pulmonary lymphatics. Am Rev Respir Dis 115:625-683, 1977.
263. Hendin AS, Greenspan RH: Ventilatory pumping of human pulmonary lymphatic vessels. Radiology 108:553-557, 1973.
264. Rosenberger A, Abrams HL: Radiology of the thoracic duct. AJR Am J Roentgenol 111:807-820, 1971.
265. Mountain CF, Dresler CM: Regional lymph node classification for lung cancer staging. Chest 111:1718-1723, 1997.
266. Ko JP, Drucker EA, Shepard JA, et al: CT depiction of regional nodal stations for lung cancer staging. AJR Am J Roentgenol 174:775-782, 2000.
267. Cymbalista M, Waysberg A, Zacharias C, et al: CT demonstration of the 1996 AJCC-UICC regional lymph node classification for lung cancer staging [poster]. Radiographics 19:899-900, 1999.
268. Glazer GM, Orringer MB, Gross BH, et al: The mediastinum in non–small cell lung cancer: CT-surgical correlation. AJR Am J Roentgenol 142:1101-1105, 1984.
269. Quint LE, Glazer GM, Orringer MB, et al: Mediastinal lymph node detection and sizing at CT and autopsy. AJR Am J Roentgenol 147:469-472, 1986.
270. Rouvière H: Anatomy of the Human Lymphatic System [translated by MJ Tobias]. Ann Arbor, MI, Edwards, 1983.
271. Baird JA: The pathways of lymphatic spread of carcinoma of the lung. Br J Surg 52:868-875, 1965.
272. Felson B: The mediastinum. Semin Roentgenol 4:31, 1969.
273. Bannister LH: The respiratory system. In Williams P (ed): Gray's Anatomy. New York, Churchill Livingstone, 1995, pp 1627-1682.
274. Baron RL, Lee JK, Sagel SS, et al: Computed tomography of the normal thymus. Radiology 142:121-125, 1982.
275. Nicolaou S, Muller NL, Li DK, et al: Thymus in myasthenia gravis: Comparison of CT and pathologic findings and clinical outcome after thymectomy. Radiology 201:471-474, 1996.
276. Francis IR, Glazer GM, Bookstein FL, et al: The thymus: Reexamination of age-related changes in size and shape. AJR Am J Roentgenol 145:249-254, 1985.
277. Savoca CJ, Austin JH, Goldberg HI: The right paratracheal stripe. Radiology 122:295-301, 1977.
278. Muller NL, Webb WR, Gamsu G: Paratracheal lymphadenopathy: Radiographic findings and correlation with CT. Radiology 156:761-765, 1985.
279. Proto AV, Simmons JD, Zylak CJ: The posterior junction anatomy. Crit Rev Diagn Imaging 20:121-173, 1983.
280. Heitzman ER, Scrivani JV, Martino J, et al: The azygos vein and its pleural reflections. I. Normal roentgen anatomy. Radiology 101:249-258, 1971.
281. Heitzman ER, Scrivani JV, Martino J, et al: The azygos vein and its pleural reflections. II. Applications in the radiological diagnosis of mediastinal abnormality. Radiology 101:259-266, 1971.
282. Onitsuka H, Kuhns LR: Dextroconvexity of the mediastinum in the azygoesophageal recess: A normal CT variant in young adults. Radiology 135:126, 1980.
283. Gammill SL, Krebs C, Meyers P, et al: Cardiac measurements in systole and diastole. Radiology 94:115-120, 1970.
284. Heath D: The human carotid body in health and disease. J Pathol 164:1-8, 1991.
285. Bonham AC: Neurotransmitters in the CNS control of breathing. Respir Physiol 101:219-230, 1995.
286. Biscoe T, Willshaw P: Stimulus-response relationships of the peripheral arterial chemoreceptors. In Hornbein T, Lenfant CJ (eds): Regulation of Breathing, Part One. Lung Biology in Health and Disease. New York, Marcel Dekker, 1981.
287. Gozal D, Hathout GM, Kirlew KA, et al: Localization of putative neural respiratory regions in the human by functional magnetic resonance imaging. J Appl Physiol 76:2076-2083, 1994.
288. Sant'Ambrogio G, Tsubone H, Sant'Ambrogio FB: Sensory information from the upper airway: Role in the control of breathing. Respir Physiol 102:1-16, 1995.
289. Widdicombe J: Nervous receptors in the respiratory tract and lungs. In Hornbein T, Lenfant CJ (eds): Regulation of Breathing. Part One. Lung Biology in Health and Disease. New York, Marcel Dekker, 1981, p 429.
290. Ford GT, Whitelaw WA, Rosenal TW, et al: Diaphragm function after upper abdominal surgery in humans. Am Rev Respir Dis 127:431-436, 1983.
291. Duron B: Intercostal and diaphragmatic muscle endings and afferents. In Hornbein T, Lenfant CJ (eds): Regulation of Breathing. Part One. Lung Biology in Health and Disease. New York, Marcel Dekker, 1981, p 473.
292. Bianchi AL, Denavit-Saubie M, Champagnat J: Central control of breathing in mammals: Neuronal circuitry, membrane properties, and neurotransmitters. Physiol Rev 75:1-45, 1995.
293. Berger AJ, Mitchell RA, Severinghaus JW: Regulation of respiration (second of three parts). N Engl J Med 297:138-143, 1977.
294. Martin J, Aubier M, Engel LA: Effects of inspiratory loading on respiratory muscle activity during expiration. Am Rev Respir Dis 125:352-358, 1982.
295. Phillipson EA, McClean PA, Sullivan CE, et al: Interaction of metabolic and behavioral respiratory control during hypercapnia and speech. Am Rev Respir Dis 117:903-909, 1978.
296. Milic-Emili J: Recent advances in clinical assessment of control of breathing. Lung 160:1, 1962.
297. Leitch AG: The hypoxic drive to breathing in man. Lancet 1:428-430, 1981.
298. Schoene RB: Control of ventilation in climbers to extreme altitude. J Appl Physiol 53:886-890, 1982.

299. Mateika JH, Duffin J: A review of the control of breathing during exercise. Eur J Appl Physiol Occup Physiol 71:1-27, 1995.
300. Cherniak N, Altos M: Respiratory responses in ventilatory loading. In Hornbein T, Lenfant CJ (eds): Regulation of Breathing, Part Two. Lung Biology in Health and Disease. New York, Marcel Dekker, 1981.
301. Killian KJ, Campbell EJ: Dyspnea and exercise. Annu Rev Physiol 45:465-479, 1983.
302. Henke KG, Badr MS, Skatrud JB, et al: Load compensation and respiratory muscle function during sleep. J Appl Physiol 72:1221-1234, 1992.
303. Remmers JE, Lahiri S: Regulating the ventilatory pump: A splendid control system prone to fail during sleep. Am J Respir Crit Care Med 157:S95-S100, 1998.
304. Joseph V, Pequignot JM, Van Reeth O: Neurochemical perspectives on the control of breathing during sleep. Respir Physiol Neurobiol 130:253-263, 2002.
305. Roussos C: The thorax. In Lenfant C (ed): Lung Biology in Health and Disease. New York, Marcel Dekker, 1995.
306. Strohl KP: Upper airway muscles of respiration. Am Rev Respir Dis 124:211-213, 1981.
307. Tangel DJ, Mezzanotte WS, White DP: Respiratory-related control of palatoglossus and levator palatini muscle activity. J Appl Physiol 78:680-688, 1995.
308. Wheatley JR, Tangel DJ, Mezzanotte WS, et al: Influence of sleep on alae nasi EMG and nasal resistance in normal men. J Appl Physiol 75:626-632, 1993.
309. Krol RC, Knuth SL, Bartlett D Jr: Selective reduction of genioglossal muscle activity by alcohol in normal human subjects. Am Rev Respir Dis 129:247-250, 1984.
310. Sharp JT: Respiratory muscles: A review of old and newer concepts. Lung 157:185-199, 1980.
311. De Troyer A, Sampson M, Sigrist S, et al: The diaphragm: Two muscles. Science 213:237-238, 1981.
312. Belman MJ, Sieck GC: The ventilatory muscles. Fatigue, endurance and training. Chest 82:761-766, 1982.
313. Comtois A, Gorczyca W, Grassino A: Microscopic anatomy of the arterial diaphragmatic circulation. Clin Invest Med 7:81, 1984.
314. Rochester DF, Briscoe AM: Metabolism of the working diaphragm. Am Rev Respir Dis 119:101-106, 1979.
315. Lennon EA, Simon G: The height of the diaphragm in the chest radiograph of normal adults. Br J Radiol 38:937-943, 1965.
316. Wittenborg MH, Aviad I: Organ influence on the normal posture of the diaphragm: A radiological study of inversions and heterotaxies. Br J Radiol 36:280-288, 1963.
317. Wechsler RJ, Steiner RM: Cross-sectional imaging of the chest wall. J Thorac Imaging 4:29-40, 1989.
318. Loh L, Goldman M, Davis JN: The assessment of diaphragm function. Medicine (Baltimore) 56:165-169, 1977.
319. Im JG, Webb WR, Rosen A, et al: Costal pleura: Appearances at high-resolution CT. Radiology 171:125-131, 1989.
320. Bhalla M, McCauley DI, Golimbu C, et al: Counting ribs on chest CT. J Comput Assist Tomogr 14:590-594, 1990.
321. Navani S, Shah JR, Levy PS: Determination of sex by costal cartilage calcification. AJR Am J Roentgenol 108:771-774, 1970.
322. Vix VA: Extrapleural costal fat. Radiology 112:563-565, 1974.
323. Shauffer IA, Collins WV: The deep clavicular rhomboid fossa. Clinical significance and incidence in 10,000 routine chest photofluorograms. JAMA 195:778-779, 1966.
324. Hogg JC, Nepszy S: Regional lung volume and pleural pressure gradient estimated from lung density in dogs. J Appl Physiol 27:198-203, 1969.
325. Altman P, Dittmer D: Respiration and Circulation. Bethesda, MD, Federation of American Societies for Experimental Biology, 1971, p 27.
326. Staub NC: Pulmonary edema. Physiol Rev 54:678-811, 1974.
327. Wandtke JC, Hyde RW, Fahey PJ, et al: Measurement of lung gas volume and regional density by computed tomography in dogs. Invest Radiol 21:108-117, 1986.
328. Goldman HI, Becklake MR: Respiratory function tests; normal values at median altitudes and the prediction of normal results. Am Rev Tuberc 79:457-467, 1959.
329. Joseph AE, de Lacey GJ, Bryant TH, et al: The hypertransradiant hemithorax: The importance of lateral decentring, and the explanation for its appearance due to rotation. Clin Radiol 29:125-131, 1978.
330. Glazier JB, DeNardo GL: Pulmonary function studied with the xenon-133 scanning technique. Normal values and a postural study. Am Rev Respir Dis 94:188-194, 1966.
331. Murata K, Itoh H, Todo G, et al: Centrilobular lesions of the lung: Demonstration by high-resolution CT and pathologic correlation. Radiology 161:641-645, 1986.
332. Itoh H, Murata K, Konishi J, et al: Diffuse lung disease: Pathologic basis for the high-resolution computed tomography findings. J Thorac Imaging 8:176-188, 1993.
333. Kim JS, Muller NL, Park CS, et al: Cylindrical bronchiectasis: Diagnostic findings on thin-section CT. AJR Am J Roentgenol 168:751-754, 1997.
334. Kim SJ, Im JG, Kim IO, et al: Normal bronchial and pulmonary arterial diameters measured by thin section CT. J Comput Assist Tomogr 19:365-369, 1995.
335. Webb WR, Gamsu G, Wall SD, et al: CT of a bronchial phantom. Factors affecting appearance and size measurements. Invest Radiol 19:394-398, 1984.
336. McNamara AE, Muller NL, Okazawa M, et al: Airway narrowing in excised canine lungs measured by high-resolution computed tomography. J Appl Physiol 73:307-316, 1992.
337. Kim JS, Muller NL, Park CS, et al: Bronchoarterial ratio on thin section CT: Comparison between high altitude and sea level. J Comput Assist Tomogr 21:306-311, 1997.
338. Herold CJ, Wetzel RC, Robotham JL, et al: Acute effects of increased intravascular volume and hypoxia on the pulmonary circulation: Assessment with high-resolution CT. Radiology 183:655-662, 1992.
339. Hedlund L, Vock P, Effmann E: Evaluating lung density by computed tomography. Semin Respir Med 5:76, 1983.
340. Hedlund L, Vock P, Effmann E: Computed tomography of the lung: Densitometric studies. Radiol Clin North Am 21:775, 1983.
341. Rosenblum LJ, Mauceri RA, Wellenstein DE, et al: Density patterns in the normal lung as determined by computed tomography. Radiology 137:409-416, 1980.
342. Webb WR, Stern EJ, Kanth N, et al: Dynamic pulmonary CT: Findings in healthy adult men. Radiology 186:117-124, 1993.
343. Verschakelen JA, Van Fraeyenhoven L, Laureys G, et al: Differences in CT density between dependent and nondependent portions of the lung: Influence of lung volume. AJR Am J Roentgenol 161:713-717, 1993.
344. Park CS, Muller NL, Worthy SA, et al: Airway obstruction in asthmatic and healthy individuals: Inspiratory and expiratory thin-section CT findings. Radiology 203:361-367, 1997.
345. Worthy SA, Park CS, Kim JS, et al: Bronchiolitis obliterans after lung transplantation: High-resolution CT findings in 15 patients. AJR Am J Roentgenol 169:673-677, 1997.
346. Rhodes CG, Wollmer P, Fazio F, et al: Quantitative measurement of regional extravascular lung density using positron emission and transmission tomography. J Comput Assist Tomogr 5:783-791, 1981.
347. Muller NL, Staples CA, Miller RR, et al: "Density mask." An objective method to quantitate emphysema using computed tomography. Chest 94:782-787, 1988.
348. Zerhouni EA, Boukadoum M, Siddiky MA, et al: A standard phantom for quantitative CT analysis of pulmonary nodules. Radiology 149:767-773, 1983.

METHODS OF RADIOLOGIC INVESTIGATION

As a general rule, establishing the *presence* of a disease process on the radiograph should constitute the first step in radiologic diagnosis of chest disease. If this examination does not clearly show the nature and extent of the abnormality, additional studies such as CT or MR imaging can be carried out to *complement* the radiograph.

RADIOGRAPHY

Projections

The most satisfactory routine radiographic views for evaluation of the chest are posteroanterior (PA) and lateral projections with the patient standing; such projections provide the essential requirement for proper three-dimensional assessment. In patients who are too ill to stand, anteroposterior upright or supine projections offer alternative but considerably less satisfactory views. The anteroposterior projection is of inferior quality because of the shorter focal-film distance, the greater magnification of the heart, and the restricted ability of many such patients to suspend respiration or achieve full inspiration.

Situations in which the performance of routine radiography is likely to be cost-effective have been the subject of considerable study.[1] Table 2–1 summarizes our recommendations on the use of chest radiographs based on a review of the literature and recommendations of the American College of Radiology[2] and the American Thoracic Society.[3]

Basic Radiographic Techniques

Diagnostic accuracy in chest disease is related partly to the quality of the radiographic images themselves. Careful attention to several variables is necessary to ensure such quality.
Patient Positioning. Positioning must be such that the x-ray beam is centered properly, the patient's body is not rotated, and the scapulas are rotated sufficiently anteriorly that they are projected away from the lungs. On properly centered radiographs, the medial ends of the clavicles are projected equidistant from the spinous processes of the thoracic vertebrae.

Patient Respiration. Respiration must be suspended, preferably at full inspiration.
Exposure. Exposure factors should be such that there is faint visualization of the thoracic spine *and* the intervertebral disks on the PA radiograph so that lung markings behind the heart are clearly visible; exposure should be as short as possible, consistent with the production of adequate contrast.
Kilovoltage. A high-kilovoltage technique appropriate to the film speed should be used[2] for PA and lateral chest radiographs; we recommend using 115 to 150 kVp. (The abbreviation kVp is the peak voltage applied across the x-ray tube.)

Conventional Film-Screen Radiography

Conventional chest radiography uses film to record the images. Film has several advantages, including easy handling, high sensitivity, and good uniformity; however, it is limited by the small exposure range over which it provides diagnostic information. Because x-ray attenuation in the thorax ranges from the nearly radiotransparent lung to the highly attenuating mediastinum, rib cage, and spine, several techniques have been developed to allow adequate visualization of the various structures. These techniques include wide-latitude film, the use of customized patient-specific filters,[4] and scanning equalization radiography.[5,6] The latter technique incorporates a feedback system that modulates the x-ray beam intensity according to the patient's body habitus.

Digital Radiography

Digital radiography has many advantages over conventional screen-film systems.[7,8] One of the most important is its wide exposure latitude, which is 10 to 100 times greater than the widest dynamic range of screen-film systems. During digital image processing, the systems automatically determine the range of clinically appropriate gray levels and produce an image within that range. As a result, the final image is virtually independent of absolute x-ray exposure levels. (A potential disadvantage is that patients may receive unnecessarily high radiation doses, which may not be detected because they do not result in perceivable alterations in image quality.)

TABLE 2–1. Recommendations for the Use of Chest Radiography

Indications for chest radiography:
  Signs and symptoms related to the respiratory and cardiovascular systems
  Follow-up of previously diagnosed thoracic disease for the evaluation of improvement, resolution, or progression
  Staging of intrathoracic and extrathoracic tumors
  Preoperative assessment of patients scheduled for intrathoracic surgery
  Preoperative evaluation of patients who have cardiac or respiratory symptoms or patients who have a significant potential for thoracic pathology that may lead to increased perioperative morbidity or mortality
  Monitoring of patients who have life support devices and patients who have undergone cardiac or thoracic surgery or other interventional procedures
Routine chest radiographs are not indicated in the following situations:
  Routine screening of unselected populations
  Routine prenatal chest radiographs for the detection of unsuspected disease
  Routine radiographs solely because of hospital admission
  Mandated radiographs for employment
  Repeated radiograph examinations after admission to a long-term facility

Based on recommendations from American College of Radiology: ACR Standard for the Performance of Pediatric and Adult Chest Radiography. Reston, VA, American College of Radiology, 1997, p 27; and American Thoracic Society: Chest x-ray screening statements. Am Thorac News 10:14, 1984.

The wider latitude of digital systems allows them to be used under a much broader range of exposure conditions than possible with conventional systems and makes them an ideal choice for applications in which exposure is highly variable or difficult to control, such as bedside radiography. Another major advantage of digital radiography is that it produces what are essentially electronic images; as a result, an image may be transmitted to any location, displayed at multiple sites simultaneously, and efficiently archived for later reference. The images can be distributed widely by using picture archiving and communications systems (PACS), displayed on video monitors (soft copy), or printed onto film or paper (hard copy). Two main types of digital radiography systems are available commercially: systems based on photostimulable storage phosphor image receptors and systems based on selenium-coated receptors.

Storage Phosphor Radiography. Storage phosphor imaging (computed radiography) has been used mainly for bedside chest radiography because its wide dynamic range allows it to achieve consistent images over a wide range of x-ray exposure (Fig. 2–1).[9] Storage phosphor systems have a dynamic range of approximately 1:10,000 as opposed to 1:100 for standard films[10]; that is, they are capable of producing diagnostic images over a much broader range of exposure, which results in a considerable decrease in the repeat rate for bedside chest radiographs.[11]

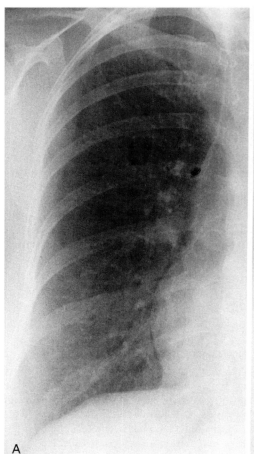
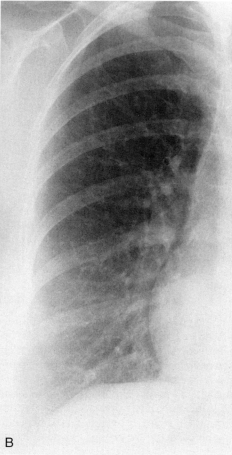

A

B

FIGURE 2–1

Storage phosphor and conventional radiography. Views of a normal right lung in a 54-year-old woman obtained with storage phosphor technology (**A**) and conventional radiography (**B**) demonstrate comparable visualization of parenchymal detail. *(From Müller NL, Fraser RS, Colman NC, Paré PD: Radiologic Diagnosis of Diseases of the Chest. Philadelphia, WB Saunders, 2001.)*

With storage phosphor technology, a reusable photostimulable phosphor rather than film is used to record the image. Plates coated with the phosphor are loaded into special cassettes that are outwardly similar to screen-film cassettes. During exposure, the receptor stores the x-ray energy and is then scanned by a laser beam, which results in the creation of visible or infrared radiation, the intensity of which corresponds to the absorbed x-ray energy. The resultant luminescence is measured and recorded digitally.[12]

Selenium Detector Digital Radiography. As with storage phosphor systems, selenium-based chest imaging systems use a receptor that allows production of a digital image that can be adjusted after processing and displayed on a monitor or on film. The main advantage of selenium-based detectors is considerably greater quantum efficiency than with conventional screen-film systems and photostimulable phosphor detectors.[13,14]

COMPUTED TOMOGRAPHY

The CT image is a two-dimensional representation of a three-dimensional cross-sectional slice, the third dimension being the section or slice thickness. The CT image is composed of multiple picture elements (typically 512 × 512) known as *pixels*. A pixel is a unit area (i.e., each square on the image matrix); it reflects the attenuation of a unit volume of tissue, or voxel, which corresponds to the area of the pixel multiplied by the section thickness. The x-ray attenuation of the structures within a given voxel is averaged to produce the image.

Technical Considerations

Several operator-dependent parameters greatly influence the information provided by chest CT. The main ones are slice thickness, slice spacing, field of view, the reconstruction algorithm, and image display settings (window width and level). In selected cases, intravenous contrast medium may be used to distinguish vessels from soft tissue lesions or detect intravascular abnormalities such as thromboemboli (Fig. 2–2).

The optimal slice thickness is determined by the size of the structure being assessed and by the number of scans required to evaluate the patient. It has been well established that thin sections (1- to 1.5-mm collimation) are required for adequate assessment of the pulmonary parenchyma and peripheral bronchi.[15,16] Adequate assessment of diffuse interstitial and airway abnormalities can be obtained by performing these scans at 10-mm intervals. Although only 10% to 20% of the lung parenchyma is sampled, the improved spatial resolution allows better assessment of normal and abnormal findings than is possible with thicker sections.[17] This approach is not acceptable in all situations, however; for example, when assessing pulmonary metastases, it is essential to evaluate the entire chest, preferably by using continuous (volumetric) spiral CT through the chest with 1- to 5-mm-thick sections. Volumetric scanning at 1- to 3-mm collimation during a single breath-hold is recommended for the assessment of abnormalities involving the trachea and central bronchi. The optimal slice thickness is dictated by the indication for performing the CT scan.

CT numbers in the thorax range from approximately −1000 Hounsfield units (HU) for air in the trachea to

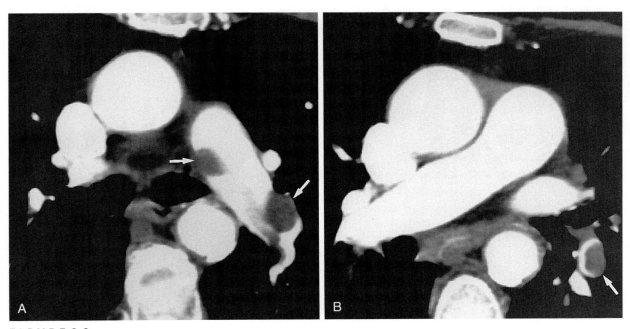

FIGURE 2–2

Spiral CT in pulmonary thromboembolism. A 3-mm-collimation spiral CT scan after the intravenous administration of contrast medium (**A** and **B**) shows several emboli in the left main and interlobar pulmonary arteries (*arrows*). The patient was an 84-year-old woman with acute shortness of breath. (*From Müller NL, Fraser RS, Colman NC, Paré PD: Radiologic Diagnosis of Diseases of the Chest. Philadelphia, WB Saunders, 2001.*)

approximately 700 HU for dense bones. The display of the CT image on the monitor (soft copy) or film (hard copy) is determined by the window level and width and is limited to 256 shades of gray. No single window setting can adequately display all of the information available on a chest CT scan. To display the large number of attenuation values (HU) within a limited number of shades of gray, a CT number is selected that approximately corresponds to the mean attenuation value of the tissue being examined. This center CT attenuation value is called the *window level*. The computer is instructed to assign one shade of gray to a certain number of CT attenuation values above and below the window level. The range of CT numbers above and below the window level is called the *window width*. To depict the lungs adequately, a window level of −600 to −700 HU and a window width of 1000 to 1500 HU are most commonly recommended.[18] Window levels of 30 to 50 HU and window widths of 350 to 500 HU usually provide the best assessment of the mediastinum, hila, and pleura. These figures represent guidelines only, and there are no universally accepted ideal window settings for the lung parenchyma or the mediastinum; different windows may provide optimal assessment of particular abnormalities in individual cases.

High-Resolution Computed Tomography

In most cases, CT scan data are reconstructed by using a standard or soft tissue algorithm that smoothes the image and reduces visible image noise; such an algorithm is preferred in the assessment of abnormalities of the mediastinum and chest wall. However, use of a high–spatial frequency reconstruction algorithm is required for optimal assessment of the lung parenchyma.[19,20] This algorithm reduces image smoothing and increases spatial resolution, thereby allowing better depiction of normal and abnormal parenchymal interfaces and better visualization of small vessels, airways, and subtle interstitial abnormalities.[2,20] The combination of thin-section CT scanning (1-mm collimation) and a high–spatial frequency reconstruction algorithm provides for optimal assessment of interstitial and air space lung disease and is referred to as HRCT (Fig. 2–3).[15,18]

Spiral Computed Tomography

The earliest (conventional) CT scans of the chest consisted of a series of cross-sectional slices obtained during

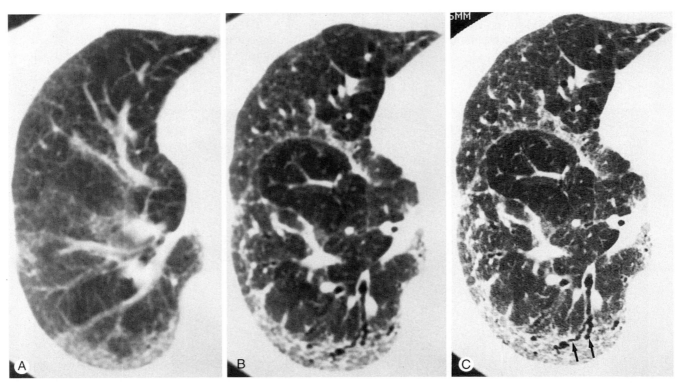

FIGURE 2–3

Influence of section thickness and reconstruction algorithm on image quality. A 10-mm-collimation CT scan (**A**) in a 71-year-old patient shows poorly defined areas of increased attenuation in the right lung. The pattern and distribution of abnormalities are visualized better on the 1.5-mm-collimation CT scan (**B**). Both images (**A** and **B**) were reconstructed with a standard reconstruction algorithm. HRCT scanning (1.5-mm-collimation CT scan reconstructed by using a high–spatial frequency algorithm) (**C**) allows optimal assessment of fine parenchymal detail. The edges of vessels and bronchi are defined more sharply than with the standard algorithm. The abnormalities consist of a fine reticular pattern and areas of ground-glass attenuation involving mainly the subpleural regions. Note the irregular dilation of the posterior basal bronchi of the right lower lobe as they enter an area of fibrosis (traction bronchiectasis *[arrows]*). The diagnosis of idiopathic pulmonary fibrosis was confirmed by open lung biopsy. *(From Müller NL, Fraser RS, Colman NC, Paré PD: Radiologic Diagnosis of Diseases of the Chest. Philadelphia, WB Saunders, 2001.)*

suspended respiration. After each slice was obtained, the patient was allowed to breathe while the table was moved to the next scanning position. Although each image could be obtained in approximately 1 second, there was a delay of 5 to 10 seconds between the images recorded. The development of spiral (helical) CT in the 1980s allowed continuous scanning while the patient is moved through the CT gantry.[21] With this procedure, the x-ray beam traces a helical or spiral curve in relation to the patient. Cross-sectional images can be reconstructed after the data specific to each plane of section have been estimated.[22] The position and spacing of these images can be chosen retrospectively for arbitrary table positions and at small increments.

Until the 1990s, CT scanners had only one row of detectors. These devices are being replaced by scanners with multiple rows of detectors (multidetector row CT). Such arrays allow simultaneous acquisition of data from each of several detectors, which results in improved temporal resolution, improved spatial resolution in the z-axis, increased efficiency in x-ray tube use, and decreased image noise.[23] The improved temporal resolution permits imaging of the entire chest with thin sections during a single breath-hold. The increased spatial resolution in the z-axis (cephalocaudal plane) allows the production of high-quality multiplanar and three-dimensional reformations without additional radiation exposure (Fig. 2–4). The use of graphics-based software systems and volume-rendering techniques allows a depiction of the luminal surface of the airways that resembles the images seen by bronchography ("CT bronchography")[24,25] or during bronchoscopy ("virtual bronchoscopy") (Fig. 2–5).[26,27]

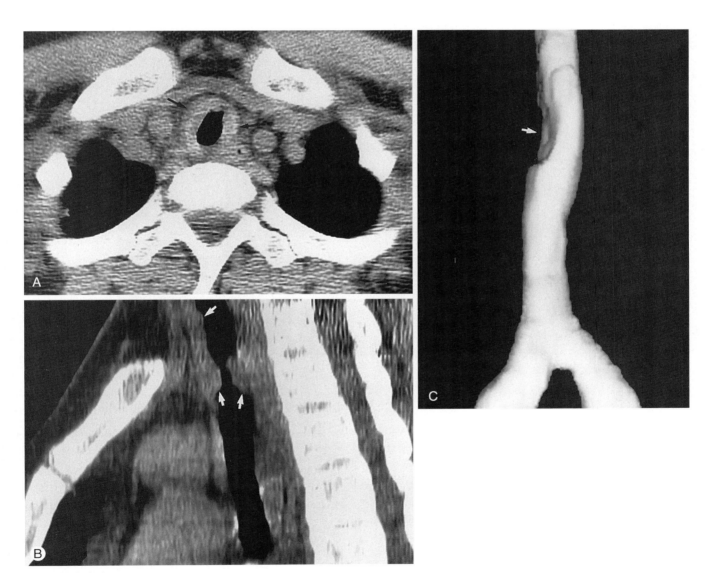

FIGURE 2–4

Spiral CT with sagittal and three-dimensional reconstruction in endotracheal tuberculosis. A 3-mm-collimation spiral CT scan (**A**) shows circumferential thickening of the trachea *(arrows)*. The sagittal reconstruction (**B**) allows better assessment of the focal nature of the thickening with narrowing of the lumen *(arrows)*. The narrowing is also well seen on a coronal three-dimensional reconstruction *(arrow in* **C***)*. The patient was a 27-year-old woman who had endotracheal tuberculosis. *(Case courtesy of Dr. Kyung Soo Lee, Department of Radiology, Samsung Medical Center, Seoul, South Korea. From Müller NL, Fraser RS, Colman NC, Paré PD: Radiologic Diagnosis of Diseases of the Chest. Philadelphia, WB Saunders, 2001.)*

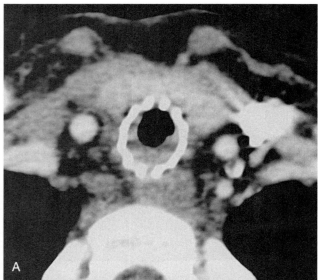

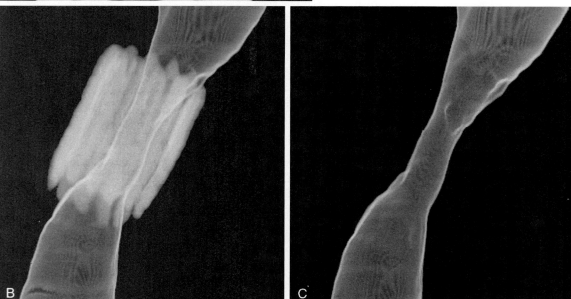

FIGURE 2–5

CT tracheobronchography. Progressive shortness of breath developed in a patient previously treated with a tracheal endoprosthesis for post-tracheotomy stenosis. A spiral CT scan (**A**) shows the prosthesis and recurrent narrowing resulting from soft tissue internal to the prosthesis. CT tracheobronchography performed with a volume-rendering technique (**B**) shows the extent of narrowing and the relationship to the prosthesis. Electronic subtraction of the prosthesis (**C**) allows better assessment of the extent of stenosis. *(Case courtesy of Dr. Martine Remy-Jardin, Department of Radiology, Hôpital Calmette, Lille, France.)*

Indications

Table 2–2 summarizes the most common indications for the use of CT as based on published data.[28,29] HRCT is the imaging modality of choice for the diagnosis of bronchiectasis and is useful in assessing patients who have symptoms or pulmonary function abnormalities suggestive of parenchymal lung disease but normal or questionable radiographic findings (Fig. 2–6).[15,18] It is also recommended in the assessment of patients in whom the combination of clinical and radiographic findings does not provide a confident diagnosis and further radiologic assessment is considered warranted. This indication in particular includes patients who have chronic interstitial and air space disease and immunocompromised patients who have acute parenchymal abnormalities; in such patients, the differential diagnosis can be narrowed or a specific diagnosis often made on HRCT when the radiographic findings are nonspecific.

TABLE 2–2. Most Common Indications for Chest Computed Tomography

Evaluation of suspected mediastinal abnormalities identified on standard chest radiographs

Determination of the presence and extent of neoplastic disease

Search for diffuse or central calcification in a pulmonary nodule

Diagnosis of pulmonary thromboembolism

Guide to percutaneous biopsy of mediastinal, pleural, or pulmonary nodules or masses

Localization of loculated collections of fluid within the pleural space when standard radiographic or ultrasonic techniques prove inadequate

Assessment of abnormalities of the thoracic aorta

Diagnosis of bronchiectasis and assessment of the nature and extent of interstitial lung disease, small-airway disease, and emphysema with HRCT

From Müller NL, Fraser RS, Colman NC, Paré PD: Radiologic Diagnosis of Diseases of the Chest. Philadelphia, WB Saunders, 2001.

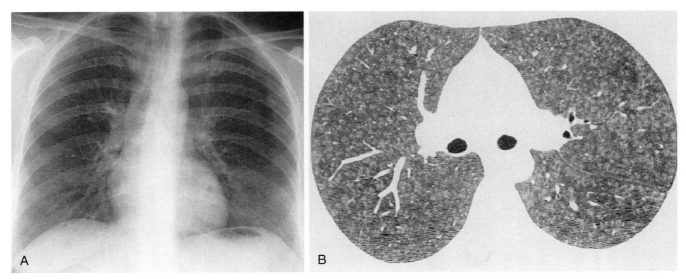

FIGURE 2–6

HRCT in chronic diffuse lung disease. A posteroanterior chest radiograph (**A**) in a 35-year-old woman with progressive shortness of breath shows subtle bilateral areas of increased opacity. An HRCT scan (**B**) shows small rounded opacities in a centrilobular distribution. Although the radiographic findings were nonspecific, the HRCT appearance is most suggestive of hypersensitivity pneumonitis. The diagnosis was proved by open lung biopsy. *(From Müller NL, Fraser RS, Colman NC, Paré PD: Radiologic Diagnosis of Diseases of the Chest. Philadelphia, WB Saunders, 2001.)*

MAGNETIC RESONANCE IMAGING

When certain atomic nuclei are placed in a magnetic field and stimulated by radio waves of a particular sequence, they emit some of the absorbed energy in the form of radio signals. Currently, most medical MR imaging uses hydrogen protons as the nuclei of interest because of their abundance in the body. The greater the number of hydrogen protons present, the more intense the MR signal. Several factors influence the nature of the energy emitted during MR imaging, the most important being relaxation time and motion.

The signal strength during MR imaging diminishes exponentially with a characteristic *relaxation time* that is determined, in part, by the general environment of the nuclei. There are two such relaxation times, designated *T1* and *T2*. T1 represents the time required for the component of the net magnetization vector parallel to the external field to return to its initial value after it has been perturbed by the radio frequency pulse. The T1 relaxation time tends to be long for fluids (e.g., cerebrospinal fluid or hydatid cyst contents) and shorter for fat. Any process that increases tissue water content (e.g., edema) lengthens T1.

The T2 relaxation time is related to the exponential decay of the magnetization *perpendicular* to the external field. It is the result of random molecular motion, which leads to signal dephasing. The latter in turn is related to the local molecular environment, with T2 times being characteristically long for homogeneous environments (e.g., fluid) and short for complex tissues (e.g., muscle). An increase in tissue water as a result of congestive heart failure or a pulmonary neoplasm results in lengthening of the T2 relaxation time.[30]

The MR signal is influenced by the motion of water or blood during the imaging sequence. Depending on the velocity of blood flow and the image sequence used, the signal of flowing blood may be increased (*white blood* signal), decreased (*black blood* signal), or intermediate. Many specialized MR pulse sequences have been devised that have special sensitivity to flow and may allow quantification of the flow.[31,32]

The depiction of blood vessels on MR imaging can be improved by using gadolinium enhancement (MR angiography) and specialized MR sequences.[33,34] The use of gadolinium enhancement and high-speed imaging gradients makes it possible to obtain three-dimensional images of the mediastinal and pulmonary vessels during a single breath-hold.[33,34] On these images, flowing blood results in high signal intensity (white blood MR angiography) (Fig. 2–7). Visualization of the vessel walls is optimized by using sequences in which flowing blood results in signal void (black blood angiography).[28]

MR imaging has several advantages over CT, including (1) a lack of ionizing radiation; (2) direct coronal, sagittal, or oblique as well as transverse imaging; (3) intrinsic contrast in blood vessels as a result of flow; and (4) increased soft tissue contrast because of multiple MR parameters versus only electron density on CT (Fig. 2–8). The main limitation of MR imaging in the assessment of chest disease is the presence of physiologic motion, which severely degrades image quality. Although quality has improved greatly with the use of cardiac gating and respiratory compensation, the use of MR imaging for assessment of the lung parenchyma is still hampered by the low signal-to-noise ratio related to the low proton density of the lungs and the loss of signal caused by the magnetic field inhomogeneity created by the difference in diamagnetic susceptibilities between air and water.

Indications

Evaluation of the Heart and Great Vessels. MR imaging has a well-established role in the assessment of congenital abnormalities of the heart and great vessels. It is superior to

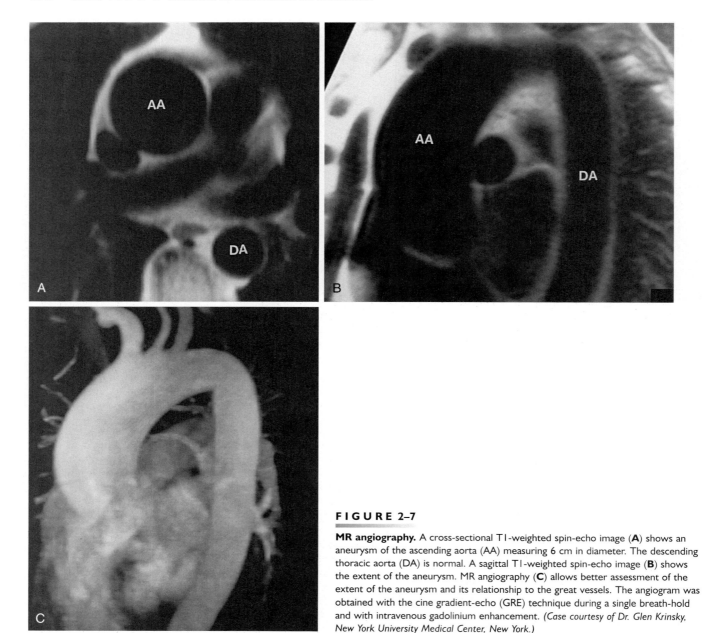

FIGURE 2–7

MR angiography. A cross-sectional T1-weighted spin-echo image (**A**) shows an aneurysm of the ascending aorta (AA) measuring 6 cm in diameter. The descending thoracic aorta (DA) is normal. A sagittal T1-weighted spin-echo image (**B**) shows the extent of the aneurysm. MR angiography (**C**) allows better assessment of the extent of the aneurysm and its relationship to the great vessels. The angiogram was obtained with the cine gradient-echo (GRE) technique during a single breath-hold and with intravenous gadolinium enhancement. *(Case courtesy of Dr. Glen Krinsky, New York University Medical Center, New York.)*

echocardiography in the assessment of adult congenital heart disease because it permits unobstructed views of all atrial, ventricular, and great-vessel abnormalities.[35,36] However, it is usually reserved for patients who have nondiagnostic or equivocal findings on echocardiography.[36] MR imaging also allows excellent evaluation of central pulmonary artery abnormalities. Cine gradient-echo sequences permit assessment of cardiac wall motion and can detect high-velocity jets related to ventricular septal defects, valvular regurgitation, or focal stenosis.[35,37] Velocity-encoded cine sequences can be used to calculate blood flow.[38]

Evaluation of the Mediastinum and Hila. Currently, MR imaging is a secondary imaging modality for assessment of the mediastinum and hila; it is used mainly as a problem-solving technique in cases in which the CT findings are equivocal.

Nonetheless, it has been shown to be superior to CT in the assessment of mediastinal and vascular invasion by pulmonary carcinoma.[39] It can also be helpful in the diagnosis of bronchogenic cysts in cases in which the CT findings are not diagnostic (see Fig. 2–8)[40]; these lesions characteristically show homogeneous high signal intensity on T2-weighted MR images as a result of their fluid content.

Evaluation of the Chest Wall. MR imaging allows excellent assessment of primary chest wall tumors,[41] as well as chest wall invasion by lymphoma[42] and pulmonary carcinoma, particularly tumors located in the superior sulcus region.[43,44] It is also the imaging modality of choice for the assessment of paraspinal lesions such as neurogenic tumors because it provides assessment of the tissue characteristics of the mass, as well as the presence or absence of intraspinal extension.[45,46]

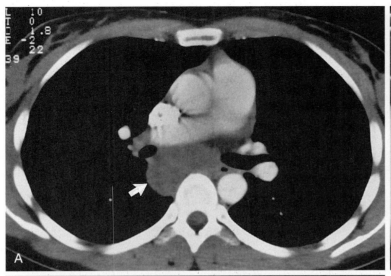

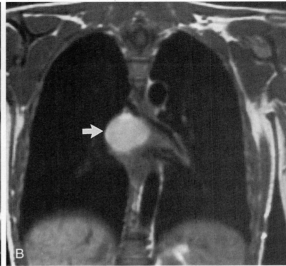

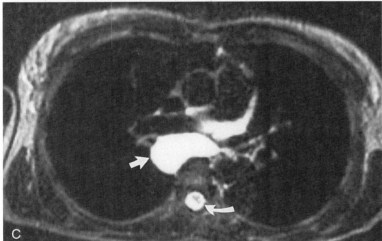

FIGURE 2–8

Soft tissue and fluid characterization on CT and MR imaging. A contrast-enhanced CT scan (**A**) shows a large, smoothly marginated subcarinal lesion *(arrow)*. The attenuation value is consistent with either a soft tissue lesion or a cyst filled with proteinaceous material. A coronal T1-weighted (TR/TE 923/20) spin-echo MR image (**B**) shows a subcarinal mass with high signal intensity *(arrow)*. A transverse T2-weighted (TR/TE 2769/100) spin-echo MR image obtained at the same level as the CT scan (**C**) shows an area of homogeneous high signal intensity *(straight arrow)*. The high signal intensity on the T2-weighted image is diagnostic of fluid. The signal in the subcarinal mass *(straight arrow)* on the T2-weighted image (**C**) is identical to that of cerebrospinal fluid *(curved arrow)*. *(From Müller NL, Fraser RS, Colman NC, Paré PD: Radiologic Diagnosis of Diseases of the Chest. Philadelphia, WB Saunders, 2001.)*

RADIONUCLIDE IMAGING

The most commonly used scintigraphic technique in pulmonary nuclear medicine is the ventilation-perfusion ($\dot{V}/\dot{Q}$) lung scan. Positron emission tomography (PET) with 2-[^{18}F]-fluoro-2-deoxy-D-glucose (FDG) is playing an increasing role the diagnosis and staging of pulmonary carcinoma and other malignant tumors.

Ventilation-Perfusion Scanning

The radiopharmaceuticals of choice for perfusion lung scanning are ^{99m}Tc-labeled human albumin microspheres (technetium Tc 99m HAM) and macroaggregated albumin (technetium Tc 99m MAA). Most experience with ventilation imaging has been with xenon 133 and technetium 99m aerosols.

Perfusion scintigraphy is sensitive, but nonspecific for diagnosing pulmonary disease. Virtually all conditions that affect the parenchyma and/or airways, including neoplasms, infections, COPD, and asthma, can cause decreased pulmonary arterial blood flow within the affected lung zone.

Thromboemboli characteristically cause abnormal perfusion with preserved ventilation (mismatched defects) (Fig. 2–9), whereas parenchymal lung disease most often causes ventilation and perfusion abnormalities in the same lung region (matched defects). Combined ventilation and perfusion scintigraphy is performed routinely to improve diagnostic specificity.

The $\dot{V}/\dot{Q}$ lung scan has been shown to be a safe, noninvasive technique to evaluate regional pulmonary perfusion and ventilation and has been used widely in the evaluation of patients who have suspected thromboembolism (Tables 2–3 and 2–4).[47,48] Quantitative $\dot{V}/\dot{Q}$ lung scanning has been shown to be a useful method for determining regional lung function in patients who are to undergo pulmonary resection or lung transplantation. Its major use is in the prediction of postoperative function after lobectomy or pneumonectomy. The predicted postoperative FEV$_1$ after these two procedures is calculated by multiplying the preoperative value by the percentage of radionuclide activity in the lobes or lung that will remain after surgery.[49] An expected postoperative FEV$_1$ less than 0.8 L or 35% of predicted usually precludes lung resection.

Positron Emission Tomography

PET is a functional imaging technique in which tomographic images are obtained after the administration of positron-emitting radiopharmaceuticals. Similar to CT and MR imaging, PET is based on the principle that a three-dimensional representation of an object can be obtained from multiple annular projections. However, rather than the anatomic information obtained by CT, PET provides functional information.

Malignant cells have increased glucose transport and metabolism related to their rapid proliferation and increased content of messenger RNA.[50,51] These biochemical alterations can be imaged by PET after administration of the glucose analogue FDG, whose mechanism of uptake and initial phosphorylation are similar to that of glucose. Once FDG is phosphorylated (FDG-6-phosphate), it is not metabolized further and remains within the cell. The amount of FDG-6-phosphate within the cell can be assessed with PET systems and is proportional to glucose uptake and metabolism.

Current indications for FDG-PET imaging include distinction of benign from malignant pulmonary nodules, assessment of the presence or absence of metastases in patients known to have pulmonary carcinoma, and differentiation between parenchymal scarring and recurrent tumor in

Right Posterior

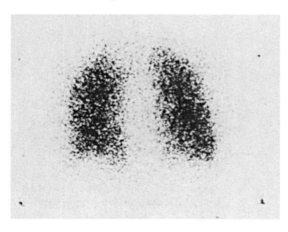

WASH-IN ⟶

Right Posterior

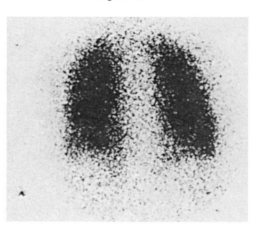

EQUILIBRIUM

Right Posterior

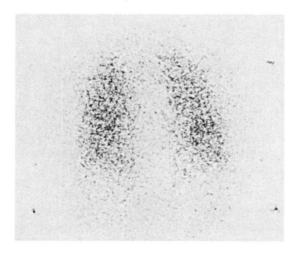

WASH-OUT

A

FIGURE 2–9

Value of ventilation-perfusion lung scans in the diagnosis of thromboembolism. A xenon inhalation lung scan (**A**) discloses normal ventilation parameters during the wash-in, equilibrium, and wash-out phases.

patients who have had previous therapy for pulmonary carcinoma (Fig. 2–10).[52]

The reported sensitivity and specificity of FDG-PET imaging for distinguishing malignant from benign lesions range from approximately 80% to 100% and 50% to 97%, respectively.[53,54] False-positive results have been reported in conditions of active inflammation, such as aspergillosis, tuberculosis, and sarcoidosis. Several investigators have shown that PET imaging is superior to CT in the detection of mediastinal nodal metastases from non–small cell pulmonary carcinoma.[55,56] In one meta-analytic comparison of the diagnostic performance of PET imaging and CT, the mean sensitivity

Anterior

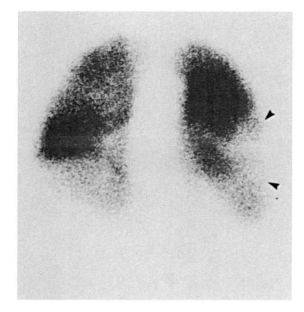

Posterior

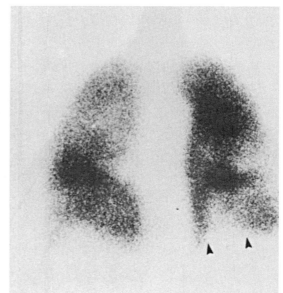

Right Posterior Oblique

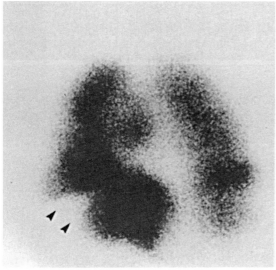

Left Posterior Oblique

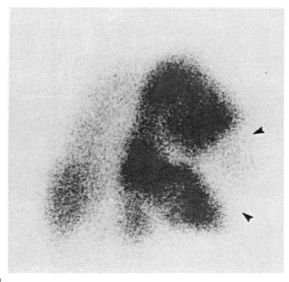

B

FIGURE 2–9—cont'd

Corresponding technetium 99m–labeled macroaggregated albumin perfusion lung scans (**B**) in the anterior, posterior, and right and left posterior oblique projections identify multiple segmental filling defects throughout both lungs *(arrowheads)*. These findings, in concert with the ventilation study, are virtually diagnostic (high probability) of pulmonary thromboembolism. The patient was a 65-year-old man with acute dyspnea. *(From Müller NL, Fraser RS, Colman NC, Paré PD: Radiologic Diagnosis of Diseases of the Chest. Philadelphia, WB Saunders, 2001.)*

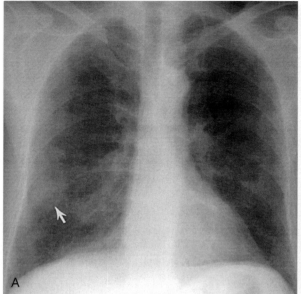

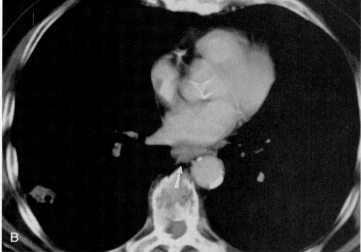

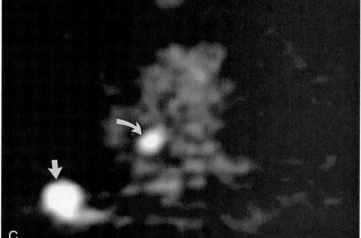

FIGURE 2–10

Positron emission tomography (PET). A posteroanterior chest radiograph (**A**) shows a poorly defined right lower lobe nodule (*arrow*). A CT scan (**B**) confirms the presence of the right lower lobe nodule and shows an enlarged paraesophageal lymph node (*arrow*). A PET image (**C**) shows marked 2-[^{18}F]-fluoro-2-deoxy-D-glucose (FDG) uptake in the right lower lobe nodule (*straight arrow*) and in the paraesophageal node (*curved arrow*). This case was biopsy-proven large cell carcinoma. (*Case courtesy of Dr. Ned Patz, Duke University Medical Center, Durham, NC.*)

TABLE 2–3. Sensitivity, Specificity, and Positive Predictive Value of Ventilation-Perfusion Lung Scanning for Detecting Acute Pulmonary Thromboembolism Using the Original PIOPED Interpretation Criteria

Ventilation-Perfusion Interpretation	Sensitivity (%)	Specificity (%)	PPV (%)
High	40	98	87
High, intermediate	82	64	49
High, intermediate, low	98	12	32

PIOPED, Prospective Investigation of Pulmonary Embolism Diagnosis; PPV, positive predictive value.
Data from Value of the ventilation/perfusion scan in acute pulmonary embolism.
Results of the Prospective Investigation of Pulmonary Embolism Diagnosis (PIOPED).

TABLE 2–4. Effect of Selected Risk Factors on the Prevalence of Pulmonary Thromboembolism

Ventilation-Perfusion	0 Risk Factors*	1 Risk Factor*	≥2 Risk Factors*
High	63/77 (82%)	41/49 (84%)	56/58 (97%)
Intermediate	52/207 (25%)	40/107 (37%)	77/173 (45%)
Low, very low	14/315 (4%)	19/155 (12%)	37/179 (21%)

*Risk factors include immobilization, trauma to the lower extremities, surgery, and central venous instrumentation within 3 months of enrollment. Results are based on data published in Worsley DF, Alavi, A, Palevsky HI: Comparison of diagnostic performance with ventilation-perfusion lung imaging in different patient populations. Radiology 199:481, 1996.

and specificity of PET in detecting mediastinal nodal metastases were 79% and 91%, respectively, versus 60% and 77%, respectively, for CT.[56] A number of investigators have also shown that whole-body PET imaging is superior to CT and bone scintigraphy in the detection of extrathoracic metastases.[52,57,58]

The main limitation of PET imaging is low spatial resolution and lack of anatomic landmarks, which impedes precise localization of lesions. This problem has been overcome recently with the introduction of scanners that allow the acquisition of PET and CT images during the same session. On these PET-CT scanners, the PET images are coregistered (fused) with the CT images to allow simultaneous depiction of metabolic or functional information (PET) and anatomic information (CT).[59,60] Such imaging is superior to either PET or CT alone for assessment of the primary tumor, mediastinal nodal involvement, and extrathoracic metastases.[61,62]

ULTRASONOGRAPHY

With respect to thoracic disease, ultrasonography has its greatest value in the assessment of congenital and acquired heart disease, particularly in establishing the nature of valvular deformity, the volume of cardiac chambers, the thickness of their walls, the effectiveness of cardiac contraction (ejection fraction), and the presence of a right-to-left shunt. The role of ultrasound in the assessment of abnormalities of the aorta has increased considerably with the advent of transesophageal echocardiography. The procedure is also valuable for detecting pericardial effusion, assessing its size, and differentiating it from cardiomegaly and has been used to detect intravascular air bubbles in cases of pulmonary air embolism.

Because it is portable, does not use ionizing radiation, and frequently provides useful diagnostic information, ultrasound is also used commonly in the diagnosis of pleural, diaphragmatic, and infradiaphragmatic abnormalities. Except for these applications, the role of ultrasound in the diagnosis of non-cardiovascular chest disease is limited by the physical composition of the intrathoracic structures. Neither air nor bone transmits sound; instead, they reflect or absorb incoming sonic energy and prevent the collection of information about acoustic interfaces behind ribs or lung tissue. Thus, the technique is limited to assessment of pulmonary masses or consolidation abutting the mediastinum, chest wall, or diaphragm and documentation of the presence and nature of pleural fluid.

Indications

Assessment of Pleural Effusion. Because of its portability, bedside sonography has become a major imaging modality for determination of the presence of pleural fluid and for guidance during aspiration and drainage.[63,64] Most pleural fluid collections are readily identified at ultrasound as anechoic or hypoechoic collections, often delineated by echogenic aerated lung (Fig. 2–11). Although transudates and exudates have similar radiologic appearances, they may have different ultrasound characteristics.[65,66] In one study of 50 patients, 15 of 19 (79%) effusions containing septations at ultrasound represented exudates.[65] In another investigation of 320 patients, effusions that had complex septated, complex nonseptated, or homogeneously echogenic patterns were always exudates.[66] Other findings indicative of exudative effusion include the presence of a thickened pleura or an associated pulmonary parenchymal lesion. Although these findings are helpful in diagnosis, hypoechoic effusions may be either transudates or exudates.[65,66]

Assessment of the Diaphragm. Ultrasonography provides excellent assessment of diaphragmatic and peridiaphragmatic masses and fluid collections and allows easy distinction of small pleural effusions from infradiaphragmatic fluid collections. Because the liver provides an optimal acoustic window to assess the right hemidiaphragm, the procedure is also helpful in the diagnosis of traumatic tears of the right hemidiaphragm.[67] The presence of bowel gas usually precludes optimal sonographic assessment of the left hemidiaphragm.

Guide to Needle Biopsy and Catheter Placement. Ultrasonography allows excellent visualization of pulmonary, pleural, or mediastinal lesions in contact with the chest wall or in a juxtadiaphragmatic location and permits real-time

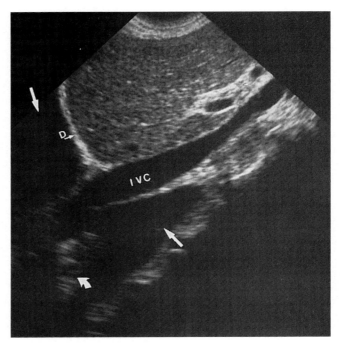

FIGURE 2–11

Pleural effusion on ultrasound. Ultrasound shows a large echo-free right pleural effusion (*straight arrows*). Also noted are an atelectatic right lung (*curved arrow*), the diaphragm (D), the inferior vena cava (IVC), and the liver. The effusion was shown on needle aspiration to be a transudate. (*From Müller NL, Fraser RS, Colman NC, Paré PD: Radiologic Diagnosis of Diseases of the Chest. Philadelphia, WB Saunders, 2001.*)

monitoring while performing fine-needle biopsy.[68] As such, the procedure is used frequently as a guide to placement of a catheter for pleural sclerotherapy or drainage of empyema.[69,70] Ultrasonography also allows pleural drainage to be performed at the bedside in critically ill patients.

Endoscopic Ultrasound-Guided Biopsy. Transesophageal endoscopic ultrasound allows visualization and characterization of abnormalities situated in the posterior mediastinum, particularly those adjacent to the esophagus, and in the aortopulmonary window.[71,72] The procedure is also useful in assessing abnormalities of the tracheobronchial wall, including the presence of intramural or extraluminal tumor.[73,74] In combination with fine-needle aspiration biopsy, it is being used with increasing frequency in the diagnosis of mediastinal tumors and in the staging of pulmonary carcinoma.[72,75] For example, it has been shown to improve staging by allowing identification of N2 and N3 nodal involvement.[74,76] It may also be helpful in biopsy of parenchymal nodules located next to bronchi.[73]

REFERENCES

1. Robin ED, Burke CM: Routine chest x-ray examinations. Chest 90:258-262, 1986.
2. American College of Radiology: ACR Standard for the Performance of Pediatric and Adult Chest Radiography. Reston, VA, American College of Radiology, 1997, p 27.
3. American Thoracic Society: Chest x-ray screening statements. Am Thorac News 10:14, 1984.
4. Hasegawa BH, Naimuddin S, Dobbins JT 3rd, et al: Digital beam attenuator technique for compensated chest radiography. Radiology 159:537-543, 1986.

5. Plewes DB: A scanning system for chest radiography with regional exposure control: Theoretical considerations. Med Phys 10:646-654, 1983.
6. Plewes DB, Vogelstein E: A scanning system for chest radiography with regional exposure control: Practical implementation. Med Phys 10:655-663, 1983.
7. MacMahon H, Vyborny C: Technical advances in chest radiography. AJR Am J Roentgenol 163:1049-1059, 1994.
8. Ravin CE, Chotas HG: Chest radiography. Radiology 204:593-600, 1997.
9. Wandtke JC: Bedside chest radiography. Radiology 190:1-10, 1994.
10. Schaefer CM, Greene R, Llewellyn HJ, et al: Interstitial lung disease: Impact of post-processing in digital storage phosphor imaging. Radiology 178:733-738, 1991.
11. Sagel SS, Jost RG, Glazer HS, et al: Digital mobile radiography. J Thorac Imaging 5:36-48, 1990.
12. Sonoda M, Takano M, Miyahara J, Kato H: Computed radiography utilizing scanning laser stimulated luminescence. Radiology 148:833-838, 1983.
13. Chotas HG, Floyd CE Jr, Ravin CE: Technical evaluation of a digital chest radiography system that uses a selenium detector. Radiology 195:264-270, 1995.
14. Garmer M, Hennigs SP, Jager HJ, et al: Digital radiography versus conventional radiography in chest imaging: Diagnostic performance of a large-area silicon flat-panel detector in a clinical CT-controlled study. AJR Am J Roentgenol 174:75-80, 2000.
15. Muller NL: Clinical value of high-resolution CT in chronic diffuse lung disease. AJR Am J Roentgenol 157:1163-1170, 1991.
16. McGuinness G, Naidich DP: Bronchiectasis: CT/clinical correlations. Semin Ultrasound CT MR 16:395-419, 1995.
17. Leung AN, Staples CA, Muller NL: Chronic diffuse infiltrative lung disease: Comparison of diagnostic accuracy of high-resolution and conventional CT. AJR Am J Roentgenol 157:693-696, 1991.
18. Webb W, Muller N, Naidich D (eds): High Resolution CT of the Lung. Philadelphia, Lippincott-Raven, 2001.
19. Mayo JR, Webb WR, Gould R, et al: High-resolution CT of the lungs: An optimal approach. Radiology 163:507-510, 1987.
20. Zwirewich CV, Terriff B, Muller NL: High-spatial-frequency (bone) algorithm improves quality of standard CT of the thorax. AJR Am J Roentgenol 153:1169-1173, 1989.
21. Kalender WA, Seissler W, Klotz E, Vock P: Spiral volumetric CT with single-breath-hold technique, continuous transport, and continuous scanner rotation. Radiology 176:181-183, 1990.
22. Crawford CR, King KF: Computed tomography scanning with simultaneous patient translation. Med Phys 17:967-982, 1990.
23. Rydberg J, Buckwalter KA, Caldemeyer KS, et al: Multisection CT: Scanning techniques and clinical applications. Radiographics 20:1787-1806, 2000.
24. Remy-Jardin M, Remy J, Artaud D, et al: Volume rendering of the tracheobronchial tree: Clinical evaluation of bronchographic images. Radiology 208:761-770, 1998.
25. Higgins WE, Ramaswamy K, Swift RD, et al: Virtual bronchoscopy for three-dimensional pulmonary image assessment: State of the art and future needs. Radiographics 18:761-778, 1998.
26. Johnson CD, Hara AK, Reed JE: Virtual endoscopy: What's in a name? AJR Am J Roentgenol 171:1201-1202, 1998.
27. Hopper KD, Iyriboz TA, Mahraj RP, et al: CT bronchoscopy: Optimization of imaging parameters. Radiology 209:872-877, 1998.
28. Naidich D, Webb W, Muller N, et al (eds): Computed Tomography and Magnetic Resonance of the Thorax. Philadelphia, Lippincott-Raven, 1999.
29. Remy-Jardin M, Remy J: Spiral CT angiography of the pulmonary circulation. Radiology 212:615-636, 1999.
30. Mayo JR: Magnetic resonance imaging of the chest. Where we stand. Radiol Clin North Am 32:795-809, 1994.
31. Firmin DN, Nayler GL, Kilner PJ, Longmore DB: The application of phase shifts in NMR for flow measurement. Magn Reson Med 14:230-241, 1990.
32. Boxerman JL, Mosher TJ, McVeigh ER, et al: Advanced MR imaging techniques for evaluation of the heart and great vessels. Radiographics 18:543-564, 1998.
33. Ho VB, Prince MR: Thoracic MR aortography: Imaging techniques and strategies. Radiographics 18:287-309, 1998.
34. Alley MT, Shifrin RY, Pelc NJ, Herfkens RJ: Ultrafast contrast-enhanced three-dimensional MR angiography: State of the art. Radiographics 18:273-285, 1998.
35. Higgins CB, Sakuma H: Heart disease: Functional evaluation with MR imaging. Radiology 199:307-315, 1996.
36. Higgins CB, Caputo GR: Role of MR imaging in acquired and congenital cardiovascular disease. AJR Am J Roentgenol 161:13-22, 1993.
37. Sechtem U, Pflugfelder PW, White RD, et al: Cine MR imaging: Potential for the evaluation of cardiovascular function. AJR Am J Roentgenol 148:239-246, 1987.
38. Kondo C, Caputo GR, Semelka R, et al: Right and left ventricular stroke volume measurements with velocity-encoded cine MR imaging: In vitro and in vivo validation. AJR Am J Roentgenol 157:9-16, 1991.
39. Webb WR, Gatsonis C, Zerhouni EA, et al: CT and MR imaging in staging non-small cell bronchogenic carcinoma: Report of the radiologic diagnostic oncology group. Radiology 178:705, 1991.
40. Nakata H, Egashira K, Watanabe H, et al: MRI of bronchogenic cysts. J Comput Assist Tomogr 17:267-270, 1993.
41. Fortier M, Mayo JR, Swensen SJ, et al: MR imaging of chest wall lesions. Radiographics 14:597-606, 1994.
42. Bergin CJ, Healy MV, Zincone GE, Castellino RA: MR evaluation of chest wall involvement in malignant lymphoma. J Comput Assist Tomogr 14:928-932, 1990.
43. Heelan RT, Demas BE, Caravelli JF, et al: Superior sulcus tumors: CT and MR imaging. Radiology 170:637-641, 1989.
44. McLoud TC, Filion RB, Edelman RR, Shepard JA: MR imaging of superior sulcus carcinoma. J Comput Assist Tomogr 13:233-239, 1989.
45. Flickinger FW, Yuh WT, Behrendt DM: Magnetic resonance imaging of mediastinal paraganglioma. Chest 94:652-654, 1988.
46. Siegel MJ, Jamroz GA, Glazer HS, Abramson CL: MR imaging of intraspinal extension of neuroblastoma. J Comput Assist Tomogr 10:593-595, 1986.
47. Value of the ventilation/perfusion scan in acute pulmonary embolism. Results of the Prospective Investigation of Pulmonary Embolism Diagnosis (PIOPED). The PIOPED Investigators. JAMA 263:2753-2759, 1990.
48. Hull RD, Raskob GE, Ginsberg JS, et al: A noninvasive strategy for the treatment of patients with suspected pulmonary embolism. Arch Intern Med 154:289-297, 1994.
49. Ali MK, Mountain CF, Ewer MS, et al: Predicting loss of pulmonary function after pulmonary resection for bronchogenic carcinoma. Chest 77:337-342, 1980.
50. Weber G: Enzymology of cancer cells (first of two parts). N Engl J Med 296:486-492, 1977.
51. Weber G: Enzymology of cancer cells (second of two parts). N Engl J Med 296:541-551, 1977.
52. Hagge RJ, Coleman RE: Positron emission tomography: Lung cancer. Semin Roentgenol 37:110-117, 2002.
53. Gupta NC, Frank AR, Dewan NA, et al: Solitary pulmonary nodules: Detection of malignancy with PET with 2-[F-18]-fluoro-2-deoxy-D-glucose. Radiology 184:441-444, 1992.
54. Sazon DA, Santiago SM, Soo Hoo GW, et al: Fluorodeoxyglucose-positron emission tomography in the detection and staging of lung cancer. Am J Respir Crit Care Med 153:417-421, 1996.
55. Wahl RL, Quint LE, Greenough RL, et al: Staging of mediastinal non–small cell lung cancer with FDG PET, CT, and fusion images: Preliminary prospective evaluation. Radiology 191:371-377, 1994.
56. Dwamena BA, Sonnad SS, Angobaldo JO, Wahl RL: Metastases from non–small cell lung cancer: Mediastinal staging in the 1990s—meta-analytic comparison of PET and CT. Radiology 213:530-536, 1999.
57. Valk PE, Pounds TR, Hopkins DM, et al: Staging non–small cell lung cancer by whole-body positron emission tomographic imaging. Ann Thorac Surg 60:1573-1581, discussion 1581-1582, 1995.
58. Marom EM, McAdams HP, Erasmus JJ, et al: Staging non–small cell lung cancer with whole-body PET. Radiology 212:803-809, 1999.
59. Townsend DW: A combined PET/CT scanner: The choices. J Nucl Med 42:533-534, 2001.
60. Kluetz PG, Meltzer CC, Villemagne VL, et al: Combined PET/CT imaging in oncology. Impact on patient management. Clin Positron Imaging 3:223-230, 2000.
61. Aquino SL, Asmuth JC, Alpert NM, et al: Improved radiologic staging of lung cancer with 2-[^{18}F]-fluoro-2-deoxy-D-glucose-positron emission tomography and computed tomography registration. J Comput Assist Tomogr 27:479-484, 2003.
62. Lardinois D, Weder W, Hany TF, et al: Staging of non–small-cell lung cancer with integrated positron-emission tomography and computed tomography. N Engl J Med 348:2500-2507, 2003.
63. Lipscomb DJ, Flower CD, Hadfield JW: Ultrasound of the pleura: An assessment of its clinical value. Clin Radiol 32:289-290, 1981.
64. O'Moore PV, Mueller PR, Simeone JF, et al: Sonographic guidance in diagnostic and therapeutic interventions in the pleural space. AJR Am J Roentgenol 149:1-5, 1987.
65. Hirsch JH, Rogers JV, Mack LA: Real-time sonography of pleural opacities. AJR Am J Roentgenol 136:297-301, 1981.
66. Yang PC, Luh KT, Chang DB, et al: Value of sonography in determining the nature of pleural effusion: Analysis of 320 cases. AJR Am J Roentgenol 159:29-33, 1992.
67. Somers JM, Gleeson FV, Flower CD: Rupture of the right hemidiaphragm following blunt trauma: The use of ultrasound in diagnosis. Clin Radiol 42:97-101, 1990.
68. Ikezoe J, Morimoto S, Arisawa J, et al: Percutaneous biopsy of thoracic lesions: Value of sonography for needle guidance. AJR Am J Roentgenol 154:1181-1185, 1990.
69. Morrison MC, Mueller PR, Lee MJ, et al: Sclerotherapy of malignant pleural effusion through sonographically placed small-bore catheters. AJR Am J Roentgenol 158:41-43, 1992.
70. Klein JS, Schultz S, Heffner JE: Interventional radiology of the chest: Image-guided percutaneous drainage of pleural effusions, lung abscess, and pneumothorax. AJR Am J Roentgenol 164:581-588, 1995.
71. Catalano MF, Rosenblatt ML, Chak A, et al: Endoscopic ultrasound-guided fine needle aspiration in the diagnosis of mediastinal masses of unknown origin. Am J Gastroenterol 97:2559-2565, 2002.
72. Fritscher-Ravens A: Endoscopic ultrasound evaluation in the diagnosis and staging of lung cancer. Lung Cancer 41:259-267, 2003.
73. Falcone F, Fois F, Grosso D: Endobronchial ultrasound. Respiration 70:179-194, 2003.
74. Herth F, Ernst A, Schulz M, Becker H: Endobronchial ultrasound reliably differentiates between airway infiltration and compression by tumor. Chest 123:458-462, 2003.
75. LeBlanc JK, Espada R, Ergun G: Non–small cell lung cancer staging techniques and endoscopic ultrasound: Tissue is still the issue. Chest 123:1718-1725, 2003.
76. Herth FJ, Becker HD, Ernst A: Ultrasound-guided transbronchial needle aspiration: An experience in 242 patients. Chest 123:604-607, 2003.

RADIOLOGIC SIGNS OF CHEST DISEASE

The differential diagnosis of radiologic abnormalities is based on considerations such as density, size, number, homogeneity, sharpness of definition, anatomic location, and the presence or absence of calcification or cavitation. In this chapter, we describe the basic radiologic signs that are seen in chest disease and that are useful in the differential diagnosis. These signs can be considered in four major categories: increased lung density, decreased lung density, atelectasis, and pleural abnormalities.

INCREASED LUNG DENSITY

Most diseases that increase lung density involve the air spaces and interstitial tissue to a variable extent; however, it is helpful to recognize three general radiographic patterns, depending on which component is affected: (1) *air space disease,* the air being replaced by liquid, cells, or a combination of the two (consolidation); (2) *interstitial disease;* and (3) *combined air space and interstitial disease.* This division is useful if one accepts the proviso that the term *air space pattern* indicates predominant involvement of the parenchymal air spaces, and that a *linear, reticular, or nodular pattern* indicates predominant involvement of the interstitium.

Predominantly Air Space Disease

Parenchymal consolidation is defined as replacement of gas within the air spaces by liquid, cells, or a combination of the two. Such air space disease is characterized on radiographs and CT scans by the presence of one or more fairly homogeneous opacities associated with obscuration of the pulmonary vessels and little or no volume loss (Fig. 3–1).[1,2] The margins of the opacities are poorly defined except in areas where the consolidation abuts the pleura. Air-containing bronchi (air bronchograms) are frequently evident; localized small lucencies corresponding to patent membranous bronchioles (air bronchiolograms) or nonconsolidated lung parenchyma and localized round areas of consolidation measuring 10 mm in diameter or less (air space nodules) may also be identified.

Distribution Characteristics

Consolidation may be focal, patchy, or distributed widely throughout both lungs (Table 3–1). Focal consolidation may be segmental or nonsegmental in distribution; occasionally, it involves an entire lobe or lung. Segmental consolidation with or without associated volume loss typically results from endobronchial obstruction (e.g., from pulmonary carcinoma) or from pulmonary infarction (e.g., thromboembolism or invasive aspergillosis) (Fig. 3–2). Segmental distribution can be seen after aspiration and with pneumonia caused by *Staphylococcus aureus, Streptococcus pyogenes,* or a variety of gram-negative bacteria; however, infection by these organisms is more commonly associated with multifocal or patchy bilateral consolidation (bronchopneumonia). A similar distribution may be seen in severe fungal pneumonia, particularly in immunocompromised patients (Fig. 3–3).

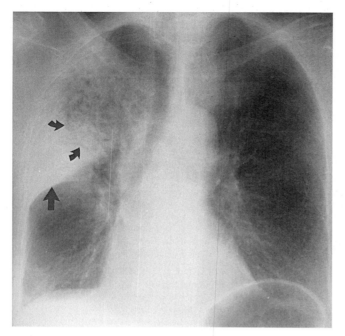

FIGURE 3–1

Air space consolidation. A posteroanterior chest radiograph in a 64-year-old woman shows extensive air space consolidation in the right upper lobe. The findings consist of confluent fluffy opacities with poorly defined margins except where the consolidation abuts the horizontal fissure (*straight arrow*). Note the presence of air bronchograms (*curved arrows*). Incidental note is made of a small right pleural effusion. The patient had lobar pneumonia caused by *Streptococcus pneumoniae*. (From Müller NL, Fraser RS, Colman NC, Paré PD: Radiologic Diagnosis of Diseases of the Chest. Philadelphia, WB Saunders, 2001.)

On HRCT scan, areas of air space consolidation are often marginated by interlobular septa (Fig. 3–4).[3] Single or multiple spared lobules may be present within areas of massive consolidation.[3] Involvement of a secondary lobule or a cluster of lobules with adjacent normal parenchyma is particularly common in bronchopneumonia[4] and is also known as *lobular pneumonia.*

Causes of nonsegmental consolidation include pneumonia, focal hemorrhage, neoplasm, irradiation, Löffler's syndrome, and chronic eosinophilic pneumonia. Nonsegmental pneumonia is caused most commonly by *Streptococcus pneumoniae* and less often by *Klebsiella pneumoniae, Legionella* species, and *Mycobacterium tuberculosis* (see Fig. 3–1). The consolidation in Löffler's syndrome is typically migratory, whereas that in chronic eosinophilic pneumonia characteristically involves the peripheral lung regions. Nonsegmental consolidation that progresses over a period of several months should raise the possibility of bronchioloalveolar carcinoma or lymphoma. Consolidation of an entire lobe may be secondary to bronchial obstruction (e.g., pulmonary carcinoma), in which case it is usually associated with atelectasis and a lack of air bronchograms, or it may be secondary to bacterial pneumonia (typically from *S. pneumoniae* or *K. pneumoniae*), in which case it is associated with normal or, occasionally, increased lung volume and air bronchograms.

Extensive or diffuse bilateral consolidation is seen most commonly in hydrostatic pulmonary edema, acute respiratory

TABLE 3–1. Air-Space Consolidation

Common Causes	Helpful Diagnostic Features
Acute	
Pulmonary edema	Hydrostatic pulmonary edema tends to involve mainly the central lung regions (butterfly distribution) and is commonly associated with cardiomegaly and septal (Kerley B) lines. Pulmonary edema with increased permeability (adult respiratory distress syndrome) tends to be patchy or to involve mainly the peripheral lung regions. Cardiomegaly and septal lines are uncommon
Pneumonia	Consolidation may be homogeneous and lobar (nonsegmental) in distribution (e.g., *Streptococcus pneumoniae*), inhomogeneous and patchy (segmental) in distribution (e.g., gram-negative organisms, *Staphylococcus aureus*), or diffuse (e.g., *Pneumocystis jiroveci* pneumonia)
Hemorrhage	May be focal (e.g., pulmonary contusion, bronchiectasis) or diffuse (e.g., Goodpasture's syndrome, bleeding diathesis). When secondary to pulmonary embolism, may resemble a truncated cone (Hampton's hump)
Aspiration	Aspiration of gastric contents (aspiration pneumonia) tends to involve mainly the dependent lung regions. Aspiration of lipids (lipid pneumonia) can usually be diagnosed on HRCT by the presence of localized areas of fat density
Chronic	
Cryptogenic organizing pneumonia	Findings consist of patchy, nonsegmental, unilateral or bilateral areas of consolidation that progress over several weeks or months. Frequently has a predominantly peribronchial or subpleural distribution on HRCT
Chronic eosinophilic pneumonia	Characteristic homogeneous nonsegmental peripheral consolidation pneumonia involving mainly the upper lobes
Neoplasm	Postobstructive pneumonitis involving a segment, lobe, or entire lung is a common manifestation of endobronchial pulmonary carcinoma. Nonsegmental consolidation is seen with bronchioloalveolar carcinoma and lymphoma
Alveolar proteinosis	An uncommon cause of chronic air space consolidation that may be patchy or involve mainly the perihilar regions. HRCT shows ground-glass attenuation with associated smooth thickening of interlobular septa (crazy-paving pattern)

Adapted from Müller NL, Fraser RS, Colman NC, Paré PD: Radiologic Diagnosis of Diseases of the Chest. Philadelphia, WB Saunders, 2001.

distress syndrome, diffuse pulmonary hemorrhage, and pneumocystis pneumonia. In the first of these conditions, the consolidation tends to involve mainly the perihilar regions (*butterfly* distribution) and is commonly associated with thickening of the interlobular septa (septal lines) and cardiomegaly. The consolidation in acute respiratory distress syndrome tends to have a patchy and predominantly peripheral distribution and is typically associated with a normal heart size. Pneumocystis pneumonia often progresses from a subtle perihilar haze to diffuse bilateral consolidation.

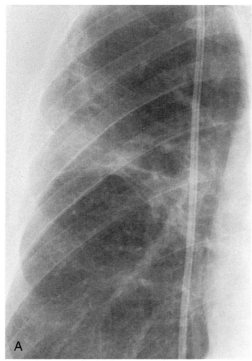

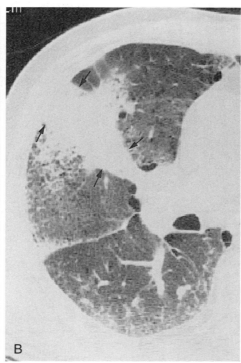

FIGURE 3–2

Subsegmental consolidation. A view of the right lung from a posteroanterior chest radiograph (**A**) shows a wedge-shaped, pleural-based area of consolidation in the right upper lobe. An HRCT scan (**B**) also shows a subsegmental area of dense consolidation *(arrows)* that extends into the adjacent parenchyma. The appearance is consistent with an infarct. The patient was an immunocompromised 54-year-old woman with angioinvasive aspergillosis. *(From Müller NL, Fraser RS, Colman NC, Paré PD: Radiologic Diagnosis of Diseases of the Chest. Philadelphia, WB Saunders, 2001.)*

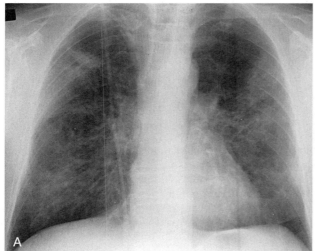

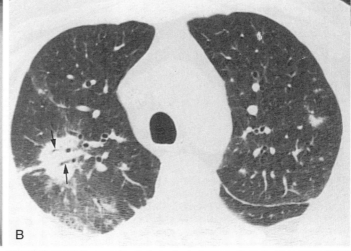

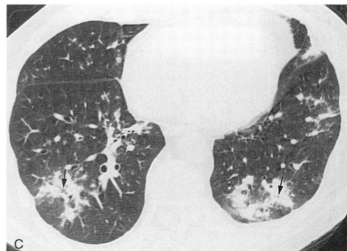

FIGURE 3–3

Bronchopneumonia. A posteroanterior chest radiograph (**A**) shows patchy bilateral areas of consolidation. HRCT scans (**B** and **C**) show the predominant peribronchial distribution of the areas of consolidation. Air bronchograms are clearly evident within the areas of consolidation *(arrows)*. The patient was a 55-year-old man with acute myelogenous leukemia and *Aspergillus* bronchopneumonia. *(From Müller NL, Fraser RS, Colman NC, Paré PD: Radiologic Diagnosis of Diseases of the Chest. Philadelphia, WB Saunders, 2001.)*

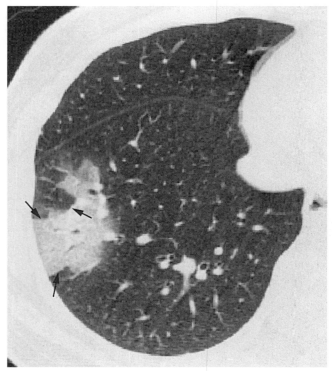

FIGURE 3–4

Pulmonary hemorrhage. An HRCT scan in a 29-year-old woman shows a focal area of consolidation in the right lower lobe as a result of pulmonary hemorrhage. Several of the margins are clearly outlined by interlobular septa *(arrows)*, a feature leading to sharp demarcation between involved and uninvolved secondary pulmonary lobules. *(From Müller NL, Fraser RS, Colman NC, Paré PD: Radiologic Diagnosis of Diseases of the Chest. Philadelphia, WB Saunders, 2001.)*

TABLE 3–2. Septal Pattern

Common Causes	Characteristic Radiographic and HRCT Findings
Hydrostatic pulmonary edema	Most common cause. Predominantly lower lung zone distribution. Smooth interlobular septal thickening on HRCT
Lymphangitic carcinomatosis	May be focal or diffuse. Smooth or nodular septal thickening. Lymph node enlargement seen at initial evaluation in 30% of cases
Sarcoidosis	Septal thickening seldom evident on radiograph but commonly seen on HRCT. Septal involvement usually mild compared with peribronchovascular nodularity. Thickening may be smooth or nodular. Usually associated with bilateral hilar and mediastinal lymph node enlargement
Idiopathic pulmonary fibrosis	Irregular septal thickening usually mild and associated with other findings of fibrosis, including intralobular lines, traction bronchiectasis, and honeycombing
Asbestosis	Irregular septal thickening usually mild and associated with other findings of fibrosis and pleural plaques or diffuse pleural thickening

From Müller NL, Fraser RS, Colman NC, Paré PD: Radiologic Diagnosis of Diseases of the Chest. Philadelphia, WB Saunders, 2001.

Predominantly Interstitial Disease

Radiologic Patterns of Diffuse Interstitial Disease

Interstitial lung disease is associated with five radiologic patterns: septal, reticular, nodular, reticulonodular, and ground-glass. Although each of these patterns can be visualized on HRCT and correlated with specific histopathologic findings,[5-7] superimposition of structures makes interpretation considerably more difficult on the chest radiograph.

Septal Pattern

A septal pattern results from thickening of the interlobular septa (i.e., the tissue that separates the secondary pulmonary lobules). Normally, no septal lines can be identified on the radiograph, and only a few can be seen on HRCT, mostly in the anterior and lower aspects of the lower lobes.[8,9] When thickened, interlobular septa (septal lines) are visualized on the radiograph as short (1 to 2 cm) lines perpendicular to and continuous with the pleura (Kerley B lines) or as longer (2 to 6 cm) lines oriented toward the hila (Kerley A lines) (Fig. 3–5). On HRCT scan, septal lines can be seen as short lines that extend to the pleura in the lung periphery and as polygonal arcades outlining one or more pulmonary lobules in more central lung regions (Fig. 3–6).[8,9]

The presence of septal lines as the predominant radiologic abnormality effectively restricts the diagnostic considerations to hydrostatic pulmonary edema or malignancy (either lymphangitic spread of carcinoma or lymphoma), usually with simultaneous involvement of the bronchoarterial interstitium. Distinction between edema and cancer can often be determined on the basis of clinical findings. In cases in which there is doubt, the HRCT appearance may be helpful in differentiation: interlobular septal thickening as a result of edema is usually smooth, whereas malignancy frequently has a nodular component (Fig. 3–7).[5,10] Although septal thickening may also be seen in a number of other disorders, such as idiopathic pulmonary fibrosis, sarcoidosis, and alveolar proteinosis, it is not usually the main abnormality.[9] Apparent thickening of interlobular septa on HRCT scan may result from disease affecting the parenchyma on both sides of a normal septum, particularly in idiopathic pulmonary fibrosis, acute respiratory distress syndrome, and alveolar proteinosis.[10,11] The most common causes of interlobular septal thickening are listed in Table 3–2.

Reticular Pattern

A reticular pattern is characterized by innumerable interlacing line shadows that suggest a mesh (Fig. 3–8).[2] On a chest radiograph the pattern may be the result of summation of smooth or irregular linear opacities, cystic spaces, or both. Although distinction between these abnormalities is often difficult on a radiograph, it can be made readily on HRCT scan. The most common causes of a reticular pattern are listed in Table 3–3.

Even though pulmonary edema often leads to a predominant linear pattern characterized by the presence of septal (Kerley B) lines, a fine reticular pattern is also seen frequently.

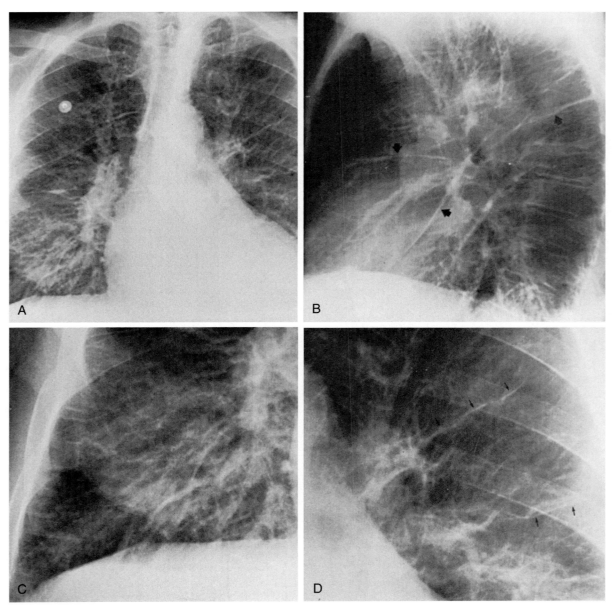

FIGURE 3–5

Interstitial pulmonary edema. Posteroanterior (**A**) and lateral (**B**) radiographs reveal multiple linear opacities throughout both lungs that are seen to better advantage on magnified views of the lower right (**C**) and upper left (**D**) lungs. These lines consist of a combination of long septal lines (Kerley A), predominantly in the midlung zones (*arrows* in **D**), and shorter peripheral septal lines (Kerley B). In lateral projection (**B**), the interlobar fissures are prominent (*arrows*) and represent pleural edema. *(From Müller NL, Fraser RS, Colman NC, Paré PD: Radiologic Diagnosis of Diseases of the Chest. Philadelphia, WB Saunders, 2001.)*

Other causes of a reticular pattern that develops acutely are viral and mycoplasmal pneumonia.

Chronic diseases with a fine reticular pattern include interstitial pulmonary edema associated with mitral stenosis, asbestosis, idiopathic pulmonary fibrosis, and pulmonary fibrosis associated with connective tissue disease. The last two conditions are initially characterized on the chest radiograph by a fine reticular pattern involving mainly the lower lung zones. As disease progresses, the reticular pattern becomes coarser and the process more diffuse. HRCT scan shows intralobular linear opacities (reflecting thickening of the interstitium within the secondary lobule), irregular thickening of the interlobular septa, and honeycombing predominantly in the subpleural lung regions and in the lower lung zones (Fig. 3–9).[5 7]

Cystic air spaces can be defined as enlarged foci of air-containing lung surrounded by walls of variable thickness and composition.[2] Such spaces may be present without associated fibrosis, as in lymphangioleiomyomatosis (Fig. 3–10),[12] or with prominent collagen deposition and parenchymal remodeling (honeycombing), as in idiopathic pulmonary fibrosis, Langerhans cell histiocytosis, asbestosis,

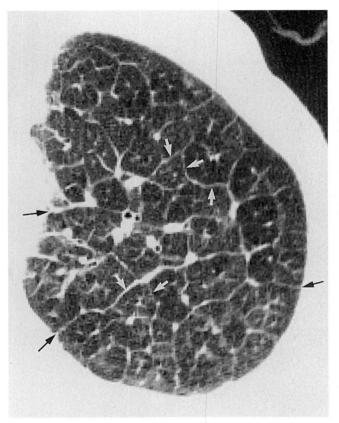

FIGURE 3-6

Interlobular septal thickening. An HRCT scan targeted to the left upper lobe shows interlobular septal thickening. The thickened septa can be identified as lines (*black arrows*) perpendicular to the pleura and extending to it and, more centrally, as polygonal arcades (*white arrows*) outlining the secondary pulmonary lobules. The patient was a 77-year-old woman with interstitial pulmonary edema secondary to left heart failure. (*From Müller NL, Fraser RS, Colman NC, Paré PD: Radiologic Diagnosis of Diseases of the Chest. Philadelphia, WB Saunders, 2001.*)

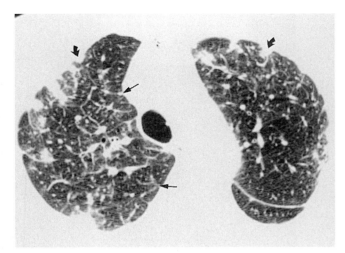

FIGURE 3-7

Lymphangitic carcinomatosis. An HRCT scan shows thickening of the interlobular septa (*straight arrows*) and several nodules (*curved arrows*) with irregular margins, predominantly in the subpleural lung regions. (*From Müller NL, Fraser RS, Colman NC, Paré PD: Radiologic Diagnosis of Diseases of the Chest. Philadelphia, WB Saunders, 2001.*)

TABLE 3-3. Reticular Pattern of Interstitial Disease

Common Causes	Characteristic Radiographic and HRCT Findings
Acute	
Hydrostatic pulmonary edema	Reticular pattern usually seen in association with septal (Kerley) lines. Prominence of upper lobe vessels, pleural effusions, and cardiomegaly common
Mycoplasma pneumonia	Often in association with segmental consolidation. HRCT shows centrilobular nodules and branching linear opacities (*tree-in-bud* pattern)
Chronic	
Idiopathic pulmonary fibrosis and pulmonary fibrosis associated with connective tissue disease	Lower lung zone predominance. HRCT shows intralobular linear opacities, irregular thickening of interlobular septa, and honeycombing involving mainly the subpleural regions and lower lung zones
Asbestosis	Lower lung zone predominance. Almost always in association with pleural plaques or diffuse pleural thickening. HRCT shows subpleural lines, intralobular lines, and irregular interlobular septal thickening in a predominantly subpleural distribution
Chronic extrinsic allergic alveolitis	Usually has middle or lower lung zone predominance. HRCT commonly shows intralobular lines, poorly defined centrilobular nodules, and extensive areas of ground-glass attenuation
Sarcoidosis	Coarse reticulation is seen with chronic fibrosis. Involves mainly the perihilar region of the middle and upper lung zones

From Müller NL, Fraser RS, Colman NC, Paré PD: Radiologic Diagnosis of Diseases of the Chest. Philadelphia, WB Saunders, 2001.

and sarcoidosis.[2,13] Common causes of a cystic pattern are listed in Table 3–4.

Honeycombing refers to the presence of cystic spaces 0.3 to 1 cm in diameter whose walls consist of a variable amount of fibrous tissue (see Fig. 3–8). The most common diseases in which the abnormality is identified are idiopathic pulmonary fibrosis, connective tissue disease, and sarcoidosis[14]; however, the process can be seen in advanced pulmonary fibrosis of any cause.[13,14] The spaces represent mainly respiratory bronchioles and alveolar ducts that have become dilated as a result of traction by fibrous tissue in the adjacent parenchyma.[3,15] The presence, distribution, and extent of honeycombing are assessed much more readily on HRCT than on the chest radiograph.[16]

The presence and severity of honeycombing vary considerably in different regions of the lung with different diseases. Langerhans cell histiocytosis and sarcoidosis usually show a predilection for the middle and upper lung zones, whereas idiopathic pulmonary fibrosis and pulmonary fibrosis associated with connective tissue disease generally involve mainly the lower lung zones. On HRCT scan, the cystic spaces in Langerhans cell histiocytosis have a random or diffuse

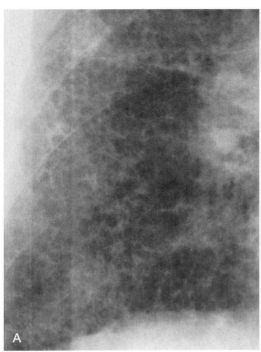
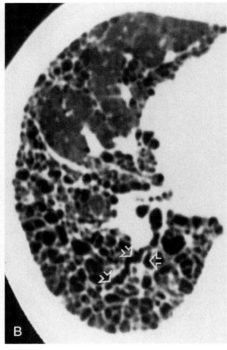

FIGURE 3–8

Reticular pattern. A close-up view of the right lower lung zone from a posteroanterior chest radiograph (**A**) shows a reticular pattern. An HRCT scan (**B**) shows honeycombing throughout the right lower lobe. Note the associated dilation and distortion of the bronchi (traction bronchiectasis) *(arrows)*. Although the honeycombing is diffuse in the right lower lobe, it shows a subpleural predominance in the right middle lobe. This pattern and distribution are consistent with idiopathic pulmonary fibrosis. *(From Müller NL, Fraser RS, Colman NC, Paré PD: Radiologic Diagnosis of Diseases of the Chest. Philadelphia, WB Saunders, 2001.)*

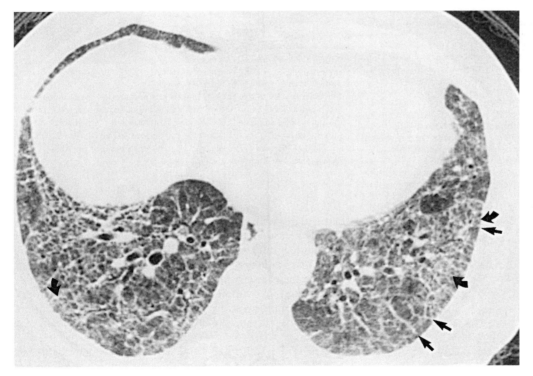

FIGURE 3–9

Reticular pattern on HRCT. An HRCT scan through the lower lung zones shows a diffuse fine reticular pattern from a combination of irregular thickening of interlobular septa and intralobular lines. The interlobular septa are 1 to 2 cm in length and separated by 1 to 2 cm *(straight arrows)*, which corresponds to the diameter of the secondary lobule, whereas the intralobular linear opacities are smaller and separated by only a few millimeters *(curved arrows)*. The patient was a 58-year-old woman with idiopathic pulmonary fibrosis. *(From Müller NL, Fraser RS, Colman NC, Paré PD: Radiologic Diagnosis of Diseases of the Chest. Philadelphia, WB Saunders, 2001.)*

distribution in the middle and upper lung zones with relative sparing of the lung bases, whereas the cysts in sarcoidosis have a predominantly peribronchovascular and perihilar distribution.[13] The honeycombing in idiopathic pulmonary fibrosis and connective tissue diseases involves mainly the subpleural lung regions and the lower lung zones.[13] In lymphangioleiomyomatosis, the cysts are thin walled and surrounded by normal lung parenchyma.[13,17] They are usually distributed diffusely throughout the lungs, thereby allowing ready distinction from Langerhans cell histiocytosis and idiopathic pulmonary fibrosis.[13]

Nodular Pattern

A nodular pattern is produced when the parenchymal interstitium is expanded in a roughly spherical fashion by a

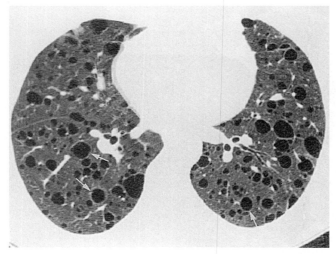

FIGURE 3–10

Cystic spaces in lymphangioleiomyomatosis. An HRCT scan through the lung bases shows numerous cystic spaces with thin walls *(arrows)*. The lung parenchyma between the cysts is normal, and there is no evidence of fibrosis. *(From Müller NL, Fraser RS, Colman NC, Paré PD: Radiologic Diagnosis of Diseases of the Chest. Philadelphia, WB Saunders, 2001.)*

TABLE 3–4. Cystic Pattern of Interstitial Disease

Common Causes	Characteristic Radiographic and HRCT Findings
Idiopathic pulmonary fibrosis and pulmonary fibrosis associated with connective tissue disease	Cystic pattern characteristic of end-stage fibrosis (honeycombing). Lower lung zone and subpleural predominance
Langerhans pulmonary histiocytosis	Cysts often have bizarre shapes. Commonly associated with nodules. Diffuse but shows relative sparing of costophrenic angles on radiographs and basal regions on HRCT
Sarcoidosis	Cystic spaces are seen in association with extensive fibrosis and usually represent central conglomeration of ectatic bronchi (traction bronchiectasis). Middle and upper lung zone predominance. Subpleural honeycombing may occasionally be present
Lymphangioleiomyomatosis	Smooth thin-walled cysts. Diffuse distribution on radiograph and HRCT
Bronchiectasis	Bronchial dilation readily diagnosed on HRCT
Lymphocytic interstitial pneumonia	Cysts random in distribution, usually few in number, and associated with areas of ground-glass attenuation

From Müller NL, Fraser RS, Colman NC, Paré PD: Radiologic Diagnosis of Diseases of the Chest. Philadelphia, WB Saunders, 2001.

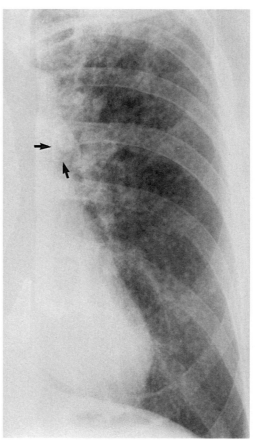

FIGURE 3–11

Silicosis. A view of the left lung from a posteroanterior chest radiograph in a patient with silicosis shows well-defined nodules, most numerous in the upper lobes. Eggshell calcification of the hilar and mediastinal nodes *(arrows)* is a finding virtually diagnostic of silicosis. *(From Müller NL, Fraser RS, Colman NC, Paré PD: Radiologic Diagnosis of Diseases of the Chest. Philadelphia, WB Saunders, 2001.)*

cellular infiltrate, fibrous tissue, or both (Fig. 3–11). In the setting of interstitial lung disease, nodules are defined as round opacities less than 1 cm in diameter.[7,18] The most common causes of a nodular pattern are listed in Table 3–5.

A purely nodular pattern in a febrile patient with acute disease is most suggestive of hematogenous infection, particularly miliary tuberculosis (Fig. 3–12). The nodules usually measure less than 3 mm in diameter and are typically distributed diffusely throughout the lungs (although they may have a lower lung zone predominance).[19] A similar pattern may be seen in miliary fungal disease (e.g., histoplasmosis and coccidioidomycosis), silicosis, coal workers' pneumoconiosis, intravenous talcosis, metastatic carcinoma (particularly from the thyroid), and bronchioloalveolar carcinoma.[7,20,21]

The nodules in silicosis and coal workers' pneumoconiosis tend to involve mainly the middle and upper lung zones (see Fig. 3–11),[18] whereas those resulting from hematogenous processes, such as miliary tuberculosis and metastatic carcinoma, are diffuse or involve mainly the lower lung zones (where blood flow is greater).[8,19] On HRCT scan, nodules resulting from hematogenous processes tend to have a random distribution in relation to lobular structures.[8,20] By contrast, the nodules in silicosis and coal workers' pneumoconiosis frequently show a predominantly centrilobular distribution, a localization that corresponds to the accumulation of dust

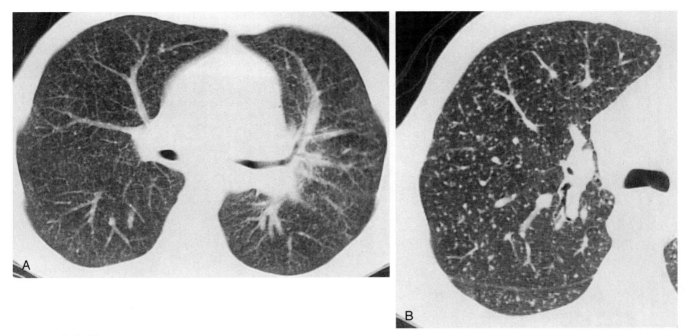

FIGURE 3–12

Miliary nodules on CT. A conventional 10-mm-collimation CT scan (**A**) in a patient with miliary tuberculosis shows 1- to 2-mm-diameter nodules throughout both lungs. An HRCT scan (**B**) targeted to the right lung in the same patient shows the sharp margins of the miliary nodules better. *(From Müller NL, Fraser RS, Colman NC, Paré PD: Radiologic Diagnosis of Diseases of the Chest. Philadelphia, WB Saunders, 2001.)*

TABLE 3–5. Small Nodular Pattern of Interstitial Disease

Common Causes	Characteristic Radiographic and HRCT Findings
Acute	
Miliary tuberculosis or histoplasmosis	Diffuse throughout both lungs. Random distribution on HRCT
Endobronchial spread of tuberculosis	Patchy or asymmetrical bilateral distribution. Centrilobular nodules and branching lines (*tree-in-bud* appearance) on HRCT
Viral infection	Diffuse or patchy. Centrilobular nodules on HRCT
Subacute or Chronic	
Sarcoidosis	Usually has perihilar and upper lobe predominance. Generally associated with bilateral hilar and mediastinal lymphadenopathy. HRCT shows nodular thickening along bronchial and perivascular interstitium
Extrinsic allergic alveolitis	Generalized or middle and lower lung zone predominance. HRCT shows poorly defined centrilobular nodules and areas of ground-glass attenuation
Silicosis and coal workers' pneumoconiosis	Upper lung zone predominance. HRCT often shows centrilobular predominance
Metastatic carcinoma	Diffuse or lower lung zone predominance. HRCT shows random distribution in relation to lobular structures

From Müller NL, Fraser RS, Colman NC, Paré PD: Radiologic Diagnosis of Diseases of the Chest. Philadelphia, WB Saunders, 2001.

and fibrous tissue adjacent to respiratory bronchioles (Fig. 3–13).[21,22]

Centrilobular nodules reflect the presence of a bronchiolocentric process and are seen in various forms of bronchiolitis (Fig. 3–14). In extrinsic allergic alveolitis, such nodules have ill-defined margins and are distributed diffusely throughout the lungs. Centrilobular nodules that have a patchy distribution and are associated with branching linear opacities (tree-in-bud pattern) are most suggestive of infectious bronchiolitis, including viral, mycoplasmal, and bacterial etiology, and endobronchial spread of tuberculosis (Fig. 3–15).[23-25]

Nodules in sarcoidosis are characteristically located predominantly in the central peribronchovascular region of the upper and middle lung zones.[6,26] They are also seen along interlobular septa and in the subpleural regions, including the interlobar fissures (albeit usually to a lesser extent than in the peribronchovascular interstitium) (Fig. 3–16). Such a perilymphatic distribution is also characteristic of lymphangitic carcinomatosis; however, as distinct from sarcoidosis, the predominant abnormality is thickening of the interlobular septa.[8,27]

The value of anatomic localization in the differential diagnosis of small nodules on HRCT scan was assessed in a study of 58 patients.[25] Four radiologists categorized the nodules according to their location and distribution into four groups: perilymphatic, random, centrilobular and diffuse throughout the lungs, and centrilobular but patchy in distribution. All four observers agreed in 79% of cases (46 of 58) with regard to nodule localization, and three of the four agreed in an additional 17% (10 of 58). The observers were correct in 218

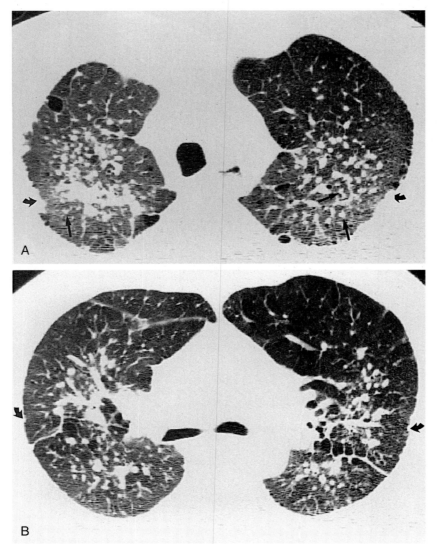

FIGURE 3–13

Silicosis. HRCT scans at the level of the upper (**A**) and middle (**B**) lung zones show numerous sharply defined nodules. Many have a centrilobular distribution *(straight arrows)*. Subpleural nodules *(curved arrows)* and evidence of emphysema are also present. The patient was a 58-year-old man with long-standing silicosis. *(From Müller NL, Fraser RS, Colman NC, Paré PD: Radiologic Diagnosis of Diseases of the Chest. Philadelphia, WB Saunders, 2001.)*

(94%) of 232 localizations in the 58 cases. Diseases were associated with the following distributions: perilymphatic—sarcoidosis and lymphangitic carcinomatosis; random—miliary infection and metastatic carcinoma; diffuse centrilobular—hypersensitivity pneumonitis and respiratory bronchiolitis; and centrilobular but patchy—infectious bronchiolitis.

Reticulonodular Pattern

The presence of interconnecting linear opacities results in a reticular pattern.[2] Orientation of some linear opacities parallel to the x-ray beam causes an additional nodular component that results in a reticulonodular pattern. The latter can also be produced by the presence of nodules superimposed on a reticular pattern, as in sarcoidosis (Fig. 3–16), Langerhans cell histiocytosis, and lymphangitic carcinomatosis.

Ground-Glass Pattern

A ground-glass pattern is considered to be present when there is a hazy increase in opacity unassociated with obscuration of the underlying vascular markings.[2] (If vessels are obscured, the term *consolidation* should be used.) The abnormality is a frequent and important finding on HRCT scan, but it is often difficult to recognize and can readily be missed on the chest radiograph.[28] With HRCT, ground-glass attenuation reflects the presence of abnormalities below the resolution limit. It can be seen in a number of situations, including interstitial disease, air space disease, and increased capillary blood volume from congestive heart failure or blood flow redistribution.[29-31]

Acute lung diseases characteristically associated with a ground-glass pattern include *Pneumocystis jiroveci* pneumonia (Fig. 3–17),[32] pulmonary hemorrhage,[33] and acute interstitial pneumonia.[34] The first of these diseases is particularly associated with the pattern, and in an individual infected with HIV, the abnormality is highly suggestive of this diagnosis.[35] Ground-glass opacification is also frequently the main abnormality seen in the subacute phase of extrinsic allergic alveolitis (Fig. 3–18).[36] The areas of ground-glass attenuation in pulmonary alveolar proteinosis usually have a patchy or geographic distribution[37]; interlobular septal thickening is also

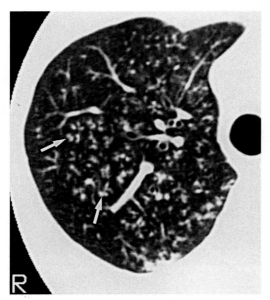

FIGURE 3–14

Centrilobular nodules caused by bronchiolitis. An HRCT (1.5-mm-collimation) scan shows small nodules and branching structures *(arrows)*. These abnormalities are situated approximately 5 mm away from vessels that are too large to be within the secondary pulmonary lobule and represent borders of secondary pulmonary lobules. Structures and abnormalities located 5 mm away from these borders must be centrilobular in location. The patient was a 28-year-old man with bronchiolitis related to inhalation of foreign material. *(From Müller NL, Fraser RS, Colman NC, Paré PD: Radiologic Diagnosis of Diseases of the Chest. Philadelphia, WB Saunders, 2001.)*

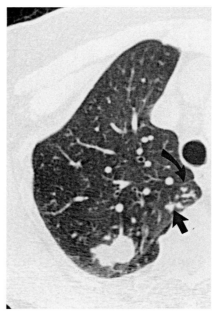

FIGURE 3–15

Centrilobular nodules in tuberculosis. An HRCT scan shows a lobulated, 2-cm-diameter nodule in the posterior segment of the right upper lobe. Note the centrilobular distribution of smaller nodules *(straight arrow)* and normal interlobular septum *(curved arrow)*. The patient was an 80-year-old woman with reactivation tuberculosis (large nodule) and endobronchial spread (smaller nodules). *(From Müller NL, Fraser RS, Colman NC, Paré PD: Radiologic Diagnosis of Diseases of the Chest. Philadelphia, WB Saunders, 2001.)*

TABLE 3–6. Ground-Glass Opacification

Common Causes	Helpful Diagnostic Features
Pneumocystis jiroveci pneumonia	Patchy or diffuse ground-glass attenuation in a patient with AIDS is highly suggestive
Extrinsic allergic alveolitis	May be diffuse or have a lower lung zone predominance. Often associated with lobular areas of decreased attenuation and air trapping as a result of bronchiolar obstruction. Often associated with poorly defined centrilobular nodules
Idiopathic interstitial pneumonias	Ground-glass attenuation may be the predominant or only abnormality seen in patients with desquamative interstitial pneumonia, nonspecific interstitial pneumonia, or acute interstitial pneumonia. In patients with usual interstitial pneumonia, it is generally seen in association with a predominantly subpleural and lower lung zone reticular pattern and honeycombing
Pulmonary hemorrhage	May be focal (e.g., caused by bronchiectasis) or diffuse (e.g., caused by Goodpasture's syndrome)

From Müller NL, Fraser RS, Colman NC, Paré PD: Radiologic Diagnosis of Diseases of the Chest. Philadelphia, WB Saunders, 2001.

commonly identified in the areas of ground-glass attenuation on HRCT scan.[37,38] The most common causes of a ground-glass pattern are listed in Table 3–6. The combination of ground-glass attenuation and superimposed reticulation is known as a "crazy-paving" pattern.[38]

Limitations of the Pattern Approach

Modifying Factors

The pattern of parenchymal abnormality seen on a chest radiograph and HRCT may be modified by associated underlying parenchymal lung disease, particularly emphysema, and by the secondary effects sometimes produced by the diffuse interstitial disease itself. For example, on radiographs, lobar pneumonia superimposed on emphysema may simulate interstitial lung disease (Fig. 3–19), whereas conglomerate interstitial fibrosis may simulate air space disease.

Nonspecific Radiographic Findings

In the appropriate clinical context, identification of a particular pattern of disease on the chest radiograph, whether air space, linear, reticular, nodular, or reticulonodular, often allows one to narrow the differential diagnosis to a relatively small number of entities and, occasionally, to make a specific diagnosis with a high degree of confidence. In some instances, however, it is impossible to determine the main pattern of abnormality, in which case it is preferable to recognize the nonspecificity of the radiologic findings than to choose the wrong pattern for differential diagnosis. Experienced readers may disagree in the interpretation of a radiographic pattern; for example, in one review of 360 chest radiographs from patients who had biopsy-proven diffuse "infiltrative" disease,

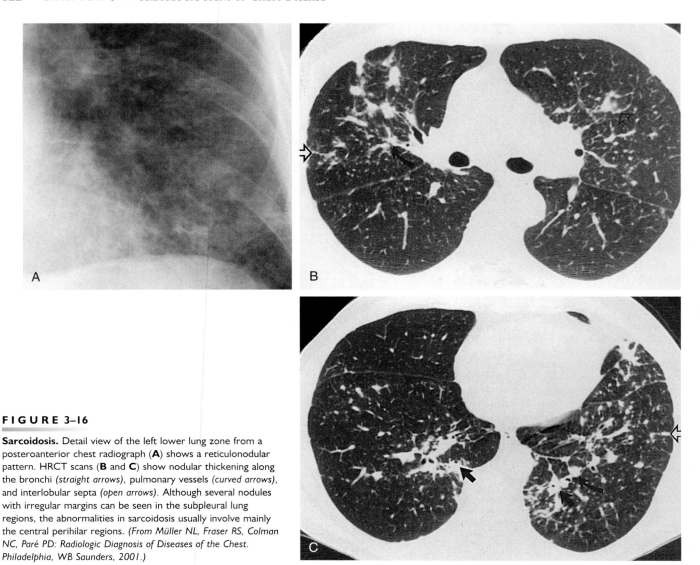

FIGURE 3–16

Sarcoidosis. Detail view of the left lower lung zone from a posteroanterior chest radiograph (**A**) shows a reticulonodular pattern. HRCT scans (**B** and **C**) show nodular thickening along the bronchi *(straight arrows)*, pulmonary vessels *(curved arrows)*, and interlobular septa *(open arrows)*. Although several nodules with irregular margins can be seen in the subpleural lung regions, the abnormalities in sarcoidosis usually involve mainly the central perihilar regions. *(From Müller NL, Fraser RS, Colman NC, Paré PD: Radiologic Diagnosis of Diseases of the Chest. Philadelphia, WB Saunders, 2001.)*

two expert readers agreed that the predominant pattern was either nodular or linear in only 70% of cases.[18]

Comparison of Chest Radiography and High-Resolution Computed Tomography

Several groups of investigators have compared the diagnostic accuracy of HRCT with that of chest radiography in the differential diagnosis of chronic diffuse interstitial and air space lung disease.[39-41] In one investigation of 118 patients, radiographs and CT scans were assessed independently by three observers without knowledge of clinical or pathologic data.[39] The observers made a confident diagnosis in 23% of radiographic and 49% of CT interpretations, the diagnosis being correct in 77% and 93% of readings, respectively. A confident diagnosis was made more than twice as often on the basis of HRCT scans than chest radiographs, and the CT-based diagnosis was correct more often. In a second study of 140 patients, three independent observers listed the three most likely diagnoses and recorded the degree of confidence they

had in their choice.[40] The percentages of high-confidence diagnosis by each of the three observers that were correct with chest radiography were 29%, 34%, and 19%, as compared with 57%, 55%, and 47% with HRCT. Interobserver agreement for the proposed diagnosis was also significantly better with HRCT than with conventional radiography.[40]

The diagnostic accuracy of radiography and CT improves considerably when the findings are analyzed in the context of clinical findings, pulmonary function test results, and laboratory data. The value of such combined information in classifying chronic diffuse lung disease was assessed in an investigation of 208 patients.[41] When findings were evaluated independently, a correct diagnosis with a high degree of confidence was made in 29% of cases on the basis of clinical data, 9% on the basis of radiographic images, and 36% on the basis of HRCT findings. Combining the clinical and radiographic data allowed a correct diagnosis with a high degree of confidence in 54% of cases. When the information provided by the clinical, radiographic, and CT findings was considered together, a high-confidence diagnosis was made in 84% of cases and a correct one in 95%.

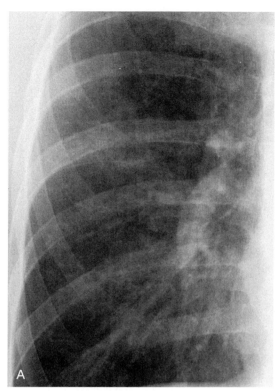

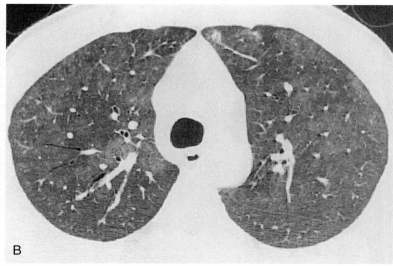

FIGURE 3–17

Pneumocystis jiroveci **pneumonia.** A view of the right lung from a posteroanterior chest radiograph (**A**) in a 28-year-old patient with AIDS shows a mild hazy increase in opacity (ground-glass opacity). An HRCT scan (**B**) reveals extensive bilateral areas of ground-glass attenuation. The latter can readily be recognized by comparing the attenuation of the involved lung with the attenuation within the bronchi (black bronchus sign). *(From Müller NL, Fraser RS, Colman NC, Paré PD: Radiologic Diagnosis of Diseases of the Chest. Philadelphia, WB Saunders, 2001.)*

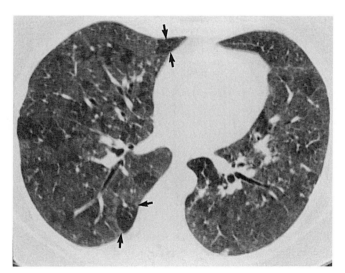

FIGURE 3–18

Extrinsic allergic alveolitis. An HRCT scan in a 59-year-old woman shows extensive bilateral areas of ground-glass attenuation. Focal areas of lung parenchyma without ground-glass attenuation have the size and configuration of secondary pulmonary lobules *(arrows)*. This pattern of diffuse ground-glass attenuation with sparing of individual secondary pulmonary lobules is characteristic of the subacute stage of allergic alveolitis. *(From Müller NL, Fraser RS, Colman NC, Paré PD: Radiologic Diagnosis of Diseases of the Chest. Philadelphia, WB Saunders, 2001.)*

General Signs in Diseases That Increase Lung Density

In addition to the basic patterns and signs already described, several additional radiologic features may aid in determining the nature of a pathologic process within the lungs.

Characteristics of the Border of a Pulmonary Lesion

The margin of a pulmonary nodule may be smooth, lobulated, or spiculated (Fig. 3–20). These characteristics are helpful in predicting whether the nodule is benign or malignant. In general, smooth margins suggest benignity, and spiculation suggests malignancy; lobulation is seen with approximately equal frequency in benign and malignant nodules.[42,43] For example, in one review of the CT findings of 634 solitary pulmonary nodules, 52 of 66 (79%) that had sharply defined, smooth, nonlobulated margins were benign, and 14 (21%) were malignant.[44] Of 218 nodules that had spiculated margins, 184 (84%) represented primary pulmonary carcinoma and 9 (4%) a metastasis; only 25 (11%) were benign. Of 359 nodules that had smooth but lobulated margins, 202 (56%) were benign and 157 were malignant (either primary pulmonary carcinoma or metastasis). Correlation of HRCT with pathologic findings has shown that spiculation usually relates to fibrosis or infiltration of carcinoma in the interstitial tissue/lymphatics of interlobular septa, airways, and vessels adjacent to the tumor.[42]

A discussion of *satellite lesions* is included here because they are closely related to the margins of a pulmonary lesion. These abnormalities can be defined as small nodular opacities in

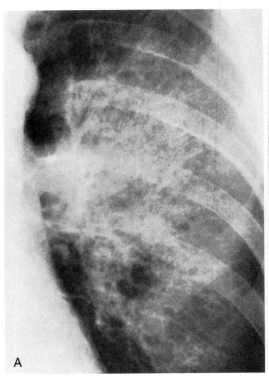
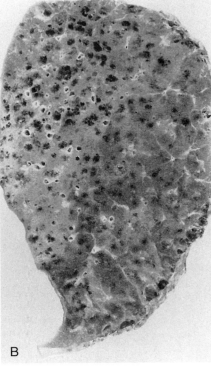

FIGURE 3–19

Acute air space pneumonia superimposed on emphysema. A view of the left midlung zone from a posteroanterior radiograph (**A**) reveals a poorly defined opacity in the superior segment of the left lower lobe. Instead of the homogeneous opacity characteristic of acute air space pneumonia, this consolidation contains many small radiolucencies. A slice of an upper lobe (**B**) from another patient shows essentially homogeneous consolidation of the apical and posterior lung parenchyma. Within this region are numerous well-defined emphysematous spaces unaffected by the pneumonia. Such incomplete consolidation is responsible for the appearance of the radiograph in the first patient (**A**). (*From Müller NL, Fraser RS, Colman NC, Paré PD: Radiologic Diagnosis of Diseases of the Chest. Philadelphia, WB Saunders, 2001.*)

close proximity to a larger lesion, usually a solitary peripheral nodule. They generally indicate an infectious cause; in two studies they were observed in about 10% of patients who had tuberculomas,[45,46] as compared with only 1% of patients who had carcinoma.

When considering these margin features in diagnosis, it is important to remember that the ability of any single sign to predict the benign or malignant nature of a pulmonary nodule depends in part on the prevalence of malignancy in the population under study. For example, a nodule in an adolescent patient is likely to be benign regardless of its margin characteristics, whereas a noncalcified nodule increasing in size in an older patient who smokes is likely to be malignant even if it has a well-defined, smooth border.

The contour of an opacity that relates to the pleura, either over the convexity of the thorax or contiguous to the mediastinum or diaphragm, can provide a useful clue regarding whether the process is intrapulmonary or extrapulmonary in origin. A mass that originates within the pleural space or extrapleurally displaces the pleura and underlying lung inward such that the angle formed by the margins of the mass and the chest wall is obtuse; by contrast, an intrapulmonary mass tends to form an acute angle with the contiguous pleura (Fig. 3–21). When viewed en face, the extrapulmonary mass is indistinctly defined because of the obtuse angle of its margins, whereas an intrapulmonary mass tends to be more sharply defined. As with other radiologic signs, this sign is fallible; occasionally, an extrapulmonary mass relates to the lung with an acute angle and an intrapulmonary mass with an obtuse angle.

Silhouette Sign

The mediastinal and diaphragmatic contours are rendered radiographically visible by their contrast with contiguous air-containing lung. When a soft tissue opacity is situated in any portion of lung adjacent to a mediastinal or diaphragmatic border, that border can no longer be seen radiographically (Fig. 3–22). This situation constitutes a positive silhouette sign.[47] The corollary is that an opacity within the lungs that does *not* obliterate the mediastinal or diaphragmatic contour cannot be situated within lung contiguous to these structures (Fig. 3–23). These contours are apparent only when structures have been exposed adequately; for example, in an underexposed radiograph, massive consolidation of the right lower lobe may prevent identification of the right border of the heart, merely because the x-ray photons have insufficient penetration to reproduce the heart shadow through the lower lobe density, despite the presence of air-containing lung contiguous to the heart.

The silhouette sign is most useful in differentiation of disease in the middle lobe and lingula from that in the lower lobe. However, it may provide precise anatomic information in a variety of other situations, including obliteration of the aortic arch on the left side by airlessness of the apical-posterior segment of the left upper lobe, obliteration of the ascending arch of the aorta and the superior vena cava by consolidation of the anterior segment of the right upper lobe, and obliteration of the posterior paraspinal line by contiguous airless lung in the left posterior gutter.

Cavitation

A cavity is defined radiologically as a gas-containing space within the lung surrounded by a wall whose thickness is greater than 1 mm.[1] In most cases, it is formed by necrosis of the central portion of a lesion and drainage of the resultant, partially liquefied material via communicating airways.[1] Neither the presence of a fluid level nor the size of the cavity

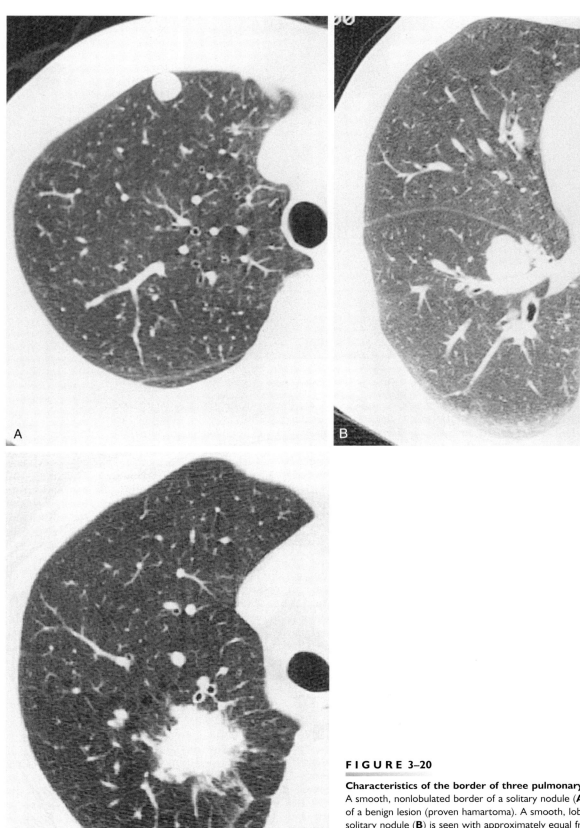

FIGURE 3–20

Characteristics of the border of three pulmonary nodules on HRCT.
A smooth, nonlobulated border of a solitary nodule (**A**) is most suggestive
of a benign lesion (proven hamartoma). A smooth, lobulated contour of a
solitary nodule (**B**) is seen with approximately equal frequency in benign and
malignant lesions (proven adenocarcinoma). A spiculated border of a nodule
(**C**) is most suggestive of a malignant lesion (proven adenocarcinoma). *(From
Müller NL, Fraser RS, Colman NC, Paré PD: Radiologic Diagnosis of Diseases of
the Chest. Philadelphia, WB Saunders, 2001.)*

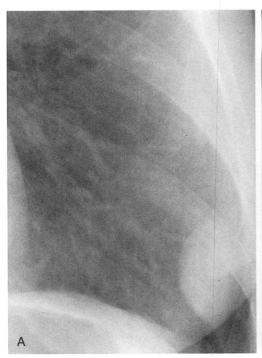

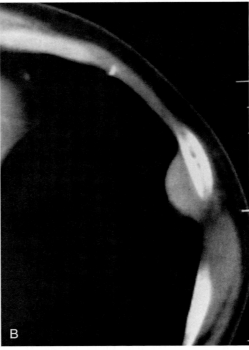

FIGURE 3–2I

Extrapulmonary sign. A view of the left lower hemithorax from a posteroanterior chest radiograph (**A**) shows the characteristic features of an extrapulmonary mass: a smooth convex border at the area where it abuts the lung and tapering superiorly and inferiorly; the lateral margin, where it abuts the soft tissues of the chest wall, is obscured. A CT scan (**B**) shows tapering anterior and posterior margins. The patient was a 46-year-old woman with a benign fibrous tumor of the pleura. *(From Müller NL, Fraser RS, Colman NC, Paré PD: Radiologic Diagnosis of Diseases of the Chest. Philadelphia, WB Saunders, 2001.)*

is necessary to the definition of cavity. The terms *cavity* and *abscess* are not synonymous: an intrapulmonary abscess without communication with the bronchial tree is radiographically opaque; only when the abscess communicates with the airways and allows air to replace necrotic material should the term *cavity* be applied.

In many cases, the radiologic appearance of the cavity gives some indication of its cause, particularly whether it is benign or malignant (Fig. 3–24). The specific radiologic features that should be noted with respect to this distinction include the thickness of the cavity wall, the character of its inner lining (whether irregular or smooth), the presence and nature of its contents, the number of lesions, and when multiple, the number that have cavitated. The following discussion indicates the findings that are suggestive of a specific cause for each of these features; there are occasional exceptions to the rule in each category.

Cavity Wall. The cavity wall is usually thick in an acute lung abscess (Fig. 3–25), primary and metastatic carcinoma, and Wegener's granulomatosis and often thin in chronic infection such as coccidioidomycosis. Assessment of cavity wall thickness is most useful in distinguishing between a benign and a malignant lesion. In one study of 65 solitary cavities in the lung, all lesions in which the thickest part of the cavity wall was 1 mm or less were benign[48]; of the lesions whose thickest measurement was 4 mm or less, 92% were benign; of those that were 5 to 15 mm in their thickest part, benign and malignant lesions were equally divided; and 92% of lesions whose cavity wall was greater than 15 mm in thickness were malignant.

Character of the Inner Lining. The inner lining is usually nodular in carcinoma, shaggy in acute lung abscess, and smooth in most other cavitary lesions.

Nature of the Cavitary Contents. When material is identified within a cavity, it usually represents pus or partially liquefied necrotic neoplasm and appears as a flat, smooth air-fluid level without specific radiologic features. Occasionally, intracavitary material has characteristics that are strongly suggestive of a specific disease. Examples include an intracavitary fungus ball, which may form a mobile mass (Fig. 3–26), and the collapsed membranes of a ruptured *Echinococcus* cyst, which float on top of the fluid within the cyst and create the characteristic *water lily sign* or the *sign of the camalote* (a water plant found in South American rivers).[49] Another rare but characteristic intracavitary mass is that associated with pulmonary gangrene, in which irregular pieces of sloughed necrotic lung parenchyma float like icebergs in the cavity fluid; although this complication can be seen with infection by virtually any organism, it is most common with *K. pneumoniae*.[50]

Multiplicity of Lesions. Some cavitary disease is characteristically solitary (e.g., primary pulmonary carcinoma, acute lung abscess, and post-traumatic lung cyst). Other diseases are characteristically multiple (e.g., metastatic carcinoma, Wegener's granulomatosis, and septic thromboemboli).[51,52]

Bubble Lucencies (Pseudocavitation). Round or oval areas of low attenuation usually measuring 5 mm or less in diameter may be visible within a pulmonary nodule on CT scan, particularly HRCT (Fig. 3–27).[42] Such *bubble lucencies* (pseudocavitation) can be identified on HRCT in approximately 60% of bronchioloalveolar carcinomas, 30% of acinar adenocarcinomas, and less commonly in other malignant lung tumors.[42] They are uncommonly identified in benign lesions. Correlation with pathologic findings has shown that the lucencies usually represent patent airways, often ectatic, or foci of emphysema surrounded by carcinoma.[42]

Calcification and Ossification

The presence or absence of calcification plus its location on either the radiograph or CT scan is an important diagnostic

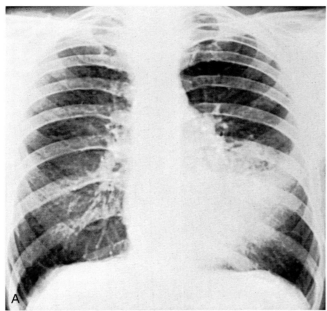

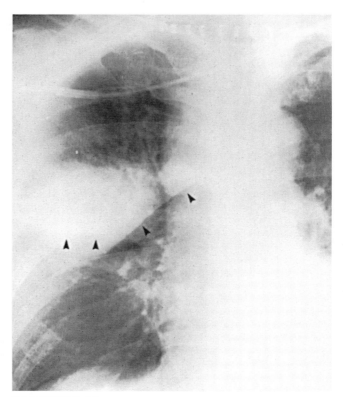

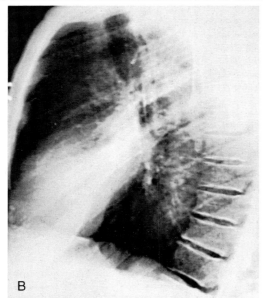

FIGURE 3–23

Application of the silhouette sign for disease localization. A detail view of the right hemithorax from an anteroposterior chest radiograph shows an area of air space consolidation in the right lung caused by acute bacterial pneumonia. The process does not obliterate any portion of the right mediastinal contour and is sharply delineated by the superomedial portion of the right major fissure *(oblique arrowheads)* and the lateral aspect of the minor fissure *(vertical arrowheads)*. These three features localize the pneumonia to the posterior and lateral portions of the right upper lobe. *(From Müller NL, Fraser RS, Colman NC, Paré PD: Radiologic Diagnosis of Diseases of the Chest. Philadelphia, WB Saunders, 2001.)*

FIGURE 3–22

Silhouette sign. Posteroanterior (**A**) and lateral (**B**) radiographs reveal obliteration of the left heart border by a shadow of homogeneous density situated within the lingula; such obliteration inevitably indicates lingular disease (provided that the radiographic exposure is adequate). Squamous cell carcinoma of the lingular bronchus with distal obstructive pneumonitis was diagnosed. *(From Müller NL, Fraser RS, Colman NC, Paré PD: Radiologic Diagnosis of Diseases of the Chest. Philadelphia, WB Saunders, 2001.)*

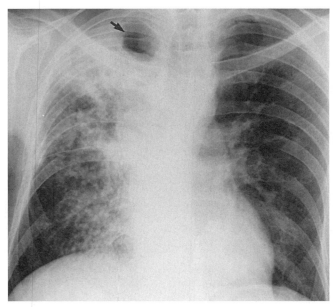

FIGURE 3–24

Tuberculous cavity with bronchogenic spread. A posteroanterior chest radiograph shows a 3-cm-diameter cavity in the apical segment of the right upper lobe *(arrow)*, extensive consolidation in the right upper lobe, and 3- to 7-mm-diameter nodules throughout the right lung. The findings are characteristic of tuberculosis with endobronchial spread. *(From Müller NL, Fraser RS, Colman NC, Paré PD: Radiologic Diagnosis of Diseases of the Chest. Philadelphia, WB Saunders, 2001.)*

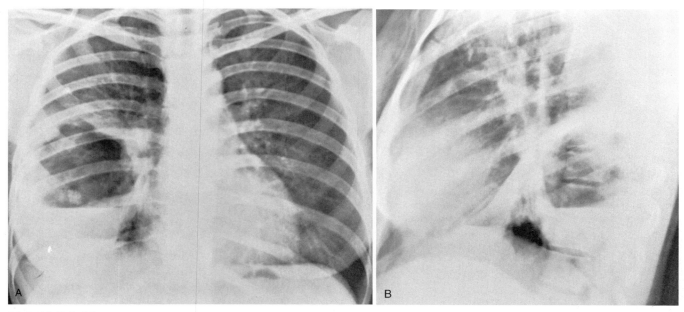

FIGURE 3–25

Acute staphylococcal lung abscess. Radiographs in posteroanterior (**A**) and lateral (**B**) projection reveal a large cavity in the right lower lobe. The thickness of its wall and the shaggy irregular nature of its inner lining suggest an acute lung abscess. *(From Müller NL, Fraser RS, Colman NC, Paré PD: Radiologic Diagnosis of Diseases of the Chest. Philadelphia, WB Saunders, 2001.)*

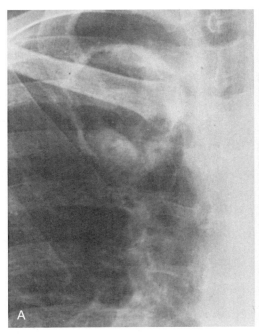
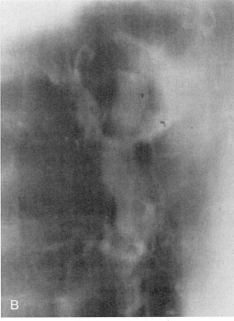

FIGURE 3–26

Intracavitary fungus ball. Views of the upper half of the right lung with the patient upright (**A**) and supine (**B**) reveal a thin-walled, but irregular cavity in the paramediastinal zone. Situated within it is a smooth oblong shadow of homogeneous density whose relationship to the wall of the cavity changes from the erect (**A**) to the supine (**B**) position. The cavity was of tuberculous origin, and the loose body was composed of a conglomeration of fungal hyphae. *(From Müller NL, Fraser RS, Colman NC, Paré PD: Radiologic Diagnosis of Diseases of the Chest. Philadelphia, WB Saunders, 2001.)*

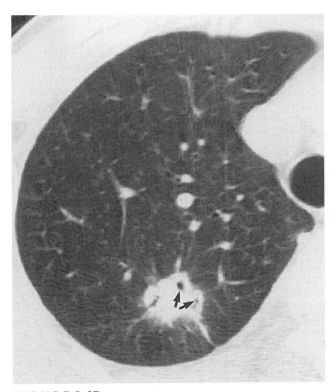

FIGURE 3–27

Bubble lucencies. An HRCT scan through a 2-cm-diameter nodule in the right upper lobe shows focal lucencies measuring less than 5 mm in diameter *(arrows)*. Pathologic assessment showed bronchioloalveolar carcinoma. *(From Müller NL, Fraser RS, Colman NC, Paré PD: Radiologic Diagnosis of Diseases of the Chest. Philadelphia, WB Saunders, 2001.)*

sign. In fact, calcification within a solitary pulmonary nodule is the most reliable radiologic evidence that a lesion is benign.[53,54] Moreover, even though calcification may be present in a malignant tumor, its pattern allows distinction from a benign nodule in most cases.[54,55]

Four patterns of calcification are associated with benign lesions: diffuse, central, laminated, and popcorn (Fig. 3–28).[55] The diffuse and laminated forms are virtually diagnostic of a granuloma. A small central nidus of calcification is seen most commonly with granulomatous lesions, although it also occurs in some hamartomas. Popcorn calcification is characteristic of hamartoma. Such benign patterns of calcification are rarely seen in malignant tumors. In a study of 634 nodules assessed with CT, 153 were diagnosed correctly as benign based on the presence of central or diffuse calcification[44]; although focal areas of calcification were identified in 13% of the primary lung tumors, only one carcinoid tumor had a benign pattern of calcification. The other malignant tumors had neither central nor diffuse calcification.

Calcification in malignant tumors can be seen in several circumstances. The most important from a differential diagnosis point of view is the occasional case in which a peripheral primary carcinoma engulfs a calcified granuloma, in which case the calcification is usually eccentric. Additional situations include a solitary metastasis of osteogenic sarcoma or chondrosarcoma and some primary pulmonary carcinoid tumors, in which there is ossification of the stroma.[56,57]

Lymph node calcification is generally amorphous and irregular in distribution. It results most commonly from a healed granulomatous infection, usually tuberculosis or histoplasmosis, in which case it constitutes part of Ranke's complex. A ring of calcification around the periphery of a lymph node ("eggshell" calcification) is an uncommon pattern seen most often after silica (see Fig. 3–11) or coal dust exposure; rare causes include sarcoidosis, Hodgkin's lymphoma (after mediastinal irradiation), histoplasmosis, amyloidosis, and tuberculosis (Fig. 3–29).

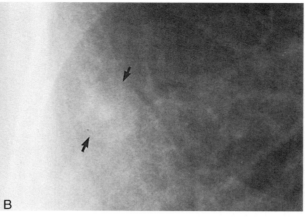

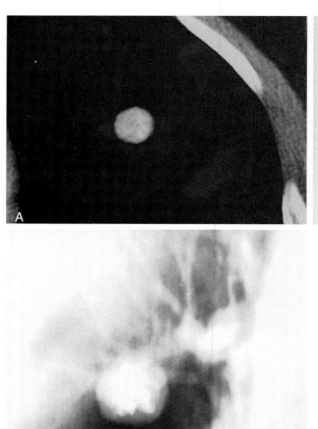

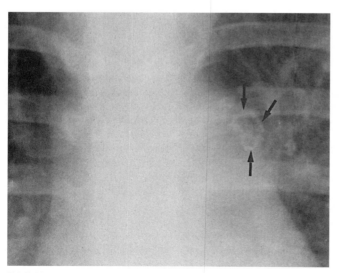

FIGURE 3–28

Benign patterns of calcification. A CT scan (**A**) shows diffuse calcification in a tuberculoma. A magnified view of the right lung from another patient (**B**) shows a tuberculoma *(arrows)* with a central nidus of calcification. A view from the right upper lobe (**C**) shows a large central area of so-called popcorn ball calcification characteristic of a hamartoma. *(From Müller NL, Fraser RS, Colman NC, Paré PD: Radiologic Diagnosis of Diseases of the Chest. Philadelphia, WB Saunders, 2001.)*

FIGURE 3–29

Eggshell calcification in tuberculosis. A view from an anteroposterior chest radiograph in a 4-year-old girl shows eggshell calcification in an aortopulmonary window node *(arrows)*. Smaller calcified nodes can be seen lateral to the aortic arch and in the left hilum. The patient had been treated for primary tuberculosis 2 years previously. *(From Müller NL, Fraser RS, Colman NC, Paré PD: Radiologic Diagnosis of Diseases of the Chest. Philadelphia, WB Saunders, 2001.)*

DECREASED LUNG DENSITY

Diseases that cause a decrease in lung density result in increased radiolucency (hyperlucency) on the chest radiograph and decreased attenuation on CT scan. Here we are dealing only with diseases of the lung that cause increased radiolucency. Any assessment of chest radiographs must take into consideration the contribution that abnormalities of extrapulmonary tissue might make to reduced density. Certain pleural diseases (e.g., pneumothorax) and some congenital and acquired abnormalities of the chest wall (e.g., congenital absence of the pectoral muscles and mastectomy) produce unilateral radiolucency that might easily be mistaken for pulmonary disease. Because it eliminates the influence of superimposition of density from the chest wall, CT is superior to the chest radiograph in showing focal and diffuse reductions in lung density.

Decreased lung density may be explained by several mechanisms, including (1) obstructive overinflation without lung destruction (e.g., asthma), (2) increased gas with decreased blood and tissue (e.g., emphysema), (3) reduction in the quantity of blood and tissue in the absence of pulmonary overinflation (e.g., Swyer-James syndrome and pulmonary thromboembolism without infarction), and (4) a combination of the three mechanisms (e.g., proximal interruption [absence] of the right or left pulmonary artery).

Alteration in Pulmonary Volume

General Excess of Air

Lung diseases that cause decreased density are characterized by overinflation, with the exception of unilateral interruption (absence) of the pulmonary artery, unilateral hyperlucent lung (Swyer-James syndrome), partly obstructing endobronchial lesions, and pulmonary thromboembolism without infarction. Radiologic signs that may be observed in association with a general increase in intrapulmonary air relate to the diaphragm, the retrosternal space, and the cardiovascular silhouette (Fig. 3–30); the most important of these are signs related to the diaphragm.

In patients who have severe emphysema, the diaphragm is depressed, often to the level of the 7th rib anteriorly and the 11th interspace or 12th rib posteriorly; the normal dome configuration is concomitantly flattened. Although such flattening is often evaluated subjectively, direct measurement is more accurate. Direct measurement is best done on the lateral radiograph by drawing a straight line from the sternophrenic junction to the posterior costophrenic junction. The dome of the hemidiaphragm should be 2.6 cm or more above this line; a measurement less than 2.6 cm indicates overinflation.[58] Flattening of the diaphragm can also be assessed on the posteroanterior (PA) radiograph by drawing a line from the costophrenic to the costovertebral angle and measuring the height of the dome of each hemidiaphragm[58]; however, this measurement is less sensitive than one performed on a lateral radiograph.[58,59]

The severity of diaphragmatic flattening is valuable in differential diagnosis. It is invariably most marked in emphysema; in fact, overinflation in this disease may render the diaphragmatic contour concave rather than convex upward (see Fig. 3–30). By contrast, the upper diaphragmatic surface is nearly always convex in asthma. (It should be remembered, however, that this applies in adults only; severe air trapping in infants and children may be associated with remarkable depression and flattening of the diaphragmatic domes).

Another helpful sign in the detection of overinflation is an increase in the retrosternal air space on the lateral chest radiograph.[60] Direct measurement is again more sensitive than subjective assessment; a distance greater than 2.5 cm between the posterior aspect of the sternum and the most anterior margin of the ascending aorta is indicative of overinflation.[60,61]

Local Excess of Air

Isolated overinflation of a segment or of one or more lobes occurs in two circumstances: with and without air trapping. Distinction between the two is of major diagnostic importance.

Overinflation *with air trapping* results from obstruction of the egress of air from affected lung parenchyma. It may be seen in neonatal lobar hyperinflation (congenital lobar emphysema),[62] in congenital bronchial atresia,[63] or in association with an endobronchial lesion that causes check-valve obstruction of the airway. The last-named condition may be seen with

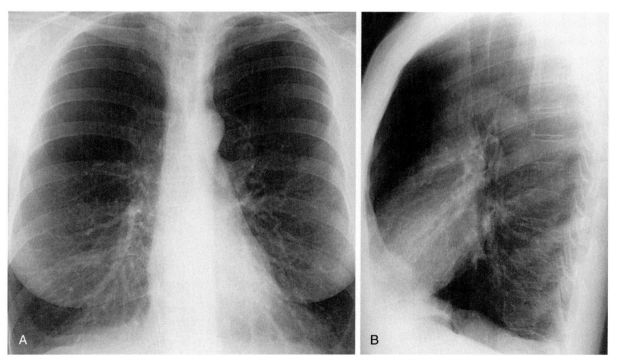

FIGURE 3–30

Diffuse emphysema. A posteroanterior chest radiograph (**A**) shows a low position and flattened contour of both hemidiaphragms. The lungs are oligemic. In the lateral projection (**B**), the superior aspect of the diaphragm is concave rather than convex, and the retrosternal air space is deepened. (*From Müller NL, Fraser RS, Colman NC, Paré PD: Radiologic Diagnosis of Diseases of the Chest. Philadelphia, WB Saunders, 2001.*)

tumors of the main, lobar, or segmental bronchi; although recognition of such obstruction may be useful in its diagnosis,[64] it is a rare manifestation. For example, in a study of the radiographic patterns of 600 cases of bronchogenic carcinoma, overinflation distal to a partly obstructing endobronchial lesion was not seen in any case.[65,66] In fact, in our experience, the volume of lung behind a partly obstructing endobronchial lesion is almost invariably reduced at TLC. Despite this smaller volume, the density of affected parenchyma is typically *less* than that of the opposite lung as a result of decreased perfusion (oligemia) secondary to hypoventilation-mediated hypoxic vasoconstriction. The overall effect is an increase in radiolucency despite the reduction in volume (Fig. 3–31).

Overinflation *without air trapping* is a compensatory process: parts of the lung assume a larger volume than normal in response to the loss of volume elsewhere in the thorax. This process may occur after surgical removal of lung tissue or as a result of atelectasis (Fig. 3–32) or parenchymal scarring. The remaining lung contains more than its normal amount of air.

Bullae, Blebs, and Pneumatoceles

Bullae. A bulla is a sharply demarcated, air-containing space that measures 1 cm or more in diameter and possesses a smooth wall 1 mm or less in thickness. The space may be unilocular or separated into several compartments by thin septa (Fig. 3–33).

Blebs. A bleb is a localized collection of air in the immediate subpleural lung or within the pleura. It develops most frequently over the lung apices and seldom exceeds 1 cm in diameter. Its pathogenesis has been hypothesized to be dissection of gas from ruptured alveoli into the adjacent interstitial tissue and into the interstitial layer of the visceral pleura, where it accumulates in the form of a cyst.[67,68]

Pneumatoceles. A pneumatocele is a thin-walled, gas-filled space within the lung that characteristically increases in size over a period of days to weeks and almost invariably resolves; it typically occurs in association with infection. The pathogenesis is believed to relate to check-valve obstruction of an airway lumen or to local necrosis of a bronchial wall with dissection of air into the adjacent bronchovascular interstitial

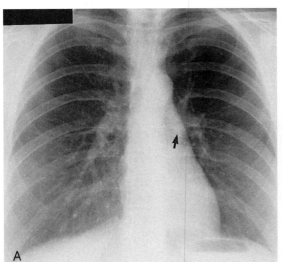
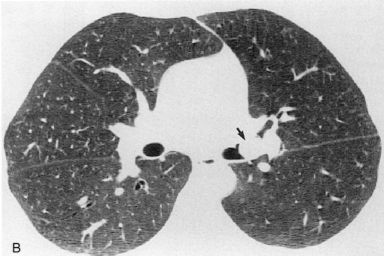
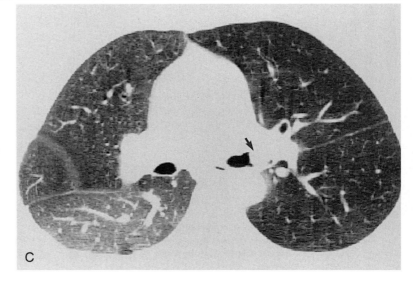

FIGURE 3–31

Decreased vascularity and lung volume caused by endobronchial tumor. A posteroanterior chest radiograph (**A**) reveals increased radiolucency of the left hemithorax and decreased vascularity. An endobronchial tumor *(arrow)* is present in the distal left main bronchus. Also note the decrease in size of the left lung. An HRCT scan (**B**) shows the tumor *(arrow)*, decreased vascularity of the left lung, and a slight decrease in attenuation. Note the decrease in size of the left lung with shift of the mediastinum and anterior junction line to the left. An HRCT scan at end expiration (**C**) shows air trapping in the left lung with a shift of the mediastinum and anterior junction line to the right. *(From Müller NL, Fraser RS, Colman NC, Paré PD: Radiologic Diagnosis of Diseases of the Chest. Philadelphia, WB Saunders, 2001.)*

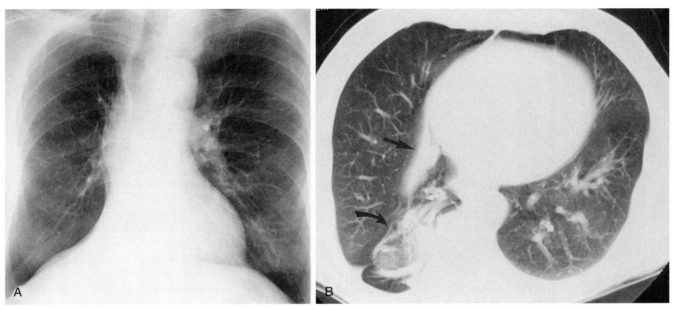

FIGURE 3–32

Overinflation without air trapping. A posteroanterior chest radiograph (**A**) shows increased radiolucency of the right hemithorax as a result of compensatory overinflation of the right upper lobe secondary to combined atelectasis of the right middle and lower lobes. A CT scan (**B**) shows right middle (*straight arrow*) and lower (*curved arrow*) lobe atelectasis and hyperinflation of the right upper lobe. There is decreased vascularity and attenuation of the right lung when compared with the left. The patient was a 69-year-old man with long-standing atelectasis of unknown cause. *(From Müller NL, Fraser RS, Colman NC, Paré PD: Radiologic Diagnosis of Diseases of the Chest. Philadelphia, WB Saunders, 2001.)*

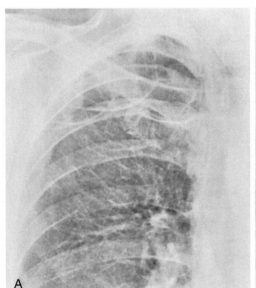

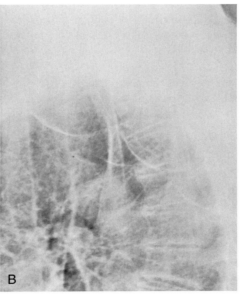

FIGURE 3–33

Bullae. Views of the upper half of the right lung in posteroanterior (**A**) and lateral (**B**) projections reveal several spaces in the lung apex sharply separated from contiguous lung by curvilinear, hairline shadows. The appearance suggests multiple bullae rather than a single space separated into compartments by thin septa. *(From Müller NL, Fraser RS, Colman NC, Paré PD: Radiologic Diagnosis of Diseases of the Chest. Philadelphia, WB Saunders, 2001.)*

tissue (Fig. 3–34).[69] It is usually caused by *S. aureus* infection in infants and children or *P. jiroveci* in patients who have AIDS (Fig. 3–35). The abnormality can also occur after trauma.

Alteration in Pulmonary Vasculature

Just as overinflation may reflect an abnormality of the conducting airways, so may an alteration in the vascular pattern indicate an abnormality of perfusion. Vascular loss may be central or peripheral. In the former instance the loss is produced by vascular obstruction (e.g., massive pulmonary thromboembolism), and in the latter, by peripheral vascular obliteration (e.g., emphysema). Other causes include congenital cardiac malformations (e.g., tetralogy of Fallot) and diseases that affect the peripheral pulmonary vasculature (e.g., primary pulmonary hypertension).

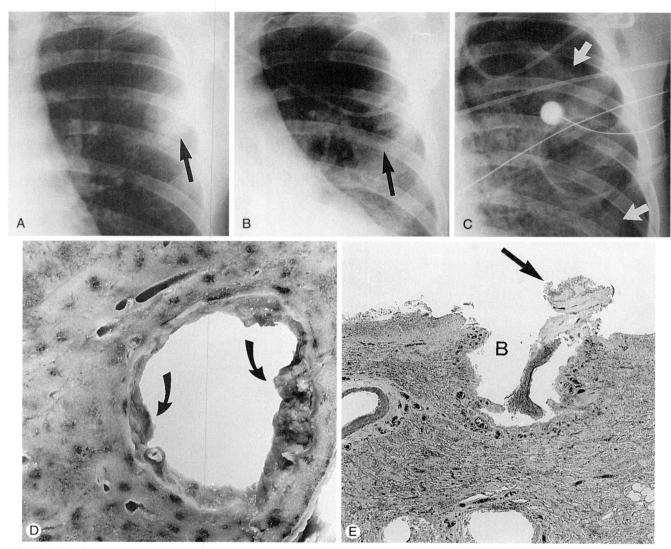

FIGURE 3–34

Pulmonary pneumatocele. A chest radiograph (**A**) from a 28-year-old man with acute myelocytic leukemia and leukopenia shows an ill-defined opacity in the peripheral parenchyma of the left upper lobe *(arrow)*. Twelve days later (**B**), the opacity has been replaced by a smooth, thin-walled cavity approximately 4 cm in diameter *(arrow)*. The following day (**C**), the lesion measured 5.5 cm even in the presence of partial collapse of the left lung as a result of pneumothorax *(arrows)*. At autopsy (**D**), the cavity was seen to have a shaggy inner lining related to the presence of necrotic tissue *(arrows)*. A section through an airway (bronchus [B]) entering the cavity (**E**) showed a partially obstructing flap of mucus and inflammatory exudate *(arrow)*; this flap was mobile in the gross specimen and was hypothesized to permit entry of air into the cavity during inspiration and prevent its egress on expiration. The cause of the cavity was believed to be anaerobic organisms related to aspiration. *(From Quigley MJ, Fraser RS: Pulmonary pneumatocele: Pathology and pathogenesis. AJR Am J Roentgenol 150:1275-1277, 1988.)*

ATELECTASIS

The term *atelectasis* is derived from the Greek words *ateles* (incomplete) and *ektasis* (stretching). In this text, we use it specifically to denote diminished gas within the lung associated with reduced lung volume. (Although the term *collapse* is often used synonymously with atelectasis, it should be reserved for complete atelectasis.[1])

Mechanisms of Atelectasis

Atelectasis can be classified into five types: resorption, passive, compressive, adhesive, and cicatrization (Table 3–7).

Resorption Atelectasis

Resorption atelectasis occurs when airflow to a region of lung is interrupted as a result of airway obstruction (Fig. 3–36). The end result of such obstruction is not necessarily a collapsed lobe or lung, particularly if the obstructing process is prolonged (e.g., as with pulmonary carcinoma). In this situation, *obstructive pneumonitis* frequently leads to consolidation severe enough to limit the loss of volume. The characteristic radiographic picture of obstructive pneumonitis (i.e., homogeneous opacification of a segment, lobe, or lung without air bronchograms) is highly suggestive of an obstructing endobronchial lesion (Fig. 3–37).

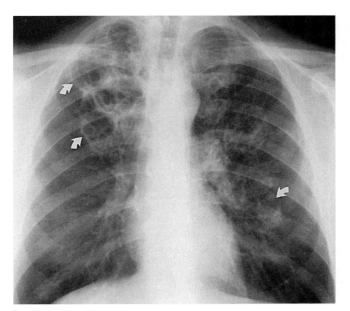

FIGURE 3–35

Pneumatoceles in *Pneumocystis jiroveci* pneumonia. A posteroanterior chest radiograph in a 53-year-old man with AIDS shows numerous cystic lesions *(arrows)* involving mainly the right upper lobe. The pneumatoceles had not been present on a chest radiograph taken 3 months previously when *P. carinii* was identified in BAL fluid. *(From Müller NL, Fraser RS, Colman NC, Paré PD: Radiologic Diagnosis of Diseases of the Chest. Philadelphia, WB Saunders, 2001.)*

TABLE 3–7. Mechanisms of Atelectasis

Atelectasis	Mechanisms
Resorption atelectasis	Occurs when communication between the trachea and alveoli is obstructed; the obstruction may be in a major bronchus or in multiple small bronchi or bronchioles
Passive atelectasis	Denotes the loss of volume as a result of lung elastic recoil in the presence of a nonloculated pneumothorax
Compressive atelectasis	Denotes loss of volume accompanying an intrathoracic space-occupying process such as pleural effusion, pulmonary mass, or bulla
Adhesive atelectasis	Adhesive atelectasis is related to a deficiency of surfactant. As with passive, compressive, and cicatrization atelectasis, it is associated with patent large airway communications
Cicatrization atelectasis	Results from contraction of interstitial fibrous tissue as it matures. Can be focal (e.g., tuberculosis) or diffuse (e.g., idiopathic pulmonary fibrosis)

From Müller NL, Fraser RS, Colman NC, Paré PD: Radiologic Diagnosis of Diseases of the Chest. Philadelphia, WB Saunders, 2001.

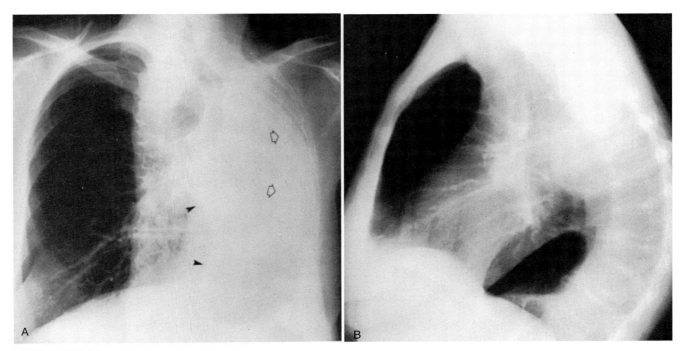

FIGURE 3–36

Total atelectasis of the left lung. Posteroanterior **(A)** and lateral **(B)** chest radiographs disclose an opaque and shrunken left hemithorax. The right lung is markedly overinflated and has displaced the mediastinum to the left posteriorly *(arrowheads)* and anteriorly *(open arrows)*. The cardiac silhouette is obscured except for its anterior surface, which is visible in lateral projection; curvilinear calcification in the upper left hemithorax identifies the aortic arch. The patient was a 73-year-old woman with carcinoma. *(From Müller NL, Fraser RS, Colman NC, Paré PD: Radiologic Diagnosis of Diseases of the Chest. Philadelphia, WB Saunders, 2001.)*

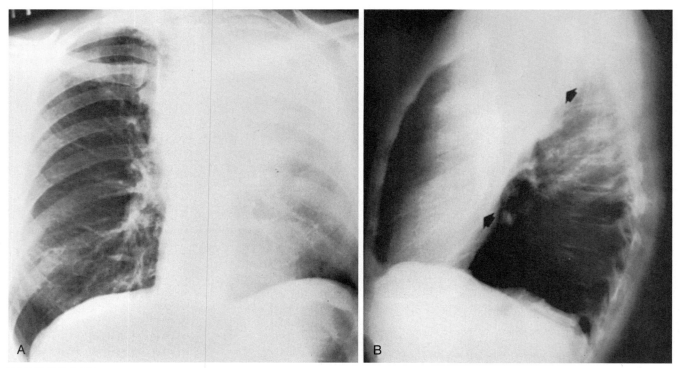

FIGURE 3–37

Obstructive pneumonitis—left upper lobe. Posteroanterior (**A**) and lateral (**B**) radiographs show homogeneous opacification of the left upper lobe; there is no air bronchogram. The major fissure *(arrows)* is not displaced forward, and the only signs indicating loss of volume are a slight mediastinal shift and hemidiaphragmatic elevation. Collapse was prevented by the accumulation of fluid and alveolar macrophages within the distal air spaces and chronic inflammatory cells and fibrous tissue within the interstitium—obstructive pneumonitis. The patient had squamous cell carcinoma originating in the left upper lobe bronchus. *(From Müller NL, Fraser RS, Colman NC, Paré PD: Radiologic Diagnosis of Diseases of the Chest. Philadelphia, WB Saunders, 2001.)*

Passive Atelectasis

Passive atelectasis denotes loss of volume as the lung retracts in the presence of pneumothorax (Fig. 3–38). Provided that the pleural space is free (i.e., without adhesions), atelectasis of any portion of lung is proportional to the amount of air in the adjacent pleural space.

Compressive Atelectasis

Compressive atelectasis results from compression of the lung by an adjacent space-occupying abnormality or by contraction of fibrous tissue in the adjacent pleura. Any space-occupying intrathoracic lesion, such as a bronchogenic cyst, a bulla, or a peripheral neoplasm, induces airlessness of a thin layer of contiguous lung parenchyma (Fig. 3–39). This atelectasis is local rather than general, as in pneumothorax. Although some authors have considered the presence of atelectasis in patients with pleural effusion a form of passive atelectasis,[70] it seems more reasonable to consider it a form of compressive atelectasis.

On CT scan, atelectasis is commonly seen in healthy individuals in the dependent lung regions as an ill-defined area of increased attenuation or subpleural curvilinear opacities (Fig. 3–40).[71,72] The former measures from a few millimeters to 1 cm or more in thickness and has been called *dependent opacity* or *dependent density*.[71,73] Subpleural curvilinear opacities, also known as *subpleural lines,* are linear areas of increased attenuation measuring several centimeters in length and located

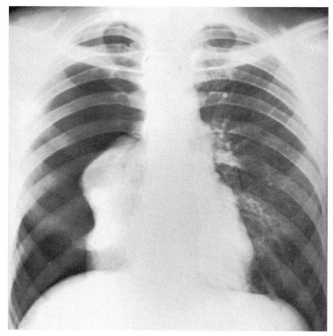

FIGURE 3–38

Passive atelectasis—spontaneous pneumothorax. A posteroanterior radiograph after spontaneous pneumothorax reveals the small volume occupied by a whole lung when totally collapsed. The well-defined air bronchogram indicates airway patency. *(From Müller NL, Fraser RS, Colman NC, Paré PD: Radiologic Diagnosis of Diseases of the Chest. Philadelphia, WB Saunders, 2001.)*

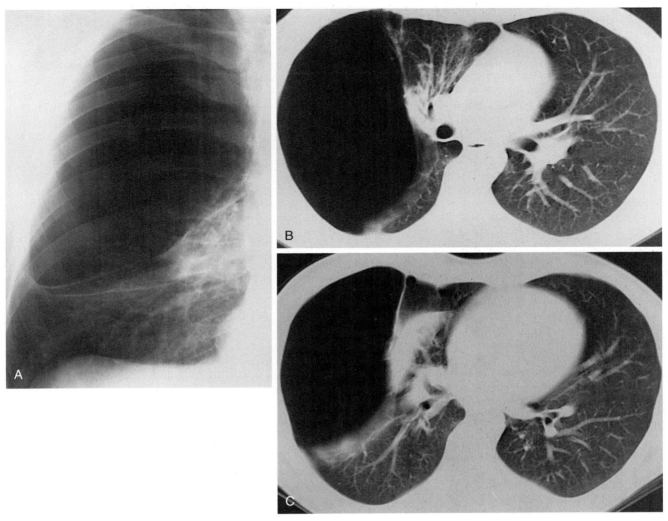

FIGURE 3–39

Compressive atelectasis. A magnified view of the right lung (**A**) shows almost complete replacement of the upper lobe by a large bulla. Note the associated compression of the adjacent lung. A CT scan at the level of the bronchus intermedius (**B**) shows a large bulla and associated compressive atelectasis in the right upper lobe. A CT scan at a more caudal level (**C**) shows areas of atelectasis in the right middle and lower lobes; the left lung is normal. *(From Müller NL, Fraser RS, Colman NC, Paré PD: Radiologic Diagnosis of Diseases of the Chest. Philadelphia, WB Saunders, 2001.)*

within 1 cm of the pleura and parallel to it.[74] Both manifestations of dependent atelectasis characteristically disappear when the patient changes position (see Fig. 3–40); differentiation of dependent atelectasis from true interstitial or air space disease can easily be established by scanning the patient in the supine and prone positions.[71,75]

Round Atelectasis

Round atelectasis (rounded atelectasis, folded lung) is a distinct form of compressive atelectasis that is characteristically associated with focal or diffuse pleural thickening.[76] On conventional radiographs, the lesion appears as a fairly homogeneous, round, oval, wedge-shaped, or less commonly, irregularly shaped subpleural mass.[76] It usually measures 2.5 to 5 cm in greatest diameter, although it may attain a size as large as 10 cm[77] and involve an entire lobe.[78]

The characteristic CT features consist of bronchi and vessels curving and converging toward a round or oval mass that abuts an area of pleural thickening and is associated with evidence of volume loss in the affected lobe (Fig. 3–41).[79,80] The hilar (central) aspect of the mass usually has indistinct margins as a result of blurring by the entering vessels. Air bronchograms are identified within the mass in approximately 60% of cases. Vessels and bronchi curve into the periphery of the mass, thus forming the basis for the *comet tail* sign. Although this sign is seen commonly, bronchi and blood vessels are sometimes oriented obliquely or in the cephalo-caudal plane and are not readily apparent on conventional cross-sectional CT images. Multiplanar spiral CT reconstructions or multiplanar MR imaging may be helpful in better determining the course of the vessels and airways in these cases.[77]

Most cases of round atelectasis are seen in patients who have been exposed to asbestos.[81] Other causes include pleural effusion secondary to tuberculosis, therapeutic pneumothorax, congestive heart failure, infections other than tuberculosis, pulmonary infarction, and malignancy.

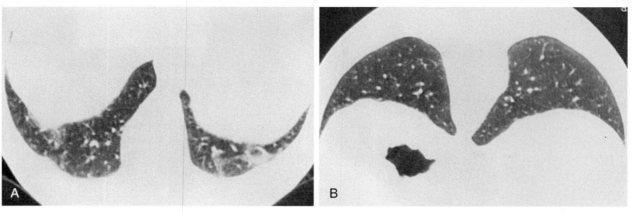

FIGURE 3–40

Dependent atelectasis. A CT scan with the patient supine (**A**) shows localized areas of ground-glass attenuation in the dependent portions of both lower lobes. A repeat scan with the patient prone (**B**) is normal. Reversibility from the supine to the prone positions allows distinction of passive dependent atelectasis from air space or interstitial lung disease. *(From Müller NL, Fraser RS, Colman NC, Paré PD: Radiologic Diagnosis of Diseases of the Chest. Philadelphia, WB Saunders, 2001.)*

Adhesive Atelectasis

The term *adhesive atelectasis* is used to describe atelectasis caused, at least in part, by a deficiency of surfactant.[82] The best examples of this form of disease are the respiratory distress syndrome of newborn infants and acute radiation pneumonitis (Fig. 3–42); other causes include acute respiratory distress syndrome, pneumonia, prolonged shallow breathing, and pulmonary thromboembolism.[82,83]

Cicatrization Atelectasis

The volume attained by the lung depends on the balance between the force applied to the lung by outward recoil of the chest wall and the inward elastic recoil of the lung parenchyma. It follows that when the lung is stiffer than normal (i.e., when compliance is decreased), lung volume is decreased. This situation classically occurs with pulmonary fibrosis and is termed *cicatrization atelectasis.*

Localized cicatrization atelectasis is best exemplified by chronic infection, often granulomatous in nature, and is epitomized by long-standing fibrocaseous tuberculosis (Fig. 3–43). The bronchi and bronchioles within the affected lung are dilated as a result of the increased elastic recoil from the surrounding pulmonary fibrosis, a phenomenon known as *traction bronchiectasis/bronchiolectasis.*[84] The radiologic signs are as might be expected—a segment or lobe occupying a volume smaller than normal, having inhomogeneous density as a result of dilated air-containing airways, and showing irregular thickened strands extending from the atelectatic segment to the hilum. Compensatory signs of chronic loss of volume are usually evident, including a local mediastinal shift (frequently manifested by sharp deviation of the trachea when segments of the upper lobe are involved), displacement of the hilum (which may be severe in upper lobe disease), and compensatory overinflation of the remainder of the affected lung.

Generalized fibrotic disease of the lungs may be associated with loss of volume. For example, elevation of the diaphragm and an overall reduction in lung size are commonly seen in idiopathic pulmonary fibrosis. A gradual reduction in thoracic volume in cases of diffuse interstitial disease is a useful indicator of the fibrotic nature of the underlying pathologic process.

Radiologic Signs of Atelectasis

Radiologic signs of atelectasis may be classified into direct and indirect types (Table 3–8). The former includes displacement of the interlobar fissures and crowding of bronchi and vessels within the area of atelectasis; indirect signs include pulmonary opacification and signs related to shift of other structures to compensate for the loss of volume.

Direct Signs

Displacement of Interlobar Fissures. Displacement of the fissures that form the boundary of an atelectatic lobe is one of the most dependable and easily recognized signs of atelectasis (Fig. 3–44). For each lobe, the position and configuration of the displaced fissures are predictable for a given loss of volume; these factors are considered later in relation to patterns of specific lobar and segmental atelectasis.

TABLE 3–8. Radiologic Signs of Atelectasis

Direct
    Displacement of interlobar fissures
    Crowding of vessels and bronchi
Indirect
    Local increase in opacity
    Elevation of a hemidiaphragm
    Displacement of the mediastinum
    Compensatory overinflation of the remaining lung
    Displacement of hila
    Approximation of ribs
    Absence of an air bronchogram (in cases of resorption atelectasis only)
    Absence of visibility of the interlobar artery (in cases of lower lobe atelectasis only)

From Müller NL, Fraser RS, Colman NC, Paré PD: Radiologic Diagnosis of Diseases of the Chest. Philadelphia, WB Saunders, 2001.

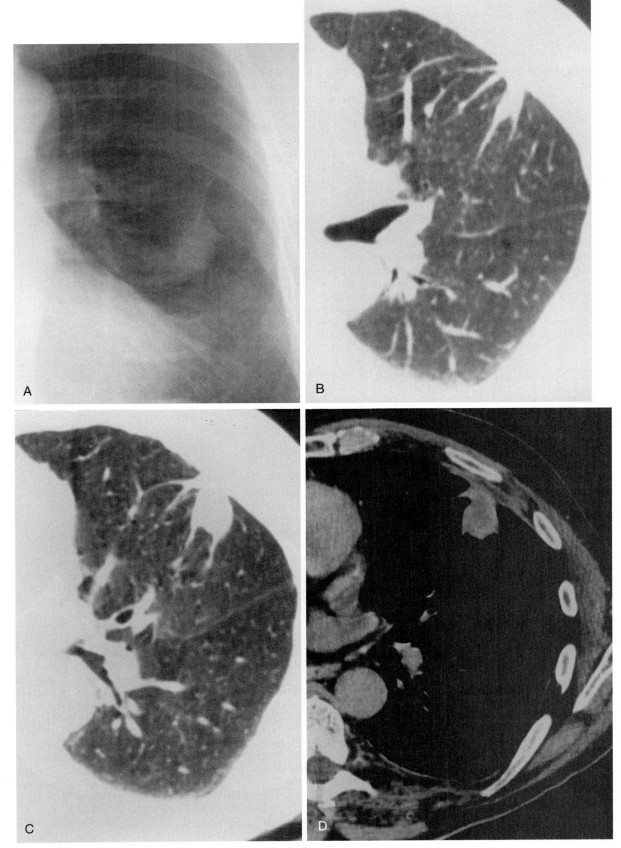

FIGURE 3–41

Round atelectasis. A view of the left lung from a posteroanterior chest radiograph (**A**) shows an oval soft tissue nodule measuring 3 cm in maximal diameter. CT scans (**B** and **C**) show vessels converging toward the nodule. There is evidence of volume loss, with the vessels and the left major fissure curving toward the area of round atelectasis. A CT scan photographed at soft tissue windows (**D**) shows that the nodule abuts a focal area of pleural thickening. The patient was a 70-year-old man who had a history of asbestos exposure. *(From Müller NL, Fraser RS, Colman NC, Paré PD: Radiologic Diagnosis of Diseases of the Chest. Philadelphia, WB Saunders, 2001.)*

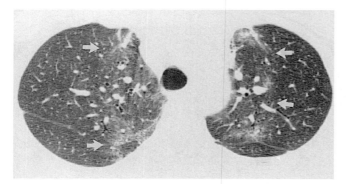

FIGURE 3–42

Adhesive atelectasis in radiation pneumonitis. An HRCT scan shows areas of ground-glass attenuation in a distribution conforming to the radiation portals for the treatment of Hodgkin's lymphoma *(arrows)*. Evidence of loss of volume is present, with bronchi and vessels closer to the mediastinum than normal, particularly on the left side. The patient was a 28-year-old woman who had undergone radiation therapy 5 months previously. *(From Müller NL, Fraser RS, Colman NC, Paré PD: Radiologic Diagnosis of Diseases of the Chest. Philadelphia, WB Saunders, 2001.)*

Crowding of Vessels and Bronchi. As the lung loses volume, the vessels and bronchi in the atelectatic area become crowded together. This finding is one of the earliest signs of atelectasis and can be recognized most readily when comparison is made with previous radiographs.[85] Increased opacification of the atelectatic lobe may result in obscuration of the vessels; however, except in patients who have resorptive atelectasis, crowded air bronchograms are visible within the area of atelectasis on the radiograph or CT scan (see Fig. 3–44).

Indirect Signs

Apart from the presence of a local opacity, the main indirect signs of atelectasis are related to mechanisms that compensate for the reduction in intrapleural pressure—diaphragmatic elevation, mediastinal shift, approximation of ribs, and overinflation of the remainder of the lung (see Fig. 3–44).

Patterns of Atelectasis

Total Pulmonary Atelectasis

Atelectasis of an entire lung is usually secondary to complete obstruction of a main bronchus and is associated with increased opacity of the atelectatic lung (see Fig. 3–36). In patients who have partial obstruction or pneumothorax, however, loss of volume may occur with normal or increased radiolucency of the atelectatic lung.

Lobar Atelectasis

The patterns created by atelectasis of the right and left upper lobes differ and are described separately. The lower lobes have almost identical patterns and are considered together.

Right Upper Lobe

The minor fissure and the upper half of the major fissure approximate by shifting upward and forward (Fig. 3–45). On lateral projection, both fissures appear gently curved, the minor fissure assuming a concave configuration inferiorly, whereas the major fissure may be convex, concave, or flat[86]; the

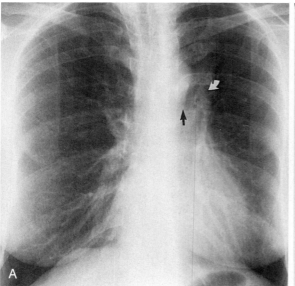
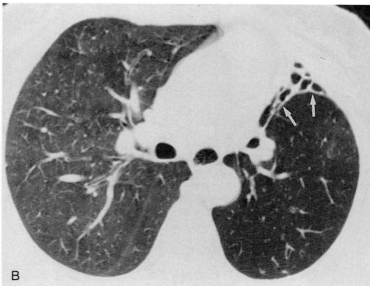

FIGURE 3–43

Severe cicatrization atelectasis caused by tuberculosis. A posteroanterior chest radiograph (**A**) in a 41-year-old woman shows loss of volume of the left upper lobe with elevation of the left main bronchus *(straight black arrow)* and left hilum *(curved white arrow)* and a shift of the mediastinum. The left lung has decreased vascularity in comparison to the right. Although the left upper lobe is collapsed, it has not resulted in any increase in opacity. An HRCT scan (**B**) confirms the presence of complete atelectasis of the left upper lobe. All that remains are markedly ectatic bronchi outlined by the major fissure *(arrows)*, which is displaced cephalad, anteriorly, and medially. Marked hyperinflation of the left lower lobe and decreased size of the left hemithorax are apparent. The findings are the result of previous tuberculosis. *(From Müller NL, Fraser RS, Colman NC, Paré PD: Radiologic Diagnosis of Diseases of the Chest. Philadelphia, WB Saunders, 2001.)*

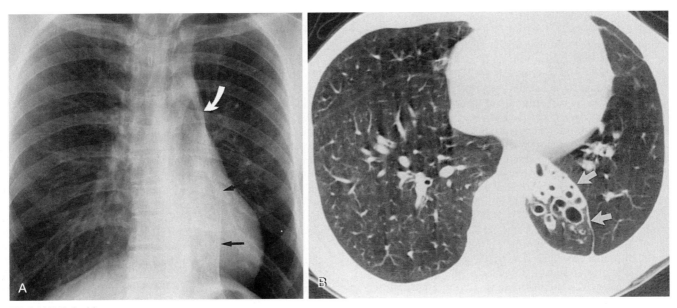

FIGURE 3–44

Left lower lobe atelectasis. A posteroanterior chest radiograph (**A**) shows caudal and medial displacement of the left major fissure *(black arrows)* characteristic of left lower lobe atelectasis. Crowding of ectatic bronchi within the atelectatic lobe can also be seen. Indirect signs of left lower lobe atelectasis include overinflation of the left upper lobe, overinflation of the right lung with displacement of the anterior junction line *(curved white arrow)* to the left, and a shift of the mediastinum. An HRCT scan (**B**) shows caudal and medial displacement of the major fissure *(arrows)* and left lower lobe bronchiectasis. Although the lobe is markedly atelectatic, there is little opacification of the lung parenchyma, presumably because of reflex vasoconstriction. The patient was a 23-year-old man who had a history of childhood viral pneumonia. *(From Müller NL, Fraser RS, Colman NC, Paré PD: Radiologic Diagnosis of Diseases of the Chest. Philadelphia, WB Saunders, 2001.)*

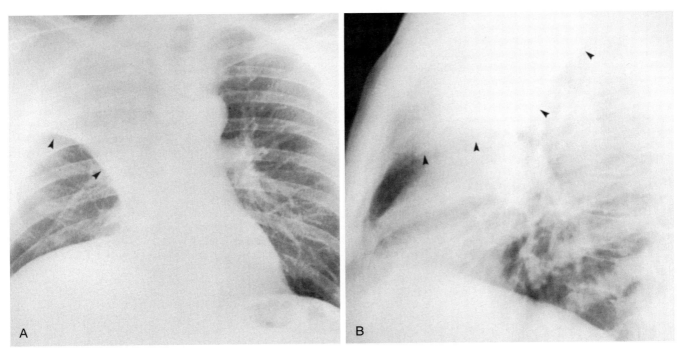

FIGURE 3–45

Right upper lobe atelectasis (moderate). Posteroanterior (**A**) and lateral (**B**) radiographs show a homogeneous opacity *(arrowheads)* occupying the anterosuperior portion of the right hemithorax. In lateral projection, the opacity is sharply defined on its posterior and anteroinferior margins. The right hemidiaphragm is elevated, and the trachea is slightly displaced to the right. The patient was a 51-year-old man with a large squamous cell carcinoma in the right upper lobe. The atelectasis was caused by bronchial compression from involved lymph nodes. *(From Müller NL, Fraser RS, Colman NC, Paré PD: Radiologic Diagnosis of Diseases of the Chest. Philadelphia, WB Saunders, 2001.)*

minor fissure shows roughly the same curvature in PA projection.

Another sign commonly associated with right or left upper lobe atelectasis (less commonly with middle lobe atelectasis) is the *juxtaphrenic peak*.[87] This peak consists of a small, sharply defined triangular opacity that projects upward from the medial half of the hemidiaphragm at or near the highest point of the dome (Fig. 3–46). The peak is usually related to cephalic displacement of an inferior accessory fissure.[88,89]

Right upper lobe atelectasis caused by large hilar tumors may be associated with a characteristic downward bulge in the medial portion of the minor fissure. This feature, combined with the concave appearance of the lateral aspect of the minor fissure, results in a reverse S configuration of the minor fissure and is known as the Golden's S sign (Fig. 3–47).[90] On the radiograph[82] and CT scan,[91] this sign strongly suggests the presence of pulmonary carcinoma as the cause of atelectasis. Though initially described for right upper lobe atelectasis, Golden's S sign is applicable to atelectasis of any lobe.[82]

On CT scan, the medial margin of the atelectatic right upper lobe abuts the mediastinum and is associated with superior and medial displacement of the minor fissure (see Fig. 3–47). With elevation of the minor fissure, the overinflated middle lobe shifts upward laterally alongside the atelectatic upper lobe. Compensatory overinflation of the right lower lobe results in superior, anterior, and medial displacement of the major fissure.[78]

Left Upper Lobe

The major difference between atelectasis of the left and right upper lobes is related to the absence of a minor fissure on the left; all lung tissue anterior to the major fissure is involved (Fig. 3–48). This fissure, which is slightly more vertical than the major fissure on the right, is displaced forward in a plane roughly parallel to the anterior chest wall, a relationship particularly evident on the lateral radiograph. As volume loss increases, the fissure moves further anteriorly and medially, until on lateral projection the shadow of the lobe is no more than a broad linear opacity contiguous with and parallel to the anterior chest wall. The contiguity of the atelectatic lobe with the anterior mediastinum obliterates the left cardiac border in frontal projection (the *silhouette sign*).

As the apical segment moves downward and forward, the space that it vacates is occupied by the overinflated superior segment of the lower lobe; the apex of the hemithorax contains aerated lung (see Fig. 3–48).[92] Sometimes, this lower lobe segment inserts itself medially between the apex of the atelectatic upper lobe and the mediastinum and thereby creates a sharp interface with the medial edge of the atelectatic lobe and allows visualization of the aortic arch. The overinflated superior segment is seen as a crescent of hyperlucency, hence the term *Luftsichel (air crescent)* in the German literature.[93] This finding is seen more often on the left (see Fig. 3–48) than on the right.

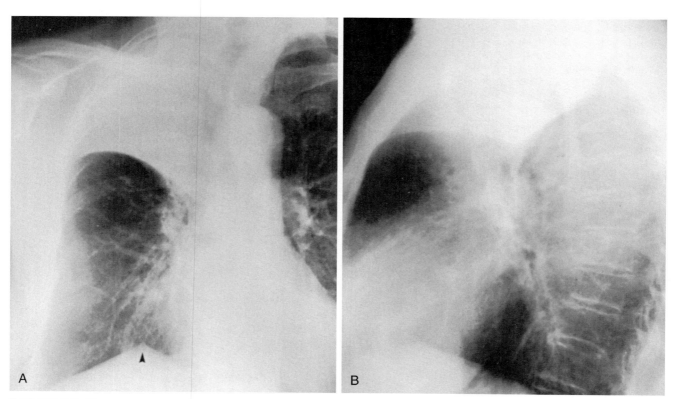

FIGURE 3–46

Juxtaphrenic peak in upper lobe atelectasis. Posteroanterior (**A**) and lateral (**B**) chest radiographs in a patient with right upper lobe atelectasis show the normally smooth contour of the right hemidiaphragm to be interrupted by a triangular opacity *(arrowhead),* the apex pointing cephalad. This juxtaphrenic peak is due to an inferior accessory fissure that can be seen extending obliquely cephalad and medially from the juxtaphrenic peak. *(From Müller NL, Fraser RS, Colman NC, Paré PD: Radiologic Diagnosis of Diseases of the Chest. Philadelphia, WB Saunders, 2001.)*

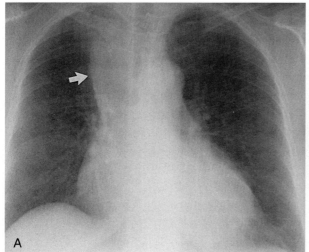

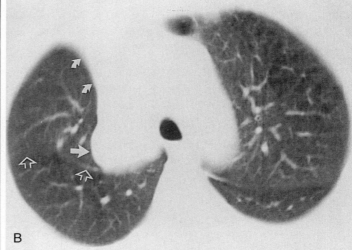

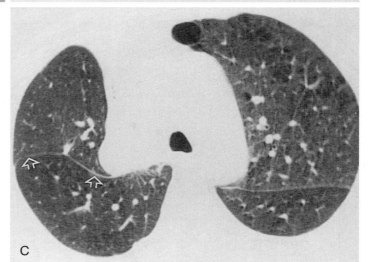

FIGURE 3–47

Right upper lobe atelectasis with Golden's S sign. A posteroanterior chest radiograph (**A**) shows right upper lobe atelectasis with elevation and medial displacement of the minor fissure. Note the focal convexity resulting from a central tumor (Golden's S sign) *(arrow).* A CT scan at the level of the tracheal carina (**B**) shows upward and medial displacement of the minor fissure *(curved arrows)* with a localized convexity (Golden's S sign) *(straight arrow)* and upward and forward displacement of the right major fissure *(open arrows).* The reorientation of the major fissure is easier to appreciate on HRCT scan (**C,** *open arrows).* The patient was a 55-year-old woman with squamous cell carcinoma. *(From Müller NL, Fraser RS, Colman NC, Paré PD: Radiologic Diagnosis of Diseases of the Chest. Philadelphia, WB Saunders, 2001.)*

On CT scan, the atelectatic left upper lobe can be seen to abut the anterior chest wall and mediastinum (Fig. 3–49). The major fissure is shifted cephalad and anteriorly. The posterior margin of the atelectatic left upper lobe has a V-shaped contour or a small peak from the lung apex to the hilum as a result of tethering of the major fissure by the hilum. A focal convexity in the hilar region indicates the presence of a central obstructing tumor (Golden's S sign) (see Fig. 3–49).

Right Middle Lobe

The diagnosis of right middle lobe atelectasis is one of the easiest to make on a lateral radiograph and one of the most difficult to make on a PA projection (Fig. 3–50). With progressive loss of volume, the minor fissure and the lower half of the major fissure approximate and are almost in contact when collapse is complete. On a PA projection, there may be no discernible increase in opacity, the only evidence of disease being obliteration of part of the right cardiac border as a result of contiguity of the right atrium with the medial segment of the atelectatic lobe (the *silhouette sign*). The difficulty in detecting atelectasis in this projection is related to the obliquity of the atelectatic lobe in a superoinferior plane and the

thickness of the collapsed lobe itself. The CT appearance of right middle lobe atelectasis is characteristic and consists of a broad triangular or trapezoidal opacity with the apex directed toward the hilum (see Fig. 3–50).

Lower Lobes

The configuration of atelectatic lower lobes is modified by the fulcrum-like effect exerted on the lung by the hilum and pulmonary ligament,[94] the fissures approximating in such a manner that the upper half of the major fissure swings downward and the lower half backward (Fig. 3–51; see Fig. 3–44). This displacement is best appreciated in lateral projection when the lobe is only partly atelectatic and the major fissure is tangential to the x-ray beam and visible as a well-defined interface. During its downward displacement, the upper half of the fissure usually becomes clearly evident on a PA projection as a well-defined interface extending obliquely downward and laterally from the region of the hilum (see Figs. 3–44 and 3–51).[95,96] On CT scan, an atelectatic lower lobe can be seen to lose volume in a posteromedial direction, thereby pulling the major fissure down (see Fig. 3–44). The lateral portion of the major fissure shows a greater degree of mobility because

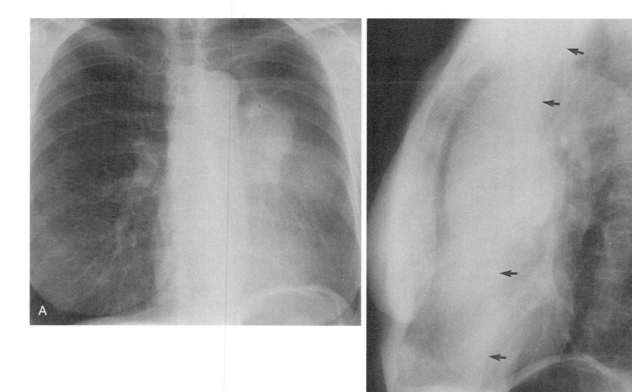

FIGURE 3–48

Left upper lobe atelectasis with the Luftsichel sign. A posteroanterior chest radiograph (**A**) shows elevation of the left hilum and left main bronchus and a poorly defined opacity in the left perihilar region. A crescent of aerated lung outlines the aortic arch (the Luftsichel sign). A lateral radiograph (**B**) reveals anterior displacement of the major fissure *(arrows)*. The overinflated superior segment of the left lower lobe outlines the aortic arch and accounts for the area of increased lucency lateral to the aortic arch on the posteroanterior radiograph. *(From Müller NL, Fraser RS, Colman NC, Paré PD: Radiologic Diagnosis of Diseases of the Chest. Philadelphia, WB Saunders, 2001.)*

the medial aspect is fixed to the mediastinum by the hilar structures and the pulmonary ligament.

Segmental Atelectasis

Segmental atelectasis usually results from bronchial obstruction and is associated with obstructive pneumonitis. A homogeneous opacity that conforms to the anatomic distribution of a bronchopulmonary segment and in which no air bronchogram is identifiable should alert the physician immediately to the presence of an obstructing endobronchial lesion (Fig. 3–52).

Linear (Platelike) Atelectasis

Linear (platelike) atelectasis is characterized by linear opacities ranging from 1 to 3 mm in thickness and 4 to 10 cm in length; they are situated in the mid and lower lung zones, most commonly the latter (Fig. 3–53). Though usually oriented in a roughly horizontal plane, the opacities may be oriented obliquely, depending on the zone of lung affected; in midlung zones particularly, they may be angled more than 45 degrees to the horizontal. The opacities may be single or multiple, unilateral or bilateral. Almost invariably, they are associated with

conditions that diminish diaphragmatic excursion, such as intra-abdominal surgery and systemic lupus erythematosus.

PLEURAL ABNORMALITIES

Pleural Effusion

Conventional PA and lateral chest radiographs are considerably less sensitive than the lateral decubitus view in the detection of pleural effusion. Although 10 mL of fluid can be detected on the lateral decubitus view, accumulation of at least 175 mL of fluid is necessary to cause blunting of the lateral costophrenic sulcus on a PA radiograph.[97] Moreover, although most effusions greater than 200 mL are evident on the PA radiograph, 500 mL of fluid may be present without any blunting of the costophrenic sulcus on this view (Fig. 3–54).[97] Because the posterior costophrenic sulcus is deeper than the lateral sulcus, small effusions are detected more readily on a lateral radiograph than on the frontal view.[98,99]

Ultrasonography, CT, and MR imaging allow more effective detection of small or loculated effusions, as well as distinction of effusions from pleural thickening.[100] Because of its ready

Text continued on p. 150

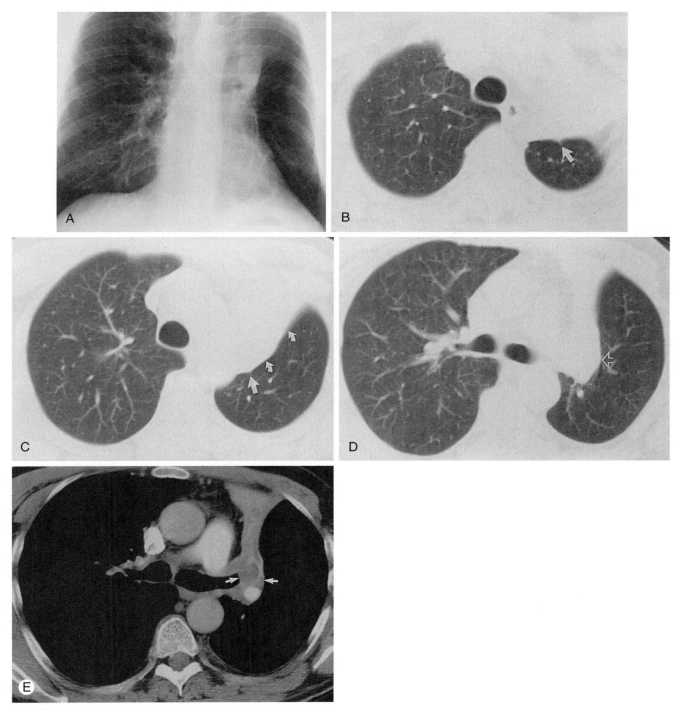

FIGURE 3–49

Left upper lobe atelectasis. A posteroanterior radiograph (**A**) shows elevation of the left hilum and opacification of the left upper lobe. A CT scan near the lung apex (**B**) reveals anterior and cephalic displacement of the major fissure. The slightly peaked appearance of the posterior surface of the major fissure *(arrow)* is caused by tethering from the hilar structures. A CT scan at the level of the aortic arch (**C**) shows anterior and medial displacement of the interlobar fissure *(curved arrows)* with a focal peak *(straight arrow)*. The peaked appearance of the posterior fissural surface *(straight arrow)* and lack of air bronchograms are indicative of resorptive atelectasis. A CT scan at the level of the left main bronchus (**D**) shows a focal convexity *(arrow)* characteristic of a central obstructive tumor (Golden's S sign). A CT scan photographed at soft tissue windows (**E**) shows the tumor *(arrows)* associated with complete obstruction of the left upper lobe bronchus. The patient was a 58-year-old man with squamous cell carcinoma. *(From Müller NL, Fraser RS, Colman NC, Paré PD: Radiologic Diagnosis of Diseases of the Chest. Philadelphia, WB Saunders, 2001.)*

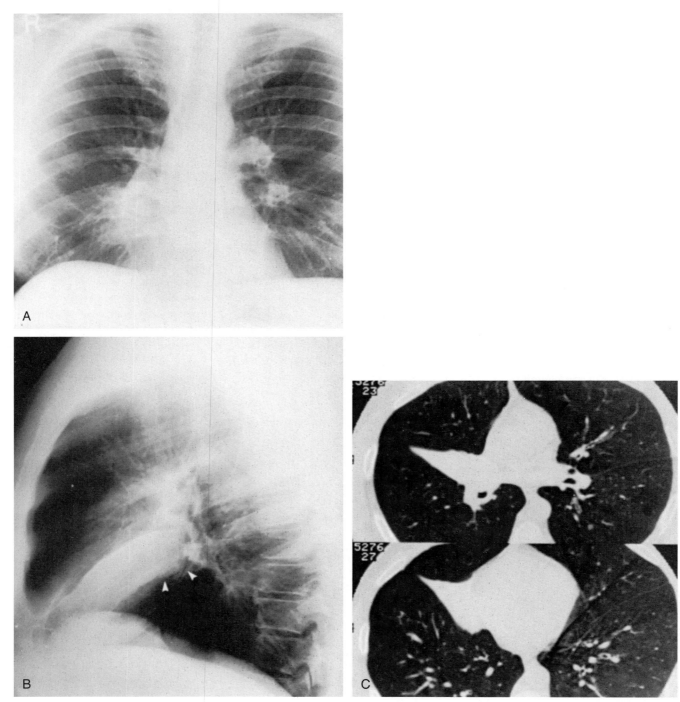

FIGURE 3–50

Right middle lobe atelectasis. A posteroanterior radiograph (**A**) shows a vague opacity in the right lower hemithorax obliterating the right cardiac border. A lateral projection in the same patient (**B**) shows the characteristic triangular opacity of middle lobe atelectasis. The convex inferior configuration of the major fissure at the hilum *(arrowheads)* is indicative of an underlying mass. The opacity of the middle lobe possesses a sharp oblique orientation downward. CT scans (**C**) show the typical triangular opacity with its apex pointing peripherally. Contiguity between the visceral and parietal pleura over the anterolateral aspect of the lobe has been lost. The right middle lobe bronchus was obstructed by carcinoma. *(From Müller NL, Fraser RS, Colman NC, Paré PD: Radiologic Diagnosis of Diseases of the Chest. Philadelphia, WB Saunders, 2001.)*

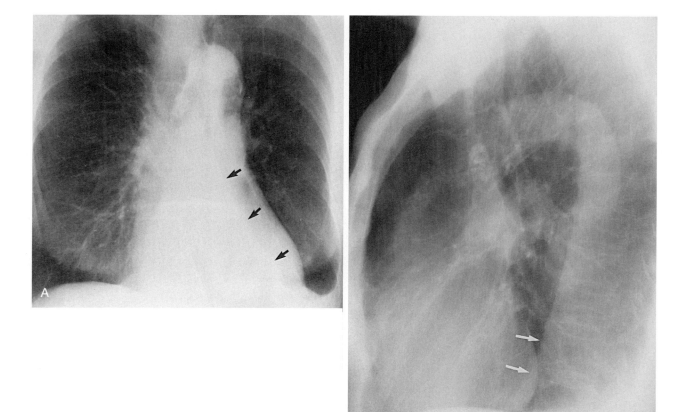

FIGURE 3–51

Left lower lobe atelectasis. A posteroanterior chest radiograph (**A**) shows a caudal and medial shift of the left major interlobar fissure (*arrows*). Note also the caudal displacement of the left hilum, compensatory overinflation of the left upper lobe and right lung, and shift of the mediastinum. A lateral radiograph (**B**) reveals posterior displacement of the interlobar fissure (*arrows*). The atelectatic left lower lobe is associated with increased opacity in the paravertebral region. A small left pleural effusion is also evident. The patient was a 74-year-old man with left lower lobe atelectasis secondary to a mucus plug. (*From Müller NL, Fraser RS, Colman NC, Paré PD: Radiologic Diagnosis of Diseases of the Chest. Philadelphia, WB Saunders, 2001.*)

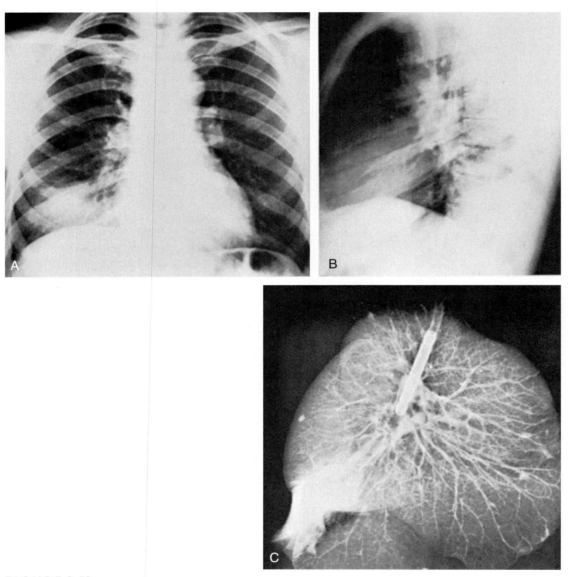

FIGURE 3–52

Segmental atelectasis and consolidation, posterior basal segment, right lower lobe. Posteroanterior (**A**) and lateral (**B**) radiographs show a homogeneous opacity localized to the posterior bronchopulmonary segment of the right lower lobe; no air bronchogram is present. The process is consolidative and atelectatic, the latter evidenced by posterior displacement of the major fissure. A lateral radiograph of the resected lung (**C**) shows the precise segmental nature of the disease; as a result of preoperative chemotherapy, the bronchial obstruction had been partly relieved, so the operative specimen shows a well-defined air bronchogram. Squamous cell carcinoma of the posterior basal bronchus was diagnosed. *(From Müller NL, Fraser RS, Colman NC, Paré PD: Radiologic Diagnosis of Diseases of the Chest. Philadelphia, WB Saunders, 2001.)*

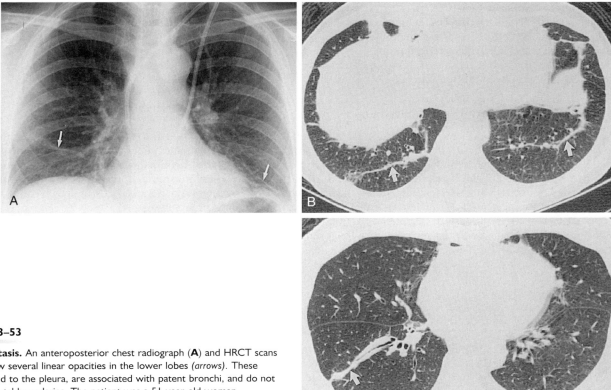

FIGURE 3–53

Linear atelectasis. An anteroposterior chest radiograph (**A**) and HRCT scans (**B** and **C**) show several linear opacities in the lower lobes *(arrows)*. These opacities extend to the pleura, are associated with patent bronchi, and do not respect segmental boundaries. The patient was a 51-year-old woman undergoing chemotherapy for acute leukemia. The abnormalities resolved spontaneously. *(From Müller NL, Fraser RS, Colman NC, Paré PD: Radiologic Diagnosis of Diseases of the Chest. Philadelphia, WB Saunders, 2001.)*

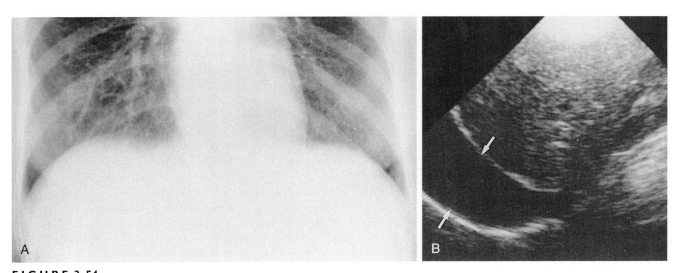

FIGURE 3–54

Right pleural effusion. A view of the lower part of the thorax from an anteroposterior chest radiograph (**A**) is essentially normal except for questionable minimal blunting of the right costophrenic sulcus. Ultrasound (**B**) shows right pleural effusion *(arrows)*. *(From Müller NL, Fraser RS, Colman NC, Paré PD: Radiologic Diagnosis of Diseases of the Chest. Philadelphia, WB Saunders, 2001.)*

---

availability and utility for bedside imaging, ultrasonography has become a particularly important imaging modality, not only for determining the presence of pleural fluid but also as a guide to therapeutic and diagnostic aspiration (see Fig. 3–54).[101] The procedure has also been shown to be superior to lateral decubitus radiography in the quantification of pleural fluid.[102]

Typical Configuration of Free Pleural Fluid

Normally, the opacity produced by an effusion on a PA radiograph is high laterally and curves gently downward and medially with a smooth, meniscus-shaped upper border; it terminates along the midcardiac border (Fig. 3–55). In lateral projection, because the fluid has ascended along the anterior and posterior thoracic wall to roughly an equal extent, the upper surface of the fluid density is semicircular, being high anteriorly and posteriorly and curving smoothly downward to its lowest point in the midaxillary line. Comparison of the maximal height of the fluid density on PA and lateral projections shows that this height is identical posteriorly, laterally, and anteriorly (i.e., the top of the fluid accumulation is *horizontal*); the meniscus shape is caused by the fact that the layer of fluid is of insufficient depth to cast a discernible shadow when viewed en face.[103,104]

The first place that fluid accumulates in an erect patient is between the inferior surface of the lower lobe and the diaphragm; in effect, the lung floats on a layer of fluid. A subpulmonary location of fluid is *usual* in the normal pleural space (although it would be reasonable to consider subpulmonary accumulation of a large amount of fluid atypical).[98] Subpulmonary effusion causes a configuration in an erect patient that closely simulates diaphragmatic elevation (thus the designation *pseudodiaphragmatic contour*). It may be unilateral or bilateral, the former more commonly on the right.[105] Several signs are helpful in its detection:

1. In PA projection (Fig. 3–56), the peak of the pseudodiaphragmatic configuration is lateral to that of the normal hemidiaphragm, being situated near the junction of the middle and lateral thirds rather than near the center, and it slopes down sharply toward the lateral costophrenic sulcus.[98,103]
2. On the left side, the pseudodiaphragmatic contour is separated farther than normal from the gastric air bubble, and effusion should be suspected when the distance between the two is greater than 2 cm. Care is needed to detect interposition of the spleen or the left lobe of the liver and to exclude the presence of gross ascites.[106]
3. On lateral projection, a characteristic configuration is frequently seen anteriorly where the convex upper margin of the fluid meets the major fissure. In these cases, the contour anterior to the fissure is flattened, this portion of the pseudodiaphragmatic contour descending abruptly to the anterior costophrenic sulcus.[98,103]

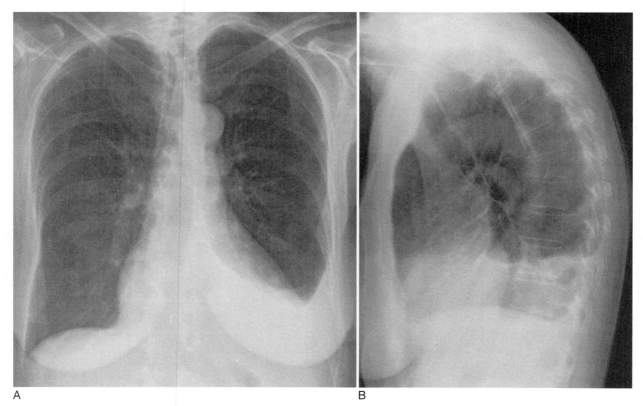

A   B

FIGURE 3–55

Pleural effusion. Posteroanterior (**A**) and lateral (**B**) radiographs show uniform opacification of the lower left hemithorax. The upper aspect of the fluid is meniscus shaped in both projections. Only the right hemidiaphragm is seen on lateral projections, the left being obscured by fluid (the silhouette sign).

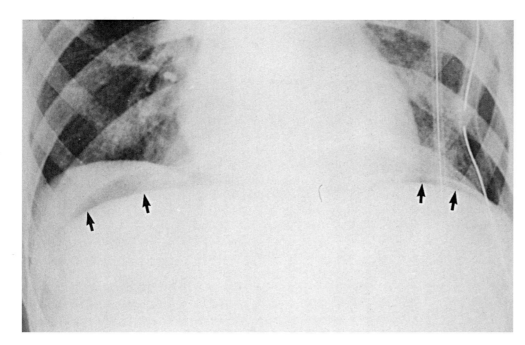

FIGURE 3–56

Subpulmonic effusion. A view of the lower part of the chest from an upright anteroposterior chest radiograph reveals the presence of pneumoperitoneum *(arrows)* and a small right subpulmonic pleural effusion. Note the characteristic distribution of subpulmonic effusion with a flat upper surface medially and a steep lateral drop-off. On the left side, the normal thickness of the hemidiaphragm is approximately 1 mm. *(From Müller NL, Fraser RS, Colman NC, Paré PD: Radiologic Diagnosis of Diseases of the Chest. Philadelphia, WB Saunders, 2001.)*

4. Pulmonary vessels, which are normally visible below the diaphragmatic contour, cannot be seen through the pseudodiaphragmatic contour of a subpulmonic effusion. Care should be taken to exclude underexposed radiographs, lower lobe consolidation, and ascites, all of which may cause similar findings.[107]

Distribution of Pleural Effusion in Supine Patients

In a supine patient, free pleural fluid layers posteriorly and produces a hazy increase in opacity without obscuration of the bronchovascular markings.[103] With small pleural effusions, the increase in opacity is limited to the lower lung zones; as the amount of fluid increases, there is progressive cephalic extension of the increased opacity until the entire hemithorax is involved (Fig. 3–57).[108] An apical fluid cap is seen on supine radiographs in approximately 50% of patients who have large effusions.[108]

When compared with lateral decubitus radiographs, supine radiographs have relatively low sensitivity and specificity in the diagnosis of pleural effusions.[109] In one prospective analysis of anteroposterior radiographs, pleural effusions were correctly identified on supine views in 24 of 36 cases (sensitivity of 67%) and excluded correctly in 18 of 26 cases (specificity of 69%).[109] The most helpful diagnostic findings were increased opacity of the hemithorax, blunting of the costophrenic angle, and obscuration of the hemidiaphragm.

Pleural effusions are characterized on CT scan by attenuation values between those of water (0 HU) and soft tissue (approximately 100 HU); except when small,[110] effusions can usually be readily distinguished from pleural thickening or masses (Fig. 3–58).[111] On CT scan of a supine patient, free pleural fluid accumulates first in the posterior pleural recesses. Because the lung tends to maintain its shape as it loses volume, the fluid has a concave or meniscoid anterior margin. As the effusion increases in size, fluid extends

cephalad and anteriorly and may involve the major and right minor fissures.

Loculation of Pleural Fluid

A loculated effusion may occur anywhere in the pleural space—between the parietal and visceral pleura over the periphery of the lung or between visceral layers in the interlobar fissures. Loculation is caused by adhesions between contiguous pleural surfaces and tends to occur during or after episodes of pleuritis; it is often associated with pyothorax or hemothorax. Over the convexity of the thorax, a loculated effusion appears as a smooth, sharply demarcated, homogeneous opacity protruding into the hemithorax and compressing contiguous lung (Fig. 3–59).

Interlobar loculated effusions are typically elliptical when viewed tangentially on the chest radiograph, their extremities blending imperceptibly with the normal interlobar fissure (Fig. 3–60). In some conditions, particularly cardiac failure, the effusion may simulate a mass and be misdiagnosed as a pulmonary neoplasm; however, its distinctive configuration on PA or lateral projection should establish the diagnosis in most cases. Occasionally, CT or ultrasonography is required for definitive diagnosis (Fig. 3–61). These fluid accumulations tend to be absorbed spontaneously when the heart failure resolves and have been called *vanishing tumor (phantom tumor, pseudotumor).*

Radiologic Signs of Pleural Thickening

Several radiologic features are helpful in differentiating the various causes of pleural thickening on radiographs and CT scans.[112] Evidence of underlying parenchymal disease is usually seen in patients who have had tuberculosis or empyema. Extensive calcification of the fibrothorax also favors

Text continued on p. 155

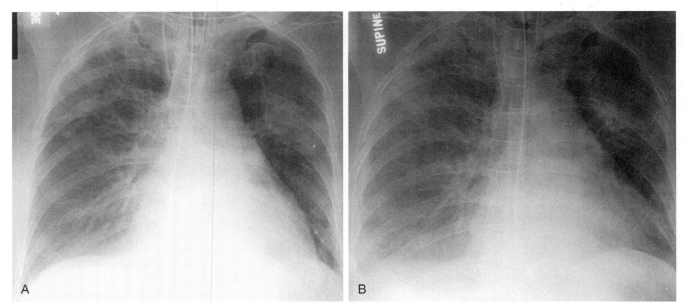

FIGURE 3–57

Pleural effusion in a supine patient. An anteroposterior supine view (**A**) shows hazy opacification of the right hemithorax. A view of the chest 24 hours later (**B**) shows a further increase in the opacity, obscuration of the lateral border of the right hemidiaphragm, blunting of the right costophrenic sulcus, and fluid extending cephalad along the lateral chest wall. The patient was a 60-year-old woman in whom a large right pleural effusion developed after liver transplantation. *(From Müller NL, Fraser RS, Colman NC, Paré PD: Radiologic Diagnosis of Diseases of the Chest. Philadelphia, WB Saunders, 2001.)*

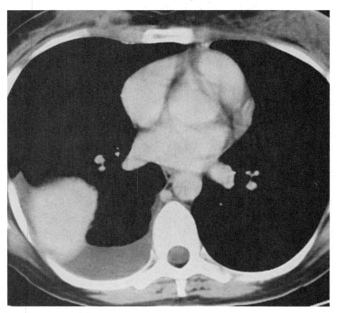

FIGURE 3–58

Pleural effusion. A contrast-enhanced CT scan shows a small right pleural effusion. The near-water density of pleural fluid allows ready distinction from the pleural-based mass. The patient was a 35-year-old woman with a fibrous tumor of the pleura. *(From Müller NL, Fraser RS, Colman NC, Paré PD: Radiologic Diagnosis of Diseases of the Chest. Philadelphia, WB Saunders, 2001.)*

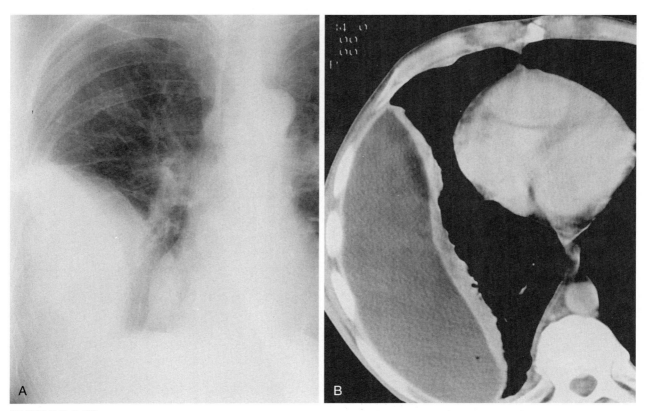

FIGURE 3–59

Loculated pleural effusion. A view of the right hemithorax from a posteroanterior chest radiograph (**A**) shows a sharply demarcated, homogeneous opacity that has convex borders with the lung and displaces the adjacent parenchyma. A contrast-enhanced CT scan (**B**) shows right pleural effusion associated with enhancement and thickening of the visceral and parietal pleura and compressive atelectasis of the adjacent lung. The findings are characteristic of a loculated empyema. Visualization of enhancing thickened visceral and parietal pleura surrounding pleural fluid is known as the split-pleura sign. *(From Müller NL, Fraser RS, Colman NC, Paré PD: Radiologic Diagnosis of Diseases of the Chest. Philadelphia, WB Saunders, 2001.)*

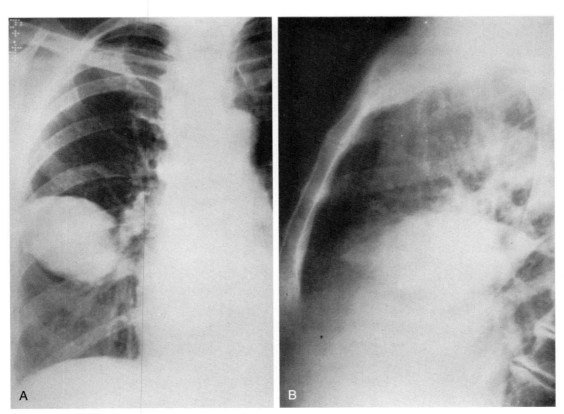

FIGURE 3–60

Pleural effusion localized to the minor fissure. A view of the right hemithorax from a posteroanterior radiograph (**A**) shows a sharply circumscribed, homogeneous opacity in the right midlung zone. In lateral projection (**B**), the true nature of the opacity can be appreciated: the mass is elliptical in shape, its pointed extremities being situated anteriorly and posteriorly in keeping with the position of the minor fissure. This unusual collection of pleural fluid developed during a recent episode of cardiac decompensation. With appropriate therapy, it disappeared completely in 3 weeks (vanishing tumor). (*From Müller NL, Fraser RS, Colman NC, Paré PD: Radiologic Diagnosis of Diseases of the Chest. Philadelphia, WB Saunders, 2001.*)

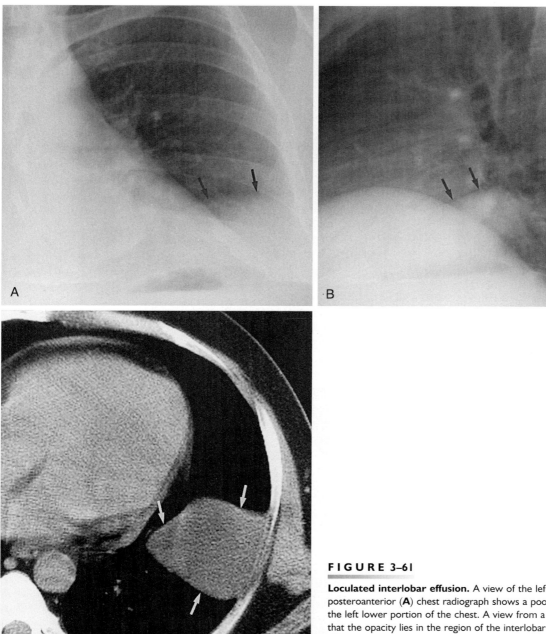

FIGURE 3–61

Loculated interlobar effusion. A view of the left hemithorax from a posteroanterior (**A**) chest radiograph shows a poorly defined opacity *(arrows)* in the left lower portion of the chest. A view from a lateral radiograph (**B**) reveals that the opacity lies in the region of the interlobar fissure *(arrows)*. A CT scan (**C**) shows the characteristic appearance of fluid within the left major fissure *(arrows)*. The fluid collection tapers medially. Follow-up chest radiographs 6 months later showed resolution of the fluid collection. *(From Müller NL, Fraser RS, Colman NC, Paré PD: Radiologic Diagnosis of Diseases of the Chest. Philadelphia, WB Saunders, 2001.)*

these conditions and is seldom seen with asbestos-related diffuse pleural thickening.[113] Pleural plaques are identified radiologically as circumscribed areas of pleural thickening, typically 3 to 10 mm in thickness and 1 to 5 cm in length (Fig. 3–62). They are usually associated with a history of asbestos exposure. Diffuse asbestos-related pleural thickening is considered to be present when there is a smooth uninterrupted pleural opacity extending over at least a fourth of the chest wall with or without associated obliteration of the costophrenic sulci (Fig. 3–63).[100,114] Pleural thickening secondary to hemorrhagic effusion, tuberculosis, and empyema

is generally unilateral, whereas that related to asbestos is usually bilateral, whether manifested as diffuse thickening or as plaques.[71,112,115]

When pleural fibrosis is extensive, it seldom involves the mediastinal pleura (see Fig. 3–63).[112] This feature is helpful in the differential diagnosis of benign from malignant causes of pleural thickening. For example, in one study, only 1 (12%) of 8 patients with fibrothorax had mediastinal pleural thickening as opposed to 8 (73%) of 11 with mesothelioma (Fig. 3–64).[112] (The *mediastinal pleura* is defined as the pleura that abuts the mediastinum, the posterior extent of which is

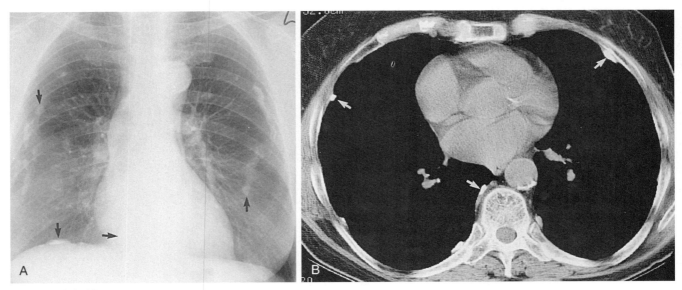

FIGURE 3–62

Calcified asbestos-related pleural plaques. A posteroanterior chest radiograph (**A**) and CT scan (**B**) show multiple bilateral, discrete, calcified pleural plaques *(arrows)* involving the costal, diaphragmatic, and paravertebral pleura. The patient was a 79-year-old man with occupational asbestos exposure. *(From Müller NL, Fraser RS, Colman NC, Paré PD: Radiologic Diagnosis of Diseases of the Chest. Philadelphia, WB Saunders, 2001.)*

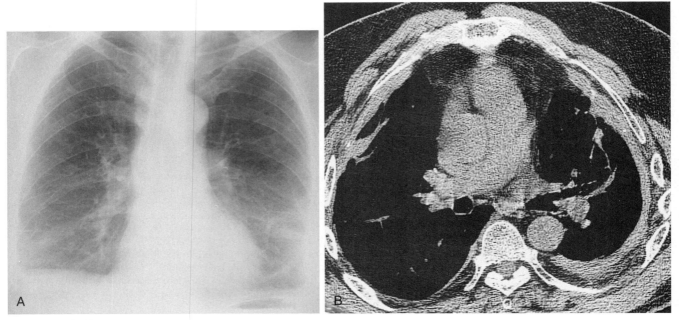

FIGURE 3–63

Pleural fibrosis. A posteroanterior chest radiograph (**A**) shows extensive bilateral pleural thickening. The blunted costophrenic angles are sharply angulated rather than meniscus shaped, a finding helpful in distinguishing pleural thickening from effusion. Curved bands of increased opacity extend from the left lung to the pleural thickening, a feature most commonly related to asbestos. A CT scan (**B**) reveals marked thickening of the costal and paravertebral pleura with small foci of calcification. The patient was a 53-year-old man with a history of exposure to asbestos. *(From Müller NL, Fraser RS, Colman NC, Paré PD: Radiologic Diagnosis of Diseases of the Chest. Philadelphia, WB Saunders, 2001.)*

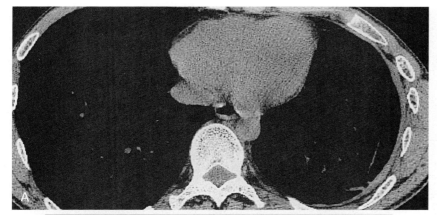

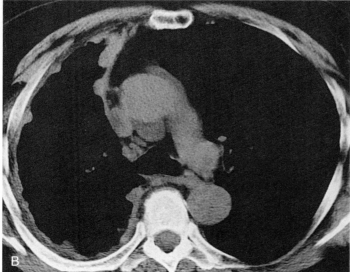

FIGURE 3–64

Benign versus malignant pleural thickening.
A, Benign pleural thickening. A CT scan reveals smooth thickening of the left costal pleura with no associated pleural effusion or involvement of the mediastinal pleura. The patient was a 32-year-old man with surgically proven benign fibrothorax, presumably caused by previous pleurisy. **B,** Malignant pleural thickening. A CT scan shows right pleural thickening that is diffuse and nodular, shown on biopsy to represent mesothelioma. In both cases, the size of the affected hemithorax is decreased, a finding that is not helpful in distinguishing benign from malignant pleural thickening. *(From Müller NL, Fraser RS, Colman NC, Paré PD: Radiologic Diagnosis of Diseases of the Chest. Philadelphia, WB Saunders, 2001.)*

demarcated by the anterior aspect of the vertebrae.[100,116]) The parietal pleura abutting the paravertebral sulci is not part of the anatomic mediastinal pleura and is most commonly referred to as the *paravertebral pleura.*[112,117]

Radiologic Signs of Pneumothorax

Pneumothorax in Upright Patients

A radiologic diagnosis of pneumothorax can be made only by identifying the visceral pleural line. This line is visualized as a sharply defined line of increased opacity that can readily be distinguished from the black line attributable to the Mach effect, which may be seen outlining a skin fold (Fig. 3–65).

In an erect patient, pneumothorax is first evident near the apex of the chest; a subpulmonic location has been reported occasionally in patients who have COPD[118] or penetrating thoracic injury.[119] The visceral pleural line is usually readily identifiable, even on radiographs exposed at TLC. In most cases, the inspiratory chest radiograph is the only imaging modality required for diagnosis. When pneumothorax is strongly suspected clinically but a pleural line is not identified, gas in the pleural space can be detected by one of two procedures: (1) radiography in the erect position in full expiration (the rationale being that lung volume is reduced while the volume of gas in the pleural space is constant, thus making it easier to detect the pneumothorax) or (2) radiography in the lateral decubitus position with a horizontal x-ray beam (the rationale being that air rises to the highest point in the hemithorax and is more clearly visible over the lateral chest wall than over the apex, where overlying bone shadows may obscure fine linear shadows). Although upright expiratory radiographs are obtained in most patients in whom pneumothorax is suspected clinically, the lateral decubitus view provides an excellent alternative when an upright view cannot be obtained or when it provides equivocal findings.[120-122.]

Pneumothorax in Supine Patients

When patients who have suspected pneumothorax must be examined in the supine position, as is often the case in the intensive care unit, gas within the pleural space rises to the vicinity of the diaphragm, the highest point in the hemithorax in this position. Depending on the size of the pneumothorax, the result can be an exceptionally deep radiolucent costophrenic sulcus (*deep sulcus sign*) (Fig. 3–66),[119] a lucency over the right or left upper quadrant,[123] or a much sharper than normal appearance of the hemidiaphragm with or without the presence of a visceral pleural line visible above it.[119] Other findings include visualization of the anterior

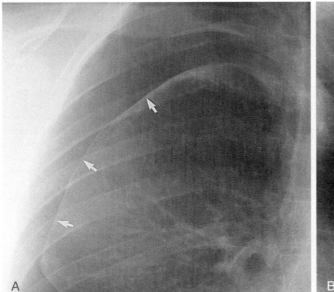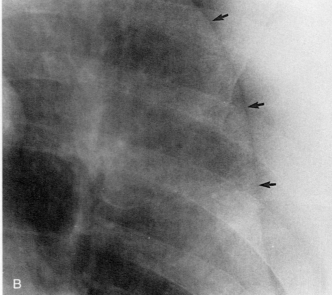

FIGURE 3–65

Pneumothorax versus skin fold. A view of the right side of the chest from a posteroanterior radiograph (**A**) shows a sharply defined pleural line *(arrows)* characteristic of pneumothorax. A view of the left side of the chest from an anteroposterior radiograph (**B**) shows a skin fold. The black line *(arrows)* seen at the edge of the skin fold is due to the Mach effect. *(From Müller NL, Fraser RS, Colman NC, Paré PD: Radiologic Diagnosis of Diseases of the Chest. Philadelphia, WB Saunders, 2001.)*

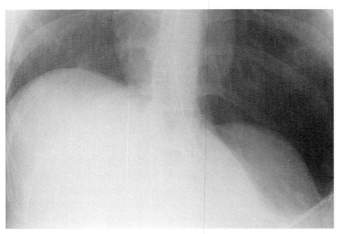

FIGURE 3–66

Pneumothorax with the deep sulcus sign. A view of the lower portion of the chest from an anteroposterior chest radiograph with the patient supine shows a radiolucent left costophrenic sulcus and a sharply defined left hemidiaphragm. These findings are characteristic of pneumothorax in a supine patient. *(From Müller NL, Fraser RS, Colman NC, Paré PD: Radiologic Diagnosis of Diseases of the Chest. Philadelphia, WB Saunders, 2001.)*

costophrenic sulcus, increased sharpness of the cardiac border, collection of air within the minor fissure, and depression of the ipsilateral hemidiaphragm.[119,124,125] When a pneumothorax is suspected in a supine patient, confirmation can be obtained most readily by performing a lateral decubitus view with the involved hemithorax uppermost.[120-122] CT has also been shown to be useful and is superior to frontal chest radiography.[124]

REFERENCES

1. Tuddenham WJ: Glossary of terms for thoracic radiology: Recommendations of the Nomenclature Committee of the Fleischner Society. AJR Am J Roentgenol 143:509-517, 1984.
2. Austin JH, Müller NL, Friedman PJ, et al: Glossary of terms for CT of the lungs: Recommendations of the Nomenclature Committee of the Fleischner Society. Radiology 200:327-331, 1996.
3. Itoh H, Murata K, Konishi J, et al: Diffuse lung disease: Pathologic basis for the high-resolution computed tomography findings. J Thorac Imaging 8:176-188, 1993.
4. Heitzman ER, Markarian B, Berger I, Dailey E: The secondary pulmonary lobule: A practical concept for interpretation of chest radiographs. II. Application of the anatomic concept to an understanding of roentgen pattern in disease states. Radiology 93:513-519, 1969.
5. Müller NL, Miller RR: Computed tomography of chronic diffuse infiltrative lung disease. Part 1. Am Rev Respir Dis 142:1206-1215, 1990.
6. Müller NL, Miller RR: Computed tomography of chronic diffuse infiltrative lung disease. Part 2. Am Rev Respir Dis 142:1440-1448, 1990.
7. Webb WR, Müller NL, Naidich DP: High-Resolution CT of the Lung. Philadelphia, Lippincott-Raven, 2001, pp 71-192.
8. Hirakata K, Nakata H, Nakagawa T: CT of pulmonary metastases with pathological correlation. Semin Ultrasound CT MR 16:379-394, 1995.
9. Johkoh T, Müller NL, Ichikado K, et al: Perilobular pulmonary opacities: High-resolution CT findings and pathologic correlation. J Thorac Imaging 14:172-177, 1999.
10. Johkoh T, Itoh H, Müller NL, et al: Crazy-paving appearance at thin-section CT: Spectrum of disease and pathologic findings. Radiology 211:155-160, 1999.
11. Kang EY, Grenier P, Laurent F, Müller NL: Interlobular septal thickening: Patterns at high-resolution computed tomography. J Thorac Imaging 11:260-264, 1996.
12. Müller NL, Chiles C, Kullnig P: Pulmonary lymphangiomyomatosis: Correlation of CT with radiographic and functional findings. Radiology 175:335-339, 1990.
13. Primack SL, Hartman TE, Hansell DM, Müller NL: End-stage lung disease: CT findings in 61 patients. Radiology 189:681-686, 1993.
14. Genereux GP: The end-stage lung: Pathogenesis, pathology, and radiology. Radiology 116:279-289, 1975.
15. Hogg J: Chronic interstitial lung disease of unknown cause: A new classification based on pathogenesis. AJR Am J Roentgenol 156:225, 1991.
16. Staples CA, Müller NL, Vedal S, et al: Usual interstitial pneumonia: Correlation of CT with clinical, functional, and radiologic findings. Radiology 162:377-381, 1987.
17. Templeton PA, McLoud TC, Müller NL, et al: Pulmonary lymphangioleiomyomatosis: CT and pathologic findings. J Comput Assist Tomogr 13:54-57, 1989.
18. McLoud TC, Carrington CB, Gaensler EA: Diffuse infiltrative lung disease: A new scheme for description. Radiology 149:353-363, 1983.

19. Kwong JS, Carignan S, Kang EY, et al: Miliary tuberculosis. Diagnostic accuracy of chest radiography. Chest 110:339-342, 1996.
20. Murata K, Takahashi M, Mori M, et al: Pulmonary metastatic nodules: CT-pathologic correlation. Radiology 182:331-335, 1992.
21. Remy-Jardin M, Degreef JM, Beuscart R, et al: Coal worker's pneumoconiosis: CT assessment in exposed workers and correlation with radiographic findings. Radiology 177:363-371, 1990.
22. Begin R, Bergeron D, Samson L, et al: CT assessment of silicosis in exposed workers. AJR Am J Roentgenol 148:509-514, 1987.
23. Im JG, Itoh H, Shim YS, et al: Pulmonary tuberculosis: CT findings—early active disease and sequential change with antituberculous therapy. Radiology 186:653-660, 1993.
24. Aquino SL, Gamsu G, Webb WR, Kee ST: Tree-in-bud pattern: Frequency and significance on thin section CT. J Comput Assist Tomogr 20:594-599, 1996.
25. Gruden JF, Webb WR, Naidich DP, McGuinness G: Multinodular disease: Anatomic localization at thin-section CT—multireader evaluation of a simple algorithm. Radiology 210:711-720, 1999.
26. Müller NL, Kullnig P, Miller RR: The CT findings of pulmonary sarcoidosis: Analysis of 25 patients. AJR Am J Roentgenol 152:1179-1182, 1989.
27. Munk PL, Müller NL, Miller RR, Ostrow DN: Pulmonary lymphangitic carcinomatosis: CT and pathologic findings. Radiology 166:705-709, 1988.
28. Müller NL: Clinical value of high-resolution CT in chronic diffuse lung disease. AJR Am J Roentgenol 157:1163-1170, 1991.
29. Remy-Jardin M, Remy J, Giraud F, et al: Computed tomography assessment of ground-glass opacity: Semiology and significance. J Thorac Imaging 8:249-264, 1993.
30. Bergin CJ, Wirth RL, Berry GJ, Castellino RA: Pneumocystis carinii pneumonia: CT and HRCT observations. J Comput Assist Tomogr 14:756-759, 1990.
31. Leung AN, Miller RR, Müller NL: Parenchymal opacification in chronic infiltrative lung diseases: CT-pathologic correlation. Radiology 188:209-214, 1993.
32. Moskovic E, Miller R, Pearson M: High resolution computed tomography of Pneumocystis carinii pneumonia in AIDS. Clin Radiol 42:239-243, 1990.
33. Primack SL, Miller RR, Müller NL: Diffuse pulmonary hemorrhage: Clinical, pathologic, and imaging features. AJR Am J Roentgenol 164:295-300, 1995.
34. Müller NL, Coiby TV: Idiopathic interstitial pneumonias: High-resolution CT and histologic findings. Radiographics 17:1016-1022, 1997.
35. Hartman TE, Primack SL, Müller NL, Staples CA: Diagnosis of thoracic complications in AIDS: Accuracy of CT. AJR Am J Roentgenol 162:547-553, 1994.
36. Hansell DM, Moskovic E: High-resolution computed tomography in extrinsic allergic alveolitis. Clin Radiol 43:8-12, 1991.
37. Godwin JD, Müller NL, Takasugi JE: Pulmonary alveolar proteinosis: CT findings. Radiology 169:609-613, 1988.
38. Murch CR, Carr DH: Computed tomography appearances of pulmonary alveolar proteinosis. Clin Radiol 40:240-243, 1989.
39. Mathieson JR, Mayo JR, Staples CA, Müller NL: Chronic diffuse infiltrative lung disease: Comparison of diagnostic accuracy of CT and chest radiography. Radiology 171:111-116, 1989.
40. Grenier P, Valeyre D, Cluzel P, et al: Chronic diffuse interstitial lung disease: Diagnostic value of chest radiography and high-resolution CT. Radiology 179:123-132, 1991.
41. Grenier P, Chevret S, Beigelman C, et al: Chronic diffuse infiltrative lung disease: Determination of the diagnostic value of clinical data, chest radiography, and CT and Bayesian analysis. Radiology 191:383-390, 1994.
42. Zwirewich CV, Vedal S, Miller RR, Müller NL: Solitary pulmonary nodule: High-resolution CT and radiologic-pathologic correlation. Radiology 179:469-476, 1991.
43. Zerhouni EA, Stitik FP, Siegelman SS, et al: CT of the pulmonary nodule: A cooperative study. Radiology 160:319-327, 1986.
44. Siegelman SS, Khouri NF, Leo FP, et al: Solitary pulmonary nodules: CT assessment. Radiology 160:307-312, 1986.
45. Bleyer JM, Marks JH: Tuberculosis and hamartomas of the lung: Comparative study of 66 proved cases. AJR Am J Roentgenol 77:1013, 1957.
46. Steele JD: The Solitary Pulmonary Nodule. Springfield, IL, Charles C Thomas, 1964.
47. Felson B: Chest Roentgenology. Philadelphia, WB Saunders, 1973.
48. Woodring JH, Fried AM, Chuang VP: Solitary cavities of the lung: Diagnostic implications of cavity wall thickness. AJR Am J Roentgenol 135:1269-1271, 1980.
49. Lewall DB, McCorkell SJ: Rupture of echinococcal cysts: Diagnosis, classification, and clinical implications. AJR Am J Roentgenol 146:391-394, 1986.
50. Penner C, Maycher B, Long R: Pulmonary gangrene. A complication of bacterial pneumonia. Chest 105:567-573, 1994.
51. Cordier JF, Valeyre D, Guillevin L, et al: Pulmonary Wegener's granulomatosis. A clinical and imaging study of 77 cases. Chest 97:906-912, 1990.
52. Huang RM, Naidich DP, Lubat E, et al: Septic pulmonary emboli: CT-radiographic correlation. AJR Am J Roentgenol 153:41-45, 1989.
53. Good CA: The solitary pulmonary nodule: A problem of management. Radiol Clin North Am 1:429, 1963.
54. Gurney JW: Determining the likelihood of malignancy in solitary pulmonary nodules with Bayesian analysis. Part I. Theory. Radiology 186:405-413, 1993.
55. O'Keefe MEJ, Good CA, McDonald JR: Calcification in solitary nodules of the lung. AJR Am J Roentgenol 77:1023, 1957.
56. Maile CW, Rodan BA, Godwin JD, et al: Calcification in pulmonary metastases. Br J Radiol 55:108-113, 1982.
57. Zwiebel BR, Austin JH, Grimes MM: Bronchial carcinoid tumors: Assessment with CT of location and intratumoral calcification in 31 patients. Radiology 179:483-486, 1991.

58. Reich SB, Weinshelbaum A, Yee J: Correlation of radiographic measurements and pulmonary function tests in chronic obstructive pulmonary disease. AJR Am J Roentgenol 144:695-699, 1985.
59. Kilburn KH, Warshaw RH, Thornton JC: Do radiographic criteria for emphysema predict physiologic impairment? Chest 107:1225-1231, 1995.
60. Sutinen S, Christoforidis AJ, Klugh GA, et al: Roentgenologic criteria for the recognition of nonsymptomatic pulmonary emphysema: Correlation between roentgenologic findings and pulmonary pathology. Am Rev Respir Dis 91:69, 1965.
61. Pratt PC: Role of conventional chest radiography in diagnosis and exclusion of emphysema. Am J Med 82:998-1006, 1987.
62. Kennedy CD, Habibi P, Matthew DJ, Gordon I: Lobar emphysema: Long-term imaging follow-up. Radiology 180:189-193, 1991.
63. Jederlinic PJ, Sicilian LS, Baigelman W, Gaensler EA: Congenital bronchial atresia. A report of 4 cases and a review of the literature. Medicine (Baltimore) 66:73-83, 1987.
64. Woodring JH: Pitfalls in the radiologic diagnosis of lung cancer. AJR Am J Roentgenol 154:1165-1175, 1990.
65. Byrd RB, Miller WE, Carr DT, et al: The roentgenographic appearance of squamous cell carcinoma of the bronchus. Mayo Clin Proc 43:327-332, 1968.
66. Byrd RB, Miller WE, Carr DT, et al: The roentgenographic appearance of small cell carcinoma of the bronchus. Mayo Clin Proc 43:337-341, 1968.
67. Grimes OF, Farber SM: Air cysts of the lung. Surg Gynecol Obstet 113:720, 1961.
68. Feraru F, Morrow CS: Surgery of subpleural blebs: Indications and contraindications. Am Rev Respir Dis 79:577, 1959.
69. Quigley MJ, Fraser RS: Pulmonary pneumatocele: Pathology and pathogenesis. AJR Am J Roentgenol 150:1275-1277, 1988.
70. Reed JC: Chest Radiology: Plain Film Patterns and Differential Diagnoses. St Louis, Mosby–Year Book, 1997, pp 185-210.
71. Aberle DR, Gamsu G, Ray CS, Feuerstein IM: Asbestos-related pleural and parenchymal fibrosis: Detection with high-resolution CT. Radiology 166:729-734, 1988.
72. Lynch DA, Webb WR, Gamsu G, et al: Computed tomography in pulmonary sarcoidosis. J Comput Assist Tomogr 13:405-410, 1989.
73. Gamsu G, Aberle DR, Lynch D: Computed tomography in the diagnosis of asbestos-related thoracic disease. J Thorac Imaging 4:61-67, 1989.
74. Yoshimura H, Hatakeyama M, Otsuji H, et al: Pulmonary asbestosis: CT study of subpleural curvilinear shadow. Work in progress. Radiology 158:653-658, 1986.
75. Primack SL, Remy-Jardin M, Remy J, Müller NL: High-resolution CT of the lung: Pitfalls in the diagnosis of infiltrative lung disease. AJR Am J Roentgenol 167:413-418, 1996.
76. Schneider HJ, Felson B, Gonzalez LL: Rounded atelectasis. AJR Am J Roentgenol 134:225-232, 1980.
77. Batra P, Brown K, Hayashi K, Mori M: Rounded atelectasis. J Thorac Imaging 11:187-197, 1996.
78. Lee KS, Ahn JM, Im JG, et al: Lobar atelectasis: Typical and atypical radiographic and CT findings. Postgrad Radiol 15:203, 1995.
79. McHugh K, Blaquiere RML: CT features of rounded atelectasis. AJR Am J Roentgenol 153:257-260, 1989.
80. Carvalho PM, Carr DH: Computed tomography of folded lung. Clin Radiol 41:86-91, 1990.
81. Hillerdal G: Rounded atelectasis. Clinical experience with 74 patients. Chest 95:836-841, 1989.
82. Woodring JH, Reed JC: Types and mechanisms of pulmonary atelectasis. J Thorac Imaging 11:92-108, 1996.
83. Iannuzzi M, Petty TL: The diagnosis, pathogenesis, and treatment of adult respiratory distress syndrome. J Thorac Imaging 1:1-10, 1986.
84. Westcott JL, Cole SR: Traction bronchiectasis in end-stage pulmonary fibrosis. Radiology 161:665-669, 1986.
85. Proto AV, Tocino I: Radiographic manifestations of lobar collapse. Semin Roentgenol 15:117-173, 1980.
86. Khoury MB, Godwin JD, Halvorsen RA Jr, Putman CE: CT of obstructive lobar collapse. Invest Radiol 20:708-716, 1985.
87. Kattan KR, Eyler WR, Felson B: The juxtaphrenic peak in upper lobe collapse. Semin Roentgenol 15:187-193, 1980.
88. Cameron DC: The juxtaphrenic peak (Katten's sign) is produced by rotation of an inferior accessory fissure. Australas Radiol 37:332-335, 1993.
89. Davis SD, Yankelevitz DF, Wand A, Chiarella DA: Juxtaphrenic peak in upper and middle lobe volume loss: Assessment with CT. Radiology 198:143-149, 1996.
90. Golden R: The effect of bronchostenosis upon the roentgen-ray shadows in carcinoma of the bronchus. Am J Roentgenol Radiat Ther 13:21, 1925.
91. Reinig JW, Ross P: Computed tomography appearance of Golden's "S" sign. J Comput Tomogr 8:219-223, 1984.
92. Zdansky E: Bemerkung zur atelektatischen Retraktion des linken Oberlappens. [Atelectatic retraction of the left upper lobe.] Fortschr Roentgenstr 100:725, 1964.
93. Webber M, Davies P: The Luftsichel: An old sign in upper lobe collapse. Clin Radiol 32:271-275, 1981.
94. Rabinowitz JG, Cohen BA, Mendleson DS: Symposium on Nonpulmonary Aspects in Chest Radiology. The pulmonary ligament. Radiol Clin North Am 22:659-672, 1984.
95. Fisher MS: Significance of a visible major fissure on the frontal chest radiograph. AJR Am J Roentgenol 137:577-580, 1981.
96. Friedman PJ: Radiology of the superior segment of the lower lobe: A regional perspective introducing the B6 bronchus sign. Radiology 144:15-25, 1982.
97. Colins JD, Burwell D, Furmanski S, et al: Minimal detectable pleural effusions. A roentgen pathology model. Radiology 105:51-53, 1972.

98. Raasch BN, Carsky EW, Lane EJ, et al: Pleural effusion: Explanation of some typical appearances. AJR Am J Roentgenol 139:899-904, 1982.
99. Henschke CI, Davis SD, Romano PM, Yankelevitz DF: The pathogenesis, radiologic evaluation, and therapy of pleural effusions. Radiol Clin North Am 27:1241-1255, 1989.
100. Müller NL: Imaging of the pleura. Radiology 186:297-309, 1993.
101. O'Moore PV, Mueller PR, Simeone JF, et al: Sonographic guidance in diagnostic and therapeutic interventions in the pleural space. AJR Am J Roentgenol 149:1-5, 1987.
102. Eibenberger KL, Dock WI, Ammann ME, et al: Quantification of pleural effusions: Sonography versus radiography. Radiology 191:681-684, 1994.
103. Fleischner FG: Atypical arrangement of free pleural effusion. Radiol Clin North Am 1:347, 1963.
104. Davis S: The Shape of a pleural effusion. BMJ 1:436, 1963.
105. Dunbar JS, Favreau M: Infrapulmonary pleural effusion with particular reference to its occurrence in nephrosis. J Can Assoc Radiol 10:24, 1959.
106. Kafura PJ, Barnhard HJ: Ascites simulating subpulmonary pleural effusion. Radiology 101:525-526, 1971.
107. Schwarz MI, Marmorstein BL: A new radiologic sign of subpulmonic effusion. Chest 67:176-178, 1975.
108. Woodring JH: Recognition of pleural effusion on supine radiographs: How much fluid is required? AJR Am J Roentgenol 142:59-64, 1984.
109. Ruskin JA, Gurney JW, Thorsen MK, Goodman LR: Detection of pleural effusions on supine chest radiographs. AJR Am J Roentgenol 148:681-683, 1987.
110. Pugatch RD, Faling LJ, Robbins AH, Snider GL: Differentiation of pleural and pulmonary lesions using computed tomography. J Comput Assist Tomogr 2:601-606, 1978.
111. Maffessanti M, Tommasi M, Pellegrini P: Computed tomography of free pleural effusions. Eur J Radiol 7:87-90, 1987.
112. Leung AN, Müller NL, Miller RR: CT in differential diagnosis of diffuse pleural disease. AJR Am J Roentgenol 154:487-492, 1990.
113. Friedman AC, Fiel SB, Radecki PD, Lev-Toaff AS: Computed tomography of benign pleural and pulmonary parenchymal abnormalities related to asbestos exposure. Semin Ultrasound CT MR 11:393-408, 1990.
114. McLoud TC, Woods BO, Carrington CB, et al: Diffuse pleural thickening in an asbestos-exposed population: Prevalence and causes. AJR Am J Roentgenol 144:9-18, 1985.
115. Lynch DA, Gamsu G, Ray CS, Aberle DR: Asbestos-related focal lung masses: Manifestations on conventional and high-resolution CT scans. Radiology 169:603-607, 1988.
116. Platzer W: Pernkopf Anatomy: Atlas of Topographic and Applied Human Anatomy. Vol 2, Thorax, Abdomen, and Extremities. Baltimore, Urban & Schwarzenberg, 1989, p 63.
117. Im JG, Webb WR, Rosen A, Gamsu G: Costal pleura: Appearances at high-resolution CT. Radiology 171:125-131, 1989.
118. Christensen EE, Dietz GW: Subpulmonic pneumothorax in patients with chronic obstructive pulmonary disease. Radiology 121:33-37, 1976.
119. Schulman A, Dalrymple RB: Subpulmonary pneumothorax. Br J Radiol 51:494-497, 1978.
120. Carr JJ, Reed JC, Choplin RJ, et al: Conventional film and computed radiography of experimentally induced pneumothoraces in cadavers: Implications for detection in patients. Radiology 183:193, 1992.
121. Beres RA, Goodman LR: Pneumothorax: Detection with upright versus decubitus radiography. Radiology 186:19-22, 1993.
122. Beres RA, Goodman LR: Pneumothorax detection: Clarifications and additional thoughts. Radiology 186:25, 1993.
123. Rhea JT, vanSonnenberg E, McLoud TC: Basilar pneumothorax in the supine adult. Radiology 133:593-595, 1979.
124. Tocino IM, Miller MH, Fairfax WR: Distribution of pneumothorax in the supine and semirecumbent critically ill adult. AJR Am J Roentgenol 144:901-905, 1985.
125. Spizarny DL, Goodman LR: Air in the minor fissure: A sign of right-sided pneumothorax. Radiology 160:329-331, 1986.

DIAGNOSTIC METHODS IN CHEST DISEASE

THE CLINICAL HISTORY

The most important part of any clinical history is the patient's description of the symptoms, which should be listened to and recorded with care. When the patient has finished reporting symptoms, the physician should ask for any pertinent information about the family history, past illnesses and personal habits, where the patient has lived and traveled, the patient's occupational history, any history of exposure to allergens, medication use, and HIV risk factors. Finally, because lung disease is frequently only one manifestation of a more general process or is secondary to a disease involving other organs, an account of the function of other body systems is essential.

Symptoms of Respiratory Disease

The principal symptoms of respiratory disease are cough (with or without expectoration), hemoptysis, chest pain, and shortness of breath (dyspnea).

Cough and Expectoration

Cough is a defense mechanism that protects against the inhalation of noxious substances and rids the conducting airways of aspirated foreign material and excessive respiratory tract secretions. The prevalence of chronic cough is high, particularly in cigarette smokers, in whom more than 30% of men and 25% of women have the symptom.[1] It is also surprisingly frequent in people who do not smoke; approximately 5% of individuals in the general nonsmoking population complain of the symptom.[2] Epidemiologic surveys have implicated exposure to indoor or outdoor air pollution in some of these individuals.[3] There is evidence that the presence of chronic cough and sputum production is associated with a subsequent decline in lung function and the development of dyspnea,[4,5] as well as an increased risk for myocardial infarction,[6] possibly as a consequence of accompanying systemic inflammation.[7] Cough is also a symptom of more than 100 diseases,[8] ranging from the trivial to the most serious; however, clinically stable patients subjected to obvious irritant exposure such as tobacco smoke should avoid exposure (e.g., quit smoking) as the first diagnostic and therapeutic maneuver.

The etiology of a patient's cough can often be deduced from the history alone. Patients who have chronic postnasal drip frequently describe a hacking cough that originates from a need to "clear the throat"; this type of cough can easily be distinguished from the deep, "loose" cough of patients who have disease in the bronchi or lung parenchyma. A prolonged change in the character of a cough in a current or previous smoker should raise the possibility of an endobronchial neoplasm. Some coughs, particularly those associated with acute bacterial infection, are productive of purulent secretions in the early stage of disease. A patient with chronic bronchitis usually expectorates mucoid material, but with "colds" it may be yellow or green and sometimes slightly blood streaked. Saccular bronchiectasis gives rise to daily copious, purulent, and often blood-streaked expectoration. A foul or fetid odor indicates infection with anaerobic organisms and is often associated with abscess formation. Expectoration of casts of the bronchial tree consisting of inspissated mucus may be seen in bronchitis, asthma, or mucoid impaction, the last often in association with allergic aspergillosis.

Knowledge of the time of occurrence of the cough may also be helpful in diagnosis. Most people who have a chronic cough complain that it is worse when they lie down at night; this is particularly true of those who have bronchiectasis, postnasal drip from chronic sinusitis, or cough secondary to acid reflux. A patient who has chronic bronchitis or bronchiectasis characteristically expectorates on arising in the morning. Spasms of cough caused by asthma or left-sided heart failure frequently occur at night and may awaken the patient. A cough during or shortly after eating suggests aspiration.

The etiology of cough is best considered in two categories—acute and chronic. The cause of acute cough is usually apparent from the clinical context. However, the cause of chronic cough may remain obscure even after obtaining a history, physical examination, chest radiograph, and lung function studies. In about 90% of such patients, cough can be explained by postnasal drip, asthma, gastroesophageal reflux, bronchiectasis, or eosinophilic bronchitis.[9] It is important to remember, however, that many patients have more than one cause of cough. Detailed investigation and management of these patients have been described in other publications.[9,10]

It should be remembered that *Bordetella pertussis* infection is the cause of cough in up to 10% to 20% of adults who have the symptom for more than 2 to 3 weeks.[11] Those who have contact with infected children are particularly at risk.[12] Cough is mostly paroxysmal and may disturb sleep. The diagnosis can be established by detection of *Bordetella* DNA by polymerase chain reaction (PCR) or by serologic investigation; culture lacks sensitivity.[13]

Hemoptysis

Hemoptysis (expectoration of blood) is an alarming symptom to the patient and physician alike and often indicates serious underlying pathology. It always warrants a careful history and chest radiographs; many patients also require more extensive investigation.

It is important as a first consideration to differentiate a pulmonary source of bleeding from one outside the lung, including the nose, nasopharynx, esophagus, or upper gastrointestinal tract. Blood originating from the lung is usually bright red, is often frothy, and generally provokes cough. It may be mixed with sputum or purulent secretions and often occurs in the context of a history of known lung disease. By contrast, blood originating in the esophagus or gastrointestinal tract is usually dark red or black and never frothy. It may be associated with nausea and vomiting and may be mixed with food particles. A history of upper gastrointestinal tract or hepatic disease, such as duodenal ulcer or cirrhosis, should increase the suspicion of such nonpulmonary bleeding. Difficulty in diagnosis is particularly likely when vomited blood is aspirated into the airways or expectorated blood is swallowed. When there is doubt about the source of bleeding, the patient should be assumed to have lung disease.

The differential diagnosis of hemoptysis divorced from any clinical and radiographic context is extensive (Table 4–1). Common causes include bronchitis, bronchiectasis, lung abscess, pneumonia, and pulmonary carcinoma[14,15]; tuberculosis is an important consideration in patients from populations in which the background prevalence is high.[16] The character of expectorated blood may sometimes suggest the underlying disease process. Although simple streaking of mucoid material can occur in bronchitis, it may also denote a more serious condition such as tuberculosis or carcinoma. When sputum is frankly bloody and does not contain mucoid or purulent material, it is more likely to be the result of pulmonary infarction than pneumonia, particularly if it persists unchanged for several days. Bloody material mixed with pus should suggest pneumonia or lung abscess in acute illness and bronchiectasis in chronic disease. When the blood is diluted so that it has a pink and sometimes frothy appearance, pulmonary edema secondary to left-sided heart failure should be suspected.

Hemoptysis, even when minor, is an indication for a chest radiograph; in most cases, culture of expectorated sputum for mycobacteria is likewise appropriate. Although bronchoscopy is also indicated in many patients, it is reasonable to forgo this procedure in those who have a strong clinical history of a nonneoplastic disease process that can explain the bleeding, those who have a demonstrated site of extrapulmonary bleeding, those whose clinical status is so poor that no action would be taken regardless of the bronchoscopic findings, and those who are nonsmokers and who have no findings on chest radiography suggesting a neoplasm.[17] However, if hemoptysis recurs despite antibiotic therapy for presumed infection, direct visualization of the airways is indicated.

When the chest radiograph is normal or does not demonstrate any findings suggestive of malignancy, certain clinical features indicate a higher risk of undetected pulmonary carcinoma, including a history of smoking, age older than 40 years, and recurrent bleeding.[18] HRCT and bronchoscopy are indicated in such patients and are complementary in establishing the etiology of hemoptysis.[19] The prognosis of patients who have hemoptysis in the setting of a normal chest radiograph and nondiagnostic bronchoscopic findings is generally good; however, carcinoma will ultimately develop in a significant number of those who have the risk factors just mentioned.[20]

The definition of massive hemoptysis varies from 100 mL/day[21] to more than 1000 mL/day[22]; it is not surprising that the prognosis varies accordingly. Massive hemoptysis

TABLE 4–1. Causes of Hemoptysis*

Infectious

Lung abscess
Bronchitis
Tuberculosis
Bronchiectasis (including cystic fibrosis)
Fungus ball (mycetoma)
Paragonimiasis (in endemic areas)

Cardiovascular

Left ventricular failure
Pulmonary thromboembolism with infarction
Mitral stenosis
Tricuspid endocarditis with septic embolism
Pulmonary hypertension
Aneurysms
   Aortic aneurysm
   Subclavian artery aneurysm
   Left ventricular pseudoaneurysm
Vascular prostheses
Arteriovenous malformation
Absence of the inferior vena cava
Pulmonary artery agenesis with lung systemic vascularization

Neoplastic

Pulmonary carcinoma
Carcinoid tumor
Tracheobronchial gland tumors
Metastatic carcinoma/sarcoma

Traumatic

Aortic tear
Lung contusion
Ruptured bronchus
Bronchoscopy
Swan-Ganz catheterization
Lung biopsy
Transtracheal aspirate
Lymphangiography

Immunologic

Wegener's granulomatosis
Systemic lupus erythematosus
Goodpasture's syndrome
Idiopathic pulmonary hemorrhage

Drugs and Toxins

Anticoagulants
Cocaine
Penicillamine
Trimellitic anhydride
Amiodarone

Miscellaneous

Coagulopathy
Thrombocytopenia
Amyloidosis
Broncholithiasis
Endometriosis
Aspirated foreign body
Intralobar sequestration
Radiation
Lymphangioleiomyomatosis
Factitious
Cryptogenic organizing pneumonia (COP, BOOP)
Lipid pneumonia
Dieulafoy's disease

*Most common causes indicated in **bold** type.
BOOP, bronchiolitis obliterans with organizing pneumonia.

is seen most commonly with tuberculosis (both active and bacteriologically inactive), bronchiectasis, carcinoma, abscess, and fungus ball.[23] In most cases it is not the actual quantity of blood lost that causes death, the mechanism probably being asphyxiation as a result of bronchial occlusion by clot.

Chest Pain

Pain within the thorax can be conveniently discussed according to its three principal sites of origin: pleura, mediastinum, and chest wall.

Pleural Pain. Because both the lung and the visceral pleura lack sensory nerves to detect pain, pulmonary disease may progress to an advanced stage without producing even minor chest pain. The parietal pleura, on the other hand, is richly supplied with nerves that can be stimulated by inflammation or stretching. Pain may vary from lancinating discomfort during slight inspiratory effort to a less severe, but still sharp pain that may "catch" the patient at the end of a maximal inspiration. Pleural pain often disappears or is reduced to a dull ache during expiration or breath-holding. Pressure over the intercostal muscles in the area of pain may or may not elicit discomfort; when it does, the pain is typically mild in comparison to the sensation during breathing. This is in contrast to chest wall pain, which is usually associated with a region of tenderness, often over a very small area.

Except when it involves the diaphragm, the diseased area of pleura (which is often secondary to a pulmonary parenchymal lesion) typically underlies the area in which pain is perceived. The central part of the diaphragm is innervated by the phrenic nerve, and the sensory afferent fibers enter the cervical cord mainly in the third and fourth cervical posterior nerve roots; hence, irritation of this portion of the pleura is referred to the neck and the upper part of the shoulder. The lower intercostal nerves, which enter the thoracic cord in the 7th to 12th dorsal posterior nerve roots, supply the outer parts of the diaphragmatic pleura; thus, irritation of this portion causes referred pain in the lower part of the thorax.

Mediastinal Pain. The trachea, esophagus, heart, aorta, and many lymph nodes are situated in the mediastinum, and disease involving any of these organs may be manifested as pain in that region. Inflammation or neoplastic infiltration of the mediastinal soft tissue itself may also cause discomfort. The most common retrosternal pain is the result of myocardial ischemia; typically, it is described as "squeezing," "pressing," or "choking" and may extend to the neck or down the left arm or both arms. The pain may simulate that experienced in other conditions, including massive pulmonary thromboembolism, pulmonary hypertension, acute pericarditis, and dissecting aortic aneurysm.

Esophageal disease may give rise to "burning" pain and is usually clearly related to the ingestion of food. Those who have regurgitation of gastric secretions may complain that the pain is worse when they recline and relieved when they stand. A common retrosternal sensation, which presumably originates in sensory nerve endings of the tracheal mucosa, is the painful rawness experienced with infection of the upper respiratory tract and dry, hacking cough.

Chest Wall Pain. Pain originating in or referred to the chest wall that is not the result of parietal pleural irritation is common. Each year, approximately 10% to 20% of the

200,000 patients in the United States who have normal angiograms undertaken for investigation of presumed cardiac disease are eventually considered to have chest wall pain.[24] Such pain may be caused by disease in muscles, nerves, or bones. When it appears to originate in intercostal muscle, there may be a history of trauma that produced strain or even tearing; in our experience, such trauma is frequently caused by the dry, often paroxysmal cough that accompanies acute infectious tracheobronchitis. Often, however, no obvious precipitating cause can be found. Pain related to muscle injury may be differentiated from parietal pleural pain by limited exacerbation (if any) during deep inspiration, tenderness to palpation in the painful area, aggravation by coughing or trunk movement, and persistence between paroxysms of coughing.

Radicular pain is caused by pressure on or inflammation of the posterior nerve root. It follows the specific intercostal nerve distribution and radiates around the chest from behind or, in some cases, is localized to one area. Usually, it is described as dull and aching and is made worse by movement, particularly coughing. It may be caused by a protruding intervertebral disk, rheumatoid spondylitis, a malignant neoplasm involving the vertebrae, or inflammatory or neoplastic disease within the spinal cord. A variety of intercostal nerve root pain whose origin may be difficult to identify in the early stages is that due to herpes zoster; it is generally described as "burning," most often over a wide area unilaterally in the distribution of one or more intercostal nerves.

After muscle, the skeleton is probably the most common source of chest wall pain. When the pain is confined to the vertebral and paravertebral areas, it is usually caused by inflammatory or neoplastic disease, and percussion over the vertebral spines may elicit local tenderness. Rib fractures caused by accidental trauma or prolonged episodes of severe coughing are a common cause of chest wall pain. The costochondral junctions of the ribs may be the site of perichondritis, often associated with tenderness and swelling (Tietze's syndrome); usually, the pain is persistent and described as "gnawing" or "aching." Rib pain caused by malignancy is often appreciable before a mass develops; at first, it tends to be poorly localized but later becomes a dull, boring ache over the affected area.

A relatively innocuous transitory pain of undetermined origin has been described by the name "precordial catch." It is a severe, sharp pain over the left side of the chest, usually at the cardiac apex, that occurs at rest or during mild activity and lasts from 30 seconds to 5 minutes.[25] It comes on suddenly during inspiration, and the invariable reaction is a brief suspension of respiration; subsequently, breathing is maintained at a shallow level while the pain gradually disappears. Its onset is often associated with poor posture, improvement of which sometimes relieves the pain. The condition is very common, and its importance lies solely in its differentiation from chest pain of more serious consequence.

Dyspnea

Dyspnea is a common respiratory symptom that should be distinguished from tachypnea (a rapid respiratory rate) and hyperpnea (breathing more deeply and/or more rapidly). A dictionary definition of dyspnea as "difficult or labored breathing"[26] does little to illuminate the wide variety of sensations experienced by patients who have this symptom. In fact, attempts have been made to quantify the language of breathlessness and correlate patients' descriptions with specific diagnoses.[27] Such work suggests that the quality and intensity of respiratory sensations vary with different diseases; however, no particular sensation or set of sensations has sufficient sensitivity or specificity to have diagnostic value in isolation.

A detailed description by the patient of the specific features of the dyspnea is useful in differentiating organic causes of shortness of breath from a functional disorder. The latter is related to anxiety and is believed to be responsible for approximately 20% of cases of chronic dyspnea unexplained by the history, physical examination, chest radiography, and spirometry.[28] It is usually described as an inability to take a deep breath or to adequately "fill the lungs with air." In dyspnea of organic cause, on the other hand, the sensation is more difficult to describe; patients may say that they are "short-winded" or "puff" and on request will demonstrate hyperpnea rather than the deep sighing respirations of functional dyspnea. Shortness of breath only during exertion is the hallmark of organic disease. By contrast, patients who are short of breath at rest and not during exercise almost invariably have functional dyspnea; they may also describe symptoms that are consistent with hyperventilation or a panic disorder.[29,30] It should be remembered, however, that such symptoms do not exclude the presence of significant pulmonary disease; both hyperventilation and panic disorder are more common in patients who have lung disease than they are in the general population.[29]

Quantification of the severity of dyspnea and elucidation of the circumstances that provoke it may be helpful in arriving at a correct etiologic diagnosis. A number of formal scales have been devised to express this quantification in a precise manner[31-33]; they attempt to describe the severity of dyspnea provoked by a defined activity and are a refinement of the key components of history taking. For example, patients with COPD usually have a history of slowly progressive dyspnea that parallels the irrevocable decline in lung function; the severity of dyspnea increases when performing the same activity, and activities requiring less effort come to provoke dyspnea. Both aspects are important and often require clarification by the clinician.

The quality of the dyspnea may also provide some general diagnostic clues. A sense of increased effort or work of breathing characterizes the breathlessness resulting from an increased mechanical load or from neuromuscular weakness, whereas a sense of air hunger or suffocation is seen most often in patients who have heart failure.[34]

An acute onset of dyspnea may also be related to several disease processes. A young patient who has been in good health may well have pneumothorax, particularly if there is associated chest pain. Uncommonly, such dyspnea is the initial episode of asthma or the first indication of mitral stenosis or myocardial infarction. Acute dyspnea may also occur with pneumonia or diffuse bronchiolitis; however, the patient generally has premonitory symptoms of fever and cough, with or without infection of the upper respiratory tract, which readily differentiates these symptoms from other conditions. The sudden onset of dyspnea, particularly in association with hyperpnea and tachycardia, in an ill or a postoperative patient should raise the possibility of thromboembolism.

Some degree of dyspnea is normal during pregnancy,[35] probably as a result of the hyperventilation produced by increased blood progesterone and the restriction of diaphragmatic descent. However, dyspnea that is acute, severe, and progressive, that occurs at rest, or that is associated with other signs and symptoms of cardiopulmonary disease is abnormal and warrants further careful evaluation.

The inability to lie flat because of a feeling of suffocation or shortness of breath (*orthopnea*) or a history of waking during the night with shortness of breath (*paroxysmal nocturnal dyspnea*) strongly suggests the presence of organic disease. These symptoms are usually associated with left ventricular failure, but they may also occur in patients who have asthma, COPD, or bilateral diaphragmatic paralysis in the absence of heart disease. *Platypnea* is dyspnea worsened by assuming an erect position and is associated with postural arterial oxygen desaturation (*orthodeoxia*); it is generally related to a cardiac or pulmonary shunt.[36,37]

Evaluation of the symptoms that accompany dyspnea is also important in establishing a correct diagnosis. For example, patients who have dyspnea accompanied by angina pectoris may also have chest tightness, sweatiness, nausea, or faintness. Similarly, dyspneic asthmatic patients frequently complain of chest tightness, wheezing, and cough.

Miscellaneous Symptoms

A sudden onset of *hoarseness* almost always indicates intrinsic laryngeal disease, most often the result of viral infection, trauma, allergic edema, or inhalation of noxious fumes. Chronic hoarseness is also most likely to be caused by primary laryngeal disease and should prompt examination of the vocal cords to exclude serious conditions such as carcinoma. The most common pulmonary cause of persistent hoarseness is unilateral abductor paralysis, usually the result of extension of carcinoma into the aortopulmonary window with involvement of the recurrent laryngeal nerve. Hoarseness is also common in patients who use high-dose inhaled corticosteroids for the management of asthma and is due to vocal cord myopathy or thrush.

Fever should suggest infectious pneumonia, particularly when the chest radiograph reveals an air space or segmental opacity; if the pneumonia is accompanied by a single shaking chill, it is probably pneumococcal in origin. However, it must be remembered that fever may also occur with a variety of noninfectious pulmonary diseases, including extrinsic allergic alveolitis, connective tissue disease, and infarction.

Confusion, irrationality, and even *coma* may be seen in patients who have chronic pulmonary disease, particularly those who are elderly; precipitating causes include pneumonia, fat embolism or thromboembolism, and carcinoma. The central nervous system (CNS) symptoms in these conditions may be due to hypoperfusion, arterial blood gas abnormalities (increased $PaCO_2$ and/or decreased PaO_2), metabolic abnormalities (hyponatremia, hypercalcemia), or direct CNS involvement (metastatic disease, cryptococcosis, fat emboli). In the appropriate clinical setting, it is important to rule out infection or metastatic carcinoma involving the meninges or cerebrum.

Halitosis is most commonly caused by some disorder of the oral cavity; however, in the appropriate setting, it should suggest the possibility of anaerobic pulmonary infection.

Quality-of-Life Evaluation

The impact of symptom intensity and the level of lung dysfunction on perceived quality of life is highly variable. For example, mild airflow obstruction or lung restriction may impose a large burden on an active individual, whereas the same level of impairment may have little influence on someone who has a sedentary lifestyle. A number of generic quality-of-life questionnaires are available to assess this aspect of disease; several questionnaires specifically designed for patients who have respiratory disease have also been developed and validated.[38,39] Even more targeted are quality-of-life assessment questionnaires for individual respiratory diseases such as asthma[40] and COPD.[41,42]

Past Medical and Personal History

Thorough questioning about the patient's medical history and personal habits is an essential part of the initial evaluation of any lung disease. Knowledge derived from such examination may greatly alter the differential diagnosis; for example, respiratory symptoms or an abnormal chest radiograph may simply represent sequelae of previous lung disease, or a lung lesion may be a metastasis from a previously recognized primary malignancy. In addition to careful questioning of the patient about prior illness, it is mandatory that previous chest radiographs be obtained for comparison with current studies, a task that should always be assumed by the treating physician.

Patients should be thoroughly questioned about their use of medications. It is important to remember that almost any clinical syndrome can be secondary to the effects of a drug. Examples of conditions that might be associated with such therapy include infectious pneumonia in patients who are receiving immunosuppressive therapy, lipoid pneumonia after the use of nose drops or laxatives containing mineral oil, and respiratory failure as a result of recent sedation.

The duration and intensity of a patient's cigarette smoke exposure are clearly of significance in assessing suspected cases of pulmonary carcinoma or COPD. It is important to remember that a history of smoking cessation does not always hold up to objective confirmation.[43] Because of the potential importance of "secondhand" smoking, knowledge of the personal tobacco use of people with whom the patient lives, and has lived, is also relevant. Heavy alcohol intake may result in decreased resistance to infection and an increased risk of aspiration. All patients should be questioned about risk factors for infection with HIV, including sexual practices, intravenous drug use, and history of blood transfusion or the use of blood products. Inquiry about contact with animals, both domestic and wild, may be very helpful in diagnosis, as exemplified by bronchospasm related to a household pet, psittacosis from a sick bird in the home, hantavirus pneumonia after exposure to mouse droppings, or Q fever from the inhalation of dust contaminated by sheep or cattle.

Family History

In pulmonary disease, this aspect is important with respect to a potential source of infection, as well as for inherited disorders. Tuberculosis is the most serious of the pulmonary diseases that spread in the home; however, *Mycoplasma* infection, pertussis, severe acute respiratory syndrome (SARS), and many other viral infections may also be disseminated throughout the household. Some pulmonary diseases show familial clustering and a clearly defined dominant or recessive pattern of inheritance. Such diseases include cystic fibrosis, emphysema associated with α_1-protease inhibitor deficiency, some forms of interstitial pulmonary fibrosis, pulmonary hypertension, and bronchiectasis related to ciliary dyskinesia (immotile ciliary syndrome). Most of these conditions are rare, and they may be recognized only when a family history of one of them is revealed. A variety of other pulmonary diseases are also influenced by heredity, although their expression is strongly affected by environmental factors. Asthma and COPD are the most important of these diseases. These conditions, which have been termed "complex genetic disorders," are not inherited in simple mendelian fashion and are probably related to a variety of gene variants with variable penetrance. Several groups have also reported an association between pulmonary carcinoma and a family history of lung cancer.

Residence and Travel History

Questioning about recent travel and country of origin is also necessary, particularly in the assessment of possible pneumonia; the diagnosis of many fungal and parasitic diseases, as well as SARS, is aided by the discovery that a patient has lived or traveled in an endemic area.

Occupational History

As with medications, virtually any pulmonary syndrome can be the result of exposure to noxious agents in the workplace, and an occupational history should therefore be part of every clinical history. In addition to aiding in the identification of a specific disease, recognition of the relationship of the work environment to the patient's illness prevents further potentially damaging exposure to the harmful agent, allows for suitable compensation to be considered, identifies potential risk for other workers, and may lead to the application of preventive public health measures. Knowledge of the occupational history is particularly important in the evaluation of patients who have interstitial lung disease, asthma, malignancy, and COPD. The physician should appreciate that different jobs may be associated with exposure to a specific agent and that an individual in a specific occupation may come in contact with many potentially harmful substances.

Systemic Inquiry

A description of the association between pulmonary disease and diseases of other organs would be a description of most of the field of internal medicine. The mere fact that certain other organs or tissues are involved may suggest a specific condition; for example, a patient with diffuse lung disease who has Raynaud's phenomenon and difficulty swallowing almost certainly has progressive systemic sclerosis. In some instances the pulmonary disease is secondary to disease of another organ; for example, inquiry may reveal symptoms indicating a primary site for multiple nodules of metastatic carcinoma

in the lung. In other cases, systemic symptoms are secondary to the pulmonary disease itself. For example, small cell carcinoma of the lung may be associated with several forms of neuromuscular disease, whereas the diagnosis of ventilatory failure may be suggested by a history of headache, confusion, tremor, twitching, or somnolence.

PHYSICAL EXAMINATION

Significant disagreement can be demonstrated between physicians in the appreciation of physical signs.[44] However, those who demonstrate better competence in physical examination are more likely to establish a correct clinical diagnosis based on examination alone,[44] a fact that attests both to the importance of the procedure and to lack of skill as an important cause of the disagreement.

Information obtained by physical examination can be complementary to that derived from chest radiography and physiologic and laboratory testing. For example, a breathless patient who has a normal chest radiograph may be pale or may have findings of pulmonary hypertension or thyrotoxicosis on physical examination; in these circumstances, the examination provides the direction for further investigation. In addition, physical examination may be the only tool immediately available for assessment of the patient; for example, appreciation of tension pneumothorax in a mechanically ventilated patient may be necessary long before a chest radiograph can be obtained.

Methods of Examination and Signs of Disease

The front of the thorax is best examined when the patient is supine, and the back is best examined when the patient is sitting or standing; patients who are too weak to sit upright unaided should be supported by someone standing at the foot of the bed and holding their hands. It is important to keep in mind that examination of the chest is a comparative exercise, each region of one side being compared with the corresponding area on the other side; this rule applies equally for inspection, palpation, percussion, and auscultation.

Inspection

Even before obtaining the clinical history, the physician has an opportunity to learn much about the patient on cursory inspection alone. Does the patient appear sick or well, oriented or disoriented, thin or fat, blue or yellow, sober or drunk? Does the patient smell of tobacco smoke? Are the fingers clubbed or yellow with nicotine? Are there abnormalities such as hoarseness, stridor, and wheezing?

The thoracic cage should be inspected first for evidence of deformity and the skin for color, evidence of collateral venous circulation, and scars. The respiratory rate may be a valuable indicator of early respiratory dysfunction and should be recorded. Movement of the chest wall should also be observed, particularly with respect to asymmetry between the two sides. A local lag during inspiration may not be obvious during quiet breathing, and the patient should be asked to take a deep breath while movements of the chest cage on the two sides are compared. A lag during inspiration or an area of diminished movement, seen or felt, that involves all or part of a hemithorax may be the only physical sign of disease of the lung or pleura. It may indicate localized airway obstruction, loss of elasticity of the underlying tissues, or reflex spasm of the intercostal and diaphragmatic musculature in an attempt to reduce pain on movement. This sign is present in acute diseases such as atelectasis, pneumonia, and pleuritis; it may also indicate chronic (usually fibrotic) disease of the lung or pleura, in which case it is often associated with scoliosis of the thoracic spine (with the concavity to the diseased side).

When the loss of volume is considerable, whether the result of an acute or chronic process, there may also be a shift of the mediastinum, detectable as displacement of the apical cardiac impulse and the trachea toward the involved side. With fibrosis and particularly with atelectasis, the lower intercostal spaces may be abnormally sucked in during inspiration. Paradoxical inward movement of the lateral rib margin during inspiration (Hoover's sign) is commonly seen in patients who have severe COPD.[45]

It is also important to assess respiratory muscle function. Such assessment is best done by observing the relative contribution of diaphragmatic and intercostal muscles in the normal breathing cycle with the patient in the supine position. In this situation, in-drawing of the abdominal wall on inspiration or sequential rather than simultaneous abdominal and thoracic movement suggests paralysis or fatigue of the diaphragm and constitutes a clear indication of the cause of dyspnea or impending ventilatory failure.

Palpation

A suspected ventilatory lag detected on inspection of the chest may be confirmed when a hand is placed on each hemithorax while the patient breathes deeply. The relative contribution of the respiratory muscles can also be assessed by palpation of the abdominal, intercostal, and accessory muscles during inspiration. The apical cardiac impulse and the trachea should be palpated, a shift from normal position indicating loss of volume or a relative increase in the volume of one hemithorax in comparison to the other. Palpation of the left parasternal region may demonstrate a heave, indicative of possible right ventricular hypertrophy. When indicated, the intercostal spaces and ribs should be palpated to identify tumors and elicit any tenderness to pressure. The axillae and the cervical region should also be explored carefully to detect enlarged lymph nodes, particularly in patients who have suspected malignancy or infection.

Tactile or vocal fremitus is the feeling of vibration of the chest wall with the spoken voice. The palm or side of the hand is placed on alternating sides of the chest in a symmetrical manner as the patient says "ninety-nine," and asymmetry in vibration is noted. Increased vibration is felt in conditions in which sound transmission is increased, such as pneumonia; decreased vibration is felt when sound transmission is reduced, such as with pleural effusion, lobar atelectasis, pneumothorax, or fibrothorax. In common practice, signs such as altered fremitus and regional chest wall lag are looked for only when pathology is strongly suspected or in an attempt to distinguish one abnormality (such as consolidation) from another (such as effusion). They should not be part of the routine examination of a healthy individual who has normal chest auscultation.

Percussion

Except in a "ceremonial" sense, percussion is also not generally part of the routine physical examination of a healthy patient. Nevertheless, it may provide valuable clues to the presence of disease; for example, it may indicate the presence of small amounts of subpulmonic fluid in situations in which the chest radiograph is equivocal. It should be stressed that the percussing finger assesses only the superficial 5 cm of lung tissue; no matter how much force is used, the central portion of the lung remains "silent." In addition, the differences in percussion note are perceived not only by the ears but also by touch; over solid tissue, the examining fingers appreciate a difference in vibration as well as a sensation of resistance that can be distinguished from the elasticity felt over air-containing areas.

As with inspection, the chest wall should be percussed in an orderly fashion, with corresponding areas compared on each side. Since the degree of resonance is influenced by the thickness of the chest wall and the volume of lung underlying the percussing finger, "normal" percussion differs both from patient to patient and from area to area in the same patient. The percussion note in disease and in health may vary from tympanitic (over the stomach gas bubble) to flat (over the liver), sounds readily detectable by even the inexperienced. Between these extremes are degrees of hyper-resonance and dullness, whose significance can be evaluated only with experience.

In the presence of lung disease, the percussion note varies from the impaired resonance heard over an area of pneumonia that is partially consolidated, to the dullness over a completely consolidated or collapsed segment or lobe, to the extreme dullness or flatness associated with a large accumulation of pleural fluid. At the other end of the scale, the note is hyper-resonant in cases of emphysema and pneumothorax and is sometimes tympanitic over large superficial cavities or a particularly large pneumothorax.

Auscultation

The quality and intensity of the breath sounds, as well as the presence or absence of adventitious noises, are ascertained by listening with the bell or diaphragm held firmly against the chest while the patient breathes quietly and then deeply.

The quality and intensity of breath sounds vary from region to region, even in normal subjects, depending on the thickness of the chest wall, the proximity of larger bronchi to the chest wall, and the depth of respiration. In the axillae or at the lung bases, a vesicular sound that has been likened to the rustle of wind in trees is heard during inspiration and often early in expiration. The sound of flowing air has a somewhat different quality over the trachea and upper retrosternal area; the pitch is higher, and expiration is clearly audible and lasts longer than the inspiratory phase. Between the scapulas and anteriorly under the clavicles, particularly on the right side, the breath sounds assume the characteristics of both vesicular and bronchial airflow and are described as bronchovesicular.

Many factors contribute to a reduction or abolition of vesicular breathing. In some patients, it may be difficult to hear breath sounds because of an excess of subcutaneous fat, the presence of fluid or air in the pleural cavity, or shallow breathing as a result of weakness or neuromuscular disease. In others, there is significant bronchopulmonary disease, such as obstruction of a lobar or segmental bronchus. Destruction of pulmonary parenchyma, as in emphysema, or diminished flow under conditions of generalized airflow obstruction may also be associated with very faint breath sounds.

The quality of breath sounds changes from vesicular to bronchovesicular or bronchial when the underlying parenchyma partly or completely loses its air content, *but the airways remain patent.* This change in breath sound quality occurs in pneumonia and nonobstructive atelectasis and is explained by the observation that consolidated or airless lung tissue is an excellent conductor of the high-pitched, prolonged expiratory sounds that emanate from patent bronchi.

Voice sounds may also provide clues to the presence and nature of pulmonary disease. During quiet speech, a soft, "confused," barely audible sound can be heard normally over lung tissue distant from large bronchi. In the presence of consolidation or nonobstructive atelectasis, these sounds become more distinct and produce a noise known as *bronchophony*. In many cases, words are distinctly audible over the involved area when the patient whispers "one, two, three"; this "whispering pectoriloquy" does not occur in the absence of bronchial breath sounds and is a useful confirmatory sign of pneumonic consolidation. Consolidation of lung tissue or its compression by a large pleural effusion may also result in *egophony* (a change in timbre of the spoken voice [e.g., *ee* as in bee to an *a*-like sound resembling a bleating goat] but not in pitch or volume).[46] When a large accumulation of fluid compresses the lower portion of the lung, the voice sounds sometimes have a nasal quality over the upper part of the lung. When they are loud in comparison to the opposite side and breath sounds in the same region are reduced, bronchial stenosis is probably present on that side.[47]

Several attempts have been made to standardize the terminology of abnormal (adventitious) lung sounds.[48,49] Discontinuous sounds are known as *crackles*. Continuous sounds that are high pitched are called *wheezes*; when of lower pitch, they are known as *rhonchi*. Use of this terminology in practice is inconsistent and variable, a deficiency that confounds the inherent inaccuracy in physical examination related to expected interobserver variability in the description of subtle events. To avoid these problems, we stress the necessity of using this terminology in a consistent fashion. Adventitious sounds may be divided into those having their origin in the airways and lung parenchyma, those related to the pulmonary vasculature, and those originating in the pleura.

Crackles may be fine (relatively high-pitched sounds usually heard at the end of inspiration as air enters the acinar unit) or coarse (the low-pitched, bubbling sounds that result from the accumulation of secretions in larger bronchi and the trachea).[48] Fine crackles are probably best appreciated when the patient takes slow deep breaths that generate quiet breath sounds.[50] They are sometimes detected at the lung bases at the end of a deep inspiration in individuals without pulmonary disease; such individuals are likely to be obese, and the crackles may diminish in intensity or even disappear after several deep inspirations. More frequently, fine crackles are indicative of pulmonary disease, in which case they are usually persistent and often occur in "showers." Such crackles may be present in several conditions, most commonly pulmonary edema, pneumonia, and interstitial fibrosis.

Other adventitious sounds that originate in the bronchopulmonary tree are continuous. The presence of wheezes or rhonchi indicates partial obstruction of a bronchial lumen; although they may also be heard in inspiration, they are louder during expiration when the airways are narrower. Wheezes may be heard at a distance without the aid of a stethoscope. Sounds produced by turbulent flow in the lower part of the trachea or a main bronchus as a result of partial obstruction may also be audible without the aid of a stethoscope. Rhonchi or wheezes not appreciated during quiet breathing may become audible when the rate of airflow is increased during fast, deep breathing or when the airways are narrowed during maximal expiration; however, this finding has little diagnostic importance.[51] Focal wheezes or rhonchi that do not disappear with coughing should suggest the possibility of an endobronchial neoplasm. *Stridor* is a specific form of continuous sound characterized by an especially loud "musical" sound of constant pitch. It is caused by obstruction of the larynx or trachea and may be heard during inspiration, during expiration, or throughout the entire respiratory cycle.

Another group of adventitious sounds can be heard in association with pleural disease. A *friction rub* is caused by a fibrinous exudate rubbing on adjacent parietal and visceral pleural surfaces. It may be secondary to trauma, neoplastic infiltration, or inflammation of the pleura itself or by an underlying pulmonary neoplasm, infarct, or pneumonia. Characteristically, it disappears when fluid forms and separates the two pleural surfaces. During both inspiration and expiration and particularly in areas where excursion of the thoracic cage is greatest, a rubbing, rasping, or leathery sound may be heard as the visceral lining moves against the parietal one. The noise is usually associated with pain. Its disappearance during breath-holding but not after coughing distinguishes it from rhonchi associated with partial bronchial obstruction, which it may closely resemble.

Hamman described a crunching or clicking sound over the lower retrosternal area that is synchronous with the heartbeat.[52] This sound is audible with a stethoscope and may be noticed by the patient when lying on the left side. Although Hamman believed the sound to be pathognomonic of air in the mediastinum, it is in fact more commonly associated with a left pneumothorax. The sound is of diagnostic importance in that it may be present with small (radiographically undetectable) collections of air.

Clinical examination of the heart is essential in every case of suspected pulmonary disease. Abnormalities affecting either the parenchyma or the pulmonary vasculature may cause pulmonary arterial hypertension, which may be manifested as right ventricular heave, an accentuated pulmonic component of the second heart sound, or pulmonic or tricuspid regurgitant murmurs. In a minority of cases of diffuse pulmonary edema secondary to mitral stenosis or acute left ventricular decompensation, convincing radiographic evidence of cardiac enlargement is absent; in such cases, a mitral valve murmur or left ventricular gallop suggests the cause of the edema. Pulsus paradoxus, an exaggeration of the normal inspiratory decrease in systolic pressure to greater than 10 mm Hg and usually associated with cardiac tamponade, may be observed in patients who have obstructive pulmonary disease, particularly severe asthma, or massive thromboembolism. It may also be found when the intrathoracic pressure swing is excessive, as may occur with obstruction of either the upper or lower airways; it should be remembered, however, that pulsus paradoxus can be seen in some young healthy individuals.

Extrathoracic Manifestations of Pulmonary Disease

The potential for diseases of the chest to have manifestations outside the lungs has been mentioned previously. Specific findings are discussed in the sections dealing with the relevant diseases. The following discussion deals with clubbing and cyanosis, abnormalities that should be sought in all patients with disease of the lungs or pleura.

Clubbing and Hypertrophic Osteoarthropathy

Clubbing refers to swelling of the soft tissue of the distal portions of the fingers and toes. Hypertrophic osteoarthropathy (HOA) is localized principally to the periosteum of the phalanges and distal portions of the arms and legs. The terms are not synonymous: clubbing frequently occurs in the absence of full-blown osteoarthropathy, and the latter occasionally occurs without clubbing.[53] Although the disorders are usually secondary (most often to cardiac or pulmonary disease), they may be idiopathic, in which case they are known as *pachydermoperiostosis*.[54]

The pathogenesis of clubbing is not completely understood. Blood flow to the digits appears to be increased,[55] possibly as a result of an increase in the number of small vessels.[56] Although various inflammatory mediators, vasoactive compounds, and growth factors have been implicated in this proliferation,[57,58] there is no convincing evidence to incriminate one of them in all cases.

Four criteria are generally accepted for a diagnosis of clubbing: (1) increased bulk of the terminal digital tuft, (2) change in the angle between the nail and the proximal skin to greater than 180 degrees, (3) sponginess of the nail bed and periungual erythema, and (4) increased nail curvature. When all these changes are present or when at least one is severe, clubbing is readily recognizable. However, detection of clubbing at an early stage is difficult and subject to considerable interobserver variation. The clinical diagnosis of HOA requires the presence of deep-seated pain and/or joint symptoms, including arthralgia with swelling and stiffness, affecting mainly the fingers, wrists, ankles, and knees. Radiographs usually show subperiosteal new bone formation in the long bones of the extremities. Changes may be apparent on bone scan before radiographic change.

Except in the rare idiopathic form, clubbing or HOA is virtually pathognomonic of visceral disease, the primary organ of involvement having either vagal or glossopharyngeal innervation.[59] Malignant neoplasms account for 90% of the typical cases of HOA associated with lung disease, with the vast majority being primary non–small cell carcinoma.[60] Clubbing is common in patients who have cyanotic congenital heart disease, idiopathic pulmonary fibrosis, and subacute bacterial endocarditis; however, HOA is rare.[59]

Cyanosis

Cyanosis is a blue or bluish-gray discoloration of the skin and mucous membranes caused by an excessive blood concentration of reduced hemoglobin. Cyanosis is most obvious in the nail beds or buccal mucosa and is best appreciated in full daylight; it is virtually unrecognizable under a fluorescent lamp. The estimated concentration of reduced hemoglobin that must be present before cyanosis is visible is 50 g/L; therefore, this sign is never present in patients who have severe anemia. Cyanosis may be central (hypoxemic), in which case it is associated with pulmonary or cardiac disease, or peripheral, when the mechanism is related to sluggish blood flow and excessive removal of oxygen by tissues. In patients who have a normal hemoglobin concentration and normal perfusion, central cyanosis can be appreciated by most observers under appropriate lighting conditions when arterial oxygen saturation is about 75%.[61] Since a PaO_2 of 40 can yield a saturation of 75%, central cyanosis is generally a marker of severe hypoxemia.

The pathogenesis of central cyanosis is related to the development of hypoxemia. As discussed elsewhere (see page 45), ventilation-perfusion abnormality is responsible for hypoxemia in most parenchymal lung disease. Hypoventilation can also contribute to it in patients who have severe chronic airflow obstruction. In other lung diseases, such as severe acute air space pneumonia associated with circulatory collapse, both central and peripheral factors contribute to cyanosis.

Cardiac disease associated with a right-to-left shunt may also cause central cyanosis, but it can be distinguished from pulmonary conditions by clinical findings and the results of pulmonary function tests. A right-to-left cardiac shunt may become evident when an increase in pulmonary vascular resistance results in pulmonary hypertension sufficient to cause blood to flow from the right to the left atrium through a patent foramen ovale; this can occur in pulmonary thromboembolic disease, in which case it may be associated with systemic arterial emboli. Similar shunting can occasionally occur in the absence of pulmonary hypertension and may be associated with platypnea and orthodeoxia. Arterial oxygen desaturation as a result of intrapulmonary shunting also occurs in association with cirrhosis of the liver; however, the desaturation is rarely severe enough to cause cyanosis. Isolated peripheral cyanosis may be either paroxysmal and precipitated by cold, as in Raynaud's disease, or general and prolonged, in which case it is often associated with systemic hypotension and physical signs of circulatory collapse.

When the pathogenesis of cyanosis is obscure, methemoglobinemia or sulfhemoglobinemia should be considered. The former is rarely primary and congenital; more commonly, it results from the ingestion of drugs, including nitrates, chlorates, quinones, aniline dyes, sulfonamide derivatives, and phenacetin. Sulfhemoglobinemia and methemoglobinemia may occur simultaneously, usually from ingestion of the same drugs, in which case the cyanosis is lead colored. When either of these conditions is present, the venous blood is brownish even after being shaken in air for 15 minutes. The diagnosis can be confirmed by spectroscopic analysis.

PATHOLOGIC AND ENDOSCOPIC INVESTIGATION

Endoscopy

Laryngoscopy

The larynx can be examined indirectly with the use of a mirror or directly; direct examination may be combined with bronchoscopy. Laryngoscopy should be performed in any patient who complains of a persistent, dry, hacking or brassy cough, particularly when the cough is associated with hoarseness. The vocal cords should be well seen, not only to exclude an intrinsic abnormality but also to detect paralysis that would account for the hoarseness. In the latter situation, chest radiography or CT may reveal a mediastinal lesion.

Esophagoscopy and Upper Gastrointestinal Endoscopy

Pulmonary disease may occur in association with several esophageal abnormalities, and the diagnosis may be facilitated by direct endoscopic examination of the esophagus. Aspiration pneumonia may be secondary to esophageal diverticula, achalasia, or stenosis from peptic ulceration or neoplasia. When the origin of expectorated blood is not known, direct viewing of the upper gastrointestinal tract may detect bleeding esophageal varices or peptic ulceration. Diffuse pulmonary disease can also occur in association with dysphagia in patients who have progressive systemic sclerosis, in which case esophagoscopy and esophageal motility studies may be required to confirm the diagnosis.

Bronchoscopy

Flexible fiberoptic bronchoscopy (FFB) is a safe and relatively easy procedure that has proved extremely useful in the diagnosis and management of many pulmonary diseases (Table 4–2).[62-65] Among the more common uses are the diagnosis and staging of pulmonary carcinoma, the diagnosis of suspected pulmonary infection, and the investigation of diffuse interstitial lung disease (especially sarcoidosis and lymphangitic carcinomatosis). Although the procedure is suitable for examining the lower respiratory tract in most situations, rigid bronchoscopy may be preferable for the management of massive hemoptysis, stent placement, and laser resection of endobronchial tissue, especially when airway compromise is severe.[66,67]

Attention to a number of factors is important to optimize the safety of FFB, including (1) assessment of underlying COPD and institution of appropriate therapy if necessary, (2) administration of antibiotics to patients at risk for the consequences of transient bacteremia or endocarditis, (3) measurement of coagulation parameters (and their correction if necessary) for patients at risk of excessive bleeding or those in whom transbronchial biopsy is anticipated, (4) administration of bronchodilator therapy to patients who have asthma, (5) avoidance of the procedure in the 6 weeks immediately after myocardial infarction, (6) maintenance of intravenous access, and (7) absence of food for 4 hours and clear fluids for 2 hours before the procedure.

A sedative (usually midazolam) should be provided for most patients[68]; atropine is not required routinely.[69] Lidocaine is well tolerated for anesthesia; however, special care is required in the elderly and in patients who have liver or heart disease, in whom toxicity develops more easily as a result of slower drug metabolism. Supplemental oxygen should be given routinely and arterial oxygen saturation monitored during the procedure. Resuscitation equipment should be readily available.

The procedure is relatively safe in experienced hands: mortality in several large series has ranged from 0% to 0.1%,[70] and the procedure has been performed without problem in the elderly, in acutely ill mechanically ventilated patients, and in patients who have asthma or significant thrombocytopenia. Major complications occur in less than 3% of patients[71] and include pneumonia, aspiration of gastric contents, septic shock with acute respiratory distress syndrome (ARDS), pneumothorax, and hemorrhage (the last two almost always associated with transbronchial biopsy).

Cytology

The practice of cytology is concerned primarily with the morphologic features of individual cells or small clusters of cells and is most useful in the diagnosis of malignancy. Interpretation of cytologic abnormalities varies with the origin of the material being examined and the technique by which it is obtained. Four categories of such material can be defined in relation to chest disease: (1) sputum, bronchial washings, and bronchial brushings (sampling the airway surface and, to a lesser extent, the lung parenchyma); (2) BAL fluid (sampling primarily the lung parenchyma); (3) pleural fluid; and (4) pulmonary or mediastinal material aspirated via a thin needle.

Sputum and Bronchial Washings and Brushings

Cells and other material suitable for cytologic examination are most often obtained from the lungs by spontaneous or induced expectoration of sputum, by bronchial washing or brushing performed during endoscopy, and by BAL.[72]

Spontaneous samples of sputum are best collected by having patients rinse their mouth with water and then expectorate a deep cough specimen into a wide-mouthed collecting jar. The optimal time is considered to be early morning, just after rising. Inadequate samples because of insufficient sputum are fairly common[73]; in this situation, it may be helpful to induce deep expectoration by having the patient inhale an aerosolized heated solution of saline or another irritating substance. It is also useful to obtain sputum specimens for analysis after bronchoscopy; the procedure itself leads to repeated deep coughing that may produce diagnostic specimens.

Once collected, sputum is usually processed in one of two ways. In the first, a freshly expectorated sample is brought to the laboratory, where it is smeared evenly over glass slides, fixed, and stained. In the second (Saccomanno) method,[74] sputum is expectorated into a jar containing alcohol, which acts as a fixative that permits the collection of specimens over a period of several days. In the laboratory, the material is mixed in a household-type food blender for a short time, which effectively emulsifies the mucus and produces a fluid that can be centrifuged. When the supernatant is discarded, the residual concentrated cellular material is smeared on glass slides and stained.

Specimens derived by direct brushing of a bronchial lesion should be taken before biopsy to diminish the degree of blood contamination. They can be smeared directly onto glass slides and rapidly fixed in the endoscopy room. Bronchial washing specimens (typically consisting of about 5 mL of fluid instilled and aspirated through the bronchoscope) can be processed in a cytospin apparatus or centrifuged to yield a cell-rich

TABLE 4–2. Guidelines for Fiberoptic Bronchoscopy in Adults

A. **Diagnostic Uses**
1. To evaluate lung lesions of unknown etiology that appear on the chest roentgenogram as a density, infiltrate, atelectasis, or localized hyperlucency
2. To assess airway patency
3. To investigate unexplained hemoptysis, unexplained cough (or change in the nature of a cough), localized wheeze, or stridor
4. To search for the origin of suspicious or positive sputum cytology
5. To investigate the etiology of unexplained paralysis of a vocal cord or hemidiaphragm, superior vena cava syndrome, chylothorax, or unexplained pleural effusion
6. To evaluate problems associated with endotracheal tubes such as tracheal damage, airway obstruction, or tube placement
7. To stage lung cancer preoperatively and subsequently to evaluate, when appropriate, the response to therapy
8. To obtain material for microbiologic studies in suspected pulmonary infections
9. To evaluate the airways for suspected bronchial tear or other injury after thoracic trauma
10. To determine a suspected tracheoesophageal fistula
11. To determine the location and extent of respiratory tract injury after acute inhalation of noxious fumes or aspiration of gastric contents
12. To obtain material for study from the lungs of patients with diffuse or focal lung diseases

B. **Therapeutic Uses**
1. To remove retained secretions or mucus plugs not mobilized by conventional noninvasive techniques
2. To remove foreign bodies
3. To remove abnormal endobronchial tissue or foreign material by the use of forceps or laser techniques
4. To perform difficult intubations, e.g., in patients with cervical spondylitis, dental problems, myasthenia gravis, acromegaly, achalasia, full stomach, small bowel obstruction, and trauma to the head, neck, larynx, or trachea

C. **Research Applications**
Multiple and varied applications include, but are not limited to, the study of tracheal mucus velocity, regional gas exchange, cilial structure and function, and the chemical and cellular nature of material obtained by bronchoalveolar lavage

D. **Conditions Involving Increased Risk**
As in all clinical situations, the risk of bronchoscopy must be weighed against the potential benefit for the patient. Sound clinical judgment and careful assessment of each patient must predominate, especially in decisions regarding the need for hospitalization. Increased-risk situations include
1. Lack of patient cooperation
2. Recent myocardial infarction or unstable angina
3. Partial tracheal obstruction
4. Unstable bronchial asthma
5. Respiratory insufficiency associated with moderate to severe hypoxemia or any degree of hypercapnia
6. Uremia and pulmonary hypertension (possibility of serious hemorrhage after biopsy)
7. Lung abscess (danger of flooding the airway with purulent material)
8. Immunosuppression (danger of postbronchoscopy infection)
9. Obstruction of the superior vena cava (possibility of bleeding and laryngeal edema)
10. Debility, advanced age, and malnutrition
11. Unstable cardiac arrhythmia
12. Respiratory failure requiring mechanical ventilation
13. Disorders requiring laser therapy, biopsy of lesions obstructing large airways, or multiple transbronchial lung biopsies
The danger of a serious complication from bronchoscopy is especially high in patients with the following conditions:
1. Malignant arrhythmia
2. Profound refractory hypoxemia
3. Severe bleeding diathesis that cannot be corrected when biopsy is anticipated
In most situations involving increased risk, patient safety requires hospitalization and overnight observation after the procedure

E. **Contraindications**
1. Absence of consent from the patient or the patient's representative
2. Bronchoscopy by an inexperienced person without direct supervision
3. Bronchoscopy without adequate facilities and personnel to care for such emergencies as cardiopulmonary arrest, pneumothorax, or bleeding
4. Inability to adequately oxygenate the patient during the procedure

F. **Additional Comments**
1. In most patients with undiagnosed pulmonary disorders and in those requiring therapeutic intervention, bronchoscopy is but one component of their overall evaluation or treatment
2. The fiberoptic bronchoscope is the instrument of choice when bronchoscopy is needed for patients on mechanical ventilators or for those with disease or trauma involving the skull, jaws, or cervical spine
3. The rigid open-tube bronchoscope is the instrument of choice during massive hemoptysis
4. Outpatients may undergo bronchoscopy in the hospital in a daycare setting
5. When out-of-hospital bronchoscopy is performed, there should be adequate facilities and personnel to care for emergencies and to properly handle specimens
6. Bronchoscopy should not be used routinely as a substitute for conventional noninvasive techniques for mobilizing pulmonary secretions
7. Bronchoscopy is not a routine initial procedure in the evaluation of unexplained cough
8. Bronchoscopy is not routinely necessary to obtain sputum for diagnostic study in cases of pneumonia or acute bronchitis

From Burgher LW, Jones FL, Patterson JR, et al: Guidelines for fiberoptic bronchoscopy in adults. Am Rev Respir Dis 136:1066, 1987. Official Statement of the American Thoracic Society. © American Lung Association.

"button" that can be smeared on slides and further processed for histologic examination. The latter procedure increases the likelihood of a positive diagnosis and enables immunocytochemistry to be performed.[75,76]

The principal purpose of cytologic examination of sputum and specimens obtained by bronchial washing and brushing is the detection of malignancy. In large series of patients with confirmed pulmonary carcinoma, true-positive diagnoses have been reported in 50% to 90% of cases.[77] Because bronchoscopy is usually indicated in patients who have suspected pulmonary carcinoma and because the diagnostic yield of the procedure is greater than that of sputum cytology, it has been argued that sputum analysis should be limited to individuals in whom surgery is not contemplated or bronchoscopy has been unsuccessful.[78,79] In fact, largely because of the availability and high yield of bronchoscopy and transthoracic needle aspiration (TTNA), sputum cytology is now a relatively uncommon means of establishing a diagnosis of pulmonary carcinoma.[80] Nevertheless, it has been argued that it is still a cost-effective initial procedure in patients who have central lesions.[81]

False-positive diagnoses are uncommon in experienced laboratories. The reasons for such diagnoses include evaluation of poorly preserved or inadequately prepared specimens and misinterpretation of reactive epithelial atypia as neoplasia. The latter is most frequently seen in association with pneumonia,[82] infarction,[83] or cytotoxic drugs.[84] Although malignant cells can be found in sputum specimens in the absence of radiologic abnormality (e.g., in carcinoma in situ), this situation should always be viewed with suspicion and the diagnostic slides reviewed in consultation with the cytopathologist.

False-negative results occur in 10% to 50% of proven cases of carcinoma and are related most commonly to inadequate collection and preparation of specimens or to sampling. As might be expected, the yield of malignant cells (and hence the likelihood of diagnosis) increases with the number of specimens examined.[77] The diagnosis is also more likely with central than with peripheral neoplasms and with large than with small tumors.[73,77] The use of ancillary techniques such as fluorescence in situ hybridization (FISH), high-resolution image cytometry, and PCR may prove valuable in increasing sensitivity.[85-87] Metastatic neoplasms are less commonly detected than primary lung carcinomas, probably because they involve the pulmonary parenchyma more frequently than the proximal airways; nevertheless, discovery has been reported in about 30% to 50% of cases.[88]

The reliability of cytologic examination in identifying specific histologic types of carcinoma is good for well-differentiated tumors[73]; however, as might be expected, it is poor for poorly differentiated forms. From a practical point of view, the distinction between small cell and non–small cell carcinoma can be made with confidence in the vast majority of cases.

There is increasing interest in and standardization of examination of sputum for benign conditions. The type and number of inflammatory cells in the induced sputum of patients who have obstructive lung disease may be of diagnostic and prognostic value.[89] A more widely used application is the detection of infectious organisms, particularly *Pneumocystis jiroveci (carinii)* and some other fungi.[90] In the appropriate clinical setting, the presence of macrophages containing lipid supports a diagnosis of lipid pneumonia or fat embolism.[91,92] The identification of asbestos bodies virtually ensures a history of occupational exposure to the mineral.[93]

Though clearly different from sputum cytologic examination, a promising new and similarly noninvasive diagnostic method involves the analysis of expired breath condensate. When large volumes of expired gas are collected and cooled, the volatile substances condense and can be quantified. A variety of substances potentially involved in pulmonary disease are detectable, including hydrogen peroxide, thiobarbituric acid–reactive substances, isoprostanes, prostaglandins, leukotrienes, and products of nitric oxide (NO).[94,95]

Bronchoalveolar Lavage

BAL is a relatively noninvasive procedure for sampling both cells and noncellular material located in the lung parenchyma.[96] The procedure involves the instillation of saline into the peripheral lung via a wedged fiberoptic bronchoscope.[97] For clinical purposes, 20- to 50-mL aliquots are injected and recovered by gentle suction to avoid airway trauma and collapse. A total of 100 to 300 mL of normal saline can be instilled; about 40% to 60% of the injected volume is usually recovered. When disease is focal, lavage should be directed to the site of greatest abnormality; when diffuse, lavage of the middle lobe, lingula, or lower lobes allows for better fluid recovery than does lavage of the upper lobes.

Approximately 95% of normal individuals have fewer than 25×10^4 cells per milliliter of lavage fluid.[98] About 80% to 90% are macrophages; most of the remainder are lymphocytes (5% to 15%), with neutrophils and eosinophils accounting for less than 1%.

With appropriate precautions, the procedure is generally well tolerated, even in patients who have asthma or COPD[99,100] or who are critically ill and mechanically ventilated.[101] Complications are uncommon and include fever,[102] pneumonitis, hemorrhage, pneumothorax,[103] and bronchospasm.[104] A moderate impairment in gas exchange may be seen in sicker patients.[105] Foci of consolidation corresponding to the region undergoing lavage are common on chest radiographs[106]; clearing generally occurs within 24 hours.

BAL is most useful in the diagnosis of infection, particularly in immunocompromised patients such as those who have AIDS[107,108]; in the latter situation, it is especially valuable in the diagnosis of *P. jiroveci* pneumonia. The procedure is also useful in the diagnosis of neoplasia, particularly peripheral tumors that are not visualized endoscopically,[109] and in a variety of less common pulmonary abnormalities such as lipid pneumonia, fat embolism, and alveolar proteinosis. It is also an important therapeutic modality in the last-named condition[110] and has been used extensively in the study of many diseases.

Pleural Fluid

If sufficient fluid is available, one portion can be passed through a membrane filter or processed by cytospin technique and another centrifuged to yield a cell-rich residue from which smears or a cell block can be made. The latter procedure frequently yields small tissue fragments on which histochemical and immunohistochemical investigations can be performed, thereby greatly facilitating diagnosis.

As with the cytologic investigation of bronchial secretions, the primary diagnostic objective is identification of carcinoma. Most investigators report positive results in about 50% of cases proved to be malignant[111]; repeated examinations increase the yield. It should be remembered that an absence of malignant cells in an effusion from a patient known to have cancer may be explained by pneumonia distal to an obstructing carcinoma or lymphatic obstruction. The false-positive rate is less than 0.5% in most series.[112]

In addition to malignant cells, the number and nature of inflammatory and other cells in an effusion may provide valuable clues to its cause. Red blood cell counts of more than 10,000 cells/mm³ are common to all types of effusion and are therefore of no discriminatory value.[111] However, a count exceeding 100,000 cells/mm^3 is often associated with malignancy, infarction, or trauma. A grossly bloody effusion is suggestive of a "bloody tap"; in such cases, the count is high only in the first portion of the aspirate.

A large number of neutrophils usually indicates the presence of bacterial pneumonia, although it can also occur in association with infarction, malignancy, and tuberculosis.[111] An effusion containing 50% lymphocytes or more is almost certainly associated with tuberculosis or neoplasia. Most malignant effusions contain an admixture of other cell types and thus exhibit a polymorphous cell population. By contrast, the lymphocyte-rich effusion of tuberculosis typically contains a paucity of mesothelial and other mononuclear or polymorphonuclear inflammatory cells.[111] In fact, the cellular uniformity may be so marked that it suggests well-differentiated lymphoma.[113]

Pleural eosinophilia occurs in a variety of conditions and may or may not be associated with an elevated eosinophil count in the blood. Probably the most common cause is pleural trauma, such as that encountered in surgery, spontaneous pneumothorax, or TTNA. The pathogenesis of eosinophilia in these situations may be related to the presence of air in the pleural space. Other conditions occasionally associated with pleural fluid eosinophilia include infections (both fungal and parasitic), benign asbestos effusion, immunologic abnormalities such as rheumatoid disease, pulmonary infarction, and drug hypersensitivity.[114] Tuberculous and neoplastic effusions uncommonly contain a large number of eosinophils; however, up to 20% of eosinophilic effusions have been associated with a malignant neoplasm in some reviews.[114]

Needle Aspiration

Unlike procedures such as transthoracic needle biopsy and closed chest needle biopsy of the pleura, which typically produce tissue fragments visible with the naked eye, fine-needle aspiration results in a specimen that consists predominantly of single cells or small clusters of cells. It is associated with high reliability, minimal patient discomfort, and few and relatively minor complications and has thus become an important method in the diagnosis of chest disease, particularly pulmonary carcinoma. Aspirates can be taken across the chest wall (TTNA), across the bronchial wall (transbronchial needle aspiration [TBNA]), across the esophagus (endoscopic ultrasound-guided needle aspiration), or directly during mediastinoscopy or thoracotomy (intraoperative needle aspiration). The relative merits of needle biopsy versus needle aspiration are considered on page 175.

Transthoracic Needle Aspiration. TTNA consists of sucking fluid and cells into a syringe through a narrow-gauge needle inserted percutaneously into a lesion in the lung, pleura, or mediastinum. Most physicians use needles of 20 to 22 gauge (equivalent to an external diameter of about 1 mm) because of the relatively low incidence of complications and good yield. However, some investigators have found that use of a 25-gauge needle provides good yield and a lower risk of complications in high-risk patients, such as those who have severe COPD.[115,116] Both single-pass needles and multiple-pass coaxial needles are available.[117] The former are inserted directly into the lesion and removed immediately after aspiration. The coaxial system consists of an outer guiding needle and an inner aspiration needle[118]; after the guide needle has been positioned adjacent to the lesion, the inner aspiration needle is advanced through it into the lesion itself. Following aspiration, the inner needle is withdrawn and the outer needle is left in place to facilitate further sampling.

The procedure may be performed under fluoroscopic, CT, or ultrasound guidance, the choice being influenced by the size and location of the lesion and the available equipment. CT guidance is recommended for biopsy of lesions adjacent to the mediastinum or hilum, for small nodules, or for situations in which an oblique or angled biopsy approach is required. Ideally, a portion of the aspirate should be stained and examined at the time of the procedure (in a manner analogous to performing frozen sections on tissue)[119]; this practice enables rapid assessment of the adequacy of the specimen so that repeat aspiration or cutting needle biopsy can be performed immediately in an attempt to increase the diagnostic yield.[120] If such assessment is not possible, multiple aspirations should be performed to increase the diagnostic yield.

Aspirated material may be evacuated directly onto glass slides, smeared, and immediately fixed. The needle contents may also be expelled into saline or 50% alcohol and transported to the laboratory, the fluid then being processed in the same manner as bronchial wash or pleural fluid specimens. As with the latter material, processing of a portion of the sample as a cell block frequently provides tissue fragments for histologic examination and histochemical and immunohistochemical analysis, procedures that significantly increase the diagnostic yield.

The two main indications for fine-needle aspiration in chest disease are the diagnosis of pulmonary malignancy and determination of the etiology of serious pneumonia when noninvasive diagnostic methods have failed.[121] Since the negative predictive value of TTNA is as low as 70% in the diagnosis of pulmonary malignancy,[122] we believe that it is not generally indicated if there is an intention to proceed with resection of a lesion regardless of the result. (An exception to this "rule" may apply in geographic regions in which TTNA yields a relatively high proportion of specific benign diagnoses, such as in areas where coccidioidomycosis is endemic.) In patients suspected of having pulmonary carcinoma, there are thus two major indications for TTNA: (1) when a cytologic diagnosis must be established in a patient with a lesion judged to be unresectable on clinical or radiologic grounds and (2) to determine the cell type in a lesion suspected of being either a metastasis or a second primary pulmonary carcinoma.

Contraindications to TTNA include a suspicion that the lesion may be an echinococcal cyst; the presence of severe pulmonary arterial hypertension, a bleeding disorder, anticoagulant therapy, or uncontrollable cough; and an inability of the patient to tolerate a complicating pneumothorax. Pneumothorax is the most common complication and occurs in about 20% to 30% of patients when 20- to 23-gauge needles are used.[123,124] The risk increases with larger needle diameter, procedures that cross more than one visceral pleural surface, an increased number of passes, and the presence of underlying chronic obstructive lung disease.[125-127] Other serious complications, including hemorrhage, air embolism, and spread of disease from the primary site along the needle tract, are rare.[128-130]

As with other cytologic techniques, the most important use of TTNA is in the establishment of a diagnosis of pulmonary carcinoma. The overall sensitivity in reported series varies from about 70% to 95% (5% to 30% false negatives)[120,124,131]; most reports are in the 85% to 95% range. The diagnostic yield is higher in peripheral than in central nodules and in larger than smaller tumors.[131] False-positive diagnoses are uncommon (probably less than 0.5% with experienced cytopathologists), the most common underlying condition being tuberculosis.[132] In a large study of performance parameters conducted by the American College of Pathologists that involved 436 institutions and almost 12,000 TTNA specimens (approximately 40% of which had histologic material for review), the overall results were as follows: sensitivity, 89%; specificity, 96%; positive predictive value, 99%; and negative predictive value, 70%.[122] As with sputum and bronchial washing/brushing specimens, the correlation between cytologic and histologic diagnoses of specific tumor types is generally good for the better-differentiated tumors and for small cell carcinoma.

Metastatic neoplasms can be differentiated from primary lung carcinoma in a substantial number of cases. In many instances, comparison of tissue fragments in the cell block with slides of a known extrathoracic primary will provide the diagnosis. In addition, the cytologic features of some neoplasms (such as renal or colorectal adenocarcinoma) are occasionally sufficiently characteristic to suggest an extrathoracic origin. Immunohistochemical examination is also useful in selected cases to identify a specific type of tumor.[133]

Although a variety of benign neoplastic and non-neoplastic nodules can also be definitely diagnosed cytologically by TTNA,[134] the procedure is relatively poor in this regard.[124,135] The most common cause of such nodules is infection, and culture of aspirated material clearly increases the diagnostic yield. In fact, material for this purpose should always be submitted to the microbiology laboratory whenever there is suspicion that a lesion might have an infectious etiology. Analysis of aspirated fluid by PCR is also useful in some cases.[136] TTNA has proved to be diagnostically useful in diffuse infection as well; for example, in one study of nonventilated patients who had nosocomial pneumonia, the procedure led to modification of the initial antibiotic therapy in 29 of 97 patients, including 12 in whom the initially chosen empirical regimen was ineffective.[137]

Transbronchial Needle Aspiration. TBNA is an underused technique that is performed by passing a thin needle through the tracheal or bronchial mucosa into an abnormality identified radiologically. The procedure has been used most often to obtain samples from metastatic carcinoma in subcarinal or paratracheal lymph nodes. It is thus most useful in the staging of non–small cell carcinoma and the diagnosis of small cell tumors.[138,139] In combination with fluoroscopic or CT fluoroscopic guidance, it has also been used to diagnose peripheral lung nodules.[140,141] It is important that aspiration be carried out before other procedures such as bronchial brushing or biopsy to minimize contamination of the aspirate by material from the airway surface or mucosa. Complications are few and generally not serious. The most common are minimal, usually transient hemoptysis and low-grade fever (occasionally associated with bacteremia); pneumothorax or significant hemorrhage caused by puncture of a large pulmonary artery or the aorta is rare.[142]

Diagnostic material has been obtained from enlarged subcarinal lymph nodes in as many as 90% of cases of proven carcinoma.[143] However, the yield is significantly less for peripheral tumors, when the main carina is bronchoscopically normal,[144] and when carcinoma is present in other lymph node groups.[145] Diagnostic material is obtained more frequently when lymph nodes appear to be increasing in size (as assessed by CT), when tumors are in the right lung, and when the underlying abnormality is small cell carcinoma.[138] CT evaluation of the mediastinum at the time of the procedure can improve the diagnostic yield dramatically.[146] The addition of ultrasound guidance may lead to more precise identification of smaller nodes that may also contain foci of carcinoma.[147]

Endoscopic Ultrasound-Guided Needle Aspiration. Transesophageal needle aspiration of mediastinal lesions has proved useful in the staging of pulmonary carcinoma and in the diagnosis of a variety of primary mediastinal abnormalities.[148,149] It can serve as the next step in mediastinal lymph node staging when transbronchial aspiration is not possible or nondiagnostic.[150]

Biopsy

Before discussing specific biopsy techniques, it is appropriate to emphasize several features that are common to all.

1. Despite the fact that reported instances of mortality are rare and morbidity is seldom serious, it must be remembered that *every* method of obtaining tissue can result in complications. Thus, biopsy is indicated only if there is at least a reasonable chance that it will provide information to guide useful therapy.
2. When considering the merits of a particular technique, it is necessary to take into account both the experience of its proponents—who will generally obtain results superior to those of less experienced investigators—and the specific expertise available in the local milieu. In fact, the various techniques have been infrequently compared by the same observer.
3. In most circumstances, the procedure chosen should be influenced by the particular diagnosis suspected clinically. For example, a lymph node in the supraclavicular fossa might simply be aspirated if the clinical situation suggests a diagnosis of metastatic pulmonary carcinoma; however, it might be excised completely if lymphoma is suspected.
4. Although biopsy is usually performed to obtain material for histologic study, in many cases it is essential that some tissue be sent to the microbiology laboratory for culture.
5. It is important to remember that most biopsies are samples of a particular abnormality. Thus, especially in diffuse pulmonary disease, the findings in one specimen cannot necessarily be extrapolated to all regions.
6. Correlation of clinical, radiologic, and pathologic findings frequently provides a more precise diagnosis than is possible with each alone, and close cooperation between specialists in the different fields should be encouraged.

Bronchial Biopsy

The principal value of bronchial biopsy is in the diagnosis of malignancy and the establishment of tumor cell type. A diagnosis of sarcoidosis can also be confirmed in many cases; other abnormalities are detected less commonly. The diagnostic yield of biopsies of tumors that are bronchoscopically visible is about 90% to 95%.[151] Multiple biopsies are useful. Although the small amount of tissue available for microscopic examination may not permit precise identification of tumor cell type, the distinction between small cell and non–small cell carcinoma is usually made easily.

Transbronchial Biopsy

The most useful and widespread application of transbronchial biopsy (TBB) is in the diagnosis of diffuse lung disease. It yields diagnostic material in a high proportion of patients who have sarcoidosis or lymphangitic carcinomatosis and has an important role in the diagnosis of rejection and the exclusion of opportunistic infection in lung transplant recipients.[97] It is not generally helpful in the diagnosis and management of idiopathic pulmonary fibrosis. Though largely supplanted by BAL, TBB has high diagnostic yield in patients who have *Pneumocystis* pneumonia.[144] The procedure can be performed safely in outpatients and without fluoroscopy in patients who have diffuse parenchymal radiographic abnormalities.[152] "Significant" bleeding or pneumothorax occurs in less than 2% of patients.[153]

Transthoracic Needle Biopsy

Transthoracic needle biopsy (TTNB) is a procedure whereby a core of lung, lymph node, or tumor tissue is obtained by the use of a cutting needle. The procedure offers no advantage over fine-needle aspiration (TTNA) in the diagnosis of pulmonary carcinoma and has a higher complication rate. However, the larger samples provided by the cutting needle are more likely to be diagnostic in benign lesions and in more diffuse disease such as vasculitis and infection.[154,155] TTNB under CT guidance is also useful in sampling hilar and mediastinal masses for the staging of lung cancer[156]; however, it is not appropriate for the evaluation of normal-size nodes.

The procedure is safer, less costly, and better tolerated than thoracotomy or mediastinoscopy.[157] The most common complications are pneumothorax and hemoptysis.[158,159] However, by careful patient selection (e.g., by avoiding uncooperative patients and those who have significant COPD or a bleeding diathesis), pneumothorax requiring chest tube drainage is uncommon and significant bleeding is rare.[160]

Thoracoscopy and Video-Assisted Thoracoscopic Surgery

Thoracoscopy is a procedure by which the visceral and parietal pleura can be directly examined by insertion of an instrument through a small incision in the chest wall.[161] The advent of video technology and the development of appropriate instrumentation have allowed video-assisted thoracoscopic surgery (VATS) to extend this minimally invasive approach to the performance of a wide variety of diagnostic and therapeutic maneuvers.[162] In contrast to "medical" thoracoscopy, VATS is usually performed under general anesthesia in the operating room with selective lung ventilation.[163] Advantages of the procedure over full thoracotomy include reduced pain, faster recovery, and the ability to operate on sicker patients.[164]

Thoracoscopic biopsy is the diagnostic method of choice in the investigation of patients who have persistent pleural effusion for which a diagnosis has not been established by closed pleural biopsy and/or fluid aspiration.[165,166] The procedure has very high sensitivity and negative predictive value for the diagnosis of malignancy in this context. Additional important uses include lung biopsy in patients who have diffuse lung disease, assessment of the mediastinum as part of the staging of pulmonary carcinoma (especially lymph nodes in stations that are not accessible by mediastinoscopy),[167] biopsy of mediastinal masses when TTNB is inappropriate or nondiagnostic,[168,169] wedge resection of pulmonary nodules, and the management of recurrent pneumothorax and chest trauma.[170]

The complications of VATS and medical thoracoscopy are similar and include bleeding, air leak, tumor seeding at the chest wall incision, fever, and wound infection.[163] Major complications occur in less than 10% of cases, and procedure-related mortality is less than 1%.[171]

Open Lung Biopsy by Thoracotomy

In this technique, the chest is opened through a standard thoracotomy incision or through a limited incision large enough to allow removal of a fragment of tissue measuring 2 to 3 cm in diameter. Selection of the appropriate site for biopsy is clearly important. Areas of discrete disease should be removed en bloc if small enough to be included in the specimen; if more extensive disease is present, the biopsy should include an area of transition between abnormal and apparently normal lung. Biopsy of only very abnormal areas may show "end-stage" disease whose etiology may be difficult to determine.[172] Several sites from the same or different lobes should be sampled if possible.

In general, biopsy specimens should be submitted to a pathologist as soon as possible after excision. Portions may then be selected for special examination, and frozen sections can be performed to provide a preliminary diagnosis or to assess the adequacy of the biopsy material. When appropriate, material should be sent for culture. In a review of 2290 cases reported in the literature, mortality and complication rates were calculated to be 1.8% and 7.0%, respectively.[173]

Mediastinoscopy and Anterior Mediastinotomy

The main indication for mediastinal biopsy is the staging of pulmonary carcinoma. Less often, the procedure is used to diagnose such carcinoma, a primary mediastinal neoplasm, or certain benign conditions such as sarcoidosis.[174] Cervical mediastinoscopy is carried out through an incision in the suprasternal notch; the soft tissue adjacent to the trachea is dissected, and biopsy material is removed under direct vision through a rigid mediastinoscope. The space explored consists of the upper half of the mediastinum, including tissue around the intrathoracic portion of the trachea, the tracheal bifurcation, and the proximal part of the main bronchi. Complications are uncommon and not usually serious; in a review of 20,000 procedures, they occurred in less than 2.5% of patients.[175] Mortality was less than 0.5%.

When the subaortic and anterior mediastinal lymph nodes need to be assessed surgically, extended cervical mediastinoscopy,[176] anterior mediastinotomy,[177] or video-assisted thoracoscopy may be used. Each has the advantage of permitting more extensive exploration of the mediastinum and more accurate assessment of neoplastic involvement of the hila than permitted by standard cervical mediastinotomy. In extended cervical mediastinoscopy, dissection through the usual cervical incision is continued between the anterior surface of the left innominate vein and the sternum. Anterior mediastinotomy is performed via a 6-cm incision in the second intercostal space lateral to the sternal border. Both techniques are useful in assessing the resectability of left upper lobe carcinomas; unresectability at thoracotomy because of mediastinal lymph node involvement that was not previously appreciated at anterior mediastinotomy has been found in less than 8% of patients.[177]

Scalene Lymph Node Biopsy

Scalene lymph node biopsy consists of the removal of tissue lying on the scalene group of muscles in the supraclavicular fossa, including the medial fat pad. The advent of sophisticated imaging techniques and the ease of other procedures such as fine-needle aspiration have markedly reduced the role of the procedure in the staging of pulmonary carcinoma and the diagnosis of nonmalignant disease. Scalene lymph nodes that are palpable usually contain pathologic tissue[178]; when they are not palpable, the diagnostic yield of biopsy is low. In this circumstance, the role of biopsy is limited to the staging of patients who appear to have N2 or N3 disease for the purpose of entry into aggressive treatment protocols.[179] Biopsy may also be required for tumor classification in patients who have known or suspected lymphoma.

Closed Pleural Biopsy

The most common method of obtaining fragments of pleural tissue for histologic examination is TTNB, a procedure that can be performed at the same time as thoracentesis. The two most commonly used needles are the Cope and the Abrams types. Some investigators have reported equivalent or better efficacy with more recently developed instruments, such as the Raja or Tru-Cut needle. The latter (and similar instruments) is particularly valuable in the diagnosis of diffuse pleural thickening when guided by ultrasound or by CT.[180] Success with these needles depends largely on the skill of the operator, the selection of patients, and the number of samples obtained. As might be expected, pneumothorax almost always accompanies the procedure, but it is typically small and does not require treatment. Other complications are rare and usually mild; they include hemorrhage into the chest wall and/or pleural cavity, mediastinal and subcutaneous emphysema, and the development of carcinoma along the needle tract.

The chief use of TTNB of the pleura is in the investigation of cancer and tuberculosis. The sensitivity for the diagnosis of tuberculosis ranges from 70% to 90%[181,182]; although only one biopsy may be required for diagnosis,[183] the yield increases with the number of samples. The diagnostic yield in patients who have neoplastic involvement of the pleura, when combined with cytologic examination, ranges from about 65% to 85%.[182]

FUNCTIONAL INVESTIGATION

Pulmonary function tests are an essential part of the investigation of many respiratory diseases. The choice of which ones should be performed in a given setting depends on the

TABLE 4–3. Tests of Lung Function

Level 1
Spirometry and peak flow (FEV_1, FVC, FEV_1/FVC)
Bronchodilator response
Oximetry
Level 2
Arterial blood gas tensions
Subdivisions of lung volume
Lung diffusing capacity
Level 3
Pulmonary and airway resistance
Lung pressure-volume curves
Measures of respiratory muscle strength ($P_{I}max$ and $P_{E}max$)
Measures of ventilatory response to hypoxia and hypercapnia
Measures of bronchial responsiveness
Stage I, II, and III exercise tests

purpose of the study, of which there are six principal types: (1) determining whether symptoms and signs such as dyspnea, cough, and cyanosis are of respiratory origin; (2) managing and monitoring the progression of disease or response to therapy in patients with recognized pulmonary disorders; (3) assessing the risk of development of pulmonary dysfunction and complications as a result of therapeutic interventions such as operative procedures and drugs; (4) quantifying the degree of disability in environmental or occupational lung disease; (5) carrying out epidemiologic surveys of population groups suspected of having acquired pulmonary disease as a result of exposure to dust or fumes; and (6) screening health status as part of a regular clinical assessment or on behalf of a third party (e.g., insurance company).

Tests that assess pulmonary function may be conveniently considered in three levels of increasing sophistication (Table 4–3). First is measurement of vital capacity and maximal expiratory flow rates by spirometry and assessment of the gas-exchanging ability of the lungs by measurement of arterial saturation by oximetry. The second level includes measurement of arterial blood gas tensions, assessment of the subdivisions of lung volume by plethysmography or the helium dilution technique, and estimation of the diffusing capacity of the lung. At the third level are more sophisticated tests for assessing lung mechanics, respiratory control, ventilation and perfusion properties of the lung, bronchial reactivity, and exercise performance.

Whatever the level of sophistication, all lung function tests must be interpreted and correlated with clinical and radiologic data; without this added information, interpretation of tests is subject to much variability among readers.[184]

Predicted Normal Values of Pulmonary Function

Interpretation of the results of pulmonary function tests is based on the degree of deviation from predicted normal values. These values are calculated from regression equations that take into account known attributes that contribute to variations in lung function, including age, sex, height, weight, and race. Genetic and environmental factors that affect lung function are responsible for much of the wide range of values among normal persons.

Ideally, the normal range for a test should encompass 95% of the values in a population; in practice, however, a difference of ±20% from the mean predicted value is used for many lung function tests. When interpreting a test result as abnormal, it is important to remember that the interindividual variation in lung function can differ greatly between tests; for example, in a normal population the forced expiratory flow ($FEF_{25\%-75\%}$) and the maximal inspiratory and expiratory pressures (measurement of which is highly effort dependent) can vary as much as 30% to 50%. Tests must also be interpreted with caution in very young and very old patients because the prediction equations for lung function are often inaccurate at these extremes.

Although one use of pulmonary function testing is to compare the values obtained from an individual with those of a normal population, monitoring the progress of a patient over time or assessing the response to short- or long-term therapy has the advantage of using the patient's own values as a control, thus permitting greater accuracy in detecting changes in lung function. The detection of a significant change, or the lack of change, in any test over time or in response to an intervention is dependent on the intrinsic variability of the test. This variability can be measured as the coefficient of variation of repeated tests, defined as the standard deviation of repeated tests divided by the mean. The coefficient of variation varies widely among lung function tests but, in general, is much narrower than the 95% confidence limits observed in the population (Table 4–4).[185]

Lung Volumes

Lung volumes and capacities may be appreciated by studying Figure 4–1. There are four volumes: (1) tidal volume (TV), the amount of gas moved in and out of the lung with each respiratory cycle; (2) residual volume (RV), the amount remaining in the lung after maximal expiration; (3) inspiratory reserve volume (IRV), the additional gas that may be inspired after the end of a quiet inspiration; and (4) expiratory reserve volume (ERV), the additional amount of gas that may be expired from the resting or end-expiratory level. There are also four capacities: (1) total lung capacity (TLC), the gas contained in the lung at the end of maximal inspiration; (2) vital capacity (VC), the amount that can be expired after a maximal inspiration or inspired after a maximal expiration; (3) inspiratory capacity (IC), the amount of gas that can be inspired from the end of a quiet expiration; and (4) functional residual capacity (FRC), the volume of gas remaining in the lung at the end of a quiet expiration.

Vital Capacity

VC is usually measured as forced vital capacity (FVC), the amount of gas that can be forcefully exhaled after complete inspiration. In patients who have obstructive pulmonary disease, FVC may be less than inspired VC by as much as 1 L as a result of dynamic compression of airways, gas trapping on expiration, and failure to detect expired volume at low flow rates.[186] Measurement of VC and FVC is most useful when combined with measurement of the volume of gas exhaled during the first second of expiration (FEV_1). The FEV_1/FVC ratio is an invaluable indicator of respiratory disease and allows separation of ventilatory abnormalities into "restrictive" or "obstructive" patterns; in patients who have obstructive pulmonary disease, FVC is relatively well maintained in relation to FEV_1, whereas in restrictive disease, FEV_1 is decreased less than FVC, so the ratio is preserved or may be higher than the predicted normal.

Functional Residual Capacity, Residual Volume, and Total Lung Capacity

FRC is determined chiefly by the balance between the outward recoil of the chest wall and the inward recoil of the lung, although both inspiratory muscle activity during expiration

TABLE 4–4. Interindividual and Intraindividual Variation in Lung Function in Normal Subjects

Test	Percentage of Variation between Individuals	Percentage of Variation within an Individual
Forced vital capacity (FVC)	±20-25	±6-16
Forced expiratory volume in 1 second (FEV_1)	±20-22	±7-18
FEV_1/FVC	±14	
Peak expiratory flow rate (PEFR)		±13-28
Forced expiratory flow between 75% and 25% (FEF_{25-75})	±40-60	
Functional residual capacity (FRC):		
By helium dilution	±20	
By body plethysmography		±4
Density dependence of maximal expiratory flow:		
$\Delta Vmax_{50}$ breathing 80% He + 20% O_2		±22
Volume of isoflow breathing 80% He + 20% O_2		±100
Pressure-volume curves:		
P_{Imax}	±19	±11
$PL_{90\%}$	±14	±9
Cstat	±9	±15
logk		±6
Diffusing capacity		
$DLCO_{SB}$	±21	±3-11
$DLCO_{SB}/VA$	±25	
Closing volume, % vital capacity	±60	
Closing capacity, % TLC	±23	

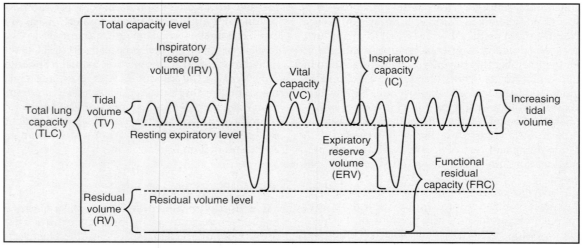

FIGURE 4–1

Lung volumes and capacities.

and flow limitation during tidal breathing can increase FRC above its static value. RV is normally determined by the balance between expiratory muscle strength and the stiffness of the chest wall, although airway closure or flow limitation may be more important in disease. TLC is determined by the balance between inspiratory muscle strength and the elastic recoil of the lung and chest wall.

FRC, RV, and TLC can be determined by either inert gas inhalation techniques or body plethysmography. In the closed-circuit inert gas method, the patient breathes from a spirometer of known volume containing helium of known concentration. At the beginning of the study, the helium concentration in the lungs is zero; as the patient breathes in and out, the gas mixes between the spirometer and lungs until the concentration of helium is the same in both. FRC is calculated by the equation:

$$FRC = \frac{Spirometer\ volume \times Initial\ He\ concentration}{Final\ He\ concentration}$$

RV and TLC are calculated by subtracting ERV and adding IC, respectively. The inert gas techniques are subject to error because they do not detect trapped gas, which does not communicate with the tracheobronchial tree; thus, they can seriously underestimate FRC, particularly in patients who have severe obstructive lung disease, bullae, or other intrathoracic noncommunicating accumulations of gas.

The other major method of measuring FRC is based on Boyle's law and uses a body plethysmograph (body box). Boyle's law states that the product of the volume and pressure of gas is constant at constant temperature ($V_1 \times P_1 = V_2 \times P_2$). To measure FRC plethysmographically, the airway is closed at FRC, and the subject pants against the closed airway, thus generating changes in mouth and pleural pressure and small increases and decreases in lung volume as a result of compression and decompression of thoracic gas. The relationship between changes in thoracic gas volume and mouth pressure ($\Delta V/\Delta P$) can be calibrated so that intrathoracic volume can be derived; in addition, RV and TLC may be obtained by having the subject perform a VC maneuver immediately after measurement of FRC. This method has the advantage that all gas subjected to the swings in intrathoracic pressure is measured, regardless of whether it communicates with the tracheobronchial tree.

Plethysmography may overestimate FRC in patients who have airway obstruction because of a failure of mouth pressure to accurately reflect mean intrathoracic pressure.[187] This artifact can be overcome if patients pant at a rate slower than 60 breaths per minute. Determination of TLC based on posteroanterior and lateral chest radiographs has been shown to be highly accurate and can be accomplished by experienced workers in less than 5 minutes.[188]

Forced Expiratory Volume and Flow

The forced expiratory maneuver is the most widely used and standardized test of lung function. Although it is relatively easy to perform, it is important to ensure that the maneuver meets technical standards, is performed with adequate patient effort, and is interpreted correctly. The American Thoracic Society has published comprehensive guidelines for performance and interpretation of the test.[189] Three to five measurements are usually obtained, and the test that has the highest sum of FEV_1 and FVC is chosen for analysis.[190,191] Expired volume is plotted against time (Fig. 4–2) to yield a typical spirogram from which FEV_1, FVC, and $FEF_{25\%-75\%}$ can be derived. Expired volume can also be plotted against the instantaneous expiratory flow rate to yield a flow-volume curve. Peak expiratory flow and flow at specific percentages of the forced expired VC, such as $\dot{V}max_{50}$ and $\dot{V}max_{25}$, can be determined from the flow-volume curve.

The usefulness of forced expiration as a test of lung function stems largely from the fact that it is relatively effort independent and is highly reproducible. Nonetheless, submaximal efforts can result in paradoxically higher values for FEV_1/FVC and $FEF_{25\%-75\%}$, especially in patients who have obstructive pulmonary disease.[192] When measured correctly, FEV_1 and FVC have an extremely narrow coefficient of variation in

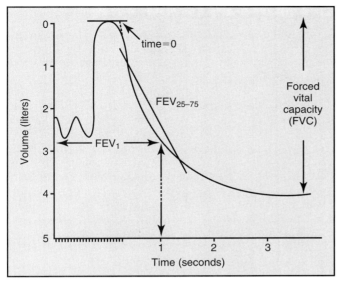

FIGURE 4–2

Measurement of ventilatory volumes. Volume in liters is plotted against time in seconds while the subject forcibly exhales from TLC. The volume-versus-time slope is back-extrapolated to 0 time, and FEV_1 is measured and compared with predicted values, as well as the measured forced vital capacity (FVC). The FEV_1/FVC ratio serves as a volume-independent measure of expiratory airflow obstruction. The average flow over the middle half of the forced expiratory volume ($FEF_{25\%-75\%}$) is obtained as the slope of the volume-time plot between 25% and 75% of FVC.

normal individuals (±5%); however, in patients who have obstructive lung disease, the coefficient of variation increases to approximately 12% when measurements are made on the same day.[185]

When compared with FVC and FEV_1, there is a much higher coefficient of variation for repeated measurements of $FEF_{25\%-75\%}$, $\dot{V}max_{50}$, and $\dot{V}max_{25}$,[193,194] variability that increases with the degree of pulmonary dysfunction.[195] There is also more variation between individuals for $FEF_{25\%-75\%}$ and $\dot{V}max_{50}$ than for FEV_1 and FVC; the 95% confidence limits for FEV_1 and FVC are generally considered to be ±20%, whereas for $FEF_{25\%-75\%}$ and $\dot{V}max_{50}$ to be judged abnormal, values should be more than 40% below predicted.[194]

Bronchodilator Response

Spirometry is used to assess bronchodilator responsiveness. A 70% increase in peak flow, a 15% increase in FEV_1, a 12% increase in FVC, and/or a 45% increase in $FEF_{25\%-75\%}$ are required to conclude that there is a beneficial effect from a bronchodilator.[196] Bronchodilator response can also be assessed by using the absolute increase in FEV_1 or the increase as a percentage of the predicted value; greater than 200 mL or 9% of predicted FEV_1 is considered significant. These measures of response have the advantage that they are uninfluenced by the baseline value. Because FVC may improve more than FEV_1, change in the FEV_1/FVC ratio is a poor estimate. Bronchodilation of smaller airways may result in a decrease in hyperinflation in patients who have airway obstruction, and measurement of IC after bronchodilator use has been advo-

cated as a useful assessment of this change; reduced hyperinflation correlates more closely with a change in symptoms than do changes in flow rates.[196a]

Diffusing Capacity

The diffusing capacity for carbon monoxide (D_{LCO}) is computed as follows:

$$D_{LCO} = \frac{\text{mL of CO taken up by capillary blood/min}}{\text{Mean alveolar } P_{CO} - \text{Mean capillary } P_{CO}}$$

The amount of CO taken up by capillary blood is calculated by subtracting the product of the expired volume and CO concentration of the expired gas from the product of the inspired volume and CO concentration of the inspired gas. Mean alveolar P_{CO} is estimated by obtaining a sample of expired gas after the dead space has been cleared, and mean capillary P_{CO} is assumed to be zero.

Several techniques for measuring diffusing capacity with carbon monoxide have been devised,[197-199] the main differences among them being the length of time that the gas is kept in the lungs and the method of determining mean alveolar P_{CO}. The single-breath method is most widely used. Guidelines for performance and interpretation have been proposed by the American Thoracic Society.[199a] The test is performed by having the subject exhale to RV and then take a greater than 90% VC breath of a gas containing 0.3% carbon monoxide, 10% helium, 21% oxygen, and the balance nitrogen. After rapid inspiration of the gas, the breath is held for about 10 seconds near TLC, the first liter of expired gas is discarded, and the next liter (representative of alveolar gas) is collected and analyzed for helium and carbon monoxide. The helium dilution is used to calculate alveolar volume (V_A), as well as the initial concentration of carbon monoxide in the alveolar space. The test can be repeated at brief intervals; two results that agree within 5% are required.[200]

D_{LCO} is dependent on lung volume. For example, after pneumonectomy or with the chest wall restriction that occurs in conditions such as kyphoscoliosis, a patient may have reduced D_{LCO} without intrinsic gas exchange abnormality in the remaining or restricted lung.[201] This has led to the suggestion that the specific diffusing capacity (diffusing capacity divided by the alveolar volume at which it is measured [D_L/V_A]) is a more accurate measurement; it is abbreviated Kco in the United Kingdom[202] and provides a useful determination of whether the reduced D_{LCO} is due solely to reduced lung volume.

Diffusing capacity is influenced by factors that alter the alveolar capillary membrane and pulmonary capillary blood volume (Table 4–5). Since the transfer of carbon monoxide is diffusion (and not perfusion) limited, pulmonary capillary blood volume (V_C) rather than pulmonary blood flow is important. To calculate the blood volume component of diffusing capacity, V_C is multiplied by the kinetic constant θ, which is the rate of combination of carbon monoxide and red blood cells. The membrane and $V_C \times \theta$ contributions to diffusing capacity can be calculated separately by measuring the diffusing capacity with different inspired partial pressures of oxygen. In normal individuals, the two components contribute approximately equally to the measured D_{LCO}.

TABLE 4–5. Factors Affecting Diffusing Capacity

Alveolar Capillary Membrane
  Lung volume
  Surface area
  "Thickness"
Pulmonary Capillary Blood Volume
  (Blood volume × Hemoglobin concentration)
  Position: increased DLCO standing → sitting → lying
  Müller or Valsalva maneuvers during breath-hold
  Hemoglobin concentration
  Hemoglobin affinity for oxygen
Distribution of Ventilation Relative to Perfusion
  Affects steady-state method especially
  Affects FCO least
Backpressure of Carbon Monoxide
  Cigarette smoking

A variety of factors influence Vc and θ and thus indirectly affect DLCO. The θ value is directly affected by the oxygen saturation of hemoglobin and the presence of carboxyhemoglobin associated with smoking or occupational exposure. Smokers can have a level of carboxyhemoglobin as high as 10%, so this must be considered when interpreting test results. Factors that increase or decrease the hemoglobin concentration also affect DLCO, and a number of correction factors for anemia and polycythemia have been suggested. One commonly used adjustment is to increase or decrease the predicted DLCO by 1.4% for each percent change in hematocrit above or below 44%.[203]

Acute changes in pulmonary capillary blood volume can also alter measured DLCO; for example, recruitment of the pulmonary vascular bed during exercise results in a substantial increase in DLCO within seconds.[204] DLCO also increases when one breathes through an inspiratory resistance, presumably as a result of increased capillary blood volume caused by negative intrathoracic pressure. It is important to recognize that increased DLCO is not caused solely by increased capillary blood; it may also be markedly increased in patients who have intra-alveolar hemorrhage, and measurement of DLCO has been recommended for the diagnosis of this condition.[205]

Arterial Blood Gas Tensions

Measurement of arterial blood gas tensions is invaluable in the assessment of cardiopulmonary disease. Specific values are used to define respiratory failure, which can be acute or chronic and can involve either or both of the ventilatory or gas-exchanging components of the respiratory system. Ventilatory failure is defined by an elevation in arterial $PaCO_2$ (>45 mm Hg) and gas exchange failure by a decrease in arterial PaO_2 (<60 mm Hg). Ventilatory failure is inevitably associated with a decrease in PaO_2, but gas exchange failure can occur with a normal or decreased $PaCO_2$. Application of the alveolar air equation to the results of blood gas analysis and comparison of calculated alveolar PAO_2 with measured PaO_2 to calculate the alveolar-arterial gradient for oxygen allows a quantitative assessment of impairment in gas exchange independent of ventilatory effects on PaO_2.

Cardiopulmonary Exercise Testing

Cardiopulmonary exercise testing (CPET) is an important method to assess the integrated function of the cardiovascular and pulmonary systems. The subject has been reviewed in a statement from the American Thoracic Society/American College of Chest Physicians, which includes a list of normal values and their variability.[205a] Tests can be performed by using submaximal or maximal exercise levels, on a cycle ergometer (preferred) or a treadmill, and by using a wide variety of physiologic responses as outcome measures. The latter include the work rate, the consumption of oxygen and production of CO_2 (and their ratio, the respiratory exchange ratio), the level and pattern of ventilation, the heart rate, blood pressure, electrocardiographic findings, arterial oxygen saturation (pulse oximetry), arterial blood gas tension, arterial lactate levels, and symptoms of dyspnea or fatigue. Measurement of IC during the test has also been advocated as a clinically useful indicator of dynamic hyperinflation in obstructive lung disease.[206]

Indications for the use of CPET include the evaluation of patients who have unexplained exercise intolerance or dyspnea and preoperative evaluation, especially for patients being considered for resection of pulmonary carcinoma, lung volume reduction surgery, or lung transplantation. Additional indications include the establishment of an exercise "prescription" for patients who have chronic pulmonary or cardiovascular disease and quantification of the degree of disability, especially in cases in which occupational exposure may warrant compensation. CPET is useful for the initial assessment and follow-up of patients who have pulmonary hypertension, heart failure, interstitial lung disease, cystic fibrosis, and COPD. Finally, assessment of the presence and severity of exercised-induced bronchoconstriction may be clinically indicated.

The 6-minute walk test is a simpler way of obtaining a quantitative assessment of the degree of functional impairment, but the test is limited in the amount of physiologic information that it provides.[207]

The integrated function of the cardiovascular-respiratory system is best evaluated by assessing relationships between the intensity of exercise or the level of O_2 consumption ($\dot{V}O_2$) and other physiologic variables (e.g., work rate versus $\dot{V}O_2$ and $\dot{V}CO_2$, $\dot{V}O_2$ versus ventilation, $\dot{V}O_2$ versus heart rate, $\dot{V}O_2$ versus $\dot{V}CO_2$, $\dot{V}O_2$ versus the dead space–tidal volume ratio, and $\dot{V}O_2$ versus arterial lactate levels). Careful interpretation of the plots of such relationships can provide evidence for a cardiac or pulmonary cause of dyspnea, give an estimate of the level of fitness, or suggest the possibility of pulmonary hypertension or a peripheral skeletal muscle abnormality.

Pressure-Volume Characteristics of the Lung

Lung compliance is the relationship between the volume of air inhaled and the pressure needed to overcome the elastic recoil of the lung. It is assessed by plotting lung volume against transpulmonary pressure (PL) over a range of volumes from TLC to FRC or lower. PL is measured by a transducer that compares mouth pressure with esophageal pressure measured with a thin-walled balloon positioned in the midesophagus. Pressure-volume data are collected during slow deflation from TLC or with stepwise interruption of expiratory flow from

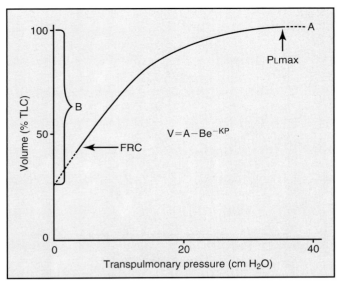

FIGURE 4–3

Elastic recoil properties of the lung. Schematic pressure-volume (P-V) curve of the lung in which lung volume as a percentage of TLC (predicted or actual) is plotted against transpulmonary pressure. The P-V behavior may be described by using various measurements from the P-V curve, including maximal elastic recoil (PLmax), elastic recoil pressure at various percentages of TLC (i.e., PL_{90}, PL_{60}, and so on), and compliance—the slope of the $\Delta V/\Delta P$ plot in the relatively linear range near FRC. These measurements all have the disadvantage of describing only a portion of the curve. The whole curve can be fitted to an exponential function[508] in which V = volume, A = the theoretical maximal lung volume at infinite transpulmonary pressure, B = the volume difference between A and the 0 transpulmonary pressure intercept, P = transpulmonary pressure, and k = the exponent that describes the shape of the P-V curve.

TLC. Compliance is calculated as the volume change divided by the transpulmonary pressure change over the relatively linear portion of the pressure-volume curve, near FRC.

$$\text{Compliance} = \frac{\Delta\,\text{Volume}}{\Delta\,\text{Pressure}}$$

Measurement of compliance has the disadvantage of being dependent on lung size, thus making comparison between individuals difficult. To circumvent this shortcoming, a number of investigators have suggested fitting the pressure-volume data to an exponential equation[208]:

$$V = A - Be^{-kP}$$

where A is the theoretical maximal lung volume achievable at infinite transpulmonary pressure, B is the difference between A and lung volume at a transpulmonary pressure of zero, P is transpulmonary pressure, and k is the shape constant that reflects the overall compliance of the lung, regardless of lung size. An increased k value correlates with the severity of emphysema measured morphologically, and a decreased k value has been reported in some cases of interstitial fibrosis.[209]

In addition to compliance, other parameters derived from the pressure-volume curve also reflect the elastic recoil properties of the lung (Fig. 4–3). The maximal elastic recoil pres-

sure that the patient can generate at TLC (PLmax) reflects the elastic recoil properties of the lung, as well as the inspiratory muscle strength. Elastic recoil pressures at various percentages of TLC (PL_{90}, PL_{80}, PL_{70}, and so on) can also be determined.

Resistance

Resistance is pressure divided by flow (R = P/V). With respect to the lungs, three forms can be measured. Airway resistance (Raw) is the difference between mouth and alveolar pressure divided by flow and is measured in a constant-volume body plethysmograph. It can also be expressed as its reciprocal, conductance (Gaw); since both measurements vary with lung volume, they can be expressed as specific resistance (SRaw = Raw × Volume) and specific conductance (SGaw = Gaw/Volume).

Pulmonary resistance (RL) is obtained by dividing the difference between mouth and esophageal pressure by flow. Since the pressure difference between the mouth and the pleural space during breathing reflects both the resistive and the elastic properties of the lung, the portion of the transpulmonary pressure swing attributable to elastic recoil must be subtracted to measure the true pressure-flow relationship.[210]

Respiratory system resistance (Rrs) is measured by forced oscillation during tidal breathing. Small pulses of flow are generated at the mouth by a loudspeaker, and the relationship between the output of the loudspeaker and the resultant flow can be analyzed to give values for total respiratory system resistance.[211]

Ventilation-Perfusion Ratios

Methods for the assessment of disturbances in ventilation-perfusion ratios are described in Chapter 1 (see page 47). The most commonly used technique involves calculation of the alveolar-arterial gradient for oxygen by using the simplified alveolar air equation. An increase in "physiologic" dead space can be measured with the Bohr equation, and venous admixture or true intrapulmonary shunt can be calculated. Radionuclides are commonly used in the study of regional ventilation-perfusion inequality; the multiple inert gas technique provides the most accurate description of the distribution of ventilation-perfusion ratios in the lung, although it does not provide regional information and is used solely as a research tool.

Respiratory Control

Alveolar hypoventilation accompanied by an elevated $PaCO_2$ and the resultant fall in PaO_2 is the final common pathway of many pulmonary disorders. The clinical challenge is to determine why hypoventilation has occurred: is the patient hypoventilating because he or she *will not* or *cannot* breathe sufficiently?[212] The first step in the investigation of "can't versus won't" is measurement of lung volumes and flow rates because hypoventilation as a result of increased work of breathing does not usually occur unless there is a reduction to less than 25% of predicted values. If hypoventilation is present with adequate ventilatory reserve, more detailed investigation of respiratory control is warranted.

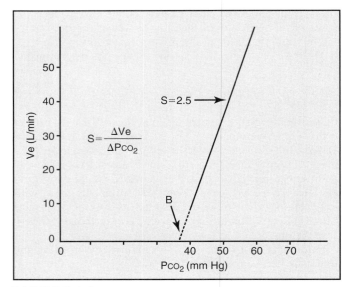

FIGURE 4–4

The CO₂ ventilatory response curve. The ventilatory response curve to increasing levels of CO_2 serves as a measure of respiratory chemosensitivity. A linear relationship between ventilation and end-tidal CO_2 is observed with the rebreathing method, and chemosensitivity is quantified as the slope of the curve $\Delta\dot{V}e/\Delta P_{CO_2}$. A normal curve in which $\Delta\dot{V}e/\Delta P_{CO_2}$ is 2.5 L/min/mm Hg is depicted. There is a wide range of normal for this slope, and the relationship can be changed by alterations in central drive, neuromuscular function, or respiratory system impedance.

It is difficult to quantify respiratory center output. The measurement that most accurately reflects central neural drive is an electrical neurogram of the phrenic nerve, but this test is difficult and invasive and is rarely used. As a result, several other techniques have been proposed.

Ventilatory Response Curves

The ventilatory response to carbon dioxide can be measured with a steady-state or rebreathing technique.[213,214] The results are expressed as the slope of the ventilatory response, $\Delta V/\Delta P_{CO_2}$, whose relationship is linear with an intercept on the CO_2 axis, reflecting the starting arterial P_{CO_2} (Fig. 4–4). The range of ventilatory response to CO_2 is remarkably wide among normal individuals (between 0.57 and 8.17 L/min/mm Hg rise in CO_2[215]).

The ventilatory response to hypoxia can be assessed by plotting changes in ventilation as a function of decreasing arterial or end-tidal P_{O_2} or as a function of arterial oxygen saturation measured with an oximeter.[215] The relationship between ventilation and P_{O_2} is curvilinear (Fig. 4–5); ventilation changes little until P_{O_2} values of approximately 50 or 60 mm Hg, and then it increases steeply. The relationship between ventilation and saturation is linear, so quantification is easier.

The range of the normal ventilatory response to hypoxemia is also extremely wide, with a mean value of 1.47 L/min per percent fall in arterial saturation; 80% of normal individuals have a slope between 0.6 and 2.75.[215]

Mouth Occlusion Pressures

The ventilatory response to CO_2 and O_2 is strongly dependent on the impedance of the respiratory system (i.e., it is not a

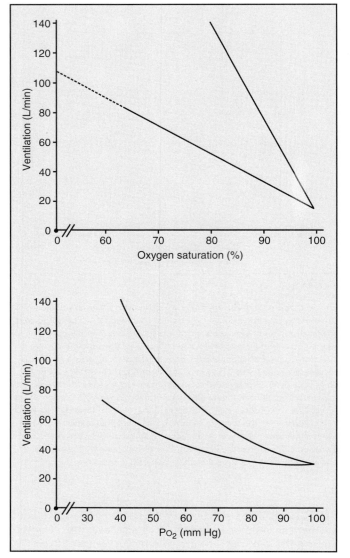

FIGURE 4–5

Ventilatory response to hypoxemia. The ventilatory response to hypoxemia is tested by plotting ventilation versus changes in oxygen saturation (*upper panel*) or P_{O_2} (*lower panel*). A wide range of normal responses is shown by these two representative curves, which are at the upper and lower limits of normal responses. The advantage of using O_2 saturation as the independent variable is that linear relationships are produced that allow easier comparison within or between subjects.

direct measure of the neural drive to breath). Thus, a patient might have a normal neural output from a normally functioning respiratory center, but the translation of that neural output to ventilation might be impaired for purely mechanical reasons. Measuring the pressure at the mouth 100 msec after occlusion represents an attempt to overcome this problem.[216] The technique is performed while the patient is breathing tidally at rest or during various stages of measuring a ventilatory response curve to hypoxia or hypercapnia. Periodically and unknown to the subject, the mouthpiece is occluded for at least 100 msec at the onset of inspiration.[216]

Although high occlusion pressure may develop in a patient who has a stiff lung or narrowed airways, that pressure would produce only a small change in volume; by contrast, only a small change in pressure is required to produce a volume change equivalent to tidal volume in a normal individual. Thus, pressure is a more direct indicator of the drive to breathe than ventilation is. Investigators using this technique have shown that patients with ventilatory impairment may have a normal or even supranormal drive, the decreased ventilation being attributable solely to the increased impedance of the respiratory system.[217]

Breathing Pattern Analysis

Ventilation at rest or during stimulated breathing can be divided into a flow component and a timing component:

$$Ve = Vt/Ti \times Ti/Ttot$$

where Vt/Ti is the mean inspiratory flow (tidal volume divided by inspiratory time), and Ti/Ttot is the duty cycle (ratio of inspiratory time to total respiratory cycle time). An increase in ventilation can be achieved by increasing the inspiratory flow rate Vt/Ti and keeping Ti/Ttot constant or by increasing Ti/Ttot and keeping Vt/Ti constant. The Vt/Ti component is thought to reflect neural output from the respiratory center, whereas the Ti/Ttot relationship reflects the timing element.[218]

Electromyography

Respiratory center output can be measured by electromyography of the diaphragm or other respiratory muscles. Recordings are made with surface electrodes placed on the fifth, sixth, and seventh intercostal spaces, close to the costochondral junctions, or with an esophageal electrode.[219] The technique has several disadvantages, in particular that it is invasive and is one step removed from the electrical output of the respiratory center.

Respiratory Muscle Performance

The final step in the assessment of respiratory control involves measurement of neurologic output as reflected in respiratory muscle performance. The simplest means of testing inspiratory and expiratory muscle strength is to measure maximal inspiratory and expiratory pressure (PImax and PEmax or MIP and MEP) at the mouth. The technique involves having a subject make maximal inspiratory and expiratory effort against a closed mouthpiece in which a small leak has been placed to avoid glottic closure and generation of pressure by the buccal and oropharyngeal muscles. The pressures generated depend on the lung volume at which the test is performed because the volume influences the length-tension relationship of various respiratory muscles. Thus, maximal inspiratory pressure is generated near RV and maximal expiratory pressure near TLC when the expiratory muscles are lengthened.[220]

Measurement of PImax and PEmax gives an overall estimate of respiratory muscle performance, but measurement of maximal transdiaphragmatic pressure (PDImax) gives a specific estimate of diaphragm strength. The latter is obtained by comparing pleural and gastric pressure during maximal inspiratory effort against a closed mouthpiece and has proved useful in the detection of bilateral or unilateral diaphragmatic paralysis.

Inhalation Challenge Tests

Inhalation challenge tests can be categorized into nonspecific and specific types. The former include those involving aerosol challenge with nebulized agonists, such as methacholine, histamine, or hypertonic saline, and those designed to produce cooling and drying of the airway mucosa by exercise and isocapnic hyperventilation. Specific challenge tests involve the inhalation of allergens to which the subject is known or suspected to be sensitive or exposure to dust or environmental agents that provoke idiosyncratic lung responses in some individuals.

Nonspecific Inhalation Challenge Tests

Most of the techniques used to measure nonspecific bronchial reactivity pharmacologically involve the inhalation of an aerosol containing a known bronchoconstrictive agent. Methacholine is the agent of choice, and its use is summarized in an American Thoracic Society statement.[221] Inhalation is begun with saline and then a weak concentration or dose of agonist. The dose is progressively increased and an index of airway narrowing is measured at each step so that a dose-response relationship can be constructed.

A variety of techniques for delivering agonists, measuring the response, and expressing the results have been developed. The most widely used and carefully standardized involves nebulized methacholine delivered with a facemask during tidal breathing; 2-minute inhalations of increasing concentrations of the agonist are followed by measurements of FEV_1. The test is stopped when there is at least a 20% fall in FEV_1 or when the highest concentration of agonist is reached. The level of nonspecific reactivity is calculated as the concentration of inhaled agonist that results in a 20% fall in FEV_1 (PC_{20}).[222] In stable patients, measurements show remarkable reproducibility over time.

PC_{20} is lower than 8 mg/mL in currently symptomatic asthmatic patients, whereas in individuals who have normal pulmonary function and no history of pulmonary disease, it is usually greater than 16 mg/mL. These values allow clear separation of patients who have reactive airway disease from normal individuals, although patients who have chronic COPD, cystic fibrosis, or other chronic airway diseases may have intermediate values. Thus, in doubtful cases, the test can substantiate a diagnosis of asthma and is particularly helpful in patients whose baseline spirometry is normal or whose primary complaint is cough. In patients who have asthma, measurements of bronchial reactivity correlate well with the severity of symptoms and the need for medication.[222]

Bronchial reactivity can change over time; for example, intensive therapy can result in a decrease in nonspecific bronchial reactivity, whereas exposure to allergens or occupational sensitizers can increase it. Serial measurements of PC_{20} can be obtained to adjust the intensity of treatment, assess its efficacy, and gauge the detrimental effect of exposure.[223]

An alternative method of measuring airway responsiveness is to use an indirect stimulus, that is, an agent that releases bronchoconstricting mediators from airway cells. In addition to testing the responsiveness of smooth muscle, this test assesses the intermediate cells that mediate its action. Agents used for this purpose include ultrasonically nebulized hypertonic or hypotonic saline aerosols, mannitol, and adenosine monophosphate.[224,225,225a]

Specific Inhalation Challenge Tests

Specific inhalation challenge tests are performed in individuals who have or are suspected of having allergy or sensitivity to specific agents. They are less well standardized than nonspecific tests; in addition, they are time-consuming and can induce severe and prolonged responses that can be hazardous. For these reasons, these tests are rarely indicated in clinical practice and should be reserved for special cases being investigated in larger centers with experts in the methods. Inhalation challenge testing with agents suspected of causing allergic alveolitis or occupational asthma, however, may be important in establishing proof of specific sensitivity to these agents and may be required for compensation purposes.

Exercise-Induced Bronchoconstriction and Isocapnic Hyperventilation

With the demonstration that the bronchoconstriction associated with exercise is caused by breathing cool, dry air, techniques have been developed to measure the bronchial responsiveness to such air during isocapnic hyperventilation.[226] Patients are asked to hyperventilate from a source of dry air, either cold or at room temperature, and isocapnia is maintained by adding carbon dioxide to the inspired gas to maintain a constant end-tidal carbon dioxide content. Expiratory flow is measured with progressively increasing levels of hyperventilation, and the level of ventilation or the calculated respiratory heat loss that produces a given drop in FEV_1 can be calculated in a fashion similar to the way PC_{20} is calculated.

Expired Nitric Oxide Concentration

Analysis of expired concentrations of gases other than O_2 and CO_2 is a "lung function" test that has recently been developed. Most promising is the use of expired concentrations of NO. Standards for the measurement of expired NO have been proposed by the American Thoracic Society.[226a] Expired NO is elevated in asthmatic patients and decreases to normal levels when treatment brings asthma under control. It has been suggested that expired NO is a marker of the activity of the allergic inflammatory reaction characteristic of asthma.[227]

REFERENCES

1. Lundback B, Stjernberg N, Nystrom L, et al: Epidemiology of respiratory symptoms, lung function and important determinants. Report from the Obstructive Lung Disease in Northern Sweden Project. Tuber Lung Dis 75:116-126, 1994.
2. Brown CA, Crombie IK, Smith WC, et al: The impact of quitting smoking on symptoms of chronic bronchitis: Results of the Scottish Heart Health Study. Thorax 46:112-116, 1991.
3. Xu X, Wang L: Association of indoor and outdoor particulate level with chronic respiratory illness. Am Rev Respir Dis 148:1516-1522, 1993.
4. Sherman CB, Xu X, Speizer FE, et al: Longitudinal lung function decline in subjects with respiratory symptoms. Am Rev Respir Dis 146:855-859, 1992.
5. Cullinan P: Persistent cough and sputum: Prevalence and clinical characteristics in south east England. Respir Med 86:143-149, 1992.
6. Haider AW, Larson MG, O'Donnell CJ, et al: The association of chronic cough with the risk of myocardial infarction: The Framingham Heart Study. Am J Med 106:279-284, 1999.
7. Sin DD, Man SF: Why are patients with chronic obstructive pulmonary disease at increased risk of cardiovascular diseases? The potential role of systemic inflammation in chronic obstructive pulmonary disease. Circulation 107:1514-1519, 2003.
8. Leith D, Butler J, Sneddon S, et al: Cough. In Fishman A, Macklem P, Meade J (eds): Handbook of Physiology. Section 3, The Respiratory System. Vol 3, Mechanics of Breathing, Part 1. Bethesda, MD, American Physiological Society, 1986.
9. Irwin RS, Madison JM: The persistently troublesome cough. Am J Respir Crit Care Med 165:1469-1474, 2002.
10. Irwin RS, Boulet LP, Cloutier MM, et al: Managing cough as a defense mechanism and as a symptom. A consensus panel report of the American College of Chest Physicians. Chest 114:133S-181S, 1998.
11. Gonzales R, Sande MA: Uncomplicated acute bronchitis. Ann Intern Med 133:981-991, 2000.
12. Postels-Multani S, Schmitt HJ, Wirsing von Konig CH, et al: Symptoms and complications of pertussis in adults. Infection 23:139-142, 1995.
13. von Konig CH, Halperin S, Riffelmann M, et al: Pertussis of adults and infants. Lancet Infect Dis 2:744-750, 2002.
14. Santiago S, Tobias J, Williams AJ: A reappraisal of the causes of hemoptysis. Arch Intern Med 151:2449-2451, 1991.
15. Hirshberg B, Biran I, Glazer M, et al: Hemoptysis: Etiology, evaluation, and outcome in a tertiary referral hospital. Chest 112:440-444, 1997.
16. Yaacob I, Harun Z, Ahmad Z: Fibreoptic bronchoscopy—a Malaysian experience. Singapore Med J 32:26-28, 1991.
17. Weaver LJ, Solliday N, Cugell DW: Selection of patients with hemoptysis for fiberoptic bronchoscopy. Chest 76:7-10, 1979.
18. O'Neil KM, Lazarus AA: Hemoptysis. Indications for bronchoscopy. Arch Intern Med 151:171-174, 1991.
19. McGuinness G, Beacher JR, Harkin TJ, et al: Hemoptysis: Prospective high-resolution CT/bronchoscopic correlation. Chest 105:1155-1162, 1994.
20. Lederle FA, Nichol KL, Parenti CM: Bronchoscopy to evaluate hemoptysis in older men with nonsuspicious chest roentgenograms. Chest 95:1043-1047, 1989.
21. Bobrowitz ID, Ramakrishna S, Shim YS: Comparison of medical v surgical treatment of major hemoptysis. Arch Intern Med 143:1343-1346, 1983.
22. Corey R, Hla KM: Major and massive hemoptysis: Reassessment of conservative management. Am J Med Sci 294:301-309, 1987.
23. Stoller J: Diagnosis and management of massive hemoptysis: A review. Respir Care 37:564, 1992.
24. Wise CM: Chest wall syndromes. Curr Opin Rheumatol 6:197-202, 1994.
25. Miller AJ, Texidor TA: The "precordial catch," a syndrome of anterior chest pain. Ann Intern Med 51:461-467, 1959.
26. Dorland's Illustrated Medical Dictionary. Philadelphia, WB Saunders, 1994.
27. Mahler DA, Harver A, Lentine T, et al: Descriptors of breathlessness in cardiorespiratory diseases. Am J Respir Crit Care Med 154:1357-1363, 1996.
28. DePaso WJ, Winterbauer RH, Lusk JA, et al: Chronic dyspnea unexplained by history, physical examination, chest roentgenogram, and spirometry. Analysis of a seven-year experience. Chest 100:1293-1299, 1991.
29. Smoller JW, Pollack MH, Otto MW, et al: Panic anxiety, dyspnea, and respiratory disease. Theoretical and clinical considerations. Am J Respir Crit Care Med 154:6-17, 1996.
30. Saisch SG, Wessely S, Gardner WN: Patients with acute hyperventilation presenting to an inner-city emergency department. Chest 110:952-957, 1996.
31. Mahler DA, Wells CK: Evaluation of clinical methods for rating dyspnea. Chest 93:580-586, 1988.
32. Guyatt GH, Townsend M, Keller J, et al: Measuring functional status in chronic lung disease: Conclusions from a randomized control trial. Respir Med 85(Suppl B):17-21, discussion 33-37, 1991.
33. Stoller JK, Ferranti R, Feinstein AR: Further specification and evaluation of a new clinical index for dyspnea. Am Rev Respir Dis 134:1129-1134, 1986.
34. Meek P, Schwartzman R, Adams L, et al: Dyspnea: Mechanisms, assessment, and management: A consensus statement. Am J Respir Crit Care Med 159:321, 1999.
35. Zeldis SM: Dyspnea during pregnancy. Distinguishing cardiac from pulmonary causes. Clin Chest Med 13:567-585, 1992.
36. Mercho N, Stoller JK, White RD, et al: Right-to-left interatrial shunt causing platypnea after pneumonectomy. A recent experience and diagnostic value of dynamic magnetic resonance imaging. Chest 105:931-933, 1994.
37. Byrd RP Jr, Lopez PR, Joyce BW, et al: Platypnea, orthodeoxia and cirrhosis. J Ky Med Assoc 90:189-192, 1992.
38. Guyatt GH, Berman LB, Townsend M, et al: A measure of quality of life for clinical trials in chronic lung disease. Thorax 42:773-778, 1987.
39. Guyatt GH, King DR, Feeny DH, et al: Generic and specific measurement of health-related quality of life in a clinical trial of respiratory rehabilitation. J Clin Epidemiol 52:187-192, 1999.
40. Juniper EF, Guyatt GH, Epstein RS, et al: Evaluation of impairment of health related quality of life in asthma: Development of a questionnaire for use in clinical trials. Thorax 47:76-83, 1992.
41. Jones PW, Quirk FH, Baveystock CM, et al: A self-completed measure of health status for chronic airflow limitation. The St. George's Respiratory Questionnaire. Am Rev Respir Dis 145:1321-1327, 1992.
42. Van Der Molen T, Willemse BW, Schokker S, et al: Development, validity and responsiveness of the Clinical COPD Questionnaire. Health Qual Life Outcomes 1:13, 2003.
43. Harber P, Tashkin D, Shimozaki S, et al: Veracity of disability claimants' self-reports of current smoking status. Comparison of carboxyhemoglobin levels from disability claimant and reference population. Chest 93:561-563, 1988.

44. Spiteri MA, Cook DG, Clarke SW: Reliability of eliciting physical signs in examination of the chest. Lancet 1:873-875, 1988.

45. Garcia-Pachon E: Paradoxical Movement of the Lateral Rib Margin (Hoover Sign) for Detecting Obstructive Airway Disease. Chest 122:651-655, 2002.

46. Sapira JD: About egophony. Chest 108:865-867, 1995.

47. Jones FL Jr: Poor breath sounds with good voice sounds. A sign of bronchial stenosis. Chest 93:312-313, 1988.

48. Mikami R, Murao M, Cugell DW, et al: International Symposium on Lung Sounds. Synopsis of proceedings. Chest 92:342-345, 1987.

49. Pulmonary terms and symbols. A report of the ACCP-STS Joint Committee on Pulmonary Nomenclature. Chest 67:583-593, 1975.

50. Kiyokawa H, Greenberg M, Shirota K, et al: Auditory Detection of Simulated Crackles in Breath Sounds. Chest 119:1886, 2001.

51. King DK, Thompson BT, Johnson DC: Wheezing on maximal forced exhalation in the diagnosis of atypical asthma. Lack of sensitivity and specificity. Ann Intern Med 110:451-455, 1989.

52. Hamman L: Spontaneous mediastinal emphysema. Bull Johns Hopkins Hosp 64:1, 1939.

53. Clarke S, Barnsley L, Peters M, et al: Hypertrophic pulmonary osteoarthropathy without clubbing of the digits. Skeletal Radiol 30:652, 2001.

54. Carcassi U: History of hypertrophic osteoarthropathy (HOA). Clin Exp Rheumatol 10(Suppl 7):3-7, 1992.

55. Racoceanu SN, Mendlowitz M, Suck AF, et al: Digital capillary blood flow in clubbing. ^{85}Kr studies in hereditary and acquired cases. Ann Intern Med 75:933-935, 1971.

56. Fara EF, Baughman RP: A study of capillary morphology in the digits of patients with acquired clubbing. Am Rev Respir Dis 140:1063-1066, 1989.

57. Martinez-Lavin M: Pathogenesis of hypertrophic osteoarthropathy. Clin Exp Rheumatol 10(Suppl 7):49-50, 1992.

58. Hojo S, Fujita J, Yamadori I, et al: Hepatocyte growth factor and digital clubbing. Intern Med 36:44-46, 1997.

59. Shneerson JM: Digital clubbing and hypertrophic osteoarthropathy: The underlying mechanisms. Br J Dis Chest 75:113-131, 1981.

60. Sridhar KS, Lobo CF, Altman RD: Digital clubbing and lung cancer. Chest 114:1535-1537, 1998.

61. Martin L, Khalil H: How much reduced hemoglobin is necessary to generate central cyanosis? Chest 97:182-185, 1990.

62. Honeybourne D, Babb J, Bowie P, et al: British Thoracic Society guidelines on diagnostic flexible bronchoscopy. Thorax 56(Suppl 1):i11, 2001.

63. Wood-Baker R, Burdon J, McGregor A, et al: Fibre-optic bronchoscopy in adults: A position paper of the Thoracic Society of Australia and New Zealand. Intern Med J 31:479-487, 2001.

64. Seijo LM, Sterman DH: Interventional pulmonology. N Engl J Med 344:740-749, 2001.

65. Burgher L, Jones F, Patterson J, et al: Guidelines for fiberoptic bronchoscopy in adults. Am Rev Respir Dis 136:1066, 1987.

66. Seijo LM, Sterman DH: Interventional Pulmonology. New Engl J Med 344:740, 2001.

67. Dweik RA, Stoller JK: Role of Bronchoscopy in Massive Hemoptysis. Clin Chest Med 20:89-105, 1999.

68. Matot I, Kramer MR: Sedation in outpatient bronchoscopy. Resp Med 94:1145-1153, 2000.

69. Cowl CT, Prakash UB, Kruger BR: The Role of Anticholinergics in Bronchoscopy. Chest 118:188-192, 2000.

70. Pue CA, Pacht ER: Complications of fiberoptic bronchoscopy at a university hospital. Chest 107:430-432, 1995.

71. Prakash UB, Offord KP, Stubbs SE: Bronchoscopy in North America: The ACCP Survey. Chest 100:1668-1675, 1991.

72. Young JA: ACP Broadsheet No 140: July 1993. Techniques in pulmonary cytopathology. J Clin Pathol 46:589-595, 1993.

73. Ng AB, Horak GC: Factors significant in the diagnostic accuracy of lung cytology in bronchial washing and sputum samples. II. Sputum samples. Acta Cytol 27:397-402, 1983.

74. Saccomanno G, Saunders RP, Ellis H, et al: Concentration of carcinoma or atypical cells in sputum. Acta Cytol 63:305-310, 1963.

75. Calabretto ML, Giol L, Sulfaro S: Diagnostic utility of cell-block from bronchial washing in pulmonary neoplasms. Diagn Cytopathol 15:191-192, 1996.

76. Bardales RH, Powers CN, Frierson HF Jr, et al: Exfoliative respiratory cytology in the diagnosis of leukemias and lymphomas in the lung. Diagn Cytopathol 14:108-113, 1996.

77. Ng AB, Horak GC: Factors significant in the diagnostic accuracy of lung cytology in bronchial washing and sputum samples. I. Bronchial washings. Acta Cytol 27:391-396, 1983.

78. Gledhill A, Bates C, Henderson D, et al: Sputum cytology: A limited role. J Clin Pathol 50:566-568, 1997.

79. Goldberg-Kahn B, Healy JC, Bishop JW: The cost of diagnosis: A comparison of four different strategies in the workup of solitary radiographic lung lesions. Chest 111:870-876, 1997.

80. Steffee CH, Segletes LA, Geisinger KR: Changing cytologic and histologic utilization patterns in the diagnosis of 515 primary lung malignancies. Cancer 81:105-115, 1997.

81. Raab SS, Hornberger J, Raffin T: The importance of sputum cytology in the diagnosis of lung cancer: A cost-effectiveness analysis. Chest 112:937-945, 1997.

82. Johnston WW: Ten years of respiratory cytopathology at Duke University Medical Center. III. The significance of inconclusive cytopathologic diagnoses during the years 1970 to 1974. Acta Cytol 26:759-766, 1982.

83. Lawther RE, Graham AN, McCluggage WG, et al: Pulmonary infarct cytologically mimicking adenocarcinoma of the lung. Ann Thorac Surg 73:1964-1965, 2002.

84. Koss LG, Melamed MR, Mayer K: The effect of busulfan on human epithelia. Am J Clin Pathol 44:385-397, 1965.

85. Sokolova IA, Bubendorf L, O'Hare A, et al: A fluorescence in situ hybridization–based assay for improved detection of lung cancer cells in bronchial washing specimens. Cancer 96:306-315, 2002.

86. Arvanitis DA, Papadakis E, Zafiropoulos A, et al: Fractional allele loss is a valuable marker for human lung cancer detection in sputum. Lung Cancer 40:55-66, 2003.

87. Palcic B, Garner DM, Beveridge J, et al: Increase of sensitivity of sputum cytology using high-resolution image cytometry: Field study results. Cytometry 50:168-176, 2002.

88. Kern WH, Schweizer CW: Sputum cytology of metastatic carcinoma of the lung. Acta Cytol 20:514-520, 1976.

89. Pavord ID, Sterk PJ, Hargreave FE, et al: Clinical applications of assessment of airway inflammation using induced sputum. Eur Respir J Suppl 37:40S-43S, 2002.

90. Tarrand JJ, Lichterfeld M, Warraich I, et al: Diagnosis of invasive septate mold infections. A correlation of microbiological culture and histologic or cytologic examination. Am J Clin Pathol 119:854-858, 2003.

91. Corwin RW, Irwin RS: The lipid-laden alveolar macrophage as a marker of aspiration in parenchymal lung disease. Am Rev Respir Dis 132:576-581, 1985.

92. Mimoz O, Edouard A, Beydon L, et al: Contribution of bronchoalveolar lavage to the diagnosis of posttraumatic pulmonary fat embolism. Intensive Care Med 21:973-980, 1995.

93. Wheeler TM, Johnson EH, Coughlin D, et al: The sensitivity of detection of asbestos bodies in sputa and bronchial washings. Acta Cytol 32:647-650, 1988.

94. Paredi P, Kharitonov SA, Barnes PJ: Analysis of expired air for oxidation products. Am J Respir Crit Care Med 166:S31-S37, 2002.

95. Effros RM, Biller J, Foss B, et al: A simple method for estimating respiratory solute dilution in exhaled breath condensates. Am J Respir Crit Care Med 168:1500-1505, 2003.

96. Taskinen EI, Tukiainen PS, Alitalo RL, et al: Bronchoalveolar lavage. Cytological techniques and interpretation of the cellular profiles. Pathol Annu 29(Pt 2):121-155, 1994.

97. Kvale PA: Bronchoscopic biopsies and bronchoalveolar lavage. Chest Surg Clin N Am 6:205-222, 1996.

98. Merchant RK, Schwartz DA, Helmers RA, et al: Bronchoalveolar lavage cellularity. The distribution in normal volunteers. Am Rev Respir Dis 146:448-453, 1992.

99. Smith DL, Deshazo RD: Bronchoalveolar lavage in asthma. An update and perspective. Am Rev Respir Dis 148:523-532, 1993.

100. Hattotuwa K, Gamble EA, O'Shaughnessy T, et al: Safety of bronchoscopy, biopsy, and BAL in research patients with COPD. Chest 122:1909-1912, 2002.

101. Heyland DK, Cook DJ, Marshall J, et al: The Clinical Utility of Invasive Diagnostic Techniques in the Setting of Ventilator-Associated Pneumonia. Chest 115:1076-1084, 1999.

102. Krause A, Hohberg B, Heine F, et al: Cytokines derived from alveolar macrophages induce fever after bronchoscopy and bronchoalveolar lavage. Am J Respir Crit Care Med 155:1793-1797, 1997.

103. Krueger JJ, Sayre VA, Karetzky MS: Bronchoalveolar lavage–induced pneumothorax. Chest 94:440-441, 1988.

104. Strumpf IJ, Feld MK, Cornelius MJ, et al: Safety of fiberoptic bronchoalveolar lavage in evaluation of interstitial lung disease. Chest 80:268-271, 1981.

105. Montravers P, Gauzit R, Dombret MC, et al: Cardiopulmonary effects of bronchoalveolar lavage in critically ill patients. Chest 104:1541-1547, 1993.

106. Gurney JW, Harrison WC, Sears K, et al: Bronchoalveolar lavage: Radiographic manifestations. Radiology 163:71-74, 1987.

107. Breuer R, Lossos IS, Lafair JS, et al: Utility of bronchoalveolar lavage in the assessment of diffuse pulmonary infiltrates in non-AIDS immunocompromised patients. Respir Med 84:313-316, 1990.

108. Rust M, Albera C, Carratu L, et al: The clinical use of BAL in patients with pulmonary infections. Eur Respir J 3:954-955, 961-969, 1990.

109. Pirozynski M: Bronchoalveolar lavage in the diagnosis of peripheral, primary lung cancer. Chest 102:372-374, 1992.

110. Bingisser R, Kaplan V, Zollinger A, et al: Whole-lung lavage in alveolar proteinosis by a modified lavage technique. Chest 113:1718-1719, 1998.

111. Light RW, Erozan YS, Ball WC Jr: Cells in pleural fluid. Their value in differential diagnosis. Arch Intern Med 132:854-860, 1973.

112. Kutty CP, Remeniuk E, Varkey B: Malignant-appearing cells in pleural effusion due to pancreatitis: Case report and literature review. Acta Cytol 25:412-416, 1981.

113. Spieler P: The cytologic diagnosis of tuberculosis in pleural effusions. Acta Cytol 23:374-379, 1979.

114. Rubins JB, Rubins HB: Etiology and prognostic significance of eosinophilic pleural effusions. A prospective study. Chest 110:1271-1274, 1996.

115. vanSonnenberg E, Goodacre BW, Wittich GR, et al: Image-guided 25-gauge needle biopsy for thoracic lesions: Diagnostic feasibility and safety. Radiology 227:414-418, 2003.

116. Oikonomou A, Matzinger FR, Seely JM, et al: Ultrathin needle (25 G) aspiration lung biopsy: Diagnostic accuracy and complication rates. Eur Radiol 14:375-382, 2004.

117. Tarver RD, Conces DJ Jr: Interventional chest radiology. Radiol Clin North Am 32:689-709, 1994.

118. Klein JS, Salomon G, Stewart EA: Transthoracic needle biopsy with a coaxially placed 20-gauge automated cutting needle: Results in 122 patients. Radiology 198:715-720, 1996.

119. Yang GC, Alvarez II: Ultrafast Papanicolaou stain. An alternative preparation for fine needle aspiration cytology. Acta Cytol 39:55-60, 1995.

120. Logrono R, Kurtycz DF, Sproat IA, et al: Multidisciplinary approach to deep-seated lesions requiring radiologically-guided fine-needle aspiration. Diagn Cytopathol 18:338-342, 1998.

121. Sokolowski JW Jr, Burgher LW, Jones FL Jr, et al: Guidelines for percutaneous transthoracic needle biopsy. Am Rev Respir Dis 140:255-256, 1989.

122. Zarbo RJ, Fenoglio-Preiser CM: Interinstitutional database for comparison of performance in lung fine-needle aspiration cytology. A College of American Pathologists Q-Probe Study of 5264 cases with histologic correlation. Arch Pathol Lab Med 116:463-470, 1992.

123. Li H, Boiselle PM, Shepard JO, et al: Diagnostic accuracy and safety of CT-guided percutaneous needle aspiration biopsy of the lung: Comparison of small and large pulmonary nodules. AJR Am J Roentgenol 167:105-109, 1996.

124. Westcott JL, Rao N, Colley DP: Transthoracic needle biopsy of small pulmonary nodules. Radiology 202:97-103, 1997.

125. Perlmutt LM, Johnston WW, Dunnick NR: Percutaneous transthoracic needle aspiration: A review. AJR Am J Roentgenol 152:451-455, 1989.

126. Moore EH, Shepard JA, McLoud TC, et al: Positional precautions in needle aspiration lung biopsy. Radiology 175:733-735, 1990.

127. Miller KS, Fish GB, Stanley JH, et al: Prediction of pneumothorax rate in percutaneous needle aspiration of the lung. Chest 93:742-745, 1988.

128. Omenaas E, Moerkve O, Thomassen L, et al: Cerebral air embolism after transthoracic aspiration with a 0.6 mm (23 gauge) needle. Eur Respir J 2:908-910, 1989.

129. Nagasaka T, Nakashima N, Nunome H: Needle tract implantation of thymoma after transthoracic needle biopsy. J Clin Pathol 46:278-279, 1993.

130. Cazzadori A, Di Perri G, Marocco S, et al: Tuberculous pleurisy after percutaneous needle biopsy of a pulmonary nodule. Respir Med 88:477-478, 1994.

131. Layfield LJ, Coogan A, Johnston WW, et al: Transthoracic fine needle aspiration biopsy. Sensitivity in relation to guidance technique and lesion size and location. Acta Cytol 40:687-690, 1996.

132. Silverman JF: Inflammatory and neoplastic processes of the lung: Differential diagnosis and pitfalls in FNA biopsies. Diagn Cytopathol 13:448-462, 1995.

133. Raab SS, Slagel DD, Hughes JH, et al: Sensitivity and cost-effectiveness of fine-needle aspiration with immunocytochemistry in the evaluation of patients with a pulmonary malignancy and a history of cancer. Arch Pathol Lab Med 121:695-700, 1997.

134. Fraser RS: Transthoracic needle aspiration. The benign diagnosis. Arch Pathol Lab Med 115:751-761, 1991.

135. Moulton JS, Moore PT: Coaxial percutaneous biopsy technique with automated biopsy devices: Value in improving accuracy and negative predictive value. Radiology 186:515-522, 1993.

136. Shim JJ, Cheong HJ, Kang EY, et al: Nested polymerase chain reaction for detection of Mycobacterium tuberculosis in solitary pulmonary nodules. Chest 113:20-24, 1998.

137. Dorca J, Manresa F, Esteban L, et al: Efficacy, safety, and therapeutic relevance of transthoracic aspiration with ultrathin needle in nonventilated nosocomial pneumonia. Am J Respir Crit Care Med 151:1491-1496, 1995.

138. Harrow EM, Abi-Saleh W, Blum J, et al: The utility of transbronchial needle aspiration in the staging of bronchogenic carcinoma. Am J Respir Crit Care Med 161:601-607, 2000.

139. Dasgupta A, Mehta AC: Transbronchial needle aspiration. An underused diagnostic technique. Clin Chest Med 20:39-51, 1999.

140. White CS, Weiner EA, Patel P, et al: Transbronchial needle aspiration: Guidance with CT fluoroscopy. Chest 118:1630-1638, 2000.

141. Reichenberger F, Weber J, Tamm M, et al: The value of transbronchial needle aspiration in the diagnosis of peripheral pulmonary lesions. Chest 116:704-708, 1999.

142. Harrow EM, Wang KP: The staging of lung cancer by bronchoscopic transbronchial needle aspiration. Chest Surg Clin N Am 6:223-235, 1996.

143. Vansteenkiste J, Lacquet LM, Demedts M, et al: Transcarinal needle aspiration biopsy in the staging of lung cancer. Eur Respir J 7:265-268, 1994.

144. Shure D: Transbronchial biopsy and needle aspiration. Chest 95:1130-1138, 1989.

145. Harrow E, Halber M, Hardy S, et al: Bronchoscopic and roentgenographic correlates of a positive transbronchial needle aspiration in the staging of lung cancer. Chest 100:1592-1596, 1991.

146. Chin R Jr, McCain TW, Lucia MA, et al: Transbronchial needle aspiration in diagnosing and staging lung cancer: How many aspirates are needed? Am J Respir Crit Care Med 166:377-381, 2002.

147. Gress FG, Savides TJ, Sandler A, et al: Endoscopic ultrasonography, fine-needle aspiration biopsy guided by endoscopic ultrasonography, and computed tomography in the preoperative staging of non–small-cell lung cancer: A comparison study. Ann Intern Med 127:604-612, 1997.

148. Kefalides PT, Savides TJ: Evaluation of mediastinal lymphadenopathy with endoscopic US-guided fine-needle aspiration biopsy. Gastrointest Endosc 55:294-296, discussion 296-297, 2002.

149. Catalano MF, Rosenblatt ML, Chak A, et al: Endoscopic ultrasound-guided fine needle aspiration in the diagnosis of mediastinal masses of unknown origin. Am J Gastroenterol 97:2559-2565, 2002.

150. Bhutani MS: Transesophageal endoscopic ultrasound-guided mediastinal lymph node aspiration: Does the end justify the means? Chest 117:298-301, 2000.

151. Popovich J Jr, Kvale PA, Eichenhorn MS, et al: Diagnostic accuracy of multiple biopsies from flexible fiberoptic bronchoscopy. A comparison of central versus peripheral carcinoma. Am Rev Respir Dis 125:521-523, 1982.

152. de Fenoyl O, Capron F, Lebeau B, et al: Transbronchial biopsy without fluoroscopy: A five year experience in outpatients. Thorax 44:956-959, 1989.

153. Hernandez Blasco L, Sanchez Hernandez IM, Villena Garrido V, et al: Safety of the transbronchial biopsy in outpatients. Chest 99:562-565, 1991.

154. Liao WY, Chen MZ, Chang YL, et al: US-guided transthoracic cutting biopsy for peripheral thoracic lesions less than 3 cm in diameter. Radiology 217:685-691, 2000.

155. Staroselsky AN, Schwarz Y, Man A, et al: Additional information from percutaneous cutting needle biopsy following fine-needle aspiration in the diagnosis of chest lesions. Chest 113:1522-1525, 1998.

156. Zwischenberger JB, Savage C, Alpard SK, et al: Mediastinal transthoracic needle and core lymph node biopsy: Should it replace mediastinoscopy? Chest 121:1165-1170, 2002.

157. Salazar AM, Westcott JL: The role of transthoracic needle biopsy for the diagnosis and staging of lung cancer. Clin Chest Med 14:99-110, 1993.

158. Dennie CJ, Matzinger FR, Marriner JR, et al: Transthoracic needle biopsy of the lung: Results of early discharge in 506 outpatients. Radiology 219:247-251, 2001.

159. Morgenroth A, Pfeuffer HP, Austgen M, et al: Six years' experience with perthoracic core needle biopsy in pulmonary lesions. Thorax 44:177-183, 1989.

160. Niden AH, Salem F: A safe high-yield technique for cutting needle biopsy of the lung in patients with diffuse lung disease. Chest 111:1615-1621, 1997.

161. Mathur PN, Astoul P, Boutin C: Medical thoracoscopy. Technical details. Clin Chest Med 16:479-486, 1995.

162. Walker WS, Craig SR: Video-assisted thoracoscopic pulmonary surgery—current status and potential evolution. Eur J Cardiothorac Surg 10:161-167, 1996.

163. Harris RJ, Kavuru MS, Rice TW, et al: The diagnostic and therapeutic utility of thoracoscopy. A review. Chest 108:828-841, 1995.

164. Colt HG: Thoracoscopy: Window to the pleural space. Chest 116:1409-1415, 1999.

165. Loddenkemper R: Thoracoscopy—state of the art. Eur Respir J 11:213-221, 1998.

166. Menzies R, Charbonneau M: Thoracoscopy for the diagnosis of pleural disease. Ann Intern Med 114:271-276, 1991.

167. Mouroux J, Venissac N, Alifano M: Combined video-assisted mediastinoscopy and video-assisted thoracoscopy in the management of lung cancer. Ann Thorac Surg 72:1698-1704, 2001.

168. Kern JA, Daniel TM, Tribble CG, et al: Thoracoscopic diagnosis and treatment of mediastinal masses. Ann Thorac Surg 56:92-96, 1993.

169. Roviaro G, Varoli F, Nucca O, et al: Videothoracoscopic approach to primary mediastinal pathology. Chest 117:1179-1183, 2000.

170. Liu DW, Liu HP, Lin PJ, et al: Video-assisted thoracic surgery in treatment of chest trauma. J Trauma 42:670-674, 1997.

171. Jaklitsch MT, DeCamp MM Jr, Liptay MJ, et al: Video-assisted thoracic surgery in the elderly. A review of 307 cases. Chest 110:751-758, 1996.

172. Gaensler EA, Carrington CB: Open biopsy for chronic diffuse infiltrative lung disease: Clinical, roentgenographic, and physiological correlations in 502 patients. Ann Thorac Surg 30:411-426, 1980.

173. Wall CP, Gaensler EA, Carrington CB, et al: Comparison of transbronchial and open biopsies in chronic infiltrative lung diseases. Am Rev Respir Dis 123:280-285, 1981.

174. Hammoud ZT, Anderson RC, Meyers BF, et al: The current role of mediastinoscopy in the evaluation of thoracic disease. J Thorac Cardiovasc Surg 118:894-899, 1999.

175. Kirschner PA: Cervical mediastinoscopy. Chest Surg Clin N Am 6:1-20, 1996.

176. Freixinet Gilart J, Garcia PG, de Castro FR, et al: Extended cervical mediastinoscopy in the staging of bronchogenic carcinoma. Ann Thorac Surg 70:1641-1643, 2000.

177. Olak J: Parasternal mediastinotomy (Chamberlain procedure). Chest Surg Clin N Am 6:31-40, 1996.

178. Brantigan JW, Brantigan CO, Brantigan OC: Biopsy of nonpalpable scalene lymph nodes in carcinoma of the lung. Am Rev Respir Dis 107:962-974, 1973.

179. Lee JD, Ginsberg RJ: Lung cancer staging: The value of ipsilateral scalene lymph node biopsy performed at mediastinoscopy. Ann Thorac Surg 62:338-341, 1996.

180. Hsu WH, Chiang CD, Hsu JY, et al: Value of ultrasonically guided needle biopsy of pleural masses: An under-utilized technique. J Clin Ultrasound 25:119-125, 1997.

181. Kirsch CM, Kroe DM, Jensen WA, et al: A modified Abrams needle biopsy technique. Chest 108:982-986, 1995.

182. Escudero Bueno C, Garcia Clemente M, Cuesta Castro B, et al: Cytologic and bacteriologic analysis of fluid and pleural biopsy specimens with Cope's needle. Study of 414 patients. Arch Intern Med 150:1190-1194, 1990.

183. Jimenez D, Perez-Rodriguez E, Diaz G, et al: Determining the optimal number of specimens to obtain with needle biopsy of the pleura. Respir Med 96:14-17, 2002.

184. Cary J, Huseby J, Culver B, et al: Variability in interpretation of pulmonary function tests. Chest 76:389-390, 1979.

185. Pennock BE, Rogers RM, McCaffree DR: Changes in measured spirometric indices. What is significant? Chest 80:97-99, 1981.

186. Hughes JA, Hutchison DC: Errors in the estimation of vital capacity from expiratory flow-volume curves in pulmonary emphysema. Br J Dis Chest 76:279-285, 1982.

187. Begin P, Peslin R: Plethysmographic measurements of thoracic gas volume. Back to the hypotheses. Bull Eur Physiopathol Respir 19:247-251, 1983.

188. O'Brien R, Drizd T: Roentgenographic determination of total lung capacity: Normal values from a national population survey. Am Rev Respir Dis 128:949-952, 1983.

189. Standardization of Spirometry, 1994 Update. American Thoracic Society. Am J Respir Crit Care Med 152:1107-1136, 1995.

190. ATS statement—Snowbird workshop on standardization of spirometry. Am Rev Respir Dis 119:831-838, 1979.

191. Peslin R, Bohadana A, Hannhart B, et al: Comparison of various methods for reading maximal expiratory flow-volume curves. Am Rev Respir Dis 119:271-277, 1979.
192. Suratt PM, Hooe DM, Owens DA, et al: Effect of maximal versus submaximal expiratory effort on spirometric values. Respiration 42:233-236, 1981.
193. Whitaker CJ, Chinn DJ, Lee WR: The statistical reliability of indices derived from the closing volume and flow volume traces. Bull Physiopathol Respir (Nancy) 14:237-247, 1979.
194. Lam S, Abboud RT, Chan-Yeung M, et al: Use of maximal expiratory flow-volume curves with air and helium-oxygen in the detection of ventilatory abnormalities in population surveys. Am Rev Respir Dis 123:234-237, 1981.
195. Rossoff LJ, Csima A, Zamel N: Reproducibility of maximum expiratory flow in severe chronic obstructive pulmonary disease. Bull Eur Physiopathol Respir 15:1129-1136, 1979.
196. Sourk RL, Nugent KM: Bronchodilator testing: Confidence intervals derived from placebo inhalations. Am Rev Respir Dis 128:153-157, 1983.
196a. O'Donnell DE, Lam M, Webb KA: Spirometric correlates of improvement in exercise performance after anticholinergic therapy in chronic obstructive pulmonary disease. Am J Respir Crit Care Med 160:542-549, 1999.
197. Russell NJ, Bagg LR, Dobrzynski J, et al: Clinical assessment of a rebreathing method for measuring pulmonary gas transfer. Thorax 38:212-215, 1983.
198. Cotton DJ, Newth CJ, Portner PM, et al: Measurement of single-breath CO diffusing capacity by continuous rapid CO analysis in man. J Appl Physiol 46:1149-1156, 1979.
199. Graham BL, Mink JT, Cotton DJ: Improved accuracy and precision of single-breath CO diffusing capacity measurements. J Appl Physiol 51:1306-1313, 1981.
199a. American Thoracic Society: Single-breath carbon monoxide diffusing capacity (transfer factor). Recommendations for a standard technique—1995 update. Am J Respir Crit Care Med 152:2185-2198, 1995.
200. Make B, Miller A, Epler G, et al: Single breath diffusing capacity in the industrial setting. Chest 82:351-356, 1982.
201. Siegler D, Zorab PA: The influence of lung volume on gas transfer in scoliosis. Br J Dis Chest 76:44-50, 1982.
202. Ayers LN, Ginsberg ML, Fein J, et al: Diffusing capacity, specific diffusing capacity and interpretation of diffusion defects. West J Med 123:255-264, 1975.
203. Mohsenifar Z, Brown HV, Schnitzer B, et al: The effect of abnormal levels of hematocrit on the single breath diffusing capacity. Lung 160:325-330, 1982.
204. Fisher JT, Cerny FJ: Characteristics of adjustment of lung diffusing capacity to work. J Appl Physiol 52:1124-1127, 1982.
205. Hallenborg C, Holden W, Menzel T, et al: The clinical usefulness of a screening test to detect static pulmonary blood using a multiple-breath analysis of diffusing capacity. Am Rev Respir Dis 119:349-356, 1979.
205a. ATS/ACCP statement on cardiopulmonary exercise testing. Am J Respir Crit Care Med 167:211-277, 2003.
206. O'Donnell DE, Revill SM, Webb KA: Dynamic hyperinflation and exercise intolerance in chronic obstructive pulmonary disease. Am J Respir Crit Care Med 164:770-777, 2001.
207. ATS statement: Guidelines for the six-minute walk test. Am J Respir Crit Care Med 166:111-117, 2002.
208. Knudson RJ, Kaltenborn WT: Evaluation of lung elastic recoil by exponential curve analysis. Respir Physiol 46:29-42, 1981.
209. Paré PD, Brooks LA, Bates J, et al: Exponential analysis of the lung pressure-volume curve as a predictor of pulmonary emphysema. Am Rev Respir Dis 126:54-61, 1982.
210. Mead J, Whittenberger J: Physical properties of human lungs measured during spontaneous respiration. J Appl Physiol 5:779, 1953.

211. Oostveen E, MacLeod D, Lorino H, et al: The forced oscillation technique in clinical practice: Methodology, recommendations and future developments. Eur Respir J 22:1026-1041, 2003.
212. Lopata M, Lourenco RV: Evaluation of respiratory control. Clin Chest Med 1:33-45, 1980.
213. Cherniack NS, Dempsey J, Fencl V, et al: Workshop on assessment of respiratory control in humans. I. Methods of measurement of ventilatory responses to hypoxia and hypercapnia. Am Rev Respir Dis 115:177-181, 1977.
214. Read DJ: A clinical method for assessing the ventilatory response to carbon dioxide. Australas Ann Med 16:20-32, 1967.
215. Rebuck AS, Slutsky A: Measurement of ventilatory responses to hypercapnia and hypoxia. In Hornbein T, Lenfant C (eds): Regulation of Breathing. Part II. Lung Biology in Health and Disease. New York, Marcel Dekker, 1981, p 745.
216. Whitelaw WA, Derenne JP, Milic-Emili J: Occlusion pressure as a measure of respiratory center output in conscious man. Respir Physiol 23:181-199, 1975.
217. Zackon H, Despas PJ, Anthonisen NR: Occlusion pressure responses in asthma and chronic obstructive pulmonary disease. Am Rev Respir Dis 114:917-927, 1976.
218. Milic-Emili J: Recent advances in clinical assessment of control of breathing. Lung 160:1, 1982.
219. Milic-Emili J, Whitelaw WA, Grassino A: Measurement and testing of respiratory drive. In Hornbein T, Lenfant C (eds): Regulation of Breathing. Part II. Lung Biology in Health and Disease. New York, Marcel Dekker, 1981, p 675.
220. Ringqvist T: The ventilatory capacity in healthy subjects. An analysis of causal factors with special reference to the respiratory forces. Scand J Clin Lab Invest Suppl 88:5-179, 1966.
221. Crapo RO, Casaburi R, Coates AL, et al: Guidelines for methacholine and exercise challenge testing—1999. This official statement of the American Thoracic Society was adopted by the ATS Board of Directors, July 1999. Am J Respir Crit Care Med 161:309-329, 2000.
222. Cockcroft DW, Killian DN, Mellon JJ, et al: Bronchial reactivity to inhaled histamine: A method and clinical survey. Clin Allergy 7:235-243, 1977.
223. Sont JK, Willems LN, Bel EH, et al: Clinical control and histopathologic outcome of asthma when using airway hyperresponsiveness as an additional guide to long-term treatment. The AMPUL Study Group. Am J Respir Crit Care Med 159:1043-1051, 1999.
224. Anderson SD, Schoeffel RE, Finney M: Evaluation of ultrasonically nebulised solutions for provocation testing in patients with asthma. Thorax 38:284-291, 1983.
225. Anderson SD, Brannan JD: Methods for "indirect" challenge tests including exercise, eucapnic voluntary hyperpnea, and hypertonic aerosols. Clin Rev Allergy Immunol 24:27-54, 2003.
225a. Spicuzza L, Polosa R: The role of adenosine as a novel bronchoprovocant in asthma. Curr Opin Allergy Clin Immunol 3:65-69, 2003.
226. O'Byrne PM, Ryan G, Morris M, et al: Asthma induced by cold air and its relation to nonspecific bronchial responsiveness to methacholine. Am Rev Respir Dis 125:281-285, 1982.
226a. Recommendations for standardized procedures for the on-line and off-line measurement of exhaled lower respiratory nitric oxide and nasal nitric oxide in adults and children—1999. This official statement of the American Thoracic Society was adopted by the ATS Board of Directors, July 1999. Am J Respir Crit Care Med 160:2104-2117, 1999.
227. Smith AD, Cowan JO, Filsell S, et al: Diagnosing asthma: Comparisons between exhaled nitric oxide measurements and conventional tests. Am J Respir Crit Care Med 169:473-478, 2004.

DEVELOPMENTAL AND METABOLIC LUNG DISEASE

For purposes of discussion, developmental anomalies of the trachea, lungs, and major pulmonary vessels can be divided into two groups, depending on the predominant anlage affected: (1) those originating in the primitive foregut or its derivative the lung bud (*bronchopulmonary or foregut anomalies*) and (2) those arising from the sixth aortic arch or venous radicles and their derivatives (*pulmonary vascular anomalies*). Despite the convenience of this division and the use of specific terms for various anatomic patterns of disease, it should be appreciated that considerable overlap exists between conditions in both groups[1,2] and that multiple lesions are occasionally identified in the same patient.[3-5] The presence of significant pathogenetic differences and the reliability of precise morphologic classification can thus be questioned.

For obvious reasons, most developmental abnormalities that affect the lungs are manifested at or soon after birth. However, occasional examples of most anomalies have been reported in adolescents or adults, and it is important for respiratory physicians to be aware of them, even if their practice does not include children. It is also important to recognize that abnormalities of pulmonary development and growth during childhood may have significant effects on pulmonary function in adult life.[6]

BRONCHOPULMONARY ANOMALIES

Pulmonary Agenesis, Aplasia, and Hypoplasia

Arrested development of the lung can be classified into three types: (1) *agenesis,* in which one or both lungs are completely absent, with no trace of bronchial or vascular supply or parenchymal tissue; (2) *aplasia,* in which all but a rudimentary bronchus that ends in a blind pouch is suppressed, with no evidence of pulmonary vasculature or parenchyma; and (3) *hypoplasia,* in which the gross morphology of the lung is essentially unremarkable but the number or size of airways, vessels, and alveoli is decreased. In practice, an etiologic, pathogenetic, and clinical distinction between agenesis and aplasia is seldom apparent, and the two conditions are usually considered together.[7] By contrast, hypoplasia is often associated with other congenital anomalies, many of which are thought to be important in pathogenesis, and it is likely that most of these cases represent a disease state that is qualitatively different from either agenesis or aplasia.

Pulmonary hypoplasia can be regarded as *primary* (without obvious associated etiologic factors) or *secondary* (when it occurs with other congenital anomalies that may be implicated in its pathogenesis). Typically, it involves the whole lung; when it affects only one lobe, it is often accompanied by anomalies of the ipsilateral pulmonary artery and anomalous pulmonary venous drainage (hypogenetic lung syndrome; see page 202).

Etiology and Pathogenesis

Agenesis/Aplasia. Unilateral pulmonary agenesis (aplasia) has occasionally been described in twins and infants who have chromosomal abnormalities, thus suggesting a genetic basis for the anomaly.[8] The abnormality has also been described in association with anomalies of the chest wall and skeleton or the ipsilateral aspect of the face,[8-10] which has led some to hypothesize an underlying abnormality in development of the aortic arches.[8,10]

Secondary Hypoplasia. Decreased volume of the ipsilateral hemithorax is the most frequent associated abnormality and can itself have several causes. The most common is a space-occupying mass within the pleural cavity, usually abdominal contents displaced through a congenital diaphragmatic hernia.[11] In addition, a variety of musculoskeletal deformities of the thoracic cage,[12] diaphragm,[13] and abdominal wall[14] have been associated; although these deformities may also act by reducing the size of the thoracic cavity, it is possible that decreased intrauterine respiratory movements caused by diminished chest wall compliance or decreased muscle mass may be important as well (see later).

Another relatively common group of developmental anomalies associated with pulmonary hypoplasia involves the kidney and urinary tract. Of these, Potter's syndrome (renal agenesis, abnormal facies, limb abnormalities, and pulmonary hypoplasia) is the most frequent. It has been suggested that the presence of oligohydramnios in these conditions leads to hypoplasia as a result of thoracic compression by the closely applied uterine wall.[12] Although this mechanism is theoretically possible, the occasional cases in which both renal and pulmonary abnormalities are present and amniotic fluid is either normal or excessive in amount suggest that other factors, such as loss of the ability of the lungs to retain their normally produced fluid, may be more important.[15,16] Because such fluid normally exerts positive pressure within the developing lung, deficiency of this fluid could theoretically result in the loss of an internal template about which the lung can form.

Pulmonary hypoplasia has also been shown to occur in animals subjected to intrauterine cervical cord injury[15] and bilateral section of the phrenic nerve.[17] As a result, it has been speculated that the central nervous system (CNS) may play an important role in lung development, possibly by maintaining normal fetal respiratory movements[18]; it is therefore conceivable that some neurologic abnormality could result in human pulmonary hypoplasia. It is also possible that a decrease in respiratory muscle movement is important in the hypoplasia associated with a deformed chest wall or diaphragmatic muscle dysfunction.

Primary Hypoplasia. The pathogenesis of primary hypoplasia is less clear than the secondary form.[12] By definition unassociated with other anomalies, it most likely represents an intrinsic defect in lung development. Conceivably, unrecognized abnormalities in CNS control of fetal respiratory movements might also be involved in some cases.

Pathologic Characteristics

Although the severity and type of changes vary among different cases, the most consistent finding in secondary pulmonary hypoplasia is a decrease in the number of airway generations, from about 50% to 75% of normal.[19-21] In addition, the number of alveoli is frequently decreased, estimated by one group of investigators to be about a third of normal.[21] This decreased number is often associated with a decrease in alveolar size. Some investigators have shown normal airway and alveolar maturation for gestational age; others have found an immature appearance.[19,22] Abnormalities of the pulmonary arterial system have also been identified and consist of decreased elastic tissue in the larger arteries, increased muscle in normally muscular arteries, and extension of muscle into normally nonmuscular arteries. The basis for the variation in morphologic findings may be related to the severity and cause of the hypoplasia, as well as the timing of the etiologic events that led to the anomaly.[23]

Radiologic Manifestations

The radiographic findings in cases of agenesis, aplasia, or severe hypoplasia are similar and principally characterized by total or almost total absence of aerated lung in one hemithorax (Fig. 5-1). The markedly reduced volume is indicated by approximation of the ribs, elevation of the ipsilateral hemidiaphragm, and shift of the mediastinum. In most cases, the contralateral lung is greatly overinflated and displaced, along with the anterior mediastinum, into the involved hemithorax[24]; this displacement of air-containing lung to the side of the agenesis may lead to some confusion in diagnosis. CT may be required to establish the degree of underdevelopment[25] or to differentiate agenesis from other conditions that may mimic it closely radiographically, including total atelectasis from any cause, severe bronchiectasis with collapse, and

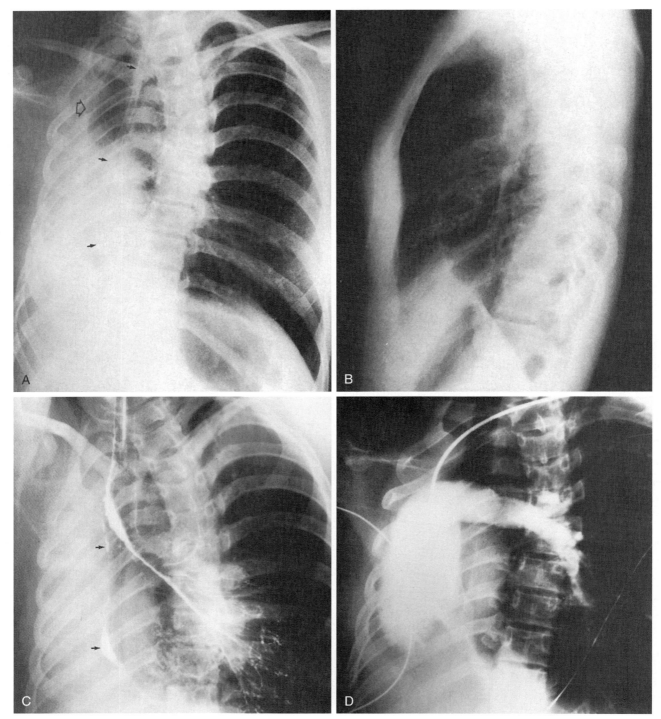

FIGURE 5–1

Agenesis of the right lung. A posteroanterior chest radiograph (**A**) shows marked displacement of the mediastinum to the right, both the heart and the esophagus being entirely within the right hemithorax (the latter indicated by the position of the nasogastric tube—*solid arrows*). The left lung is severely overinflated, as indicated by the displaced anterior mediastinal junction line in posteroanterior projection (*open arrow*), and by the large retrosternal air space in lateral projection (**B**). A bronchogram (**C**) shows no vestige of a right main bronchus (*arrows* point to contrast medium in the displaced esophagus). A pulmonary angiogram (**D**) reveals total absence of a right pulmonary artery. *(Courtesy of Dr. David Stephen, Royal Prince Albert Hospital, Sydney, Australia.)*

advanced fibrothorax.[26] The diagnosis of agenesis can also be made with MR imaging.[27] In patients with aplasia, CT can show the rudimentary bronchus as well as absence of the ipsilateral pulmonary artery[25]; in patients with hypoplasia, CT can show the patent bronchus, the pulmonary artery, and the hypoplastic lung.[25]

Clinical Manifestations

Clinical findings depend on the degree of pulmonary abnormality and the presence of congenital malformations elsewhere, particularly malformations of the kidneys, diaphragm, and chest wall. In asymptomatic patients, physical examination characteristically reveals asymmetry of the two sides of the thorax, a reduction in respiratory movement, and absence of air entry into the affected side. Patients with aplasia manifest similar findings.

Although most evidence suggests that patients with unilateral pulmonary agenesis usually die in the neonatal period, survival into adulthood, sometimes without symptoms, is clearly possible.[9] The number of individuals who survive with hypoplasia is undoubtedly much greater. Nonetheless, the anomaly appears to predispose to respiratory infections,[12] and some patients die of this complication before they reach their teens. Among those who survive, many have mild pulmonary function abnormalities, including increased residual volume and airway responsiveness to methacholine.[28]

Bronchopulmonary Sequestration

Bronchopulmonary sequestration is a pulmonary malformation in which a portion of lung parenchyma is detached from the remaining normal lung and receives its blood supply via a systemic artery. The anomaly may be *intralobar* or *extralobar*: the first type is contiguous with normal lung parenchyma and located within the same visceral pleural envelope; the latter is enclosed within its own pleural membrane, usually close to a normal lung but sometimes within or below the diaphragm. Although it is discussed here as a specific entity, sequestration possesses anatomic features that overlap with those of a variety of other congenital anomalies, and the distinctiveness of the condition has been questioned.[2,29]

Pathogenesis

The most widely accepted pathogenetic theory considers sequestration to be a developmental anomaly of tracheobronchial branching with persistence and localized development of a separated branch fragment and retention of its embryonic systemic vascular supply. The location of the sequestration may reflect the time at which the developmental aberration occurs. Fragments of the developing bronchial tree that separate at an early stage from the primitive lung bud or from a separate foregut diverticulum may acquire a separate pleural investment and develop within the mediastinum or outside the thorax, thus forming an extralobar sequestration. By contrast, separated bronchial fragments of the partially developed lung might be expected to continue their development within the lung itself, thus becoming the intralobar form.

The developmental mechanisms that underlie the abnormal blood supply to the sequestered lung are not clear. Normally, when the pulmonary artery elaborates from the sixth embryonic arch and invaginates its branches into the primitive pulmonary anlage, the branches of the splanchnic plexus that initially supply the lung bud regress and remain only as the bronchial arteries. According to standard theory, additional branches persist and result in the anomalous systemic arterial supply to the sequestered lung. The reason for this hypothesized persistence may be failure of normal pulmonary vascular ingrowth caused by the abnormal position of the sequestered branch fragment.

Although most investigators believe that bronchopulmonary sequestration represents a developmental anomaly, some have proposed that the intralobar form is in fact an acquired lesion, pathogenetically distinct from the extralobar variety.[30,31] According to this view, the initial event in the formation of intralobar sequestration is focal bronchial obstruction, possibly caused by infection or aspiration of a foreign body. Persistence of the obstruction (or perhaps the effects of an associated infectious pneumonitis) leads to the characteristic cystic and fibrotic changes in lung parenchyma. The initial inflammatory process is also thought to interrupt pulmonary blood flow to the affected lung segment; hypertrophy of systemic arteries (small branches of which are normally present in the pulmonary ligament of some individuals) then results in the "anomalous" vascular supply.

Intralobar Sequestration

The incidence of intralobar sequestration is low; in one review of the literature to 1975, only 400 cases were identified.[29] In approximately two thirds of cases, the sequestered lung is situated in the paravertebral gutter within the posterior bronchopulmonary segment of the left lower lobe; in most others, it occupies the same anatomic region of the right lower lobe. The abnormality is infrequently associated with other anomalies, the most common being esophageal diverticula, diaphragmatic hernia, and a variety of skeletal and cardiac defects.[32]

Pathologic Characteristics

Grossly, the abnormal tissue is usually well demarcated from surrounding lung parenchyma and consists of one or more cystic spaces with a variable amount of intervening, more solid tissue (see Color Fig. 5–1). The cysts are filled with mucus or, when infection is present, with pus. Microscopically, they resemble dilated bronchi with respiratory epithelium and occasional mural cartilage plates. The amount of intervening parenchymal tissue varies from scanty to abundant and in uncomplicated cases shows changes of obstructive pneumonitis.

The abnormal tissue invariably derives its arterial supply from the aorta or one of its branches, most commonly the descending thoracic aorta; though usually solitary, multiple tributary vessels can be seen. Typically, the anomalous vessel enters the lung by way of the lower part of the pulmonary ligament and is much larger than would be expected for the volume of tissue supplied. Venous drainage is almost always via the pulmonary venous system, thus creating a left-to-left shunt.

Radiologic Manifestations

The most common radiographic manifestation is a homogeneous opacity in the posterior basal segment of a lower lobe (usually the left and almost invariably contiguous with the hemidiaphragm) (Fig. 5–2); less commonly, the appearance is that of a cystic mass or prominent vessels.[31,33,34] Definitive diagnosis is based on demonstration of the anomalous arterial supply. Traditionally, such demonstration has been achieved with aortography, a procedure that allows assessment of the origin of the arterial supply, identification of one or more tributary vessels, and evaluation of venous drainage.[31] Identification of the systemic arterial supply can also be accomplished by CT (see Fig. 5–2).[31,34] Demonstration of the origin and course of the anomalous systemic vessel supplying the sequestered lung has improved considerably with the advent of spiral CT, particularly multidetector CT, and the use of multiplanar reformation.[31,35,36]

Although MR imaging has been performed in only a few cases, it allows excellent visualization of vessels in multiple imaging planes and may obviate the need for angiography.[31,37] The procedure may show vessels not visualized at arteriography.[38]

Clinical Manifestations

Most patients are asymptomatic until an acute respiratory infection develops, which in many cases does not happen until adulthood.[32] Signs and symptoms are then usually those of acute lower lobe pneumonia, the basic defect becoming apparent only through radiologic observation of the sequence of changes during resolution of the infection. Infections are generally caused by pyogenic bacteria. The differential diagnosis includes bronchiectasis, lung abscess, and hernia of Bochdalek.

Extralobar Sequestration

Extralobar pulmonary sequestration is less common than the intralobar variety; in the review of sequestration cited previously, only 123 cases were identified up to 1975.[29] The abnormality was related to the left hemidiaphragm in 90% of cases; it may be situated between the inferior surface of the lower lobe and the diaphragm, below the diaphragm, or within the substance of the diaphragm; occasionally, it is located in the retroperitoneum or mediastinum.

As with intralobar sequestration, the systemic arterial supply is commonly from the aorta, usually the abdominal portion or one of its branches. In contrast to the intralobar variety, however, venous drainage is generally via the systemic venous system—the inferior vena cava, the azygos or hemiazygos veins, or the portal system—and a left-to-right shunt is created. Also in contrast to intralobar sequestration, the extralobar anomaly is seen most often in neonates and in many cases is associated with other congenital anomalies, particularly eventration or paralysis of the ipsilateral hemidiaphragm (in approximately 60% of cases[12]) and left diaphragmatic hernia (in approximately 30%[32]).

Morphologically, the sequestered tissue is completely enclosed in a pleural sac. The cut surface reveals spongy, tan-colored tissue with irregularly arranged vessels, often more prominent at one end of the specimen. Airways are usually few in number, and parenchymal tissue often appears immature.

Radiographic findings typically consist of a sharply defined, triangular opacity in the posterior costophrenic angle, usually adjacent to the left hemidiaphragm.[32,39] Aortography generally shows the anomalous systemic arterial supply; multiple feeding vessels are evident in about 20% of cases.[39] Identification of the venous drainage, usually into a systemic vein, may require selective catheterization of the feeding vessels. The CT findings consist most commonly of a homogeneous opacity or well-circumscribed mass[34,39]; cystic areas are seen occasionally.

Because the sequestered pulmonary tissue is enveloped in its own pleural sac, the chance of its becoming infected is very small, unless there is communication with the gastrointestinal tract.[40] Consequently, the chief mode of manifestation in patients without other significant congenital anomalies is a homogeneous soft tissue mass in an asymptomatic individual. As with intralobar sequestration, the systemic arterial supply to this anomaly should be determined before surgery is undertaken.

Bronchogenic Cysts

Like bronchopulmonary sequestration, bronchogenic cysts are believed to represent localized portions of the tracheobronchial tree that become separated from adjacent airways during the branching process. Unlike the latter, however, they do not undergo further development and thus have no associated parenchyma or distinctive vascular supply. They are thought by some authors to represent one end of a spectrum of pathogenetically similar conditions, including sequestration and (possibly) congenital cystic bronchiectasis.[41,42] About 75% to 85% of cysts are located in the mediastinum and 15% to 25% in the lung.[43,44]

Histologically, the cyst wall is typically lined by respiratory or metaplastic squamous epithelium and contains cartilage, smooth muscle, and sometimes seromucinous bronchial-type glands (Fig. 5–3).[45] The presence of these structures, especially cartilage, is essential to establishment of the developmental nature of the cyst. Although intrapulmonary cysts that do not contain cartilage and glands in their wall may represent bronchogenic cysts, the walls of healed abscess cavities may contain very little fibrous tissue and have the capacity to epithelialize with a ciliated pseudostratified epithelium. On the other hand, the epithelium and portions of the wall of a true congenital cyst may be destroyed if the cyst becomes secondarily infected, so their absence does not exclude a congenital origin in the presence of inflammation. In practice, therefore, it may be impossible to differentiate an infected intrapulmonary congenital cyst from an acquired infected bulla or abscess solely on morphologic criteria; in such cases, radiologic evidence of previous disease may be helpful in diagnosis.

Although the morphologic features of mediastinal bronchial cysts are much less likely to be altered by infection, a precise histologic diagnosis may also be difficult. Since esophageal epithelium is ciliated and pseudostratified in early development and seromucinous glands similar to bronchial glands can be found in the normal esophagus, it is possible that a mediastinal cyst that does not contain cartilage and that

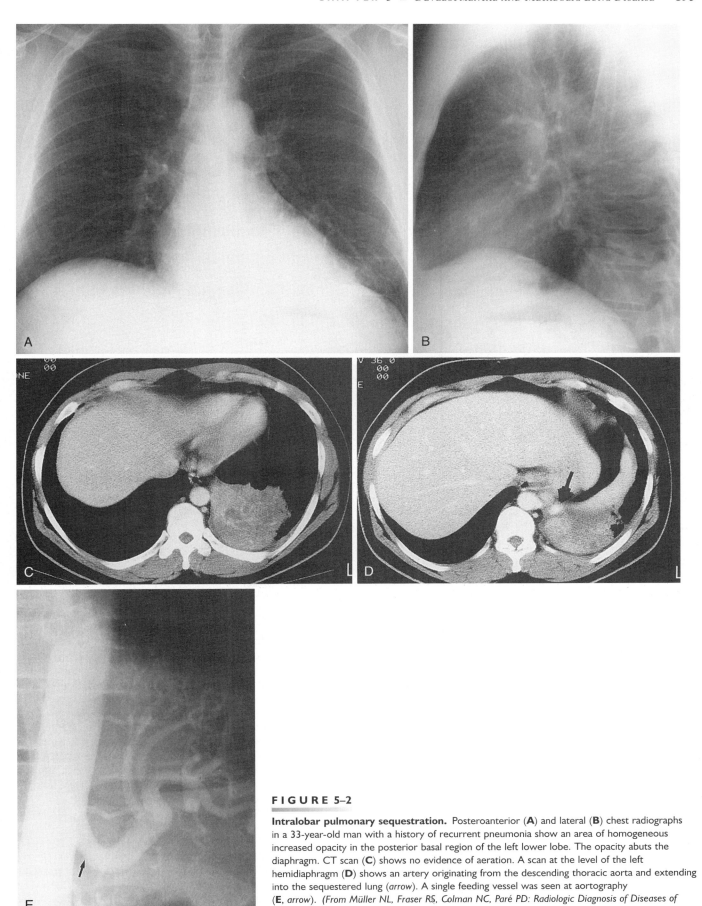

FIGURE 5–2

Intralobar pulmonary sequestration. Posteroanterior (**A**) and lateral (**B**) chest radiographs in a 33-year-old man with a history of recurrent pneumonia show an area of homogeneous increased opacity in the posterior basal region of the left lower lobe. The opacity abuts the diaphragm. CT scan (**C**) shows no evidence of aeration. A scan at the level of the left hemidiaphragm (**D**) shows an artery originating from the descending thoracic aorta and extending into the sequestered lung (*arrow*). A single feeding vessel was seen at aortography (**E**, *arrow*). *(From Müller NL, Fraser RS, Colman NC, Paré PD: Radiologic Diagnosis of Diseases of the Chest. Philadelphia, WB Saunders, 2001.)*

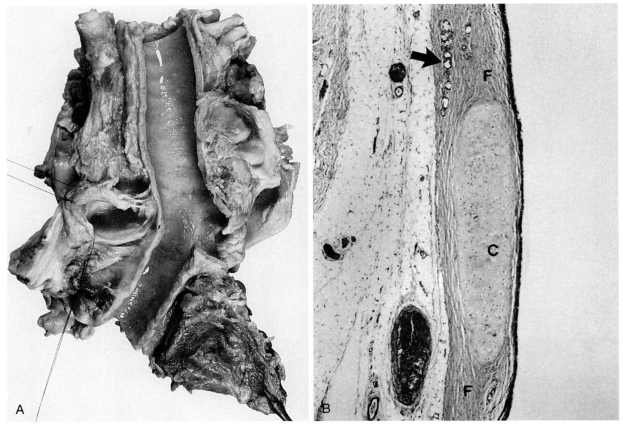

FIGURE 5–3

Mediastinal bronchogenic cyst. A unilocular cyst approximately 2 cm in greatest dimension is present in the connective tissue adjacent to the trachea just above the origin of the left main bronchus (**A**). A histologic section of cyst wall (**B**) shows cartilage (C), seromucinous glands (*arrow*), and fibrous tissue (F). At this magnification, the respiratory epithelial lining is evident only as a dark line to the right of the cartilage. The cyst was an incidental finding in a 65-year-old woman. *(From Fraser RS, Müller NL, Colman NC, Paré PD: Fraser and Paré's Diagnosis of Diseases of the Chest, 4th ed. Philadelphia, WB Saunders, 1999.)*

is situated posteriorly may be of esophageal derivation.[45] Because of these potential diagnostic difficulties, mediastinal cysts that contain only respiratory-type epithelium without additional structures that indicate bronchial origin are probably best classified imprecisely as simple cysts.

Pulmonary Bronchogenic Cysts

The typical radiographic appearance is a sharply circumscribed, round or oval opacity of unit density in the medial third of a lower lobe. Serial radiographs usually show little change in size and shape with time, although slow growth can sometimes be observed over a period of years. Characteristically, the lesions do not communicate with the tracheobronchial tree until they become infected, an outcome that occurs eventually in about 75% of cases. When communication is established, the cyst contains air, with or without fluid (Fig. 5–4)[46]; in such cases, the usual sharp definition of the shadow may be obscured by consolidation of surrounding parenchyma, and the true nature of the cyst becomes apparent only when the pneumonitis has resolved. Confident diagnosis can be made on CT scan based on the presence of nonenhancing homogeneous attenuation at or near water density (0 to 20 Hounsfield units [HU]) and a smooth, thin

wall.[25,47,48] In approximately 50% of cases, the cysts have higher than water density as a result of proteinaceous material or calcium in the cyst contents.[49,50] CT frequently demonstrates areas of scarring and decreased attenuation and vascularity in the adjacent lung.[48] When infected, the cysts may have inhomogeneous enhancement and resemble an abscess.[51] Occasionally, they are air filled and multilocular.[44] MR imaging is superior to CT in diagnosis, the characteristic finding being homogeneous high-signal intensity (approximating that of cerebrospinal fluid) on T2-weighted spin-echo images.[51,52]

In adults, most uninfected pulmonary bronchogenic cysts cause no symptoms and are discovered by accident on a screening chest radiograph. Symptoms, of which hemoptysis is the most common, almost invariably relate to infection in and around the cyst. Communication between a cyst and the tracheobronchial tree may incorporate a check-valve mechanism that may result in rapid expansion of the cyst.[53]

Mediastinal Bronchogenic Cysts

Mediastinal bronchogenic cysts are usually seen as clearly defined masses of homogeneous density in the right paratracheal region (Fig. 5–5) or just inferior to and slightly to the right of the carina, overlapping the right hilar shadow. Most

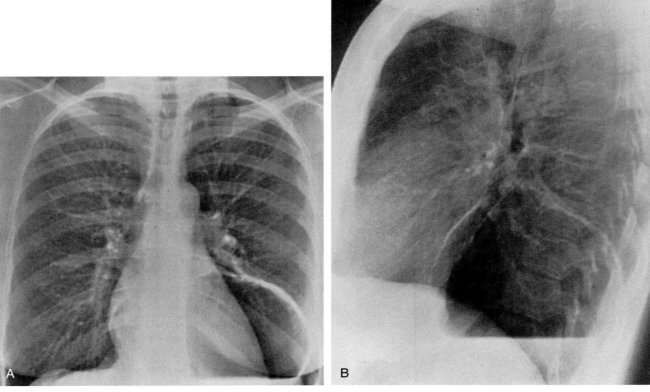

FIGURE 5–4

Congenital bronchogenic cyst. Posteroanterior (**A**) and lateral (**B**) radiographs reveal a large cystic space in the left lower lobe containing a prominent fluid level. The cyst wall measured a maximum of 3 mm in width. *(From Fraser RS, Müller NL, Colman NC, Paré PD: Fraser and Paré's Diagnosis of Diseases of the Chest, 4th ed. Philadelphia, WB Saunders, 1999.)*

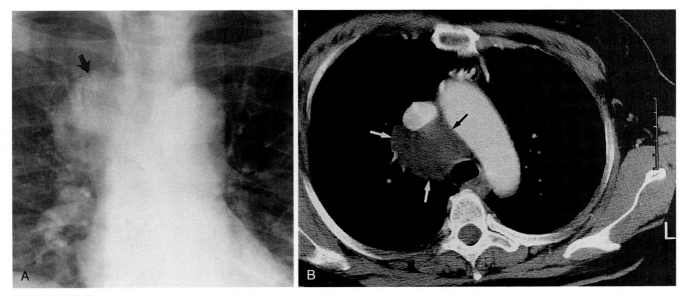

FIGURE 5–5

Mediastinal bronchogenic cyst. A view from a posteroanterior chest radiograph (**A**) in a 60-year-old woman shows a right paratracheal mass (*arrow*). A contrast-enhanced CT scan (**B**) shows that the lesion (*arrows*) has homogeneous water density characteristic of a bronchogenic cyst. The attenuation value was 9 HU. *(From Müller NL, Fraser RS, Colman NC, Paré PD: Radiologic Diagnosis of Diseases of the Chest. Philadelphia, WB Saunders, 2001.)*

are oval or round; the shape may vary with inspiration and expiration. In contrast to pulmonary bronchogenic cysts, the mediastinal variety rarely communicates with the tracheobronchial tree.[54]

A diagnosis of benign cyst can be made confidently on CT scan when it shows homogeneous attenuation at or near water density (0 to 20 HU) (see Fig. 5–5).[44,49] In approximately 50% of patients, the cysts have higher attenuation (130 HU) and are indistinguishable from soft tissue lesions. Similar to pulmonary cysts, this increase in attenuation is the result of a high protein level or calcium oxalate in the cyst contents.[49,55] As with pulmonary cysts, difficulty in distinguishing a soft tissue lesion from a cystic one may be resolved by MR imaging.[51,52]

Many individuals are asymptomatic[56]; however, in one surgical review of 69 patients, almost two thirds complained of a symptom attributable to the cyst.[57] The location of the cyst appears to be more important than size in this respect, with those in the carinal area sometimes causing symptoms related to airway compression even when quite small. Symptomatic compression of the heart or great vessels can also occur, as exemplified by cysts that caused paroxysmal atrial fibrillation or pulmonary artery stenosis.[58,59] Although surgical excision is usually curative, a cyst may recur after partial resection, sometimes after many years.[60]

Congenital Adenomatoid Malformation

The term *congenital cystic adenomatoid malformation* refers to a group of several pathologically distinctive abnormalities characterized by architecturally abnormal pulmonary tissue with or without gross cyst formation. When present, the cysts can usually be shown to communicate with normal airways. Most often, the vascular supply is via the pulmonary circulation. As might be expected, most cases are discovered in the very young. In a review of 142 cases from the literature and 17 new cases, the malformation was diagnosed in 62% of patients between birth and 1 month of age[61]; an additional 24% of cases became manifested after 1 month, mostly in the first 5 years of life. Cases have also been detected in adults up to about 60 years of age.[62,63]

The condition has been divided into five morphologic subtypes that are thought to consist of a spectrum of abnormalities affecting the trachea and main bronchi (type 0) to the distal acinus (type 4).[64] Because not all types are cystic or adenomatoid, it has been proposed that the lesions be known collectively as "congenital pulmonary airway malformation."[64] The *type 1* form is the most common (60% to 70% of cases) and consists of a large, often multiloculated cyst lined mostly by bronchiolar-type epithelium and sometimes associated with several smaller cysts in the adjacent parenchyma. Other forms are composed of small (0.5 to 1.5 cm) cysts (type 2), more or less solid masses (types 0 and 3), and large multicystic structures lined by alveolar epithelium (type 4).

In older children and adults, the lesion usually appears radiologically as a lower lobe soft tissue mass containing numerous air-containing cysts. It is a space-occupying lesion that expands the ipsilateral hemithorax and shifts the mediastinum to the contralateral side. Occasionally, one cyst expands preferentially, thereby creating a single lucent area.[63,65] The cysts may contain fluid, air, or both (Fig. 5–6). Fluid levels are seen occasionally; only rarely does fluid fill the cysts completely and result in complete radiographic opacification.[65] CT is superior to chest radiography in showing the cystic and solid components of the abnormality.[63,66]

Most patients initially seek medical attention for increasing respiratory distress, the severity being related chiefly to the volume of lung involved. A minority initially have cough and fever, with or without recurrent respiratory infections[63]; most of these patients are older than 1 month. Spontaneous pneumothorax occurs occasionally, particularly in patients who have type 4 lesions. Some cases, particularly the type 1 form, are complicated by mucin-secreting bronchioloalveolar carcinoma.[67]

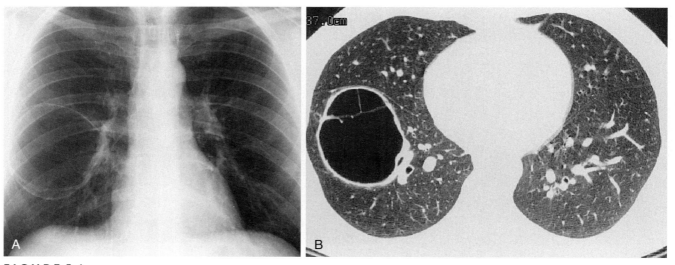

FIGURE 5–6

Congenital cystic adenomatoid malformation. A posteroanterior chest radiograph (**A**) in a 31-year-old man shows a large cystic lesion in the right lower lobe. An HRCT scan (**B**) shows a few septations within the thin-walled cyst. At surgery, the lesion was shown to be a type 1 malformation. *(From Müller NL, Fraser RS, Colman NC, Paré PD: Radiologic Diagnosis of Diseases of the Chest. Philadelphia, WB Saunders, 2001.)*

Congenital Bronchial Atresia

This anomaly consists of atresia or stenosis of a lobar, segmental, or subsegmental bronchus at or near its origin; the apicoposterior segmental bronchus of the left upper lobe is most commonly affected.[68] The mean age at the time of diagnosis is 17 years, and approximately two thirds of patients are male. Two pathogenetic theories have been proposed[69]: (1) an island of multiplying cells at the tip of a bronchial bud loses its connection with the bud itself but continues to branch independently, thereby resulting in a normal distal bronchial branch pattern without a connection between the distal and central airways; and (2) intrauterine interruption of the bronchial artery blood supply results in localized bronchial wall ischemia and secondary luminal obliteration. Whatever the mechanism of airway interruption, mucus secreted within the patent airways distal to the point of atresia cannot pass the stenosis and accumulates in the form of a plug or mucocele.

Because air can enter the affected bronchopulmonary segments only via collateral channels, overinflation and expiratory air trapping result.[70,71]

Chest radiographs typically show an area of pulmonary hyperlucency associated with a hilar mass (Fig. 5–7).[68] The hyperlucency results from a combination of oligemia and an increase in the volume of air within the affected segment. The adjacent normal lung is compressed and displaced; the mediastinum may or may not show displacement. Accumulation of secretions and mucoid impaction distal to the bronchial atresia result in ovoid or round branching opacities near the hilum in most cases.[72] CT is the best imaging technique for confirming the diagnosis because it allows excellent visualization of the mucoid impaction, segmental hyperlucency, and decreased vascularity.[47,73] The former is readily recognized by the presence of branching soft tissue densities in a bronchial distribution, usually associated with bronchial dilation.[74] A similar appearance has been reported on MR images.[75,76]

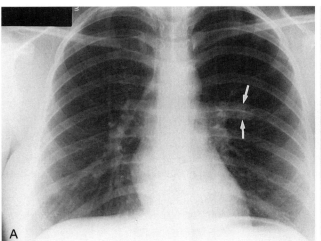

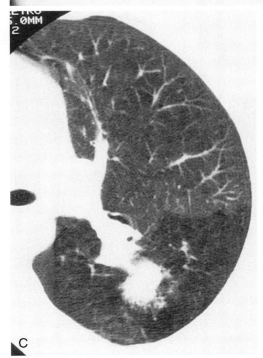

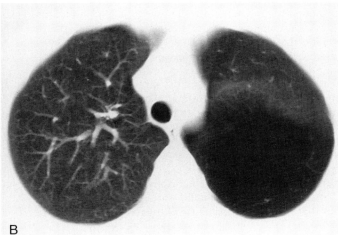

FIGURE 5–7

Bronchial atresia. A posteroanterior chest radiograph (**A**) in a 14-year-old girl shows marked lucency and decreased vascularity in the left upper lobe. An ill-defined opacity is visible near the left hilum (*arrows*). A conventional 10-mm-collimation CT scan (**B**) shows a marked decrease in attenuation and vascularity in the region of the apicoposterior segment of the left upper lobe. An HRCT scan (**C**) shows a focal opacity near the origin of the apicoposterior segmental bronchus and decreased attenuation of the adjacent lung. *(From Müller NL, Fraser RS, Colman NC, Paré PD: Radiologic Diagnosis of Diseases of the Chest. Philadelphia, WB Saunders, 2001.)*

The majority of patients are asymptomatic. Some have a history of recurrent pneumonia,[68] and pectus excavatum has been noted in some individuals.[77]

Anomalous Tracheobronchial Branching

Many variations in the tracheobronchial branching pattern have been described.[78,79] Some represent an isolated alteration of normal bronchial development, whereas others are associated with anomalies in other organs or tissues and are discovered in early neonatal life or in stillbirths or abortions as part of a spectrum of abnormalities. Although most of these abnormal branches are of no radiologic, functional, or clinical consequence, pathologic effects are occasionally produced, usually related to recurrent infection.

Abnormal Bronchial Number. This variation is generally characterized by more than one lobar or segmental bronchus[79,80]; occasionally, an airway branch is absent.

Abnormal Origin of Lobar or Segmental Bronchi. The most common of these variations is tracheal origin of the right upper lobe bronchus, sometimes known as a "pig" bronchus. The airway usually arises from the right lateral wall of the trachea less than 2 cm above the carina (Fig. 5–8).[81] Typically, it is discovered incidentally at bronchoscopy, chest radiography, or CT[82]; occasionally, it is associated with recurrent infection or dyspnea.[83,84] Some patients have been identified in whom the left apicoposterior bronchus arises directly from the left main bronchus.[85] Some of these individuals have developed emphysema, bronchiectasis, and chronic pneumonia in the apicoposterior segment, possibly as a result of extrinsic compression of the anomalous airway by the left pulmonary artery.

Bronchial Isomerism. Bronchial isomerism is characterized by a pattern of bronchial branching and pulmonary lobe formation that is identical in the two lungs. Although it can be an isolated finding, it is frequently associated with a variety of cardiac, splenic, and other anomalies.[86]

Tracheobronchial Diverticula. The most common location of an airway diverticulum is probably the inferior medial wall of the right main or intermediate bronchus. The abnormality (sometimes termed the *accessory cardiac bronchus*) may end blindly or be associated with small amounts of abnormal pulmonary parenchyma. The frequency of the anomaly ranges from 0.09% to 0.5% in the general population.[80] The diagnosis can be readily made with CT, which demonstrates a distinct airway originating in the medial wall of the main bronchus or bronchus intermedius cephalic to the origin of the middle lobe bronchus (Fig. 5–9).[87] Although usually an incidental finding in an asymptomatic patient, the bronchus can serve as a reservoir of infectious organisms and result in hemorrhage, productive cough, or recurrent pneumonia.

Tracheoesophageal and Bronchoesophageal Fistulas

Extralaryngeal communication of the normal tracheobronchial tree is most often seen as a tracheoesophageal fistula. Two clinicopathologic subtypes have been described. In the first, which accounts for approximately 85% of cases, the esophagus ends blindly in a dilated pouch (esophageal atresia).[88] The trachea can communicate with the proximal or distal esophageal segments (or both). Other congenital anomalies, particularly of the gastrointestinal and cardiovascular systems, are present in approximately 50% of patients.[89] The presence of a blind (proximal) esophageal ending leads to regurgitation and aspiration of oropharyngeal secretions and milk, thereby resulting in cough and pneumonia. The condition is thus invariably detected in the neonatal period.

Congenital tracheoesophageal and bronchoesophageal communications can also occur in association with an

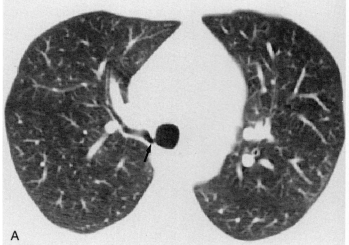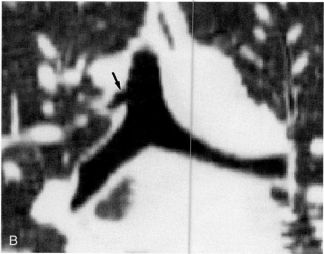

FIGURE 5–8

Tracheal bronchus. A 3-mm-collimation spiral CT scan at the level of the aortic arch (**A**) demonstrates the right upper lobe bronchus (*arrow*) originating directly from the trachea. A coronal reconstruction (**B**) demonstrates the lower part of the trachea and right upper lobe bronchus (*arrow*) originating from the trachea rather than from the right main bronchus. The patient was a 42-year-old man with no symptoms related to the airways or lung parenchyma. (*From Fraser RS, Müller NL, Colman NC, Paré PD: Fraser and Paré's Diagnosis of Diseases of the Chest, 4th ed. Philadelphia, WB Saunders, 1999.*)

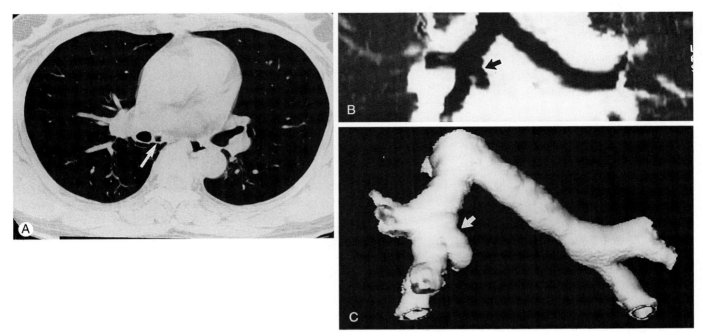

FIGURE 5–9

Accessory cardiac bronchus—spiral CT with coronal and three-dimensional reconstruction. A cross-sectional spiral CT image (**A**) demonstrates a localized area of air density (*arrow*) medial to the bronchus intermedius. A coronal reconstruction (**B**) demonstrates that this localized abnormality communicates with the distal right main bronchus (*arrow*). Three-dimensional reconstruction (**C**) more clearly defines the bronchial anatomy and the cardiac bronchus. The patient was a 39-year-old woman with recurrent respiratory infections. *(Case courtesy of Dr. Kyung Soo Lee, Department of Radiology, Samsung Medical Center, Seoul, South Korea.)*

otherwise normal esophagus. In this situation, survival into adult life is possible because of the lack of early signs and symptoms related to regurgitation and aspiration.[88,90] Of the bronchi, the right main bronchus is most commonly affected; however, the left main bronchus and even segmental airways are sometimes involved.[91] Anatomically, the fistulas are usually obliquely oriented, the esophageal end being distal to the upper airway communication. It has been proposed that this arrangement—possibly aided by contraction of mural smooth muscle during swallowing—explains the frequent mildness of respiratory symptoms and the delay in diagnosis until adulthood.[92] Occlusive membranes and mucosal folds at the esophageal origin of the fistulas may act as check-valves and provide further protection against aspiration.[93]

Chest radiographs of neonates who have tracheoesophageal fistula and esophageal atresia frequently show acute air space pneumonia consistent with aspiration. Total opacification of the right lung associated with deviation of the esophagus to the right and a normal position of the trachea should lead to the suspicion of "esophageal lung," in which the right main bronchus originates from the esophagus.[94] In older patients without esophageal atresia, evidence of bronchiectasis may be present. The diagnosis of fistula is best confirmed by identification of contrast medium within the tracheobronchial tree after ingestion.

Although the diagnosis of fistulas unassociated with esophageal atresia is frequently not made until adulthood, careful questioning often reveals a history of coughing when eating or drinking or recurrent pneumonia, sometimes for many years.[92] Bronchoscopy may reveal the orifice of the

communication. The prognosis is good after reparative surgery.[90]

ANOMALIES OF THE PULMONARY ARTERIES

Absence of the Main Pulmonary Artery

Absence of the main pulmonary artery can be manifested by a variety of anatomic patterns.[95] In some cases, the artery is atretic, either in its proximal portion or over its entire length, with a residual fibrous cord marking its usual position. In such cases, the right and left main pulmonary arteries persist in their normal sites and are connected to the aorta by a ductus.

In other cases, all morphologic evidence of a main pulmonary artery is lost, and a single great artery arises from a common semilunar heart valve, invariably in association with a ventricular septal defect (persistent truncus arteriosus).[96] Independent pulmonary arteries are thus absent, and the pulmonary blood supply is derived from branches of the single trunk vessel at systemic pressure.[96] Several anatomic subtypes have been defined.[97] In the first three, one or two pulmonary vessels arise from the common trunk in its early portion. Type IV, believed to represent complete failure of development of the sixth aortic arch, lacks all evidence of pulmonary arterial growth, and the pulmonary blood supply is derived solely from bronchial arteries. The majority of patients die in infancy unless they undergo successful corrective surgery.[98] However, some patients survive into middle age without intervention with minimal or no dyspnea.[99]

Proximal Interruption of the Pulmonary Artery

Although rare examples of complete absence of both intrapulmonary and extrapulmonary artery branches have been described,[100] this anomaly is better designated proximal "interruption" of the right or left pulmonary artery since the vessels in the lung are usually intact and patent. Interruption of the right pulmonary artery is more common.[96] The vast majority of affected patients have a left aortic arch, and substantial bronchial collateral circulation develops during childhood. Patients can be classified into four groups[96]: (1) proximal interruption without pulmonary arterial hypertension, in which case patients are usually asymptomatic and the diagnosis is made on the basis of radiologic findings; (2) proximal interruption with pulmonary arterial hypertension, which in the majority of cases is associated with symptoms in early childhood; (3) proximal interruption with recurrent pulmonary infection or hemoptysis, often secondary to associated malformations of the lung parenchyma; and (4) proximal interruption with a left patent ductus arteriosus or congenital heart disease.

The radiographic findings consist of a decreased size of the right lung associated with small right and enlarged left hila.[96] Enlargement of the intercostal arteries may result in rib notching. Despite its reduced volume, the lung is usually hyperlucent; when taken in conjunction with the diminutive hilar shadow, this finding may lead to the erroneous diagnosis of Swyer-James syndrome. Differentiation is generally possible with radiography in full expiration: patients who have Swyer-James syndrome show ipsilateral air trapping as a result of bronchiolar obstruction, a sign that is absent in cases of proximal pulmonary artery interruption. The diagnosis may also be confirmed by echocardiography and perfusion lung scans.[96] Chronic thromboembolic occlusion of a pulmonary artery may also mimic proximal interruption, even on angiography.[101] Contrast-enhanced CT and MR imaging allows demonstration of the absent proximal artery and the patent intrapulmonary arteries, which are typically decreased in caliber.[102,103] They may also allow demonstration of bronchial collaterals or the less common transpleural intercostal collaterals.[102,104]

Proximal interruption of the left pulmonary artery is less common than right-sided interruption and has a high incidence of associated congenital cardiovascular anomalies, particularly tetralogy of Fallot. The distal left pulmonary artery may be supplied by a patent ductus arteriosus, by acquired bronchial artery collaterals, or by a vessel originating in the ascending aorta.[96] Though usually diagnosed in infancy, the abnormality is occasionally undetected until adulthood, and then on the basis of an abnormal chest radiograph.[104] The radiologic findings are similar to those of the right-sided anomaly.

Anomalous Origin of the Left Pulmonary Artery

In this condition, an aberrant left pulmonary artery passes posteriorly and to the right until it reaches the right side of the distal end of the trachea or the right main bronchus; it then turns sharply to the left and passes between the esophagus and trachea in its course to the left hilum (thus the designation "pulmonary sling").[105] The intimate relationship of this vessel to the right main bronchus and trachea results in compression of these structures and various obstructive effects on the right or both lungs. The pathogenic mechanism has been hypothesized to be faulty development or reabsorption of the ventral portion of the left sixth aortic arch, which leaves the developing left pulmonary plexus to connect with the right sixth aortic arch (subsequently the right pulmonary artery).[106]

Conventional chest radiographs may reveal an anterior impression on the distal part of the trachea and a paratracheal opacity.[107] The demonstration of local posterior displacement of the barium-filled esophagus in the region of the lower part of the trachea makes the diagnosis virtually certain. The diagnosis can be confirmed by CT or MR imaging, both of which demonstrate the origin and course of the anomalous artery, as well as the presence of associated airway abnormalities.[108]

Affected infants usually have stridor and feeding problems shortly after birth. Occasional patients are asymptomatic, and the anomaly is detected as an incidental finding on a chest radiograph in adulthood.[109] The abnormality is commonly associated with tracheobronchial anomalies such as tracheal stenosis ("funnel trachea") and anomalous origin of the right upper lobe bronchus from the trachea; cardiovascular malformations are also frequent.

Pulmonary Artery Stenosis

Stenosis (coarctation) of the pulmonary artery may be single or multiple, short or long, or unilateral or bilateral and may occur anywhere from the pulmonary valve to small pulmonary arteries.[110] Stenosis affecting the main branch or proximal branches of the pulmonary artery is often associated with cardiovascular anomalies, most frequently infundibular, valvular, or supravalvular pulmonic stenosis (60% of cases) and atrial septal defect. Some cases are associated with Ehlers-Danlos or Down's syndrome, thus suggesting a genetic defect[110,111]; others occur after maternal rubella.[112]

Radiographically, the pulmonary vasculature may appear normal, diminished, or increased, depending on the presence and nature of associated malformations.[113] In instances in which the pulmonary artery stenosis is the only or the major anomaly, the chest radiograph may reveal poststenotic dilation of affected pulmonary artery branches, diffuse oligemia, and signs of pulmonary artery hypertension and cor pulmonale.

Physical examination may reveal an accentuated pulmonic second sound and a grade 2 to 4/6 murmur over the upper part of the chest anteriorly that radiates to the neck and back; however, when the stenosis is severe, flow may be so reduced that the lesions are acoustically silent.

Congenital Aneurysms of the Pulmonary Artery

Congenital aneurysms of the pulmonary arteries are usually seen with other pulmonary abnormalities (such as arteriovenous malformations or bronchopulmonary sequestration[114]) or congenital cardiac defects (such as pulmonic stenosis, tetralogy of Fallot, and ventricular septal defect).[115] They are generally the result of disturbed hemodynamics associated with pulmonary valve stenosis. Such poststenotic dilatation affects the left pulmonary artery much more commonly than the right; in fact, enlargement of the main pulmonary artery and its left branch in conjunction with a normal right hilum should strongly suggest the diagnosis of pulmonary valve stenosis. The abnormality may be confused radiographically with a central or peripheral neoplasm.[116,117] Definitive diagnosis may be made with contrast-enhanced CT, MR imaging, or angiography.

Clinical manifestations include asymmetry of the thorax (the left side usually being more prominent), a systolic ejection murmur (attributable to stenosis of the pulmonary valve orifice in relation to the increased caliber of the main pulmonary artery), and accentuation of the second pulmonic sound (possibly caused by the proximity of the dilated pulmonary artery to the anterior chest wall rather than by pulmonary hypertension). The abnormality is compatible with a normal life span.[118]

Direct Communication of the Right Pulmonary Artery with the Left Atrium

This rare congenital malformation is characterized by direct communication between a branch of the right pulmonary artery and the left atrium without intervening lung parenchyma.[119] Aneurysmal dilation of the anomalous branch is common. In some cases, the right lung itself is normal, the anomalous artery behaving as a supernumerary vessel arising from an otherwise unremarkable right pulmonary artery. In others, there is aplasia or severe hypoplasia of the lower lobe,[120] in which case the vessel appears to represent a residual interlobar or lower lobe artery that persists in the absence of peripheral portions of the pulmonary vascular bed. The chest radiograph most often reveals a round opacity 2 to 3 cm in diameter in the right hemithorax adjacent to the left atrium.[121] Definitive diagnosis may be made by angiography or MR imaging.[122] Patients have dyspnea, and cyanosis and clubbing may be present.

ANOMALIES OF THE PULMONARY VEINS

Congenital Pulmonary Venous Stenosis or Atresia

Congenital obstruction of one or more pulmonary veins can be caused by compression by an intrathoracic mass or by intrinsic abnormalities of the veins themselves. In addition, some cardiac anomalies such as cor triatriatum can result in venous obstruction that is clinically indistinguishable from the other two forms. The intrinsic anomaly is characterized by stenosis or atresia of one or more pulmonary veins, typically localized at the venoatrial junction.[123] The stenosis can be caused by a primary abnormality of either the atrium or the veins themselves, the former consisting of endocardial thickening at the mouth of the vein and the latter of medial muscular hypertrophy, intimal fibrosis, or a combination of the two.

In patients without associated cardiovascular anomalies, radiographic manifestations consist of signs of pulmonary venous hypertension, with or without arterial hypertension and right ventricular enlargement. Confirmation can be obtained by arteriography.[124] In most cases of isolated stenosis, the condition is recognized in the first 3 years of life; occasional individuals have survived to adolescence before the diagnosis is made.[125] As might be expected, common vein atresia is invariably recognized in the neonatal period.

Varicosities of the Pulmonary Veins

This abnormality consists of abnormal tortuosity and dilation of one or more pulmonary veins just before their entrance into the left atrium. It may be congenital or acquired.[126] The former is thought to occur during the period of transition from splanchnic to pulmonary venous drainage, although the reason for the localized dilation at that time is not understood. The majority of cases in which the vein has been studied have shown normal structure,[127] and an intrinsic defect of the vessel wall does not seem likely. In most cases, the lesion is apparent radiologically as one or more round or oval homogeneous opacities, somewhat lobulated but well defined, in the medial third of either lung. On the left, the lingular vein is usually affected; on the right, it is most often a branch of the inferior pulmonary vein in the region of the medial basal segment of the right lower lobe.[128] The abnormality is not generally recognized until the patient reaches adulthood.

Acquired varicosities of the pulmonary veins are invariably associated with disease of the mitral valve, most commonly regurgitation.[129] They typically occur on the right side, a striking unilaterality that can be attributed to the anatomy of the mitral valve, whose plane is directed posteriorly, superiorly, and to the right.

The radiographic differential diagnosis includes all masses in the lungs. A definitive diagnosis can be readily made with contrast-enhanced CT, MR imaging, or angiography.[126,130] The varicosities themselves seldom give rise to symptoms.

Anomalous Pulmonary Venous Drainage

Anomalous pulmonary venous drainage occurs when pulmonary venous blood flows directly into the right side of the heart or the systemic veins. It may be partial (involving part or all of one lung) or total (both lungs); the special situation in which an anomalous vein drains the right lung and is associated with other right-sided anomalies is considered separately (see later under "Hypogenetic Lung Syndrome").

Although the anatomy of the anomalous connections is highly variable,[131] drainage may be considered in four groups: (1) supracardiac, usually to a persistent left superior vena cava and thence to the left innominate vein (approximately 50% of cases); (2) cardiac, in which a direct connection is established with the right atrium or coronary sinus (30% of cases); (3) infradiaphragmatic, in which a common vein extends below the diaphragm to join the portal vein or one of its radicles (15% of cases); and (4) mixed (approximately 5% of cases). In most cases, the pathogenesis is probably a failure of connection between the primitive pulmonary splanchnic plexus and the common pulmonary vein derived from the atrium.

Partial Anomalous Drainage. The anomalous vein may be visible on plain radiographs, although more precise depiction can be achieved with CT.[132] The most common site in adults is the left upper lobe.[133] In this situation, the anomalous vein courses cephalad lateral to the aortic arch and usually drains into the left brachiocephalic vein, a course that is particularly well demonstrated with contrast-enhanced dynamic or spiral CT and multiplanar or three-dimensional reconstructions.[133] MR imaging or pulmonary angiography may be required to confirm the diagnosis.[134,135] MR imaging also allows identification of associated cardiac abnormalities, the most common being atrial septal defect.[134,136]

Since there is generally no significant obstruction to blood flow, pulmonary vascular changes and congestive heart failure develop late in the course of the disease, if at all.[137] When present, symptoms and signs are identical to those of atrial septal defect and include a widely split second heart sound, a systolic ejection murmur, and a gallop rhythm. Because pulmonary venous blood mixes with systemic venous blood at or before the right atrium, oxygen saturation tends to be identical in all heart chambers and the two major vessels; in the absence of severe pulmonary hypertension, this finding may be a clue to the presence of the anomaly.

Total Anomalous Drainage. In this relatively uncommon abnormality, an atrial septal defect or patent ductus arteriosus is necessary for survival. Other cardiovascular anomalies, syndromes of deranged bronchial anatomy, and splenic abnormalities are also frequent.[138] Typically, the pulmonary veins join directly behind the heart to form a common, somewhat dilated sac before communicating with the systemic venous system. Clinical and pathologic manifestations can result from the large left-to-right shunt (in which case pulmonary arterial and right ventricular dilatation is frequently present) or from obstruction to venous blood flow.

Radiographic features are variable. Cases with communication at the supracardiac or cardiac level are usually characterized by severe pulmonary pleonemia;[139] those with significant pulmonary venous obstruction and hypertension show a characteristic radiographic combination of interstitial pulmonary edema and a normal-sized heart.

As might be expected, many patients die in infancy. Those who survive to adulthood characteristically have a large septal defect and a short anomalous pathway, drainage being directly into the superior vena cava or right atrium.[140]

ANOMALIES OF BOTH ARTERIES AND VEINS

Hypogenetic Lung Syndrome

Hypogenetic lung (scimitar) syndrome is a rare congenital anomaly characterized by hypoplasia and anomalous pulmonary venous drainage of the right lung.[5,141,142] The anomalous pulmonary vein most commonly drains into the inferior vena cava below the level of the right hemidiaphragm. Hypoplasia of the right pulmonary artery, partial or complete arterial supply to the right lung by systemic arteries originating in the aorta, anomalies of the right bronchial tree (commonly mirror image), and bronchial diverticula are commonly present.[143,144] Associated cardiovascular anomalies are also frequent, the most common being atrial septal defect.[139]

Although the pathogenesis is unclear, the multiple associated pulmonary anomalies suggest that the condition most likely represents a basic developmental derangement of the entire lung bud early in embryogenesis. The occurrence in some families suggests a genetic abnormality[142]; however, most cases are sporadic. Why the combination of changes is so consistently located on the right side is unknown.

The diagnosis can often be made on the chest radiograph, the characteristic findings consisting of a small right lung with a small hilum and diminished vascularity, shift of the heart and mediastinum to the right, and the characteristic appearance of the anomalous draining vein coursing parallel to the right atrium.[139] The anomalous vein typically has a curved appearance, likened to the shape of a Turkish sword or scimitar (Fig. 5–10). If the radiographic findings are not definitive, the diagnosis can usually be made with CT.[144-146] In addition,

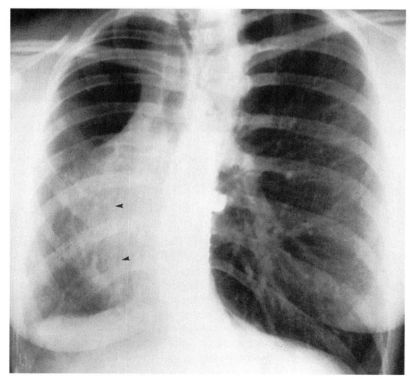

FIGURE 5–10

Hypogenetic lung (scimitar) syndrome. A posteroanterior radiograph reveals a small right hemithorax. The pulmonary vasculature of the right lung is diminutive and disorganized, whereas that of the left lung is normal. A large vascular shadow (*arrowheads*) coursing caudally from the midlung zone toward the cardiophrenic angle can be identified through a dextroposed cardiac silhouette. (*From Fraser RS, Müller NL, Colman NC, Paré PD: Fraser and Paré's Diagnosis of Diseases of the Chest, 4th ed. Philadelphia, WB Saunders, 1999.*)

CT allows identification of associated abnormalities, such as a bilobed right lung with absence of the minor fissure and a horseshoe lung.[142,146] The diagnosis may also be made with MR imaging.[147]

Most patients have cardiorespiratory symptoms, similar in many respects to those of large left-to-right shunts with pulmonary arterial hypertension.[148] Some patients have repeated bronchopulmonary infections or hemoptysis. A systolic murmur of moderate intensity is usually heard along the left sternal border. Patients without pulmonary arterial hypertension or symptoms in infancy have a good prognosis and often lead a normal life without surgical correction of the abnormalities.[142]

Congenital Arteriovenous Fistula

The term *pulmonary arteriovenous malformation* (arteriovenous fistula, arteriovenous aneurysm) is used here to describe a spectrum of abnormal vascular communications between pulmonary arteries and pulmonary veins that range from those that are too small to be visualized radiologically to complex aneurysms with multiple feeding arteries and draining veins that may involve the entire blood supply of a segment or lobe.[149] Many patients have multiple lesions in the lungs, and it has been estimated that approximately 60% of patients with pulmonary lesions have arteriovenous communications in the skin, mucous membranes, or other organs.[150] The latter condition, known as *hereditary hemorrhagic telangiectasia* (Rendu-Osler-Weber disease), has an autosomal dominant pattern of inheritance.[151] Most pulmonary fistulas are not recognized until the twenties or thirties[152]; they occur twice as frequently in women as men.

Pathologic Characteristics

Grossly, pulmonary arteriovenous fistulas appear as more or less spherical, vascular masses ranging in diameter from 1 mm to several centimeters, often just beneath the pleura or adjacent to bronchovascular bundles (Fig. 5–11). Examination of some fistulas by the corrosion cast technique has shown them to be supplied and drained by several vessels, the draining veins usually being somewhat larger than the feeding arteries.[153] The intervening vessels may be few and markedly ectatic, resembling a cyst, or numerous and more or less uniform in diameter, resulting in a complex branching mass resembling a Medusa's head. The vascular walls are typically thin, especially in larger vessels, a characteristic that is presumably related to parenchymal hemorrhage.

Radiologic Manifestations

The malformations are seen most commonly in the lower lobes and are multiple in about a third of cases.[154] The characteristic radiographic appearance is a round or oval homogeneous mass of unit density, somewhat lobulated in contour but sharply defined, in the medial third of the lung that ranges from less than 1 cm to several centimeters in diameter (Fig. 5–12). A feeding artery and draining vein can often be identified, the artery relating to the hilum and the vein deviating from the course of the artery toward the left atrium.

The characteristic CT finding consists of a homogeneous, circumscribed nodule or serpiginous mass connected with blood vessels.[155,156] Optimal investigation requires the use of

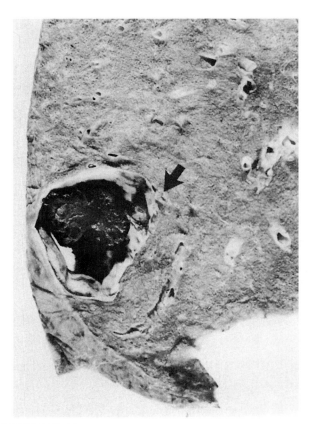

FIGURE 5-11

Pulmonary arteriovenous malformation. A magnified view of a lower lobe shows a well-circumscribed, subpleural cystic space filled with blood clot. A portion of the feeder pulmonary artery is evident at the right (*arrow*). Histologic sections showed the cyst wall to have a variable appearance, focally resembling the pulmonary artery and pulmonary vein. (*From Fraser RS, Müller NL, Colman NC, Paré PD: Fraser and Paré's Diagnosis of Diseases of the Chest, 4th ed. Philadelphia, WB Saunders, 1999.*)

spiral volumetric CT, which permits assessment of the entire lung in one or two breath-holds and thus minimizes the risk of missing small lesions. The procedure also enables image reconstruction of various levels within the lesion, thereby facilitating depiction of the center of the malformation (Fig. 5–13).[155,156] Despite the value of spiral CT, pulmonary angiography is routinely performed before treatment to confirm the presence of the malformation, assess the feeding arterial and draining venous structures, and detect other malformations.[155,157]

Clinical Manifestations

As might be expected, hemoptysis is the most common initial complaint. Dyspnea is present in as many as 60% of patients in some series.[158] Signs suggestive of the abnormality include cyanosis, finger clubbing, and a continuous murmur or bruit audible over the lesion or lesions. Because of the strong association with hereditary telangiectasia, extrathoracic manifestations of disease are also fairly common. Epistaxis, telangiectasis in the skin or mucous membranes, and upper or lower gastrointestinal tract hemorrhage can be seen, and symptoms referable to the CNS are present in many patients. Although the latter are attributable to intracerebral aneurysms in some cases, in many they are related to complications of the pulmonary

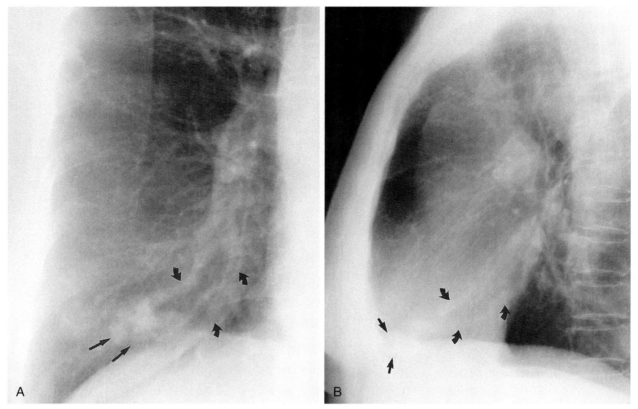

FIGURE 5–12

Pulmonary arteriovenous malformation. Views of the right lung from posteroanterior (**A**) and lateral (**B**) chest radiographs in a 71-year-old woman show a serpiginous soft tissue opacity in the right middle lobe (*straight arrows*). The associated large feeding artery and draining vein (*curved arrows*) are diagnostic of an arteriovenous malformation. *(From Müller NL, Fraser RS, Colman NC, Paré PD: Radiologic Diagnosis of Diseases of the Chest. Philadelphia, WB Saunders, 2001.)*

aneurysms, such as metastatic abscess, hypoxemia, cerebral embolism, and cerebral thrombosis from secondary polycythemia.

Arterial blood gas analysis and cardiac catheterization may provide useful data to confirm the diagnosis: PO_2 and arterial oxygen saturation are decreased, cardiac output is increased, and pulmonary artery pressure is normal. The electrocardiogram is generally normal, a sign useful in distinguishing it from congenital heart disease. Although the majority of patients have polycythemia, repeated hemorrhage from the nose or lungs may cause anemia.

The prognosis is generally good. Transcatheter embolization has become a safe, effective means of vascular occlusion and is widely considered to be the procedure of choice for standard treatment.[149,159]

ANOMALIES OF THE PULMONARY LYMPHATICS

Diffuse Pulmonary Lymphangiomatosis

Lymphangiomatosis is a rare pulmonary abnormality that has sometimes been confused with lymphangiectasia. To obviate this confusion, it has been proposed that the latter term be confined to lesions characterized by dilation of existing lymphatic vessels, without an increase in number or complexity[160]; by

contrast, lymphangiomatosis is used to refer to lesions in which the primary abnormality is an increase in the number of lymphatics. The condition is most commonly recognized in infancy and childhood, during which time it has been estimated to account for approximately 5% of all chronic interstitial disease.[161] Pathologically, there is a proliferation of variably sized, anastomosing lymphatic vessels in pleural, interlobular septal, and peribronchovascular connective tissue.

Chest radiographs show bilateral interstitial disease, sometimes with a lower lobe predominance.[160,162] Pleural effusion (chylothorax), either unilateral or bilateral, is common[163]; chylopericardium is seen occasionally.[163] The main CT abnormality is smooth thickening of the interlobular septa and bronchoarterial bundles[164]; patchy bilateral areas of ground-glass attenuation (presumed to represent pulmonary edema) are also commonly seen.

Clinical manifestations of "asthma" have been noted in a number of patients.[160] Concomitant mediastinal, skeletal, and other visceral lymphangiomatous malformations are present in some individuals.[164,165] Pulmonary function tests often show combined restrictive and obstructive features.

Congenital Pulmonary Lymphangiectasia

Congenital pulmonary lymphangiectasia is an almost invariably fatal abnormality that usually becomes manifest at

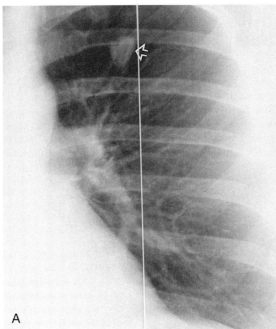

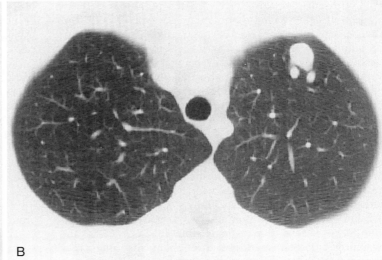

FIGURE 5–13

Arteriovenous malformation. A view of the left lung from a posteroanterior chest radiograph (**A**) in a 33-year-old man with Rendu-Osler-Weber disease shows a slightly lobulated soft tissue opacity in the left upper lobe (*arrow*). A 5-mm-collimation spiral CT scan performed without intravenous contrast material (**B**) shows the opacity with the associated feeding artery and draining vein. A maximal-intensity projection reconstruction obtained by using volumetric spiral CT data (**C**) allows better depiction of the vascular nature of the lesion with demonstration of the feeding artery and draining vein (*arrows*). *(From Müller NL, Fraser RS, Colman NC, Paré PD: Radiologic Diagnosis of Diseases of the Chest. Philadelphia, WB Saunders, 2001.)*

birth.[166] It has been classified into three subtypes based on the presence or absence of congenital cardiac malformations, involvement of other viscera, and early or late expression. The most common form (group II) is thought to result from abnormal development of the lung between the 14th and 20th weeks of gestation. Many patients have congenital abnormalities of other structures, usually polycystic or other renal disease or congenital ichthyosis.[167] The radiographic changes are highly variable; most commonly, there is a marked prominence of interstitial markings in the form of Kerley A and B lines simulating interstitial pulmonary edema.

Patients in group I have cardiac anomalies, and the pathogenesis is at least partly related to obstruction of pulmonary venous return.[166] Patients in group III have a combination of pulmonary disease and lymphangiectasia in other viscera, especially the intestine.[168] Pulmonary involvement is less severe than in groups I and II and is associated with a better prognosis. HRCT shows interlobular septal thickening, peribronchial cuffing, bilateral pleural effusions, and increased attenuation within the mediastinum with obliteration of the mediastinal fat planes because of edema.[169]

MISCELLANEOUS VASCULAR ANOMALIES

Anomalies of the Heart and Great Vessels Resulting in Increased Pulmonary Blood Flow

These anomalies include atrial and ventricular septal defect, patent ductus arteriosus, and an aorticopulmonary window. The left-to-right shunt results in some degree of increased pulmonary blood flow, which may be recognizable radiologically as increased size and amplitude of pulsation in the central and peripheral pulmonary arteries.

Anomalies of the Heart and Great Vessels Resulting in Decreased Pulmonary Blood Flow

By far the most common cause of general pulmonary oligemia as a result of diminished flow is a congenital anomaly of the right ventricular outflow tract (isolated pulmonic stenosis, tetralogy of Fallot with pulmonary atresia, type IV persistent truncus arteriosus, or Ebstein's anomaly). The caliber of the pulmonary vessels generally reflects the severity of the decrease in flow, the hila usually being diminutive and the peripheral vessels correspondingly small (except with valvular pulmonic stenosis, in which case poststenotic dilatation may enlarge the main or left pulmonary artery shadow). The reduction in flow throughout the lungs is more or less uniform.

Because decreased pulmonary circulation always increases bronchial collateral flow, the pulmonary vascular pattern throughout the lungs may be formed partly or wholly by a greatly hypertrophied bronchial arterial system. This extensive systemic arterial supply is particularly evident in the tetralogy of Fallot and in type IV pulmonary artery atresia. Although pulmonary arterial flow is negligible in these cases, the diminutive vascular markings throughout the lungs may represent the pulmonary arterial tree being filled through systemic–pulmonary artery anastomoses.

Systemic Arterial Supply to the Lung

A portion of lung, which may be normal or abnormal, may be supplied by a systemic artery arising from the aorta or one of its branches. The abnormality may be congenital or acquired.[170] The former is usually seen as part of another pulmonary anomaly, such as bronchopulmonary sequestration, hypogenetic lung syndrome, congenital cystic adenomatoid malformation, absence of the main pulmonary artery, and proximal interruption of a pulmonary artery.

A systemic artery may also supply a portion of lung in the absence of these conditions, either in the form of a systemic-pulmonary vascular fistula or as a localized blood supply of otherwise normal lung.[171-173] In the latter situation, a large systemic artery supplies a portion of one lung, invariably the basal segments of one of the lower lobes, either partly or completely. Examination of the bronchial tree shows normal architecture, by definition excluding sequestration. Additional pulmonary artery supply to the affected segments may or may not be present, but the main pulmonary artery and its branches to other lobes are normal. The anomalous artery is usually solitary and arises from the descending aorta. The cause and pathogenesis are unknown.

The chest radiograph shows normal or increased vascular markings.[173] The increased blood flow from the systemic artery causes dilation of the draining inferior pulmonary veins, which may result in a tubular shadow visible radiographically in the left lower lobe.[172,174] The dilated vein and the increased vascularity in the lower lobe are readily recognized on CT scan (Fig. 5–14). Pulmonary angiography, CT, or MR imaging can be used to determine whether there is an absence of pulmonary arterial supply to the involved lung.

Congenital systemic-pulmonary vascular fistulas may involve either normal or anomalous systemic arterial branches, and communication may be with either pulmonary veins or arteries, usually in the basal segment of one of the lower lobes.[175] Affected patients may be asymptomatic or may suffer from recurrent hemoptysis; a murmur may be audible over the defect.[171,175] Morphologic and angiographic studies have shown a complex arrangement of intercommunicating vessels. When communication exists with a pulmonary artery, catheterization of this vessel may reveal increased oxygen saturation, thereby providing evidence of a left-to-right shunt.

Similar systemic-pulmonary vascular fistulas may be secondary to infection, trauma, or surgery. Although the incidence of such acquired systemic arterialization of the lung is unknown, it is probably much higher than commonly realized, particularly when there is obliteration of the pleural space by fibrous tissue as a result of pleuritis. Occasionally, significant symptoms result from the subsequent shunt.[176]

METABOLIC PULMONARY DISEASE

Pulmonary Calcification and Ossification

Abnormal calcification may occur in normal tissue (metastatic calcification) or in tissue that is degenerating or dead (dystrophic calcification).[177] The latter is by far the more common

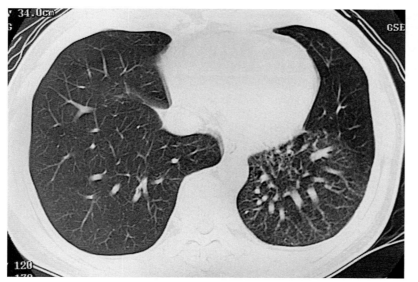

FIGURE 5–14

Systemic arterial supply to the lung. A CT scan shows increased vascularity of the left lower lobe caused by enlargement of the pulmonary veins. The systemic arterial supply to the left lower lobe originated from the descending thoracic aorta. The patient was a 54-year-old woman. *(From Müller NL, Fraser RS, Colman NC, Paré PD: Radiologic Diagnosis of Diseases of the Chest. Philadelphia, WB Saunders, 2001.)*

and in the lung is associated most often with foci of remote granulomatous inflammation. Dystrophic calcification may also occur in fibrous tissue in association with many underlying disorders, in which case there may be bone formation in addition to the deposition of calcium salts. The process is probably mediated by growth factors and cytokines that stimulate differentiation of fibroblasts into osteoblasts.[177] Two morphologic variants have been described, one nodular and the other linear (branching or "dendriform").[178]

Metastatic Calcification

Metastatic calcification typically occurs in patients who have hypercalcemia, usually associated with chronic renal failure[179] and less often with an intraosseous malignancy such as multiple myeloma[180]; it has also been reported after kidney and liver transplantation.[181,182] The abnormality is especially common in patients undergoing maintenance hemodialysis. For example, in one investigation of 23 such patients, 14 (61%) had pulmonary uptake on technetium 99m (^{99m}Tc)-diphosphonate scanning.[179]

Pathologically, deposits of calcium phosphate are seen in a more or less linear fashion in alveolar septa and the walls of small pulmonary vessels and bronchi (Fig. 5–15).[183] Interstitial fibrosis may or may not be present. Air spaces are typically unaffected.

The radiographic manifestations usually consist of numerous 3- to 10-mm-diameter fluffy, poorly defined nodular opacities mimicking air space nodules.[184] The calcific nature of the opacities can be confirmed by scanning with bone-imaging agents such as ^{99m}Tc-diphosphonate[185] or by HRCT (Fig. 5–16).[184,186] The latter procedure may also show calcification of arteries in the chest wall or, less commonly, calcification of the pulmonary arteries, superior vena cava, or myocardium.[184,187] Few patients in whom metastatic calcification is pathologically demonstrable show evidence of its presence on radiographs. For example, in one study of the chest

radiographs and CT scans of seven patients who had biopsy-proven disease, calcification was evident on radiographs in only two cases and on CT scans in four.[184]

The abnormality has a predilection for the apical and subapical lung zones, a feature attributable to regional differences in pulmonary ventilation and perfusion.[184] Because the $\dot{V}/\dot{Q}$ ratio is higher at the apex than at the base of the lung, the local milieu at the former site has a higher partial pressure of oxygen, a lower partial pressure of carbon dioxide, and a higher pH (approximately 7.50 versus 7.39 at the base).[177] This relative alkalinity favors the precipitation of calcium salts in the apical region.

Clinical manifestations of metastatic calcification are typically absent. However, pulmonary function abnormalities may be seen—primarily a decrease in carbon monoxide diffusing capacity (DLCO).[179,188]

Pulmonary Alveolar Proteinosis

Pulmonary alveolar proteinosis (PAP, alveolar lipoproteinosis, alveolar phospholipidosis) is an uncommon disease characterized by the accumulation of protein- and lipid-rich material resembling surfactant within the parenchymal air spaces.[189,190] Although the disease occurs predominantly in patients between the ages of 20 and 50 years (the mean age at diagnosis being about 38), very young children constitute a subgroup at increased risk.[191] There is a male-to-female preponderance of about 2.5:1.[189]

Etiology and Pathogenesis

Ultrastructural,[192] immunohistochemical,[193] and biochemical[194] observations indicate that the material that accumulates in the alveoli in PAP consists predominantly of surfactant. The cause of the accumulation varies and can be conveniently discussed under three headings—acquired, congenital, and secondary.[189]

Acquired. Acquired disease is the most common form of PAP and accounts for more than 90% of all cases. There is now substantial evidence that it is related to the presence of an antibody to granulocyte-macrophage colony-stimulating factor (GM-CSF).[189,190] As its name suggests, an important feature of this substance is stimulation of hematopoiesis; however, it is also produced by pulmonary epithelial cells, and receptors for it are present in alveolar macrophages and alveolar type II epithelial cells. Experiments in genetically altered mice that lack either GM-CSF or a component of its receptor have shown impaired surfactant clearance that results in disease similar to that seen in humans who have PAP.[189] Thus, it appears that the abnormality is basically one of autoimmunity. The reason for the development of an antibody to GM-CSF is unclear. Approximately 75% of patients have a history of smoking at the onset of symptoms, and it has been speculated that cigarette-induced toxicity may be important[189]; however, in view of the rarity of the disease, it is clear that additional factors must be involved.

Congenital. Most cases of this form of PAP are the result of an abnormality in the gene coding for surfactant B, which leads to both reduced levels of this substance and a disturbance in the processing of surfactant C.[189] An intrinsic abnormality in the receptor for GM-CSF may be present in other individuals.

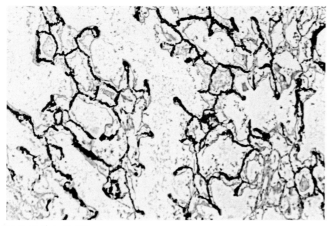

FIGURE 5–15

Metastatic pulmonary calcification. The section shows extensive deposition of calcium phosphate (stained black) in alveolar septa. The tissue was from the upper lobe of a patient with chronic renal failure; no corresponding radiographic abnormality was detected. *(From Fraser RS, Müller NL, Colman NC, Paré PD: Fraser and Paré's Diagnosis of Diseases of the Chest, 4th ed. Philadelphia, WB Saunders, 1999.)*

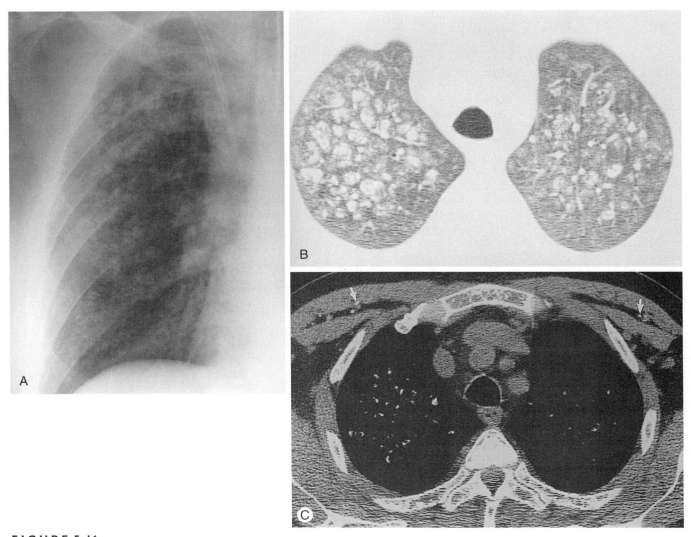

FIGURE 5–16

Metastatic pulmonary calcification. A close-up view of the right lung from a posteroanterior chest radiograph (**A**) in a 42-year-old patient who had chronic renal failure shows poorly defined nodular opacities involving mainly the upper lobe. Similar findings were present in the left lung. A hemodialysis catheter is in place. An HRCT scan through the lung apices (**B**) shows nodular areas of increased attenuation. Soft tissue windows (**C**) demonstrate the presence of calcification within the opacities. Vascular calcification in the chest wall is also evident (*arrows*). *(From Fraser RS, Müller NL, Colman NC, Paré PD: Fraser and Paré's Diagnosis of Diseases of the Chest, 4th ed. Philadelphia, WB Saunders, 1999.)*

Secondary. This variant of PAP is seen in association with other disease, including inorganic dust inhalation (particularly acute silicosis[195]), immunodeficiency syndromes (such as AIDS[196] or immunoglobulin deficiency[197]), and hematologic malignancies such as acute myelogenous leukemia. The pathogenesis of surfactant accumulation is varied and depends on the particular underlying abnormality. For example, in acute myelogenous leukemia it may be related to derivation of alveolar macrophages from a clone of malignant cells that lack the GM-CSF receptor.[189]

Pathologic Characteristics

On microscopic examination, the alveoli can be seen to be filled with finely granular, proteinaceous material that is rich in lipids and stains eosinophilic with hematoxylin and eosin and purple with periodic acid–Schiff (PAS) (see Color

Fig. 5–2). Acicular (needle shaped) crystals and laminated bodies believed to be cell fragments can also be seen. Macrophages are present within the granular material but are not usually abundant except (sometimes) focally at the border between normal and affected lung. Alveolar septa are usually normal or at most slightly thickened by a lymphocytic infiltrate. Ultrastructural examination shows the intraalveolar material to consist of amorphous granular debris containing numerous, relatively discrete osmiophilic granules or lamellar bodies, some of which resemble tubular myelin (Fig. 5–17).[192]

Radiologic Manifestations

The characteristic radiographic pattern consists of bilateral and symmetric areas of air space consolidation that have a vaguely nodular appearance and a predominantly perihilar or

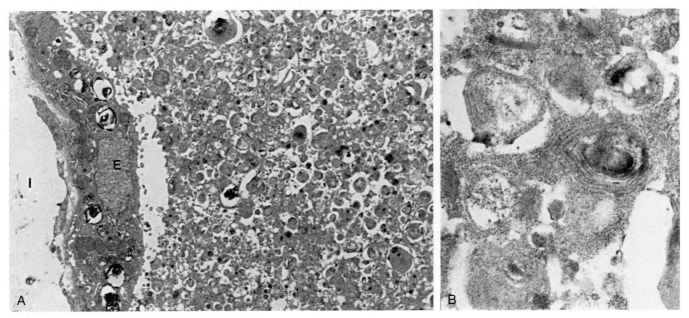

FIGURE 5–17

Pulmonary alveolar proteinosis. A transmission electron micrograph (**A**) shows a type II pneumocyte (E) overlying a somewhat fibrotic interstitium (I). The adjacent alveolar air space is filled with numerous, variably electron-dense bodies; at greater magnification (**B**), some can be seen to have distinct lamellations resembling those of the normal type II cell osmiophilic body. (**A**, ×9500; **B**, ×56,000.) *(From Fraser RS, Müller NL, Colman NC, Paré PD: Fraser and Paré's Diagnosis of Diseases of the Chest, 4th ed. Philadelphia, WB Saunders, 1999.)*

lower lobe distribution (Fig. 5–18).[198,199] In patients who have less severe disease, the appearance may be one of ground-glass opacities.[200] Occasionally, the parenchymal involvement is asymmetric or unilateral.[201,202] In some patients, a linear interstitial pattern can be seen superimposed on the areas of consolidation or ground-glass opacities; rarely, it is the predominant or only abnormality seen on radiographs.[201]

HRCT is superior to conventional CT and chest radiography in assessment of the pattern and distribution of abnormalities[201,203] and may show lesions even when radiography is normal.[202] The predominant abnormality typically consists of bilateral ground-glass opacities, although consolidation may also be present (particularly in the dorsal lung regions).[198,201,204] The ground-glass opacities tend to involve all lung zones to a similar extent but can have a predominant lower zone distribution. In most cases, a fine linear pattern forming polygonal shapes measuring 3 to 10 mm in diameter can be seen superimposed on the areas of ground-glass attenuation (*crazy-paving*, see Fig. 5–18).[200,203,204] The pattern reflects the presence of interstitial edema or the accumulation of lipoproteinaceous material in the air spaces adjacent to the interlobular septa.[203,205] Though characteristic of PAP, it can also be seen in a variety of other conditions, including bronchioloalveolar carcinoma, lipid pneumonia, pulmonary hemorrhage and/or edema, and bacterial pneumonia.[206-208]

Clinical Manifestations

The most frequent symptom is shortness of breath on exertion that is usually progressive and unassociated with orthopnea. Cough, usually nonproductive, is also common. Fatigue, weight loss, and pleuritic pain may be present. A low-grade fever develops or is evident at initial evaluation in some

patients and should suggest concomitant infection. Although this fever may be related to "common" community and hospital bacteria, opportunists such as *Nocardia*, *Aspergillus*, and *Cryptococcus* species are not infrequently the cause.[189] The incidence of such infections appears to be decreased after lavage.[190] Fine or coarse crackles can sometimes be heard on auscultation. Clubbing of the fingers has been identified in about a third of patients.[190]

Laboratory Findings and Diagnosis

Laboratory investigation reveals a normal or slightly elevated white blood cell count and, not uncommonly, polycythemia. An increase in the level of serum lactate dehydrogenase is common.[209] Analysis of BAL fluid and serum has shown an increase in some tumor markers such as carcinoembryonic antigen,[210] as well as an increase in surfactant proteins.[211,212] The degree of elevation of these substances seems to reflect the severity of disease.

Pulmonary function studies can be completely normal but usually show a restrictive defect associated with a reduction in diffusing capacity and lung volumes.[213] Hypoxemia is common and often severe (mean ± SD of 58.6 ± 15.8 mm Hg in a review of published cases to 2002).[189] Although ventilation-perfusion inequality may be partly responsible, intrapulmonary shunting of blood through consolidated parenchyma is probably more important. The hypoxemia may be associated with pulmonary hypertension.[214] The results of follow-up function studies of patients managed successfully with BAL correlate well with clinical improvement.[215]

The diagnosis can usually be confirmed by analysis of BAL fluid. Features suggestive of the diagnosis include (1) a grossly opaque or milky effluent; (2) relatively few inflammatory

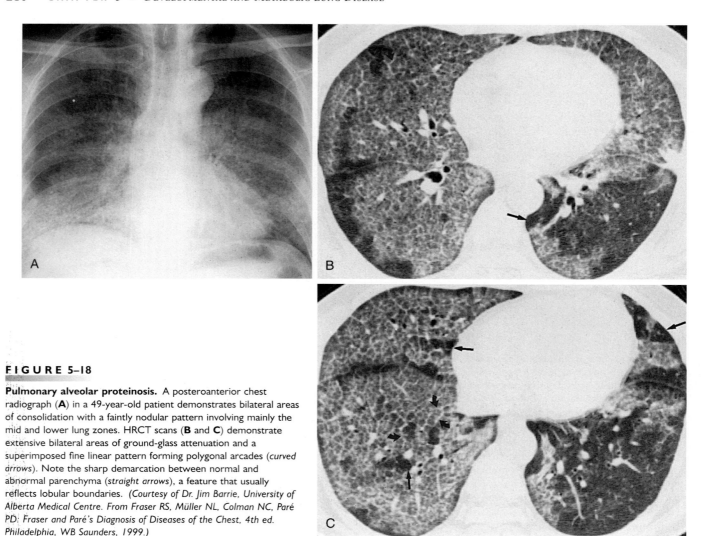

FIGURE 5–18

Pulmonary alveolar proteinosis. A posteroanterior chest radiograph (**A**) in a 49-year-old patient demonstrates bilateral areas of consolidation with a faintly nodular pattern involving mainly the mid and lower lung zones. HRCT scans (**B** and **C**) demonstrate extensive bilateral areas of ground-glass attenuation and a superimposed fine linear pattern forming polygonal arcades (*curved arrows*). Note the sharp demarcation between normal and abnormal parenchyma (*straight arrows*), a feature that usually reflects lobular boundaries. *(Courtesy of Dr. Jim Barrie, University of Alberta Medical Centre. From Fraser RS, Müller NL, Colman NC, Paré PD: Fraser and Paré's Diagnosis of Diseases of the Chest, 4th ed. Philadelphia, WB Saunders, 1999.)*

cells, including alveolar macrophages; (3) large acellular eosinophilic bodies in a diffuse background of granular basophilic material; (4) PAS staining of the proteinaceous material; (5) elevated levels of surfactant proteins; and (6) characteristic ultrastructural features. If it is deemed necessary to confirm the diagnosis by tissue examination, transbronchial biopsy is likely to be sufficient.

Prognosis and Natural History

Analysis of cases documented in the literature before the widespread use of therapeutic BAL shows the disease to have been fatal in about a third of patients, death resulting either from respiratory failure caused by the proteinosis or from superimposed infection.[216] In occasional patients, clinically significant pulmonary fibrosis develops as a late complication. Actuarial survival rates in the literature review mentioned previously were 79%, 75%, and 68% at 2, 5, and 10 years.[189] Irrigation of the lung parenchyma by BAL (whole-lung lavage) has greatly improved this prognosis, with most patients experiencing improvement in symptomatology, exercise tolerance, and arterial oxygenation.[190] Some patients require only one or two procedures,[217] whereas a few require that lavage be

repeated semiannually or annually. As might be expected in view of the pathogenesis, the condition has been documented to recur after lung transplantation.[218] Spontaneous resolution without treatment has been observed in about 25% of patients in some series.[219]

Amyloidosis

Though originally thought to represent a single substance, amyloid is now known to consist of several proteins, each of which resembles the others morphologically but is distinctive biochemically.[220] Over 15 such proteins have been identified, several of which have been implicated in respiratory disease. The most important in this respect are *amyloid L* (AL) and *amyloid A* (AA). AL is derived from immunoglobulin light chains and is thus usually associated with abnormal plasma cell function, either localized to the lungs or as part of a systemic disease such as multiple myeloma or macroglobulinemia. AA is derived from a serum acute phase reactant (SAA) synthesized in the liver. The latter can be formed in several settings, including connective tissue disease (particularly rheumatoid disease), chronic infection (particularly tuberculosis), bronchiectasis, and certain neoplasms (such as

Hodgkin's lymphoma). Other precursor proteins of amyloid include *transthyretin* (prealbumin), a serum protein that normally transports thyroxine and is associated with heart and pulmonary deposits in so-called senile amyloidosis[221]; β_2-*microglobulin*, a normal serum protein that is often increased in chronic renal failure[222]; and *endocrine-related amyloid* (AE), derived from local hormone deposition in the stroma of some neuroendocrine tumors of the lung and other organs.[223]

Because of its great variety of clinical and pathologic manifestations, amyloidosis has been classified by schema other than that related to biochemical origin.[224] The most widely used of these classifications includes four major forms that depend on the underlying clinical features: (1) *primary amyloidosis*, in which no associated disease is recognized or in which there is an underlying plasma cell disorder (most commonly multiple myeloma); (2) *secondary amyloidosis*, in which there is an underlying chronic inflammatory abnormality such as bronchiectasis or rheumatoid disease; (3) *familial amyloidosis*, a relatively uncommon form that may be localized to a specific tissue such as nerve; and (4) so-called *senile amyloidosis*, which affects many organs and tissues and is usually seen in individuals older than 70.

Although these classifications are useful in understanding the nature of amyloidosis, from the point of view of diagnosis and the clinical consequences of thoracic involvement, it is often more useful to consider the disease in terms of its anatomic location. According to this concept, there are three major forms of amyloidosis in the lower respiratory tract: tracheobronchial, nodular parenchymal, and diffuse parenchymal (interstitial). Although these forms can occur in combination, in many cases the amyloid is deposited predominantly in one site, thus providing some rationale for classification on this basis. In addition to airway and pulmonary parenchymal disease, amyloidosis can also affect the pleura,[225] pulmonary arteries,[221] hilar and mediastinal lymph nodes,[226,227] and diaphragm.[228]

In considering a diagnosis of thoracic amyloidosis, it must be remembered that pulmonary diseases such as chronic tuberculosis, bronchiectasis, and cystic fibrosis can themselves result in amyloidosis. Though rare, this secondary phenomenon may occasionally alter the radiologic appearance of the underlying pulmonary abnormality.

Pathogenesis

A detailed description of the pathogenetic features of amyloidosis is beyond the scope of this text; however, certain features related to pulmonary disease deserve mention. Although most localized deposits of amyloid in the lung consist of AL,[229] the great majority of patients have no evidence of systemic disease such as multiple myeloma or serologic immunoglobulin abnormality.[230,231] Thus, it has been speculated that local immunoglobulin deposition, possibly related to either overproduction or impaired clearance secondary to chronic inflammation, may be responsible for the amyloid accumulation.[231] Immunohistochemical and gene rearrangement studies of some pulmonary amyloid nodules have shown evidence of clonal plasma cell expansion, thus suggesting that a localized neoplastic process may be involved.[232] The validity of this mechanism is supported by the observation that occasional foci of nodular pulmonary lymphoma are associated with AL amyloid derived from the same light chain as found in the tumor cells.[233]

Pathologic Characteristics

Airway involvement occurs most commonly in the trachea and proximal bronchi. Although overlap does occur, it is usually manifested in one of two ways: a localized nodule or (more commonly) multiple discrete or confluent intramural plaques that distort the airway wall and cause stenosis of its lumen.[229,234] Histologically, the amyloid is situated in the subepithelial interstitial tissue and often surrounds tracheobronchial gland ducts and acini, some of which may show atrophy.

The parenchymal nodules of localized pulmonary amyloid can be solitary or multiple and are usually fairly well defined and gray.[234] Amyloid is often identifiable in the alveolar interstitium at the periphery of the nodule; however, in the central region, the normal parenchymal architecture is generally obscured by a more or less solid mass of amyloid that typically contains fairly numerous multinucleated giant cells and variable numbers of lymphocytes and plasma cells (see Color Fig. 5–3). Calcification and ossification are not uncommon.

In diffuse interstitial disease, amyloid is present in the media of small blood vessels and in the parenchymal interstitium (Fig. 5–19; see Color Fig. 5–3). In the latter site, it is typically located adjacent to endothelial and epithelial basement

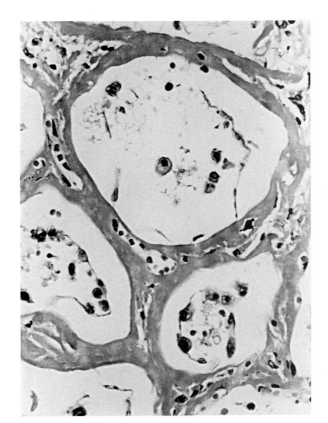

FIGURE 5–19

Amyloidosis: diffuse interstitial. A highly magnified view of lung parenchyma shows mild thickening of the alveolar septal interstitium by amyloid. Its location between the capillary wall and alveolar epithelial surface can be clearly seen. (*From Fraser RS, Müller NL, Colman NC, Paré PD: Fraser and Paré's Diagnosis of Diseases of the Chest, 4th ed. Philadelphia, WB Saunders, 1999.*)

membranes and can appear in a uniform and more or less linear pattern or as multiple small nodules.[235] Inflammatory cells and ossification or calcification are typically absent.

Radiologic Manifestations

Tracheobronchial amyloidosis results in focal or diffuse thickening of the airway wall or, rarely, a localized intraluminal nodule.[236,237] The abnormality is generally confined to the trachea but can extend to the main, lobar, and segmental bronchi.[238] CT demonstrates thickening of the airway wall, narrowing of the lumen, and in some cases, foci of calcification (Fig. 5–20).[236,238]

Nodular primary parenchymal amyloidosis is manifested as solitary or, less commonly, multiple nodules usually ranging from 0.5 to 5 cm in diameter (Fig. 5–21).[237,239] Calcification is seldom evident on radiographs[240] but is seen in 20% to 50% of nodules on CT scans.[239,241] The nodules occur most commonly in the lower lobes and are typically located peripherally. Cysts can be seen adjacent to the nodules in some cases. Disease may progress slowly over a period of several years, with a slight increase in size of the nodules and the development of additional nodules.[242]

Radiographic findings in interstitial parenchymal disease consist of a reticular, nodular, or reticulonodular pattern that may be diffuse or involve mainly the lower lobes.[237] The nodules may be small, similar to miliary tuberculosis, but can be as large as 2.5 cm in diameter. Interlobular septal thickening and areas of ground-glass attenuation or consolidation may also be evident.[239] Punctate calcification may be seen in some of the nodules and areas of consolidation.

Clinical Manifestations

The plaque-like form of tracheobronchial amyloidosis is often manifested by recurrent hemoptysis, bronchitis, and pneumonia.[243] Occasionally, it causes symptoms that simulate asthma. Discrete tracheal and endobronchial nodules seldom cause symptoms and are usually discovered incidentally at bronchoscopy; however, they can be large enough to cause airway obstruction with distal atelectasis or bronchiectasis. Symptoms and signs in such cases depend on the volume of lung affected and whether infection is present. The presence of amyloid in other sites is rare.[244]

The nodular parenchymal form of amyloidosis usually provokes no symptoms and is discovered on a screening chest radiograph.[245] New lesions have occasionally been reported to appear after the surgical excision of nodules,[246] but whether this finding represents the effect of inadequate resection or the development of independent lesions is unclear. The majority of patients have no evidence of extrathoracic disease (either amyloidosis or otherwise).

Progressive dyspnea and respiratory insufficiency are frequent in diffuse interstitial disease.[245] Although the former may be secondary to pulmonary disease itself, it is important to remember that it may be related to cardiac amyloidosis. Diffuse involvement is most often seen as part of multisystem disease (primary amyloidosis), in which circumstance AL is

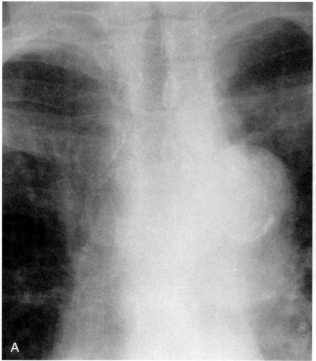

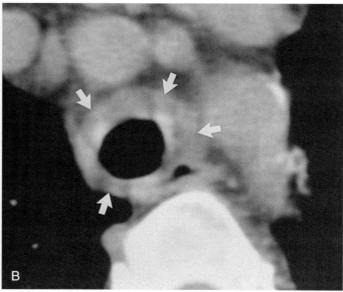

FIGURE 5-20

Diffuse tracheal amyloidosis. A view from a posteroanterior chest radiograph (**A**) demonstrates irregular narrowing of the trachea. A CT scan immediately above the level of the aortic arch (**B**) demonstrates marked circumferential thickening of the trachea (*arrows*). On CT and at bronchoscopy, the entire trachea was abnormal. The diagnosis was proved by endoscopic biopsy. *(From Fraser RS, Müller NL, Colman NC, Paré PD: Fraser and Paré's Diagnosis of Diseases of the Chest, 4th ed. Philadelphia, WB Saunders, 1999.)*

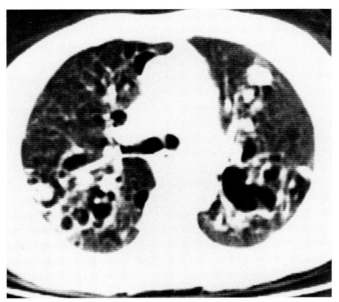

FIGURE 5–21

Amyloidosis: nodular parenchymal. A CT scan at the level of the carina reveals multiple nodules and cystic spaces. The patient was an elderly woman who complained of dyspnea. *(From Fraser RS, Müller NL, Colman NC, Paré PD: Fraser and Paré's Diagnosis of Diseases of the Chest, 4th ed. Philadelphia, WB Saunders, 1999.)*

typically present and may be associated with multiple myeloma.[237]

Laboratory Findings

Circulating monoclonal light chains, more often λ than κ, are frequently present in patients who have primary amyloidosis.[247,248] Nonspecific immunoglobulin abnormalities may be observed, with serum levels of IgA, IgG, and IgM being either increased or decreased, in patients who have the secondary form of disease. Biopsy of rectal tissue or abdominal wall fat may confirm the diagnosis in both conditions. When disease is localized to the lungs, transbronchial or transthoracic needle biopsy often yields diagnostic tissue. Pulmonary function tests may show evidence of restriction and impaired gas transfer in patients who have diffuse interstitial disease[249] and air trapping and fixed upper airway obstruction in those who have proximal tracheobronchial involvement.[244]

Prognosis and Natural History

The prognosis in patients who have nodular parenchymal amyloidosis is generally good: in most cases, the nodules remain stationary in size or grow slowly and cause no symptoms. By contrast, progression of disease is frequent in the tracheobronchial and diffuse interstitial forms of disease. Bronchoscopic or surgical excision of localized airway deposits may provide relief of obstruction; however, recurrence is common, and approximately 30% of patients have been reported to die of the disease.[244] The natural history and prognosis of disease in patients who have diffuse interstitial pulmonary involvement may be determined by the presence of amyloid elsewhere in the body, particularly the heart and

kidneys; however, many patients die of respiratory failure.[250] In one series of 35 patients, the median survival time after diagnosis was only 16 months.[237]

Pulmonary Alveolar Microlithiasis

Pulmonary alveolar microlithiasis is a rare disease characterized by the presence of innumerable tiny calculi ("calcospherites") within alveolar air spaces.[251,252] Although it can occur at any age, most reported cases have been in patients between the ages of 20 and 50 years.[253]

The etiology and pathogenesis are unknown. The abnormality has been documented in twins, and a familial occurrence has been noted in approximately 35% of reported cases,[254] thus implying a genetic factor. In many of these cases, a high rate of consanguinity has been found in the parents of affected individuals, thus suggesting an autosomal recessive pattern of inheritance. Despite these observations, there is evidence that environmental factors are important in at least some cases. For example, in one report of a family of seven siblings, the disease developed in the four sisters who lived together but not in the three who had left home at an early age.[255] Because serum calcium and phosphorus levels are generally normal, a systemic metabolic abnormality is unlikely to be involved in most cases.[256]

Microliths range in size from about 250 to 750 μm in diameter; are round, oval, or irregular in shape; and have a concentric laminated appearance.[257,258] Chemical analysis and energy-dispersive x-ray microanalysis have shown them to be composed principally of calcium phosphate.[259,260] In early disease, the alveolar walls are normal; eventually, interstitial fibrosis develops, sometimes associated with multinucleated giant cell formation.[259]

The characteristic radiographic pattern is one of a fine micronodulation diffusely involving both lungs (Fig. 5–22).[261] Regardless of the effect of superimposition or summation of shadows, individual deposits are usually identifiable as sharply defined nodules measuring less than 1 mm in diameter. The overall density is greater over the lower than the upper zone. Occasionally, there is a reticular pattern or septal lines superimposed on the characteristic "sandstorm" appearance.[262] Other findings that may be seen include bullae in the lung apices, a zone of increased lucency between the lung parenchyma and the ribs (known as a "black pleural line"), and pleural calcification.[255,263,264]

HRCT manifestations consist of calcific nodules measuring 1 mm or less in diameter, sometimes confluent, and distributed predominantly along the cardiac borders and dorsal portions of the lower lung zones.[265,266] The higher attenuation in the dorsal portion of the lungs persists when scans are obtained with the patient in the prone position. Calcific interlobular septal thickening is commonly seen. Other features noted on HRCT scans include apical bullae and thin-walled subpleural cysts.[265] Correlation of HRCT with radiographic findings has shown that the "black pleural line" can be caused by subpleural cysts along the costal and mediastinal pleura or by a layer of extrapleural fat.[265,267]

Many patients are asymptomatic when the disease is first discovered, the diagnosis being made on the basis of the typical radiographic pattern seen on a screening chest film or on a film obtained in an individual whose sibling is known to have the

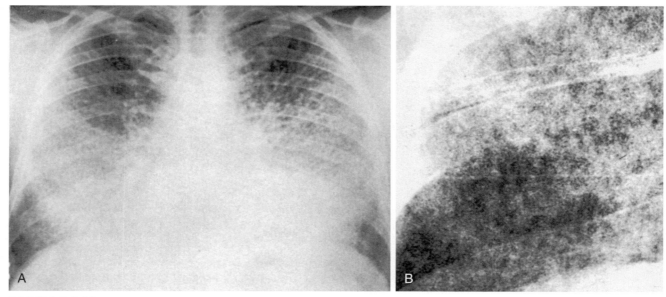

FIGURE 5-22

Alveolar microlithiasis. A posteroanterior radiograph (**A**) of this 40-year-old asymptomatic man reveals a remarkably uniform opacification of both lungs. On close scrutiny (**B**), this uniform opacification can be seen to be produced by a multitude of tiny, discrete opacities of calcific density. Pulmonary function test results were normal except for an 800-mL reduction in residual volume, representing displacement of pulmonary volume by the calcospherites. *(From Fraser RS, Müller NL, Colman NC, Paré PD: Fraser and Paré's Diagnosis of Diseases of the Chest, 4th ed. Philadelphia, WB Saunders, 1999.)*

disease. The most common symptom is dyspnea on exertion; cough develops occasionally.[268] Pectus excavatum and hypertrophic pulmonary osteoarthropathy have been noted in some patients.[253] As the disease progresses, respiratory insufficiency may develop in association with cyanosis, clubbing of the fingers, and evidence of pulmonary hypertension.[269]

The diagnosis can generally be made with confidence from the classic radiographic pattern and the striking radiologic-clinical disparity in severity of disease. Values from chemical analysis of blood are invariably within the normal range. Microliths can be identified in sputum, BAL fluid,[260] and transbronchial biopsy specimens.[270] The course of the disease is variable; however, it appears to progress slowly in many patients.

Lipid Storage Disease

Gaucher's Disease

Gaucher's disease is an autosomal recessive abnormality characterized by a deficiency of β-glucosidase, the enzyme that catabolizes glucosylceramide. This deficiency results in an accumulation of glucosylceramide, predominantly in the reticuloendothelial cells (Gaucher cells) of the liver, spleen, lymph nodes, bones, and in the infantile form of the disease, the brain. The majority of patients are female, and more than 95% are Ashkenazi Jews.

Histologically, Gaucher cells may be found in the peribronchovascular or alveolar interstitium, alveolar air spaces, or alveolar capillary lumina.[271] Their presence in the last-named site has been speculated to underlie the pulmonary hypertension seen in some individuals.[272] Radiologic

manifestations consist of a reticulonodular or miliary pattern affecting both lungs diffusely.[273] Lytic lesions are occasionally seen in the ribs.

Symptomatic pulmonary involvement is uncommon[273] and usually manifested by dyspnea; signs of pulmonary hypertension are seen occasionally. Gaucher cells can be detected in BAL fluid.[274] In an investigation of 95 patients who had the adult form of disease, approximately two thirds had pulmonary function abnormalities (most commonly, reduced FRC and DLCO).[275]

Niemann-Pick Disease

Niemann-Pick disease is caused by an inherited defect in the production of sphingomyelinase, a deficiency that results in the deposition of sphingomyelin in the liver, spleen, lung, bone marrow, and brain. Five clinical variants have been described that depend on the age at onset and the predominant organs affected. Many patients die in infancy or childhood; however, some survive into adulthood, occasionally exhibiting the first manifestations of their disease at that time.[276]

Pathologically, aggregates of large multivacuolated "foam" cells are present in the parenchyma of many organs, including the lungs. The radiographic manifestations consist of a reticular or reticulonodular pattern involving mainly the lower lung zones.[277,278] HRCT demonstrates patchy bilateral ground-glass opacities and smooth thickening of the interlobular septa involving primarily the lower lobes.[278,279] Hepatomegaly and peripheral lymph node enlargement are common. Pulmonary involvement can be asymptomatic or (rarely) severe enough to cause respiratory failure.[280]

Hermansky-Pudlak Syndrome

Hermansky-Pudlak syndrome is an autosomal recessive disease characterized by tyrosinase-positive oculocutaneous albinism, a defect in platelet function, and the accumulation of ceroid pigment in macrophages throughout the body.[281,282] It has been documented most often in persons from Puerto Rico and southern Holland.[283] Ceroid is a complex chromolipid that appears histologically as a brown pigment that is PAS positive, diastase resistant, and acid-fast. The substance appears to accumulate within lysosomes, thus suggesting an enzymatic defect[284,285]; however, the nature of such a defect is unknown.

Involvement of the pulmonary interstitium has been documented in a number of reports.[284,286] Histologically, it consists of variably severe parenchymal fibrosis associated with variable numbers of ceroid-laden macrophages. The most common radiographic manifestation is a bilateral reticular or reticulonodular pattern.[287] Less frequent findings include perihilar fibrosis and pleural thickening.[286,287] The earliest manifestations on HRCT consist of septal thickening, ground-glass opacities, and mild reticulation.[287] HRCT findings in the more advanced stages of disease include moderate to severe reticulation, traction bronchiectasis, honeycombing, and peribronchovascular thickening. The abnormalities tend to involve mainly the subpleural lung regions and the middle and lower zones.

Patients experience progressive dyspnea and appear to be susceptible to infection and to have a bleeding tendency. Pulmonary function studies reveal a restrictive pattern; hypoxemia at rest is characteristic.

Erdheim-Chester Disease

This rare abnormality is characterized by the deposition of lipid-laden macrophages in a variety of tissues, particularly bones. Pulmonary involvement was documented in 13 patients in a 1998 review[288]; mediastinal fibrosis and pleural thickening or effusion have also been reported.[288] The most common radiographic manifestations consist of bilateral reticular opacities and pleural thickening.[289] HRCT demonstrates interlobular septal thickening, subpleural micronodules, and areas of ground-glass attenuation.[289,290] Clinical manifestations include dyspnea and cough. Progression to respiratory failure and death has been seen in a number of patients.

Glycogen and Mucopolysaccharide Storage Disease

Involvement of thoracic structures other than the heart is only rarely detectable either clinically or radiologically in glycogen storage disease. *Pompe's disease* (acid maltase deficiency) usually affects infants and is fatal; involvement of the diaphragm and respiratory muscles of the chest wall can cause dyspnea and respiratory failure.[291]

Patients who have mucopolysaccharide storage diseases such as Hurler's, Hunter's, and Morquio's syndrome may survive into adulthood. Respiratory complications in these individuals include kyphoscoliosis, respiratory failure, pneumonia, and sleep apnea.[292]

Heritable Diseases of Connective Tissue

More than 100 distinct heritable disorders of connective tissue exist, each presumed to be caused by mutation in a single gene that controls the structure or metabolism of one or more macromolecules. Several of these disorders are complicated by abnormalities of the thoracic cage and pleuropulmonary interstitium.[293]

Marfan's Syndrome

Marfan's syndrome is an inherited connective tissue disorder characterized by a variety of cardiovascular, skeletal, and ocular abnormalities, including long extremities (particularly the fingers and toes), scoliosis, subluxation of the lens, and aortic dilation and dissection.[294] It is inherited in an autosomal dominant fashion (although about 25% of patients have no family history). The diagnosis is based on clinical findings and requires anomalies in two major organs and involvement of a third organ in an index case.[295] The disorder is the result of mutations in the gene responsible for production of fibrillin, a protein that is a part of the microfibrillary array that surrounds elastic and other connective tissue fibers.[294]

The most common chest radiograph manifestations are a long thin thorax, scoliosis, and pectus excavatum[296]; in one series of 50 patients, 34 (68%) had pectus deformity and 22 (44%) had scoliosis.[297] The most frequently reported pleuropulmonary abnormality is pneumothorax,[296,298] a complication that arises in about 5% to 10% of patients.[296,299] Other pulmonary manifestations include apical bullae and, less commonly, diffuse emphysema, bronchiectasis, and upper lobe fibrosis.[296,298]

Cardiovascular disease develops in most patients who have Marfan's syndrome and is the cause of death in more than 90%.[300] The most common abnormalities are aortic aneurysm, aortic dissection, and aortic and mitral valve insufficiency. Aortic aneurysm and aortic dissection usually involve the ascending aorta (Fig. 5–23). Serial chest radiographs may reveal progressive aortic enlargement and commonly show cardiomegaly as a result of aortic regurgitation.[301] The diagnosis can usually be confirmed by CT. Diagnostic features of aortic dissection include the presence of an intimal flap and a false lumen.[300,301] Aortic aneurysms and dissection, as well as the associated cardiovascular abnormalities, can also be recognized readily on MR imaging and echocardiography.[302,303]

Ehlers-Danlos Syndrome

Ehlers-Danlos syndrome consists of a group of inherited disorders of connective tissue that can be divided into several different types on the basis of clinical, genetic, and biochemical features.[304] Structural abnormalities of collagen are probably the cause of most apparent clinical findings. Pleuropulmonary and thoracic skeletal abnormalities consist most commonly of emphysema, often associated with bullae, pneumothorax, and scoliosis. Easy bruisability is also a prominent feature in some patients, and rupture of pulmonary vessels can be associated with significant pulmonary hemorrhage.[305] Other pulmonary abnormalities include tracheobronchomegaly,[306] fibrous pseudotumors, and cysts.[306,307]

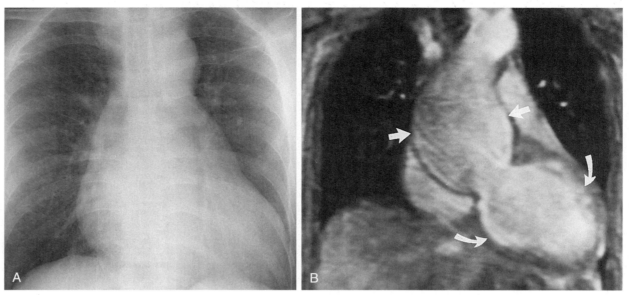

FIGURE 5–23

Marfan's syndrome. A posteroanterior chest radiograph (**A**) reveals dilation of the ascending aorta and cardiomegaly. A coronal MR image (**B**) demonstrates marked focal dilation of the ascending aorta (*straight arrows*) and dilation of the left ventricle (*curved arrows*) as a result of aortic regurgitation. The patient was a 32-year-old man. (*From Fraser RS, Müller NL, Colman NC, Paré PD: Fraser and Paré's Diagnosis of Diseases of the Chest, 4th ed. Philadelphia, WB Saunders, 1999.*)

Pulmonary Abnormalities in Systemic Endocrine Disease

Diabetes Mellitus

A variety of pulmonary complications have been associated with diabetes, the most common and serious being infection. Disease caused by organisms such as *Mycobacterium tuberculosis*, *Mucorales* species, *Staphylococcus aureus*, and a variety of gram-negative bacteria appears to have an increased incidence.[308] There is also evidence that infection caused by some organisms (e.g., *Streptococcus pneumoniae*, *Legionella* species, gram-negative organisms, and influenza virus) is associated with increased morbidity and mortality.[308]

As in other organs, the thickness of the pulmonary alveolar epithelial and capillary basement membranes is greater in diabetic patients than in age-matched controls.[309] It has been hypothesized that this greater membrane thickness may underlie, at least partly, the reduction in DLCO that has been observed in a number of investigations.[310,311] Other abnormalities in pulmonary function that have been identified include reductions (usually mild) in lung elastic recoil, forced vital capacity, and FEV_1.[312,313] In addition, there is evidence that diabetic autonomic neuropathy may result in functional or clinical abnormalities (such as an increased threshold for cough) in some patients.[314,315] Sleep-disordered breathing and diabetes also appear to have a complex relationship in that the disorder may increase insulin resistance and insulin resistance may, in turn, worsen breathing during sleep.[316] Finally, a number of cases of acute respiratory distress syndrome (ARDS) apparently unassociated with pulmonary infection have been reported in patients who have diabetes, usually in the setting of ketoacidosis.[317]

Hypopituitarism and Acromegaly

Several pulmonary function abnormalities have been demonstrated in patients who have either hypopituitarism or growth hormone excess (i.e., acromegaly). Hypopituitarism has been found to be associated with a restrictive type of ventilatory impairment, TLC being approximately 75% of normal.[318] By contrast, patients who have acromegaly have large lungs with a TLC greater than that in matched controls by 25% or more.[319] Another relatively common finding in patients who have acromegaly is upper airway obstruction, in some patients associated with sleep apnea and significant nocturnal hypoxemia.[320] Abnormal small airway function has also been described by some investigators.[321]

Hypothyroidism

Abnormal accumulations of fluid can be seen in the pleural spaces of patients who have myxedema in the absence of cardiovascular, renal, or other causes of fluid retention.[322] Patchy air space disease has been described as well; in one study it was presumed to be edema, although there was no dyspnea or cardiomegaly.[323]

Hypoxemia and reduced lung volumes can also occur in patients who have myxedema, usually in association with obesity and hypoventilation and often with coma.[324] However, some of these patients are not obese, and their blood gas values have been shown to return to normal with thyroid therapy despite little or no change in body weight.[325] Some patients have sleep apnea.[326]

Hyperthyroidism

Pulmonary function studies in some patients who have hyperthyroidism have shown a decrease in vital capacity and an increase in minute ventilation during exercise.[327] Some investigators have also found evidence of inspiratory and expiratory muscle weakness,[328] an increase in hypoxic and hypercapnic ventilatory drive,[329] and pulmonary artery hypertension.[330]

Hyperparathyroidism

As discussed elsewhere (see page 207), hypercalcemia associated with hyperparathyroidism can result in diffuse metastatic calcification of the lungs. Though usually detectable only by histologic examination, it is sometimes severe enough to be visible radiologically and rarely causes symptoms.

REFERENCES

1. Clements BS, Warner JO, Shinebourne EA: Congenital bronchopulmonary vascular malformations: Clinical application of a simple anatomical approach in 25 cases. Thorax 42:409-416, 1987.
2. Clements BS, Warner JO: Pulmonary sequestration and related congenital bronchopulmonary-vascular malformations: Nomenclature and classification based on anatomical and embryological considerations. Thorax 42:401-408, 1987.
3. Grewal RG, Yip CK: Intralobar pulmonary sequestration and mediastinal bronchogenic cyst. Thorax 49:615-616, 1994.
4. Vevecka E, De Boeck K, Moerman P, et al: Tracheal bronchus associated with congenital cystic adenomatoid malformation. Pediatr Pulmonol 20:413-416, 1995.
5. Panicek DM, Heitzman ER, Randall PA, et al: The continuum of pulmonary developmental anomalies. Radiographics 7:747-772, 1987.
6. Helms PJ: Lung growth: Implications for the development of disease. Thorax 49:440-441, 1994.
7. Landing BH, Dixon LG: Congenital malformations and genetic disorders of the respiratory tract (larynx, trachea, bronchi, and lungs). Am Rev Respir Dis 120:151-185, 1979.
8. Lurie IW, Ilyina HG, Gurevich DB, et al: Trisomy 2p: Analysis of unusual phenotypic findings. Am J Med Genet 55:229-236, 1995.
9. Mardini MK, Nyhan WL: Agenesis of the lung. Report of four patients with unusual anomalies. Chest 87:522-527, 1985.
10. Cunningham ML, Mann N: Pulmonary agenesis: A predictor of ipsilateral malformations. Am J Med Genet 70:391-398, 1997.
11. Vanamo K: A 45-year perspective of congenital diaphragmatic hernia. Br J Surg 83:1758-1762, 1996.
12. Page DV, Stocker JT: Anomalies associated with pulmonary hypoplasia. Am Rev Respir Dis 125:216-221, 1982.
13. Goldstein JD, Reid LM: Pulmonary hypoplasia resulting from phrenic nerve agenesis and diaphragmatic amyoplasia. J Pediatr 97:282-287, 1980.
14. Argyle JC: Pulmonary hypoplasia in infants with giant abdominal wall defects. Pediatr Pathol 9:43-55, 1989.
15. Adzick NS, Harrison MR, Glick PL, et al: Experimental pulmonary hypoplasia and oligohydramnios: Relative contributions of lung fluid and fetal breathing movements. J Pediatr Surg 19:658-665, 1984.
16. Harding R, Hooper SB: Regulation of lung expansion and lung growth before birth. J Appl Physiol 81:209-224, 1996.
17. Fewell JE, Lee CC, Kitterman JA: Effects of phrenic nerve section on the respiratory system of fetal lambs. J Appl Physiol 51:293-297, 1981.
18. Liggins GC, Vilos GA, Campos GA, et al: The effect of spinal cord transection on lung development in fetal sheep. J Dev Physiol 3:267-274, 1981.
19. Chamberlain D, Hislop A, Hey E, Reid L: Pulmonary hypoplasia in babies with severe rhesus isoimmunisation: A quantitative study. J Pathol 122:43-52, 1977.
20. Hislop A, Hey E, Reid L: The lungs in congenital bilateral renal agenesis and dysplasia. Arch Dis Child 54:32-38, 1979.
21. Kitagawa M, Hislop A, Boyden EA, Reid L: Lung hypoplasia in congenital diaphragmatic hernia. A quantitative study of airway, artery, and alveolar development. Br J Surg 58:342-346, 1971.
22. Cooney TP, Thurlbeck WM: Lung growth and development in anencephaly and hydranencephaly. Am Rev Respir Dis 132:596-601, 1985.
23. Hislop A, Sanderson M, Reid L: Unilateral congenital dysplasia of lung associated with vascular anomalies. Thorax 28:435-441, 1973.
24. Soulen RL, Cohen RV: Plain film recognition of pulmonary agenesis in the adult. Chest 60:185-187, 1971.
25. Mata JM, Caceres J, Lucaya J, Garcia-Conesa JA: CT of congenital malformations of the lung. Radiographics 10:651-674, 1990.
26. Wu CT, Chen MR, Shih SL, et al: Case report: Agenesis of the right lung diagnosed by three-dimensional reconstruction of helical chest CT. Br J Radiol 69:1052-1054, 1996.
27. Newman B, Gondor M: MR evaluation of right pulmonary agenesis and vascular airway compression in pediatric patients. AJR Am J Roentgenol 168:55-58, 1997.

28. Ijsselstijn H, Tibboel D, Hop WJ, et al: Long-term pulmonary sequelae in children with congenital diaphragmatic hernia. Am J Respir Crit Care Med 155:174-180, 1997.
29. Sade RM, Clouse M, Ellis FH Jr: The spectrum of pulmonary sequestration. Ann Thorac Surg 18:644-658, 1974.
30. Stocker JT, Malczak HT: A study of pulmonary ligament arteries. Relationship to intralobar pulmonary sequestration. Chest 86:611-615, 1984.
31. Frazier AA, Rosado de Christenson ML, Stocker JT, Templeton PA: Intralobar sequestration: Radiologic-pathologic correlation. Radiographics 17:725-745, 1997.
32. Savic B, Birtel FJ, Tholen W, et al: Lung sequestration: Report of seven cases and review of 540 published cases. Thorax 34:96-101, 1979.
33. Felker RE, Tonkin IL: Imaging of pulmonary sequestration. AJR Am J Roentgenol 154:241-249, 1990.
34. Ikezoe J, Murayama S, Godwin JD, et al: Bronchopulmonary sequestration: CT assessment. Radiology 176:375-379, 1990.
35. Frush DP, Donnelly LF: Pulmonary sequestration spectrum: A new spin with helical CT. AJR Am J Roentgenol 169:679-682, 1997.
36. Konen E, Raviv-Zilka L, Cohen RA, et al: Congenital pulmonary venolobar syndrome: Spectrum of helical CT findings with emphasis on computerized reformatting. Radiographics 23:1175-1184, 2003.
37. Naidich DP, Rumancik WM, Lefleur RS, et al: Intralobar pulmonary sequestration: MR evaluation. J Comput Assist Tomogr 11:531-533, 1987.
38. Doyle AJ: Demonstration of blood supply to pulmonary sequestration by MR angiography. AJR Am J Roentgenol 158:989-990, 1992.
39. Rosado-de-Christenson ML, Frazier AA, Stocker JT, Templeton PA: From the archives of the AFIP. Extralobar sequestration: Radiologic-pathologic correlation. Radiographics 13:425-441, 1993.
40. Gerle RD, Jaretzki A 3rd, Ashley CA, Berne AS: Congenital bronchopulmonary-foregut malformation. Pulmonary sequestration communicating with the gastrointestinal tract. N Engl J Med 278:1413-1419, 1968.
41. Heithoff KB, Sane SM, Williams HJ, et al: Bronchopulmonary foregut malformations. A unifying etiological concept. AJR Am J Roentgenol 126:46-55, 1976.
42. Wesley JR, Heidelberger KP, DiPietro MA, et al: Diagnosis and management of congenital cystic disease of the lung in children. J Pediatr Surg 21:202-207, 1986.
43. St-Georges R, Deslauriers J, Duranceau A, et al: Clinical spectrum of bronchogenic cysts of the mediastinum and lung in the adult. Ann Thorac Surg 52:6-13, 1991.
44. Suen HC, Mathisen DJ, Grillo HC, et al: Surgical management and radiological characteristics of bronchogenic cysts. Ann Thorac Surg 55:476-481, 1993.
45. Salyer DC, Salyer WR, Eggleston JC: Benign developmental cysts of the mediastinum. Arch Pathol Lab Med 101:136-139, 1977.
46. Rogers LF, Osmer JC: Bronchogenic cyst. A review of 46 cases. Am J Roentgenol Radium Ther Nucl Med 91:273-290, 1964.
47. Rappaport DC, Herman SJ, Weisbrod GL: Congenital bronchopulmonary diseases in adults: CT findings. AJR Am J Roentgenol 162:1295-1299, 1994.
48. Yoon YC, Lee KS, Kim TS, et al: Intrapulmonary bronchogenic cyst: CT and pathologic findings in five adult patients. AJR Am J Roentgenol 179:167-170, 2002.
49. Nakata H, Nakayama C, Kimoto T, et al: Computed tomography of mediastinal bronchogenic cysts. J Comput Assist Tomogr 6:733-738, 1982.
50. Mendelson DS, Rose JS, Efremidis SC, et al: Bronchogenic cysts with high CT numbers. AJR Am J Roentgenol 140:463-465, 1983.
51. Naidich DP, Rumancik WM, Ettenger NA, et al: Congenital anomalies of the lungs in adults: MR diagnosis. AJR Am J Roentgenol 151:13-19, 1988.
52. Nakata H, Egashira K, Watanabe H, et al: MRI of bronchogenic cysts. J Comput Assist Tomogr 17:267-270, 1993.
53. Dahmash NS, Chen JT, Ravin CE, et al: Unusual radiologic manifestations of bronchogenic cyst. South Med J 77:762-764, 1984.
54. De Nunzio MC, Evans AJ: Case report: The computed tomographic features of mediastinal bronchogenic cyst rupture into the bronchial tree. Br J Radiol 67:589-590, 1994.
55. Yernault JC, Kuhn G, Dumortier P, et al: "Solid" mediastinal bronchogenic cyst: Mineralogic analysis. AJR Am J Roentgenol 146:73-74, 1986.
56. Patel SR, Meeker DP, Biscotti CV, et al: Presentation and management of bronchogenic cysts in the adult. Chest 106:79-85, 1994.
57. Ribet ME, Copin MC, Gosselin B: Bronchogenic cysts of the mediastinum. J Thorac Cardiovasc Surg 109:1003-1010, 1995.
58. Aktogu S, Yuncu G, Halilcolar H, et al: Bronchogenic cysts: Clinicopathological presentation and treatment. Eur Respir J 9:2017-2021, 1996.
59. Johnston SR, Adam A, Allison DJ, et al: Recurrent respiratory obstruction from a mediastinal bronchogenic cyst. Thorax 47:660-662, 1992.
60. Metersky ML, Moskowitz H, Thayer JO: Recurrent mediastinal bronchogenic cyst. Respiration 62:234-236, 1995.
61. Miller RK, Sieber WK, Yunis EJ: Congenital adenomatoid malformation of the lung. A report of 17 cases and review of the literature. Pathol Annu 15:387-402, 1980.
62. Avitabile AM, Greco MA, Hulnick DH, Feiner HD: Congenital cystic adenomatoid malformation of the lung in adults. Am J Surg Pathol 8:193-202, 1984.
63. Patz EF Jr, Müller NL, Swensen SJ, Dodd LG: Congenital cystic adenomatoid malformation in adults: CT findings. J Comput Assist Tomogr 19:361-364, 1995.
64. Stocker JT: Congenital pulmonary airway malformation—a new name for and an expanded classification of congenital cystic adenomatoid malformation of the lung. Histopathology 41:424-458, 2002.
65. Stocker JT, Madewell JE, Drake RM: Congenital cystic adenomatoid malformation of the lung. Classification and morphologic spectrum. Hum Pathol 8:155-171, 1977.
66. Kim WS, Lee KS, Kim IO, et al: Congenital cystic adenomatoid malformation of the lung: CT-pathologic correlation. AJR Am J Roentgenol 168:47-53, 1997.

67. Ribet ME, Copin MC, Soots JG, Gosselin BH: Bronchioloalveolar carcinoma and congenital cystic adenomatoid malformation. Ann Thorac Surg 60:1126-1128, 1995.
68. Jederlinic PJ, Sicilian LS, Baigelman W, Gaensler EA: Congenital bronchial atresia. A report of 4 cases and a review of the literature. Medicine (Baltimore) 66:73-83, 1987.
69. Reid L: The Pathology of Emphysema. London, Lloyd-Luke (Medical Books), 1967.
70. Haller JA Jr, Tepas JJ 3rd, White JJ, et al: The natural history of bronchial atresia. Serial observations of a case from birth to operative correction. J Thorac Cardiovasc Surg 79:868-872, 1980.
71. Robotham JL, Menkes HA, Chipps BE, et al: A physiologic assessment of segmental bronchial atresia. Am Rev Respir Dis 121:533-540, 1980.
72. Kinsella D, Sissons G, Williams MP: The radiological imaging of bronchial atresia. Br J Radiol 65:681-685, 1992.
73. al-Nakshabandi N, Lingawi S, Müller NL: Residents' corner. Answer to case of the month #72. Congenital bronchial atresia. Can Assoc Radiol J 51:47-48, 2000.
74. Cohen AM, Solomon EH, Alfidi RJ: Computed tomography in bronchial atresia. AJR Am J Roentgenol 135:1097-1099, 1980.
75. Finck S, Milne EN: A case report of segmental bronchial atresia: Radiologic evaluation including computed tomography and magnetic resonance imaging. J Thorac Imaging 3:53-57, 1988.
76. Rossoff LJ, Steinberg H: Bronchial atresia and mucocele: A report of two cases. Respir Med 88:789-791, 1994.
77. van Klaveren RJ, Morshuis WJ, Lacquet LK, et al: Congenital bronchial atresia with regional emphysema associated with pectus excavatum. Thorax 47:1082-1083, 1992.
78. Warkany J: The trachea and bronchi. In Warkany J (ed): Congenital Malformations. Chicago, Year Book, 1971, p 599.
79. Atwell SW: Major anomalies of the tracheobronchial tree: With a list of the minor anomalies. Dis Chest 52:611-615, 1967.
80. Mangiulea VG, Stinghe RV: The accessory cardiac bronchus. Bronchologic aspect and review of the literature. Dis Chest 54:433-436, 1968.
81. Jackson GD, Littleton JT: Simultaneous occurrence of anomalous cardiac and tracheal bronchi: A case study. J Thorac Imaging 3:59-60, 1988.
82. Shipley RT, McLoud TC, Dedrick CG, Shepard JA: Computed tomography of the tracheal bronchus. J Comput Assist Tomogr 9:53-55, 1985.
83. Ritsema GH: Ectopic right bronchus: Indication for bronchography. AJR Am J Roentgenol 140:671-674, 1983.
84. Hosker HS, Clague HW, Morritt GN: Ectopic right upper lobe bronchus as a cause of breathlessness. Thorax 42:473-474, 1987.
85. Remy J, Smith M, Marache P, Nuyts JP: [Pathogenetic left tracheal bronchus. A review of the literature in connection with four cases (author's transl)]. J Radiol Electrol Med Nucl 58:621-630, 1977.
86. Soto B, Pacifico AD, Souza AS Jr, et al: Identification of thoracic isomerism from the plain chest radiograph. AJR Am J Roentgenol 131:995-1002, 1978.
87. McGuinness G, Naidich DP, Garay SM, et al: Accessory cardiac bronchus: CT features and clinical significance. Radiology 189:563-566, 1993.
88. Black RJ: Congenital tracheo-oesophageal fistula in the adult. Thorax 37:61-63, 1982.
89. Holden MP, Wooler GH: Tracheo-oesophageal fistula and oesophageal atresia: Results of 30 years' experience. Thorax 25:406-412, 1970.
90. Ramo OJ, Salo JA, Mattila SP: Congenital bronchoesophageal fistula in the adult. Ann Thorac Surg 59:887-889, discussion 890, 1995.
91. Moreno Azcoita M, Ruiz de Adana JC, Sanchez Urdazpal L, et al: Congenital oesophagobronchial fistula in an adult involving left main bronchus. Thorax 49:835-836, 1994.
92. Osinowo O, Harley HR, Janigan D: Congenital broncho-oesophageal fistula in the adult. Thorax 38:138-142, 1983.
93. Kameya S, Umeda Y, Mizuno K, et al: Congenital esophagobronchial fistula in the adult. Am J Gastroenterol 79:589-592, 1984.
94. Leithiser RE Jr, Capitanio MA, Macpherson RI, Wood BP: "Communicating" bronchopulmonary foregut malformations. AJR Am J Roentgenol 146:227-231, 1986.
95. Edwards JE, McGoon DC: Absence of anatomic origin from heart of pulmonary arterial supply. Circulation 47:393-398, 1973.
96. Ellis K: Fleischner lecture. Developmental abnormalities in the systemic blood supply to the lungs. AJR Am J Roentgenol 156:669-679, 1991.
97. Collett RW, Edwards JE: Persistent truncus arteriosus: A classification according to anatomic types. Surg Clin North Am 29:1245, 1949.
98. Marcelletti C, McGoon DC, Mair DD: The natural history of truncus arteriosus. Circulation 54:108-111, 1976.
99. Hicken P, Evans D, Heath D: Persistent truncus arteriosus with survival to the age of 38 years. Br Heart J 28:284-286, 1966.
100. Spencer H: Pathology of the Lung (Excluding Pulmonary Tuberculosis), vol 1, 4th ed. New York, Pergamon Press, 1985.
101. Moser KM, Olson LK, Schlusselberg M, et al: Chronic thromboembolic occlusion in the adult can mimic pulmonary artery agenesis. Chest 95:503-508, 1989.
102. Morgan PW, Foley DW, Erickson SJ: Proximal interruption of a main pulmonary artery with transpleural collateral vessels: CT and MR appearances. J Comput Assist Tomogr 15:311-313, 1991.
103. Lynch DA, Higgins CB: MR imaging of unilateral pulmonary artery anomalies. J Comput Assist Tomogr 14:187-191, 1990.
104. Bouros D, Paré P, Panagou P, et al: The varied manifestation of pulmonary artery agenesis in adulthood. Chest 108:670-676, 1995.
105. Berdon WE, Baker DH: Vascular anomalies and the infant lung: Rings, slings, and other things. Semin Roentgenol 7:39-64, 1972.

106. Gallo P, Fazzari F, La Magra C, et al: Facio-auriculo-vertebral anomalad and pulmonary artery sling. A hitherto undescribed but probably non-casual association. Pathol Res Pract 173:172-179, 1981.
107. Gumbiner CH, Mullins CE, McNamara DG: Pulmonary artery sling. Am J Cardiol 45:311-315, 1980.
108. Vogl TJ, Diebold T, Bergman C, et al: MRI in pre- and postoperative assessment of tracheal stenosis due to pulmonary artery sling. J Comput Assist Tomogr 17:878-886, 1993.
109. Stone DN, Bein ME, Garris JB: Anomalous left pulmonary artery: Two new adult cases. AJR Am J Roentgenol 135:1259-1263, 1980.
110. McCue C, Robertson L, Lester R, et al: Pulmonary artery coarctations: A report of 20 cases with review of 319 cases from the literature. J Pediatr 67:222, 1965.
111. Lees MH, Menashe VD, Sunderland CO, et al: Ehlers-Danlos syndrome associated with multiple pulmonary artery stenoses and tortuous systemic arteries. J Pediatr 75:1031-1036, 1969.
112. Rowe RD: Maternal rubella and pulmonary artery stenoses. Report of eleven cases. Pediatrics 32:180-185, 1963.
113. Hoeffel JC, Henry M, Jimenez J, Pernot C: Congenital stenosis of the pulmonary artery and its branches. Clin Radiol 25:481-490, 1974.
114. Ellis K, Seaman W, Griffiths S, et al: Some congenital anomalies of the pulmonary arteries. Semin Roentgenol 2:325, 1967.
115. Bartter T, Irwin RS, Nash G: Aneurysms of the pulmonary arteries. Chest 94:1065-1075, 1988.
116. Buckingham WB, Sutton GC, Meszaros WT: Abnormalities of the pulmonary artery resembling intrathoracic neoplasms. Dis Chest 40:698-704, 1961.
117. Silverman JM, Julien PJ, Herfkens RJ, Pelc NJ: Magnetic resonance imaging evaluation of pulmonary vascular malformations. Chest 106:1333-1338, 1994.
118. Trell E: Pulmonary arterial aneurysm. Thorax 28:644-649, 1973.
119. Jimenez M, Fournier A, Choussat A: Pulmonary artery to the left atrium fistula as an unusual cause of cyanosis in the newborn. Pediatr Cardiol 10:216-220, 1989.
120. Ohara H, Ito K, Kohguchi N, et al: Direct communication between the right pulmonary artery and the left atrium. A case report and review of the literature. J Thorac Cardiovasc Surg 77:742-747, 1979.
121. Krause DW, Kuehn HJ, Sellers RD, Wilson WJ: Roentgen sign associated with an aberrant vessel connecting right main pulmonary artery to left atrium. Radiology 111:177-178, 1974.
122. Stuckey S: Direct communication between the right pulmonary artery and the left atrium: Magnetic resonance findings. Australas Radiol 37:216-220, 1993.
123. Mortenson W, Lundstrom NR: Congenital obstruction of the pulmonary veins at their atrial junctions. Review of the literature and a case report. Am Heart J 87:359-362, 1974.
124. Belcourt CL, Roy DL, Nanton MA, et al: Stenosis of individual pulmonary veins: Radiologic findings. Radiology 161:109-112, 1986.
125. Vogel M, Ash J, Rowe RD, et al: Congenital unilateral pulmonary vein stenosis complicating transposition of the great arteries. Am J Cardiol 54:166-171, 1984.
126. Asayama J, Shiguma R, Katsume H, Ijichi H: Pulmonary varix. Angiology 35:735-739, 1984.
127. Ben-menachem Y, Kuroda K, Kyger ER 3rd, et al: The various forms of pulmonary varices. Report of three cases and review of the literature. Am J Roentgenol Radium Ther Nucl Med 125:881-889, 1975.
128. Steinberg I: Pulmonary varices mistaken for pulmonary and hilar disease. Am J Roentgenol Radium Ther Nucl Med 101:947-952, 1967.
129. Shida T, Ohashi H, Nakamura K, Morimoto M: Pulmonary varices associated with mitral valve disease: A case report and survey of the literature. Ann Thorac Surg 34:452-456, 1982.
130. Borkowski GP, O'Donovan PB, Troup BR: Pulmonary varix: CT findings. J Comput Assist Tomogr 5:827-829, 1981.
131. Blake HA, Hall RJ, Manion WC: Anomalous pulmonary venous return. Circulation 32:406-414, 1965.
132. Greene R, Miller SW: Cross-sectional imaging of silent pulmonary venous anomalies. Radiology 159:279-281, 1986.
133. Dillon EH, Camputaro C: Partial anomalous pulmonary venous drainage of the left upper lobe vs duplication of the superior vena cava: Distinction based on CT findings. AJR Am J Roentgenol 160:375-379, 1993.
134. Vesely TM, Julsrud PR, Brown JJ, Hagler DJ: MR imaging of partial anomalous pulmonary venous connections. J Comput Assist Tomogr 15:752-756, 1991.
135. White CS, Baffa JM, Haney PJ, et al: Anomalies of pulmonary veins: Usefulness of spin-echo and gradient-echo MR images. AJR Am J Roentgenol 170:1365-1368, 1998.
136. Wang ZJ, Reddy GP, Gotway MB, et al: Cardiovascular shunts: MR imaging evaluation. Radiographics 23(Spec No):S181-S194, 2003.
137. Kissner DG, Sorkin RP: Anomalous pulmonary venous connection. Medical therapy. Chest 89:752-754, 1986.
138. Petersen RC, Edwards WD: Pulmonary vascular disease in 57 necropsy cases of total anomalous pulmonary venous connection. Histopathology 7:487-496, 1983.
139. Kiely B, Filler J, Stone S, et al: Syndrome of anomalous venous drainage of the right lung to the inferior vena cava: A review of 67 reported cases and three new cases in children. Am J Cardiol 20:102, 1967.
140. Singh R, Weisinger B, Carpenter M, et al: Total anomalous pulmonary venous return, surgically corrected in two patients beyond 40 years of age. Chest 60:38-43, 1971.
141. Woodring JH, Howard TA, Kanga JF: Congenital pulmonary venolobar syndrome revisited. Radiographics 14:349-369, 1994.
142. Dupuis C, Charaf LA, Breviere GM, et al: The "adult" form of the scimitar syndrome. Am J Cardiol 70:502-507, 1992.

143. Cukier A, Kavakama J, Teixeira LR, et al: Scimitar sign with normal pulmonary venous drainage and systemic arterial supply. Scimitar syndrome or bronchopulmonary sequestration? Chest 105:294-295, 1994.

144. Godwin JD, Tarver RD: Scimitar syndrome: Four new cases examined with CT. Radiology 159:15-20, 1986.

145. Olson MA, Becker GJ: The scimitar syndrome: CT findings in partial anomalous pulmonary venous return. Radiology 159:25-26, 1986.

146. Gilkeson RC, Basile V, Sands MJ, Hsu JT: Chest case of the day. Scimitar syndrome. AJR Am J Roentgenol 169:267-270, 1997.

147. Baran R, Kir A, Tor MM, et al: Scimitar syndrome: Confirmation of diagnosis by a noninvasive technique (MRI). Eur Radiol 6:92-94, 1996.

148. Mathey J, Galey JJ, Logeais Y, et al: Anomalous pulmonary venous return into inferior vena cava and associated bronchovascular anomalies (the scimitar syndrome). Thorax 23:398-407, 1968.

149. Burke CM, Safai C, Nelson DP, Raffin TA: Pulmonary arteriovenous malformations: A critical update. Am Rev Respir Dis 134:334-339, 1986.

150. Dines DE, Arms RA, Bernatz PE, et al: Pulmonary arteriovenous fistulas. Mayo Clin Proc 49:460-465, 1974.

151. Guttmacher AE, Marchuk DA, White RI Jr: Hereditary hemorrhagic telangiectasia. N Engl J Med 333:918-924, 1995.

152. Gomes MM, Bernatz PE: Arteriovenous fistulas: A review and ten-year experience at the Mayo Clinic. Mayo Clin Proc 45:81-102, 1970.

153. Steinberg I, Maisel B, Vogel FS: Pulmonary arteriovenous fistula associated with capillary telangiectasia (Rendu-Osler-Weber disease); report of a case illustrating use of metal casting for demonstrating the lesion. J Thorac Surg 35:517-522, 1958.

154. Gossage JR, Kanj G: Pulmonary arteriovenous malformations. A state of the art review. Am J Respir Crit Care Med 158:643-661, 1998.

155. Remy J, Remy-Jardin M, Wattinne L, Deffontaines C: Pulmonary arteriovenous malformations: Evaluation with CT of the chest before and after treatment. Radiology 182:809-816, 1992.

156. Remy J, Remy-Jardin M, Giraud F, Wattinne L: Angioarchitecture of pulmonary arteriovenous malformations: Clinical utility of three-dimensional helical CT. Radiology 191:657-664, 1994.

157. Coley SC, Jackson JE: Pulmonary arteriovenous malformations. Clin Radiol 53:396-404, 1998.

158. Moyer JH, Glantz G, Brest AN: Pulmonary arteriovenous fistulas; physiologic and clinical considerations. Am J Med 32:417-435, 1962.

159. Dutton JA, Jackson JE, Hughes JM, et al: Pulmonary arteriovenous malformations: Results of treatment with coil embolization in 53 patients. AJR Am J Roentgenol 165:1119-1125, 1995.

160. Tazelaar HD, Kerr D, Yousem SA, et al: Diffuse pulmonary lymphangiomatosis. Hum Pathol 24:1313-1322, 1993.

161. Fan LL, Mullen AL, Brugman SM, et al: Clinical spectrum of chronic interstitial lung disease in children. J Pediatr 121:867-872, 1992.

162. Canny GJ, Cutz E, MacLusky IB, Levison H: Diffuse pulmonary angiomatosis. Thorax 46:851-853, 1991.

163. Ramani P, Shah A: Lymphangiomatosis. Histologic and immunohistochemical analysis of four cases. Am J Surg Pathol 17:329-335, 1993.

164. Swensen SJ, Hartman TE, Mayo JR, et al: Diffuse pulmonary lymphangiomatosis: CT findings. J Comput Assist Tomogr 19:348-352, 1995.

165. Takahashi K, Takahashi H, Maeda K, et al: An adult case of lymphangiomatosis of the mediastinum, pulmonary interstitium and retroperitoneum complicated by chronic disseminated intravascular coagulation. Eur Respir J 8:1799-1802, 1995.

166. Felman AH, Rhatigan RM, Pierson KK: Pulmonary lymphangiectasia. Observation in 17 patients and proposed classification. Am J Roentgenol Radium Ther Nucl Med 116:548-558, 1972.

167. Rhatigan RM, Hobin FP: Congenital pulmonary lymphangiectasis and ichthyosis congenita. A case report. Am J Clin Pathol 53:95-99, 1970.

168. Noonan JA, Walters LR, Reeves JT: Congenital pulmonary lymphangiectasis. Am J Dis Child 120:314-319, 1970.

169. Nobre LF, Müller NF, de Souza AS Jr, et al: Congenital pulmonary lymphangiectasia. CT and pathologic findings. J Thorac Imaging 19:56-59, 2004.

170. Tadavarthy SM, Klugman J, Castaneda-Zuniga WR, et al: Systemic-to-pulmonary collaterals in pathological states: A review. Radiology 144:55-59, 1982.

171. Brundage BH, Gomez AC, Cheitlin MD, Gmelich JT: Systemic artery to pulmonary vessel fistulas: Report of two cases and a review of the literature. Chest 62:19-23, 1972.

172. Hirai T, Ohtake Y, Mutoh S, et al: Anomalous systemic arterial supply to normal basal segments of the left lower lobe. A report of two cases. Chest 109:286-289, 1996.

173. Miyake H, Hori Y, Takeoka H, et al: Systemic arterial supply to normal basal segments of the left lung: Characteristic features on chest radiography and CT. AJR Am J Roentgenol 171:387-392, 1998.

174. Matzinger FR, Bhargava R, Peterson RA: Systemic arterial supply to the lung without sequestration: An unusual cause of hemoptysis. Can Assoc Radiol J 45:44-47, 1994.

175. Currarino G, Willis K, Miller W: Congenital fistula between an aberrant systemic artery and a pulmonary vein without sequestration. A report of three cases. J Pediatr 87:554-557, 1975.

176. Syme J: Systemic to pulmonary arterial fistula of the chest wall and lung following lobectomy. Australas Radiol 19:326-333, 1975.

177. Chan ED, Morales DV, Welsh CH, et al: Calcium deposition with or without bone formation in the lung. Am J Respir Crit Care Med 165:1654-1669, 2002.

178. Joines RW, Roggli VL: Dendriform pulmonary ossification. Report of two cases with unique findings. Am J Clin Pathol 91:398-402, 1989.

179. Faubert PF, Shapiro WB, Porush JG, et al: Pulmonary calcification in hemodialyzed patients detected by technetium-99m diphosphonate scanning. Kidney Int 18:95-102, 1980.

180. Weber CK, Friedrich JM, Merkle E, et al: Reversible metastatic pulmonary calcification in a patient with multiple myeloma. Ann Hematol 72:329-332, 1996.

181. Breitz HB, Sirotta PS, Nelp WB, et al: Progressive pulmonary calcification complicating successful renal transplantation. Am Rev Respir Dis 136:1480-1482, 1987.

182. Raisis IP, Park CH, Yang SL, Maddrey W: Lung uptake of technetium-99m phosphate compounds after liver transplantation. Clin Nucl Med 13:188-189, 1988.

183. Bestetti-Bosisio M, Cotelli F, Schiaffino E, et al: Lung calcification in long-term dialysed patients: A light and electron microscopic study. Histopathology 8:69-79, 1984.

184. Hartman TE, Müller NL, Primack SL, et al: Metastatic pulmonary calcification in patients with hypercalcemia: Findings on chest radiographs and CT scans. AJR Am J Roentgenol 162:799-802, 1994.

185. Rosenthal DI, Chandler HL, Azizi F, Schneider PB: Uptake of bone imaging agents by diffuse pulmonary metastatic calcification. AJR Am J Roentgenol 129:871-874, 1977.

186. Johkoh T, Ikezoe J, Nagareda T, et al: Metastatic pulmonary calcification: Early detection by high-resolution CT. J Comput Assist Tomogr 17:471-473, 1993.

187. Lingam RK, Teh J, Sharma A, Friedman E: Case report. Metastatic pulmonary calcification in renal failure: A new HRCT pattern. Br J Radiol 75:74-77, 2002.

188. Akmal M, Barndt RR, Ansari AN, et al: Excess PTH in CRF induces pulmonary calcification, pulmonary hypertension and right ventricular hypertrophy. Kidney Int 47:158-163, 1995.

189. Seymour JF, Presneill JJ: Pulmonary alveolar proteinosis: Progress in the first 44 years. Am J Respir Crit Care Med 166:215-235, 2002.

190. Shah PL, Hansell D, Lawson PR, et al: Pulmonary alveolar proteinosis: Clinical aspects and current concepts on pathogenesis. Thorax 55:67-77, 2000.

191. Mahut B, Delacourt C, Scheinmann P, et al: Pulmonary alveolar proteinosis: Experience with eight pediatric cases and a review. Pediatrics 97:117-122, 1996.

192. Gilmore LB, Talley FA, Hook GE: Classification and morphometric quantitation of insoluble materials from the lungs of patients with alveolar proteinosis. Am J Pathol 133:252-264, 1988.

193. Singh G, Katyal SL: Surfactant apoprotein in nonmalignant pulmonary disorders. Am J Pathol 101:51-62, 1980.

194. Satoh K, Arai H, Yoshida T, et al: Glycosaminoglycans and glycoproteins in bronchoalveolar lavage fluid from patients with pulmonary alveolar proteinosis. Inflammation 7:347-353, 1983.

195. Buechner HA, Ansari A: Acute silico-proteinosis. A new pathologic variant of acute silicosis in sandblasters, characterized by histologic features resembling alveolar proteinosis. Dis Chest 55:274-278, 1969.

196. Ruben FL, Talamo TS: Secondary pulmonary alveolar proteinosis occurring in two patients with acquired immune deficiency syndrome. Am J Med 80:1187-1190, 1986.

197. Bedrossian CW, Luna MA, Conklin RH, Miller WC: Alveolar proteinosis as a consequence of immunosuppression. A hypothesis based on clinical and pathologic observations. Hum Pathol 11:527-535, 1980.

198. Wang BM, Stern EJ, Schmidt RA, Pierson DJ: Diagnosing pulmonary alveolar proteinosis. A review and an update. Chest 111:460-466, 1997.

199. Goldstein LS, Kavuru MS, Curtis-McCarthy P, et al: Pulmonary alveolar proteinosis: Clinical features and outcomes. Chest 114:1357-1362, 1998.

200. Lee KN, Levin DL, Webb WR, et al: Pulmonary alveolar proteinosis: High-resolution CT, chest radiographic, and functional correlations. Chest 111:989-995, 1997.

201. Godwin JD, Müller NL, Takasugi JE: Pulmonary alveolar proteinosis: CT findings. Radiology 169:609-613, 1988.

202. Zimmer WE, Chew FS: Pulmonary alveolar proteinosis. AJR Am J Roentgenol 161:26, 1993.

203. Murch CR, Carr DH: Computed tomography appearances of pulmonary alveolar proteinosis. Clin Radiol 40:240-243, 1989.

204. Holbert JM, Costello P, Li W, et al: CT features of pulmonary alveolar proteinosis. AJR Am J Roentgenol 176:1287-1294, 2001.

205. Kang EY, Grenier P, Laurent F, Müller NL: Interlobular septal thickening: Patterns at high-resolution computed tomography. J Thorac Imaging 11:260-264, 1996.

206. Johkoh T, Itoh H, Müller NL, et al: Crazy-paving appearance at thin-section CT: Spectrum of disease and pathologic findings. Radiology 211:155-160, 1999.

207. Tan RT, Kuzo RS: High-resolution CT findings of mucinous bronchioloalveolar carcinoma: A case of pseudopulmonary alveolar proteinosis. AJR Am J Roentgenol 168:99-100, 1997.

208. Franquet T, Gimenez A, Bordes R, et al: The crazy-paving pattern in exogenous lipoid pneumonia: CT-pathologic correlation. AJR Am J Roentgenol 170:315-317, 1998.

209. Hoffman RM, Rogers RM: Serum and lavage lactate dehydrogenase isoenzymes in pulmonary alveolar proteinosis. Am Rev Respir Dis 143:42-46, 1991.

210. Fujishima T, Honda Y, Shijubo N, et al: Increased carcinoembryonic antigen concentrations in sera and bronchoalveolar lavage fluids of patients with pulmonary alveolar proteinosis. Respiration 62:317-321, 1995.

211. Honda Y, Kuroki Y, Shijubo N, et al: Aberrant appearance of lung surfactant protein A in sera of patients with idiopathic pulmonary fibrosis and its clinical significance. Respiration 62:64-69, 1995.

212. Honda Y, Kuroki Y, Matsuura E, et al: Pulmonary surfactant protein D in sera and bronchoalveolar lavage fluids. Am J Respir Crit Care Med 152:1860-1866, 1995.

213. Selecky PA, Wasserman K, Benfield JR, Lippmann M: The clinical and physiological effect of whole-lung lavage in pulmonary alveolar proteinosis: A ten-year experience. Ann Thorac Surg 24:451-461, 1977.

214. Oliva PB, Vogel JH: Reactive pulmonary hypertension in alveolar proteinosis. Chest 58:167-168, 1970.

215. Yeh SD, White DA, Stover-Pepe DE, et al: Abnormal gallium scintigraphy in pulmonary alveolar proteinosis (PAP). Clin Nucl Med 12:294-297, 1987.

216. Davidson JM, Macleod WM: Pulmonary alveolar proteinosis. Br J Dis Chest 63:13-28, 1969.

217. Wilson JW, Rubinfeld AR, White A, Mullerworth M: Alveolar proteinosis treated with a single bronchial lavage. Med J Aust 145:158-160, 1986.

218. Parker LA, Novotny DB: Recurrent alveolar proteinosis following double lung transplantation. Chest 111:1457-1458, 1997.

219. Kariman K, Kylstra JA, Spock A: Pulmonary alveolar proteinosis: Prospective clinical experience in 23 patients for 15 years. Lung 162:223-231, 1984.

220. Westermark P: The pathogenesis of amyloidosis: Understanding general principles. Am J Pathol 152:1125-1127, 1998.

221. Smith RR, Hutchins GM, Moore GW, Humphrey RL: Type and distribution of pulmonary parenchymal and vascular amyloid. Correlation with cardiac amyloid. Am J Med 66:96-104, 1979.

222. Fernandez-Alonso J, Rios-Camacho C, Valenzuela-Castano A, Hernanz-Mediano W: Mixed systemic amyloidosis in a patient receiving long term haemodialysis. J Clin Pathol 47:560-561, 1994.

223. Abe Y, Utsunomiya H, Tsutsumi Y: Atypical carcinoid tumor of the lung with amyloid stroma. Acta Pathol Jpn 42:286-292, 1992.

224. Amyloid and the lower respiratory tract [editorial]. Thorax 38:84, 1983.

225. Kavuru MS, Adamo JP, Ahmad M, et al: Amyloidosis and pleural disease. Chest 98:20-23, 1990.

226. Hsiu JG, Stitik FP, D'Amato NA, et al: Primary amyloidosis presenting as a unilateral hilar mass. Report of a case diagnosed by fine needle aspiration biopsy. Acta Cytol 30:55-58, 1986.

227. Melato M, Antonutto G, Falconieri G, Manconi R: Massive amyloidosis of mediastinal lymph nodes in a patient with multiple myeloma. Thorax 38:151-152, 1983.

228. Streeten EA, de la Monte SM, Kennedy TP: Amyloid infiltration of the diaphragm as a cause of respiratory failure. Chest 89:760-762, 1986.

229. Toyoda M, Ebihara Y, Kato H, Kita S: Tracheobronchial AL amyloidosis: Histologic, immunohistochemical, ultrastructural, and immunoelectron microscopic observations. Hum Pathol 24:970-976, 1993.

230. Cordier JF, Loire R, Brune J: Amyloidosis of the lower respiratory tract. Clinical and pathologic features in a series of 21 patients. Chest 90:827-831, 1986.

231. da Costa P, Corrin B: Amyloidosis localized to the lower respiratory tract: Probable immunoamyloid nature of the tracheobronchial and nodular pulmonary forms. Histopathology 9:703-710, 1985.

232. Miyamoto T, Kobayashi T, Makiyama M, et al: Monoclonality of infiltrating plasma cells in primary pulmonary nodular amyloidosis: Detection with polymerase chain reaction. J Clin Pathol 52:464-467, 1999.

233. Lim JK, Lacy MQ, Kurtin PJ, et al: Pulmonary marginal zone lymphoma of MALT type as a cause of localised pulmonary amyloidosis. J Clin Pathol 54:642-646, 2001.

234. Chen KT: Amyloidosis presenting in the respiratory tract. Pathol Annu 24(Pt 1):253-273, 1989.

235. Monreal FA: Pulmonary amyloidosis: Ultrastructural study of early alveolar septal deposits. Hum Pathol 15:388-390, 1984.

236. Kwong JS, Müller NL, Miller RR: Diseases of the trachea and main-stem bronchi: Correlation of CT with pathologic findings. Radiographics 12:645-657, 1992.

237. Utz J, Swensen S, Gertz M: Pulmonary amyloidosis. The Mayo Clinic experience from 1980 to 1993. Ann Intern Med 124:407-413, 1996.

238. Kirchner J, Jacobi V, Kardos P, Kollath J: CT findings in extensive tracheobronchial amyloidosis. Eur Radiol 8:352-354, 1998.

239. Pickford HA, Swensen SJ, Utz JP: Thoracic cross-sectional imaging of amyloidosis. AJR Am J Roentgenol 168:351-355, 1997.

240. Bhate DV: Case of the spring season: Diffuse primary amyloidosis with nodular calcified lung lesions. Semin Roentgenol 14:81-82, 1979.

241. Urban BA, Fishman EK, Goldman SM, et al: CT evaluation of amyloidosis: Spectrum of disease. Radiographics 13:1295-1308, 1993.

242. Gross BH, Felson B, Birnberg FA: The respiratory tract in amyloidosis and the plasma cell dyscrasias. Semin Roentgenol 21:113-127, 1986.

243. Hodge DS, Anderson WR, Tsai SH: Primary diffuse bronchial amyloidosis. Arch Pathol Lab Med 101:615-616, 1977.

244. O'Regan A, Fenlon HM, Beamis JF Jr, et al: Tracheobronchial amyloidosis. The Boston University experience from 1984 to 1999. Medicine (Baltimore) 79:69-79, 2000.

245. Hui AN, Koss MN, Hochholzer L, Wehunt WD: Amyloidosis presenting in the lower respiratory tract. Clinicopathologic, radiologic, immunohistochemical, and histochemical studies on 48 cases. Arch Pathol Lab Med 110:212-218, 1986.

246. Dundore PA, Aisner SC, Templeton PA, et al: Nodular pulmonary amyloidosis: Diagnosis by fine-needle aspiration cytology and a review of the literature. Diagn Cytopathol 9:562-564, 1993.

247. Jimenez C, Vital C, Merlio JP, et al: Plasmacytoma and gastric amyloidosis associated with nodular pulmonary amyloidosis. Ann Pathol 8:155, 1988.

248. Cathcart ES, Ritchie RF, Cohen AS, Brandt K: Immunoglobulins and amyloidosis. An immunologic study of sixty-two patients with biopsy-proved disease. Am J Med 52:93-101, 1972.

249. Crosbie WA, Lewis ML, Ramsay ID, Doyle D: Pulmonary amyloidosis with impaired gas transfer. Thorax 27:625-630, 1972.

250. Lee SC, Johnson H: Multiple nodular pulmonary amyloidosis. A case report and comparison with diffuse alveolar-septal pulmonary amyloidosis. Thorax 30:175-185, 1975.

251. Prakash UB, Barham SS, Rosenow EC 3rd, et al: Pulmonary alveolar microlithiasis. A review including ultrastructural and pulmonary function studies. Mayo Clin Proc 58:290-300, 1983.

252. Mariotta S, Guidi L, Papale M, et al: Pulmonary alveolar microlithiasis: Review of Italian reports. Eur J Epidemiol 13:587-590, 1997.

253. Ucan ES, Keyf AI, Aydilek R, et al: Pulmonary alveolar microlithiasis: Review of Turkish reports. Thorax 48:171-173, 1993.

254. Castellana G, Gentile M, Castellana R, et al: Pulmonary alveolar microlithiasis: Clinical features, evolution of the phenotype, and review of the literature. Am J Med Genet 111:220-224, 2002.

255. Gomez G, Lichtenberger E, Santamaria A, et al: Familial pulmonary alveolar microlithiasis: Four cases from Colombia, S.A. Is microlithiasis also an environmental disease? Radiology 72:550, 1959.

256. O'Neill RP, Cohn JE, Pellegrino ED: Pulmonary alveolar microlithiasis—a family study. Ann Intern Med 67:957-967, 1967.

257. Moran CA, Hochholzer L, Hasleton PS, et al: Pulmonary alveolar microlithiasis. A clinicopathologic and chemical analysis of seven cases. Arch Pathol Lab Med 121:607-611, 1997.

258. Tao LC: Microliths in sputum specimens and their relationship to pulmonary alveolar microlithiasis. Am J Clin Pathol 69:482-485, 1978.

259. Barnard NJ, Crocker PR, Blainey AD, et al: Pulmonary alveolar microlithiasis. A new analytical approach. Histopathology 11:639-645, 1987.

260. Pracyk JB, Simonson SG, Young SL, et al: Composition of lung lavage in pulmonary alveolar microlithiasis. Respiration 63:254-260, 1996.

261. Helbich TH, Wojnarovsky C, Wunderbaldinger P, et al: Pulmonary alveolar microlithiasis in children: Radiographic and high-resolution CT findings. AJR Am J Roentgenol 168:63-65, 1997.

262. Balikian JP, Fuleihan FJ, Nucho CN: Pulmonary alveolar microlithiasis. Report of five cases with special reference to roentgen manifestations. Am J Roentgenol Radium Ther Nucl Med 103:509-518, 1968.

263. Cheong W, Wang Y, Tan L, et al: Pulmonary alveolar microlithiasis. Australas Radiol 32:401-404, 1988.

264. Felson B: The roentgen diagnosis of disseminated pulmonary alveolar diseases. Semin Roentgenol 2:3, 1967.

265. Korn MA, Schurawitzki H, Klepetko W, Burghuber OC: Pulmonary alveolar microlithiasis: Findings on high-resolution CT. AJR Am J Roentgenol 158:981-982, 1992.

266. Melamed JW, Sostman HD, Ravin CE: Interstitial thickening in pulmonary alveolar microlithiasis: An underappreciated finding. J Thorac Imaging 9:126-128, 1994.

267. Hoshino H, Koba H, Inomata S, et al: Pulmonary alveolar microlithiasis: High-resolution CT and MR findings. J Comput Assist Tomogr 22:245-248, 1998.

268. Turktas I, Saribas S, Balkanci F: Pulmonary alveolar microlithiasis presenting with chronic cough. Postgrad Med J 69:70-71, 1993.

269. Stamatis G, Zerkowski HR, Doetsch N, et al: Sequential bilateral lung transplantation for pulmonary alveolar microlithiasis. Ann Thorac Surg 56:972-975, 1993.

270. Cale WF, Petsonk EL, Boyd CB: Transbronchial biopsy of pulmonary alveolar microlithiasis. Arch Intern Med 143:358-359, 1983.

271. Amir G, Ron N: Pulmonary pathology in Gaucher's disease. Hum Pathol 30:666-670, 1999.

272. Alan E, Bakst M, Sean P, et al: Continuous intravenous epoprostenol therapy for pulmonary hypertension in Gaucher's disease. Am Coll Chest Physicians 116:1127-1129, 1999.

273. Goitein O, Elstein D, Abrahamov A, et al: Lung involvement and enzyme replacement therapy in Gaucher's disease. Q J Med 94:407-415, 2001.

274. Carson KF, Williams CA, Rosenthal DL, et al: Bronchoalveolar lavage in a girl with Gaucher's disease. A case report. Acta Cytol 38:597-600, 1994.

275. Kerem E, Elstein D, Abrahamov A, et al: Pulmonary function abnormalities in type I Gaucher disease. Eur Respir J 9:340-345, 1996.

276. Long RG, Lake BD, Pettit JE, et al: Adult Niemann-Pick disease: Its relationship to the syndrome of the sea-blue histiocyte. Am J Med 62:627-635, 1977.

277. Ferretti GR, Lantuejoul S, Brambilla E, Coulomb M: Case report. Pulmonary involvement in Niemann-Pick disease subtype B: CT findings. J Comput Assist Tomogr 20:990-992, 1996.

278. Duchateau F, Dechambre S, Coche E: Imaging of pulmonary manifestations in subtype B of Niemann-Pick disease. Br J Radiol 74:1059-1061, 2001.

279. Rodrigues R, Marchiori E, Müller NL: Niemann-Pick disease: High-resolution CT findings in two siblings. J Comput Assist Tomogr 28:52-54, 2004.

280. Niggemann B, Rebien W, Rahn W, Wahn U: Asymptomatic pulmonary involvement in 2 children with Niemann-Pick disease type B. Respiration 61:55-57, 1994.

281. Garay SM, Gardella JE, Fazzini EP, Goldring RM: Hermansky-Pudlak syndrome. Pulmonary manifestations of a ceroid storage disorder. Am J Med 66:737-747, 1979.

282. Schinella RA, Greco MA, Garay SM, et al: Hermansky-Pudlak syndrome: A clinicopathologic study. Hum Pathol 16:366-376, 1985.

283. DePinho RA, Kaplan KL: The Hermansky-Pudlak syndrome. Report of three cases and review of pathophysiology and management considerations. Medicine (Baltimore) 64:192-202, 1985.

284. Takahashi A, Yokoyama T: Hermansky-Pudlak syndrome with special reference to lysosomal dysfunction. A case report and review of the literature. Virchows Arch A Pathol Anat Histopathol 402:247-258, 1984.

285. Sakuma T, Monma N, Satodate R, et al: Ceroid pigment deposition in circulating blood monocytes and T lymphocytes in Hermansky-Pudlak syndrome: An ultrastructural study. Pathol Int 45:866-870, 1995.

286. Reynolds SP, Davies BH, Gibbs AR: Diffuse pulmonary fibrosis and the Hermansky-Pudlak syndrome: Clinical course and postmortem findings. Thorax 49:617-618, 1994.

287. Shimizu K, Matsumoto T, Miura G, et al: Hermansky-Pudlak syndrome with diffuse pulmonary fibrosis: Radiologic-pathologic correlation. J Comput Assist Tomogr 22:249-251, 1998.

288. Devouassoux G, Lantuejoul S, Chatelain P, et al: Erdheim-Chester disease: A primary macrophage cell disorder. Am J Respir Crit Care Med 157:650-653, 1998.

289. Rush WL, Andriko JA, Galateau-Salle F, et al: Pulmonary pathology of Erdheim-Chester disease. Mod Pathol 13:747-754, 2000.

290. Remy-Jardin M, Gosselin B, Remy J: Pulmonary involvement in Erdheim-Chester disease: High-resolution CT findings. Eur Radiol 3:389, 1993.

291. Lightman NI, Schooley RT: Adult-onset acid maltase deficiency. Case report of an adult with severe respiratory difficulty. Chest 72:250-252, 1977.

292. Semenza GL, Pyeritz RE: Respiratory complications of mucopolysaccharide storage disorders. Medicine (Baltimore) 67:209-219, 1988.

293. Pyeritz RE: Connective tissue in the lung: Lessons from the Marfan syndrome. Ann Intern Med 103:289-290, 1985.

294. Hasham SN, Guo DC, Milewicz DM: Genetic basis of thoracic aortic aneurysms and dissections. Curr Opin Cardiol 17:677-683, 2002.

295. De Paepe A, Devereux RB, Dietz HC, et al: Revised diagnostic criteria for the Marfan syndrome. Am J Med Genet 62:417-426, 1996.

296. Tanoue LT: Pulmonary involvement in collagen vascular disease: A review of the pulmonary manifestations of the Marfan syndrome, ankylosing spondylitis, Sjögren's syndrome, and relapsing polychondritis. J Thorac Imaging 7:62-77, 1992.

297. Pyeritz RE, McKusick VA: The Marfan syndrome: Diagnosis and management. N Engl J Med 300:772-777, 1979.

298. Wood JR, Bellamy D, Child AH, Citron KM: Pulmonary disease in patients with Marfan syndrome. Thorax 39:780-784, 1984.

299. Hall JR, Pyeritz RE, Dudgeon DL, Haller JA Jr: Pneumothorax in the Marfan syndrome: Prevalence and therapy. Ann Thorac Surg 37:500-504, 1984.

300. Posniak HV, Olson MC, Demos TC, et al: CT of thoracic aortic aneurysms. Radiographics 10:839-855, 1990.

301. Fisher ER, Stern EJ, Godwin JD 2nd, et al: Acute aortic dissection: Typical and atypical imaging features. Radiographics 14:1263-1271, discussion 1271-1274, 1994.

302. Sommer T, Fehske W, Holzknecht N, et al: Aortic dissection: A comparative study of diagnosis with spiral CT, multiplanar transesophageal echocardiography, and MR imaging. Radiology 199:347-352, 1996.

303. Mayo JR: Magnetic resonance imaging of the chest. Where we stand. Radiol Clin North Am 32:795-809, 1994.

304. Mao JR, Bristow J: The Ehlers-Danlos syndrome: On beyond collagens. J Clin Invest 107:1063-1069, 2001.

305. Yost BA, Vogelsang JP, Lie JT: Fatal hemoptysis in Ehlers-Danlos syndrome. Old malady with a new curse. Chest 107:1465-1467, 1995.

306. Franquet T, Gimenez A, Caceres J, et al: Imaging of pulmonary-cutaneous disorders: Matching the radiologic and dermatologic findings. Radiographics 16:855-869, 1996.

307. Murray RA, Poulton TB, Saltarelli MG, et al: Rare pulmonary manifestation of Ehlers-Danlos syndrome. J Thorac Imaging 10:138-141, 1995.

308. Koziel H, Koziel MJ: Pulmonary complications of diabetes mellitus. Pneumonia. Infect Dis Clin North Am 9:65-96, 1995.

309. Vracko R, Thorning D, Huang TW: Basal lamina of alveolar epithelium and capillaries: Quantitative changes with aging and in diabetes mellitus. Am Rev Respir Dis 120:973-983, 1979.

310. Guazzi M, Brambilla R, De Vita S, Guazzi MD: Diabetes worsens pulmonary diffusion in heart failure, and insulin counteracts this effect. Am J Respir Crit Care Med 166:978-982, 2002.

311. Mori H, Okubo M, Okamura M, et al: Abnormalities of pulmonary function in patients with non–insulin-dependent diabetes mellitus. Intern Med 31:189-193, 1992.

312. Sandler M, Bunn AE, Stewart RI: Cross-section study of pulmonary function in patients with insulin-dependent diabetes mellitus. Am Rev Respir Dis 135:223-229, 1987.

313. Walter RE, Beiser A, Givelber RJ, et al: Association between glycemic state and lung function: The Framingham Heart Study. Am J Respir Crit Care Med 167:911-916, 2003.

314. Vianna LG, Gilbey SG, Barnes NC, et al: Cough threshold to citric acid in diabetic patients with and without autonomic neuropathy. Thorax 43:569-571, 1988.

315. Antonelli Incalzi R, Fuso L, Giordano A, et al: Neuroadrenergic denervation of the lung in type I diabetes mellitus complicated by autonomic neuropathy. Chest 121:443-451, 2002.

316. Bottini P, Tantucci C: Sleep apnea syndromes in endocrine diseases. Respiration 70:320, 2003.

317. Young MC: Simultaneous acute cerebral and pulmonary edema complicating diabetic ketoacidosis. Diabetes Care 18:1288-1290, 1995.

318. De Troyer A, Desir D, Copinschi G: Regression of lung size in adults with growth hormone deficiency. Q J Med 49:329-340, 1980.

319. Harrison BD, Millhouse KA, Harrington M, Nabarro JD: Lung function in acromegaly. Q J Med 47:517-532, 1978.

320. Trotman-Dickenson B, Weetman AP, Hughes JM: Upper airflow obstruction and pulmonary function in acromegaly: Relationship to disease activity. Q J Med 79:527-538, 1991.

321. Kitabara L: Airway difficulties associated with anesthesia in acromegaly. Br J Anaesth 43:1187, 1971.

322. Brown SD, Brashear RE, Schnute RB: Pleural effusion in a young woman with myxedema. Arch Intern Med 143:1458-1460, 1983.

323. Sadiq MA, Davies JC: Unusual lung manifestations of myxoedema. Br J Clin Pract 31:224, 1977.

324. Menendez CE, Rivlin RS: Thyrotoxic crisis and myxedema coma. Med Clin North Am 57:1463-1470, 1973.

325. Domm BM, Vassallo CL: Myxedema coma with respiratory failure. Am Rev Respir Dis 107:842-845, 1973.

326. Orr WC, Males JL, Imes NK: Myxedema and obstructive sleep apnea. Am J Med 70:1061-1066, 1981.

327. Stein M, Kimball P, Johnson R: Pulmonary function in hyperthyroidism. J Clin Invest 40:348, 1961.

328. Siafakas NM, Milona I, Salesiotou V, et al: Respiratory muscle strength in hyperthyroidism before and after treatment. Am Rev Respir Dis 146:1025-1029, 1992.

329. Zwillich CW, Matthay M, Potts DE, et al: Thyrotoxicosis: Comparison of effects of thyroid ablation and beta-adrenergic blockade on metabolic rate and ventilatory control. J Clin Endocrinol Metab 46:491-500, 1978.

330. Thurnheer R, Jenni R, Russi EW, et al: Hyperthyroidism and pulmonary hypertension. J Intern Med 242:185-188, 1997.

C H A P T E R   **SIX**

INFECTIOUS DISEASE OF THE LUNGS

GENERAL CONSIDERATIONS

Epidemiologic Considerations

Infection of the lower respiratory tract is one of the most common and important causes of human disease from the points of view of morbidity, mortality, and economic cost to society. It has been estimated that approximately 4 million cases of community-acquired pneumonia occur annually in the United States,[1,2] with 600,000 hospitalizations; both mortality and the proportion of hospitalizations attributed to such infection seem to be increasing.[3] The overall incidence has ranged from 2.6 to 16.8 cases per 1000 adults per year in various community studies[4]; however, the incidence varies considerably with age, sex, race, and socioeconomic status.[5-7] For example, it is more common in blacks than whites,[8] in women than men,[8] and in older than younger individuals.[8] As might be expected, it is particularly prevalent in nursing home residents.[9]

In the United States, pneumonia is the sixth leading cause of death and the number one cause of death from infection.[5] The authors of an extensive meta-analysis of the prognosis and outcome of 33,148 patients who had community-acquired pneumonia found an overall mortality rate of 13.7%.[10] In "developed" countries, the annual death rate is approximately 50 to 60 per 100,000.[11] As with incidence figures, however, those related to mortality also vary considerably in specific groups of patients. As might be expected, the mortality rate in patients not requiring hospitalization is generally low, in the range of 0.1%.[1] However, reported mortality rates in patients who have pneumonia of sufficient severity to require admission to the hospital range from 4% to almost 40%.[7,10,12] Age is also a very important variable: pneumonia has been estimated to account for nearly half of all deaths resulting from infectious disease in the geriatric population.[13]

Overall, hospital-acquired pneumonia develops in about 0.5% to 1.0% of patients.[14] However, in specific situations the incidence is considerably greater. For example, it has been found to complicate the course of as many as 18% of patients who have undergone surgery[15] and 6% to 52% of those undergoing mechanical ventilation.[16] In this latter group it accounts for almost half of all infections.[17,18] Among nosocomial infections, pneumonia has the highest mortality and morbidity[19]; its presence increases length of stay in survivors by an average of 7 to 9 days per patient,[20] with an attendant increase in cost.[21,22] Mortality in such patients is high, estimated at 30% to 70% by different investigators,[23] but the mortality attributable to pneumonia in this setting of substantial comorbidity is considerably less.[17,24]

Pathogenesis and Patterns of Infection

Organisms can enter the lung and cause infection by three routes: the tracheobronchial tree, the pulmonary vasculature, and directly from the mediastinum or neck or across the diaphragm or chest wall. Although there is overlap, infection acquired by each of these routes results in fairly characteristic pulmonary abnormalities that may be recognized both pathologically and radiologically.

Infection via the Tracheobronchial Tree

Infection acquired via the tracheobronchial tree occurs most commonly by aspiration or inhalation of microorganisms; occasionally, it follows direct physical implantation from an infected source, such as a bronchoscope,[25] or extension of disease into the airway from a peribronchial lymph node (e.g., in tuberculosis). With respect to pulmonary infection, we use the terms *inhalation* to refer to the breathing of air that contains potentially infectious material, such as fungal spores or droplet nuclei harboring bacteria or viral particles, and *aspiration* to refer to the introduction of solid or liquid material into the lungs. When the latter material consists of a foreign body or is copious (as is often the case with aspirated gastric contents), it usually causes pulmonary damage directly by chemical or physical mechanisms (see page 744); we use the term *aspiration pneumonia* to refer to such damage. Aspiration of smaller amounts of nasal or oral secretions that contain microorganisms is also a common cause of pneumonia, in this case as a result of the organisms themselves. Although such a process has also been termed "aspiration pneumonia," we prefer to refer to this form of disease by the specific type of causative organism (e.g., anaerobic pneumonia, actinomycosis).

Coughing or sneezing by an individual whose respiratory tract is either colonized or infected produces a myriad of minute droplets that are laden with microorganisms. On exposure to air, the droplets lose water and become droplet nuclei, which, because of their extremely small size, can remain suspended in air for an extended period; exposure to such contaminated air by another individual can then result in spread of organisms.[26] Inhaled droplet nuclei measuring 1 to 2 μm are likely to affect peripheral airway epithelium, where they may proliferate and cause disease. Depending on their virulence, a substantial number of organisms may be necessary for disease to occur because small numbers may be effectively cleared by host defenses[27]; however, some organisms (e.g., *Mycobacterium tuberculosis*) are capable of producing disease with only a small inoculum. In addition to the inhalational transmission of organisms from person to person, products of some microorganisms, such as the microconidia of *Histoplasma capsulatum,* are inhaled as airborne particles originating in contaminated soil.

As indicated, aspiration of oropharyngeal secretions is also a common mechanism by which pathogenic organisms gain access to the lungs. The normal adult oropharyngeal flora consists of a variety of aerobic and anaerobic microorganisms.[28] Most are commensals of low virulence that never cause pulmonary infection; however, some (e.g., *Actinomyces israelii* and a variety of anaerobic bacteria) can cause pulmonary disease if aspirated in sufficient quantity by a susceptible host. In addition, it is not uncommon for the upper airways to be colonized by pathogenic organisms such as *Streptococcus pneumoniae* or *Staphylococcus aureus* (in otherwise healthy individuals) or by potentially virulent gram-negative bacteria (in hospitalized or chronically ill patients). In both situations, aspiration of contaminated saliva or nasal secretions may deliver a bacterial inoculum sufficient to cause infection. The importance of this mechanism is underlined by observations that asymptomatic aspiration occurs occasionally in many healthy individuals and with even greater frequency in patients who are comatose, who have ingested excessive alcohol, or whose nasopharyngeal secretions are increased as a result of upper respiratory tract viral infection.[29]

Deposition of bacteria and fungi on the airway or alveolar epithelial surface by inhalation or aspiration may be followed by one of three events: (1) destruction and clearance of organisms with restoration of the original sterile lung; (2) limited but prolonged proliferation of organisms on the epithelial surface, unassociated with transepithelial invasion (colonization); and (3) more marked proliferation of organisms associated with an acute inflammatory reaction and, often, tissue necrosis. Which of these events ensues depends on a number of factors, including the size of the inoculum, the virulence of the organism, the status of the host inflammatory and immune reactions, and the presence or absence of underlying lung disease.[30]

Many substances are produced by microorganisms to enhance the likelihood of colonization or invasion, including proteases and other chemicals that directly damage epithelial cells or connective tissue[31]; substances that cause a reduction in mucociliary clearance, such as pyocyanin[32]; adhesion molecules, which promote attachment to the epithelial surface; and substances that inhibit the host inflammatory reaction.[33]

The pathogenesis of lower respiratory tract infection by viruses is somewhat different from that of bacteria and fungi. Once deposited on the mucosa of the respiratory tract, a virus must gain access to the underlying epithelial cells to propagate. It does so by means of molecules that interact with specific receptors on the surface of the host cells; the presence and nature of these molecules and receptors are important in determining the infectivity of the virus and the site at which it causes disease. After penetration of the cell membrane, viral DNA (or newly constituted DNA in the case of RNA viruses) acts as a template for the production of various molecules required for the formation of new viruses. Several outcomes may ensue: (1) the host cell may die and release its newly formed viruses to infect other cells; (2) the host cell may remain viable with continuing production and release of new virions, a process that may be associated with an immune reaction to viral antigens expressed on the cell surface; and (3) the virus may remain within the cell in a latent state for extended periods (e.g., after incorporation of viral DNA with host DNA) and then reappear to cause disease only when the general immunity of the host is impaired.

The course of viral infection of the lower respiratory tract, particularly that caused by influenza virus, can be complicated by superimposed bacterial pneumonia. The propensity for the development of such superinfection is probably related to several factors,[34,35] including (1) a deficiency of mucociliary clearance caused by either the loss of airway and alveolar lining cells or ciliary abnormalities, (2) the presence of intra-

alveolar edema fluid containing nutrients that can be used for bacterial growth, (3) impairment of alveolar macrophage phagocytosis and bactericidal efficiency, (4) interference with polymorphonuclear leukocyte chemotaxis, and (5) enhancement of bacterial adherence to damaged epithelium.

Underlying lung disease is an important risk factor for pulmonary infection. For example, patients with COPD have an increased susceptibility to viral and chlamydial disease. The pathogenesis of this increased susceptibility is unclear but may be related to structural changes in airway epithelium (e.g., squamous metaplasia and goblet cell hyperplasia), abnormal mucociliary clearance, or impairment of the local inflammatory reaction. Another example is a fungus ball (aspergilloma), which almost always develops in a preexisting pulmonary cavity or focus of bronchiectasis.

Clinical considerations that are helpful in the etiologic diagnosis of pneumonia include the age of the patient, the presence and severity of comorbid disease, the rapidity of progression, and whether the infection is hospital (nosocomial) or community acquired. For example, a community-acquired pneumonia that is abrupt in onset and associated with rigor and a white blood count greater than 20,000/mm³ may well be pneumococcal in origin; however, these features are not specific enough to reliably distinguish this infection from pneumonia caused by *Legionella* species or other organisms in any given patient.[36] The severity and cause of pneumonia are profoundly influenced by immunologic status, with immunosuppressed patients being prone to widespread pneumonia, often by opportunistic organisms. Age is also an important variable in prediction; for example, pneumonia is more likely to be caused by viruses, *Chlamydia pneumoniae*, or *Mycoplasma pneumoniae* in younger than in older patients. The severity and pattern of infection caused by a particular organism are also related to age in some cases; for example, although rhinovirus usually causes only coryza in adults, it may produce croup, bronchitis, bronchiolitis, and bronchopneumonia in children.[37]

Although it is occasionally possible to detect pneumonia on the basis of physical examination of the chest when the chest radiograph is normal, more often, physical signs of lung disease are completely absent in patients who have significant areas of parenchymal consolidation.[38] In addition, there may be radiographic evidence of pneumonia without accompanying physical signs in one area and vice versa in other areas. Similarly, no single feature of the clinical history accurately predicts the presence or absence of radiographically detectable pneumonia.[39]

Infection of the lower respiratory tract acquired via the airways may be predominantly confined to the airways themselves (tracheitis, bronchitis, or bronchiolitis) or to the lung parenchyma (pneumonia). Pneumonia in turn can be subdivided into three types, each with fairly typical pathologic and radiologic characteristics: nonsegmental air space (lobar) pneumonia, bronchopneumonia (lobular pneumonia), and interstitial pneumonia. Despite some overlap among these patterns with respect to their underlying etiologies,[40,41] they can be recognized with sufficient frequency and are associated with specific etiologic organisms in enough cases that recognition of these types is diagnostically useful in the appropriate clinical context. For example, nonsegmental air space pneumonia is usually of bacterial origin, most commonly *S. pneumoniae*, whereas diffuse interstitial pneumonia often results from infection by viruses and *Pneumocystis jiroveci* (*P. carinii*).[42,43] It should be remembered, however, that a number of factors can modify the typical radiologic manifestations of pulmonary infection,[44] including underlying disease (such as emphysema[45]) and the age and immunologic status of the patient. As might be expected, the correlation between radiologic and pathologic/microbiologic findings is better with HRCT than with radiography.[46,47]

Tracheitis, Bronchitis, and Bronchiolitis. Infection involving predominantly the airways may be limited to the trachea, bronchi, or bronchioles or may affect two or three of these sites simultaneously. Viruses (particularly respiratory syncytial virus [RSV] and parainfluenza virus) and mycoplasmal organisms are the most frequent pathogenic agents. Of greatest importance in terms of morbidity is bronchiolitis, which is seen particularly in children and is clinically characterized by wheezing, dyspnea, and in the most severely affected, cyanosis, prostration, and death.[48,49] Viral bronchiolitis in children is also well recognized as a precursor of adult bronchiectasis and unilateral hyperlucent lung (Swyer-James syndrome) and has been implicated in both the pathogenesis and exacerbation of asthma.[50]

Though relatively uncommon, localized bacterial tracheitis is potentially a serious infection, particularly in children and occasionally in adults.[51] *S. aureus* and *Haemophilus influenzae* are the most common causative agents.[52] The condition is often seen after viral upper airway infection and can lead to life-threatening airway obstruction as a result of granulation tissue and inflammatory exudate in the tracheal lumen. As in viral respiratory tract infection, bacterial bronchitis can be an isolated abnormality or can be seen with tracheitis, bronchiolitis, or both. In children, concomitant involvement of both the proximal and distal airways is a relatively common manifestation of pertussis. In adults, bronchial infection occurs most often in patients who have underlying airway disease, usually COPD, bronchiectasis, or cystic fibrosis. In patients who have cystic fibrosis, chronic infection by *Pseudomonas aeruginosa* or *Burkholderia cepacia* is likely to be important in pathogenesis of the progressive bronchiectasis seen in many individuals.

Acute bronchitis is usually associated with a normal radiograph or nonspecific radiographic findings; occasionally, bronchial wall thickening or bronchial dilation, or both, may be noted.[53] Bronchiolitis may also be associated with a normal radiograph or may result in accentuation of lung markings or a reticulonodular pattern. On HRCT, inflammation of the bronchiolar wall and filling of the bronchiolar lumen by exudate result in small centrilobular nodules and branching lines ("tree-in-bud" pattern, Fig. 6–1).[54]

Air Space Pneumonia. Nonsegmental air space pneumonia is most commonly caused by *S. pneumoniae* but can occur with other organisms such as *Klebsiella pneumoniae*. The most important pathogenetic feature of this form of disease appears to be the rapid production of edema fluid with relatively minimal cellular reaction. The pneumonic consolidation tends to occur initially in the periphery of the lung beneath the visceral pleura.[55] As it increases in amount, edema fluid flows directly from acinus to acinus; because it usually contains abundant organisms, infection spreads concomitantly. Thus, the infection does not localize in discrete foci, as in bronchopneumonia, but instead comes to occupy a confluent portion of the lung parenchyma (see Color Fig. 6–1) limited only by pleural boundaries and, eventually, by the host's cellular inflammatory reaction.

Radiographically, nonsegmental air space pneumonia appears as a homogeneous consolidation that is relatively sharply demarcated from adjacent uninvolved parenchyma (Fig. 6–2). As the term implies, the consolidation characteristically crosses segmental boundaries, a finding of major importance in distinguishing it from bronchopneumonia. It usually abuts an interlobar fissure but rarely may involve the entire lobe (hence the preference for the term acute air space rather than lobar pneumonia). The larger bronchi often remain patent and air containing, thereby resulting in an air bronchogram. The amount of inflammatory exudate may be such that it results in expansion of a lobe and a bulging fissure sign (Fig. 6–3).[56]

A clinical diagnosis of acute air space pneumonia caused by *S. pneumoniae* is often suggested by the presence of cough, expectoration, chills, fever, and (particularly) pleural pain. In

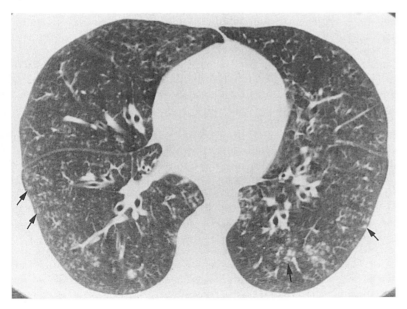

FIGURE 6–1

Acute bronchiolitis—*Mycoplasma pneumoniae*. An HRCT scan shows small nodular opacities (*arrows*) in a centrilobular distribution involving mainly the lower lobes. The patient was a 40-year-old woman. (*From Müller NL, Fraser RS, Colman NC, Paré PD: Radiologic Diagnosis of Diseases of the Chest. Philadelphia, WB Saunders, 2001.*)

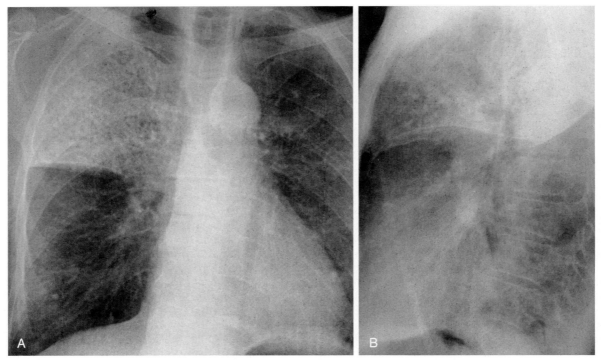

FIGURE 6–2

Acute air space pneumonia. Posteroanterior (**A**) and lateral (**B**) chest radiographs in a 79-year-old man show diffuse consolidation of the right upper lobe. Small foci of consolidation are present in the right lower lobe and in the left lung. Sputum cultures grew *Streptococcus pneumoniae*. *(From Müller NL, Fraser RS, Colman NC, Paré PD: Radiologic Diagnosis of Diseases of the Chest. Philadelphia, WB Saunders, 2001.)*

many cases, physical signs indicate the location of the disease, although the classic signs of parenchymal consolidation—inspiratory lag, impaired percussion, bronchial breathing, fine crackles, and whispering pectoriloquy—are heard much less often than formerly, probably because of increased access to medical care and the prompt institution of antibiotic therapy. In fact, physical examination of the chest usually reveals only fine crackles and decreased breath sounds.

Bronchopneumonia. Bronchopneumonia is exemplified by infection with *S. aureus*, most gram-negative bacteria, and some fungi. It differs pathogenetically from nonsegmental air space pneumonia by the production of a relatively small amount of fluid and the rapid exudation of numerous polymorphonuclear leukocytes, typically in relation to small membranous and respiratory bronchioles (Fig. 6–4). The neutrophils appear to limit the spread of organisms, at least initially, and the disease therefore has a patchy appearance (see Color Fig. 6–2); extension of infection within secondary lobules results in confluent pneumonia, a process frequently associated with necrosis and hemorrhage.

The pattern of healing of bronchopneumonia also differs from that of acute air space pneumonia caused by *S. pneumoniae*. Since the latter is not usually associated with tissue destruction, restoration of normal lung architecture is the rule once host defenses are in control. By contrast, bronchopneumonia is typically associated with virulent organisms and some degree of tissue destruction. Thus, if the patient survives the infection, organization of the inflammatory focus is inevitable and is manifested in the early stage as foci of fibroblastic tissue in airway and alveolar air spaces

(organizing pneumonia) and later as mature fibrous tissue associated with a variable degree of loss of normal lung architecture.

The radiologic manifestations of bronchopneumonia can range from focal peribronchial and peribronchiolar areas of consolidation involving one or more segments of a single lobe to multilobar, bilateral consolidation (Fig. 6–5).[57] Inflammation of small bronchioles and adjacent alveoli results in poorly defined centrilobular nodular opacities measuring 4 to 10 mm in diameter (air space nodules) or may extend to involve the entire secondary lobule (lobular consolidation).[43,58] Confluence of pneumonia in adjacent lobules may result in a pattern simulating nonsegmental air space pneumonia; distinction from the latter can be made in most cases by the presence of a segmental or lobular distribution of the abnormalities in other areas. Because it involves the airways, bronchopneumonia frequently results in loss of volume of the affected segments or lobes.

As indicated, bronchopneumonia is typically caused by highly pathogenic organisms and is associated with the exudation of abundant neutrophils; the combined action of microbial toxins and leukocyte enzymes leads to tissue destruction,[59] which may result in several complications, including abscess formation, pneumatocele, and pulmonary gangrene.

Pulmonary Abscess. Pulmonary abscesses vary in size from those that can be seen only with the microscope to those that occupy a large portion of a lobe. Larger ones often erode into an airway and result in drainage of necrotic material and the formation of a cavity. These abscesses may be solitary or mul-

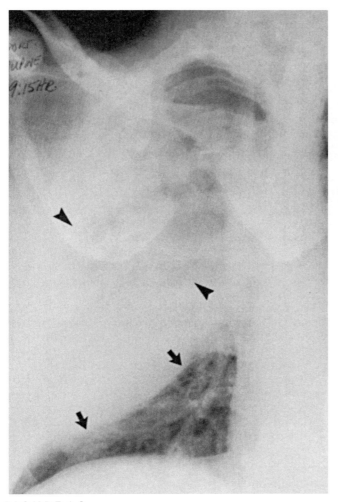

FIGURE 6–3

Acute *Klebsiella* pneumonia—bulging fissure. A view of the right lung from a posteroanterior chest radiograph reveals massive air space consolidation involving most of the upper lobe. The downward-displaced minor fissure (*arrows*) indicates lobar expansion; central radiolucencies (between *arrowheads*) suggest parenchymal necrosis. *(From Müller NL, Fraser RS, Colman NC, Paré PD: Radiologic Diagnosis of Diseases of the Chest. Philadelphia, WB Saunders, 2001.)*

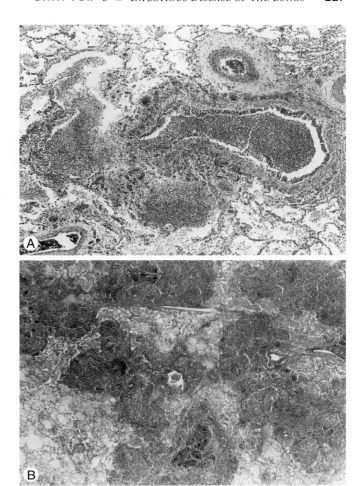

FIGURE 6–4

Acute bronchopneumonia. A histologic section (**A**) shows early disease consisting of an acute inflammatory exudate within the lumen of a terminal bronchiole and immediately adjacent lung parenchyma; the surrounding air spaces are unaffected. More advanced disease is shown in **B**; although there is confluence of inflammation originating in several bronchioles, the patchy nature of the process is still identifiable. Postmortem lung culture grew *Pseudomonas aeruginosa*. *(From Fraser RS, Müller NL, Colman NC, Paré PD: Fraser and Paré's Diagnosis of Diseases of the Chest, 4th ed. Philadelphia, WB Saunders, 1999.)*

tiple and, in cases of relatively long-standing disease, may be associated with considerable pulmonary destruction and fibrosis (see Color Fig. 6–3).

The radiologic manifestations consist of single or multiple masses that are often cavitated (Fig. 6–6). They may be isolated or occur within areas of consolidation. In a review of the radiographic findings in 50 patients, the internal margins of the abscesses were smooth in almost 90% and shaggy in the remainder.[60] Air-fluid levels were present in about 70% and adjacent parenchymal consolidation in 50%. Maximal wall thickness was 4 mm or less in about 5% of cases, between 5 and 15 mm in about 80%, and greater than 15 mm in approximately 15%.

Clinically, a pulmonary abscess may develop in the course of known pneumonia or may be the initial manifestation of disease. Many are caused by anaerobic bacteria,[61] in which case the patient is often elderly and has poor oral hygiene and an underlying condition predisposing to aspiration; signs and symptoms of the disease may be remarkably mild, although fever is common. Other relatively common agents are *S. aureus* and *P. aeruginosa*. Hemoptysis is seen in some cases and may be the initial and sometimes fatal manifestation.[62]

Pulmonary Gangrene. A relatively uncommon complication of pneumonia is the development of fragments of necrotic lung within an abscess cavity (pulmonary sequestrum or gangrene) (Fig. 6–7). The pathogenesis of the pulmonary necrosis in these cases may be related to a direct action of bacterial toxins, to ischemia secondary to thrombosis of pulmonary vessels adjacent to the focus of pneumonia, or to a combination of the two.[63] Whatever the mechanism, it is likely that separation of necrotic from adjacent viable lung tissue is mediated at least partly by leukocyte enzymes. Radiologic manifestations initially consist of small lucencies within an area of consolidated lung, usually in a lobe that is enlarged and shows outward bulging of the fissure.[64] The lucencies rapidly coalesce into a large cavity containing fluid and

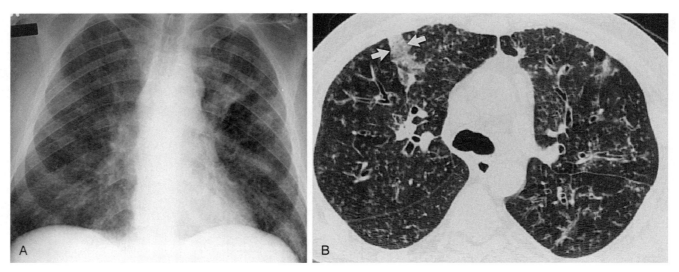

FIGURE 6–5

Haemophilus influenzae **pneumonia.** An anteroposterior chest radiograph (**A**) shows poorly defined nodular opacities and patchy areas of consolidation. An HRCT scan (**B**) shows that the small nodules have a centrilobular distribution, consistent with bronchiolitis. An area of lobular consolidation (*arrows*) characteristic of early bronchopneumonia is also present. Sputum and blood cultures grew *H. influenzae*. *(From Müller NL, Fraser RS, Colman NC, Paré PD: Radiologic Diagnosis of Diseases of the Chest. Philadelphia, WB Saunders, 2001.)*

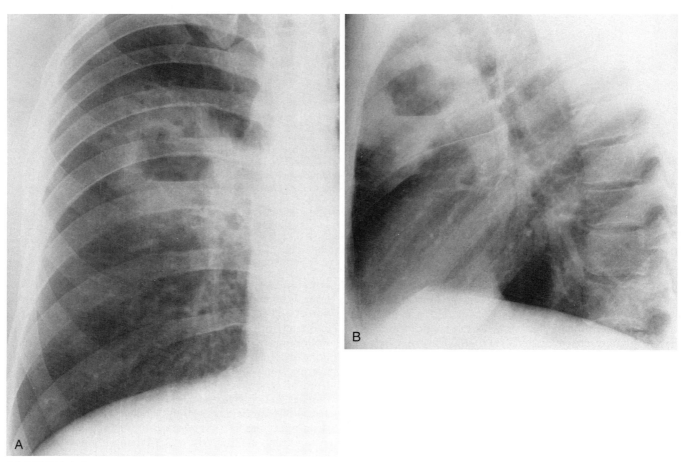

FIGURE 6–6

Lung abscess. Views of the right lung from posteroanterior (**A**) and lateral (**B**) chest radiographs show a large abscess with an air-fluid level in the anterior segment of the right upper lobe. The internal margin of the abscess is irregular, and there is minimal surrounding consolidation. The patient was a 38-year-old alcoholic man who customarily slept on his stomach. Gram stain of sputum revealed gram-positive and gram-negative bacteria. *(From Fraser RS, Müller NL, Colman NC, Paré PD: Fraser and Paré's Diagnosis of Diseases of the Chest, 4th ed. Philadelphia, WB Saunders, 1999.)*

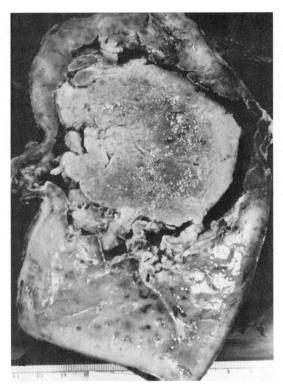

FIGURE 6–7

Pulmonary sequestrum. A slice of left lung shows a large fragment of the necrotic lung within a cavity in the upper lobe. *Klebsiella pneumoniae* was isolated from the patient's sputum premortem. *(From Fraser RS, Müller NL, Colman NC, Paré PD: Fraser and Paré's Diagnosis of Diseases of the Chest, 4th ed. Philadelphia, WB Saunders, 1999.)*

sloughed lung. Lateral decubitus views demonstrate the necrotic lung fragment to be freely mobile within the cavity.

Pneumatocele. A pneumatocele is a thin-walled, gas-filled space that usually develops in association with infection; characteristically, it increases in size over a period of days to weeks and almost invariably resolves (Fig. 6–8). Of the several mechanisms proposed for their formation, the most likely is drainage of a focus of necrotic lung parenchyma followed by check-valve obstruction of the airway subtending it. The "valve," which may be inflammatory exudate or necrotic airway wall (or both), enables air to enter the parenchymal space during inspiration but prevents its egress during expiration.[65] The complication is caused most often by *S. aureus* in infants and children and *P. jiroveci* in patients who have AIDS.[66]

Interstitial Pneumonia. Interstitial pneumonia is typically seen in association with infection by viruses, *M. pneumoniae*, and *P. jiroveci*. Two pathologic patterns occur, depending to some extent on the virulence of the organism and the rapidity with which the infection develops: (1) relatively long-standing or insidious infection, manifested predominantly by lymphocytic infiltration of alveolar septa without significant air space abnormality (Fig. 6–9A), and (2) more rapidly progressive or virulent disease, characterized by diffuse alveolar damage (Fig. 6–9B). The underlying pathogenetic mechanism in the latter form of disease is related to damage to the alveolar-capillary membrane. Histologic features include interstitial thickening by edema fluid, capillary congestion, and an inflammatory cellular infiltrate; type II cell hyperplasia; and a proteinaceous exudate within air spaces. In alveolar ducts and respiratory bronchioles, the exudate typically appears concentrated and flattened (hyaline membranes).

The radiographic manifestations of interstitial pneumonia resulting from viral or mycoplasmal infection consist of a reticular or reticulonodular pattern (Fig. 6–10).[67] Associated bronchiolitis may result in centrilobular linear and nodular opacities[54]; bronchitis may be manifested by peribronchial thickening and accentuation of lung markings. Pneumonia caused by *P. jiroveci* is typically manifested radiographically as

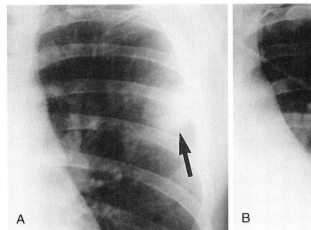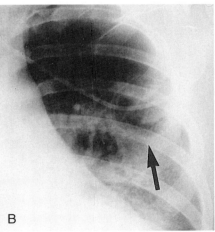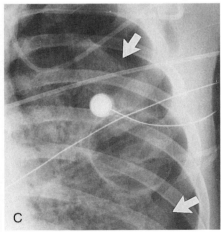

FIGURE 6–8

Pulmonary pneumatocele. A chest radiograph (**A**) from a 28-year-old man shows an ill-defined opacity in the peripheral parenchyma of the left upper lobe *(arrow)*. Twelve days later (**B**), the opacity has been replaced by a smooth, thin-walled cavity approximately 4 cm in diameter. The following day (**C**), the lesion measured 5.5 cm, even in the presence of partial collapse of the left lung as a result of pneumothorax *(arrows)*. *(From Quigley MF, Fraser RS: Pulmonary pneumatocele: Pathology and pathogenesis. AJR Am J Roentgenol 150:1275, 1988.)*

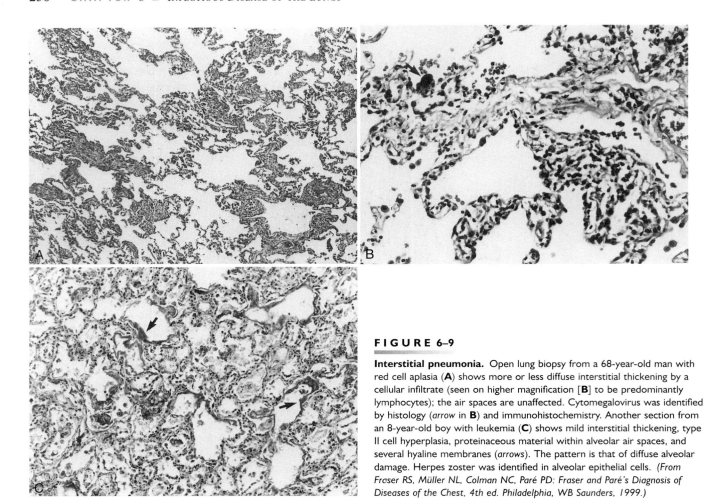

FIGURE 6–9

Interstitial pneumonia. Open lung biopsy from a 68-year-old man with red cell aplasia (**A**) shows more or less diffuse interstitial thickening by a cellular infiltrate (seen on higher magnification [**B**] to be predominantly lymphocytes); the air spaces are unaffected. Cytomegalovirus was identified by histology (*arrow* in **B**) and immunohistochemistry. Another section from an 8-year-old boy with leukemia (**C**) shows mild interstitial thickening, type II cell hyperplasia, proteinaceous material within alveolar air spaces, and several hyaline membranes (*arrows*). The pattern is that of diffuse alveolar damage. Herpes zoster was identified in alveolar epithelial cells. *(From Fraser RS, Müller NL, Colman NC, Paré PD: Fraser and Paré's Diagnosis of Diseases of the Chest, 4th ed. Philadelphia, WB Saunders, 1999.)*

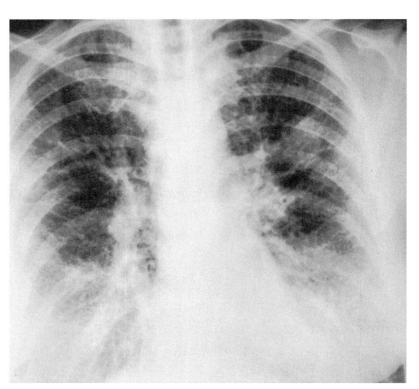

FIGURE 6–10

Acute interstitial pneumonia—*Mycoplasma pneumoniae*. A posteroanterior chest radiograph shows thickening of the bronchovascular bundles and a ground-glass opacity throughout both lungs. Focal consolidation in the left upper lobe and bilateral hilar lymph node enlargement are also evident. The patient was a previously healthy 17-year-old girl. *(From Müller NL, Fraser RS, Colman NC, Paré PD: Radiologic Diagnosis of Diseases of the Chest. Philadelphia, WB Saunders, 2001.)*

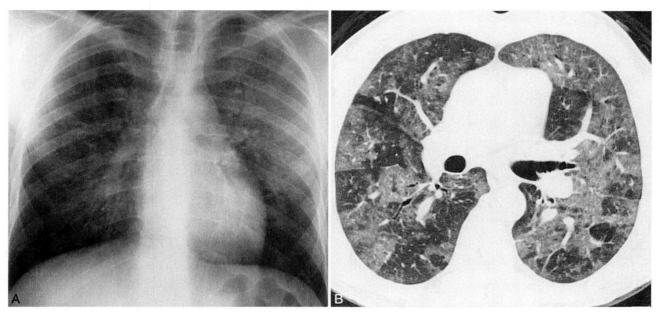

FIGURE 6–11

Pneumocystis pneumonia. A posteroanterior chest radiograh (**A**) shows bilateral ground-glass opacities and a poorly defined reticulonodular pattern. An HRCT scan from another patient (**B**) shows bilateral areas of ground-glass attenuation and areas of normal-appearing lung causing a geographic pattern. Both patients had AIDS. *(From Müller NL, Fraser RS, Colman NC, Paré PD: Radiologic Diagnosis of Diseases of the Chest. Philadelphia, WB Saunders, 2001.)*

a bilateral, symmetrical, fine granular or poorly defined reticulonodular pattern (Fig. 6–11A).[68] With more severe infection, the findings progress to more homogeneous parenchymal opacification ranging from ground-glass opacities to consolidation; a heterogeneous reticulonodular pattern is often apparent at the periphery of the homogeneous opacity.[69] On HRCT, the predominant abnormality consists of extensive bilateral areas of ground-glass attenuation (Fig. 6–11B); small nodules, reticular opacities, and interlobular septal thickening are seen in 20% to 40% of patients.[70]

Many viral infections that involve the lungs begin insidiously with fever, headache, and malaise, although other features (e.g., rash, pharyngitis, arthralgia) are not infrequently seen in association with specific organisms. The major symptom of lower respiratory tract involvement is cough; though initially nonproductive, it may become associated with mucoid or frankly purulent sputum if infection is prolonged. The latter feature should raise the possibility of bacterial superinfection. More severe disease may be manifested by dyspnea and, rarely, respiratory failure. Distinction of infection by viruses from that caused by bacteria or other organisms is not generally possible on a clinical basis alone.

Infection via the Pulmonary Vasculature

Infection via the pulmonary vasculature usually occurs in association with an extrapulmonary focus of infection. In many cases, the source of such infection is evident from the clinical findings. Sometimes, however, as in endocarditis or minute foci of infection in the skin or an internal organ, it is not apparent. The organisms responsible for the infection may be found free in the blood (sepsis) or may be associated with thrombus (septic emboli). A nodular appearance of the indi-

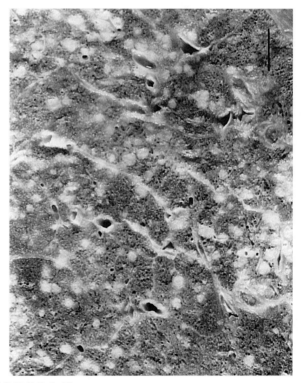

FIGURE 6–12

Miliary tuberculosis. A magnified view of a lower lobe shows numerous randomly distributed nodules approximately 1 to 3 mm in diameter representing hematogenous spread of tubercle bacilli. *(Bar = 1 cm.) (From Fraser RS, Müller NL, Colman NC, Paré PD: Fraser and Paré's Diagnosis of Diseases of the Chest, 4th ed. Philadelphia, WB Saunders, 1999.)*

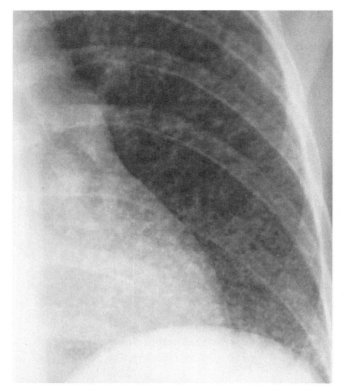

FIGURE 6–13

Miliary tuberculosis. A view of the left lung from an anteroposterior chest radiograph demonstrates numerous sharply defined nodules measuring 1 to 3 mm in diameter, most abundant in the lung base. *(From Fraser RS, Müller NL, Colman NC, Paré PD: Fraser and Paré's Diagnosis of Diseases of the Chest, 4th ed. Philadelphia, WB Saunders, 1999.)*

vidual foci of disease is typical. When pulmonary disease is associated with sepsis, it typically takes the form of innumerable nodules 1 to 5 mm in diameter (miliary infection) (Fig. 6–12); because the organisms probably "seed out" from alveolar capillaries, arterioles, and venules, disease tends to be more or less randomly distributed within the lobule. Such a pattern is most commonly encountered with tuberculosis, but it is occasionally seen with fungal infection (particularly in immunocompromised patients). Pulmonary disease associated with septic emboli is also manifested by multiple, but usually less numerous nodules; in addition, occlusion of pulmonary arteries by thrombus may result in hemorrhage or infarction (or both) and less well defined or wedge-shaped foci of disease.

The radiologic appearance of miliary infection consists of discrete, pinpoint opacities usually evenly distributed throughout both lungs[71]; sometimes, there is a slight basal predominance reflecting gravity-induced increased blood flow (Fig. 6–13). When first visible, the nodules measure 1 to 2 mm in diameter (hence the term miliary, which refers to the similarly sized millet seed); in the absence of adequate therapy, they may increase to 3 to 5 mm in diameter.[71] Septic emboli are characterized by the presence of nodules usually measuring 1 to 3 cm in diameter, which are frequently cavitated (Fig. 6–14). As indicated, CT also frequently shows subpleural wedge-shaped areas of consolidation, often with central areas of necrosis or frank cavitation (see Fig. 6–14).[72]

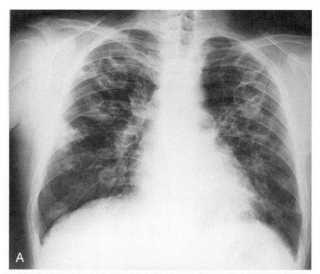

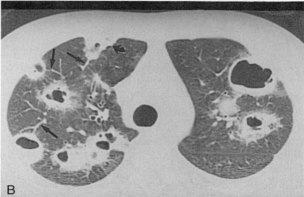

FIGURE 6–14

Septic embolism. A chest radiograph (**A**) shows multiple bilateral cavitated nodules. A CT scan (**B**) shows that several of the nodules are in a subpleural location; some have vessels leading into them *(feeding vessel sign)* *(straight arrows)*. A wedge-shaped focus of subpleural consolidation *(curved arrow)* is also evident. Blood cultures grew *Nocardia*. The patient was HIV positive. *(Case courtesy of Dr. Tomàs Franquet, Department of Radiology, Hospital de Sant Pau, Barcelona, Spain.)*

Infection by Direct Spread from an Extrapulmonary Site

Direct spread across the chest wall or diaphragm or from the mediastinum may occur in contaminated thoracic wounds or by extension of infection from an extrapulmonary source, such as an abdominal abscess or a focus of mediastinitis secondary to esophageal rupture. In these cases, the pulmonary disease is generally localized to an area contiguous with the extrapulmonary infection and often takes the form of an abscess. The source of such infections is sometimes not immediately apparent.[73]

Microbiologic and Other Diagnostic Considerations

A diagnosis of pneumonia is usually made on the basis of the clinical history and radiographic findings. In a previously healthy individual who has a new onset of fever, systemic symptoms, cough, purulent sputum production, neutrophilia, and air space consolidation on the chest radiograph, such diagnosis can be made with a high degree of confidence.[74] However, all these findings are not evident in every case, and care must be taken to not underdiagnose or overdiagnose the abnormality, particularly in certain situations. For example, a number of the typical signs and symptoms of pneumonia are not infrequently absent or altered in the elderly.[75,76] In addition, the presence of underlying cardiopulmonary disease may cause diagnostic problems with respect to differentiation from infarction, hemorrhage, and edema.[6,77]

Mechanical ventilation is also a setting in which diagnosis may be difficult. For example, in a mechanically ventilated patient who has acute respiratory distress syndrome (ARDS), clinical assessment may fail to recognize the proliferative (organizing) phase of ARDS, empyema, nosocomial sinusitis,[78] or catheter-related infection as sources of fever and wrongly attribute them to the presence of "pneumonia."[79,80] Similarly, purulent tracheal secretions originating from either the upper or the lower respiratory tract are seldom caused by pneumonia in patients receiving prolonged mechanical ventilation.[81,82] Interobserver variability aside,[16] the radiographic diagnosis of ventilator-associated pneumonia also lacks sensitivity and specificity[77]: although the presence of an air bronchogram correlates with pneumonia in most cases, the usefulness of this finding is confined to patients who do not have underlying ARDS.

Identification of a specific microorganism responsible for a pneumonia is hampered by the lack of sensitivity and specificity of commonly used laboratory tests. However, there is little evidence that the results of microbiologic investigation influence the choice of treatment in most patients who have community-acquired pneumonia that does not require admission to the hospital; moreover, mortality in this setting does not seem to be related to the determination of a specific cause for the pneumonia.[83] In all probability, patients in whom an organism cannot be identified have pneumonia caused by *S. pneumoniae* or *M. pneumoniae*, viruses, and "atypical" organisms such as *Chlamydia* species. Most such patients probably receive antibiotics suitable for therapy or have not required antibiotics because the infection is of viral origin.[84,85]

In contrast to a mildly ill patient who has community-acquired pneumonia, early identification of the organism responsible for the pneumonia probably improves the prognosis in severely ill patients, especially those who have nosocomial ventilator-associated pneumonia.[86,87] The unnecessary empirical treatment of patients who do not have pneumonia also has a significant risk: patients receiving such treatment may later become infected with resistant organisms, and such infections are associated with higher mortality than infections in patients who have not received previous antibiotic therapy.[88,89] Despite these observations, many investigators have found that after correcting for confounding variables that contribute independently to death, the role played by pneumonia in causing death seems to be relatively modest or is absent altogether in patients who have ventilator-acquired nosocomial pneumonia.[17,24,89,90] It is possible that attributable death in such patients is confined to those whose infection is caused by certain "high-risk" pathogens such as *P. aeruginosa*, *Acinetobacter* species, and *Xanthomonas maltophilia*.[91]

These inconsistencies account at least partly for the diverse approaches that have been proposed for the management of patients who have ventilator-acquired pneumonia[92,93] and for the investigation of patients who have community-acquired pneumonia.[94] We favor attempting to establish a diagnosis as firmly as possible and to define the cause of the infection in patients who have severe disease, in those whose condition progresses despite initial therapy, and in patients at risk for opportunistic or unusual infection as a result of an immunocompromised status or a particular environmental exposure.[94,95] A variety of techniques have been described to do so; their use depends on the expertise and inclination of consultants in any given institution.

Sputum Culture and Gram Stain. In the absence of appropriate measures to ensure a good-quality specimen, sputum Gram stain and culture are neither sensitive nor specific for identification of the causative organism of pneumonia.[85,94] In fact, many sputum specimens are unsatisfactory for diagnostic study because of contamination by upper airway flora, failure to produce secretions from the lower airways, or eradication of pathogens from sputum by the previous use of antibiotics.[94] When purulent sputum uncontaminated by upper airway secretions can be obtained before the institution of antibiotics, however, its examination may be very helpful in diagnosis. For example, the sensitivity of Gram stain for the diagnosis of bacteremic pneumococcal pneumonia is as high as 85%.[96] The value of this information will no doubt increase with increasing prevalence of penicillin-resistant organisms in the community (see page 237).[95] Gram staining of sputum also has a high negative predictive value with respect to culture.[97]

Information derived from sputum studies is unlikely to influence management in most patients who have community-acquired pneumonia.[85] However, we favor performing Gram stain and culture before initiating antibiotic therapy in any patient whose illness is of sufficient severity to warrant admission to the hospital,[98] provided that obtaining the sample does not lead to delay in initiating therapy.[95] The results of such investigation may allow modification of antibiotic therapy to include coverage for an unanticipated infection,[99,100] have prognostic importance, influence the duration of therapy, and provide information concerning the local epidemiology of infection.[101]

Blood Culture. Although culture of blood taken before the institution of antibiotics has poor sensitivity for identification of the organism responsible for pneumonia, cultures should be performed in any patient requiring admission to the hospital for community-acquired pneumonia. The specificity of a positive culture is high (although some patients have mixed infections), and the finding has prognostic importance.[94] In the setting of suspected ventilator-associated pneumonia, blood culture can also be useful in identifying another source of infection.[102]

Endotracheal Aspiration. Lower respiratory tract secretions can be obtained easily by endotracheal aspiration in patients who are intubated. Nonquantitative analysis of such specimens is a sensitive, albeit nonspecific means of determining the cause of pneumonia.[80,103] Quantitative culture improves specificity such that its performance may be comparable to that of more invasive methods of bacteriologic diagnosis.[104,105]

Protected Brush Specimens. In an attempt to improve the sensitivity and specificity of culture or Gram stain for the diagnosis of pneumonia, material has been obtained bronchoscopically by protected specimen brush.[20] Quantification of the growth of the bacteria recovered has been used to help define the presence or absence of pneumonia and to aid in identification of the causative pathogen.[106] The wide application and utility of such testing, however, have been limited by lack of standardization of the tests; by the paucity of studies demonstrating improvement in mortality, morbidity, or other outcome variables in comparison to less invasive methods of diagnosis[104,107]; and by the concern that no test is sufficiently sensitive to exclude pneumonia in patients for whom clinical suspicion is high.[108]

The reported sensitivity of protected brush specimen analysis has varied from about 50% to 80%.[109,110] The specificity of the test has generally been in excess of 80%.[109,111] In a study of 147 ventilated patients suspected of having nosocomial pneumonia in which a threshold of 10^3 colony-forming units per milliliter was used for the diagnosis, only 45 had confirmation of pneumonia.[81] Culture was falsely positive in only four patients, and no patient who had less than the diagnostic colony count showed evidence of pneumonia on follow-up. Although most other investigators have not attained this degree of success, some have demonstrated similar favorable findings.[112]

In fact, it may be inappropriate to establish definitive threshold values of quantitative culture for the diagnosis of pneumonia by protected brush. The significance of a positive result should be interpreted in light of the pretest probability of disease, and consideration should be given to both the potential harm that could be done by not treating the pneumonia and the risk of unnecessary therapy.[113] Although quantitative data concerning the risks and benefits of giving or withholding treatment are largely unavailable in the setting of critically ill patients, given a fixed risk-to-benefit ratio for antibiotic therapy, it is evident that as the pretest probability for pneumonia increases, the threshold used to define an abnormal test result should decrease (i.e., fewer organisms would be necessary before one would embark on a course of therapy).[113]

Bronchoalveolar Lavage. BAL, including protected lavage with quantitative culture of distal lung secretions, has been found to yield results for the diagnosis of pneumonia similar to those derived from protected brush specimens.[114] Optimal performance of the test depends on using an adequate lavage volume and on performing the test before a change or institution of antibiotics.[115] Identification of intracellular organisms in phagocytic cells has a specificity for pneumonia of greater than 95% in most studies; although some investigators have reported a markedly lower yield,[111] the reported sensitivity has generally varied from 60% to greater than 90%.[109,116,117] The appearance of organisms on Gram stain has been found to be closely related to the results of culture and therefore allows early and appropriate antibiotic selection.[117] Assessment of BAL neutrophilia may also be helpful in diagnosis; for example, absence of neutrophilia predicted the absence of pneumonia within 2 days of specimen collection in 97% of patients in one study,[118] and the finding of less than 50% neutrophils in lavage fluid had a negative predictive value of 100% in another.[80]

Transthoracic Needle Aspiration. Percutaneous fine-needle aspiration of the lung with an ultrathin needle has been used for the identification of pathogens in nonventilated and (occasionally) ventilated patients who have pneumonia.[119,120] As might be expected, the specificity and positive predictive value of a positive culture have been reported to be as high as 100%,[121] whereas the sensitivity and negative predictive value are poor (approximately 61% and 34%, respectively). Results are better when the radiographic opacity is more extensive and the patient has not yet received antibiotics.[122] Whether outcome is favorably altered has not been determined.

Whether the aforementioned methods should be the standard of care for patients who are severely ill with pneumonia, especially those who have ventilator-acquired pneumonia, is a controversial issue; in addition, if used at all, it is uncertain which of the tests is best.[92,93,123] Most importantly, it is not known whether application of any of the techniques results in a reduction in mortality and morbidity in a cost-effective fashion in comparison to a less invasive and simplified approach (e.g., clinical assessment and quantitative culture and Gram stain of endotracheal aspirates).[124]

Pneumonia in Specific Patient Groups

Community-Acquired Pneumonia

The reported frequency of different organisms responsible for community-acquired pneumonia varies widely in different series.[6] This variation is the result of several factors, including the techniques used for diagnosis, the age of the patients, the presence or absence of additional significant disease, and the severity of the pneumonia.[125] Moreover, even with rigorous effort, the causative organism can be established in no more than 50% of patients who have community-acquired pneumonia.[126] Despite these limitations, some general observations may be made.

S. pneumoniae is the most commonly identified pathogen in most investigations[126,127] and accounts for about 35% of identified organisms. In patients admitted to the hospital for pneumonia, anaerobic bacteria have been isolated in approximately 20% to 35%.[128] Between 2% and 8% of patients have *H. influenzae* infection[6]; most have underlying chronic airflow obstruction or are elderly. *Moraxella catarrhalis* is a not uncommon cause of pneumonia in the same settings.[129] Community-acquired *S. aureus* pneumonia is uncommon and usually follows influenza virus infection; it is often associated with bacteremia and high mortality and should be considered in all severely ill patients admitted to the intensive care unit (ICU) for the management of pneumonia.[130] Methicillin-resistant *S. aureus* can be a particularly serious cause of pneumonia in residents of nursing homes.[131]

The frequency with which *Legionella* species are identified as a cause of community-acquired pneumonia shows marked regional variation. Although they account for only 2% or less of cases overall, in some series they are much more common, particularly in patients sick enough to require hospitalization and care in an ICU.[132] Gram-negative enteric organisms are an uncommon cause of pneumonia in the general population, but they should also be considered in severely ill patients, especially those who are older, who have aspirated, or who have significant underlying disease.[133,134] Though often not considered among the causes of community-acquired pneumonia in epidemiologic surveys, it is clear that tuberculosis must also be considered in outpatients who have pneumonia;

its prevalence is greater in certain populations, such as residents of nursing homes, alcoholics, the homeless, drug addicts, and HIV-infected individuals, as well as in individuals from populations in which tuberculosis has a high prevalence.[135]

When analysis is confined to ambulatory patients who do not require hospitalization, the proportion of bacterial species identified as the cause of community-acquired pneumonia decreases dramatically; for example, in a study of 149 such patients, only 3 (2%) were found to have bacterial pneumonia.[136] Many of these patients have "atypical pneumonia" caused by *M. pneumoniae* (identified in almost 30% of patients in some series)[2,137] or *C. pneumoniae* (approximately 20%).[2,138] Other chlamydia-like organisms have also been recognized as a cause of community-acquired pneumonia.[139,140] Q fever pneumonia (caused by *Coxiella burnetii*) shows significant geographic variation in incidence, its discovery generally being confined to rural settings.[2] In adults, influenza virus is the most important cause of community-acquired viral pneumonia.[139,140]

The severity of pneumonia influences the necessity for admission (whether to a ward or to the ICU), the use of diagnostic techniques, and the choice of antibiotics. Severe pneumonia has been defined as that requiring admission to an ICU.[141] Short of this, the presence of certain clinical features of pneumonia mandates serious consideration for admission to the hospital, at least until a favorable response to therapy can be established.[142,143] These features include any history of significant underlying disease, age older than 65 years, altered mental status, previous splenectomy, suspicion of aspiration, elevation of temperature to greater than 38.3°C, and evidence of infection elsewhere. A variety of laboratory findings have also been associated with increased morbidity and mortality, including a white blood cell count less than 4×10^9 or greater than 30×10^9, an absolute neutrophil count less than 1×10^9, PaO_2 less than 60 or $PaCO_2$ greater than 50 mm Hg while breathing room air, elevated blood urea nitrogen and creatinine, serum hemoglobin less than 90 g/L, metabolic acidosis, and findings of disseminated intravascular coagulation (DIC). Radiographic findings that warrant extra vigilance include multilobar involvement, cavitation, and pleural effusion.

In the absence of these risk factors, a complicated clinical course is unlikely.[1] Based on an analysis of clinical and laboratory data from 14,199 adult inpatients who had community-acquired pneumonia, a prediction rule that stratified patients into five classes with respect to risk for death within 30 days was developed and applied to an additional 40,236 patients.[1] The mortality rate among patients in the first three classes was found to be sufficiently low that outpatient treatment could reasonably be considered. This was especially true for class I patients (<50 years of age, absence of comorbid disease, normal mental status, heart rate <125 beats/min, respiratory rate <30 breaths/min, systolic blood pressure >90 mm Hg, and temperature between 35°C and 40°C). These findings imply that simple clinical and laboratory observations are of value in assessing the risk of death in patients who have community-acquired pneumonia. No single criterion or group of criteria, however, can replace overall clinical judgment; social factors and clinical circumstances such as persistent vomiting should also influence a decision for hospitalization in the individual patient.[144,145]

Hospital-Acquired Pneumonia

Hospital-acquired (nosocomial) pneumonia can be defined as pneumonia occurring 48 hours or more after admission, thus excluding infection that is incubating at the time of admission.[20] Bacteria are the most frequently identified cause. Early in the hospital course (within the first 4 days), the more common organisms are *S. pneumoniae*, *M. catarrhalis*, methicillin-sensitive *S. aureus*, and *H. influenzae*.[146] Later on, enteric gram-negative organisms, such as *Enterobacter* species, *Escherichia coli*, *Klebsiella* species, *Proteus* species, and *S. aureus*, including methicillin-resistant species, predominate.[20] The presence of specific risk factors increases the likelihood that certain organisms are responsible. For example, anaerobic bacteria are more likely to be found in patients in whom pneumonia develops after witnessed aspiration or who have poor dentition or altered consciousness.[147] *P. aeruginosa* infection should be considered in patients who have received corticosteroids or broad-spectrum antibiotics, those who have had a prolonged stay in the ICU, or patients who have underlying lung disease such as bronchiectasis.[148] *S. aureus* is more common in patients who have coma,[149] head injury, recent influenza infection, renal failure, or a history of intravenous drug abuse. *Legionella* species are endemic in some hospitals[150]; pneumonia caused by them is associated with corticosteroid therapy. Prolonged hospitalization or previous use of antibiotics also favors the development of nosocomial pneumonia caused by antibiotic-resistant organisms such as *S. aureus*, *Acinetobacter* species, *Serratia marcescens*, and *P. aeruginosa*.[151] Similar organisms should be suspected when pneumonia is severe (e.g., in patients undergoing mechanical ventilation or in the ICU).[152]

Risk factors for the development of nosocomial pneumonia have been assessed by many investigators[146,153,154] and have been grouped into five general categories: (1) host factors, such as age and degree of immunosuppression; (2) factors that favor microbial colonization of the upper airway or stomach (previous use of antibiotics being especially important in this regard); (3) factors that favor aspiration of upper airway or gastric secretions; (4) duration of mechanical ventilation (prolonged ventilation being associated with an increased risk of exposure to contaminated equipment or to the colonized hands of health care workers); and (5) factors that prevent adequate clearance of airway secretions, such as recent surgery or immobilization as a result of trauma or illness. As might be expected, multiple risk factors are often present in patients who contract pneumonia.

Pneumonia in the Compromised Host

Abnormal immune or inflammatory function is an important manifestation of many diseases and is a complication of the therapy used in numerous others. For obvious reasons, both the incidence and severity of infection, including that of the lungs, is increased in patients who have these disorders. In addition, the organisms responsible for infection often differ from those associated with infection in a "normal" host. For example, invasive aspergillosis, *Pneumocystis jiroveci (carinii)* pneumonia (PCP), and cytomegalovirus (CMV) pneumonia are relatively common diseases in patients who have acute myelogenous leukemia, AIDS, and organ transplants, respectively; however, these conditions are seen rarely in patients whose immune and inflammatory systems are normal.

Disorders of immune or inflammatory function can be inherited or acquired, the latter being by far the most common. Discussion of the various clinical, radiologic, and pathologic features of pulmonary infection associated with most acquired abnormalities of host defense can be found in the appropriate chapters elsewhere in the text; particular attention is given to infections in patients who have had organ transplants (see page 531) or who have AIDS (see page 423).

Congenital disorders of immune function, either cell mediated or humoral, are often associated with an increased incidence of pulmonary infection. One of the most frequently encountered is common variable immunodeficiency, which is associated with B-cell dysfunction.[155] Bronchiectasis was once an inevitable feature of this disease[156]; however, early recognition of bronchiectasis and prompt institution of intravenous gamma globulin therapy have prevented both this complication and the recurrent lung infection that causes it.[157] For unknown reasons, about 20% of patients who have symptoms associated with the disorder have been found to have interstitial lung disease.[158]

AEROBIC AND FACULTATIVE BACTERIA

Streptococcus pneumoniae

S. pneumoniae is a gram-positive bacterium that is oval or lancet shaped and usually arranged in pairs. It is surrounded by a well-defined polysaccharide capsule whose structure permits typing with specific antisera.[159] It has been estimated to be present as a normal commensal in up to 20% of the population.[160] In certain groups, such as patients who have asthma or COPD, colonization rates may be substantially higher. As indicated previously, *S. pneumoniae* is the most common pathogenic organism identified in patients admitted to the hospital for pneumonia; it accounts for about 40% of all isolated species.[161] Important risk factors include age, current cigarette smoking, drug and alcohol abuse, chronic disease, and underlying immunosuppression.[162,163] The emergence of drug resistance has become an important feature of the organism, with up to 35% of strains having been found to be resistant to penicillin in various parts of the United States, Europe, and East Asia.[164]

Pathogenesis and Pathologic Characteristics. Infection of the lower respiratory tract usually follows aspiration of organisms from a focus of colonization in the nasopharynx.[165] Virulence depends in part on the polysaccharide capsule, which helps protect the organism from phagocytosis,[165] and the ability of the bacteria to adhere to bronchopulmonary epithelial cells by surface macromolecules (adhesins).[166] The latter is enhanced by a variety of cytokines induced by the organism's cell wall, by cigarette smoking, and (sometimes) by antecedent viral infection.[167,168] Adherence of the organism to epithelial cells has several consequences, including the production of cytokines and toxins that are capable of initiating an inflammatory reaction.[168] The bacterium also affects endothelial cells by causing an increase in alveolar-capillary membrane permeability and initiation of the procoagulant cascade.[168] These processes are associated with the development of edema fluid, which spreads from alveolus to alveolus and results in more

or less uniform consolidation of the lung parenchyma (see Color Fig. 6–1).

Under the influence of cytokines,[169] leukocytes subsequently emigrate from the capillaries into the air spaces.[165] Although these cells can kill the organism, they may not control the infection completely, and resolution is often associated with the appearance of anticapsular antibodies, which facilitate phagocytosis of the organism by alveolar macrophages. The high incidence of resolution is probably related to the lack of toxins produced by the organism, a feature also reflected by the absence of tissue necrosis. Although experimental studies have shown that a considerable increase in proteolytic activity accompanies the accumulation of neutrophils in the air spaces, a simultaneous and comparable rise in serum and lung fluid antiproteases seems to protect the lung parenchyma from damage.[170] As a result, abscess formation is uncommon and probably occurs only in association with particularly virulent strains or with concomitant infection by anaerobic organisms.[171]

Radiologic Manifestations. The characteristic radiographic pattern consists of homogeneous, nonsegmental consolidation involving one lobe (Fig. 6–15). Because the consolidation begins in the peripheral air spaces, it almost invariably abuts a visceral pleural surface, either interlobar or over the convexity of the lung. Occasionally, infection is manifested as a round (spherical) focus of consolidation that simulates a mass,[172] patchy areas of consolidation, or mixed air space and interstitial opacities.[43] Complications such as cavitation, pulmonary gangrene, and pneumatocele formation are rare; it is probable that many of these complications are related to mixed infections.[171]

The reported incidence of pleural effusion varies with the radiographic technique used to detect it, the severity of infection, and the presence or absence of bacteremia. Pleural effusion is evident on posteroanterior and lateral radiographs in about 10% of patients overall,[173] in approximately 30% of those who have severe pneumonia requiring treatment in the ICU,[174] and in about 50% of those who have bacteremia.[175]

Clinical Manifestations. The usual clinical manifestation is abrupt, with fever, shaking chills, cough, slight expectoration, and intense pleural pain. Cough may be nonproductive at first but soon produces bloody, "rusty," or greenish material. Debilitated or alcoholic patients may be deeply cyanosed, and shock may ensue rapidly. In the elderly, these classic features of disease may be absent and pneumonia may be confused with or confounded by other disease, such as congestive heart failure, thromboembolism, or malignancy.[176] Clinical examination reveals findings of consolidation; a friction rub may be audible. There are no particular clinical features of the infection that distinguish it from pneumonia caused by *Legionella* species or other organisms in any given patient.[177] Metastatic foci of infection may occur in any tissue but are usually clinically evident only in the heart, meninges, or joints. Perhaps the most important complication of pneumococcal infection is superinfection, usually by gram-negative organisms in patients who have received broad-spectrum antibiotics.

Laboratory Findings and Diagnosis. Isolation of the organism or the demonstration of a specific polysaccharide antigen is necessary for definitive diagnosis. The sensitivity of a good Gram stain for the diagnosis of pneumococcal pneumonia is only about 15%, in part because sputum samples are often not obtained in timely fashion.[178] However, the finding

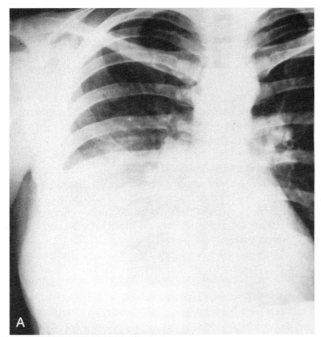

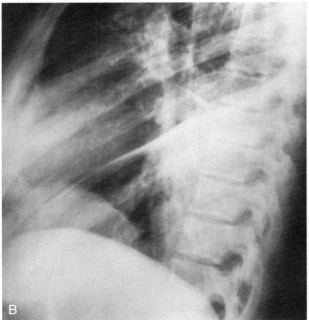

FIGURE 6–15

Acute air space pneumonia—*Streptococcus pneumoniae*.
Posteroanterior (**A**) and lateral (**B**) radiographs reveal extensive consolidation of the right lower lobe, a portion of the anterior segment being the only lung tissue unaffected. An air bronchogram is visible in the lateral projection. There is little loss of volume. *(From Müller NL, Fraser RS, Colman NC, Paré PD: Radiologic Diagnosis of Diseases of the Chest. Philadelphia, WB Saunders, 2001.)*

as counterimmunoelectrophoresis,[180] coagglutination,[181] and enzyme-linked immunosorbent assay (ELISA)[182] also suggests the presence of infection.[6] In addition, polymerase chain reaction (PCR) has been used to detect streptococcal DNA in blood, pleural fluid, and lung aspirates[183-185]; however, the procedure cannot distinguish colonization from infection in samples taken from the throat and sputum.[186]

The white cell count is usually higher than 20,000/mm³, but leukopenia often develops in extremely ill patients. Hyponatremia and hypobilirubinemia may be seen.[187] Analysis of arterial blood gas may show mild or even severe hypoxemia; in most cases, PCO_2 is also reduced.

Prognosis and Natural History. A number of risk factors have been associated with an increased risk of death from pneumonia in general and from *S. pneumoniae* pneumonia in particular.[12] These risk factors can be related to demographic factors (increasing age, ethnicity, and residence in a nursing home), clinical features (see page 235), and laboratory abnormalities (see page 235).[188] In the absence of these risk factors, a good outcome can be anticipated. Somewhat surprisingly, the increasing prevalence of antibiotic-resistant organisms has not been associated with an appreciable increase in mortality.[189] The explanation is presumably related to the fact that most strains have intermediate-grade resistance rather than high-grade resistance, and high doses of antibiotics can still achieve effective tissue-killing levels. In addition, antibiotics to which the organism is sensitive are sometimes chosen as part of the initial empirical regimen for treatment of a severely ill patient.[164]

Streptococcus pyogenes

S. pyogenes is a gram-positive organism that appears on smear in short chains. It used to be one of the most common causes of bronchopneumonia, predominantly in the young and the elderly. With the advent of antibiotics, however, it has become uncommon. Nevertheless, it appears to be increasing in importance as a cause of severe pneumonia, both sporadically and in outbreaks.[190,191]

In most respects the radiographic characteristics are indistinguishable from those of acute staphylococcal pneumonia: homogeneous or patchy consolidation in a segmental distribution and some loss of volume that typically affects the lower lobes and is sometimes bilateral.[192] The tendency to form pneumatoceles or pyopneumothorax as in acute staphylococcal pneumonia is absent, although lung abscesses and cavities may develop and empyema is common. The onset of pneumonia is usually abrupt, with pleural pain, shaking chills, fever, and cough productive of purulent and often blood-tinged material; signs of pleural effusion are generally detectable. Complications include residual pleural thickening[193] and bronchiectasis (especially in children in whom the disease develops in conjunction with an exanthem).

Staphylococcus aureus

S. aureus is a gram-positive coccus that appears on smear in pairs, short chains, tetrads, or clusters.[194] It is distinguished from other staphylococcal species by its production of coagulase, a plasma-clotting enzyme. Methicillin-resistant strains of *S. aureus* (MRSA) have become particularly important and

of a predominant organism in a good-quality specimen does have high specificity for diagnosis.[179] Infection can be proved by culture of the organism from normally sterile sources, such as lung (via transthoracic needle aspiration), blood, or pleura.[178] The finding of capsular antigen in sputum, BAL fluid, or pleural fluid by techniques such account for almost 40% of staphylococcal isolates in some American hospitals.[131] Although colonization with organisms of this strain is also common in long-care treatment institutions, in only a small percentage of affected people does frank infection develop.

The organism is an uncommon cause of community-acquired pneumonia; it accounts for only about 3% of all cases and about 3% to 12% of those severe enough to require admission to the hospital and management in an ICU.[12] Such severe infection rarely occurs in healthy adults. Risk factors include very young or old age, alcoholism, chronic disease such as COPD, AIDS, malnutrition, bacteremia associated with soft tissue infection or endocarditis,[149,194] residence in an institution, debilitation, intravenous drug abuse, and recent influenza infection.[195,196] S. aureus is more important as a cause of nosocomial pneumonia, especially in the ICU, in which setting it is one of the most common pathogenic organisms.[194] The organism is also extremely common in the sputum of patients who have cystic fibrosis.

The most common pathologic pattern is acute bronchopneumonia, frequently associated with abscess formation. Some degree of parenchymal fibrosis is common as a residuum. Occasionally (usually in association with influenza infection and a rapidly fatal outcome), there is extensive intra-alveolar edema and hemorrhage, relatively sparse neutrophil infiltration, and little or no evidence of tissue necrosis. Pneumonia associated with hematogenous spread of organisms is characterized by well- or ill-defined nodules, mostly 0.5 to 3 cm in diameter.

The parenchymal consolidation in acute staphylococcal bronchopneumonia is typically segmental in distribution. Depending on the severity of involvement, the process may be patchy or homogeneous, the latter representing confluent bronchopneumonia. The consolidation involves more than one lobe in approximately 60% of patients and is bilateral in approximately 40%.[57,197] Because an inflammatory exudate fills the airways, segmental atelectasis may accompany the consolidation; for the same reason, an air bronchogram is seldom observed, and its presence should cast some doubt on the diagnosis. With HRCT, bronchiolar involvement is manifested by centrilobular nodular and branching linear opacities (tree-in-bud pattern).

Abscesses develop in 15% to 30% of patients (Fig. 6–16).[57,197] Pneumatocele formation is also common and occurs in about 50% of children and 15% of adults.[57,198] Pneumatoceles usually appear during the first week of the pneumonia and disappear spontaneously within weeks or months. Pleural effusions develop in 30% to 50% of patients; of these, approximately half represent empyemas.[57,197] Spontaneous pneumothorax occurs occasionally.

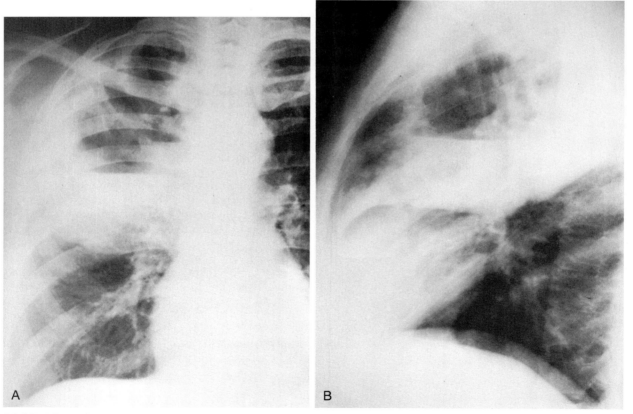

FIGURE 6–16

Acute lung abscess—*Staphylococcus aureus*. Posteroanterior (**A**) and lateral (**B**) radiographs reveal massive consolidation of the whole of the right upper lobe, a large ragged cavity being evident in the center. The volume of the lobe is increased, as indicated by posterior bulging of the major fissure. *(From Müller NL, Fraser RS, Colman NC, Paré PD: Radiologic Diagnosis of Diseases of the Chest. Philadelphia, WB Saunders, 2001.)*

In pneumonia related to hematogenous spread of organisms, the radiologic appearance is one of multiple nodules or masses throughout the lungs. Sometimes the nodules have poorly defined borders or are confluent. Abscesses may erode into bronchi and produce air-containing cavities, frequently with fluid levels.[199] On CT scan, most abnormalities are in a subpleural location. In approximately two thirds of cases, some of the nodules have a vessel coursing into their substance (feeding vessel sign).[72,200] Septic infarcts result in subpleural wedge-shaped areas of consolidation.[200]

The clinical picture of *S. aureus* pneumonia is variable and depends on the patient's age and degree of debilitation and whether the pneumonia is superimposed on influenza infection. In children and adults who acquire the infection after influenza, the onset is usually abrupt, with pleural pain, cough, and expectoration of purulent yellow or brown sputum, sometimes streaked with blood.[201] When the infection develops in the hospital, the clinical signs and symptoms are similar to those that occur with other virulent hospital-acquired bacterial infections.

The diagnosis should be considered whenever pneumonia develops in association with influenza or in a hospitalized patient. A positive sputum culture is a sensitive indicator of infection; however, it lacks specificity.[194] The white blood cell count is usually elevated, but leukopenia may be present in severely ill patients. Positive blood cultures are obtained in many patients; however, it is important to remember that these may represent either bacteremia secondary to the pneumonia or hematogenous spread of organisms from an extrapulmonary source.

Complications of staphylococcal pneumonia include meningitis, metastatic abscesses (particularly to the brain and kidneys), and acute endocarditis, which may develop in patients who do not have antecedent valvular disease. Pleural effusion is fairly common and may be complicated by empyema. Given the common association of *S. aureus* pneumonia with underlying disease and the hospital setting, it is not surprising that the mortality rate is very high, varying from about 20% to 85% in several series.[131,202]

Moraxella catarrhalis

M. catarrhalis (*Branhamella catarrhalis, Neisseria catarrhalis*) is an intracellular gram-negative, kidney-shaped diplococcus.[203] Known for a long time as a commensal in the oral cavity, it has been increasingly recognized as an important pathogen in the upper and lower respiratory tract.[204] Infection usually occurs in patients who have underlying pulmonary disease, particularly those who with COPD who are receiving corticosteroid therapy.[205] Patients who are deficient in immunoglobulins also appear to be susceptible.[206] Nosocomial outbreaks of infection have been described.[207]

Clinically, the disease takes the form of an acute febrile tracheobronchitis or bronchopneumonia.[208] In most patients, the infection is mild; however, it may be severe in those who are immunocompromised.[203] Complications such as pleural effusion, empyema, or septicemia are uncommon. Although positive blood cultures have been reported,[206] the diagnosis is usually based on the identification of typical organisms on a good-quality Gram stain of sputum accompanied by heavy growth on culture.[203]

Neisseria meningitidis

N. meningitidis is a gram-negative diplococcus that in disease is found largely intracellularly. The organism has been isolated from blood[209] and other nominally sterile sources[210] in patients who have pneumonia without meningitis and in pure growth from patients with purulent exacerbations of chronic bronchitis.[211] Viral infection (such as adenoviral pneumonia or influenza) appears to be an important risk factor.[212,213] Young adults in military service also appear to be particularly susceptible, perhaps because of their close contact with carriers of *N. meningitidis* and the greater likelihood of their acquiring viral infection. Published reproductions of chest radiographs show a pattern of acute air space pneumonia. The typical history is of gradually increasing fever for 2 to 3 weeks, followed by pleural pain.[214]

Bacillus anthracis (Anthrax)

B. anthracis is an encapsulated, gram-positive rod that typically occurs in chains.[159] Spores are found in decaying soil and organic matter, in which they germinate under appropriate conditions and are ingested by herbivorous livestock such as goats, sheep, and cattle. Humans are infected most commonly by direct contact, which results in cutaneous disease; less often, infection develops after the ingestion of contaminated meat or inhalation of contaminated soil. In industrialized societies, anthrax has traditionally been an occupational disease affecting individuals involved in handling hides in the textile, tannery, and wool industries. A major concern today is potential use of the organism for bioterrorism.[215,216]

Spores of the organism are taken up by alveolar macrophages and transported to the mediastinal lymph nodes within hours, with no specific pulmonary lesion developing. In the lymph nodes, the spores germinate and form vegetative bacilli that multiply and produce various virulence factors.[217] The latter include capsular polypeptide, which confers resistance to phagocytosis, and anthrax toxin, which promotes edema and the formation of proinflammatory cytokines within tissue macrophages.[218] Toxin released into the bloodstream can cause edema, hemorrhage, necrosis, and shock.[216] Pathologically, the earliest abnormality is hemorrhagic mediastinitis, which may be followed by direct spread of the organism to the pleura[215] and the subsequent development of large pleural effusions. Diffuse alveolar damage may be seen in the lungs as a complication of sepsis or toxemia; true infectious pneumonia is uncommon.[216]

The most common radiographic manifestations are bilateral pleural effusions, widening of the mediastinum, and unilateral or bilateral interstitial opacities or areas of consolidation.[219-221] CT typically demonstrates edema of mediastinal fat and high-attenuation mediastinal and hilar lymph nodes as a result of hemorrhage.[220-222] The nodes show marked enhancement after the intravenous administration of contrast, a finding highly suggestive of the diagnosis in a patient who has a history of possible exposure.[221]

The initial symptoms are nonspecific and consist of mild fever, malaise, myalgia, nonproductive cough, nausea, vomiting, and chest discomfort.[215] Severe dyspnea, hypotension, and hemorrhage can follow within days of exposure. Evidence of meningitis is common.[215] Mediastinal lymph node enlargement may cause tracheal compression and stridor.[216] Physical examination may reveal widespread crackles and signs of pleural effusion. If treatment is not initiated, death within 24 hours is not uncommon.[218]

In the absence of a specific occupational exposure or an association with other recently diagnosed patients, the non-specific nature of the initial symptoms makes diagnosis difficult. Consideration of the infection should occur in any previously healthy person who has an acute febrile illness that rapidly leads to shock. Widening of the mediastinum radiographically significantly increases the likelihood of its presence in this setting.[216] The findings of nausea and vomiting, dyspnea, neurologic symptoms, abnormal auscultation, tachycardia, high hematocrit, high transaminase, low albumin, normal white blood cell count, and low serum sodium values strengthen diagnostic suspicion, whereas the findings of rhinorrhea, sore throat, myalgia, and headache weaken it.[223,224] Positive culture and Gram stain of blood or another appropriate specimen confirm the diagnosis; examination of sputum is seldom useful.

Listeria monocytogenes

L. monocytogenes is a short, gram-positive rod that can be found in soil, water, sewage, many domestic animals, and (occasionally) the upper airways, genitalia, or lower gastrointestinal tract of asymptomatic human carriers. Most cases of adult human infection are sporadic and not associated with an identifiable infectious source. Transmission is believed to occur by ingestion or direct contact with contaminated food, especially pâté and unpasteurized cheese[225] or animal products, or after contact with human carriers. Listeriosis occurs predominantly in neonates, pregnant women, immunocompromised individuals, and older patients who have underlying chronic debilitating disease; many patients have lymphoreticular malignancies. In adults, disease usually takes the form of meningitis, frequently associated with septicemia. Pulmonary or pleural infection supervenes in a minority of cases.[226]

Corynebacterium Species

Corynebacteria are gram-positive bacilli or coccobacilli that possess irregular swellings at one end that result in a club-shaped appearance.[159] *Corynebacterium diphtheriae* (the cause of diptheria) is the most important member of the genus to cause human disease. Diphtheria is typically manifested as pharyngitis associated with a classic membrane that can extend to the larynx and result in upper airway obstruction[227]; the organism has not been reported to cause pneumonia. Although members of the genus other than *C. diphtheriae* are usually judged to be commensals or contaminants when cultured, some have been documented to cause significant pulmonary disease, especially in immunocompromised individuals.[228]

Rhodococcus equi

R. equi is a gram-positive, weakly acid-fast coccobacillus. Infection has been documented most often in patients who have AIDS (see page 424). However, it has also been seen in other immunocompromised patients[229] and, rarely, in

otherwise healthy individuals. Radiologic findings consist of a round opacity or area of consolidation, often in an upper lobe. Cavitation is common.[230] Pneumonia is usually insidious in onset and accompanied by fatigue, fever, and nonproductive cough.

GRAM-NEGATIVE BACTERIA

Gram-negative bacilli can be divided into three major groups: (1) Enterobacteriaceae, including the *Klebsiella-Enterobacter-Serratia* group, *E. coli, Yersinia pestis,* and the various species of *Morganella, Proteus, Shigella,* and *Salmonella;* (2) non-Enterobacteriaceae that ferment sugars, including species of *Aeromonas, Pasteurella,* and *Vibrio;* and (3) non-Enterobacteriaceae that do not ferment sugars, including *Stenotrophomonas maltophilia* and species of *Acinetobacter, Alcaligenes, Burkholderia, Chryseobacterium,* and *Pseudomonas.*

Klebsiella, Enterobacter, and Serratia Species

The Enterobacteriaceae are a large group of gram-negative rods, often referred to as coliforms, whose natural habitat is the intestinal tract of humans and animals.[159] They are an important cause of nosocomial pneumonia and community-acquired pneumonia in certain groups such as the elderly and patients who have underlying chronic disease.[99] The most important member of the group from a clinical point of view is *K. pneumoniae,* an encapsulated and nonmotile organism that is ubiquitous in the environment, particularly in water; it is also found in the normal human gastrointestinal tract.[231] The bacterium is a common cause of serious infection and has been identified in more than 10% of patients who have bacteremia; up to 25% of these individuals have nosocomial pneumonia.[232] In addition, about 1% to 5% of all cases of community-acquired pneumonia are due to *Klebsiella.*[233] Pneumonia occurs predominantly in men in the sixth decade of life, many of whom are chronic alcoholics.[234] Chronic bronchopulmonary disease and, to a lesser extent, diabetes mellitus and debilitation also appear to predispose to infection.[12]

The genus *Enterobacter* contains motile species but is otherwise similar to *Klebsiella* and can be grouped with the latter in routine laboratory testing. Pathogenic organisms (most often *Enterobacter aerogenes* and sometimes *Enterobacter cloacae*) usually cause nosocomial pneumonia.[235] *S. marcescens* is a common saprophyte of soil, water, and sewage. Most infections are acquired in the hospital by elderly, debilitated patients, the majority of whom have been receiving antibiotic therapy. Outbreaks associated with improperly sterilized bronchoscopes have also been described.[236]

K. pneumoniae usually gains entry to the lung by aspiration of oral secretions, the areas most commonly affected being the posterior portion of an upper lobe and the superior portion of a lower lobe. Homogeneous consolidation resembling that of acute air space pneumonia secondary to *S. pneumoniae* is seen in some cases; a patchy distribution with abscess formation and cavitation may also be seen. Vascular occlusion can result in the formation of large cavities containing fragments of necrotic lung (pulmonary gangrene).[237] Extension of infection to the pleura with resultant empyema is common. *Enterobacter* and *Serratia* species usually cause necrotizing hemorrhagic bronchopneumonia, frequently with abscess formation.[238]

Klebsiella pneumonia is characteristically manifested radiographically as homogeneous parenchymal consolidation containing an air bronchogram. When compared with pneumococcal pneumonia, it has a greater tendency for the formation of voluminous inflammatory exudate leading to lobar expansion with resultant bulging of interlobar fissures (see Fig. 6–3, page 227),[56] a greater tendency for abscess and cavity formation (Fig. 6–17),[239] and a greater frequency of pleural effusion and empyema.[240] Occasionally, the pneumonia undergoes only partial resolution and passes into a chronic phase with cavitation and persistent positive cultures; in this circumstance, the radiographic picture simulates that of tuberculosis.

The onset of acute *Klebsiella* pneumonia is usually abrupt, with prostration, pain on breathing, cyanosis, moderate fever, and severe dyspnea. Expectoration is often greenish, purulent, and blood streaked and, occasionally, brick red and gelatinous ("currant jelly sputum").[12] Malaise, chills, and shortness of breath may be present for some time,[241] but on admission to the hospital, many patients are in shock. Physical signs are generally those of parenchymal consolidation. The white blood cell count is usually moderately elevated; when it is normal or reduced, the prognosis is unfavorable. Bacteremia has been reported to occur in about 25% of cases.[239]

The mortality from *Klebsiella-Enterobacter-Serratia* infection associated with bacteremia is approximately 50%, death usually occurring within 48 hours of onset of the disease.

Escherichia coli

E. coli is an important commensal of the small and large bowel. Pneumonia occurs chiefly in debilitated patients. It is the cause of about 5% to 20% of pneumonias acquired in the hospital or in a nursing home[242] and about 1% to 5% of community-acquired infections severe enough to require admission to the hospital.[243] Most cases are probably acquired by aspiration of contaminated secretions from colonized airways.

The radiographic manifestations are usually those of bronchopneumonia. Involvement is generally multilobar, with a strong lower lobe anatomic bias. Cavitation is uncommon whereas pleural effusion is frequent.[244] Clinically, infection is characterized by the abrupt onset of fever, chills, dyspnea, pleuritic pain, cough, and expectoration of yellow sputum. Gastrointestinal symptoms, including nausea, abdominal pain, dysphagia, diarrhea, and vomiting, may be present. A presumptive diagnosis requires a predominant or pure growth of *E. coli* on sputum culture; occasional colonies are of little significance, particularly in patients receiving antibiotic therapy.

Salmonella Species

Pleuropulmonary infection caused by *Salmonella* species is uncommon. That caused by nontyphoid strains generally occurs in immunosuppressed individuals.[245,246] Pneumonia can occur secondary to aspiration of infected gastrointestinal contents or by seeding during bacteremia. Empyema is most

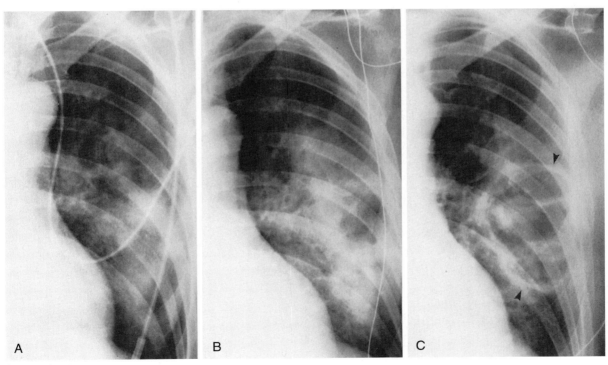

FIGURE 6–17

Acute lung abscess—*Klebsiella pneumoniae*. A view of the left lung from a posteroanterior chest radiograph (**A**) shows a poorly defined area of air space consolidation in the lower lobe. Three days later (**B**), the consolidation is more extensive, and several radiolucencies have appeared, indicative of necrosis and bronchial communication. Five days later (**C**), the cavities have coalesced to form a smoothly contoured, multiloculated abscess (*arrowheads*). The patient was a 45-year-old alcoholic man. *(From Müller NL, Fraser RS, Colman NC, Paré PD: Radiologic Diagnosis of Diseases of the Chest. Philadelphia, WB Saunders, 2001.)*

often secondary to pulmonary disease, but it may also develop by transdiaphragmatic spread from an abdominal focus.[247] Pulmonary manifestations include bronchopneumonia, abscess formation, and ARDS.[248] The course of the disease is usually prolonged, with chills, fever, and pleural pain; cough is often nonproductive, but purulent sputum may be expectorated eventually.

Proteus and Morganella Species

Organisms of the *Proteus* and *Morganella* genera are widely distributed in nature and may be isolated from the feces of healthy humans. The most common organism associated with human infection is *Proteus mirabilis*. Like *E. coli*, *Proteus* is more often implicated in urinary tract and wound infections and only occasionally is the cause of pulmonary disease. Infection usually occurs in a background of chronic respiratory disease, such as bronchiectasis, or in patients who have tracheostomies.[249] The typical radiologic appearance is nonsegmental homogeneous consolidation, predominantly in the posterior portion of the upper lobes or the superior portion of the lower lobes; abscess formation is frequent. Clinically, the onset and course of the pneumonia are more insidious than that seen in other gram-negative pneumonias.

Yersinia pestis

Y. pestis is a small, somewhat pleomorphic nonmotile rod that takes up stains more avidly at its two ends, which gives it a bipolar appearance. It is the cause of plague, a disease that is endemic in many parts of the world.[250] Between 1988 and 2002, a total of 112 human cases were reported from 11 western states in the United States.[250]

Pathogenesis and Pathologic Characteristics. The bacillus is primarily a parasite of wild rodents; however, domestic animals such as dogs and cats can also be infected.[251] In the United States, ground squirrels are the most important reservoir. Transmission of the disease occurs from animal to animal and from animal to humans by fleas or ticks that abandon their host on its death. In endemic areas, sporadic disease (sylvatic plague) occurs in people such as small-animal veterinarians and farmers or trappers who come in contact with rural animals.[252] Occasionally and far more ominously, the disease spreads to urban rats from which epidemics of human infection can result. Though usually acquired from a tick bite or flea bite, disease can also be transmitted to carnivores by the ingestion of infected rodents and (rarely) to humans by inhalation from patients with pneumonic plague or from laboratory exposure.[253] If aerosolized, it is also a potential weapon of bioterrorism.[254,255]

When the flea bites another animal, organisms become mixed with ingested blood and are regurgitated into the wound. In humans, the initial site of infection gives rise within 1 to 5 days to a local skin lesion, usually on the legs. Regional lymph nodes become enlarged and extremely tender, and the overlying skin becomes firm and purplish and forms the characteristic buboes of bubonic plague. The disease may then enter a septicemic phase with involvement of the lungs (secondary pneumonic plague), from which airborne person-to-person transmission of organisms can lead directly to pneumonia (primary pneumonic plague). The latter is pathologically characterized initially by severe bronchitis and bronchiolitis, followed by hemorrhagic bronchopneumonia that rapidly becomes confluent and forms large areas of homogeneous consolidation. Microscopically, necrosis is usually prominent and organisms are abundant. Regional lymph nodes are enlarged and edematous. Secondary plague pneumonia lacks the lobular distribution of the primary disease and affects the lung parenchyma more or less diffusely; however, histologic changes are identical to those of the primary form.

Radiologic Manifestations. The radiographic pattern is one of nonsegmental, homogeneous consolidation, which may be extensive and occasionally simulates diffuse bilateral pulmonary edema; cavitation does not occur. Severe disease may simulate ARDS.[256] Pleural effusion may be present. Occasionally, radiographic manifestations within the thorax are restricted to hilar and paratracheal lymph node enlargement.[257]

Clinical Manifestations. Primary pneumonic plague is fulminating, with high fever, dyspnea, cyanosis, and a rapid downhill course. Coughing and the expectoration of bloody, frothy material may occur, and pleural pain is common. Most patients have mild to moderate leukocytosis. DIC often develops terminally and is manifested by cutaneous petechiae and eventually by massive ecchymoses (the Black Death). The diagnosis should be suspected when there is a combination of confluent pneumonia and enlarged mediastinal lymph nodes on the chest radiograph, enlarged and tender lymph nodes on physical examination, and a history of contact with rodents or cats in an endemic area. It can be confirmed by Gram stain and culture of sputum, blood, or material aspirated from an enlarged lymph node. Antibodies are present during the second week of the illness and may be demonstrated by agglutination or by ELISA.[255] The diagnosis can also be confirmed by PCR.[255]

The death rate of cases reported to the World Health Organization between 1980 and 1994 was approximately 10%.[258] Public health authorities should be promptly notified of any diagnosis.

Pasteurella multocida

Pasteurellae are nonmotile bacilli that have a bipolar appearance on Gram stain. *P. multocida* infects principally animals and is an important cause of disease in domestic animals.[259] Infected patients usually give a history of animal contact, and disease is especially common in farmers.[260] The organism is an uncommon respiratory pathogen, and isolation of *P. multocida* from sputum usually occurs in the presence of chronic lung disease such as bronchiectasis, chronic bronchitis, and/or emphysema.[259] Sometimes, such isolation is simply a reflection of colonization of the abnormal lung; however, occasional cases have been associated with exacerbation of these conditions, presumably by causing acute bronchitis. The organism can also cause acute bronchopneumonia, often associated with empyema and sometimes with abscess formation.[259] The pathologic, radiologic, and clinical features of any of these forms of infection are nonspecific.

Burkholderia pseudomallei

B. pseudomallei is the cause of melioidosis, an endemic glanders-like disease of animals and humans. It is a natural saprophyte that has been cultured from soil, fresh water, rice paddies, and vegetable produce. Disease occurs principally in rodents, cats, and dogs and is endemic throughout Southeast Asia and northern Australia.[261] Human infection occurs predominantly in adult men during the wet season, presumably by contact of damaged skin with infected soil or ground water.[262] In endemic regions, melioidosis is a relatively common cause of community-acquired sepsis, pneumonia, or both. Underlying disease, particularly diabetes mellitus and alcoholism, increases susceptibility.[263] The incubation period of acute infection may be as short as 3 days; however, the disease is more typically latent, with reactivation occurring months to years later, often concomitant with other illnesses or surgical procedures.[261]

Acute melioidosis is characterized pathologically by abscesses that vary in size from microscopic to 3 cm in diameter. Although they can involve virtually any organ, they most frequently affect the lungs, liver, and spleen.[264] Organisms are usually abundant. Chronic disease is manifested as foci of granulomatous inflammation similar to those found in lymphogranuloma venereum; organisms are typically difficult to identify.

Acute disease is characterized radiographically by irregular nodular opacities 3 to 15 mm in diameter that are widely disseminated throughout both lungs or by segmental or lobar areas of consolidation.[265] The consolidation may be multilobar or limited to a single lobe and can be patchy or confluent. The nodules tend to enlarge, coalesce, and cavitate as they progress; though seldom seen at initial evaluation, cavitation eventually develops in 40% to 60% of patients. CT and ultrasound frequently demonstrate abscesses in the liver and spleen.[266] Pleural effusion or empyema is seen at the time of admission or within the first week thereafter in approximately 15% of patients.[265] The chronic form of disease is characterized by nodular opacities, irregular linear opacities, areas of consolidation, and cavitation.[265] It usually involves the upper lobes predominantly or exclusively; in contrast to tuberculosis, however, it tends to spare the lung apex, is seldom associated with superior retraction of the hila, and rarely calcifies.

The clinical spectrum of melioidosis is broad and includes acute fulminant septicemia and subacute and chronic disease; subclinical infection also occurs in many people.[261] The condition has been labeled a "medical time bomb" because of its propensity to recrudesce with a decrease in host defense after a prolonged and asymptomatic carrier state.[261] Disease may be localized or disseminated. The onset of acute melioidosis is usually abrupt but may be preceded by a brief period of malaise, anorexia, and diarrhea. Symptoms can include high fever, chills, cough, expectoration of purulent blood-streaked material, dyspnea, and pleuritic pain, followed rapidly by evidence of bacteremic dissemination, including miliary visceral and osseous abscesses. The clinical picture of chronic melioidosis mimics pulmonary tuberculosis, and patients usually present with fever, productive cough, and weight loss.[267] Pleuritic chest pain and hemoptysis are frequent.

A positive culture is diagnostic. A positive serologic test constitutes evidence for either current or past infection; although the specificity of the finding for active disease declines with age, very high titers are diagnostically useful.[268] Use of ELISA on blood or urine samples enhances the sensitivity and specificity of serologic tests and provides a means for rapid diagnosis.[269,270] PCR has also been used to provide rapid identification of the organism in buffy coat specimens and pus.

Burkholderia cepacia

The major importance of B. cepacia is as a cause of opportunistic infection in patients who have cystic fibrosis (see page 676).[271,272] There is good evidence that the organism is transmitted between patients with this disease and that its presence worsens the prognosis.[273] The organism is also responsible for increased morbidity and mortality in patients who have undergone lung transplantation[274] and has been documented to cause nosocomial pneumonia in immunocompromised individuals via contaminated nebulizing devices.[275]

Pseudomonas aeruginosa

P. aeruginosa is a motile, gram-negative rod that may occur as a single bacterium, in pairs, and (occasionally) in short chains. It is distributed widely in soil, water, plants, and animals and is frequently present in small numbers in the intestine and on the skin of healthy individuals.

P. aeruginosa pneumonia is the most common and most lethal form of nosocomial pulmonary infection.[276] It causes approximately 20% of cases of nosocomial pneumonia in adult patients in the ICU[277] and is the most common cause of nosocomial tracheobronchitis in mechanically ventilated patients.[278] The organism thrives in moist environments such as sinks, water baths, nebulizers, and showers, and many infections are believed to be derived from such sources[159]; outbreaks of infection have also been traced to contaminated respiratory therapy and bronchoscopy equipment.[236,279] A number of risk factors increase the likelihood of development of P. aeruginosa pneumonia in the ICU, including extended ICU care because of the severity of underlying disease, prolonged mechanical ventilation, and previous antimicrobial therapy.[280] The organism is also responsible for about 5% to 10% of cases of community-acquired pneumonia of sufficient severity to warrant admission to the hospital.[281]

Pneumonia usually results from aspiration of the organism from a colonized upper airway. Leakage of subglottic secretions into the lower airways has also been strongly linked to the risk for pneumonia in intubated patients.[282] Colonization of the oropharynx is preceded by increased adherence of the organism to airway epithelium, a process that is also promoted by the organism's pili that extend from its surface[159] and by the increased affinity of the organism for epithelial cells undergoing repair.[283] P. aeruginosa produces a number of potent enzymes and toxic substances that promote local invasion and systemic disease by their inhibition of mucociliary clearance and the pulmonary inflammatory reaction.[31,159,282,284] Lipopolysaccharide derived from the organism's capsule (endotoxin) is particularly important in causing fever, shock, oliguria, leukocytosis, DIC, and ARDS.[159] The pathologic appearance is typically one of acute bronchopneumonia.

Radiologic manifestations are usually those of bronchopneumonia and consist of multifocal bilateral areas of consolidation.[285] These areas may be lobular, subsegmental, or segmental in distribution and patchy or confluent (Fig. 6–18).[285] The consolidation frequently involves all lobes,[285] although it tends to involve the lower ones predominantly.

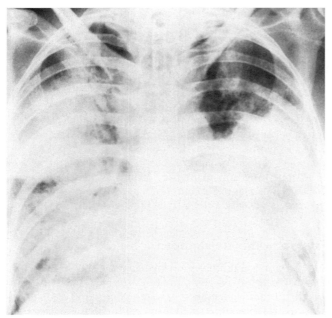

FIGURE 6–18

Acute bronchopneumonia—*Pseudomonas aeruginosa*. This 38-year-old-woman was admitted to the hospital in a deep coma as a result of an overdose of barbiturates. Several days after admission, an anteroposterior radiograph showed massive consolidation of all lobes of both lungs, the superior portion of the left upper lobe being the least involved. An air bronchogram was present in all areas. *(From Müller NL, Fraser RS, Colman NC, Paré PD: Radiologic Diagnosis of Diseases of the Chest. Philadelphia, WB Saunders, 2001.)*

Abscess formation, cavitation, and unilateral or bilateral pleural effusions, usually small, are evident in approximately 20% to 25% of patients.[285] Multiple nodular opacities are seen occasionally, generally in association with bacteremia.[286,287]

An upper respiratory tract infection may precede the pneumonia, whose onset is typically abrupt, with chills, fever, severe dyspnea, and cough productive of copious yellow or green, occasionally blood-streaked sputum. Although empyema is common, pleural pain is infrequent. There are no special features that distinguish this pneumonia from that caused by other bacteria.[276] The white blood cell count is usually normal in the early stage but commonly rises to an average of about 20,000/mm³; however, leukopenia with neutropenia is not uncommon.[287] The diagnosis is generally made by positive culture of sputum or blood. The mortality rate in ventilated patients is very high.

Stenotrophomonas maltophilia

S. maltophilia (*X. maltophilia*, *Pseudomonas maltophilia*) is a gram-negative rod that is widely distributed in the environment. It has become an important nosocomial pathogen in immunocompromised patients who have cancer or organ transplants.[288] It also colonizes the airways of patients with severe cystic fibrosis[289]; as with *B. cepacia*, such colonization may worsen the course of the disease.

Acinetobacter Species

Acinetobacter species are encapsulated, nonmotile coccobacilli that are widely distributed in soil and water.[159] Though usually considered a contaminant or commensal when cultured in clinical specimens, the organism can cause an acute bacteremic pneumonia that is often fatal.[290] Transmission in the ICU is often by hand-to-hand contact.

Bartonella henselae

B. henselae causes cat-scratch disease. Although the abnormality is usually confined to the skin, pneumonia has been reported occasionally.[291] The organism also causes bacillary angiomatosis, a condition characterized by localized vascular proliferation in the skin and mucous membranes (including the tracheobronchial tree) in patients who have AIDS.[292]

Bordetella Species

Bordetella pertussis and *Bordetella parapertussis* are the agents responsible for whooping cough (pertussis).[293] The former is encapsulated and is the most important cause; *B. parapertussis* causes a relatively mild form of disease that is often subclinical. Although it was generally assumed that pertussis had largely been eradicated through immunization, it is now appreciated that immunity may not be long lasting and that the disease is occurring more frequently in adults.[294,295]

The organism produces a number of virulence factors that promote adhesion to the respiratory epithelium, cause damage to ciliated cells, help evade host defense, and produce a variety of systemic effects.[296] Pathologically, disease is characterized by tracheobronchitis and bronchiolitis and is associated with patchy (sometimes extensive) epithelial necrosis. Intraluminal mucus is usually abundant and results in partial or complete airway obstruction and patchy areas of hyperinflation and atelectasis. Organisms can be identified by Gram stain adjacent to epithelial cilia. Bronchopneumonia caused by superimposed bacterial infection may alter the typical pathologic appearance.

Reported radiographic findings consist of atelectasis, segmental consolidation (usually in the lower lobes or middle lobe), and hilar lymph node enlargement.[297] However, some of these abnormalities may be caused by bacterial superinfection.

Acute pertussis is most common in children younger than 2 years, in whom it is frequently prolonged and debilitating. The characteristic clinical picture consists of a paroxysmal cough ending in a "whoop." The diagnosis may be difficult to make in adults since they are less likely to have the full-blown whoop and vomiting and often manifest little more than a short-lived, mild paroxysmal cough. In fact, some investigators have found the infection to be a common cause of prolonged coughing in adults who have no other apparent source of cough on initial evaluation.[298] Coughing spasms are also less severe and the course less prolonged in vaccinated patients.[299]

Acute pertussis causes moderate to severe lymphocytosis. Definitive diagnosis depends on positive culture from nasopharyngeal swabbing, which is most readily accomplished during the initial catarrhal phase of the illness[296] if an epidemiologic link to a known case is made.[294] A direct fluorescent antibody test has been found to be useful in questionable cases; however, culture, serology (especially ELISA), or PCR is required for confirmation.[295,296]

The disease can have serious consequences; more than 500,000 deaths occur yearly, mainly in children in "developing" countries.[296] Saccular bronchiectasis was a relatively common complication in patients before the availability of antibiotics; however, follow-up studies of patients treated with these agents have found this complication to be relatively infrequent.[300]

Francisella tularensis

F. tularensis is a nonmotile, pleomorphic bacillus that is the cause of tularemia.[301] The disease is most common in rodents and small mammals; insects (such as ticks, deer flies, and mosquitoes) act as both reservoirs and vectors. Humans can be infected by several mechanisms, including (1) penetration of the organism into an open sore on the hands while skinning infected animals such as rabbits or muskrats, (2) transmission of the organism from animal to human through the bite of insect vectors or directly from cat scratches or bites, (3) ingestion of contaminated water or meat from infected animals,[302] and (4) inhalation of organisms derived from culture material in the laboratory or from an environmental source.[303] It is this last mechanism that is related to placement of *F. tularensis* on the list of organisms that are potential weapons of bioterrorism. Because of the mechanism of transmission, most cases occur in rural endemic areas; however, a surprising number are detected in cities by astute observers who question the possibility of recent animal contact in parks, zoos, and adjacent wooded suburbs.

Pulmonary disease usually develops as a result of hematogenous dissemination of organisms from other sites; occasionally, it is caused by aspiration of pharyngeal organisms or by inhalation. Pathologically, the lungs have multiple gray-white nodules that show coagulative necrosis associated with a largely mononuclear inflammatory infiltrate.[303] Organisms are typically difficult to identify.

The most common radiographic manifestation consists of air space consolidation, which is patchy in approximately 80% of patients and segmental or nonsegmental in the remainder.[304] Hilar lymph node enlargement occurs in 25% to 50% of cases and pleural effusions at about the same frequency. The former is usually ipsilateral to the areas of consolidation. Cavitation occurs in approximately 15% to 20% of patients who have consolidation.[304]

Exposure to the organism is followed by the development of peripheral cutaneous ulcers, enlarged regional lymph nodes, and/or typhoid-like symptoms. Findings related to pleuropulmonary infection appear within 1 to 14 days of exposure and consist of high fever (usually >40°C), chills, malaise, weakness, and headaches. The throat is frequently affected, with manifestations ranging from simple pharyngitis to ulcerative tonsillitis.[301] Physical findings in the chest are minimal in most patients. Laboratory findings are nonspecific.[301]

The diagnosis is made by positive culture. A rise in agglutination titers taken 2 weeks apart also confirms recent infection. A presumptive diagnosis can be made by finding a single titer of 1:160 or greater or by detecting antigen by fluorescent assay.[301]

Haemophilus influenzae

H. influenzae is a pleomorphic, nonmotile coccobacillus that sometimes occurs in pairs or short chains and is by far the most important species of the genus to cause respiratory tract infection.[305] In adults, the organism is isolated most commonly from patients who have COPD.[306] Other chronic underlying diseases such as alcoholism and diabetes mellitus[305] are also important risk factors. It has been reported to be responsible for about 5% to 40% of community-acquired pneumonias in which an organism is successfully identified.[307-309] *H. influenzae* is also an important cause of nosocomial pneumonia of mild to moderate severity in patients who have no particular risk factors for pneumonia, as well as an important cause of pneumonia of marked severity in recently hospitalized patients in whom no antibiotics have been administered.[243]

Chronic infection by *H. influenzae* may be more common than generally appreciated. For example, in a series of 115 patients who had symptoms of at least 1 month's duration and radiographic abnormalities, the organism was identified by quantitative culture of protected brush samples in 53 (46%)[310]; two thirds of these patients had significant comorbidity, but a third were otherwise healthy. As a pathogen in the lower respiratory tract, *H. influenzae* often causes acute bronchitis only. It is also an occasional cause of life-threatening epiglottitis in adults.[311]

The radiologic manifestations of pulmonary *H. influenzae* infection are variable. In 50% to 60% of patients, the pattern is that of bronchopneumonia with areas of consolidation in a patchy or segmental distribution.[312] The consolidation may be unilateral or bilateral and tends to involve mainly the lower lobes. In 30% to 50% of patients, the pattern is that of acute nonsegmental air space consolidation similar to *S. pneumoniae*; this pattern may be seen alone or in combination with a pattern of bronchopneumonia.[312] A reticular or reticulonodular interstitial pattern, by itself or in combination with air space consolidation, occurs in 15% to 30% of cases. Cavitation has been reported occasionally. Pleural effusion develops in approximately 50% of patients; empyema is uncommon.

Clinical features are not specific. The mortality rate from bacteremic *H. influenzae* pneumonia has been estimated to be as high as 57%, a reflection of the common severity of underlying comorbid disease.[313]

Legionella Species

Legionella organisms are weakly staining, gram-negative coccobacilli that are responsible for legionnaires' disease. *Legionella pneumophila* serogroup 1 accounts for the great majority of cases, a conclusion based partly on lack of testing to detect other species and serogroups.[314] After the recognition of legionnaires' disease in Philadelphia in 1976, many common-source outbreaks[315,316] and sporadic cases[317] have been identified throughout the world. Pneumonia develops in most patients. It is often severe and may be associated with evidence of liver, renal, or central nervous system disturbance[318]; this combination of clinical findings has been referred to as legionnaires' disease. A flulike syndrome unaccompanied by evidence of lower respiratory tract involvement is sometimes seen; this manifestation is commonly referred to as Pontiac fever because it was first recognized in an epidemic in Pontiac, Michigan.[319]

The precise incidence of *L. pneumophila* pneumonia in the United States is uncertain, estimates having ranged from 13,000[320] to 250,000 cases per year.[321] Prospective studies have documented the organism in 2% to 25% of patients hospitalized with pneumonia,[322,323] which makes it one of the more common in this setting; as a consequence, therapy for the organism is mandatory in patients who have severe pneumonia of undetermined cause.[324] The reported incidence of *Legionella* species has varied from 1% to 40% in patients with nosocomial pneumonia; this variation depends partly on the techniques used to diagnose the infection and partly on the presence or absence of an environmental source of infection. Despite its high frequency as a cause of nosocomial infection in some studies, the organism appears to be a distinctly uncommon cause of pneumonia in patients receiving mechanical ventilation.[14] Major risk factors for the development of *Legionella* pneumonia include cigarette smoking, chronic lung disease, and immunosuppression (especially by corticosteroids).[325]

The natural habitat of *Legionella* appears to be biofilms or protozoa within water.[326] Some investigators have shown a peak incidence of disease in the summer and early fall, a finding that might be explained by the organism's preference for warm water.[326] When disease occurs in outbreaks, bacteria are frequently recovered from air-conditioning cooling towers and evaporative condensers,[327] the presumed mechanism of infection being aerosolization of infected water particles. However, the association of nosocomial *Legionella* infection with potable water suggests that aspiration after upper airway colonization may be important in this setting.[328]

Pathogenesis and Pathologic Characteristics. Once organisms gain access to the lungs, they enter the cytoplasm of various cells, predominantly alveolar macrophages, via phagosomes. Such entry may be partly mediated by complement or immunoglobulin receptors on the macrophage surface[329]; however, bacteria-directed cell invasion of epithelial cells is also important.[330] Once inside the cell, it appears that the organism has the ability to prevent fusion of phagosomes with lysosomes, thus preventing effective macrophage killing; the phagosomes subsequently become intimately associated with cell endoplasmic reticulum, after which the bacteria begin replicating. The organisms undergo a variety of morphologic and, probably, functional alterations that favor their ability to invade other cells and perpetuate infection after their release.[330] Once invasion of new cells has occurred, the bacteria resume a "vegetative" form and undergo further intracellular replication.

In addition to being a target cell of the bacterium, the alveolar macrophage is also an important effector cell in host resistance. Resistance to infection in experimental animals is related to macrophage activation and the resulting increased ability to inhibit replication of the organism.[331] T_H1 helper cells are particularly important in this cellular immune response. The role of neutrophils in containing the infection is unclear, and neutropenia does not appear to be associated with an increased risk of pneumonia.[324]

The typical gross appearance is that of bronchopneumonia, which when seen in autopsy specimens, is usually extensive and confluent.[332] Abscess formation is not uncommon.[333] Microscopically, alveolar air spaces are more or less uniformly filled with a mixture of polymorphonuclear leukocytes, red blood cells, macrophages, fibrin, and necrotic debris; leukocytoclasis is typically prominent. Vasculitis and thrombosis of small vessels can be seen. Although the identification of gram-negative coccobacilli in respiratory secretions or tissue may be an important clue to the diagnosis,[334] the organisms are more reliably identified by direct immunofluorescent or immunohistochemical techniques.[335]

Radiologic Manifestations. The characteristic radiographic pattern is one of air space consolidation that is initially peripheral and sublobar, similar to that seen in acute *S. pneumoniae* pneumonia (Fig. 6–19). In many cases, the area of consolidation subsequently enlarges to occupy all or a large portion of a lobe or to involve contiguous lobes on the ipsilateral side.[336,337] Progression of the pneumonia is usually rapid, most of a lobe becoming involved within 3 or 4 days, often despite the institution of appropriate antibiotic therapy; such behavior is seldom seen in acute air space pneumonia caused by *S. pneumoniae*.[336,338] There is a tendency for bilateral involvement as the disease progresses.

In immunocompetent patients, abscess formation with subsequent cavitation is seen in approximately 5% of patients.[339] By contrast, cavitation is noted fairly frequently in immunocompromised patients (Fig. 6–20).[340,341] Pleural effusion may occur, usually at the peak of the illness. Hilar lymph node enlargement is very uncommon. The radiographic pattern associated with infection by various *Legionella* species is similar to that of *L. pneumophila*.[342,343]

Clinical Manifestations. The incubation period for pneumonia has been estimated to range from 2 to 10 days.[344] The usual initial symptoms are fever (sometimes high and unremitting), malaise, myalgia, rigor, confusion, headache, and diarrhea. The most common respiratory complaints are a nonproductive cough without previous upper respiratory tract symptoms and, as the pneumonia progresses, dyspnea.[345] In time, cough may become productive and associated with hemoptysis. Pleural pain develops in about a third of patients.[346] Fever may persist for more than 2 weeks, and the chest radiograph does not usually begin to clear until the end of the second week.[344] *Legionella* pneumonia shows a greater tendency to organize than other bacterial pneumonias do,[347] and patients may be left with permanent sequelae.[348]

Symptoms reflecting the involvement of other organs, notably the gastrointestinal, renal, and central nervous systems, are much more common in legionnaires' disease than in pneumonia caused by other organisms. Patients often complain of watery diarrhea and occasionally of abdominal pain. Many patients become confused and even obtunded; in addition to this encephalopathy, other neuromuscular disturbances include myositis, cerebellar dysfunction, neurogenic bladder, and peripheral neuropathy. Hematuria and proteinuria may be present; renal failure is usually associated with shock. The bilirubin level may be elevated. The white blood cell count is usually below 15,000/mm³ with a shift to the left. Lymphopenia is frequent, the count often being 1000/mm³ or less.[349]

Although some of these symptoms and signs are typical of legionellosis, none reliably distinguishes it from other community-acquired or nosocomial pneumonias.[324,350] However, the constellation of hyponatremia, a high creatine phosphokinase level (as a result of rhabdomyolysis), failure to

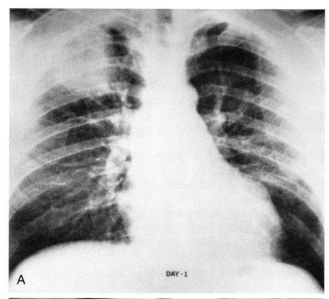

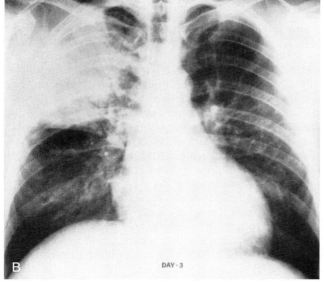

FIGURE 6–19

Acute legionnaires' pneumonia. A posteroanterior radiograph
(**A**) shows homogeneous consolidation of the axillary portion of the
right upper lobe; an air bronchogram is apparent. Radiographs 2 days
later (**B**) show marked worsening. *Legionella pneumophilia* was recovered
from sputum. (*From Müller NL, Fraser RS, Colman NC, Paré PD: Radiologic
Diagnosis of Diseases of the Chest. Philadelphia, WB Saunders, 2001.*)

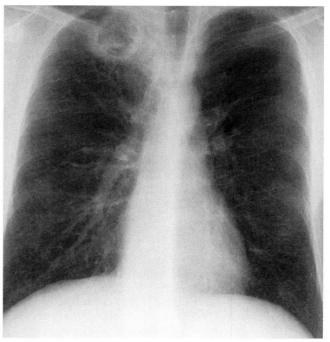

FIGURE 6–20

Abscess formation—*Legionella pneumophila.* A posteroanterior chest
radiograph in a 25-year-old renal transplant patient shows a 3-cm-diameter
cavity in the right lung apex. (*From Müller NL, Fraser RS, Colman NC, Paré
PD: Radiologic Diagnosis of Diseases of the Chest. Philadelphia, WB Saunders,
2001.*)

Legionella pneumonia is a serious disease; many patients
require assisted ventilation, and the mortality rate in early
series varied from 10% to 25%.[5,352] However, mortality has
decreased substantially in the 1990s, perhaps as a result of the
application of guidelines that include effective antibiotics for
the empirical treatment of community-acquired and nosocomial pneumonia.[353,354]

SPIROCHETES

The Treponemataceae are motile, spiral-shaped organisms
that are usually quite thin and are seen to best advantage by
darkfield microscopy, fluorescent antibody techniques, or
silver staining of tissue sections. Two genera—*Leptospira*
and *Treponema*—are associated with pulmonary disease in
humans.

Leptospira interrogans

L. interrogans is an aerobic, very slender spirochete that is
widely distributed in nature, primarily as a saprophyte or parasite of rodents and many domestic animals. Human infection
most often results from contact with contaminated water or
damp soil and is most prevalent in the tropics. The clinical
manifestations of leptospirosis are usually associated with
symptoms and signs of kidney and liver failure (Weil's
disease).[355] Although pulmonary involvement can be demonstrated in 20% to 70% of patients,[356] severe disease is rare.[357]
Patients often have conjunctivitis and muscle tenderness,

respond to a β-lactam antibiotic, and the presence of diarrhea
and headache are features that should suggest the diagnosis.[351]

Confirmation of the diagnosis requires a positive culture,
a positive immunofluorescent test, a positive hemagglutination test for antibody, or the detection of antigen by DNA
probe or radioimmunoassay. Urinary antigen testing has
insufficient sensitivity to guide clinical management because
it can reliably detect only *L. pneumophila* serogroup 1 infections.[314] Similarly, sputum culture is poorly sensitive and
requires special laboratory techniques that are not widely
available. The time required for results to be available also
makes this test of little use in guiding treatment.[314]

features considered by some to be valuable clues to the diagnosis.[358] Other manifestations include headaches, chills, nausea and vomiting, pyuria, hematuria, and hepatomegaly. Respiratory symptoms include cough and (occasionally) hemoptysis; the latter may be severe.[359] ARDS may develop. The diagnosis can be confirmed by culture of organisms from blood and urine and by ELISA.[356]

Treponema pallidum

T. pallidum is a slender spirochete that is responsible for syphilis, a disease of protean clinical manifestations that is usually acquired through sexual contact with an infected person and classically progresses through primary, secondary, and tertiary stages. Pulmonary syphilis occurs in both the congenital and acquired forms of disease. The former (pneumonia alba) occurs as part of a spectrum of syphilitic involvement of multiple organs and is generally associated with stillbirth or early death. Acquired disease is rarely associated with pulmonary involvement and is most often seen in the tertiary stage. It has two major manifestations: fibrogummatous parenchymal disease and pulmonary arteritis. Pleural effusion[360] and subacute pneumonitis with a radiographic pattern of reticulonodular infiltration[360] have also been described in patients with HIV infection and AIDS, respectively.

ANAEROBIC BACTERIA

More than 30 genera and 200 species of anaerobes have been identified in human infection, and in fact, such infection of the lung is usually polymicrobial.[159] Among the most important agents are the gram-negative bacilli *Bacteroides*, *Fusobacterium*, *Porphyromonas*, and *Prevotella*; the gram-positive bacilli *Actinomyces*, *Eubacterium*, and *Clostridium*; the gram-positive cocci *Peptostreptococcus* and *Peptococcus*; and the gram-negative coccus *Veillonella*.[361] Mixed anaerobic-aerobic infections are common, especially in nosocomial infection.[362]

Because of the requirements for special sampling and microbiologic technique, the precise incidence of anaerobic lung infection is uncertain. However, when particular efforts have been made, the organisms have been found in 20% to 35% of patients who have either nosocomial or community-acquired pneumonia.[128] There is a significant male preponderance (3 or 4:1).[363] Many cases are believed to be related to aspiration of contaminated oral secretions. As a result, clinical situations that increase the number of organisms in such secretions (such as gingivitis or periodontitis) and that result in an increased risk of aspiration (such as stroke, dysphagia, seizure disorder, drug abuse, or alcoholism) are risk factors for the disease.[364] Patients who have disease despite good oral hygiene may have an endobronchial lesion that interferes with clearance of organisms previously aspirated in the distal parenchyma.[365]

Lemierre's syndrome is an uncommon form of anaerobic infection in which the primary focus occurs in the pharynx, with secondary septic thrombophlebitis of the internal jugular vein resulting in metastatic infection to bones, joints, lungs, and pleura.[366] The causative agent is a member of either the *Fusobacterium* or *Bacteroides* genus; young adults appear to be particularly susceptible. *Bacteroides fragilis* bacteremia is more commonly associated with abdominal surgery or with gynecologic or obstetric conditions.[367] Early invasion of regional veins is a hallmark of such infections, with consequent thrombophlebitis and, in many cases, pulmonary thromboemboli.[368]

Members of the *Clostridium* genus, usually *Clostridium perfringens*, are sometimes causes of pleuropulmonary infection, either as primary disease or in association with bacteremia after attempted abortion under nonantiseptic conditions.[369] The former usually occurs in patients who have underlying pulmonary or cardiac disease or after pulmonary thromboembolism.[370] Empyema is relatively common; although it often follows thoracentesis, it can occur spontaneously in an otherwise healthy person. Gas formation can result in pyopneumothorax.[370]

Anaerobic bacteria are a particularly common cause of empyema. For example, in one study at three hospitals equipped with anaerobic research laboratories, they were recovered from pleural fluid in 63 (76%) of 83 adult patients who had not received antimicrobial therapy or undergone thoracic surgery.[371] Most of these infections are polymicrobial.

The typical radiographic pattern is that of bronchopneumonia ranging from localized segmental areas of consolidation to patchy bilateral consolidation to extensive confluent multilobar consolidation (Fig. 6–21). The distribution reflects gravitational flow; the posterior segments of the upper lobes or the superior segments of the lower lobes tend to be involved with aspiration in the recumbent position and the basal segments of the lower lobes with aspiration in the erect position.[372] Abscess formation and cavitation are relatively common.[373,374] Empyema may occur with or without apparent parenchymal abnormalities.[373] Occasionally, hilar or mediastinal lymph node enlargement is associated with an abscess, a combination of findings resembling that seen in patients who have pulmonary carcinoma.[375]

The clinical features are variable. In some cases, pneumonia is acute and indistinguishable from that caused by *S. pneumoniae*[374]; in others, it is complicated by abscess formation or empyema and has an insidious onset and protracted course. In the initial stage of infection, cough is frequently nonproductive, and the expectorated material, if any, is seldom putrid. When cavitation occurs—usually 7 to 10 or more days after the onset of pneumonia—expectoration increases and becomes putrid in 40% to 75% of cases.[376] Foul-smelling sputum always indicates the presence of anaerobic organisms; however, in the absence of abscess formation, such putrid expectoration is present in only 5% of patients.[377] Pleural pain occurs in approximately 50% of patients and hemoptysis in 25%.[378] Physical findings are not specific; clubbing is common when the infection is chronic.[379]

In most cases, the leukocyte count is mildly to moderately elevated. Anemia and weight loss may be seen with chronic disease.[362] A definitive diagnosis can be made only with special effort, and the diagnosis is usually presumptive.[380] Culture of expectorated material is of little value in diagnosis since it is invariably contaminated by mouth flora. To be considered conclusively pathogenic, organisms must be isolated from a closed space, such as the pleural or peritoneal cavity, or other sterile source, such as blood.

The prognosis is good with early diagnosis and prompt institution of therapy.[381] Antibiotic therapy markedly decreases the incidence of abscess formation. However, the mortality rate of patients in whom a lung abscess develops is

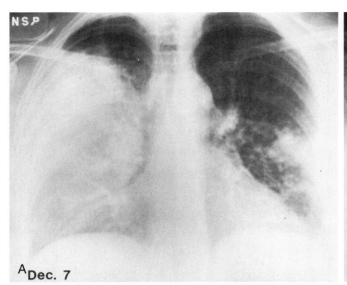

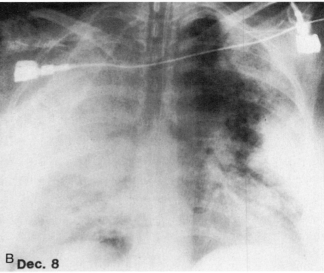

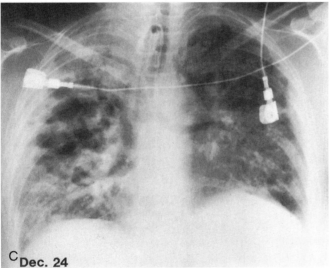

FIGURE 6–21

Anaerobic pneumonia—air space pneumonia with abscess formation. The first examination (**A**) in this 45-year-old alcoholic woman revealed massive homogeneous consolidation of the right lower lobe and patchy consolidation of the left lung. Twenty-four hours later (**B**), pneumonia had extended throughout most of the right lung and much of the left. During the next 2 weeks while receiving antibiotic therapy, most of the pneumonia in the left lung had resolved (**C**); however, a thick-walled cavity had appeared in the right lung. *(From Müller NL, Fraser RS, Colman NC, Paré PD: Radiologic Diagnosis of Diseases of the Chest. Philadelphia, WB Saunders, 2001.)*

about 5% to 10%, with most deaths occurring in those who have serious underlying disease.[382] In patients who respond to therapy, cavity closure occurs steadily but may require a prolonged period to be complete. Long-term follow-up may show a residual cyst, bronchiectasis, or both.[383]

MYCOBACTERIA

Mycobacterium tuberculosis

Epidemiology

Tuberculosis is a disease of great social and economic importance. It has been estimated that a third of the world's population has been infected with tubercle bacilli. Current trends suggest that active disease will develop in almost 12 million individuals in 2006[384] and lead to over 2 million deaths.[385,386]

Tuberculosis has been considered to be a pandemic whose time scale spans centuries.[386] As discussed later, certain social and environmental factors favor the spread of disease once it

involves a susceptible population. The epidemic peaks in approximately 50 to 100 years, then declines over the next several hundred years as natural selection affects the population's intrinsic (genetic) resistance. In populations on the ascending limb of the epidemic, tuberculosis affects predominantly young individuals and is manifested as progressive primary disease. On the descending limb, primary infection is controlled by an effective immune response and disease is much more common in older patients, in whom it has features characteristic of reactivation. (This concept of the disease does not negate the importance of specific programs in nutrition and housing that have been instituted to limit its development and spread.)

In the 19th and early 20th century, declines in tuberculosis morbidity and mortality were seen in many areas of the world, a process that was accelerated by the advent of effective chemotherapy in the 1950s. However, the gutting of tuberculosis control and surveillance mechanisms in many regions, the emergence of HIV infection, and development of drug resistance have been associated with a significant resurgence of the disease on a global scale. Approximately 80% of cases are seen in 22 high-burden countries that have about two thirds of the world's population. In absolute terms, the annual incidence of tuberculosis exceeds 1 million in China and India, 500,000 in Indonesia, and 200,000 in Bangladesh, Pakistan, Nigeria, and the Philippines.[386] In the United States, the number of newly diagnosed patients was about 26,000 in 1992 (10.5 per 100,000 population). After a vigorous public health response, the incidence had declined significantly (43.5%) by 2002.[387]

A discussion of the epidemiologic features of disease caused by *M. tuberculosis* is best considered in two parts, that associated with the development of infection alone and that with the development of clinically evident disease (tuberculosis). (The particular features of tuberculosis associated with HIV infection are discussed on page 425.)

Development of Infection. In most cases, infection is acquired by the inhalation of droplet nuclei carrying the organisms.[388] The risk of infection is related to the degree of contagiousness of the primarily infected individual, the adequacy of antimicrobial defense of the exposed individual, the frequency of contact between the two, and the environment in which the contact takes place. The degree of source contagiousness is itself associated with several variables, including the extent and nature of the tuberculous disease, the frequency of coughing, and the virulence of the infecting organism.[389] The development of cavitary disease is important in contagiousness, both by creating a more favorable local environment for bacterial growth and by forming a relatively easy exit route out of the lung. The extent of pulmonary involvement, whether associated with cavitation or not, is also related to the risk of disease spread—the more extensive the disease, the larger the number of organisms and the more severe the cough.[390] The last of these factors is particularly important as a means of creating bacteria-laden droplet nuclei.[391] As might be expected, smear-positive patients are more contagious than those who are smear negative (as a result of a greater number of organisms in sputum), and the greater the number of organisms in smear-positive specimens, the greater the degree of infectiousness.[392] The organism load is also related to the rate at which sputum becomes culture negative after antituberculous therapy.

Because the organism is transferred from person to person via droplets suspended in air, contact between contagious and noninfected individuals is clearly a risk factor, particularly if it occurs in a poorly ventilated location. In fact, individuals who have had close contact with an infectious person have been shown to be twice as likely to be tuberculin positive as those who have only a casual acquaintance.[393] The increased incidence of infection in people who live in relatively crowded areas, such as prisons, hostels, slums of large metropolitan centers, and refugee camps, is at least partly explained by this observation. Workers in contact with individuals in these environments are also at increased risk.[394] Not surprisingly, transmission of the organism occurs frequently in the home, and infection, sometimes widespread, can develop from a single active case in school or a daycare center.[395] Health care workers constitute another group at increased risk[396]; in some settings, the incidence of purified protein derivative (PPD) conversion appears to be quite high.[397]

The effect of host factors on the acquisition of infection is poorly understood. Heredity appears to play an important role, as indicated by experimental animal studies in which strains have been bred that are either resistant or sensitive to disease.[398] Certain ethnic groups, such as African Americans and native North Americans, have long been noted to have an increased rate of infection and disease in comparison to white individuals.

Although it is likely that these observations are influenced to some extent by socioeconomic or other environmental factors, there is evidence that at least some of the difference is the result of heredity.[399,400] Whatever the pathogenetic basis, it is clear that immigrants to North America and Western Europe from "developing" countries are much more likely to be infected than individuals among the general population in these regions and that they represent an important potential source of future illness.

Development of Disease. Tuberculosis has been estimated to develop in only 10% of individuals infected with *M. tuberculosis*.[384] Although the possibility of development of the disease exists for the lifetime of an infected individual, the risk is highest during the 2 years after initial infection, during which time the incidence has been estimated to be as high as 4% per year.[401] Disease may be associated either with progression of the primary focus of infection (*primary* or *progressive primary tuberculosis*) or with the development of new disease months or years after "healing" of the initial infection has occurred (*postprimary tuberculosis*). The latter is often the result of reactivation of an endogenous focus of infection acquired in earlier life[402]; however, for some settings an exogenous source (i.e., reinfection) is responsible for as many as 50% of cases.[403,404]

Although the precise mechanisms by which infection develops into clinically evident disease are not well understood, a number of risk factors have been identified.[393,405] Clearly, these risk factors are not all independent, and in many cases a combination of several factors is likely to be involved.[406] It is also likely that many factors that are associated with an increased risk for infection also confer an increased risk for disease.

Tuberculosis remains a disease predominantly of the poor and marginalized.[407] High prevalence rates are found among the homeless,[408] in prison populations,[409] and in refugees originating in war zones.[410] HIV coinfection is an important factor in some of these situations.[386] As might be expected, drug or alcohol abuse is also associated with adverse socioeconomic conditions that favor both infection and an increased risk of disease.[406,411] There is also evidence that alcohol can influence the response to infection by its effect on the immune response.[412]

Although tuberculosis can develop at any age, case rates vary markedly in different groups. Rates are generally relatively high in the early years of life, decrease during adolescence, and increase markedly in middle and old age.[413] The reason for the relatively high proportion of cases in the elderly is complex and probably related to several factors, including the higher prevalence of infection 50 to 70 years ago in some populations, decreased immunity, malnutrition, coexistent diseases such as diabetes and malignancy and their therapies, and communal living in nursing homes.[413] There is evidence that the last-named is particularly important; some investigators have found the case rate in this setting to be as high as 14 times that of the general population and 4 times that of non-institutionalized patients of the same age.[414] Compounding the problem is the observation that tuberculosis in the elderly tends to be advanced at the time of diagnosis, more commonly associated with miliary disease, manifested by atypical clinical features, and associated with a poor tolerance of therapy.[415]

The reasons for the increased incidence of tuberculosis in certain ethnic groups is complex and probably multifactorial. Although socioeconomic factors undoubtedly have an important influence,[416] it is likely that genetically related susceptibility is also important.[417] In North America, case rates are highest in African Americans, Native Americans, and recent immigrants from parts of the world with a high prevalence of the disease.[418]

The emigration from "developing" countries to North America and Europe that has occurred in the recent past has had an important influence on the case rate in these regions. Although most affected patients have been in their adopted country for 5 years or less when the disease develops, the potential for onset well after this time period cannot be overlooked[419]; for example, of the 500,000 refugees who immigrated to the United States from Southeast Asia during the 1970s, 60% had a positive PPD reaction.[420] Compounding this problem is the fact that a significant number of immigrants in whom tuberculosis develops are infected by drug-resistant organisms.[421]

A variety of epidemiologic observations also suggest that inherited susceptibility is an important risk factor. For example, the development of tuberculosis has been found to be significantly higher in monozygotic than dizygotic twin pairs,[422] and a number of groups have shown a relationship between HLA phenotype or gene abnormalities and the presence of tuberculosis in selected groups of patients.[423,424]

A number of disorders have been associated with an increased risk for the development of tuberculosis.[425] The increased incidence in patients who have diabetes mellitus is on the order of 2 to 3.5[426]; it is paralleled by an increased incidence of diabetes in those who have tuberculosis.[427] There is also little question that silicosis predisposes to tuberculosis,[428] probably via an effect of the mineral on alveolar macrophage function.[429] The prevalence of the complication in affected workers depends to a large extent on the prevalence of tuberculosis in the population from which they come.[430] A small increase in the risk for tuberculosis has been found in patients who have undergone partial gastrectomy for peptic ulcer disease or jejunoileal bypass for the treatment of obesity.[431,432] Hypothesized mechanisms include malnutrition and decreased immune function. Another well-established condition associated with tuberculosis is chronic renal failure. Although patients who do not require dialysis are at increased risk, a much greater effect is seen in those on hemodialysis, in whom the incidence has been estimated to be 6 to 16 times that expected.[433]

Immunocompromised patients are also clearly at increased risk for mycobacterial disease.[434] By far the most important underlying immunosuppressive condition is HIV infection, which has a major influence on the incidence and course of tuberculosis throughout the world.[435] The presence of the virus increases the likelihood that primary infection will progress to clinically evident disease and that latent disease will undergo reactivation.[436] Compounding these effects is the relatively high incidence of drug-resistant organisms in some areas and an increased risk of disseminated and extrapulmonary disease. Patients who have organ transplants are also at increased risk for tuberculosis, rates of up to 8% to 12%

having been documented in regions in which the local prevalence of tuberculosis is high.[437]

Immunosuppressive therapy is likewise associated with the development of tuberculosis. Corticosteroid administration is a well-established risk factor, and there is evidence that the use of nonsteroidal anti-inflammatory drugs may have the same effect.[438] Patients receiving infliximab for the treatment of chronic inflammatory disorders also have an increased risk of reactivation disease.[439] Although the pathogenesis is probably complex, immunosuppression related to either therapy or underlying disease is likely to be involved in the increased incidence of tuberculosis in patients who have malignant neoplasms.[440]

M. tuberculosis has the capacity to develop resistance to the effects of antituberculous drugs.[441] Such resistance may be primary (i.e., developing in individuals who have not received previous drug therapy) or secondary (acquired as a result of a patient's not following appropriate therapy). Multidrug resistance is defined as resistance to two or more first-line medications (usually isoniazid and rifampin).[421] Historically, it has been a problem associated with "developing" countries, in which the cost and availability of medication and public health care programs have been such that resistance was almost certain to develop in a significant number of patients.[442] However, immigrants from these countries may bring resistant organisms with them to "developed" regions, thereby resulting in an increase in primary resistance in these areas.[386] In fact, although there is a significant variation in the presence of resistant organisms in different age groups, ethnic populations, and hospital centers, in certain regions and population groups in the United States the incidence of drug resistance, particularly to multiple agents, is now alarmingly high.[386,404] The most important risk factor is previous treatment of tuberculosis[386]; many patients also have a history of drug abuse and HIV infection.[443]

Primary Pulmonary Tuberculosis

Patients who become ill immediately after their first exposure to *M. tuberculosis* have traditionally been thought to have pathologic, radiologic, and clinical features that differ from those associated with reactivation of previous disease or reinfection; consequently, it has been customary to consider tuberculosis under the headings of *primary* and *postprimary* disease. It should be remembered, however, that the pathologic and radiologic abnormalities associated with postprimary disease are probably related, at least partly, to hypersensitivity and acquired immunity; because these features generally develop within 1 to 3 weeks of the onset of the initial infection, a "postprimary" form of disease can develop during the primary infection itself if the latter is not checked by the body's defense mechanisms. Moreover, there is evidence from DNA fingerprinting studies that the radiologic features of tuberculosis are similar in patients who have apparently acquired the infection recently and those who have evidence of remote infection (and, by inference, reactivation [postprimary] disease).[444] The descriptions that follow should be considered with these points in mind.

Primary pulmonary tuberculosis has traditionally been thought to occur predominantly in children and to be particularly prevalent in regions in which the annual risk of infection is high. With the reduction in incidence of the disease since the early part of the 20th century in many regions, however, and the resulting increase in the number of nonsensitized individuals, the primary form of disease appears to have become more common in adults than it was previously.[445]

Pathogenesis and Pathologic Characteristics

Two factors appear to be particularly important in the development of tuberculosis: (1) the ability of the organism to survive and multiply within macrophages and to persist for many years in unfavorable conditions in an inactive but viable state within necrotic tissue and superficially normal cells (latency)[446] and (2) the ability of the host to mount an effective cell-mediated immune response.[447] The interplay between these two processes largely determines whether infection is established and, once established, the extent and nature of the ensuing disease.[384,448] The development of such disease, as manifested pathologically by necrosis and eventually fibrosis, appears to be related principally to a delayed hypersensitivity reaction mediated by sensitized T lymphocytes.[449] There is also evidence that cytotoxic T cells are directly involved in the immunologic response.[450] On the other hand, *M. tuberculosis* has evolved a number of properties for evading the host immune response, including its well-developed capsule, virulence factors such as catalase and sulfatides,[451,452] inhibition of recognition of infected cells by immune effector cells, and resistance to the antimicrobial properties of alveolar and tissue macrophages.[448,453]

As discussed previously, primary infection usually develops in humans by inhalation of droplet nuclei laden with bacilli. The organisms are deposited on the surface of transitional airways and alveoli, where they are phagocytosed by alveolar macrophages. Although the latter may destroy some bacilli,[454] many are able to survive, multiply, and eventually kill the macrophage. Blood-borne monocytes are attracted to the region, where they differentiate into macrophages, ingest free bacilli, and interact with T lymphocytes to release a variety of mediators such as interferon-γ and tumor necrosis factor-α, which are involved in both differentiation of macrophages into epithelioid histiocytes and granuloma formation.[455,456] Dendritic cells also contribute to the development of granulomas by means of their antigen-presenting properties and promote both acquired and innate immunity against persisting organisms.[457,458]

After several weeks (coinciding with the development of hypersensitivity), granulomas are well formed, and their central portions undergo necrosis (Fig. 6–22).[459] As the disease progresses, individual necrotic foci tend to enlarge and coalesce, thereby resulting in relatively large foci of necrotic debris surrounded by a layer of epithelioid histiocytes and multinucleated giant cells. These cells in turn are surrounded by layers of mononuclear cells—both lymphocytes and blood-derived monocytes—and fibroblasts. These three zones—epithelioid cells, mononuclear cells, and fibroblasts—serve to isolate the tubercle bacilli within a relatively discrete region of the lung parenchyma and, in most cases, prevent further spread of the disease. At this point, the inflammatory focus may be grossly visible, the central necrotic material being white and somewhat crumbly (similar to goat cheese); this appearance is known as *caseation necrosis* and is characteristic (albeit not diagnostic) of tuberculous necrosis. Although the result of these reactions is clearly beneficial to

the host in that they localize and destroy a substantial number of bacteria, they also possess the major disadvantage of causing tissue destruction.

The initial focus of parenchymal disease is termed the *Ghon focus*. It either enlarges as disease progresses or, much more commonly, undergoes healing. In the latter event, fibroblasts at the periphery of the necrotic foci proliferate and form collagen. Although this process sometimes results in conversion of the entire area into a dense fibrous scar, more often the central necrotic material persists and becomes separated from the surrounding lung parenchyma by a well-developed fibrous capsule (see Color Fig. 6–4). Dystrophic calcification is common in the necrotic material at this stage and is often of sufficient degree to be visible radiographically. Despite the fact that the disease is inactive, viable organisms may remain within the encapsulated necrotic areas and serve as a focus for reactivation in later life.

During the early stage of infection, organisms commonly spread to regional lymph nodes, the combination of the Ghon focus and affected nodes being known as the *Ranke complex*. The course of the disease in lymph nodes is similar to that in parenchyma and initially consists of granulomatous inflammation and necrosis followed by fibrosis and calcification; however, the degree of inflammatory reaction is typically greater in lymph nodes than in the parenchyma, which makes this site of infection more obvious radiographically. Because of their anatomic location, such lymph nodes can be associated with a variety of complications, including enlargement sufficient to compress the adjacent bronchus (resulting in atelectasis) and extranodal extension of the inflammatory reaction (resulting in localized airway mucosal swelling or ulceration).

In addition to lymphatic dissemination to regional lymph nodes, organisms also gain access to the bloodstream (and thus extrapulmonary tissues) via efferent nodal lymphatics or vessels in the vicinity of the Ghon focus. Although such hematogenous dissemination is probably common,[460] clinical manifestations of miliary or localized extrapulmonary tuberculosis in primary disease are usually absent, presumably as a result of the limited number of disseminated organisms and the adequacy of host defense. Nevertheless, this systemic dispersal of organisms is important because the minute areas of infection that it establishes remain as potential foci for subsequent reactivation of disease.

In a small number of patients with primary tuberculosis, local parenchymal disease progresses, either at the site of the initial Ghon focus or elsewhere in the lung (usually the apical or posterior segments of the upper lobes). Such evolution is termed *progressive primary tuberculosis* and is similar in both its morphology and course to postprimary disease (see Color Fig. 6–5).

Radiologic Manifestations

The largest study of the radiologic manifestations of primary tuberculosis in children is based on a review of 252 consecutive cases, for which chest radiographs were available in 191.[461] Air space consolidation was identified in approximately 70% of these cases; it affected the right lung more often than the left, was bilateral in 15% of cases, and showed no significant predilection for any particular lung region. Air space consolidation is also the most common manifestation of disease in

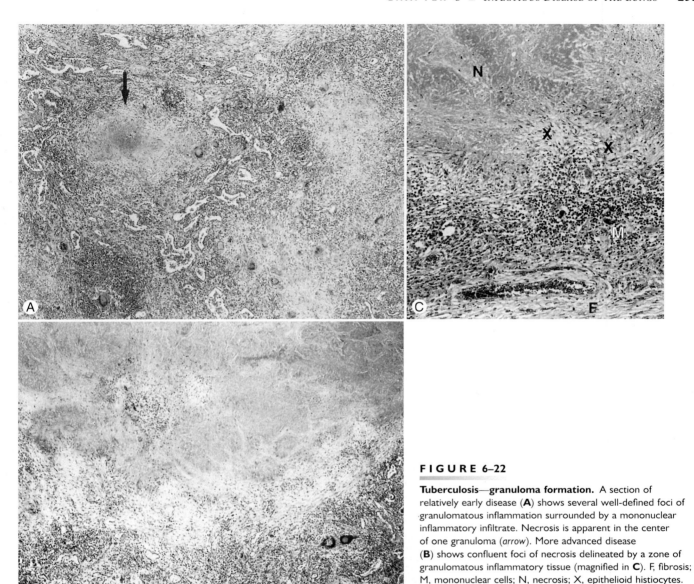

FIGURE 6–22

Tuberculosis—granuloma formation. A section of relatively early disease (**A**) shows several well-defined foci of granulomatous inflammation surrounded by a mononuclear inflammatory infiltrate. Necrosis is apparent in the center of one granuloma (*arrow*). More advanced disease (**B**) shows confluent foci of necrosis delineated by a zone of granulomatous inflammatory tissue (magnified in **C**). F, fibrosis; M, mononuclear cells; N, necrosis; X, epithelioid histiocytes. (*From Fraser RS, Müller NL, Colman NC, Paré PD: Fraser and Paré's Diagnosis of Diseases of the Chest, 4th ed. Philadelphia, WB Saunders, 1999.*)

adults.[462] It is usually homogeneous, dense, and anatomically confined to a segment (Fig. 6–23) or, more commonly, a lobe.[463] In approximately 25% of cases it is multifocal, and in 10% it is bilateral.[461,462] Cavitation or miliary disease (or both) develop in about 2% to 5% of cases.[461,462]

Evidence of lymph node enlargement is identified on the chest radiograph in about 90% to 95% of children who have primary disease.[461,464] Most have hilar involvement, most commonly on the right; approximately 50% have both hilar and mediastinal disease (usually the right paratracheal region).[461] Lymph node enlargement is seen less commonly in adults, being reported in about 10% to 30% of patients.[462,465] As with children, it is most commonly unilateral and hilar or paratracheal (see Fig. 6–23). It may be the only abnormality; in fact, such an appearance should suggest the disease. Although bilateral lymph node enlargement or lymph node enlargement

without parenchymal consolidation does not exclude the diagnosis, this picture is uncommon in adults (with the exception of patients who have AIDS).[462]

On CT scan, approximately 50% of affected nodes have low attenuation (<30 Hounsfield units [HU]), and 50% have soft tissue attenuation (>35 HU).[466] After the intravenous administration of contrast, approximately 60% of affected lymph nodes have relatively low attenuation of the central region and show peripheral (rim) enhancement (Fig. 6–24), 20% show inhomogeneous enhancement, and 20% show homogeneous enhancement or nonenhancement.[466]

Follow-up chest radiographs in children who have had primary tuberculosis have shown evidence of calcification in the pulmonary lesion in about 10% to 15% of cases and in the lymph nodes in about 5% to 35%.[461,464] Although a calcified Ranke complex constitutes reasonable evidence of primary

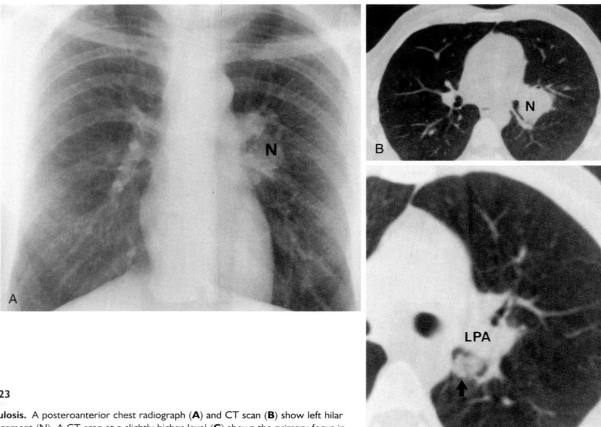

FIGURE 6–23

Primary tuberculosis. A posteroanterior chest radiograph (**A**) and CT scan (**B**) show left hilar lymph node enlargement (N). A CT scan at a slightly higher level (**C**) shows the primary focus in the superior segment of the lower lobe (*arrow*) behind the left pulmonary artery (LPA). The patient was a 25-year-old man. (*From Müller NL, Fraser RS, Colman NC, Paré PD: Radiologic Diagnosis of Diseases of the Chest. Philadelphia, WB Saunders, 2001.*)

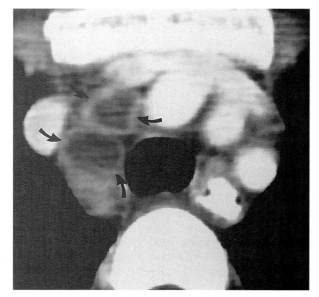

FIGURE 6–24

Primary tuberculosis. A contrast-enhanced CT scan 2 cm above the level of the aortic arch shows enlarged right paratracheal lymph nodes (*curved arrows*) with a low-attenuation center and rim enhancement. (*From Müller NL, Fraser RS, Colman NC, Paré PD: Radiologic Diagnosis of Diseases of the Chest. Philadelphia, WB Saunders, 2001.*)

tuberculosis (Fig. 6–25), the same radiographic finding can occur as a sequela of fungal infection.

Atelectasis, usually lobar and right sided, has been reported in 10% to 30% of children.[461,464] It is usually the result of bronchial compression by enlarged lymph nodes; less commonly, endobronchial disease is responsible.[464] The complication is less common in adults; it tends to involve the anterior segment of an upper lobe and may simulate pulmonary carcinoma.[467]

Pleural effusion has been reported in 5% to 10% of children and 30% to 40% of adults.[461,462,464] It is usually seen in association with parenchymal abnormalities; however, it is the only radiographic manifestation of the disease in about 5% of adult cases.[462]

Clinical Manifestations

The decision to categorize a case of tuberculosis as primary is often based on the observation of young age, recent tuberculin conversion, and radiographic evidence of hilar or mediastinal lymph node enlargement, or pleural effusion.[462,468] As discussed previously, however, the clinical and radiologic distinction between primary and postprimary disease is not always clear-cut.

The majority of patients who have primary infection are asymptomatic. This fact was well illustrated in a study of 715

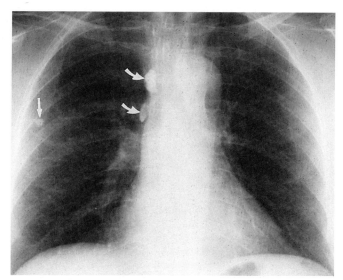

FIGURE 6–25

Calcified Ghon's focus and lymph nodes (Ranke's complex). A posteroanterior chest radiograph shows a calcified right upper lobe nodule (*straight arrow*) and calcified right paratracheal lymph nodes (*curved arrows*). (*From Müller NL, Fraser RS, Colman NC, Paré PD: Radiologic Diagnosis of Diseases of the Chest. Philadelphia, WB Saunders, 2001.*)

children whose tuberculin reaction became positive between birth and 5 years of age[469]; only 136 of the 611 children with adequate follow-up studies showed radiographic changes in the chest. Tuberculosis developed in only 55 (9%); the remaining patients were clinically well. Cough and fever are the most prominent symptoms related to the chest. Weight loss, hemoptysis, sweating, chest pain, erythema nodosum, and lethargy may also be evident.[464] Additional manifestations may develop as a result of spread of disease to extrapulmonary locations, such as the meninges or pericardium.

Postprimary Tuberculosis

Pathogenesis and Pathologic Characteristics. Postprimary tuberculosis tends to be initially localized to the apical and posterior segments of the upper lobes. It has been postulated that such localization is related to the relatively high PO_2 in these zones as a result of a high ventilation-perfusion ratio[470] or to impaired lymphatic drainage from decreased pulmonary arterial blood flow.[471] Whatever the mechanism, it is believed that the majority of cases that arise in these locations are caused by organisms transmitted hematogenously during primary infection.

Pathologically, the sequence of events is similar to that of the primary infection, except that necrosis probably occurs more rapidly because of the presence of hypersensitivity. In addition, in contrast to primary tuberculosis, in which fibrosis and healing are the rule, postprimary disease tends to progress, with foci of inflammation and necrosis enlarging to occupy ever-greater portions of lung parenchyma. During this process, communication with airways is frequent and results in drainage of necrotic material and cavity formation (see Color Fig. 6–6). The formation of cavities depends on liquefaction of caseous material, a process that may be mediated by enzymes derived from inflammatory cells in the vicinity of the

necrotic tissue.[472] The significance of cavity formation lies in the communication with the outside environment that it provides the organisms. This communication has two important effects: first, it leads to a continuous supply of well-oxygenated air to the interior of the cavity, which can theoretically result in increased extracellular bacterial multiplication; second, it provides a means for spread of organisms to other parts of the lung and to other individuals.

As in primary tuberculosis, the course of the disease from this point on depends largely on the interplay between host response and the virulence of the organism. When host factors prevail, there is gradual healing with the formation of localized or extensive, often calcified parenchymal scars, sometimes accompanied by emphysema, bronchiectasis, and/or residual cavities (see Color Fig. 6–7). Such abnormalities can occur alone but are seen most often in association with well-demarcated foci of necrotic parenchyma. The latter vary from 1 mm to several centimeters in diameter and either develop and maintain communication with the tracheobronchial tree (thus forming a chronic cavity) or fail to communicate and are filled with caseous material (forming a "tuberculoma").[473] The development of a fungus ball (usually caused by *Aspergillus* species) within a chronic cavity is a rather frequent complication (see page 282).

When host defense is insufficient, disease progresses, either locally by gradual expansion of the region of necrosis and inflammation or remotely in other parts of the lung or body by spread of bacteria via the airways, lymphatics, or bloodstream. Endobronchial spread of liquefied necrotic material from a cavity may result in tuberculous infection in the same lobe or in other lobes of either lung. Such infection initially occurs in the region of the transitional airways and usually causes a typical granulomatous inflammatory reaction that results in the appearance of multiple parenchymal nodules (see Color Fig. 6–8). In some individuals, the large amounts of tuberculoprotein that suddenly occupy the acini may cause an exudative inflammatory reaction in the absence of a significant granulomatous component; this reaction can be associated with widespread parenchymal necrosis and rapid destruction of whole lobules.

Dissemination of organisms by way of the lymphatics or pulmonary vasculature may result in miliary tuberculosis of the lungs, liver, spleen, bone marrow, and many other organs. In the lungs, the appearance is that of a multitude of nodules measuring 1 to 2 mm in diameter and scattered more or less randomly throughout the parenchyma and on the pleura (see Color Fig. 6–9). The nodules tend to be slightly larger in the apices than in the bases and are usually about the same size and of the same histologic age, which implies a single episode of dissemination. Sometimes, however, both active and partly or completely healed foci may be observed at the same time, thus suggesting repeated or protracted episodes of hematogenous spread.[474] It is important to remember that the lungs may be the site of miliary tuberculosis without evidence of a pulmonary source of the infection, dissemination having occurred from an extrapulmonary location; the frequency of such an event has increased since the advent of antituberculous chemotherapy.[474]

Involvement of the tracheobronchial tree is frequent and may be seen in association with either acute or chronic disease. The former is characterized by typical necrotizing granulomatous inflammation in the airway wall and occurs especially when the infection is rapidly progressive or extensive. In most cases, it develops by spread of organisms within the airway lumen or along peribronchial lymphatic channels from an area of cavitation or localized pneumonia. Although such airway involvement is usually associated with obvious parenchymal disease, bronchial infection occasionally persists as peripheral disease heals, thus providing a potential source of bacteria-laden sputum in the absence of significant radiographic abnormality. Chronic airway disease is manifested principally by bronchiectasis and may develop by two mechanisms: (1) most commonly by destruction and fibrosis of lung parenchyma, which results in retraction and irreversible bronchial dilatation, and (2) by mural fibrosis and bronchostenosis secondary to localized endobronchial infection. Since the vast majority of cases of postprimary tuberculosis affect the apical and posterior segments of an upper lobe, bronchiectasis is usually found in these sites; because of adequate bronchial drainage, symptoms are usually minimal ("bronchiectasis sicca").

Vascular disease is also common in postprimary tuberculosis. Pulmonary arteries and veins in an area of active tuberculous infection may show vasculitis and thrombosis, and an acid-fast stain should be performed on any necrotizing granulomatous pulmonary vasculitis to exclude a tuberculous etiology. Occasionally, a small to medium-sized artery is contiguous with the fibrous capsule of a cavity wall, usually in a tangential fashion, and undergoes localized dilatation (Rasmussen's aneurysm). Subsequent rupture may result in hemoptysis and, occasionally, death.

Radiologic Manifestations. Focal areas of consolidation are seen on the chest radiograph and HRCT scan in approximately 50% to 70% of patients who have postprimary tuberculosis.[475,476] In most cases, the consolidation is limited to one segment or portions of several segments of a lobe, typically the apical and posterior segments of an upper lobe.[477] Occasionally, disease evolves to affect an entire lobe (tuberculous lobar pneumonia) or, after endobronchial spread of disease, several lobes.[465,477] Rarely, disease affects all lobes and leads to respiratory failure.[478]

On radiographs, the areas of consolidation have ill-defined margins and show a tendency to coalesce, often with small satellite foci in the adjacent lung (Fig. 6–26). Frequently, there is an accentuation of the bronchovascular markings leading to the ipsilateral hilum. Associated hilar or mediastinal lymph node enlargement is identified on radiographs in about 5% to 10% of patients.[465,475] Mediastinal lymph node enlargement (defined as a lymph node >10 mm in short-axis diameter) is more commonly seen on HRCT scan[476,479]; as in primary disease, such nodes usually show inhomogeneous enhancement or low-attenuation centers with rim enhancement after intravenous administration of contrast material.[480]

Cavitation is identified on the chest radiograph in 20% to 45% of patients (Fig. 6–27)[475,481] and somewhat more frequently on HRCT scan.[481,482] Most cavities are located in the apical or posterior segments of the upper lobes or the superior segments of the lower lobes.[477] They may be single or multiple and have thin or thick walls. Approximately 20% have an air-fluid level. After adequate therapy, a cavity may disappear or remain evident as an air-filled cystic space with a paperthin wall.

The presence of a single nodule greater than 1 cm in diameter (tuberculoma), with or without adjacent smaller nodules,

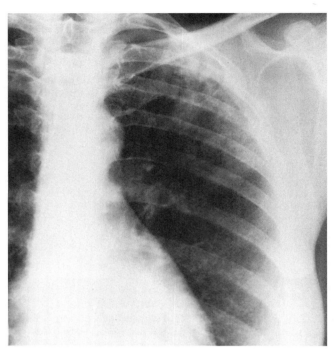

FIGURE 6–26

Postprimary tuberculosis. A view of the upper left hemithorax from a posteroanterior radiograph shows poorly defined focal areas of consolidation and small satellite foci in the upper left lobe. *(From Müller NL, Fraser RS, Colman NC, Paré PD: Radiologic Diagnosis of Diseases of the Chest. Philadelphia, WB Saunders, 2001.)*

has been described as the main or only abnormality seen on the chest radiograph in about 5% of patients.[465,475] The lesion appears as a round or oval opacity situated most commonly in an upper lobe.[483] It usually measures 1 to 4 cm in diameter and is typically smooth and sharply defined; occasionally, it has an indistinct, lobulated, or spiculated margin (Fig. 6–28).[484] Small discrete nodules in the immediate vicinity of the main lesion—*satellite* lesions—can be identified in most cases.[483] Similar to granulomas caused by other infectious organisms, tuberculomas often show little or no enhancement on CT scan after the intravenous administration of contrast material.[485] Most lesions remain stable for a long time, and many calcify. The calcification is usually diffuse but may be central or punctate.[463,486]

Nodular opacities measuring 2 to 10 mm in diameter and localized to one or two regions of the lungs, usually the apical or posterior segments of the upper lobes or the superior segment of the lower lobes, have been described as the main or only radiologic manifestation in about 20% to 25% of patients (Fig. 6–29).[465,475] More commonly, such opacities are seen in association with focal areas of consolidation.[465,476] On HRCT scan, they are centrilobular in distribution and often associated with branching linear opacities (Fig. 6–30), an appearance that has been likened to a tree-in-bud.[479] The abnormalities have been shown to reflect the presence of necrotic material within the lumina of terminal and respiratory bronchioles and an inflammatory exudate in their walls and the adjacent parenchyma.[479,481] More extensive endobronchial spread of disease can be inferred when multiple nodules measuring 2 to 10 mm in diameter are seen in two or

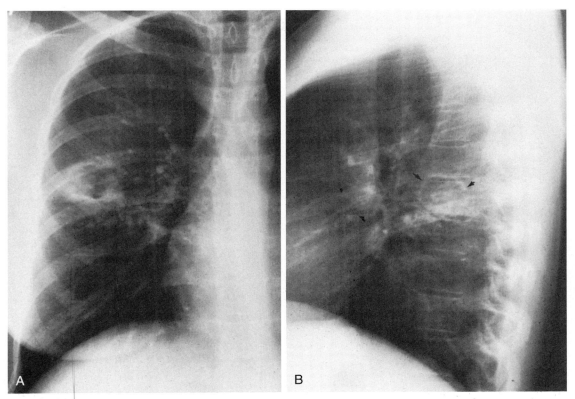

FIGURE 6–27

Cavitary tuberculosis. Posteroanterior (**A**) and lateral (**B**) radiographs show a poorly defined, thin-walled cavity in the superior segment of the right lower lobe (*arrows* in **B**). Both lungs were otherwise normal. *(From Müller NL, Fraser RS, Colman NC, Paré PD: Radiologic Diagnosis of Diseases of the Chest. Philadelphia, WB Saunders, 2001.)*

more lobes or in a lobe other than the one containing a cavity or area of consolidation. Such spread can be seen in 10% to 20% of patients on the chest radiograph and in almost all on HRCT.[465,475,487] Other abnormalities, in decreasing order of frequency, are 4- to 8-mm-diameter nodules with poorly defined margins (also commonly located in a centrilobular distribution), lobular areas of consolidation, and thickening of the interlobular septa.[477,479]

When first visible, miliary tuberculosis is manifested radiographically as innumerable nodules measuring 1 to 2 mm in diameter (Fig. 6–31A); in the absence of adequate therapy, these nodules may grow to 3 to 5 mm in diameter.[71] On HRCT, the nodules are usually sharply defined and measure 1 to 4 mm in diameter (Fig. 6–31B).[488,489] Although some may be seen in relation to vessels, interlobular septa, or pleural surfaces, most have a random distribution in relation to the structures of the secondary pulmonary lobule.[197] Other abnormalities that may be seen include nodular thickening of the interlobular septa and interlobar fissures, nodular irregularity of vessels, and areas of ground-glass attenuation.[42,488-490]

Bronchiectasis is seen on HRCT in many patients, most often those who have healed disease.[487] It is bilateral in approximately 60% of cases and unilateral in the remainder.[482] The upper lobes are most often affected.[482] In most patients, the abnormality is not readily apparent on radiography.

Clinical Manifestations. The most frequent symptoms of postprimary tuberculosis are nonspecific and include the insidious onset of fatigue, weakness, anorexia, weight loss, and a low-grade fever (sometimes associated with rigor).[491] Cough is the most common pulmonary manifestation. Typically, it is associated with sputum production and has persisted since a presumed upper respiratory tract infection.[492] Hemoptysis is usually minor but is of concern because it suggests cavitation or airway ulceration and an increased risk of infectivity. As might be expected, cough is particularly common and troublesome in patients who have tracheobronchial involvement.[493]

In some patients, the initial complaint is pleuritic chest pain, frequently associated with fever. Such pain is most commonly seen in young adults, a majority of whom are believed to have primary disease. Rarely, pleuritic chest pain is related to the presence of pneumothorax. Hoarseness is usually a manifestation of laryngeal involvement; as might be expected, it is typically associated with positive sputum smear and culture and a high degree of contagiousness.[425] Shortness of breath is uncommon and generally indicates extensive disease, most often as a result of tuberculous bronchopneumonia or miliary disease complicated by ARDS.[478] Occasionally, there is an acute onset of high fever, sweating, productive cough, pleuritic pain, and tachycardia that is suggestive of nontuberculous bacterial pneumonia.

Examination of the chest rarely provides information helpful in diagnosis. If an apical lesion is identified on the chest radiograph, post-tussive crackles on auscultation strongly suggest activity. Crackles and rhonchi may be heard over the affected areas in patients who have experienced recent

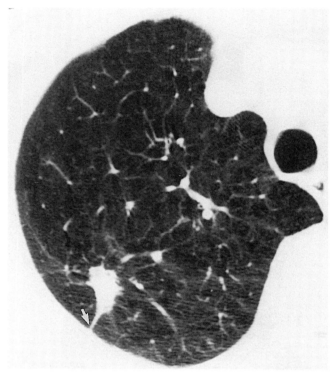

FIGURE 6–28

Tuberuloma. A view of the right upper lobe in a 59-year-old smoker shows a 1.5-cm-diameter nodule with spiculated margins and a pleural tag (*arrow*). Emphysema is also present. The resected nodule was found to be a granuloma from which cultures grew *Mycobacterium tuberculosis*. (*From Müller NL, Fraser RS, Colman NC, Paré PD: Radiologic Diagnosis of Diseases of the Chest. Philadelphia, WB Saunders, 2001.*)

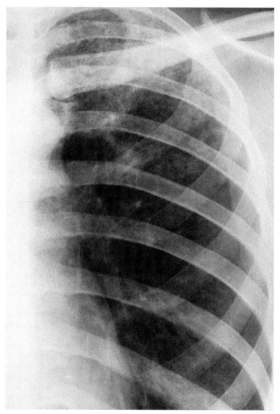

FIGURE 6–29

Tuberculosis—small nodular opacities. A view of the left upper aspect of the chest from a posteroanterior radiograph shows poorly defined, small nodular opacities involving the apicoposterior segment of the left upper lobe. (*From Müller NL, Fraser RS, Colman NC, Paré PD: Radiologic Diagnosis of Diseases of the Chest. Philadelphia, WB Saunders, 2001.*)

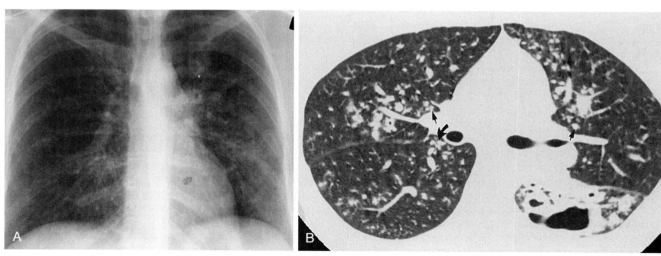

FIGURE 6–30

Tuberculosis—endobronchial spread. A posteroanterior chest radiograph (**A**) shows poorly defined nodular opacities in both lungs. An HRCT scan (**B**) shows a cavity in the superior segment of the left lower lobe and nodular opacities that are 2 to 8 mm in diameter and have a centrilobular distribution (*straight arrows*). A few branching linear opacities, combined with the centrilobular nodules, give an appearance that has been likened to a *tree-in-bud* (*curved arrow*). (*From Müller NL, Fraser RS, Colman NC, Paré PD: Radiologic Diagnosis of Diseases of the Chest. Philadelphia, WB Saunders, 2001.*)

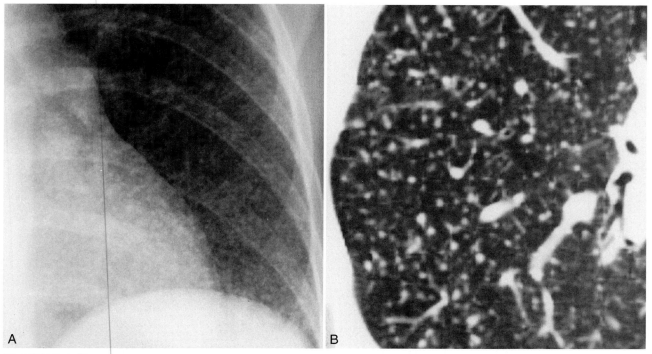

FIGURE 6–31

Miliary tuberculosis. A view of the left lung from an anteroposterior chest radiograph (**A**) shows numerous sharply defined nodules 1 to 3 mm in diameter. An HRCT scan from another patient (**B**) shows multiple nodules measuring approximately 2 mm in diameter in random distribution throughout the lung. *(From Müller NL, Fraser RS, Colman NC, Paré PD: Radiologic Diagnosis of Diseases of the Chest. Philadelphia, WB Saunders, 2001.)*

bronchial dissemination. A localized wheeze should suggest the possibility of bronchial wall involvement. When onset of the disease is characterized by pain on respiration, a friction rub or signs of pleural effusion or pneumothorax may be heard. Sometimes, physical findings suggest compression of mediastinal structures by enlarged lymph nodes.

In North America, miliary tuberculosis usually occurs in elderly patients who have a concomitant chronic disease such as alcoholism, diabetes mellitus, renal failure, or hematologic or solid malignancies.[494] In younger individuals, HIV infection is an important risk factor. The onset of miliary disease is usually insidious; most patients have had nonspecific symptoms such as fever, weight loss, weakness, anorexia, and night sweats for more than 8 weeks.[495] Headache and abdominal pain should suggest involvement of the meninges and peritoneum. Funduscopic examination reveals choroidal tubercles in 30% to 60% of patients.[496] Hepatomegaly, with or without splenomegaly, is not uncommon.[494] Although miliary disease can occur in association with other types of pulmonary tuberculosis, in the majority of patients it is the sole manifestation of the disease. When considering the diagnosis, it is important to remember that 10% to 30% of patients do not have nodules on standard radiographs, even in retrospect.[71] In addition, tuberculin testing with 5 tuberculin units (TU) is negative in at least 25% to 50% of patients.[494]

As discussed previously, hematogenous dissemination is a frequent complication of primary tuberculosis; although clinical evidence of involvement of extrapulmonary tissues and organs is rare during the initial infection, symptoms and signs may develop subsequently, sometimes many years after the initial seeding. Such reactivation can occur in any tissue or organ in the body, but most often involves the kidneys, adrenal glands, fallopian tubes, epididymis, and bones (particularly the thoracic spine). In up to 75% of cases, the chest radiograph shows an abnormality compatible with remote tuberculosis. Before the onset of the AIDS epidemic, approximately 15% of cases of tuberculosis involved extrapulmonary sites in the absence of pulmonary disease.[497] Because the risk for extrapulmonary disease is much greater in patients who have AIDS,[498] the incidence of this form of infection is increasing. In fact, patients who have extrapulmonary tuberculosis in the United States are often elderly or black or have AIDS; they commonly have fever of unknown origin, and many have miliary disease.

Although involvement of extramediastinal lymph nodes is much less common than involvement of hilar and mediastinal nodes, it is still the most frequent form of extrapulmonary tuberculosis in the non-AIDS population, in whom it accounts for approximately 20% to 25% of cases.[499] It appears to be more common in children and young adult immigrants from "developing" countries.[499] Patients usually have painless swelling in the neck or supraclavicular region. Though most often localized to one side, involvement of both sides of the neck or other lymph node groups is not uncommon.[500] Progression of disease may be followed by extension into the skin with the formation of a sinus tract. Rapid lymph node enlargement may occur; sometimes, such enlargement is seen during therapy, in which case it has been speculated to represent an immunologic reaction.[501] Chest radiographs often show no evidence of current or previous tuberculosis.[502]

The next most frequent site of extrapulmonary tuberculosis in adults is the genitourinary system. The discovery of pyuria, hematuria, and albuminuria in a patient who has had pulmonary tuberculosis or who shows radiographic evidence of a healed pulmonary lesion should suggest renal involvement.[503] Tuberculosis of the female genital system usually occurs as salpingitis and oophoritis and is manifested clinically as pelvic pain and menstrual disturbance. It should be noted, however, that menstrual disorders are frequent in pulmonary tuberculosis without genital involvement, and their presence does not necessarily mean extension of the disease.

Involvement of the bones and joints occurs in about 10% of cases of non–AIDS-related extrapulmonary tuberculosis, most often in elderly patients.[497] Tuberculosis of the spine

(Pott's disease) is the most common form of skeletal disease and usually affects the lower thoracic or upper lumbar vertebrae.[504] Early radiographic manifestations consist of irregularity of the vertebral end plates, decreased height of the intervertebral disk space, and sclerosis of the adjacent bone. With progression of disease, there is a tendency to anterior wedging of the vertebral body and the subsequent development of kyphosis and paravertebral abscesses (the latter associated with displacement of the paraspinal interface[505]) (Fig. 6–32). CT is superior to radiography in assessing the presence of paraspinal abscesses and involvement of the spinal canal.[506,507]

Tuberculous meningitis is seen most often in children who have progressive primary or miliary disease and in patients

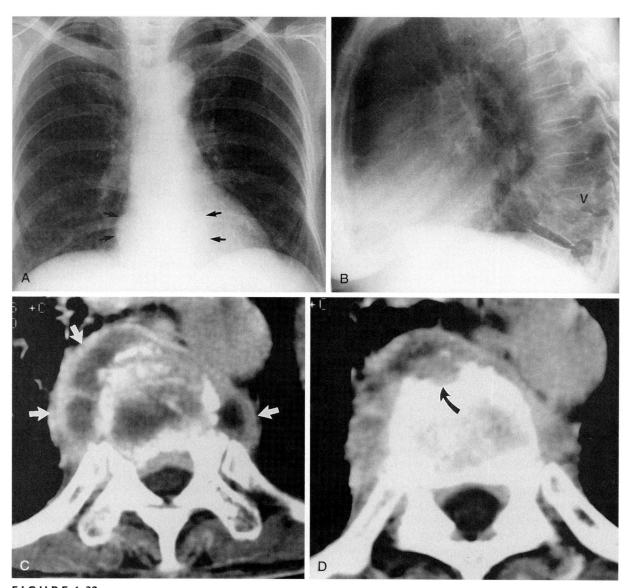

FIGURE 6–32

Tuberculous spondylitis. A posteroanterior chest radiograph (**A**) shows miliary nodules in the lung and displacement of the paraspinal interfaces (*arrows*). A lateral radiograph (**B**) shows destruction of the T10 vertebral body (V) leading to localized kyphosis. Contrast-enhanced CT scans (**C** and **D**) show destruction of the T10 vertebral body, paraspinal abscess formation with low-attenuation centers and rim enhancement (*straight arrows*), and cortical erosion of the adjacent T9 vertebral body (*curved arrow*). (*From Müller NL, Fraser RS, Colman NC, Paré PD: Radiologic Diagnosis of Diseases of the Chest. Philadelphia, WB Saunders, 2001.*)

who have AIDS.[508] Symptoms include headache, somnolence, irritability, vomiting, and (sometimes) neck stiffness. The diagnosis is best made by culture of the tubercle bacillus from cerebrospinal fluid, which has been reported to be positive in about 50% to 80% of cases.[509]

The most common cardiac complication of tuberculosis is pericarditis. In areas of the world with a high background prevalence, it is relatively frequent.[510] It can be manifested as an accumulation of fluid with relatively little pericardial thickening and can lead to tamponade; alternatively (usually in long-standing disease), there is marked pericardial fibrosis, often with dystrophic calcification, accompanied by clinical manifestations of constrictive pericarditis.

Involvement of the upper respiratory and gastrointestinal tracts used to be fairly common in patients who had advanced pulmonary disease, but such involvement has now largely been eradicated by chemotherapy. Nevertheless, tuberculous laryngitis continues to be reported.[511] The gastrointestinal tract is usually affected in the ileocecal area or the rectum, the latter being associated with perianal or ischiorectal abscesses; peritonitis occurs occasionally. Biopsy of the liver reveals granulomas in about 25% of patients who have tuberculosis, usually in association with miliary disease; however, this finding is seldom associated with clinical or biochemical evidence of hepatic dysfunction.[512]

Laboratory Findings and Diagnosis

Techniques for the diagnosis of tuberculosis are numerous and possess varying degrees of complexity and expense, as well as sensitivity and specificity. With the use of modern techniques it has been suggested that identification of M. tuberculosis and reporting of drug sensibility data should be possible in at least 10 to 14 days and 15 to 30 days, respectively[513]; as molecular biologic techniques become more standardized and available, these times may be significantly shortened.

Tuberculin Skin Test

Numerous investigators have studied the indications for and limitations of the tuberculin skin test in the diagnosis of tuberculosis; summary reviews of their results and guidelines for use and interpretation of the test have been reported by groups such as the American Thoracic Society and the Centers for Disease Control and Prevention.[514,515]

The material used is a protein precipitate derived from filtrates of heat-killed cultures of bacilli grown in a synthetic medium.[516] Intermediate-strength PPD (5 TU) is the form that is used for diagnostic testing and should be administered by the Mantoux method. The latter is carried out by injecting 0.1 mL of the solution intradermally in the forearm (usually the volar aspect) through a 26- or 27-gauge, short-beveled needle with the needle bevel pointing upward. A discrete 5- to 10-mm-diameter wheal is produced with proper injection. In the case of improper injection, a second test dose can be administered immediately at a site several centimeters away from the first. The test should be read on the second or third day after injection,[517] the diameter of induration being measured at a right angle to the line of injection (i.e., transversely to the long axis of the forearm) and recorded in millimeters. Interpretation of a test as positive depends on the degree of induration as well as a number of clinical variables, such as the likelihood of previous contact with M. tuberculosis and the presence of diseases or situations associated with an increased risk of tuberculosis. Thus, depending on the circumstance, a positive reaction may be considered to be as small as 5 mm or as large as 15 mm (Table 6–1). Within this framework, the size of the reaction has no particular diagnostic significance.[518]

It is important to remember that a positive skin test does not necessarily signify active disease. Once a patient has been infected by M. tuberculosis and hypersensitivity has developed, the reaction is generally positive, although it may decrease

TABLE 6–1. Criteria for Tuberculin Positivity by Risk Group

Reaction ≥5 mm of Induration	Reaction ≥10 mm of Induration	Reaction ≥15 mm of Induration
HIV-positive persons	Recent immigrants (i.e., within the last 5 yr) from high-prevalence countries	Persons with no risk factors for tuberculosis (TB)
Recent contacts of TB case patients	Injection drug users	
Fibrotic changes on chest radiograph consistent with previous TB	Residents and employees* of the following high-risk congregate settings: prisons and jails, nursing homes and other long-term facilities for the elderly, hospitals and other health care facilities, residential facilities for patients with AIDS, and homeless shelters	
Patients with organ transplants and other immunosuppressed patients (receiving the equivalent of ≥15 mg/day of prednisone for 1 mo or more)†	Mycobacteriology laboratory personnel Persons with the following clinical conditions that place them at high risk: silicosis, diabetes mellitus, chronic renal failure, some hematologic disorders (e.g., leukemias and lymphomas), other specific malignancies (e.g., carcinoma of the head or neck and lung), weight loss of ≥10% of ideal body weight, gastrectomy, and jejunoileal bypass Children younger than 4 yr or infants, children, and adolescents exposed to adults at high risk	

*For persons who are otherwise at low risk and are tested at the start of employment, a reaction of 15-mm induration or greater is considered positive.
†The risk of TB in patients treated with corticosteroids increases with higher dose and longer duration.
Adapted from Centers for Disease Control and Prevention. Screening for tuberculosis and tuberculosis infection in high-risk populations: Recommendations of the Advisory Council for the Elimination of Tuberculosis. MMWR Recomm Rep 44(RR-11):19-34, 1995; from Al Zahrani K, Al Jahdali H, Menzies D: Does size matter? Utility of size of tuberculin reactions for the diagnosis of mycobacterial disease. Am J Respir Crit Care Med 162:1419-1422, 2000.

with time. Thus, interpretation of a test result with respect to disease activity must always be made in the light of clinical and radiologic findings.

A false-positive PPD test result may represent cross-reaction as a result of infection with nontuberculous mycobacteria or a response to previous vaccination with bacille Calmette-Guérin (BCG). Although a large reaction to PPD can develop in some patients who have been vaccinated with BCG,[519] it has been recommended that such a reaction be considered an indication of infection by M. tuberculosis, particularly in an individual from an area in which the prevalence is high or who has an increased risk because of concomitant disease.[520]

A false-negative reaction may be related to errors in performance and interpretation of the test or to a deficient cell-mediated immunologic response.[521] A variety of conditions are responsible for the latter, including acute infections (particularly viral infections such as measles, but also many bacterial disorders), sarcoidosis, chronic renal failure, malignancy, HIV infection, and immunosuppressive therapy.[522] The reaction to tuberculin also tends to decrease with increasing age.[523] A number of patients who have tuberculosis are totally anergic; selective anergy to PPD also appears to occur in some patients.[524] Overall, a negative reaction to 5 TU occurs in as many as 10% to 20% of patients who have relatively mild tuberculous infection and a positive sputum culture.[525]

In contrast to the loss of sensitivity to tuberculin that may occur with aging, treatment, or disease, some patients show an enhanced reaction with repeated testing. This "booster phenomenon" can be defined as an increase in tuberculin reaction size of at least 6 mm on repeated testing in the absence of new mycobacterial infection or BCG vaccination.[520] The reaction is believed to occur in patients who have had remote tuberculous or nontuberculous mycobacterial infection or BCG vaccination; the immune stimulus engendered in such patients by the administered tuberculoprotein results in an increased reaction on subsequent testing.[519] As a result of these observations, it has been recommended that a second skin test be given 1 week after the first in patients in whom repeated monitoring of skin testing is anticipated, such as health care workers. If the second test is positive (booster effect), the patient should be considered to have had mycobacterial infection and be managed according to the results of other clinical, radiologic, and laboratory findings; if it is again negative, a positive reaction to a third test within the next few years probably represents new infection. When a test becomes positive after a previously negative result, the greater the magnitude of induration, the greater the likelihood that the result represents conversion (i.e., recent infection) rather than a booster phenomenon.[520]

Bacteriologic Investigation

Material for bacteriologic diagnosis can come from a variety of sources, including spontaneously produced and induced sputum; bronchial lavage, pleural, peritoneal, or cerebrospinal fluid; and tissue specimens. Sputum is generally the easiest to obtain and the most valuable source of organisms in the setting of pulmonary disease. In patients who do not expectorate spontaneously, inhalation of a warmed solution of hypertonic saline (3%) administered by ultrasonic nebulizer induces the production of material sufficient for analysis in almost all patients.[526] Specimens of sputum obtained immediately after bronchoscopy are also valuable because of the deep coughing that often ensues after the procedure. A pooled specimen collected over a period of 12 to 48 hours may be helpful when other methods are not effective or appropriate.[527]

When a diagnosis of pulmonary tuberculosis is suspected and sputum is not available or is nondiagnostic, bronchoscopy may be indicated. The technique can be highly productive for both smear and culture diagnosis,[528] usually from brushings or lavage and sometimes from biopsy specimens[529]; overall, the diagnostic yield in patients whose sputum specimens are smear negative is about 75% on culture.[526]

Depending on the clinical situation, other fluid specimens are more likely to be diagnostic. Urine specimens are best obtained in the morning after rising, preferably during midstream; multiple samples are advised.[515] Pleural, pericardial, cerebrospinal, and peritoneal fluid should undergo biochemical and cytologic analysis in addition to smear and culture. The frequency of positive culture results from these fluids is variable: in pleural fluid, it is approximately 15%[530]; in cerebrospinal fluid, 50% to 80%[509]; and in pericardial fluid, 20% to 30%.[510]

Biopsy specimens from patients with suspected tuberculosis should be submitted for both pathologic and bacteriologic study. The latter is necessary both for assessing antibiotic sensitivity and for diagnosis; although identification of necrotizing granulomatous inflammation strongly supports a diagnosis of tuberculosis, fungal and some nonmycobacterial bacterial infections, as well as reactions to some foreign materials and drugs, can have a similar histologic appearance. Nonetheless, the finding of granulomas in a pleural biopsy specimen almost always indicates tuberculosis; a positive culture of such tissue is found in about 55% to 80% of cases of tuberculous effusion.[531] The likelihood that tuberculosis is the cause of a granulomatous reaction is less for liver biopsy specimens because many other diseases give rise to hepatic granulomas. Transbronchial, liver, and bone marrow biopsy specimens frequently show granulomatous inflammation in miliary tuberculosis, reported rates being about 45% to 75%,[532] 75% to 100%,[533] and 35% to 100%,[533] respectively. The use of more sensitive techniques for the detection of mycobacteria, such as PCR, may increase the likelihood of a definite diagnosis.[534] Although the diagnostic yield of transbronchial biopsy is probably highest in cases of miliary tuberculosis, there is evidence that it is also useful in patients who have other forms of the disease, particularly those who reside in areas with a high background prevalence.[535,536] When endobronchial abnormalities are apparent bronchoscopically, bronchial biopsy specimens are often diagnostic.[537]

Many techniques have been used to identify and characterize mycobacteria in clinical specimens and to determine which particular species is present. The techniques vary considerably in sensitivity and specificity, as well as availability and cost. Although routine culture remains the gold standard, the time involved for its completion (6 to 8 weeks in many cases) is an important limitation. In addition, sputum, body fluid, or tissue samples containing the organism are not always easily available for culture or other analysis. As a result, several techniques have been investigated in an attempt to identify the organism more rapidly in infected specimens and to confirm its presence elsewhere by indirect means, such as serology.

Material from a variety of specimens can be smeared on a glass slide and examined after Ziehl-Neelsen (acid-fast) staining or fluorochrome techniques[538]; because of shorter processing time and greater sensitivity, the latter is preferred by many laboratories.[539] A smear showing the organisms is virtually diagnostic of tuberculosis in a patient who has clinical and radiographic findings suggestive of the disease. However, the number of organisms required for a smear to be assessed as positive is substantial, and overall, only 50% to 80% of patients who have pulmonary tuberculosis have positive smears.[515] Identification of organisms on smears during the course of therapy may represent the presence of nonviable bacilli or contamination by nontuberculous mycobacteria[540]; however, the possibility of noncompliance or drug-resistant organisms should be considered.

Culture is much more sensitive than microscopic examination of smears for establishing a diagnosis of tuberculosis and is the only widely available test that can establish the sensitivity of the organism to antibiotics. False-positive culture results are uncommon and generally due to cross-contamination of laboratory specimens.[541] A more important technical limitation is time: culture on standard media may take up to 6 to 8 weeks to provide a result. One of the most widely used methods to reduce this time is radiometry. In this technique, a concentrated specimen is inoculated into a liquid culture medium to which ^{14}C-labeled palmitic acid has been added. Mycobacteria metabolize this substance and produce $^{14}CO_2$, which can be detected in a BACTEC instrument and quantified as a growth index. After this procedure, the organism can be detected in as few as 7 to 8 days in smear-positive patients and 16 to 20 days in those who are smear negative.[542] By using the BACTEC method as a base, M. tuberculosis can be distinguished from other mycobacterial species by either biochemical[543] or nucleic acid probe[544] techniques. In addition to its rapidity, the BACTEC method results in an increased sensitivity of mycobacterial detection (approximately 70% to 95% versus 60% to 80% for routine culture),[545] an attribute that is particularly valuable in smear-negative patients.

As in other infectious diseases, the use of serology to diagnose tuberculosis has been extensively investigated.[546] Performance of the tests varies with the antigen used and the specific diagnostic cutoff level; sensitivities and specificities in several studies have ranged from 70% to 80% and 90% to 98%, respectively.[547] The routine use of serology in the diagnosis of tuberculosis is somewhat limited by these findings, and the procedure probably has its greatest value in specific situations such as extrapulmonary disease.[548] As might be expected, the value of the test is limited in patients who are immunosuppressed.[549]

A whole-blood interferon-γ release assay that assesses cell-mediated immunity to tuberculin has also been used. Responses are unaffected by BCG vaccination[456,550] and can provide a tool for screening in populations at increased risk for tuberculosis, such as immigrants from high-prevalence areas and contacts of active cases.

Techniques such as DNA hybridization, restriction fragment length analysis, and PCR offer great promise for more rapid and reliable identification and characterization of mycobacteria.[551] By amplifying the DNA present in clinical specimens, PCR can greatly increase the likelihood of detecting organisms[539,552] and has allowed some investigators to identify them in almost all smear-positive patients and in more than half of those who are culture negative.[456,539] In addition, because the DNA probe used can be specific for particular mycobacteria, a negative test is useful for rapidly

determining that acid-fast organisms identified on a smear are or are not M. tuberculosis. Despite these advantages, PCR has significant limitations. It is relatively costly and is of limited value in distinguishing between active and recently treated or remote disease.[553,554] Moreover, false-positive results have been estimated by some investigators to occur in as many as 5% of specimens.[456] Finally, the sensitivity of PCR is lower in smear-negative cases than in smear-positive ones. Its use in this setting should thus be confined to patients in whom the clinical suspicion for tuberculosis is high.[539,553]

Restriction fragment length polymorphism (RFLP) analysis (genetic fingerprinting) has become a particularly useful technique in the epidemiologic investigation of tuberculosis.[555] The procedure is based on the use of specific DNA insertion sequences (the most extensively investigated being IS6110) that occur in a variable number of copies and in different positions in different mycobacterial strains. By detecting different sequence patterns in clinical isolates, reliable information can be acquired concerning the origin of local outbreaks of disease.[556] Similar information can also be obtained by spoligotyping,[557] a procedure in which spacer sequences within the M. tuberculosis genome are amplified by a PCR technique and then identified by using synthetic oligomeric DNA sequences. Although this technique has less discriminatory power than RFLP does, it has the advantage of not requiring culture of the organism.

Cytology

Cytologic examination of specimens obtained by transthoracic needle aspiration can be useful in diagnosis.[558] However, false-positive results can occur based solely on cytologic abnormalities, and definitive diagnosis is dependent on culture of the organisms or identification of them within tissue fragments.[559] When interpreting the results of transthoracic needle aspiration, it must be remembered that one of the most frequent causes of false-positive diagnosis of malignancy in these specimens is tuberculosis.[560] Fine-needle aspiration has also been used effectively in the diagnosis of extrapulmonary tuberculosis.[561]

Hematologic and Biochemical Investigation

The white blood cell count in pulmonary tuberculosis is usually within normal limits but may be increased to 10,000 to 15,000/mm^3. Anemia is common in chronic pulmonary or miliary disease, possibly related to lymphokine-induced blunting of the erythropoietin response.[562] A leukemoid reaction, lymphopenia,[563] and pancytopenia have also been described in miliary disease.[564]

Hypercalcemia is likewise frequent, the incidence varying from about 5% to 50% in different reviews.[565] The likelihood of hypercalcemia probably depends on several factors, including sun exposure, vitamin D intake, and the form of tuberculous disease.[566] It may be associated with hypokalemia, presumably as the result of distal tubular damage caused by an excess of calcium permitting increased renal excretion of potassium.[567] Hyponatremia develops in some cases of pulmonary tuberculosis[568] but is more common in tuberculous meningitis[496]; it probably represents the effect of inappropriate antidiuretic hormone secretion. In a study of 50 patients who had advanced pulmonary tuberculosis, 92% were found to have evidence of sick euthyroid syndrome and 73% of males to have hypogonadotropic hypogonadism.[569] Evidence of hypoadrenalism has been found in 0% to 55% of patients in various studies.[569]

Pulmonary Function Tests

In the absence of chronic bronchitis and emphysema, most patients who have pulmonary tuberculosis show little impairment in respiratory function, even in the presence of advanced disease. Because the disease interferes equally with ventilation and perfusion, $\dot{V}/\dot{Q}$ abnormalities do not develop.[570] An exception to this general rule is miliary tuberculosis, in which pulmonary function tests not uncommonly show a restrictive pattern and a reduction in diffusing capacity; despite treatment and restoration of the chest radiograph to normal, diffusing capacity may remain considerably below predicted normal values.[571]

Prognosis and Natural History

In "developed" countries in the pre-AIDS era, patients who died with active tuberculosis were often elderly and chronically ill from associated disease; they were equally likely to succumb from the tuberculosis (often not recognized) as from the underlying illness.[572] After the appearance of AIDS, the demographics have changed somewhat, with peak mortality in the 25- to 55-year-old age group in the United States, particularly among African and Hispanic Americans.[406] Although this change is largely related to HIV infection, whose progression appears to be accelerated by tuberculosis,[573] the presence of alcohol or drug abuse in the absence of AIDS also appears to be an important risk factor for death.[406]

Overall, the 4- to 5-year mortality rate of *untreated* tuberculosis is said to be about 50%.[574] However, timely diagnosis and adequate chemotherapy can reduce this rate dramatically (by at least 95%); in the United States, the rate has decreased progressively in the 20th century from 12.4 per 100,000 in 1953 to 0.6 in 1993.[575] The cause of death is variable. Some patients die suddenly of massive pulmonary hemorrhage or respiratory failure related to extensive tuberculous bronchopneumonia or ARDS (or both).[478,576] In others, a definite cause of death is not found, even at autopsy; in this group, cardiac arrhythmias are a likely mechanism.[577]

The development of miliary tuberculosis is associated with a particularly poor prognosis; for example, in one study approximately 25% of patients died a median of 6 days after the initiation of treatment.[494] In a significant number of cases, the abnormality is first identified at autopsy.[578] The cause of death in these patients is variable; in some, complicating disease such as ARDS or DIC develops.[579]

In "developing" areas of the world, such as sub-Saharan Africa, where the treatment of both HIV and tuberculosis may be suboptimal, about 30% of HIV-positive patients die within 12 months of therapy for tuberculosis.[580] However, many of these deaths are the result of HIV-related diseases other than tuberculosis.[581]

Bacille Calmette-Guérin

BCG is an avirulent strain of *Mycobacterium bovis* that has been widely used in the preparation of a prophylactic vaccine against *M. tuberculosis*. It has been estimated that approximately 3 billion doses of the vaccine have been given since the strain was developed.[582] Although its effectiveness is not uniform, it is still advocated as a means of prevention in some individuals and populations at high risk.[583] In fact, on the basis of a meta-analysis of published reports in 1994, one group estimated that the vaccine reduces the risk of tuberculosis by approximately 50%.[584]

Systemic complications and fatal disease as a result of disseminated BCG are uncommon but have been documented in a number of patients, especially children with immunodeficiency syndromes.[585] Preparations of both BCG vaccine and the methanol-extracted residue of killed bacilli have also been used as nonspecific immunostimulants in the treatment of neoplastic disease, most commonly carcinoma of the bladder.[586] Because these preparations are administered to patients who may have immunodeficiency related to either chemotherapy or neoplasia and because they are usually given repeatedly and in relatively large doses, the incidence of complications, notably BCG pneumonitis, is significantly greater than after antituberculous vaccination.[587]

Disease may be caused by direct infection by the organism,[588] by reactivation of latent infection,[587] or by a hypersensitivity phenomenon.[589] BCG therapy has also been associated with radiographic and HRCT changes indistinguishable from those of miliary tuberculosis.[590] Histologic examination of biopsy specimens from affected patients has shown necrotizing granulomas similar in all respects to miliary tuberculosis, but in which organisms are rarely identified.[591] When disease occurs within 3 months of intravesical therapy, patients develop fever and generalized symptoms of systemic illness.[592] Among patients who have late manifestations, most have localized disease that suggests reactivation of infection in the genitourinary tract, vertebrae, or retroperitoneal soft tissue.[592]

Nontuberculous Mycobacteria

A small but increasing proportion of mycobacterial infection is caused by nontuberculous mycobacteria (NTM). Overall, approximately 20 species have been associated with human disease[593]; however, a number of these species may represent examples of colonization or specimen contamination rather than true infection.[594] Of the several classification schemes developed to categorize these bacilli, that of Runyon has come to be almost universally accepted.[595] According to this scheme, organisms can be considered in four groups on the basis of cultural characteristics (principally, the presence or absence of pigment and the rate of growth).

The majority of NTM pulmonary infections are caused by a few species, including *Mycobacterium kansasii*, *Mycobacterium chelonae* complex, and *Mycobacterium avium-intracellulare*; however, new or previously nonpathogenic species are being seen more frequently, particularly in immunocompromised patients,[596] and specific organisms may assume prominence in particular geographic regions. Most infections can be considered in one of four clinical groups: pulmonary disease or cervical lymphadenitis in immunocompetent individuals, disseminated disease in immunocompromised patients, and localized skin disease.[597]

Epidemiology

As with tuberculosis, the incidence of disease caused by NTM varies considerably throughout the world. As a result of the AIDS epidemic, the proportion of tuberculous disease caused by NTM—particularly *M. avium* complex—has increased significantly in the last 20 years. There is also evidence that the number of cases is increasing in the non-AIDS population, at least in some areas of the world[598,599]; possible reasons include an aging population, improved methods for detecting organisms in clinical specimens, increased physician awareness of the disease, and increased exposure of patients to the source of the organism.[600] Data concerning the incidence of disease caused by specific organisms are also influenced by marked variability in their own geographic distribution.

Many patients in whom NTM pulmonary disease is diagnosed have underlying lung disease. The most common associated conditions are COPD, healed tuberculosis or fungal disease, bronchiectasis, alveolar proteinosis, pneumoconiosis (particularly silicosis), and cystic fibrosis.[601-603] An increased risk of NTM infection has also been observed in patients with rheumatoid disease, diabetes mellitus, heart disease, alcoholism, and achalasia and in those who have had a partial gastrectomy.[604] Immunocompromised patients are at increased risk for NTM infection as well; although this increased risk is particularly pertinent with respect to patients with AIDS (see page 428), those who have an underlying malignant neoplasm (particularly hairy cell leukemia[605]) or an organ transplant[606] or who are receiving corticosteroid or other immunosuppressive therapy are also affected.

NTM infection can be acquired by a variety of mechanisms, including inhalation, ingestion, direct inoculation after trauma, and iatrogenically.[607] Although animal-to-human transmission may occur with some species (e.g., *Mycobacterium simiae*), it is probably uncommon, and human-to-human transmission has not been convincingly documented.[608] Because many of the organisms are found in water, contamination of hospital water supplies can result in true nosocomial infection and "pseudoinfection" (the latter sometimes related to bronchoscopy).[609]

Pathologic Characteristics

In most cases, the gross and histologic characteristics of pulmonary disease caused by NTM are identical to those of *M. tuberculosis* and are characterized by a variable degree of fibrosis, cavitation, granulomatous inflammation, and caseation necrosis.[610] Bronchial spread and miliary disease can occur, albeit less often than in tuberculosis. Because of the relatively frequent association with underlying chronic pulmonary disease, gross abnormalities attributable to the infection may be difficult to identify, particularly in early infection. A definitive histologic diagnosis of the nontuberculous nature of the disease is not usually possible,[611] with the exception of disseminated *M. avium* complex infection in children with immunodeficiency syndromes and patients with AIDS.[612] In these individuals, infection is typically manifested as aggregates of macrophages stuffed with organisms, often with minimal or no granulomatous reaction and necrosis.

Occasionally, lung biopsy specimens from patients who apparently are not immunocompromised reveal nonspecific chronic inflammation without a granulomatous component and yet grow an NTM species on culture[610]; although the significance of this finding is not clear, it is probably best to consider the positive culture a result of colonization or contamination while recognizing the possibility that the histologic reaction itself may be atypical.

Radiologic Manifestations

The considerable overlap between the radiologic patterns of pulmonary disease caused by NTM and *M. tuberculosis* precludes confident distinction between the two in any particular case (Fig. 6–33).[482,613] In fact, one of the more common patterns consists of single or multiple cavities, often associated with radiographic evidence of endobronchial spread.[482,613] Nevertheless, certain patterns are seen more commonly in the former and may be helpful in suggesting the diagnosis in the appropriate clinical setting.[614,615]

A second, somewhat more distinctive pattern, seen particularly in nonimmunocompromised women infected with *M. avium* complex, consists of bilateral small nodules that are usually well circumscribed, measure less than 1 cm in diameter, and have a centrilobular distribution.[616,617] The nodules often have a patchy distribution in all lobes,[482] although they occasionally predominantly involve the upper lobes or middle lobe and lingula.[616,618] On HRCT, most patients have bronchiectasis, usually involving several lobes and occasionally only the middle lobe and lingula (Fig. 6–34).[619] The extent of bronchiectasis and the number of nodules tend to be greater in patients who have *M. avium-intracellulare* infection than in those who have other NTM infections or tuberculosis.[482,615]

Clinical Manifestations

The usual clinical features of NTM infection are similar to those of tuberculosis and, in a specific patient, are indistinguishable from this disease. Some patients have no evidence of previous pulmonary disease[620]; as described earlier, many of these patients are older women who have a radiographic pattern of focal bronchiectasis and patchy nodules without cavitation (the Lady Windermere syndrome).[621,622]

Apart from patients with AIDS—in whom the incidence of disseminated *M. avium* complex infection is as high as 15% to 25%—disseminated NTM disease is rare. Virtually all affected patients are immunocompromised as a result of therapy or underlying disease.[623] In patients infected with *M. avium* complex, the initial clinical finding tends to be fever of unknown origin; disease related to *M. kansasii* and *M. chelonae* tends to be manifested as subcutaneous nodules or draining abscesses.[624] Pulmonary involvement is common in disseminated disease, with a miliary radiographic pattern in most patients and parenchymal consolidation in roughly 25%.[625]

In contrast to *M. tuberculosis*, whose identification signifies disease, isolation of NTM from sputum not uncommonly represents environmental contamination of culture material or colonization of the respiratory tract.[626] Diagnosis is made even more difficult by the fact that both the diseased and the colonized states are commonly associated with underlying pulmonary abnormalities.[627] As a result, interpretation of a positive smear or culture must be done carefully and in the light of underlying clinical and radiologic features. Guidelines for diagnosis have been published by the American Thoracic Society on the basis of three categories of clinical manifestations (Table 6–2). By using strict criteria such as these, only a minority of NTM isolates are associated with clinically important disease.[628]

Pulmonary disease caused by NTM tends to progress if untreated.[629] As might be expected, the prognosis also varies with the importance of any underlying lung disease.[630] The

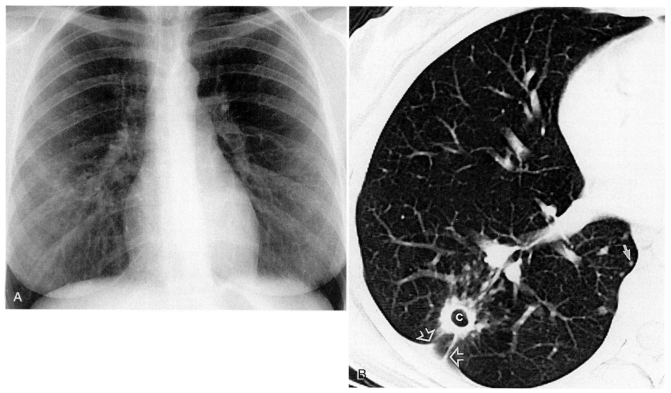

FIGURE 6–33

Pulmonary *Mycobacterium avium* complex infection. A posteroanterior chest radiograph (**A**) in a 28-year-old woman shows poorly defined small nodular opacities in the right lower lobe. An HRCT scan (**B**) shows a cavity (c) in the right lower lobe and associated pleural tags (*open arrows*) and several centrilobular nodular opacities (*closed arrow*). Sputum culture grew *M. avium* complex. The radiologic findings are indistinguishable from those of tuberculosis. (*From Müller NL, Fraser RS, Colman NC, Paré PD: Radiologic Diagnosis of Diseases of the Chest. Philadelphia, WB Saunders, 2001.*)

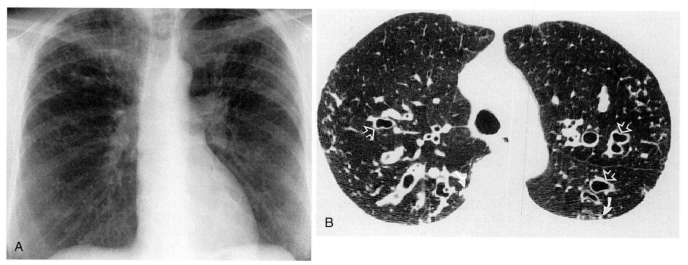

FIGURE 6–34

Pulmonary *Mycobacterium avium* complex infection. A posteroanterior chest radiograph (**A**) in a 52-year-old woman shows poorly defined small nodular opacities and evidence of bronchiectasis in the upper lung zones. An HRCT scan (**B**) demonstrate bronchiectasis (*open arrows*) and several centrilobular and subpleural nodules (*closed arrow*). (*From Fraser RS, Müller NL, Colman NC, Paré PD: Fraser and Paré's Diagnosis of Diseases of the Chest, 4th ed. Philadelphia, WB Saunders, 1999.*)

TABLE 6–2. Recommended Diagnostic Criteria for Pulmonary Disease Caused by Nontuberculous Mycobacteria (NTM)

Patients with Cavitary Lung Disease

Presence of two or more sputum specimens (or sputum and a bronchial washing) that are acid-fast bacilli smear positive and/or result in moderate to heavy growth of NTM on culture
Other reasonable causes for the disease process have been excluded (e.g., tuberculosis, fungal disease)

Patients with Noncavitary Lung Disease

Presence of two or more sputum specimens (or sputum and a bronchial washing) that are acid-fast bacilli smear positive and/or produce moderate to heavy growth on culture
If the isolate is *Mycobacterium kansasii* or *Mycobacterium avium* complex, failure of the sputum cultures to clear with bronchial toilet or within 2 weeks of institution of specific mycobacterial drug therapy (although studied only for these two species, this criterion is probably valid for other species of NTM)
Other reasonable causes for the disease process have been excluded

Patients with Cavitary or Noncavitary Lung Disease Whose Sputum Evaluation is Nondiagnostic or in Whom Another Disease Cannot Be Excluded

A transbronchial or open lung biopsy yields the organism and shows mycobacterial histopathologic features (i.e., granulomatous inflammation, with or without acid-fast bacilli). No other criteria needed
A transbronchial or open lung biopsy that fails to reveal the organism but shows mycobacterial histopathologic features in the absence of a previous history of other granulomatous or mycobacterial disease plus (1) presence of two or more positive cultures of sputum or bronchial washings; (2) other reasonable causes for granulomatous disease have been excluded

Adapted from Wallace RJ Jr, O'Brien R, Glassroth J, et al: Diagnosis and treatment of disease caused by nontuberculous mycobacteria. Am Rev Respir Dis 142:940, 1990.

cause of death in affected patients is variable; many, particularly those who have obstructive airway disease, die of cor pulmonale. As might be expected, disseminated disease in an immunocompromised patient is often fatal.[623]

FUNGI AND ACTINOMYCES

Fungi can cause pulmonary disease by several mechanisms and in a variety of clinical settings. Some organisms (such as *Histoplasma capsulatum* and *Coccidioides immitis*) are primary pathogens that most frequently infect healthy individuals. They are found in specific geographic areas—hence the term *endemic* is often used to describe the infections—and typically dwell in the soil. In appropriate climatic conditions, they germinate and produce spores, which when inhaled by a susceptible host change form (a process known as *dimorphism*) and proliferate. In an individual who has an intact inflammatory response and adequate cell-mediated immunity, such proliferation is almost invariably limited, the resulting disease being subclinical or mild and manifested only by the development of a positive skin test. In a few apparently "normal" individuals, however, fulminant primary infection or chronic pulmonary disease, with or without systemic dissemination, can cause significant morbidity and is occasionally fatal. Such complications are much more common in patients who have an underlying immune deficiency such as AIDS.[631]

A second group of organisms (such as *Aspergillus* and *Candida* species) are opportunistic invaders that chiefly affect patients who are immunocompromised or have underlying pulmonary disease. These organisms are not dimorphic and are usually ubiquitous in the environment. Intact mucosal barriers and adequate phagocytic function are the major host factors that determine whether colonization progresses to clinically evident disease. In the latter situation, the fungi may be present as saprophytes (e.g., a mycetoma) or, more commonly, as invasive organisms that cause tissue destruction.

In addition to saprophytic and invasive infection, some fungi (particularly *Aspergillus* species) can cause disease by an exaggerated hypersensitivity reaction without actually invading tissue (see page 282). Furthermore, inhalation of massive amounts of fungi occasionally provokes a toxic, nonallergic pulmonary reaction (mycotoxicosis, organic dust toxic syndrome) (see page 511).

The Actinomycetaceae, which include microorganisms such as *Actinomyces israelii* and *Nocardia* species, are classified as bacteria. Because many of their clinical and pathologic characteristics are similar to those of fungi, however, they can be conveniently considered together with true mycotic infections.

Histoplasma capsulatum (Histoplasmosis)

Histoplasmosis is an endemic fungal disease usually caused by the dimorphic organism *H. capsulatum*.[632] Its natural habitat is soil that contains a high nitrogen content, usually derived from the guano of birds or bats. Thus, areas such as chicken houses, blackbird and pigeon roosts, bat-infested caves or attics, and other sites where bird guano accumulates are the most common sources for outbreaks of infection. Situations in which clouds of dust are raised, such as bulldozing of roosting sites, are particularly likely to be associated with disease because of aerosolization of the spores. Animal-to-human and person-to-person transmission is not known to occur.

Although the organism is of worldwide distribution, most reports of disease have come from North America, particularly the Ohio, Mississippi, and St. Lawrence River valleys, where the organism is considered endemic. Infection is common in such areas, positive histoplasmin skin tests having been found in as many as 70% to 80% of the population in some studies.[633] Even in endemic areas, however, cases are unevenly distributed, probably reflecting point sources of heavily contaminated soil.[634] Although clinically evident disease can develop in individuals of any age, it is more common and of greater significance in infants, the elderly, and the immunosuppressed.[635]

Pathogenesis and Pathologic Characteristics. In appropriate environmental conditions, the mycelia of *H. capsulatum* produce microconidia measuring 2 to 5 μm in diameter that are inhaled and deposited in peripheral alveolar air spaces. The earliest host response is an infiltrate of polymorphonuclear leukocytes.[636] These cells are unable to kill the organism effectively and are soon replaced by lymphocytes and macrophages.[637] Lymphocyte-mediated cellular immunity accompanied by granulomatous inflammation, necrosis, and fibrosis develops about 1 to 2 weeks after the initial infection.[638] The appearance at this stage is identical, both macroscopically and histologically, to primary tuberculosis. In most cases, the ensuing focus of parenchymal disease is too small to be detected radiographically; occasionally, individual foci of necrosis coalesce and enlarge to form one or more foci of disease large enough to be identifiable.

Spread of organisms to regional lymph nodes is invariable and results in enlargement that is often more prominent than that observed in primary tuberculosis. Complications related to nodal disease are similar to those of the latter condition and include atelectasis and obstructive pneumonitis caused by airway compression (see Color Fig. 6–10) and, in long-standing disease, broncholithiasis.[639] Blood-borne dissemination of organisms also occurs early in the course of disease, in many cases resulting in small extrapulmonary foci of granulomatous inflammation, particularly in the liver and spleen. As in primary tuberculosis, such hematogenous spread is seldom clinically significant; however, the foci of disease that are established can undergo dystrophic calcification and serve as radiographic markers of previous disease.

Healing of parenchymal disease is rapid in the vast majority of cases. The morphologic appearance is again similar to that of tuberculosis and consists of foci of necrotic parenchyma surrounded by a fibrous capsule (see Color Fig. 6–11); dystrophic calcification is frequent. In tissue sections, organisms can be identified in necrotic tissue by silver stain as small (3 to 5 μm) round to oval yeasts.

Despite the many similarities in the pathogenesis and pathology of tuberculosis and histoplasmosis, there are also fundamental differences.[640] As in tuberculosis, the initial infection results in the development of cell-mediated immunity, as reflected by the acquisition of enhanced fungicidal properties by alveolar macrophages. In contrast to tuberculosis, however, this immunity appears to be more ephemeral. For example, in one investigation of histoplasmin-positive individuals, 15% to 20% reverted to negative when re-examined 2 years after the initial test[641]; moreover, most of these individuals subsequently become positive once again, presumably as a result of reinfection. In view of these findings, the terms *primary* and *postprimary* as applied to tuberculosis may not be suitable to a classification of histoplasmosis. Furthermore, in contrast to the endogenous reactivation of disease in postprimary tuberculosis, recurrent pneumonia caused by *H. capsulatum* has been hypothesized to be related most commonly to infection from an exogenous source.[640]

The nomenclature that has been proposed for types of disease caused by *H. capsulatum* is variable. We use a simple division into asymptomatic and symptomatic; asymptomatic can in turn be subdivided into acute, chronic, and disseminated histoplasmosis. It is likely that these clinical categories are dependent on a combination of the size and virulence of the initial inoculum and the status of the host's immunity.[640]

Asymptomatic Histoplasmosis

Most infections (probably 95% to 99%) are not associated with symptoms.[640] However, chest radiographs of converters have revealed pulmonary parenchymal opacities, with or without hilar lymph node enlargement, in as many as 10% to 25% of cases. The lack of symptoms may reflect a low-exposure dose in a nonimmunized person or a moderate-sized inoculum in one who is immunized.

Acute Histoplasmosis

Symptoms of flulike disease are perhaps the most common clinical manifestation of acute histoplasmosis. They consist of fever, headache, chills, cough, and retrosternal discomfort, the last-named symptom probably being related to mediastinal node involvement.[640] In most of these cases, physical examination of the chest is normal. Hepatosplenomegaly may develop, usually in children. Erythema nodosum or erythema multiforme is occasionally present, generally in young women and sometimes associated with arthralgia[640]; in such cases the diagnosis often becomes evident through awareness of a local outbreak of disease. Occasionally, a patient presents with more severe disease consisting of cough productive of mucopurulent sputum, hemoptysis, and musculoskeletal pain.[650] Crackles, a friction rub, and signs of consolidation may be evident. The differential diagnosis includes acute viral or bacterial pneumonia; however, because hilar lymph node enlargement is uncommon in these infections, this finding should suggest acute histoplasmosis in endemic areas.

The chest radiograph is normal in most patients.[651] The most common radiographic findings consist of single or multiple, poorly defined areas of air space consolidation.[652] Severe disease is characterized by homogeneous, nonsegmental, parenchymal consolidation simulating acute bacterial air space pneumonia (Fig. 6–35). In contrast to the latter, the disease tends to clear in one area and appear in another. Hilar lymph node enlargement is common and pleural effusion is rare.[651,652] After heavy exposure, the radiograph may show widely disseminated, fairly discrete nodular shadows, with individual lesions measuring 3 or 4 mm in diameter[653]; such abnormalities may not be apparent for a week or more after the onset of symptoms. Hilar lymph node enlargement is present in most such cases.[652]

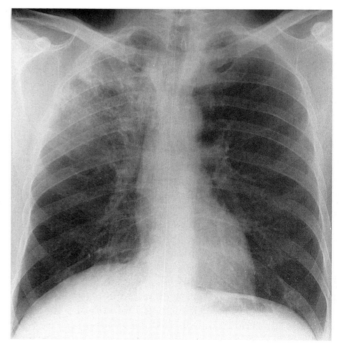

FIGURE 6–35

Acute histoplasmosis. A 48-year-old man related a 3-week history of right-sided pleuritic chest pain. A posteroanterior chest radiograph shows extensive consolidation in the right upper lobe and small areas of consolidation in the apex of the left lung. Sputum cultures grew *Histoplasma capsulatum.* (*Courtesy of Dr. Thomas Hartman, Mayo Clinic, Rochester MN.*)

Histoplasmoma. This relatively common form of pulmonary histoplasmosis may or may not be associated with a history of previous symptomatic disease.[654] The abnormality typically appears radiographically as a sharply defined nodule between 0.5 and 3 cm in diameter, in most cases in a lower lobe.[655] Although the lesion may be solitary, smaller satellite lesions are often seen.[649] The nodules may have a central focus of calcification in which a characteristic "target" lesion is produced or be diffusely calcified (Fig. 6–36); such calcification is frequently identified on CT even when it is not apparent on the radiograph.[656] Serial radiographs over a period of months or years may reveal moderate growth, even to a point where the diagnosis of neoplasia may be considered.[657] Even the presence of calcification does not necessarily mean that a histoplasmoma is "healed": such lesions may also increase in size, and histologic examination has shown apparently active fibrosis 10 years or more after they are first discovered. Although the pathogenesis of this phenomenon is not certain, it has been postulated to represent a reaction similar to that seen in fibrosing mediastinitis (see page 850)

Calcification of lymph nodes is also common in healed infection and may be seen in isolation or in association with a histoplasmoma. Broncholithiasis is an occasional complication (Fig. 6–37)[651]; in many cases, CT reveals parabronchial calcification and clarifies the nature of the abnormality.[658]

Chronic Histoplasmosis

Chronic Pulmonary Histoplasmosis. In contrast to most individuals who have acute disease, which typically subsides clinically and radiographically without treatment in weeks to months, rare patients have chronic progressive pulmonary disease. Some of these cases are virtually identical to postprimary tuberculosis, with affected patients having predominantly upper lobe disease characterized by fibrosis, necrosis, cavitation, and granulomatous inflammation. A background of pulmonary emphysema is usually present, and the infection may spread to involve the mediastinum or sites outside the thorax, in a fashion similar to the chronic disseminated form of disease. Some have suggested that the infective load in this situation is limited and that most of the changes are due to an immunologic response to a small number of organisms.[644]

The radiographic appearance (Fig. 6–38) simulates postprimary tuberculosis,[651] the earliest manifestations consisting of segmental or subsegmental areas of consolidation in the apices of the lungs, frequently outlining areas of centrilobular

FIGURE 6–36

Calcified histoplasmoma. A posteroanterior chest radiograph (**A**) shows a 1.5-cm-diameter nodule in the right lower lobe (*arrow*); calcification is not apparent. HRCT scans (**B** and **C**) show diffuse calcification of the nodule, as well as calcified right hilar and subcarinal nodes. (*From Müller NL, Fraser RS, Colman NC, Paré PD: Radiologic Diagnosis of Diseases of the Chest. Philadelphia, WB Saunders, 2001.*)

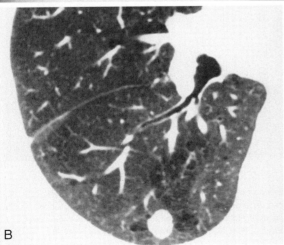

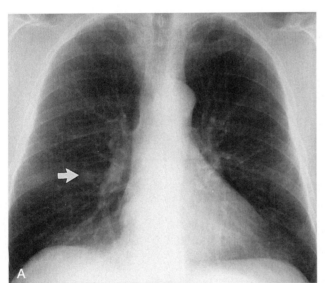

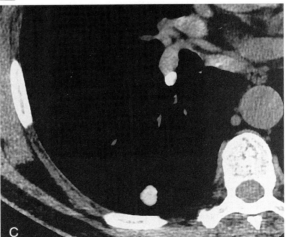

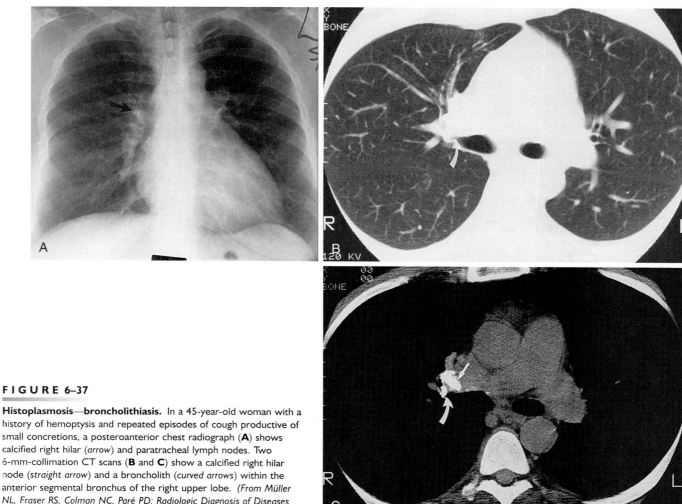

FIGURE 6–37

Histoplasmosis—broncholithiasis. In a 45-year-old woman with a history of hemoptysis and repeated episodes of cough productive of small concretions, a posteroanterior chest radiograph (**A**) shows calcified right hilar (*arrow*) and paratracheal lymph nodes. Two 6-mm-collimation CT scans (**B** and **C**) show a calcified right hilar node (*straight arrow*) and a broncholith (*curved arrows*) within the anterior segmental bronchus of the right upper lobe. (*From Müller NL, Fraser RS, Colman NC, Paré PD: Radiologic Diagnosis of Diseases of the Chest. Philadelphia, WB Saunders, 2001.*)

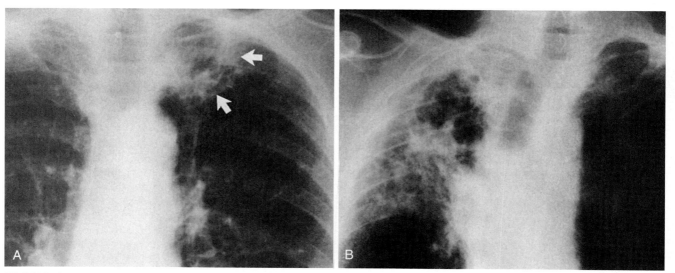

FIGURE 6–38

Chronic progressive histoplasmosis. A view of the upper half of the left lung (**A**) reveals a poorly defined, inhomogeneous opacity (*arrows*) containing a central radiolucency representing a cavity. The right lung was clear at that time. Approximately 1 year later (**B**), the left apical lesion had resolved almost completely, but there was now extensive disease throughout the right upper lobe associated with considerable loss of volume (note the tracheal shift to the right). The appearance is similar to that of chronic tuberculosis. (*From Müller NL, Fraser RS, Colman NC, Paré PD: Radiologic Diagnosis of Diseases of the Chest. Philadelphia, WB Saunders, 2001.*)

emphysema. Thick-walled bullae sometimes contain fluid levels; with time, the bullae can disappear completely or can increase gradually in size. Serial chest radiographs tend to show progressive loss of volume associated with increased prominence of linear opacities.

Chronic pulmonary histoplasmosis tends to be associated with cough and expectoration, which in some cases are probably the result of underlying COPD, with which it is inevitably associated.[659] Spillage of necrotic material from affected cavities or bullae may be accompanied by fever. Patients may complain of weight loss, deep-seated chest pain, hemoptysis, and general malaise; however, they can also remain asymptomatic.[644] The prognosis is variable; however, disease usually progresses and requires treatment.[659] Widespread dissemination is uncommon.

Chronic Mediastinal Histoplasmosis. A variety of clinical and radiologic abnormalities can result from involvement of the mediastinum by histoplasmosis. Sometimes they are related to one or more enlarged mediastinal lymph nodes.[660] Rarely, there is more or less diffuse deposition of fibrous tissue that is hypothesized to be caused by an immunologic reaction (fibrosing mediastinitis; see page 850).

Disseminated Histoplasmosis

With the exception of patients who have AIDS (see page 433), clinically apparent disseminated histoplasmosis is a rare occurrence. Approximately a third of patients are infants younger than 2 years; another 20% are adults who are immunosuppressed.[661] Symptomatic disseminated histoplasmosis has been subdivided into acute, subacute, and chronic types based on clinical and pathologic features. The first is characterized clinically by persistent high fever, prominent hepatosplenomegaly, anemia, leukopenia, and thrombocytopenia; interstitial pneumonia also develops in some patients. The radiographic and HRCT findings are usually similar to those of miliary tuberculosis.[490]

Subacute disseminated histoplasmosis has a clinical course that runs for months. Symptoms and signs include moderate fever, mild to moderate hepatosplenomegaly, and abdominal pain (caused by gastrointestinal ulceration); sometimes there is evidence of Addison's disease, meningitis, focal cerebritis, or endocarditis. Anemia, leukopenia, and thrombocytopenia may be present.

Chronic disseminated histoplasmosis is a relatively mild form of disease that is associated with little or no fever, absence of hepatosplenomegaly, and no evidence of bone marrow suppression. Patients are characteristically older adults, and the course is one of months to years.[659] The diagnosis is often made after the discovery and biopsy of an oropharyngeal ulcer. Specific organ involvement may result in Addison's disease, meningitis, endocarditis, or laryngitis.[662]

Laboratory Findings and Diagnosis

The white cell count is usually normal but may increase to 15,000/mm³ in patients who have acute "epidemic" disease[642] and to 20,000/mm³ in those who have cavitary disease.[643] Leukopenia, anemia, and thrombocytopenia develop in approximately 50% of patients who have symptomatic disseminated disease, but rarely in those with other varieties.

Examination of smears of expectorated material, pleural fluid, or bone marrow for the presence of organisms is seldom useful in patients who have acute histoplasmosis. Cultures are seldom positive in asymptomatic individuals or in the presence of self-limited disease, even in patients who are acutely ill from exposure to a heavy inoculum[644]; during more severe disease or in the presence of thin-walled cavities, growth is successful in no more than a third of patients. In patients with thick-walled cavities, positive sputum culture has been reported in 50% to 70% of cases (provided that multiple specimens are collected). The use of *Histoplasma*-specific DNA probes promises to be more sensitive than culture in many of these situations.[645] Positive results on smear and culture in disseminated histoplasmosis vary with the severity of the disease. In the acute, relatively severe form, blood and bone marrow smears, appropriately stained, are often diagnostic; culture results are generally even better, and blood, bone marrow, liver, and even urine should be sampled for this purpose when disseminated disease is suspected.

Though useful in epidemiologic studies, skin testing has little or no role in diagnosis in individual patients because a positive reaction indicates only previous exposure and does not prove the presence of disease.

A number of different methods can be used to detect serum antibodies to *H. capsulatum*; most experts agree that using multiple tests, with both mycelial and yeast antigens, increases diagnostic accuracy.[646] A fourfold rise in titer in serial determinations or a single determination of greater than 1:32 constitutes strong evidence of recent infection. In regions where the prevalence of positive skin test reactors is relatively low, some investigators accept yeast-phase titers of 1:32 and mycelial titers of 1:8 or more as highly suggestive evidence of active disease[647]; yeast titers of 1:8 and 1:16 have been regarded as presumptive evidence of the diagnosis. The value of the test is hampered by the delay in forming antibodies and by the tests' lack of sensitivity in patients who are immunocompromised[648] or who suffer from indolent or chronic disease.[649]

Coccidioides immitis (Coccidioidomycosis)

Coccidioidomycosis is caused by the dimorphic fungus *C. immitis*.[663,664] In its natural habitat (soil), it grows as a mycelium of septate hyphae that produces numerous 2- to 5-μm arthrospores. These spores are quite resistant to drying and are highly virulent. Within tissue, the organisms exist as large (mostly 20 to 40 μm) spherules that have a thick capsule and reproduce by endosporulation (i.e., the cytoplasm of the spherule undergoes cleavage rather than budding to produce spores).

Within the United States, infection is found mostly in California, especially in the San Joaquin Valley. In areas in which the organism is endemic, the incidence of infection is high: a positive skin test develops in approximately 25% of newly arrived persons at the end of 1 year and 50% at the end of 4 years. The majority of infections that appear outside endemic areas are believed to be related to travel within them[665]; although most examples of such travel are recent,[666] cases of reactivation have been documented many years after initial exposure. The risk of acquiring the infection is greatest during dry and windy conditions in which soil is disturbed. Although coccidioidomycosis commonly affects a variety of domestic animals, animal-to-animal and animal-to-human spread is not generally believed to occur; the disease is also probably not transmitted from person to person.

Approximately 20% to 40% of patients who acquire the infection have clinical manifestations, of whom about 2% to 3% have illness lasting weeks or months[667]; clinical evidence of disseminated disease occurs in less than 0.1%. There is evidence that disseminated disease is more likely to occur in Filipinos and African Americans than in whites, although the epidemiologic data supporting such evidence have been questioned.[668] An increased risk of infection has been documented in Native Americans[669] and in individuals who are older, who have diabetes, and who smoke.[670] Patients who are immunocompromised as a result of conditions such as AIDS or organ transplants also have increased susceptibility to both pulmonary and disseminated disease.[671,672]

Skin reactivity to *C. immitis* is long-lived but wanes with time, thus suggesting that exogenous reinfection may occur in some individuals who reside in endemic areas. Reactivation of quiescent disease in nonendemic areas has been well documented,[669] however, and it is likely that some cases of late-onset, disseminated disease in endemic areas are the result of loss of immunocompetence in individuals who experienced asymptomatic dissemination during primary infection. Acute or chronic progressive disease can also develop after a period of remission following the primary infection, possibly as a consequence of an impairment in host defenses.[673]

Pathogenesis and Pathologic Characteristics. Within the lung, inhaled arthrospores develop into sporangia (spherules) that rapidly induce a neutrophilic exudate. Although this reaction often persists, granulomatous inflammation consisting of both granulomas and isolated multinucleated giant cells containing spherules also develops with time. The combination of exudative and granulomatous inflammation is seen in other forms of coccidioidomycosis and is characteristic of the disease.[674] As might be expected, the development of a granulomatous reaction can be deficient in patients who are immunocompromised.[675]

In most cases, the pneumonic focus remains relatively small and undergoes resolution, with only a small scar remaining. In some, however, disease progresses to involve a whole lobe or lung in a pattern resembling confluent bacterial bronchopneumonia. In these cases, necrosis may be extensive and can be associated with cavitation. Ulcerative bronchitis and bronchiolitis are often prominent, and bronchiectasis may develop if the patient survives. Hilar and mediastinal lymph nodes may be enlarged and contain a substantial amount of necrotic tissue and organisms; erosion of the capsule and spread of infected material into adjacent structures such as bronchi or mediastinum can result in dissemination of disease in a fashion similar to tuberculosis.

Coccidioidomycosis can occur in several clinicopathologic patterns, often termed primary, persistent primary, chronic progressive, and disseminated.

Primary Coccidioidomycosis

As indicated previously, most patients who acquire the infection for the first time are asymptomatic.[667,676] When present, symptoms of primary infection are often nonspecific and flulike. A more specific syndrome known as *valley fever* occurs in 5% to 20% of patients who have symptomatic disease. It may be seen in isolated cases or in miniepidemics and consists of erythema nodosum or erythema multiforme, arthralgia, and (sometimes) eosinophilia. This combination of findings may also be associated with flulike symptoms and should suggest the diagnosis in an endemic area.

The most common radiologic manifestation consists of single or multiple foci of air space consolidation (Fig. 6–39).[677] Sometimes, these foci evolve into thin-walled cavities that may persist or resolve spontaneously.[678] Small pleural effusions occur in approximately 20% of cases[679]; large effusions are rare. Lymph node enlargement occurs in approximately 20% of cases, seldom in the absence of parenchymal involvement.

Persistent Primary Coccidioidomycosis

Primary disease that persists longer than 6 weeks is designated *persistent primary coccidioidomycosis*.[668] It can be associated with progressive pneumonia involving large portions of the lungs and is sometimes associated with miliary dissemination and death. More commonly, it is manifested as one or more nodules pathologically similar to tuberculomas[680]; these nodules may persist indefinitely and occasionally serve as a focus for reactivation. Cavitation can occur either within an area of pneumonia or by evacuation of necrotic material within a nodule.

Radiographically, a nodule typically develops over a period of approximately 5 to 6 weeks as a focus of consolidation becomes smaller, denser, and better defined.[679] Occasionally, nodular opacities result from filling in of a cavity.[677] The nodules are generally solitary, 0.5 to 5 cm in diameter, and located in the lung periphery.[677] In the majority of patients, they have homogeneous attenuation on CT scan; however, central areas of low attenuation resulting from necrosis and foci of calcification are seen in some cases.[681] Cavitation has been reported in about 10% to 15% of cases.[681,682] The cavities are usually single and located in the upper lobes and may be thin or thick walled (Fig. 6–40)[683]; the former have a tendency to change size, possibly as a result of check-valve bronchiolar communication.

Most patients who have nodular disease are asymptomatic, even in the presence of cavitation. In fact, nodules may not be discovered for months or years after a patient has left an endemic area. They are most often found incidentally and investigated to exclude the possibility of malignancy. Transthoracic needle aspiration may provide the diagnosis by revealing the spherules on Papanicolaou-stained specimens.[584] In contrast to the nodular form of disease, persistent coccidioidal pneumonia is commonly accompanied by hemoptysis, fever, cough, and expectoration, especially when cavitation is present. Pneumothorax and empyema develop in about 2% of patients who have acute cavitary disease and usually require surgical intervention.

Chronic Progressive Coccidioidomycosis

Chronic progressive coccidioidomycosis accounts for less than 1% of cases of coccidioidal pulmonary disease.[685] Some investigators have recognized two varieties—chronic fibronodular and chronic necrotizing, the latter associated with cavitation.[676] Disease can occur either in temporal continuity with primary coccidioidomycosis or after a variable time interval during which the infection has apparently been stable and unaccompanied by clinical evidence of activity. It usually develops insidiously and has a prolonged course of up to 15 years. Although dissemination can occur, the disease generally

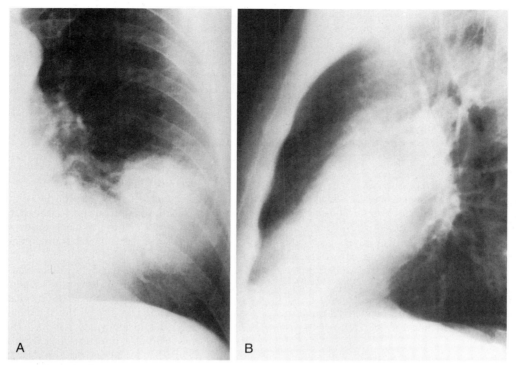

FIGURE 6–39

Primary coccidioidomycosis. Views of the left lung from posteroanterior (**A**) and lateral (**B**) radiographs show homogeneous consolidation of much of the lingular segment of the left upper lobe. A faint air bronchogram could be identified on the original radiographs but does not reproduce well here. The upper border of the consolidation is sharply circumscribed and resembles a mass. *(From Müller NL, Fraser RS, Colman NC, Paré PD: Radiologic Diagnosis of Diseases of the Chest. Philadelphia, WB Saunders, 2001.)*

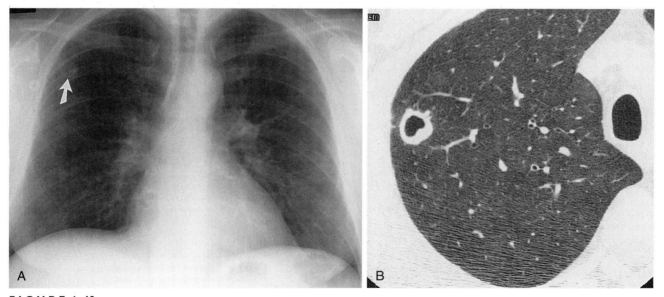

FIGURE 6–40

Cavitary coccidioidomycosis. A posteroranterior chest radiograph (**A**) shows a sharply circumscribed cavitated nodule in the right upper lobe (*arrow*). An HRCT scan (**B**) shows uneven thickness of the wall and smooth outer margins. *(From Müller NL, Fraser RS, Colman NC, Paré PD: Radiologic Diagnosis of Diseases of the Chest. Philadelphia, WB Saunders, 2001.)*

remains confined to the lungs. Radiographic abnormalities resemble those of chronic cavitary tuberculosis.

Disseminated Coccidioidomycosis

Disseminated coccidioidomycosis is rare; it may occur as a complication of the primary illness or after reactivation of latent disease in susceptible individuals. It shows a considerable male preponderance and a predilection for African Americans and Filipinos. The course may be chronic and insidious or rapidly fatal, the latter usually in association with primary disease. As might be expected, patients who have underlying immunodeficiency disease (particularly AIDS[686]) or are receiving immunosuppressive therapy are at increased risk.

Although disseminated disease can affect any organ of the body, either alone or in combination, the principal sites of involvement are the skin, bones, joints, kidneys, and central nervous system (particularly the meninges). Pulmonary involvement, usually extensive, is the rule in patients who die.[674] Hematogenous dissemination resulting in miliary disease can occur early in the course of the infection or at an advanced stage of chronic illness in the context of widespread dissemination.[687] The latter situation may be complicated by ARDS.

Laboratory Findings and Diagnosis

The hemoglobin value is decreased in many patients who have disseminated disease. The white blood cell count is normal or moderately elevated in most patients, often with a significant degree of eosinophilia,[688] particularly in those who have erythema nodosum.

Wet mounts of sputum or exudates derived from cutaneous or other sites treated with 10% potassium hydroxide may reveal typical endospore-containing spherules. When sputum is unavailable or examination is not diagnostic, flexible fiberoptic bronchoscopy has proved to be a valuable procedure for obtaining material.[689] Culture of the organism is not difficult; however, proper methods are important to prevent laboratory acquisition of the disease, for which there is a significant risk.

Serologic tests using tube precipitation (TP), latex particle agglutination (LPA), and immunodiffusion (using heated coccidioidin, IDTP) are invaluable for screening and become positive 1 to 3 weeks after exposure. An ELISA that gives results comparable to these methods has also been developed.[690] The LPA test is more sensitive but less specific than TP; however, neither provides positive results in the cerebrospinal fluid of patients who have meningitis.[669] A complement fixation reaction becomes positive in the cerebrospinal fluid of most patients in whom meningitis develops and is diagnostic of dissemination; seropositivity occurs in 50% of patients within 4 weeks and in 90% within 8 weeks. Serum complement fixation titers sustained above 1:16 to 1:32 are unusual in uncomplicated primary coccidioidomycosis and indicate a high risk for progressive primary or disseminated disease.[691]

Skin testing can be performed with either spherulin or coccidioidin, the former being the more sensitive.[692] In the relatively benign nondisseminated form of disease, the skin test is positive in virtually all patients within 3 weeks of the onset of infection; it may revert to negative within 2 years but can remain positive for as long as 10 years. Patients who have disseminated disease are often anergic, and the skin test reaction

may be negative. A combination of a negative skin test and a complement fixation titer greater than 1:16 is practically pathognomonic of disseminated disease.

Blastomyces dermatitidis (North American Blastomycosis)

North American blastomycosis is caused by the dimorphic fungus B. dermatitidis, which occurs as a mycelium in culture and presumably in its natural habitat and as a yeast at 37°C. In tissue, the yeasts are round or oval in shape, measure about 10 to 15 μm in diameter, and possess thick walls; they reproduce by broad-based buds.

The disease occurs most commonly in the Western Hemisphere, mainly in the central and southeastern United States[693] and south central Canada.[694] The organism may be associated with miniepidemics after point-source infection or sporadic endemic infection.[695]

The lack of sensitivity and specificity of skin tests and serology for the detection of infection by B. dermatitidis and the inability to uncover point sources of outbreaks have prevented an accurate determination of the incidence of the disease; however, in vitro lymphocyte studies have shown that the likelihood of subclinical infection developing is significantly greater than the likelihood of contracting symptomatic disease.[696] Middle-aged men are most often affected, the male preponderance being about 5:1 to 15:1.[695] Infection is believed to occur most often by inhalation of airborne spores. Although the natural habitat of the organism is not certain, reports of individual patients and clusters of cases implicate wooded areas containing decaying vegetation or wood as a source of many infections.[697] Occasional cases appear to represent endogenous reactivation.[698]

The gross appearance of acute blastomycosis is usually that of bronchopneumonia. As in coccidioidomycosis, exudative and granulomatous forms of inflammation frequently coexist. The relative proportion of each pattern is quite variable, both among individual patients and at different sites in the same patient at the same time.[699] Foci of ulcerative bronchitis are not uncommon.[700]

The most common radiographic finding consists of acute air space consolidation.[701,702] It may be patchy or confluent and subsegmental, segmental, or nonsegmental (Fig. 6–41). The next most common abnormality is a mass, either single or multiple.[703] Cavitation occurs in approximately 15% to 20% of cases.[701] Hilar and mediastinal lymph node enlargement is uncommon, even on CT.[704] Pleural effusion has been identified on chest radiographs in 10% to 15% of cases and is almost invariably associated with parenchymal disease. Overwhelming infection is usually accompanied by a radiographic pattern of miliary dissemination.[705]

Although pulmonary infection may be associated with only flulike symptoms, it is more commonly manifested by symptoms of acute pneumonia, including the abrupt onset of fever, chills, productive cough, and pleuritic chest pain.[697] Arthralgias and myalgias are not uncommon, and erythema nodosum develops occasionally. Crackles and rhonchi can be heard in some patients, but signs of parenchymal consolidation are seldom apparent. Pulmonary disease may be rapidly progressive and complicated by miliary spread, ARDS, or both.[706] A more indolent variant resembling tuberculosis sometimes follows the initial pulmonary infection and is occasionally the

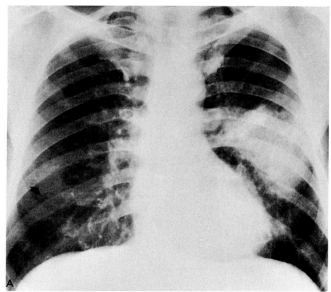

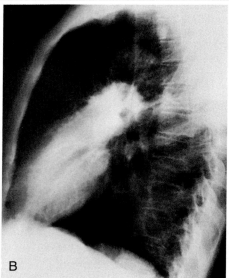

FIGURE 6–41

North American blastomycosis. Posteroanterior (**A**) and lateral (**B**) chest radiographs show a large, poorly defined shadow of homogeneous density in the lingula; the consolidation is nonsegmental and shows no evidence of an air bronchogram. The posteroanterior radiograph also reveals destruction of the anterior portion of the right fifth rib (*arrow*). *Blastomyces dermatitidis* was cultured from a 24-hour sputum collection and from fluid aspirated from the swelling over the right fifth rib. *(From Müller NL, Fraser RS, Colman NC, Paré PD: Radiologic Diagnosis of Diseases of the Chest. Philadelphia, WB Saunders, 2001.)*

first manifestation.[707] Such disease can remain confined to the lungs or can spread locally in the thorax or elsewhere. Dissemination occurs most commonly to skin, bone, and the genitourinary tract; recognition of involvement of these sites may provide the first clue to the diagnosis.[708] Bone lesions develop in about 25% of sporadic cases.[693] The leukocyte count is normal or only moderately raised in most patients, but it may exceed 30,000/mm³ when disease is extensive.[709]

Identification of the organism on smear, culture, or both provides the basis of diagnosis in most patients. It can be detected by microscopic examination of sputum or secretions obtained from dermal, subcutaneous, or other lesions after digestion in 10% potassium hydroxide or with Papanicolaou stain. Probably because of the frequency of airway involvement, *B. dermatitidis* is particularly likely to be identified in sputum specimens. Growth in culture media takes from 1 to several weeks.[710] Skin tests have no practical value in diagnosis.[711] Standard serologic tests have low sensitivity (varying from about 40% to 85%), cross-react with other fungi (particularly *H. capsulatum*), and lack availability, factors that severely limit their usefulness.[695]

The case fatality rate in patients reported to the Wisconsin Department of Health between 1986 and 1995 was 4.3% (29 of 670 patients).[712] As might be expected, disease is more aggressive in immunocompromised patients; in one series of such patients, the mortality rate was about 30%.[713]

Paracoccidioides brasiliensis (South American Blastomycosis)

South American blastomycosis (paracoccidioidomycosis) is caused by the dimorphic fungus *P. brasiliensis*. In tissue, the organism consists predominantly of yeasts that are round to oval in shape and quite variable in diameter, ranging from 2 μm for recently separated buds up to 60 μm for mature mother cells. Characteristically, reproduction is by multiple, narrow-necked buds that appear around the perimeter of the mother cells (*pilot wheel* arrangement).

The disease is found principally in Latin America but ranges from Mexico to Argentina.[714] Clinically evident disease shows a striking male preponderance and is seen most commonly in persons between 25 and 45 years of age. The natural habitat of the organism is believed to be soil, and farmers, manual laborers, and other workers engaged in rural occupations are particularly affected. Many cases, however, have been reported in city dwellers and professionals who have not had direct or continued contact with soil. The majority of infections are probably caused by inhalation, which results in primary pneumonia and secondary systemic dissemination. Animal-to-human and person-to-person transmission has not been documented.

Pathologically, pulmonary disease can take a variety of forms,[715,716] including (1) multiple smooth or lobulated nodules that may become confluent and resemble postprimary tuberculosis, with or without cavitation; (2) solitary nodules (paracoccidioidomas); (3) foci of necrosis and inflammation similar to acute bacterial pneumonia, usually in patients receiving corticosteroid or immunosuppressive therapy; and (4) miliary nodules representing hematogenous spread. Histologic findings consist of a combination of granulomatous and exudative inflammation.

In the primary form of the disease, transient air space opacities may be seen in the midlung zones. Paracoccidioidomas—single or multiple, solid or cavitary—are the principal manifestation in other cases.[717] Progressive pulmonary disease may resemble tuberculosis; however, the lower lobes are more frequently involved than the upper ones, and cavitation is less commonly seen radiographically (Fig. 6–42).[718] Hilar lymph node enlargement can occur by itself or in association with any form of pulmonary disease. The HRCT manifestations of chronic disease consist of interlobular septal thickening,

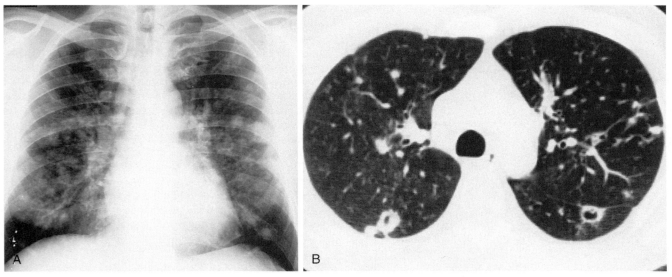

FIGURE 6–42

South American blastomycosis. A 52-year-old man presented with fever and severe headache but no respiratory symptoms. CT demonstrated intracerebral granulomas. An admission posteroanterior chest radiograph (**A**) shows numerous bilateral nodules measuring 0.5 to 2 cm in diameter, as well as paratracheal and right hilar lymphadenopathy. A CT scan (**B**) shows that some of the nodules are cavitated. Fine-needle aspiration biopsy of one of the nodules demonstrated *Paracoccidioides brasiliensis*. (*Case courtesy of Dr. Arthur Soares Souza Jr, Instituto de Radiodiagnostico Rio Preto, Sao Paulo, Brazil.*)

traction bronchiectasis, multiple variably sized (1 to 25 mm) and sometimes cavitated nodules, peribronchovascular interstitial thickening, centrilobular opacities, and intralobular lines (see Fig. 6–42).[719] These abnormalities are usually bilateral and symmetrical and involve all lung zones.

The results of studies of skin test reactivity indicate that infection is often asymptomatic or associated with mild, nonspecific complaints.[714] Such infection usually resolves; uncommonly, it is followed by progressive pneumonia and dissemination. Most clinically important disease appears to be associated with reactivation of a focus of primary infection[714] and is typically associated with dissemination to the skin or oronasal mucosa and significant pulmonary involvement.[720]

Cryptococcus neoformans

In the vast majority of cases, cryptococcosis is caused by *C. neoformans*, a unimorphic fungus that exists in yeast form both in its natural habitat and in animals and humans. Though rather pleomorphic, the organisms are usually round to oval in shape and 5 to 10 μm in diameter in tissue. Most strains possess a well-defined capsule that becomes visible as a pericellular halo with India ink preparations and standard tissue mucin stains.

The organism is found in a variety of natural habitats, one of the most important of which is dried pigeon excreta. Although it is believed that many cases of disease are acquired by inhalation of the organism from this source, a history of repeated exposure to pigeons is uncommonly associated with an increased risk of cryptococcal disease. There is no evidence of animal-to-human or person-to-person transmission. Although cryptococcosis can occur in otherwise normal hosts, it is seen much more frequently in patients who have chronic pulmonary disease, AIDS, or lymphoproliferative or autoim-

mune disorders being treated by chemotherapy or corticosteroid therapy.[721]

Pulmonary involvement can have several pathologic appearances,[722] including (1) relatively well defined, solitary or multiple nodules; (2) ill-defined areas of parenchymal consolidation that have a mucoid appearance resembling mucin-secreting bronchioloalveolar carcinoma or pneumococcal pneumonia as a result of the presence of large numbers of encapsulated organisms; (3) miliary nodules; and (4) predominantly interstitial proliferation of organisms accompanied by minimal cellular reaction (particularly in patients who have AIDS[723]). As with other fungal infections, the inflammatory reaction to *Cryptococcus* is variable and may consist of exudative or granulomatous reactions.

The most common radiographic manifestations of pulmonary infection consist of single or multiple nodules and areas of consolidation.[724,725] The nodules are most commonly subpleural in location and measure 0.5 to 4 cm in diameter.[726,727] The areas of consolidation can be segmental, nonsegmental, patchy, or masslike (Fig. 6–43). Cavitation is uncommon in otherwise healthy individuals but is frequently present in immunocompromised patients, particularly those who have AIDS.[727] The latter also have a higher incidence of disseminated disease. Such disease can be manifested as a miliary pattern or diffuse, ill-defined opacities.[726,728] Hilar and mediastinal lymph node enlargement has been reported in approximately 40% of patients who have AIDS and 10% to 25% of those who do not.[725,729] Pleural effusion is uncommon and usually connotes dissemination of the organism.[729]

In otherwise healthy individuals, disease is generally confined to the lungs. The initial infection often does not result in symptoms, may be self-limited, and is probably recognized infrequently.[730,731] When symptoms occur, they are nonspecific. Acute respiratory failure requiring mechanical ventilation is seen occasionally.[732] Dissemination occurs to

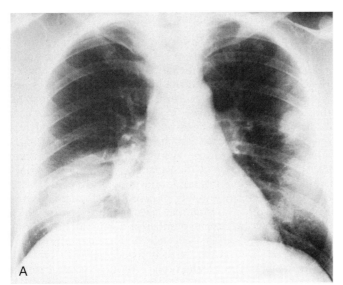

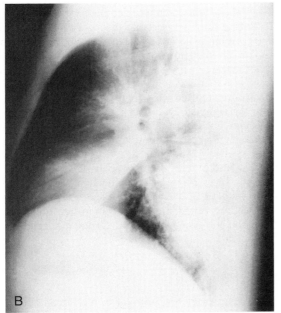

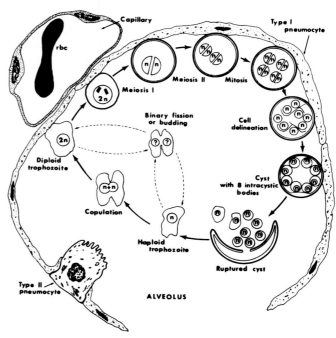

FIGURE 6–44

Pneumocystis jiroveci (carinii)—**hypothesized reproductive cycle.**
Diagrammatic representation of an alveolus illustrating potential mechanisms of cyst development and organism reproduction. *(From Gutierrez Y: The biology of* Pneumocystis carinii. *Semin Diagn Pathol 6:203, 1989.)*

FIGURE 6–43

Acute cryptococcal pneumonia. Posteroanterior (**A**) and lateral (**B**) radiographs show nonsegmental homogeneous consolidation of both lower lobes and the right middle lobe. *(From Müller NL, Fraser RS, Colman NC, Paré PD: Radiologic Diagnosis of Diseases of the Chest. Philadelphia, WB Saunders, 2001.)*

open lung biopsy or by detection of cryptococcal antigen in serum, pleural fluid, or BAL fluid in the context of a compatible clinical picture.[731] Skin tests are not very helpful because of cross-reactivity with other fungi.

Pneumocystis jiroveci (P. carinii)

P. jiroveci (P. carinii) is a ubiquitous organism at first thought to be a protozoan but now considered to be properly classified as a fungus.[734] In vivo, the organism can be identified in two forms[735,736]: (1) thick-walled, round or crescent-shaped cysts measuring 3 to 6 μm in diameter and (2) extracystic "trophozoites" that range from 1 to 5 μm, are pleomorphic, and often show pseudopod-like surface projections. It has been proposed that the life cycle of the organism in the lung begins with trophozoites, which enlarge extracellularly, become mature, and encyst (Fig. 6–44). Individual cysts then undergo maturation by developing intracystic sporozoites that are liberated when the cyst ruptures and develop into trophozoites. The possibility that trophozoites can reproduce by binary fission has also been suggested.[735]

Although *Pneumocystis* infection is common in humans (as evidenced by the presence of antibodies to the organism in a high proportion of healthy individuals at an early age[737]), it results in clinically significant pneumonia almost uniquely in individuals who have underlying disease, the most important of which is AIDS (see page 428); other patients at risk include those who have received organ transplants[738] and those who have lymphoreticular or other hematologic malignancies (usually associated with concomitant cytotoxic therapy),[739] systemic vasculitis or connective tissue disorders (usually in

the central nervous system (commonly causing a low-grade meningitis, sometimes with a normal chest radiograph), cutaneous and mucocutaneous tissues, bones, and less commonly, the viscera. As might be expected, such dissemination is more likely in immunocompromised patients and generally occurs weeks to months after the onset of pneumonia; few patients survive without therapy.[733]

A presumptive diagnosis can be made when *C. neoformans* is identified in sputum or bronchial lavage fluid in association with radiologic evidence of disease. A positive diagnosis is made by appropriate staining and culture of material obtained by transbronchial biopsy, transthoracic needle aspiration, or association with corticosteroid and cytotoxic therapy),[740] congenital immunodeficiency diseases, and (rarely) adrenocorticotropic hormone–producing neoplasms.[741] Symptoms or a radiographic abnormality may become apparent for the first time in patients in whom corticosteroid therapy is being reduced while other immunosuppressive therapy is being maintained.[742]

The mode of transmission of the organism has not been conclusively demonstrated; however, because of its almost invariable presence within the lungs, it is presumed to be by inhalation. The results of some serologic and molecular studies,[743,744] as well as the documentation of occasional clusters of PCP,[745] have suggested that disease may be acquired directly from another affected individual. However, most investigators have failed to find evidence for such spread,[746,747] and it is generally thought that the majority of cases of clinical disease result from reactivation of previously acquired asymptomatic (latent) infection.[748]

Pathogenesis

The factors involved in the transformation from a state of symbiosis to one of disease and the mechanisms by which *P. jiroveci* produces tissue damage and clinical disease are incompletely understood.[749] It is clear that an alteration in immune function is of prime importance. In addition to clinical observations indicating that immunosuppression is strongly associated with pneumonia in humans, experimental studies have shown that the disease can develop in isolated animals treated with corticosteroids.[750] This effect is most closely associated with T-cell function, particularly CD4+ cells.[751] It has been most clearly demonstrated in patients with AIDS, in whom a CD4+ count of less than 200 cells/μL is not uncommonly associated with PCP; moreover, there is a more or less linear relationship between the CD4+ blood count and the risk of contracting the disease.[752]

Other immune and inflammatory cells, particularly CD8+ T cells and alveolar macrophages, also have an important role in pathogenesis.[751] For example, experimental evidence has shown that CD8+ lymphocytes are recruited into the lung during the infection, where they provide a supportive role in defense.[753] Alveolar macrophages bind and phagocytose the organisms,[754] after which they are stimulated to release a variety of proinflammatory substances, of which tumor necrosis factor-α appears to be particularly important.[755] A protective role for polymorphonuclear leukocytes has been suggested by the results of animal studies and observations in patients who have AIDS.[756] It is also possible that humoral immunity has an effect; for example, in one investigation, a relative deficiency of IgG antibodies in BAL fluid was found in patients with AIDS plus PCP as opposed to AIDS patients without PCP.[757]

Both quantitative and qualitative abnormalities of surfactant have been documented in the BAL fluid of patients with AIDS before the development of PCP,[758] and it has been speculated that such alterations may be related to the saprophyte-pathogen transformation of the organism. In most cases of active disease, the organisms are found predominantly within alveolar air spaces; they are seldom identified in the alveolar interstitium or elsewhere in the body, thus suggesting limited invasive capability. The trophozoites produce no known toxins.

Pathologic Characteristics

In the typical case of PCP, histologic examination shows an alveolar interstitial infiltrate of lymphocytes and plasma cells, proliferation of type II epithelial cells, and a finely vacuolated ("foamy"), eosinophilic exudate in the alveolar air spaces (see Color Fig. 6–12). The latter consists of cysts and trophozoites admixed with host-derived material, including surfactant, fibrin, and matrix proteins such as fibronectin and vitronectin.[759] This exudate is highly characteristic of *Pneumocystis* infection and can be identified in tissue sections and BAL specimens stained by the Papanicolaou method.[760] Other pathologic abnormalities are found in addition or by themselves in a significant number of cases[761] and include diffuse alveolar damage,[762] granulomatous inflammation (in which organisms may be few in number and difficult to identify in BAL fluid),[763] interstitial and/or vascular invasion,[764] parenchymal calcification (usually associated with previous treatment),[765] and cyst formation.[761] All these atypical pathologic manifestations are more common in patients with AIDS, particularly those who have received prophylactic therapy for the infection. Fibrosis is variable in occurrence and severity and can be present in a focal or diffuse distribution and within the alveolar interstitium, air spaces, or both.[766] It can be evident at the time of the initial diagnosis but is usually more prominent in patients who have been treated.

Cysts are most often identified by staining with a silver technique, by which they are seen as typical round, oval, or crescent-shaped structures (the latter representing an effete cyst that has discharged its sporozoites) (see Color Fig. 6–12). Intracystic sporozoites and free trophozoites can be identified with Giemsa and Wright stains. When present in BAL fluid in clusters of 10 to 30 cysts, as in the typical case, confident identification of *P. jiroveci* is possible. If the cysts are few in number, however, distinction from other fungi such as *H. capsulatum*, *C. neoformans*, and *Candida* species may be difficult.[767,768]

Radiologic Manifestations

In the early stage of PCP, a granular or hazy opacity (ground-glass pattern) is apparent, particularly in the perihilar areas (Fig. 6–45).[769] In more advanced disease, the pattern is usually one of air space consolidation (although a granular or reticulogranular pattern may still be present at the periphery of the consolidated area).[68] Terminally, the lungs may be massively consolidated, to the point of almost complete airlessness; in fact, in some patients the acute onset and diffuse involvement are characteristic of ARDS.[770] Pneumonia is generally bilateral and most prominent in the lower lobes; less commonly, it involves the upper lobes predominantly or exclusively.[771]

Solitary or multiple, solid or cavitary nodular opacities are occasionally the principal manifestation.[772,773] Though seen most often in patients who have AIDS, they have also been described in patients with lymphoma.[774] Additional uncommon findings include pleural effusion[775] and enlarged noncalcified or calcified hilar and mediastinal lymph nodes.[776,777] A more common radiographic manifestation, seen in patients who have AIDS, is parenchymal cysts (see page 431).

The predominant CT finding in PCP consists of bilateral areas of ground-glass attenuation, which may be diffuse or

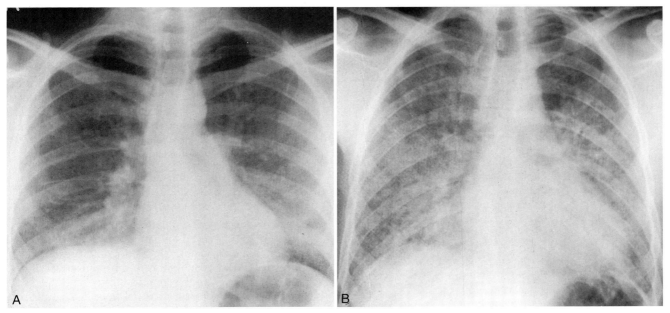

FIGURE 6–45

Pneumocystis pneumonia. A posteroanterior chest radiograph (**A**) shows a diffuse hazy increase in lung opacity (ground-glass opacity) throughout both lungs, worse in the lower lobes. Several days lateral (**B**), the disease had progressed to consolidation. *(From Müller NL, Fraser RS, Colman NC, Paré PD: Radiologic Diagnosis of Diseases of the Chest. Philadelphia, WB Saunders, 2001.)*

have a distinct mosaic pattern consisting of areas of normal lung intervening between the foci of ground-glass attenuation (Fig. 6–46).[70] Associated thickening of interlobular septa and parenchymal consolidation are each seen in approximately 20% to 50% of cases.[778] With time, the areas of ground-glass attenuation progress to consolidation; eventually, interstitial abnormalities such as thickened interlobular septa or irregular lines of attenuation become evident and may predominate.[68] Occasionally, there is a pattern of diffuse fibrosis or peripheral bronchiectasis and bronchiolectasis.[68,779]

Clinical Manifestations

The clinical course of PCP has significant differences in patients with and without AIDS. In the latter, the duration of prodromal symptoms tends to be short, and patients often have a relatively acute manifestation of fever and hypoxemia.[780,781] By contrast, patients who have AIDS frequently have a prodrome of fever, malaise, cough, and breathlessness of several weeks' duration before the infection is recognized. Dyspnea is the most common symptom; in many patients, a dry hacking cough and substernal tightness are also present.[782] Physical signs are usually minimal and include a few scattered crackles and wheezes. In severe infection, patients may show a hemodynamic profile similar to that of patients with bacterial sepsis.[783] In patients who have AIDS, the clinical picture may be complicated by the presence of other infectious or neoplastic disease or (rarely) by disseminated disease; in the latter situation, signs and symptoms of infection relate to the specific organ or tissue affected.[784] The development of sudden onset of shortness of breath in a patient with AIDS should raise the possibility of pneumothorax. Pneumomediastinum may also be seen.[785]

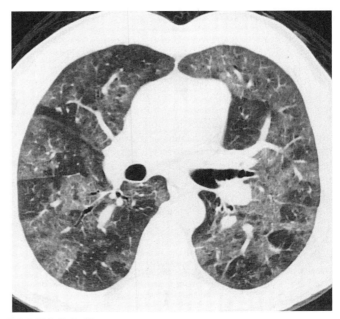

FIGURE 6–46

Pneumocystis pneumonia. An HRCT scan shows bilateral areas of ground-glass attenuation interspersed with areas of normal-appearing lung causing a mosaic pattern. The patient was a 46-year-old man with AIDS. *(From Müller NL, Fraser RS, Colman NC, Paré PD: Radiologic Diagnosis of Diseases of the Chest. Philadelphia, WB Saunders, 2001.)*

Laboratory Findings and Diagnosis

In most patients, the white blood cell count is slightly to moderately increased, with polymorphonuclear leukocytes predominating. However, leukopenia may occur and is associated with a worse prognosis. Lymphopenia is found in approximately 50% of patients.[786] Immunosuppressed patients, both transplant recipients and those who have AIDS, usually show a reversal of the helper-to-suppressor T-cell ratio.

Serum lactate dehydrogenase (LDH) is frequently elevated.[787] However, the diagnostic utility of this finding is limited since the enzyme is also elevated in patients who have other infections, particularly disseminated tuberculosis but also other bacterial pneumonia.[788] In fact, in the setting of PCP, changes in LDH levels are better considered to be a reflection of the extent of radiographic disease than an indicator of *Pneumocystis* infection per se.[789] As a corollary, a diagnosis other than PCP should be considered in a patient who has a normal LDH value in the face of significant radiographic abnormalities. Many patients also have an elevation of other serum enzymes, such as aspartate aminotransferase (AST), alanine aminotransferase (ALT), and alkaline phosphatase.[788] Patients who have PCP almost always have a reduced D$_{LCO}$.[790] A significant increase in the alveolar-arterial gradient for oxygen is also typical, and desaturation on exertion is a sensitive indicator of the disease.[791]

Diagnostic techniques for PCP are outlined in Chapter 8 (see page 432).

Prognosis and Natural History

The overall 30-day survival rate of patients who have AIDS and PCP in the United States is about 85% (see page 432). There is evidence that the prognosis is worse in patients who have non–AIDS-related disease[792]; in some investigations, as many as a third of such patients do not survive.[739] The use of prophylactic therapy, in both patients with and patients without AIDS, has clearly been shown to reduce the incidence of pneumonia. Most individuals who survive a single episode of PCP have little evidence of residual clinical disability. A degree of expiratory airflow obstruction and diminished diffusing capacity for carbon monoxide are common long-term sequelae.[793] Occasionally, the residual fibrosis is severe enough to be manifested as restrictive lung disease.[794]

Candida Species

Candidiasis is caused by fungi of the genus *Candida*, of which *Candida albicans* is the most common pathogen. However, other species are implicated fairly frequently in immunocompromised patients, and their incidence appears to be increasing.[795] In tissue, all species occur as pseudohyphae and yeasts, the latter measuring about 2 to 4 μm in diameter.

C. albicans is found in the gastrointestinal tract and mucocutaneous regions, and a variety of non-*albicans* species are found on the skin in healthy individuals. Their numbers are held in check naturally by saprophytic bacteria. Conditions in which the composition of the normal flora is altered are thus likely to lead to overgrowth of *Candida* species and an increased risk of infection. Such conditions exist in adults receiving antibiotic therapy or inhaled corticosteroids (the latter related to overgrowth in the upper airways). Other situations or diseases associated with an increased risk of colonization include diabetes mellitus, chronic debilitation, use of indwelling urinary and intravenous catheters, immunodeficiency (e.g., by congenital thymic deficiencies and AIDS), and prolonged hospital stay.[277,796] In such situations, the development of localized mucocutaneous candidiasis is not infrequent.

Fortunately, dissemination and visceral involvement, including that in the lungs, are uncommon.[731] Specific conditions that favor the development of visceral infection include malignancy (usually in association with immunosuppressive chemotherapy or the granulocytopenia associated with acute leukemia or lymphoma),[797] extensive burns, major abdominal or open heart surgery,[798] intravenous drug abuse (with a propensity for the development of endocarditis), organ transplantation,[799] parenteral hyperalimentation, central venous catheters, and extended antibiotic therapy.

Pulmonary disease can be manifested as a primary infection (bronchopneumonia), which in many cases is probably acquired by aspiration of organisms from the oral cavity, or as blood-borne miliary disease, the latter often associated with a primary focus in the gastrointestinal tract.[800] The inflammatory cellular response in both situations is related to the integrity of host defense, there being little or none in granulocytopenic patients and a variably intense polymorphonuclear infiltrate in other individuals. Granulomas are rarely seen.[801]

The most common radiographic manifestations consist of unilateral or bilateral areas of segmental or nonsegmental consolidation (Fig. 6–47).[802] Less commonly, a diffuse nodular or miliary pattern is seen.[803] Nodules may range from a few millimeters to 3 cm in diameter. Pleural effusions occur in approximately 20% of patients. HRCT findings include a bilateral, predominantly nodular pattern or bilateral areas of ground-glass attenuation and consolidation (see Fig. 6–47).[46]

The diagnosis should be considered in patients who have radiographic evidence of pulmonary disease and repeated, heavy growth of *Candida* in sputum that is otherwise free of pathogens. Because the organism is commonly a saprophyte of the oropharynx and occasionally the lower respiratory tract, conclusive diagnosis usually requires its demonstration in tissue.[804]

Aspergillus Species

Aspergillosis is a disease of worldwide distribution caused by the dimorphic fungus *Aspergillus*. Although over 300 species have been described, only a few have been associated with human disease, the most important being *Aspergillus fumigatus*. Other *Aspergillus* species occasionally pathogenic for humans are *A. niger*, *A. flavus*, and *A. glaucus*. In the mycelial phase, the organisms occur as septate, rather uniform hyphae that branch dichotomously at an angle of 45 degrees (Fig. 6–48). They are usually visible in tissue specimens stained with hematoxylin and eosin but are particularly well seen with periodic acid–Schiff (PAS) and Grocott methenamine stains. However, definite identification of a particular fungus as *Aspergillus* usually requires culture and immunohistochemical or molecular confirmation, particularly if only small amounts of tissue or fluid are available for examination.

Aspergillus organisms are ubiquitous in the environment, having been found in soil, water, and decaying organic

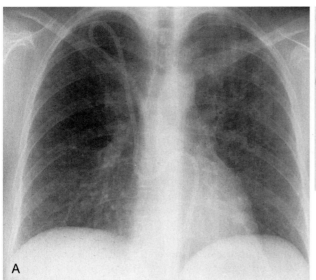

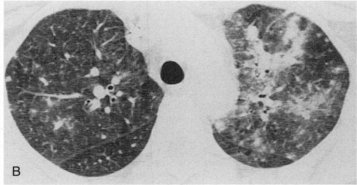

FIGURE 6–47

***Candida* pneumonia.** A posteroanterior chest radiograph (**A**) shows poorly defined areas of consolidation and a few nodular opacities in the upper lobes. An HRCT scan (**B**) shows nodules of various sizes, focal areas of consolidation, and ground-glass attenuation. The patient was a 27-year-old woman who had undergone bone marrow transplantation. *(From Müller NL, Fraser RS, Colman NC, Paré PD: Radiologic Diagnosis of Diseases of the Chest. Philadelphia, WB Saunders, 2001.)*

material of many types. In most instances, infection is believed to occur by inhalation of airborne conidia from a contaminated area. Colonization of the nasal mucosa not uncommonly precedes either disseminated or pulmonary infection.[805] There is no evidence of transmission from animal to human or from person to person.

Pathogenesis. The pathogenesis of the various types of *Aspergillus* infection is complex and incompletely understood. As might be expected, the quantity and virulence of inhaled organisms and the adequacy of host defense are the principal factors.[806,807]

Although *Aspergillus* species produce a variety of enzymes and toxins,[808] the precise mechanisms by which these substances are involved in the production of pulmonary disease are unclear. Intravenous injection of mycelial extracts from *A. fumigatus* and *A. flavus* is lethal in several animals and is capable of producing lung hemorrhage in dogs.[809] Several proteases are produced by *Aspergillus* organisms[810,811]; although the results of experimental studies provide evidence that some are involved in tissue invasion,[812] those of other investigations suggest that others have little role, if any.[813]

The presence of intact host defense, including that related to macrophage, neutrophil, and T-cell function, is clearly important in limiting the proliferation and spread of *Aspergillus* organisms.[814,815] For example, the results of some experimental studies suggest that alveolar macrophages may prevent germination of conidia by phagocytosing and killing them and that defense against invasion is dependent on this mechanism, at least initially.[816] Surfactant proteins A and D may have an important facilitatory role in such phagocytosis and killing.[817] *Aspergillus* organisms produce several substances that appear to be able to decrease the effectiveness of these cellular reactions. For example, there is evidence that spores of *A. fumigatus* secrete chemicals that inhibit phagocytosis,[818] the production of reactive

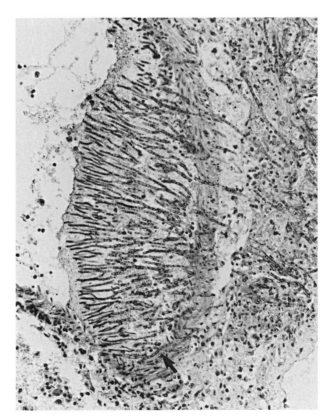

FIGURE 6–48

***Aspergillus* species.** A fan-shaped mass of septate hyphae is shown branching at an angle of approximately 45 degrees (*arrow*). Note how the fungi traverse the pulmonary artery wall with minimal inflammatory reaction or necrosis. *(From Fraser RS, Müller NL, Colman NC, Paré PD: Fraser and Paré's Diagnosis of Diseases of the Chest, 4th ed. Philadelphia, WB Saunders, 1999.)*

oxygen intermediates,[819] and the development of T-cell cytotoxicity.[820]

Disease caused by *Aspergillus* species can be manifested in three ways, each with distinctive clinical, radiologic, and pathologic features: (1) *saprophytic infestation*, in which the fungus colonizes airways, cavities (aspergilloma), or necrotic tissue; (2) *allergic disease*, characterized by such entities as allergic bronchopulmonary aspergillosis and extrinsic allergic alveolitis; and (3) *invasive disease*, a form that is usually acute in onset and rapidly fatal. Although these three varieties are not mutually exclusive—for example, occasional cases of saprophytic or allergic disease progress to invasive aspergillosis—as a rule, crossover does not occur.

Saprophytic Aspergillosis

Saprophytic aspergillosis is characterized by growth of the organism unassociated with invasion of viable tissue. Within the lungs, it may take three forms: (1) colonization of the tracheobronchial tree without the formation of macroscopically visible colonies, (2) invasion of necrotic tissue (such as an infarct or a necrotic neoplasm[821,822]), and (3) the development of a grossly identifiable colony within a preexisting cavity or ectatic bronchus (fungus ball, aspergilloma). Although these three forms do not usually have any clinical consequences, the latter may be associated with local tissue damage and hemoptysis. In addition, the saprophytic colonies can serve as a source for invasive disease when local or systemic defenses become compromised.

Airway Colonization

Airway colonization usually occurs in patients who have underlying airway disease, such as asthma, bronchiectasis, or chronic bronchitis. In these abnormalities, the organism has been cultured in 2% to 3% of patients in some series.[823] Colonization is particularly common in patients who have cystic fibrosis, in whom positive sputum cultures have been reported in as many as 50% to 55% of individuals.[824] The factors that aid *Aspergillus* organisms in colonizing the airways are not clear; however, there is experimental evidence that they produce several substances that cause epithelial damage and inhibit ciliary function.[825]

Fungus Ball

A fungus ball (mycetoma, aspergilloma) can be defined as a conglomeration of fungal hyphae admixed with mucus and cellular debris within a pulmonary cavity or ectatic bronchus. The disorders most commonly associated with this complication are tuberculosis and sarcoidosis.[826,827] The common factor in these and other less frequent underlying conditions is the presence of an enlarged cystic space in which normal clearance mechanisms are impaired. Although many fungal organisms inhaled within such spaces are probably killed by inflammatory cells, defective clearance presumably favors the establishment of colonies, which can then enlarge and form the grossly visible fungus ball.

Pathologically, an aspergilloma characteristically consists of a round to oval-shaped mass of tan-colored, somewhat friable material situated within a cavity having a fibrous wall of variable thickness (see Color Fig. 6–13). Histologically, the

wall is composed of mature fibrous tissue containing a variable number of chronic inflammatory cells and blood vessels; the latter, which mostly represent branches of the bronchial arteries and veins, may be abundant and are the source of hemoptysis in most cases.[828] An acute inflammatory or (rarely) granulomatous reaction can be present at the junction of the wall and the fungus ball; however, invasion of tissue by the organism is not usually seen.

Certain *Aspergillus* species, notably *A. niger*, are sometimes associated with local tissue deposition of crystals of calcium oxalate.[829] It has been speculated that the oxalic acid derived from these crystals may cause local tissue damage and result in intracavitary hemorrhage.[830]

Radiographically, a fungus ball consists of a solid, more or less round mass of soft tissue density within a spherical or ovoid cavity, usually in an upper lobe.[831] Typically, the mass is separated from the wall of the cavity by an air space of variable size and shape—the distinctive air crescent sign (Fig. 6–49). A fluid level is seldom present.[832] Most cavities are thin walled and contiguous with a pleural surface, which may be thickened.[833] In fact, thickening of the wall of a tuberculous cavity or the adjacent pleura has been described as an early radiographic sign of colonization that antedates detection of the fungus ball.

The fungus ball usually moves when the patient changes position[834]; however, some are irregular in shape and conform, for example, to an elongated bronchiectatic cavity, in which case change in position of the patient may not be accompanied by a concomitant movement of the fungus ball.

Similar to the radiograph, the most characteristic finding of an aspergilloma on CT scan consists of an ovoid or round soft tissue intracavitary mass that moves when the patient is turned from the supine to the prone position (see Fig. 6–49).[835] Areas of increased attenuation, presumably representing calcium deposits, are relatively common.[836] CT may show fungal fronds situated on the cavity wall that intersect with each other and form an irregular spongelike network that antedates development of the mature fungus ball.[836]

Although the abnormality may be discovered incidentally, cough and expectoration are common complaints; hemoptysis has been reported in 50% to 95% of cases.[837] The latter varies from relatively minor streaking of the sputum to life-threatening hemorrhage. There is evidence that serious bleeding may be more frequent in patients who have AIDS.[838] Most often, the diagnosis is readily apparent from the typical radiologic features; in the few patients in whom confirmation is necessary, transthoracic needle aspiration or bronchial washing of the affected lobe usually yields sufficient material for corroborative culture or cytologic identification. The diagnosis is supported by a positive precipitin test to fungal antigen[839] or by an elevated level of *Aspergillus*-specific IgE.[840]

The prognosis is generally good. The lesions undergo spontaneous lysis in 5% to 10% of cases,[841] and some disappear when bacterial infection develops within the cavity.[839] Nonetheless, as indicated previously, there may be massive hemoptysis, sometimes sufficient to result in death. Rarely, the fungus extends through the cavity wall into adjacent tissue,[842] where it may cause pneumonia or pleural effusion.

Allergic Aspergillosis

Hypersensitivity reactions to *Aspergillus* organisms can take three forms: (1) *extrinsic allergic alveolitis*, most likely the

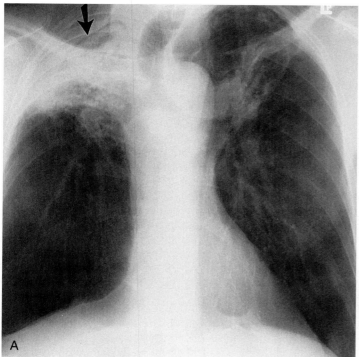

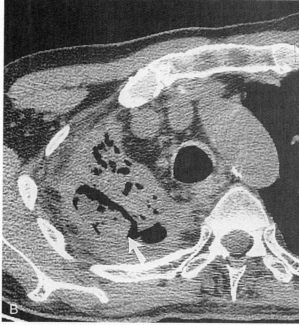

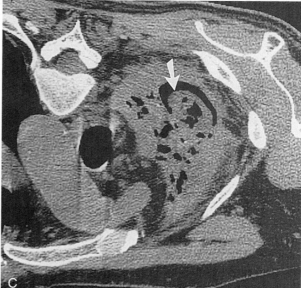

FIGURE 6–49

Aspergillus **with an air crescent sign and change in position.** A 65-year-old man with previous tuberculosis was evaluated for hemoptysis. A posteroanterior chest radiograph (**A**) shows extensive scarring in the upper lobes. A large fungus ball in the right upper lobe shows a characteristic crescent of air between it and the cavity wall (*arrow*). Marked pleural thickening surrounds the cavity. An HRCT scan with the patient supine (**B**) and prone (**C**) shows a change in position of the aspergilloma (*arrows*) despite its large size. Bronchiectasis and marked pleural thickening are also seen. *Aspergillus fumigatus* was recovered at bronchoscopy. *(From Müller NL, Fraser RS, Colman NC, Paré PD: Radiologic Diagnosis of Diseases of the Chest. Philadelphia, WB Saunders, 2001.)*

result of hypersensitivity to inhaled conidia and usually seen in an occupational setting[843]; (2) a *Löffler-like* syndrome[844]; and (3) allergic bronchopulmonary aspergillosis (ABPA). ABPA is by far the most common of the three and is the subject of the remainder of the discussion in this section. It is characterized by mucus plugging and bronchiectasis of the proximal airways and is usually seen in patients who have a history of asthma. The condition is also prevalent in patients who have cystic fibrosis.[845]

The pathogenesis is not clear. The fungus is able to proliferate in mucus in the airway lumen, which theoretically results in the production of a continual supply of antigen that may lead to chronic inflammation of the airway wall and the development of antibodies in the blood, skin sensitivity, and tissue and blood eosinophilia. However, why the condition develops in some individuals and not others remains a mystery. There is experimental evidence that spores of *A. fumigatus* show enhanced binding to activated epithelial cells and basement membrane components, a feature that may be related to colonization of the airways of patients with asthma, in whom such mucosal abnormalities are not uncommon.[846] Attempts to correlate attacks of ABPA with heavy exposure to spores have usually proved unsuccessful.[847] Nonetheless, it is generally accepted that episodes of ABPA are more common during periods of high atmospheric *Aspergillus* spore counts, which tend to occur during the winter months.[847]

Pathologically, the segmental and proximal subsegmental airways are characteristically dilated and filled with plugs of inspissated mucus that contain numerous eosinophils.[848] The bronchial walls adjacent to the mucus plugs contain an inflammatory infiltrate composed of eosinophils, lympho-cytes, and plasma cells. Scattered fragments of fungal hyphae can be identified within the mucus by special stains; tissue invasion is seen rarely. Although granulomas are usually absent in the walls of the ectatic airways, necrotizing granu-lomatous inflammation can sometimes be seen centered about distal bronchioles and small bronchi (bronchocentric granulomatosis).[849] Although this histologic pattern can be caused by other conditions (e.g., infections such as tubercu-losis and immunologic abnormalities such as rheumatoid disease[850,851]), it is most commonly associated with ABPA.

The typical radiographic pattern consists of homogeneous, finger-like shadows of unit density lying in a precise bronchial distribution, usually involving the upper lobes and almost always in the more central segmental bronchi rather than peripheral branches (Fig. 6–50). These bifurcating opacities have been described as having a *gloved-finger*, an *inverted Y or V*, or a *cluster-of-grapes* appearance. The shadows tend to be transient, but they may persist unchanged for weeks or even months or may enlarge. Bronchiectasis may be evident after expectoration of a mucus plug; when severely dilated, affected bronchi may contain a fluid level or an aspergilloma.[852] As with radiographs, the CT findings of ABPA consist principally of mucoid impaction and bronchiectasis involving predominantly the segmental and subsegmental airways (Fig. 6–51).[853] The bronchiectasis tends to be varicose and involve more than two lobes (the upper lobes predomi-nately). High attenuation of the mucus plugs, presumably related to the presence of calcium, may be evident on HRCT.[854]

Less common abnormalities include atelectasis and areas of consolidation.

Many patients have a variety of allergic manifestations in addition to asthma, including rhinitis, conjunctivitis, eczema, urticaria, and food allergy.[855] Acute episodes of ABPA are sometimes associated with increased cough, hemoptysis, fever, pleuritic pain, wheezing, and dyspnea[856]; however, there is often little change in the clinical state of the patient, and the incident is not recognized unless a chest radiograph is obtained or serum IgE levels are monitored.[857]

In a particular patient, confidence in diagnosis depends on the number and type of abnormalities that are identified, including (in approximate order of diagnostic importance) radiographic or CT manifestations of mucoid impaction or ectasia of proximal bronchi, asthma, eosinophilia of blood (>1000/mm^3) and sputum, an elevated serum IgE level (both total and specifically related to *Aspergillus*),[858] characteristic histologic findings on specimens obtained by bronchoscopy,[859] positive sputum culture for *Aspergillus* species, and an imme-diate or delayed skin reaction to intracutaneous injection of *Aspergillus* antigen.

Many patients whose disease remits with steroid therapy show subsequent exacerbations.[860] With recurrent attacks, almost half the patients expectorate mucus plugs,[856] and a slightly lesser number produce sufficient sputum to suggest the development of bronchiectasis.[861] Despite these find-ings, the long-term prognosis is good. Functional disability has been shown to be related to the chronicity of the disease.[861]

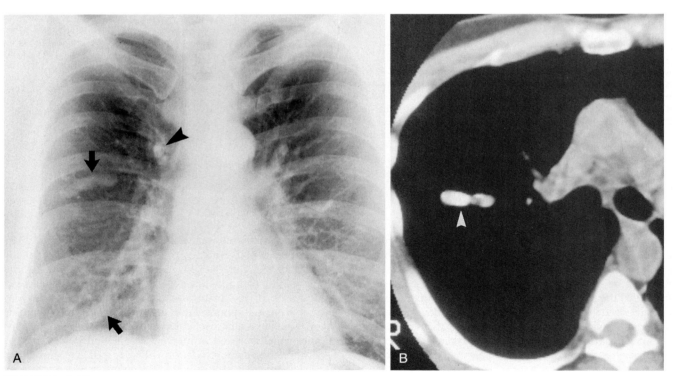

FIGURE 6–50

Allergic bronchopulmonary aspergillosis. A posteroanterior radiograph (**A**) shows branching, bandlike opacities in the right lower lobe (*oblique arrow*) and right upper lobe (*vertical arrow*); an end-on opacity (*arrowhead*) is seen in the upper part of the hilum. A CT scan (**B**) shows one of the opacities to be calcified (*arrowhead*). (*From Müller NL, Fraser RS, Colman NC, Paré PD: Radiologic Diagnosis of Diseases of the Chest. Philadelphia, WB Saunders, 2001.*)

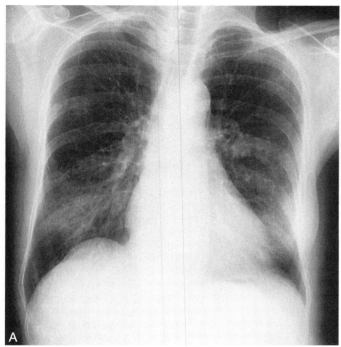

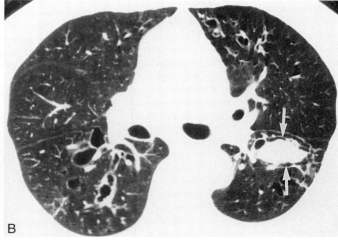

FIGURE 6–51

Allergic bronchopulmonary aspergillosis. A posteroanterior radiograph (**A**) reveals focal nodular opacities in the superior segment of the left lower lobe. An HRCT scan (**B**) demonstrates mucoid impaction in this segment (arrows), as well as extensive bronchiectasis. (From Fraser RS, Müller NL, Colman NC, Paré PD: Fraser and Paré's Diagnosis of Diseases of the Chest, 4th ed. Philadelphia, WB Saunders, 1999.)

Invasive Aspergillosis

Invasive aspergillosis is characterized by extension of *Aspergillus* organisms into viable tissue, usually associated with tissue destruction. Major risk factors for the complication include prolonged neutropenia (>3 weeks) or neutrophil dysfunction, corticosteroid therapy (particularly prolonged and high dose), transplantation (especially lung and bone marrow), hematologic malignancy (especially leukemia), cytotoxic therapy, and AIDS (the risk increasing with lower CD4+ counts).[862-864] Invasive disease also develops occasionally in patients with COPD (including emphysema, asthma, and cystic fibrosis)[865] or idiopathic pulmonary fibrosis[865]; corticosteroid therapy seems to be particularly important in this situation. Many patients who contract invasive aspergillosis are already hospitalized, and a variety of nosocomial sources of the organism have been identified, including central venous catheters and dust created during hospital renovation.[866,867]

Clinicopathologic Forms

Invasive pulmonary aspergillosis is manifested by four major clinicopathologic forms of disease that are useful to consider separately: acute bronchopneumonia, angioinvasive aspergillosis, acute tracheobronchitis, and chronic necrotizing aspergillosis.[868] The first two encompass the majority of cases; other uncommon forms of invasive disease within the thorax include bronchiolitis,[869] miliary disease[870] fibrosing mediastinitis,[871] and pleural infiltration with or without effusion.[872]

Acute Bronchopneumonia. Acute bronchopneumonia may develop secondary to bronchitis, as described later, or more commonly in a fashion analogous to bacterial bronchopneumonia (see Color Fig. 6–14). Pathologically, the inflammatory reaction is patchy in distribution and centered about the terminal airways.[868] Vascular permeation can occur but is not often apparent. Occasionally, the process becomes confluent (simulating acute air space pneumonia[873]) or nodular (resembling an abscess or angioinvasive disease[874]).

The radiographic pattern is one of patchy or homogeneous air space consolidation without specific features.[875,876] CT findings include foci of bilateral, predominantly peribronchial consolidation (Fig. 6–52) or poorly defined centrilobular nodular opacities measuring 2 to 5 mm in diameter.[877] Clinically, patients characteristically have unremitting fever that responds poorly to antibiotic therapy. Dyspnea and tachypnea occur in patients with more extensive disease.

Angioinvasive Aspergillosis. This form of disease is probably the most common manifestation of invasive pulmonary aspergillosis. Although it can be found in association with any of the other forms, it is frequently the sole abnormality. It is typically seen in patients who have acute leukemia.

Angioinvasive aspergillosis has two pathologic patterns[868,878]: (1) a relatively well defined nodule with a pale or yellowish center and a hemorrhagic rim (see Color Fig. 6–15) and (2) a less well defined, roughly wedge-shaped, pleural-based hemorrhagic area resembling a typical thromboembolic infarct. Although the latter probably reflects vascular occlusion and air space hemorrhage with or without ischemic necrosis, it is likely that the former is the result of locally produced toxins diffusing into the adjacent lung parenchyma.[868] Histologic examination of the central portion of the nodules shows necrotic lung parenchyma infiltrated by numerous fungal hyphae (see Color Fig. 6–15); the adjacent parenchyma shows intra-alveolar hemorrhage. Characteristically, there is also extensive vascular permeation and apparent occlusion of small to medium arteries by fungal hyphae; thrombus may or may not be present. Fragments of necrotic lung infiltrated by fungus (sequestra) may become separated from viable parenchyma (see Color Fig. 6–16), the space between the two

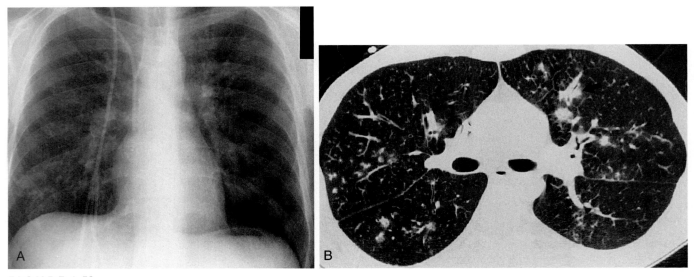

FIGURE 6–52

Aspergillus **bronchopneumonia.** In a 36-year-old man with fever and cough after allogeneic bone marrow transplantation, an anteroposterior chest radiograph (**A**) demonstrates poorly defined nodular opacities in both lungs. An HRCT scan (**B**) reveals focal areas of consolidation in a predominantly peribronchial distribution (*arrows*). *(From Fraser RS, Müller NL, Colman NC, Paré PD: Fraser and Paré's Diagnosis of Diseases of the Chest, 4th ed. Philadelphia, WB Saunders, 1999.)*

representing the air crescents seen radiologically (see farther on). It has been speculated that this separation of necrotic lung from viable parenchyma is related to enzymatic liquefaction of pulmonary tissue at the junction of tissue invaded and not invaded by fungus.[879]

The radiographic pattern consists of nodules or single or multiple areas of homogeneous consolidation (Fig. 6–53).[803,874] Cavitation is common and sometimes manifested by an air crescent partly or completely surrounding a central homogeneous mass (see Fig. 6–53).[880] This air crescent sign can develop 1 day to 3 weeks after the appearance of the initial radiographic abnormality.[881] Occasionally, the characteristic consolidation extends to involve an entire lobe and radiographically simulates acute bacterial pneumonia.[873] Pleural involvement is rare but may result in effusion or pneumothorax because of a bronchopleural fistula.[882]

CT may show a rim of ground-glass attenuation surrounding a soft tissue nodule (Fig. 6–54, "halo sign")[876,883] as a result of air space hemorrhage surrounding the nodule of necrotic lung tissue.[884,885] With time, these lesions may develop air crescents or progress to frank cavitation.[883] Vascular obstruction may result in homogeneous subsegmental, segmental, or lobar consolidation as a consequence of infarction or hemorrhage.[886]

Patients with angioinvasive aspergillosis commonly have fever, dyspnea, nonproductive cough, and pleuritic chest pain at initial evaluation; the combination of such pain with sinus tenderness, epistaxis, and nasal discharge is a useful clue to the diagnosis.[887] Hemoptysis may develop; when massive, it tends to occur during cavity/sequestrum formation,[881] often shortly after recovery from chemotherapy-induced neutropenia. In situ thrombosis of a large pulmonary artery may suggest acute thromboembolic disease.[888] Mediastinal and chest wall vessels are also affected occasionally and result in the superior vena cava syndrome or an absent peripheral pulse from subclavian

artery occlusion.[889] Invasion of the pleura[882] or the chest wall[890] can result in effusion, fistulas, or osteomyelitis, with corresponding signs and symptoms. Dissemination outside the thorax occurs in 25% to 50% of patients; involvement of the gastrointestinal tract (often associated with hemorrhage) or the central nervous system, or both, is frequently a terminal event.[874]

Acute Tracheobronchitis. Acute tracheobronchitis is a relatively uncommon manifestation of invasive aspergillosis in which infection is limited principally to the larger airways with little, if any, extension of organisms into surrounding pulmonary parenchyma or blood vessels.[868] Although it can be seen in any immunocompromised patient, acute tracheobronchitis has a particular predilection for the anastomotic site of lung or heart-lung transplants,[891] probably related to trauma and/or interruption of the bronchial vascular supply as a result of the surgery.

Pathologic findings consist of focal or diffuse mucosal ulceration, often associated with pseudomembranes or occlusive plugs composed of mucus, sloughed epithelial cells, and hyphae.[892] Patchy areas of atelectasis related to the mucus/mycelial plugs may be the only radiographic clue to the diagnosis.[835] Occasionally, tracheal or bronchial wall thickening is seen on HRCT.[877]

Patients may complain of dyspnea, cough, and/or hemoptysis; sputum production is generally scanty. Localized or generalized wheezing may be apparent.[893] If extensive enough or if located in a strategic site such as the trachea, the intraluminal mucus/mycelial plugs can lead to respiratory failure. Occasionally, fungi extend through the airway wall and cause fistulas[894] or sudden massive hemorrhage (as a result of infiltration of a major pulmonary artery).

Chronic Necrotizing Aspergillosis. This form (sometimes known as "semi-invasive" aspergillosis) is a rare and usually slowly progressive type of aspergillosis that often affects

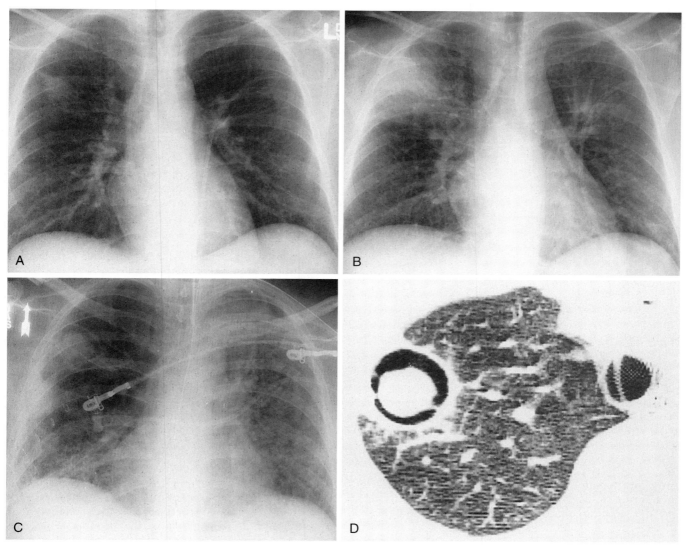

FIGURE 6–53

Angioinvasive aspergillosis—progression of radiographic findings. A 23-year-old patient with acute leukemia presented with fever and cough. An anteroposterior (AP) chest radiograph (**A**) demonstrates a rounded area of consolidation in the right upper lobe that showed considerable progression 1 week later (**B**). The following day, open lung biopsy demonstrated pulmonary hemorrhage but failed to identify any organisms. An AP chest radiograph 2 weeks after biopsy (**C**) and HRCT (**D**) demonstrates a smoothly marginated cavity in the right upper lobe containing a soft tissue mass. Repeat biopsy performed under CT guidance confirmed the diagnosis of invasive aspergillosis, the soft tissue mass within the cavity representing necrotic lung (sequestrum). *(From Fraser RS, Müller NL, Colman NC, Paré PD: Fraser and Paré's Diagnosis of Diseases of the Chest, 4th ed. Philadelphia, WB Saunders, 1999.)*

patients who have underlying chronic pulmonary disease.[895] Although conditions associated with abnormalities in host defense may also be present (e.g., diabetes, poor nutrition, connective tissue disorders), they are typically relatively mild in comparison to those associated with the more virulent forms of invasive disease. A history of intensive immunosuppressive therapy is usually absent; however, some patients have been taking low doses of corticosteroids.

In most patients, histologic examination shows a combination of necrosis, fibrosis, and granulomatous inflammation resembling chronic fibrocaseous tuberculosis[896]; vascular invasion by fungal hyphae is seen occasionally. A less common manifestation is the presence of an ectatic airway containing abundant fungal hyphae similar to a fungus ball; in contrast

to the latter, however, focal necrosis of the airway wall is associated with invasive hyphae.

The radiographic and CT manifestations consist of unilateral or bilateral areas of consolidation, with or without cavitation, and single or multiple nodules.[876,897] The areas of consolidation may have a segmental or lobar distribution.[897,898] The abnormalities are most commonly limited to the upper lobes but can also involve the lower lobes predominantly or exclusively.[897,898] The cavitation may be associated with an intracavitary mycetoma. Adjacent pleural thickening is common, and the infection may extend to involve the chest wall and mediastinum.[835]

Clinically, the disease has an indolent course (typically months and sometimes years).[864,896] Cough, expectoration

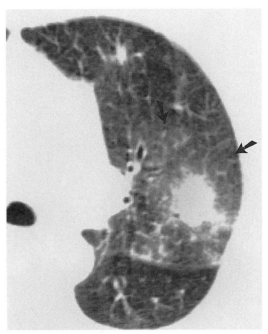

FIGURE 6–54

Angioinvasive aspergillosis—CT halo sign. HRCT of the left upper lobe demonstrates a nodule that is surrounded by a halo of ground-glass attenuation (*arrow*) (halo sign). The patient was a 72-year-old woman with acute leukemia. *(From Fraser RS, Müller NL, Colman NC, Paré PD: Fraser and Paré's Diagnosis of Diseases of the Chest, 4th ed. Philadelphia, WB Saunders, 1999.)*

(sometimes bloody), fever, and weight loss are the usual features. An increased white blood cell count is not infrequent. Spread of infection outside the thorax is uncommon.

Laboratory Findings and Diagnosis

The diagnosis of invasive aspergillosis should be suspected in any patient who is immunocompromised or has acute leukemia or other lymphoreticular or hematologic disease associated with granulocytopenia when fever does not respond to broad-spectrum antibiotics. Short of demonstrating hyphae in lung tissue by histologic examination, it may be difficult to prove. Sputum is unavailable for culture in many patients; even when it can be obtained, the sensitivity of culture (which depends on the number of specimens and the nature of the underlying disease) is probably no more than 50% to 60%.[899] Similar values have been found for culture of respiratory tract secretions sampled by BAL. To compound matters, a positive culture may reflect simple colonization. Nevertheless, in the appropriate clinical setting, a positive sputum or BAL fluid culture has been found to be a reliable method of diagnosis.[864,899] Because it has a high negative predictive value for pulmonary disease, surveillance culture of the nose may also be useful.[900] Blood cultures are infrequently positive.[837]

Serology is not helpful in diagnosis since infection may progress rapidly before the development of antibodies; moreover, antibody response is often poor in the clinical settings commonly associated with invasive disease.[864] Though not

widely available, a monoclonal antibody test to detect galactomannan (an antigen related to *Aspergillus*) has been reported to have a sensitivity and specificity of more than 90%.[901] The usefulness of PCR testing of lung secretions is limited to its high negative predictive value; the positive predictive value is relatively poor because of the inability to distinguish invasive disease from airway colonization.[902,903]

Prognosis

The prognosis of invasive aspergillosis is generally poor. Recovery is associated with early diagnosis, appropriate therapy, and reversal of the underlying immunosuppression.[904]

Zygomycosis

Zygomycosis (mucormycosis, phycomycosis) is caused by fungi of the orders Entomophthorales and Mucorales. In tissue, the organisms typically appear as broad (5 to 20 μm) nonseptate hyphae that branch at a 90-degree angle. They are worldwide in distribution and are commonly found in decaying organic material. They are also frequent laboratory contaminants. In culture and in nature, hyphae produce large sporangia that liberate sporangiospores into the air; inhalation of the latter is believed to cause most cases of human infection.

The disease can be divided into several clinicopathologic varieties, the main forms of which are rhinocerebral, pulmonary, cutaneous and subcutaneous (including sternotomy wound infection), and gastrointestinal. Usually, there is only local progression of disease at these sites; dissemination occasionally results in multiorgan involvement.[905] *Rhizopus* species are responsible for the rhinocerebral form of the disease, whereas a variety of species of other genera, as well as *Rhizopus*, are the cause of pulmonary disease.[906] Rhinocerebral zygomycosis is a fulminant disease that involves the nose and paranasal sinuses and frequently extends into the orbits and cranium[907]; occasionally, it also involves the lungs, presumably by aspiration. Primary pulmonary disease occurs most often in patients who have undergone transplantation or who have lymphoproliferative or hematologic disorders or diabetes.[908,909] The incidence of the disease has been found to range from 1% to 9% after organ transplantation, as opposed to only 1% after bone marrow transplantation.[731]

The inflammatory reaction to the fungi is variable and ranges from none to an intense neutrophil infiltrate. Multinucleated giant cells are sometimes present, but well-formed granulomas are uncommon.[905] Fungal hyphae are often seen within vascular lumina and extending through their walls into the adjacent pulmonary parenchyma; concomitant necrosis and hemorrhage are common.

The most common radiographic findings consist of focal or multifocal, unilateral or bilateral air space consolidation.[910] The consolidation is frequently segmental and homogeneous as a result of vascular obstruction.[911,912] The consolidation may be round and rapidly progressive[913] (Fig. 6–55); occasionally, lobar expansion is noted.[910] Another common finding consists of solitary or multiple small or large nodules.[910] Cavitation of the areas of consolidation or nodules is seen in approximately 40% of patients. As with angioinvasive aspergillosis, CT scan may show a halo of ground-glass attenuation surrounding the

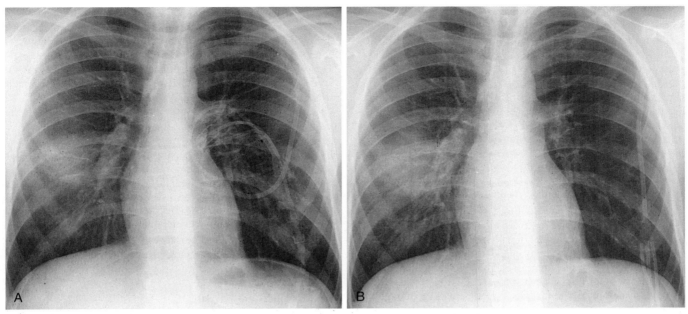

FIGURE 6–55

Mucormycosis. A posteroanterior (**A**) chest radiograph demonstrates a rounded area of consolidation in the superior segment of the right lower lobe. A follow-up radiograph obtained the next day (**B**) shows a considerable increase in size of the consolidation. The patient was a 15-year-old boy with severe neutropenia secondary to chemotherapy for acute leukemia. (*Case courtesy of Dr. James Barrie, University of Alberta Hospital, Edmonton, Canada.*)

nodule (halo sign).[911] Associated hilar or mediastinal lymph node enlargement occurs in approximately 10% of patients and unilateral or bilateral pleural effusion in 20%.[910]

Patients are usually ill with fever, cough, chest pain, dyspnea, and bloody sputum.[909] Massive pulmonary hemorrhage, commonly fatal, can occur as a result of erosion of a pulmonary artery.[914] In most instances, this complication is preceded by radiographic opacities, often with cavitation or air crescents. Definitive diagnosis can be difficult and generally requires histologic confirmation. The prognosis is grave; in one review of the literature published in 1999, only 38 (44%) of 87 patients who had pulmonary mucormycosis survived[909]; mortality is almost uniform in disseminated disease.[915]

Geotrichum candidum

Geotrichosis is a rare disease caused by *G. candidum*, a ubiquitous yeastlike fungus that is found in soil, sewage, animal excreta, and a variety of dairy and other spoiled food products. It can also be a normal inhabitant of the human gastrointestinal tract and is sometimes isolated from the sputum of healthy individuals.[916]

G. candidum is detected most frequently as a saprophyte in the sputum of patients who have chronic pulmonary disease. Most cases of clinically evident disease are believed to develop once such colonization has been established. Both bronchial and bronchopulmonary forms may be seen. The former is characterized by symptoms of bronchitis or asthma, sometimes associated with eosinophilia.[917] Bronchoscopic or gross pathologic examination reveals yellow-white plaques adherent to the airway mucosa, similar to the plaques of oral candidiasis[916]; invasion of underlying parenchyma does not occur. By

contrast, in the bronchopulmonary form, tissue invasion is characteristic and may be extensive. Fever and hemoptysis are present in most cases, and crackles, rhonchi, and signs of consolidation may be detected. In both the bronchial and bronchopulmonary forms, purulent expectoration may be copious, and the sputum may be gelatinous.[918]

Radiographic findings are not distinctive. The bronchial form of the disease may be associated with no abnormalities or with accentuation of the basal pulmonary markings.[917,919] The bronchopulmonary form is usually manifested as parenchymal consolidation, predominantly in the upper lobes and frequently associated with thin-walled cavities.[920]

Because colonization is relatively more common than infection, tissue confirmation of the presence of fungus and an inflammatory reaction to it is necessary for definitive diagnosis.

Sporothrix schenckii

Sporotrichosis is caused by *S. schenckii*, a dimorphic fungus that is a common saprophyte of worldwide distribution. The organism has been found in soil, peat moss, and decaying vegetable matter, on thorns, and in a variety of other substances; rarely, it can be isolated from secretions derived from the normal human respiratory tract.[921] Disease is acquired most often by direct inoculation of organisms into the skin from thorns, splinters, or other contaminated objects. Respiratory disease is usually primary and presumably results from inhalation of airborne spores; occasionally, it represents dissemination from a cutaneous lesion. Most affected individuals have no evidence of immunodeficiency, particularly when the infection is confined to the skin; however, alcoholics appear to be susceptible to both cutaneous and pulmonary disease,[922] and cell-mediated immunity is often abnormal in patients in whom it is disseminated.[923]

Pathologic findings in the lung usually consist of solitary or multiple thin-walled cavities. The typical histologic appearance consists of multifocal areas of necrosis surrounded by a granulomatous inflammatory infiltrate containing numerous giant cells[922]; well-defined granulomas tend to be sparse. Fibrosis is frequently present and may be prominent. Organisms can be seen with PAS and Grocott stains but may be few in number and difficult to identify with certainty; in fact, immunohistochemical study is considerably more sensitive than routine histochemistry.[924]

Radiographically, the disease also closely resembles postprimary tuberculosis and, as a result, is probably frequently misdiagnosed.[922] Findings include isolated nodular masses that may cavitate and leave thin-walled cavities and a diffuse reticulonodular pattern.[922] Hilar lymph node enlargement occurs in many cases and may cause bronchial obstruction.[925] Bronchopulmonary and mediastinal lymph node enlargement can be present in the absence of parenchymal disease.[926] In some cases, pulmonary disease spreads through the pleura into the chest wall and thereby creates a sinus tract.[925]

The most common clinical form of disease is lymphocutaneous; extracutaneous or disseminated disease is uncommon and pulmonary disease is rare. Pulmonary involvement may be associated with malaise, cough, and fever. The diagnosis should be considered in any patient with chronic cavitary disease suspected of being tuberculosis in which acid-fast organisms are not found. Such disease may progress slowly over a period of several years.[927]

The organism can be readily isolated from sputum and may be seen in sputum specimens submitted for cytologic examination.[927] However, as indicated previously, it can exist as a simple saprophyte, and its presence in these specimens does not necessarily indicate disease. Serologic investigation using the direct fluorescent antibody technique appears to be highly specific.[928]

Miscellaneous Fungal Infections

Adiaspiromycosis is a disease of worldwide distribution that is found in many animals but only rarely in humans.[929] It is caused by the dimorphic fungus *Chrysosporium parvum* (*Emmonsia crescens*). Infection is believed to be acquired by inhalation of spores (aleuriospores) measuring 3 to 4 μm in diameter that are produced by mycelia in the soil.[930] Such infection is variably severe and ranges from a solitary granuloma discovered as an incidental finding at autopsy[931] to extensive bilateral pneumonia.[932]

Pseudallescheriasis (allescheriasis, monosporidiosis, petriellidiosis) is caused by a ubiquitous soil- or sewage-inhabiting fungus that in its perfect form is known as *Pseudallescheria boydii*. In tissue, the organism appears as septate hyphae similar to *Aspergillus* species, from which it cannot usually be confidently distinguished by morphology alone. Many of the reported cases have involved farmers or other individuals from rural areas.[933] In the lungs, the organism is found most frequently as a colonizer in association with chronic fibrotic disease such as tuberculosis, sarcoidosis, or ankylosing spondylitis[934,935]; immunosuppressive or corticosteroid therapy is also a risk for colonization and disease. Cases of allergic bronchopulmonary disease and bronchopneumonia similar to those caused by *Aspergillus* have also been documented.[936,937] Patients may be asymptomatic or may suffer repeated episodes of hemoptysis; sometimes, the only symptoms and signs are those of the underlying disease. Symptoms of asthma associated with peripheral eosinophilia and an elevated serum IgE level are seen in patients with allergic disease.[936] The organism must be cultured for certain diagnosis.

Penicilliosis is caused by a variety of *Penicillium* species, the most commonly implicated of which in human disease is *Penicillium marneffei*.[938] The organisms are ubiquitous inhabitants of soil and decomposing organic matter. They are also common airborne contaminants of culture media, and care must be exercised when interpreting a positive culture result as definitive evidence of disease. Most cases have been reported in individuals residing in Southeast Asia.[939,940] Although the disease can also develop elsewhere, there is often a history of residence in or travel to an endemic region.[938] Many patients have underlying immunodeficiency; in fact, in endemic areas, the organism has been found to be a common cause of opportunistic infection in patients who have AIDS.[939]

Pathologic findings are those of necrotizing pneumonia, sometimes associated with multinucleated giant cell and/or true granuloma formation.[938,941]

Clinical features include fever, weight loss, anemia, and leukocytosis.[939] Skin lesions (usually papules with or without central necrosis) occur in about two thirds of patients.[942] Pleural effusion has been reported with absence of disease elsewhere.[943] Cough is the principal manifestation of pulmonary involvement.

Actinomyces Species

Actinomycosis is caused by a variety of species, but *A. israelii* is the most important cause of human disease. The organisms are non–spore forming and consist of branching filaments about 0.2 to 0.3 μm in diameter that are pleomorphic in shape. They are anaerobic or microaerophilic and form mycelia that fragment into bacillary or coccobacillary forms. Within tissue, mycelia are characteristically aggregated in clusters (sometimes termed "sulfur granules" because of their yellow color, although their sulfur content is minimal).

The organisms are normal inhabitants of the human oropharynx and are frequently found in the crypts of surgically excised tonsils, in dental caries, and at the gingival margins of persons who have poor oral hygiene.[944] In most cases, disease is believed to be acquired by spread of the organisms from these sites,[945] usually directly from the oropharynx into the lungs by aspiration or into the gastrointestinal tract by swallowing. The condition is worldwide in distribution; men are affected somewhat more often than women.[946]

Before the advent of antibiotics, actinomycosis was the most commonly diagnosed "fungal" disease of the lungs; it presented a fairly typical clinical picture of empyema and sinus tracts in the chest wall. Nowadays, it is seen most commonly in the cervicofacial region after dental extraction, usually in the form of osteomyelitis of the mandible or a soft tissue abscess that often drains spontaneously through the skin. Pulmonary disease, with or without chest wall involvement, is uncommon.

Grossly, the lungs typically contain one or more abscesses, the latter often interconnected by sinus tracts.[944] Sulfur

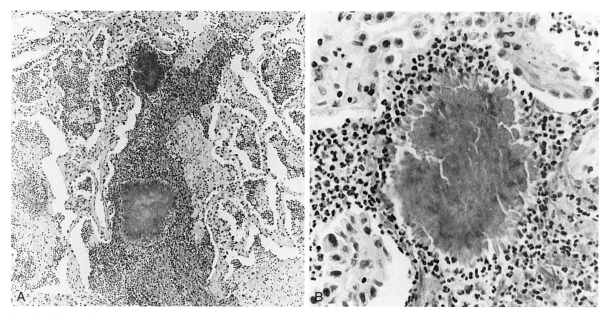

FIGURE 6–56

Actinomycosis. A section of lung parenchyma (**A**) shows a mild degree of alveolar interstitial fibrosis and extensive air space filling by alveolar macrophages. A neutrophilic exudate is also evident, probably in a respiratory bronchiole; it contains two small actinomycotic colonies (one of which is magnified in **B**). *(From Fraser RS, Müller NL, Colman NC, Paré PD: Fraser and Paré's Diagnosis of Diseases of the Chest, 4th ed. Philadelphia, WB Saunders, 1999.)*

granules can be seen within neutrophil aggregates on histologic examination (Fig. 6–56). Organisms are usually easily identified by Gram and silver stains. The characteristic granules can also be seen in sputum and in specimens obtained by transthoracic needle aspiration.[947,948]

The most common radiologic manifestation consists of patchy or confluent unilateral air space consolidation.[949,950] Occasionally, a patient has a nodule or mass, sometimes cavitated. The areas of consolidation usually measure between 2 and 12 cm in diameter and tend to involve the lower lobes predominantly or exclusively (Fig. 6–57). Pleural thickening adjacent to the consolidation is evident on radiographs in approximately 50% of patients and on CT in 75% to 100%.[949,950] CT often demonstrates central areas of low attenuation within the consolidation and rim enhancement after intravenous administration of contrast material (see Fig. 6–57). Hilar or mediastinal lymphadenopathy is evident on CT scan in most cases.[950] Chest wall invasion is uncommon.

The initial clinical manifestations of pulmonary involvement are cough, sputum production, and hemoptysis.[951] Progression of infection may be manifested as one or more sinus tracts through the skin or, rarely, a bronchocutaneous fistula or a fistula into the mediastinum, liver, or neck. Dissemination to extrapulmonary sites may simulate metastatic pulmonary carcinoma.[952] The prognosis is generally good, provided that the infection is recognized and appropriate antibiotic therapy is instituted.

Nocardia Species

The most important species with respect to human pulmonary nocardiosis is *N. asteroides*,[953] an aerobic, non–

spore-forming bacterium that in tissue consists of thin, branching filaments. The latter are gram positive and usually acid-fast, although many show this property only with weak decolorizing agents. The organism may be identified on smears or cultures of exudate from the lung and extrathoracic abscesses; however, prolonged culture on selective media may be necessary for successful isolation.[954]

Nocardia species are common natural inhabitants of soil throughout the world, and most cases of pulmonary disease are believed to be acquired by inhalation from this source. Person-to-person transmission is rare, but has been well documented.[955] The organism can be found as a saprophyte in the sputum of patients who have chronic obstructive or other lung disease.[956] Most cases of disease are seen in patients who are immunocompromised.[957,958] Nonetheless, it is a relatively uncommon cause of opportunistic infection in AIDS.[954] For unclear reasons, patients with alveolar proteinosis appear to be particularly susceptible.[959]

Pulmonary disease is manifested pathologically as microabscesses or macroabscesses, usually associated with granulation tissue and fibrosis in the more long-standing cases. Organisms can be identified admixed with neutrophils on silver stain.

The most frequent radiographic abnormality is air space consolidation, usually homogeneous and nonsegmental, but sometimes patchy and inhomogeneous (Fig. 6–58).[960,961] The consolidation is most commonly multilobar.[962] Another common finding is the presence of nodules or masses.[963] CT frequently demonstrates localized areas of low attenuation with rim enhancement suggestive of abscess formation within both the areas of consolidation and the nodules.[963,964] Cavitation is seen on CT in approximately 80% of patients with AIDS and in 20% of those without AIDS.[963] The infection may

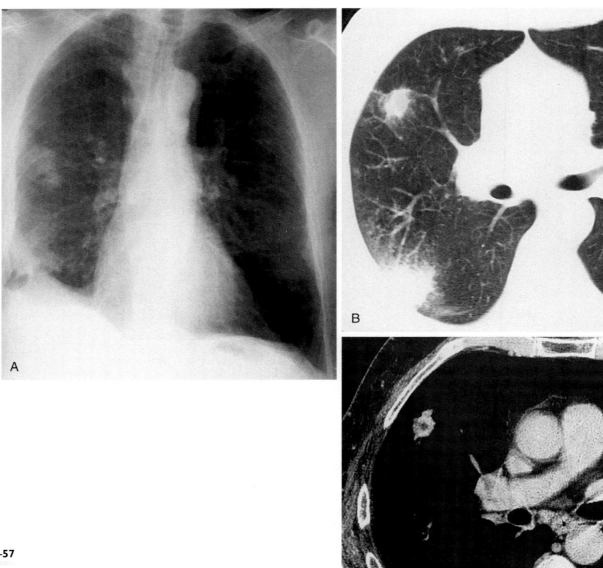

FIGURE 6–57

Pleuropulmonary actinomycosis. A posteroanterior chest radiograph (**A**) and a 10-mm-collimation CT scan (**B**) reveal patchy areas of consolidation in the right upper and lower lobes and associated right pleural thickening. HRCT (**C**) performed after the intravenous administration of contrast material demonstrates localized areas of low attenuation within the consolidation consistent with abscess formation. The patient was a 59-year-old alcoholic man. *(From Fraser RS, Müller NL, Colman NC, Paré PD: Fraser and Paré's Diagnosis of Diseases of the Chest, 4th ed. Philadelphia, WB Saunders, 1999.)*

extend into the pleural space and cause effusion or empyema and, less commonly, into the chest wall.[964]

Cough, purulent sputum, pleural pain, and fever are the usual symptoms; hemoptysis occurs occasionally.[957,965] Physical examination may reveal crackles, signs of consolidation, or pleural effusion.[966] The course is usually chronic; however, acute fulminating pneumonia can occur.[967] Infection occasionally spreads to extrathoracic sites, most often the brain or subcutaneous tissue.[968] The white blood cell count is usually moderately elevated, with neutrophilia.[957] The organism can be identified in fine-needle aspirates and bronchial wash specimens, but it can easily be missed during screening if not specifically looked for.[969]

The prognosis of pulmonary nocardiosis is not good; for example, in a review of 35 patients, the case fatality rate was 40%.[953] Once dissemination has occurred, the prognosis is even worse.[970]

VIRUSES

Many respiratory infections caused by viruses begin in the upper respiratory tract. Some organisms, including certain enteroviruses and the chickenpox and measles viruses, propagate there and then disseminate throughout the body, usually without producing lower respiratory tract symptoms. Others

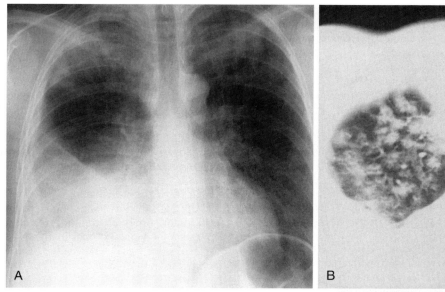

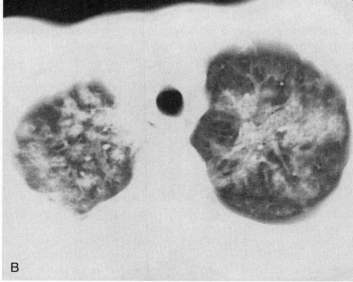

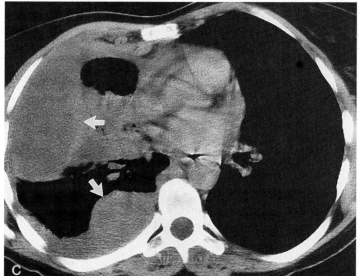

FIGURE 6–58

Pleuropulmonary nocardiosis. A 36-year-old previously healthy man was evaluated for severe pleuritic chest pain. A posteroanterior chest radiograph (**A**) demonstrates areas of consolidation in the upper lobes and right middle lobe and a right pleural effusion. A CT scan (**B**) shows extensive consolidation in the upper lobes. A CT scan photographed with soft tissue windows (**C**) demonstrates a large right pleural effusion with evidence of loculation anterolaterally and posteromedially (*arrows*). Consolidation in the right middle lobe is also evident. *Nocardia asteroides* was recovered from both BAL and pleural fluid. *(From Fraser RS, Müller NL, Colman NC, Paré PD: Fraser and Paré's Diagnosis of Diseases of the Chest, 4th ed. Philadelphia, WB Saunders, 1999.)*

typically remain confined to the respiratory mucosa, where they cause a spectrum of disease that includes rhinitis, pharyngitis, laryngotracheitis (croup), bronchitis, bronchiolitis, and pneumonia ("primary atypical pneumonia"). Although specific respiratory viruses tend to produce fairly well defined clinical syndromes, each can cause several forms of upper or lower respiratory tract disease, depending on the virulence and dose of the organism and host resistance.[37,971] Lower respiratory tract disease caused by these organisms, particularly pneumonia, is relatively uncommon; however, in certain populations such as infants or patients who are immunocompromised, the incidence of such infection, as well as clinically significant disease, is significant.

In addition to these acute complications, viral infection can have important long-term sequelae for the lungs. For example, experimental evidence suggests that neonatal infection may impair subsequent lung development,[972] and viral-induced childhood bronchiolitis is well recognized as a precursor of adult bronchiectasis. Airway infection can clearly induce

symptoms of asthma in patients who have this disease, and there is evidence that such infection in childhood is involved in the pathogenesis of asthma in later life.[50,973] Finally, several viruses such as Epstein-Barr virus (EBV), herpesvirus 8, and papillomavirus are implicated in the development of some pleural and pulmonary neoplasms.

The diagnosis of viral pneumonia is often one of exclusion and is based on an absence of sputum production, failure to culture pathogenic bacteria, relatively benign clinical findings, a white blood cell count that is normal or only slightly elevated, a chest radiograph that reveals bronchopneumonia or localized interstitial disease, and a lack of response to antibiotic therapy. Confirmation of the diagnosis and identification of the specific causative virus can be accomplished by a variety of means, including standard culture (which has the disadvantage of taking up to several weeks), shell-vial culture (in which centrifugation and the use of monoclonal antibodies can decrease the identification time to a few days), serology (again limited by the time taken for seroconversion to occur), detection of viral antigens within respiratory tract secretions or blood by monoclonal antibodies, detection of virus-associated molecules by in situ hybridization or PCR, and observation of virus-induced changes cytologically or histologically.[974] As might be expected, the sensitivity and specificity of these tests and their cost-effectiveness are variable and related to some extent to the underlying organism and the pattern of disease that it causes.

Influenza Virus

Influenza viruses are subdivided into types A, B, and C on the basis of internal membrane and nucleoprotein antigens. Group A can be subdivided into a variety of antigenic subtypes related to the presence of two distinct surface glycoproteins, hemagglutinin (H) and neuraminidase (N).[975,976] The former is necessary for binding to and penetration of the host cell membrane by the virus[977,978]; antibody to it is protective against infection. Neuraminidase is involved in the release and spread of replicated virus particles; although antibody against it is not as important in immunity as anti-H antibody is, it is capable of limiting the severity of the disease.

Influenza viruses have the important ability to change the structural (and hence antigenic) nature of these glycoproteins spontaneously, the variant forms possessing a virulence different from that of their progenitors. Types A, B, and C can all undergo minor structural changes; however, only type A has been found to produce immunologically distinct forms, which are designated by numerical subscripts in the H and N loci. Because immunity to infection is conferred by antibodies to the H and N glycoproteins, such antigenic changes are of major importance in explaining the pathogenesis of disease; they may be relatively minor (antigenic drift) or major (antigenic shift) in degree.

Epidemiology

Influenza can occur in pandemics, epidemics, or sporadically in individual or small clusters of patients. Type A viruses cause almost all severe epidemics and all pandemics. Even though outbreaks can also occur with type B, they are less frequent, more localized, and clinically less serious and often cause only a brief coryza-like illness. Although the type A virus is generally transmitted from person to person by droplet infection, antigenically similar viruses also infect swine, horses, and wild and domesticated birds, and human disease is occasionally derived from these sources. In fact, it is believed that these animals serve as a milieu for genetic recombination whereby new and sometimes more virulent strains capable of causing human disease are created.[979] Whatever the source, it is clear that influenza is an important infection: worldwide, it has been estimated to result in symptomatic disease in approximately 20% of children and 5% of adults each year.[975]

Influenza outbreaks tend to occur on an annual basis, typically during the winter in temperate climates; in tropical and subtropical areas they occur either during the rainy season or throughout the year, depending on the particular location.[975] Attack rates are especially high in schoolchildren; complications and hospitalization are also more likely in these individuals and in the elderly (particularly those residing in nursing homes). The 24- to 48-hour incubation period allows rapid spread of the disease. It is highly contagious, and a large proportion of individuals may contract the disease to some degree in closed environments such as cruise ships and airplanes.[980] Nosocomial transmission of disease is well documented.[981]

Pneumonia is an uncommon but serious complication of influenza infection that is usually caused by type A and occasionally type B organisms.[982] Although it is often localized and of only mild to moderate severity, it can be overwhelming and rapidly fatal. Most cases are recognized during epidemics or pandemics. In approximately a third of cases of severe pneumonia, the illness develops abruptly in apparently healthy persons.[983] Most of the remainder have a predisposing condition such as cardiac disease,[982] pregnancy,[984] cystic fibrosis,[985] or immunodeficiency. Infants and the elderly are at particular risk for serious disease.[986] Although the virus is the only pathogen recovered from the lungs in some patients at autopsy, thus implying that it can cause fatal pneumonia, in many cases death is related to superinfection by bacteria such as S. aureus, S. pneumoniae, H. influenzae, and M. catarrhalis.[982]

Pathogenesis and Pathologic Characteristics

Experimental studies have shown that viruses adhere to the cilia and microvilli of epithelial cells, from which they enter the cell cytoplasm.[987] Subsequent replication plus release of new virions is accompanied by degeneration and sloughing of epithelial cells that line bronchi, bronchioles, and alveoli.[988] Host defense against the organism is related to a variety of factors, including interferon-mediated production of Mx proteins, which appear to inhibit viral replication[989]; an appropriate immune response, particularly locally produced IgA[976]; and the presence of surfactant-related lectins capable of mediating viral aggregation.[990]

The typical histologic appearance of fatal influenza pneumonia is diffuse alveolar damage, the parenchyma showing a variably severe interstitial mononuclear inflammatory infiltrate; consolidation of alveolar air spaces by hemorrhage, edema, and fibrin; type II cell hyperplasia; and hyaline membranes.[991,992] Though not usually prominent except in association with bacterial superinfection, a polymorphonuclear infiltrate may also be seen in apparently pure viral infection.[993] The virus can be cultured or seen by immunofluorescence in a high proportion of cases.[994] Inclusions representing viral aggregates cannot be detected with light microscopy.

Radiologic Manifestations

Involvement may be local or general. The former is usually in the form of lower lobe segmental consolidation that may be either homogeneous or patchy and unilateral or bilateral.[995] Serial radiographs may show poorly defined, patchy areas of consolidation 1 to 2 cm in diameter that rapidly become confluent (Fig. 6–59). Pleural effusion is comparatively rare. Resolution averages about 3 weeks.

Clinical Manifestations

Clinical findings depend to some extent on the age and underlying health of the patient. In young adults, a flulike syndrome without significant pulmonary complaints is the most common manifestation. The syndrome has a rapid onset and consists of dry cough, myalgia, chills, headache,

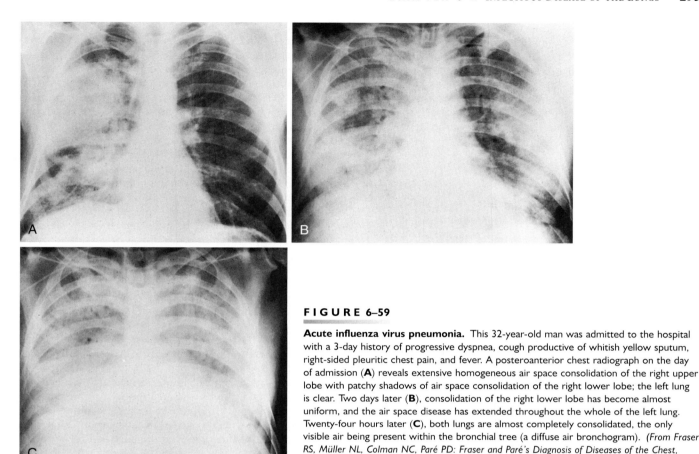

FIGURE 6–59

Acute influenza virus pneumonia. This 32-year-old man was admitted to the hospital with a 3-day history of progressive dyspnea, cough productive of whitish yellow sputum, right-sided pleuritic chest pain, and fever. A posteroanterior chest radiograph on the day of admission (**A**) reveals extensive homogeneous air space consolidation of the right upper lobe with patchy shadows of air space consolidation of the right lower lobe; the left lung is clear. Two days later (**B**), consolidation of the right lower lobe has become almost uniform, and the air space disease has extended throughout the whole of the left lung. Twenty-four hours later (**C**), both lungs are almost completely consolidated, the only visible air being present within the bronchial tree (a diffuse air bronchogram). *(From Fraser RS, Müller NL, Colman NC, Paré PD: Fraser and Paré's Diagnosis of Diseases of the Chest, 4th ed. Philadelphia, WB Saunders, 1999.)*

conjunctivitis, and a temperature of 38.5°C or higher. Substernal burning pain and signs of otitis media and/or sinusitis may be apparent. Significant rhinorrhea and pharyngitis are seldom seen.[996] Older patients have a tendency for the development of lower respiratory tract disease in addition to the flulike symptoms. Bronchitis/bronchiolitis may be manifested only by mild hemoptysis, with or without local or diffuse crackles and rhonchi. Patients who have pneumonia, however, may be extremely ill, with rapid progression of tachypnea, dyspnea, cyanosis, and hypoxemia. As indicated, many of these patients are elderly or have underlying cardiopulmonary disease. Airway or parenchymal involvement may also cause exacerbation of underlying disease in patients who have asthma, cystic fibrosis, and COPD.[997-999] Additional uncommon complications include seizures and encephalitis, myocarditis, pericarditis, myositis, and Reye's syndrome.[982]

Bacterial superinfection develops within 2 weeks (most often within a few days) after the initial viral infection. The patient—who may have been improving—begins to expectorate purulent sputum, which may be rusty or bloody, and may complain of pleural pain. Complications of such superinfection include all those normally associated with bacteria, such as abscess formation, sepsis, and empyema.

Laboratory Findings

The white blood cell count is usually normal in uncomplicated influenza; however, leukopenia develops in some cases, and overwhelming infection may result in neutrophilia of 20,000/mm³ or more. Bacterial superinfection is manifested by the production of purulent sputum and similar neutrophilia.

The virus can be isolated from respiratory tract secretions in monkey kidney cells or chick embryo; however, culture takes several days, and the yield decreases rapidly after the initial infection. More efficient and rapid methods of diagnosis include PCR and the detection of virus-associated antigens. A number of commercial tests that measure the latter are now available for office use[1000]; these tests are usually performed on nasal washes, give rapid results (often in 15 to 30 minutes), and depending on the particular test and study, have been associated with sensitivities and specificities in the range of 60% to 95% and 50% to 100%, respectively.[980,1000] Infection can also be confirmed by measurement of acute and convalescent antibody titers to components of a viral strain known to be epidemic at the time that a patient is ill.

Prognosis and Natural History

Most cases of uncomplicated influenza resolve spontaneously in days to weeks and are associated with complete recovery. The development of pneumonia, either primary or bacterial, is a serious sequela, particularly in the very young or very old and in patients who have underlying cardiac or pulmonary disease. Mortality rates in such populations may be as high as 3% to 5%.[975] Patients who survive the pulmonary infection may have residual, functionally significant fibrosis.[1001]

Epidemiologic studies performed during influenza epidemics and in cases of sporadic infection have revealed increased morbidity and mortality from both nonviral respiratory and cardiovascular disease.[1002,1003] The cause of the excess mortality is age related and is often cerebrovascular disease in patients older than 65 years and myocardial infarction in those 40 to 64 years of age.[1004] Patients at greatest risk are elderly residents of nursing homes, in which setting the mortality rate can be as high as 30%.[1005]

Parainfluenza Virus

Parainfluenza viruses can be classified into types 1, 2, 3, and 4, the first three of which are responsible for the vast majority of respiratory tract disease.[1006] Infections caused by types 1 and 2 occur predominantly in the autumn and early winter.[1007] They can achieve epidemic proportions and can account for a high proportion of cases of pneumonia, croup, and acute bronchiolitis in young children. Lower respiratory tract infection in adults is uncommon. Parainfluenza type 3 infection tends to occur in the spring and is an important cause of bronchiolitis or pneumonia in infants and children. Immunocompromised individuals of any age, particularly those who have received transplants, are also at increased risk.[1008,1009] In otherwise healthy adults, the organisms are responsible for pharyngitis and a small percentage of cases of coryza.

Respiratory Syncytial Virus

RSV is especially well known as a cause of disease in infants and small children,[980] in whom it has been estimated to be responsible for about 90,000 hospitalizations and 4500 deaths per year in the United States.[1010] It is being recognized increasingly in adults, particularly those who have underlying cardiopulmonary disease, malignancy, or immunodeficiency or those who are institutionalized[1011,1012] but also in individuals who are otherwise healthy.[1013] In fact, outbreaks in persons residing in nursing homes and in the general population have been found to have case rates close to those seen with influenza.[980,1013]

The virus can be separated into types A and B on the basis of antigenic differences in the surface glycoproteins F and G, which are responsible for adherence to and penetration of the organism into the host cell membrane.[1013] Infection may occur sporadically, as localized outbreaks, or in epidemics. It is highly contagious, and infection rates in relatively enclosed places such as daycare centers, nursing homes, and hospital pediatric wards may be high.[1014] Transmission is by airborne droplets or hand-to-hand or hand-to-surface contact. Immunity is associated with both cell-mediated and humoral responses and is usually incomplete (i.e., additional infections may occur throughout life).[1015] Surfactant proteins A and D appear to be important in innate defense against infection.

Pathologically, pulmonary RSV infection may involve the airways or the parenchyma predominantly.[1016] In the latter situation, disease is manifested as interstitial pneumonitis, sometimes as a pattern of giant cell pneumonia or diffuse alveolar damage.[1017,1018] When airway involvement predominates, the most severe changes occur in small membranous and respiratory bronchioles and consist of epithelial degeneration and desquamation accompanied by a variably intense inflammatory cell infiltrate. Cytoplasmic inclusions can be seen in some of the degenerated epithelial cells.[1016]

In infants, the chest radiograph shows patchy areas of consolidation interspersed with zones of overinflation.[1019] HRCT findings were reviewed in a series of 20 patients who had allogeneic bone marrow transplants.[1019a] The predominant abnormalities were small centrilobular nodules, air space consolidation, ground-glass opacities, and bronchial wall thickening. In most cases these abnormalities were bilateral and asymmetrical in distribution and present in both central and peripheral areas of the lungs. Rarely, patients experience an acute onset of pneumonia with rapid progression to ARDS.[1020]

Symptoms of RSV infection in adults are usually those of a "cold" (rhinitis, pharyngitis, and conjunctivitis, sometimes accompanied by otitis media or sinusitis). However, manifestations of lower respiratory tract involvement (most often cough) are seen in an appreciable number of patients. Some cases resemble influenza. In contrast to influenza and measles virus, infection by RSV seems to be associated with relatively little risk of bacterial superinfection.[1021] The organism can be propagated in cell culture, but slowly and with some difficulty; shell-vial culture has been shown to be both more rapid and more sensitive.[1022] Antigen detection by enzyme-linked immunoassay or immunofluorescence is even more rapid and as reliable.[1023]

Infection is mild and self-limited in the vast majority of patients. However, in adults who are immunocompromised or who have underlying cardiopulmonary disease and in infants and young children, it may be severe and rapidly fatal. The results of studies of the long-term sequelae of RSV bronchiolitis vary, with some investigators finding evidence of residual airway hyperresponsiveness[1024] and others no change in pulmonary function.[1025]

Coronaviruses

Coronaviruses typically cause coryza, most commonly during the winter and spring in temperate climates. Studies on volunteers inoculated intranasally with the organism suggest that disease is limited to the upper respiratory tract in the vast majority of cases.[1026] Nonetheless, the virus has been associated with exacerbations of asthma and COPD, presumably as a result of infection of the lower respiratory tract airways.[999]

More important from a clinical point of view was the discovery in 2003 that a form of coronavirus is the cause of severe acute respiratory syndrome (SARS).[1027] This highly contagious disease appears to have originated in China in 2002 and rapidly spread to affect patients in a number of countries around the world.[1028,1029] Within approximately 8 months, almost 8500 cases had been reported, over 800 of which proved to be fatal.[1027] The natural reservoir of the organism is thought to be wild animals such as ferrets, badgers, and civets.

Infection is believed to be transmitted by droplets or fomites in association with close interpersonal contact. Hospitals, laboratories involved in diagnosis or research on the organism, and nursing homes have been the most common sources of infection. Extensive spread has also been documented in confined environments such as airplanes. The pathologic findings are those of diffuse alveolar damage, sometimes with evidence of superimposed bacterial bronchopneumonia.[1030]

The most common radiographic manifestations consist of focal unilateral or multifocal unilateral or bilateral areas of consolidation.[1031,1032] The consolidation tends to predominantly involve the peripheral lung regions and the middle and lower lung zones. Less frequent findings include focal or diffuse ground-glass opacities and, rarely, lobar consolidation. Approximately 20% to 40% of patients have normal radiographs at initial evaluation.[1032,1033] HRCT demonstrates parenchymal abnormalities in virtually all these patients, the most common being focal, multifocal, or diffuse ground-glass opacities or areas of consolidation.[1035] Interlobular septal and intralobular interstitial thickening ("crazy-paving" pattern) is often seen superimposed on the ground-glass opacities. HRCT findings commonly seen in other pneumonias, such as branching nodular and linear opacities (tree-in-bud pattern), hilar and mediastinal lymph node enlargement, and pleural effusion, are uncommon.[1033,1035]

The incubation period is about 5 to 7 days. Initial symptoms include fever, chills with or without rigor, dry cough, myalgia, headache, and dizziness.[1029] Gastrointestinal and upper respiratory tract symptoms are seen less often. In some patients, the initial illness improves over a period of several days but is then followed by recurrent fever and radiologic progression of disease associated with a fall in serum viral load. In approximately 20% of cases the illness develops into full-blown ARDS. Laboratory findings include lymphopenia, evidence of DIC, and elevated blood levels of LDH and creatine kinase.

As indicated, the disease is serious, with a case fatality rate of approximately 10%.[1027] Risk factors associated with a relatively bad prognosis include older age, high peak LDH level, high neutrophil count at initial evaluation, chronic hepatitis B infection, and the presence of comorbid disease such as diabetes.

Measles Virus

Measles (rubeola) is a highly contagious viral disease that is seen most frequently in highly populated areas, where sporadic cases and small epidemics occur. Since the introduction of active immunization programs in the 1960s, there has been a remarkable reduction in the number of reported cases. Nonetheless, miniepidemics are still reported in "developed" countries,[1036] and the disease remains a significant problem in "developing" countries that lack effective immunization programs.[1037]

In its natural form, measles is found principally in small children. In countries that have active immunization programs, however, a significant number of older individuals contract the illness,[1038] presumably because of a combination of nonimmunization, vaccine failure (which occurs in about 5% of individuals), and decreased likelihood of childhood exposure to the organism. The infection is highly contagious and is probably spread largely by airborne droplets. The incubation period is about 10 days to 2 weeks.

Although some investigators have estimated that only about 5% of patients suffer a complication other than the typical rash,[1039] others have reported the occurrence of other complications in almost 45%.[1036] Pulmonary disease is the most common complication (3% to 4% of cases) and can occur as primary measles virus pneumonia or as secondary

bacterial pneumonia. The latter is the more common and is caused most often by S. pneumoniae, K. pneumoniae, H. influenzae, or N. meningitidis.[1040,1041] The risk of primary measles pneumonia appears to be higher in pregnant women and individuals who are immunocompromised.[1042,1043]

The pathologic findings of fatal measles pneumonia without bacterial superinfection are those of diffuse alveolar damage.[1044] Characteristically, this damage is associated with numerous multinucleated giant cells that contain eosinophilic nuclear and cytoplasmic viral inclusions (hence, giant cell pneumonia, Fig. 6–60). The giant cells may be seen in expectorated sputum or BAL specimens on cytologic examination before and concurrent with the rash.[1045]

In children, the most common findings are patchy air space consolidation, bronchial wall thickening, peribronchial infiltrates, perihilar linearity, small nodules, and lymph node enlargement.[1046,1047] In contrast to its frequency in children, radiologic evidence of lymph node enlargement in adults is uncommon.[1041] CT abnormalities include areas of ground-glass attenuation, small nodular opacities, and consolidation.[1048]

In the typical case, prodromal symptoms of fever, malaise, myalgia, headache, conjunctivitis, sneezing, coughing, and nasal discharge are present for 2 to 6 days before the characteristic maculopapular, erythematous rash appears. Primary measles pneumonia characteristically develops before or coincident with the peak of the measles exanthem and is manifested as cough and, in severe cases, hemoptysis, dyspnea, and features of ARDS.[1047] Bacterial superinfection usually occurs several days after the rash, when the patient's condition has begun to improve. It should be suspected when cough, purulent expectoration, tachycardia, rise in temperature, and pleural pain develop during early convalescence.

The white blood cell count in primary measles pneumonia may be normal but is often low, particularly in the early stage; in the presence of secondary bacterial infection, polymorphonuclear leukocytosis commonly develops. The diagnosis is usually evident from the clinical picture, including the characteristic rash. In atypical cases, the virus can be isolated on tissue cultures of throat washings or blood or identified by immunohistochemical means in biopsy or cytology specimens.[1049]

The overall fatality rate in "developed" countries is probably less than 0.1%; however, it is significantly greater in "developing" countries, in which many thousands of infants and children succumb each year. Most deaths are caused by pneumonia.[1037]

Enteroviruses

The enteroviruses include polioviruses, coxsackieviruses, and echoviruses. They are transmitted predominantly by the fecal-oral route and because of acid resistance are able to pass through the stomach and replicate in the lower intestinal tract. Children and young adults are most commonly affected. The incubation period ranges from 7 to 12 days.

Polioviruses

The effects of polioviruses on the thorax are usually indirect, paralysis of the muscles of respiration sometimes resulting in

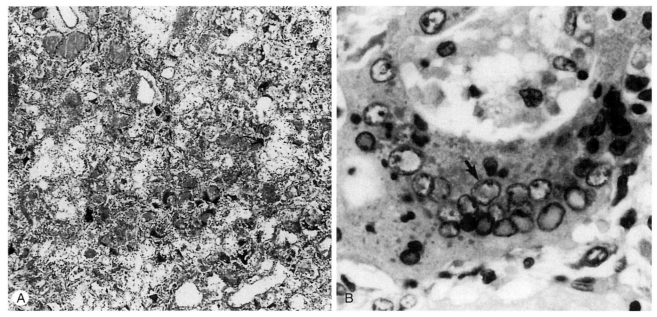

FIGURE 6–60

Measles (giant cell) pneumonia. A low-power view (**A**) shows extensive air space consolidation by proteinaceous fluid, macrophages, and red blood cells. Irregularly shaped giant cells are clearly visible. A magnified view (**B**) of one giant cell shows numerous nuclei, some of which contain lightly stained, but well-defined viral inclusions (*arrow*). *(From Fraser RS, Müller NL, Colman NC, Paré PD: Fraser and Paré's Diagnosis of Diseases of the Chest, 4th ed. Philadelphia, WB Saunders, 1999.)*

respiratory failure in acute disease and often in pulmonary function abnormalities in patients who have postpolio syndrome.[1050]

Coxsackieviruses

These viruses can be divided into *group A*, which is distinguished by its ability to induce flaccid paralysis in mice, and *group B*, which causes spastic paralysis. The former (particularly type A10) typically produce vesicular and ulcerative lesions on the soft palate and (occasionally) a coryza-like illness. Group B viruses cause a great variety of clinical diseases, including pharyngitis and pleurodynia.[1051] The latter consists of severe aching and gripping pain in the lower thoracic and upper abdominal regions, usually accompanied by difficulty breathing and fever. Remissions and exacerbations may occur over a period of several weeks. It may be associated with meningitis (evidenced by headache), myocarditis, pericarditis, and orchitis.

Rhinoviruses

Rhinoviruses are the cause of the common cold in approximately 40% to 50% of cases. Clinically significant lower respiratory tract infection is uncommon, but includes croup, acute bronchitis, bronchiolitis, and bronchopneumonia in both children and adults. There is evidence that children who have bronchopulmonary dysplasia and elderly adults with COPD are at increased risk for clinically significant disease.[1052,1053] The radiographic and clinical findings are identical to those of other viral pneumonias. Some investigators have shown a correlation between the severity of infection and

both lymphopenia, particularly of T4 cells, and polymorphonuclear leukocytosis.[1054]

Perhaps more important than direct infection is the indirect effect that rhinovirus may have on patients who have asthma. Although some studies of experimentally infected asthmatic volunteers have shown a minority to experience clinical exacerbation associated with only a mild decrease in flow rates,[1055] there is little doubt that the virus can cause clinically significant airway narrowing in some patients.[1056] Rhinovirus infection has also been associated with exacerbation of clinical symptoms and worsening pulmonary function in some patients who have COPD.[1057]

Retroviruses

Retroviruses are characterized by a unique mode of replication in which viral RNA is converted to DNA by the process of reverse transcription; the latter is then incorporated into the host cell DNA and acts as a template for the formation of new virions. Human retroviruses can be categorized in two groups: human T-cell leukemia viruses (HTLV) and human immunodeficiency viruses (HIV). Viruses in both groups share a pronounced tropism for cells expressing CD4 receptors (particularly lymphocytes) and the ability to persist for prolonged periods as clinically latent infection. Although each is more closely associated with extrathoracic or systemic disease—leukemia and degenerative neurologic disease in the former and AIDS in the latter—there is also evidence that they may have a direct pathogenic effect in the lungs in some patients. For example, analysis of BAL fluid from some patients who have HTLV-1–associated myelopathy has shown an increased cell count associated with an increased proportion of lymphocytes.[1058] In addition, histologic examination of the lungs has revealed nonspecific interstitial pneumonitis or bronchiolitis.[1059,1060]

The vast majority of the pulmonary manifestations associated with HIV-1 infection are secondary to viral-induced immunodeficiency. However, there is evidence that the virus also directly affects the lungs, most likely via circulating monocytes or lymphocytes emigrating from the blood into the alveolar interstitium and air spaces.[1061] The infection is manifested in BAL fluid by an increased number of lymphocytes, mostly CD8+; this increase is associated with a decreased number of CD4+ lymphocytes, the ratio of the two increasing with the development of clinical disease and with increasing severity of such disease.[1062] A variety of other abnormalities in BAL fluid cell type and function have also been documented.[1063,1064] It has been hypothesized that the presence of infected cells in the lung parenchyma may increase the likelihood of opportunistic infections by interfering with normal cellular defense mechanisms.[1061] It has also been suggested that HIV may be directly involved in the pathogenesis of lymphocytic interstitial pneumonitis and pulmonary emphysema in patients who have AIDS.[1065,1066]

Hantaviruses

Hantaviruses are lipid-enveloped, single-stranded RNA viruses that typically cause a symptom complex referred to as *hemorrhagic fever with renal syndrome*. Several antigenically different viruses from various parts of the world have been found to cause the syndrome, which is variable in severity and clinically characterized by fever, hypotension, and renal failure. In the early 1990s, Sin Nombre virus was identified as the agent responsible for a disease that was frequently fulminant and clinically severe and had prominent pulmonary involvement—the hantavirus pulmonary syndrome.[1067] Additional varieties of the virus, such as the Bayou and Black Creek Canal viruses, have since been recognized to cause similar disease.[1068,1069]

The natural reservoir of all hantaviruses is wild rodents, the deer mouse being the most important animal harboring the Sin Nombre variant in the United States.[1070] Climatic or other environmentally driven changes in the local rodent population are believed to be at least partly responsible for variations in the incidence of disease and the development of local outbreaks. The organism is thought to be transmitted by the inhalation of dried rodent excreta, and activities associated with an increased risk of such exposure, such as cleaning barns, trapping, and plowing with hand tools, have been associated with the development of infection. Presumably because of this association, most cases have been identified in rural areas. The majority of cases of Sin Nombre virus infection have been identified in the southwestern United States; infections with the Black Creek and Bayou viruses have occurred in Texas and southeastern states such as Florida. Most patients have been between the ages of 20 and 40 years.

Pathologic examination of the lungs of patients dying of hantavirus pulmonary syndrome show interstitial and air space edema with a mild to moderate interstitial infiltrate of cytologically mature and activated lymphocytes.[1071] Evidence of viral-induced tissue damage, such as epithelial necrosis, vascular thrombosis, or hyaline membranes, is typically sparse or absent. Virus-like particles can be identified in endothelial cells and alveolar macrophages by electron microscopic examination.

The initial chest radiograph often reveals changes indicative of interstitial pulmonary edema, including septal (Kerley B) lines, hilar indistinctness, and peribronchial cuffing (Fig. 6–61).[1072] Air space consolidation may also be evident and may rapidly become extensive. Pleural effusions are common and may be large. The time to resolution of the radiographic findings ranges from about 1 to 3 weeks in most cases.

The disease typically begins with a 2- to 3-day prodrome of fever, myalgia, and (sometimes) abdominal pain and headache; rash and features of coryza and pharyngitis are usually absent.[1070] The prodrome is followed after 3 to 6 days by progressive cough and dyspnea, tachypnea, and tachycardia. Respiratory failure with worsening hypoxemia and

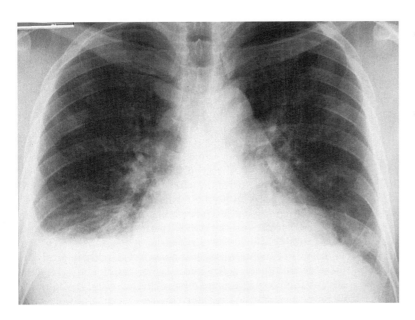

FIGURE 6–61

Hantavirus pneumonia. A chest radiograph demonstrates mild cardiomegaly with prominence of the pulmonary vascular markings and small bilateral pleural effusions. These findings resolved rapidly after renal dialysis. *(Case courtesy of Dr. Eun-Young Kang, Department of Radiology, Korea University Medical Center, Guro Hospital, Seoul, South Korea.)*

intractable hypotension may ensue. DIC develops in some cases. Patients who survive these acute events enter a convalescent phase, which may be remarkably rapid. The case fatality rate is about 50%.[1070] However, long-term sequelae in patients who survive appear to be slight, presumably reflecting minimal pulmonary tissue damage.

Laboratory findings include leukocytosis (sometimes to 25,000 cells/mm³ and often with a shift to the left), thrombocytopenia, increased LDH and AST, and hemoconcentration. The diagnosis can be confirmed by the demonstration of virus-specific IgM antibodies or a fourfold rise in IgG antibodies.[1073] The virus can also be detected in tissue samples by immunohistochemical examination or PCR.

Rubella Virus

Postnatal infection with rubella virus is characterized by fever, a maculopapular rash, and lymph node enlargement; lower respiratory tract involvement has not been reported. However, approximately 10% to 15% of infants born to mothers infected during the first trimester of pregnancy have congenital teratogenic anomalies that not uncommonly include the respiratory system. The most frequent abnormalities are pulmonary artery stenosis and interstitial pneumonitis.[1074] The former may affect the main pulmonary artery, its major branches, or less commonly, the muscular arteries in either isolated or multiple locations.[1075] The overall effect may be mild and unassociated with clinical evidence of stenosis or may be severe enough to result in pulmonary hypertension. Survival into adulthood can occur, sometimes with the development of cor pulmonale.[1076]

Adenovirus

Adenoviruses cause a small proportion of viral-induced respiratory disease.[1077] Infections may occur sporadically or as outbreaks in specific groups, such as military populations recently removed from civilian life, individuals in geriatric or psychiatric care centers, or children attending summer camp.[1078,1079] Immunocompromised patients, particularly those who have transplants or AIDS, appear to be particularly susceptible.[1080] Most cases of severe lower respiratory tract disease are associated with infection by types 3, 7, and 35.[1080-1082] Disease may be manifested as pharyngitis, pharyngoconjunctivitis, laryngotracheobronchitis, bronchiolitis, pneumonia, or a nonspecific acute respiratory syndrome.

Pathologic findings in severe cases include necrotizing bronchitis and bronchiolitis and/or diffuse alveolar damage; interstitial inflammation with little evidence of tissue necrosis may be present in milder disease. The virus can be seen as a homogeneous, basophilic inclusion occupying most of the nucleus of alveolar and airway epithelial cells.

The radiographic manifestations of adenovirus pneumonia in infants and young children usually consist of bilateral segmental or nonsegmental consolidation.[1083] Overinflation is seen in the majority of cases. Other common findings are lobar atelectasis and pleural effusion.[1083]

Adenoviruses are one of the more common causes of an acute respiratory syndrome characterized by fever, pharyngitis, cough, hoarseness, chest pain, and conjunctivitis. Chills and myalgia may be present and simulate influenza infection.

Tracheobronchitis is prominent in some cases and may resemble pertussis clinically. The pneumonia is generally mild and associated with upper respiratory symptoms.[1084] Patients usually have fever and nonproductive cough for several days before the onset of dyspnea.[1079] A transient fall in the white blood cell count and an elevation in transaminases, LDH, and creatine phosphokinase may be seen. A septic shocklike picture, sometimes associated with ARDS, may develop in more severely affected patients.[1079]

Complications of the primary infection are relatively uncommon. Bacterial superinfection occurs occasionally. As might be expected, disseminated infection is most frequent in immunocompromised patients. Pneumonia is rarely fatal in otherwise healthy adult patients. Long-term sequelae include bronchiectasis, bronchiolitis obliterans, and hyperlucent lung syndrome.[1085,1086] It has also been proposed that chronic (subclinical) airway infection may be involved in the pathogenesis COPD.[1087]

Herpesviruses

Herpesviruses are double-stranded DNA viruses that are surrounded by a lipid envelope derived from the host nuclear membrane. The organisms (genomes) are able to remain dormant within infected cells without causing recognizable disease, often for the lifetime of the individual. In certain circumstances, often associated with an alteration in immune function but sometimes without obvious clinical correlate, reactivation occurs and clinically evident disease ensues. Such disease is usually localized and well tolerated in otherwise healthy individuals; however, in immunocompromised patients, it is frequently disseminated and severe.

The organisms can be subdivided antigenically into more than 70 subtypes, only a small number of which have been implicated in adult human pleuropulmonary disease, including herpes simplex type 1 (HSV-1, herpesvirus hominis), herpesvirus 6, herpesvirus 8, varicella virus (varicella-zoster virus), CMV, and EBV.

Herpes Simplex Type I

HSV-1 is transmitted in situations of close personal contact through saliva or vesicle fluid and is most commonly associated with oral disease such as acute gingivostomatitis in children or recurrent coldsores (herpes labialis) in older individuals. Infection of the lower respiratory tract may be more common than generally appreciated: in an investigation of 308 consecutive patients who had severe lower respiratory tract infection, it was the most frequent microorganism identified.[1088] Such infection often involves only the tracheobronchial mucosa. Many such cases develop by extension from a focus of disease in the oropharynx or esophagus, either via aspiration or by direct mucosal spread; in some patients, extension appears to be the result of tracheal intubation.[1089] Many patients have an underlying predisposing condition such as severe burns, AIDS, malignancy, or an organ transplant.[1088-1090]

Tracheobronchial disease is manifested pathologically by focal or diffuse epithelial ulcers (Fig. 6–62).[1090,1091] Infected cells at the ulcer margins contain characteristic eosinophilic intranuclear inclusions or appear as single or multinucleated

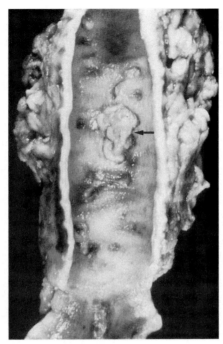

FIGURE 6–62

Herpes simplex tracheitis. The trachea of this 40-year-old burn patient has been opened posteriorly and reveals multiple foci of ulceration, some covered with a pyogenic membrane *(arrow)*. *(From Fraser RS, Müller NL, Colman NC, Paré PD: Fraser and Paré's Diagnosis of Diseases of the Chest, 4th ed. Philadelphia, WB Saunders, 1999.)*

cells that have ground-glass nuclei. Such cells may be detected in expectorated sputum or in bronchial washings or brushings and constitute strong evidence of lower respiratory tract HSV infection in the absence of oropharyngeal herpetic disease (which can cause specimen contamination).[1092] Pneumonia is usually characterized by alveolar necrosis and a proteinaceous exudate with a variable polymorphonuclear inflammatory response.

Radiologic manifestations of pneumonia consist most commonly of bilateral areas of air space consolidation.[1091] Occasionally, there are poorly defined nodular opacities corresponding on HRCT to small (3- to 20-mm-diameter) soft tissue nodules associated with areas of ground-glass attenuation.[886]

Tracheobronchial infection is manifested clinically by fever, productive cough, and in some patients, signs of bronchospasm[1088,1093]; hemoptysis occurs occasionally. Pseudomembranes related to tracheal ulcers may be large enough to cause upper airway obstruction.[1088] Symptoms of pneumonia are nonspecific and depend on the extent of disease. ARDS supervenes in some patients.[1094,1095]

The diagnosis of HSV tracheobronchitis or pneumonia is usually based on cytologic and histologic findings in specimens obtained by tracheobronchial brushing or biopsy; confirmation can be obtained by viral culture or by immunofluorescent or immunohistochemical studies. Bronchoscopy is valuable for identifying ulceration in the trachea and proximal bronchi and for improving the sensitivity and specificity of the cytologic diagnosis.[1091] The presence of mucocutaneous coldsores should raise suspicion of the disease; however, these lesions are often absent and may be seen in association with other diseases.

Herpesvirus 6

Herpesvirus 6 has been identified in BAL fluid or pulmonary tissue in a high proportion of transplant patients in some studies.[1096] Although evidence of clinically significant disease caused by the virus is not usually apparent in these patients, its presence has been associated with increased mortality, and it has been speculated that the infection may enhance the pathogenicity of other opportunistic organisms.[1096,1097] It is also possible that the virus causes interstitial pneumonitis in some patients.[1098]

Herpesvirus 8

Herpesvirus 8 has been implicated in the pathogenesis of a number of pleuropulmonary disorders, including hypertension, idiopathic pulmonary fibrosis, primary serosal (pleural) lymphoma, and Kaposi's sarcoma.[1099-1101] In fact, measurement of sequences of the organism in BAL fluid specimens by PCR has been found by some investigators to be a sensitive and specific technique for the diagnosis of pulmonary Kaposi's sarcoma.[1102]

Varicella Virus

Varicella virus (varicella-zoster virus) infection is seen in two clinical forms: (1) chickenpox (varicella), which represents primary and usually disseminated disease in previously uninfected individuals, and (2) zoster (shingles), which represents reactivation of latent virus, typically as a unilateral dermatomal skin eruption. Although either form may be associated with pneumonia, the majority of cases occur after chickenpox. In addition, zoster may be complicated by unilateral diaphragmatic paralysis, presumably as a result of extension of infection from the dorsal root to the adjacent posterior and lateral spinal cord and anterior horn cells.[1103]

Chickenpox is a highly contagious, predominantly mucocutaneous disease that tends to occur during the colder months in temperate climates.[1104] It is thought to be transmitted by droplet infection. In "developed" countries, most cases are recognized in childhood; in "developing" countries, disease is more common in adolescents and young adults. The overall incidence of pneumonia is about 10% to 15%; however, in adults admitted to the hospital in some older reviews, the incidence had been as high as 50%.[1105] Pneumonia is most common in adults who have severe cutaneous involvement. Preexisting neoplastic disease—particularly leukemia and lymphoma—and immunodeficiency are predisposing factors.[1106,1107] Both the incidence and the severity of pneumonia are also significantly greater in pregnant women.[1108]

Histologic findings in the more severe cases of pneumonia consist of diffuse alveolar damage. Angular, eosinophilic intranuclear inclusions surrounded by a halo can be seen in alveolar epithelial cells. Vesicles similar to those on the skin and mucous membranes may be seen in the trachea and larger bronchi and on the pleural and peritoneal surfaces.[1109] Pathologic features of healed infection (see later) consist of foci of hyalinized collagen or necrotic tissue surrounded by a fibrous capsule.[1110]

The characteristic radiographic pattern of acute pneumonia consists of multiple 5- to 10-mm-diameter nodular opacities (Fig. 6–63). Smaller nodular opacities and miliary-like nodules may also be seen but are uncommon.[1111] The opacities are usually fairly discrete in the lung periphery but tend to coalesce near the hila and in the lung bases.[1112] Progression to extensive air space consolidation can occur rapidly. Hilar lymph node enlargement occurs but may be difficult to appreciate because of contiguity of the consolidation in the parahilar parenchyma.[1109,1111-1113] Pleural effusion is uncommon and virtually never large.[1114]

Radiographic clearing usually takes from 10 days to several months.[1111] However, residual nodules, either calcified or not, may remain for many years after the pneumonia has resolved clinically.[1112,1115] The foci of calcification vary in size and number but seldom exceed 2 to 3 mm in diameter; they predominate in the lower half of the lungs. Hilar lymph nodes do not calcify.

The onset of chickenpox is often marked by high fever, which may precede the rash by 2 to 3 days. The rash itself may be scarlatiniform in its early stages but rapidly becomes maculopapular, vesicular, and pustular. It is often preceded by pain and, at least initially, has a distinct dermatomal distribution. Thoracic dermatomes are affected in approximately half the cases. Most patients have a history of contact with an affected child 3 to 21 days before onset of the acute illness. Symptoms and signs of pneumonia usually develop 2 to 3 days after appearance of the skin eruption and consist of cough, dyspnea, tachypnea, pleuritic chest pain, and in severe cases, hemoptysis and cyanosis. The temperature may be high. Expectoration is not purulent unless there is secondary bacterial infection (a relatively uncommon complication in comparison to influenza virus infection).

In approximately a third of cases, the white blood cell count exceeds 10,000/mm³ and is associated with polymorphonuclear leukocytosis. The virus can be cultured from fluid derived from early vesicles. Cytologic examination of vesicle scrapings for the presence of viral inclusions is a more rapid and frequently diagnostic procedure.

Cytomegalovirus

CMV is a common human pathogen that has been associated with a wide variety of illnesses, the manifestations of which depend largely on the immunologic status of the host. In children and older individuals, the virus is believed to be transmitted predominantly by direct contact with body secretions (e.g., saliva, tears, urine, semen) of an infected individual.[1116] Such infection is common, with seropositivity rates varying from 40% to 100% in different adult populations around the world.[1117] Higher rates tend to occur in groups with lower socioeconomic status. Most infections are unassociated with

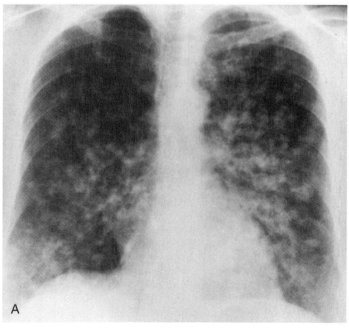
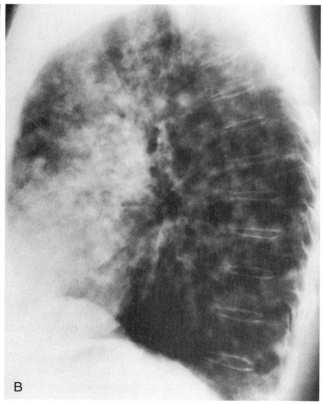

FIGURE 6–63

Acute varicella-zoster pneumonia. Posteroanterior (**A**) and lateral (**B**) radiographs reveal widespread pulmonary disease with a pattern characteristic of patchy air space consolidation. Also seen are multiple, poorly defined nodular opacities. The patient was a 42-year-old woman who had non-Hodgkin's lymphoma. *(From Fraser RS, Müller NL, Colman NC, Paré PD: Fraser and Paré's Diagnosis of Diseases of the Chest, 4th ed. Philadelphia, WB Saunders, 1999.)*

symptoms, the only significant effect being the presence of latent virus as a potential source of reinfection. As a corollary, CMV is an uncommon cause of community-acquired pneumonia.[1118] By contrast, pneumonia and other clinical manifestations of active infection are much more frequent in patients who have underlying disease, particularly immunodeficiency related to organ transplantation (see page 536).[1119]

Serologic studies indicate that many patients in whom clinical disease develops have had previous exposure to CMV (i.e., the disorder represents reactivation of latent virus).[1120] As with primary disease, this *secondary* form of infection can elicit an antibody response, and patients may remain asymptomatic, the principal manifestation of the infection being asymptomatic shedding of virus in various body secretions.[1120] It is also clear that seropositive patients can be reinfected from an exogenous source and that infection with two strains can occur at the same time.[1121] From a practical point of view, clinically evident disease tends to be more common and more severe in immunosuppressed patients who have primary disease (e.g., seronegative recipients of an organ transplant from a seropositive donor).[1117]

The pathologic characteristics of pulmonary CMV infection are variable and reflect the complex interaction between viral reproduction and host immunologic control. The organism may be cultured from the lung or BAL fluid of individuals who have no clinical symptoms and who show neither histologic evidence of disease nor the typical cytologic inclusions associated with presence of the virus.[1119] In other patients (particularly those who have AIDS), such inclusions can be identified focally in occasional cells or diffusely throughout the parenchyma, without evidence of pulmonary injury or inflammation.[1122,1123]

The pathogenesis of CMV-induced pulmonary disease is complex and not completely understood. It is clear from a variety of experimental and pathologic observations that the virus causes direct tissue damage in many cases.[1124] Clinical and experimental animal studies have provided evidence that an immunologically mediated mechanism may also be involved in the pathogenesis of disease in some cases.[1124] Pneumonia may be manifested pathologically as multiple, relatively well defined hemorrhagic nodules 0.1 to 1.5 cm in diameter scattered randomly throughout the parenchyma or as more diffuse disease (either diffuse alveolar damage or interstitial pneumonitis).[1125] Infected cells are significantly enlarged and contain round to oval, homogeneous, basophilic inclusions that fill most of the nucleus and are separated from its membrane by a distinct halo (*owl eye nucleus*) (Fig. 6–64). Intracytoplasmic inclusions, which appear after the nuclear inclusions are well developed, may also be seen.

The most common radiographic findings are bilateral linear opacities (reticular pattern), ground-glass opacities, and parenchymal consolidation (Fig. 6–65).[1126] Less frequent manifestations include small nodular opacities, a reticulonodular pattern, and lobar consolidation.[46,1127] HRCT findings usually consist of a combination of areas of ground-glass attenuation, parenchymal consolidation, and nodular or reticulonodular opacities (Fig. 6–66).[1128,1129] The abnormalities are bilateral and symmetrical and tend to involve all lung zones. Pleural effusion is seen in approximately 50% of cases.

In older children and adults without immunodeficiency, the only symptom of CMV infection may be prolonged fever.[1130] Some patients have features resembling infectious

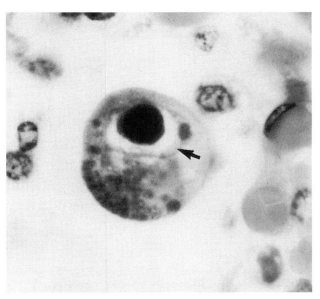

FIGURE 6–64

Cytomegalovirus. An infected pulmonary epithelial cell shows a deeply basophilic round nuclear inclusion surrounded by a clear halo (the nuclear membrane is indicated by an *arrow*). Several intracytoplasmic inclusions are also present. *(From Fraser RS, Müller NL, Colman NC, Paré PD: Fraser and Paré's Diagnosis of Diseases of the Chest, 4th ed. Philadelphia, WB Saunders, 1999.)*

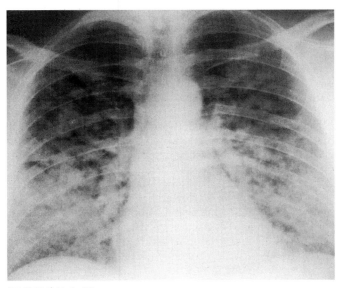

FIGURE 6–65

Acute cytomegalovirus pneumonia. A posteroanterior chest radiograph shows widespread patchy air space consolidation, more marked in the lower lobes. There is mild left ventricular enlargement. The patient had undergone renal transplantation. *(From Fraser RS, Müller NL, Colman NC, Paré PD: Fraser and Paré's Diagnosis of Diseases of the Chest, 4th ed. Philadelphia, WB Saunders, 1999.)*

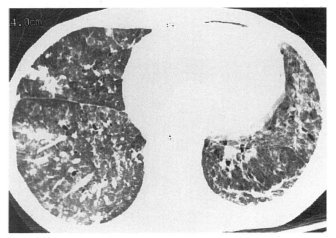

FIGURE 6–66

Cytomegalovirus pneumonia. An HRCT scan demonstrates bilateral nodular opacities with irregular margins and areas of ground-glass attenuation. Irregular linear opacities are present in the left lower lobe. The patient was a 38-year-old man who had undergone bilateral lung transplantation. *(From Fraser RS, Müller NL, Colman NC, Paré PD: Fraser and Paré's Diagnosis of Diseases of the Chest, 4th ed. Philadelphia, WB Saunders, 1999.)*

mononucleosis[1131]; pneumonia is an uncommon complication.[1132] CMV is a rare cause of community-acquired pneumonia without associated mononucleosis symptoms.[1118] Signs and symptoms of pulmonary involvement in immunocompromised individuals are nonspecific and include nonproductive cough, progressive dyspnea, and cyanosis.

As with other organisms, several techniques are available to detect CMV, each with its own advantages and limitations.[1133] The virus can be isolated from various body secretions, blood, or tissue, most efficiently by the shell-vial technique. Additional tests include immunostaining with monoclonal antibodies, in situ hybridization, and PCR, all of which have been evaluated in BAL fluid, blood, and tissue specimens.[1119,1134] A major limitation of these techniques is that identification of CMV in specimens other than tissue does not necessarily indicate concomitant disease. As a result, in some cases it is necessary to document tissue damage in biopsy specimens to be certain that the virus is truly pathogenic. Complement fixation, agglutination, ELISA, and radioimmunoassay methods have also been used to diagnose CMV infection serologically; as with other viral infections, a fourfold rise in titer is considered to be a positive test result. However, the time delay limits use of the technique in practice.

Epstein-Barr Virus

EBV infects B lymphocytes and pharyngeal epithelial cells, in which it can remain dormant for prolonged periods; clinical manifestations of disease are largely related to organs and tissues containing these cells. Infection usually occurs by direct person-to-person spread.

EBV is perhaps best known as the cause of infectious mononucleosis, a syndrome that affects predominantly young adults and consists of pharyngitis, fever, more or less diffuse lymph node enlargement, splenomegaly, and an increase in lymphocytes, often cytologically atypical, in peripheral blood.

Intrathoracic disease is uncommon and is manifested most often by lymph node enlargement (Fig. 6–67), interstitial pneumonitis, or both.[1135] Patients typically complain of the insidious onset of weakness, malaise, fever, and sore throat. Spasmodic cough productive of small amounts of sputum and dyspnea are manifestations of lower respiratory tract involvement.

EBV has been implicated in the development of several lymphoproliferative disorders, particularly high-grade lymphoma in association with AIDS or organ transplants (post-transplant lymphoproliferative disorders), some primary pleural lymphomas associated with chronic pyothorax, and lymphomatoid granulomatosis.[1136,1137] There is also evidence that it has a role in the pathogenesis of lymphocytic interstitial pneumonitis,[1138] idiopathic pulmonary fibrosis,[1100] and rare cases of pulmonary carcinoma.[1139]

Papillomaviruses

Papillomaviruses are the cause of squamous papillomas in the larynx and (less often) the lower respiratory tract (see page 374). There is evidence that the viruses are responsible for the development of pulmonary carcinoma in some patients who have this condition and, possibly, in those who have de novo bronchial squamous cell carcinoma.[1140,1141] As mentioned elsewhere (see page 836), there is also evidence that iatrogenic infection by simian virus 40 (a papovavirus that does not normally infect humans) may be involved in the pathogenesis of mesothelioma.

MYCOPLASMAS, CHLAMYDIAE, AND RICKETTSIAE

Mycoplasma pneumoniae

The mycoplasmas are the smallest free-living organisms that can be cultured on artificial media. Although they share a number of bacterial attributes, their small size, absence of a cell wall, and genetic features set them apart from most bacteria, and they are usually considered a separate group. Although the organisms are pleomorphic, they tend to be filamentous or rod shaped in tissue. At one end is a specialized terminal structure that is believed to be necessary for attachment of the organism to epithelial surfaces.

Of the various *Mycoplasma* species that have been isolated from the respiratory tract, *M. pneumoniae* is by far the most frequent cause of human disease. In fact, it is one of the more common causes of community-acquired pneumonia: it has been estimated to account for 10% to 15% of cases in the population as a whole[1142,1143] and up to 30% to 50% of cases in specific groups such as military recruits.[1144] Infections occur throughout the year, with a peak during the autumn and early winter in temperate regions. Disease is most common in individuals between 5 and 20 years of age. Transmission of the organism is usually from person to person by droplet inhalation secondary to coughing.

Despite the high incidence of pneumonia in the general population, the organism does not appear to be particularly contagious, with disease usually being transmitted after prolonged contact in families or close communities. In these

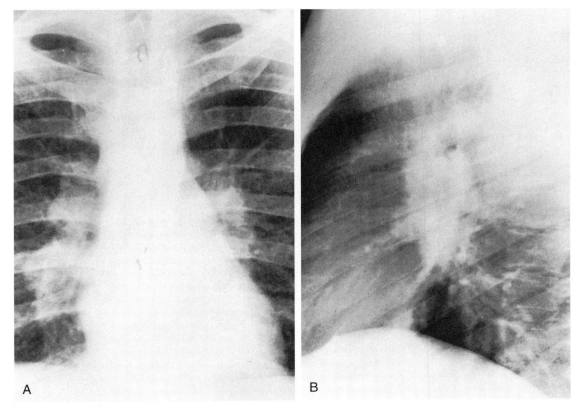

FIGURE 6–67

Infectious mononucleosis. This 17-year-old had a clinical history and laboratory findings compatible with infectious mononucleosis. Views from posteroanterior (**A**) and lateral (**B**) radiographs demonstrate marked enlargement of both hila, the lobulated contour being typical of lymph node enlargement. There is no evidence of mediastinal lymphadenopathy or pulmonary or pleural disease. One month later, a chest radiograph was normal. (*From Fraser RS, Müller NL, Colman NC, Paré PD: Fraser and Paré's Diagnosis of Diseases of the Chest, 4th ed. Philadelphia, WB Saunders, 1999.*)

settings, however, the infection rate is high; careful inquiry into family groups usually reveals symptoms of upper or lower respiratory tract involvement in most individuals.[1145] Local outbreaks of relatively severe infection can occur, again usually in families or community groups.[1146]

Pathogenesis and Pathologic Characteristics

In experimental and natural human infection, the organism is initially localized along the tracheobronchial epithelium, where it is in intimate contact with the surface of ciliated cells,[1147] apparently by attachment to its terminal unit. The pathogenesis of subsequent tissue damage may be related to several mechanisms, including (1) a direct cytotoxic effect of the organism, (2) the host immune reaction, and (3) cytotoxic and inflammatory changes resulting from contact of macrophages with the organism.

Pathologic findings consist principally of a peribronchial and peribronchiolar mononuclear inflammatory infiltrate (Fig. 6–68); epithelial ulceration and a neutrophilic infiltrate occur in more severe cases.[1148] Inflammation and type II cell hyperplasia occur to a variable degree in the adjacent parenchyma. Other histologic patterns reported occasionally include diffuse alveolar damage, organizing pneumonia, alveolar hemorrhage, and an alveolar proteinosis–like

picture.[1148,1149] To what extent these findings represent a direct effect of the *Mycoplasma* organism or are secondary to other mechanisms is not clear. Interstitial fibrosis may develop as a long-term complication.[1150]

Radiologic Manifestations

The typical radiographic pattern is indistinguishable from that of many viral pneumonias and consists of interstitial or air space opacities or a combination of both (Fig. 6–69).[1151] In the early stages, the interstitial inflammation causes a fine reticular pattern,[1152] followed by signs of patchy air space consolidation that tends to be segmental, in contrast to the nonsegmental distribution of acute bacterial air space pneumonia (e.g., caused by *S. pneumoniae*).[1153] Disease is manifested predominantly in the lower lobes.[1154] Hilar lymph node enlargement is rare in adults[1155] but occurs in approximately 30% of children.[1156] Pleural effusions are usually small and unilateral.[1157]

The main HRCT findings consist of centrilobular nodular and branching linear opacities in a patchy distribution, thickening of the bronchovascular bundles, and areas of groundglass attenuation and lobular or segmental consolidation (Fig. 6–70).[1158] In many patients, the areas of consolidation have a lobular distribution.

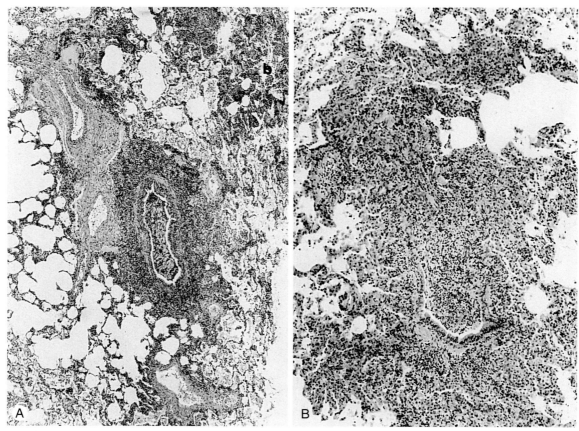

FIGURE 6–68

***Mycoplasma pneumoniae*—bronchiolitis and pneumonitis.** A section of an open lung biopsy specimen from a 23-year-old man with rapidly progressive respiratory failure (**A**) shows patchy, mild to moderate interstitial pneumonitis and severe inflammation centered about a membranous bronchiole and a respiratory bronchiole (b). A mild degree of alveolar interstitial inflammation is also evident. Another view from the same biopsy specimen (**B**) shows the same reaction in a proximal respiratory bronchiole. *(From Fraser RS, Müller NL, Colman NC, Paré PD: Fraser and Paré's Diagnosis of Diseases of the Chest, 4th ed. Philadelphia, WB Saunders, 1999.)*

Clinical Manifestations

The typical case of *Mycoplasma* infection begins insidiously with fever, nonproductive cough, headache, malaise, and (rarely) chills.[1159,1160] Myalgia, arthralgia, and gastrointestinal symptoms are usually mild or absent. Upper respiratory tract involvement, characterized predominantly by sore throat and symptoms of rhinitis, is present in about 50% of cases; bullous myringitis occurs occasionally.[1161]

The major symptom of lower respiratory tract involvement is cough, which may be hacking and paroxysmal. Though initially nonproductive, it may become associated with mucoid or frankly purulent sputum if infection is prolonged. Hemoptysis and pleuritic chest pain are uncommon. ARDS develops occasionally.[1162] Particularly severe disease consisting of multiple lobe involvement, prolonged fever, respiratory distress, and pleural effusion has been described in some patients who have sickle cell disease.[1163]

Complications and extrapulmonary manifestations of *M. pneumoniae* infection are not uncommon and are often more serious than the respiratory tract disease.[1159] They include meningoencephalitis, meningitis, transverse myelitis, and cranial nerve palsies[1164]; hemagglutination, hemolysis (related to the presence of cold agglutinins), thrombocytopenic purpura, and peripheral venous thrombosis; pericarditis and myocarditis[1165]; and rash associated with high fever, stomatitis, and ophthalmia (Stevens-Johnson syndrome).[1156]

Laboratory Findings and Diagnosis

The white blood cell count in mycoplasmal pneumonia is usually normal; however, levels above 10,000/mm³ have been recorded in a quarter to a third of patients in some reviews.[1167] Cold agglutinins are present in a titer of greater than 1:32 in most patients. Nonetheless, their presence is of little diagnostic value because approximately a quarter of cold agglutinin–positive pneumonias are caused by organisms other than *M. pneumoniae* (usually viruses).

Because isolation takes 1 week or longer, at which time clinical recovery is well under way in most patients, culture is generally useful only to confirm the diagnosis. Similarly, a fourfold rise in specific IgG antibody titer or in cold agglutinins is of little diagnostic value during the acute phase of the disease. Demonstration of the presence of *Mycoplasma*-specific IgA or IgM antibodies has been advocated as a more rapid and reliable test for early diagnosis.[1168] As with other

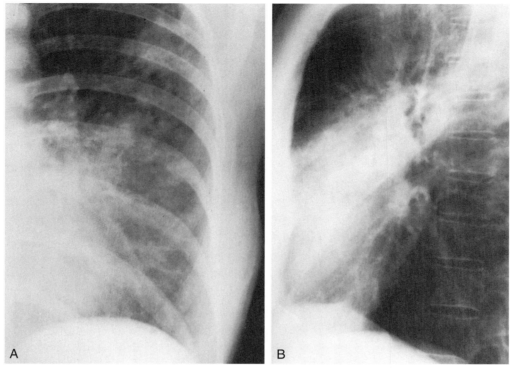

FIGURE 6–69

Acute pneumonia caused by *Mycoplasma pneumoniae*. Views of the left lung from posteroanterior (**A**) and lateral (**B**) radiographs demonstrate patchy air space consolidation in the distribution of the lingular and posterior segments of the left upper lobe. *(From Fraser RS, Müller NL, Colman NC, Paré PD: Fraser and Paré's Diagnosis of Diseases of the Chest, 4th ed. Philadelphia, WB Saunders, 1999.)*

pulmonary infections, molecular diagnostic techniques can be particularly useful. For example, by using a probe to mycoplasmal RNA, sensitivities and specificities of 75% to 100% and 85% to 95% have been reported.[1169] PCR also yields rapid results and is highly sensitive.[1170]

Prognosis and Natural History

Although nearly all infections caused by *M. pneumoniae* are mild, pneumonia is usually more prolonged and severe than that caused by viruses. Rarely, disease is fulminant and fatal. In a few patients, diffuse pulmonary disease results in residual dysfunction, either restrictive or obstructive.[1171,1172]

Chlamydiae

Chlamydiae are small, obligate intracellular organisms that are properly classified as bacteria. They differ from the latter (including intracellular forms such as rickettsiae) chiefly by their unique mode of reproduction and by their inability to synthesize high-energy compounds such as adenosine triphosphate (ATP) and guanosine triphosphate (GTP). The organisms exist in an extracellular form as *elementary bodies* measuring 0.2 to 0.3 μm in diameter.[1173] These elementary bodies attach to and enter susceptible cells, within which they convert to large *reticulate bodies* measuring 0.5 to 1.0 μm that undergo division to form intracellular colonies. The reticulate

bodies themselves are noninfectious and eventually undergo conversion into numerous elementary bodies, at which point the phagosome membrane disrupts, the cell dies, and the elementary bodies are released. On disruption of the membrane, the release of phagolysosomal enzymes is believed to be responsible for cell lysis.

Three species—*Chlamydia trachomatis*, *Chlamydia pneumoniae*, and *Chlamydia psittaci*—can cause pulmonary disease in humans.

Chlamydia trachomatis

This organism is best known as a cause of genitourinary infections in adults and conjunctivitis and pneumonia in infants born to infected mothers. However, it has also been found to cause pneumonia occasionally in both immunocompromised and immunocompetent adults.[1174] Clinical manifestations are nonspecific and range from those associated with acute bronchitis to those of severe diffuse interstitial pneumonia.[1175]

Chlamydia pneumoniae

In the mid-1980s, a new strain of *Chlamydia* was isolated from patients with pneumonia and labeled TWAR because of its similarity to isolates previously designated TW-183 and AR-39. Subsequent genetic analysis showed the organism to be distinct from *C. trachomatis* and *C. psittaci*, and it was renamed *C. pneumoniae*. Epidemiologic studies have since found it to be

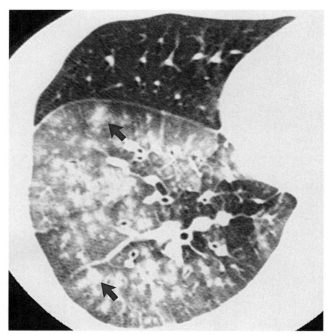

FIGURE 6–70

Mycoplasma pneumoniae **pneumonia.** An HRCT scan at the level of the right lower lobe reveals small nodules (*arrows*) in a predominantly centrilobular distribution and areas of ground-glass attenuation. Sharp demarcation between normal and abnormal secondary pulmonary lobules is consistent with lobular pneumonia. (*From Reittner P, Müller NL, Heyneman L, et al: Mycoplasma pneumoniae pneumonia: Radiographic and high-resolution CT features in 28 patients. AJR Am J Roentgenol 174:37-41, 2000.*)

one of the more common causes of community-acquired pneumonia. In fact, clinically evident disease appears to account for about 5% to 10% of cases of nonbacterial lower respiratory tract infection.[1176,1177] Although it usually occurs sporadically, outbreaks of disease in families and local communities have been described.[1178] Patients who have AIDS, COPD, or cystic fibrosis appear to have an increased risk of infection.[1179-1181] Pathologic features of the infection are poorly documented because the disease is rarely fatal.

The most frequent radiologic manifestations consist of air space consolidation or interstitial opacities.[1182] The consolidation can be unilateral or bilateral, focal, multifocal, or less commonly, lobar. Less common findings include areas of atelectasis and small nodules. The radiographic abnormalities tend to progress to bilateral, mixed interstitial and air space opacities during the course of infection. Pleural effusions, typically of small to medium size, are seen in approximately 25% of patients.

The most common clinical manifestations are sore throat, nonproductive cough, and fever[1183]; hoarseness occurs in some patients. The organism can be isolated on tissue culture and identified with specific antibodies.[1184] A direct immunofluorescence test is both sensitive and specific and has been widely used for diagnosis.[1185] The use of PCR as a diagnostic tool is likely to become even more important in the future.[1186] Disease is usually mild, self-limited, and without sequelae. However, fatalities have been reported in some patients who have underlying disease.

Chlamydia psittaci

This organism is a common pathogen of many birds and mammals that only occasionally infects humans. Because human illness was initially associated with parrots and other members of the order Psittaciformes, it has been widely known as *psittacosis*, although the presence of disease in many other birds suggests that the term *ornithosis* is more appropriate. Most human cases in which a history of exposure can be obtained are acquired from parakeets, pigeons, or poultry.[1187,1188] The organisms are excreted in the birds' feces and urine and remain viable for at least a month at ambient temperature; in most cases, human infection results from the inhalation of such dried excreta. Disease can occur sporadically or in epidemics, the latter usually among poultry workers.[1188]

Pathologic features of fatal human disease consist of diffuse alveolar damage.[1189] Intracytoplasmic, somewhat rod-shaped inclusions can be identified, but usually with difficulty.

The chest radiographic pattern has been described as a homogeneous ground-glass opacity, sometimes containing small areas of radiolucency,[1190] a patchy reticular pattern radiating from the hilar areas or involving the lung bases,[1191] and segmental or nonsegmental consolidation with or without atelectasis. Enlargement of hilar lymph nodes may be seen.[1191] Radiographic resolution is often delayed for many weeks after clinical cure.

Ornithosis varies in intensity from a mild febrile episode to severe pneumonia indistinguishable from an acute bacterial infection[1192]; it can also be manifested as chronic, recurrent disease. Its onset may be insidious or abrupt. In more severe cases, features of the disease tend to simulate those of typhoid and include bradycardia and even "rose spots."[1193] Headaches, fever, and chills are almost invariable. The most prominent respiratory symptom is cough, which is usually dry but may be productive of nonpurulent mucoid material; hemoptysis occurs occasionally. Pleuritic pain and dyspnea may develop in cases of overwhelming infection. Systemic symptoms and signs include malaise, anorexia, nausea and vomiting, pharyngitis, polyarthritis, myalgia, and abdominal pain. Hepatosplenomegaly and superficial lymph node enlargement may be present.

When considering the potential risk of avian exposure in the clinical history, several features must be remembered. Although the bird or birds responsible may have been obviously ill or may have died of the disease, this is not invariable.[1194] In addition, infection may be acquired from a recently purchased bird that remains healthy after having acquired immunity. Finally, a history of avian exposure is not always obtained.[1195]

The white blood cell count ranges from normal to moderately increased, with or without eosinophilia. The organism can be isolated by culture of spleen or liver tissue in the intraperitoneal cavity of mice, in chicken embryos, and on tissue; growth occurs in 5 to 30 days.

Rickettsiae

Rickettsiae are small, obligate intracellular organisms that are properly classified as bacteria. They are found naturally in a variety of arthropods and are transmitted to humans and animals by their bites. Four groups cause disease in humans, but the major organism responsible for respiratory disease is *Coxiella burnetii*. Though not usually clinically prominent, pulmonary involvement in Rocky Mountain spotted fever is also evident in some patients.

Coxiella burnetii

C. burnetii is the cause of Q fever. Its natural reservoir appears to be ticks, from which it is transmitted to a variety of animal, insect, and avian hosts by bites. It is exceptionally resistant to drying and can survive for many months in a hostile extracellular environment. Such resistance favors transmission by inhalation, and most infections have emanated from laboratory cultures[1196] or from infected animals used in research or slaughtered in abattoirs.[1197,1198] Animals are especially contagious after parturition (the organism grows well in the reproductive tract of cows and can be recovered from the placenta).

Q fever is worldwide in distribution; it was originally described in Australia (Queensland fever) and subsequently in the United States, Europe, and elsewhere. Pneumonia has been estimated to occur in about 5% of cases in Australia, in contrast to an incidence of approximately 50% in patients in the United States and the United Kingdom,[1198] a finding that may reflect a difference in the virulence of strains of the organism. There is a strong occupational association, with farmers, abattoir and stockyard workers, and veterinary and medical laboratory personnel being at particular risk.

The pathologic characteristics of Q fever pneumonia consist of mild interstitial inflammation and alveolar air space filling by a combination of blood, edema fluid, fibrin, and mononuclear inflammatory cells[1199]; necrosis may be present. Airways contain a similar exudate, and their walls may show focal areas of epithelial ulceration and a mononuclear inflammatory infiltrate.

The radiographic findings typically consist of multiple areas of rounded consolidation measuring 5 to 20 cm in diameter or multiple areas of segmental consolidation.[1200,1201] Some patients have lobar or sublobar consolidation associated with loss of volume.[1202] The areas of consolidation usually involve the lower lobes. A small pleural effusion is present in approximately 10% of patients.[1202] Resolution tends to be slow, averaging 30 days and sometimes taking several months.

Onset of the disease is usually insidious, with malaise for several days followed by headache (sometimes severe), chills, myalgia, and arthralgia; nausea, vomiting, and diarrhea occur in a minority of cases.[1197] Pulmonary involvement is characterized by dry cough and, in severe cases, dyspnea and chest pain. Fever is frequently remittent and may last for several weeks. Extrapulmonary disease is common and includes hepatitis, endocarditis, myocarditis, meningoencephalitis, and phlebitis. The illness may have a chronic progressive course or relapse and recur[1203]; in most such cases the heart is the principal site of disease.

The organism can be isolated from urine, blood, sputum, or pleural fluid. The disease is usually self-limited, and long-term sequelae develop in few patients.

Rickettsia rickettsii

This organism is the cause of Rocky Mountain spotted fever. It is found exclusively in North and South America and, despite its name, is most prevalent in the eastern United States. Humans are infected by the bite of several species of tick, so the majority of cases occur during the warm months. From the initial site of inoculation, the organisms disseminate via the bloodstream and invade capillary endothelial cells, where they multiply and eventually cause endothelial necrosis, vasculitis, and thrombosis; the result is widespread tissue necrosis and hemorrhage. The skin, subcutaneous tissues, and central nervous system are most severely affected.

Although respiratory involvement is not usually a prominent clinical feature, evidence of lower respiratory tract involvement was observed in about 40% of patients in one series at some time in the course of the illness.[1204] Radiologic manifestations are variable. In one study the predominant abnormalities were focal or diffuse air space consolidation, diffuse interstitial disease, and pleural effusion.[1205]

Clinically, patients have fever, rash, headaches, and myalgia. Involvement of the respiratory tract is typically manifested by cough.[1204] Patients with radiologic evidence of diffuse interstitial and air space disease have been found to have a mortality rate of about 50%, whereas patients with focal disease tend to recover.[1205]

PROTOZOA

Entamoeba histolytica

Although human infestation is sometimes caused by other amebae, the term "amebiasis" is reserved for that caused by *E. histolytica*, a species usually associated with colonic disease (amebic dysentery). The latter is of worldwide distribution, with areas of high endemicity in regions where hygiene and therapeutic measures are inadequate. Cysts are passed in the feces of affected individuals (who are frequently asymptomatic) and are usually ingested in contaminated water or food. Most cases in the United States develop in immigrants from endemic regions who have been in the country for less than 2 years[1206]; institutionalized individuals such as prisoners and the mentally ill are also at increased risk.[1206a]

Whereas amebic dysentery shows no age or sex predominance, pleuropulmonary disease develops most frequently between the ages of 20 and 40 years and is 10 to 15 times more common in men than women.[1207] Such involvement has been estimated to occur in approximately 1 in 1000 patients who have amebic dysentery[1208]; however, when the liver is involved, the incidence has been reported to be as high as 6 to 40 per 100.[1206a]

The cysts of *E. histolytica* are acid resistant and able to travel through the stomach to the small intestine, where trophozoites excyst. The trophozoites migrate to the colon, where they multiply and pass through the epithelium into the submucosa. Penetration of the mucosa is associated with necrosis and ulceration and the characteristic symptoms of amebic dysentery. Organisms may subsequently spread to the liver and induce the development of microabscesses and, eventually, macroabscesses.

Pleuropulmonary disease can occur by several mechanisms, the most frequent of which is extension from a hepatic abscess, usually located in the right lobe. Such abscesses may extend into the subphrenic space and form a separate subdiaphragmatic abscess, in which case a sterile pleural effusion may ensue. In other cases, empyema or a basal pulmonary abscess develops by transdiaphragmatic extension of infection, either in association with a hepatic abscess alone or in conjunction with combined hepatic and subphrenic abscesses. Sections of lung infected by *E. histolytica* show poorly defined areas of necrosis that are frequently soft to semifluid in consistency and possess a characteristic mucinous, hemorrhagic appearance likened to anchovy paste or chocolate sauce. Histologically, there is a variable degree of necrosis, fibrosis, and mononuclear inflammatory infiltrate. Trophozoites may be identified at the margins of necrotic areas contiguous with normal lung.

The most common radiographic manifestations in the chest consist of elevation of the right hemidiaphragm, pleural effusion, and atelectasis or consolidation in the right lower lobe (Fig. 6–71).[1206a] The consolidation can progress to abscess formation. The presence of a hepatic abscess and its extension across the hemidiaphragm can be assessed by CT or ultrasound.[1209]

The possibility of pleuropulmonary amebiasis should be considered in a patient who is or has been a resident of an endemic area and complains of right upper quadrant abdominal pain and a dry cough, particularly if the patient has a history of diarrhea (although this is uncommon). The dry cough characterizes the early stage of disease; later, it may become productive of the characteristic "chocolate sauce." Hemoptysis is common with pulmonary involvement. Expectoration of bile (biloptysis) may also occur, most often as a result of a bronchohepatic or, less often, a bronchobiliary fistula.[1210] Physical examination may reveal a palpable, tender liver, lower intercostal tenderness, or both.

Leukocytosis is usually moderate and may be associated with eosinophilia and anemia. Antineutrophil cytoplasmic antibodies (c-ANCAs) were found in a large proportion of patients in one investigation.[1211] A positive diagnosis can be made by the demonstration of organisms in sputum, pleural fluid, or material obtained by needle aspiration; however, they are often few in number, and both overdiagnosis and underdiagnosis are said to be common.[1206a] Tests using

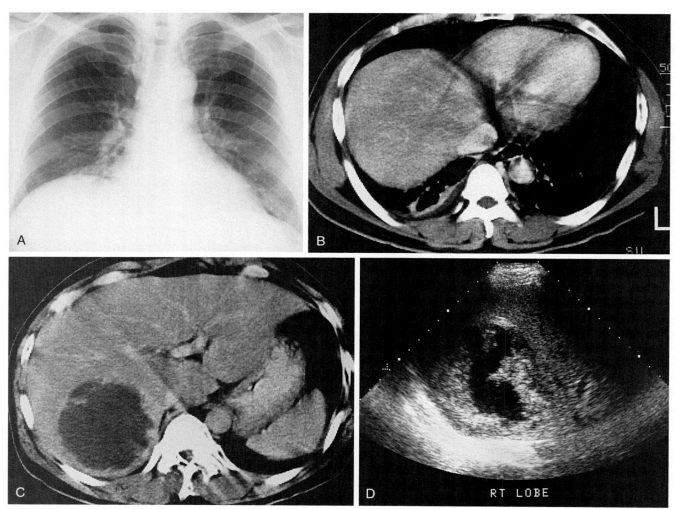

FIGURE 6–71

Amebiasis. A posteroanterior chest radiograph (**A**) demonstrates elevation of the right hemidiaphragm. A CT scan after the intravenous administration of contrast (**B**) demonstrates a small right pleural effusion and areas of atelectasis in the right lower lobe. A scan through the liver (**C**) reveals a large cystic lesion in the right lobe of the liver. Ultrasonographic examination (**D**) demonstrates echogenic material within the lesion consistent with an abscess. The diagnosis of amebiasis was proved by fine-needle aspiration under ultrasound guidance. The patient was a 42-year-old South Korean man with a 1-week history of fever and chills. (*Case courtesy of Dr. Soon Ju Cha, Inje University Hospital, Seoul, South Korea.*)

monoclonal antibodies and PCR are under development. A presumptive diagnosis can be made if trophozoites or cysts are identified in stool. The overall mortality rate associated with thoracic amebiasis has been estimated to be about 10% to 15%.[1207]

Toxoplasma gondii

Toxoplasmosis is caused by *Toxoplasma gondii*, an intracellular protozoan that causes widespread infestation that is rarely manifested clinically. The organism is found in many wild and domestic animals throughout the world. Humans usually acquire infection by ingestion of material contaminated by oocyst-infected stool or poorly cooked, cyst-containing meat.

On ingestion, the oocysts are disrupted by digestive enzymes and release trophozoites that enter the intestinal mucosa and disseminate via the bloodstream. In immunologically competent persons the disease is usually limited, intracellular infestation and minimal cell death occurring predominantly in cardiac and skeletal muscle and the brain. The organisms encyst in these organs and occasionally other sites, where they remain viable and can serve as a source of disease in individuals who subsequently lose their immunologic competence.

Disease occurs in several clinicopathologic forms.[1212] Lymph node enlargement, with or without symptoms similar to infectious mononucleosis, is the most common clinically recognized form of the disease in adults; a variety of lymph node groups may be affected, including those in the mediastinum. Generalized disease in adults usually occurs in immunocompromised hosts. Histologically, the lungs show interstitial pneumonitis with or without an adjacent air space exudate; parenchymal necrosis is seen in severe cases.

Organisms can be identified free in necrotic tissue or in alveolar epithelial and capillary endothelial cells.

In immunocompetent individuals, pulmonary toxoplasmosis usually results in a focal reticular pattern resembling acute viral pneumonia; air space consolidation occurs in some cases. Occasionally, poorly defined areas of ground-glass opacity may be seen that are easier to appreciate on HRCT scans than on radiographs (Fig. 6–72). Hilar lymph node enlargement is common.[1213] In patients who have AIDS, the radiographic manifestations consist of a bilateral, predominantly coarse nodular pattern or, less commonly, a diffuse fine reticulonodular pattern indistinguishable from that seen in PCP.[1214]

Clinical manifestations of toxoplasmosis in adults usually resemble infectious mononucleosis.[1212] Patients may be asymptomatic or may manifest low-grade fever and lymph node enlargement, with or without a rash, over a period of several weeks or months. Anemia and lymphocytosis are common. Disseminated disease is characterized by fever, disorientation, confusion, headache, and manifestations of myocarditis. Pneumonia is associated with nonproductive cough, tachypnea, dyspnea, and cyanosis. An IgM titer of 1:160 or greater is the best indicator of an infestation acquired during the previous 2 to 4 months.[1215]

Plasmodium falciparum

Clinically evident pulmonary disease is not uncommon in patients who have malaria, particularly those infested with *P. falciparum*.[1216] Findings range from mild cough, sometimes with evidence of airflow obstruction, to fulminant respiratory failure, the latter usually associated with ARDS.[1217,1218] Histologic findings in the latter cases are those of diffuse alveolar damage.

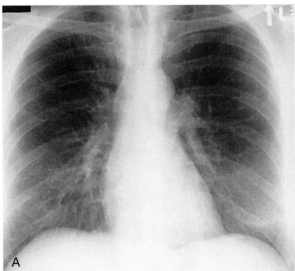
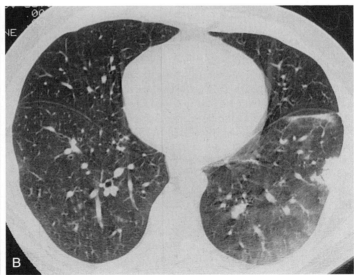

FIGURE 6–72

Toxoplasmosis. A 45-year-old man without an evident immune disturbance had a 1-month history of spiking fevers. A chest radiograph (**A**) demonstrates a poorly defined increased opacity in the left lower lobe. An HRCT scan (**B**) reveals areas of ground-glass attenuation in both lower lobes and a focal area of consolidation in the left lower lobe. The diagnosis was first suggested on the basis of pathologic findings in an excised lymph node and confirmed by positive serology. *(From Fraser RS, Müller NL, Colman NC, Paré PD: Fraser and Paré's Diagnosis of Diseases of the Chest, 4th ed. Philadelphia, WB Saunders, 1999.)*

HELMINTHS

Ascaris lumbricoides

In the great majority of cases, human ascariasis is caused by
A. lumbricoides. The adult female worm lives in the small
intestine, where it produces up to 250,000 eggs per day. These
eggs are passed in feces to the external environment, where
they are resistant to drying and freezing and can remain viable
for many years. When ingested, the ovum hatches in the small
intestine, and the larvae enter the portal veins or intestinal
lymphatics. From there they pass by way of the right side of
the heart to the lungs, where they are trapped by the alveolar
capillaries and exit into the air spaces. At this point they molt
and develop into third-stage larvae. These larvae migrate up
the airways to the larynx, where they are swallowed, and they
complete their odyssey by developing into mature worms in
the small intestine.

The radiologic findings consist of patchy areas of homogeneous consolidation; in many cases, these areas are transient
and without clear-cut segmental distribution. The areas of
consolidation may be several centimeters in diameter and, in
moderately severe cases, tend to be rather discrete and concentrated in the perihilar regions; with more severe involvement, they tend to coalesce and assume a lobular pattern.[1219]

Pulmonary symptoms consist of nonproductive cough, retrosternal chest pain, and in more severe cases, hemoptysis and
dyspnea. A transient, intensely pruritic skin eruption may
appear within 4 or 5 days after the onset of respiratory symptoms.[1219] Low-grade fever may be present. Leukocytosis of
20,000 to 25,000 cells/mm³ is common, with an eosinophilia
of 30% to 70%. The diagnosis can be confirmed by the identification of larvae in sputum or gastric aspirates; identification of adult worms or ova in stool is strongly supportive.

Strongyloides stercoralis

The great majority of cases of strongyloidiasis are caused by
the nematode *S. stercoralis*, a parasite prevalent in tropical and
temperate climates throughout the world. The life cycle of the
organism is complex. Free-living filariform larvae penetrate
the undamaged skin and pass via the bloodstream to the lung,
where they migrate from the capillaries into the alveoli and
thence up the airways to the larynx and down the esophagus
to the gut. Within the small intestine, they develop into adult
females that take up residence and lay eggs in the mucosal
crypts. In their subsequent passage through the gut, the eggs
develop into noninfectious rhabditiform larvae; these larvae
in turn may be passed in stool and develop directly into filariform larvae in the soil or may transform directly into filariform larvae within the gut, thereby leading to autoinfection
through direct penetration of the intestinal mucosa or perianal skin. This ability of the organism to migrate through the
lungs without a soil cycle permits persistence of chronic and
recurrent infestation for years, long after residence in an
endemic area has terminated.

The disease is endemic in rural tropical areas where the
climate is warm and the soil moist (including the southern
United States); in these regions, infestation has been estimated
to affect up to 35% of the population.[1220] Since the larvae par-
asitize humans through penetration of skin, the disease is seen
most frequently in areas where people walk barefoot on soil
contaminated by feces. In the majority of cases, infestation is
accompanied by mild or no clinical symptoms. However,
severe disease (so-called hyperinfection) can occur, particularly in immunocompromised hosts[1221] and patients receiving
corticosteroid therapy for asthma or COPD.[1222]

Radiographic manifestations consist of nonsegmental,
patchy areas of consolidation, presumably caused by an allergic reaction to migration of the filariform larvae through the
lungs. Hyperinfection may be associated with air space consolidation,[1223] focal opacities,[1224] or diffuse reticulonodular or
nodular patterns.[1225,1226] The nodules may have poorly defined
or well-defined margins and generally measure 2 to 5 mm in
diameter, an appearance that may simulate miliary tuberculosis.[1227] Pleural effusions may be seen, usually in association
with parenchymal abnormalities but occasionally as the only
radiographic manifestation.[1228]

In most cases, pulmonary symptoms are mild or absent; in
more severe disease, there may be dyspnea, hemoptysis, and
bronchospasm. Abdominal pain and diarrhea or diarrhea
alternating with constipation is common.[1229] IgE and total
blood eosinophil levels are usually increased. The diagnosis
can be made by finding larvae in sputum, gastric washings, or
BAL fluid[1230]; a presumptive diagnosis can be based on their
detection in stool. An ELISA using antigen extracted from
filariform larvae has been found to have a sensitivity of 85%
to 90% and a specificity of almost 100%.[1231]

Trichinella spiralis

Trichinosis results from the ingestion of larvae of the round
worm *T. spiralis*.[1232] It is worldwide in distribution and is
found wherever contaminated meat, particularly pork, is eaten
raw or undercooked. Live encysted larvae in the meat reach
the small intestine, where they mature, mate, and produce
eggs. When the eggs hatch, the larvae penetrate the duodenal
wall and are carried to the lungs, from which they pass via the
pulmonary circulation into the systemic circulation and are
distributed to striated muscles throughout the body. Although
any muscle may be parasitized, the diaphragm is perhaps
the most frequently involved. Within muscle, the coiled
Trichinella larvae encyst and become surrounded by a thick
refractile hyaline layer that frequently calcifies 6 to 18 months
after infestation.

Radiologically, there are no abnormalities related to the
lungs since the larvae produce minimal reaction in their
passage through the pulmonary circulation. Calcified walls of
larval cysts within the respiratory muscles may be visible as
oval opacities 1.0 cm in their longest diameter.

Clinically, no symptoms result from passage of the parasite
through the lungs. Diarrhea develops 2 to 4 days after the ingestion of contaminated meat; fever, muscular pain, facial edema,
and central nervous system symptoms may develop by the
seventh day. Deposition of the larvae in skeletal muscles occurs
by the 10th day and may result in dyspnea and tachypnea.
Leukocytosis with some degree of eosinophilia is common.

Tropical Eosinophilia

As the name suggests, this disease is confined largely to the
tropics and is associated with moderate to severe leukocytosis

and eosinophilia. The cause is believed to be the parasitic microfilariae *Wuchereria bancrofti*, *Brugia malayi*, and *Brugia timori*. It has been speculated that adult worms somewhere in the body release into the bloodstream microfilariae that are trapped largely in the lungs, where they cause a local inflammatory reaction[1233]; such a mechanism would explain the prominence of respiratory symptoms and the relative absence of circulating systemic microfilariae (in contrast to the typical forms of filariasis). The disease is confined to regions in which appropriate mosquito vectors live—the Indian subcontinent, Malaysia, southern Asia, northern Africa, and certain areas of South America. Most patients are adult men between the ages of 20 and 40 years.

Pathologic findings consist of a prominent eosinophilic leukocyte infiltrate located within the alveolar interstitium and air spaces and around bronchovascular structures.[1234]

Radiographically, lung involvement is diffuse and symmetrical and characterized by a reticulonodular pattern, sometimes accompanied by nodules 2 to 5 mm in diameter (Fig. 6–73); the mid and lower lung zones are predominantly affected. Hilar lymph node enlargement occurs in some cases, and pleural effusion is rare.[1235,1236]

The main symptom is cough, usually productive of small amounts of mucoid or mucopurulent material. It tends to be particularly bothersome at night when it occurs in paroxysms, sometimes with the production of blood-streaked sputum. Attacks of coughing and dyspnea may be so severe that they suggest status asthmaticus. Weight loss, fatigue, low-grade fever, and slight enlargement of the liver and spleen are frequent.

Leukocytosis is usually marked—60,000 white blood cells/mm^3 is not unusual—with eosinophilia sometimes as high as 60%. Very high levels of serum and BAL fluid IgE and filarial-specific antibodies are also found in acute disease.[1237] Microfilariae may be identified in specimens of pulmonary secretions submitted for cytologic examination[1238] and in pleural fluid.[1239] Confirmation of the diagnosis may be provided by complement fixation and skin tests using *Dirofilaria immitis* antigen. Pulmonary function test results show either a restrictive pattern or a combined restrictive and obstructive pattern. Occasionally, such aberrations become irreversible.[1240]

Dirofilaria immitis

Pulmonary dirofilariasis is caused most often by *D. immitis*, a natural parasite of dogs and, less commonly, cats and a variety of wild carnivores. In these animals it is initially present in subcutaneous tissue; from there it migrates to the right heart chambers and main pulmonary artery, where one or several worms take up residence and release microfilariae into the blood. Mosquitos subsequently transmit filariae both to the definitive host and to humans. Since humans are not a natural host, the organism does not complete its life cycle and dies before reaching sexual maturity; it is then carried into the pulmonary circulation, where it lodges in a peripheral vessel and causes necrosis of surrounding tissue.

Most reports of human disease come from the eastern and southern coastal United States.[1241] Although the condition is rare, serologic studies in areas of endemic heartworm infestation suggest that the incidence of human infection is much greater than the number of reported cases of dirofilariasis

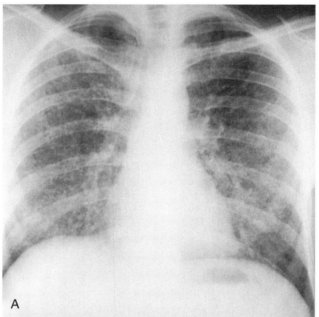

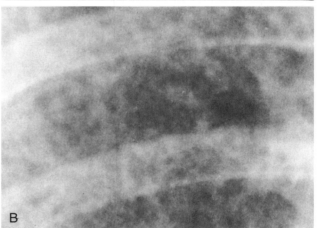

FIGURE 6–73

Tropical eosinophilia. A posteroanterior chest radiograph (**A**) and a magnified view of the right upper lobe (**B**) reveal multiple discrete and confluent nodular opacities throughout both lungs ranging in diameter from 3 to 5 mm. There is no evidence of hilar or mediastinal lymph node enlargement. The patient was a young man from East India with a gradual onset of nocturnal cough, fever, and high blood eosinophilia. Recovery was complete after appropriate chemotherapy. *(From Fraser RS, Müller NL, Colman NC, Paré PD: Fraser and Paré's Diagnosis of Diseases of the Chest, 4th ed. Philadelphia, WB Saunders, 1999.)*

would suggest.[1242] It seems likely that a large proportion of these clinically undetected cases are the result of death of microfilariae at the site of their initial inoculation. The vast majority of patients are adults, an age group in which there is a greater likelihood that chest radiography will be performed and in which a malignancy will be suspected when a solitary nodule is found.

Pulmonary disease is characterized pathologically by a more or less well circumscribed, spherical or lobulated nodule, usually located in the subpleural parenchyma.[1243] Histologically, a central region of coagulative or caseous-like necrosis is surrounded by a variable amount of fibrous tissue and inflammatory infiltrate. One or more usually degenerated worms can be identified within a pulmonary artery in the central portion of the nodule. This pathologic appearance probably results from an inflammatory reaction to antigen released by the degenerating worm rather than vascular occlusion and ischemia.

Radiologically, the typical manifestation is a solitary spherical or somewhat wedge-shaped, well-circumscribed nodule 1 to 2 cm in diameter.[1244] Multiple nodules are seen occasionally.[1245] The majority of patients are asymptomatic, the diagnosis being made after pulmonary resection because of suspicion of pulmonary carcinoma. Systemic eosinophilia is not uncommon, but usually mild (about 5% in most cases).[1246] Immunologic tests, including indirect hemagglutination and ELISA,[1247] may prove to be helpful but have not yet been shown to permit confident distinction of dirofilariasis from carcinoma.

Echinococcus granulosus

Echinococcosis (hydatid disease) is caused by larvae of the class Cestoda, of which *E. granulosus* is responsible for the vast majority of human pulmonary infestations.[1248,1249] The adult worm consists of four segments: a head (scolex), which is composed of four suckers and a rostellum that contains a double row of hooklets for attachment to the intestinal mucosa, and three proglottids, the last of which is the egg-laying organ.

Disease occurs in two forms. The *pastoral variety* is the more common and, as the name implies, occurs in rural settings in which sheep, cows, or pigs are the intermediate hosts and dogs the usual definitive hosts. Humans usually acquire the disease by direct contact with infested dogs or by ingestion of egg-contaminated water, food, or soil; humans thus become accidental intermediate hosts. The disease is particularly common in the sheep-raising Mediterranean regions and in Russia, Argentina, Chile, Uruguay, Australasia, and portions of Africa. The *sylvatic variety* is very likely caused by a different strain of the tapeworm, the definitive hosts being species of the Canidae family, including the dog, wolf, arctic fox, and coyote. A variety of herbivores, including moose, deer, reindeer, elk, caribou, and bison, serve as intermediate hosts. The disease is seen primarily in Alaska and northern Canada. It is acquired by the same mechanism as the pastoral variety.

Pathogenesis and Pathologic Characteristics

The mature adult worms live in the small intestine of the definitive host. Eggs are passed in feces to grazing land or water and are ingested by the intermediate hosts. In these hosts, larvae develop in the duodenum, penetrate the wall, and pass into the portal bloodstream to the liver, where most are trapped in the sinusoids. Of those that escape, most are caught in the alveolar capillaries. The majority of such entrapped larvae die, but the few that survive develop into cysts that produce brood capsules containing immature worms. The life cycle of the parasite is completed when the definitive host feeds on the remains of an intermediate host that harbors the cysts, with subsequent intra-intestinal development of adult worms.

The ability of the hepatic and pulmonary capillary sieves to contain the larvae is largely responsible for the preponderance of disease in these organs. In the pastoral variety, approximately 65% to 70% of cysts occur in the liver and 15% to 30% in the lungs. For reasons that are unclear, however, lung cysts appear to show a preponderance over liver cysts in sylvatic disease.[1250] Although an increase in size of the cysts of 0.5 to 1 cm/yr is considered typical, rates up to 5 cm/yr have been recorded.[1249] It has been speculated that the organism may be able to produce a substance homologous to human cyclophilin (a molecule that interacts with cyclosporine to induce T-cell suppression) and thereby induce local depression of host defense.[1249]

Within the lung, hydatid cysts are typically spherical or oval (see Color Fig. 6–17) and are surrounded by a layer of fibrous tissue containing a nonspecific chronic inflammatory infiltrate (the pericyst). The cyst itself is composed of two layers: (1) a laminated, outer chitinous membrane (the exocyst) that serves to protect the developing organisms from the host inflammatory cells and (2) a thin, inner layer formed by a syncytium of cells (the endocyst) that constitutes the germinal layer. The latter produces the intracystic fluid and gives origin to numerous brood capsules (daughter cysts) within which larval scolices develop.

Although intrapulmonary hydatid cysts can cause symptoms by direct compression of surrounding structures, the disease most often becomes clinically evident as a result of rupture into contiguous bronchi. Rupture may occur in two ways: (1) through the pericyst, exocyst, and endocyst, the contents being expelled into the airway and replaced by air; this is commonly followed by secondary bacterial infection; and (2) through the pericyst only, thereby establishing communication between the bronchial tree and the potential space between the exocyst and pericyst. Uncommonly, a cyst ruptures directly into lung parenchyma and results in pneumonitis or into the pleural cavity and produces pyopneumothorax. Pulmonary or pleural echinococcosis can also occur secondary to hepatic disease as a result of extension of an intrahepatic cyst across the diaphragm with the formation of a hepatobronchial fistula, parenchymal abscess, or empyema.[1251]

Radiologic Manifestations

Cysts are characteristically visualized radiologically as solitary, sharply circumscribed, spherical or oval masses surrounded by normal lung (Fig. 6–74).[1252] They are multiple in 20% to 30% of patients. Their size ranges from 1 to greater than 20 cm in diameter[1253]; the larger cysts are usually seen in the pastoral type of disease, those in the sylvatic variety rarely exceeding 10 cm.[1249] Most are located in the lower lobes, more often posteriorly than anteriorly and somewhat more commonly on the right.[1254] Though often spherical or oval, they may have an irregular shape, attributed by some to the fact that they impinge on relatively rigid structures such as bronchovascular bundles as they grow and become indented and lobulated.[1252]

When communication develops between the cyst and the bronchial tree, air may enter the space between the pericyst and exocyst and produce a thin crescent around the periphery of the cyst—the *meniscus* or *crescent* sign.[1255] After the cyst has ruptured into an airway, its membrane may float on residual fluid within the cyst and give rise to the classic *water lily sign* or *sign of the camalote* (Fig. 6–75).[1256] This finding is rare in the sylvatic form of the disease.[1250]

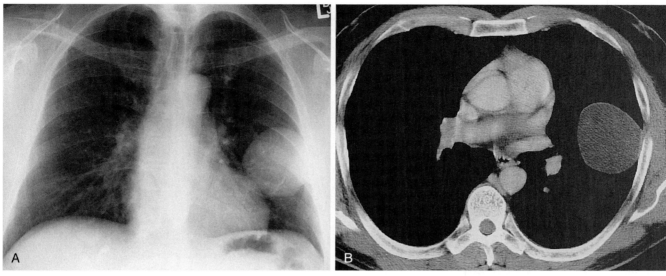

FIGURE 6–74

Hydatid cyst. A posteroanterior chest radiograph (**A**) shows a smoothly marginated, 6-cm-diameter mass in the left lung. A CT scan (**B**) shows a cystic lesion containing fluid with attenuation values similar to water (0 HU). The patient was a 51-year-old asymptomatic man who hunted for several years in northern Canada. *(From Müller NL, Fraser RS, Colman NC, Paré PD: Radiologic Diagnosis of Diseases of the Chest. Philadelphia, WB Saunders, 2001.)*

CT can be helpful in identifying detached or collapsed endocyst membranes, collapsed daughter cyst membranes, and intact daughter cysts.[1257] The cyst fluid has attenuation values close to 0 HU (see Fig. 6–74).[1258] MR imaging also allows reliable differentiation of the fluid-filled cysts from solid tumors,[1259,1260] the cysts having low signal intensity on T1-weighted MR images and homogeneous high signal intensity on T2-weighted images.

Clinical Manifestations and Laboratory Findings

The majority of intact pulmonary hydatid cysts—particularly those of the sylvatic form—cause no symptoms. Occasionally, an unruptured cyst causes nonproductive cough and minimal hemoptysis.[1261] When a cyst ruptures, there is often an abrupt onset of cough, expectoration, and fever; an acute hypersensitivity reaction consisting of urticaria, pruritus, and in some cases, hypotension may develop. The patient may complain of chest pain, and the sputum may become purulent.

Laboratory aids in diagnosis include indirect hemagglutination, latex agglutination, complement fixation, and ELISA; these tests have a sensitivity ranging from 80% to 100% and a specificity of 88% to 98% for hepatic cysts[1249]; however, their sensitivity for the detection of pulmonary cysts is only 50% to 55%. In addition, their specificity is limited by cross-reactions with antigens of other parasites. Blood eosinophilia, usually mild, occurs in 25% to 50% of cases[1262]; it may be severe when associated with anaphylaxis after cyst rupture. Specimens of pleural fluid or sputum may reveal scolices, hooklets, or fragments of exocyst, thereby confirming the diagnosis.

Paragonimus Species

Paragonimiasis is caused by flukes of the genus *Paragonimus*, of which *P. westermani* is the most frequent; *P. mexicanus* can

be found in Mexico and Central America and *P. kellicotti* in the United States.[1263,1264] The disease is most common in Southeast Asia, and immigration of refugees from this region has resulted in an increased incidence of the disease in the western world.[1265] Humans acquire the disease by ingesting raw or undercooked crabs or crayfish or by drinking water contaminated by them. As a result, the disease tends to occur in families because of the common dietary exposure.

The life cycle of *P. westermani* is one of the most fascinating of all parasites. Within the lungs of humans or animals, the larval forms develop into adult flukes that possess oral and ventral suckers for attachment to adjacent tissue. Eggs are deposited in burrows in the lung parenchyma and are coughed up or swallowed and excreted in feces. Under suitable moist conditions, they develop into ciliated miracidia, which infest freshwater snails. Within the snail, further larval forms develop and, after about 2 months, are liberated as cercariae. These cercariae are actively motile parasites that penetrate the soft periarticular tissues of certain species of crayfish and crabs. When ingested by the definitive host, metacercariae are liberated in the jejunum, from which they penetrate the wall of the small bowel into the peritoneal cavity, burrow through the diaphragm into the pleural space, and finally invade the lung. The mature parasite lives for many years in the lung and produces ova continuously.

Pathologic examination of the lungs shows single or multiple, 1- to 3-cm cystic spaces containing reddish brown mucinous fluid and usually a single adult parasite.[1264] The cysts are frequently located near larger bronchioles or bronchi. Microscopically, the parasites are surrounded by a cellular infiltrate composed largely of eosinophils. Fibrosis eventually develops. When erosion occurs into a draining airway, the contents of the cyst may spread to other portions of the lung and cause bronchopneumonia.

The chest radiograph is normal in approximately 20% of patients in whom *Paragonimus* eggs are identified in

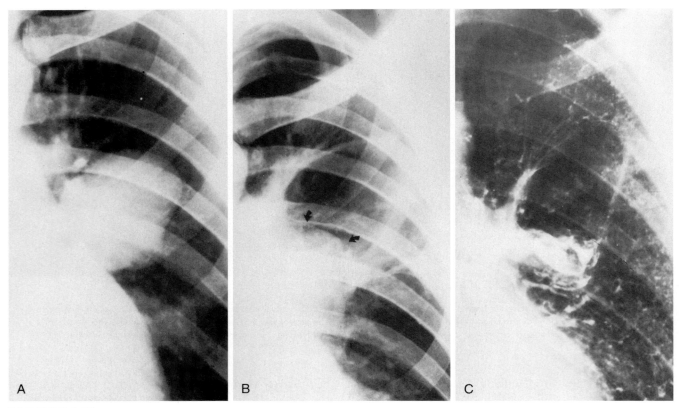

FIGURE 6–75

Hydatid cyst with rupture. A sharply circumscribed homogeneous mass (**A**) in the left midlung has a smooth but somewhat lobulated contour. Four years later (**B**), the cyst contains air; the irregular mass present at the bottom of the cyst (*arrows*) represents collapsed membranes. A bronchogram (**C**) shows contrast material within the cyst outlining the membranes. *(Courtesy of Alfred Hospital, Melbourne, Australia.)*

sputum.[1266] The most common abnormalities consist of parenchymal opacities and cystic lesions, each seen in approximately 50% of patients.[1267] The parenchymal opacities may be poorly defined or homogeneous, single or multiple, and nodular, subsegmental, or segmental (Fig. 6–76). The cystic lesions usually measure between 0.5 and 5 cm in diameter and are thin walled. They may be seen in areas of consolidation or as isolated ring shadows. The lesions often have a crescent-shaped or oval opacity along one aspect of the inner lining; this opacity has soft tissue attenuation on CT and presumably represents the worm.[1267] Communication between the cysts and a bronchus can be demonstrated by CT and may mimic bronchiectasis.[1267] Irregular tracks or burrows measuring up to 5 mm in diameter and connecting adjacent cysts have been identified on both radiographs and CT in a small number of patients. Studies of immigrants to the United States who have resided in an endemic area have shown a somewhat different chest radiographic pattern in which the opacities mimic postprimary tuberculosis.[1265] Pleural abnormalities include unilateral or bilateral effusion, hydropneumothorax, and thickening.[1267]

Symptoms do not develop for 1 year or longer after the presumed time of infestation. Although hemoptysis has been considered to be an almost invariable symptom, it was noted in only 64% in one series of 25 patients.[1265] It tends to occur sporadically for months or even years in the absence of other signs of illness. Dyspnea, low-grade fever, anorexia, and weight

loss may be present; if pleural effusion or pneumothorax develops, there may be pleural pain.

Eosinophilia (absolute level greater than 500 cells/mm^3) is seen in about two thirds of cases.[1268] Pleural fluid has also been reported to show eosinophilia, a low glucose level and pH, and high protein and LDH levels.[1269] Some patients are anemic. The diagnosis can be made in most patients by identifying the eggs in sputum or stool.[1270] The sensitivity of a single sputum examination is about 30% to 40%[1268]; it increases to 50% to 90% with repeated examinations. An indirect ELISA has been found by one group of investigators to be highly sensitive and specific for the detection of circulating antibody to the organism.[1271] Another group has documented similar results with an ELISA in which fluke cysteine proteinases were used as antigens.[1272]

Schistosoma Species

Schistosomiasis is caused by flukes of the class Trematoda, of which three (*S. mansoni*, *S. japonicum*, and *S. haematobium*) are the most important in human infestation. *S. mekongi* and *S. intercalatum* are also seen in parts of Southeast Asia and Africa, respectively.[1273] Acquisition of disease is limited to areas inhabited by the intermediate host, the snail. The geographic distribution of these and thus of schistosomiasis itself varies considerably. Infestation by *S. mansoni* and *S. haematobium* is

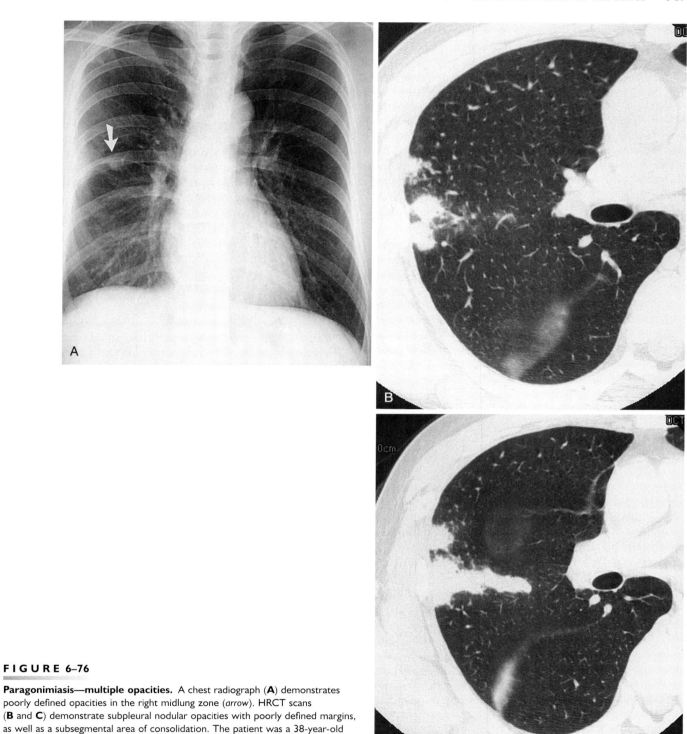

FIGURE 6–76

Paragonimiasis—multiple opacities. A chest radiograph (**A**) demonstrates poorly defined opacities in the right midlung zone (*arrow*). HRCT scans (**B** and **C**) demonstrate subpleural nodular opacities with poorly defined margins, as well as a subsegmental area of consolidation. The patient was a 38-year-old South Korean man evaluated for vague chest pain and cough. *(Case courtesy of Dr. Kyung Soo Lee, Samsung Medical Center, Seoul, South Korea.)*

endemic in the Middle East (especially Egypt and parts of Saudi Arabia) and in large areas of central and southern Africa; *S. mansoni* is also found in the Caribbean islands and in South America, particularly Brazil. *S. japonicum* is predominant in China, Japan, and the Philippines.

Although disease is most commonly identified in these regions, increased emigration from them means that it is likely to be more frequently encountered elsewhere; for example, it has been estimated that approximately 400,000 infected immigrants reside in the United States.[1274] Acute schistosomiasis ("Katayama fever"), which can be seen during migration of larvae through the lungs, is also increasingly being recognized in travelers to regions where the disease is endemic.[1275,1276]

Pathogenesis and Pathologic Characteristics

Humans acquire the infestation by drinking, swimming, or working in fresh water containing the infective cercariae. The larvae penetrate the skin or, less commonly, the oral mucosa and travel as schistosomula via the venous circulation to the pulmonary capillaries. They pass through these vessels to the systemic circulation and traverse the mesenteric vessels into the intrahepatic portion of the portal system. There they develop into adolescent worms, which migrate against portal blood flow to the superior mesenteric (*S. japonicum* and *S. mekongi*), inferior mesenteric (*S. mansoni*), or vesical (*S. haematobium*) venules. The adult male and female worms copulate in these vessels, and the females then migrate to smaller venous channels in the submucosa and mucosa of the bowel or bladder and lay their eggs. Many of these eggs are extruded into the lumen of the bowel or urinary bladder and are excreted in feces or urine; those that reach fresh water develop into larvae, which enter snails. Several transformations take place within the snail, with infective cercariae eventually emerging. Penetration of the skin of a person in contact with contaminated water completes the odyssey.

Tissue damage occurs as a result of a reaction to antigens derived from the eggs.[1277] Such damage may be localized to the gastrointestinal or vesical mucosa. However, some eggs are also released directly into venous blood. In the case of *S. mansoni*, *S. japonicum*, and *S. mekongi*, release usually occurs into the portal system with deposition in the liver; with *S. haematobium*, release is into the inferior vena cava with direct embolization to the lungs. Eggs of the former three species may also reach the lungs via portal-systemic vein anastomoses once the liver has become cirrhotic as a result of *Schistosoma*-related fibrosis. Once they reach the lungs, most embolized eggs become impacted in small pulmonary arteries and arterioles, after which they are extruded into the surrounding perivascular tissue. As in the bowel and bladder, the eggs incite an inflammatory reaction and fibrosis that when widespread, results in obliterative arteritis and pulmonary hypertension.

Histologic findings in transbronchial biopsy specimens from patients with "Katayama fever" have been consistent with eosinophilic pneumonia.[1273]

Radiologic Manifestations

The radiographic appearance varies considerably, depending on the number of eggs that reach the lung and the interval since the formation of perivascular granulomas after extrusion of the eggs. Some cases—perhaps the majority—show a diffuse miliary or reticulonodular pattern presumably caused by the migration of ova through vessel walls and subsequent reaction to these foreign bodies.[1278] Foci of pneumonic consolidation can develop around embolized dead adult worms. Pleural effusion does not occur, although focal pleural thickening may develop. Pulmonary arterial hypertension is indistinguishable from that resulting from any other cause, there being a marked degree of dilatation of the main pulmonary artery and its branches with rapid tapering toward the periphery.

Clinical Manifestations and Laboratory Findings

Clinical manifestations occur in three very distinct time intervals after parasitization. Disease that occurs during the migration of schistosomula from the skin through the pulmonary circulation is manifested by fever, cough, diarrhea, arthralgia, anorexia, malaise, and urticaria; leukocytosis and eosinophilia are almost invariable. It is at this stage that transitory opacities may be found on the chest radiograph. This form of schistosomiasis is seldom seen in inhabitants of endemic areas and is instead characteristic of the reaction in visitors.

Somewhat later, after the deposition of eggs in the intestinal and bladder venules, cough, dyspnea, hypoxemia, and pulmonary edema may develop acutely, findings that are believed to constitute an allergic reaction to the sudden mobilization of many eggs to the lungs. A similar syndrome may be observed when chemotherapy is instituted in patients who have documented schistosomiasis.[1279]

In the third and most important group, the clinical manifestations are those of pulmonary hypertension, usually after years of persistent disease. Evidence of cirrhosis (in cases of *S. mansoni* and *S. japonicum* infestation) or dysuria and hematuria (*S. haematobium*) may be present. Moderate leukocytosis and eosinophilia are usual, the latter sometimes as high as 33%.

In patients suspected of having schistosomiasis, concentrated specimens of stool and urine should be examined repeatedly for ova. Infestation may also be demonstrated in many cases by finding eggs in biopsy specimens of the rectal and bladder mucosa. Examination of sputum seldom reveals ova; however, they have been identified in BAL fluid.[1280] Specific IgE against soluble egg antigen is found in high titer during the acute, but not the chronic stages. Levels of IgM and IgG antibody to cercarial antigen are increased in acute disease, and levels of IgG to the adult worm are increased in chronic disease.[1281] Specific skin tests and precipitin tests are available for individual species.[1282]

REFERENCES

1. Fine MJ, Auble TE, Yealy DM, et al: A prediction rule to identify low-risk patients with community-acquired pneumonia. N Engl J Med 336:243-250, 1997.
2. Marrie TJ, Peeling RW, Fine MJ, et al: Ambulatory patients with community-acquired pneumonia: The frequency of atypical agents and clinical course. Am J Med 101:508-515, 1996.
3. File TM: The epidemiology of respiratory tract infections. Semin Respir Infect 15:184-194, 2000.
4. Bochud PY, Moser F, Erard P, et al: Community-acquired pneumonia. A prospective outpatient study. Medicine (Baltimore) 80:75-87, 2001.
5. Mandell LA: Community-acquired pneumonia. Etiology, epidemiology, and treatment. Chest 108:35S-42S, 1995.
6. Macfarlane J: An overview of community acquired pneumonia with lessons learned from the British Thoracic Society Study. Semin Respir Infect 9:153-165, 1994.
7. Kaplan V, Angus DC, Griffin MF, et al: Hospitalized community-acquired pneumonia in the elderly: Age- and sex-related patterns of care and outcome in the United States. Am J Respir Crit Care Med 165:766-772, 2002.
8. Marston BJ, Plouffe JF, File TM Jr, et al: Incidence of community-acquired pneumonia requiring hospitalization. Results of a population-based active surveillance Study in Ohio. The Community-Based Pneumonia Incidence Study Group. Arch Intern Med 157:1709-1718, 1997.
9. Marrie TJ: Epidemiology of community-acquired pneumonia in the elderly. Semin Respir Infect 5:260-268, 1990.
10. Fine MJ, Smith MA, Carson CA, et al: Prognosis and outcomes of patients with community-acquired pneumonia. A meta-analysis. JAMA 275:134-141, 1996.
11. Ortqvist A: Initial investigation and treatment of the patient with severe community-acquired pneumonia. Semin Respir Infect 9:166-179, 1994.
12. Leeper KV Jr: Severe community-acquired pneumonia. Semin Respir Infect 11:96-108, 1996.
13. Fein AM: Improving outcomes in pneumonia: Existing barriers and potential solutions. ATS Continuing Monograph Series, September 1997.
14. Craven DE, Steger KA: Nosocomial pneumonia in mechanically ventilated adult patients: Epidemiology and prevention in 1996. Semin Respir Infect 11:32-53, 1996.

15. Baker AM, Meredith JW, Haponik EF: Pneumonia in intubated trauma patients. Microbiology and outcomes. Am J Respir Crit Care Med 153:343-349, 1996.
16. Craven DE: Epidemiology of ventilator-associated pneumonia. Chest 117:186S-187S, 2000.
17. Hubmayr RD, Burchardi H, Elliot M, et al: Statement of the 4th International Consensus Conference in Critical Care on ICU-Acquired Pneumonia—Chicago, Illinois, May 2002. Intensive Care Med 28:1521-1536, 2002.
18. Bauer TT, Ferrer R, Angrill J, et al: Ventilator-associated pneumonia: Incidence, risk factors, and microbiology. Semin Respir Infect 15:272-279, 2000.
19. Craven DE, De Rosa FG, Thornton D: Nosocomial pneumonia: Emerging concepts in diagnosis, management, and prophylaxis. Curr Opin Crit Care 8:421-429, 2002.
20. Hospital-acquired pneumonia in adults: Diagnosis, assessment of severity, initial antimicrobial therapy, and preventive strategies. A consensus statement, American Thoracic Society, November 1995. Am J Respir Crit Care Med 153:1711-1725, 1996.
21. Warren DK, Shukla SJ, Olsen MA, et al: Outcome and attributable cost of ventilator-associated pneumonia among intensive care unit patients in a suburban medical center. Crit Care Med 31:1312-1317, 2003.
22. Rello J, Ollendorf DA, Oster G, et al: Epidemiology and outcomes of ventilator-associated pneumonia in a large US database. Chest 122:2115-2121, 2002.
23. Bassin AS, Niederman MS: New approaches to prevention and treatment of nosocomial pneumonia. Semin Thorac Cardiovasc Surg 7:70-77, 1995.
24. Heyland DK, Cook DJ, Griffith L, et al: The attributable morbidity and mortality of ventilator-associated pneumonia in the critically ill patient. The Canadian Critical Trials Group. Am J Respir Crit Care Med 159:1249-1256, 1999.
25. Nelson KE, Larson PA, Schraufnagel DE, et al: Transmission of tuberculosis by flexible fiberbronchoscopes. Am Rev Respir Dis 127:97-100, 1983.
26. Riley R: Indoor spread of respiratory infection by recirculation of air. Bull Eur Physiopathol Respir 15:699, 1979.
27. Onofrio JM, Toews GB, Lipscomb MF, et al: Granulocyte-alveolar-macrophage interaction in the pulmonary clearance of Staphylococcus aureus. Am Rev Respir Dis 127:335-341, 1983.
28. Johanson WG Jr, Harris GD: Aspiration pneumonia, anaerobic infections, and lung abscess. Med Clin North Am 64:385-394, 1980.
29. Huxley EJ, Viroslav J, Gray WR, et al: Pharyngeal aspiration in normal adults and patients with depressed consciousness. Am J Med 64:564-568, 1978.
30. Stockley RA: Lung infections. 1. Role of bacteria in the pathogenesis and progression of acute and chronic lung infection. Thorax 53:58-62, 1998.
31. Pittet JF, Kudoh I, Wiener-Kronish JP: Endothelial exposure to Pseudomonas aeruginosa proteases increases the vulnerability of the alveolar epithelium to a second injury. Am J Respir Cell Mol Biol 18:129-135, 1998.
32. Wilson R, Pitt T, Taylor G, et al: Pyocyanin and 1-hydroxyphenazine produced by Pseudomonas aeruginosa inhibit the beating of human respiratory cilia in vitro. J Clin Invest 79:221-229, 1987.
33. Cundell DR, Taylor GW, Kanthakumar K, et al: Inhibition of human neutrophil migration in vitro by low-molecular-mass products of nontypeable Haemophilus influenzae. Infect Immun 61:2419-2424, 1993.
34. How does influenza virus pave the way for bacteria? Lancet 1:485-486, 1982.
35. Jakab GJ: Pulmonary defense mechanisms and the interaction between viruses and bacteria in acute respiratory infections. Bull Eur Physiopathol Respir 13:119-135, 1977.
36. Granados A, Podzamczer D, Gudiol F, et al: Pneumonia due to Legionella pneumophila and pneumococcal pneumonia: Similarities and differences on presentation. Eur Respir J 2:130-2134, 1989.
37. Denny FW Jr: The clinical impact of human respiratory virus infections. Am J Respir Crit Care Med 152:S4-S12, 1995.
38. Osmer JC, Cole BK: The stethoscope and roentgenogram in acute pneumonia. South Med J 59:75-77, 1966.
39. Metlay JP, Kapoor WN, Fine MJ: Does this patient have community-acquired pneumonia? Diagnosing pneumonia by history and physical examination. JAMA 278:1440-1445, 1997.
40. Macfarlane JT, Miller AC, Roderick Smith WH, et al: Comparative radiographic features of community acquired legionnaires' disease, pneumococcal pneumonia, Mycoplasma pneumonia, and psittacosis. Thorax 39:28-33, 1984.
41. Tew J, Calenoff L, Berlin BS: Bacterial or nonbacterial pneumonia: Accuracy of radiographic diagnosis. Radiology 124:607-612, 1977.
42. Wollschlager CM, Khan FA, Khan A: Utility of radiography and clinical features in the diagnosis of community-acquired pneumonia. Clin Chest Med 8:393-404, 1987.
43. Levy M, Dromer F, Brion N, et al: Community-acquired pneumonia. Importance of initial noninvasive bacteriologic and radiographic investigations. Chest 93:43-48, 1988.
44. Goodman LR, Goren RA, Teplick SK: The radiographic evaluation of pulmonary infection. Med Clin North Am 64:553-574, 1980.
45. Kantor HG: The many radiologic facies of pneumococcal pneumonia. AJR Am J Roentgenol 137:1213-1220, 1981.
46. Janzen DL, Padley SP, Adler BD, et al: Acute pulmonary complications in immunocompromised non-AIDS patients: Comparison of diagnostic accuracy of CT and chest radiography. Clin Radiol 47:159-165, 1993.
47. Tanaka N, Matsumoto T, Kuramitsu T, et al: High resolution CT findings in community-acquired pneumonia. J Comput Assist Tomogr 20:600-608, 1996.
48. Penn CC, Liu C: Bronchiolitis following infection in adults and children. Clin Chest Med 14:645-654, 1993.
49. Panitch HB, Callahan CW Jr, Schidlow DV: Bronchiolitis in children. Clin Chest Med 14:715-731, 1993.
50. Cohen L, Castro M: The role of viral respiratory infections in the pathogenesis and exacerbation of asthma. Semin Respir Infect 18:3-8, 2003.
51. Johnson JT, Liston SL: Bacterial tracheitis in adults. Arch Otolaryngol Head Neck Surg 113:204-205, 1987.
52. Brook I: Aerobic and anaerobic microbiology of bacterial tracheitis in children. Pediatr Emerg Care 13:16-18, 1997.
53. McGuinness G, Gruden JF, Bhalla M, et al: AIDS-related airway disease. AJR Am J Roentgenol 168:67-77, 1997.
54. Müller NL, Miller RR: Diseases of the bronchioles: CT and histopathologic findings. Radiology 196:3-12, 1995.
55. Genereux GP, Stilwell GA: The acute bacterial pneumonias. Semin Roentgenol 15:9-16, 1980.
56. Barnes D, Naraqi S, Igo J: The diagnostic and prognostic significance of bulging fissures in acute lobar pneumonia. Aust N Z J Med 18:130, 1988.
57. Macfarlane J, Rose D: Radiographic features of staphylococcal pneumonia in adults and children. Thorax 51:539-540, 1996.
58. Itoh H, Tokunaga S, Asamoto H, et al: Radiologic-pathologic correlations of small lung nodules with special reference to peribronchiolar nodules. AJR Am J Roentgenol 130:223-231, 1978.
59. Melby K, Toews GB, Pierce AK: Pulmonary elastase activity in response to Streptococcus pneumoniae and Pseudomonas aeruginosa. Am Rev Respir Dis 131:559-563, 1985.
60. Groskin SA, Panicek DM, Ewing DK, et al: Bacterial lung abscess: A review of the radiographic and clinical features of 50 cases. J Thorac Imaging 6:62-67, 1991.
61. Mori T, Ebe T, Takahashi M, et al: Lung abscess: Analysis of 66 cases from 1979 to 1991. Intern Med 32:278-284, 1993.
62. Philpott NJ, Woodhead MA, Wilson AG, et al: Lung abscess: A neglected cause of life threatening haemoptysis. Thorax 48:674-675, 1993.
63. Reich JM: Pulmonary gangrene and the air crescent sign. Thorax 48:70-74, 1993.
64. Penner C, Maycher B, Long R: Pulmonary gangrene. A complication of bacterial pneumonia. Chest 105:567-573, 1994.
65. Quigley MJ, Fraser RS: Pulmonary pneumatocele: Pathology and pathogenesis. AJR Am J Roentgenol 150:1275-1277, 1988.
66. Feurestein IM, Archer A, Pluda JM, et al: Thin-walled cavities, cysts, and pneumothorax in Pneumocystis carinii pneumonia: Further observations with histopathologic correlation. Radiology 174:697-702, 1990.
67. Rosmus HH, Paré JA, Masson AM, et al: Roentgenographic patterns of acute mycoplasma and viral pneumonitis. J Can Assoc Radiol 19:74-77, 1968.
68. Naidich DP, McGuinness G: Pulmonary manifestations of AIDS. CT and radiographic correlations. Radiol Clin North Am 29:999-1017, 1991.
69. Goodman PC: Pneumocystis carinii pneumonia. J Thorac Imaging 6:16-21, 1991.
70. Kuhlman JE, Kavuru M, Fishman EK, et al: Pneumocystis carinii pneumonia: Spectrum of parenchymal CT findings. Radiology 175:711-714, 1990.
71. Kwong JS, Carignan S, Kang EY, et al: Miliary tuberculosis. Diagnostic accuracy of chest radiography. Chest 110:339-342, 1996.
72. Kuhlman JE, Fishman EK, Teigen C: Pulmonary septic emboli: Diagnosis with CT. Radiology 174:211-213, 1990.
73. O'Brien JD, Ettinger NA: Nephrobronchial fistula and lung abscess resulting from nephrolithiasis and pyelonephritis. Chest 108:1166-1168, 1995.
74. Heckerling PS, Tape TG, Wigton RS, et al: Clinical prediction rule for pulmonary infiltrates. Ann Intern Med 113:664-670, 1990.
75. Mabie M, Wunderink RG: Use and limitations of clinical and radiologic diagnosis of pneumonia. Semin Respir Infect 18:72-79, 2003.
76. Marrie TJ: Community-acquired pneumonia in the elderly. Clin Infect Dis 31:1066-1078, 2000.
77. Wunderink RG, Woldenberg LS, Zeiss J, et al: The radiologic diagnosis of autopsy-proven ventilator-associated pneumonia. Chest 101:458-463, 1992.
78. Holzapfel L, Chastang C, Demingeon G, et al: A randomized study assessing the systematic search for maxillary sinusitis in nasotracheally mechanically ventilated patients. Influence of nosocomial maxillary sinusitis on the occurrence of ventilator-associated pneumonia. Am J Respir Crit Care Med 159:695-701, 1999.
79. Fagon JY, Chastre J, Hance AJ, et al: Evaluation of clinical judgment in the identification and treatment of nosocomial pneumonia in ventilated patients. Chest 103:547-553, 1993.
80. Kirtland SH, Corley DE, Winterbauer RH, et al: The diagnosis of ventilator-associated pneumonia: A comparison of histologic, microbiologic, and clinical criteria. Chest 112:445-457, 1997.
81. Fagon JY, Chastre J, Hance AJ, et al: Detection of nosocomial lung infection in ventilated patients. Use of a protected specimen brush and quantitative culture techniques in 147 patients. Am Rev Respir Dis 138:110-116, 1988.
82. Meduri GU: Diagnosis and differential diagnosis of ventilator-associated pneumonia. Clin Chest Med 16:61-93, 1995.
83. Theerthakarai R, El-Halees W, Ismail M, et al: Nonvalue of the initial microbiological studies in the management of nonsevere community-acquired pneumonia. Chest 119:181-184, 2001.
84. Lidman C, Burman LG, Lagergren A, et al: Limited value of routine microbiological diagnostics in patients hospitalized for community-acquired pneumonia. Scand J Infect Dis 34:873-879, 2002.
85. Ewig S, Schlochtermeier M, Goke N, et al: Applying sputum as a diagnostic tool in pneumonia: Limited yield, minimal impact on treatment decisions. Chest 121:1486-1492, 2002.
86. Kollef MH: Inadequate antimicrobial treatment: An important determinant of outcome for hospitalized patients. Clin Infect Dis 31(Suppl 4):S131-S138, 2000.

87. Iregui M, Ward S, Sherman G, et al: Clinical importance of delays in the initiation of appropriate antibiotic treatment for ventilator-associated pneumonia. Chest 122:262-268, 2002.
88. Rello J, Ausina V, Ricart M, et al: Impact of previous antimicrobial therapy on the etiology and outcome of ventilator-associated pneumonia. Chest 104:1230-1235, 1993.
89. Chastre J, Fagon JY: Ventilator-associated pneumonia. Am J Respir Crit Care Med 165:867-903, 2002.
90. Papazian L, Bregeon F, Thirion X, et al: Effect of ventilator-associated pneumonia on mortality and morbidity. Am J Respir Crit Care Med 154:91-97, 1996.
91. Kollef MH, Silver P, Murphy DM, et al: The effect of late-onset ventilator-associated pneumonia in determining patient mortality. Chest 108:1655-1662, 1995.
92. Niederman MS, Torres A, Summer W: Invasive diagnostic testing is not needed routinely to manage suspected ventilator-associated pneumonia. Am J Respir Crit Care Med 150:565-569, 1994.
93. Chastre J, Fagon JY: Invasive diagnostic testing should be routinely used to manage ventilated patients with suspected pneumonia. Am J Respir Crit Care Med 150:570-574, 1994.
94. Smith PR: What diagnostic tests are needed for community-acquired pneumonia? Med Clin North Am 85:1381-1396, 2001.
95. Mandell LA, Marrie TJ, Grossman RF, et al: Canadian guidelines for the initial management of community-acquired pneumonia: An evidence-based update by the Canadian Infectious Diseases Society and the Canadian Thoracic Society. The Canadian Community-Acquired Pneumonia Working Group. Clin Infect Dis 31:383-421, 2000.
96. Gleckman R, DeVita J, Hibert D, et al: Sputum gram stain assessment in community-acquired bacteremic pneumonia. J Clin Microbiol 26:846-849, 1988.
97. Glaister D: Early detection of lower respiratory tract infection: The value of the gram-stained sputum smear. Med Lab Sci 48:175-177, 1991.
98. Rello J, Bodi M, Mariscal D, et al: Microbiological testing and outcome of patients with severe community-acquired pneumonia. Chest 123:174-180, 2003.
99. Niederman MS, Mandell LA, Anzueto A, et al: Guidelines for the management of adults with community-acquired pneumonia. Diagnosis, assessment of severity, antimicrobial therapy, and prevention. Am J Respir Crit Care Med 163:1730-1754, 2001.
100. Bartlett JG, Dowell SF, Mandell LA, et al: Practice guidelines for the management of community-acquired pneumonia in adults. Infectious Diseases Society of America. Clin Infect Dis 31:347-382, 2000.
101. Skerrett SJ: Diagnostic testing to establish a microbial cause is helpful in the management of community-acquired pneumonia. Semin Respir Infect 12:308-321, 1997.
102. Luna CM, Videla A, Mattera J, et al: Blood cultures have limited value in predicting severity of illness and as a diagnostic tool in ventilator-associated pneumonia. Chest 116:1075-1084, 1999.
103. Rumbak MJ, Bass RL: Tracheal aspirate correlates with protected specimen brush in long-term ventilated patients who have clinical pneumonia. Chest 106:531-534, 1994.
104. Ioanas M, Ferrer R, Angrill J, et al: Microbial investigation in ventilator-associated pneumonia. Eur Respir J 17:791-801, 2001.
105. Wu CL, Yang D, Wang NY, et al: Quantitative culture of endotracheal aspirates in the diagnosis of ventilator-associated pneumonia in patients with treatment failure. Chest 122:662-668, 2002.
106. Bonten MJ, Bergmans DC, Stobberingh EE, et al: Implementation of bronchoscopic techniques in the diagnosis of ventilator-associated pneumonia to reduce antibiotic use. Am J Respir Crit Care Med 156:1820-1824, 1997.
107. Sole Violan J, Fernandez JA, Benitez AB, et al: Impact of quantitative invasive diagnostic techniques in the management and outcome of mechanically ventilated patients with suspected pneumonia. Crit Care Med 28:2737-2741, 2000.
108. Rello J, Paiva JA, Baraibar J, et al: International Conference for the Development of Consensus on the Diagnosis and Treatment of Ventilator-associated Pneumonia. Chest 120:955-970, 2001.
109. Chastre J, Fagon JY, Bornet-Lecso M, et al: Evaluation of bronchoscopic techniques for the diagnosis of nosocomial pneumonia. Am J Respir Crit Care Med 152:231-240, 1995.
110. Torres A, el-Ebiary M, Padro L, et al: Validation of different techniques for the diagnosis of ventilator-associated pneumonia. Comparison with immediate post-mortem pulmonary biopsy. Am J Respir Crit Care Med 149:324-331, 1994.
111. Marquette CH, Copin MC, Wallet F, et al: Diagnostic tests for pneumonia in ventilated patients: Prospective evaluation of diagnostic accuracy using histology as a diagnostic gold standard. Am J Respir Crit Care Med 151:1878-1888, 1995.
112. Fagon JY, Chastre J, Wolff M, et al: Invasive and noninvasive strategies for management of suspected ventilator-associated pneumonia. A randomized trial. Ann Intern Med 132:621-630, 2000.
113. Baker AM, Bowton DL, Haponik EF: Decision making in nosocomial pneumonia. An analytic approach to the interpretation of quantitative bronchoscopic cultures. Chest 107:85-95, 1995.
114. Jourdain B, Joly-Guillou ML, Dombret MC, et al: Usefulness of quantitative cultures of BAL fluid for diagnosing nosocomial pneumonia in ventilated patients. Chest 111:411-418, 1997.
115. Michaud S, Suzuki S, Harbarth S: Effect of design-related bias in studies of diagnostic tests for ventilator-associated pneumonia. Am J Respir Crit Care Med 166:1320-1325, 2002.
116. Meduri GU, Wunderink RG, Leeper KV, et al: Management of bacterial pneumonia in ventilated patients. Protected bronchoalveolar lavage as a diagnostic tool. Chest 101:500-508, 1992.
117. Timsit JF, Cheval C, Gachot B, et al: Usefulness of a strategy based on bronchoscopy with direct examination of bronchoalveolar lavage fluid in the initial antibiotic therapy of suspected ventilator-associated pneumonia. Intensive Care Med 27:640-647, 2001.
118. Garrard CS, A'Court CD: The diagnosis of pneumonia in the critically ill. Chest 108:17S-25S, 1995.
119. Torres A, Jimenez P, Puig de la Bellacasa J, et al: Diagnostic value of nonfluoroscopic percutaneous lung needle aspiration in patients with pneumonia. Chest 98:840-844, 1990.
120. Scott JA, Hall AJ: The value and complications of percutaneous transthoracic lung aspiration for the etiologic diagnosis of community-acquired pneumonia. Chest 116:1716-1732, 1999.
121. Dorca J, Manresa F, Esteban L, et al: Efficacy, safety, and therapeutic relevance of transthoracic aspiration with ultrathin needle in nonventilated nosocomial pneumonia. Am J Respir Crit Care Med 151:1491-1496, 1995.
122. Zalacain R, Llorente JL, Gaztelurrutia L, et al: Influence of three factors on the diagnostic effectiveness of transthoracic needle aspiration in pneumonia. Chest 107:96-100, 1995.
123. Timsit JF, Chevret S, Valcke J, et al: Mortality of nosocomial pneumonia in ventilated patients: Influence of diagnostic tools. Am J Respir Crit Care Med 154:116-123, 1996.
124. Sanchez-Nieto JM, Torres A, Garcia-Cordoba F, et al: Impact of invasive and noninvasive quantitative culture sampling on outcome of ventilator-associated pneumonia: A pilot study. Am J Respir Crit Care Med 157:371-376, 1998.
125. Niederman MS, Bass JB Jr, Campbell GD, et al: Guidelines for the initial management of adults with community-acquired pneumonia: Diagnosis, assessment of severity, and initial antimicrobial therapy. American Thoracic Society. Medical Section of the American Lung Association. Am Rev Respir Dis 148:1418-1426, 1993.
126. Ruiz M, Ewig S, Marcos MA, et al: Etiology of community-acquired pneumonia: Impact of age, comorbidity, and severity. Am J Respir Crit Care Med 160:397-405, 1999.
127. Woodhead M: Community-acquired pneumonia in Europe: Causative pathogens and resistance patterns. Eur Respir J Suppl 36:20s-27s, 2002.
128. Kato T, Uemura H, Murakami N, et al: Incidence of anaerobic infections among patients with pulmonary diseases: Japanese experience with transtracheal aspiration and immediate bedside anaerobic inoculation. Clin Infect Dis 23(Suppl 1):S87-S96, 1996.
129. Carr B, Walsh JB, Coakley D, et al: Prospective hospital study of community acquired lower respiratory tract infection in the elderly. Respir Med 85:185-187, 1991.
130. Soler N, Torres A, Ewig S, et al: Bronchial microbial patterns in severe exacerbations of chronic obstructive pulmonary disease (COPD) requiring mechanical ventilation. Am J Respir Crit Care Med 157:1498-1505, 1998.
131. Johnston BL: Methicillin-resistant Staphylococcus aureus as a cause of community-acquired pneumonia—a critical review. Semin Respir Infect 9:199-206, 1994.
132. El-Solh AA, Sikka P, Ramadan F, et al: Etiology of severe pneumonia in the very elderly. Am J Respir Crit Care Med 163:645-651, 2001.
133. Leroy O, Vandenbussche C, Coffinier C, et al: Community-acquired aspiration pneumonia in intensive care units. Epidemiological and prognosis data. Am J Respir Crit Care Med 156:1922-1929, 1997.
134. Leroy O, Santre C, Beuscart C, et al: A five-year study of severe community-acquired pneumonia with emphasis on prognosis in patients admitted to an intensive care unit. Intensive Care Med 21:24-31, 1995.
135. Chan CH, Cohen M, Pang J: A prospective study of community-acquired pneumonia in Hong Kong. Chest 101:442-446, 1992.
136. Marrie TJ, Peeling RW, Fine MJ, et al: Ambulatory patients with community acquired pneumonia: the frequency of atypical agents and clinical course. Am J Med 101:508-515, 1996.
137. Porath A, Schlaeffer F, Lieberman D: The epidemiology of community-acquired pneumonia among hospitalized adults. J Infect 34:41-48, 1997.
138. Maartens G, Lewis SJ, de Goveia C, et al: 'Atypical' bacteria are a common cause of community-acquired pneumonia in hospitalised adults. S Afr Med J 84:678-682, 1994.
139. Community-acquired pneumonia in adults in British hospitals in 1982-1983: A survey of aetiology, mortality, prognostic factors and outcome. The British Thoracic Society and the Public Health Laboratory Service. QJM 62:195-220, 1987.
140. Blanquer J, Blanquer R, Borras R, et al: Aetiology of community acquired pneumonia in Valencia, Spain: A multicentre prospective study. Thorax 46:508-511, 1991.
141. Ruiz M, Ewig S, Torres A, et al: Severe community-acquired pneumonia. Risk factors and follow-up epidemiology. Am J Respir Crit Care Med 160:923-929, 1999.
142. Gilbert K, Fine MJ: Assessing prognosis and predicting patient outcomes in community-acquired pneumonia. Semin Respir Infect 9:140-152, 1994.
143. Metlay JP, Fine MJ: Testing strategies in the initial management of patients with community-acquired pneumonia. Ann Intern Med 138:109-118, 2003.
144. Marras TK, Gutierrez C, Chan CK: Applying a prediction rule to identify low-risk patients with community-acquired pneumonia. Chest 118:1339-1343, 2000.
145. Fine MJ, Hough LJ, Medsger AR, et al: The hospital admission decision for patients with community-acquired pneumonia. Results from the pneumonia Patient Outcomes Research Team cohort study. Arch Intern Med 157:36-44, 1997.
146. Craven DE, Steger KA: Epidemiology of nosocomial pneumonia. New perspectives on an old disease. Chest 108:1S-16S, 1995.

147. Dore P, Robert R, Grollier G, et al: Incidence of anaerobes in ventilator-associated pneumonia with use of a protected specimen brush. Am J Respir Crit Care Med 153:1292-1298, 1996.

148. Talon D, Mulin B, Rouget C, et al: Risks and routes for ventilator-associated pneumonia with Pseudomonas aeruginosa. Am J Respir Crit Care Med 157:978-984, 1998.

149. Rello J, Quintana E, Ausina V, et al: Risk factors for Staphylococcus aureus nosocomial pneumonia in critically ill patients. Am Rev Respir Dis 142:1320-1324, 1990.

150. Carratala J, Gudiol F, Pallares R, et al: Risk factors for nosocomial Legionella pneumophila pneumonia. Am J Respir Crit Care Med 149:625-629, 1994.

151. Trouillet JL, Chastre J, Vuagnat A, et al: Ventilator-associated pneumonia caused by potentially drug-resistant bacteria. Am J Respir Crit Care Med 157:531-539, 1998.

152. Ibrahim EH, Ward S, Sherman G, et al: A comparative analysis of patients with early-onset vs late-onset nosocomial pneumonia in the ICU setting. Chest 117:1434-1442, 2000.

153. Guidelines for prevention of nosocomial pneumonia. Centers for Disease Control and Prevention. MMWR Recomm Rep 46(RR-1):1-79, 1997.

154. Markowicz P, Wolff M, Djedaini K, et al: Multicenter prospective study of ventilator-associated pneumonia during acute respiratory distress syndrome. Incidence, prognosis, and risk factors. ARDS Study Group. Am J Respir Crit Care Med 161:1942-1948, 2000.

155. Regelmann W, Filipovich A: Lung involvement in the primary immunodeficiency syndromes. Semin Respir Med 13:190, 1992.

156. Dukes RJ, Rosenow EC 3rd, Hermans PE: Pulmonary manifestations of hypogammaglobulinaemia. Thorax 33:603-607, 1978.

157. Sweinberg SK, Wodell RA, Grodofsky MP, et al: Retrospective analysis of the incidence of pulmonary disease in hypogammaglobulinemia. J Allergy Clin Immunol 88:96-104, 1991.

158. Popa V, Colby TV, Reich SB: Pulmonary interstitial disease in Ig deficiency. Chest 122:1594-1603, 2002.

159. Brooks G, Butel J, Ornston L: Javetz, Melnick & Adelberg's Medical Microbiology. Norwalk, CT, Appleton & Lange, 1995.

160. George WL, Finegold SM: Bacterial infections of the lung. Chest 81:502-507, 1982.

161. Porath A, Schlaeffer F, Pick N, et al: Pneumococcal community-acquired pneumonia in 148 hospitalized adult patients. Eur J Clin Microbiol Infect Dis 16:863-870, 1997.

162. Klugman KP, Feldman C: Streptococcus pneumoniae respiratory tract infections. Curr Opin Infect Dis 14:173-179, 2001.

163. Musher DM, Alexandraki I, Graviss EA, et al: Bacteremic and nonbacteremic pneumococcal pneumonia. A prospective study. Medicine (Baltimore) 79:210-221, 2000.

164. Garau J: Treatment of drug-resistant pneumococcal pneumonia. Lancet Infect Dis 2:404-415, 2002.

165. Tuomanen EI, Austrian R, Masure HR: Pathogenesis of pneumococcal infection. N Engl J Med 332:1280-1284, 1995.

166. Wizemann TM, Moskovitz J, Pearce BJ, et al: Peptide methionine sulfoxide reductase contributes to the maintenance of adhesins in three major pathogens. Proc Natl Acad Sci U S A 93:7985-7990, 1996.

167. Hakansson A, Kidd A, Wadell G, et al: Adenovirus infection enhances in vitro adherence of Streptococcus pneumoniae. Infect Immun 62:2707-2714, 1994.

168. Novak R, Tuomanen E: Pathogenesis of pneumococcal pneumonia. Semin Respir Infect 14:209-217, 1999.

169. Boutten A, Dehoux MS, Seta N, et al: Compartmentalized IL-8 and elastase release within the human lung in unilateral pneumonia. Am J Respir Crit Care Med 153:336-342, 1996.

170. Lonky SA, Marsh J, Steele R, et al: Protease and antiprotease responses in lung and peripheral blood in experimental canine pneumococcal pneumonia. Am Rev Respir Dis 121:685-693, 1980.

171. Leatherman JW, Iber C, Davies SF: Cavitation in bacteremic pneumococcal pneumonia. Causal role of mixed infection with anaerobic bacteria. Am Rev Respir Dis 129:317-321, 1984.

172. Hershey CO, Panaro V: Round pneumonia in adults. Arch Intern Med 148:1155-1157, 1988.

173. Brewin A, Arango L, Hadley WK, et al: High-dose penicillin therapy and pneumococcal pneumonia. JAMA 230:409-413, 1974.

174. Moine P, Vercken JB, Chevret S, et al: Severe community-acquired pneumonia. Etiology, epidemiology, and prognosis factors. French Study Group for Community-Acquired Pneumonia in the Intensive Care Unit. Chest 105:1487-1495, 1994.

175. Lippmann ML, Goldberg SK, Walkenstein MD, et al: Bacteremic pneumococcal pneumonia. A community hospital experience. Chest 108:1608-1613, 1995.

176. Musgrave T, Verghese A: Clinical features of pneumonia in the elderly. Semin Respir Infect 5:269-275, 1990.

177. Fernandez-Sabe N, Roson B, Carratala J, et al: Clinical diagnosis of Legionella pneumonia revisited: Evaluation of the Community-Based Pneumonia Incidence Study Group scoring system. Clin Infect Dis 37:483-489, 2003.

178. Austrian R: Pneumococcal pneumonia. Diagnostic, epidemiologic, therapeutic and prophylactic considerations. Chest 90:738-743, 1986.

179. Roson B, Carratala J, Verdaguer R, et al: Prospective study of the usefulness of sputum Gram stain in the initial approach to community-acquired pneumonia requiring hospitalization. Clin Infect Dis 31:869-874, 2000.

180. Jimenez P, Meneses M, Saldias F, et al: Pneumococcal antigen detection in bronchoalveolar lavage fluid from patients with pneumonia. Thorax 49:872-874, 1994.

181. Menendez Villanueva R: The diagnostic evaluation of rapid sputum technics for Pneumonococcus in community-acquired pneumonia: The usefulness of Bayes theorem for clinical application. Arch Bronchopneumol 31:317, 1995.

182. Gillespie SH, Smith MD, Dickens A, et al: Diagnosis of Streptococcus pneumoniae pneumonia by quantitative enzyme linked immunosorbent assay of C-polysaccharide antigen. J Clin Pathol 47:749-751, 1994.

183. Salo P, Ortqvist A, Leinonen M: Diagnosis of bacteremic pneumococcal pneumonia by amplification of pneumolysin gene fragment in serum. J Infect Dis 171:479-482, 1995.

184. Scott JA, Marston EL, Hall AJ, et al: Diagnosis of pneumococcal pneumonia by psaA PCR analysis of lung aspirates from adult patients in Kenya. J Clin Microbiol 41:2554-2559, 2003.

185. Falguera M, Lopez A, Nogues A, et al: Evaluation of the polymerase chain reaction method for detection of Streptococcus pneumoniae DNA in pleural fluid samples. Chest 122:2212-2216, 2002.

186. Murdoch DR, Anderson TP, Beynon KA, et al: Evaluation of a PCR assay for detection of Streptococcus pneumoniae in respiratory and nonrespiratory samples from adults with community-acquired pneumonia. J Clin Microbiol 41:63-66, 2003.

187. Torres JM, Cardenas O, Vasquez A, et al: Streptococcus pneumoniae bacteremia in a community hospital. Chest 113:387-390, 1998.

188. Watanakunakorn C, Greifenstein A, Stroh K, et al: Pneumococcal bacteremia in three community teaching hospitals from 1980 to 1989. Chest 103:1152-1156, 1993.

189. Moroney JF, Fiore AE, Harrison LH, et al: Clinical outcomes of bacteremic pneumococcal pneumonia in the era of antibiotic resistance. Clin Infect Dis 33:797-805, 2001.

190. O'Brien KL, Beall B, Barrett NL, et al: Epidemiology of invasive group A streptococcus disease in the United States, 1995-1999. Clin Infect Dis 35:268-276, 2002.

191. Outbreak of group A streptococcal pneumonia among Marine Corps recruits—California, November 1–December 20, 2002. MMWR Morb Mortal Wkly Rep 52(6):106-109, 2003.

192. Basiliere JL, Bistrong HW, Spence WF: Streptococcal pneumonia. Recent outbreaks in military recruit populations. Am J Med 44:580-589, 1968.

193. Welch CC, Tombridge TL, Baker WJ, et al: β-Hemolytic streptococcal pneumonia: Report of an outbreak in a military population. Am J Med Sci 242:157-165, 1961.

194. al-Ujayli B, Nafziger DA, Saravolatz L: Pneumonia due to Staphylococcus aureus infection. Clin Chest Med 16:111-120, 1995.

195. El-Solh AA, Pietrantoni C, Bhat A, et al: Microbiology of severe aspiration pneumonia in institutionalized elderly. Am J Respir Crit Care Med 167:1650-1654, 2003.

196. Gonzalez C, Rubio M, Romero-Vivas J, et al: Staphylococcus aureus bacteremic pneumonia: Differences between community and nosocomial acquisition. Int J Infect Dis 7:102-108, 2003.

197. Kaye MG, Fox MJ, Bartlett JG, et al: The clinical spectrum of Staphylococcus aureus pulmonary infection. Chest 97:788-792, 1990.

198. Chartrand SA, McCracken GH Jr: Staphylococcal pneumonia in infants and children. Pediatr Infect Dis 1:19-23, 1982.

199. Naraqi S, McDonnell G: Hematogenous staphylococcal pneumonia secondary to soft tissue infection. Chest 79:173-175, 1981.

200. Huang RM, Naidich DP, Lubat E, et al: Septic pulmonary emboli: CT-radiographic correlation. AJR Am J Roentgenol 153:41-45, 1989.

201. Kuperman AS, Fernandez RB: Subacute staphylococcal pneumonia. Am Rev Respir Dis 101:95-100, 1970.

202. Bergmans D, Bonten M, Gaillard C, et al: Clinical spectrum of ventilator-associated pneumonia caused by methicillin-sensitive Staphylococcus aureus. Eur J Clin Microbiol Infect Dis 15:437-445, 1996.

203. Wright PW, Wallace RJ Jr: Pneumonia due to Moraxella (Branhamella) catarrhalis. Semin Respir Infect 4:40-46, 1989.

204. Verduin CM, Hol C, Fleer A, et al: Moraxella catarrhalis: From emerging to established pathogen. Clin Microbiol Rev 15:125-144, 2002.

205. Barreiro B, Esteban L, Prats E, et al: Branhamella catarrhalis respiratory infections. Eur Respir J 5:675-679, 1992.

206. Sugiyama H, Ogata E, Shimamoto Y, et al: Bacteremic Moraxella catarrhalis pneumonia in a patient with immunoglobulin deficiency. J Infect Chemother 6:61-62, 2000.

207. Richards SJ, Greening AP, Enright MC, et al: Outbreak of Moraxella catarrhalis in a respiratory unit. Thorax 48:91-92, 1993.

208. Wallace RJ Jr, Musher DM: In honor of Dr. Sarah Branham, a star is born. The realization of Branhamella catarrhalis as a respiratory pathogen. Chest 90:447-450, 1986.

209. Winstead JM, McKinsey DS, Tasker S, et al: Meningococcal pneumonia: Characterization and review of cases seen over the past 25 years. Clin Infect Dis 30:87-94, 2000.

210. Lambotte O, Timsit JF, Garrouste-Orgeas M, et al: The significance of distal bronchial samples with commensals in ventilator-associated pneumonia: Colonizer or pathogen? Chest 122:1389-1399, 2002.

211. Davies BI, Spanjaard L, Dankert J: Meningococcal chest infections in a general hospital. Eur J Clin Microbiol Infect Dis 10:399-404, 1991.

212. Ellenbogen C, Graybill JR, Silva J Jr, et al: Bacterial pneumonia complicating adenoviral pneumonia. A comparison of respiratory tract bacterial culture sources and effectiveness of chemoprophylaxis against bacterial pneumonia. Am J Med 56:169-178, 1974.

213. Young LS, LaForce FM, Head JJ, et al: A simultaneous outbreak of meningococcal and influenza infections. N Engl J Med 287:5-9, 1972.

214. Witt D, Olans RN: Bacteremic W-135 meningococcal pneumonia. Am Rev Respir Dis 125:255-257, 1982.

215. Guarner J, Jernigan JA, Shieh WJ, et al: Pathology and pathogenesis of bioterrorism-related inhalational anthrax. Am J Pathol 163:701-709, 2003.

216. Shafazand S: When bioterrorism strikes: Diagnosis and management of inhalational anthrax. Semin Respir Infect 18:134-145, 2003.

217. Quintiliani R Jr, Quintiliani R: Inhalational anthrax and bioterrorism. Curr Opin Pulm Med 9:221-226, 2003.

218. Shafazand S, Doyle R, Ruoss S, et al: Inhalational anthrax: Epidemiology, diagnosis, and management. Chest 116:1369-1376, 1999.

219. Brown K: Anthrax. A 'sure killer' yields to medicine. Science 294:1813-1814, 2001.

220. Earls JP, Cerva D Jr, Berman E, et al: Inhalational anthrax after bioterrorism exposure: Spectrum of imaging findings in two surviving patients. Radiology 222:305-312, 2002.

221. Wood B, DeFranco B, Ripple M, et al: Inhalational anthrax: Radiologic and pathologic findings in two cases. AJR Am J Roentgenol 181:1071, 2003.

222. Krol CM, Uszynski M, Dillon EH, et al: Dynamic CT features of inhalational anthrax infection. AJR Am J Roentgenol 178:1063-1066, 2002.

223. Hupert N, Bearman GM, Mushlin AI, et al: Accuracy of screening for inhalational anthrax after a bioterrorist attack. Ann Intern Med 139:337-345, 2003.

224. Kuehnert MJ, Doyle TJ, Hill HA, et al: Clinical features that discriminate inhalational anthrax from other acute respiratory illnesses. Clin Infect Dis 36:328-336, 2003.

225. Farber JM, Ross WH, Harwig J: Health risk assessment of *Listeria monocytogenes* in Canada. Int J Food Microbiol 30:145-156, 1996.

226. Ananthraman A, Israel RH, Magnussen CR: Pleural-pulmonary aspects of *Listeria monocytogenes* infection. Respiration 44:153-157, 1983.

227. Dobie RA, Tobey DN: Clinical features of diphtheria in the respiratory tract. JAMA 242:2197-201, 1979.

228. Stamm WE, Tompkins LS, Wagner KF, et al: Infection due to *Corynebacterium* species in marrow transplant patients. Ann Intern Med 91:167-173, 1979.

229. Perez MG, Vassilev T, Kemmerly SA: *Rhodococcus equi* infection in transplant recipients: A case of mistaken identity and review of the literature. Transpl Infect Dis 4:52-56, 2002.

230. Verville TD, Huycke MM, Greenfield RA, et al: *Rhodococcus equi* infections of humans. 12 cases and a review of the literature. Medicine (Baltimore) 73:119-132, 1994.

231. Gorzynski E: Enterobacteriaceae: II. In Milgrom F, Flanagan T (eds): Medical Microbiology. New York, Churchill Livingstone, 1982, p 309.

232. Yinnon AM, Butnaru A, Raveh D, et al: *Klebsiella* bacteraemia: Community versus nosocomial infection. QJM 89:933-941, 1996.

233. Bouza E, Cercenado E: *Klebsiella* and *Enterobacter:* Antibiotic resistance and treatment implications. Semin Respir Infect 17:215-230, 2002.

234. Ko WC, Paterson DL, Sagnimeni AJ, et al: Community-acquired *Klebsiella pneumoniae* bacteremia: Global differences in clinical patterns. Emerg Infect Dis 8:160-166, 2002.

235. Karnad A, Alvarez S, Berk SL: *Enterobacter* pneumonia. South Med J 80:601-604, 1987.

236. Kirschke DL, Jones TF, Craig AS, et al: *Pseudomonas aeruginosa* and *Serratia marcescens* contamination associated with a manufacturing defect in bronchoscopes. N Engl J Med 348:214-220, 2003.

237. Reed WP: Indolent pulmonary abscess associated with *Klebsiella* and *Enterobacter*. Am Rev Respir Dis 107:1055-1059, 1973.

238. Goldstein JD, Godleski JJ, Balikian JP, et al: Pathologic patterns of *Serratia marcescens* pneumonia. Hum Pathol 13:479-484, 1982.

239. Pierce AK, Sanford JP: Aerobic gram-negative bacillary pneumonias. Am Rev Respir Dis 110:647-658, 1974.

240. Moon WK, Im JG, Yeon KM, et al: Complications of *Klebsiella* pneumonia: CT evaluation. J Comput Assist Tomogr 19:176-181, 1995.

241. Holmes RB: Friedlander's pneumonia. Am J Roentgenol Radium Ther Nucl Med 75:728-745, discussion, 745-747, 1956.

242. Crossley KB, Thurn JR: Nursing home-acquired pneumonia. Semin Respir Infect 4:64-72, 1989.

243. Mundy LM, Auwaerter PG, Oldach D, et al: Community-acquired pneumonia: Impact of immune status. Am J Respir Crit Care Med 152:1309-1315, 1995.

244. Tillotson JR, Lerner AM: Pneumonias caused by gram negative bacilli. Medicine (Baltimore) 45:65-76, 1966.

245. Aguado JM, Obeso G, Cabanillas JJ, et al: Pleuropulmonary infections due to nontyphoid strains of *Salmonella*. Arch Intern Med 150:54-56, 1990.

246. Casado JL, Navas E, Frutos B, et al: *Salmonella* lung involvement in patients with HIV infection. Chest 112:1197-1201, 1997.

247. Burney DP, Fisher RD, Schaffner W: *Salmonella* empyema: A review. South Med J 70:375-377, 1977.

248. Sharma AM, Sharma OP: Pulmonary manifestations of typhoid fever. Two case reports and a review of the literature. Chest 101:1144-1146, 1992.

249. Adler JL, Burke JP, Martin DF, et al: *Proteus* infections in a general hospital. II. Some clinical and epidemiological characteristics. With an analysis of 71 cases of *Proteus* bacteremia. Ann Intern Med 75:531-536, 1971.

250. Centers for Disease Control and Prevention (CDC): Imported plague—New York City, 2002. MMWR Morb Mortal Wkly Rep 52(31):725-728, 2003.

251. Gage KL, Dennis DT, Orloski KA, et al: Cases of cat-associated human plague in the Western US, 1977-1998. Clin Infect Dis 30:893-900, 2000.

252. Plague pneumonia—California. MMWR Morb Mortal Wkly Rep 33:481-3, 1984.

253. Burmeister RW, Tigertt WD, Overholt EL: Laboratory-acquired pneumonic plague. Report of a case and review of previous cases. Ann Intern Med 56:789-800, 1962.

254. Chang MH, Glynn MK, Groseclose SL: Endemic, notifiable bioterrorism-related diseases, United States, 1992-1999. Emerg Infect Dis 9:556-564, 2003.

255. Krishna G, Chitkara RK: Pneumonic plague. Semin Respir Infect 18:159-167, 2003.

256. Alsofrom DJ, Mettler FA Jr, Mann JM: Radiographic manifestations of plague in New Mexico, 1975-1980. A review of 42 proved cases. Radiology 139:561-565, 1981.

257. Sites VR, Poland JD: Mediastinal lymphadenopathy in bubonic plague. Am J Roentgenol Radium Ther Nucl Med 116:567-570, 1972.

258. Dennis DT, Hughes JM: Multidrug resistance in plague. N Engl J Med 337:702-704, 1997.

259. Klein NC, Cunha BA: *Pasteurella multocida* pneumonia. Semin Respir Infect 12:54-56, 1997.

260. Hubbert WT, Rosen MN: *Pasteurella multocida* infections. II. *Pasteurella multocida* infection in man unrelated to animal bite. Am J Public Health Nations Health 60:1109-1117, 1970.

261. Ip M, Osterberg LG, Chau PY, et al: Pulmonary melioidosis. Chest 108:1420-1424, 1995.

262. Suputtamongkol Y, Hall AJ, Dance DA, et al: The epidemiology of melioidosis in Ubon Ratchatani, northeast Thailand. Int J Epidemiol 23:1082-1090, 1994.

263. Currie BJ, Fisher DA, Howard DM, et al: Endemic melioidosis in tropical northern Australia: A 10-year prospective study and review of the literature. Clin Infect Dis 31:981-986, 2000.

264. Piggott JA, Hochholzer L: Human melioidosis. A histopathologic study of acute and chronic melioidosis. Arch Pathol 90:101-111, 1970.

265. Dhiensiri T, Puapairoj S, Susaengrat W: Pulmonary melioidosis: Clinical-radiologic correlation in 183 cases in northeastern Thailand. Radiology 166:711-715, 1988.

266. Chong VF, Fan YF: The radiology of melioidosis. Australas Radiol 40:244-249, 1996.

267. Everett ED, Nelson RA: Pulmonary melioidosis. Observations in thirty-nine cases. Am Rev Respir Dis 112:331-340, 1975.

268. Kanaphun P, Thirawattanasuk N, Suputtamongkol Y, et al: Serology and carriage of *Pseudomonas pseudomallei:* A prospective study in 1000 hospitalized children in northeast Thailand. J Infect Dis 167:230-233, 1993.

269. Phung LV, Han Y, Oka S, et al: Enzyme-linked immunosorbent assay (ELISA) using a glycolipid antigen for the serodiagnosis of melioidosis. FEMS Immunol Med Microbiol 12:259-264, 1995.

270. Desakorn V, Smith MD, Wuthiekanun V, et al: Detection of *Pseudomonas pseudomallei* antigen in urine for the diagnosis of melioidosis. Am J Trop Med Hyg 51:627-633, 1994.

271. Taylor RF, Gaya H, Hodson ME: *Pseudomonas cepacia:* Pulmonary infection in patients with cystic fibrosis. Respir Med 87:187-192, 1993.

272. Soni R, Marks G, Henry DA, et al: Effect of *Burkholderia cepacia* infection in the clinical course of patients with cystic fibrosis: A pilot study in a Sydney clinic. Respirology 7:241-245, 2002.

273. Muhdi K, Edenborough FP, Gumery L, et al: Outcome for patients colonised with *Burkholderia cepacia* in a Birmingham adult cystic fibrosis clinic and the end of an epidemic. Thorax 51:374-377, 1996.

274. Aris RM, Routh JC, LiPuma JJ, et al: Lung transplantation for cystic fibrosis patients with *Burkholderia cepacia* complex. Survival linked to genomovar type. Am J Respir Crit Care Med 164:2102-2106, 2001.

275. Yamagishi Y, Fujita J, Takigawa K, et al: Clinical features of *Pseudomonas cepacia* pneumonia in an epidemic among immunocompromised patients. Chest 103:1706-1709, 1993.

276. Dunn M, Wunderink RG: Ventilator-associated pneumonia caused by *Pseudomonas* infection. Clin Chest Med 16:95-109, 1995.

277. Richards MJ, Edwards JR, Culver DH, et al: Nosocomial infections in medical intensive care units in the United States. National Nosocomial Infections Surveillance System. Crit Care Med 27:887-892, 1999.

278. Nseir S, Di Pompeo C, Pronnier P, et al: Nosocomial tracheobronchitis in mechanically ventilated patients: Incidence, aetiology and outcome. Eur Respir J 20:1483-1489, 2002.

279. Cobben NA, Drent M, Jonkers M, et al: Outbreak of severe *Pseudomonas aeruginosa* respiratory infections due to contaminated nebulizers. J Hosp Infect 33:63-70, 1996.

280. Chastre J, Trouillet JL: Problem pathogens (*Pseudomonas aeruginosa* and *Acinetobacter*). Semin Respir Infect 15:287-298, 2000.

281. Arancibia F, Bauer TT, Ewig S, et al: Community-acquired pneumonia due to gram-negative bacteria and *Pseudomonas aeruginosa:* Incidence, risk, and prognosis. Arch Intern Med 162:1849-1858, 2002.

282. Rello J, Sonora R, Jubert P, et al: Pneumonia in intubated patients: Role of respiratory airway care. Am J Respir Crit Care Med 154:111-115, 1996.

283. de Bentzmann S, Roger P, Puchelle E: *Pseudomonas aeruginosa* adherence to remodelling respiratory epithelium. Eur Respir J 9:2145-2150, 1996.

284. Azghani AO: *Pseudomonas aeruginosa* and epithelial permeability: Role of virulence factors elastase and exotoxin A. Am J Respir Cell Mol Biol 15:132-140, 1996.

285. Winer-Muram HT, Jennings SG, Wunderink RG, et al: Ventilator-associated *Pseudomonas aeruginosa* pneumonia: Radiographic findings. Radiology 195:247-252, 1995.

286. Joffe N: Roentgenologic aspects of primary *Pseudomonas aeruginosa* pneumonia in mechanically ventilated patients. Am J Roentgenol Radium Ther Nucl Med 107:305-312, 1969.

287. Iannini PB, Claffey T, Quintiliani R: Bacteremic *Pseudomonas* pneumonia. JAMA 230:558-561, 1974.

288. Gopalakrishnan R, Hawley HB, Czachor JS, et al: *Stenotrophomonas maltophilia* infection and colonization in the intensive care units of two community hospitals: A study of 143 patients. Heart Lung 28:134-141, 1999.

289. Goss CH, Otto K, Aitken ML, et al: Detecting *Stenotrophomonas maltophilia* does not reduce survival of patients with cystic fibrosis. Am J Respir Crit Care Med 166:356-361, 2002.

290. Baraibar J, Correa H, Mariscal D, et al: Risk factors for infection by *Acinetobacter baumannii* in intubated patients with nosocomial pneumonia. Chest 112:1050-1054, 1997.

291. Abbasi S, Chesney PJ: Pulmonary manifestations of cat-scratch disease; a case report and review of the literature. Pediatr Infect Dis J 14:547-548, 1995.

292. Moore EH, Russell LA, Klein JS, et al: Bacillary angiomatosis in patients with AIDS: Multiorgan imaging findings. Radiology 197:67-72, 1995.

293. Bruckner DA, Colonna P: Nomenclature for aerobic and facultative bacteria. Clin Infect Dis 21:263-272, 1995.

294. Hoey J: Pertussis in adults. CMAJ 168:453-454, 2003.

295. Pertussis—United States, 1997-2000. MMWR Morb Mortal Wkly Rep 51(4):73-76, 2002.

296. Keitel WA, Edwards KM: Pertussis in adolescents and adults: Time to reimmunize? Semin Respir Infect 10:51-57, 1995.

297. Fawcett J, Parry HE: Lung changes in pertussis and measles in childhood; a review of 1894 cases with a follow-up study of the pulmonary complications. Br J Radiol 30:76-82, 1957.

298. Gilberg S, Njamkepo E, Du Chatelet IP, et al: Evidence of *Bordetella pertussis* infection in adults presenting with persistent cough in a french area with very high whole-cell vaccine coverage. J Infect Dis 186:415-418, 2002.

299. Grob PR, Crowder MJ, Robbins JF: Effect of vaccination on severity and dissemination of whooping cough. Br Med J (Clin Res Ed) 282:1925-1928, 1981.

300. Respiratory sequele of whooping cough: Swansea Research Unit of the Royal College of General Practitioners. BMJ 290:1937, 1985.

301. Jensen WA, Kirsch CM: Tularemia. Semin Respir Infect 18:146-158, 2003.

302. Reintjes R, Dedushaj I, Gjini A, et al: Tularemia outbreak investigation in Kosovo: Case control and environmental studies. Emerg Infect Dis 8:69-73, 2002.

303. Feldman KA, Enscore RE, Lathrop SL, et al: An outbreak of primary pneumonic tularemia on Martha's Vineyard. N Engl J Med 345:1601-1606, 2001.

304. Rubin SA: Radiographic spectrum of pleuropulmonary tularemia. AJR Am J Roentgenol 131:277-281, 1978.

305. Trollfors B, Brorson JE, Claesson B, et al: Invasive infections caused by *Haemophilus* species other than *Haemophilus influenzae*. Infection 13:12-14, 1985.

306. Johnson SR, Thompson RC, Humphreys H, et al: Clinical features of patients with beta-lactamase producing *Haemophilus influenzae* isolated from sputum. J Antimicrob Chemother 38:881-884, 1996.

307. Zalacain R, Torres A, Celis R, et al: Community-acquired pneumonia in the elderly: Spanish multicentre study. Eur Respir J 21:294-302, 2003.

308. Pfaller MA, Ehrhardt AF, Jones RN: Frequency of pathogen occurrence and antimicrobial susceptibility among community-acquired respiratory tract infections in the respiratory surveillance program study: Microbiology from the medical office practice environment. Am J Med 111(Suppl 9A):4S-12S, discussion 36S-38S, 2001.

309. Neill AM, Martin IR, Weir R, et al: Community acquired pneumonia: Aetiology and usefulness of severity criteria on admission. Thorax 51:1010-1016, 1996.

310. Kirtland SH, Winterbauer RH, Dreis DF, et al: A clinical profile of chronic bacterial pneumonia. Report of 115 cases. Chest 106:15-22, 1994.

311. Khilanani U, Khatib R: Acute epiglottitis in adults. Am J Med Sci 287:65-70, 1984.

312. Pearlberg J, Haggar AM, Saravolatz L, et al: *Hemophilus influenzae* pneumonia in the adult. Radiographic appearance with clinical correlation. Radiology 151:23-26, 1984.

313. Quinones CA, Memon MA, Sarosi GA: Bacteremic *Hemophilus influenzae* pneumonia in the adult. Semin Respir Infect 4:12-18, 1989.

314. Waterer GW, Baselski VS, Wunderink RG: *Legionella* and community-acquired pneumonia: A review of current diagnostic tests from a clinician's viewpoint. Am J Med 110:41-48, 2001.

315. Conwill DE, Werner SB, Dritz SK, et al: Legionellosis—the 1980 San Francisco outbreak. Am Rev Respir Dis 126:666-669, 1982.

316. Nechwatal R, Ehret W, Klatte OJ, et al: Nosocomial outbreak of legionellosis in a rehabilitation center. Demonstration of potable water as a source. Infection 21:235-240, 1993.

317. England AC III, Fraser AW, Plikayhs BD, et al: Sporadic legionellosis in The United States: The first thousand cases. Ann Intern Med 94:164-170, 1981.

318. Van Arsdall JA 2nd, Wunderlich HF, Melo JC, et al: The protean manifestations of legionnaires' disease. J Infect 7:51-62, 1983.

319. Fraser DW: Legionnaires' disease: Four summers' harvest. Am J Med 68:1-2, 1980.

320. Breiman RF, Butler JC: Legionnaires' disease: Clinical, epidemiological, and public health perspectives. Semin Respir Infect 13:84-89, 1998.

321. Bartlett JG: New developments in infectious diseases for the critical care physician. Crit Care Med 11:563-573, 1983.

322. Lieberman D, Schlaeffer F, Boldur I, et al: Multiple pathogens in adult patients admitted with community-acquired pneumonia: A one year prospective study of 346 consecutive patients. Thorax 51:179-184, 1996.

323. Bohte R, van Furth R, van den Broek PJ: Aetiology of community-acquired pneumonia: A prospective study among adults requiring admission to hospital. Thorax 50:543-547, 1995.

324. Roig J, Domingo C, Morera J: Legionnaires' disease. Chest 105:1817-1825, 1994.

325. Stout JE, Yu VL: Legionellosis. N Engl J Med 337:682-687, 1997.

326. Muder RR, Yu VL, Fang GD: Community-acquired legionnaires' disease. Semin Respir Infect 4:32-39, 1989.

327. Friedman S, Spitalny K, Barbaree J, et al: Pontiac fever outbreak associated with a cooling tower. Am J Public Health 77:568-572, 1987.

328. Blatt SP, Parkinson MD, Pace E, et al: Nosocomial legionnaires' disease: Aspiration as a primary mode of disease acquisition. Am J Med 95:16-22, 1993.

329. Bellinger-Kawahara C, Horwitz MA: Complement component C3 fixes selectively to the major outer membrane protein (MOMP) of *Legionella pneumophila* and mediates phagocytosis of liposome-MOMP complexes by human monocytes. J Exp Med 172:1201-1210, 1990.

330. Hoffman P: Invasion of eukaryotic cells by *Legionella pneumophila*: A common strategy for all hosts? Can J Infect Dis 8:139, 1997.

331. Friedman H, Yamamoto Y, Newton C, et al: Immunologic response and pathophysiology of *Legionella* infection. Semin Respir Infect 13:100-108, 1998.

332. Winn WC Jr, Glavin FL, Perl DP, et al: The pathology of legionnaires' disease. Fourteen fatal cases from the 1977 outbreak in Vermont. Arch Pathol Lab Med 102:344-350, 1978.

333. Winn WC Jr, Myerowitz RL: The pathology of the *Legionella* pneumonias. A review of 74 cases and the literature. Hum Pathol 12:401-422, 1981.

334. Baptiste-Desruisseaux D, Duperval R, Marcoux JA: Legionnaires' disease in the immunocompromised host: Usefulness of Gram's stain. Can Med Assoc J 133:117-118, 1985.

335. Theaker JM, Tobin JO, Jones SE, et al: Immunohistological detection of *Legionella pneumophila* in lung sections. J Clin Pathol 40:143-146, 1987.

336. Kroboth FJ, Yu VL, Reddy SC, et al: Clinicoradiographic correlation with the extent of Legionnaire disease. AJR Am J Roentgenol 141:263-268, 1983.

337. Pedro-Botet ML, Sabria-Leal M, Haro M, et al: Nosocomial and community-acquired *Legionella* pneumonia: Clinical comparative analysis. Eur Respir J 8:1929-1933, 1995.

338. Meyers R: Legionnaires' disease update: Be prepared for this summer. J Respir Dis 1:12, 1980.

339. Fairbank JT, Mamourian AC, Dietrich PA, et al: The chest radiograph in legionnaires' disease. Further observations. Radiology 147:33-34, 1983.

340. Moore EH, Webb WR, Gamsu G, et al: Legionnaires' disease in the renal transplant patient: Clinical presentation and radiographic progression. Radiology 153:589-593, 1984.

341. Meenhorst PL, Mulder JD: The chest x-ray in *Legionella* pneumonia (legionnaires' disease). Eur J Radiol 3:180-186, 1983.

342. Muder RR, Reddy SC, Yu VL, et al: Pneumonia caused by Pittsburgh pneumonia agent: Radiologic manifestations. Radiology 150:633-637, 1984.

343. Mehta P, Patel JD, Milder JE: *Legionella micdadei* (Pittsburgh pneumonia agent). Two infections with unusual clinical features. JAMA 249:1620-1623, 1983.

344. Davis GS, Winn WC Jr, Beaty HN: Legionnaires Disease. Infections caused by *Legionella pneumophila* and *Legionella*-like organisms. Clin Chest Med 2:145-166, 1981.

345. Tsai TF, Finn DR, Plikaytis BD, et al: Legionnaires' disease: Clinical features of the epidemic in Philadelphia. Ann Intern Med 90:509-517, 1979.

346. Kirby BD, Snyder KM, Meyer RD, et al: Legionnaires' disease: Report of sixty-five nosocomially acquired cases of review of the literature. Medicine (Baltimore) 59:188-205, 1980.

347. Blackmon JA, Harley RA, Hicklin MD, et al: Pulmonary sequelae of acute legionnaires' disease pneumonia. Ann Intern Med 90:552-554, 1979.

348. Lattimer GL, Rhodes LV 3rd, Salventi JS, et al: The Philadelphia epidemic of legionnaire's disease: Clinical, pulmonary, and serologic findings two years later. Ann Intern Med 90:522-526, 1979.

349. Fraser DW, Tsai TR, Orenstein W, et al: Legionnaires' disease: Description of an epidemic of pneumonia. N Engl J Med 297:1189-1197, 1977.

350. Gupta SK, Imperiale TF, Sarosi GA: Evaluation of the Winthrop-University Hospital criteria to identify *Legionella* pneumonia. Chest 120:1064-1071, 2001.

351. Sopena N, Sabria-Leal M, Pedro-Botet ML, et al: Comparative study of the clinical presentation of *Legionella* pneumonia and other community-acquired pneumonias. Chest 113:1195-1200, 1998.

352. Falco V, Fernandez de Sevilla T, Alegre J, et al: *Legionella pneumophila*. A cause of severe community-acquired pneumonia. Chest 100:1007-1011, 1991.

353. Benin AL, Benson RF, Besser RE: Trends in legionnaires disease, 1980-1998: Declining mortality and new patterns of diagnosis. Clin Infect Dis 35:1039-1046, 2002.

354. Gacouin A, Le Tulzo Y, Lavoue S, et al: Severe pneumonia due to *Legionella pneumophila*: Prognostic factors, impact of delayed appropriate antimicrobial therapy. Intensive Care Med 28:686-691, 2002.

355. Heath CW Jr, Alexander AD, Galton MM: Leptospirosis in the United States. Analysis of 483 cases in man, 1949, 1961. N Engl J Med 273:915-922, 1965.

356. Hill MK, Sanders CV: Leptospiral pneumonia. Semin Respir Infect 12:44-49, 1997.

357. Teglia OF, Battagliotti C, Villavicencio RL, et al: Leptospiral pneumonia. Chest 108:874-875, 1995.

358. Maze SS, Kirsch RE: Leptospirosis experience at Groote Schuur Hospital, 1969-1979. S Afr Med J 59:33-36, 1981.

359. Burke BJ, Searle JF, Mattingly D: Leptospirosis presenting with profuse haemoptysis. BMJ 2:982, 1976.

360. Zaharopoulos P, Wong J: Cytologic diagnosis of syphilitic pleuritis: A case report. Diagn Cytopathol 16:35-38, 1997.
361. Bartlett J: Anaerobic bacterial infections of the lung and pleural space. Clin Infect Dis 16:248, 1993.
362. Gorbach SL, Bartlett JG: Anaerobic infections (second of three parts). N Engl J Med 290:1237-1245, 1974.
363. Hagan JL, Hardy JD: Lung abscess revisited. A survey of 184 cases. Ann Surg 197:755-762, 1983.
364. Marik PE: Aspiration pneumonitis and aspiration pneumonia. N Engl J Med 344:665-671, 2001.
365. Bartlett JG, Finegold SM: Anaerobic infections of the lung and pleural space. Am Rev Respir Dis 110:56-77, 1974.
366. Gowan RT, Mehran RJ, Cardinal P, et al: Thoracic complications of Lemierre syndrome. Can Respir J 7:481-485, 2000.
367. Leigh DA: Clinical importance of infections due to *Bacteroides fragilis* and role of antibiotic therapy. BMJ 3:225-228, 1974.
368. Felner JM, Dowell VR Jr: "*Bacteroides*" bacteremia. Am J Med 50:787-796, 1971.
369. Goldberg NM, Rifkind D: Clostridial empyema. Arch Intern Med 115:421-425, 1965.
370. Raff MJ, Johnson JD, Nagar D, et al: Spontaneous clostridial empyema and pyopneumothorax. Rev Infect Dis 6:715-719, 1984.
371. Bartlett JG, Gorbach SL, Thadepalli H, et al: Bacteriology of empyema. Lancet 1:338-340, 1974.
372. Gorbach SL, Bartlett JG: Anaerobic infections. 1. N Engl J Med 290:1177-1184, 1974.
373. Landay MJ, Christensen EE, Bynum LJ, et al: Anaerobic pleural and pulmonary infections. AJR Am J Roentgenol 134:233-240, 1980.
374. Bartlett JG: Anaerobic bacterial pneumonitis. Am Rev Respir Dis 119:19-23, 1979.
375. Rohlfing BM, White EA, Webb WR, et al: Hilar and mediastinal adenopathy caused by bacterial abscess of the lung. Radiology 128:289-293, 1978.
376. Clinical conferences at the Johns Hopkins Hospital: Lung abscess. Johns Hopkins Med J 150:141-147, 1982.
377. Bartlett J: Anaerobic bacterial pleuropulmonary infections. Semin Respir Med 13:158, 1992.
378. Gopalakrishna KV, Lerner PI: Primary lung abscess: Analysis of 66 cases. Cleve Clin Q 42:3-13, 1975.
379. Schweppe HI, Knowles JH, Kane L: Lung abscess. An analysis of the Massachusets General Hospital cases from 1943 through 1956. N Engl J Med 265:1039-1043, 1961.
380. Levison ME: Anaerobic pleuropulmonary infection. Curr Opin Infect Dis 14:187-191, 2001.
381. Abernathy RS: Antibiotic therapy of lung abscess: Effectiveness of penicillin. Dis Chest 53:592-598, 1968.
382. Pohlson EC, McNamara JJ, Char C, et al: Lung abscess: A changing pattern of the disease. Am J Surg 150:97-101, 1985.
383. Barnett TB, Herring CL: Lung abscess. Initial and late results of medical therapy. Arch Intern Med 127:217-227, 1971.
384. Tufariello JM, Chan J, Flynn JL: Latent tuberculosis: Mechanisms of host and bacillus that contribute to persistent infection. Lancet Infect Dis 3:578-590, 2003.
385. Corbett EL, Watt CJ, Walker N, et al: The growing burden of tuberculosis: Global trends and interactions with the HIV epidemic. Arch Intern Med 163:1009-1021, 2003.
386. Cegielski JP, Chin DP, Espinal MA, et al: The global tuberculosis situation. Progress and problems in the 20th century, prospects for the 21st century. Infect Dis Clin North Am 16:1-58, 2002.
387. Trends in tuberculosis morbidity—United States, 1992-2002. MMWR Morb Mortal Wkly Rep 52(11):217-220, 222, 2003.
388. Riley RL: Disease transmission and contagion control. Am Rev Respir Dis 125:16-19, 1982.
389. Bloom BR, Small PM: The evolving relation between humans and *Mycobacterium tuberculosis*. N Engl J Med 338:677-678, 1998.
390. Loudon RG, Spohn SK: Cough frequency and infectivity in patients with pulmonary tuberculosis. Am Rev Respir Dis 99:109-111, 1969.
391. Loudon RG, Bumgarner LR, Lacy J, et al: Aerial transmission of mycobacteria. Am Rev Respir Dis 100:165-171, 1969.
392. Liippo KK, Kulmala K, Tala EO: Focusing tuberculosis contact tracing by smear grading of index cases. Am Rev Respir Dis 148:235-236, 1993.
393. Bloch AB, Rieder HL, Kelly GD, et al: The epidemiology of tuberculosis in the United States. Implications for diagnosis and treatment. Clin Chest Med 10:297-313, 1989.
394. Jochem K, Tannenbaum TN, Menzies D: Prevalence of tuberculin skin test reactions among prison workers. Can J Public Health 88:202-206, 1997.
395. Hoge CW, Fisher L, Donnell HD Jr, et al: Risk factors for transmission of *Mycobacterium tuberculosis* in a primary school outbreak: Lack of racial difference in susceptibility to infection. Am J Epidemiol 139:520-530, 1994.
396. Menzies D, Fanning A, Yuan L, et al: Factors associated with tuberculin conversion in Canadian microbiology and pathology workers. Am J Respir Crit Care Med 167:599-602, 2003.
397. Sokolove PE, Mackey D, Wiles J, et al: Exposure of emergency department personnel to tuberculosis: PPD testing during an epidemic in the community. Ann Emerg Med 24:418-421, 1994.
398. Forget A, Skamene E, Gros P, et al: Differences in response among inbred mouse strains to infection with small doses of *Mycobacterium bovis* BCG. Infect Immun 32:42-47, 1981.

399. Bellamy R, Beyers N, McAdam KP, et al: Genetic susceptibility to tuberculosis in Africans: A genome-wide scan. Proc Natl Acad Sci U S A 97:8005-8009, 2000.
400. Delgado JC, Baena A, Thim S, et al: Ethnic-specific genetic associations with pulmonary tuberculosis. J Infect Dis 186:1463-1468, 2002.
401. Glassroth J, Robins AG, Snider DE Jr: Tuberculosis in the 1980s. N Engl J Med 302:1441-1450, 1980.
402. Stead WW: Pathogenesis of a first episode of chronic pulmonary tuberculosis in man: Recrudescence of residuals of the primary infection or exogenous reinfection? Am Rev Respir Dis 95:729-745, 1967.
403. Barnes PF, Cave MD: Molecular epidemiology of tuberculosis. N Engl J Med 349:1149-1156, 2003.
404. Espinal MA: The global situation of MDR-TB. Tuberculosis (Edinb) 83:44-51, 2003.
405. Buskin SE, Gale JL, Weiss NS, et al: Tuberculosis risk factors in adults in King County, Washington, 1988 through 1990. Am J Public Health 84:1750-1756, 1994.
406. Friedman LN, Williams MT, Singh TP, et al: Tuberculosis, AIDS, and death among substance abusers on welfare in New York City. N Engl J Med 334:828-833, 1996.
407. Grange J, Story A, Zumla A: Tuberculosis in disadvantaged groups. Curr Opin Pulm Med 7:160-164, 2001.
408. Schieffelbein CW Jr, Snider DE Jr: Tuberculosis control among homeless populations. Arch Intern Med 148:1843-1846, 1988.
409. Jones TF, Craig AS, Valway SE, et al: Transmission of tuberculosis in a jail. Ann Intern Med 131:557-563, 1999.
410. Barr RG, Menzies R: The effect of war on tuberculosis. Results of a tuberculin survey among displaced persons in El Salvador and a review of the literature. Tuber Lung Dis 75:251-259, 1994.
411. Kline SE, Hedemark LL, Davies SF: Outbreak of tuberculosis among regular patrons of a neighborhood bar. N Engl J Med 333:222-227, 1995.
412. Nelson S, Mason C, Bagby G, et al: Alcohol, tumor necrosis factor, and tuberculosis. Alcohol Clin Exp Res 19:17-24, 1995.
413. Couser JI Jr, Glassroth J: Tuberculosis. An epidemic in older adults. Clin Chest Med 14:491-499, 1993.
414. Stead WW: Special problems in tuberculosis. Tuberculosis in the elderly and in residents of nursing homes, correctional facilities, long-term care hospitals, mental hospitals, shelters for the homeless, and jails. Clin Chest Med 10:397-405, 1989.
415. Rajagopalan S: Tuberculosis and aging: A global health problem. Clin Infect Dis 33:1034-1039, 2001.
416. Cantwell MF, McKenna MT, McCray E, et al: Tuberculosis and race/ethnicity in the United States: Impact of socioeconomic status. Am J Respir Crit Care Med 157:1016-1020, 1998.
417. Stead WW: Genetics and resistance to tuberculosis. Could resistance be enhanced by genetic engineering? Ann Intern Med 116:937-941, 1992.
418. Rivest P, Tannenbaum T, Bedard L: Epidemiology of tuberculosis in Montreal. CMAJ 158:605-609, 1998.
419. Nolan CM, Elarth AM: Tuberculosis in a cohort of Southeast Asian refugees. A five-year surveillance study. Am Rev Respir Dis 137:805-809, 1988.
420. Vu DM, Prendergast TJ, Engle P: Tuberculosis in refugees from Southeast Asia. Chest 82:133-135, 1982.
421. Kent JH: The epidemiology of multidrug-resistant tuberculosis in the United States. Med Clin North Am 77:1391-1409, 1993.
422. Comstock GW: Tuberculosis in twins: A re-analysis of the Prophit survey. Am Rev Respir Dis 117:621-624, 1978.
423. Bellamy R, Ruwende C, Corrah T, et al: Variations in the *NRAMP1* gene and susceptibility to tuberculosis in West Africans. N Engl J Med 338:640-644, 1998.
424. Dubaniewicz A, Moszkowska G, Szczerkowska Z, et al: Analysis of *DQB1* allele frequencies in pulmonary tuberculosis: Preliminary report. Thorax 58:890-891, 2003.
425. Leff A, Geppert EF: Public health and preventive aspects of pulmonary tuberculosis. Infectiousness, epidemiology, risk factors, classification, and preventive therapy. Arch Intern Med 139:1405-1410, 1979.
426. Koziel H, Koziel MJ: Pulmonary complications of diabetes mellitus. Pneumonia. Infect Dis Clin North Am 9:65-96, 1995.
427. Zack MB, Fulkerson LL, Stein E: Glucose intolerance in pulmonary tuberculosis. Am Rev Respir Dis 108:1164-1169, 1973.
428. Rosenman KD, Hall N: Occupational risk factors for developing tuberculosis. Am J Ind Med 30:148-154, 1996.
429. Corbett EL, Churchyard GJ, Clayton T, et al: Risk factors for pulmonary mycobacterial disease in South African gold miners. A case-control study. Am J Respir Crit Care Med 159:94-99, 1999.
430. Becklake MR: The mineral dust diseases. Tuber Lung Dis 73:13-20, 1992.
431. Buskin SE, Weiss NS, Gale JL, et al: Tuberculosis in relation to a history of peptic ulcer disease and treatment of gastric hyperacidity. Am J Epidemiol 141:218-224, 1995.
432. Snider DE Jr: Jejunoileal bypass for obesity: A risk factor for tuberculosis. Chest 81:531, 1982.
433. Tuberculosis in patients having dialysis. BMJ 280:349, 1980.
434. Abbott MR, Smith DD: Mycobacterial infections in immunosuppressed patients. Med J Aust 1:351-353, 1981.
435. Godfrey-Faussett P, Ayles H: Can we control tuberculosis in high HIV prevalence settings? Tuberculosis (Edinb) 83:68-76, 2003.
436. Murray JF: Tuberculosis and HIV infection worldwide. Pneumologie 49(Suppl 3):653-656, 1995.

437. Sakhuja V, Jha V, Varma PP, et al: The high incidence of tuberculosis among renal transplant recipients in India. Transplantation 61:211-215, 1996.

438. Tomasson HO, Brennan M, Bass MJ: Tuberculosis and nonsteroidal anti-inflammatory drugs. Can Med Assoc J 130:275-278, 1984.

439. Keane J, Gershon S, Wise RP, et al: Tuberculosis associated with infliximab, a tumor necrosis factor alpha–neutralizing agent. N Engl J Med 345:1098-1104, 2001.

440. Kaplan MH, Armstrong D, Rosen P: Tuberculosis complicating neoplastic disease. A review of 201 cases. Cancer 33:850-858, 1974.

441. Cole ST, Telenti A: Drug resistance in Mycobacterium tuberculosis. Eur Respir J Suppl 20:701s-713s, 1995.

442. Iseman MD, Sbarbaro JA: The increasing prevalence of resistance to antituberculosis chemotherapeutic agents: Implications for global tuberculosis control. Curr Clin Top Infect Dis 12:188-207, 1992.

443. Neville K, Bromberg A, Bromberg R, et al: The third epidemic—multidrug-resistant tuberculosis. Chest 105:45-48, 1994.

444. Jones BE, Ryu R, Yang Z, et al: Chest radiographic findings in patients with tuberculosis with recent or remote infection. Am J Respir Crit Care Med 156:1270-1273, 1997.

445. Colice GL: Pulmonary tuberculosis. Is resurgence due to reactivation or new infection? Postgrad Med 97:35-38, 44, 47-48, 1995.

446. Rook GA, Zumla A: Advances in the immunopathogenesis of pulmonary tuberculosis. Curr Opin Pulm Med 7:116-123, 2001.

447. Schluger NW, Rom WN: The host immune response to tuberculosis. Am J Respir Crit Care Med 157:679-691, 1998.

448. Boom WH, Canaday DH, Fulton SA, et al: Human immunity to M. tuberculosis: T cell subsets and antigen processing. Tuberculosis (Edinb) 83:98-106, 2003.

449. Munk ME, Emoto M: Functions of T-cell subsets and cytokines in mycobacterial infections. Eur Respir J Suppl 20:668s-675s, 1995.

450. Pithie AD, Lammas DA, Fazal N, et al: CD4+ cytolytic T cells can destroy autologous and MHC-matched macrophages but fail to kill intracellular Mycobacterium bovis-BCG. FEMS Immunol Med Microbiol 11:145-154, 1995.

451. Goren MB: Immunoreactive substances of mycobacteria. Am Rev Respir Dis 125:50-69, 1982.

452. Diaz GA, Wayne LG: Isolation and characterization of catalase produced by Mycobacterium tuberculosis. Am Rev Respir Dis 110:312-319, 1974.

453. Flynn JL, Chan J: Immune evasion by Mycobacterium tuberculosis: Living with the enemy. Curr Opin Immunol 15:450-455, 2003.

454. van Crevel R, Ottenhoff TH, van der Meer JW: Innate immunity to Mycobacterium tuberculosis. Clin Microbiol Rev 15:294-309, 2002.

455. Botha T, Ryffel B: Reactivation of latent tuberculosis infection in TNF-deficient mice. J Immunol 171:3110-3118, 2003.

456. Frieden TR, Sterling TR, Munsiff SS, et al: Tuberculosis. Lancet 362:887-899, 2003.

457. Tsuchiya T, Chida K, Suda T, et al: Dendritic cell involvement in pulmonary granuloma formation elicited by bacillus Calmette-Guérin in rats. Am J Respir Crit Care Med 165:1640-1646, 2002.

458. Dreher D, Nicod LP: Dendritic cells in the mycobacterial granuloma are involved in acquired immunity. Am J Respir Crit Care Med 165:1577-1578, 2002.

459. Dannenberg AM Jr: Pathogenesis of pulmonary tuberculosis. Am Rev Respir Dis 125:25-29, 1982.

460. Stead WW, Bates JH: Evidence of a "silent" bacillemia in primary tuberculosis. Ann Intern Med 74:559-561, 1971.

461. Leung AN, Müller NL, Pineda PR, et al: Primary tuberculosis in childhood: Radiographic manifestations. Radiology 182:87-91, 1992.

462. Choyke PL, Sostman HD, Curtis AM, et al: Adult-onset pulmonary tuberculosis. Radiology 148:357-362, 1983.

463. Lee KS, Im JG: CT in adults with tuberculosis of the chest: Characteristic findings and role in management. AJR Am J Roentgenol 164:1361-1367, 1995.

464. Weber AL, Bird KT, Janower ML: Primary tuberculosis in childhood with particular emphasis on changes affecting the tracheobronchial tree. Am J Roentgenol Radium Ther Nucl Med 103:123-132, 1968.

465. Woodring JH, Vandiviere HM, Fried AM, et al: Update: The radiographic features of pulmonary tuberculosis. AJR Am J Roentgenol 146:497-506, 1986.

466. Pombo F, Rodriguez E, Mato J, et al: Patterns of contrast enhancement of tuberculous lymph nodes demonstrated by computed tomography. Clin Radiol 46:13-17, 1992.

467. Matthews JI, Matarese SL, Carpenter JL: Endobronchial tuberculosis simulating lung cancer. Chest 86:642-644, 1984.

468. Stead WW, Dutt AK: What's new in tuberculosis? Am J Med 71:1-4, 1981.

469. Myers JA, Bearman JE, Dixon HG: The natural history of the tuberculosis in the human body. V. Prognosis among tuberculin-reactor children from birth to five years of age. Am Rev Respir Dis 87:354-369, 1963.

470. West J: Localization of Disease: Pulmonary Tuberculosis, Regional Differences in the Lung. New York, Academic Press, 1977, p 236.

471. Goodwin RA, Des Prez RM: Apical localization of pulmonary tuberculosis, chronic pulmonary histoplasmosis, and progressive massive fibrosis of the lung. Chest 83:801-805, 1983.

472. Converse PJ, Dannenberg AM Jr, Estep JE, et al: Cavitary tuberculosis produced in rabbits by aerosolized virulent tubercle bacilli. Infect Immun 64:4776-4787, 1996.

473. Ishida T, Yokoyama H, Kaneko S, et al: Pulmonary tuberculoma and indications for surgery: Radiographic and clinicopathological analysis. Respir Med 86:431-436, 1992.

474. Slavin RE, Walsh TJ, Pollack AD: Late generalized tuberculosis: A clinical pathologic analysis and comparison of 100 cases in the preantibiotic and antibiotic eras. Medicine (Baltimore) 59:352-366, 1980.

475. Krysl J, Korzeniewska-Kosela M, Müller NL, et al: Radiologic features of pulmonary tuberculosis: An assessment of 188 cases. Can Assoc Radiol J 45:101-107, 1994.

476. Lee KS, Hwang JW, Chung MP, et al: Utility of CT in the evaluation of pulmonary tuberculosis in patients without AIDS. Chest 110:977-984, 1996.

477. Lee KS, Song KS, Lim TH, et al: Adult-onset pulmonary tuberculosis: Findings on chest radiographs and CT scans. AJR Am J Roentgenol 160:753-758, 1993.

478. Penner C, Roberts D, Kunimoto D, et al: Tuberculosis as a primary cause of respiratory failure requiring mechanical ventilation. Am J Respir Crit Care Med 151:867-872, 1995.

479. Im JG, Itoh H, Shim YS, et al: Pulmonary tuberculosis: CT findings—early active disease and sequential change with antituberculous therapy. Radiology 186:653-660, 1993.

480. Im JG, Song KS, Kang HS, et al: Mediastinal tuberculous lymphadenitis: CT manifestations. Radiology 164:115-119, 1987.

481. Im JG, Itoh H, Han MC: CT of pulmonary tuberculosis. Semin Ultrasound CT MR 16:420-434, 1995.

482. Primack SL, Logan PM, Hartman TE, et al: Pulmonary tuberculosis and Mycobacterium avium-intracellulare: A comparison of CT findings. Radiology 194:413-417, 1995.

483. Sochocky S: Tuberculoma of the lung. Am Rev Tuberc 78:403-410, 1958.

484. Zwirewich CV, Vedal S, Miller RR, et al: Solitary pulmonary nodule: High-resolution CT and radiologic-pathologic correlation. Radiology 179:469-476, 1991.

485. Swensen SJ, Brown LR, Colby TV, et al: Pulmonary nodules: CT evaluation of enhancement with iodinated contrast material. Radiology 194:393-398, 1995.

486. Winer-Muram HT, Rubin SA: Thoracic complications of tuberculosis. J Thorac Imaging 5:46-63, 1990.

487. Hatipoglu ON, Osma E, Manisali M, et al: High resolution computed tomographic findings in pulmonary tuberculosis. Thorax 51:397-402, 1996.

488. Oh YW, Kim YH, Lee NJ, et al: High-resolution CT appearance of miliary tuberculosis. J Comput Assist Tomogr 18:862-866, 1994.

489. Hong SH, Im JG, Lee JS, et al: High resolution CT findings of miliary tuberculosis. J Comput Assist Tomogr 22:220-224, 1998.

490. McGuinness G, Naidich DP, Jagirdar J, et al: High resolution CT findings in miliary lung disease. J Comput Assist Tomogr 16:384-390, 1992.

491. Harvey C, Eykyn S, Davidson C: Rigors in tuberculosis. Postgrad Med J 69:724-725, 1993.

492. Wallis RS, Johnson JL: Adult tuberculosis in the 21st century: Pathogenesis, clinical features, and management. Curr Opin Pulm Med 7:124-132, 2001.

493. Mariotta S, Masullo M, Guidi L, et al: Tracheobronchial involvement in 84 cases of pulmonary tuberculosis. Monaldi Arch Chest Dis 50:356-359, 1995.

494. Maartens G, Willcox PA, Benatar SR: Miliary tuberculosis: Rapid diagnosis, hematologic abnormalities, and outcome in 109 treated adults. Am J Med 89:291-296, 1990.

495. Mert A, Bilir M, Tabak F, et al: Miliary tuberculosis: Clinical manifestations, diagnosis and outcome in 38 adults. Respirology 6:217-224, 2001.

496. Munt PW: Miliary tuberculosis in the chemotherapy era: With a clinical review in 69 American adults. Medicine (Baltimore) 51:139-155, 1972.

497. Farer LS, Lowell AM, Meador MP: Extrapulmonary tuberculosis in the United States. Am J Epidemiol 109:205-217, 1979.

498. Small PM, Schecter GF, Goodman PC, et al: Treatment of tuberculosis in patients with advanced human immunodeficiency virus infection. N Engl J Med 324:289-294, 1991.

499. Summers GD, McNicol MW: Tuberculosis of superficial lymph nodes. Br J Dis Chest 74:369-373, 1980.

500. Kent DC: Tuberculous lymphadenitis: Not a localized disease process. Am J Med Sci 254:866-74, 1967.

501. Carter EJ, Mates S: Sudden enlargement of a deep cervical lymph node during and after treatment for pulmonary tuberculosis. Chest 106:1896-1898, 1994.

502. Manolidis S, Frenkiel S, Yoskovitch A, et al: Mycobacterial infections of the head and neck. Otolaryngol Head Neck Surg 109:427-433, 1993.

503. Christensen WI: Genitourinary tuberculosis: Review of 102 cases. Medicine (Baltimore) 53:377-390, 1974.

504. Turgut M: Spinal tuberculosis (Pott's disease): Its clinical presentation, surgical management, and outcome. A survey study on 694 patients. Neurosurg Rev 24:8-13, 2001.

505. Weaver P, Lifeso RM: The radiological diagnosis of tuberculosis of the adult spine. Skeletal Radiol 12:178-186, 1984.

506. Whelan MA, Naidich DP, Post JD, et al: Computed tomography of spinal tuberculosis. J Comput Assist Tomogr 7:25-30, 1983.

507. Coppola J, Müller NL, Connell DG: Computed tomography of musculoskeletal tuberculosis. Can Assoc Radiol J 38:199-203, 1987.

508. Yechoor VK, Shandera WX, Rodriguez P, et al: Tuberculous meningitis among adults with and without HIV infection. Experience in an urban public hospital. Arch Intern Med 156:1710-1716, 1996.

509. Weir MR, Thornton GF: Extrapulmonary tuberculosis. Experience of a community hospital and review of the literature. Am J Med 79:467-478, 1985.

510. Hugo-Hamman CT, Scher H, De Moor MM: Tuberculous pericarditis in children: A review of 44 cases. Pediatr Infect Dis J 13:13-18, 1994.

511. Shin JE, Nam SY, Yoo SJ, et al: Changing trends in clinical manifestations of laryngeal tuberculosis. Laryngoscope 110:1950-1953, 2000.

512. Bowry S, Chan CH, Weiss H, et al: Hepatic involvement in pulmonary tuberculosis. Histologic and functional characteristics. Am Rev Respir Dis 101:941-948, 1970.

513. Shinnick TM, Good RC: Diagnostic mycobacteriology laboratory practices. Clin Infect Dis 21:291-299, 1995.

514. Targeted tuberculin testing and treatment of latent tuberculosis infection. This official statement of the American Thoracic Society was adopted by the ATS Board of Directors, July 1999. This is a Joint Statement of the American Thoracic Society (ATS) and the Centers for Disease Control and Prevention (CDC). This statement was endorsed by the Council of the Infectious Diseases Society of America. (IDSA), September 1999, and the sections of this statement. Am J Respir Crit Care Med 161:S221-S247, 2000.

515. Diagnostic Standards and Classification of Tuberculosis in Adults and Children. This official statement of the American Thoracic Society and the Centers for Disease Control and Prevention was adopted by the ATS Board of Directors, July 1999. This statement was endorsed by the Council of the Infectious Disease Society of America, September 1999. Am J Respir Crit Care Med 161:1376-1395, 2000.

516. Huebner RE, Schein MF, Bass JB Jr: The tuberculin skin test. Clin Infect Dis 17:968-975, 1993.

517. Singh D, Sutton C, Woodcock A: Tuberculin test measurement: Variability due to the time of reading. Chest 122:1299-1301, 2002.

518. Al Zahrani K, Al Jahdali H, Menzies D: Does size matter? Utility of size of tuberculin reactions for the diagnosis of mycobacterial disease. Am J Respir Crit Care Med 162:1419-1422, 2000.

519. Miret-Cuadras P, Pina-Gutierrez JM, Juncosa S: Tuberculin reactivity in bacillus Calmette-Guérin vaccinated subjects. Tuber Lung Dis 77:52-58, 1996.

520. Menzies D: Interpretation of repeated tuberculin tests. Boosting, conversion, and reversion. Am J Respir Crit Care Med 159:15-21, 1999.

521. Kendig EL Jr, Kirkpatrick BV, Carter WH, et al: Underreading of the tuberculin skin test reaction. Chest 113:1175-1177, 1998.

522. Bovornkitti S, Kangsadal P, Sathirapat P, et al: Reversion and reconversion rate of tuberculin skin reactions in correction with the use of prednisone. Dis Chest 38:51-55, 1960.

523. Slutkin G, Perez-Stable EJ, Hopewell PC: Time course and boosting of tuberculin reactions in nursing home residents. Am Rev Respir Dis 134:1048-1051, 1986.

524. Montecalvo MA, Wormser GP: Selective tuberculin anergy: Case report and review. Mt Sinai J Med 61:363-365, 1994.

525. Jasmer RM, Nahid P, Hopewell PC: Clinical practice. Latent tuberculosis infection. N Engl J Med 347:1860-1866, 2002.

526. Anderson C, Inhaber N, Menzies D: Comparison of sputum induction with fiberoptic bronchoscopy in the diagnosis of tuberculosis. Am J Respir Crit Care Med 152:1570-1574, 1995.

527. Diagnostic Standards and Classification of Tuberculosis and Other Mycobacterial Diseases. New York, American Lung Association, 1974.

528. Mohan A, Pande JN, Sharma SK, et al: Bronchoalveolar lavage in pulmonary tuberculosis: A decision analysis approach. QJM 88:269-276, 1995.

529. Wallace JM, Deutsch AL, Harrell JH, et al: Bronchoscopy and transbronchial biopsy in evaluation of patients with suspected active tuberculosis. Am J Med 70:1189-1194, 1981.

530. Light RW: Pleural diseases. Dis Mon 38:261-331, 1992.

531. Kumar S, Seshadri MS, Koshi G, et al: Diagnosing tuberculous pleural effusion: Comparative sensitivity of mycobacterial culture and histopathology. Br Med J (Clin Res Ed) 283:20, 1981.

532. Pant K, Chawla R, Mann PS, et al: Fiberbronchoscopy in smear-negative miliary tuberculosis. Chest 95:1151-1152, 1989.

533. Kinoshita M, Ichikawa Y, Koga H, et al: Re-evaluation of bone marrow aspiration in the diagnosis of miliary tuberculosis. Chest 106:690-692, 1994.

534. Lombard EH, Victor T, Jordaan A, et al: The detection of *Mycobacterium tuberculosis* in bone marrow aspirate using the polymerase chain reaction. Tuber Lung Dis 75:65-69, 1994.

535. Lai RS, Lee SS, Ting YM, et al: Diagnostic value of transbronchial lung biopsy under fluoroscopic guidance in solitary pulmonary nodule in an endemic area of tuberculosis. Respir Med 90:139-143, 1996.

536. Charoenratanakul S, Dejsomritrutai W, Chaiprasert A: Diagnostic role of fiberoptic bronchoscopy in suspected smear negative pulmonary tuberculosis. Respir Med 89:621-623, 1995.

537. Altin S, Cikrikcioglu S, Morgul M, et al: 50 endobronchial tuberculosis cases based on bronchoscopic diagnosis. Respiration 64:162-164, 1997.

538. Martin G, Lazarus A: Epidemiology and diagnosis of tuberculosis. Recognition of at-risk patients is key to prompt detection. Postgrad Med 108:42-44, 47-50, 53-54, 2000.

539. Woods GL: The mycobacteriology laboratory and new diagnostic techniques. Infect Dis Clin North Am 16:127-144, 2002.

540. Vidal R, Martin-Casabona N, Juan A, et al: Incidence and significance of acid-fast bacilli in sputum smears at the end of antituberculous treatment. Chest 109:1562-1565, 1996.

541. Burman WJ, Stone BL, Reves RR, et al: The incidence of false-positive cultures for *Mycobacterium tuberculosis*. Am J Respir Crit Care Med 155:321-326, 1997.

542. Kirihara JM, Hillier SL, Coyle MB: Improved detection times for *Mycobacterium avium* complex and *Mycobacterium tuberculosis* with the BACTEC radiometric system. J Clin Microbiol 22:841-845, 1985.

543. Siddiqi SH, Hwangbo CC, Silcox V, et al: Rapid radiometric methods to detect and differentiate *Mycobacterium tuberculosis/M. bovis* from other mycobacterial species. Am Rev Respir Dis 130:634-640, 1984.

544. Lumb R, Lanser JA, Lim IS: Rapid identification of mycobacteria by the Gen-Probe Accuprobe system. Pathology 25:313-315, 1993.

545. Morgan MA, Horstmeier CD, DeYoung DR, et al: Comparison of a radiometric method (BACTEC) and conventional culture media for recovery of mycobacteria from smear-negative specimens. J Clin Microbiol 18:384-388, 1983.

546. Bothamley GH: Serological diagnosis of tuberculosis. Eur Respir J Suppl 20:676s-688s, 1995.

547. Charpin D, Herbault H, Gevaudan MJ, et al: Value of ELISA using A60 antigen in the diagnosis of active pulmonary tuberculosis. Am Rev Respir Dis 142:380-384, 1990.

548. Baig SM: Anti-purified protein derivative cell-enzyme-linked immunosorbent assay, a sensitive method for early diagnosis of tuberculous meningitis. J Clin Microbiol 33:3040-3041, 1995.

549. Pouthier F, Perriens JH, Mukadi Y, et al: Anti-A60 immunoglobulin G in the serodiagnosis of tuberculosis in HIV-seropositive and seronegative patients. AIDS 8:1277-1280, 1994.

550. Lalvani A, Pathan AA, McShane H, et al: Rapid detection of *Mycobacterium tuberculosis* infection by enumeration of antigen-specific T cells. Am J Respir Crit Care Med 163:824-828, 2001.

551. Richeldi L, Barnini S, Saltini C: Molecular diagnosis of tuberculosis. Eur Respir J Suppl 20:689s-700s, 1995.

552. Salian NV, Rish JA, Eisenach KD, et al: Polymerase chain reaction to detect *Mycobacterium tuberculosis* in histologic specimens. Am J Respir Crit Care Med 158:1150-1155, 1998.

553. Schluger NW: Changing approaches to the diagnosis of tuberculosis. Am J Respir Crit Care Med 164:2020-2024, 2001.

554. Choi YJ, Hu Y, Mahmood A: Clinical significance of a polymerase chain reaction assay for the detection of *Mycobacterium tuberculosis*. Am J Clin Pathol 105:200-204, 1996.

555. Laszlo A: Tuberculosis: 7. Laboratory aspects of diagnosis. CMAJ 160:1725-1729, 1999.

556. Genewein A, Telenti A, Bernasconi C, et al: Molecular approach to identifying route of transmission of tuberculosis in the community. Lancet 342:841-844, 1993.

557. Hayward AC, Watson JM: Typing of mycobacteria using spoligotyping. Thorax 53:329-330, 1998.

558. Dahlgren SE, Ekstrom P: Aspiration cytology in the diagnosis of pulmonary tuberculosis. Scand J Respir Dis 53:196-201, 1972.

559. Robicheaux G, Moinuddin SM, Lee LH: The role of aspiration biopsy cytology in the diagnosis of pulmonary tuberculosis. Am J Clin Pathol 83:719-722, 1985.

560. Pappolla MA, Mehta VT: PAS reaction stains phagocytosed atypical mycobacteria in paraffin sections. Arch Pathol Lab Med 108:372-373, 1984.

561. Mondal A, Patra DK: Efficacy of fine needle aspiration cytology in the diagnosis of tuberculosis of the thyroid gland: A study of 18 cases. J Laryngol Otol 109:36-38, 1995.

562. Ebrahim O, Folb PI, Robson SC, et al: Blunted erythropoietin response to anaemia in tuberculosis. Eur J Haematol 55:251-254, 1995.

563. Lombard EH, Mansvelt EP: Haematological changes associated with miliary tuberculosis of the bone marrow. Tuber Lung Dis 74:131-135, 1993.

564. Demiroglu H, Ozcebe OI, Ozdemir L, et al: Pancytopenia with hypocellular bone marrow due to miliary tuberculosis: An unusual presentation. Acta Haematol 91:49-51, 1994.

565. Roussos A, Lagogianni I, Gonis A, et al: Hypercalcaemia in Greek patients with tuberculosis before the initiation of anti-tuberculosis treatment. Respir Med 95:187-190, 2001.

566. Chan TY, Chan CH, Shek CC: The prevalence of hypercalcaemia in pulmonary and miliary tuberculosis—a longitudinal study. Singapore Med J 35:613-615, 1994.

567. Bradley GW, Sterling GM: Hypercalcaemia and hypokalaemia in tuberculosis. Thorax 33:464-467, 1978.

568. Vorherr H, Massry SG, Fallet R, et al: Antidiuretic principle in tuberculous lung tissue of a patient with pulmonary tuberculosis and hyponatremia. Ann Intern Med 72:383-387, 1970.

569. Post FA, Soule SG, Willcox PA, et al: The spectrum of endocrine dysfunction in active pulmonary tuberculosis. Clin Endocrinol (Oxf) 40:367-371, 1994.

570. Simpson DG, Uschner M, McClement J: Respiratory function in pulmonary tuberculosis. Am Rev Respir Dis 87:1-16, 1963.

571. Williams NH Jr, Kane C, Yoo OH: Pulmonary function in miliary tuberculosis. Am Rev Respir Dis 107:858-860, 1973.

572. Davis CE Jr, Carpenter JL, McAllister CK, et al: Tuberculosis. Cause of death in antibiotic era. Chest 88:726-729, 1985.

573. Maartens G: Advances in adult pulmonary tuberculosis. Curr Opin Pulm Med 8:173-177, 2002.

574. Medical Section of the American Lung Association: Control of tuberculosis in the United States. Am Rev Respir Dis 146:1623, 1992.

575. Centers for the Disease Control and Prevention: Reported Tuberculosis in the United States, 1995. Atlanta, Center for Disease Control and Prevention, 1996.

576. Alkhuja S, Miller A: Tuberculosis and sudden death: A case report and review. Heart Lung 30:388-391, 2001.

577. Ellis ME, Webb AK: Cause of death in patients admitted to hospital for pulmonary tuberculosis. Lancet 1:665-667, 1983.

578. Selby C, Thomson D, Leitch AG: Death in notified cases of tuberculosis in Edinburgh: 1983-1992. Respir Med 89:369-371, 1995.

579. Kim JY, Park YB, Kim YS, et al: Miliary tuberculosis and acute respiratory distress syndrome. Int J Tuberc Lung Dis 7:359-364, 2003.

580. Harries AD, Hargreaves NJ, Kemp J, et al: Deaths from tuberculosis in sub-Saharan African countries with a high prevalence of HIV-1. Lancet 357:1519-1523, 2001.
581. Mukadi YD, Maher D, Harries A: Tuberculosis case fatality rates in high HIV prevalence populations in sub-Saharan Africa. AIDS 15:143-152, 2001.
582. Roche PW, Triccas JA, Winter N: BCG vaccination against tuberculosis: Past disappointments and future hopes. Trends Microbiol 3:397-401, 1995.
583. Brewer TF, Colditz GA: Bacille Calmette-Guérin vaccination for the prevention of tuberculosis in health care workers. Clin Infect Dis 20:136-142, 1995.
584. Colditz GA, Brewer TF, Berkey CS, et al: Efficacy of BCG vaccine in the prevention of tuberculosis. Meta-analysis of the published literature. JAMA 271:698-702, 1994.
585. Abramowsky C, Gonzalez B, Sorensen RU: Disseminated bacillus Calmette-Guérin infections in patients with primary immunodeficiencies. Am J Clin Pathol 100:52-56, 1993.
586. Crawford ED: Diagnosis and treatment of superficial bladder cancer: An update. Semin Urol Oncol 14:1-9, 1996.
587. Izes JK, Bihrle W 3rd, Thomas CB: Corticosteroid-associated fatal mycobacterial sepsis occurring 3 years after instillation of intravesical bacillus Calmette-Guérin. J Urol 150:1498-1500, 1993.
588. Palayew M, Briedis D, Libman M, et al: Disseminated infection after intravesical BCG immunotherapy. Detection of organisms in pulmonary tissue. Chest 104:307-309, 1993.
589. LeMense GP, Strange C: Granulomatous pneumonitis following intravesical BCG. What therapy is needed? Chest 106:1624-1626, 1994.
590. Jasmer RM, McCowin MJ, Webb WR: Miliary lung disease after intravesical bacillus Calmette-Guérin immunotherapy. Radiology 201:43-44, 1996.
591. Sampson MG, Colman NC: Pulmonary complications of oral BCG. Chest 80:655-656, 1981.
592. Gonzalez OY, Musher DM, Brar I, et al: Spectrum of bacille Calmette-Guérin (BCG) infection after intravesical BCG immunotherapy. Clin Infect Dis 36:140-148, 2003.
593. Gangadharam PR: Microbiology of nontuberculosis mycobacteria. Semin Respir Infect 11:231-243, 1996.
594. Wayne LG, Sramek HA: Agents of newly recognized or infrequently encountered mycobacterial diseases. Clin Microbiol Rev 5:1-25, 1992.
595. Runyon EH: Anonymous mycobacteria in pulmonary disease. Med Clin North Am 43:273-290, 1959.
596. Tortoli E, Piersimoni C, Kirschner P, et al: Characterization of mycobacterial isolates phylogenetically related to, but different from Mycobacterium simiae. J Clin Microbiol 35:697-702, 1997.
597. Horsburgh CR Jr: Epidemiology of disease caused by nontuberculous mycobacteria. Semin Respir Infect 11:244-251, 1996.
598. O'Brien DP, Currie BJ, Krause VL: Nontuberculous mycobacterial disease in northern Australia: A case series and review of the literature. Clin Infect Dis 31:958-967, 2000.
599. Marras TK, Daley CL: Epidemiology of human pulmonary infection with nontuberculous mycobacteria. Clin Chest Med 23:553-567, 2002.
600. Rosenzweig DY: Nontuberculous mycobacterial disease in the immunocompetent adult. Semin Respir Infect 11:252-261, 1996.
601. Sonnenberg P, Murray J, Glynn JR, et al: Risk factors for pulmonary disease due to culture-positive M. tuberculosis or nontuberculous mycobacteria in South African gold miners. Eur Respir J 15:291-296, 2000.
602. Witty LA, Tapson VF, Piantadosi CA: Isolation of mycobacteria in patients with pulmonary alveolar proteinosis. Medicine (Baltimore) 73:103-109, 1994.
603. Tomashefski JF Jr, Stern RC, Demko CA, et al: Nontuberculous mycobacteria in cystic fibrosis. An autopsy study. Am J Respir Crit Care Med 154:523-528, 1996.
604. Karsell PR: Achalasia, aspiration, and atypical mycobacteria. Mayo Clin Proc 68:1025-1026, 1993.
605. Castor B, Juhlin I, Henriques B: Septic cutaneous lesions caused by Mycobacterium malmoense in a patient with hairy cell leukemia. Eur J Clin Microbiol Infect Dis 13:145-148, 1994.
606. Patel R, Roberts GD, Keating MR, et al: Infections due to nontuberculous mycobacteria in kidney, heart, and liver transplant recipients. Clin Infect Dis 19:263-273, 1994.
607. Hoy JF, Rolston KV, Hopfer RL, et al: Mycobacterium fortuitum bacteremia in patients with cancer and long-term venous catheters. Am J Med 83:213-217, 1987.
608. Penny ME, Cole RB, Gray J: Two cases of Mycobacterium kansasii infection occurring in the same household. Tubercle 63:129-131, 1982.
609. Maloney S, Welbel S, Daves B, et al: Mycobacterium abscessus pseudoinfection traced to an automated endoscope washer: Utility of epidemiologic and laboratory investigation. J Infect Dis 169:1166-1169, 1994.
610. Marchevsky A, Damsker B, Gribetz A, et al: The spectrum of pathology of nontuberculous mycobacterial infections in open-lung biopsy specimens. Am J Clin Pathol 78:695-700, 1982.
611. Corpe RF, Stergus I: Is the histopathology of nonphotochromogenic mycobacterial infections distinguishable from that caused by Mycobacterium tuberculosis? Am Rev Respir Dis 87:289-291, 1963.
612. Chester A, Winn W: Unusual and newly recognized patterns of nontuberculous myobacterial infection with emphasis on the immunocompromised host. In Sommers S, Rosen P, Fechner R (eds): Pathology Annual. Part 1. Norwalk, CT, Appleton-Century-Croft, 1986.
613. Albelda SM, Kern JA, Marinelli DL, et al: Expanding spectrum of pulmonary disease caused by nontuberculous mycobacteria. Radiology 157:289-296, 1985.
614. Evans AJ, Crisp AJ, Hubbard RB, et al: Pulmonary Mycobacterium kansasii infection: Comparison of radiological appearances with pulmonary tuberculosis. Thorax 51:1243-1247, 1996.
615. Hollings NP, Wells AU, Wilson R, et al: Comparative appearances of non-tuberculous mycobacteria species: A CT study. Eur Radiol 12:2211-2217, 2002.
616. Miller WT Jr: Spectrum of pulmonary nontuberculous mycobacterial infection. Radiology 191:343-350, 1994.
617. Prince DS, Peterson DD, Steiner RM, et al: Infection with Mycobacterium avium complex in patients without predisposing conditions. N Engl J Med 321:863-868, 1989.
618. Lynch DA, Simone PM, Fox MA, et al: CT features of pulmonary Mycobacterium avium complex infection. J Comput Assist Tomogr 19:353-360, 1995.
619. Hartman TE, Swensen SJ, Williams DE: Mycobacterium avium-intracellulare complex: Evaluation with CT. Radiology 187:23-26, 1993.
620. Rosenzweig DY: Pulmonary mycobacterial infections due to Mycobacterium intracellulare-avium complex. Clinical features and course in 100 consecutive cases. Chest 75:115-119, 1979.
621. Reich JM, Johnson RE: Mycobacterium avium complex pulmonary disease presenting as an isolated lingular or middle lobe pattern. The Lady Windermere syndrome. Chest 101:1605-1609, 1992.
622. Zumla AI, Grange J: Non-tuberculous mycobacterial pulmonary infections. Clin Chest Med 23:369-376, 2002.
623. Wallace RJ Jr, Swenson JM, Silcox VA, et al: Spectrum of disease due to rapidly growing mycobacteria. Rev Infect Dis 5:657-679, 1983.
624. Diagnosis and treatment of disease caused by nontuberculous mycobacteria. Am Rev Respir Dis 142:940-953, 1990.
625. Saito H, Tasaka H, Osasa S, et al: Disseminated Mycobacterium intracellulare infection. Am Rev Respir Dis 109:572-576, 1974.
626. Ahn CH, Lowell JR, Onstad GD, et al: Elimination of Mycobacterium intracellulare from sputum after bronchial hygiene. Chest 76:480-482, 1979.
627. Iseman MD, Corpe RF, O'Brien RJ, et al: Disease due to Mycobacterium avium-intracellulare. Chest 87:139S-149S, 1985.
628. Choudhri S, Manfreda J, Wolfe J, et al: Clinical significance of nontuberculous mycobacteria isolates in a Canadian tertiary care center. Clin Infect Dis 21:128-133, 1995.
629. Francis PB, Jay SJ, Johanson WG Jr: The course of untreated Mycobacterium kansasii disease. Am Rev Respir Dis 111:477-487, 1975.
630. Johanson WG Jr, Nicholson DP: Pulmonary disease due to Mycobacterium kansasii. An analysis of some factors affecting prognosis. Am Rev Respir Dis 99:73-85, 1969.
631. Stansell JD: Pulmonary fungal infections in HIV-infected persons. Semin Respir Infect 8:116-123, 1993.
632. Bradsher RW: Histoplasmosis and blastomycosis. Clin Infect Dis 22(Suppl 2):S102-S111, 1996.
633. Leggiadro RJ, Luedtke GS, Convey A, et al: Prevalence of histoplasmosis in a mid-southern population. South Med J 84:1360-1361, 1991.
634. Storch G, Burford JG, George RB, et al: Acute histoplasmosis. Description of an outbreak in northern Louisiana. Chest 77:38-42, 1980.
635. Torres HA, Rivero GA, Kontoyiannis DP: Endemic mycoses in a cancer hospital. Medicine (Baltimore) 81:201-212, 2002.
636. Reynolds RJ 3rd, Penn RL, Grafton WD, et al: Tissue morphology of Histoplasma capsulatum in acute histoplasmosis. Am Rev Respir Dis 130:317-320, 1984.
637. Wu-Hsieh BA: Resistance mechanisms in murine experimental histoplasmosis. Arch Med Res 24:233-238, 1993.
638. Allendoerfer R, Magee DM, Deepe GS Jr, et al: Transfer of protective immunity in murine histoplasmosis by a CD4+ T-cell clone. Infect Immun 61:714-718, 1993.
639. Bhagavan BS, Rao DR, Weinberg T: Histoplasmosis producing broncholithiasis. Arch Pathol 91:577-579, 1971.
640. Goodwin RA, Loyd JE, Des Prez RM: Histoplasmosis in normal hosts. Medicine (Baltimore) 60:231-266, 1981.
641. Zeidberg LD, Dillon A, Gass RS: Some factors in the epidemiology of histoplasmin sensitivity in Williamson County, Tennessee. Am J Public Health 41:80-89, 1951.
642. Houston S: Tropical respiratory medicine. 3. Histoplasmosis and pulmonary involvement in the tropics. Thorax 49:598-601, 1994.
643. Rubin H, Furcolow ML, Yates JL, et al: The course and prognosis of histoplasmosis. Am J Med 27:278-288, 1959.
644. Goodwin RA Jr, Des Prez RM: State of the art: Histoplasmosis. Am Rev Respir Dis 117:929-956, 1978.
645. Huffnagle KE, Gander RM: Evaluation of Gen-Probe's Histoplasma capsulatum and Cryptococcus neoformans AccuProbes. J Clin Microbiol 31:419-421, 1993.
646. Jacobson ES, Straus SE: Reevaluation of diagnostic histoplasma serologies. Am J Med Sci 281:143-151, 1981.
647. Wheat J, French ML, Kohler RB, et al: The diagnostic laboratory tests for histoplasmosis: Analysis of experience in a large urban outbreak. Ann Intern Med 97:680-685, 1982.
648. Kauffman CA, Israel KS, Smith JW, et al: Histoplasmosis in immunosuppressed patients. Am J Med 64:923-932, 1978.
649. Richert JH, Campbell CC: The significance of skin and serologic tests in the diagnosis of pulmonary residuals of histoplasmosis. A review of 123 cases. Am Rev Respir Dis 86:381-384, 1962.
650. Wynne JW, Olsen GN: Acute histoplasmosis presenting as the adult respiratory distress syndrome. Chest 66:158-161, 1974.
651. Gurney JW, Conces DJ: Pulmonary histoplasmosis. Radiology 199:297-306, 1996.
652. Conces DJ Jr: Histoplasmosis. Semin Roentgenol 31:14-27, 1996.

653. Furcolow ML, Grayston JT: Occurrence of histoplasmosis in epidemics: Etiologic studies. Am Rev Tuberc 68:307-320, 1953.

654. Prager RL, Burney DP, Waterhouse G, et al: Pulmonary, mediastinal, and cardiac presentations of histoplasmosis. Ann Thorac Surg 30:385-390, 1980.

655. Goodwin RA Jr, Snell JD Jr: The enlarging histoplasmoma. Concept of a tumor-like phenomenon encompassing the tuberculoma and coccidioidoma. Am Rev Respir Dis 100:1-12, 1969.

656. Siegelman SS, Khouri NF, Leo FP, et al: Solitary pulmonary nodules: CT assessment. Radiology 160:307-312, 1986.

657. Palayew MJ, Frank H: Benign progressive multinodular pulmonary histoplasmosis. A radiological and clinical entity. Radiology 111:311-314, 1974.

658. Conces DJ Jr, Tarver RD, Vix VA: Broncholithiasis: CT features in 15 patients. AJR Am J Roentgenol 157:249-253, 1991.

659. Kauffman CA: Fungal infections in older adults. Clin Infect Dis 33:550-555, 2001.

660. Savides TJ, Gress FG, Wheat LJ, et al: Dysphagia due to mediastinal granulomas: Diagnosis with endoscopic ultrasonography. Gastroenterology 109:366-373, 1995.

661. Wood KL, Hage CA, Knox KS, et al: Histoplasmosis after treatment with anti–tumor necrosis factor-alpha therapy. Am J Respir Crit Care Med 167:1279-1282, 2003.

662. Sataloff RT, Wilborn A, Prestipino A, et al: Histoplasmosis of the larynx. Am J Otolaryngol 14:199-205, 1993.

663. Stevens DA: Coccidioidomycosis. N Engl J Med 332:1077-1082, 1995.

664. Galgiani JN: Coccidioidomycosis. Curr Clin Top Infect Dis 17:188-204, 1997.

665. Standaert SM, Schaffner W, Galgiani JN, et al: Coccidioidomycosis among visitors to a *Coccidioides immitis*–endemic area: An outbreak in a military reserve unit. J Infect Dis 171:1672-1675, 1995.

666. Coccidioidomycosis in travelers returning from Mexico—Pennsylvania, 2000. MMWR Morb Mortal Wkly Rep 49(44):1004-1006, 2000.

667. From the Centers for Disease Control and Prevention. Coccidioidomycosis—Arizona, 1990-1995. JAMA 277:104-105, 1997.

668. Drutz DJ, Catanzaro A: Coccidioidomycosis. Part II. Am Rev Respir Dis 117:727-771, 1978.

669. Drutz DJ, Catanzaro A: Coccidioidomycosis. Part I. Am Rev Respir Dis 117:559-585, 1978.

670. Rosenstein NE, Emery KW, Werner SB, et al: Risk factors for severe pulmonary and disseminated coccidioidomycosis: Kern County, California, 1995-1996. Clin Infect Dis 32:708-715, 2001.

671. Ampel NM, Dols CL, Galgiani JN: Coccidioidomycosis during human immunodeficiency virus infection: Results of a prospective study in a coccidioidal endemic area. Am J Med 94:235-240, 1993.

672. Holt CD, Winston DJ, Kubak B, et al: Coccidioidomycosis in liver transplant patients. Clin Infect Dis 24:216-221, 1997.

673. Walker MP, Brody CZ, Resnik R: Reactivation of coccidioidomycosis in pregnancy. Obstet Gynecol 79:815-817, 1992.

674. Huntington RJ, Waldmann W, Sargent J, et al: Pathologic and clinical observations on 142 cases of fatal coccidioidomycosis with necropsy. In Ajello L (ed): Coccidioidomycosis. Tucson, University of Arizona Press, 1965, p 143.

675. Graham AR, Sobonya RE, Bronnimann DA, et al: Quantitative pathology of coccidioidomycosis in acquired immunodeficiency syndrome. Hum Pathol 19:800-806, 1988.

676. Catanzaro A: Pulmonary coccidioidomycosis. Med Clin North Am 64:461-473, 1980.

677. Batra P, Batra RS: Thoracic coccidioidomycosis. Semin Roentgenol 31:28-44, 1996.

678. Klein EW, Griffin JP: Coccidioidomycosis: (Diagnosis outside the Sonoran zone). The roentgen features of acute multiple pulmonary cavities. Am J Roentgenol Radium Ther Nucl Med 94:653-659, 1965.

679. Batra P: Pulmonary coccidioidomycosis. J Thorac Imaging 7:29-38, 1992.

680. Deppisch LM, Donowho EM: Pulmonary coccidioidomycosis. Am J Clin Pathol 58:489-500, 1972.

681. Kim KI, Leung AN, Flint JD, et al: Chronic pulmonary coccidioidomycosis: Computed tomographic and pathologic findings in 18 patients. Can Assoc Radiol J 49:401-407, 1998.

682. Greendyke WH, Resnick DL, Harvey WC: The varied roentgen manifestations of primary coccidioidomycosis. Am J Roentgenol Radium Ther Nucl Med 109:491-499, 1970.

683. Winn WA: A long term study of 300 patients with cavitary-abscess lesions of the lung of coccidioidal origin. An analytical study with special reference to treatment. Dis Chest 54(Suppl 1):268, 1968.

684. Raab SS, Silverman JF, Zimmerman KG: Fine-needle aspiration biopsy of pulmonary coccidiodomycosis. Spectrum of cytologic findings in 73 patients. Am J Clin Pathol 99:582-587, 1993.

685. Bayer AS, Yoshikawa TT, Guze LB: Chronic progressive coccidioidal pneumonitis. Report of six cases with clinical, roentgenographic, serologic, and therapeutic features. Arch Intern Med 139:536-540, 1979.

686. Jones JL, Fleming PL, Ciesielski CA, et al: Coccidioidomycosis among persons with AIDS in the United States. J Infect Dis 171:961-966, 1995.

687. Arsura EL, Kilgore WB: Miliary coccidioidomycosis in the immunocompetent. Chest 117:404-409, 2000.

688. Harley WB, Blaser MJ: Disseminated coccidioidomycosis associated with extreme eosinophilia. Clin Infect Dis 18:627-629, 1994.

689. Wallace JM, Catanzaro A, Moser KM, et al: Flexible fiberoptic bronchoscopy for diagnosing pulmonary coccidioidomycosis. Am Rev Respir Dis 123:286-290, 1981.

690. Martins TB, Jaskowski TD, Mouritsen CL, et al: Comparison of commercially available enzyme immunoassay with traditional serological tests for detection of antibodies to *Coccidioides immitis*. J Clin Microbiol 33:940-943, 1995.

691. Bayer AS: Fungal pneumonias; pulmonary coccidioidal syndromes (Part I). Primary and progressive primary coccidioidal pneumonias—diagnostic, therapeutic, and prognostic considerations. Chest 79:575-583, 1981.

592. Levine HB, Gonzalez-Ochoa A, Ten Eyck DR: Dermal sensitivity to *Coccidioides immitis*. A comparison of responses elicited in man by spherulin and coccidioidin. Am Rev Respir Dis 107:379-386, 1973.

693. Witorsch P, Utz JP: North American blastomycosis: A study of 40 patients. Medicine (Baltimore) 47:169-200, 1968.

694. St-Germain G, Murray G, Duperval R: Blastomycosis in Quebec (1981-90): Report of 23 cases and review of published cases from Quebec. Can J Infect Dis 4:89, 1993.

695. Bradsher RW, Chapman SW, Pappas PG: Blastomycosis. Infect Dis Clin North Am 17:21-40, vii, 2003.

696. Vaaler AK, Bradsher RW, Davies SF: Evidence of subclinical blastomycosis in forestry workers in northern Minnesota and northern Wisconsin. Am J Med 89:470-476, 1990.

697. Klein BS, Vergeront JM, Weeks RJ, et al: Isolation of *Blastomyces dermatitidis* in soil associated with a large outbreak of blastomycosis in Wisconsin. N Engl J Med 314:529-534, 1986.

698. Kravitz GR, Davies SF, Eckman MR, et al: Chronic blastomycotic meningitis. Am J Med 71:501-505, 1981.

699. Vanek J, Schwarz J, Hakim S: North American blastomycosis: A study of ten cases. Am J Clin Pathol 54:384-400, 1970.

700. Schwarz J, Salfelder K: Blastomycosis. A review of 152 cases. Curr Top Pathol 65:165-200, 1977.

701. Sheflin JR, Campbell JA, Thompson GP: Pulmonary blastomycosis: Findings on chest radiographs in 63 patients. AJR Am J Roentgenol 154:1177-1180, 1990.

702. Kuzo RS, Goodman LR: Blastomycosis. Semin Roentgenol 31:45-51, 1996.

703. Brown LR, Swensen SJ, Van Scoy RE, et al: Roentgenologic features of pulmonary blastomycosis. Mayo Clin Proc 66:29-38, 1991.

704. Winer-Muram HT, Beals DH, Cole FH Jr: Blastomycosis of the lung: CT features. Radiology 182:829-832, 1992.

705. Griffith JE, Campbell GD: Acute miliary blastomycosis presenting as fulminating respiratory failure. Chest 75:630-632, 1979.

706. Lemos LB, Baliga M, Guo M: Acute respiratory distress syndrome and blastomycosis: Presentation of nine cases and review of the literature. Ann Diagn Pathol 5:1-9, 2001.

707. Frean J, Blumberg L, Woolf M: Disseminated blastomycosis masquerading as tuberculosis. J Infect 26:203-206, 1993.

708. Lemos LB, Baliga M, Guo M: Blastomycosis: The great pretender can also be an opportunist. Initial clinical diagnosis and underlying diseases in 123 patients. Ann Diagn Pathol 6:194-203, 2002.

709. Guha PK, Thompson JR: Acute pulmonary blastomycosis. A diagnostic challenge in a tuberculosis sanatorium. Am Rev Respir Dis 86:640-647, 1962.

710. Martynowicz MA, Prakash UB: Pulmonary blastomycosis: An appraisal of diagnostic techniques. Chest 121:768-773, 2002.

711. Campbell CC: Use and interpretation of serologic and skin tests in the respiratory mycoses: Current considerations. Dis Chest 54(Suppl 1):305, 1968.

712. Blastomycosis—Wisconsin, 1986-1995. From the Centers for Disease Control and Prevention. JAMA 276:444, 1996.

713. Pappas PG, Threlkeld MG, Bedsole GD, et al: Blastomycosis in immunocompromised patients. Medicine (Baltimore) 72:311-325, 1993.

714. Bethlem EP, Capone D, Maranhao B, et al: Paracoccidioidomycosis. Curr Opin Pulm Med 5:319-325, 1999.

715. Pena CE: Deep mycotic infections in Colombia. A clinicopathologic study of 162 cases. Am J Clin Pathol 47:505-520, 1967.

716. Salfelder K, Doehnert G, Doehnert HR: Paracoccidioidomycosis. Anatomic study with complete autopsies. Virchows Arch A Pathol Pathol Anat 348:51-76, 1969.

717. Butka BJ, Bennett SR, Johnson AC: Disseminated inoculation blastomycosis in a renal transplant recipient. Am Rev Respir Dis 130:1180-1183, 1984.

718. Londero AT, Ramos CD, Lopes JO: Progressive pulmonary paracoccidioidomycosis: A study of 34 cases observed in Rio Grande do Sul (Brazil). Mycopathologia 63:53-56, 1978.

719. Funari M, Kavakama J, Shikanai-Yasuda MA, et al: Chronic pulmonary paracoccidioidomycosis (South American blastomycosis): High-resolution CT findings in 41 patients. AJR Am J Roentgenol 173:59-64, 1999.

720. Angulo-Ortega A, Pollak L: Paracoccidioidomycosis. In Baker R (ed): Human Infection with Fungi, Actinomycetes and Algae. New York, Springer-Verlag, 1971.

721. Pappas PG, Perfect JR, Cloud GA, et al: Cryptococcosis in human immunodeficiency virus–negative patients in the era of effective azole therapy. Clin Infect Dis 33:690-699, 2001.

722. McDonnell JM, Hutchins GM: Pulmonary cryptococcosis. Hum Pathol 16:121-128, 1985.

723. Gal AA, Koss MN, Hawkins J, et al: The pathology of pulmonary cryptococcal infections in the acquired immunodeficiency syndrome. Arch Pathol Lab Med 110:502-507, 1986.

724. Roebuck DJ, Fisher DA, Currie BJ: Cryptococcosis in HIV negative patients: Findings on chest radiography. Thorax 53:554-557, 1998.

725. Lacomis JM, Costello P, Vilchez R, et al: The radiology of pulmonary cryptococcosis in a tertiary medical center. J Thorac Imaging 16:139-148, 2001.

726. Patz EF Jr, Goodman PC: Pulmonary cryptococcosis. J Thorac Imaging 7:51-55, 1992.

727. Woodring JH, Ciporkin G, Lee C, et al: Pulmonary cryptococcosis. Semin Roentgenol 31:67-75, 1996.

728. Miller WT Jr, Edelman JM, Miller WT: Cryptococcal pulmonary infection in patients with AIDS: Radiographic appearance. Radiology 175:725-728, 1990.

729. Zinck SE, Leung AN, Frost M, et al: Pulmonary cryptococcosis: CT and pathologic findings. J Comput Assist Tomogr 26:330-334, 2002.

730. Rozenbaum R, Goncalves AJ: Clinical epidemiological study of 171 cases of cryptococcosis. Clin Infect Dis 18:369-380, 1994.

731. Wheat LJ, Goldman M, Sarosi G: State-of-the-art review of pulmonary fungal infections. Semin Respir Infect 17:158-181, 2002.

732. Vilchez RA, Linden P, Lacomis J, et al: Acute respiratory failure associated with pulmonary cryptococcosis in non-AIDS patients. Chest 119:1865-1869, 2001.

733. Perla EN, Maayan S, Miller SN, et al: Disseminated cryptococcosis presenting as the adult respiratory distress syndrome. N Y State J Med 85:704-706, 1985.

734. Stringer JR, Beard CB, Miller RF, et al: A new name *(Pneumocystis jiroveci)* for *Pneumocystis* from humans. Emerg Infect Dis 8:891-896, 2002.

735. Hasleton PS, Curry A, Rankin EM: *Pneumocystis carinii* pneumonia: A light microscopical and ultrastructural study. J Clin Pathol 34:1138-1146, 1981.

736. Cushion MT, Ruffolo JJ, Walzer PD: Analysis of the developmental stages of *Pneumocystis carinii*, in vitro. Lab Invest 58:324-331, 1988.

737. Meuwissen JH, Tauber I, Leeuwenberg AD, et al: Parasitologic and serologic observations of infection with *Pneumocystis* in humans. J Infect Dis 136:43-49, 1977.

738. Ballardie FW, Winearls CG, Cohen J, et al: *Pneumocystis carinii* pneumonia in renal transplant recipients—clinical and radiographic features, diagnosis and complications of treatment. QJM 57:729-747, 1985.

739. Zahar JR, Robin M, Azoulay E, et al: *Pneumocystis carinii* pneumonia in critically ill patients with malignancy: A descriptive study. Clin Infect Dis 35:929-934, 2002.

740. Godeau B, Coutant-Perronne V, Le Thi Huong D, et al: *Pneumocystis carinii* pneumonia in the course of connective tissue disease: Report of 34 cases. J Rheumatol 21:246-251, 1994.

741. Fulkerson WJ, Newman JH: Endogenous Cushing's syndrome complicated by *Pneumocystis carinii* pneumonia. Am Rev Respir Dis 129:188-189, 1984.

742. van der Lelie J, Venema D, Kuijper EJ, et al: *Pneumocystis carinii* pneumonia in HIV-negative patients with haematologic disease. Infection 25:78-81, 1997.

743. Leigh TR, Millett MJ, Jameson B, et al: Serum titres of *Pneumocystis carinii* antibody in health care workers caring for patients with AIDS. Thorax 48:619-621, 1993.

744. Latouche S, Poirot JL, Bernard C, et al: Study of internal transcribed spacer and mitochondrial large-subunit genes of *Pneumocystis carinii* hominis isolated by repeated bronchoalveolar lavage from human immunodeficiency virus–infected patients during one or several episodes of pneumonia. J Clin Microbiol 35:1687-1690, 1997.

745. Hennequin C, Page B, Roux P, et al: Outbreak of *Pneumocystis carinii* pneumonia in a renal transplant unit. Eur J Clin Microbiol Infect Dis 14:122-126, 1995.

746. Manoloff ES, Francioli P, Taffe P, et al: Risk for *Pneumocystis carinii* transmission among patients with pneumonia: A molecular epidemiology study. Emerg Infect Dis 9:132-134, 2003.

747. Wohl AR, Simon P, Hu YW, et al: The role of person-to-person transmission in an epidemiologic study of *Pneumocystis carinii* pneumonia. AIDS 16:1821-1825, 2002.

748. Maskell NA, Waine DJ, Lindley A, et al: Asymptomatic carriage of *Pneumocystis jiroveci* in subjects undergoing bronchoscopy: A prospective study. Thorax 58:594-759, 2003.

749. Martin WJ 2nd: Pathogenesis of *Pneumocystis carinii* pneumonia. Am J Respir Cell Mol Biol 8:356-357, 1993.

750. Frenkel JK, Good JT, Shultz JA: Latent *Pneumocystis* infection of rats, relapse, and chemotherapy. Lab Invest 15:1559-1577, 1966.

751. Shellito JE: Host defense against *Pneumocystis carinii:* More than the CD4$^+$ lymphocyte. J Lab Clin Med 128:448-449, 1996.

752. Masur H, Ognibene FP, Yarchoan R, et al: CD4 counts as predictors of opportunistic pneumonias in human immunodeficiency virus (HIV) infection. Ann Intern Med 111:223-231, 1989.

753. Beck JM, Newbury RL, Palmer BE, et al: Role of CD8$^+$ lymphocytes in host defense against *Pneumocystis carinii* in mice. J Lab Clin Med 128:477-487, 1996.

754. Fraser IP, Takahashi K, Koziel H, et al: *Pneumocystis carinii* enhances soluble mannose receptor production by macrophages. Microbes Infect 2:1305-1310, 2000.

755. Limper AH: Tumor necrosis factor alpha–mediated host defense against *Pneumocystis carinii*. Am J Respir Cell Mol Biol 16:110-111, 1997.

756. Laursen AL, Rungby J, Andersen PL: Decreased activation of the respiratory burst in neutrophils from AIDS patients with previous *Pneumocystis carinii* pneumonia. J Infect Dis 172:497-505, 1995.

757. Laursen AL, Jensen BN, Andersen PL: Local antibodies against *Pneumocystis carinii* in bronchoalveolar lavage fluid. Eur Respir J 7:679-685, 1994.

758. Escamilla R, Prevost MC, Hermant C, et al: Surfactant analysis during *Pneumocystis carinii* pneumonia in HIV-infected patients. Chest 101:1558-1562, 1992.

759. Limper AH, Thomas CF Jr, Anders RA, et al: Interactions of parasite and host epithelial cell cycle regulation during *Pneumocystis carinii* pneumonia. J Lab Clin Med 130:132-138, 1997.

760. Tregnago R, Xavier RG, Pereira RP, et al: The diagnosis of *Pneumocystis carinii* pneumonia by cytologic evaluation of Papanicolaou and Leishman-stained bronchoalveolar specimens in patients with the acquired immunodeficiency syndrome. Cytopathology 4:77-84, 1993.

761. Travis WD, Pittaluga S, Lipschik GY, et al: Atypical pathologic manifestations of *Pneumocystis carinii* pneumonia in the acquired immune deficiency syndrome. Review of 123 lung biopsies from 76 patients with emphasis on cysts, vascular invasion, vasculitis, and granulomas. Am J Surg Pathol 14:615-625, 1990.

762. Askin FB, Katzenstein AL: *Pneumocystis* infection masquerading as diffuse alveolar damage: A potential source of diagnostic error. Chest 79:420-422, 1981.

763. Wakefield AE, Miller RF, Guiver LA, et al: Granulomatous *Pneumocystis carinii* pneumonia: DNA amplification studies on bronchoscopic alveolar lavage samples. J Clin Pathol 47:664-666, 1994.

764. Murry CE, Schmidt RA: Tissue invasion by *Pneumocystis carinii:* A possible cause of cavitary pneumonia and pneumothorax. Hum Pathol 23:1380-1387, 1992.

765. Lee MM, Schinella RA: Pulmonary calcification caused by *Pneumocystis carinii* pneumonia. A clinicopathological study of 13 cases in acquired immune deficiency syndrome patients. Am J Surg Pathol 15:376-380, 1991.

766. Saldana MJ, Mones JM, Martinez GR: The pathology of treated *Pneumocystis carinii* pneumonia. Semin Diagn Pathol 6:300-312, 1989.

767. Chan JK, Tsang DN, Wong DK: *Penicillium marneffei* in bronchoalveolar lavage fluid. Acta Cytol 33:523-526, 1989.

768. Silletti RP, Glezerov V, Schwartz IS: Pulmonary paracoccidioidomycosis misdiagnosed as *Pneumocystis* pneumonia in an immunocompromised host. J Clin Microbiol 34:2328-2330, 1996.

769. Cohen BA, Pomeranz S, Rabinowitz JG, et al: Pulmonary complications of AIDS: Radiologic features. AJR Am J Roentgenol 143:115-122, 1984.

770. Maxfield RA, Sorkin IB, Fazzini EP, et al: Respiratory failure in patients with acquired immunodeficiency syndrome and *Pneumocystis carinii* pneumonia. Crit Care Med 14:443-449, 1986.

771. Chaffey MH, Klein JS, Gamsu G, et al: Radiographic distribution of *Pneumocystis carinii* pneumonia in patients with AIDS treated with prophylactic inhaled pentamidine. Radiology 175:715-719, 1990.

772. Barrio JL, Suarez M, Rodriguez JL, et al: *Pneumocystis carinii* pneumonia presenting as cavitating and noncavitating solitary pulmonary nodules in patients with the acquired immunodeficiency syndrome. Am Rev Respir Dis 134:1094-1096, 1986.

773. Bleiweiss IJ, Jagirdar JS, Klein MJ, et al: Granulomatous *Pneumocystis carinii* pneumonia in three patients with the acquired immune deficiency syndrome. Chest 94:580-583, 1988.

774. Hartz JW, Geisinger KR, Scharyj M, et al: Granulomatous pneumocystosis presenting as a solitary pulmonary nodule. Arch Pathol Lab Med 109:466-469, 1985.

775. Lubat E, Megibow AJ, Balthazar EJ, et al: Extrapulmonary *Pneumocystis carinii* infection in AIDS: CT findings. Radiology 174:157-160, 1990.

776. Mayor B, Schnyder P, Giron J, et al: Mediastinal and hilar lymphadenopathy due to *Pneumocystis carinii* infection in AIDS patients: CT features. J Comput Assist Tomogr 18:408-411, 1994.

777. Groskin SA, Massi AF, Randall PA: Calcified hilar and mediastinal lymph nodes in an AIDS patient with *Pneumocystis carinii* infection. Radiology 175:345-346, 1990.

778. Hartman TE, Primack SL, Müller NL, et al: Diagnosis of thoracic complications in AIDS: Accuracy of CT. AJR Am J Roentgenol 162:547-553, 1994.

779. McGuinness G, Naidich DP, Garay S, et al: AIDS associated bronchiectasis: CT features. J Comput Assist Tomogr 17:260-266, 1993.

780. Nuesch R, Bellini C, Zimmerli W: *Pneumocystis carinii* pneumonia in human immunodeficiency virus (HIV)-positive and HIV-negative immunocompromised patients. Clin Infect Dis 29:1519-1523, 1999.

781. Kovacs JA, Hiemenz JW, Macher AM, et al: *Pneumocystis carinii* pneumonia: A comparison between patients with the acquired immunodeficiency syndrome and patients with other immunodeficiencies. Ann Intern Med 100:663-671, 1984.

782. Kovacs JA, Gill VJ, Meshnick S, et al: New insights into transmission, diagnosis, and drug treatment of *Pneumocystis carinii* pneumonia. JAMA 286:2450-2460, 2001.

783. Parker MM, Ognibene FP, Rogers P, et al: Severe *Pneumocystis carinii* pneumonia produces a hyperdynamic profile similar to bacterial pneumonia with sepsis. Crit Care Med 22:50-54, 1994.

784. Ragni MV, Dekker A, DeRubertis FR, et al: *Pneumocystis carinii* infection presenting as necrotizing thyroiditis and hypothyroidism. Am J Clin Pathol 95:489-493, 1991.

785. Rumbak MJ, Winer-Muram HT, Beals DH, et al: Tension pneumomediastinum complicating *Pneumocystis carinii* pneumonia in acquired immunodeficiency syndrome. Crit Care Med 20:1492-1494, 1992.

786. Bradshaw M, Myerowitz RL, Schneerson R, et al: *Pneumocystis carinii* pneumonitis. Ann Intern Med 73:775-777, 1970.

787. Roblot F, Le Moal G, Godet C, et al: *Pneumocystis carinii* pneumonia in patients with hematologic malignancies: A descriptive study. J Infect 47:19-27, 2003.

788. Quist J, Hill AR: Serum lactate dehydrogenase (LDH) in *Pneumocystis carinii* pneumonia, tuberculosis, and bacterial pneumonia. Chest 108:415-418, 1995.

789. Boldt MJ, Bai TR: Utility of lactate dehydrogenase vs radiographic severity in the differential diagnosis of *Pneumocystis carinii* pneumonia. Chest 111:1187-1192, 1997.

790. Mitchell DM, Fleming J, Harris JR, et al: Serial pulmonary function tests in the diagnosis of *P. carinii* pneumonia. Eur Respir J 6:823-827, 1993.

791. Levine SJ: *Pneumocystis carinii*. Clin Chest Med 17:665-695, 1996.

792. Sepkowitz KA: *Pneumocystis carinii* pneumonia among patients with neoplastic disease. Semin Respir Infect 7:114-121, 1992.

793. Morris AM, Huang L, Bacchetti P, et al: Permanent declines in pulmonary function following pneumonia in human immunodeficiency virus–infected persons. The Pulmonary Complications of HIV Infection Study Group. Am J Respir Crit Care Med 162:612-616, 2000.

794. Suffredini AF, Owens GR, Tobin MJ, et al: Long-term prognosis of survivors of *Pneumocystis carinii* pneumonia. Structural and functional correlates. Chest 89:229-233, 1986.

795. Meunier-Carpentier F, Kiehn TE, Armstrong D: Fungemia in the immunocompromised host. Changing patterns, antigenemia, high mortality. Am J Med 71:363-370, 1981.
796. Whimbey E, Gold JW, Polsky B, et al: Bacteremia and fungemia in patients with the acquired immunodeficiency syndrome. Ann Intern Med 104:511-514, 1986.
797. Myerowitz RL, Pazin GJ, Allen CM: Disseminated candidiasis. Changes in incidence, underlying diseases, and pathology. Am J Clin Pathol 68:29-38, 1977.
798. Hogevik H, Alestig K: Fungal endocarditis—a report on seven cases and a brief review. Infection 24:17-21, 1996.
799. Grossi P, Farina C, Fiocchi R, et al: Prevalence and outcome of invasive fungal infections in 1,963 thoracic organ transplant recipients: A multicenter retrospective study. Italian Study Group of Fungal Infections in Thoracic Organ Transplant Recipients. Transplantation 70:112-116, 2000.
800. Dubois PJ, Myerowitz RL, Allen CM: Pathoradiologic correlation of pulmonary candidiasis in immunosuppressed patients. Cancer 40:1026-1036, 1977.
801. Parker JC Jr, McCloskey JJ, Knauer KA: Pathobiologic features of human candidiasis. A common deep mycosis of the brain, heart and kidney in the altered host. Am J Clin Pathol 65:991-1000, 1976.
802. Buff SJ, McLelland R, Gallis HA, et al: *Candida albicans* pneumonia: Radiographic appearance. AJR Am J Roentgenol 138:645-648, 1982.
803. Pagani JJ, Libshitz HI: Opportunistic fungal pneumonias in cancer patients. AJR Am J Roentgenol 137:1033-1039, 1981.
804. Chen KY, Ko SC, Hsueh PR, et al: Pulmonary fungal infection: Emphasis on microbiological spectra, patient outcome, and prognostic factors. Chest 120:177-184, 2001.
805. Aisner J, Murillo J, Schimpff SC, et al: Invasive aspergillosis in acute leukemia: Correlation with nose cultures and antibiotic use. Ann Intern Med 90:4-9, 1979.
806. Mondon P, Thelu J, Lebeau B, et al: Virulence of *Aspergillus fumigatus* strains investigated by random amplified polymorphic DNA analysis. J Med Microbiol 42:299-303, 1995.
807. Henwick S, Hetherington SV, Patrick CC: Complement binding to *Aspergillus conidia* correlates with pathogenicity. J Lab Clin Med 122:27-35, 1993.
808. Bardana EJ Jr: The clinical spectrum of aspergillosis—part 1: Epidemiology, pathogenicity, infection in animals and immunology of *Aspergillus*. Crit Rev Clin Lab Sci 13:21-83, 1981.
809. Tilden EB, Hatton EH, Freeman S, et al: Preparation and properties of the endotoxins of *Aspergillus fumigatus* and *Aspergillus flavus*. Mycopathologia 14:325-346, 1961.
810. Markaryan A, Morozova I, Yu H, et al: Purification and characterization of an elastinolytic metalloprotease from *Aspergillus fumigatus* and immunoelectron microscopic evidence of secretion of this enzyme by the fungus invading the murine lung. Infect Immun 62:2149-2157, 1994.
811. Moutaouakil M, Monod M, Prevost MC, et al: Identification of the 33-kDa alkaline protease of *Aspergillus fumigatus* in vitro and in vivo. J Med Microbiol 39:393-399, 1993.
812. Tomee JF, Wierenga AT, Hiemstra PS, et al: Proteases from *Aspergillus fumigatus* induce release of proinflammatory cytokines and cell detachment in airway epithelial cell lines. J Infect Dis 176:300-303, 1997.
813. Tang CM, Cohen J, Krausz T, et al: The alkaline protease of *Aspergillus fumigatus* is not a virulence determinant in two murine models of invasive pulmonary aspergillosis. Infect Immun 61:1650-1656, 1993.
814. Levitz SM, Selsted ME, Ganz T, et al: In vitro killing of spores and hyphae of *Aspergillus fumigatus* and *Rhizopus oryzae* by rabbit neutrophil cationic peptides and bronchoalveolar macrophages. J Infect Dis 154:483-489, 1986.
815. Hebart H, Bollinger C, Fisch P, et al: Analysis of T-cell responses *to Aspergillus fumigatus* antigens in healthy individuals and patients with hematologic malignancies. Blood 100:4521-4528, 2002.
816. Schaffner A, Douglas H, Braude A: Selective protection against conidia by mononuclear and against mycelia by polymorphonuclear phagocytes in resistance to *Aspergillus*. Observations on these two lines of defense in vivo and in vitro with human and mouse phagocytes. J Clin Invest 69:617-631, 1982.
817. Madan T, Eggleton P, Kishore U, et al: Binding of pulmonary surfactant proteins A and D to *Aspergillus fumigatus* conidia enhances phagocytosis and killing by human neutrophils and alveolar macrophages. Infect Immun 65:3171-3179, 1997.
818. Murayama T, Amitani R, Ikegami Y, et al: Suppressive effects of *Aspergillus fumigatus* culture filtrates on human alveolar macrophages and polymorphonuclear leucocytes. Eur Respir J 9:293-300, 1996.
819. Robertson MD, Seaton A, Milne LJ, et al: Suppression of host defences by *Aspergillus fumigatus*. Thorax 42:19-25, 1987.
820. Mullbacher A, Eichner RD: Immunosuppression in vitro by a metabolite of a human pathogenic fungus. Proc Natl Acad Sci U S A 81:3835-3837, 1984.
821. McGregor DH, Papasian CJ, Pierce PD: Aspergillosis within cavitating pulmonary adenocarcinoma. Am J Clin Pathol 91:100-103, 1989.
822. Buchanan DR, Lamb D: Saprophytic invasion of infarcted pulmonary tissue by *Aspergillus* species. Thorax 37:693-698, 1982.
823. Kahanpaa A: Bronchopulmonary occurrence of fungi in adults especially according to cultivation material. Acta Pathol Microbiol Scand [B] Microbiol Immunol 227:1-147, 1972.
824. Paradowski LJ: Saprophytic fungal infections and lung transplantation—revisited. J Heart Lung Transplant 16:524-531, 1997.
825. Amitani R, Taylor G, Elezis EN, et al: Purification and characterization of factors produced by *Aspergillus fumigatus* which affect human ciliated respiratory epithelium. Infect Immun 63:3266-3271, 1995.
826. Kawamura S, Maesaki S, Tomono K, et al: Clinical evaluation of 61 patients with pulmonary aspergilloma. Intern Med 39:209-212, 2000.
827. Chatzimichalis A, Massard G, Kessler R, et al: Bronchopulmonary aspergilloma: A reappraisal. Ann Thorac Surg 65:927-929, 1998.
828. Awe RJ, Greenberg SD, Mattox KL: The source of bleeding in pulmonary aspergillomas. Tex Med 80:58-61, 1984.
829. Kurrein F, Green GH, Rowles SL: Localized deposition of calcium oxalate around a pulmonary *Aspergillus niger* fungus ball. Am J Clin Pathol 64:556-563, 1975.
330. Lee SH, Barnes WG, Schaetzel WP: Pulmonary aspergillosis and the importance of oxalate crystal recognition in cytology specimens. Arch Pathol Lab Med 110:1176-1179, 1986.
831. Golberg B: Radiological appearances in pulmonary aspergillosis. Clin Radiol 13:106-114, 1962.
832. Levin EJ: Pulmonary intracavitary fungus ball. Radiology 66:9-16, 1956.
833. Libshitz HI, Atkinson GW, Israel HL: Pleural thickening as a manifestation of aspergillus superinfection. Am J Roentgenol Radium Ther Nucl Med 120:883-886, 1974.
834. Irwin A: Radiology of the aspergilloma. Clin Radiol 18:432-438, 1967.
835. Gefter WB: The spectrum of pulmonary aspergillosis. J Thorac Imaging 7:56-74, 1992.
836. Roberts CM, Citron KM, Strickland B: Intrathoracic aspergilloma: Role of CT in diagnosis and treatment. Radiology 165:123-128, 1987.
837. Pennington JE: *Aspergillus* lung disease. Med Clin North Am 64:475-490, 1980.
838. Addrizzo-Harris DJ, Harkin TJ, McGuinness G, et al: Pulmonary aspergilloma and AIDS. A comparison of HIV-infected and HIV-negative individuals. Chest 111:612-618, 1997.
839. Pulmonary aspergilloma. BMJ 2:124, 1971.
840. Jaques D, Bonzon M, Polla BS: Serological evidence of *Aspergillus* type I hypersensitivity in a subgroup of pulmonary aspergilloma patients. Int Arch Allergy Immunol 106:263-270, 1995.
841. Butz RO, Zvetina JR, Leininger BJ: Ten-year experience with mycetomas in patients with pulmonary tuberculosis. Chest 87:356-358, 1985.
842. Rafferty P, Biggs BA, Crompton GK, et al: What happens to patients with pulmonary aspergilloma? Analysis of 23 cases. Thorax 38:579-583, 1983.
843. Hinojosa M, Fraj J, De la Hoz B, et al: Hypersensitivity pneumonitis in workers exposed to esparto grass (*Stipa tenacissima*) fibers. J Allergy Clin Immunol 98:985-991, 1996.
844. Bardana EJ Jr: The clinical spectrum of aspergillosis—part 2: Classification and description of saprophytic, allergic, and invasive variants of human disease. Crit Rev Clin Lab Sci 13:85-159, 1981.
845. Stevens DA, Moss RB, Kurup VP, et al: Allergic bronchopulmonary aspergillosis in cystic fibrosis—state of the art: Cystic Fibrosis Foundation Consensus Conference. Clin Infect Dis 37(Suppl 3):S225-S264, 2003.
846. Bromley IM, Donaldson K: Binding of *Aspergillus fumigatus* spores to lung epithelial cells and basement membrane proteins: Relevance to the asthmatic lung. Thorax 51:1203-1209, 1996.
847. Vernon DR, Allan F: Environmental factors in allergic bronchopulmonary aspergillosis. Clin Allergy 10:217-227, 1980.
848. Bosken CH, Myers JL, Greenberger PA, et al: Pathologic features of allergic bronchopulmonary aspergillosis. Am J Surg Pathol 12:216-222, 1988.
849. Koss MN, Robinson RG, Hochholzer L: Bronchocentric granulomatosis. Hum Pathol 12:632-638, 1981.
850. Maguire GP, Lee M, Rosen Y, et al: Pulmonary tuberculosis and bronchocentric granulomatosis. Chest 89:606-608, 1986.
851. Hellems SO, Kanner RE, Renzetti AD Jr: Bronchocentric granulomatosis associated with rheumatoid arthritis. Chest 83:831-832, 1983.
852. Buckingham SJ, Hansell DM: *Aspergillus* in the lung: Diverse and coincident forms. Eur Radiol 13:1786-1800, 2003.
853. Ward S, Heyneman L, Lee M, et al: Accuracy of CT in the diagnosis of allergic bronchopulmonary aspergillosis in asthmatic patients. AJR Am J Roentgenol 173:937, 1999.
854. Logan PM, Müller NL: High-attenuation mucous plugging in allergic bronchopulmonary aspergillosis. Can Assoc Radiol J 47:374-377, 1996.
855. Ricketti AJ, Greenberger PA, Patterson R: Immediate-type reactions in patients with allergic bronchopulmonary aspergillosis. J Allergy Clin Immunol 71:541-545, 1983.
856. Glimp RA, Bayer AS: Fungal pneumonias. Part 3. Allergic bronchopulmonary aspergillosis. Chest 80:85-94, 1981.
857. Patterson R, Greenberger PA, Radin RC, et al: Allergic bronchopulmonary aspergillosis: Staging as an aid to management. Ann Intern Med 96:286-291, 1982.
858. Imbeau SA, Nichols D, Flaherty D, et al: Relationships between prednisone therapy, disease activity, and the total serum IgE level in allergic bronchopulmonary aspergillosis. J Allergy Clin Immunol 62:91-95, 1978.
859. Aubry MC, Fraser R: The role of bronchial biopsy and washing in the diagnosis of allergic bronchopulmonary aspergillosis. Mod Pathol 11:607-611, 1998.
860. Breslin AB, Jenkins CR: Experience with allergic bronchopulmonary aspergillosis: Some unusual features. Clin Allergy 14:21-28, 1984.
861. Malo JL, Hawkins R, Pepys J: Studies in chronic allergic bronchopulmonary aspergillosis. 1. Clinical and physiological findings. Thorax 32:254-261, 1977.
862. Allam MF, Del Castillo AS, Diaz-Molina C, et al: Invasive pulmonary aspergillosis: Identification of risk factors. Scand J Infect Dis 34:819-822, 2002.
863. Singh N, Husain S: *Aspergillus* infections after lung transplantation: Clinical differences in type of transplant and implications for management. J Heart Lung Transplant 22:258-266, 2003.
864. Soubani AO, Chandrasekar PH: The clinical spectrum of pulmonary aspergillosis. Chest 121:1988-1999, 2002.

865. Palmer LB, Greenberg HE, Schiff MJ: Corticosteroid treatment as a risk factor for invasive aspergillosis in patients with lung disease. Thorax 46:15-20, 1991.

866. Berner R, Sauter S, Michalski Y, et al: Central venous catheter infection by Aspergillus fumigatus in a patient with B-type non-Hodgkin lymphoma. Med Pediatr Oncol 27:202-204, 1996.

867. Dewhurst AG, Cooper MJ, Khan SM, et al: Invasive aspergillosis in immunosuppressed patients: Potential hazard of hospital building work. BMJ 301:802-804, 1990.

868. Fraser R: Pulmonary aspergillosis: Pathologic and pathogenic features. In Rosen P, Fechner R (eds): Pathology Annual Part 1. Norwalk, CT, Appleton & Lange, 1993, p 231.

869. Sieber SC, Cole SR, McNab JM, et al: Bronchiolitis associated with the finding of the fungus aspergillus. Report of two cases. Conn Med 58:13-17, 1994.

870. Young RC, Bennett JE, Vogel CL, et al: Aspergillosis. The spectrum of the disease in 98 patients. Medicine (Baltimore) 49:147-173, 1970.

871. Cohen DM, Goggans EA: Sclerosing mediastinitis and terminal valvular endocarditis caused by fungus suggestive of Aspergillus species. Am J Clin Pathol 56:91-96, 1971.

872. Meredith HC, Cogan BM, McLaulin B: Pleural aspergillosis. AJR Am J Roentgenol 130:164-166, 1978.

873. Young RC, Vogel CL, DeVita VT: Aspergillus lobar pneumonia. JAMA 208:1156-1162, 1969.

874. Herbert PA, Bayer AS: Fungal pneumonia (Part 4): Invasive pulmonary aspergillosis. Chest 80:220-225, 1981.

875. Logan PM, Primack SL, Miller RR, et al: Invasive aspergillosis of the airways: Radiographic, CT, and pathologic findings. Radiology 193:383-388, 1994.

876. Franquet T, Müller NL, Gimenez A, et al: Spectrum of pulmonary aspergillosis: Histologic, clinical, and radiologic findings. Radiographics 21:825-837, 2001.

877. Franquet T, Müller NL, Oikonomou A, et al: Aspergillus infection of the airways: Computed tomography and pathologic findings. J Comput Assist Tomogr 28:10-16, 2004.

878. Orr DP, Myerowitz RL, Dubois PJ: Patho-radiologic correlation of invasive pulmonary aspergillosis in the compromised host. Cancer 41:2028-2039, 1978.

879. Kibbler CC, Milkins SR, Bhamra A, et al: Apparent pulmonary mycetoma following invasive aspergillosis in neutropenic patients. Thorax 43:108-112, 1988.

880. Curtis AM, Smith GJ, Ravin CE: Air crescent sign of invasive aspergillosis. Radiology 133:17-21, 1979.

881. Albelda SM, Talbot GH, Gerson SL, et al: Pulmonary cavitation and massive hemoptysis in invasive pulmonary aspergillosis. Influence of bone marrow recovery in patients with acute leukemia. Am Rev Respir Dis 131:115-120, 1985.

882. Albelda SM, Gefter WB, Epstein DM, et al: Bronchopleural fistula complicating invasive pulmonary aspergillosis. Am Rev Respir Dis 126:163-165, 1982.

883. Kuhlman JE, Fishman EK, Siegelman SS: Invasive pulmonary aspergillosis in acute leukemia: Characteristic findings on CT, the CT halo sign, and the role of CT in early diagnosis. Radiology 157:611-614, 1985.

884. Primack SL, Hartman TE, Lee KS, et al: Pulmonary nodules and the CT halo sign. Radiology 190:513-515, 1994.

885. Hruban RH, Meziane MA, Zerhouni EA, et al: Radiologic-pathologic correlation of the CT halo sign in invasive pulmonary aspergillosis. J Comput Assist Tomogr 11:534-536, 1987.

886. Brown MJ, Miller RR, Müller NL: Acute lung disease in the immunocompromised host: CT and pathologic examination findings. Radiology 190:247-254, 1994.

887. Gerson SL, Talbot GH, Lusk E, et al: Invasive pulmonary aspergillosis in adult acute leukemia: Clinical clues to its diagnosis. J Clin Oncol 3:1109-1116, 1985.

888. Kirshenbaum JM, Lorell BH, Schoen FJ, et al: Angioinvasive pulmonary aspergillosis: Presentation as massive pulmonary saddle embolism in an immunocompromised patient. J Am Coll Cardiol 6:486-489, 1985.

889. Vlasveld LT, Delemarre JF, Beynen JH, et al: Invasive aspergillosis complicated by subclavian artery occlusion and costal osteomyelitis after autologous bone marrow transplantation. Thorax 47:136-137, 1992.

890. Caligiuri P, MacMahon H, Courtney J, et al: Opportunistic pulmonary aspergillosis with chest wall invasion. Plain film and computed tomographic findings. Arch Intern Med 143:2323-2324, 1983.

891. Herrera JM, McNeil KD, Higgins RS, et al: Airway complications after lung transplantation: Treatment and long-term outcome. Ann Thorac Surg 71:989-993, discussion 993-994, 2001.

892. Clarke A, Skelton J, Fraser RS: Fungal tracheobronchitis. Report of 9 cases and review of the literature. Medicine (Baltimore) 70:1-14, 1991.

893. Tait RC, O'Driscoll BR, Denning DW: Unilateral wheeze caused by pseudomembranous aspergillus tracheobronchitis in the immunocompromised patient. Thorax 48:1285-1287, 1993.

894. Mineur P, Ferrant A, Wallon J, et al: Bronchoesophageal fistula caused by pulmonary aspergillosis. Eur J Respir Dis 66:360-366, 1985.

895. Binder RE, Faling LJ, Pugatch RD, et al: Chronic necrotizing pulmonary aspergillosis: A discrete clinical entity. Medicine (Baltimore) 61:109-124, 1982.

896. Yousem SA: The histological spectrum of chronic necrotizing forms of pulmonary aspergillosis. Hum Pathol 28:650-656, 1997.

897. Franquet T, Müller NL, Gimenez A, et al: Semiinvasive pulmonary aspergillosis in chronic obstructive pulmonary disease: Radiologic and pathologic findings in nine patients. AJR Am J Roentgenol 174:51-56, 2000.

898. Kim SY, Lee KS, Han J, et al: Semiinvasive pulmonary aspergillosis: CT and pathologic findings in six patients. AJR Am J Roentgenol 174:795-798, 2000.

899. Horvath JA, Dummer S: The use of respiratory-tract cultures in the diagnosis of invasive pulmonary aspergillosis. Am J Med 100:171-178, 1996.

900. Nucci M, Biasoli I, Barreiros G, et al: Predictive value of a positive nasal swab for Aspergillus sp. in the diagnosis of invasive aspergillosis in adult neutropenic cancer patients. Diagn Microbiol Infect Dis 35:193-196, 1999.

901. Verweij PE, Dompeling EC, Donnelly JP, et al: Serial monitoring of Aspergillus antigen in the early diagnosis of invasive aspergillosis. Preliminary investigations with two examples. Infection 25:86-89, 1997.

902. Raad I, Hanna H, Huaringa A, et al: Diagnosis of invasive pulmonary aspergillosis using polymerase chain reaction–based detection of aspergillus in BAL. Chest 121:1171-1176, 2002.

903. Rantakokko-Jalava K, Laaksonen S, Issakainen J, et al: Semiquantitative detection by real-time PCR of Aspergillus fumigatus in bronchoalveolar lavage fluids and tissue biopsy specimens from patients with invasive aspergillosis. J Clin Microbiol 41:4304-4311, 2003.

904. Aisner J, Wiernik PH, Schimpff SC: Treatment of invasive aspergillosis: Relation of early diagnosis and treatment to response. Ann Intern Med 86:539-543, 1977.

905. Marchevsky AM, Bottone EJ, Geller SA, et al: The changing spectrum of disease, etiology, and diagnosis of mucormycosis. Hum Pathol 11:457-464, 1980.

906. Rippon S: The Pathogenic Fungi and the Pathogenic Actinomycetes, 3rd ed. Philadelphia, WB Saunders, 1988.

907. Rangel-Guerra RA, Martinez HR, Saenz C, et al: Rhinocerebral and systemic mucormycosis. Clinical experience with 36 cases. J Neurol Sci 143:19-30, 1996.

908. Nosari A, Oreste P, Montillo M, et al: Mucormycosis in hematologic malignancies: An emerging fungal infection. Haematologica 85:1068-1071, 2000.

909. Lee FY, Mossad SB, Adal KA: Pulmonary mucormycosis: The last 30 years. Arch Intern Med 159:1301-1309, 1999.

910. McAdams HP, Rosado de Christenson M, Strollo DC, et al: Pulmonary mucormycosis: Radiologic findings in 32 cases. AJR Am J Roentgenol 168:1541-1548, 1997.

911. Jamadar DA, Kazerooni EA, Daly BD, et al: Pulmonary zygomycosis: CT appearance. J Comput Assist Tomogr 19:733-738, 1995.

912. Kim N, Barrie J, Raymond G: Residents' corner. Answer to case of the month #87: Pulmonary mucormycosis with angioinvasion of the left subclavian artery. Can Assoc Radiol J 53:312-314, 2002.

913. Rubin SA, Chaljub G, Winer-Muram HT, et al: Pulmonary zygomycosis: A radiographic and clinical spectrum. J Thorac Imaging 7:85-90, 1992.

914. Dykhuizen RS, Kerr KN, Soutar RL: Air crescent sign and fatal haemoptysis in pulmonary mucormycosis. Scand J Infect Dis 26:498-501, 1994.

915. Tedder M, Spratt JA, Anstadt MP, et al: Pulmonary mucormycosis: Results of medical and surgical therapy. Ann Thorac Surg 57:1044-1050, 1994.

916. Morenz J: Geotrichosis. In Baker R (ed): Human Infection with Fungi, Actinomycetes and Algae. New York, Springer-Verlag, 1971, p 919.

917. Bell D, Brodie J, Henderson A: A case of pulmonary geotrichosis. Br J Dis Chest 56:26-29, 1962.

918. Fishbach RS, White ML, Finegold SM: Bronchopulmonary geotrichosis. Am Rev Respir Dis 108:1388-1392, 1973.

919. Ross JD, Reid KD, Speirs CF: Bronchopulmonary geotrichosis with severe asthma. BMJ 5500:1400-1402, 1966.

920. Conant N, Martin D, Smith D, et al: Manual of Clinical Mycology. (Prepared under the auspices of the Division of Medical Sciences of the National Research Council.) Philadelphia, WB Saunders, 1971.

921. Evers RH, Whereatt RR: Pulmonary sporotrichosis. Chest 66:91-92, 1974.

922. England DM, Hochholzer L: Primary pulmonary sporotrichosis. Report of eight cases with clinicopathologic review. Am J Surg Pathol 9:193-204, 1985.

923. Heller HM, Fuhrer J: Disseminated sporotrichosis in patients with AIDS: Case report and review of the literature. AIDS 5:1243-1246, 1991.

924. Marques ME, Coelho KI, Sotto MN, et al: Comparison between histochemical and immunohistochemical methods for diagnosis of sporotrichosis. J Clin Pathol 45:1089-1093, 1992.

925. Trevathan RD, Phillips S: Primary pulmonary sporotrichosis. Case report. JAMA 195:965-967, 1966.

926. Boehm D, Lynch JM, Hodges GR, et al: Case report. Disseminated sporotrichosis presenting as sarcoidosis: Electron microscopic and immunologic studies. Am J Med Sci 283:71-78, 1982.

927. Farley ML, Fagan MF, Mabry LC, et al: Presentation of Sporothrix schenckii in pulmonary cytology specimens. Acta Cytol 35:389-395, 1991.

928. Pluss JL, Opal SM: Pulmonary sporotrichosis: Review of treatment and outcome. Medicine (Baltimore) 65:143-153, 1986.

929. Turner D, Burke M, Bashe E, et al: Pulmonary adiaspiromycosis in a patient with acquired immunodeficiency syndrome. Eur J Clin Microbiol Infect Dis 18:893-895, 1999.

930. Nuorva K, Pitkanen R, Issakainen J, et al: Pulmonary adiaspiromycosis in a two year old girl. J Clin Pathol 50:82-85, 1997.

931. Salfelder K, Fingerland A, de Mendelovici M, et al: Two cases of adiaspiromycosis. Beitr Pathol 148:94-100, 1973.

932. Kodousek R, Vortel V, Fingerland A, et al: Pulmonary adiaspiromycosis in man caused by Emmonsia crescens: Report of a unique case. Am J Clin Pathol 56:394-399, 1971.

933. Saadah HA, Dixon T: Petriellidium boydii (Allescheria boydii). Necrotizing pneumonia in a normal host. JAMA 245:605-606, 1981.

934. McCarthy DS, Longbottom JL, Riddell RW, et al: Pulmonary mycetoma due to Allescheria boydii. Am Rev Respir Dis 100:213-216, 1969.

935. Travis LB, Roberts GD, Wilson WR: Clinical significance of Pseudallescheria boydii: A review of 10 years' experience. Mayo Clin Proc 60:531-537, 1985.

936. Miller MA, Greenberger PA, Amerian R, et al: Allergic bronchopulmonary mycosis caused by Pseudallescheria boydii. Am Rev Respir Dis 148:810-812, 1993.

937. Alture-Werber E, Edberg SC, Singer JM: Pulmonary infection with *Allescheria boydii*. Am J Clin Pathol 66:1019-1024, 1976.

938. Tsang DN, Chan JK, Lau YT, et al: *Penicillium marneffei* infection: An underdiagnosed disease? Histopathology 13:311-318, 1988.

939. Duong TA: Infection due to *Penicillium marneffei*, an emerging pathogen: Review of 155 reported cases. Clin Infect Dis 23:125-130, 1996.

940. Phillips P: *Penicillium marneffei* part of Southeast Asian AIDS. JAMA 276:86-87, 1996.

941. Deng ZL, Connor DH: Progressive disseminated penicilliosis caused by *Penicillium marneffei*. Report of eight cases and differentiation of the causative organism from *Histoplasma capsulatum*. Am J Clin Pathol 84:323-327, 1985.

942. Cooper CR Jr, McGinnis MR: Pathology of *Penicillium marneffei*. An emerging acquired immunodeficiency syndrome–related pathogen. Arch Pathol Lab Med 121:798-804, 1997.

943. Fenech FF, Mallia CP: Pleural effusion caused by *Penicillium lilacinum*. Br J Dis Chest 66:284-290, 1972.

944. Brown JR: Human actinomycosis. A study of 181 subjects. Hum Pathol 4:319-330, 1973.

945. Apotheloz C, Regamey C: Disseminated infection due to *Actinomyces meyeri*: Case report and review. Clin Infect Dis 22:621-625, 1996.

946. Snape PS: Thoracic actinomycosis: An unusual childhood infection. South Med J 86:222-224, 1993.

947. Lazzari G, Vineis C, Cugini A: Cytologic diagnosis of primary pulmonary actinomycosis: Report of two cases. Acta Cytol 25:299-301, 1981.

948. Das DK: Actinomycosis in fine needle aspiration cytology. Cytopathology 5:243-250, 1994.

949. Kwong JS, Müller NL, Godwin JD, et al: Thoracic actinomycosis: CT findings in eight patients. Radiology 183:189-192, 1992.

950. Cheon JE, Im JG, Kim MY, et al: Thoracic actinomycosis: CT findings. Radiology 209:229-233, 1998.

951. Baik JJ, Lee GL, Yoo CG, et al: Pulmonary actinomycosis in Korea. Respirology 4:31-35, 1999.

952. Kuijper EJ, Wiggerts HO, Jonker GJ, et al: Disseminated actinomycosis due to *Actinomyces meyeri* and *Actinobacillus actinomycetemcomitans*. Scand J Infect Dis 24:667-672, 1992.

953. Georghiou PR, Blacklock ZM: Infection with *Nocardia* species in Queensland. A review of 102 clinical isolates. Med J Aust 156:692-697, 1992.

954. Coker RJ, Bignardi G, Horner P, et al: *Nocardia* infection in AIDS: A clinical and microbiological challenge. J Clin Pathol 45:821-822, 1992.

955. Stevens DA, Pier AC, Beaman BL, et al: Laboratory evaluation of an outbreak of nocardiosis in immunocompromised hosts. Am J Med 71:928-934, 1981.

956. Rosett W, Hodges GR: Recent experiences with nocardial infections. Am J Med Sci 276:279-285, 1978.

957. Hui CH, Au VW, Rowland K, et al: Pulmonary nocardiosis re-visited: Experience of 35 patients at diagnosis. Respir Med 97:709-717, 2003.

958. Menendez R, Cordero PJ, Santos M, et al: Pulmonary infection with *Nocardia* species: A report of 10 cases and review. Eur Respir J 10:1542-1546, 1997.

959. Andriole VT, Ballas M, Wilson GL: The association of nocardiosis and pulmonary alveolar proteinosis. A case study. Ann Intern Med 60:266-275, 1964.

960. Hathaway BM, Mason KN: Nocardiosis. Study of fourteen cases. Am J Med 32:903-909, 1962.

961. Raich RA, Casey F, Hall WH: Pulmonary and cutaneous nocardiosis. The significance of the laboratory isolation of *Nocardia*. Am Rev Respir Dis 83:505-509, 1961.

962. Feigin DS: Nocardiosis of the lung: Chest radiographic findings in 21 cases. Radiology 159:9-14, 1986.

963. Buckley JA, Padhani AR, Kuhlman JE: CT features of pulmonary nocardiosis. J Comput Assist Tomog 19:726-732, 1995.

964. Yoon HK, Im JG, Ahn JM, et al: Pulmonary nocardiosis: CT findings. J Comput Assist Tomogr 19:52-55, 1995.

965. van Kralingen KW, Hekker TA, Bril H, et al: Haemoptysis and an abnormal x-ray after prolonged treatment in the ICU. Eur Respir J 7:419-420, 1994.

966. Murray JF, Finegold SM, Froman S, et al: The changing spectrum of nocardiosis. A review and presentation of nine cases. Am Rev Respir Dis 83:315-330, 1961.

967. Neu HC, Silva M, Hazen E, et al: Necrotizing nocardial pneumonitis. Ann Intern Med 66:274-284, 1967.

968. Krick JA, Stinson EB, Remington JS: *Nocardia* infection in heart transplant patients. Ann Intern Med 82:18-26, 1975.

969. Busmanis I, Harney M, Hellyar A: Nocardiosis diagnosed by lung FNA: A case report. Diagn Cytopathol 12:56-58, 1995.

970. Mok CC, Yuen KY, Lau CS: Nocardiosis in systemic lupus erythematosus. Semin Arthritis Rheum 26:675-683, 1997.

971. Andersen P: Pathogenesis of lower respiratory tract infections due to *Chlamydia*, *Mycoplasma*, *Legionella* and viruses. Thorax 53:302-307, 1998.

972. Castleman WL, Sorkness RL, Lemanske RF, et al: Neonatal viral bronchiolitis and pneumonia induces bronchiolar hypoplasia and alveolar dysplasia in rats. Lab Invest 59:387-396, 1988.

973. Folkerts G, Busse WW, Nijkamp FP, et al: Virus-induced airway hyperresponsiveness and asthma. Am J Respir Crit Care Med 157:1708-1720, 1998.

974. Shelhamer JH, Gill VJ, Quinn TC, et al: The laboratory evaluation of opportunistic pulmonary infections. Ann Intern Med 124:585-599, 1996

975. Nicholson KG, Wood JM, Zambon M: Influenza. Lancet 362:1733-1745, 2003.

976. Moorman JP: Viral characteristics of influenza. South Med J 96:758-61, 2003

977. Skehel JJ, Wiley DC: Influenza viruses and cell membranes. Am J Respir Crit Care Med 152:S13-S15, 1995.

978. Rott R, Klenk HD, Nagai Y, et al: Influenza viruses, cell enzymes, and pathogenicity. Am J Respir Crit Care Med 152:S16-S19, 1995.

979. Webster RG, Sharp GB, Claas EC: Interspecies transmission of influenza viruses. Am J Respir Crit Care Med 152:S25-S30, 1995.

980. Greenberg SB: Respiratory viral infections in adults. Curr Opin Pulm Med 8:201-208, 2002.

981. Stott DJ, Kerr G, Carman WF: Nosocomial transmission of influenza. Occup Med (Lond) 52:249-253, 2002.

982. Khater F, Moorman JP: Complications of influenza. South Med J 96:740-743, 2003.

983. Louria DB, Blumenfeld HL, Ellis JT, et al: Studies on influenza in the pandemic of 1957-1958. II. Pulmonary complications of influenza. J Clin Invest 38:213-265, 1959.

984. Mullooly JP, Barker WH, Nolan TF Jr: Risk of acute respiratory disease among pregnant women during influenza A epidemics. Public Health Rep 101:205-211, 1986.

985. Conway SP, Simmonds EJ, Littlewood JM: Acute severe deterioration in cystic fibrosis associated with influenza A virus infection. Thorax 47:112-114, 1992.

986. Bradley SF: Influenza in the elderly. Prevention is the best strategy in high-risk populations. Postgrad Med 99:138-139, 143-149, 1996.

987. Dourmashkin RR, Tyrrell DA: Attachment of two myxoviruses to ciliated epithelial cells. J Gen Virol 9:77-88, 1970.

988. Stinson SF, Ryan DP, Hertweck S, et al: Epithelial and surfactant changes in influenzal pulmonary lesions. Arch Pathol Lab Med 100:147-153, 1976.

989. Horisberger MA: Interferons, Mx genes, and resistance to influenza virus. Am J Respir Crit Care Med 152:S67-S71, 1995.

990. Benne CA, Kraaijeveld CA, van Strijp JA, et al: Interactions of surfactant protein A with influenza A viruses: Binding and neutralization. J Infect Dis 171:335-341, 1995.

991. Oseasohn R, Adelson L, Kaji M: Clinicopathologic study of thirty-three fatal cases of Asian influenza. N Engl J Med 260:509-518, 1959.

992. Yeldandi AV, Colby TV: Pathologic features of lung biopsy specimens from influenza pneumonia cases. Hum Pathol 25:47-53, 1994.

993. Noble RL, Lillington GA, Kempson RL: Fatal diffuse influenzal pneumonia: Premortem diagnosis by lung biopsy. Chest 63:644-646, 1973.

994. Hers JF, Masurel N, Mulder J: Bacteriology and histopathology of the respiratory tract and lungs in fatal Asian influenza. Lancet 2:1141-1143, 1958.

995. Fry J: Influenza A (Asian) 1957; clinical and epidemiological features in a general practice. BMJ 14:259-261, 1958.

996. Taylor R, Nemaia H, Tukuitonga C, et al: An epidemic of influenza in the population of Niue. J Med Virol 16:127-136, 1985.

997. Roldaan AC, Masural N: Viral respiratory infections in asthmatic children staying in a mountain resort. Eur J Respir Dis 63:140-150, 1982.

998. Wang EE, Prober CG, Manson B, et al: Association of respiratory viral infections with pulmonary deterioration in patients with cystic fibrosis. N Engl J Med 311:1653-1658, 1984.

999. Smith CB, Golden CA, Kanner RE, et al: Association of viral and *Mycoplasma pneumoniae* infections with acute respiratory illness in patients with chronic obstructive pulmonary diseases. Am Rev Respir Dis 121:225-232, 1980.

1000. Storch GA: Rapid diagnostic tests for influenza. Curr Opin Pediatr 15:77-84, 2003.

1001. Laraya-Cuasay LR, DeForest A, Huff D, et al: Chronic pulmonary complications of early influenza virus infection in children. Am Rev Respir Dis 116:617-625, 1977.

1002. Tillett HE, Smith JW, Clifford RE: Excess morbidity and mortality associated with influenza in England and Wales. Lancet 1:793-795, 1980.

1003. Cameron AS, Roder DM, Esterman AJ, et al: Mortality from influenza and allied infections in South Australia during 1968-1981. Med J Aust 142:14-17, 1985.

1004. Tillett HE, Smith JW, Gooch CD: Excess deaths attributable to influenza in England and Wales: Age at death and certified cause. Int J Epidemiol 12:344-352, 1983.

1005. Horman JT, Stetler HC, Israel E, et al: An outbreak of influenza A in a nursing home. Am J Public Health 76:501-504, 1986.

1006. Henrickson KJ: Parainfluenza viruses. Clin Microbiol Rev 16:242-264, 2003.

1007. Herrmann EC Jr, Hable KA: Experiences in laboratory diagnosis of parainfluenza viruses in routine medical practice. Mayo Clin Proc 45:177-188, 1970.

1008. Wendt CH, Weisdorf DJ, Jordan MC, et al: Parainfluenza virus respiratory infection after bone marrow transplantation. N Engl J Med 326:921-926, 1992.

1009. Vilchez RA, Dauber J, McCurry K, et al: Parainfluenza virus infection in adult lung transplant recipients: An emergent clinical syndrome with implications on allograft function. Am J Transplant 3:116-120, 2003.

1010. From the Centers for Disease Control and Prevention. Update: Respiratory syncytial virus activity—United States, 1994-95 season. JAMA 273:282, 1995.

1011. Falsey AR, Walsh EE: Respiratory syncytial virus infection in adults. Clin Microbiol Rev 13:371-384, 2000.

1012. Whimbey E, Ghosh S: Respiratory syncytial virus infections in immunocompromised adults. Curr Clin Top Infect Dis 20:232-255, 2000.

1013. Hashem M, Hall CB: Respiratory syncytial virus in healthy adults: The cost of a cold. J Clin Virol 27:14-21, 2003.

1014. Hall CB: The nosocomial spread of respiratory syncytial viral infections. Annu Rev Med 34:311-319, 1983.

1015. Harris J, Werling D: Binding and entry of respiratory syncytial virus into host cells and initiation of the innate immune response. Cell Microbiol 5:671-680, 2003.

1016. Aherne W, Bird T, Court SD, et al: Pathological changes in virus infections of the lower respiratory tract in children. J Clin Pathol 23:7-18, 1970.

1017. Parham DM, Bozeman P, Killian C, et al: Cytologic diagnosis of respiratory syncytial virus infection in a bronchoalveolar lavage specimen from a bone marrow transplant recipient. Am J Clin Pathol 99:588-592, 1993.

1018. Delage G, Brochu P, Robillard L, et al: Giant cell pneumonia due to respiratory syncytial virus. Occurrence in severe combined immunodeficiency syndrome. Arch Pathol Lab Med 108:623-625, 1984.

1019. Sterner G, Wolontis S, Bloth B, et al: Respiratory syncytial virus. An outbreak of acute respiratory illnesses in a home for infants. Acta Paediatr Scand 55:273-279, 1966.

1019a. Gasparetto EL, Escuissato DL, Marchiori E, et al: High-resolution CT findings of respiratory syncytial virus pneumonia after bone marrow transplantation. AJR Am J Roentgenol 182:1133-1137, 2004.

1020. Zaroukian MH, Kashyap GH, Wentworth BB: Respiratory syncytial virus infection: A cause of respiratory distress syndrome and pneumonia in adults. Am J Med Sci 295:218-222, 1988.

1021. Hall CB, Powell KR, Schnabel KC, et al: Risk of secondary bacterial infection in infants hospitalized with respiratory syncytial viral infection. J Pediatr 113:266-271, 1988.

1022. Reina J, Ros MJ, Del Valle JM, et al: Evaluation of direct immunofluorescence, dot-blot enzyme immunoassay, and shell-vial culture for detection of respiratory syncytial virus in patients with bronchiolitis. Eur J Clin Microbiol Infect Dis 14:1018-1020, 1995.

1023. Halstead DC, Todd S, Fritch G: Evaluation of five methods for respiratory syncytial virus detection. J Clin Microbiol 28:1021-1025, 1990.

1024. Vikerfors T, Grandien M, Olcen P: Respiratory syncytial virus infections in adults. Am Rev Respir Dis 136:561-564, 1987.

1025. McConnochie KM, Mark JD, McBride JT, et al: Normal pulmonary function measurements and airway reactivity in childhood after mild bronchiolitis. J Pediatr 107:54-58, 1985.

1026. Reed SE: The behaviour of recent isolates of human respiratory coronavirus in vitro and in volunteers: Evidence of heterogeneity among 229E-related strains. J Med Virol 13:179-192, 1984.

1027. Kuiken T, Fouchier RA, Schutten M, et al: Newly discovered coronavirus as the primary cause of severe acute respiratory syndrome. Lancet 362:263-270, 2003.

1028. Low DE, McGeer A: SARS—one year later. N Engl J Med 349:2381-2382, 2003.

1029. Hui DS, Sung JJ: Severe acute respiratory syndrome. Chest 124:12-15, 2003.

1030. Franks TJ, Chong PY, Chui P, et al: Lung pathology of severe acute respiratory syndrome (SARS): A study of 8 autopsy cases from Singapore. Hum Pathol 34:743-748, 2003.

1031. Müller NL, Ooi GC, Khong PL, et al: Severe acute respiratory syndrome: Radiographic and CT findings. AJR Am J Roentgenol 181:3-8, 2003.

1032. Wong KT, Antonio GE, Hui DS, et al: Severe acute respiratory syndrome: Radiographic appearances and pattern of progression in 138 patients. Radiology 228:401-406, 2003.

1033. Grinblat L, Shulman H, Glickman A, et al: Severe acute respiratory syndrome: Radiographic review of 40 probable cases in Toronto, Canada. Radiology 228:802-809, 2003.

1034. Wong KT, Antonio GE, Hui DS, et al: Thin section CT of severe acute respiratory syndrome. Radiology 228:395-400, 2003.

1035. Müller NL, Ooi GC, Khong PL, et al: High-resolution CT findings of severe acute respiratory syndrome at presentation and after admission. AJR Am J Roentgenol 182:39-44, 2004.

1036. Mason WH, Ross LA, Lanson J, et al: Epidemic measles in the postvaccine era: Evaluation of epidemiology, clinical presentation and complications during an urban outbreak. Pediatr Infect Dis J 12:42-48, 1993.

1037. Duke T, Mgone CS: Measles: Not just another viral exanthem. Lancet 361:763-773, 2003.

1038. Hinman AR, Orenstein WA, Bloch AB, et al: Impact of measles in the United States. Rev Infect Dis 5:439-444, 1983.

1039. Barkin RM: Measles mortality. Analysis of the primary cause of death. Am J Dis Child 129:307-309, 1975.

1040. Loukides S, Panagou P, Kolokouris D, et al: Bacterial pneumonia as a suprainfection in young adults with measles. Eur Respir J 13:356-360, 1999.

1041. Gremillion DH, Crawford GE: Measles pneumonia in young adults. An analysis of 106 cases. Am J Med 71:539-542, 1981.

1042. Atmar RL, Englund JA, Hammill H: Complications of measles during pregnancy. Clin Infect Dis 14:217-226, 1992.

1043. Kaplan LJ, Daum RS, Smaron M, et al: Severe measles in immunocompromised patients. JAMA 267:1237-1241, 1992.

1044. Vargas PA, Bernardi FD, Alves VA, et al: Uncommon histopathological findings in fatal measles infection: Pancreatitis, sialoadenitis and thyroiditis. Histopathology 37:141-146, 2000.

1045. Harboldt SL, Dugan JM, Tronic BS: Cytologic diagnosis of measles pneumonia in a bronchoalveolar lavage specimen. A case report. Acta Cytol 38:403-406, 1994.

1046. Osborne D: Radiologic appearance of viral disease of the lower respiratory tract in infants and children. AJR Am J Roentgenol 130:29-33, 1978.

1047. Abramson O, Dagan R, Tal A, et al: Severe complications of measles requiring intensive care in infants and young children. Arch Pediatr Adolesc Med 149:1237-1240, 1995.

1048. Tanaka H, Honma S, Yamagishi M, et al: [Clinical features of measles pneumonia in adults: Usefulness of computed tomography.] Nihon Kyobu Shikkan Gakkai Zasshi 31:1129-1133, 1993.

1049. Minnich LL, Goodenough F, Ray CG: Use of immunofluorescence to identify measles virus infections. J Clin Microbiol 29:1148-1150, 1991.

1050. Stanghelle JK, Festvag LV: Postpolio syndrome: A 5 year follow-up. Spinal Cord 35:503-508, 1997.

1051. Hable KA, O'Connell EJ, Herrmann EC Jr: Group B coxsackieviruses as respiratory viruses. Mayo Clin Proc 45:170-176, 1970.

1052. Chidekel AS, Rosen CL, Bazzy AR: Rhinovirus infection associated with serious lower respiratory illness in patients with bronchopulmonary dysplasia. Pediatr Infect Dis J 16:43-47, 1997.

1053. Wald TG, Shult P, Krause P, et al: A rhinovirus outbreak among residents of a long-term care facility. Ann Intern Med 123:588-593, 1995.

1054. Levandowski RA, Ou DW, Jackson GG: Acute-phase decrease of T lymphocyte subsets in rhinovirus infection. J Infect Dis 153:743-748, 1986.

1055. Halperin SA, Eggleston PA, Beasley P, et al: Exacerbations of asthma in adults during experimental rhinovirus infection. Am Rev Respir Dis 132:976-980, 1985.

1056. Gern JE, Calhoun W, Swenson C, et al: Rhinovirus infection preferentially increases lower airway responsiveness in allergic subjects. Am J Respir Crit Care Med 155:1872-1876, 1997.

1057. Smith CB, Kanner RE, Golden CA, et al: Effect of viral infections on pulmonary function in patients with chronic obstructive pulmonary diseases. J Infect Dis 141:271-280, 1980.

1058. Sugimoto M, Nakashima H, Watanabe S, et al: T-lymphocyte alveolitis in HTLV-I–associated myelopathy. Lancet 2:1220, 1987.

1059. Kuwabara H, Katanaka J, Nagai M, et al: Human T lymphotropic virus type I associated myelopathy with pulmonary and cutaneous lesions. J Clin Pathol 46:273-275, 1993.

1060. Kikuchi T, Saijo Y, Sakai T, et al: Human T-cell lymphotropic virus type I (HTLV-I) carrier with clinical manifestations characteristic of diffuse panbronchiolitis. Intern Med 35:305-309, 1996.

1061. Chayt KJ, Harper ME, Marselle LM, et al: Detection of HTLV-III RNA in lungs of patients with AIDS and pulmonary involvement. JAMA 256:2356-2359, 1986.

1062. Agostini C, Zambello R, Trentin L, et al: Prognostic significance of the evaluation of bronchoalveolar lavage cell populations in patients with HIV-1 infection and pulmonary involvement. Chest 100:1601-1606, 1991.

1063. Twigg HL 3rd, Soliman DM, Spain BA: Impaired alveolar macrophage accessory cell function and reduced incidence of lymphocytic alveolitis in HIV-infected patients who smoke. AIDS 8:611-618, 1994.

1064. Sadat-Sowti B, Parrot A, Quint L, et al: Alveolar CD8$^+$CD57$^+$ lymphocytes in human immunodeficiency virus infection produce an inhibitor of cytotoxic functions. Am J Respir Crit Care Med 149:972-980, 1994.

1065. Travis WD, Fox CH, Devaney KO, et al: Lymphoid pneumonitis in 50 adult patients infected with the human immunodeficiency virus: Lymphocytic interstitial pneumonitis versus nonspecific interstitial pneumonitis. Hum Pathol 23:529-541, 1992.

1066. Diaz PT, Clanton TL, Pacht ER: Emphysema-like pulmonary disease associated with human immunodeficiency virus infection. Ann Intern Med 116:124-128, 1992.

1067. Moolenaar RL, Breiman RF, Peters CJ: Hantavirus pulmonary syndrome. Semin Respir Infect 12:31-39, 1997.

1068. Hjelle B, Goade D, Torrez-Martinez N, et al: Hantavirus pulmonary syndrome, renal insufficiency, and myositis associated with infection by Bayou hantavirus. Clin Infect Dis 23:495-500, 1996.

1069. Khan AS, Gaviria M, Rollin PE, et al: Hantavirus pulmonary syndrome in Florida: Association with the newly identified Black Creek Canal virus. Am J Med 100:46-48, 1996.

1070. Butler JC, Peters CJ: Hantaviruses and hantavirus pulmonary syndrome. Clin Infect Dis 19:387-394, quiz 395, 1994.

1071. Zaki SR, Greer PW, Coffield LM, et al: Hantavirus pulmonary syndrome. Pathogenesis of an emerging infectious disease. Am J Pathol 146:552-579, 1995.

1072. Ketai LH, Williamson MR, Telepak RJ, et al: Hantavirus pulmonary syndrome: Radiographic findings in 16 patients. Radiology 191:665-668, 1994.

1073. Jenison S, Yamada T, Morris C, et al: Characterization of human antibody responses to Four Corners hantavirus infections among patients with hantavirus pulmonary syndrome. J Virol 68:3000-3006, 1994.

1074. Esterly JR, Oppenheimer EH: Pathological lesions due to congenital rubella. Arch Pathol 87:380-388, 1969.

1075. Esterly JR, Oppenheimer EH: Vascular lesions in infants with congenital rubella. Circulation 36:544-554, 1967.

1076. Waller BF, Smith FA, Kerwin DM, et al: Fetal rubella 27 years later. Chest 81:735-738, 1982.

1077. Glezen P, Denny FW: Epidemiology of acute lower respiratory disease in children. N Engl J Med 288:498-505, 1973.

1078. Martone WJ, Hierholzer JC, Keenlyside RA, et al: An outbreak of adenovirus type 3 disease at a private recreation center swimming pool. Am J Epidemiol 111:229-237, 1980.

1079. Klinger JR, Sanchez MP, Curtin LA, et al: Multiple cases of life-threatening adenovirus pneumonia in a mental health care center. Am J Respir Crit Care Med 157:645-649, 1998.

1080. Carrigan DR: Adenovirus infections in immunocompromised patients. Am J Med 102:71-74, 1997.

1081. Murtagh P, Cerqueiro C, Halac A, et al: Adenovirus type 7h respiratory infections: A report of 29 cases of acute lower respiratory disease. Acta Paediatr 82:557-561, 1993.

1082. Brummitt CF, Cherrington JM, Katzenstein DA, et al: Nosocomial adenovirus infections: Molecular epidemiology of an outbreak due to adenovirus 3a. J Infect Dis 158:423-432, 1988.

1083. Han BK, Son JA, Yoon HK, et al: Epidemic adenoviral lower respiratory tract infection in pediatric patients: Radiographic and clinical characteristics. AJR Am J Roentgenol 170:1077-1080, 1998.

1084. George RB, Ziskind MM, Rasch JR, et al: *Mycoplasma* and adenovirus pneumonias. Comparison with other atypical pneumonias in a military population. Ann Intern Med 65:931-942, 1966.

1085. Becroft DM: Bronchiolitis obliterans, bronchiectasis, and other sequelae of adenovirus type 21 infection in young children. J Clin Pathol 24:72-82, 1971.

1086. Spigelblatt L, Rosenfeld R: Hyperlucent lung: Long-term complication of adenovirus type 7 pneumonia. Can Med Assoc J 128:47-49, 1983.

1087. Elliott WM, Hayashi S, Hogg JC: Immunodetection of adenoviral E1A proteins in human lung tissue. Am J Respir Cell Mol Biol 12:642-648, 1995.

1088. Prellner T, Flamholc L, Haidl S, et al: Herpes simplex virus—the most frequently isolated pathogen in the lungs of patients with severe respiratory distress. Scand J Infect Dis 24:283-292, 1992.

1089. Schuller D, Spessert C, Fraser VJ, et al: Herpes simplex virus from respiratory tract secretions: Epidemiology, clinical characteristics, and outcome in immunocompromised and nonimmunocompromised hosts. Am J Med 94:29-33, 1993.

1090. Nash G, Foley FD: Herpetic infection of the middle and lower respiratory tract. Am J Clin Pathol 54:857-863, 1970.

1091. Graham BS, Snell JD Jr: Herpes simplex virus infection of the adult lower respiratory tract. Medicine (Baltimore) 62:384-393, 1983.

1092. Vernon SE: Cytologic features of nonfatal herpesvirus tracheobronchitis. Acta Cytol 26:237-242, 1982.

1093. Sherry MK, Klainer AS, Wolff M, et al: Herpetic tracheobronchitis. Ann Intern Med 109:229-233, 1988.

1094. Lheureux P, Verhest A, Vincent JL, et al: Herpes virus infection, an unusual source of adult respiratory distress syndrome. Eur J Respir Dis 67:72-77, 1985.

1095. Tuxen DV, Cade JF, McDonald MI, et al: Herpes simplex virus from the lower respiratory tract in adult respiratory distress syndrome. Am Rev Respir Dis 126:416-419, 1982.

1096. Jacobs F, Knoop C, Brancart F, et al: Human herpesvirus-6 infection after lung and heart-lung transplantation: A prospective longitudinal study. Transplantation 75:1996-2001, 2003.

1097. Russler SK, Tapper MA, Knox KK, et al: Pneumonitis associated with coinfection by human herpesvirus 6 and *Legionella* in an immunocompetent adult. Am J Pathol 138:1405-1411, 1991.

1098. Cone RW: Human herpesvirus 6 as a possible cause of pneumonia. Semin Respir Infect 10:254-258, 1995.

1099. Cool CD, Rai PR, Yeager ME, et al: Expression of human herpesvirus 8 in primary pulmonary hypertension. N Engl J Med 349:1113-1122, 2003.

1100. Tang YW, Johnson JE, Browning PJ, et al: Herpesvirus DNA is consistently detected in lungs of patients with idiopathic pulmonary fibrosis. J Clin Microbiol 41:2633-2640, 2003.

1101. Cesarman E, Knowles DM: Kaposi's sarcoma–associated herpesvirus: A lymphotropic human herpesvirus associated with Kaposi's sarcoma, primary effusion lymphoma, and multicentric Castleman's disease. Semin Diagn Pathol 14:54-66, 1997.

1102. Benfield TL, Dodt KK, Lundgren JD: Human herpes virus-8 DNA in bronchoalveolar lavage samples from patients with AIDS-associated pulmonary Kaposi's sarcoma. Scand J Infect Dis 29:13-16, 1997.

1103. Soler JJ, Perpina M, Alfaro A: Hemidiaphragmatic paralysis caused by cervical herpes zoster. Respiration 63:403-406, 1996.

1104. Weller TH: Varicella and herpes zoster. Changing concepts of the natural history, control, and importance of a not-so-benign virus. N Engl J Med 309:1434-1440, 1983.

1105. Mermelstein RH, Freireich AW: Varicella pneumonia. Ann Intern Med 55:456-463, 1961.

1106. Jura E, Chadwick EG, Josephs SH, et al: Varicella-zoster virus infections in children infected with human immunodeficiency virus. Pediatr Infect Dis J 8:586-590, 1989.

1107. Locksley RM, Flournoy N, Sullivan KM, et al: Infection with varicella-zoster virus after marrow transplantation. J Infect Dis 152:1172-1181, 1985.

1108. Esmonde TF, Herdman G, Anderson G: Chickenpox pneumonia: An association with pregnancy. Thorax 44:812-815, 1989.

1109. Triebwasser JH, Harris RE, Bryant RE, et al: Varicella pneumonia in adults. Report of seven cases and a review of literature. Medicine (Baltimore) 46:409-423, 1967.

1110. Knyvett AF: The pulmonary lesions of chickenpox. QJM 35:313-323, 1966.

1111. Kaufman SA, Levene G, Tan DY: Primary chickenpox pneumonia. Am J Roentgenol Radium Ther Nucl Med 76:527-532, 1956.

1112. Sargent EN, Carson MJ, Reilly ED: Roentgenographic manifestations of varicella pneumonia with postmortem correlation. Am J Roentgenol Radium Ther Nucl Med 98:305-317, 1966.

1113. Burton GG, Sayer WJ, Lillington GA: Varicella pneumonia in adults: Frequency of sudden death. Dis Chest 50:179-185, 1966.

1114. Charles RE, Katz RL, Ordonez NG, et al: Varicella-zoster infection with pleural involvement. A cytologic and ultrastructural study of a case. Am J Clin Pathol 85:522-526, 1986.

1115. Brunton FJ, Moore ME: A survey of pulmonary calcification following adult chicken-pox. Br J Radiol 42:256-259, 1969.

1116. Nankervis GA, Kumar ML: Diseases produced by cytomegaloviruses. Med Clin North Am 62:1021-1035, 1978.

1117. Ho M: Epidemiology of cytomegalovirus infections. Rev Infect Dis 12(Suppl 7):S701-S710, 1990.

1118. Marrie TJ, Janigan DT, Haldane EV, et al: Does cytomegalovirus play a role in community-acquired pneumonia? Clin Invest Med 8:286-295, 1985.

1119. Tamm M, Traenkle P, Grilli B, et al: Pulmonary cytomegalovirus infection in immunocompromised patients. Chest 119:838-843, 2001.

1120. Meyers JD, Flournoy N, Thomas ED: Risk factors for cytomegalovirus infection after human marrow transplantation. J Infect Dis 153:478-488, 1986.

1121. Chou SW: Reactivation and recombination of multiple cytomegalovirus strains from individual organ donors. J Infect Dis 160:11-15, 1989.

1122. Craighead JE: Pulmonary cytomegalovirus infection in the adult. Am J Pathol 63:487-500, 1971.

1123. Smith TF, Holley KE, Keys TF, et al: Cytomegalovirus studies of autopsy tissue. I. Virus isolation. Am J Clin Pathol 63:854-858, 1975.

1124. Grundy JE: Virologic and pathogenetic aspects of cytomegalovirus infection. Rev Infect Dis 12(Suppl 7):S711-S719, 1990.

1125. Beschorner WE, Hutchins GM, Burns WH, et al: Cytomegalovirus pneumonia in bone marrow transplant recipients: Miliary and diffuse patterns. Am Rev Respir Dis 122:107-114, 1980.

1126. Olliff JF, Williams MP: Radiological appearances of cytomegalovirus infections. Clin Radiol 40:463-467, 1989.

1127. Schulman LL: Cytomegalovirus pneumonitis and lobar consolidation. Chest 91:558-561, 1987.

1128. Kang EY, Patz EF Jr, Müller NL: Cytomegalovirus pneumonia in transplant patients: CT findings. J Comput Assist Tomogr 20:295-299, 1996.

1129. McGuinness G, Scholes JV, Garay SM, et al: Cytomegalovirus pneumonitis: Spectrum of parenchymal CT findings with pathologic correlation in 21 AIDS patients. Radiology 192:451-459, 1994.

1130. Cohen JI, Corey GR: Cytomegalovirus infection in the normal host. Medicine (Baltimore) 64:100-114, 1985.

1131. Pannuti CS, Vilas Boas LS, Angelo MJ, et al: Cytomegalovirus mononucleosis in children and adults: Differences in clinical presentation. Scand J Infect Dis 17:153-156, 1985.

1132. Idell S, Johnson M, Beauregard L, et al: Pneumonia associated with rising cytomegalovirus antibody titres in a healthy adult. Thorax 38:957-958, 1983.

1133. Chou S: Newer methods for diagnosis of cytomegalovirus infection. Rev Infect Dis 12(Suppl 7):S727-S736, 1990.

1134. Bewig B, Haacke TC, Tiroke A, et al: Detection of CMV pneumonitis after lung transplantation using PCR of DNA from bronchoalveolar lavage cells. Respiration 67:166-172, 2000.

1135. Garten AJ, Mendelson DS, Halton KP: CT manifestations of infectious mononucleosis. Clin Imaging 16:114-116, 1992.

1136. Martin A, Capron F, Liguory-Brunaud MD, et al: Epstein-Barr virus–associated primary malignant lymphomas of the pleural cavity occurring in longstanding pleural chronic inflammation. Hum Pathol 25:1314-1318, 1994.

1137. Katzenstein AL, Peiper SC: Detection of Epstein-Barr virus genomes in lymphomatoid granulomatosis: Analysis of 29 cases by the polymerase chain reaction technique. Mod Pathol 3:435-441, 1990.

1138. Barbera JA, Hayashi S, Hegele RG, et al: Detection of Epstein-Barr virus in lymphocytic interstitial pneumonia by in situ hybridization. Am Rev Respir Dis 145:940-946, 1992.

1139. Butler AE, Colby TV, Weiss L, et al: Lymphoepithelioma-like carcinoma of the lung. Am J Surg Pathol 13:632-639, 1989.

1140. Byrne JC, Tsao MS, Fraser RS, et al: Human papillomavirus-11 DNA in a patient with chronic laryngotracheobronchial papillomatosis and metastatic squamous-cell carcinoma of the lung. N Engl J Med 317:873-878, 1987.

1141. Bejui-Thivolet F, Liagre N, Chignol MC, et al: Detection of human papillomavirus DNA in squamous bronchial metaplasia and squamous cell carcinomas of the lung by in situ hybridization using biotinylated probes in paraffin-embedded specimens. Hum Pathol 21:111-116, 1990.

1142. Karalus NC, Cursons RT, Leng RA, et al: Community acquired pneumonia: Aetiology and prognostic index evaluation. Thorax 46:413-418, 1991.

1143. Almirall J, Morato I, Riera F, et al: Incidence of community-acquired pneumonia and *Chlamydia pneumoniae* infection: A prospective multicentre study. Eur Respir J 6:14-18, 1993.

1144. Amundson DE, Weiss PJ: Pneumonia in military recruits. Mil Med 159:629-631, 1994.

1145. Noah ND: *Mycoplasma pneumoniae* infection in the United Kingdom—1967-73. BMJ 2:544-546, 1974.

1146. Khatib R, Schnarr D: Point-source outbreak of *Mycoplasma pneumoniae* infection in a family unit. J Infect Dis 151:186-187, 1985.

1147. Murphy GF, Brody AR, Craighead JE: Exfoliation of respiratory epithelium in hamster tracheal organ cultures infected with *Mycoplasma pneumoniae*. Virchows Arch A Pathol Anat Histol 389:93-102, 1980.

1148. Rollins S, Colby T, Clayton F: Open lung biopsy in *Mycoplasma pneumoniae* pneumonia. Arch Pathol Lab Med 110:34-41, 1986.

1149. Benisch BM, Fayemi A, Gerber MA, et al: Mycoplasmal pneumonia in a patient with rheumatic heart disease. Am J Clin Pathol 58:343-348, 1972.

1150. Kaufman JM, Cuvelier CA, Van der Straeten M: *Mycoplasma* pneumonia with fulminant evolution into diffuse interstitial fibrosis. Thorax 35:140-144, 1980.

1151. Brolin I, Wernstedt L: Radiographic appearance of mycoplasmal pneumonia. Scand J Respir Dis 59:179-189, 1978.

1152. Borthwick RC, Cameron DC, Philp T: Radiographic patterns of pulmonary involvement in acute mycoplasmal infections. Scand J Respir Dis 59:190-193, 1978.

1153. Alexander ER, Foy HM, Kenny GE, et al: Pneumonia due to *Mycoplasma pneumoniae*. Its incidence in the membership of a co-operative medical group. N Engl J Med 275:131-136, 1966.

1154. Grayston JT, Alexander ER, Kenny GE, et al: *Mycoplasma pneumoniae* infections. Clinical and epidemiologic studies. JAMA 191:369-374, 1965.

1155. Izumikawa K, Hara K: Clinical features of mycoplasmal pneumonia in adults. Yale J Biol Med 56:505-510, 1983.

1156. Niitu Y: M. pneumoniae respiratory diseases: Clinical features—children. Yale J Biol Med 56:493-503, 1983.

1157. Dean NL: Mycoplasmal pneumonias in the community hospital. The "unusual" manifestations become common. Clin Chest Med 2:121-131, 1981.

1158. Reittner P, Müller NL, Heyneman L, et al: *Mycoplasma pneumoniae* pneumonia: Radiographic and high-resolution CT features in 28 patients. AJR Am J Roentgenol 174:37-41, 2000.

1159. Lind K: Manifestations and complications of *Mycoplasma pneumoniae* disease: A review. Yale J Biol Med 56:461-468, 1983.

1160. Ali NJ, Sillis M, Andrews BE, et al: The clinical spectrum and diagnosis of *Mycoplasma pneumoniae* infection. QJM 58:241-251, 1986.

1161. Evatt BL, Dowdle WR, Johnson M Jr, et al: Epidemic mycoplasma pneumonia. N Engl J Med 285:374-378, 1971.

1162. Fischman RA, Marschall KE, Kislak JW, et al: Adult respiratory distress syndrome caused by *Mycoplasma pneumoniae*. Chest 74:471-473, 1978.

1163. Solanki DL, Berdoff RL: Severe mycoplasma pneumonia with pleural effusions in a patient with sickle cell-hemoglobin C(SC) disease. Case report and review of the literature. Am J Med 66:707-710, 1979.

1164. Hely MA, Williamson PM, Terenty TR: Neurological complications of *Mycoplasma pneumoniae* infection. Clin Exp Neurol 20:153-160, 1984.

1165. Sands MJ Jr, Rosenthal R: Progressive heart failure and death associated with *Mycoplasma pneumoniae* pneumonia. Chest 81:763-765, 1982.

1166. Teisch JA, Shapiro L, Walzer RA: Vesiculopustular eruption with mycoplasma infection. JAMA 211:1694-1697, 1970.

1167. Levine DP, Lerner AM: The clinical spectrum of *Mycoplasma pneumoniae* infections. Med Clin North Am 62:961-978, 1978.

1168. Granstrom M, Holme T, Sjogren AM, et al: The role of IgA determination by ELISA in the early serodiagnosis of *Mycoplasma pneumoniae* infection, in relation to IgG and mu-capture IgM methods. J Med Microbiol 40:288-292, 1994.

1169. Kleemola SR, Karjalainen JE, Raty RK: Rapid diagnosis of *Mycoplasma pneumoniae* infection: Clinical evaluation of a commercial probe test. J Infect Dis 162:70-75, 1990.

1170. Falguera M, Nogues A, Ruiz-Gonzalez A, et al: Detection of *Mycoplasma pneumoniae* by polymerase chain reaction in lung aspirates from patients with community-acquired pneumonia. Chest 110:972-976, 1996.

1171. Tablan OC, Reyes MP: Chronic interstitial pulmonary fibrosis following *Mycoplasma pneumoniae* pneumonia. Am J Med 79:268-270, 1985.

1172. Reyes de la Rocha S, Leonard JC, Demetriou E: Potential permanent respiratory sequela of Stevens-Johnson syndrome in an adolescent. J Adolesc Health Care 6:220-223, 1985.

1173. Campbell S, Larsen J, Knight ST, et al: Chlamydial elementary bodies are translocated on the surface of epithelial cells. Am J Pathol 152:1167-1170, 1998.

1174. Komaroff AL, Aronson MD, Schachter J: *Chlamydia trachomatis* infection in adults with community-acquired pneumonia. JAMA 245:1319-1322, 1981.

1175. Tack KJ, Peterson PK, Rasp FL, et al: Isolation of *Chlamydia trachomatis* from the lower respiratory tract of adults. Lancet 1:116-120, 1980.

1176. Herrmann B, Salih MA, Yousif BE, et al: Chlamydial etiology of acute lower respiratory tract infections in children in the Sudan. Acta Paediatr 83:169-172, 1994.

1177. Thom DH, Grayston JT, Campbell LA, et al: Respiratory infection with *Chlamydia pneumoniae* in middle-aged and older adult outpatients. Eur J Clin Microbiol Infect Dis 13:785-792, 1994.

1178. Blasi F, Cosentini R, Denti F, et al: Two family outbreaks of *Chlamydia pneumoniae* infection. Eur Respir J 7:102-104, 1994.

1179. Blasi F, Boschini A, Cosentini R, et al: Outbreak of *Chlamydia pneumoniae* infection in former injection-drug users. Chest 105:812-815, 1994.

1180. Von Hertzen L, Alakarppa H, Koskinen R, et al: *Chlamydia pneumoniae* infection in patients with chronic obstructive pulmonary disease. Epidemiol Infect 118:155-164, 1997.

1181. Emre U, Bernius M, Roblin PM, et al: *Chlamydia pneumoniae* infection in patients with cystic fibrosis. Clin Infect Dis 22:819-823, 1996.

1182. McConnell CT Jr, Plouffe JF, File TM, et al: Radiographic appearance of *Chlamydia pneumoniae* (TWAR strain) respiratory infections. CBPIS Study Group. Community-based Pneumonia Incidence Study. Radiology 192:819-824, 1994.

1183. Wright SW, Edwards KM, Decker MD, et al: Prevalence of positive serology for acute *Chlamydia pneumoniae* infection in emergency department patients with persistent cough. Acad Emerg Med 4:179-183, 1997.

1184. Montalban GS, Roblin PM, Hammerschlag MR: Performance of three commercially available monoclonal reagents for confirmation of *Chlamydia pneumoniae* in cell culture. J Clin Microbiol 32:1406-1407, 1994.

1185. Garnett P, Brogan O, Lafong C, et al: Comparison of throat swabs with sputum specimens for the detection of *Chlamydia pneumoniae* antigen by direct immunofluorescence. J Clin Pathol 51:309-311, 1998.

1186. Gaydos CA, Roblin PM, Hammerschlag MR, et al: Diagnostic utility of PCR-enzyme immunoassay, culture, and serology for detection of *Chlamydia pneumoniae* in symptomatic and asymptomatic patients. J Clin Microbiol 32:903-905, 1994.

1187. McKendrick GD, Davies J, Dutta T: A small outbreak of psittacosis. Lancet 2:1255, 1973.

1188. Andrews BE, Major R, Palmer SR: Ornithosis in poultry workers. Lancet 1:632-634, 1981.

1189. Barnes MG, Brainerd H: Pneumonitis with alveolar-capillary block in a cattle rancher exposed to epizootic bovine abortion. N Engl J Med 271:981-985, 1964.

1190. Barrett PK, Greenberg MJ: Outbreak of ornithosis. BMJ 5507:206-207, 1966.

1191. Stenstrom R, Jansson E, Wager O: Ornithosis pneumonia with special reference to roentgenological lung findings. Acta Med Scand 171:349-356, 1962.

1192. van Berkel M, Dik H, van der Meer JW, et al: Acute respiratory insufficiency from psittacosis. Br Med J (Clin Res Ed) 290:1503-1504, 1985.

1193. Editorial: Psittacosis. Lancet 2:1246, 1973.

1194. Byrom NP, Walls J, Mair HJ: Fulminant psittacosis. Lancet 1:353-356, 1979.

1195. Macfarlane JT, Macrae AD: Psittacosis. Br Med Bull 39:163-167, 1983.

1196. Johnson JE, Kadull PJ: Laboratory-acquired Q fever. A report of fifty cases. Am J Med 41:391-403, 1966.

1197. Rauch AM, Tanner M, Pacer RE, et al: Sheep-associated outbreak of Q fever, Idaho. Arch Intern Med 147:341-344, 1987.

1198. Spelman DW: Q fever: A study of 111 consecutive cases. Med J Aust 1:547-548, 551, 553, 1982.

1199. Urso FP: The pathologic findings in rickettsial pneumonia. Am J Clin Pathol 64:335-342, 1975.

1200. Gordon JD, MacKeen AD, Marrie TJ, et al: The radiographic features of epidemic and sporadic Q fever pneumonia. J Can Assoc Radiol 35:293-296, 1984.

1201. Pickworth FE, el-Soussi MA, Wells IP, et al: The radiological appearances of "Q" fever pneumonia. Clin Radiol 44:150-153, 1991.

1202. Millar JK: The chest film findings in "Q" fever—a series of 35 cases. Clin Radiol 29:371-375, 1978.

1203. Brouqui P, Dupont HT, Drancourt M, et al: Chronic Q fever. Ninety-two cases from France, including 27 cases without endocarditis. Arch Intern Med 153:642-648, 1993.

1204. Donohue JF: Lower respiratory tract involvement in Rocky Mountain spotted fever. Arch Intern Med 140:223-227, 1980.

1205. Martin W 3rd, Choplin RH, Shertzer ME: The chest radiograph in Rocky Mountain spotted fever. AJR Am J Roentgenol 139:889-893, 1982.

1206. Lyche KD, Jensen WA: Pleuropulmonary amebiasis. Semin Respir Infect 12:106-112, 1997.

1206a. Shamsuzzaman SM, Hashiguchi Y: Thoracic amebiasis. Clin Chest Med 23:479-492, 2002.

1207. Ibarra-Perez C: Thoracic complications of amebic abscess of the liver: Report of 501 cases. Chest 79:672-677, 1981.

1208. Barrett-Connor E: Parasitic pulmonary disease. Am Rev Respir Dis 126:558-563, 1982.

1209. Radin DR, Ralls PW, Colletti PM, et al: CT of amebic liver abscess. AJR Am J Roentgenol 150:1297-1301, 1988.

1210. Roy DC, Ravindran P, Padmanabhan R: Bronchobiliary fistula secondary to amebic liver abscess. Chest 62:523-524, 1972.

1211. Pudifin DJ, Duursma J, Gathiram V, et al: Invasive amoebiasis is associated with the development of anti-neutrophil cytoplasmic antibody. Clin Exp Immunol 97:48-51, 1994.

1212. Quinn EL, Fisher EJ, Cox F, et al: The clinical spectrum of toxoplasmosis in the adult. Cleve Clin Q 42:71-81, 1975.

1213. Theologides A, Kennedy BJ: Clinical manifestations of toxoplasmosis in the adult. Arch Intern Med 117:536-540, 1966.

1214. Goodman PC, Schnapp LM: Pulmonary toxoplasmosis in AIDS. Radiology 184:791-793, 1992.

1215. Welch PC, Masur H, Jones TC, et al: Serologic diagnosis of acute lymphadenopathic toxoplasmosis. J Infect Dis 142:256-264, 1980.

1216. Anstey NM, Jacups SP, Cain T, et al: Pulmonary manifestations of uncomplicated falciparum and vivax malaria: Cough, small airways obstruction, impaired gas transfer, and increased pulmonary phagocytic activity. J Infect Dis 185:1326-1334, 2002.

1217. Lichtman AR, Mohrcken S, Engelbrecht M, et al: Pathophysiology of severe forms of falciparum malaria. Crit Care Med 18:666-668, 1990.

1218. Bruneel F, Hocqueloux L, Alberti C, et al: The clinical spectrum of severe imported falciparum malaria in the intensive care unit: Report of 188 cases in adults. Am J Respir Crit Care Med 167:684-689, 2003.

1219. Gelpi AP, Mustafa A: Ascaris pneumonia. Am J Med 44:377-389, 1968.

1220. Humpherys K, Hieger LR: *Strongyloides stercoralis* in routine Papanicolaou-stained sputum smears. Acta Cytol 23:471-476, 1979.

1221. Stone WJ, Schaffner W: *Strongyloides* infections in transplant recipients. Semin Respir Infect 5:58-64, 1990.

1222. Chu E, Whitlock WL, Dietrich RA: Pulmonary hyperinfection syndrome with *Strongyloides stercoralis*. Chest 97:1475-1477, 1990.

1223. Weller IV, Copland P, Gabriel R: *Strongyloides stercoralis* infection in renal transplant recipients. Br Med J (Clin Res Ed) 282:524, 1981.

1224. Gompels MM, Todd J, Peters BS, et al: Disseminated strongyloidiasis in AIDS: Uncommon but important. AIDS 5:329-332, 1991.

1225. Kramer MR, Gregg PA, Goldstein M, et al: Disseminated strongyloidiasis in AIDS and non-AIDS immunocompromised hosts: Diagnosis by sputum and bronchoalveolar lavage. South Med J 83:1226-1229, 1990.

1226. Venizelos PC, Lopata M, Bardawil WA, et al: Respiratory failure due to *Strongyloides stercoralis* in a patient with a renal transplant. Chest 78:104-106, 1980.

1227. Krysl J, Müller NL, Miller RR, et al: Patient with miliary nodules and diarrhea. Can Assoc Radiol J 42:363-366, 1991.

1228. Woodring JH, Halfhill H 2nd, Reed JC: Pulmonary strongyloidiasis: Clinical and imaging features. AJR Am J Roentgenol 162:537-542, 1994.

1229. Grove DI: Strongyloidiasis in Allied ex-prisoners of war in south-east Asia. BMJ 280:598-601, 1980.

1230. Williams J, Nunley D, Dralle W, et al: Diagnosis of pulmonary strongyloidiasis by bronchoalveolar lavage. Chest 94:643-644, 1988.

1231. Wehner JH, Kirsch CM: Pulmonary manifestations of strongyloidiasis. Semin Respir Infect 12:122-129, 1997.

1232. Ribas-Mujal D: Trichinosis. In Marcial-Rojas R (ed): Pathology of Protozoal and Helminthic Diseases with Clinical Correlation. Baltimore, Williams & Williams, 1971, p 677.

1233. Udwadia F: Pulmonary eosinophilia, Chapter III: Tropical eosinophilia. In Herzog H (ed): Progress in Respiratory Research. New York, SA Karger, 1975.

1234. Udwadia FE, Joshi VV: A study of tropical eosinophilia. Thorax 19:548-554, 1964.

1235. Boornazian JS, Fagan MJ: Tropical pulmonary eosinophilia associated with pleural effusions. Am J Trop Med Hyg 34:473-475, 1985.

1236. Sandhu M, Mukhopadhyay S, Sharma SK: Tropical pulmonary eosinophilia: A comparative evaluation of plain chest radiography and computed tomography. Australas Radiol 40:32-37, 1996.

1237. Nutman TB, Vijayan VK, Pinkston P, et al: Tropical pulmonary eosinophilia: Analysis of antifilarial antibody localized to the lung. J Infect Dis 160:1042-1050, 1989.

1238. Anupindi L, Sahoo R, Rao RV, et al: Microfilariae in bronchial brushing cytology of symptomatic pulmonary lesions. A report of two cases. Acta Cytol 37:397-399, 1993.

1239. Aggarwal J, Kapila K, Gaur A, et al: Bancroftian filarial pleural effusion. Postgrad Med J 69:869-870, 1993.

1240. Rom WN, Vijayan VK, Cornelius MJ, et al: Persistent lower respiratory tract inflammation associated with interstitial lung disease in patients with tropical pulmonary eosinophilia following conventional treatment with diethylcarbamazine. Am Rev Respir Dis 142:1088-1092, 1990.

1241. Asimacopoulos PJ, Katras A, Christie B: Pulmonary dirofilariasis. The largest single-hospital experience. Chest 102:851-855, 1992.

1242. Cordero M, Muro A, Simon F, et al: Are transient pulmonary solitary nodules a common event in human dirofilariosis? Clin Invest 70:437-440, 1992.

1243. Flieder DB, Moran CA: Pulmonary dirofilariasis: A clinicopathologic study of 41 lesions in 39 patients. Hum Pathol 30:251-256, 1999.

1244. Levinson ED, Ziter FM Jr, Westcott JL: Pulmonary lesions due to *Dirofilaria immitis* (dog heartworm). Report of four cases with radiologic findings. Radiology 131:305-307, 1979.

1245. Awe RJ, Mattox KL, Alvarez BA, et al: Solitary and bilateral pulmonary nodules due to *Dirofilaria immitis*. Am Rev Respir Dis 112:445-449, 1975.

1246. Ciferri F: Human pulmonary dirofilariasis in the United States: A critical review. Am J Trop Med Hyg 31:302-308, 1982.

1247. Perera L, Muro A, Cordero M, et al: Evaluation of a 22 kDa *Dirofilaria immitis* antigen for the immunodiagnosis of human pulmonary dirofilariosis. Trop Med Parasitol 45:249-252, 1994.

1248. Gottstein B, Reichen J: Hydatid lung disease (echinococcosis/hydatidosis). Clin Chest Med 23:397-408, ix, 2002.

1249. Bhatia G: Echinococcus. Semin Respir Infect 12:171-186, 1997.

1250. Wilson JF, Diddams AC, Rausch RL: Cystic hydatid disease in Alaska. A review of 101 autochthonous cases of *Echinococcus granulosus* infection. Am Rev Respir Dis 98:1-15, 1968.

1251. Kilani T, El Hammami S, Horchani H, et al: Hydatid disease of the liver with thoracic involvement. World J Surg 25:40-45, 2001.

1252. McElvaney G, Müller NL, Pitman RG, et al: Clinical-radiologic-pathologic conference: A family with lung nodules discovered by radiographic survey. Can Assoc Radiol J 39:17-20, 1988.

1253. Halezeroglu S, Celik M, Uysal A, et al: Giant hydatid cysts of the lung. J Thorac Cardiovasc Surg 113:712-717, 1997.

1254. Ozdemir IA, Kalaycioglu E: Surgical treatment and complications of thoracic hydatid disease. Report of 61 cases. Eur J Respir Dis 64:217-221, 1983.

1255. McPhail JL, Arora TS: Intrathoracic hydatid disease. Dis Chest 52:772-781, 1967.

1256. Ozer Z, Cetin M, Kahraman C: Pleural involvement by hydatid cysts of the lung. Thorac Cardiovasc Surg 33:103-105, 1985.

1257. von Sinner WN: New diagnostic signs in hydatid disease; radiography, ultrasound, CT and MRI correlated to pathology. Eur J Radiol 12:150-159, 1991.

1258. von Sinner W: Radiographic, CT, and MRI spectrum of hydatid disease of the chest: Pictorial essay. Eur Radiol 3:62, 1993.

1259. von Sinner WN, Rifai A, te Strake L, et al: Magnetic resonance imaging of thoracic hydatid disease. Correlation with clinical findings, radiography, ultrasonography, CT and pathology. Acta Radiol 31:59-62, 1990.

1260. von Sinner WN, Linjawi T, Al Watban J: Mediastinal hydatid disease: Report of three cases. J Can Assoc Radiol 41:79, 1990.

1261. Sadrieh M, Dutz W, Navabpoor MS: Review of 150 cases of hydatid cyst of the lung. Dis Chest 52:662-666, 1967.

1262. Jerray M, Benzarti M, Garrouche A, et al: Hydatid disease of the lungs. Study of 386 cases. Am Rev Respir Dis 146:185-189, 1992.

1263. Nakamura-Uchiyama F, Mukae H, Nawa Y: Paragonimiasis: A Japanese perspective. Clin Chest Med 23:409-420, 2002.

1264. Velez ID, Ortega JE, Velasquez LE: Paragonimiasis: A view from Columbia. Clin Chest Med 23:421-431, ix-x, 2002.

1265. Johnson RJ, Johnson JR: Paragonimiasis in Indochinese refugees. Roentgenographic findings with clinical correlations. Am Rev Respir Dis 128:534-538, 1983.

1266. Ogakwu M, Nwokolo C: Radiological findings in pulmonary paragonimiasis as seen in Nigeria: A review based on one hundred cases. Br J Radiol 46:699-705, 1973.

1267. Im JG, Whang HY, Kim WS, et al: Pleuropulmonary paragonimiasis: Radiologic findings in 71 patients. AJR Am J Roentgenol 159:39-43, 1992.

1268. Kagawa FT: Pulmonary paragonimiasis. Semin Respir Infect 12:149-158, 1997.

1269. Romeo DP, Pollock JJ: Pulmonary paragonimiasis: Diagnostic value of pleural fluid analysis. South Med J 79:241-243, 1986.

1270. Johnson RJ, Jong EC, Dunning SB, et al: Paragonimiasis: Diagnosis and the use of praziquantel in treatment. Rev Infect Dis 7:200-206, 1985.

1271. Maleewong W, Intapan PM, Priammuenwai M, et al: Monoclonal antibodies to *Paragonimus heterotremus* and their potential for diagnosis of paragonimiasis. Am J Trop Med Hyg 56:413-417, 1997.

1272. Ikeda T, Oikawa Y, Nishiyama T: Enzyme-linked immunosorbent assay using cysteine proteinase antigens for immunodiagnosis of human paragonimiasis. Am J Trop Med Hyg 55:435-437, 1996.

1273. Schwartz E: Pulmonary schistosomiasis. Clin Chest Med 23:433-443, 2002.

1274. Morris W, Knauer CM: Cardiopulmonary manifestations of schistosomiasis. Semin Respir Infect 12:159-170, 1997.

1275. Schwartz E, Rozenman J, Perelman M: Pulmonary manifestations of early schistosome infection among nonimmune travelers. Am J Med 109:718-722, 2000.

1276. Cooke GS, Lalvani A, Gleeson FV, et al: Acute pulmonary schistosomiasis in travelers returning from Lake Malawi, sub-Saharan Africa. Clin Infect Dis 29:836-839, 1999.

1277. Cheever AW: Schistosomiasis. Infection versus disease and hypersensitivity versus immunity. Am J Pathol 142:699-702, 1993.

1278. Farid Z, Greer JW, Ishak KG, et al: Chronic pulmonary schistosomiasis. Am Rev Tuberc 79:119-133, 1959.

1279. Davidson BL, el-Kassimi F, Uz-Zaman A, et al: The "lung shift" in treated schistosomiasis. Bronchoalveolar lavage evidence of eosinophilic pneumonia. Chest 89:455-457, 1986.

1280. Abdulla MA, Hombal SM, al-Juwaiser A: Detection of *Schistosoma mansoni* in bronchoalveolar lavage fluid. A case report. Acta Cytol 43:856-858, 1999.

1281. Lunde MN, Ottesen EA: Enzyme-linked immunosorbent assay (ELISA) for detecting IgM and IgE antibodies in human schistosomiasis. Am J Trop Med Hyg 29:82-85, 1980.

1282. Kagan IG, Rairigh DW, Kaiser RL: A clinical, parasitologic, and immunologic study of schistosomiasis in 103 Puerto Rican males residing in the United States. Ann Intern Med 56:457-470, 1962.

PULMONARY NEOPLASMS

P ulmonary neoplasms are among the most common conditions encountered in respiratory medicine and enter
into the differential diagnosis of many lesions seen on
chest radiographs. Partly because of the many cell types that
exist in the normal lung and the associated range of histogenetic possibilities, there are numerous histologically defined
types of neoplasm. A variety of classification schemes have
been proposed to categorize these tumors. That proposed by
the World Health Organization (WHO) is one of the best
known and most widely used and, with minor modifications
(Table 7–1), is followed in this and subsequent chapters.[1]

PULMONARY CARCINOMA

Epidemiology

Pulmonary carcinoma is the most frequently diagnosed
"major" cancer in the world and the most common cause of
cancer-related death in both men and women in North

TABLE 7–1. Histologic Classification of Lung Tumors

Epithelial tumors
　Benign
　　Papillomas
　　Adenomas
　Preinvasive lesions
　　Squamous dysplasia/carcinoma in situ
　　Atypical adenomatous hyperplasia
　　Diffuse pulmonary neuroendocrine cell hyperplasia
　Malignant
　　Squamous cell carcinoma
　　Small cell carcinoma
　　　Combined small cell carcinoma
　　Adenocarcinoma
　　　Acinar
　　　Papillary
　　　Bronchioloalveolar carcinoma
　　　Solid adenocarcinoma with mucin
　　Large cell carcinoma
　　Adenosquamous carcinoma
　　Carcinomas with pleomorphic, sarcomatoid, or sarcomatous
　　　elements
　　Carcinoid tumor
　　　Typical carcinoid
　　　Atypical carcinoid
　　Carcinomas of salivary gland type
　　　Mucoepidermoid carcinoma
　　　Adenoid cystic carcinoma
　　Unclassifial carcinoma
Soft tissue tumors
Miscellaneous tumors
　Hamartoma
　Sclerosing hemangioma
　Clear cell tumour
　Pulmonary blastoma
Lymphoproliferative diseases
　Lymphoid interstitial pneumonia
　Nodular lymphoid hyperplasia
　Low-grade marginal-zone B-cell lymphoma of mucosa-associated
　　lymphoid tissue (MALT)
　Lymphomatoid granulomatosis
　Hodgkin's Lymphoma
Secondary tumors
Unclassified tumors

Modified from Brambilla E, Travis WD, Colby TV, et al: The new World Health
Organization classification of lung tumours. Eur Respir J 18:1059-1068, 2001.

America and worldwide.[2] In 2001, an estimated 169,500
deaths in the United States were due to pulmonary carcinoma—more than a third of all cancer deaths in men and
close to a quarter in women.[3] Because many of these individuals are between 50 and 70 years of age at the time of death,
the neoplasm is responsible for the most years of life lost of
any cancer. Among current smokers, the estimated lifetime
risk for the development of lung cancer is 17.2% in men and
11.6% in women.[4]

The incidence of the tumor has increased progressively
during the 20th century. In the United States, the overall incidence rose from 38.5 per 100,000 person-years in 1969 to 1971
to 62.6 in 1996 to 2000.[5] A variety of factors, such as ethnicity, age, gender, geographic location, and socioeconomic
status, influence the rate in specific groups. For example, the
rate in men exceeds that in women, and the rate in African
American men exceeds that in white men.[6] In the United
States, the incidence in men peaked in 1981 and declined by
1.8% per year from 1991 through 2000.[5] Death rates have
shown a similar decline, decreasing by 1.7% per year since
1991 in white men and by 2.5% per year since 1993 in black
men.[5] By contrast, the incidence rates in white and African
American women are similar and have continued to rise at a
rate of 0.7% per year since 1991.[5] Such differences are reflected
in the current proportion of cases seen in the two sexes: the
ratio of men to women was reported to be 6.8:1 in a series
reported from the Lahey Clinic in 1957 to 1960,[7] whereas it is
now about 1.5:1.[8]

As discussed later, the declining incidence rate in men and
the increasing rate in women are largely related to parallel
trends in smoking prevalence before the development of carcinoma.[9] However, factors other than tobacco smoke are likely
to be important as well. For example, although pulmonary
carcinoma develops in African Americans at an earlier age
than in white Americans,[6] the risk cannot be accounted for
entirely by differences in tobacco consumption. There is also
evidence, after controlling for the amount smoked and body
size, that women are more susceptible to the development of
pulmonary carcinoma than men.[9,10]

There are unexplained differences in the incidence of specific types of carcinoma. For example, when compared with
the 1970s, an increased proportion of adenocarcinoma has
been documented by several groups of investigators.[2] By contrast, squamous cell carcinoma has been decreasing in both
African American and white men younger than 75 years and
in white women younger than 65 years. The proportion of
cases of small cell carcinoma is higher in white than African
American men, a difference that is particularly marked in
younger individuals.[11] This difference does not seem to be
related to smoking habits or diet.[8]

The incidence of pulmonary carcinoma increases with age
among both smokers and nonsmokers, a finding more likely
related to cumulative exposure to carcinogens than to aging
itself.[12] Nonetheless, nearly 3% of pulmonary carcinomas
occur in patients younger than 40 years.[13] There is an inverse
relationship between the risk for pulmonary carcinoma and
increasing socioeconomic status.[14] Although variations in
smoking behavior probably account for a significant part of
this difference, some investigators have shown that it persists
after smoking is taken into account;[15] differences in occupational exposure to potential carcinogens also do not appear to
be involved.[16]

Etiology

Tobacco Smoke

The most important cause of pulmonary carcinoma is tobacco smoke, a statement amply demonstrated by the observation that approximately 90% of all cases in North America and Europe are the result of cigarette consumption.[2,17] The relationship between smoking and pulmonary carcinoma meets virtually all the criteria for causality as outlined by Hill in 1965, including strength of association, consistency of data, identification of a specific causative agent, and the presence of both biologic and temporal plausibility.[18]

The epidemiologic features of pulmonary carcinoma largely parallel those of tobacco use. For example, in a study in which the prevalence of cigarette smoking from 1920 to 1990 was plotted against the age-adjusted mortality rates of pulmonary carcinoma from 1930 to 1992, a strong temporal relationship was found for both men and women with an approximately 30-year latency period between smoking and the development of carcinoma.[9] By contrast, the results of a variety of retrospective and prospective studies have shown that pulmonary carcinoma occurs infrequently in nonsmokers in the general population.[19]

A clear-cut dose-response relationship between the amount of tobacco smoked and the risk for pulmonary carcinoma has been shown by many investigators.[20,21] The duration of smoking appears to be an important variable in this regard—specifically, there is evidence that smoking one pack per day for 40 years is associated with greater risk than smoking two packs per day for 20 years.[22] It has also been well established that stopping the habit or appreciably reducing the number of cigarettes smoked results in a decreased risk for pulmonary carcinoma; however, although the relative risk declines exponentially after the first year, a complete return to the incidence rates of never-smokers has not been documented.[23] It is important to note that changes in the design and composition of cigarettes over the past 50 years have not led to any benefit in public health.[2]

The risk of development of carcinoma is present even with relatively low levels of tobacco exposure. For example, men and women who smoke only one to nine cigarettes a day have a clear increase in risk in comparison to nonsmokers.[24] Moreover, there is abundant data that exposure to secondhand (environmental) smoke is also hazardous. On the basis of a review of 30 epidemiologic studies conducted worldwide, members of the U.S. Environmental Protection Agency concluded that environmental tobacco smoke is responsible for approximately 3000 pulmonary carcinoma deaths per year in lifelong nonsmoking Americans.[25] Other groups have also demonstrated a small but consistent increase in risk for pulmonary carcinoma in nonsmokers exposed to environmental tobacco smoke (usually nonsmokers whose spouses smoke) in comparison to those who are not exposed[26-29]; some have found a dose-response relationship. Even childhood exposure may be associated with an increased risk,[30] although assessment of such risk is confounded by possible inheritable risk factors.[31]

The plausibility of the association between environmental tobacco smoke and pulmonary carcinoma in nonsmokers is reinforced by the recognition that such smoke contains carcinogens[32] and that tobacco metabolites can be found in the urine and saliva of individuals exposed to environmental tobacco smoke.[33]

More than 4000 constituents of cigarette smoke have been identified; tobacco itself accounts for 2550 of these substances, with additives, pesticides, and other organic and metallic compounds accounting for the rest.[34] More than 60 are established carcinogens[35]; radioactive elements in tobacco smoke include radon, lead, bismuth, and polonium. Which of these numerous constituents or elements is responsible for the development of neoplasia has not been identified; however, it is clear from experiments in several animal species that both epithelial atypia and invasive cancer can develop from either inhalation of tobacco smoke or direct intrapulmonary inoculation of tobacco condensates. Dysplastic changes in airway epithelium can also be found in the lungs of nonsmokers who have been exposed to environmental tobacco smoke and have died of nonrespiratory disease.[36]

Other Inhaled Particulate and Chemical Substances

Exposure to a variety of inorganic particulate materials and organic chemicals is associated with an increased risk for the development of pulmonary carcinoma.[37] Such agents include asbestos, crystalline silica, polycyclic aromatic hydrocarbons (PAHs), arsenic, nickel, cadmium, chromium compounds, bis(chloromethyl)ether, chloromethyl methyl ether, mustard gas, beryllium, and vinyl chloride. The greatest risk lies in specific work environments where exposure can occur over long periods and the concentration of noxious materials can reach dangerous levels. It has been estimated that at least 10,000 to 12,000 cases of pulmonary carcinoma per year can be attributed to exposure to carcinogens in the workplace in the United States[38]; of these, more than half are related to asbestos.

Asbestos. The association between asbestos exposure and pulmonary carcinoma has been conclusively demonstrated in workers who have been involved in mining and milling of the mineral, as well as those who have had secondary contact with it in a variety of industries.[39] Several variables are important in this relationship. Amphibole fibers (crocidolite, amosite, and anthophyllite) are associated with a significantly greater risk than chrysotile fibers are.[40] The intensity and duration of asbestos exposure are also important:[41] in most series in which an increased incidence of carcinoma has been demonstrated, workers have been exposed for at least 20 years. The relationship between malignancy risk and asbestos exposure is linear[42]; although there may or may not be a threshold below which there is no risk, in practical terms, it may be impossible to prove any measurable increase in the risk for carcinoma with low-level exposure to asbestos.[43]

The increased risk of asbestos-associated pulmonary carcinoma is strongly associated with cigarette smoking, a relationship that is likely to be synergistic.[44] For example, asbestos exposure is associated with a risk of 20:1 in heavy smokers versus exposed nonsmokers and a risk as high as 100:1 for heavy smokers versus unexposed nonsmokers.[45] Exposed nonsmokers also have an increased risk for pulmonary carcinoma (albeit small in absolute numbers) when compared with unexposed nonsmokers.[46]

The elevated risk for the development of pulmonary carcinoma in asbestos-exposed individuals has also been associated with the presence of asbestosis. In fact, pleuropulmonary malignancy develops in approximately 50% of patients who have this disease[47]; this figure is particularly remarkable in light of the fact that some patients die of respiratory failure or cor pulmonale before a neoplastic complication has the opportunity to develop. Whether asbestos-exposed individuals have an increased risk for pulmonary carcinoma in the *absence* of pathologic evidence of asbestosis has been a matter of considerable debate.[48-50]

A strong argument has been made that the excess risk for pulmonary carcinoma in asbestos-exposed workers is confined to individuals who have, at a minimum, histologic evidence of asbestosis.[51] Theoretical support for such an association is provided by animal models of malignancy and fibrotic lung disease and the observation that patients who have diffuse interstitial fibrosis of other causes are at risk for the development of pulmonary carcinoma (see page 341). On the other hand, several observations suggest that the association between asbestosis and pulmonary carcinoma may be neither absolute nor causal, and it is possible that this abnormality is no more than a marker of more intense exposure to asbestos.[52] For instance, asbestos has been shown to act as both a promoter and inducer of carcinogenesis,[53,54] and there is evidence that it can reduce the immune surveillance of cancer by natural killer (NK) cells.[55] These effects argue against the necessity for asbestosis in the pathogenesis of asbestos-related pulmonary carcinoma.

Accurate information on dose, radiographic abnormalities, and smoking history is required to give a definitive answer to the asbestosis-carcinoma question; in addition, large populations are required to confirm the negative hypothesis—that those who do not have fibrosis are not at excess risk for lung cancer.[38] However, it seems reasonable to conclude that if there is an increased risk for pulmonary carcinoma in asbestos-exposed workers who do not have asbestosis *histologically*, it is small. At the same time, the hypothesis that asbestosis is a necessary prerequisite for the development of carcinoma cannot be considered to have been definitively proved. From a practical point of view, however, it is important to remember that an excess risk for pulmonary carcinoma exists in asbestos-exposed workers in the absence of *radiographic* evidence of asbestosis.[56]

The relationship between the presence of pleural plaques alone and pulmonary carcinoma has also been somewhat controversial; however, careful review of the literature has led to the conclusion that in the absence of asbestosis, there is no increase in risk for pulmonary carcinoma in patients who have plaques.[57]

Silica. In a 1996 publication, members of the International Agency for Research on Cancer (IARC) concluded that crystalline silica inhaled in the form of quartz or cristobalite from occupational sources is carcinogenic to humans.[58] Excess risk has since been reported in workers in industries unassociated with exposure to other occupational carcinogens and has been shown to be independent of cigarette smoking.[59,60] The strength of the association has been found to be much greater in workers who have silicosis than in workers who have been exposed to silica but have no evidence of the disease. The relative risk for pulmonary carcinoma among the former often exceeds 3.0 and is as high as 6.0; by contrast, the relative risk for carcinoma in the absence of silicosis is modest, being estimated at 1.3.[38] As a consequence, the conclusion of the IARC

that silica exposure in the *absence* of silicosis can cause lung cancer has been controversial.[61]

Polycyclic Aromatic Hydrocarbons. PAHs are a group of carcinogenic chemicals formed during the incomplete combustion of organic matter. Depending on the specific occupation, workers may be exposed to a variety of PAHs, such as coke oven and coal gasification fumes and soot. An increased risk for the development of pulmonary carcinoma has been demonstrated in a number of such occupations,[62,63] including aluminum, rubber, and steel production plants. Diesel exhaust is also considered a probable but not proven pulmonary carcinogen by the IARC.[64] Concern regarding possible carcinogenicity from exposure to the low level of PAHs found in the atmosphere is magnified in workers exposed to diesel fumes, such as railroad workers, taxi drivers, and dockworkers. In two meta-analyses of case-control and cohort studies in which the relationship between occupational exposure to diesel exhaust and pulmonary carcinoma was examined, evidence for an association was found even in studies in which there was adequate control for the effect of cigarette smoking[65,66]; a duration-response effect was also evident.

Radiation

Exposure to radiation may be from an external source or by inhalation of radioactive gases. The latter is related primarily to radon, a substance formed during the decay of uranium to stable lead. The radioactive decay of radon gas itself releases a number of radioactive isotopes known as radon daughters that adhere to particles suspended in air. When inhaled, they are deposited in the respiratory tract, where they are able to irradiate the surrounding tissue with alpha particles. In 1988, members of the IARC concluded that radon should be classified as a human carcinogen.[67] Studies of the risk for pulmonary carcinoma in uranium miners have shown a consistent increase when compared with nonexposed individuals, the risk being greater in association with younger age at first exposure, as well as with longer duration and intensity of exposure. The risk is greatly increased by concomitant cigarette smoking; nevertheless, exposed nonsmokers have a risk for lung cancer similar to that of nonexposed active smokers.[68] Although the incidence of all histologic types is increased, the predominant one is small cell carcinoma.[69]

Radon is also found frequently in the indoor environment of human habitations. It can be derived from water or natural gas, in which case it may enter buildings through cracks in the foundation or from building materials themselves.[70] The observation that levels of radon found in some homes—especially those that have poorly ventilated basements—approach those in mines in which an association with carcinoma has been documented has led to concern that radon may also be carcinogenic in the nonoccupational setting. This concern is supported by the results of an analysis of 11 cohort studies of radon-exposed miners in which a linear relative risk for pulmonary carcinoma was consistently found across the range of exposures, thus suggesting that even low exposure is dangerous.[71] The authors of a meta-analysis of eight case-control studies concluded that the risk from domestic radon exposure was real, albeit small (relative risk, 1.14), and that the magnitude of the risk was consistent with that predicted by extrapolation of data available from radon-exposed miners.[72]

Viral Infection

Despite the abundant evidence linking viral infection with human cancer, there is little to suggest that it is an important factor in most carcinomas of the lung. However, it is likely that the rare cases of pulmonary squamous cell carcinoma that develop in association with laryngotracheobronchial papillomas are caused by human papillomavirus (see page 374).[73] There is also an association between lymphoepithelioma-like carcinoma and Epstein-Barr virus.[74]

Pulmonary Fibrosis

The term *scar carcinoma* refers to a pulmonary carcinoma that is intimately related to a localized area of parenchymal fibrosis. Early investigators who studied this association postulated that the scars preceded the carcinoma and were pathogenetically related to its development, and the term has since come to encompass this concept. In addition to the parenchymal scarring itself, other factors have been implicated in carcinogenesis, the most important being the epithelial metaplasia and hyperplasia that are frequently present at the junction of the fibrotic and unscarred lung.[75] However, the validity of a causal relationship has been questioned, and most observers now believe that the cancer induces the fibrosis rather than the other way around.[76]

A pathogenetic association between diffuse interstitial pulmonary fibrosis and carcinoma has been more convincingly documented.[77] The former include a variety of abnormalities, such as progressive systemic sclerosis, rheumatoid disease, and idiopathic pulmonary fibrosis. In contrast to carcinoma associated with focal scars, it is often possible to be certain on clinical and radiologic grounds that the fibrosis preceded the development of carcinoma in all these diseases, thus suggesting that the fibrosis is truly pathogenic. The cellular/molecular basis for the association is unclear.[78] However, as with focal scars, epithelial metaplasia and hyperplasia are frequently present in association with the areas of fibrosis and have been shown to have high proliferative activity and, occasionally, cytologic atypia.[79] It is possible that growth factors elaborated by epithelial cells and macrophages adjacent to the fibrotic region, such as transforming growth factor-β_1, enhance tumor development in such proliferating cells.[80]

Other Lung Disease

The association of tuberculosis and carcinoma in the same area of the lung has been reported with sufficient frequency to suggest that the combination may be more than coincidental. For example, in a cytologic screening study of 800 men 40 years or older who had been admitted to an urban sanatorium, malignant cells were found in 57 (10%) of those who provided satisfactory sputum specimens[81]; in 50 of these men, follow-up examinations confirmed the diagnosis of carcinoma. Retrospective review of their chest radiographs revealed no evidence of malignancy in 25. However, although it is not possible to exclude that tuberculosis predisposes to the development of carcinoma in some patients, it is likely that it is the cancer and its attendant systemic effects that result in the appearance of the infection in the vast majority of cases.

Several investigators have shown a small increase in the risk for pulmonary carcinoma in nonsmokers who have a history of asthma or pneumonia.[82] A significantly higher incidence of pulmonary carcinoma has also been documented in smoking patients who have chronic bronchitis than in those who do not have chronic bronchitis.[83] In addition, abnormalities in lung function are associated with increased risk after correction for the amount smoked.[84] The association of impaired lung function and chronic bronchitis with pulmonary carcinoma risk seems to be robust. However, whether impaired lung function and chronic bronchitis are more accurate representations of the amount smoked (intensity, cigarette type, breath-hold) than pack-years are, whether COPD and carcinoma are related to a common susceptibility, and whether chronic mucus hypersecretion or emphysema (or both) plays a pathogenic role in pulmonary carcinoma have not been determined.

Diet

There has been a great deal of interest in the potential benefit of antioxidant vitamins, such as β-carotene (provitamin A) and α-tocopherol (vitamin E), in the prophylaxis of pulmonary carcinoma in both smokers and nonsmokers.[85] A number of investigators have shown a small but important inverse relationship between the consumption of fruits and vegetables high in vitamin content and pulmonary carcinoma, even after controlling for the amount smoked.[86] This association is supported by the results of experimental studies in animals and cell cultures.[87] Unexpectedly, two large randomized, controlled trials examining the use of these vitamins in lung cancer prevention reported a small increase in the incidence of lung cancer in the treated groups.[88] Many foods contain a variety of substances in addition to β-carotene and vitamin E that are anticarcinogens.[2,89] It is conceivable that these substances underlie the discrepancy in the results of these preventive trials. If this interpretation is correct, a high blood carotene level is best considered to be a marker of healthy intake of fruits and vegetables rather than a suppressor of carcinoma.

Genetic Factors

Although tobacco smoke and the various occupational carcinogens discussed previously are responsible for most cases of pulmonary carcinoma, it is clear that cancer develops in only a minority of individuals exposed to these agents. Such individual susceptibility may be explained, at least in part, by host-specific factors that confer sensitivity or resistance to disease. The results of a number of epidemiologic studies suggest that at least some such factors are inherited. In fact, individuals who smoke and who have a family history of pulmonary carcinoma have a 30- to 35-fold increased risk for pulmonary carcinoma when compared with nonsmokers who have no family history.[90] This and other related observations could be explained by inherited variations in the metabolism of environmental carcinogens that confer sensitivity or resistance to their effects by influencing processes such as DNA repair, cell cycle, apoptosis, and signal transduction.[91,92] It is also possible that genetic variation might influence the risk for carcinoma via an effect on smoking behavior and nicotine addiction.[93,94]

Pathogenesis

Genetic and Molecular Factors

As with cancer at other sites, pulmonary carcinoma occurs by a multistep process in which progressive accumulation of mutations leads to a loss of normal mechanisms for control of cellular growth.[94] Genes involved in DNA repair, cell growth, angiogenesis, signal transduction, and cell cycle control may all be damaged during the course of progression of carcinoma.[95] Exposure to carcinogens causes both initiating events (mutations) and tumor promotion, which results in the growth of cells containing such mutations.[96] DNA damage can result in the activation of growth-stimulating genes or the inactivation of growth-suppressing genes (oncogenes).[97] Under the influence of carcinogens, these oncogenes develop from nuclear proto-oncogenes, which are components of the normal cellular genome with important functions in non-neoplastic cellular processes.[98] Oncogenes can be either recessive or dominant.[96] For dominant oncogenes (such as *ras* and *myc*), activation of only one of the two copies of the gene results in oncogenesis; in the case of recessive oncogenes (also known as *tumor suppressor genes*), two different lesions involving both copies of the gene are required.[96] Two well-described tumor suppressor genes are the retinoblastoma gene (*Rb*) and p53.[99]

Dominant oncogenes may cause cancer by the production of functional but abnormal proteins or by the overexpression of an otherwise normal gene and its cognate receptors[94]; in both circumstances, the gene product drives cell growth in an unrestrained fashion. The loss and inactivation of the protein products of tumor suppressor genes, which normally modulate cellular proliferation and are involved in the response to and repair of DNA damage,[94] may permit the accelerated growth of neoplastic tissue.[100] Biallelic loss of function is the result of point mutations, deletions, and promoter hypermethylation.[101]

Growth factors, which are mostly the products of proto-oncogenes,[102] are a group of signaling molecules that are involved in the control of cell proliferation.[103] When secreted by tumor cells or adjacent stromal cells, they augment cell growth in an autocrine or paracrine fashion and thereby assume a promoter function for neoplastic cells. They require specific receptors and intracellular signal transduction pathways to stimulate cell division.[103] The best known of these growth factors are the autocrine polypeptide gastrin-releasing peptide/bombesin[95] (which is active in small cell carcinoma), transforming growth factor-α, and the ErbB family of transmembrane receptor tyrosine kinases (found in non–small cell carcinoma).[94]

Immunologic Factors

Cell-mediated immunity has an important role in the host response to neoplastic cells. Convincing evidence for such a role is provided by observing the consequence of deficiencies in cell-mediated immunity, such as the development of Kaposi's sarcoma and lymphoma in patients who have AIDS. Evidence that this process may also be important in the development of pulmonary carcinoma has been documented by a number of investigators.[104] However, it is not clear which, if any, of the immunologic abnormalities that have been found are related to this effect and which are simply a reaction to the carcinoma without significance from a pathogenetic point of view.

NK cells are important in the immune surveillance of tumors in general.[105] Their activity is decreased in the peripheral blood and resected lung specimens of patients who have pulmonary carcinoma.[106] However, the significance of this decreased activity is unclear because decreased numbers of

NK cells have also been described in smokers who do not have carcinoma.[107] Lymphokine-activated killer cells have a significant antitumor effect when activated by interleukin-2 in clinical trials[108]; analysis of BAL fluid has shown these cells to have lytic activity in some patients with pulmonary carcinoma,[109] thus suggesting that a variation in their number may have an effect on tumor progression in some cases.

Cytotoxic T cells are probably responsible for in vitro cytotoxicity directed against autologous tumor. Whether these lymphocytes are active against and help control carcinoma in vivo is less clear; however, their presence has significant prognostic value in patients who have had resected non–small cell carcinoma,[110] and preliminary work using expanded clones of these cells for adoptive immunotherapy suggests that they might be therapeutically useful.[111] The precise role of macrophages in the host reaction to pulmonary carcinoma is uncertain, but they are found in many tumors, and some have suggested that the effectiveness of their cytostatic function correlates positively with resectability.[112]

Most evidence suggests that humoral immunity is relatively unimportant in the pathogenesis of pulmonary carcinoma[105]; however, the presence of antibodies against a variety of tumor antigens has been associated with a favorable prognosis in small cell carcinoma.[113]

Pathologic Characteristics

The WHO classification (see Table 7–1) subdivides pulmonary carcinoma into nine categories. The first five account for more than 95% of all malignant epithelial tumors and consist of squamous cell carcinoma (approximately 30% to 35% of cases), small cell carcinoma (10% to 15%), adenocarcinoma (40% to 45%), large cell carcinoma (10%), and adenosquamous carcinoma (1% to 2%).

Most studies of interobserver and intraobserver agreement have shown a high degree of reproducibility in the diagnosis of small cell carcinoma and well-differentiated forms of squamous cell carcinoma and adenocarcinoma[114,115]; however, that for poorly differentiated tumors and for large cell carcinoma is considerably worse, with values ranging from 20% to 40% in some studies.[116] Nonetheless, the distinction between small cell and non–small cell tumors can be made reliably in the vast majority of cases.[117]

The WHO classification recognizes the possibility of different degrees and types of differentiation in any particular tumor, and the portion that is most "highly differentiated" is the one that defines the specific categorization. Although this guideline is certainly practical, it is clear that such a "final" diagnosis depends, in part, on the amount of tissue examined. This proviso is particularly relevant when only small tissue fragments are available for examination, such as those obtained by endoscopy or transthoracic needle biopsy.[118] For example, in a study of 107 pulmonary carcinomas diagnosed initially by fiberoptic bronchoscopy, 41 (38%) were given a different diagnosis on subsequent examination of tissue in lymph nodes or excised lung.[119]

Squamous Cell Carcinoma

This tumor originates most frequently in segmental or lobar bronchi. Early lesions, which consist of carcinoma in situ or minimally invasive carcinoma, may be grossly undetectable or may be recognized as a white, plaquelike swelling or a fine granularity of the bronchial mucosa.[120] More advanced carcinomas characteristically appear as polypoid or papillary tumors within the bronchial lumen (see Color Fig. 7–1). Because of this, airway obstruction is almost invariable, and distal atelectasis, bronchiectasis, and obstructive pneumonitis are present to some degree in most surgically resected tumors (see Color Fig. 7–2). In large neoplasms, necrosis is frequent and may be extensive; drainage of necrotic material leads to cavitation in many cases.

Histologically, squamous cell carcinoma is defined by the presence of intercellular bridges and/or keratinization (see Color Fig. 7–3). The tumors vary from well-differentiated forms that show obvious and abundant keratinization to poorly differentiated forms that may be difficult to distinguish with confidence from small or large cell carcinoma.

Small Cell Carcinoma

This form is typically found in relation to the proximal airways, particularly the lobar and main bronchi (see Color Fig. 7–4).[121] In the early stages, it appears as a poorly delimited tumor located predominantly in the submucosa and peribronchovascular connective tissue. With growth, it becomes a poorly circumscribed mass that obliterates the underlying airways and vessels. The endobronchial extension that is characteristic of squamous cell carcinoma is uncommon; when airway obstruction does occur, it is usually a result of compression by the expanding tumor rather than intraluminal obstruction. Invasion of small blood vessels and lymphatics is evident in most tumors at an early stage, and local lymphangitic spread is not uncommon in the adjacent lung. In addition, regional bronchopulmonary and hilar lymph nodes are almost invariably enlarged as a result of metastatic or invasive carcinoma (see Color Fig. 7–4).

Histologically, the tumor consists of cells approximately two to three times the size of a mature lymphocyte. Cytoplasm is scanty, a feature that is often reflected in molding of adjacent cell nuclei (see Color Fig. 7–3). The latter may be small and hyperchromatic (corresponding to the oat cell pattern of previous histologic classifications) or somewhat vesicular with finely stippled and dispersed chromatin. Artifactual tumor crushing is common, especially in tissue obtained by endoscopic biopsy; although diagnosis can be difficult in this circumstance, the presence of areas of crushed, hyperchromatic cells is in itself suggestive of small cell carcinoma,[122] and examination of multiple tissue sections almost invariably reveals one or more clusters that are sufficiently preserved to provide a definitive diagnosis.

Minute foci of glandular or squamous differentiation or undifferentiated (large cell) carcinoma may be identified in some tumors, a finding that does not alter the classification. Occasionally, such foci account for a significant proportion of the tumor, in which case it is classified as *combined small cell carcinoma*.[123] Although a number of investigators have found these combined tumors to have the same natural history as that of histologically "pure" small cell tumors, some have found the prognosis to be better[115] and others worse.[124]

A number of observations indicate that small cell carcinoma has neuroendocrine differentiation, including the ultrastructural demonstration of neurosecretory granules and the presence of positive immunohistochemical reactions to a variety of neuropeptides.[125,126] A variety of such neuropeptides have been identified, including gastrin-releasing peptide (bombesin), vasoactive intestinal polypeptide, serotonin, and adrenocorticotropic hormone (ACTH).[127]

Adenocarcinoma

Adenocarcinoma is a neoplasm of variable histologic appearance that has been subdivided into a number of subtypes, including acinar carcinoma, papillary carcinoma, solid carcinoma with mucin formation, and bronchioloalveolar carcinoma. Although the histologic patterns corresponding to these subgroups are usually easily identifiable, the distinctiveness of the subgroups themselves is open to question for several reasons.[128,129] In fact, many investigators consider the most useful division to be into two types—bronchioloalveolar carcinoma and nonbronchioloalveolar carcinoma.

The majority of pulmonary adenocarcinomas appear as nodules located in the periphery of the lung, frequently in a subpleural location.[128] They are often well circumscribed, although a spiculated or ill-defined appearance is grossly evident in some tumors. Focal fibrosis is frequently present in the central portion of the tumor and imparts a puckered appearance to the overlying pleura. Adenocarcinoma that arises in relation to a major airway is uncommon[128]; when it does occur in this location, it is grossly indistinguishable from squamous cell carcinoma. Tumors that show a pure or predominant bronchioloalveolar pattern histologically may also be manifested as a solitary nodule (see Color Fig. 7–5) or (less commonly) as a poorly defined area of parenchymal consolidation (see Color Fig. 7–6).[130] They can be recognized grossly by their characteristic nondestructive growth; underlying structures such as airways and interlobular septa are readily identified despite being surrounded by tumor.

As indicated, the histologic pattern of nonbronchioloalveolar carcinoma is variable and consists of acini or tubules (with or without intraluminal mucin formation, see Color Fig. 7–3), papillary structures, or sheets of cells without structural evidence of glandular differentiation. The latter can be distinguished from large cell carcinoma only by the presence of intracellular mucin in a significant proportion of tumor cells.[131]

Histologically, a bronchioloalveolar growth pattern is characterized by tumor cell spread along the framework of the lung parenchyma without its destruction (see Color Fig. 7–7). The alveolar interstitium adjacent to the tumor may be virtually normal, but it is commonly thickened by a combination of fibrous tissue and a chronic inflammatory infiltrate.[132] Intra-alveolar secretions derived from the tumor cells may be absent or may be so abundant that they form the major proportion of the tumor's volume and fill air spaces a considerable distance from the tumor cells. Such secretions may consist of proteinaceous material or (more commonly) mucus.

Careful examination of the lung parenchyma at a distance from a resected adenocarcinoma (either bronchioloalveolar or nonbronchioloalveolar in type) may show small (1- to 5-mm), variably shaped gray nodules.[133] Histologically, these nodules correspond to foci of alveolar epithelial proliferation, usually associated with a mild degree of interstitial fibrosis (Fig. 7–1).[134] The epithelial cells resemble alveolar type II cells and may have uniform nuclei or show varying degrees of atypia;

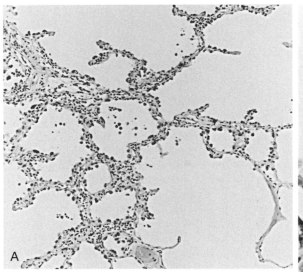
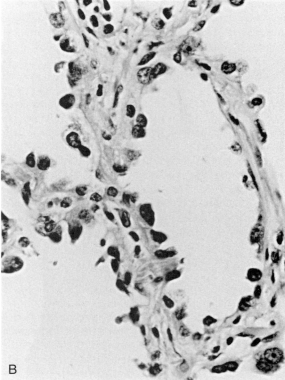

FIGURE 7–1

Alveolar epithelial hyperplasia. A focus of lung parenchyma (**A**) shows a moderate degree of interstitial fibrosis associated with type II cell hyperplasia. A magnified view (**B**) shows a moderate degree of nuclear atypia (atypical hyperplasia). The patient had a 2.5-cm bronchioloalveolar carcinoma in the resected lobe. *(From Fraser RS, Miller NL, Colman NC, Paré PD: Fraser and Paré's Diagnosis of Diseases of the Chest, 4th ed. Philadelphia, WB Saunders, 1999.)*

in some cases, the latter may be so marked that distinction from bronchioloalveolar carcinoma is not possible. This observation, as well as the results of DNA ploidy analysis and molecular biologic studies, strongly suggests that these foci are the result of hyperplasia and dysplasia and are analogous to the squamous metaplasia and dysplasia that occur in bronchi in association with squamous cell carcinoma.[135,136]

Large Cell Carcinoma

A diagnosis of large cell carcinoma is applied to tumors that do not possess the typical appearance of small cell carcinoma and have no evidence at the light microscopic level of either squamous or glandular differentiation. Grossly, they tend to be bulky tumors located in the peripheral parenchyma (see Color Fig. 7–8).[137] Although multiple foci of necrosis are characteristic, cavitation is uncommon. Histologically, the tumors consist of sheets of cells that usually contain abundant eosinophilic cytoplasm (see Color Fig. 7–3). Nuclei are large and often vesicular with prominent nucleoli.

The WHO classification consists of a number of histologic subtypes, including large cell neuroendocrine carcinoma, basaloid carcinoma, lymphoepithelioma-like carcinoma, and clear cell carcinoma. *Clear cell carcinoma* is composed of nests or sheets of large cells that have ample, somewhat foamy or clear cytoplasm; mucin stains are negative, and the cleared appearance is believed to be caused by abundant intracytoplasmic glycogen.[138] The tumor must be differentiated from metastatic renal cell carcinoma, whose histologic appearance may be similar. *Lymphoepithelioma-like carcinoma* is histologically similar to its counterpart in the nasopharynx and consists of single cells or small nests of

cells that have fairly uniform vesicular nuclei and small to moderate-sized nucleoli.[139] Numerous lymphocytes characteristically surround and infiltrate the cell nests, in some cases simulating an inflammatory lesion. As mentioned previously, there is a strong association with Epstein-Barr virus.[139]

Adenosquamous Carcinoma

As the term suggests, this histologic variant is seen in tumors that show both squamous and glandular differentiation (see Color Fig. 7–9). Its incidence varies greatly in reported series, depending on the histologic criteria used for diagnosis and whether electron microscopy is used for classification. If ultrastructural findings are used in typing, the incidence in some series is as high as 45% of all pulmonary carcinomas.[140] If only light microscopy is used, however, the number of cases is substantially less, ranging from 0.4% to 4.0%.[140a] The diagnosis also depends on the amount of squamous and glandular components within a tumor; a figure of 10% is required in the WHO classification.

Many adenosquamous carcinomas arise in the periphery of the lung and are grossly indistinguishable from large cell carcinoma or adenocarcinoma.[140a] In addition to areas of glandular and squamous differentiation, many show foci of undifferentiated (large cell) carcinoma.

Carcinomas with Pleomorphic, Sarcomatoid, or Sarcomatous Elements

This category includes a variety of tumors histologically characterized by a combination of epithelial and mesenchymal (or mesenchymal-like) elements. As the heading suggests, a number of terms have been used to describe these tumors, which has resulted in some confusion in published reports regarding their exact nature and has made comparisons between such reports difficult. The term *pleomorphic carcinoma* has been used to describe tumors that contain malignant spindle cells, giant cells, or both in association with squamous cell carcinoma, adenocarcinoma, or large cell carcinoma (Fig. 7–2A).[141] Ultrastructural or immunohistochemical features of epithelial differentiation can often be found in the spindle cells in some areas,[142,143] thus indicating that many, if not all, of these tumors represent poorly differentiated epithelial neoplasms that have a variable histologic pattern. The exceptional tumor that is composed only of spindle cells but has evidence of epithelial differentiation on immunohistochemical or ultrastructural examination has been termed *spindle cell carcinoma*.[144]

A carcinosarcoma can be defined as a neoplasm composed of an admixture of histologically malignant epithelial and mesenchymal tissues in which the latter have features of specific differentiation (such as bone, cartilage, or muscle) (Fig. 7–2B).[145] Some investigators believe that pleomorphic carcinoma and carcinosarcoma as defined here represent a spectrum of mesenchymal differentiation in pulmonary carcinoma rather than two separate entities and have advocated the use of terms such as pulmonary carcinoma with sarcoma-like lesions or sarcomatoid carcinoma, monophasic and biphasic types, to refer to both abnormalities.[142,146]

Grossly, pleomorphic carcinoma and carcinosarcoma can be manifested as a predominantly polypoid intrabronchial tumor (Fig. 7–3), with or without extension into contiguous parenchyma, or as a bulky peripheral mass without an obvious airway association. Histologically, the epithelial component is usually squamous cell carcinoma. In carcinosarcomas, the mesenchymal component is generally composed of a combination of spindle cells without obvious differentiation and malignant cartilaginous, muscular, or osteoid tissue.

Giant cell carcinoma is also considered to be part of this conglomeration of poorly differentiated neoplasms.[144] As with some other tumors, separation of this carcinoma into a specific histologic category is somewhat arbitrary, and it probably represents one end of a continuum of tumor morphology.[147] As the name suggest, this tumor is composed of sheets of cells similar to those of large cell carcinoma and numerous intermingled multinucleated giant cells; the cytoplasm of the latter cells characteristically contains polymorphonuclear leukocytes.

Radiologic Manifestations

The radiographic manifestations of pulmonary carcinoma are related to its size and anatomic location, particularly with respect to its association with an airway. Tumors have a relative frequency of 3:2 in the right versus the left lung and the upper versus the lower lobe.[148] Most squamous cell and small cell carcinomas are centrally located.[149] By contrast, adenocarcinoma occurs as an isolated peripheral lesion in approximately 50% of cases and as a peripheral lesion associated with hilar lymph node enlargement in the majority of the remainder.[149,150] Most tumors that arise in the conducting airways are situated in lobar or segmental bronchi.[151] Approximately 5% of carcinomas arise in the extreme apex of the upper lobes (Pancoast tumor).[149]

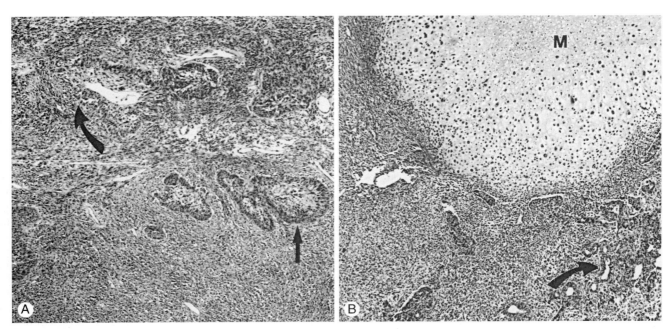

FIGURE 7–2

Pleomorphic carcinoma and carcinosarcoma. Nests of moderately differentiated squamous cell carcinoma (**A,** *short arrow*) are separated by a poorly differentiated neoplasm that has a sarcomatous appearance; there is no evidence of specific differentiation in the latter tumor. The two patterns blend imperceptibly into one another (*curved arrow*). The appearance has been designated *pleomorphic carcinoma.* In **B,** there is a mixture of adenocarcinoma (*arrow*), anaplastic neoplasm, and malignant cartilage (M), a histologic appearance designated *carcinosarcoma.* (*From Fraser RS, Müller NL, Colman NC, Paré PD: Fraser and Paré's Diagnosis of Diseases of the Chest, 4th ed. Philadelphia, WB Saunders, 1999.*)

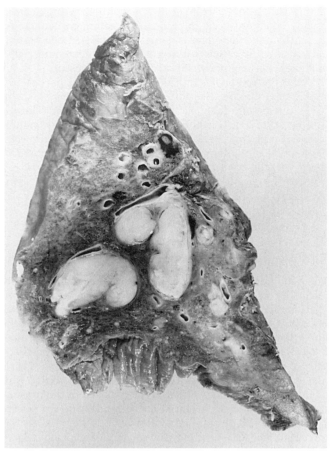

FIGURE 7–3

Pulmonary carcinosarcoma. A resected lower lobe shows a tumor almost entirely within the lumen of segmental airways. Histologic examination showed adenocarcinoma and chondrosarcoma admixed with anaplastic neoplasm. *(From Fraser RS, Müller NL, Colman NC, Paré PD: Fraser and Paré's Diagnosis of Diseases of the Chest, 4th ed. Philadelphia, WB Saunders, 1999.)*

As might be expected, the most common radiologic manifestations occur in the lungs and consist of atelectasis/obstructive pneumonitis, a solitary nodule or mass, air space consolidation, and hilar enlargement. Additional findings are seen in the mediastinum, pleura, and chest wall in some cases.

Atelectasis and Obstructive Pneumonitis

The earliest manifestation of tumors that arise in the proximal airways is frequently the result of airway obstruction rather than the tumors themselves. In fact, radiographic findings secondary to airway obstruction are present in approximately 40% of patients at initial evaluation.[149] The most frequent of these findings are related to a combination of atelectasis, bronchiectasis with mucous plugging, and consolidation. The atelectasis is usually segmental or lobar (Fig. 7–4); occasionally, an entire lung is affected. Because the airway obstruction is usually complete, air cannot pass distally, and an air bronchogram is absent; this finding is virtually pathognomonic of an obstructing endobronchial lesion and is of utmost importance in diagnosis. Parenchymal

consolidation correlates histologically with filling of alveolar air spaces by proteinaceous fluid and lipid-laden macrophages (obstructive pneumonitis). Bronchi distal to the obstruction are often somewhat dilated and filled with mucus or pus, although this feature cannot be appreciated radiographically in most cases because of surrounding parenchymal consolidation. Occasionally, a tumor is identified as a focal convexity, whereas the interlobar fissure is concave distally as a result of atelectasis, an S-shaped configuration known as *Golden's S sign* (see Fig. 7–4).[152]

Although the obstructing tumor is not often apparent on the radiograph, it can usually be seen on CT: after an intravenous bolus of contrast material, pulmonary carcinoma enhances only slightly on CT, whereas the atelectatic lung shows considerable enhancement.[153] Distinction of carcinoma from postobstructive atelectasis can also be achieved with MR imaging (Fig. 7–5).[154]

Solitary Pulmonary Nodule

There is wide variation in the criteria for designating a radiologic opacity a solitary nodule, with resultant differences in reported radiologic features and prognostic implications. The shape is usually described as round or oval. Although the defined size has varied from 1 to 6 cm in diameter, it is customary today to restrict the maximum diameter to 3 cm,[155] with larger lesions being identified as masses.

Approximately 40% of solitary nodules are malignant.[155] By using clinical and radiographic findings (Table 7–2), the distinction between benign and malignant lesions can often be established with a reasonable degree of confidence, thereby assisting in the decision regarding whether surgical intervention is warranted. For the purpose of this differential diagnosis, it is useful to divide nodules into two categories: (1) those that are clearly benign, as determined by rigidly defined radiologic signs,[156,157] and (2) those of indeterminate nature, which represent all other lesions. According to this concept, a *benign/indeterminate* categorization replaces the more traditional *benign/malignant* distinction. The main rationale for this separation is that the criteria of benignity are more certain than the radiologic signs of malignancy. The four most useful signs in assessing a solitary pulmonary nodule in everyday practice are size and change in size, calcification, and character of the tumor-lung interface. Assessment of nodule enhancement by CT or positron emission tomography (PET) holds promise of greater value in the future.

Size. The likelihood ratio for malignancy of solitary nodules has been estimated to be approximately 0.5 for nodules less than 1 cm in diameter, 0.75 for those between 1.1 and 2 cm, 3.5 for those 2.1 to 3 cm, and 5 for those greater than 3 cm.[158] When interpreting these figures, it is important to remember that the likelihood of carcinoma is influenced strongly by other factors such as age and smoking history.

Change in Size. Since uncontrolled growth is a characteristic feature of cancer, an increase in the size of a pulmonary nodule should clearly cause concern, whereas absence of such a change is comforting. However, because some benign lesions such as hamartoma and histoplasmoma can enlarge and because some bronchioloalveolar carcinomas grow slowly,[159,160] an increase in the size of a nodule by itself should not be the sole consideration governing the therapeutic approach. Nonetheless, we and others believe that a 2-year

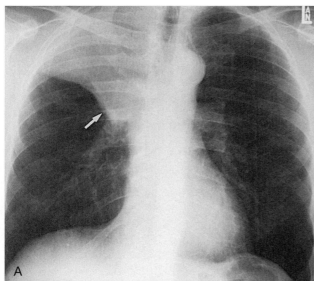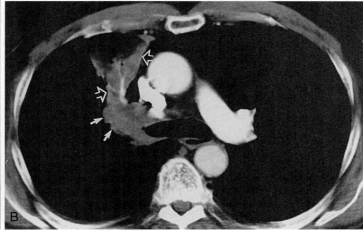

FIGURE 7–4

S sign of Golden. An anteroposterior chest radiograph (**A**) in a 67-year-old man demonstrates atelectasis and obstructive pneumonitis of the right upper lobe. The focal convexity in the hilar region (*arrow*), which indicates the location of the tumor, and the concave appearance of the interlobar fissure distally as a result of atelectasis give a configuration that resembles an S (the S sign of Golden). A contrast-enhanced CT scan (**B**) demonstrates the central tumor (*straight arrows*) and the atelectatic right upper lobe (*open arrows*). Biopsy showed squamous cell carcinoma. *(From Fraser RS, Müller NL, Colman NC, Paré PD: Fraser and Paré's Diagnosis of Diseases of the Chest, 4th ed. Philadelphia, WB Saunders, 1999.)*

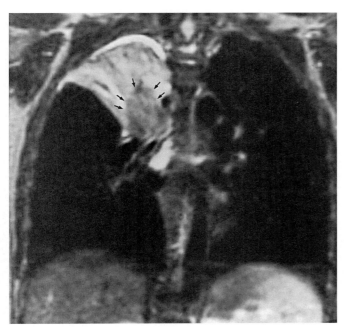

FIGURE 7–5

Obstructive pneumonitis and atelectasis. A coronal spin-echo T2-weighted MR image (TR/TE 2400/120) shows right upper lobe atelectasis and obstructive pneumonitis. The obstructing pulmonary carcinoma (*arrows*) has relatively low signal intensity in comparison to the consolidated lung. *(From Fraser RS, Müller NL, Colman NC, Paré PD: Fraser and Paré's Diagnosis of Diseases of the Chest, 4th ed. Philadelphia, WB Saunders, 1999.)*

stability in size can be considered a reasonably reliable criterion of benignity.[161,162] It should be noted, however, that the validity of this statement has been questioned,[163] particularly with respect to small nodules in which a slight change in size may be difficult to appreciate, and patients who have such nodules should continue to be monitored.

Use of the doubling time* provides a more accurate assessment of the nature of a solitary nodule than does a simple increase in size. The process requires at least two serial chest radiographs showing a roughly spherical lesion whose diameter can be averaged from measurements in at least two planes.[164] In a study of 218 pulmonary nodules (177 malignant and 41 benign), virtually all those whose doubling time was 7 days or less or 465 days or more were benign.[161] A pulmonary nodule whose rate of growth falls between these limits must be considered malignant. Perhaps the most useful application of the growth rate principle in assessing solitary nodules is in patients older than 40 years, in whom the incidence of malignancy increases markedly. In one study of individuals in this age group, almost every solitary nodule whose doubling time was less than 37 days was benign;[161] of 72 malignant nodules, the slowest-growing nodules doubled their volume in 200 days. Other investigators have quoted only slightly different figures.[164,165]

Calcification. The presence or absence of calcium is the most important feature that distinguishes benign from

---

*Doubling refers to volume, not diameter. Assuming a nodule to be spherical, its diameter must be multiplied by 1.25 to obtain the diameter of a sphere whose volume is double (e.g., the volume of a nodule 2 cm in diameter is doubled by the time its diameter reaches 2.5 cm). A doubling of diameter represents an eightfold increase in volume.

TABLE 7–2. Clinical and Radiologic Criteria in the Differentiation of Benign and Malignant Solitary Pulmonary Nodules

	Benign	Malignant
Clinical		
Age	<35 years. Exception is hamartoma	>35 years
Symptoms	Absent	Present
Past history and functional enquiry	High incidence of granuloma in area. Exposure to tuberculosis. Nonsmoker	Diagnosis of primary lesion elsewhere. Smoker. Exposure to carcinogens
Radiographic		
Size	Small (<3 cm in diameter)	Large (>3 cm in diameter)
Location	No predilection except for tuberculosis (upper lobes)	Predominantly upper lobes except for lung metastases
Contour	Margins smooth	Margins spiculated
Calcification	Almost pathognomonic of a benign lesion if laminated, diffuse, or central	Rare, may be eccentric (engulfed granuloma)
Satellite lesions	More common	Less common
Serial studies showing no change over 2 years	Almost diagnostic of benign lesion	Most unlikely
Doubling time	<30 or >490 days	Between these extremes
Computed Tomography		
Calcification	Diffuse or central	Absent or eccentric
Fat	Virtually diagnostic of hamartoma	Absent
Bubble-like lucencies	Uncommon	Common in adenocarcinomas
Enhancement with intravenous contrast material	<15 HU	>25 HU

From Fraser RS, Müller NL, Colman NC, Paré PD: Fraser and Paré's Diagnosis of Diseases of the Chest, 4th ed. Philadelphia, WB Saunders, 1999.

malignant nodules.[166,167] The identification of diffuse, laminated, or central calcification is almost certain evidence of benignity; only rare tumors that have these features prove to be malignant.[156,166] By contrast, the presence of an *eccentric* calcific opacity in a nodule or mass may represent incorporation of a calcified granuloma within the substance of a carcinoma and must be interpreted with caution.

Although calcification can be seen on thin-section CT in about 5% to 10% of pulmonary carcinomas, it usually affects tumors larger than 3 cm in diameter and is not evident on the radiograph.[168] Optimal assessment by CT requires the use of a series of thin sections (1- to 3-mm collimation) through the nodule.[169] Foci of calcification that are visible on thin-section CT usually have attenuation values of 400 Hounsfield units (HU) or higher[170]; in the absence of such foci, attenuation values of 200 HU or higher can be considered to represent calcification.

Character of the Nodule-Lung Interface. The interface between a solitary pulmonary nodule and the adjacent lung can be spiculated or smooth (Fig. 7–6). The spiculated appearance is suggestive of malignancy; for example, in a study of 283 tumors, 184 (65%) had focal or diffuse spiculation of their margins, 91 (32%) had smooth but lobulated margins, and only 8 (3%) had smooth nonlobulated margins.[166] In a review of the literature published in 1993, it was concluded that the likelihood ratio for malignancy of a nodule that has irregular or spiculated margins is approximately 5.5[158]; the corresponding figures for lobulated and smoothly marginated nodules are about 0.75 and 0.30. Radiologic-pathologic correlation has shown that spiculation may reflect the presence of fibrosis in the surrounding parenchyma, direct infiltration of carcinoma into the adjacent parenchyma, or localized lymphangitic spread.[171]

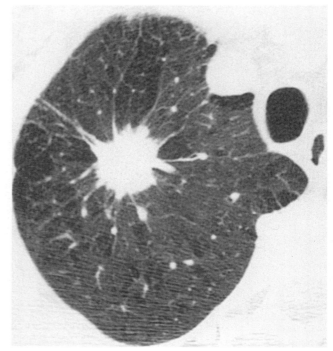

FIGURE 7–6

Pulmonary adenocarcinoma with spiculated margins. An HRCT scan in a 62-year-old man demonstrates a 2.5-cm-diameter nodule in the right upper lobe. The nodule has multiple spicules radiating from the lesion into the surrounding parenchyma (corona radiata). *(From Fraser RS, Müller NL, Colman NC, Paré PD: Fraser and Paré's Diagnosis of Diseases of the Chest, 4th ed. Philadelphia, WB Saunders, 1999.)*

The tail sign (pleural tag) consists of a linear opacity that extends from a peripheral nodule or mass to the visceral pleura. The tag can represent fibrous tissue that extends from the nodule to the visceral pleura or can result from inward retraction and apposition of a thickened visceral pleura.[171] As the visceral pleura invaginates, a small quantity of extrapleural fat is drawn into the area, thereby creating the opacity.[172] Pleural tags have been reported on thin-section CT scan in 60% to 80% of peripheral pulmonary carcinomas[171,173]; however, they can also be seen in association with metastases and granulomas, and the sign is therefore of limited value in differential diagnosis.[174,175]

Air Bronchogram. On thin-section CT scan, air bronchograms and air bronchiolograms are seen more commonly in pulmonary carcinomas than in benign nodules (Fig. 7–7).[176] For example, in a review of 132 patients, they were identified in 33 (29%) of 115 carcinomas and in only 1 (6%) of 17 benign nodules.[177] The patent airways are frequently tortuous and ectatic.[177] When cut in cross section, they are seen as focal air collections, usually measuring 5 mm or less in diameter, a finding commonly referred to as bubble-like lucency or pseudocavitation.[178] As might be expected,

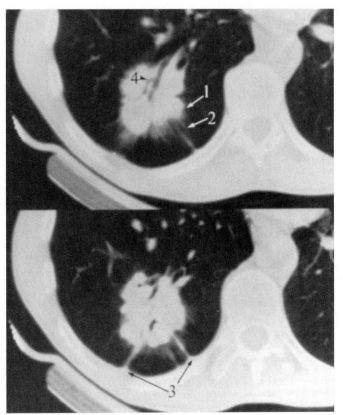

FIGURE 7–7

Air bronchogram in bronchioloalveolar carcinoma. CT scans through a right lower lobe tumor show several signs that strongly favor malignancy: marginal nodulation (1), fine spiculations (2), and pleural retraction (3). An air bronchogram (4) with narrowed, amputated airways suggests a diagnosis of bronchioloalveolar carcinoma, which was proved after surgical excision. The patient was a 55-year-old woman. (*From Fraser RS, Müller NL, Colman NC, Paré PD: Fraser and Paré's Diagnosis of Diseases of the Chest, 4th ed. Philadelphia, WB Saunders, 1999.*)

these lucencies are most common in bronchioloalveolar carcinoma.[171]

Nodule Enhancement—Computed Tomography. The potential usefulness of measuring nodule enhancement on thin-section CT scan as a means of distinguishing between benign and malignant nodules has been investigated by several groups.[179,180] The results of these studies indicate that lack of enhancement or enhancement less than 15 HU after the intravenous administration of contrast material is virtually diagnostic of a benign lesion. For example, in a prospective multicenter study of 356 nodules (185 benign and 171 malignant) in which 15 HU was used as a threshold for a positive test result, the sensitivity was 98% and the specificity was 58% in excluding malignancy.[181] From a practical point of view, the greatest value of the procedure is in providing support for conservative follow-up of noncalcified lesions that are considered likely to be benign. Because of the number of false-positive examinations, the presence of contrast enhancement is less helpful in diagnosis. It should be remembered that the results of these studies are applicable only to nodules that measure 6 to 30 mm in diameter and have homogeneous attenuation. In addition, the technique requires meticulous attention to detail.

Nodule Enhancement—Positron Emission Tomography. The use of PET after the intravenous administration of 2-(^{18}F)-fluoro-2-deoxy-D-glucose (^{18}FDG)* in distinguishing benign from malignant lung nodules has also been investigated by a number of groups (Fig. 7–8).[182,183] A comprehensive meta-analysis of studies published before 2001 indicated that the procedure had a sensitivity of 97% and specificity of 78% in the diagnosis of malignancy in nodules 10 mm or larger.[184] Because the probability of malignancy is less than 5% in patients who have negative scans, most can be monitored radiologically.[185] False-negative FDG-PET studies can be seen with carcinoid tumor, bronchioloalveolar carcinoma, and pulmonary carcinoma measuring less than 10 mm in diameter.[184] False-positive scans can occur with inflammatory conditions such as tuberculosis, histoplasmosis, and rheumatoid nodules. The main disadvantages of the technique are limited availability and high cost.

Solitary Pulmonary Mass

As discussed previously, the division of solitary opacities within the lung into nodules (measuring ≤3 cm in diameter) and masses (measuring >3 cm in diameter) serves one useful purpose—a mass is much more likely than a nodule to be malignant. Calcification in a mass does not exclude malignancy as it does in the case of a solitary nodule. For example, in a study of 353 carcinomas, 20 (6%) had calcification evident on CT scan[186]; 17 of the 20 containing calcification (85%) were larger than 3 cm in diameter. The calcification in these tumors may be punctate, chunky, or amorphous in appearance and central, peripheral, or diffuse in distribution (Fig. 7–9).[168] It is related to psammoma bodies, dystrophic calcification of necrotic carcinoma, or incorporation of a

---

*^{18}FDG is a glucose analogue labeled with a positron emitter,[18]F; it is transported through the cell membrane and phosphorylated through normal glycolytic pathways, after which it is not metabolized further and remains within the cell.

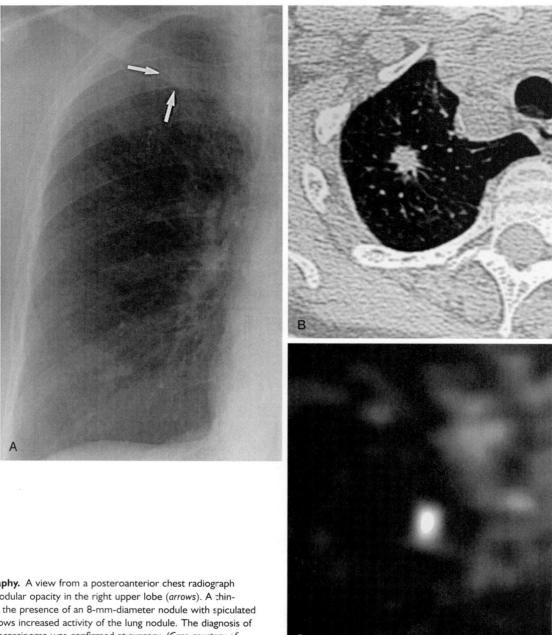

FIGURE 7–8

Positron emission tomography. A view from a posteroanterior chest radiograph
(**A**) shows a poorly defined nodular opacity in the right upper lobe (*arrows*). A thin-
section CT scan (**B**) confirms the presence of an 8-mm-diameter nodule with spiculated
margins. A PET image (**C**) shows increased activity of the lung nodule. The diagnosis of
stage I right upper lobe adenocarcinoma was confirmed at surgery. (*Case courtesy of
Dr. Ned Patz, Duke University Medical Center, Durham, NC.*)

focus of previous granulomatous inflammation or calcified
bronchial cartilage within the tumor.[168,187]

The incidence of cavitation in pulmonary carcinoma is
about 10%.[188] Although the complication can occur in tumors
of any size, most are larger than 3 cm in diameter.[189] The most
common histologic type is squamous cell carcinoma; in a
review of the radiographic findings in 600 cases, it was seen
in 22% of 263 squamous cell carcinomas, 6% of 97 large cell
carcinomas, 2% of 126 adenocarcinomas, and none of 114
small cell carcinomas.[188] Most cavities have an irregular inner
surface as a result of variably sized nodules of neoplastic tissue
projecting into the cavity and the patchy nature of necrosis

within most tumors (Fig. 7–10). The cavities may be central
or eccentric and 1 to 10 cm in diameter.

Air Space (Pneumonic) Pattern

This manifestation is restricted almost entirely to bronchioloalveolar carcinoma (Fig. 7–11). The changes may be local
or disseminated widely, the former predominating in 60% to
90% of cases.[178,190] Radiographic findings range from a hazy
increase in density (ground-glass pattern) to dense consolidation and may be seen in isolation or in conjunction with single
or multiple nodules.[190,191] In some patients in whom the

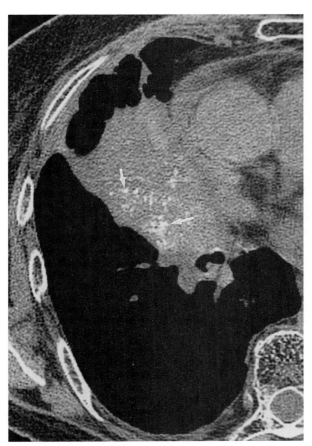

FIGURE 7–9

Calcification in pulmonary adenoarcinoma. An HRCT scan in a 70-year-old woman demonstrates a large mass in the right middle lobe containing numerous small speckled areas of calcification (*arrows*). *(From Fraser RS, Müller NL, Colman NC, Paré PD: Fraser and Paré's Diagnosis of Diseases of the Chest, 4th ed. Philadelphia, WB Saunders, 1999.)*

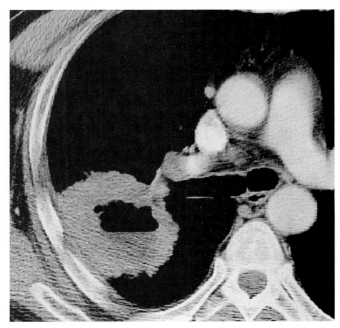

FIGURE 7–10

Cavitary squamous cell carcinoma. A view of the right lung from a contrast-enhanced CT scan in a 56-year-old man shows a 5-cm-diameter cavitated mass in the right upper lobe. The cavity has thick walls and a nodular inner contour characteristic of carcinoma. An air-fluid level within the tumor and right hilar lymphadenopathy are also evident. *(From Fraser RS, Müller NL, Colman NC, Paré PD: Fraser and Paré's Diagnosis of Diseases of the Chest, 4th ed. Philadelphia, WB Saunders, 1999.)*

disease appears to be localized, additional foci can be seen elsewhere in the lungs on CT.[192] In others, an increase in size of the initial tumor is associated with widespread dissemination on radiographs.

CT findings include areas of ground-glass opacity or consolidation as a result of the characteristic nondestructive growth of carcinoma on alveolar septa, the presence of secretions in adjacent air spaces, or both. The abnormalities can be focal (measuring less than 1 cm to several centimeters in diameter [Fig. 7–12]), patchy, or nonsegmental[178,193]; lobar consolidation can occur and may be associated with volume loss or lobar expansion. Air bronchograms or bronchiolograms and bubble-like lucencies are seen in 50% to 80% of cases.[171,194] After intravenous administration of contrast material, clear distinction of pulmonary vessels from the relatively low attenuation of the surrounding parenchyma is often present, a finding known as the *CT angiogram sign*.[195] Though characteristic of bronchioloalveolar carcinoma, the sign can also be seen in a variety of other conditions, including lymphoma, lipid pneumonia, bacterial pneumonia, infarction, and edema.[196,197] It can be considered suggestive of bronchioloalveolar carcinoma only if the mean attenuation of the consolidated lung is less than that of the chest wall musculature.[197]

Hilar Enlargement

Unilateral hilar enlargement can be the sole radiographic manifestation of pulmonary carcinoma.[149] It may represent a primary carcinoma that has arisen in a main or lobar bronchus or, more commonly, enlarged bronchopulmonary or hilar lymph nodes that are the site of direct invasion or metastasis from a small primary lesion in the adjacent bronchus or peripheral parenchyma. The pattern is particularly characteristic of small cell carcinoma.

Mediastinal Involvement

The mediastinum can be involved by metastases to lymph nodes or, less commonly, by direct invasion from a contiguous neoplasm in the lung parenchyma. In a review of the radiographic findings in 345 patients who had pulmonary carcinoma, a mediastinal mass or mediastinal lymph node enlargement was seen in 53 of 86 (62%) small cell carcinomas, in 45 of 125 (36%) adenocarcinomas, in 7 of 22 (32%) large cell carcinomas, and in 25 of 98 (26%) squamous cell carcinomas.[149] Though uncommon, enlargement of mediastinal lymph nodes can be the main or sole abnormality seen radiographically,[198] in which case it usually indicates the presence of small cell carcinoma.[149] The chief radiographic sign is

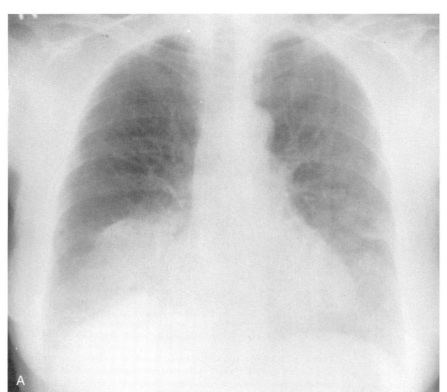

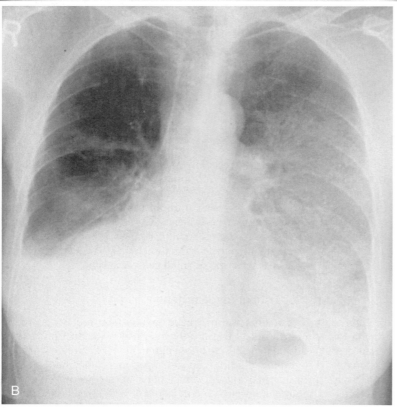

FIGURE 7–11

Progressive multicentric bronchioloalveolar carcinoma. A posterior chest radiograph (**A**) shows bilateral air space opacities involving the middle lobe and parts of both lower lobes. One year later, a radiograph (**B**) shows more extensive consolidation throughout all areas, including both upper lobes. The patient was a 56-year-old woman. (*From Fraser RS, Müller NL, Colman NC, Paré PD: Fraser and Paré's Diagnosis of Diseases of the Chest, 4th ed. Philadelphia, WB Saunders, 1999.*)

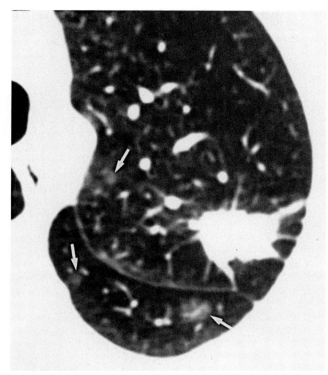

FIGURE 7–12

Bronchioloalveolar carcinoma. A view of the left lung from an HRCT scan in a 68-year-old man demonstrates a 3-cm-diameter spiculated nodule in the left upper lobe. Also noted are small focal areas of ground-glass attenuation (*arrows*). At surgery, the latter areas and the dominant nodule were shown to represent multicentric bronchioloalveolar carcinoma. (*From Fraser RS, Müller NL, Colman NC, Paré PD: Fraser and Paré's Diagnosis of Diseases of the Chest, 4th ed. Philadelphia, WB Saunders, 1999.*)

mediastinal widening, generally with an undulating or lobulated contour (Fig. 7–13).

Pleural Involvement

The reported prevalence of pleural effusion in pulmonary carcinoma ranges from about 5% to 25%.[149,188] The complication does not necessarily indicate pleural invasion by the neoplasm; serous effusion sometimes occurs as a result of lymphatic obstruction or atelectasis.[199]

Apical Neoplasms

Approximately 5% of pulmonary carcinomas arise in the apex of the lung.[149] The term *Pancoast syndrome* can be applied to the situation in which such a neoplasm is accompanied by shoulder or arm pain, which implies invasion of the adjacent chest wall. The vast majority are adenocarcinoma or squamous cell carcinoma.[200,201] MR imaging is superior to CT in assessment of these tumors.[200,202] The procedure allows direct coronal, sagittal, and oblique imaging and yields excellent anatomic detail of the thoracic inlet and brachial plexus (Fig. 7–14). It also provides better soft tissue differentiation, thereby allowing superior depiction of chest wall invasion, which is visualized as disruption of the normal extrapleural fat.

Chest Wall Involvement

The presence of rib destruction or an obvious chest wall mass on CT allows reliable diagnosis of chest wall invasion; however, these findings are present in only 20% to 40% of patients who have the complication.[203,204] Other findings, such as the presence of obtuse angles between the mass and chest wall, greater than 3-cm contact between the mass and chest wall, and focal pleural thickening, are not reliable indicators.[203,205] The reported sensitivity and specificity of CT for detecting chest wall invasion ranges from about 40% to 90%.[206]

Although MR imaging is superior to CT in the assessment of chest wall invasion in apical tumors, the procedures are equivalent in the assessment of such invasion elsewhere.[207] The earliest finding of invasion on MR imaging is disruption of the normal extrapleural fat by soft tissue (see Fig. 7–14).[208] Disruption of the pleural surface and chest wall invasion can also be assessed by ultrasonography.[209]

The skeleton may be involved in pulmonary carcinoma by direct extension or by metastasis. Rib or vertebral destruction is sometimes visible on the chest radiograph, but it is depicted best on CT scan. Although most metastases are osteolytic, purely osteoblastic lesions may occur.

Clinical Manifestations

Symptoms of pulmonary carcinoma can be the result of local bronchopulmonary disease, extension of tumor to adjacent structures, distant metastases, nonspecific constitutional effects, and immunologic reactions to or hormone secretion by the tumor (paraneoplastic syndromes). Only 10% of patients are asymptomatic when first seen, the diagnosis being suspected initially from an abnormal chest radiograph.

Bronchopulmonary Manifestations

Cough, usually mildly productive, is by far the most common symptom of pulmonary carcinoma and is seen in up to 75% of patients.[210] A change in the character of cough in a patient who has a history of smoking may be the initial feature and signals the need for further evaluation. Hemoptysis occurs in about 35% to 50% of patients and may be the only clue to the diagnosis in a patient whose chest radiograph is normal.[211] Other airway-related symptoms are less common. Partial or complete obstruction of a bronchus may result in increased shortness of breath or acute symptoms of infection in a region of obstructive pneumonitis. A local wheeze may be present when no abnormality is visible on a chest radiograph exposed at full inspiration; in this circumstance, radiography at maximal expiration may provide useful information by demonstrating local air trapping.

Neoplasms in the lung periphery seldom cause symptoms, although pain may occur after extension to the pleura. Some patients who have bronchioloalveolar carcinoma expectorate large quantities of mucoid material; this "bronchorrhea" usually indicates extensive lung involvement.[212]

Extrapulmonary Intrathoracic Manifestations

Pleura. Involvement of the pleura may be associated with pain on breathing, signs of pleural effusion, and a friction rub.

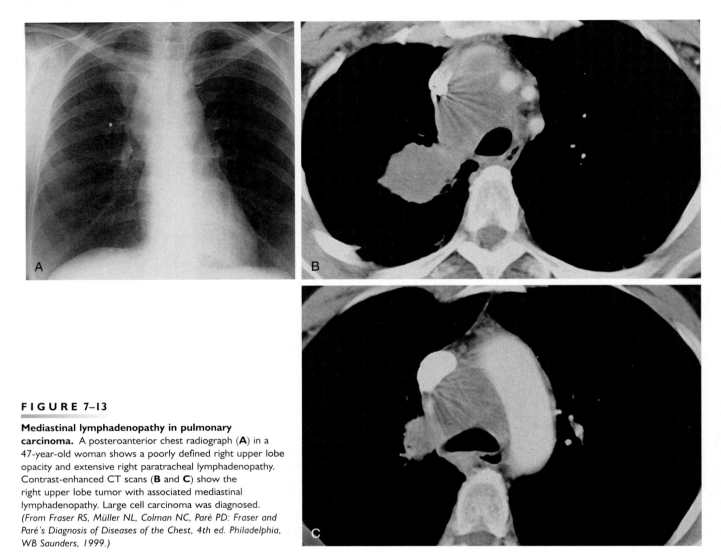

FIGURE 7–13

Mediastinal lymphadenopathy in pulmonary carcinoma. A posteroanterior chest radiograph (**A**) in a 47-year-old woman shows a poorly defined right upper lobe opacity and extensive right paratracheal lymphadenopathy. Contrast-enhanced CT scans (**B** and **C**) show the right upper lobe tumor with associated mediastinal lymphadenopathy. Large cell carcinoma was diagnosed. *(From Fraser RS, Müller NL, Colman NC, Paré PD: Fraser and Paré's Diagnosis of Diseases of the Chest, 4th ed. Philadelphia, WB Saunders, 1999.)*

Effusion may be serous or grossly hemorrhagic; the former appears to be the result of involvement of mediastinal lymph nodes by metastatic carcinoma with secondary lymphatic obstruction, whereas the latter usually results from direct invasion by malignant cells.

Mediastinum. Although mediastinal lymph node enlargement can be caused by hyperplasia as a result of a reaction either to infection in an obstructed region of lung or to the carcinoma itself, it is usually caused by metastasis. If large, it may cause a sensation of retrosternal pressure or pain. Of far greater significance is the effect of a neoplasm on the various structures that reside within the mediastinum.

Cardiac involvement is more common than generally realized. Pericardial infiltration resulting in effusion can be caused by direct invasion from a focus of intrapulmonary or mediastinal neoplasm or, more commonly, by retrograde extension of tumor along the lymphatics from nodal metastases.[213] Effusion often results in signs and symptoms of tamponade.[214] In many cases, the cause of the effusion can be confirmed by cytologic examination of pericardial fluid. Myocardial invasion usually does not cause symptoms; however, when suspected clinically, it may be confirmed by two-dimensional echocardiography or transesophageal echocardiography.

Compression or invasion of mediastinal vessels can result in occlusive thrombosis associated with prominent signs and symptoms. The most common vessels to be so affected are the superior vena cava and its major branches. The superior vena cava syndrome consists of edema of the face, neck, and upper extremities; distended neck and arm veins[215]; and (sometimes) headache and dizziness. In our experience and that of others, obstruction of the superior vena cava does not represent a complication that requires emergency treatment[216,217]; however, compression of the trachea or pericardial tamponade may coexist and requires urgent intervention.

Invasion of the recurrent laryngeal nerve can cause hoarseness, and involvement of the vagus nerve can result in dyspnea, particularly in patients who have chronic airflow obstruction (as so often accompanies pulmonary carcinoma). Although involvement of the phrenic nerve can cause hemidiaphragmatic paresis or paralysis, this complication does not usually lead to symptoms in the presence of normal ventilatory reserve. Dysphagia resulting from esophageal involvement is an uncommon initial symptom of pulmonary

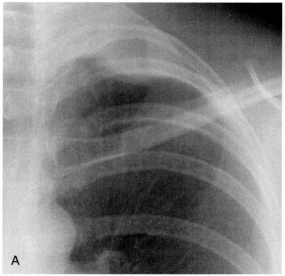

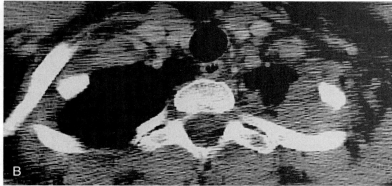

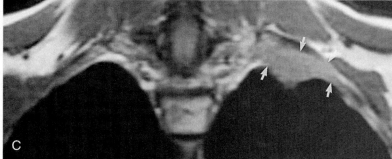

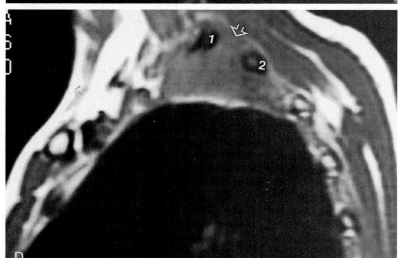

FIGURE 7–14

Pancoast tumor. A view of the upper portion of the left side of the chest from a posteroanterior radiograph (**A**) in a 36-year-old woman shows a left apical tumor. Extension of the tumor into the chest wall is difficult to appreciate on the CT scan (**B**) but can be clearly seen on a coronal T1-weighted MR image (**C**) (*arrows*). On a sagittal T1-weighted MR image (**D**), the tumor (*open arrow*) can be seen to extend between the first (1) and second (2) ribs. After radiation therapy, the patient underwent surgery, and the tumor was shown to be an adenocarcinoma with involvement of the first rib. (*From Fraser RS, Müller NL, Colman NC, Paré PD: Fraser and Paré's Diagnosis of Diseases of the Chest, 4th ed. Philadelphia, WB Saunders, 1999.*)

carcinoma.[218] Only when the esophageal wall is invaded by neoplasm is obstruction likely, in which case the primary site is commonly the left main bronchus.

Tumors of the thoracic inlet (Pancoast tumor) almost invariably result in symptoms and signs related to local invasion. Important structures within the superior thoracic inlet are (from front to back) the subclavian and jugular veins, the phrenic and vagus nerves, the subclavian and common carotid arteries, the recurrent laryngeal nerve, the eighth cervical and first thoracic nerves, the sympathetic chain and stellate ganglion, and the first four ribs and upper vertebrae. A Pancoast tumor may involve one or several of these structures and can thus result in a variety of signs and symptoms, including pain and weakness of the shoulder and arm, swelling of the arm, and Horner's syndrome.

Extrathoracic Metastatic Manifestations

Extrathoracic metastases are usually associated with a previously diagnosed or obvious synchronous pulmonary carcinoma. Occasionally, they are responsible for the initial clinical manifestations in the absence of a radiographically detectable primary lesion. Although metastases can occur in any organ or tissue, the most frequent sites are the lymph nodes, liver, adrenal gland, bone, kidney, and brain.

Lymph Nodes. The most common extrapulmonary site of metastatic pulmonary carcinoma is undoubtedly the hilar and mediastinal lymph nodes; the pattern of such metastases is discussed in the section on staging of pulmonary carcinoma (see page 360). Metastasis to the scalene group of lymph nodes, usually ipsilateral, also occurs frequently. When carcinoma is advanced, especially in patients who have extensive mediastinal lymph node involvement, spread to periaortic, mesenteric, and other intra-abdominal lymph node groups is also frequent; however, signs and symptoms caused by such spread are generally minimal or absent.

Brain and Spinal Cord. Cerebral metastases are found at autopsy in many patients who have pulmonary carcinoma; moreover, the brain is the most common site of metastasis in patients who have non–small cell carcinoma and whose manifestations are due to extrathoracic disease.[219] Though most often seen in patients who have known carcinoma, signs and symptoms of cerebral or cerebellar lesions occasionally antedate those of the primary tumor. It is important to remember that paraneoplastic neurologic syndromes (see later), cerebral infarction resulting from cancer-associated nonbacterial thrombotic endocarditis, and the late effects of chemotherapy and brain radiotherapy used in the treatment of small cell carcinoma can all mimic the signs and symptoms of cerebral metastasis. Symptoms and signs of central nervous system involvement depend on the specific location of the metastasis.

Bone. Metastatic spread to bone occurs in about 10% to 40% of patients at some time during the course of the disease.[220] More than 20% of patients who have confirmed pulmonary carcinoma have bone pain on initial evaluation. Although radionuclide bone scans are more sensitive than clinical signs and symptoms for the detection of metastases, false-negative examinations can occur.[221] Extensive bone involvement can be associated with hypercalcemia (see later).

Abdominal Viscera. The most common sites of abdominal visceral metastases are the liver and adrenal glands. Metastases to these and other intra-abdominal organs usually produce no symptoms; however, involvement of any organ can cause symptoms and signs, sometimes confusing the diagnosis. Small cell carcinoma, in particular, can cause extensive liver metastases with resultant epigastric pain and jaundice and a rapid downhill course that simulates hepatitis.[222] Metastases to the adrenal glands can generally be identified by CT and confirmed (if necessary) by thin-needle aspiration; destruction of sufficient tissue to result in Addison's disease is very uncommon.[223] Gastrointestinal metastases have been documented in 10% to 15% of patients who have pulmonary carcinoma.[224] The most common clinical manifestation is bleeding and anemia; perforation and obstruction can also occur at any level.

Extrathoracic Nonmetastatic Manifestations

Constitutional symptoms such as malaise, weakness, lassitude, fever, and weight loss are common manifestations of pulmonary carcinoma. Although they can be present in the absence of clinical evidence of extrathoracic metastases, in most cases they are associated with distant spread.[225] In addition to these relatively nonspecific features, some patients, particularly those who have small cell carcinoma, have symptoms and signs of systemic disease not directly related to the neoplastic infiltration itself.[226] Such paraneoplastic syndromes occur in up to 10% of patients and may be seen in the absence of bronchopulmonary symptoms.[227] They are mediated by hormones or peptides secreted by the tumor or by antitumor antibodies that cross-react with normal tissues.[228] The clinical manifestations of these syndromes can be considered under several headings, including neuromuscular, cutaneous, skeletal, endocrine or metabolic, hematologic or vascular, and renal.

Neuromuscular Manifestations. Paraneoplastic neuromuscular syndromes usually occur when disease is advanced; however, they occasionally precede detection of the tumor in the lung or are the first sign of its recurrence elsewhere. Small cell carcinoma is by far the most common tumor associated with the syndromes, which include myopathy, peripheral neuropathy, subacute cerebellar degeneration, encephalomyelopathy, necrotizing myelopathy, intestinal dysmotility, facial pain, and visual paraneoplastic syndrome.

Two myopathic syndromes have been associated with pulmonary carcinoma, one simulating myasthenia gravis (Lambert-Eaton myasthenic syndrome) and the other polymyositis. Lambert-Eaton myasthenic syndrome differs clinically from true myasthenia gravis by involvement of proximal rather than distal muscle groups in the extremities and by localization in the hip and lower limbs. In addition, the electromyogram in patients with paraneoplastic syndrome shows amplitude enhancement after 10 to 15 seconds of maximal voluntary contraction or during high-frequency nerve stimulation,[227] in marked contrast to the changes seen in myasthenia gravis. The syndrome is related to the development of IgG antibodies to a number of voltage-gated calcium channels involved in the release of acetylcholine at motor nerve terminals and to synaptotagmin, a synaptic vesicle protein.[229]

In most cases, peripheral neuropathy is both motor and sensory; however, only pain and paresthesia may be noted in the early stages, and sensory loss, muscle weakness, and wasting noted later on. Symptoms may precede the diagnosis of carcinoma by several months.[227] The pathogenesis is related to an antineuronal IgG nuclear antibody (*anti-Hu*) found within the neurons of the dorsal root ganglia that also reacts with tumor cells.[230] Autonomic neuropathy has been reported in association with both giant cell and small cell carcinoma[231]; it may be manifested by postural hypotension or intestinal pseudo-obstruction.[232]

Subacute cerebellar degeneration is characterized by rapidly progressive ataxia, incoordination, vertigo, nystagmus, and dysarthria. Lambert-Eaton myasthenic syndrome may occur concomitantly; antibodies to cerebellar Purkinje cells and anti-Hu antibodies are found in many patients.[226,233]

Cerebral symptoms can develop in the absence of focal neurologic signs and consist chiefly of dementia, euphoria, or a manic-depressive state; somnolence and confusion may alternate with lucid intervals.[234] A syndrome resembling limbic encephalitis has also been described in patients who have small cell carcinoma.[226]

Skeletal Manifestations. Hypertrophic pulmonary osteoarthropathy has been found in about 3% of patients who have pulmonary carcinoma (see page 169).[235] It is distinctly uncommon in patients who have small cell carcinoma[236] and should suggest the diagnosis of a non–small cell tumor.

Endocrine and Metabolic Manifestations. Cushing's syndrome associated with pulmonary carcinoma is usually related to the production of corticotropin precursors, which either have an ACTH-like action or are converted to ACTH within the tumor cells.[237] Although elevated levels of immunoreactive corticotropin can be detected in the blood of about 50% of patients who have small cell carcinoma and in a significant number of those who have non–small cell tumors,[238] associated clinical findings are quite unusual.[237] In fact, the classic picture of Cushing's syndrome is seldom seen in its entirety, probably because patients die before all the features have time to develop; however, hypokalemia or hyperglycemia develops in most patients, and they are susceptible to infection. Proximal myopathy and moon facies are seen in up to 50% of affected individuals.[237]

Pulmonary carcinoma, usually squamous cell carcinoma,[239] is the most frequent cause of tumor-induced hypercalcemia.[240] In contrast to many other paraneoplastic manifestations, hypercalcemia has not been associated with clinically occult carcinoma, and its presence is almost invariably associated with advanced disease.[241] Although it might be logical to attribute hypercalcemia to bone metastases when present and to ectopic hormone production when not present, this would be incorrect in many cases. A parathyroid hormone–related peptide appears to be the most common cause of the syndrome, both in patients who have skeletal metastases and in those who do not.[242]

The syndrome of inappropriate secretion of antidiuretic hormone (SIADH) is defined as the presence of hyponatremia with plasma hypo-osmolality and inappropriately concentrated urine.[237] It is manifested clinically by irritability, confusion, irresponsibility, and weakness, symptoms that usually appear when the serum sodium level drops below 120 mEq/L. Conditions that could also cause hyponatremia, such as renal or adrenal insufficiency, must be absent to make the diagnosis. In patients who have pulmonary carcinoma, the syndrome is confined almost entirely to those who have small cell carcinoma. Even in these patients it is uncommon; although 50% have elevated levels of ADH in their blood and approximately 10% to 15% have hyponatremia, only 1% to 5% have symptoms of SIADH.

Secretion of human chorionic gonadotropin has been said to occur in association with as many as 10% to 15% of all pulmonary carcinomas[243]; however, clinically evident disease resulting from such secretion is rare. Large cell carcinoma appears to be the most common associated cell type.[243] Affected men can have testicular atrophy and a high-pitched voice in addition to gynecomastia. It is important to remember, however, that gynecomastia is not uncommon in the absence of underlying malignancy, particularly in older and obese individuals.

The most common polypeptide hormone produced by pulmonary neoplasms may be calcitonin. The biochemical abnormality does not cause symptoms; however, levels determined by radioimmunoassay have been used as markers of response to therapy or recurrence of neoplasm.[244]

Vascular and Hematologic Manifestations. Superficial thrombophlebitis, typically migratory, has been well documented in cases of pulmonary carcinoma.[245] It may occur in unusual sites and tends to be resistant to anticoagulant therapy. The complication is seen most often with adenocarcinoma. The incidence of deep venous thrombosis and pulmonary thromboembolism is also increased in patients who have pulmonary carcinoma.[246] This finding is probably explained by the subtle procoagulant state noted in many patients, especially those who have metastatic disease.[247]

A leukemoid reaction (white blood cell count of 50,000 cells/mL or more) tends to be a late phenomenon that usually becomes manifest shortly before death; it is most frequently associated with large cell carcinoma and is related to cytokine release by the tumor.[248] An elevated platelet level is common,[249] particularly in patients who have advanced disease; it is associated with poor survival, even after controlling for stage. After lung resection, the thrombocytosis frequently resolves in the postoperative period. Anemia has been described in 5% to 10% of patients who have pulmonary carcinoma. It is most often the result of an impaired erythroid marrow response to erythropoietin, in some cases compounded by insufficient erythropoietin production.[250]

Renal Manifestations. Glomerulonephritis occurs occasionally in association with pulmonary carcinoma. In most cases it is membranous in type[251]; minimal change disease has also been reported.[252]

Investigation of the Patient Who Has Pulmonary Carcinoma

A patient who has radiographic or clinical evidence suggestive of pulmonary carcinoma requires three distinct lines of investigation. First, it is necessary to establish the diagnosis, including a determination of the specific histologic classification. Second, it is necessary to establish resectability or unresectability by a process of staging. Third (and not necessarily in this order), the ability of the patient to tolerate the anticipated surgery must be evaluated. The first two of these issues are discussed in this section.

Clinical Considerations

Although pulmonary carcinoma does not have any specific clinical features, the association of certain symptoms and signs with radiographic evidence of a pulmonary abnormality is sometimes virtually diagnostic. For example, a complaint of shoulder and arm pain in association with a lesion at the apex of a lung or a history of a recent onset of clubbing or hypertrophic osteoarthropathy associated with a peripheral spiculated pulmonary mass almost invariably indicates the presence of carcinoma. Hemoptysis associated with a pulmonary mass is also highly suggestive of malignancy; however, hemoptysis in association with a normal chest radiograph is seldom caused by pulmonary carcinoma in the absence of specific risk factors such as a smoking history or older age. Similarly, when the chest radiograph is normal, a localized wheeze may indicate the presence of pulmonary carcinoma.

Laboratory Considerations

Cytologic examination of sputum, bronchial washings and brushings, BAL fluid, and pleural fluid is a well-established method of diagnosis in patients who have suspected carcinoma (see page 170). Briefly, the sensitivity of sputum cytology has been found to be about 65% and the specificity 99%.[253] Washings and brushings performed during bronchoscopy are complementary,[254] but in such a small number of cases that routine performance of both procedures is questionable. As might be expected, positive cytologic diagnoses are made more often with central than with peripheral neoplasms and with large than with small tumors.[255,256] BAL can be useful, particularly for peripheral tumors that are not visualized endoscopically, in which situation it yields a positive diagnosis in approximately 65% to 70% of patients.[257] Most authors report a sensitivity of about 50% for the cytologic diagnosis of malignancy in pleural effusions.[258] Of particular importance from a diagnostic point of view in all these situations is the observation that the distinction between small cell and non–small cell carcinoma can be made with confidence in the vast majority of cases.

Many tumor markers produced by the carcinoma or by host cells in response to it have been identified. They can be measured in a variety of specimens, including serum, tissue, pleural fluid, sputum, and BAL fluid. Their utility in diagnosis,[259] staging,[260] identification of carcinoma type,[261] distinction of primary from metastatic disease,[262] prognostication,[263] predicting responsiveness to chemotherapy,[264] and follow-up[265] has been explored in a vast number of investigations. A major potential role for these markers is enhancement of the sensitivity of sputum analysis versus cytology for screening.[266] Markers that have been investigated for this purpose include oncogenes such as p53 and K-*ras*.[267] However, evaluation of such genes or gene products has not yet had sufficient sensitivity, specificity, or reproducibility for detection of early carcinoma to allow for its use in screening.[268] Numerous substances have also been evaluated in serum to determine whether their measurement is helpful in distinguishing benign from malignant pulmonary lesions[269]; again, however, none has been found to have sufficient sensitivity or specificity to achieve this goal or to act as a screening tool for early diagnosis.[270]

Biochemical procedures are of little value in the diagnosis of pulmonary carcinoma. However, several investigators have found that serum lactate dehydrogenase levels are increased when metastases are present and when neoplasm recurs after resection. Elevated liver enzyme levels may also be a clue to metastases to the liver, whereas hyponatremia or hypercalcemia should raise the possibility of a paraneoplastic phenomenon and give some indication of tissue type.

Radiologic Considerations

The presence of a potentially malignant lesion is almost invariably identified on conventional chest radiographs (the exceptions being the rare instance in which sputum cytology is positive for malignant cells and the chest radiograph is normal and the increasing number of patients in whom the lesion is initially detected on CT). The importance of obtaining previous radiographs for comparison cannot be overemphasized, particularly in the evaluation of a solitary pulmonary nodule but also in the assessment of possible lymph node enlargement in sites such as the hilum and the aortopulmonary window.

As discussed previously, CT plays a major role in the differentiation of benign from malignant nodules. It is also important in the staging of carcinoma (see later) and is helpful in confirming the presence of lung nodules suspected on radiographs and in distinguishing them from chest wall abnormalities or focal scars. It is important to remember, however, that pulmonary carcinomas may be missed on CT; most such tumors are endobronchial and measure between 0.2 and 2 cm in diameter.[271,272]

MR imaging plays an important role in the assessment of metastatic pulmonary carcinoma, particularly to the brain and adrenals (see later). It is also an important ancillary

imaging modality in the assessment of patients who have questionable chest wall or mediastinal invasion on CT. Perfusion scintigraphy is helpful in predicting postoperative pulmonary function. After quantitative assessment of regional lung perfusion, postoperative FEV_1 can be predicted by multiplying the preoperative FEV_1 by the percentage of perfusion to the lung that will remain after surgery.[273]

FDG-PET imaging can be helpful in the distinction of benign from malignant pulmonary nodules and in the staging of metastases to the hilar and mediastinal lymph nodes (see later). It can also demonstrate unsuspected lesions in the contralateral lung and outside the thorax[274,275] and has high sensitivity and specificity for the detection of recurrent carcinoma.[276,277] The capability of whole-body PET imaging and its high diagnostic accuracy have the potential of leading to a rapid change in the approach to diagnosis and staging of pulmonary carcinoma, in monitoring the response to treatment, and in the assessment of tumor recurrence. The main limitations of the procedure are its high cost and the need for access to a cyclotron for production of ^{18}F-deoxyglucose.

Staging

Schemes for Staging

The most widely used scheme for staging non–small cell carcinoma of the lung is the TNM classification. A variety of alterations in this scheme have been made over the years to better identify groups of patients who have similar prognosis and treatment options. The most recent revision was approved by the American Joint Committee on Cancer (AJCC) and the Union Internationale Contre le Cancer (UICC) in 1997.[278] An accompanying article outlines refinements made in regional lymph node classification.[279] Specific properties of each of the T, N, and M subtypes as defined by this revision are shown in Table 7–3, and the various combinations of T, N, and M that define different stages are presented in Table 7–4.

Patients who have small cell carcinoma are frequently staged in a simpler fashion into two categories: (1) *limited* disease, defined as carcinoma confined to a tolerable radiation port (depending on the investigators, this category has included regional mediastinal and supraclavicular lymph nodes, as well as pleural effusion), and (2) *extensive* disease, in which carcinoma has extended beyond these limits.[99,280]

Methods of Staging

A variety of techniques can be used to investigate T, N, and M parameters to determine the appropriate tumor stage.

T (Primary Tumor)

Radiography. Of the criteria that define the T categories in the TNM classification, most will already have been established during the initial diagnostic workup. For example, chest radiographs will have revealed the size of the lesion in patients in whom it is circumscribed, the presence or absence of pleural effusion (the exception being the situation in which atelectasis or obstructive pneumonitis of a lower lobe obscures its presence), and the degree of associated atelectasis or

TABLE 7–3. TNM Descriptors

Primary Tumor (T)

TX	Primary tumor cannot be assessed or tumor proven by the presence of malignant cells in sputum or bronchial washings but not visualized by imaging or bronchoscopy
T0	No evidence of primary tumor
Tis	Carcinoma *in situ*
T1	Tumor ≤3 cm in greatest dimension, surrounded by lung or visceral pleura, without bronchoscopic evidence of invasion more proximal than the lobar bronchus* (i.e., not in the main bronchus)
T2	Tumor with any of the following features of size or extent >3 cm in greatest dimension Involves the main bronchus, ≥2 cm distal to the carina Invades the visceral pleura Associated with atelectasis or obstructive pneumonitis that extends to the hilar region but does not involve the entire lung
T3	Tumor of any size that directly invades any of the following: chest wall (including superior sulcus tumors), diaphragm, mediastinal pleura, parietal pericardium; or tumor in the main bronchus <2 cm distal to the carina but without involvement of the carina; or associated atelectasis or obstructive pneumonitis of the entire lung
T4	Tumor of any size that invades any of the following: mediastinum, heart, great vessels, trachea, esophagus, vertebral body, carina; or tumor with a malignant pleural or pericardial effusion† or with satellite tumor nodule(s) within the ipsilateral primary tumor lobe of the lung

Regional Lymph Nodes (N)

NX	Regional lymph nodes cannot be assessed
N0	No regional lymph node metastasis
N1	Metastasis to ipsilateral peribronchial and/or ipsilateral hilar lymph nodes and intrapulmonary nodes involved by direct extension of the primary tumor
N2	Metastasis to ipsilateral mediastinal and/or subcarinal lymph node(s)
N3	Metastasis to contralateral mediastinal, contralateral hilar, ipsilateral or contralateral scalene, or supraclavicular lymph node(s)

Distant Metastases (M)

MX	Present of distant metastasis cannot be assessed
M0	No distant metastasis
M1	Distant metastasis present‡

*The uncommon superficial tumor of any size with its invasive component limited to the bronchial wall, which may extend proximal to the main bronchus, is also classified T1.

†Most pleural effusions associated with lung cancer are due to tumor. There are a few patients, however, in whom multiple cytopathologic examinations of pleural fluid show no tumor. In these cases, the fluid is nonbloody and is not an exudate. When these elements and clinical judgment dictate that the effusion is not related to the tumor, the effusion should be excluded as a staging element, and the patient's disease should be staged T1, T2, or T3. Pericardial effusion is classified according to the same rules.

‡Separate metastatic tumor nodule(s) in the ipsilateral nonprimary tumor lobe(s) of the lung are also classified M1.

From Mountain CF: Revisions in the International System for Staging Lung Cancer. Chest 111:1710, 1997.

TABLE 7–4. Stage Grouping—TNM Subsets*

Stage	TNM Subset
0	Carcinoma in situ
IA	T1N0M0
IB	T2N0M0
IIA	T1N1M0
IIB	T2N1M0
	T3N0M0
IIIA	T3N1M0
	T1N2M0
	T2N2M0
	T3N2M0
IIIB	T4N0M0
	T4N1M0
	T4N2M0
	T1N3M0
	T2N3M0
	T3N3M0
	T4N3M0
IV	Any T any N M1

*Staging is not relevant for occult carcinoma, designated TXN0M0.
From Mountain CF: Revisions in the International System for Staging Lung Cancer. Chest 111:1710, 1997.

established by radiographic evidence of destruction of ribs or vertebrae or by a palpable mass. Paramediastinal tumors sometimes displace or narrow the tracheal air column, thereby providing convincing evidence of mediastinal invasion. Evidence of such invasion is also suggested by marked elevation of a hemidiaphragm (related to phrenic nerve paralysis) or by clinical signs of superior vena cava syndrome or laryngeal paralysis. In the absence of signs such as these, the chest radiograph is usually unreliable in detecting invasion of the chest wall, diaphragm, or mediastinum, and it is necessary to resort to CT or MR imaging for such evaluation.

Computed Tomography. CT can reliably detect invasion of the mediastinum, provided that major mediastinal vessels or bronchi are surrounded by tumor (Fig. 7–15).[281] However, a tumor that abuts but does not obviously invade the mediastinum cannot be considered to be invasive, even when associated with obliteration of the fat plane between the mediastinum and the tumor mass.[156] CT criteria suggesting that a tumor abutting the mediastinum is likely to be resectable (albeit possibly minimally invasive) include (1) less than 3-cm contact between the tumor and the adjacent mediastinum, (2) less than 90 degrees circumferential contact between the tumor and the aorta, and (3) the presence of fat between the tumor and the adjacent mediastinal structures.[282] Carcinomas that involve the tracheal carina or that surround, encase, or abut more than 180 degrees of the aorta, main or proximal portion of the right or left pulmonary arteries, or esophagus are likely to be extensively invasive and unresectable.[156,281] Detection of a T4 status (usually considered unresectable) is one of the main indications for the use of CT in the staging of pulmonary carcinoma.[156] Although tumors that abut the mediastinum for less than 3 cm are generally resectable and tumors that encase major mediastinal vessels or bronchi are unresectable, there are no reliable criteria to predict resectability of tumors that abut the mediastinum for more than 3 cm but are not associated with major mediastinal extension.[283]

obstructive pneumonitis in the presence of airway obstruction. In the latter situation, bronchoscopy will have documented the proximal extent of the neoplasm.

In some cases, extrapulmonary spread may be evident without the results of special investigations. For example, direct extension of a neoplasm into the chest wall may be

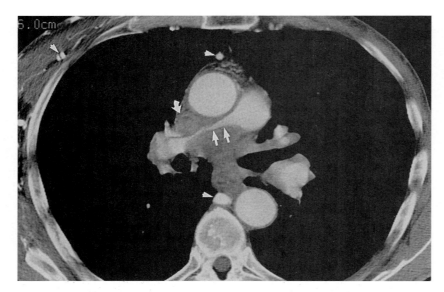

FIGURE 7–15

Unresectable large cell carcinoma. A contrast-enhanced CT scan demonstrates extensive mediastinal involvement by tumor with encasement of the right pulmonary artery (*straight arrows*) and obstruction of the superior vena cava (*curved arrow*). Note the collateral venous circulation in the chest wall and mediastinum (*arrowheads*). (From Fraser RS, Müller NL, Colman NC, Paré PD: Fraser and Paré's Diagnosis of Diseases of the Chest, 4th ed. Philadelphia, WB Saunders, 1999.)

MR Imaging. MR imaging is comparable to CT in the assessment of mediastinal invasion.[207] In an investigation of 170 patients who had non–small cell carcinoma (including 30 patients who had T3 or T4 tumors), the sensitivity of CT and MR imaging was 63% and 56%, respectively, and the specificity was 84% and 80%, respectively, for distinguishing T3 and T4 tumors from less extensive pulmonary carcinomas.[207] As with CT, the main limitation of MR imaging is its inability to distinguish tumor invasion of mediastinal fat from inflammation.[284]

N (Lymph Nodes)

Radiography. Hilar (N1) and ipsilateral (N2) or contralateral (N3) mediastinal lymph node metastases are often present at the time of initial diagnosis of pulmonary carcinoma. The following discussion outlines the most widely accepted criteria for radiologic assessment. Lymph nodes should be classified according to a standardized lymph node map, the one adopted by the AJCC and the UICC in 1997 (Fig. 7–16) being the preferred scheme at present.[279] Guides to the AJCC-UICC nodal map classification on CT have been based on the demonstration of enlarged nodes on contrast-enhanced spiral CT.[285]

The most reliable and practical measurement of lymph node size on CT is its short-axis diameter (i.e., the shortest diameter on the cross-sectional image); this parameter correlates better than the long-axis diameter with node volume and is less influenced by the spatial orientation of the node.[286] For practical reasons, we and others consider a diameter larger than 10 mm in short axis as abnormal regardless of nodal station.[287,288] The authors of a meta-analysis of 42 studies published between 1980 and 1988 found that the sensitivity of CT for the diagnosis of nodal metastases was 83% and the specificity 81% on a per-patient basis.[289] The authors of another meta-analysis of 29 studies published between 1990 and 1998 concluded that the sensitivity was 60% and the specificity was 77%.[290] The lower accuracy in the latter review may be related to more careful surgical staging, as well as greater emphasis on the accuracy of CT in the detection of specific mediastinal nodal station involvement. In spite of the limitations of CT,

the results of a prospective multicenter Canadian Lung Oncology Group study showed that CT was more cost-effective than mediastinoscopy[291]; the authors concluded that patients who have normal-sized mediastinal nodes on CT and no evidence of metastases may proceed directly to thoracotomy.[291] Because of the relative lack of specificity of enlarged nodes detected by CT alone, biopsy is usually required to confirm the presence of metastases.

Magnetic Resonance Imaging. Similar to CT, MR imaging relies on size criteria to determine nodal abnormalities and, overall, is comparable to CT.[207,292]

Positron Emission Tomography. Although CT and MR imaging rely on anatomic assessment of lymph nodes, PET relies on a biochemical difference between normal and neoplastic cells. Mediastinal nodes containing carcinoma have increased uptake and accumulation of FDG (Fig. 7–17). Several groups have shown that PET is superior to CT in the assessment of mediastinal nodal metastases.[293,294] The authors of a meta-analysis of 14 studies published between 1990 and 1998 concluded that the sensitivity of PET for the detection of mediastinal nodal metastases was 79% and the specificity was 91%[290]; as indicated earlier, comparable figures for CT were 60% and 77%, respectively. The results of another meta-analysis of 39 studies published before 2003 showed a sensitivity of 85% and a specificity of 90%[295]; FDG-PET imaging was more sensitive but less specific when CT showed enlarged lymph nodes (sensitivity, 100%; specificity, 78%) than when CT showed no lymph node enlargement (sensitivity, 82%; specificity, 93%).[295]

Endobronchial and Endoesophageal Ultrasound. Endobronchial ultrasound allows assessment of intraluminal, intramural, and peribronchial tumor growth, as well as evaluation of hilar and mediastinal lymph nodes.[296] In an investigation of 242 patients who had carcinoma and enlarged lymph nodes, successful nodal sampling by ultrasound-guided transbronchial biopsy was obtained in 207 patients (86%), and a firm diagnosis of cancer was obtained in 172 (71%)[297]; the results were independent of nodal location. The results of several studies suggest that transesophageal ultrasound with fine-needle aspiration of lymph nodes is superior to CT and

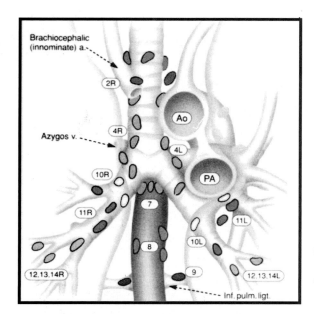

Superior Mediastinal Nodes

● **1** Highest Mediastinal

● **2** Upper Paratracheal

○ **3** Pre-vascular and Retrotracheal

● **4** Lower Paratracheal
   (including Azygos Nodes)

N_2 = single digit, ipsilateral
N_3 = single digit, contralateral or supraclavicular

Aortic Nodes

● **5** Subaortic (A-P window)

● **6** Para-aortic (ascending
   aorta or phrenic)

Inferior Mediastinal Nodes

○ **7** Subcarinal

○ **8** Paraesophageal
   (below carina)

● **9** Pulmonary Ligament

N_1 Nodes

○ **10** Hilar

● **11** Interlobar

○ **12** Lobar

○ **13** Segmental

○ **14** Subsegmental

FIGURE 7–16

Regional lymph node stations for lung cancer staging. *(From Mountain CF, Dresler CM: Regional lymph node classification for lung cancer staging. Chest 111:1719, 1997.)*

PET imaging in the staging of mediastinal nodes.[298-300] For example, in an investigation of 79 patients, the procedure had a sensitivity of 63% and a specificity of 100% as compared with 68% and 72%, respectively, for PET imaging.[300]

M (Distant Metastases)

The most widely used techniques to investigate patients who have possible extrathoracic metastases are CT (to show metastases to the adrenal glands and liver), MR imaging (to assess the brain and adrenal glands), radionuclide scans (to identify skeletal metastases), and most recently, whole-body PET imaging.

The use of these techniques should be considered in the context of the clinical picture. In patients who have non–small cell carcinoma, brain MR imaging and radionuclide scanning of bone are generally indicated only if there is clinical or laboratory evidence of metastatic disease. Such evidence includes not only organ-specific signs and symptoms (liver enlargement, bone pain) but also nonspecific symptoms of anorexia, weight loss, and fatigue. The usefulness of this proviso is demonstrated by the results of a study of 309 patients who had early-stage (T1 or T2, N0 or N1) non–small cell carcinoma, in whom routine bone, brain, and liver scans or bone scan and abdominal and brain CT performed before anticipated surgery revealed an unexpected metastasis in only 1 of 472

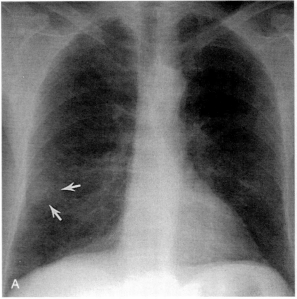

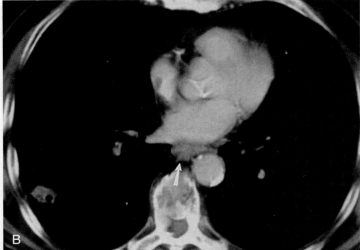

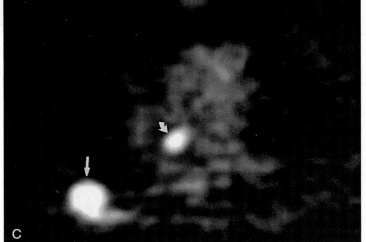

FIGURE 7–17

Positron emission tomography. A posteroanterior chest radiograph (**A**) shows a poorly defined right lower lobe nodule (*arrows*). A CT scan (**B**) confirms the presence of the nodule and shows an enlarged paraesophageal lymph node (*arrow*). A PET image (**C**) shows marked FDG uptake in the right lower lobe nodule (*straight arrow*) and in the paraesophageal node (*curved arrow*). Large cell carcinoma was diagnosed. *(Case courtesy of Dr. Ned Patz, Duke University Medical Center, Durham, NC.)*

studies (0.2%)[301]; all other detected metastatic disease was associated with clinical signs and symptoms or abnormal biochemical profiles.

In a 1995 meta-analysis of 25 studies that addressed the issue of the appropriateness of preoperative evaluation of metastatic disease, the authors concluded that a negative clinical evaluation had a high negative predictive value (consistently exceeding 90%) for finding occult metastases by bone scan and CT evaluation of the brain and abdomen.[302] These values were more impressive (>97%) when an expanded clinical evaluation that included consideration of constitutional symptoms was used. Although some investigators have reported occult brain metastases in asymptomatic individuals, especially those who have adenocarcinoma,[303] such findings must be balanced against the low cost-effectiveness of the procedure. In the meta-analysis cited previously, the prevalence of brain metastases was only 5% in asymptomatic patients. Because gadolinium-enhanced MR imaging is more sensitive than CT in the detection of such metastases, it is possible that the prevalence is higher than that suggested by the CT data.

Routine contrast-enhanced CT through the liver for the staging of lung cancer rarely changes the tumor stage and is not warranted.[206,302] Because the adrenal glands are common sites for metastatic pulmonary carcinoma and because of the ease of examination, however, most radiologists extend the chest CT scan to include the adrenal glands in patients who have a pulmonary tumor.[304] In a study of 110 patients who had pulmonary carcinoma, adrenal masses were identified in 11 (10%)[305]; in 5 patients, the adrenal glands were the only site of metastasis.

A variety of techniques have been used to help distinguish adrenal metastases from nonfunctioning adenomas, including determination of the attenuation of the mass by nonenhanced CT,[306] gadolinium-enhanced MR imagining,[307] and FDG-PET imaging.[308] Whole-body PET imaging has the advantage over other imaging modalities of showing not only adrenal metastases but also other metastases that may not be apparent on CT, MR imaging, or bone scintigraphy.[293]

Investigation of Specific Radiographic Patterns

The diagnostic approach to a patient who has pulmonary carcinoma, particularly with respect to the presence or absence of mediastinal lymph node metastases, depends in large measure on the initial radiographic appearance—a solitary pulmonary nodule or mass with or without associated adenopathy, an obstructing endobronchial lesion, or a central nonobstructing lesion. The approaches to investigation outlined in this section are meant to provide general guidelines only; specific circumstances and individual preferences may lead to legitimate deviation from these recommendations.

Solitary Pulmonary Nodule

As discussed previously (see page 346), a solitary pulmonary nodule is generally defined as a well-circumscribed lesion less than 3 cm in diameter within the lung parenchyma, without associated adenopathy, atelectasis, or pneumonia. Comparison with previous radiologic studies is an essential first step in establishing whether the lesion is new or has grown or not grown over time. Nodules that have shown no evidence of growth radiographically over at least a 2-year period can generally be considered benign.[309] In most circumstances, a new nodule should be considered malignant. The second step is to determine the presence or absence of calcification, a judgment that can sometimes be made with confidence from the chest radiograph; if not, thin-section CT is the logical next step. Localized areas of fat attenuation are virtually diagnostic of a hamartoma.[310] A nodule can also be considered almost certainly benign if it has homogeneous density and shows no enhancement or enhancement less than 15 HU after intravenous administration of contrast material.[180] In the absence of any of these features, the nodule should be considered to be of indeterminate origin.

The risk for malignancy in a patient who has an indeterminate nodule increases with age, smoking history, occupational exposure to potential carcinogens, history of previous malignancy, certain radiologic findings such as spiculation and the presence of bubble-like lucencies on CT, and increasing size of the nodule.[311] PET scanning can identify malignancy in lung nodules as small as 1 cm in diameter with a high degree of accuracy.[312] However, false-negative results can occur in patients who have bronchioloalveolar carcinoma, carcinoid tumor, or lesions less than 1 cm in diameter and in patients who are hyperglycemic, whereas false-positive results can occur with infectious or inflammatory conditions such as tuberculosis, histoplasmosis, and rheumatoid nodules.[309,313] All in all, consideration of these clinical and radiologic features leaves very few "indeterminate" nodules, and in some series, the vast majority of resected lesions prove to be malignant.[314] A watch-and-wait strategy can be used when the likelihood of pulmonary carcinoma is low and there is major surgical risk; clearly, patient preference may also influence the choice of management options.[315]

Fiberoptic bronchoscopy has little role in investigation[316]; although it can establish a diagnosis of malignancy, it cannot exclude it and, consequently, is unlikely to alter any decision regarding the advisability of surgery. Similarly, cytologic examination of sputum specimens or samples obtained by transthoracic needle aspiration is unlikely to be cost-effective or to alter decision making in this setting.[317] Mediastinal exploration for nodal metastases before resectional surgery may not be necessary in patients who have solitary pulmonary nodules and whose CT scans fail to show nodes larger than 1 cm in diameter,[291] especially when the tumor is smaller than

2 cm in diameter.[318] On the one hand, the likelihood of metastatic carcinoma in this setting is low[319]; on the other hand, patients in this group might benefit from surgical resection despite the presence of pathologically confirmed metastases in the ipsilateral mediastinum.[320] Because of its very high sensitivity for the detection of lymph node metastases,[312,321] PET scanning can improve on the results available from CT alone. Positive findings may allow confirmation of disease by directed mediastinoscopy or other surgical exploration, whereas negative findings support a decision to not undertake mediastinoscopy, either by confirming a favorable staging established by CT or by indicating that enlarged nodes seen on CT are benign.[322,323]

Peripheral Nodule or Mass with Suspected Hilar or Mediastinal Adenopathy

In this situation, the physician is dealing with the possibility of metastases in lymph nodes situated in the hilum alone, the mediastinum alone, or both. In the absence of evidence for distant metastases, patients who have radiographic signs of hilar or mediastinal lymph node enlargement usually require evaluation by CT. CT can detect small metastases in the lung not visible on radiographs, small pleural effusions, and liver and adrenal metastases. Refined information regarding the size and location of enlarged lymph nodes can also provide an indication of where to biopsy and the choice of biopsy procedure.[324] As discussed previously, the specificity of CT for the identification of malignancy in the mediastinum is imperfect, and biopsy is usually required to confirm the presence of suspected metastases. The sensitivity for the detection of lymph node metastases is less than 80%.[290] When lymph nodes are abnormal on CT, the use of PET scanning improves diagnostic accuracy and may improve the cost-effectiveness of investigation by reducing unnecessary surgery.[309] The utility of the various techniques that have been developed for biopsy of mediastinal lymph nodes is discussed elsewhere (see page 175). Although PET imaging is superior to CT, it has limited specificity. As mentioned previously, recent studies have shown that transesophageal ultrasound with fine-needle aspiration of lymph nodes allows almost 100% specificity in the diagnosis of mediastinal nodal metastases.[325,326]

Bronchoscopy is usually indicated in patients with radiologic evidence of hilar or mediastinal lymph node enlargement.[327] If a lesion is endoscopically visible, a tissue diagnosis can be obtained in more than 90% of cases. For more peripheral lesions, BAL of the involved lung segment confirms a diagnosis of carcinoma in up to 70% of cases.[257] Transbronchial needle aspiration of mediastinal lymph nodes increases the diagnostic yield of bronchoscopy, as well as provides information for staging.[324]

Lobar or Segmental Atelectasis or a Hilar Mass with Normal Lungs

Bronchoscopy has a valuable role in the diagnosis and staging of patients who have radiographic patterns of lobar or segmental atelectasis or a hilar mass with normal lungs. For example, if a lesion proves to be T3 (<2.0 cm distal to the carina), it is probably unresectable.

In patients who have non–small cell carcinoma, most pleural effusions that are discovered during the course of the initial investigation are related to pleural metastases.[278] Recovery of malignant cells from the pleural fluid of patients who have pulmonary carcinoma is generally regarded as evidence of inoperability. Because the effusions may be the result of pneumonia or other pathology, however, it is usually necessary to obtain confirmation of the diagnosis (provided that there are no other signs of unresectability).

Cytologic and Radiologic Screening

As had been shown with uterine cervical cancer, it was hypothesized in the early 1970s that screening programs to detect early pulmonary carcinoma might be the best hope to reduce mortality from this disease.[328] However, the results of studies of the usefulness of screening cytology and chest radiography to identify early carcinoma and thereby reduce mortality failed to provide direct evidence of benefit,[329] and mass screening programs were abandoned.[330] What remained poorly explained was the apparent contradiction between the more frequent identification of early-stage disease in the screened population versus controls and the failure to influence overall cancer mortality despite a high rate of cure in the screened patients.[331,332] Although "overdiagnosis bias" has been suggested as an explanation,[333] most patients who refuse surgery for suspected early-stage cancer die of the disease.

More recently, the focus of screening efforts has been on the use of low-dose spiral CT, for which a number of large and uncontrolled studies have been undertaken.[334] Overall, these studies have identified radiographically undetectable early-stage carcinoma in less than 0.5% of individuals. At the same time, lesions that are ultimately proven to be benign after surgery or further follow-up have been found in up to two thirds of patients.[335,336] Controlled studies are required to determine whether the use of this technique actually reduces the mortality from lung carcinoma and, if so, whether such a strategy is cost-effective.[337,338]

Prognosis and Natural History

Pulmonary carcinoma is one of the most important human neoplasms, not only because of its frequency but also because of its dismal prognosis: overall, only about 10% to 15% of patients survive 5 years or longer.[339] The 5-year survival rate varies from virtually nil for patients who have radiographically apparent mediastinal lymph node metastases or whose neoplasm arises in a main bronchus to about 65% for asymptomatic patients who have peripheral nodules and no lymph node metastases.[278] Although surgical resection is curative in some patients who have non–small cell carcinoma, the incidence of unresectability in general hospitals ranges from 80% to 85%, including the 5% of cases in which unresectability is determined at thoracotomy.[340] Operative mortality ranges from about 1% to 6%[341]; older patients now experience surgical results similar to[342] or only slightly worse[343] than those of younger patients.

Survival is associated with a number of factors, some so closely interrelated that it is virtually impossible to assess their relative importance. Many can be divided into factors inherent to the host and those attributable to the neoplasm itself. The latter can be further considered in three major categories: (1) *pathologic factors*, the most important of which is the

histologic classification; (2) *anatomic factors*, of which tumor stage is paramount; and (3) *clinical factors*, which relate particularly to cancer-related symptoms and whether they are local or systemic and recent or prolonged. Although each of these factors is discussed individually, it must be borne in mind that the complexity of their interrelationships necessitates their overall consideration in every patient.

Host Factors

Race, age, and sex have relatively minor prognostic influence in comparison to tumor stage and histology, patient performance status, and burden of comorbid disease. Nonetheless, most investigators have shown improved survival in women. Age also has a clear-cut (albeit not necessarily independent) influence. The prognosis is poor in patients who are younger than 40 years,[344] an observation probably related to the fact that they tend to have tumors of advanced stage at initial diagnosis. Although elderly patients appear to have relatively slower tumor growth and less metastatic disease,[345] they have a relatively poor prognosis, possibly because of the prevalence of comorbid disease.[346]

Few workers have evaluated survival according to race. However, in a study of 92,182 patients who had pulmonary carcinoma identified in hospital cancer registries in the United States, the prognosis of African Americans was found to be especially poor.[347] Whether this finding was the result of more aggressive disease or socioeconomic factors such as diminished access to health care is not certain.[348]

Histologic Classification

Although there can be little doubt that the histologic classification of a tumor is correlated with both natural history and prognosis, the degree of correlation and its significance relative to other factors are difficult to determine precisely. In fact, in some studies, tumor type has been found to exert no statistically significant independent influence on prognosis once the effect of stage is accounted for.[349] Despite these reservations, several general statements are applicable.

Squamous cell carcinoma tends to remain localized to the thorax more than other cell types do and thus causes death more frequently by local complications.[350] Most investigators have found a better prognosis, stage for stage, for squamous cell carcinoma than for adenocarcinoma or large cell carcinoma,[351] even when locally advanced tumor is treated with identical courses of radiation therapy.[352] Histologic grade and proliferative activity are also related to prognosis.[353] Although as a group their survival time is undoubtedly better, even patients who have in situ or minimally invasive squamous cell carcinoma have a guarded prognosis[354]; in these patients, death is often due to the development of a second lung malignancy.[355]

Small cell carcinoma is a fast-growing neoplasm, and in most cases, spread has occurred beyond the thorax at the time of diagnosis.[356] Although many tumors show a response to chemotherapy, it is often incomplete and of short duration. The overall median survival is about 6 to 10 months, and 5-year survival rates range from only 1% to 5%.[357] As might be expected, a better prognosis is associated with limited as opposed to extensive disease[358] and with demonstrable response to chemotherapy. Patients who have prolonged survival after a diagnosis of small cell carcinoma are at increased risk for a second malignancy, just as often acute leukemia as pulmonary carcinoma.[359]

Although some investigators have shown the prognosis for adenocarcinoma and large cell carcinoma to be similar,[360] others have found the prognosis for the former to be more favorable,[361] particularly in the absence of lymph node involvement. These observations may be related to the inclusion of peripheral bronchioloalveolar carcinoma, a subtype that has relatively good 5-year survival when resected at the solitary nodule stage. A distinction between nodular and diffuse forms of bronchioloalveolar carcinoma is of considerable prognostic importance, survival being much better in the former[362]; a number of investigators have also found a poorer prognosis in patients who have mucinous as opposed to non–mucin-secreting tumors.

Stage

The most important prognostic factor of patients who have pulmonary carcinoma is the anatomic extent of disease at the time of diagnosis as defined by the TNM staging system (Tables 7–5, 7–6, and 7–7).[278,363] The size of the primary neoplasm is of particular importance in early-stage disease; in the absence of metastases to regional lymph nodes, T1 tumors are associated with a 5-year survival rate of about 60% as opposed to 40% for T2 tumors. However, there may not be any important prognostic significance of size among T1 tumors.[354]

It is important to distinguish staging accomplished clinically and radiographically from that established pathologically, which as might be expected, is generally more accurate. The term *Will Rogers phenomenon* has been used to describe the impact of a change in stage on prognosis.[365] When patients in a more favorable stage are downgraded ("migrate") to a poorer-prognosis stage because of the application of more refined and accurate diagnostic methods, survival in both groups improves without any change in overall outcome. A specific example of this effect is provided by patients who have N2 disease that is clinically recognizable or is identified by standard radiography, transbronchial needle biopsy, or mediastinoscopy, in whom the 5-year survival rate is only 2%, even

TABLE 7–5. Clinical (Top) and Pathologic (Bottom) Stage IA and Stage IB by cTNM (Top) and pTNM (Bottom) Subset

	Months after Treatment (Cumulative Percent Surviving)				
	12 (%)	24 (%)	36 (%)	48 (%)	60 (%)
cTNM					
cT1N0M0 (n = 687)	91	79	71	67	61
cT2N0M0 (n = 1189)	72	54	46	41	38
pTNM					
pT1N0M0 (n = 511)	94	86	80	73	67
pT2N0M0 (n = 549)	87	76	67	62	57

From Mountain CF: Revisions in the International System for Staging Lung Cancer. Chest 111:1710, 1997.

TABLE 7–6. Clinical (Top) and Surgical-Pathologic (Bottom) Stage IIA and Stage IIB by cTNM (Top) and pTNM (Bottom) Subset

	Months after Treatment (Cumulative Percent Surviving)				
	12 (%)	24 (%)	36 (%)	48 (%)	60 (%)
cTNM					
cT1N1M0 (n = 29)	79	49	38	34	34
cT2N1M0 (n = 250)	61	42	34	26	24
cT3N0M0 (n = 107)	55	37	31	27	22
pTNM					
pT1N1M0 (n = 76)	89	70	64	61	55
pT2N1M0 (n = 288)	78	56	47	42	39
pT3N0M0 (n = 87)	76	55	47	40	38

From Mountain CF: Revisions in the International System for Staging Lung Cancer. Chest 111:1710, 1997.

TABLE 7–7. Clinical Stage IIIB and Stage IV by cTNM Subset

	Months after Treatment (Cumulative Percent Surviving)				
	12 (%)	24 (%)	36 (%)	48 (%)	60 (%)
cTNM					
cT4N0-1-2M0 (n = 458)	37	15	10	8	7
cAny T N3M0 (n = 572)	32	11	6	4	3
cAny T Any N M1 (n = 1,427)	20	5	2	2	1

From Mountain CF: Revisions in the International System for Staging Lung Cancer. Chest 111:1710, 1997.

when aggressive surgical resection is attempted.[366] By contrast, when N2 disease requires thoracotomy for identification, the resectability rate is higher, and the 5-year survival rate varies from about 15% to 30%.[367] Extrapolation of the relatively favorable results of aggressive surgical approaches in patients in the latter group to those in the former is thus inappropriate.

T3 tumors include those that invade the chest wall, mediastinum, or proximal portion of the main bronchus. Despite their advanced nature, they are surgically resectable by conventional criteria, and 5-year survival has been attained in a small number of patients. This is in sharp contrast to the dismal prognosis of patients who have T4 lesions, which are generally unresectable. It is likely, however, that there is important heterogeneity with respect to prognosis, even in patients who have stage IIIB and IV tumors; for example, in a study of 84 patients who had satellite nodules in a resected lobe (resulting in a T4 stage) and underwent resection (N0 to N2), the 5-year survival rate was 22%, in contrast to the 7% survival rate of all patients with T4 lesions.[368] It has also been shown that tumors that are classified as T3 by virtue of direct chest wall invasion have a better prognosis than those whose T3 designation is determined otherwise.[369] Additional flaws in the current staging scheme have been identified, and it is likely that some will be corrected in future refinements.[370]

Patients who have small cell carcinoma are usually divided simply into those who have limited disease and those who have extensive disease; as might be expected, the former typically survive longer.[371] When the brain is the sole site of metastatic disease, however, survival is similar in both groups.[372] When the bone marrow is involved (as occurs in about 30% of cases), survival time is appreciably shortened when thrombocytopenia develops.[373]

Clinical Factors

The clinical manifestations of pulmonary carcinoma and its functional effects are also important prognostic factors.[374] The performance status of the patient is the best overall measure of these effects[375]; however, performance status itself can be affected by a variety of influences, each of which could have prognostic importance individually. A sophisticated staging system has been developed for defining and evaluating clinical features of prognostic importance.[376] Such "clinical severity" staging has prognostic importance independent of TNM staging; moreover, their combined use allows a more refined estimate of prognosis than does the use of either alone. Although this clinical staging system has not been widely applied, consideration of its components is important for two reasons: (1) it calls attention to important prognostic factors that are not considered in TNM staging or in any global measure of performance status, and (2) it allows for selection and comparison of comparable patient groups in therapeutic trials.

Miscellaneous Factors

Although the aforementioned TNM and clinical staging systems separate patients into clearly different prognostic groups, considerable variability in survival exists among individual patients within any TNM or clinical stage.[377] Many investigations have been undertaken in an attempt to identify specific biologic markers in serum or tumor tissue that might help define the prognosis of such patients more precisely.[378] However, it remains to be determined whether the conclusions reached in these studies will be confirmed in larger investigations in which better-established clinical prognostic factors have been used for analysis.[374]

Multiple Primary Pulmonary Carcinomas

The criteria used to make a diagnosis of an independent carcinoma as opposed to recurrence or metastasis from an initial neoplasm can be complex and vary from investigator to investigator. It seems reasonable to conclude, however, that tumors are separate primary lesions if (1) they have a different histologic appearance or (2) the histology is the same, a disease-free interval of at least 2 years has elapsed between the two, or the tumors are located in different lobes without extrapulmonary metastases or evidence of carcinoma in common

lymphatics.[379] The reported incidence of these cases has varied from 0.2% to 4.3%.[380]

Such multiple primary carcinomas can develop synchronously (usually defined as the presence of two tumors at the time or closely after the initial diagnosis) or metachronously (the second cancer appearing after an interval, usually ≥12 months).[381] The latter occurs in at least two thirds of cases and is recognized on average 4 to 5 years after the first primary. It has been estimated that patients who undergo "curative resection" for pulmonary carcinoma have a 10% to 15% chance of developing a second lung neoplasm.[382] In patients with resectable and operable tumors, the survival rate after resection of the second tumor has been reported to be 30% or more after 5 years.[383]

Other Neoplasms Associated with Pulmonary Carcinoma

Patients who have pulmonary carcinoma are also at increased risk for the development of carcinoma elsewhere, especially in the head and neck.[384] The association of these neoplasms is probably a result of the influence of tobacco smoke on the epithelium at the different sites. This risk seems to be particularly important for supraglottic tumors, especially multicentric supraglottic tumors in the first 2 years of follow-up.[385] A smaller increased risk for pulmonary carcinoma has also been described after the diagnosis of other smoking-related tumors, such as those of the uterine cervix[386] or urinary bladder.[387] Patients who have chronic lymphocytic leukemia[388] or who smoke and have undergone thoracic irradiation for Hodgkin's lymphoma[389] or breast carcinoma also have an increased incidence of pulmonary carcinoma.[390]

In the diagnostic workup of a possible pulmonary carcinoma, malignant cells from the upper respiratory tract may be present in sputum and lead to an erroneous conclusion regarding the primary site. Distinction between a primary pulmonary carcinoma and a solitary metastasis from an upper airway carcinoma may also be problematic. Because of the relatively frequent association of the two forms of tumor, this dilemma, is not uncommon. An important differential diagnostic clue is the presence of cervical lymph node enlargement, because systemic metastases from an upper airway tumor are often preceded by metastases to this site. In the absence of this finding, a solitary lung lesion most likely represents a second primary tumor.

NEUROENDOCRINE NEOPLASMS

Several types of pulmonary neoplasm show ultrastructural and immunohistochemical features of neuroendocrine differentiation. Carcinoid tumor is the prime example of such neoplasms. Some consider small cell carcinoma to be of the same ilk and believe it to represent the most undifferentiated end of a spectrum of neuroendocrine cell tumors.[391] Although there is some logic in this viewpoint, we prefer to consider this tumor separately because of its genetic differences and its closer clinical and epidemiologic association with the other common forms of pulmonary carcinoma.[392] Some large cell carcinomas resemble carcinoid tumor histologically but have high mitotic activity and show ultrastructural and immunohistochemical evidence of neuroendocrine differentiation; some investigators believe that these tumors should be considered in a separate category (so-called large cell neuroendocrine carcinoma).

Carcinoid Tumor

Pulmonary carcinoid tumor is an uncommon malignant neoplasm derived from the surface or glandular epithelium of the conducting or transitional airways. It accounts for only about 1% to 2% of all pulmonary neoplasms.[393,394] On the basis of histologic and cytologic features, carcinoid tumors can be divided into two fairly distinct clinicopathologic types: typical and atypical, the latter representing about 10% to 20% of cases. The mean age at diagnosis is between 40 and 60,[393-395] with centrally located tumors and typical forms tending to occur earlier than peripheral or atypical ones.[396] Carcinoid tumor is the most common primary pulmonary neoplasm in children and adolescents.[397]

The etiology and pathogenesis are unclear. Although many patients with atypical tumors have a history of cigarette smoking, no association has been found between this habit and the more common typical tumor. In addition, there is no clear link of either form of tumor with other agents known to be associated with pulmonary carcinoma, such as asbestos.

Pathologic Characteristics

Typical Carcinoid Tumor. About 80% to 85% of these tumors arise in a lobar, segmental, or proximal subsegmental bronchus and grow as a polypoid mass within the lumen (see Color Fig. 7–10); they frequently cause distal atelectasis and obstructive pneumonitis. The remainder are located in the lung periphery, where they appear as well-circumscribed nodules without clear airway association on gross examination.

Histologically, the tumors typically appear to compress rather than infiltrate the adjacent normal tissue. A variety of histologic patterns can be seen, including sheets, trabeculae, or small nests of cells separated by a fibrovascular stroma (see Color Fig. 7–11A); more than one pattern is commonly present in an individual tumor. The cytoplasm of individual tumor cells is usually moderate in amount. Nuclei are oval or round and show mild pleomorphism and small nucleoli (see Color Fig. 7–11A); mitotic figures are scarce or absent, and there is no necrosis. Occasionally, the nuclei have a spindle shape, in which case the tumor may be confused with a mesenchymal neoplasm such as fibrous histiocytoma or leiomyoma.[398] Even though the fibrovascular stroma separating tumor cell nests is usually thin, it may become quite thick and contain hyalinized collagen. Foci of bone formation may develop in such thickened stroma or in adjacent cartilage plates.[399] Deposits of amyloid are present in the stroma occasionally.[400]

Although the diagnosis is usually evident with hematoxylin-eosin staining, it can be confirmed by immunohistochemical study using antibodies directed to components of the neurosecretory granule, such as chromogranin and synaptophysin.[401] Many specific neuroendocrine substances can also be identified immunohistochemically, the most common being serotonin, gastrin-releasing peptide (bombesin),

pancreatic polypeptide, vasoactive intestinal polypeptide, and leuenkephalin.[402,403]

The histologic diagnosis of typical carcinoid tumor in resected specimens is usually straightforward. However, small tissue samples obtained by bronchoscopic or transthoracic needle biopsy may be difficult to distinguish from small cell carcinoma, especially in the presence of crush artifact[404]; it is thus prudent for both the pathologist and clinician to question a diagnosis of small cell carcinoma in nonsmoking or young individuals or in patients whose sole evidence of tumor seems to be a nodule. Similarly, the diagnosis of small cell carcinoma should be reconsidered in a patient who survives 5 years or longer.[405]

Atypical Carcinoid Tumor. This term is applied to tumors that have an architectural pattern similar to that of typical carcinoid tumor but show histologic and cytologic features suggestive of an aggressive nature (see Color Fig. 7–11B).[406-408] According to the WHO classification, these features include necrosis or a mitotic rate of 2 to 10 per 10 high-power microscopic fields.[144] As with the typical form, immunohistochemical study is usually positive for neuroendocrine markers such as chromogranin and synaptophysin.[407]

Radiologic Manifestations

Radiologic manifestations depend largely on the location of the tumor. Because most are situated in lobar or segmental bronchi, evidence of airway obstruction is the most common radiographic finding. The characteristic pattern consists of a homogeneous increase in density confined precisely to a lobe or to one or more segments, usually associated with considerable loss of volume (Fig. 7–18). Patients with segmental atelectasis/obstructive pneumonitis may have periodic exacerbations and remissions, presumably reflecting intermittent relief of the obstruction. Recurrent infections distal to the neoplasm can result in bronchiectasis and lung abscesses. Occasionally, retention of mucus in airways distal to the tumor results in mucoid impaction unaccompanied by atelectasis or pneumonitis.

When a tumor partially occludes a bronchus, the reduction in ventilation of affected parenchyma can result in hypoxic vasoconstriction and a decrease in volume; the oligemia can be a subtle but highly suggestive sign of the presence of an endobronchial lesion and is an indication for bronchoscopy (Fig. 7–19).[409]

Peripheral carcinoid tumors appear radiologically as solitary nodules. They are usually homogeneous in density, sharply defined, round or oval, and slightly lobulated.[410] Most measure 1 to 3 cm in diameter, although they may grow to 10 cm.[410]

Calcification/ossification is visible on the radiograph in less than 5% of cases[411] but can be identified on CT scan in approximately 30%.[412] It is more common in central than in peripheral tumors. The pattern of calcification is variable and may include small or large, smooth or irregular, and central, eccentric, or peripheral foci.[412,413]

Because of their prominent vascular component, carcinoid tumors usually show marked enhancement on CT after the intravenous administration of contrast.[414] However, this finding does not allow reliable distinction of the neoplasm from pulmonary carcinoma. The neoplastic cells of carcinoid tumors have membrane receptors with high affinity for the

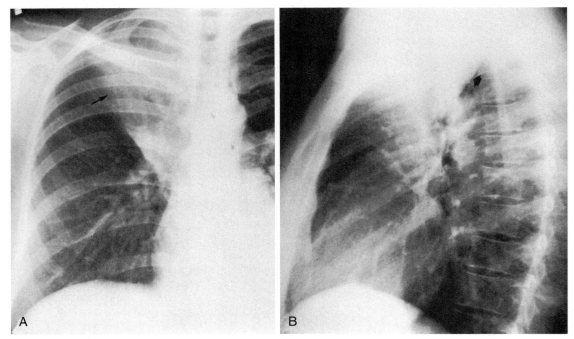

FIGURE 7–18

Carcinoid tumor. Views of the right hemithorax from posteroanterior (**A**) and lateral (**B**) radiographs demonstrate a roughly triangular shadow of homogeneous density occupying the superomedial portion of the right lung. The inferolateral border of the shadow is formed by the upwardly displaced minor fissure (*arrow* in **A**) and the posterior border of the anteriorly displaced major fissure (*arrow* in **B**). This shadow represents combined consolidation and atelectasis of the right upper lobe secondary to an endobronchial carcinoid tumor. The patient was a 30-year-old woman. (*From Fraser RS, Müller NL, Colman NC, Paré PD: Fraser and Paré's Diagnosis of Diseases of the Chest, 4th ed. Philadelphia, WB Saunders, 1999.*)

neuroregulatory peptide somatostatin.[415] Scintigraphy using a radiolabeled somatostatin analogue (^{123}I-octreotide) allows identification of both primary and metastatic tumors[415,416] and is thus a useful tool for staging and follow-up.[417] In fact, the procedure has been shown to be superior to FDG-PET imaging in assessment of these tumors.[418]

Atypical carcinoid tumors tend to be larger than typical tumors, sometimes attaining a huge size.[419] They are associated more often with hilar and mediastinal lymph node enlargement.[420]

Clinical Manifestations

The majority of central carcinoid tumors give rise to symptoms indicative of their bronchial origin,[421] the most common being cough and hemoptysis. Some patients have symptoms simulating asthma.[422] Physical signs depend on the degree of airway obstruction, the size of the bronchus obstructed, and whether infection has developed. As might be expected, peripheral tumors are not usually associated with signs and symptoms.

Despite the common presence of neuroendocrine substances on pathologic examination, clinical evidence of a paraneoplastic syndrome is distinctly uncommon. In most cases, extensive metastatic disease is necessary before signs and symptoms of such a complication appear,[423] possibly reflecting the need for adequate tumor bulk to produce sufficient amounts of active hormone. Nonetheless, serum levels of various tumor-related immunoreactive polypeptides are not

uncommonly elevated in the absence of clinical signs and symptoms.[424] Cushing's syndrome is the most frequent clinically evident paraneoplastic manifestation.[425-428] Acromegaly is also relatively common; it appears to be caused most often by tumor-related growth hormone–releasing factor acting directly on the pituitary.[429] Despite the name of the tumor, carcinoid syndrome is rare.[430] Occasional cases of pulmonary carcinoid tumor have been associated with endocrine neoplasia or hyperplasia elsewhere in the body, an association that has been considered to be part of the multiple endocrine neoplasia syndrome.[431]

Laboratory Findings and Diagnosis

In the investigation of carcinoid tumors, there is sometimes hesitancy in performing bronchoscopic biopsy because of the highly vascular nature of the lesions and the attendant risk of bleeding. However, most investigators have encountered no serious problems from hemorrhage after biopsy with either rigid or flexible bronchoscopes.[404,421] Our own inclination is generally to perform biopsy with appropriate precautions to control bleeding.

Cytologic examination of sputum or bronchial washings and brushings is often unrewarding as a result of intact bronchial epithelium overlying proximal tumors.[432] Obviously, transthoracic needle aspiration is more likely to yield cells suitable for cytologic interpretation.[433] Although the diagnosis should be suggested in both cytologic and biopsy specimens by cellular uniformity and bland nuclear features,

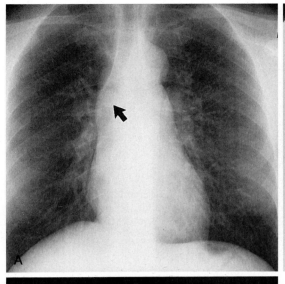

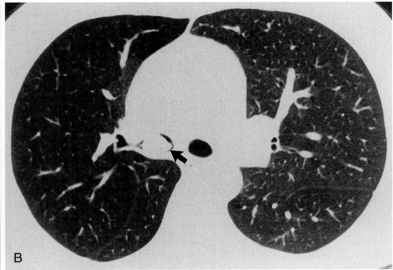

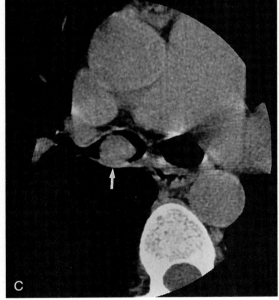

FIGURE 7–19

Typical carcinoid tumor—partial airway obstruction with hypoxic vasoconstriction. A posteroanterior chest radiograph (**A**) demonstrates a tumor in the right main bronchus (*arrow*). The right lung is slightly smaller than the left and shows decreased vascularity. HRCT (**B**) confirms the presence of tumor in the right main bronchus (*arrow*); decreased vascularity and decreased attenuation of the right lung in comparison to the left are evident, presumably as a result of reflex vasoconstriction. Soft tissue windows (**C**) demonstrate focal thickening of the posterior wall of the right main bronchus (*arrow*); there is no evidence of extrabronchial extension. *(From Fraser RS, Müller NL, Colman NC, Paré PD: Fraser and Paré's Diagnosis of Diseases of the Chest, 4th ed. Philadelphia, WB Saunders, 1999.)*

some tumors present diagnostic problems, especially the peripheral spindle cell and atypical variants. The greatest difficulty lies in the differentiation of carcinoid tumor from small cell carcinoma and in distinguishing typical from atypical forms.

Laboratory tests are helpful in the diagnosis of paraneoplastic syndromes. For example, carcinoid syndrome can be confirmed by demonstrating large amounts of 5-hydroxyindoleacetic acid (5-HIAA) and 5-hydroxytryptamine (serotonin) in urine. Intraoperative measurement of ACTH in pulmonary vessels by radioimmunoassay has been reported to be beneficial in identifying occult carcinoid tumors and ensuring adequate surgical excision.[434]

Prognosis and Natural History

The prognosis of typical carcinoid tumors is excellent. Some investigators have reported 10-year survival rates of about 90% to 95% (many patients probably dying of causes unrelated to the tumor itself),[394,404] whereas others have found 5- or 10-year survival rates of virtually 100%, even in the presence of lymph node metastases.[435,436] Even with visceral metastases, typical carcinoid tumors may be very slowly growing and associated with prolonged survival[430]; in fact, because of such slow growth, tumor recurrence may be seen many years after apparently curative resection, so follow-up must be prolonged.[437]

Despite these excellent statistics overall, it is clear that occasional histologically typical carcinoid tumors are associated with more concerning behavior. For example, in a retrospective investigation of 79 patients, the presence of an aggressive tumor (defined as one showing extension to the carina, involvement of regional lymph nodes, and/or vascular invasion) was found to be associated with a 5-year survival rate of approximately 50%[438]; 18% of these "aggressive" tumors were classified as typical according to standard histologic criteria.

As with pulmonary carcinoma, a variety of clinical and pathologic investigations have been undertaken to document criteria by which typical tumors that will metastasize can be distinguished from those that will not. Criteria that have been found to be associated with more aggressive behavior in at least some studies include a family history of cancer,[439] the presence of Cushing's syndrome,[440] aneuploidy on flow cytometric analysis,[441] and the degree of proliferative activity of a tumor as measured by the immunohistochemical reaction to Ki-67.[442]

In contrast to typical carcinoid tumor, tumors with atypical histologic features have a significantly worse prognosis. Approximately 50% to 70% of patients have lymph node metastases at the time of initial evaluation,[406,443] and the 5-year survival rate is about 40% to 70%, depending on the stage at diagnosis.[444-446]

Pulmonary Tumorlets and Neuroendocrine Cell Hyperplasia

The term *pulmonary tumorlet* refers to a minute, somewhat nodular proliferation of airway neuroendocrine cells that extends beyond the epithelium into the adjacent wall or lung parenchyma (Fig. 7–20). The term *neuroendocrine cell hyperplasia* is meant to describe a purely intraepithelial proliferation of the same cells (see Fig. 7–20). Both abnormalities are usually seen in association with concomitant pulmonary disease, the most common being bronchiectasis (tumorlet) and carcinoid tumor (neuroendocrine hyperplasia).[447,448]

Pulmonary tumorlets are generally found in older individuals,[449] although to some extent this tendency probably reflects the presence of coexistent lung disease and the fact that in many cases the lesions are discovered at autopsy. Because of

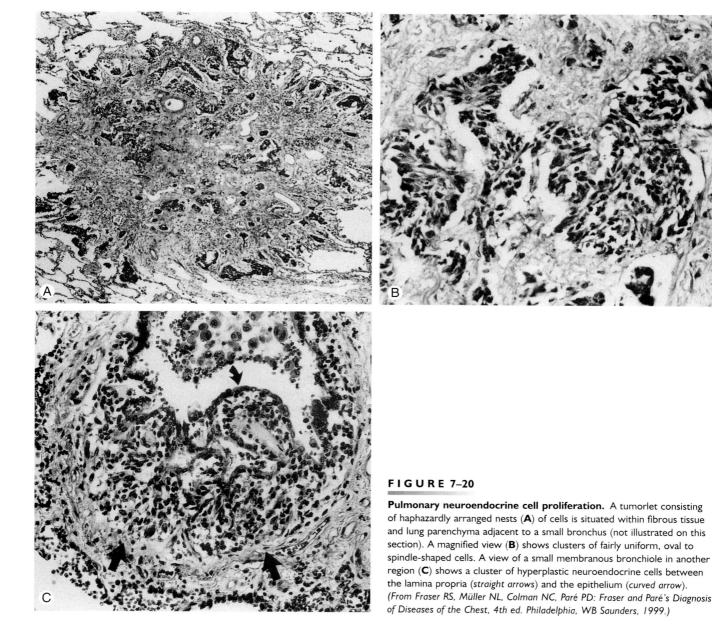

FIGURE 7–20

Pulmonary neuroendocrine cell proliferation. A tumorlet consisting of haphazardly arranged nests (**A**) of cells is situated within fibrous tissue and lung parenchyma adjacent to a small bronchus (not illustrated on this section). A magnified view (**B**) shows clusters of fairly uniform, oval to spindle-shaped cells. A view of a small membranous bronchiole in another region (**C**) shows a cluster of hyperplastic neuroendocrine cells between the lamina propria (*straight arrows*) and the epithelium (*curved arrow*). (*From Fraser RS, Müller NL, Colman NC, Paré PD: Fraser and Paré's Diagnosis of Diseases of the Chest, 4th ed. Philadelphia, WB Saunders, 1999.*)

their minute size, they are not usually apparent on the radiograph or CT scan; however, several cases have been reported in which numerous tumorlets increased sufficiently in size to be visible as minute nodules (Fig. 7–21).[450,451] In most cases, no clinical manifestations can be attributed to the neuroendocrine proliferation. However, cough and progressive dyspnea associated with obstructive pulmonary function changes have been reported in some patients.[452] Cushing's syndrome is another rare association.[453]

Miscellaneous Pulmonary Tumors Showing Neuroendocrine Differentiation

As indicated, the extent and severity of cytologic and architectural atypia vary in different neuroendocrine tumors. To maintain some semantic clarity, the term *atypical carcinoid* should be restricted to tumors that possess a focally recognizable neuroendocrine architecture but also display an increased mitotic rate and/or necrosis. However, it has been suggested that tumors with a mitotic rate greater than 10 per 10 high-power fields be separately categorized as a variant of large cell carcinoma (sometimes termed *large cell neuroendocrine carcinomas*).[454,455] It is possible that these various histologic subtypes represent a spectrum of differentiation, with large cell neuroendocrine carcinoma occupying a position between atypical carcinoid tumor and small cell carcinoma. Nevertheless, there is evidence that large and small cell tumors have molecular genetic features that differ from those of carcinoid tumors,[456] and it is possible that additional investigation may further justify separate classification. Whatever the fundamental nature of these large cell tumors, there is evidence that they have a more aggressive course than atypical carcinoid tumors have.[454,457]

MISCELLANEOUS EPITHELIAL TUMORS

Neoplasms of Tracheobronchial Glands

The observations that the morphology of the tracheobronchial mucous glands is similar to that of the oropharyngeal salivary

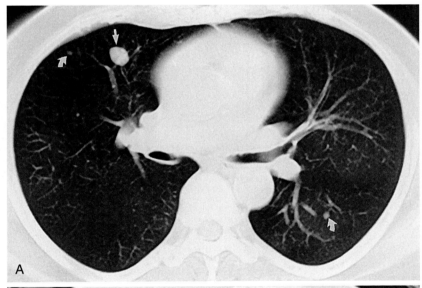

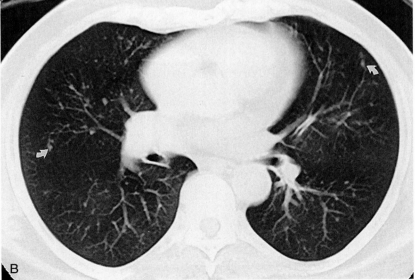

FIGURE 7–21

Carcinoid tumor associated with tumorlets and neuroendocrine cell hyperplasia. CT scans (**A** and **B**) demonstrate a 1.5-cm-diameter nodule in the right middle lobe (*straight arrow*), as well as several smaller nodules in both lungs (*curved arrows*). After a right middle lobectomy, the largest nodule was shown to represent a carcinoid tumor and the smaller nodules, tumorlets. Multiple foci of neuroendocrine cell hyperplasia were also evident and were associated with obstruction of several bronchioles. The patient was a 69-year-old woman with a history of shortness of breath. Pulmonary function tests showed an FEV$_1$/FVC ratio of 0.53 and a residual volume/TLC ratio of 0.56, but no impairment in gas transfer. (*Courtesy of Dr. R. McLean, Royal Alexandria Hospital, Edmonton, Canada.*)

glands and that neoplasms with an identical histologic appearance occur in both locations have led to the belief that a group of pulmonary tumors are derived from the glands themselves.[458] They are quite uncommon and account for no more than 0.1% to 0.2% of all tracheobronchial tumors.[459] The majority are classified as adenoid cystic or mucoepidermoid carcinoma[460]; acinic cell carcinoma, pleomorphic adenoma, oncocytoma, and mucous gland adenoma are seen rarely.

The great majority of these tumors arise in the trachea and proximal bronchi, and the diagnosis should be considered in anyone who has radiographic or endoscopic evidence of a polypoid intraluminal mass in these sites. Although the clinical features are not specific, a history of adult-onset "asthma" that has increased in severity despite adequate therapy should raise the possibility in the differential diagnosis.

The site of origin of a tracheal neoplasm strongly influences the clinical manifestations. Since the intrathoracic portion of the trachea dilates on inspiration and narrows on expiration, a lesion arising in this segment will be characterized clinically by expiratory airway obstruction and radiographically by expiratory air trapping. Conversely, the cervical portion of the trachea narrows on inspiration and dilates on expiration, so symptoms and signs of expiratory airway obstruction are lacking. A further indicator is the timing of a wheeze; with an intrathoracic tumor, a wheeze will occur on expiration, and with a cervical tumor, it will be evident on inspiration.

It is worth stressing that the presence of tracheal tumors is all too frequently overlooked on standard posteroanterior and lateral chest radiographs, the tracheal air column constituting a "blind area" for many radiologists (Fig. 17–22). Endotracheal neoplasms are frequently missed because of radiographic underexposure[461]; for this reason, the high-kilovoltage technique is strongly recommended. CT is often helpful in suspicious cases; for example, in a study of 35 patients who had focal or diffuse lesions of the trachea or main bronchi, the abnormalities were detected on the chest radiograph in 23 (66%) as opposed to 33 (94%) on CT.[462]

Adenoid Cystic Carcinoma

The most common variety of tracheobronchial gland neoplasm is adenoid cystic carcinoma, which accounts for about 75% to 80% of reported cases. In fact, along with squamous cell carcinoma, it is responsible for the vast majority of primary tumors of the trachea.[459,463] The majority arise in the lower or upper third, with a tendency to originate at the lateral and posterolateral wall near the junction of the cartilaginous and membranous portions. The mean age at diagnosis is 45 to 50 years.[464,465] Cigarette smoking does not appear to be an etiologic factor.[458]

The neoplasm characteristically grows into the airway lumen and forms a smooth-surfaced, somewhat polypoid mass (Fig. 7–23); occasionally, growth is circumferential and annular. Submucosal extension, sometimes to a considerable distance from the main tumor, is not uncommon. The overlying epithelium is usually intact. The typical histologic appearance consists of nests of uniform cells organized in a cribriform pattern.

The typical radiographic finding consists of a lobulated, polypoid mass that encroaches on the airway lumen to a variable degree (Fig. 7–24).[466] CT is superior to radiography in identifying the tumors and is particularly helpful in assessing the presence of extraluminal extent and mediastinal invasion.[462] Optimal assessment is obtained by using spiral CT with thin sections (2.5 mm or less) and multiplanar or three-dimensional reformations.[467,468]

Clinical features consist of cough, hoarseness, hemoptysis, dyspnea, wheeze, and recurrent pneumonitis. As indicated previously, a history of "asthma" is not uncommon, sometimes progressing in severity despite therapy. Endoscopy typically reveals a smooth-surfaced, sometimes lobulated tumor partly or completely occluding the airway lumen.

The prognosis is much better than that of the more common forms of pulmonary carcinoma.[459,469] For example, the overall 5-year survival rate in one relatively recent review was 80%.[470] Distant metastases are relatively uncommon, and death is usually the result of local recurrence and intrathoracic complications.

Mucoepidermoid Carcinoma

Mucoepidermoid carcinoma is the second most common form of tracheobronchial gland neoplasm.[471,472] It can develop from childhood to old age; however, a substantial number are discovered in individuals younger than 20.[471,473] Although a history of cigarette smoking has been noted by some authors,[474] it is usually absent.

The lesion is generally considered to occur in two clinicopathologic forms:[471] (1) those that have minimal nuclear pleomorphism, few mitotic figures, and a benign clinical course and (2) those that are cytologically more atypical and have a relatively aggressive course. Most tumors are situated in a main or lobar bronchus and grow within the airway lumen as a polypoid mass. Low-grade forms are often confined to the bronchial wall, whereas high-grade ones not uncommonly extend into the adjacent lung parenchyma. As the name suggests, the tumors are composed of cells that show both glandular (typically producing mucus) and "epidermoid" features.

The radiographic findings are related to tumor location and size and may consist of a solitary nodule or mass, lobar or segmental consolidation or atelectasis, or a central mass with associated obstructive pneumonitis or atelectasis.[471,475] On CT scan, the tumors are usually smoothly oval or lobulated[475]; punctate calcification within the tumor is evident in 50% of cases. Occasionally, a tumor involves the trachea rather than the bronchi and is manifested as a polypoid intraluminal nodule on radiograph and CT scan.[476]

As might be expected, symptoms are related predominantly to growth in the airway wall and lumen and include cough, hemoptysis, wheeze, recurrent pneumonia, and fever. Low-grade tumors are typically slow growing; the prognosis is usually excellent, with no evidence of local recurrence or metastases, even when treated with relatively conservative sleeve resection.[471,472] The behavior of the high-grade form, though worse than that of low-grade tumors, appears to be better than the more common forms of pulmonary carcinoma; of 13 patients with follow-up in one series, 8 were alive without evidence of disease at an average of 48 months after surgery.[471]

Tracheobronchial Papillomas

A *papilloma* can be defined as a branching or coarsely lobulated tumor composed of epithelium-lined fibrovascular

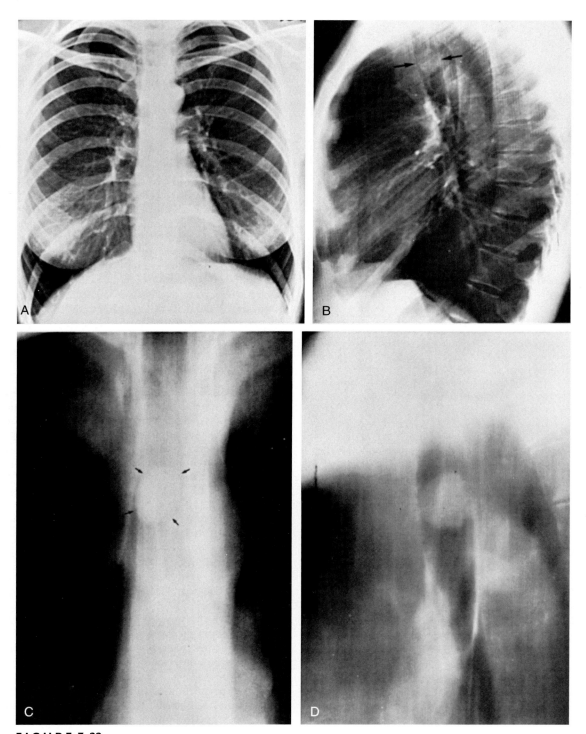

FIGURE 7–22

Mucoepidermoid carcinoma. At the time of the radiograph illustrated in **A,** this 32-year-old woman had a 4-year history of sporadic attacks of acute shortness of breath that had been diagnosed and treated by her family physician as spasmodic asthma. A number of radiographic examinations of the chest during this period had been interpreted as normal. This posteroanterior radiograph reveals mild to moderate overinflation of both lungs, consistent with a diagnosis of asthma. However, note that the mediastinum is intolerably underexposed, to a point at which the tracheal air column is not visible. In lateral projection (**B**), a smooth, sharply demarcated mass can be identified in the plane of the tracheal air column (*arrows*). Tomographic sections of the mediastinum in anteroposterior (**C**) and lateral (**D**) projection show the mass to lie within the trachea approximately 3 cm proximal to the carina (*arrows* in **C**). The mass is almost completely occluding the tracheal air column. After resection, the patient experienced an uneventful recovery. This case graphically illustrates the often-repeated observation that the tracheal air column tends to be a "blind area" for many radiologists. (*Courtesy of Dr. Michael Lefcoe, Victoria Hospital, London, Ontario.*)

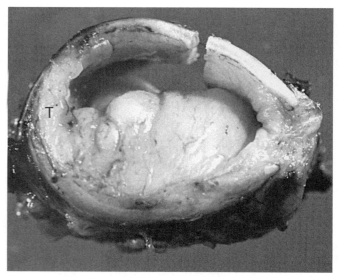

FIGURE 7–23

Adenoid cystic carcinoma. A magnified view of a cross section of the midportion of the trachea shows a somewhat lobulated tumor almost completely obstructing the lumen. The surface of the neoplasm is smooth, thus suggesting that it is composed of intact tracheal epithelium. Although tumor is present in the lateral tracheal wall (T), it does not appear to extend into the adjacent soft tissue. *(From Fraser RS, Müller NL, Colman NC, Paré PD: Fraser and Paré's Diagnosis of Diseases of the Chest, 4th ed. Philadelphia, WB Saunders, 1999.)*

papillae that arise from and project above an epithelial surface. Although such tumors within the lungs can be histologically classified into several types, depending largely on the nature of the surface lining,[477] from a clinical and radiologic point of view they are best considered under the headings "multiple" and "solitary."

Multiple Papillomas

Multiple papillomas of the respiratory tract occur most commonly in the larynx of children between 18 months and 3 years of age.[478] In the majority of patients, they remain localized to this site and eventually disappear spontaneously. In about 2% to 5% of cases, they also develop in the lower respiratory tract, where they can cause partial or complete airway obstruction.[478] Most such cases are limited to the trachea; however, extension into the bronchi, bronchioles, and even lung parenchyma can occur. In one review, the average time between the appearance of lesions in the larynx and detection of bronchopulmonary disease was 10 years.[479] Rarely, bronchial papillomas precede the appearance of laryngeal or tracheal lesions or develop in their absence.[480] The vast majority, if not all papillomas are caused by human papillomavirus, most commonly type 11.[481]

Pathologically, the tumors consist of sessile or pedunculated papillary growths lined by a flattened squamous epithelium that usually shows normal maturation.[477] Multinucleation and cytoplasmic vacuolation resembling the changes seen in condylomas of the genital tract can be found in some cases. Involvement of the distal airways or alveolar air spaces may result in solid or cavitated masses measuring up to several centimeters in diameter.[482]

Papillomas may be identified on the radiograph and CT as small nodules projecting into the lumen of the airway.[466] Larger nodules that obstruct the airway lumen may be associated with atelectasis, obstructive pneumonitis, and bronchiectasis.[483] On CT, numerous papillomas may be manifested as diffuse nodular thickening of the tracheal wall.[484] Involvement of the distal airways and parenchyma can result in multiple, sharply circumscribed nodules.[485] They may grow to several centimeters in diameter, at which point they frequently become cavitated and have walls measuring 2 to 3 mm in thickness (Fig. 7–25).[466] Many of these cavities are related to papillomatosis; however, they may be caused by a necrotic squamous cell carcinoma or an abscess secondary to obstructive pneumonitis.[486,487]

The diagnosis should be suspected in any patient with a history of laryngeal papillomas in whom cough, hemoptysis, asthma-like symptoms, recurrent pneumonia, or atelectasis develops. The prognosis is good in most patients who have solely laryngeal disease. However, it is worse in those with involvement of the lower respiratory tract, particularly when extensive; in such patients, progressive airway obstruction and parenchymal infiltration can result in increasing dyspnea, pulmonary fibrosis, and ultimately death. There is also a risk of malignant transformation, usually into squamous cell carcinoma.[478,488]

Solitary Papillomas

Solitary papillomas of the tracheobronchial tree are less common than the multiple form. They occur almost invariably in adults, often middle-aged or older and usually men.[477,489,490] Some investigators have found the presence of human papillomavirus in a large proportion of cases.[491]

Solitary papillomas are generally located in lobar or segmental bronchi, where they appear as finely corrugated tumors 0.5 to 1.5 cm in diameter (Fig. 7–26). Most are histologically identical to those seen in the multiple form and consist of mature squamous epithelium lining thin fibrovascular cores. Cytologic atypia and carcinoma in situ may also be seen, either in the papillary tumor itself or in the adjacent airway epithelium[477]; occasionally, clearly invasive squamous cell carcinoma is present.

The radiologic manifestations depend on the size and location of the papilloma. Many lesions that occur in the trachea or main bronchi measure less than 1 cm in diameter and are not detected on the chest radiograph.[462] When radiologic and CT findings are evident, they usually consist of a polypoid mass projecting into the airway lumen.[466,476] Partial bronchial obstruction may result in reflex vasoconstriction leading to decreased perfusion and hyperlucency of the affected lung or lobe. Complete obstruction is manifested by atelectasis and obstructive pneumonitis.

A history of repeated or unresolved pneumonia may be obtained; hemoptysis is seen occasionally. Sometimes the tumor appears to undergo auto-amputation at the site of its attachment to the airway wall, in which case the papilloma may be coughed up and the pneumonia cleared. As indicated, some papillomas are complicated by the development of dysplasia or carcinoma.[491]

Pulmonary Adenomas

True adenomas of the lung are rare. Some occur predominantly in the proximal airways and are believed to arise from the

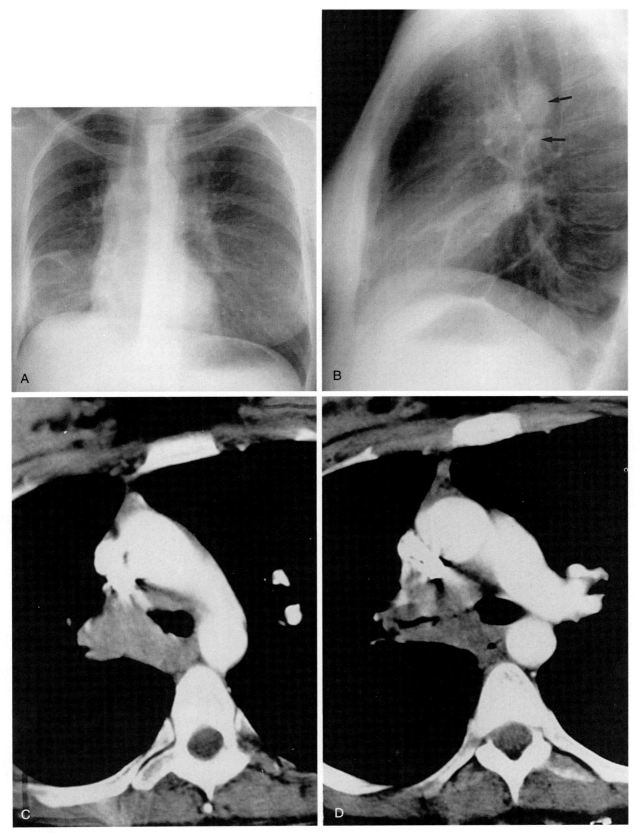

FIGURE 7–24

Adenoid cystic carcinoma. Posteroanterior and lateral chest radiographs (**A** and **B**) in a 27-year-old man with progressive shortness of breath demonstrate areas of atelectasis in the right lower and middle lobes. The lateral radiograph also shows thickening of the posterior wall of the distal end of the trachea and right main bronchus (*arrows*). Contrast-enhanced CT scans (**C** and **D**) demonstrate circumferential tumor at the level of the tracheal carina and right main and right upper lobe bronchi associated with narrowing of the lumen. Focal extension into the left main bronchus is also evident. (*From Fraser RS, Müller NL, Colman NC, Paré PD: Fraser and Paré's Diagnosis of Diseases of the Chest, 4th ed. Philadelphia, WB Saunders, 1999.*)

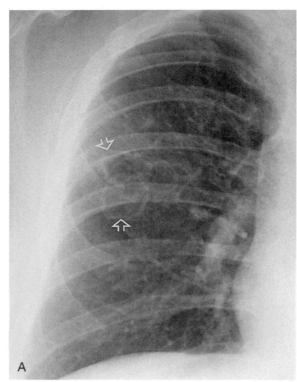

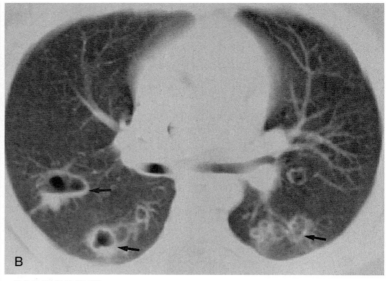

FIGURE 7–25

Tracheobronchial papillomatosis. A view of the right lung from a posteroanterior chest radiograph (**A**) reveals several thin-walled cavities (*arrows*). Similar findings were present in the left lung. A CT scan (**B**) demonstrates bilateral thin-walled cavities, several of which contain air-fluid levels (*arrows*). The patient was a 31-year-old woman with long-standing papillomatosis. (*Case courtesy of Dr. Jim Barrie, University of Alberta Hospital, Edmonton, Alberta.*)

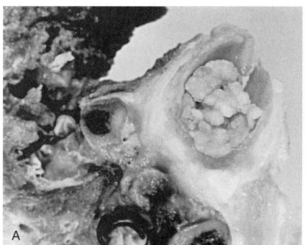

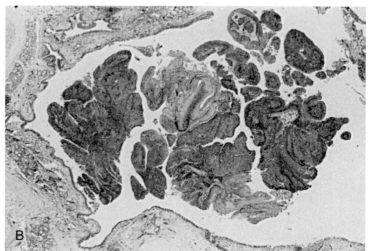

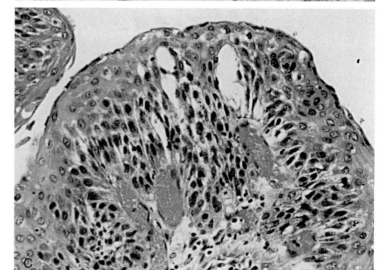

FIGURE 7–26

Solitary bronchial papilloma. A lower lobe bronchus (**A**) is almost completely occluded by a coarsely lobulated tumor confined to the airway lumen. Histologic sections at two different magnifications (**B** and **C**) show branching papillary projections lined by stratified squamous epithelium; there is mild cytologic atypia in the basal layer. Although this tumor was solitary, an identical histologic appearance is seen in the multiple form. (*From Fraser RS, Müller NL, Colman NC, Paré PD: Fraser and Paré's Diagnosis of Diseases of the Chest, 4th ed. Philadelphia, WB Saunders, 1999.*)

tracheobronchial mucous glands; such tumors include pleomorphic, oxyphilic, and mucous gland adenomas. Others are located predominantly in the lung periphery and appear to be derived from bronchiolar or alveolar epithelium. These tumors include (1) mucinous cystic tumor (mucinous cystadenoma), an unusual lesion that has been hypothesized to represent a spectrum of neoplasia analogous to mucinous tumors of the appendix and ovary[492]; (2) papillary and alveolar adenomas, probably derived from type II and/or Clara cells[493,494]; and (3) pneumocytoma (sclerosing hemangioma; see page 400).

LYMPHOPROLIFERATIVE DISORDERS AND LEUKEMIA

Pulmonary Lymphoid Hyperplasia

Focal Lymphoid Hyperplasia (Pseudolymphoma)

Focal lymphoid hyperplasia (nodular lymphoid hyperplasia, pseudolymphoma) is an uncommon abnormality characterized histologically by a localized proliferation of cytologically mature mononuclear cells (usually a mixture of lymphocytes, plasma cells, and histiocytes).[495] The biologic nature of these proliferations has been debated. At the present time, it is widely believed that the majority are neoplastic. However, occasional cases appear to be truly hyperplastic[496]; it is also possible that some are analogous to the dysplasia seen in many epithelia before the development of invasive carcinoma.

The most frequent radiologic manifestations consist of a solitary nodule or a focal area of consolidation limited to one lobe.[497,498] The tumors usually measure 2 to 5 cm in diameter,[495] although masses and areas of consolidation measuring 10 cm in diameter have been described.[499] Virtually all lesions contain air bronchograms. Less common manifestations include multiple nodules or multiple areas of consolidation and cavitation.[498] The presence of lymphadenopathy or pleural effusion should suggest the possibility of lymphoma.[497]

Most lesions are identified in adults, the majority of whom are asymptomatic.[500] Some patients have cough or hemoptysis,[496] and about 10% to 15% have evidence of an underlying autoimmune abnormality such as Sjögren's syndrome or systemic lupus erythematosus. Because of the polymorphous histologic nature of the lesion, diagnosis usually requires surgical excision with thorough histologic sampling and appropriate immunohistochemical and molecular analysis to exclude lymphoma. The prognosis of patients who have well-documented lymphoid hyperplasia is generally excellent; however, local recurrence and frank lymphoma eventually occur in some cases, and close follow-up is advisable.

Lymphoid Interstitial Pneumonia

Two varieties of diffuse pulmonary lymphoid hyperplasia have been described, depending on their anatomic localization, the first affecting predominantly the parenchymal interstitium (lymphoid or lymphocytic interstitial pneumonia [LIP]) and the second predominantly the interstitium adjacent to conducting airways (follicular bronchitis and bronchiolitis).[501] LIP is the more common of the two abnormalities. As with focal lymphoid hyperplasia, it is clear from immunologic,

immunohistochemical, and molecular studies that some lesions are in fact low-grade lymphoma.[501-503] It is not known whether cases that initially appear to be reactive and that subsequently come to be recognized as lymphoma represent a premalignant condition or a malignancy that is difficult to diagnose at the outset.[503,504]

The etiology and pathogenesis are probably varied. The possibility that it represents an immunologic disorder is supported by the observation that many cases are associated with other conditions characterized by abnormalities in immune function, the most common of which are Sjögren's syndrome and AIDS.[505,506] There is evidence that some cases may be caused by a virus, such as Epstein-Barr virus, ovine lentivirus (an organism related to HIV), or HIV itself.[507,508] It has also been speculated that some cases may represent lymphocyte-rich examples of extrinsic allergic alveolitis.[501]

Pathologically, LIP is characterized by a more or less diffuse interstitial infiltrate of mononuclear cells, in the typical case predominantly lymphocytes (Fig. 7–27).[509] Although the infiltrate is prominent in the alveolar interstitium, involvement of interstitial tissue adjacent to small vessels and airways is common. There is minimal nuclear atypia. Air spaces are uninvolved by the infiltrate, although focal bronchiolar

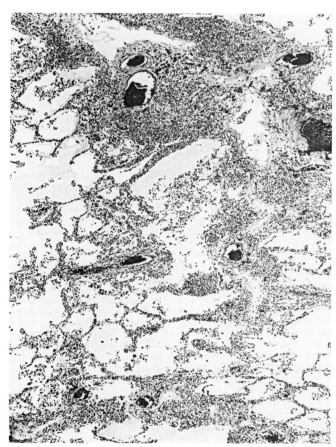

FIGURE 7–27

Lymphoid interstitial pneumonia. A variable, but overall moderately severe infiltrate of mononuclear inflammatory cells is present in perivascular and alveolar interstitial tissue. The cells were seen on higher magnification to be mostly mature lymphocytes, with occasional plasma cells. *(From Fraser RS, Müller NL, Colman NC, Paré PD: Fraser and Paré's Diagnosis of Diseases of the Chest, 4th ed. Philadelphia, WB Saunders, 1999.)*

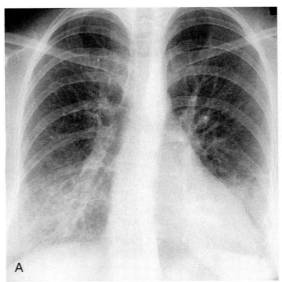
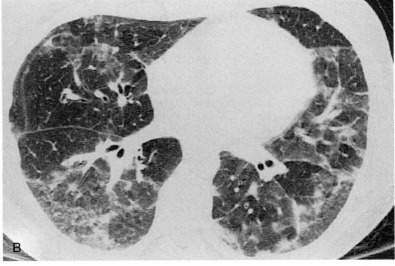

FIGURE 7–28

Lymphoid interstitial pneumonia. A posteroanterior chest radiograph (**A**) in a 26-year-old woman with rheumatoid arthritis demonstrates bilateral areas of ground-glass opacity and consolidation involving the lower lung zones. An HRCT scan at the level of the inferior pulmonary veins (**B**) demonstrates extensive bilateral areas of ground-glass attenuation and focal areas of consolidation. (*From Fraser RS, Müller NL, Colman NC, Paré PD: Fraser and Paré's Diagnosis of Diseases of the Chest, 4th ed. Philadelphia, WB Saunders, 1999.*)

obstruction can result in findings of obstructive pneumonitis. The diagnosis of a reactive process is supported by the presence of polyclonality on immunohistochemical and molecular analysis.

The most common radiographic findings consist of a reticular or reticulonodular pattern involving mainly the lower lung zones.[509,510] In some cases, branching and linear opacities consistent with interlobular septal thickening have been described in the lung periphery[511]; however, such thickening is more likely to be seen with lymphoma. Other radiographic patterns include bilateral areas of ground-glass opacity and consolidation (Fig. 7–28).[512,513] A nodular pattern may also occur,[510] most commonly in patients who have AIDS.[497,514] Hilar and mediastinal lymph node enlargement has been described in patients with AIDS,[514] but seldom in others. Pleural effusion is rare.

The most common abnormalities on HRCT consist of bilateral areas of ground-glass attenuation (see Fig. 7–28) and poorly defined centrilobular nodules; other findings include subpleural nodules, thickening of the bronchovascular bundles, and cysts.[512,515] The nodules usually measure less than 10 mm in diameter. Mediastinal lymph node enlargement has been reported in approximately two thirds of patients.[515]

The majority of patients who have LIP are adults, except in patients with AIDS, who are more often children.[509] Dyspnea and cough are the major complaints. Some patients also have systemic symptoms such as fever, weight loss, and arthralgias. Cyanosis and clubbing were present in roughly half the patients described in one study.[516] Hypergammaglobulinemia—usually both IgG and IgM—is common.[509]

The prognosis depends to some extent on the nature of the underlying disease. Patients who have AIDS often die of infectious or neoplastic abnormalities associated with their underlying disease rather than LIP itself; however, about a third experience progressive respiratory failure.[517] Some individuals not affected by AIDS also have progression of the pulmonary disease, sometimes associated with fibrosis and an evolution similar to that of idiopathic pulmonary fibrosis; in others, the disease evolves into clear-cut lymphoma.[518]

Follicular Bronchitis and Bronchiolitis

Follicular bronchitis and bronchiolitis are histologically characterized by a mononuclear cell infiltrate (again predominantly lymphocytes, with lesser numbers of plasma cells and histiocytes) in the interstitial tissue adjacent to bronchi and bronchioles. As the name suggests, germinal center formation is common and results in a distinctly nodular appearance of the abnormality (Fig. 7–29).[519] As with LIP, many patients have a history of an underlying immunodeficiency disorder or connective tissue disease, particularly Sjögren's syndrome or rheumatoid arthritis (principally the juvenile form).

The chest radiograph characteristically shows a diffuse reticular or reticulonodular pattern.[519] HRCT scan reveals small nodular opacities in a peribronchovascular, centrilobular, and subpleural distribution.[520] In most cases, these opacities measure 1 to 3 mm in diameter (Fig. 7–30), although focal opacities as large as 1 cm in diameter may be seen.

The most common clinical finding is progressive shortness of breath[519,521]; cough, fever, and recurrent pneumonia are occasionally present. Leukocytosis with prominent eosinophilia is seen in some patients.[519] Pulmonary function studies reveal evidence of obstruction, restriction, or combined restriction and obstruction.[519]

Pulmonary Lymphoma

The most frequent radiologic manifestation of thoracic involvement by lymphoma is mediastinal lymph node

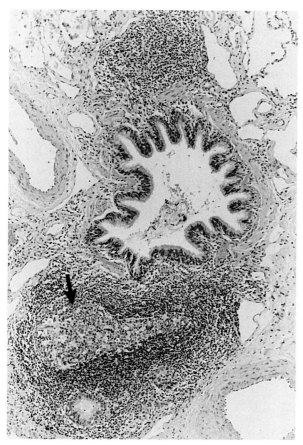

FIGURE 7–29

Follicular bronchiolitis. The interstitial tissue adjacent to a membranous bronchiole is expanded by an infiltrate of lymphoid cells, focally with germinal center formation (*arrow*). Similar disease was present in relation to many other bronchioles. The patient had rheumatoid disease. (*From Fraser RS, Müller NL, Colman NC, Paré PD: Fraser and Paré's Diagnosis of Diseases of the Chest, 4th ed. Philadelphia, WB Saunders, 1999.*)

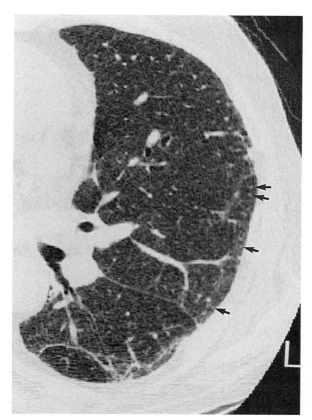

FIGURE 7–30

Follicular bronchiolitis. A view of the left lung from an HRCT scan demonstrates centrilobular subpleural nodules measuring 1 to 3 mm in diameter (*arrows*). Evidence of mild fibrosis with irregular linear opacities and thickening of interlobular septa, particularly in the left lower lobe, is also noted. The patient was a 64-year-old man with progressive systemic sclerosis. (*From Fraser RS, Müller NL, Colman NC, Paré PD: Fraser and Paré's Diagnosis of Diseases of the Chest, 4th ed. Philadelphia, WB Saunders, 1999.*)

enlargement. Although such enlargement is usually an isolated finding, evidence of pulmonary disease is also evident in some patients. Such cases, as well as those with concomitant or previous lymphoma involving lymph nodes outside the thorax, we arbitrarily designate as secondary pulmonary lymphoma. Occasionally, lymphoma appears clinically and radiologically to be limited to the lungs or to affect the lungs and extrathoracic organs with little or no evidence of lymph node involvement. Such tumors, which are sometimes termed *primary pulmonary lymphoma*, account for only 3% to 4% of all extranodal lymphomas.[522,523] Although a variety of histologic subtypes can be seen,[523] the most common are MALT lymphoma, lymphomatoid granulomatosis, and large B-cell lymphoma (the latter most commonly in patients who have AIDS or organ transplants [see pages 438 and 531]). Because these tumors are more likely to be confused with other conditions, it is useful to consider them separately.

MALT Lymphoma

Some primary extranodal lymphomas, including many that arise in the lung, are thought to be derived from mucosa-associated lymphoid tissue (MALT)—hence the terms *extranodal marginal-zone B-cell lymphoma of mucosa-associated lymphoid tissue* and *MALT lymphoma* (MALToma) that are used to describe them.[524,525] This histologic subtype is the most frequent to involve the lungs as a primary tumor, accounting for between 70% and 90% of such neoplasms in various series.[500,522,523] The vast majority occur in adults, with a mean age at diagnosis of about 55 to 60 years.

The etiology and pathogenesis are uncertain. It has been speculated that some environmental stimulus, such as cigarette smoke or infection, leads to MALT hyperplasia, which is then followed by neoplastic transformation.[526] However, many patients are nonsmokers, and histologic evidence of focal or diffuse lymphoid hyperplasia is evident only occasionally,[522] in which case there is usually a history of an immunologic abnormality such as rheumatoid disease or Sjögren's syndrome. The lymphoma does not appear to have any association with Epstein-Barr virus.[527]

Pathologic Characteristics. Grossly, MALT lymphoma usually appears as a solitary well-circumscribed nodule or an ill-defined area of consolidation involving part of a lobe (see Color Fig. 7–12).[522,526] Malignant cells are found predominantly within interstitial tissue, a feature seen most clearly at the periphery of the tumor in relation to bronchovascular bundles and interlobular septa (see Color Fig. 7–12). In the central portion of the nodule/consolidation, expansion and confluence of the interstitial infiltrate and invasion into air spaces frequently result in a more or less solid appearance. Tumor cells consist of small lymphocyte-like cells that have relatively uniform nuclei and small nucleoli; plasmacytoid differentiation may be seen. Infiltration of airway epithelium ("lymphoepithelial lesions") is common. Immunohistochemical analysis shows B-cell differentiation.[526]

Because the degree of cytologic atypia is usually slight and because of the admixture of normal inflammatory cells and germinal centers in some cases, the diagnosis may be difficult to make on the basis of the histologic appearance alone, particularly in small biopsy specimens.[522] In such cases, identification of light chain restriction by molecular study is generally accepted as an indicator of malignancy.[528,529]

Radiologic Manifestations. The most common radiologic manifestation consists of nodules or nodular areas of consolidation.[530,531] The nodules vary from 2 mm to 8 cm in diameter and may be single or, more commonly, multiple. The areas of consolidation range from a small subsegmental region to an entire lobe and may be single or multiple.[532] Both the nodules and the areas of consolidation are usually centered on the airways. Air bronchograms are visible in most cases

(Fig. 7–31).[530,533] Less common abnormalities seen on CT include peribronchovascular interstitial thickening, septal lines, and ground-glass opacities.[530] Pleural effusion is present in 10% to 20% of cases, usually in association with evidence of parenchymal involvement.[531] Lymph node enlargement is radiographically evident in less than 5% of cases[500] and on CT in as many as 10%.[534] The parenchymal abnormalities typically show an indolent course with slow growth over a period of months or years.[535]

Clinical Manifestations. Approximately 40% to 50% of patients are asymptomatic when first seen, their disease being discovered on a screening chest radiograph.[523] When present, pulmonary symptoms include cough, dyspnea, and (less commonly) chest pain and hemoptysis. Systemic symptoms such as fever, night sweats, or weight loss are present in 20% to 40% of patients[523]; although these symptoms may be seen with localized disease, they should suggest the possibility of extrathoracic involvement. Bone marrow involvement is apparent in 15% to 20% of cases.

Laboratory Findings. Fiberoptic bronchoscopy may reveal airway stenosis, and biopsy may yield sufficient tissue for diagnosis. The diagnosis can also be made by cytologic examination of bronchial washings or transthoracic needle aspiration specimens[536,537]; however, the use of flow cytometry, molecular analysis, and immunohistochemistry to characterize the lymphoid cells and demonstrate monoclonality is

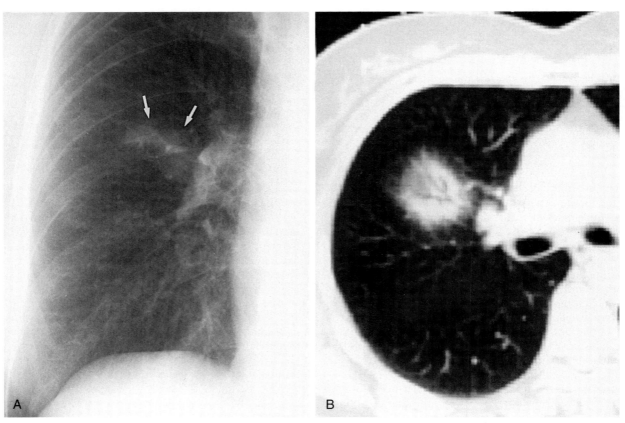

FIGURE 7–31

MALT lymphoma. Close-up views of the right lung from a posteroanterior chest radiograph (**A**) and a conventional CT scan (**B**) demonstrate a 3-cm area of consolidation in the right upper lobe (*arrows*). An air bronchogram is clearly visible on the CT scan. The patient was a 68-year-old woman. (*From Fraser RS, Müller NL, Colman NC, Paré PD: Fraser and Paré's Diagnosis of Diseases of the Chest, 4th ed. Philadelphia, WB Saunders, 1999.*)

usually necessary. Occasionally, serum immunoelectrophoresis shows a monoclonal gammopathy, typically IgM and associated with tumors that have prominent plasmacytoid differentiation.[523] The blood leukocyte count and differential are usually within normal limits.

Prognosis and Natural History. MALT lymphoma has a relatively favorable prognosis.[538,539] For example, in a study of 43 patients, the overall 5-year survival rate was 84%, a value equivalent to that of a control population[523]; however, patients who had systemic symptoms such as fever, night sweats, or weight loss had a 5-year survival rate of about 55%. Occasional cases are complicated by the development of high-grade B-cell lymphoma within or outside the lung, sometimes many years after diagnosis of the pulmonary tumor.[522,523] The development of MALT lymphoma in extrapulmonary mucosal sites, particularly the stomach and upper respiratory tract, has also been noted in a number of patients[540] either before or after appearance of the pulmonary tumor.

Lymphomatoid Granulomatosis

Lymphomatoid granulomatosis (angiocentric immunoproliferative lesion) is an uncommon disorder characterized histologically by a polymorphic lymphoreticular infiltrate that shows prominent vascular infiltration (Fig. 7–32).[525,541] The condition has been subdivided into three types (grades). Grade 1 lesions consist predominantly of small lymphocytes and rare cytologically atypical large lymphoid cells. Grade 2 lesions consist of a polymorphous infiltrate of lymphocytes, plasma cells, histiocytes, and a variable number of large, cytologically atypical cells. The last-named cells are numerous in grade 3 lesions, resulting in a more or less monomorphous infiltrate that is usually readily identifiable as lymphoma.[542] Vascular infiltration by the lymphoid cells is common and is probably responsible for the necrosis that is frequently seen in the central portion of the lesions. Immunophenotypic and molecular analysis of the atypical cells in grade 2 and 3 tumors has shown them to have a B-cell phenotype[543] and a strong association with Epstein-Barr virus infection.[543,544]

The most common radiologic manifestation is one of multiple nodules or masses 0.5 to 8 cm in diameter.[545,546] In some patients, the initial abnormality consists of poorly defined opacities, which then progress over a period of many weeks to form nodules or masses. The nodules frequently have ill-defined margins and show a tendency to coalesce (Fig. 7–33);

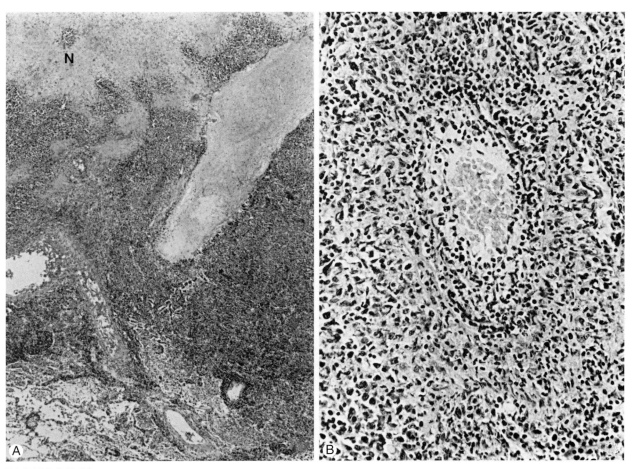

FIGURE 7–32

Lymphomatoid granulomatosis. A section of a grossly poorly defined lung nodule (**A**) shows a diffuse lymphoid infiltrate effacing the normal lung architecture. Prominent necrosis is apparent (N). The limits of the wall of a small pulmonary artery (**B**) are hardly recognizable as a result of marked cellular infiltration. *(From Fraser RS, Müller NL, Colman NC, Paré PD: Fraser and Paré's Diagnosis of Diseases of the Chest, 4th ed. Philadelphia, WB Saunders, 1999.)*

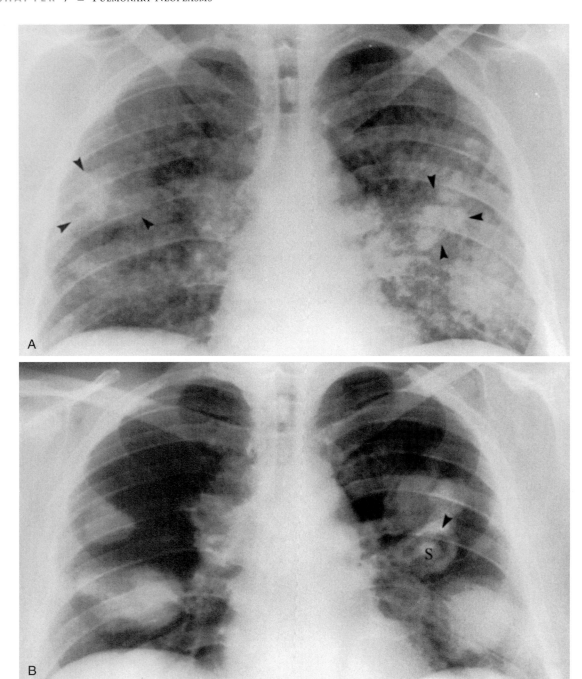

FIGURE 7–33

Lymphomatoid granulomatosis. A posteroanterior chest radiograph (**A**) demonstrates bilateral confluent and isolated nodular opacities; some of the larger opacities (*arrowheads*) possess features of air space consolidation. Bilateral hilar lymph node enlargement is present, and the aortopulmonary window is prominent, findings suggestive of mediastinal node involvement. Two months later, a repeat chest radiograph (**B**) shows that the diffuse disease has resolved but has been replaced by large cavitary and noncavitary nodules. One cavitary lesion on the left (*arrowhead*) contains a central loose body (S) that could represent necrotic tissue or a blood clot. Several of the nodules relate to the more confluent areas of consolidation identified in **A.** The patient was a 52-year-old man. *(From Fraser RS, Müller NL, Colman NC, Paré PD: Fraser and Paré's Diagnosis of Diseases of the Chest, 4th ed. Philadelphia, WB Saunders, 1999.)*

although they may be diffuse throughout both lungs, they tend to be most numerous in the lower lung zones.[545] Cavitation is present in 30% to 40% of patients.[545,547] On CT, the nodules are typically located along the bronchovascular structures and interlobular septa.[546] Other less common findings include areas of consolidation, a reticulonodular pattern, and pleural effusion.[545,547] Lymph node enlargement is seldom evident on the radiograph; however, it is not uncommon on CT.[546]

Most patients are between 40 and 60 years of age.[541,548] Thoracic symptoms (cough, dyspnea, chest pain) and systemic complaints (fever, weight loss, malaise) are present in the majority at the time of diagnosis. Neurologic manifestations—consisting of signs of cerebral involvement and cranial and peripheral neuropathies—are present in 30% of patients, and cutaneous disease—manifested by either an erythematous rash or skin nodules—is present in 40%.[541,549] Clinical evidence of involvement of lymph nodes, liver, and spleen is unusual, except in the late stage of disease.

The prognosis is variable. As might be expected, patients who have grade 1 lesions generally do well, whereas those with higher-grade lesions usually fare much worse. In one series, approximately two thirds of the latter patients died, with a median survival time of only 14 months[541]; in another, the 5-year survival rate was approximately 20%.[550] In many instances, death is related to progressive pulmonary or central nervous system disease.

Secondary Non-Hodgkin's Pulmonary Lymphoma

Pulmonary involvement by lymphoma in patients known to have disease outside the thorax is much more common than primary disease. It is radiographically apparent in about 5% of cases at initial evaluation[551]; in one series of 651 patients, 54 (8%) had histologically documented involvement.[552] As with carcinoma, such disease can develop by direct spread from involved mediastinal or hilar lymph nodes or by intravascular dissemination (metastasis). Any of the histologic subtypes of lymphoma can be responsible. Grossly, tumors can appear as solitary or multiple parenchymal nodules, segmental or lobar consolidation, or interstitial thickening resembling lymphangitic carcinomatosis (Fig. 7–34).

The typical radiographic pattern consists of solitary or multiple nodules or masses 0.5 to 8 cm in diameter.[551,553] They are usually most frequent in the lower lobes (Fig. 7–35).[554] The nodules are round, ovoid, or polyhedral and generally possess poorly defined margins, sometimes with linear strands extending into the adjacent lung parenchyma. Cavitation occurs rarely.[555] In contrast to primary pulmonary lymphoma, the secondary variety tends to affect the larger airways (in most cases probably reflecting extension from bronchopulmonary lymph nodes) and may result in atelectasis and obstructive pneumonitis. A diffuse reticulonodular pattern with thickening of the interlobar septa resembling

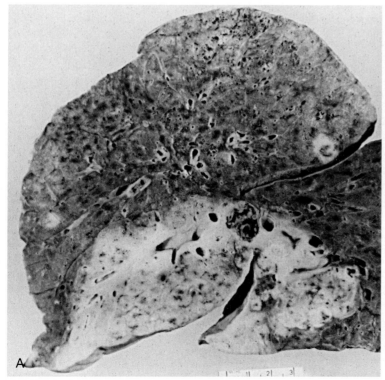
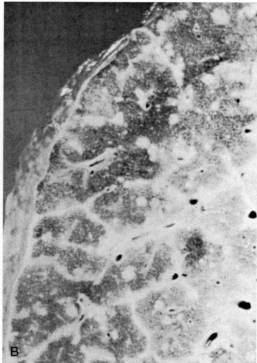

FIGURE 7–34

Secondary pulmonary lymphoma. A section of right lung removed at autopsy (**A**) reveals two small parenchymal nodules in the upper lobe and diffuse consolidation of most of the middle lobe and the anterior basal segment of the lower lobe. A magnified view of the anterior portion of a slice of upper lobe from another patient (**B**) shows thickening of interlobular septal and perivascular interstitial tissue. Both patients had disseminated large B-cell lymphoma. *(From Fraser RS, Müller NL, Colman NC, Paré PD: Fraser and Paré's Diagnosis of Diseases of the Chest, 4th ed. Philadelphia, WB Saunders, 1999.)*

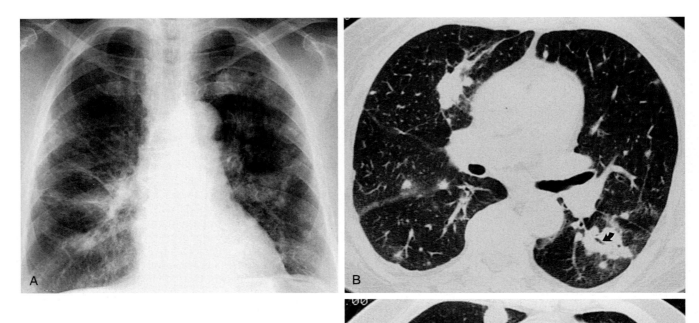

FIGURE 7–35

Secondary pulmonary lymphoma. A posteroanterior chest radiograph (**A**) in a 79-year-old woman shows poorly defined nodular opacities in both lungs. HRCT scans (**B** and **C**) reveal nodules of various sizes; most have irregular margins, and several are associated with thickening of the adjacent interlobular septa (*straight arrows*). An air bronchogram (*curved arrow*) is evident in the nodule in the superior segment of the left lower lobe. The focal areas of ground-glass attenuation, particularly evident in the left lower lobe, are due to interstitial infiltration by lymphoma. *(From Müller NL, Fraser RS, Colman NC, Paré PD: Radiologic Diagnosis of Diseases of the Chest. Philadelphia, WB Saunders, 2001.)*

lymphangitic carcinomatosis sometimes occurs.[556] Less common findings include ground-glass opacities or air space consolidation, particularly in patients with recurrent disease.

Pleural effusion alone is uncommon[557]; however, it develops in association with parenchymal lymphoma at some point in the course of the disease in many patients.[552] Pleural thickening may be seen radiologically at initial evaluation or during recurrence (occasionally as the only site).[558] The appearance may consist of plaquelike areas, focal nodules, masses, or (less commonly) diffuse thickening.

The most frequent initial complaints are fever, anorexia, weight loss, and weakness. Involvement of the upper respiratory tract, particularly the nasopharynx and tonsils, or the gastrointestinal tract may simulate carcinoma. Liver and spleen involvement may result in hepatosplenomegaly. Invasion of the spinal cord, cranial nerves, and meninges can result in pain, paresthesia, and paralysis. Pulmonary disease itself often causes no symptoms. Cough (sometimes with hemoptysis), chest pain, and dyspnea are occasionally present,[559] usually in patients with extensive disease.

The total and differential leukocyte counts are generally within normal limits, although some patients with secondary hypersplenism have hemolytic anemia, leukopenia, or thrombocytopenia. In the late stage of disease, leukemia may develop. Most pleural effusions are serous or serosanguineous. In the setting of known extrathoracic lymphoma, the diagnosis of pleuropulmonary involvement can be made by cytologic examination of sputum, bronchial washings, and pleural fluid or by transthoracic needle biopsy.

Hodgkin's Lymphoma

Intrathoracic involvement in Hodgkin's lymphoma is common, most often in the form of mediastinal and hilar lymph node enlargement. For example, in a series of 659 patients, the former was present in 405 (61%) and the latter in 193 (29%) at the time of diagnosis.[560] Evidence of pleuropulmonary involvement is present at the time of diagnosis in 10% to 15% of patients and at some time during the course of the disease in 15% to 40%.[553,560,561] Intrathoracic disease is usually associated with evidence of Hodgkin's lymphoma elsewhere in the body; for example, in a series of 1470 consecutive patients, only 44 (3%) were found to have purely intrathoracic disease after appropriate clinical and pathologic staging.[562] Primary pulmonary Hodgkin's lymphoma (unassociated with clinical or radiologic evidence of disease in lymph nodes or other tissues) is even more uncommon: a review of the literature published in 1990 documented only 60 reports.[561]

Pathologic Characteristics

The vast majority of cases of Hodgkin's lymphoma in which intrathoracic disease is evident at initial evaluation are of the nodular sclerosis subtype.[560] Pulmonary involvement probably occurs most often by direct extension from affected mediastinal or hilar lymph nodes; thus, the most common pathologic appearance is thickened peribronchovascular interstitial tissue. The infiltrate can extend from this location into adjacent bronchial mucosa and result in a plaquelike elevation or (less commonly) an endobronchial polypoid tumor, both of which can cause airway narrowing with distal atelectasis and obstructive pneumonitis. The peribronchovascular interstitial infiltrate can also extend into the adjacent lung parenchyma; enlargement and coalescence of such foci

probably account for most of the localized nodules or masses seen grossly.[563]

Radiologic Manifestations

The incidence of various intrathoracic abnormalities identifiable on plain chest radiographs was assessed in a study of 300 consecutive patients who had untreated Hodgkin's or non-Hodgkin's lymphoma.[553] The former was found to be associated with a higher incidence of intrathoracic disease at the time of diagnosis (67% versus 43%) and was manifested predominantly by bulky anterior mediastinal lymph node enlargement. In this study, lung involvement was more common in Hodgkin's lymphoma (approximately 12% versus 4%) and was always accompanied by mediastinal or hilar lymph node enlargement or both.

Mediastinal Disease. Mediastinal lymph node enlargement is seen on the initial chest radiograph in 60% to 75% of patients (Fig. 7–36).[560,564] Involvement of the anterior mediastinal and paratracheal lymph nodes is particularly frequent, being evident on the initial chest radiograph in 90% and on CT scan in almost 100% of patients who have intrathoracic disease.[553,564] Infiltration of contiguous groups of lymph nodes occurs in many patients.[565] Dystrophic calcification may be evident after mediastinal irradiation.[566,567] Although some investigators consider the complication to be unrelated to the

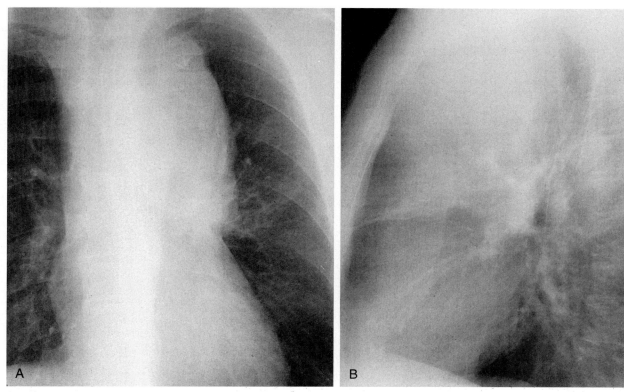

FIGURE 7–36

Hodgkin's lymphoma. A close-up view of the mediastinum from a posteroanterior chest radiograph (**A**) reveals asymmetrical widening of the mediastinum with a lobulated contour consistent with extensive anterior mediastinal lymph node enlargement. The increased soft tissue opacity in the region of the superior vena cava is consistent with paratracheal lymph node enlargement. A lateral view (**B**) confirms the presence of extensive anterior mediastinal lymphadenopathy. The patient was a 57-year-old man. (*From Fraser RS, Müller NL, Colman NC, Paré PD: Fraser and Paré's Diagnosis of Diseases of the Chest, 4th ed. Philadelphia, WB Saunders, 1999.*)

degree of irradiation,[568] others have associated it with relatively high doses.[567] The time interval between irradiation and the appearance of calcification varies from 1 to as long as 10 years.

Lymphoma can extend from lymph nodes into mediastinal interstitial tissue and invade such structures as the esophagus, superior vena cava, and pericardium with corresponding radiologic manifestations. In contrast to pulmonary carcinoma, however, it rarely results in diaphragmatic paralysis secondary to invasion of the phrenic nerve.[569] Involvement of the anterior mediastinal and internal mammary nodes may be associated with invasion of the sternum or parasternal tissue, either unilaterally or bilaterally.[570]

FDG-PET imaging has been found by several groups of investigators to be superior to CT in the evaluation of patients with Hodgkin's lymphoma.[571,572] The procedure detects more extensive disease than CT does and results in upstaging in approximately 10% to 20% of patients. In an investigation of 33 patients, the sensitivity was approximately 90% for identifying involved thoracic lymph nodes[572]; all nodes and foci of extranodal disease greater than 1 cm in diameter were detected. However, false-positive diagnoses occur in approximately 5% of cases because of increased uptake by inflammatory lesions.[573]

Pleuropulmonary Disease. Involvement of peribronchovascular tissue is manifested radiographically by a coarse reticulonodular and linear pattern that extends outward from the hila (Fig. 7–37).[574] Lymphoid tissue at the bifurcation of bronchi and vessels can also be affected, and involvement of the interlobular septa can result in Kerley lines. Consolidation of lung parenchyma remote from the mediastinum is common (Fig. 7–38).

Pleural or subpleural nodules or plaques are seen on CT in 30% of patients at some time in the course of the disease.[575] The size of such nodules ranges widely; individual foci may coalesce to form a large homogeneous nonsegmental mass, sometimes involving a whole lobe.[561,576] This type of parenchymal consolidation is unassociated with loss of volume; its borders can be shaggy and ill defined or sharply marginated. Because the airways are unaffected, an air bronchogram may be visible. Such masses can undergo necrosis and form a cavity that may be thin or thick walled; in many cases, they are multiple and situated in the lower lobes.[577] Rare manifestations include a generalized miliary or reticulonodular pattern and lobar or segmental atelectasis and obstructive pneumonitis.

Pleural effusion is seen at initial evaluation in approximately 10% of patients[564] and eventually develops in approximately 30%, most often in association with other intrathoracic manifestations of the disease.[574] The fluid can be serous, chylous, pseudochylous, or (rarely) serosanguineous. The incidence of pneumothorax is increased in patients who have Hodgkin's lymphoma[578]; radiotherapy, lung involvement, radiation fibrosis, and infection appear to be risk factors.

Chest Wall and Skeletal Involvement. Approximately 15% of patients have evidence of bone involvement radiographically.[579] Usually, such involvement occurs by direct extension of tumor from the mediastinum or lungs.[580] In such cases, destruction of ribs, vertebrae, or the sternum typically results in focal lytic areas. By contrast, vertebral involvement other than by direct extension is often purely osteoblastic ("ivory vertebra").

Follow-up. Enlarged mediastinal lymph nodes usually show slow involution after therapy. The involution may be complete, with return to a normal-appearing chest radiograph,[581] or may be associated with residual abnormalities.[582] Such abnormalities may represent only foci of fibrosis without viable tumor.[583]

Because its low water content leads to a short T2, such fibrous tissue can be readily distinguished from tumor on MR imaging, which reveals a heterogeneous pattern immediately

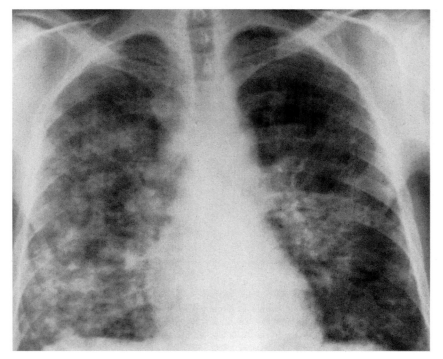

FIGURE 7–37

Hodgkin's lymphoma—mixed interstitial air space pattern. A posteroanterior chest radiograph reveals bilateral patchy air space opacities throughout both lungs, worse on the right. The bronchovascular bundles are thickened, and septal lines are present in both the upper and lower lobes. Mediastinal and hilar nodes are enlarged. (*From Fraser RS, Müller NL, Colman NC, Paré PD: Fraser and Paré's Diagnosis of Diseases of the Chest, 4th ed. Philadelphia, WB Saunders, 1999.*)

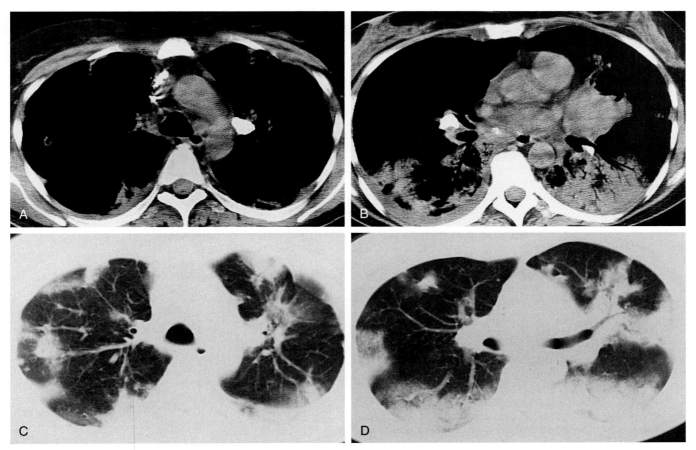

FIGURE 7–38

Hodgkin's lymphoma—parenchymal consolidation. Conventional CT scans (**A** and **B**) demonstrate calcified mediastinal and hilar lymph nodes and enlarged subcarinal and left hilar lymph nodes. Lung windows (**C** and **D**) reveal peribronchial and peripheral areas of consolidation. *(From Fraser RS, Müller NL, Colman NC, Paré PD: Fraser and Paré's Diagnosis of Diseases of the Chest, 4th ed. Philadelphia, WB Saunders, 1999.)*

after treatment that subsequently progresses to the low signal intensity on T2-weighted images that is characteristic of scar tissue.[584] Differentiation of residual tumor from necrotic tumor or fibrotic tissue can also be accomplished with gallium 67 scintigraphy.[585] However, this technique is limited by low spatial resolution and by significant variation in gallium 67 uptake between patients and between anatomic tumor sites in the same patient. FDG-PET imaging does not have the same limitations and has replaced gallium scintigraphy in the initial assessment and follow-up of patients with Hodgkin's lymphoma in institutions where it is available.[586,587]

Features of Recurrent Disease. The most frequent sites of relapse after radiation therapy are the upper mediastinum and lung parenchyma.[588] In a CT investigation in 15 patients, patterns of pulmonary involvement at relapse included nodules in 12, focal areas of consolidation in 4, and direct mediastinal extension into lung parenchyma in 3.[589] The nodules were most commonly located at a bronchial bifurcation; some were connected with thickened interlobular septa and showed cavitation.

Clinical Manifestations

Most patients who have Hodgkin's lymphoma seek the advice of a physician when they notice enlarged peripheral lymph nodes. The abnormality is discovered initially in the cervical area in the great majority. Mediastinal involvement may be manifested by retrosternal pain or a feeling of discomfort. In contrast to its occurrence in sarcoidosis, bilateral hilar node enlargement in Hodgkin's lymphoma is usually associated with symptoms, signs, or both.[590] Dry cough and chest discomfort, often described as pleuritic in character, are the most common symptoms of pleuropulmonary involvement.[561]

Systemic (B) symptoms such as fever, night sweats, and weight loss are present in about a third of patients at the time of diagnosis.[561] Although fever can be caused by the primary disease, complicating infections should be excluded. Bone involvement can produce a pain that along with other symptoms, may be induced or worsened by the ingestion of alcohol.[591] The spleen and liver are enlarged in about 50% of cases. Neurologic involvement occurs occasionally.

In its later stages, especially when the patient is receiving corticosteroids or chemotherapeutic drugs, Hodgkin's lymphoma may be complicated by infection. The lungs are frequently affected, sometimes leading to difficulty in radiologic interpretation. Tuberculosis, formerly a common complication of Hodgkin's lymphoma,[592] now has a lower incidence than other opportunistic infections. Sepsis caused by encapsulated bacteria after splenectomy develops in some patients, especially children.[593] Herpes zoster involving the skin is a relatively common accompaniment of late-stage disease[594]; involvement of the lungs is rare.

Investigation of blood usually reveals a slight leukocytosis with neutrophilia, sometimes with eosinophilia and lymphopenia. Normocytic normochromic anemia may develop early but more often is a late manifestation. A rise in the serum level of alkaline phosphatase may reflect osteoblastic bone lesions or liver disease but can also occur in their absence.

Bronchoscopy is often abnormal in patients who have pulmonary disease. In the review of 60 cases of primary disease described earlier, 17 of 35 patients undergoing the procedure had an abnormality[561]; 2 had an intraluminal mass, 5 had stenosis or external compression, 11 showed "inflammation," 5 had distortion of normal architecture, and 2 showed secretions or blood. In the case of established Hodgkin's lymphoma, bronchial biopsy specimens will often yield sufficient tissue to confirm neoplastic infiltration.

Prognosis and Natural History

The most important factors influencing prognosis are the stage of disease at the time of diagnosis and the histologic subtype. Long-term, disease-free remission is possible in the vast majority of patients who have stage I or II nodular sclerosis disease. In patients who have primary lung involvement, the prognosis appears to be related to the extent of pulmonary involvement, those with disease involving more than one lobe tending to fare worse.[561,569] Other factors that seem to portend a poorer prognosis in these patients are pleural involvement, systemic (B) symptoms, and cavitary disease.[561] A complete response to chemotherapy, radiotherapy, or both is seen in many patients; however, relapse is not uncommon (in 18 of 38 cases in the literature review cited previously).[561]

A number of investigators have examined the long-term effects of radiotherapy and chemotherapy for Hodgkin's lymphoma on pulmonary function.[595-597] Most have found a significant decrease in several parameters, including FEV_1, TLC, forced vital capacity, and diffusing capacity. However, the clinical consequences of the impaired function appear to be minor in most patients and certainly do not outweigh the benefits of the therapy. Patients are also at increased risk for the development of other malignancies after radiotherapy and chemotherapy, particularly leukemia and pulmonary carcinoma.[389,598] Risk for the latter has been shown to increase with increasing radiation dose and to have a strong (multiplicative) association with cigarette smoking.

Mediastinal Non-Hodgkin's Lymphoma

As with pulmonary disease, lymphoma involving the mediastinum may be part of a generalized process or may occur exclusively or predominantly at this site; in the latter situation, the tumor is sometimes known as *primary mediastinal lymphoma*. Although virtually any histologic type of tumor may occur in the mediastinum, the three most common forms are Hodgkin's lymphoma (see page 384), lymphoblastic lymphoma, and diffuse large cell lymphoma.

Lymphoblastic lymphoma accounts for about 60% of cases of apparently primary mediastinal non-Hodgkin's lymphoma,[599] and approximately 50% to 80% of patients with this neoplasm have a prominent mass in the mediastinum at initial evaluation.[600] Lymphoblastic leukemia is pathologically and immunologically identical to lymphoblastic lymphoma, differing from the latter tumor only by having prominent bone marrow and blood involvement (often defined as >25% marrow replacement by malignant cells); approximately 10% to 20% of affected patients are initially seen with a mediastinal mass.[601] The majority of patients with either form of tumor are children or adolescents, frequently male; immunologic studies show most tumors to have features of thymic T cells.

Signs and symptoms related to mediastinal involvement are common and include respiratory distress (as a result of airway compression) and superior vena cava syndrome. Pleural and pericardial effusions are also frequent.[601] Both the leukemic and lymphomatous forms are aggressive tumors that are usually associated with widespread dissemination, especially to extrathoracic lymph nodes and the central nervous system; a leukemic phase also commonly develops in patients who initially present with lymphoma. Despite these features, current therapy results in remission in the majority of patients and a 3-year disease-free survival rate of approximately 50%.

Diffuse large cell mediastinal lymphoma is characteristically large, in one review averaging almost 12 cm in diameter.[602] Invasion of contiguous mediastinal structures, chest wall, and lung is common at the time of diagnosis. Immunohistochemical examination shows most tumors to have features of B-cell differentiation. Sclerosis, manifested by either a diffuse increase in reticulin or a relatively broad bands of fibrous tissue, is a prominent feature in many patients. Most cases occur in young adults. A preponderance in women has been found by some investigators.[602,603] Symptoms referable to the thorax, particularly dyspnea and pain, are present in the majority of patients. Superior vena cava syndrome also occurs in many individuals. With aggressive chemotherapy and radiation therapy, a complete remission rate of about 80% and a 50% to 60% 5-year survival rate can currently be achieved.

Radiologic manifestations are similar in all histologic types. The most commonly involved lymph nodes are those in the anterior mediastinal and paratracheal regions.[551,553] Other nodal stations that may be involved include, in decreasing order of frequency, the subcarinal, hilar, internal mammary, pericardial, and posterior mediastinal regions.[551] In 40% of cases, the lymphadenopathy involves a single nodal group[553]; when multiple groups are affected, involvement may be noncontiguous. The enlarged nodes may have homogeneous soft tissue attenuation (Fig. 7–39) or, less commonly, a central area of decreased attenuation and rim enhancement. The nodes may encase major vessels and lead to obstruction of the superior vena cava. Irradiation or chemotherapy (or both) can result in rapid resolution of disease. After treatment, particularly radiotherapy, dystrophic calcification may occur, most commonly within lymph nodes in the anterior mediastinum.[566]

CT is particularly useful in staging.[551] Lymph node enlargement is seen more commonly with CT than with radiography, and CT is especially helpful in the detection of subcarinal and pericardial adenopathy. Pulmonary parenchymal involvement is also evident on CT scan in some patients in whom abnormalities are not seen on radiography. The most frequent parenchymal findings are nodules, masses, and focal areas of air space consolidation; less commonly, there is direct parenchymal infiltration from adjacent mediastinal lymph

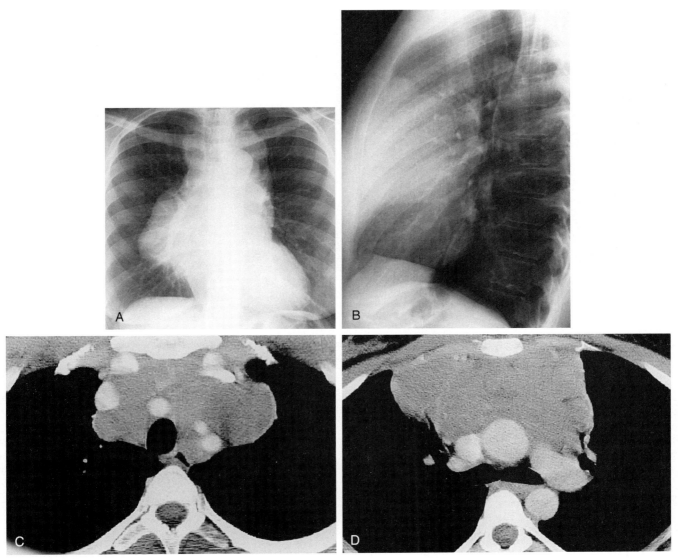

FIGURE 7–39

Mediastinal B-cell lymphoma. Posteroanterior (**A**) and lateral (**B**) chest radiographs reveal a large, lobulated anterior mediastinal mass. Note the absence of hilar lymphadenopathy, the interlobar arteries being seen clearly through the soft tissue masses (*hilum overlay* sign). Contrast-enhanced spiral CT scans (**C** and **D**) show diffuse enlargement of the anterior mediastinal and paratracheal lymph nodes with obliteration of the fat planes between them. Despite the extensive lymphadenopathy, there is no evidence of compression of the vascular structures. The patient was a 31-year-old woman. *(From Müller NL, Fraser RS, Colman NC, Paré PD: Radiologic Diagnosis of Diseases of the Chest. Philadelphia, WB Saunders, 2001.)*

nodes (Fig. 7–40). Additional findings that may be seen include pleural effusion, focal soft tissue pleural masses, and chest wall involvement.

MR imaging shows the same anatomic features as CT. Lymphoma usually has a homogeneous appearance on MR imaging, the signal intensity being slightly greater than muscle on T1- and T2-weighted images.[604] Although the procedure enables greater soft tissue contrast than CT does, it is seldom used in the initial assessment. It may be helpful, however, in patients who are allergic to intravenous contrast agents or who have superior vena cava syndrome or in the assessment of pericardial or chest wall invasion.

Gallium 67 scintigraphy is inferior to CT in the initial assessment. However, the procedure has had an important role in the evaluation of patients who have a residual mass after treatment, uptake being present in lymphoma but not in necrotic and fibrotic tissue.[605] As in Hodgkin's lymphoma, FDG-PET imaging is superior to both CT and gallium scintigraphy in both the initial evaluation and follow-up.[606] The majority of studies evaluating the procedure have been performed in patients who have large B-cell or Hodgkin's lymphoma; there is limited information available on its usefulness with other histologic types. In a retrospective review of 172 patients with various types of lymphoma, FDG-PET accurately detected disease in patients who had large B-cell, mantle cell, follicular, and Hodgkin's lymphoma[607]; it was less reliable in detecting MALT-type lymphoma, a finding that has been confirmed by other investigators.[608]

The main limitation of PET imaging is that it does not allow precise determination of the anatomic location of disease.

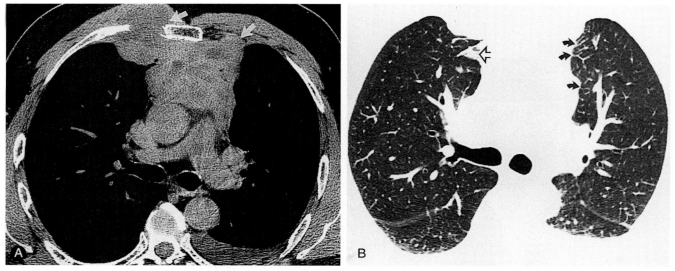

FIGURE 7–40

Mediastinal B-cell lymphoma—chest wall and pulmonary invasion. A CT scan (**A**) in a 51-year-old man shows inhomogeneous enlargement of the anterior mediastinal nodes with direct extension into the chest wall (*arrows*). A small left pleural effusion is evident. Lung windows (**B**) show thickened interlobular septa (*curved arrows*) adjacent to the enlarged lymph nodes, consistent with direct extension of lymphoma into the lungs. The focal area of consolidation in the right lung (*open arrow*) is presumed to represent secondary lymphoma. *(From Müller NL, Fraser RS, Colman NC, Paré PD: Radiologic Diagnosis of Diseases of the Chest. Philadelphia, WB Saunders, 2001.)*

Furthermore, normal uptake in the brain, myocardium, and renal collecting system can obscure the presence of lymphoma in these sites[606]; as a result, PET imaging and CT are generally considered to be complementary imaging tools in the evaluation of patients with lymphoma.

Plasma Cell Neoplasms

Multiple Myeloma

Multiple myeloma is characterized pathologically by a proliferation of plasma cells with varying degrees of atypia. Thoracic involvement is common: in a review of 958 patients, evidence of skeletal or pleuropulmonary disease was found at some time during the course of the disorder in 443 (46%)[609]; radiographic abnormalities were present in 25% at the time of diagnosis.

The usual radiographic appearance consists of one or more well-defined osteolytic lesions, diffuse osteoporosis, and/or fracture. An involved rib may show focal expansion. Extension and proliferation of tumor cells outside the ribs in the adjacent chest wall result in the typical radiologic appearance of a smooth homogeneous soft tissue mass protruding into the thorax and compressing the lung.[610] In fact, the association of an osteolytic lesion in a rib with a soft tissue mass protruding into the thorax should strongly suggest the diagnosis. Pleural or pulmonary parenchymal infiltration is very uncommon.[611] However, pleural thickening and nodularity are sometimes evident in addition to an effusion.[612]

As might be expected from the previous discussion, thoracic signs and symptoms are variable. Rib involvement can cause local tenderness and pain on respiration. Pulmonary parenchymal, bronchial, and tracheal involvement may be manifested by cough, chest pain, or dyspnea. Signs and symptoms of extrathoracic disease are common and include bone pain and hepatosplenomegaly.[613] Laboratory abnormalities are also frequent, the most common being anemia, hypercalcemia, proteinuria (Bence Jones in type in many instances), and monoclonal gammopathy. Definitive diagnosis is most often made by bone marrow biopsy. Pleuropulmonary involvement may be detected by cytologic examination of fluid or cells obtained by BAL or by biopsy.[614,615]

Plasmacytoma

A plasmacytoma can be defined as a well-delimited proliferation of neoplastic plasma cells in the absence of a generalized plasma cell disorder. As such, it excludes the far more common situation in which a localized plasma cell tumor is a manifestation of multiple myeloma. These tumors can consist of an expansile osteolytic lesion of bone or a visceral or soft tissue mass; the latter is often termed *extramedullary plasmacytoma*. The majority of the latter tumors are located in the upper respiratory tract, particularly the pharynx; about 5% occur in the lungs or trachea.[616]

Pulmonary parenchymal plasmacytomas are radiographically manifested as a nodule or somewhat lobulated mass indistinguishable from pulmonary carcinoma.[617] Large lesions can cause airway obstruction, either inspiratory or expiratory, depending on their location within the neck or thorax. Endobronchial tumors can cause atelectasis or obstructive pneumonitis.[618] Ossification is identified occasionally.[619]

Clinical symptoms depend on the location of the lesion. Parenchymal and endobronchial tumors can either cause no symptoms or be accompanied by hemoptysis, cough, dyspnea, or chest pain. Tracheal involvement can result in dyspnea and wheezing. The majority of tumors are not associated with abnormal levels of serum or urine immunoglobulins; occasionally—usually with large tumors—M protein can be detected.[620] Additional plasma cell tumors or overt multiple myeloma develops in some patients; however, prolonged survival without these complications may be seen.[616]

Leukemia

Autopsy studies show that thoracic involvement is common in leukemia of all types. Mediastinal and hilar lymph node infiltration is the most frequent finding, particularly in cases of acute lymphoblastic leukemia and chronic lymphocytic leukemia. Pleuropulmonary infiltration has been found at autopsy in 20% to 40% of cases.[621,622] Nonetheless, the likelihood that clinical and radiographic abnormalities are related to pleuropulmonary leukemic infiltration itself is low,[623] with

most abnormalities being caused by infectious pneumonia, hemorrhage, drug-induced lung damage, or heart failure.[624,625]

Acute and Chronic Myelogenous Leukemia

Pathologic Characteristics. A variety of pathologic abnormalities can be seen in association with pleuropulmonary infiltration by neoplastic myeloid cells. The most frequent is probably thickening of peribronchovascular, pleural, or (less commonly) alveolar interstitial tissue (Fig. 7–41). Though usually a microscopic finding of no clinical significance, such infiltration is occasionally severe enough to result in significant disease, such as effusion or restrictive functional impairment. Pulmonary involvement can also take the form of a

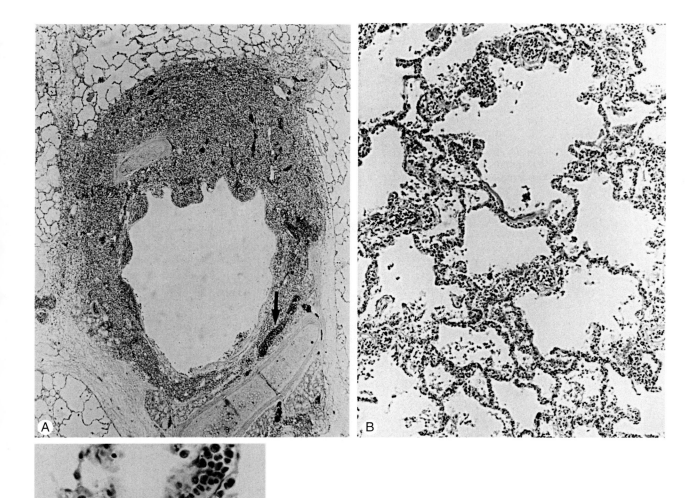

FIGURE 7–41

Acute myelogenous leukemia—histologic abnormalities. The mucosal and peribronchial interstitial tissue of a subsegmental bronchus (**A**) is diffusely infiltrated by myeloblasts. Bronchial artery branches are plugged by similar cells (*arrow*). A section from another patient (**B**) shows mild to moderate thickening of alveolar septa as a result of numerous intravascular blasts (magnified in **C**). (*From Fraser RS, Müller NL, Colman NC, Paré PD: Fraser and Paré's Diagnosis of Diseases of the Chest, 4th ed. Philadelphia, WB Saunders, 1999.*)

localized mass of myeloid cells (granulocytic sarcoma), usually located in the peripheral parenchyma and occasionally in an airway wall.[626] Such nodules can appear before a diagnosis of leukemia has been established, during clinically evident leukemia, or as a manifestation of relapse.[627]

Pulmonary leukostasis is a distinctive abnormality characterized by the presence of numerous leukemic cells within small pulmonary vessels, often unassociated with tissue invasion (see Fig. 7–41).[628] It can develop during the course of the leukemia or, less commonly, as an initial feature; in some cases it appears to be related to the institution of chemotherapy.[629] The complication usually occurs in patients who have acute myelogenous leukemia or chronic myelogenous leukemia in blast crisis. The total white blood cell count is typically between 100,000 and 500,000/mm³, with a predominance of immature forms.

The pathogenesis of the leukostasis is incompletely understood. Although blood viscosity can be increased, it is not always so, and it has been speculated that the stasis is due to mechanical obstruction by the relatively nondeformable blast cells.[628,630] The occurrence of leukostasis in some patients shortly after the induction of chemotherapy has led to speculation that the therapy itself may be important in pathogenesis, possibly by damaging the leukemic cells and causing them to agglutinate more easily or to release thromboplastic substances that can, in turn, induce local coagulation.[629]

Radiologic Manifestations. The most common intrathoracic radiologic manifestations of leukemia are mediastinal and hilar lymph node enlargement (Fig. 7–42).[631] CT may show a focal mediastinal mass or infiltration of mediastinal fat. Other findings include cardiac enlargement as a result of a focal pericardial mass or pericardial effusion, pleural effusions, pleural masses, and pulmonary opacities.

Pulmonary disease associated with leukemic cell infiltration is usually manifested as diffuse bilateral reticulation or linearity that resembles interstitial edema or lymphangitic carcinomatosis. Less common radiographic manifestations include air space consolidation and nodules.[632-634] The most common HRCT findings are interlobular septal thickening and thickening of the bronchovascular bundles (Fig. 7–43)[635]; less common findings include focal areas of ground-glass attenuation or consolidation.

Clinical Manifestations. Acute myelogenous leukemia occurs most commonly between the ages of 10 and 40 years. Its onset is typically abrupt, with major symptoms and signs related to bleeding or infection. The spleen and liver are often enlarged and bleeding; oral infection and retinal hemorrhage are frequent manifestations. Fever is almost invariable, as is pallor related to anemia. As indicated previously, pulmonary symptoms—including cough, expectoration, dyspnea, and hemoptysis—are usually the result of infection, especially by opportunistic bacteria and *Aspergillus*, rather than leukemic infiltration. Interstitial infiltration or extensive leukostasis, however, can cause dyspnea and, rarely, respiratory failure.[636]

Chronic myelogenous leukemia occurs most often in individuals between 30 and 60 years of age and typically has

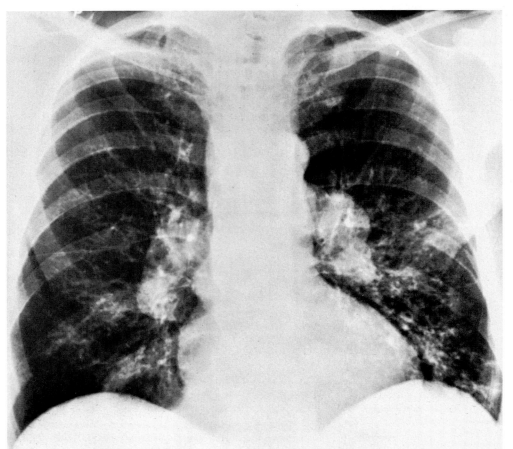

FIGURE 7–42

Chronic lymphocytic leukemia—hilar lymph node enlargement. A posteroanterior chest radiograph reveals markedly enlarged lymph nodes in both hila and (probably) slight enlargement of the nodes in the paratracheal chain bilaterally. There is no evidence of significant pulmonary or pleural disease (the minor parenchymal changes in the left lower lobe represent resolving bronchopneumonia). The patient was a 65-year-old man. *(From Fraser RS, Müller NL, Colman NC, Paré PD: Fraser and Paré's Diagnosis of Diseases of the Chest, 4th ed. Philadelphia, WB Saunders, 1999.)*

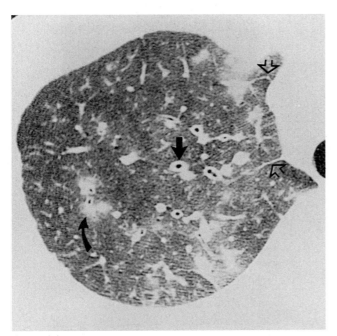

FIGURE 7–43

Chronic myelogenous leukemia. An HRCT scan targeted to the right upper lobe shows thickening of the bronchovascular bundles (*curved arrow*) and interlobular septa (*open arrows*). Poorly defined peribronchial nodules (*straight arrow*), ground-glass attenuation, and regions of peripheral consolidation are also present. (*From Heyneman LE, Johkoh T, Ward S, et al: Pulmonary leukemic infiltrates: High-resolution CT findings in 10 patients. AJR Am J Roentgenol 174:517-521, 2000.*)

a relatively indolent onset, with fatigue, weight loss, and anorexia. Lymph node enlargement and hepatosplenomegaly are present in about 50% of patients. Pulmonary signs and symptoms are even less common than in acute myelogenous leukemia, except when there is transformation to blast crisis.

The diagnosis of leukemia is made by the demonstration of neoplastic cells in peripheral blood or bone marrow. The total leukocyte count is increased in most cases but may be normal or even reduced, with few immature cells in the peripheral blood. Cytologic or immunocytochemical analysis of pulmonary secretions obtained by BAL or analysis of pleural fluid occasionally demonstrates leukemic cells,[637,638] thus revealing the cause of the pleuropulmonary manifestations.

Lymphoproliferative Disorders with Leukemia

Pulmonary involvement in leukemic lymphoproliferative disease is probably most common with chronic lymphocytic leukemia[639]; however, a significant number of cases occur in patients who have adult T-cell leukemia or hairy cell leukemia.[640,641] As with myeloproliferative disorders, the most common pathologic manifestation is an interstitial infiltrate, most often in the peribronchovascular and interlobular septal connective tissue. Infiltration of bronchiolar walls with relative sparing of the rest of the lung parenchyma is prominent in some cases.[642] Significant extension from any of these inter-

stitial locations into alveolar air spaces is uncommon; however, localized tumors of neoplastic cells similar to granulocytic sarcoma can occur.[643]

The most common radiographic sign is again mediastinal and hilar lymph node enlargement. Less common manifestations include interstitial and air space infiltrates; although these infiltrates may be diffuse, they tend to involve mainly the perihilar regions.[634] As discussed previously, an anterior mediastinal mass, representing either thymic or lymph node enlargement and sometimes associated with pleural effusion, is often the initial radiographic sign of acute lymphoblastic leukemia/lymphoma.[644,645]

Chronic lymphocytic leukemia usually develops insidiously and is manifested as painless lymph node enlargement or hepatosplenomegaly. Clinical manifestations of pulmonary involvement are uncommon; some patients have findings of chronic bronchitis or bronchiolitis.[642,646] Decreases in VC, FEV$_1$, and DLCO possibly related to leukemic infiltrates have been documented in some patients.[646] Clinical manifestations of other lymphoproliferative disorders are typically more acute and severe than those of chronic lymphocytic leukemia.[640] As might be expected, the incidence of pulmonary infection at some time during the course of the disease is high in all forms of leukemia.[640]

Pleuropulmonary involvement by chronic lymphocytic leukemia can be confirmed by detecting abnormal lymphocytes in BAL or pleural fluid or on biopsy specimens.[639]

MESENCHYMAL NEOPLASMS

Neoplasms of the lung composed of mesenchymal tissue are uncommon and account for less than 1% of all tumors at this site. With the exception of Kaposi's sarcoma in patients who have AIDS, primary sarcomas constitute only 0.01% to 0.2% of all lung tumors.[647] When considering a diagnosis of primary pulmonary sarcoma, it must be remembered that pulmonary carcinoma sometimes has a sarcomatous appearance (see page 344), and thorough sampling and immunohistochemical study of a tumor are necessary before the diagnosis of a soft tissue neoplasm can be considered definite. Moreover, other epithelial tumors (notably renal cell carcinoma and melanoma) can also have a sarcomatous appearance; metastases from such tumors, as well as from extrapulmonary sarcomas, are more common than primary pulmonary sarcoma, and they must also be considered before the diagnosis is accepted.

Neoplasms of Muscle

Leiomyoma and Leiomyosarcoma

Neoplasms of smooth muscle are among the most common primary soft tissue tumors of the lung.[648] Since smooth muscle is normally found throughout the conducting and transitional airways and the pulmonary vessels, tumors derived from this tissue can occur in any of these sites and can be conveniently discussed under the headings parenchymal, tracheobronchial, and vascular.

Parenchymal Leiomyoma and Leiomyosarcoma. The most common location of pulmonary leiomyosarcoma is in the parenchyma itself[649]; leiomyomas are equally distributed between parenchymal and endobronchial locations. Both tumors occur most commonly in adults.[650] Malignant forms are slightly more frequent in men and benign tumors more common in women. Pathologically, parenchymal tumors are typically lobulated, well-defined nodules or masses located in the periphery of the lung.[651] Necrosis and hemorrhage are frequent in the malignant forms. Microscopically, the majority of tumors consist of interlacing fascicles of spindle cells that have varying degrees of nuclear atypia.

Radiologically, these tumors are sharply defined, smooth or lobulated in contour, and homogeneous in density; cavitation occurs occasionally. Calcification may be present and presumably occurs in areas of ischemic tissue damage. More than 90% are discovered incidentally on the chest radiograph in an asymptomatic individual. Leiomyosarcoma is more likely to be associated with symptoms, including cough, chest pain, or hemoptysis.

As in smooth muscle tumors arising in other body sites, the distinction between benign and malignant tumors can be difficult pathologically. The feature that seems to best predict behavior is mitotic activity.[651,652] The possibility that a parenchymal smooth muscle neoplasm represents a metastasis should always be considered,[653] particularly in patients who have multiple tumors and in women with uterine leiomyomas or a history of hysterectomy (see page 410).

Tracheobronchial Leiomyoma and Leiomyosarcoma. These rare tumors are typically located in the trachea or a main or lobar bronchus and appear grossly as pedunculated masses that more or less completely fill the airway lumen.[648,651] Radiographic findings consist of atelectasis and obstructive pneumonitis. Defects in the air column of the trachea or bronchi may be apparent, even when the lesions are not obstructive. CT and, occasionally, conventional tomography may be useful in assessment. As might be expected, the majority of patients complain of cough, hemoptysis, or dyspnea. Provided that the tumors can be adequately excised surgically, the prognosis is excellent, even with histologically malignant tumors.[651]

Vascular Leiomyosarcoma. Discussions of sarcomas arising in the pulmonary artery usually include a variety of pathologic subtypes in addition to leiomyosarcoma.[654] However, because most tumors that have been reliably classified show smooth muscle differentiation[655,656] and because the radiologic and clinical features of all forms are more or less similar, we include all histologic varieties in the following discussion. The vast majority of tumors appear to originate in the pulmonary valve or large pulmonary arteries. They are rare, only about 140 cases having been reported by 1997.[655,657] Men and women are affected in approximately equal numbers. The average age at the time of diagnosis is about 50 years.[657]

Tumors tend to spread within the vascular lumen; although many remain confined to this site (see Color Fig. 7–13), some also extend across the vessel wall into adjacent bronchus, lymph nodes, or lung parenchyma. The affected artery is frequently occluded by tumor, with or without associated thrombus, and pulmonary infarcts are frequent. Microscopic or macroscopic metastases to the lungs are also common.

The most frequent radiographic findings are hilar pulmonary artery enlargement (Fig. 7–44), solitary or multiple lung nodules, and enlargement of the cardiopericardial contour.[657] Less common manifestations include focal areas of consolidation and areas of oligemia.[657,658] In the absence of a mass, both the clinical and radiographic findings may be those of acute pulmonary embolism, with or without infarction.[659]

The most common abnormality on CT consists of an intraluminal soft tissue mass, sometimes associated with expansion of the artery.[660] Although the mass may be indistinguishable from a thromboembolus, findings that should suggest the diagnosis of sarcoma include extension of the mass into the mediastinum or lung, peripheral pulmonary nodules, or branching soft tissue densities (corresponding to intraluminal tumor growth).[661] MR imaging findings are similar to those of CT (see Fig. 7–44). The signal characteristics do not allow distinction between a sarcoma and a thromboembolus on unenhanced conventional spin-echo images[661]; however, enhancement of sarcoma can be demonstrated after the intravenous administration of gadolinium-diethylenetriamine pentaacetic acid (Gd-DTPA), thereby permitting distinction from thrombus.[662]

Early clinical manifestations include chest pain and dyspnea; cough, hemoptysis, fever, and palpitations also occur in roughly a third of patients. Late manifestations are chiefly those of right heart failure. A heart murmur is identified in about 50% of patients. A clinical picture resembling acute or chronic thromboembolism is not uncommon.[663] As might be expected, the prognosis is poor, the median survival in patients without surgery having been reported to be only 1.5 months.[664] Death is usually related to pulmonary complications; systemic metastases occur uncommonly.[665]

Neoplasms of Vascular Tissue

Hemangiopericytoma

Hemangiopericytoma is a mesenchymal tumor that is believed to be derived from the vascular pericyte. Although some pulmonary tumors have pathologic features consistent with the diagnosis[666] and approximately 100 examples had been reported by 1993,[667] not all such cases have been convincingly proven pathologically; thus, the true incidence of the neoplasm is difficult to determine. Most reported cases have occurred in patients between 40 and 60 years of age, about equally in men and women.[666] The tumors appear as solitary, usually well-defined nodules or masses unrelated to major airways or vessels.[666] A large size is not uncommon. Microscopically, they consist of numerous vascular spaces of variable size and shape separated by aggregates of oval to spindle-shaped cells.

The radiographic appearance is that of a nodule or mass that may be round or lobulated.[667] Calcification is infrequent.[666] Tumors have been found to have an inhomogeneous appearance with central areas of low attenuation and peripheral rim enhancement on CT after the intravenous administration of contrast material.[667]

Approximately 50% of patients are asymptomatic when the tumor is discovered; sometimes, there is cough, hemoptysis, or chest pain. Although some tumors behave in a benign fashion, many are locally invasive at the time of diagnosis or recur after surgical excision; some metastasize and cause death.[668]

Kaposi's Sarcoma

Kaposi's sarcoma is believed to be derived from primitive vasoformative mesenchyme or from endothelial or pericytic cells of small vessels. It occurs in two clinicopathologic forms:

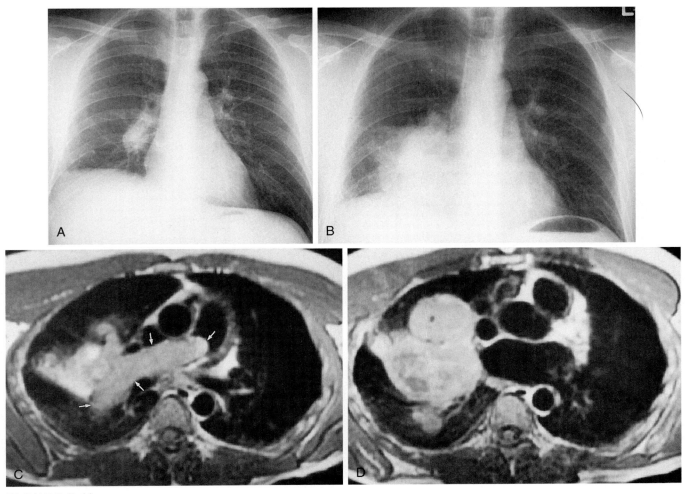

FIGURE 7–44

Leiomyosarcoma of the pulmonary artery. A posteroanterior (PA) chest radiograph (**A**) in a 38-year-old man with shortness of breath demonstrates a prominent right hilum and elevation of the right hemidiaphragm. A ventilation-perfusion scan performed at this time demonstrated no perfusion of the right lung. The findings were interpreted as being due to a large thromboembolus. A PA radiograph 1 year later (**B**) demonstrates increased size of the right hilum and a large mass in the middle lobe. MR imaging (**C**) shows tumor within the right main and interlobar pulmonary arteries (*arrows*) with growth into the adjacent lung parenchyma. MR imaging at the level of the left atrium (**D**) demonstrates extensive tumor growth in the right middle and lower lobes. The MR images were obtained by using spin-echo technique, cardiac gating, 5-mm sections, TR 2250, and TE 20. The patient underwent right pneumonectomy and complete resection of the tumor within the pulmonary artery. *(From Fraser RS, Müller NL, Colman NC, Paré PD: Fraser and Paré's Diagnosis of Diseases of the Chest, 4th ed. Philadelphia, WB Saunders, 1999.)*

(1) as an aggressive neoplasm involving the mucosal surfaces, viscera, and lymph nodes in children and young adults, especially Africans and individuals with AIDS, and (2) as a relatively indolent tumor confined predominantly to the skin in non-African individuals of advanced age. Pulmonary involvement can occur in either setting but is much more common in the former. As discussed elsewhere (see page 435), there is a strong association of the tumor with the presence of human herpesvirus 8.

Pulmonary tumors are usually multiple and are primarily located in peribronchovascular or subpleural interstitial connective tissue (Fig. 7–45). Expansion and coalescence of several tumor foci can result in nodular parenchymal involvement. Histologically, the tumors are composed of cytologically atypical spindle cells between which are numerous, slitlike vascular spaces containing hemosiderin-laden macrophages and red blood cells.

The most common radiographic findings consist of thickened bronchoarterial bundles and bilateral, poorly marginated small nodular opacities or a diffuse reticular or reticulonodular pattern.[669,670] Less common manifestations include focal, unilateral, or bilateral areas of consolidation. The latter may represent pulmonary hemorrhage and may develop suddenly in an area of previous normal lung or around a tumor nodule.[670] Hilar lymph node enlargement is identified radiographically in 10% to 20% of patients and pleural effusion in approximately 35%.[669,671]

The characteristic CT manifestations consist of bronchial wall thickening and multiple bilateral irregular lesions or nodules with poorly defined margins in a predominantly peribronchovascular distribution.[672] Other parenchymal abnormalities include interlobular septal thickening, mass lesions, and focal areas of consolidation. Pleural effusions and hilar or mediastinal lymph node enlargement have each been reported

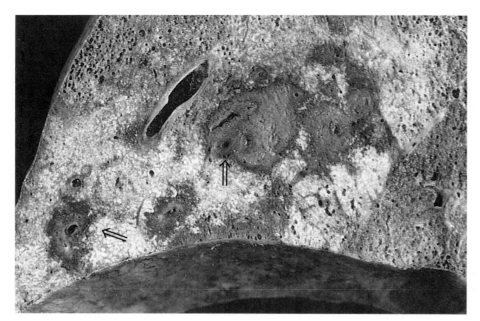

FIGURE 7–45

Kaposi's sarcoma. A magnified view of the basal aspect of a slice of lower lobe shows a patchy hemorrhagic tumor, in some areas intimately associated with a vessel (*arrows*). *(From Fraser RS, Müller NL, Colman NC, Paré PD: Fraser and Paré's Diagnosis of Diseases of the Chest, 4th ed. Philadelphia, WB Saunders, 1999.)*

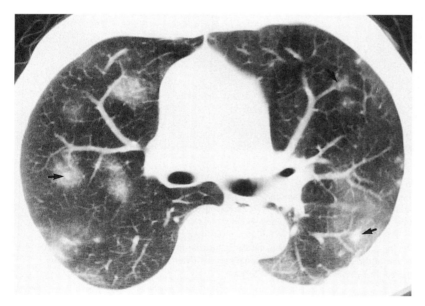

FIGURE 7–46

Kaposi's sarcoma not related to AIDS. A CT scan in an 83-year-old patient demonstrates bilateral, poorly defined nodules (*arrows*) closely related to vessels. Focal areas of ground-glass attenuation surround the nodules. On open lung biopsy, the abnormalities were shown to be due to Kaposi's sarcoma with surrounding areas of hemorrhage. The patient was HIV negative. *(From Fraser RS, Müller NL, Colman NC, Paré PD: Fraser and Paré's Diagnosis of Diseases of the Chest, 4th ed. Philadelphia, WB Saunders, 1999.)*

in 10% to 50% of cases.[673,674] Both the radiographic and CT findings are similar in patients who have and who do not have AIDS (Fig. 7–46).[675]

Pulmonary involvement is almost always associated with the presence of mucocutaneous lesions of Kaposi's sarcoma. Most patients complain of dyspnea, cough, or both[676]; occasionally, blood streaking of sputum, fever, and chest pain are present. Identification of herpesvirus DNA in BAL fluid by polymerase chain reaction (PCR) is both sensitive and specific for the abnormality, at least in patients who have AIDS.[677]

The tumor regresses in some patients who have been given intensive antiretroviral therapy,[678] and survival has improved dramatically over that in the era before the availability of highly active antiretroviral therapy (HAART).[679] Nevertheless, the prognosis of untreated or unresponsive patients who have

pulmonary Kaposi's sarcoma is poor, with median survival varying between 2 and 10 months.

Epithelioid Hemangioendothelioma

This uncommon, typically multifocal pulmonary neoplasm was initially believed to be of epithelial origin and to represent an unusual form of bronchioloalveolar neoplasm characterized by extensive intravascular spread (hence the rather cumbersome designation *intravascular bronchioloalveolar tumor* [IVBAT]). However, subsequent electron microscopic and immunohistochemical studies have indicated endothelial differentiation, and the designation *epithelioid hemangioendothelioma* is now accepted by most authors.[680,681] Approximately 80% of cases occur in women,[680] many younger than

40 years, an association that has been speculated to be related to a hormonal effect.[682]

The explanation for the multifocality of the neoplasm is unclear. The typical absence of both a dominant pulmonary tumor and an extrapulmonary primary, both at initial evaluation and over time, and the similarity in size of the pulmonary nodules suggest that the tumor originates in a multifocal fashion within the lung. Some authors, however, have found evidence of an extrapulmonary origin,[683] suggesting that the lung nodules represent metastases in at least some cases.

The usual pathologic manifestation consists of multiple well-demarcated parenchymal nodules ranging in diameter from 0.3 to 3.0 cm.[680] Light microscopic examination shows a hypocellular sclerotic central portion surrounded by a somewhat nodular, more cellular periphery. The latter consists of loose aggregates of oval to spindle-shaped cells that have small intracellular lumina believed to represent vascular differentiation.

Radiographic manifestations simulate metastases or infarcts and consist of multiple well-defined or ill-defined nodules measuring up to 2 cm in diameter.[680] Although these nodules sometimes show little or no growth on serial radiographs,[684] they can also enlarge slowly and eventually cause respiratory insufficiency.[685] There is usually no hilar or mediastinal lymph node enlargement, and pleural effusion is uncommon. Calcification may be seen on CT.[686]

Most patients are initially asymptomatic, the lesions being discovered as an incidental finding on a screening radiograph. Occasionally, there is a history of cough, chest pain, dyspnea, malaise, and weight loss. The tumors are best considered low-grade sarcomas; although metastases can occur, the tumors are often slow growing, and survival may be prolonged even with widespread pulmonary or systemic involvement.[680] Nonetheless, approximately 40% of patients for whom follow-up information has been recorded have died, usually as a result of respiratory failure.[687]

Neoplasms of Bone and Cartilage

Chondroma

It is likely that the majority of benign cartilaginous tumors in the lung represent one-sided development of neoplasms derived from a bronchial mesenchymal cell (i.e., analogous to so-called hamartomas). Tumors that might be regarded as true chondromas (i.e., composed solely of cartilage and apparently arising from tracheobronchial cartilage) are extremely rare.[688]

An exception to this interpretation is tumors that occur as part of Carney's triad, an unusual condition consisting of pulmonary chondromas, gastric epithelioid leiomyosarcoma, and extra-adrenal paraganglioma.[689] The abnormality is usually seen between the ages of 10 and 30 years; almost all patients are female. The tumors are frequently multiple and can develop synchronously or metachronously, sometimes being separated by many years.[690] Though commonly referred to as Carney's "triad," only two of the three types of tumor have been documented in approximately two thirds of cases.

Radiographic manifestations consist of single or multiple, unilateral or bilateral, smoothly marginated, round or slightly lobulated nodules.[691] Approximately 30% are calcified.[692]

Pulmonary symptoms are generally absent, the chondromas being discovered on a screening radiograph or as part of a workup or follow-up of a previously diagnosed gastric tumor. In the latter situation, they may be incorrectly interpreted as metastases. Although the follow-up period has not been long in most cases, the condition appears to have a better prognosis than the multiplicity of neoplasms might suggest.[693]

Hamartoma

A hamartoma is a tumor-like malformation composed of tissues that are normally present in the organ in which the tumor occurs but in which the tissue elements, though mature, are disorganized. In the lung, the term has traditionally been used to refer to a parenchymal tumor that is somewhat lobulated in contour and consists predominantly of cartilage and adipose tissue; similar tumors occur rarely in an endobronchial location. Despite widespread use of the term "hamartoma" to refer to such lesions, it is now widely believed that they are better regarded as benign neoplasms, probably derived from a bronchial wall mesenchymal cell.[688,694,695] The results of several clinical, radiologic and pathologic investigations support this hypothesis.

1. The tumors appear to have an onset in adult life: the peak age incidence is in the fifties, and they are identified uncommonly in individuals younger than 30 years.[696]
2. Tumors have been identified radiographically in adults whose previous chest radiographs have been normal[697]; moreover, serial radiography sometimes reveals them to increase in size.[698]
3. Foci of mesenchymal (fibroblast-like) cells are commonly present at the periphery of the cartilaginous lobules (Fig. 7–47), and transition between the two tissues is often evident.[694,699]
4. Cytogenetic analysis has shown several chromosomal abnormalities, most commonly in the q13-q15 region of chromosome 12[700]; similar abnormalities have been documented in other benign soft tissue neoplasms, thus implying that pulmonary hamartoma is also neoplastic.

On the strength of these observations, it appears likely that the diagnostic label "hamartoma" is nosologically incorrect and that these tumors are described more appropriately by a term such as *mesenchymoma*.[695] Because of widespread use of the term, however, the use of *hamartoma* is retained in this book, while recognizing that the true nature of the tumor may be other than its name implies.

Pathologic Characteristics. Approximately 90% of pulmonary hamartomas are located within the parenchyma, usually in a peripheral location. At this site, they are well-circumscribed tumors that on cut section consist of lobules of white, cartilaginous-appearing tissue (see Color Fig. 7–14). Histologically, the lobules are often composed of a central area of more or less well developed cartilage surrounded by loose (myxomatous) fibroblastic tissue. Adipose tissue, smooth muscle, seromucinous bronchial glands, and chronic inflammatory cells may also be seen in variable proportions. Calcification and ossification of the cartilage can be present and are occasionally extensive. Thin, slitlike spaces or clefts lined by ciliated columnar or cuboidal epithelium are frequently present between the lobules, most prominently at the periphery of the tumor.

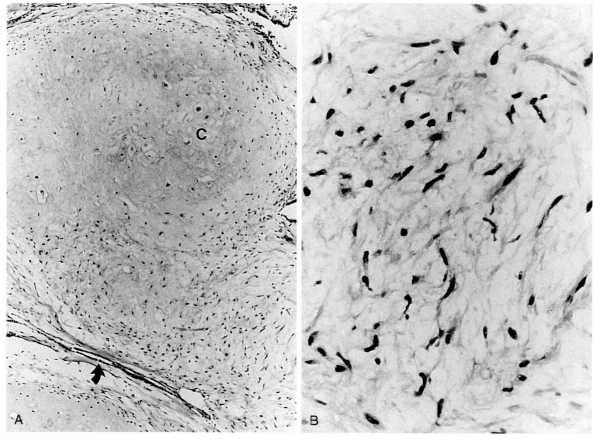

FIGURE 7–47

Pulmonary hamartoma. A magnified view (**A**) of a typical chondromatous hamartoma shows cartilage (C), an epithelium-lined cleft (*arrow*), and spindle cells within a loose stroma (seen to better advantage in **B**). A gradual transition between the spindle cells and cartilage is evident. *(From Fraser RS, Müller NL, Colman NC, Paré PD: Fraser and Paré's Diagnosis of Diseases of the Chest, 4th ed. Philadelphia, WB Saunders, 1999.)*

Although endobronchial hamartomas can be morphologically identical to the parenchymal variety,[701] more often they appear as fleshy, polypoid tumors attached to the bronchial wall by a narrow stalk. Histologically, they often lack epithelial clefts and possess a smooth or slightly undulating surface lined by normal respiratory or metaplastic squamous epithelium. The central portion is generally composed of a core of adipose tissue surrounded by somewhat compressed myxoid tissue. Cartilage is often absent or present in small amounts.[701]

Radiologic Manifestations. The radiologic manifestations of parenchymal tumors typically consist of a well-circumscribed, smoothly marginated solitary nodule without lobar predilection (Fig. 7–48).[167] Most are smaller than 4 cm in diameter. Calcification/ossification is visible on the chest radiograph in less than 10% of cases.[702] Sometimes it has a pattern that resembles popcorn; however, though virtually diagnostic, this appearance is relatively uncommon. As indicated previously, serial radiography may reveal slow or (exceptionally) rapid growth,[703] thus increasing the difficulty in differentiation from pulmonary carcinoma. In a CT study of 47 tumors, 17 showed no discernible calcium or fat, 2 showed diffuse calcification, 18 showed areas of fat, and 10 showed foci of calcium and fat (60%).[310]

As might be expected, endobronchial hamartomas are usually manifested radiographically by the effects of airway obstruction (obstructive pneumonitis and atelectasis). On CT, they may appear to be composed entirely of fat, a mixture of fat and soft tissue, or fat and calcification[704,705]; homogeneous soft tissue attenuation may also be seen.

Clinical Manifestations. Because of their predominant peripheral location, most hamartomas do not usually cause symptoms[706]; when they do, hemoptysis is the most common.[707] Endobronchial tumors may be associated with signs and symptoms of pneumonitis related to airway obstruction. In the absence of the characteristic popcorn pattern of calcification radiographically or evidence of focal areas of fat attenuation on CT, the differential diagnosis must include all other solitary pulmonary nodules, particularly carcinoma.

Although thoracotomy may be required for definitive diagnosis, transthoracic needle aspiration or biopsy can provide adequate tissue for diagnosis in many cases.[708] Bronchoscopy and biopsy usually reveal the diagnosis in the endobronchial forms. Hamartomas are benign, and adequate surgical excision results in cure in the vast majority of patients. For example, in a series of 215 patients, there were no recurrent tumors in the follow-up period of 2 to 192 months.[706]

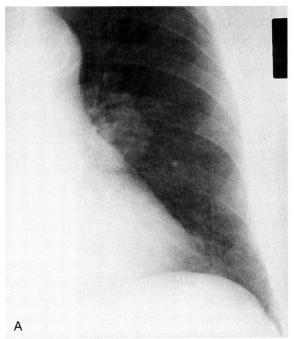

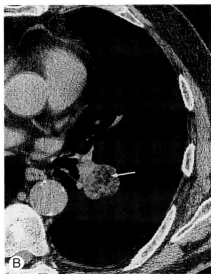

FIGURE 7–48

Pulmonary hamartoma. A view of the left lung from a posteroanterior chest radiograph (**A**) shows a 3-cm-diameter nodule adjacent to the left hilum. An HRCT scan (**B**) performed through the center of the nodule shows focal areas of fat (*arrows*). This CT appearance is diagnostic of pulmonary hamartoma. *(From Müller NL, Fraser RS, Colman NC, Paré PD: Radiologic Diagnosis of Diseases of the Chest. Philadelphia, WB Saunders, 2001.)*

Neoplasms of Neural Tissue

Neurofibroma, Schwannoma, and Neurogenic Sarcoma

Though relatively common in the mediastinum, primary neurogenic neoplasms rarely occur in the lungs.[709] Patients who have neurofibromatosis (von Recklinghausen's disease) are at increased risk. Most lesions have been classified as neurofibromas. Schwannoma (neurilemmoma) is second in frequency, and 20% to 25% have been reported as neurogenic sarcoma.[709] The tumors are usually manifested radiologically as a solitary nodule; less commonly, atelectasis or obstructive pneumonitis is present as a result of bronchial obstruction. Most patients are asymptomatic.

Granular Cell Tumor

Granular cell tumors are uncommon neoplasms believed to arise from Schwann cells. They are most often found in the tongue, skin, subcutaneous tissue, or breast; about 5% of cases originate in the lungs.[710,711] The majority of tumors arise in the larynx or main bronchi, in the latter often at or near their bifurcations. Multicentric tumors occur in 10% to 15% of patients. The neoplasms are usually 1 to 2 cm in diameter and appear as white, plaquelike thickenings of the bronchial wall or as polypoid projections in the airway lumen. Microscopically, they consist of nests of polygonal cells that contain abundant granular cytoplasm.

Radiographically, the tumors are manifested as solitary nodules or as atelectasis or obstructive pneumonitis.[712] The diagnosis is usually made by bronchoscopic biopsy. Most patients are between 30 and 49 years of age and are asymptomatic. The major symptoms are chest pain and productive cough caused by recurrent pneumonia. The prognosis is usually excellent, although neoplasms excised bronchoscopically may recur.

Neoplasms of Adipose Tissue

Lipoma

Lipomas occur only infrequently in the lower respiratory tract, usually in the tracheobronchial wall and rarely in lung parenchyma itself.[713] In fact, many benign respiratory fatty tumors do not consist purely of adipose cells but rather contain a mixture of myxomatous, fibroblastic, chondroid, or smooth muscle elements. For this reason, it has been argued that these tumors should probably be considered neoplasms derived from bronchial mesenchymal cells that exhibit multifaceted differentiation and that they are analogous to the more common chondromatous hamartoma.[688]

Radiographically, the tumor is typically manifested as atelectasis or obstructive pneumonitis as a result of airway obstruction.[714] The diagnosis can usually be made easily by CT, the low attenuation values of fat providing conclusive evidence of lipomatous differentiation. When symptoms are present, they are related to recurrent pneumonia.

Neoplasms of Fibrous Tissue

Intrapulmonary Fibrous Tumor (Fibroma)

The term *intrapulmonary fibrous tumor* has been applied to neoplasms that resemble solitary fibrous tumors of the pleura (see page 840) but are located within the lung.[715] Because many of these tumors are intimately associated with the visceral pleura, it is possible that their origin is the same as that hypothesized for the more common pleural form. Those that occur in the lung parenchyma distant from the pleura or in the airways may represent a one-sided histologic expression of a hamartoma.

Grossly, the lesions are well circumscribed and consist of spindle-shaped, fibroblast-like cells embedded in a variable amount of collagen. Their radiographic and clinical manifestations are similar to those of other benign pulmonary neoplasms: those in an endobronchial location can cause atelectasis and/or obstructive pneumonitis, whereas parenchymal lesions are usually manifested as a solitary, asymptomatic nodule. Patients whose tumors are completely excised are generally cured.

Fibrosarcoma

Fibrosarcoma is probably the second most common histologic diagnosis that has been given to soft tissue sarcomas arising in the lung (the most frequent being leiomyosarcoma).[651] However, ultrastructural and immunohistochemical studies have not been performed on many such tumors, and it is likely that some would not be classified as fibrosarcoma today. In fact, some authors have stated that true pulmonary fibrosarcoma is extremely rare.[649] The tumors can arise in the airway wall, pulmonary parenchyma, or pulmonary artery. Histologically, they are composed of fascicles of spindle-shaped cells arranged in a characteristic herringbone pattern; mitotic figures are usually evident and may be numerous.

Most endobronchial tumors occur in the lobar or main bronchi of children or young adults.[651] Patients most often present with cough, hemoptysis, or chest pain; radiologic findings are those of atelectasis, obstructive pneumonitis, or both. Intrapulmonary tumors tend to arise in middle-aged or elderly adults and often do not cause symptoms, especially when smaller[651]; radiologically, they are visualized as a smooth or lobulated mass indistinguishable from other pulmonary neoplasms. Endobronchial tumors are often amenable to local surgical excision, after which long-term survival is the rule. By contrast, intrapulmonary lesions frequently behave in a highly malignant fashion, with death occurring within 2.5 years.[651]

Malignant Fibrous Histiocytoma

By 1996, approximately 50 cases of malignant fibrous histiocytoma had been reported to arise within the lungs.[716] Because the tumor has been recognized histologically only since the 1970s, it is probable that the total number of cases is greater, some tumors previously having been designated fibrosarcoma, leiomyosarcoma, or unclassified sarcoma. Sometimes it is difficult to categorize pulmonary fibrohistiocytic tumors as benign or malignant on the basis of their histologic appearance, in which case they have been designated *borderline tumors*.[717] Pathologically, the tumors usually appear as well-circumscribed masses without an obvious site of origin from an airway or vessel wall.[718]

Radiologically, most tumors are visualized as solitary, smooth or lobulated nodules or masses within the lung parenchyma.[718,719] Approximately 20% of patients have ipsilateral pleural effusion. Most cases have been described in older adults.[718] Although many patients are asymptomatic, cough, dyspnea, hemoptysis, and chest pain may be present. When the neoplasm is limited to the thorax, the prognosis is difficult to predict; apparent cure after surgical excision has

been noted in some patients,[720] whereas survival is measured in months in others. As might be expected, extension into the chest wall or mediastinum and metastases are poor prognostic signs.[717,718]

NEOPLASMS OF UNCERTAIN HISTOGENESIS

Clear Cell Tumor

Clear cell tumors are rare pulmonary neoplasms whose histogenesis is uncertain.[721] The tumors are well-delimited but nonencapsulated nodules usually measuring 2 cm in diameter. Microscopically, they consist of sheets of polygonal cells that have minimal nuclear pleomorphism and copious, clear cytoplasm that contains abundant glycogen.[722]

Most patients are asymptomatic, the lesion being discovered as a peripheral, well-defined nodule on a screening radiograph. Almost all cases have behaved in benign fashion, unassociated with recurrence or metastases. Histologically, they must be differentiated from the more common pulmonary carcinoma with clear cell change and metastatic clear cell carcinoma from the kidney.

Sclerosing Hemangioma

Sclerosing hemangioma is an unusual pulmonary neoplasm that was originally hypothesized to originate from endothelial cells. However, more recent pathologic investigations have suggested derivation from alveolar pneumocytes or terminal bronchiolar cells, and the alternative designation "sclerosing pneumocytoma" has been proposed to emphasize this origin.[723,724] Though uncommon, the tumor has been found in a substantial proportion of cases in some series; for example, in a review of 45 surgically excised benign neoplasms, 10 (22%) were considered to be this type.[725] The neoplasm has a female-to-male preponderance of approximately 4 to 5:1, a gender difference that may be related to the presence of estrogen receptors.[726] Most lesions are discovered in patients between 30 and 50 years of age.

The tumor usually appears as a well-defined nodule 1 to 4 cm in diameter in the peripheral parenchyma, commonly in a subpleural location. Microscopically, it has a variable appearance consisting of a combination of solid or papillary areas, relatively acellular sclerotic regions, and dilated blood-filled spaces. The characteristic radiographic appearance is a well-defined, homogeneous nodule or mass without preference for any lobe. Calcification is unusual, and cavitation does not occur. Slow growth is the rule; in 14 of 51 patients reviewed in one series, the lesions had been apparent radiographically from 1 to 14 years (average, 5 years) before definitive surgery.[727] The majority of patients are asymptomatic; occasionally, a history of cough or recent or remote hemoptysis is elicited.

Pulmonary Blastoma

Pulmonary blastoma is a rare malignant tumor of uncertain histogenesis that histologically and immunohistochemically resembles the pseudoglandular lung tissue seen in early fetal life. Despite this resemblance, the appropriateness of the term "blastoma" has been questioned, and some authors consider the neoplasm to represent a variant of carcinosarcoma.[146] In fact, the tumor is grouped with pleomorphic carcinoma and carcinosarcoma in the 1999 WHO classification of pulmonary tumors.[144] To complicate matters even further, an unusual tumor that resembles pulmonary blastoma without its sarcomatous stroma has also been described.[728] Termed *well-differentiated fetal adenocarcinoma*, this lesion is believed by many observers to represent a variant of blastoma. Nonetheless, blastoma and fetal adenocarcinoma are considered by other authors to be separate entities, and the latter is grouped with other adenocarcinomas in the 1999 WHO classification.

Pathologically, the tumors are typically large masses located in the periphery of the lung.[729] Microscopically, they consist of primitive-appearing tubules or glands surrounded by polygonal or spindle-shaped stromal cells. The most common radiologic manifestation consists of a single well-circumscribed mass.[730] CT performed in a small number of cases has demonstrated homogeneous soft tissue attenuation or a heterogeneous appearance with areas of low attenuation.[730,731]

The peak incidence in an Armed Forces Institute of Pathology (AFIP) review of 52 cases was in the fourth decade.[729] Although some patients are asymptomatic, hemoptysis, cough, and chest pain are frequent complaints. The prognosis is generally poor: in a series of 39 patients, metastases developed in 17 (44%), only 2 of whom survived longer than 2 years.[732] Nonetheless, occasional patients show exceptionally long survival, even in the presence of metastatic disease.

NON-NEOPLASTIC TUMOR-LIKE LESIONS

Inflammatory Tracheobronchial Polyps

Several pathogenetic mechanisms have been proposed for inflammatory tracheobronchial polyps. In some cases, a history of chronic bronchitis or bronchiectasis has suggested that they represent an exaggerated but localized inflammatory reaction to chronic airway irritation.[733] In others, aspirated foreign material,[734] broncholithiasis,[735] or thermal injury[736] has resulted in the formation of exuberant granulation tissue that constitutes the polypoid mass. Despite these examples, most patients have no history of a concomitant pulmonary abnormality to explain the polyp formation.

The polyps are usually solitary and may be pedunculated or attached to the airway wall by a broad base. Histologically, the surface epithelium often shows squamous metaplasia and may be ulcerated. The underlying stroma has a variable appearance, depending on the number of blood vessels, the maturity of the connective tissue, and the severity of the inflammatory cellular infiltrate.

The radiographic manifestations are usually those of airway obstruction and include bronchiectasis, atelectasis, and obstructive pneumonitis. Most patients are between 30 and 60 years of age. Clinical findings include hemoptysis, cough (frequently with sputum production), and dyspnea; wheezing may simulate asthma. A history of recurrent pneumonia is common.

Plasma Cell Granuloma/Fibrous Histiocytoma (Inflammatory Pseudotumor)

Plasma cell granuloma and *fibrous histiocytoma* are terms that refer to a group of pulmonary tumors characterized histologically by a mixture of fibroblasts, histiocytes, lymphocytes, and plasma cells. Since the proportion of these cells varies considerably from tumor to tumor, a variety of terms have been used to describe them, and a dual concept of their pathogenesis has been considered. Those that have a predominance of plasma cells have been thought to represent an unusual inflammatory reaction to an unidentified agent or a reparative process secondary to a pulmonary infection and have been termed *plasma cell granuloma* or *inflammatory pseudotumor*.[737,738] By contrast, those with a relative absence of inflammatory cells have been interpreted by some authorities as being neoplastic, tumors with approximately equal numbers of fibroblasts and histiocytes having been designated *fibrous histiocytoma*, those containing predominantly histiocytic cells being called *histiocytoma*, and those composed chiefly of fibroblasts being labeled *fibroma*.

Despite these views, there is in fact considerable histologic overlap between the two "forms" of tumor, those composed predominantly of fibroblasts containing focal areas characteristic of plasma cell granuloma, and vice versa.[737] As a result, it is now widely believed that these tumors represent an unusual inflammatory reaction with a variable histologic appearance and that they should all be termed *inflammatory pseudotumor* or *inflammatory myofibroblastic tumor*.[739,740] Nevertheless, the presence of recurrence,[741] local tissue infiltration and destruction,[742] atypical histologic features,[717] and cytogenetic abnormalities[743] has suggested that some lesions may be neoplastic.

The typical radiologic manifestations consist of a solitary pulmonary nodule or a homogeneous area of consolidation that can mimic a primary or metastatic neoplasm.[744] Calcification is present occasionally[745] and cavitation rarely.[746] Endobronchial tumors can cause obstructive pneumonitis. Hilar or mediastinal lymph node enlargement and pleural effusion occur occasionally. On CT scan, the lesions have smooth or lobulated margins; homogeneous or heterogeneous attenuation; and either no enhancement or homogeneous, heterogeneous, or peripheral rim enhancement after intravenous administration of contrast medium.[744]

Although the tumors can develop at any age, most occur in children and adolescents.[746] Many patients are asymptomatic,[747] the lesion being discovered on a screening radiograph. When present, symptoms include cough, hemoptysis, and chest pain[746]; signs and symptoms of bronchial or tracheal obstruction are present in some patients.[748] Long-term follow-up usually shows no change in size or configuration of the lesions; occasionally, they increase in size[746] or regress, either with or without steroid therapy.[749,750] Despite the benign behavior in most patients, recurrence has developed after apparently complete surgical excision,[751] and locally aggressive behavior, including infiltration of pulmonary vessels, the chest wall, and/or mediastinum, can be seen.

Pulmonary Hyalinizing Granuloma

The term *hyalinizing granuloma* refers to an unusual pulmonary tumor characterized histologically by regularly spaced lamellae of hyalinized fibrous tissue associated with small numbers of plasma cells and lymphocytes.[752,753] The etiology and pathogenesis of the nodules are unclear. Some authors have speculated that they represent an exaggerated or abnormal host reaction to one of a number of agents, such as *Histoplasma capsulatum*.[753] Circulating immune complexes and a variety of autoantibodies have been identified in some patients, thus suggesting the possibility of an immunologic pathogenesis.[753] Concomitant retroperitoneal or mediastinal fibrosis, or both, have also been reported, and it is possible that the pulmonary nodules represent a similar disease process in these individuals.[752,753]

Radiographically, the nodules are usually round, homogeneous, and well defined[754]; cavitation has been noted occasionally.[752] The nodules are frequently multiple and 2 to 4 cm in diameter, and calcification is infrequent.[753] Serial radiographs may reveal slow growth[753]; when associated with multiple nodules, the appearance resembles that of metastases.

Many patients are asymptomatic; cough, dyspnea, chest pain, and hemoptysis occur occasionally. The prognosis is usually good. However, increasing dyspnea associated with enlarging nodules was noted in 6 of 19 patients in one series,[755] and retroperitoneal or mediastinal fibrosis, or both, may have significant consequences.

Endometriosis

Thoracic endometriosis is clinically manifested most often by pneumothorax (see page 830). However, in about 5% of cases the abnormality appears as a pulmonary nodule that may be confused with a neoplasm.[756] Such parenchymal involvement tends to occur at an older age than other manifestations of thoracic endometriosis (mean age of 38 years in one review[756]) and is most often on the right side. The pathogenesis of the condition is unclear. However, there is evidence that at least some cases may be related to embolization of endometrial tissue from the uterus to the lungs after labor or surgical trauma.[757]

The radiographic appearance is that of a solitary nodule measuring up to 4 cm in diameter. Cystic change may be present.[758] Occasionally, nodules can be seen to increase and decrease in size with the menstrual cycle. CT may be useful in identifying lesions that are not apparent on conventional radiographs.[759] In addition to the nodules themselves, CT may show focal areas of consolidation surrounding the nodules, presumably representing blood.

Patients usually have a history of recurrent episodes of hemoptysis (catamenial hemoptysis); occasionally, a lesion is discovered in an asymptomatic patient on a screening chest radiograph. The onset of symptoms is usually within 24 to 48 hours of the beginning of menstruation.

SECONDARY NEOPLASMS

The entire output of the right side of the heart, as well as virtually all lymphatic fluid produced by body tissues, flows through the pulmonary vascular system. It is not surprising, therefore, that secondary neoplastic involvement of the lungs is extremely common: in autopsy series of extrapulmonary cancer, the incidence of pulmonary metastases ranges from 30% to 50%. The condition is thus one of great importance because of both its serious prognostic implications and its frequency.

Pathogenesis

Secondary neoplastic involvement of the lungs, pleura, and trachea may occur by two mechanisms: (1) direct extension of tumor situated in the mediastinum, chest wall, or subphrenic space and (2) true metastasis, usually via the pulmonary arteries, less commonly via the bronchial arteries or pulmonary lymphatics or across the pleural cavity, and rarely via the airways. Although overlap does occur, each of these mechanisms and routes of spread is associated with characteristic pathologic, radiologic, and clinical features.

Direct Neoplastic Extension

Secondary involvement of the lung or trachea by direct extension is much less common than involvement by metastasis. It occurs most often by invasion from a primary neoplasm in a contiguous organ or tissue, the most common of which are thyroid[760] and esophageal carcinoma, mediastinal neoplasms such as thymoma, and chest wall sarcomas. In addition, any neoplasm metastatic to ribs or mediastinal lymph nodes can extend into the adjacent trachea or lung. Although the secondary nature of the pulmonary involvement is usually evident in these cases, the extrapulmonary source of neoplasm is occasionally inapparent, particularly in the paramediastinal region, in which encroachment or invasion of the pulmonary parenchyma can simulate primary pulmonary carcinoma extending into the mediastinum.

Metastasis

Metastasis refers to the transport of viable tumor cells from one site in the body to another. Although many consider the term to include evidence of autonomous extravascular growth as well, for purposes of this discussion we include strictly intravascular tumor emboli as constituting true metastases. With respect to the lungs and pleura, such metastases can occur by four routes.

Spread via the Pulmonary Arteries. In this situation, tumor cells are carried to the lungs in blood from the inferior or superior vena cava or in lymph draining from the main or right thoracic ducts. The details of the pathogenesis of metastases in these circumstances are incompletely understood and quite complex. The initial event must clearly be vascular invasion at the site of the primary neoplasm. In the case of venous invasion, individual cells or fragments of tumor (with or without admixed thrombus) are then dislodged and carried as tumor emboli to the lungs,[761] where they lodge chiefly within small pulmonary arteries or arterioles.

The fate of the emboli depends on several factors, including host inflammatory and immunologic reactions, the extent and rapidity of organization of any associated thrombus, the viability of the tumor cells in their new environment, and the effects on the tumor cells of physical trauma resulting from embolization.[761,762] In the majority of cases, it is probable that conditions are unsuitable for survival of malignant cells. Occasionally, however, there is proliferation within the vascular lumen and invasion of the adjacent wall. The location of this proliferation, perhaps in addition to as yet undefined properties of the tumor cells themselves,[763] determines the subsequent morphologic appearance of the metastasis. In most cases, the newly created tumor extends into the surrounding lung parenchyma and forms a relatively well defined nodule. Less often, tumor cells remain largely confined to the perivascular interstitium and spread along it and within its lymphatic channels. These are the two major morphologic manifestations of metastatic cancer in the lung and are discussed in greater detail later.

Spread via the Pulmonary and Pleural Lymphatics. Metastatic spread within the lungs and pleura via lymphatic channels may occur in two ways. As discussed earlier, the first is by hematogenous dissemination to small pulmonary arteries and arterioles, followed by invasion of the adjacent interstitial space and lymphatics and spread along these pathways toward the hilum or periphery of the lung. That this is the pathogenetic mechanism in most cases of pulmonary lymphangitic spread is suggested by the high frequency of concurrent intravascular cancer or thrombosis, or both, and by the frequent absence of neoplasm in the bronchopulmonary and hilar lymph nodes.[764]

The second mechanism is by retrograde extension along lymphatic channels. In the usual course of events, tumor first spreads from an extrathoracic site to the mediastinal lymph nodes, followed by retrograde extension to the hilar and bronchopulmonary nodes and then spread within the pleural and pulmonary lymphatics. Communicating lymphatic channels between the basal pulmonary and diaphragmatic pleura and upper abdominal lymph nodes[765] and the peritoneal cavity[766] may also provide a direct route for lymphatic spread of intra-abdominal malignancy.

Spread via the Pleural Space. Such spread occurs when individual tumor cells or small tumor fragments are liberated into the pleural space and carried within pleural fluid to another site. The precise mechanisms of tumor adherence and invasion at the secondary foci are not clear. In a histologic study of peritoneal metastases of ovarian carcinoma,[767] tumor cells were associated with focal mesothelial damage and an underlying inflammatory reaction. The tumor appeared to proliferate in the resulting exudate as it organized, eventually forming a well-developed metastatic nodule. Similar mechanisms presumably prevail in transpleural metastases.

Spread via the Airways. This method of tumor dissemination has been proposed for both extrapulmonary and primary pulmonary tumors (especially bronchioloalveolar carcinoma); however, except for the latter condition, its existence is probably rare and, in an individual patient, difficult to prove.

Patterns of Secondary Neoplastic Disease

Although metastasis by each of the routes just described frequently results in characteristic pathologic and radiologic manifestations, overlap is common. For example, tumor that metastasizes via the pulmonary artery can result in either a nodular parenchymal or an interstitial pattern of growth, or both. Accordingly, it is useful to discuss the clinicopathologic and radiologic features of pulmonary metastases in terms of patterns of disease, of which five can be recognized: parenchymal nodules, lymphatic and interstitial spread, tumor emboli,

endobronchial tumor, and pleural effusion (the last-named pattern being discussed in Chapter 20).

Parenchymal Nodules

The most common manifestation of neoplastic metastases to the lungs consists of one or more nodules within the parenchyma. These nodules are derived most often from small tumor emboli that lodge in peripheral pulmonary arteries or arterioles and subsequently extend into the adjacent lung tissue. Nodules are multiple in most cases and tend to be most numerous in the basal portions of the lungs because of the effect of gravity on blood flow (Fig. 7–49).[768,769] They range in size from barely visible to huge growths that occupy virtually the entire volume of a lung. Though most often discrete, individual deposits may enlarge, become confluent, and form a multilobulated mass. When multiple, the nodules are usually of varying size; less often, they are approximately equal and suggest a single shower of tumor emboli. Rarely, nodular deposits are so numerous and of such minute size that they suggest the diagnosis of miliary tuberculosis radiographically and pathologically.[770]

CT has considerably greater sensitivity than chest radiography for the identification of nodular metastases.[771] In a study of 13 patients who had a total of 90 surgically proven pulmonary nodules, the sensitivity of spiral CT was 95% for nodules 6 mm or larger in diameter and 69% for nodules smaller than 6 mm.[772] Detection can be improved further by using thin sections (1.5 mm or less) and cine viewing of spiral CT scans on a workstation rather than static film-based images.[773,774] Despite this increased sensitivity, nodules less than 3 mm in diameter are frequently missed.[775] Preliminary studies have shown that detection of such small nodules can be improved with the use of computer algorithms (computer-aided diagnosis).[776]

Although CT is highly sensitive in detecting pulmonary metastases, it is not specific, many of the nodules identified representing granulomas or lymphoid nodules.[771,777] As a result, specificity is greater in areas in which tuberculosis and fungal disease are less common.[778]

When pulmonary parenchymal nodules are multiple, the probability that they represent metastases is increased; conversely, although a solitary nodule can be a metastasis, the possibility that it represents a primary carcinoma is increased. From a diagnostic viewpoint, therefore, neoplastic parenchymal nodules are best discussed under the headings *solitary* and *multiple*.

Solitary Nodules

Metastatic neoplasms that occur as solitary parenchymal nodules are uncommon and account for only about 2% to 10% of cases of solitary pulmonary nodules.[156,166] Most develop in patients 45 years and older.[166] Neoplasms more likely to be associated with solitary metastases include carcinoma of the colon, kidney, testicle, and breast; sarcomas (particularly those originating in bone); and melanoma.

On HRCT, approximately 50% of nodular metastases have smooth margins and 50% have irregular margins.[171,779] They may be round or oval or have a lobulated contour (Fig. 7–50). Irregular margins with spiculation may result from a desmoplastic reaction or tumor infiltration within the adjacent

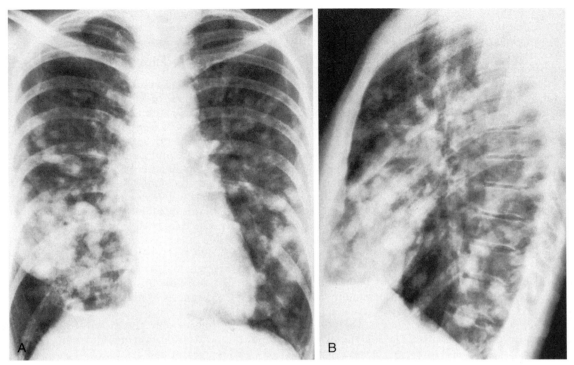

FIGURE 7–49

Metastatic adenoid cystic carcinoma of the left submaxillary gland—multiple parenchymal nodules.
Posteroanterior (**A**) and lateral (**B**) radiographs reveal multiple nodules of homogeneous density ranging in size from 5 mm to 2 cm and distributed widely throughout both lungs. The apices and bases are relatively less affected than the midzones. There is no evidence of cavitation. *(From Fraser RS, Müller NL, Colman NC, Paré PD: Fraser and Paré's Diagnosis of Diseases of the Chest, 4th ed. Philadelphia, WB Saunders, 1999.)*

bronchovascular connective tissue or lymphatics (lymphangitic spread).

It should be remembered that identification of a concomitant primary neoplasm elsewhere or a history of previous neoplasia does not necessarily indicate that a solitary nodule in the lung is a metastasis.[771] For example, in an investigation of 50 patients previously treated for a malignancy who had no evidence of metastases elsewhere, 18 had single intrathoracic lesions that proved to be unrelated pulmonary or mediastinal neoplasms[780]; 9 others had benign pulmonary lesions. In another series of 54 patients with known colonic carcinoma and a solitary pulmonary nodule, only 25 lesions were found to be metastases.[781]

With few exceptions, there are no criteria by which a solitary metastasis can be definitively distinguished from a primary pulmonary carcinoma on a chest radiograph or CT scan.[156,166] Nevertheless, certain features are associated with an increased probability of one or the other.[782] The nature of the primary extrapulmonary tumor is important: a solitary nodule in a patient who has a high-grade sarcoma or deeply invasive melanoma is much more likely to be a metastasis than a new primary. On the other hand, a nodule in a patient who has a history of squamous cell carcinoma of the oropharyngeal region is quite possibly a primary pulmonary carcinoma. The time interval between the initial tumor and appearance of the pulmonary lesion is important, though not independent of tumor type. An interval longer than 5 years in a patient who has a history of osteosarcoma is almost certain to be associated with a new pulmonary primary; however, in carcinomas originating in the breast or kidney, in which metastases can occur many years after the original tumor is identified, this conclusion is less likely to be correct. Older age and a history of cigarette smoking increase the likelihood that the tumor is primary in the lung.

Multiple Nodules

The radiographic pattern of multiple pulmonary nodules varies from diffuse micronodular shadows resembling miliary disease to large, well-defined "cannonball" masses (see Fig. 7–49). Even though most individual shadows are usually fairly sharply defined, some may be indistinct; when the latter reach 5 to 6 mm in diameter, they can simulate air space disease.[783]

On CT scan, nodular metastases are seen most commonly in the outer third of the lungs, particularly the subpleural regions of the lower zones.[290] Although those less than 2 cm in diameter are frequently round and have smooth margins (Fig. 7–51), they may have various shapes; larger nodules are often lobulated and have irregular margins.[784] Irregular margins appear to be particularly common in metastatic adenocarcinoma.[779] Occasionally, a halo of ground-glass attenuation can be seen to surround the nodules, a finding that is most common in highly vascular or hemorrhagic tumors, such as angiosarcoma.[785]

Although intravascular tumor emboli can be seen histopathologically in many patients who have nodular

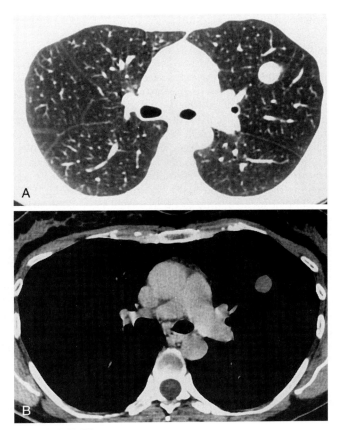

FIGURE 7–50

Single metastasis—CT findings. CT scans (**A** and **B**) demonstrate a smoothly marginated noncalcified nodule in the left upper lobe; the appearance is indistinguishable from that of a noncalcified granuloma. At thoracotomy, it was proven to be metastatic leiomyosarcoma. The primary site was subsequently determined to be the lower extremity. *(From Fraser RS, Müller NL, Colman NC, Paré PD: Fraser and Paré's Diagnosis of Diseases of the Chest, 4th ed. Philadelphia, WB Saunders, 1999.)*

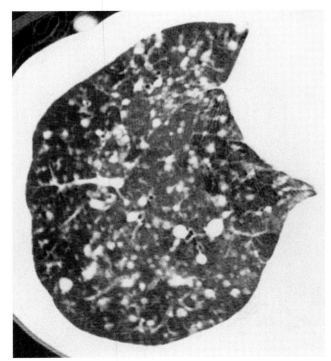

FIGURE 7–51

Metastatic carcinoma—CT appearance. A CT scan shows numerous smoothly marginated nodules 2 to 10 mm in diameter in the right lower lobe. The patient was a 70-year-old woman with metastatic adenocarcinoma from an unknown primary. *(From Müller NL, Fraser RS, Colman NC, Paré PD: Radiologic Diagnosis of Diseases of the Chest. Philadelphia, WB Saunders, 2001.)*

metastases, they tend to occur in arterioles or small arteries and are not usually apparent on CT scan.[779] Rarely, they can be identified as nodular or beaded thickening of the peripheral pulmonary arteries (Fig. 7–52).[786]

Cavitation of nodular metastases is not as common as in primary pulmonary carcinoma.[787] As with pulmonary tumors, it occurs most often in squamous cell carcinoma and is more common in the upper than the lower lobes. The site of the primary neoplasm is most frequently in the head and neck in men and the cervix in women.[787] Though uncommon, cavitation can also occur in metastatic adenocarcinoma, particularly in lesions originating in the large bowel, and in osteogenic sarcoma.[788]

Calcification of metastatic lesions is rare and almost always associated with osteogenic sarcoma, chondrosarcoma, or synovial sarcoma.[789] Calcification can also develop at the site of pulmonary metastases that persist as nodules after chemotherapy.[790] Metastatic testicular neoplasms are particularly prone to this outcome.[791]

The occurrence of spontaneous pneumothorax in association with metastatic disease to the lungs should suggest sarcoma as the primary neoplasm. Although a variety of

tumors have been reported to cause the complication, the incidence is especially high with osteogenic sarcoma.[792] It has been suggested that it is more frequent in patients undergoing chemotherapy.[793] Occasionally, it occurs before the metastasis is radiographically visible.[792]

Interstitial Thickening (Lymphangitic Carcinomatosis)

This pattern of tumor spread is frequent: in a pathologic study of 174 cases of metastatic pulmonary disease, it was seen in 97 (56%); in more than half the cases, it was the predominant mode of spread.[794] Although virtually any metastatic neoplasm can show such spread, the most common originate in the breast, stomach, and prostate.[764]

Pathologically, lymphangitic carcinomatosis varies from a slight accentuation of the interlobular septa and peribronchovascular connective tissue to obvious thickening (5 to 10 mm) of these structures (see Color Fig. 7–15). Microscopically, neoplastic cells can be present within the lymphatic spaces, in the adjacent peribronchovascular and interlobular interstitial tissue, or in both places (see Color Fig. 7–15). Edema or a desmoplastic reaction to the tumor can contribute significantly to the interstitial thickening. Tumor emboli are frequently present in adjacent arteries and arterioles, sometimes associated with thrombus.

The characteristic radiographic pattern consists of coarsened bronchovascular markings of irregular contour,

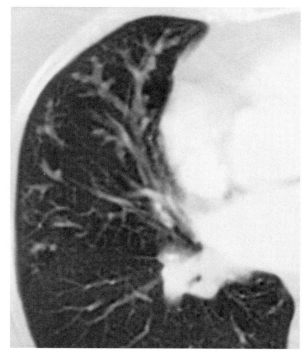

FIGURE 7–52

Intravascular tumor emboli. A detail view of the right lung shows nodular thickening of the pulmonary arteries in the right middle lobe. The appearance is characteristic of intravascular tumor emboli. The patient had metastatic carcinoma of the breast. *(Courtesy of Drs. Lynn Broderick and Robert Tarvers, Indiana University Medical Center, Indianapolis.)*

sometimes indistinctly defined, that simulate interstitial pulmonary edema. Although the appearance is uniform throughout both lungs in most patients, it tends to be more obvious in the lower zones. Septal lines (Kerley B lines) are commonly present (Fig. 7–53).[795] The linear accentuation is sometimes associated with a nodular component as a result of localized growth of tumor, in which case a coarse reticulonodular pattern is created. Though often bilateral, the abnormality may be confined to one lung or one lobe, most often in association with pulmonary carcinoma.[796] Hilar and mediastinal lymph node enlargement is seen radiographically in 20% to 40% of patients and pleural effusion in 30% to 50%.[764,797]

Lymphangitic carcinomatosis also has a characteristic HRCT appearance, consisting of smooth or nodular thickening of the interlobular septa and peribronchovascular interstitium with preservation of normal lung architecture (Fig. 7–54).[795,797] The thickened interlobular septa may be seen as peripheral lines extending to the pleural surface or centrally as polygonal arcades, frequently with a nodular or beaded appearance. This nodular thickening is highly suggestive of the diagnosis and is not seen in pulmonary edema or interstitial fibrosis.[798] It should be remembered, however, that lymphangitic carcinomatosis may be associated with interstitial edema, in which case the thickened interlobular septa may have a smooth appearance.

Thickening of the interlobular septa of adjacent lobules leads to an appearance of polygonal arcades.[795] Characteristically, the arcades are associated with a prominent central dot that represents thickening of the centrilobular

bronchovascular interstitium.[795,797] Tumor and edema in the pleural interstitial tissue lead to smooth or nodular thickening of the interlobar fissures. Discrete nodules separate from the interlobular septa may also be visualized but are relatively uncommon. Pleural effusion is seen on CT in approximately 30% of cases and hilar or mediastinal lymph node enlargement in approximately 40%.[797]

At the time of diagnosis, the HRCT findings are unilateral or markedly asymmetrical in about 50% of cases.[797,799] As indicated previously, such unilateral disease is particularly common in patients who have pulmonary carcinoma. In some, the abnormalities predominantly involve the peripheral portions of lung and lead to prominent thickening of the interlobular septa; in others, the abnormalities predominantly involve the central bronchovascular bundles.[799]

The most common clinical manifestation is dyspnea; though typically insidious in onset, this can progress rapidly and cause severe disability. In our experience, patients with dyspnea that progresses over a period of weeks to months and a with coarse linear or reticulonodular pattern on the chest radiograph frequently have lymphangitic carcinomatosis, even in the absence of a clinically recognized primary tumor. The diagnosis is usually evident in patients who have a history of carcinoma. Transbronchial biopsy is usually diagnostic and is indicated to establish the diagnosis in the absence of a known primary.

Pulmonary Hypertension and Infarction (Tumor Emboli)

Intravascular neoplasms in metastatic carcinoma to the lungs are seen most often with adenocarcinoma,[800] especially of the breast or stomach. As might be expected, the frequency and extent of vascular involvement are greater in patients with concomitant liver metastases. Probably for the same reason, an unusually high frequency of this form of metastasis is seen in hepatocellular carcinoma, out of proportion to the incidence of the neoplasm.[800] Usually, tumor is identified only histologically in small to medium-sized muscular arteries and arterioles.[801] Occasionally, emboli occur in segmental and larger arteries and may result in infarction or sudden death.[802]

Although intravascular tumor emboli are usually accompanied by radiographic evidence of another pattern of pulmonary involvement (most often lymphangitic carcinomatosis), they may be the sole manifestation of metastatic pulmonary disease. In such cases, the chest radiograph may be normal or may show dilation of central pulmonary arteries and the right ventricle as a result of pulmonary hypertension.[803] As indicated previously, emboli are identified rarely on CT scan as nodular or beaded thickening of the pulmonary arteries (see Fig. 7–52).[786] The propensity for tumor emboli to obstruct arterioles can result in an abnormal radionuclide perfusion lung scan characterized by mismatching ventilation-perfusion defects that are virtually indistinguishable from the findings seen in thromboembolic disease.[804]

Clinical symptoms caused by tumor emboli alone are usually absent. When present, the most common complaint is dyspnea; signs of cor pulmonale of relatively recent onset may be present. Rarely, pleuritic chest pain and hemoptysis indicate infarction. A past history of carcinoma or evidence of a coexisting extrathoracic primary is generally evident.

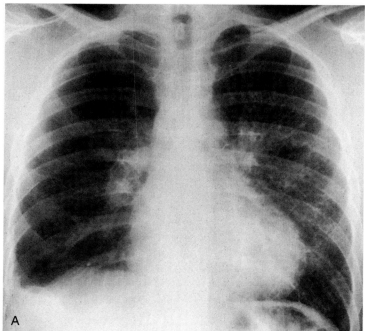

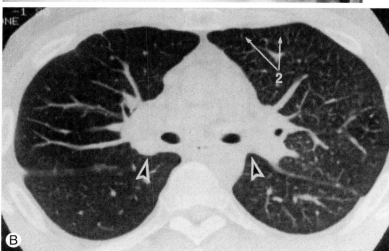

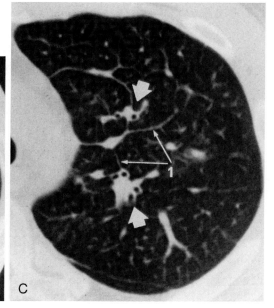

FIGURE 7–53

Lymphangitic carcinomatosis. A posteroanterior radiograph (**A**) shows an interstitial pattern with left-sided predominance consisting of Kerley A and B lines and thickened, ill-defined bronchoarterial bundles. The right hilum is moderately enlarged as a result of lymph node enlargement; the left hilum is questionably enlarged. A small right pleural effusion is present. CT scans through the hilum (**B**) and the left upper lobe (**C**) show Kerley A (1) and B (2) lines and thickened bronchoarterial bundles (*closed arrows*). Minimal lesions of a similar nature are visible in the right lung. Lymph nodes are enlarged in both hila (*arrowheads*). The patient was a 37-year-old man. An open lung biopsy of a right lung nodule several months previously had revealed adenocarcinoma, and it is possible that this was the primary lesion. (*From Müller NL, Fraser RS, Colman NC, Paré PD: Radiologic Diagnosis of Diseases of the Chest. Philadelphia, WB Saunders, 2001.*)

Differentiation between pulmonary hypertension secondary to thromboemboli and hypertension from tumor emboli may be difficult.[801,805]

Airway Obstruction (Bronchial and Tracheal Metastases)

Neoplastic infiltration of a bronchial wall is usually caused by direct extension from a parenchymal tumor or an involved lymph node or by more or less diffuse mucosal infiltration as part of lymphangitic carcinomatosis. The majority of cases are incidental microscopic findings seen by the pathologist at autopsy. Occasionally, however, considerable intraluminal growth occurs in the absence of other recognizable pulmonary metastases or primary neoplasm and leads to a consideration of primary bronchogenic carcinoma. The neoplasms most commonly manifested in this manner are breast, colorectal, and kidney carcinoma and melanoma.[806-808]

The usual radiologic findings are those of bronchial obstruction, either partial (causing oligemia and expiratory air trapping) or complete (with atelectasis and obstructive pneumonitis). Hematogenous metastases to the trachea are rare. Similar to endobronchial metastases, the most common primary sites are the kidney, breast, colon, and skin (melanoma).[476,809] Occasionally, a metastasis is detected as a polypoid soft tissue mass on the chest radiograph or CT scan.[462]

In most cases, the primary site is clinically apparent before symptoms related to endobronchial metastases develop.[810] When they occur, symptoms consist of wheezing, hemoptysis, and persistent coughing; the latter may result in expectoration of diagnostic tumor fragments.

Pleural Effusion

The most common manifestation of pleural metastases is effusion. Many such metastases occur by hematogenous spread of

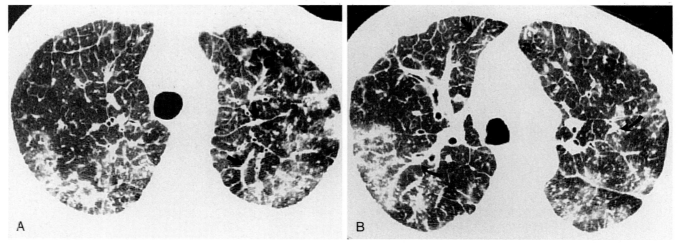

FIGURE 7–54

Lymphangitic carcinomatosis. HRCT scans (**A** and **B**) show smooth and nodular (*straight arrow*) thickening of the interlobular septa and nodular thickening along the bronchovascular bundles (*curved arrows*). The patient was a 72-year-old man with adenocarcinoma of the rectum. (*From Müller NL, Fraser RS, Colman NC, Paré PD: Radiologic Diagnosis of Diseases of the Chest. Philadelphia, WB Saunders, 2001.*)

tumor that has itself metastasized to the liver, particularly when the pleural involvement is bilateral.[811] As discussed previously, carcinoma can also reach the basal pleura directly from upper abdominal lymph nodes or the abdominal cavity via transdiaphragmatic lymphatic channels.[765,766] It must be remembered that the pleural effusion associated with carcinoma can also result from lymphatic obstruction secondary to infiltration of mediastinal lymph nodes. Effusions are usually hemorrhagic when caused by direct neoplastic involvement of the pleural surface and serous when secondary to lymphatic obstruction.

Specific Primary Sites and Tumors

Lung. Studies of patients with pulmonary carcinoma have shown lung metastases at autopsy in 7% to 50%.[812] The higher figure probably reflects a thorough pathologic search for tumor deposits, many of which are doubtless undetectable on chest radiography. As might be expected, poorly differentiated carcinomas are the most common to be complicated by pulmonary metastasis, possibly because of the frequency of concomitant systemic metastases. The exception is bronchioloalveolar carcinoma, in which bilateral and often extensive lung involvement is not uncommon as a result of spread via the airways.

Metastases to the opposite lung in small cell carcinoma have been found at the time of diagnosis in as many as 8% of patients in some studies.[812a] Apart from this tumor, radiographically detectable lung metastases at initial evaluation are uncommon. In most instances, the occurrence of such metastases can be identified with confidence only in the presence of multiple nodules; when only two tumor masses are seen and there is no evidence of systemic metastases, they most likely represent separate primaries rather than a primary and solitary metastasis.

Kidney. Because approximately 30% of all patients with renal cell carcinoma have distant metastases when first seen and because as many as 30% to 40% of patients with pulmonary metastases have no symptoms referable to the kidney, differentiation of a solitary metastasis from a primary pulmonary carcinoma can be a problem, especially if the metastasis is predominantly endobronchial. Compounding the diagnostic difficulty is the histologic variability of renal cell carcinoma; although most tumors show a classic clear cell pattern,[813] some have a sarcomatous or other histologic appearance that may not readily suggest a renal primary.

The most common radiographic manifestation of metastatic renal cell carcinoma in the thorax is solitary or multiple pulmonary nodules. Endobronchial tumors are also not uncommon, in which circumstance there may be evidence of partial or complete airway obstruction. Mediastinal and hilar node enlargement is seen in approximately 20% of patients[814]; though usually associated with pulmonary metastases, it is occasionally the sole radiographic manifestation and can result in a misdiagnosis of sarcoidosis.[815]

Although patients are usually asymptomatic, those with endobronchial metastasis may have cough and hemoptysis; in this situation, the diagnosis may be made by histologic examination of expectorated fragments of the tumor. Metastatic renal cell carcinoma should be suspected in any patient who has radiographic evidence of thoracic metastases and a history of renal cell carcinoma, however remote: occurrence up to 50 years after excision of the primary tumor has been documented.[813] The tumor is one of the more common neoplasms to undergo spontaneous regression[816]; in addition, metastatic nodules occasionally grow slowly over a long period of time.

Colorectum. Metastases to the lung in colorectal carcinoma are second in frequency only to those in the liver. They occur in approximately 5% to 45% of cases in various series[817]; the overall frequency is probably between 15% and 20%. The tumor accounts for 30% to 40% of all *solitary* metastatic neoplasms to the lung and is much more likely than other primaries to be the cause of such a nodule. Nonetheless, in a patient who has a solitary nodule and known colonic carcinoma, the metastatic nature of the nodule is not at all certain.[781]

Histologic differentiation of metastatic colorectal carcinoma from primary pulmonary carcinoma is usually straightforward in well-differentiated or moderately differentiated tumors, which represent the vast majority of cases. Symptoms and the radiologic appearance are generally identical to those of other metastatic tumors. In most patients, a primary colorectal tumor has already been recognized[818]; the majority also have evidence of concomitant liver metastases. Survival rates after resection of pulmonary metastases have been reported to be 40% at 5 years and 30% at 10 years.[819]

Liver. Pulmonary metastases in hepatocellular carcinoma have been reported in almost two thirds of patients in some series.[820] Their presence is closely related to intrahepatic vascular invasion. Tumor emboli, especially those grossly visible, are particularly common and may result in infarction, sudden death, or pulmonary hypertension.[800]

Head and Neck. The incidence of distant metastases in head and neck cancer varies with the site of the primary lesion; in a series of 169 patients who had relatively advanced disease, figures ranged from 10% to 20% for carcinomas of the floor of the mouth, tongue, and oropharynx to 30% for the hypopharynx and almost 60% for the larynx.[821] As might be expected, the lung is the most common site of such metastases; however, hilar and mediastinal lymph node involvement is also common.[822] Because carcinomas of the head and neck region and the lung often coexist[384] and because the majority show squamous differentiation histologically, distinguishing a primary from a metastatic carcinoma can be difficult. The presence of a peripheral tumor unassociated with an airway and concomitant metastases in cervical lymph nodes favors the diagnosis of metastasis; however, even in these situations, the possibility of a primary lung tumor cannot always be excluded.

Breast. Although metastases from breast carcinoma can occur both hematogenously and by lymphatic and interstitial spread, it is probable that the latter is the more common mechanism.[823] Detailed examination of mediastinal lymph nodes suggests that the mechanism of spread in many cases is metastasis from the breast to mediastinal lymph nodes and thence to the pleura and lung. Clinically significant endobronchial metastases occur with considerable frequency when compared with other tumors (a finding more likely related to the high prevalence of breast carcinoma than to its intrinsic biologic properties). Though a rare initial finding, they are sometimes the first indication of recurrence, occasionally many years after the original diagnosis.[824] Pleural effusion is common and tends to be a late manifestation; most effusions are unilateral and located on the same side as the affected breast.

Thyroid. Direct extension of tumor into the trachea is a common occurrence in patients with anaplastic thyroid carcinoma,[760] in which case it is often an important factor in causing death; pulmonary metastases are also frequent. By contrast, pulmonary metastases are rather uncommon in papillary and follicular carcinoma and occur in only 5% to 10% of patients.[825,826] Radiographically, the former tends to have a micronodular pattern (resembling miliary tuberculosis) or a reticulonodular pattern (simulating interstitial fibrosis). It is often associated with cervical lymph node metastases but not with systemic spread. By contrast, metastases from follicular carcinoma tend to develop into larger parenchymal nodules and are frequently associated with concomitant skeletal metastases. Occasionally, conventional radiographs are normal and the presence of metastasis is established by radioactive iodine imaging or CT.[827,828]

Testis. Pulmonary metastases occur with considerable frequency with any of the histologic variants of malignant testicular neoplasms and usually take the form of solitary or, more commonly, multiple parenchymal nodules.[829] Mediastinal and hilar lymph node enlargement is also common.[830] CT scans reveal enlarged, low-attenuation abdominal and pelvic lymph nodes in almost 50% of patients; low-attenuation mediastinal nodes and pulmonary parenchymal nodules are less common.[831] Clinical signs and symptoms are seldom apparent; occasionally, choriocarcinoma causes pulmonary hemorrhage and hemoptysis. A history of a previous testicular tumor can usually be obtained.

Melanoma. Pulmonary metastases from melanoma were documented in 12% of patients in one series.[832] Although many occur early in the course of disease, a substantial number are identified 10 years or more after appearance of the skin tumor. Solitary or multiple nodules are the typical radiologic manifestation.[832]

Endometrium. Endometrial adenocarcinoma metastasizes to the lungs infrequently; in a series of 470 patients, the complication developed in only 11 (2.3%) within the follow-up period of 2 to 12 years.[833] Most have concomitant disease in other viscera or lymph nodes.

Uterine Cervix. Pulmonary metastases occur in 5% to 10% of patients who have invasive cervical carcinoma.[834,835] The frequency is related to the stage of the disease with squamous cell carcinoma[835]; however, there is evidence that metastases develop in patients with adenocarcinoma regardless of the stage at diagnosis.[836] In one review, approximately 95% of metastases were detected within 2 years of identification of the primary tumor.[835] Multiple nodules are the usual radiologic manifestation.

Ovary. Thoracic metastases occur in about 25% to 50% of patients who have ovarian carcinoma.[837,838] Pleural effusion is the most common manifestation, a finding undoubtedly related to the high incidence of visceral and parietal pleural disease caused by direct spread from the peritoneal cavity via diaphragmatic lymphatics.[766] In most cases, pulmonary parenchymal tumor is contiguous with pleural metastases and probably represents direct extension from these sites rather than independent hematogenous deposits.

Prostate. The incidence of spread of prostatic carcinoma to the lungs is fairly high at autopsy[839]; however, radiographically detectable lesions are uncommon during life. As might be expected, the incidence increases with the number of organs involved; in one investigation, thoracic metastases were identified in almost 50% of patients in whom tumor was present in three or more extrathoracic sites.[840] Pleural effusion and reticular opacities (representing lymphangitic spread) are the most common radiologic abnormalities.[841] Focal or diffuse osteoblastic metastases to the thoracic skeleton may be present either with or without lung or mediastinal involvement.

Choriocarcinoma. Pulmonary metastases in gestationally related choriocarcinoma are common.[842] They are invariably hematogenous and usually manifested radiographically by multiple parenchymal nodules. Less often, there are numerous tiny opacities simulating miliary tuberculosis. Therapy generally results in complete regression of the nodules, although fibrosis (with or without dystrophic calcification) is sometimes evident at the site of previous disease. Marked vascularity is characteristic of the tumor and may be reflected pathologically by hemorrhage in the tumor itself and in the adjacent lung parenchyma.

Radiographically and on conventional CT, the nodules may have smooth margins or a characteristic fluffy appearance, the latter also the result of hemorrhage.[843] On HRCT, the hemorrhage is characterized by a halo of ground-glass attenuation.[769] Symptoms are usually absent, although dyspnea may develop and progress to respiratory failure, and hemoptysis can occur.[842]

Leiomyosarcoma. Metastatic leiomyosarcoma to the lungs may be clearly malignant histologically and clinically, in which circumstance patients usually have a well-documented history of an extrathoracic primary tumor (most often of the uterus[844]) and the diagnosis is straightforward. Sometimes, however, diagnostic difficulties arise when an excised pulmonary nodule of apparent smooth muscle origin possesses a bland histologic appearance and there is no clear-cut evidence of an extrathoracic malignancy. Several interpretations have been given for these tumors. Some have been presumed to represent primary pulmonary smooth muscle neoplasms. Others have been referred to as *pulmonary fibroleiomyomas* and have been hypothesized to represent an unusual form of hamartoma. A third group is found in association with uterine "leiomyomas" and has been thought to represent metastases from this site, hence the term *benign metastasizing leiomyoma*.[845] In fact, it is possible that the majority of these latter tumors are better considered metastatic well-differentiated leiomyosarcoma.[846]

Radiographically, the tumors are usually multiple and bilateral and range from 0.5 to 5.0 cm in diameter.[846] The nodules can increase in both size and number or can remain fairly stable over a long period.[847,848] New nodules may appear while others shrink and actually disappear; occasionally, such regression has been seen to follow termination of pregnancy or progestin withdrawal,[849] implying a hormonal effect on tumor growth.

Because the uterus is by far the most common primary tumor site, these neoplasms occur almost exclusively in women. The pulmonary lesions can be present at the same time that the uterine neoplasm is recognized but more often appear after hysterectomy, sometimes after an interval of 20 to 30 years. Metastases usually do not produce symptoms and are discovered incidentally on a screening chest radiograph. The prognosis is variable and difficult to predict. One review documented an excellent prognosis in patients who had only a few nodules; however, even with extensive pulmonary involvement, both long-term and short-term survivors were found.[850]

Other Soft Tissue Sarcomas. The lung is the most common site of metastasis from a variety of other soft tissue sarcomas.[851] In most instances, a primary source is clearly evident, and the diagnosis of metastasis can be established by plain radiography; if doubt exists, transthoracic needle aspiration should provide an answer in most cases.[852] Rarely, one or more lung nodules are evident before clinical appearance of the primary sarcoma, notably with alveolar soft tissue sarcoma.[853] As with other tumors, metastases occasionally develop many years after the primary is recognized.[854]

Sarcoma of Bone. Metastases to the lungs from sarcomas of bone are frequent, especially from osteosarcoma.[855] The typical radiographic appearance is one of multiple nodules, usually bilateral and, in the case of osteogenic sarcoma, calcified or ossified. A history of a synchronous or previous primary bone neoplasm is almost invariable. The majority of metastases do not produce symptoms; however, they can be so numerous that they cause respiratory insufficiency, and spontaneous pneumothorax is a well-recognized complication.[792]

Diagnosis

Although bronchoscopic examination is not as productive in the diagnosis of pulmonary metastases as it is in primary pulmonary carcinoma, diagnostic rates between 50% and 60% have been reported.[856,857] As might be expected, a positive yield is highest in tumors with endobronchial extension, an event that appears to be much more frequent than might be predicted by clinical and radiographic findings.[858] In a study of all patients who had pulmonary metastases and underwent bronchoscopy over a 66-month period in five community teaching hospitals, the likelihood of a positive diagnosis was highest in colorectal (79%) and breast carcinoma (57%) and lowest in genitourinary cancer (33%).[856] Biopsy, washing, and brushing are complementary procedures in diagnosis.

Malignant cells can be detected in sputum or bronchial washings in 35% to 50% of patients who have metastatic cancer to the lungs.[859] Cytologic examination of pleural fluid of malignant origin gives a somewhat higher yield, with most series obtaining an accuracy of about 50%. Of greater importance in the diagnosis of metastatic disease is transthoracic needle aspiration; with this technique, experienced practitioners can prove the malignant nature of a lesion in 85% to 90% of cases. In fact, when the site of the extrathoracic primary tumor is known, a definitive cytologic diagnosis of metastatic cancer is frequently possible.

REFERENCES

1. Brambilla E, Travis WD, Colby TV, et al: The new World Health Organization classification of lung tumours. Eur Respir J 18:1059-1068, 2001.
2. Alberg AJ, Samet JM: Epidemiology of lung cancer. Chest 123:21S-49S, 2003.
3. Bilello KS, Murin S, Matthay RA: Epidemiology, etiology, and prevention of lung cancer. Clin Chest Med 23:1-25, 2002.
4. Villeneuve PJ, Mao Y: Lifetime probability of developing lung cancer, by smoking status, Canada. Can J Public Health 85:385-388, 1994.
5. Weir HK, Thun MJ, Hankey BF, et al: Annual report to the nation on the status of cancer, 1975-2000, featuring the uses of surveillance data for cancer prevention and control. J Natl Cancer Inst 95:1276-1299, 2003.
6. Stewart JH: Lung carcinoma in African Americans: A review of the current literature. Cancer 91:2476-2482, 2001.
7. Andrews JL Jr, Bloom S, Balogh K, et al: Lung cancer in women. Lahey Clinic experience, 1957-1980. Cancer 55:2894-2898, 1985.
8. Travis WD, Lubin J, Ries L, et al: United States lung carcinoma incidence trends: Declining for most histologic types among males, increasing among females. Cancer 77:2464-2470, 1996.
9. Weiss W: Cigarette smoking and lung cancer trends. A light at the end of the tunnel? Chest 111:1414-1416, 1997.
10. Payne S: 'Smoke like a man, die like a man'?: A review of the relationship between gender, sex and lung cancer. Soc Sci Med 53:1067-1080, 2001.
11. Schwartz AG, Swanson GM: Lung carcinoma in African Americans and whites. A population-based study in metropolitan Detroit, Michigan. Cancer 79:45-52, 1997.
12. Moolgavkar SH, Dewanji A, Luebeck G: Cigarette smoking and lung cancer: Reanalysis of the British doctors' data. J Natl Cancer Inst 81:415-420, 1989.
13. Cangemi V, Volpino P, D'Andrea N, et al: Lung cancer in young patients. Panminerva Med 38:1-7, 1996.
14. van Loon AJ, Brug J, Goldbohm RA, et al: Differences in cancer incidence and mortality among socio-economic groups. Scand J Soc Med 23:110-120, 1995.
15. Mao Y, Hu J, Ugnat AM, et al: Socioeconomic status and lung cancer risk in Canada. Int J Epidemiol 30:809-817, 2001.

16. van Loon AJ, Goldbohm RA, Kant IJ, et al: Socioeconomic status and lung cancer incidence in men in The Netherlands: Is there a role for occupational exposure? J Epidemiol Community Health 51:24-29, 1997.

17. Bartecchi CE, MacKenzie TD, Schrier RW: The human costs of tobacco use (1). N Engl J Med 330:907-912, 1994.

18. Hill AB: The environment and disease: Association or causation? Proc R Soc Med 58:295-300, 1965.

19. Carbone D: Smoking and cancer. Am J Med 93:13S-17S, 1992.

20. Engeland A, Haldorsen T, Andersen A, et al: The impact of smoking habits on lung cancer risk: 28 years' observation of 26,000 Norwegian men and women. Cancer Causes Control 7:366-376, 1996.

21. Yang P, Cerhan JR, Vierkant RA, et al: Adenocarcinoma of the lung is strongly associated with cigarette smoking: Further evidence from a prospective study of women. Am J Epidemiol 156:1114-1122, 2002.

22. Peto R: Influence of dose and duration of smoking on lung cancer rates. In Zaridge D, Peto R (eds): Tobacco: A Major International Health Hazard. Lyon, France, IARC Scientific Publications No. 74, International Agency for Cancer Research, 1986, pp 23-33.

23. Samet JM: The 1990 Report of the Surgeon General: The Health Benefits of Smoking Cessation. Am Rev Respir Dis 142:993-994, 1990.

24. Fielding JE, Phenow KJ: Health effects of involuntary smoking. N Engl J Med 319:1452-1460, 1988.

25. Office of Health and Environmental Assessment of Research and Development: Respiratory Effects of Passive Smoking: Lung Cancer and Other Disorders. Washington, DC, Environment Protection Agency, 1992.

26. Boffetta P: Involuntary smoking and lung cancer. Scand J Work Environ Health 28(Suppl 2):30-40, 2002.

27. Zhong L, Goldberg MS, Parent ME, et al: Exposure to environmental tobacco smoke and the risk of lung cancer: A meta-analysis. Lung Cancer 27:3-18, 2000.

28. Fontham ET, Correa P, Reynolds P, et al: Environmental tobacco smoke and lung cancer in nonsmoking women. A multicenter study. JAMA 271:1752-1759, 1994.

29. Wells AJ: Lung cancer from passive smoking at work. Am J Public Health 88:1025-1029, 1998.

30. Janerich DT, Thompson WD, Varela LR, et al: Lung cancer and exposure to tobacco smoke in the household. N Engl J Med 323:632-636, 1990.

31. Wu AH, Fontham ET, Reynolds P, et al: Family history of cancer and risk of lung cancer among lifetime nonsmoking women in the United States. Am J Epidemiol 143:535-542, 1996.

32. Weiss ST: Passive smoking and lung cancer. What is the risk? Am Rev Respir Dis 133:1-3, 1986.

33. Hecht SS, Carmella SG, Murphy SE, et al: A tobacco-specific lung carcinogen in the urine of men exposed to cigarette smoke. N Engl J Med 329:1543-1546, 1993.

34. Burns D: Cigarete smoking. In Aisner J, Arriagada R, Green M, et al (eds): Comprehensive Textbook of Thoracic Oncology. Baltimore, Williams & Wilkins, 1996.

35. Hecht SS: Cigarette smoking and lung cancer: Chemical mechanisms and approaches to prevention. Lancet Oncol 3:461-469, 2002.

36. Agapitos E, Mollo F, Tomatis L, et al: Epithelial, possibly precancerous, lesions of the lung in relation to smoking, passive smoking, and socio-demographic variables. Scand J Soc Med 24:259-263, 1996.

37. International Agency for Research on Cancer: Monographs on the Evaluation of Carcinogenic Risk to Humans: Overall Evaluation of Carcinogenicity: An Updating of IARC Monographs, vol 1-42 (Suppl 7). Lyon, France, International Agency for Research on Cancer, 1987.

38. Steenland K, Loomis D, Shy C, et al: Review of occupational lung carcinogens. Am J Ind Med 29:474-490, 1996.

39. McDonald JC, Liddell FD, Dufresne A, et al: The 1891-1920 birth cohort of Quebec chrysotile miners and millers: Mortality 1976-88. Br J Ind Med 50:1073-1081, 1993.

40. Talcott JA, Thurber WA, Kantor AF, et al: Asbestos-associated diseases in a cohort of cigarette-filter workers. N Engl J Med 321:1220-1223, 1989.

41. Surgeon General of the United States: Asbestos Exposed Workers, The Health Consequences of Smoking: Cancer and Chronic Lung Diseases in the Workplace. U.S. Department of Health and Human Services. Washington, DC, U.S. Government Printing Office, 1985, p 228.

42. Becklake MR: Asbestos-related diseases of the lungs and pleura: Current clinical issues. Am Rev Respir Dis 126:187-194, 1982.

43. Davis JM, McDonald JC: Low level exposure to asbestos: Is there a cancer risk? Br J Ind Med 45:505-508, 1988.

44. Erren TC, Jacobsen M, Piekarski C: Synergy between asbestos and smoking on lung cancer risks. Epidemiology 10:405-411, 1999.

45. Miller A: Lung cancer. Can Lung Assoc Bull 59:3, 1980.

46. Selikoff IJ, Hammond EC: Asbestos and smoking. JAMA 242:458-459, 1979.

47. Hasan FM, Nash G, Kazemi H: Asbestos exposure and related neoplasia. The 28 year experience of a major urban hospital. Am J Med 65:649-654, 1978.

48. Cagle PT: Criteria for attributing lung cancer to asbestos exposure. Am J Clin Pathol 117:9-15, 2002.

49. Weiss W: Asbestosis: A marker for the increased risk of lung cancer among workers exposed to asbestos. Chest 115:536-549, 1999.

50. Banks DE, Wang ML, Parker JE: Asbestos exposure, asbestosis, and lung cancer. Chest 115:320-322, 1999.

51. Kipen HM, Lilis R, Suzuki Y, et al: Pulmonary fibrosis in asbestos insulation workers with lung cancer: A radiological and histopathological evaluation. Br J Ind Med 44:96-100, 1987.

52. Browne K: A threshold for asbestos related lung cancer. Br J Ind Med 43:556-558, 1986.

53. Nelson HH, Kelsey KT: The molecular epidemiology of asbestos and tobacco in lung cancer. Oncogene 21:7284-7288, 2002.

54. Janssen YM, Heintz NH, Marsh JP, et al: Induction of c-fos and c-jun proto-oncogenes in target cells of the lung and pleura by carcinogenic fibers. Am J Respir Cell Mol Biol 11:522-530, 1994.

55. Froom P, Lahat N, Kristal-Boneh E, et al: Circulating natural killer cells in retired asbestos cement workers. J Occup Environ Med 42:19-24, 2000.

56. Wilkinson P, Hansell DM, Janssens J, et al: Is lung cancer associated with asbestos exposure when there are no small opacities on the chest radiograph? Lancet 345:1074-1078, 1995.

57. Weiss W: Asbestos-related pleural plaques and lung cancer. Chest 103:1854-1859, 1993.

58. International Agency for Research on Cancer: IARC Monographs on the Evaluation of Carcinogenic Risks to Humans—Silica, Some Silicates, Coal Dust and Para-aramid Fibrils. Monograph 65. Lyon, France, International Agency for Research on Cancer, 1996.

59. Steenland K, Sanderson W: Lung cancer among industrial sand workers exposed to crystalline silica. Am J Epidemiol 153:695-703, 2001.

60. Hessel PA, Gamble JF, Gee JB, et al: Silica, silicosis, and lung cancer: A response to a recent working group report. J Occup Environ Med 42:704-720, 2000.

61. Wong O: The epidemiology of silica, silicosis and lung cancer: Some recent findings and future challenges. Ann Epidemiol 12:285-287, 2002.

62. International Agency for Research on Cancer: IARC Monographs on Polynuclear Aromatic Compounds, Part 3, Industrial Exposure in Aluminum Production, Coal Gasification, Coke Production, and Iron and Steel Founding. Monograph 34. Lyon, France, International Agency for Research on Cancer, 1984.

63. Finkelstein MM: Lung cancer among steelworkers in Ontario. Am J Ind Med 26:549-557, 1994.

64. International Agency for Research on Cancer: IARC Monographs on Diesel and Gasoline Engine Exhausts and Some Nitrosamines. Monograph 46. Lyon, France, International Agency for Research on Cancer, 1989.

65. Lipsett M, Campleman S: Occupational exposure to diesel exhaust and lung cancer: A meta-analysis. Am J Public Health 89:1009-1017, 1999.

66. Bhatia R, Lopipero P, Smith AH: Diesel exhaust exposure and lung cancer. Epidemiology 9:84-91, 1998.

67. International Agency for Research on Cancer: IARC Monographs on the Evaluation of Carcinogenic Risk to Humans: Man-made Mineral Fibres and Radon. Monograph 43. Lyon, France, International Agency for Research on Cancer, 1988.

68. Roscoe RJ, Steenland K, Halperin WE, et al: Lung cancer mortality among nonsmoking uranium miners exposed to radon daughters. JAMA 262:629-633, 1989.

69. Saccomanno G, Auerbach O, Kuschner M, et al: A comparison between the localization of lung tumors in uranium miners and in nonminers from 1947 to 1991. Cancer 77:1278-1283, 1996.

70. Samet JM: Radon and lung cancer. J Natl Cancer Inst 81:745-757, 1989.

71. Lubin JH, Boice JD Jr, Edling C, et al: Lung cancer in radon-exposed miners and estimation of risk from indoor exposure. J Natl Cancer Inst 87:817-827, 1995.

72. Lubin JH, Boice JD Jr: Lung cancer risk from residential radon: Meta-analysis of eight epidemiologic studies. J Natl Cancer Inst 89:49-57, 1997.

73. Steinberg BM, Topp WC, Schneider PS, et al: Laryngeal papillomavirus infection during clinical remission. N Engl J Med 308:1261-1264, 1983.

74. Pittaluga S, Wong MP, Chung LP, et al: Clonal Epstein-Barr virus in lymphoepithelioma-like carcinoma of the lung. Am J Surg Pathol 17:678-682, 1993.

75. Limas C, Japaze H, Garcia-Bunuel R: "Scar" carcinoma of the lung. Chest 59:219-222, 1971.

76. Barsky SH, Huang SJ, Bhuta S: The extracellular matrix of pulmonary scar carcinomas is suggestive of a desmoplastic origin. Am J Pathol 124:412-419, 1986.

77. Hubbard R, Venn A, Lewis S, et al: Lung cancer and cryptogenic fibrosing alveolitis. A population-based cohort study. Am J Respir Crit Care Med 161:5-8, 2000.

78. Bouros D, Hatzakis K, Labrakis H, et al: Association of malignancy with diseases causing interstitial pulmonary changes. Chest 121:1278-1289, 2002.

79. Nishikawa A, Furukawa F, Imazawa T, et al: Cell proliferation in lung fibrosis-associated hyperplastic lesions. Hum Exp Toxicol 14:701-705, 1995.

80. Khalil N, O'Connor RN, Flanders KC, et al: TGF-beta 1, but not TGF-beta 2 or TGF-beta 3, is differentially present in epithelial cells of advanced pulmonary fibrosis: An immunohistochemical study. Am J Respir Cell Mol Biol 14:131-138, 1996.

81. Lazo BG, Feiner LL, Seriff NS: A study of routine cytologic screening of sputum for cancer in 800 men consecutively admitted to a tuberculosis service. Chest 65:646-649, 1974.

82. Wu AH, Fontham ET, Reynolds P, et al: Previous lung disease and risk of lung cancer among lifetime nonsmoking women in the United States. Am J Epidemiol 141:1023-1032, 1995.

83. Lange P, Nyboe J, Appleyard M, et al: Ventilatory function and chronic mucus hypersecretion as predictors of death from lung cancer. Am Rev Respir Dis 141:613-617, 1990.

84. Tockman MS, Anthonisen NR, Wright EC, et al: Airways obstruction and the risk for lung cancer. Ann Intern Med 106:512-518, 1987.

85. Hennekens CH, Buring JE, Peto R: Antioxidant vitamins—benefits not yet proved. N Engl J Med 330:1080-1081, 1994.

86. Miller AB, Altenburg HP, Bueno-de-Mesquita B, et al: Fruits and vegetables and lung cancer: Findings from the European Prospective Investigation into Cancer and Nutrition. Int J Cancer 108:269-276, 2004.

87. Chung FL, Morse MA, Eklind KI, et al: Inhibition of tobacco-specific nitrosamine-induced lung tumorigenesis by compounds derived from cruciferous vegetables and green tea. Ann N Y Acad Sci 686:186-201, discussion 201-202, 1993.

88. The effect of vitamin E and beta carotene on the incidence of lung cancer and other cancers in male smokers. The Alpha-Tocopherol, Beta Carotene Cancer Prevention Study Group. N Engl J Med 330:1029-1035, 1994.

89. Holick CN, Michaud DS, Stolzenberg-Solomon R, et al: Dietary carotenoids, serum beta-carotene, and retinol and risk of lung cancer in the Alpha-Tocopherol, Beta-Carotene Cohort Study. Am J Epidemiol 156:536-547, 2002.

90. Osann KE: Lung cancer in women: The importance of smoking, family history of cancer, and medical history of respiratory disease. Cancer Res 51:4893-4897, 1991.

91. Rom WN, Hay JG, Lee TC, et al: Molecular and genetic aspects of lung cancer. Am J Respir Crit Care Med 161:1355-1367, 2000.

92. Kiyohara C, Otsu A, Shirakawa T, et al: Genetic polymorphisms and lung cancer susceptibility: A review. Lung Cancer 37:241-256, 2002.

93. Bartsch H, Nair U, Risch A, et al: Genetic polymorphism of CYP genes, alone or in combination, as a risk modifier of tobacco-related cancers. Cancer Epidemiol Biomarkers Prev 9:3-28, 2000.

94. Fong KM, Sekido Y, Gazdar AF, et al: Lung cancer. 9: Molecular biology of lung cancer: Clinical implications. Thorax 58:892-900, 2003.

95. Zochbauer-Muller S, Gazdar AF, Minna JD: Molecular pathogenesis of lung cancer. Annu Rev Physiol 64:681-708, 2002.

96. Minna JD: The molecular biology of lung cancer pathogenesis. Chest 103:449S-456S, 1993.

97. Wiencke JK: DNA adduct burden and tobacco carcinogenesis. Oncogene 21:7376-7391, 2002.

98. Hamm RD: Occupational cancer in the oncogene era. Br J Ind Med 47:217-220, 1990.

99. Filderman A, Matthay R: Bronchogenic carcinoma. In Bone R, Dantzker D, George R, et al (eds): Pulmonary and Critical Care Medicine. St Louis, CV Mosby, 1997.

100. Weintraub SJ: Inactivation of tumor suppressor proteins in lung cancer. Am J Respir Cell Mol Biol 15:150-155, 1996.

101. Sanchez-Cespedes M: Dissecting the genetic alterations involved in lung carcinogenesis. Lung Cancer 40:111-121, 2003.

102. Fong KM, Minna JD: Molecular biology of lung cancer: Clinical implications. Clin Chest Med 23:83-101, 2002.

103. Woll PJ: New perspectives in lung cancer. 2. Growth factors and lung cancer. Thorax 46:924-929, 1991.

104. Savage AM, Pritchard JA, Deeley TJ, et al: Immunological state of patients with carcinoma of the bronchus before and after radiotherapy. Thorax 35:500-505, 1980.

105. Pisani RJ: Bronchogenic carcinoma: Immunologic aspects. Mayo Clin Proc 68:386-392, 1993.

106. Feo Figarella E, Morillo F, Blanca I, et al: Failure of cell-mediated effector mechanisms in lung cancer. J Natl Cancer Inst 73:1-6, 1984.

107. Tollerud DJ, Clark JW, Brown LM, et al: Association of cigarette smoking with decreased numbers of circulating natural killer cells. Am Rev Respir Dis 139:194-198, 1989.

108. Kimura H, Yamaguchi Y: Adjuvant immunotherapy with interleukin 2 and lymphokine-activated killer cells after noncurative resection of primary lung cancer. Lung Cancer 13:31-44, 1995.

109. LeFever A, Funahashi A: Lymphokine-activated killer cell activity in lung cancer. Chest 99:292-297, 1991.

110. Fujisawa T, Yamaguchi Y: Autologous tumor killing activity as a prognostic factor in primary resected nonsmall cell carcinoma of the lung. Cancer 79:474-481, 1997.

111. Meta M, Ponte M, Guastella M, et al: Detection of oligoclonal T lymphocytes in lymph nodes draining from advanced non–small-cell lung cancer. Cancer Immunol Immunother 40:235-240, 1995.

112. Takeo S, Yasumoto K, Nagashima A, et al: Role of tumor-associated macrophages in lung cancer. Cancer Res 46:3179-3182, 1986.

113. Winter SF, Sekido Y, Minna JD, et al: Antibodies against autologous tumor cell proteins in patients with small-cell lung cancer: Association with improved survival. J Natl Cancer Inst 85:2012-2018, 1993.

114. Wagenaar SS: Preliminary results of the pathological review of a small cell lung cancer trial (EORTC 08825). Eur J Respir Dis Suppl 149:63, 1987.

115. Fraire AE, Johnson EH, Yesner R, et al: Prognostic significance of histopathologic subtype and stage in small cell lung cancer. Hum Pathol 23:520-528, 1992.

116. Feinstein AR, Gelfman NA, Yesner R: Observer variability in the histopathologic diagnosis of lung cancer. Am Rev Respir Dis 101:671-684, 1970.

117. Roggli VL, Vollmer RT, Greenberg SD, et al: Lung cancer heterogeneity: A blinded and randomized study of 100 consecutive cases. Hum Pathol 16:569-579, 1985.

118. Thomas JS, Lamb D, Ashcroft T, et al: How reliable is the diagnosis of lung cancer using small biopsy specimens? Report of a UKCCCR Lung Cancer Working Party. Thorax 48:1135-1139, 1993.

119. Chuang MT, Marchevsky A, Teirstein AS, et al: Diagnosis of lung cancer by fibreoptic bronchoscopy: Problems in the histological classification of non–small cell carcinomas. Thorax 39:175-178, 1984.

120. Nagamoto N, Saito Y, Sato M, et al: Clinicopathological analysis of 19 cases of isolated carcinoma in situ of the bronchus. Am J Surg Pathol 17:1234-1243, 1993.

121. Yesner R: Small cell tumors of the lung. Am J Surg Pathol 7:775-785, 1983.

122. Davenport RD: Diagnostic value of crush artifact in cytologic specimens. Occurrence in small cell carcinoma of the lung. Acta Cytol 34:502-504, 1990.

123. Mangum MD, Greco FA, Hainsworth JD, et al: Combined small-cell and non–small-cell lung cancer. J Clin Oncol 7:607-612, 1989.

124. Vollmer RT, Birch R, Ogden L, et al: Subclassification of small cell cancer of the lung: The Southeastern Cancer Study Group experience. Hum Pathol 16:247-252, 1985.

125. Mooi WJ, Dingemans KP, Van Zandwijk N: Prevalence of neuroendocrine granules in small cell lung carcinoma. Usefulness of electron microscopy in lung cancer classification. J Pathol 149:41-47, 1986.

126. Guinee DG Jr, Fishback NF, Koss MN, et al: The spectrum of immunohistochemical staining of small-cell lung carcinoma in specimens from transbronchial and open-lung biopsies. Am J Clin Pathol 102:406-414, 1994.

127. Gould V, Warren W, Memoli V: Neuroendocrine neoplasms of the lung. In Becker K, Gazdar A (eds): The Endocrine Lung in Health and Disease. Philadelphia, WB Saunders, 1984, p 406.

128. Edwards CW: Pulmonary adenocarcinoma: Review of 106 cases and proposed new classification. J Clin Pathol 40:125-135, 1987.

129. Rainio P, Sutinen S, Sutinen SH: Histological subtypes or grading of pulmonary adenocarcinoma. A histochemical and electron microscopic study. Acta Pathol Microbiol Immunol Scand [A] 91:227-234, 1983.

130. Dumont P, Gasser B, Rouge C, et al: Bronchoalveolar carcinoma: Histopathologic study of evolution in a series of 105 surgically treated patients. Chest 113:391-395, 1998.

131. Sorensen JB, Hirsch FR, Olsen J: The prognostic implication of histopathologic subtyping of pulmonary adenocarcinoma according to the classification of the World Health Organization. An analysis of 259 consecutive patients with advanced disease. Cancer 62:361-367, 1988.

132. Clayton F: Bronchioloalveolar carcinomas. Cell types, patterns of growth, and prognostic correlates. Cancer 57:1555-1564, 1986.

133. Miller RR: Bronchioloalveolar cell adenomas. Am J Surg Pathol 14:904-912, 1990.

134. Mori M, Tezuka F, Chiba R, et al: Atypical adenomatous hyperplasia and adenocarcinoma of the human lung: Their heterology in form and analogy in immunohistochemical characteristics. Cancer 77:665-674, 1996.

135. Ohshima S, Shimizu Y, Takahama M: Detection of c-Ki-ras gene mutation in paraffin sections of adenocarcinoma and atypical bronchioloalveolar cell hyperplasia of human lung. Virchows Arch 424:129-134, 1994.

136. Yokozaki M, Kodama T, Yokose T, et al: Differentiation of atypical adenomatous hyperplasia and adenocarcinoma of the lung by use of DNA ploidy and morphometric analysis. Mod Pathol 9:1156-1164, 1996.

137. Yesner R: Large cell carcinoma of the lung. Semin Diagn Pathol 2:255-269, 1985.

138. Yamamoto T, Yazawa T, Ogata T, et al: Clear cell carcinoma of the lung: A case report and review of the literature. Lung Cancer 10:101-106, 1993.

139. Chan JK, Hui PK, Tsang WY, et al: Primary lymphoepithelioma-like carcinoma of the lung. A clinicopathologic study of 11 cases. Cancer 76:413-422, 1995.

140. McDowell EM, McLaughlin JS, Merenyl DK, et al: The respiratory epithelium. V. Histogenesis of lung carcinomas in the human. J Natl Cancer Inst 61:587-606, 1978.

140a. Fitzgibbons PL, Kern WH: Adenosquamous carcinoma of the lung: A clinical and pathologic study of seven cases. Hum Pathol 16:463-466, 1985.

141. Fishback NF, Travis WD, Moran CA, et al: Pleomorphic (spindle/giant cell) carcinoma of the lung. A clinicopathologic correlation of 78 cases. Cancer 73:2936-2945, 1994.

142. Humphrey PA, Scroggs MW, Roggli VL, et al: Pulmonary carcinomas with a sarcomatoid element: An immunocytochemical and ultrastructural analysis. Hum Pathol 19:155-165, 1988.

143. Matsui K, Kitagawa M, Miwa A: Lung carcinoma with spindle cell components: Sixteen cases examined by immunohistochemistry. Hum Pathol 23:1289-1297, 1992.

144. Travis W, Colby T, Corrin B, et al: Histological Typing of Lung and Pleural Tumours, 3rd ed. Berlin, Springer-Verlag, 1999.

145. Berho M, Moran CA, Suster S: Malignant mixed epithelial/mesenchymal neoplasms of the lung. Semin Diagn Pathol 12:123-139, 1995.

146. Wick MR, Ritter JH, Humphrey PA: Sarcomatoid carcinomas of the lung: A clinicopathologic review. Am J Clin Pathol 108:40-53, 1997.

147. Attanoos RL, Papagiannis A, Suttinont P, et al: Pulmonary giant cell carcinoma: Pathological entity or morphological phenotype? Histopathology 32:225-231, 1998.

148. Byers TE, Vena JE, Rzepka TF: Predilection of lung cancer for the upper lobes: An epidemiologic inquiry. J Natl Cancer Inst 72:1271-1275, 1984.

149. Quinn D, Gianlupi A, Broste S: The changing radiographic presentation of bronchogenic carcinoma with reference to cell types. Chest 110:1474-1479, 1996.

150. Woodring JH, Stelling CB: Adenocarcinoma of the lung: A tumor with a changing pleomorphic character. AJR Am J Roentgenol 140:657-664, 1983.

151. Carter D: Small-cell carcinoma of the lung. Am J Surg Pathol 7:787-795, 1983.

152. Golden R: The effect of bronchostenosis upon the roentgen-ray shadows in carcinoma of the bronchus. AJR Am J Roentgenol 13:21, 1952.

153. Onitsuka H, Tsukuda M, Araki A, et al: Differentiation of central lung tumor from postobstructive lobar collapse by rapid sequence computed tomography. J Thorac Imaging 6:28-31, 1991.

154. Herold CJ, Kuhlman JE, Zerhouni EA: Pulmonary atelectasis: Signal patterns with MR imaging. Radiology 178:715-720, 1991.

155. Erasmus JJ, Connolly JE, McAdams HP, et al: Solitary pulmonary nodules: Part I. Morphologic evaluation for differentiation of benign and malignant lesions. Radiographics 20:43-58, 2000.

156. Primack SL, Lee KS, Logan PM, et al: Bronchogenic carcinoma: Utility of CT in the evaluation of patients with suspected lesions. Radiology 193:795-800, 1994.

157. Cummings SR, Lillington GA, Richard RJ: Managing solitary pulmonary nodules. The choice of strategy is a "close call." Am Rev Respir Dis 134:453-460, 1986.

158. Gurney JW: Determining the likelihood of malignancy in solitary pulmonary nodules with Bayesian analysis. Part I. Theory. Radiology 186:405-413, 1993.

159. Jensen KG, Schiodt T: Growth conditions of hamartoma of the lung: A study based on 22 cases operated on after radiographic observation for from one to 18 years. Thorax 13:233-237, 1958.

160. Weisel W, Glicklich M, Landis FB: Pulmonary hamartoma, an enlarging neoplasm. AMA Arch Surg 71:128-135, 1955.
161. Nathan MH, Collins VP, Adams RA: Differentiation of benign and malignant pulmonary nodules by growth rate. Radiology 79:221-232, 1962.
162. Good CA, Wilson TW: The solitary circumscribed pulmonary nodule; study of seven hundred five cases encountered roentgenologically in a period of three and one-half years. JAMA 166:210-215, 1958.
163. Yankelevitz DF, Henschke CI: Does 2-year stability imply that pulmonary nodules are benign? AJR Am J Roentgenol 168:325-328, 1997.
164. Garland LH: The rate of growth and natural duration of primary bronchial cancer. Am J Roentgenol Radium Ther Nucl Med 96:604-611, 1966.
165. Weiss W, Boucot KR, Cooper DA: The survival of men with measurable proved lung cancer in relation to growth rate. Am J Roentgenol Radium Ther Nucl Med 98:404-415, 1966.
166. Siegelman SS, Khouri NF, Leo FP, et al: Solitary pulmonary nodules: CT assessment. Radiology 160:307-312, 1986.
167. Bateson EM: An Analysis of 155 solitary lung lesions illustrating the differential diagnosis of mixed tumours of the lung. Clin Radiol 16:51-65, 1965.
168. Grewal RG, Austin JH: CT demonstration of calcification in carcinoma of the lung. J Comput Assist Tomogr 18:867-871, 1994.
169. Khan A, Herman PG, Vorwerk P, et al: Solitary pulmonary nodules: Comparison of classification with standard, thin-section, and reference phantom CT. Radiology 179:477-481, 1991.
170. Webb WR: Radiologic evaluation of the solitary pulmonary nodule. AJR Am J Roentgenol 154:701-708, 1990.
171. Zwirewich CV, Vedal S, Miller RR, et al: Solitary pulmonary nodule: High-resolution CT and radiologic-pathologic correlation. Radiology 179:469-476, 1991.
172. Sone S, Sakai F, Takashima S, et al: Factors affecting the radiologic appearance of peripheral bronchogenic carcinomas. J Thorac Imaging 12:159-172, 1997.
173. Kuriyama K, Tateishi R, Doi O, et al: CT-pathologic correlation in small peripheral lung cancers. AJR Am J Roentgenol 149:1139-1143, 1987.
174. Webb WR: The pleural tail sign. Radiology 127:309-313, 1978.
175. Hill CA: "Tail" signs associated with pulmonary lesions: Critical reappraisal. AJR Am J Roentgenol 139:311-316, 1982.
176. Kuriyama K, Tateishi R, Doi O, et al: Prevalence of air bronchograms in small peripheral carcinomas of the lung on thin-section CT: Comparison with benign tumors. AJR Am J Roentgenol 156:921-924, 1991.
177. Kui M, Templeton PA, White CS, et al: Evaluation of the air bronchogram sign on CT in solitary pulmonary lesions. J Comput Assist Tomogr 20:983-986, 1996.
178. Lee KS, Kim Y, Han J, et al: Bronchioloalveolar carcinoma: Clinical, histopathologic, and radiologic findings. Radiographics 17:1345-1357, 1997.
179. Yamashita K, Matsunobe S, Tsuda T, et al: Intratumoral necrosis of lung carcinoma: A potential diagnostic pitfall in incremental dynamic computed tomography analysis of solitary pulmonary nodules? J Thorac Imaging 12:181-187, 1997.
180. Swensen SJ, Brown LR, Colby TV, et al: Lung nodule enhancement at CT: Prospective findings. Radiology 201:447-455, 1996.
181. Swensen SJ, Viggiano RW, Midthun DE, et al: Lung nodule enhancement at CT: Multicenter study. Radiology 214:73-80, 2000.
182. Patz EF Jr, Lowe VJ, Hoffman JM, et al: Focal pulmonary abnormalities: Evaluation with F-18 fluorodeoxyglucose PET scanning. Radiology 188:487-490, 1993.
183. Lowe VJ, Fletcher JW, Gobar L, et al: Prospective investigation of positron emission tomography in lung nodules. J Clin Oncol 16:1075-1084, 1998.
184. Gould MK, Maclean CC, Kuschner WG, et al: Accuracy of positron emission tomography for diagnosis of pulmonary nodules and mass lesions: A meta-analysis. JAMA 285:914-924, 2001.
185. Erasmus JJ, McAdams HP, Patz EF Jr: Non–small cell lung cancer: FDG-PET imaging. J Thorac Imaging 14:247-256, 1999.
186. Mahoney MC, Shipley RT, Corcoran HL, et al: CT demonstration of calcification in carcinoma of the lung. AJR Am J Roentgenol 154:255-258, 1990.
187. Nakata H, Hirakata K, Watanabe H, et al: Lung cancer associated with punctate calcification: CT and histological correlation. Radiat Med 15:91-97, 1997.
188. Byrd RB, Carr DT, Miller WE, et al: Radiographic abnormalities in carcinoma of the lung as related to histological cell type. Thorax 24:573-575, 1969.
189. Mack MJ, Hazelrigg SR, Landreneau RJ, et al: Thoracoscopy for the diagnosis of the indeterminate solitary pulmonary nodule. Ann Thorac Surg 56:825-830, discussion 830-832, 1993.
190. Hill CA: Bronchioloalveolar carcinoma: A review. Radiology 150:15-20, 1984.
191. Gaeta M, Caruso R, Barone M, et al: Ground-glass attenuation in nodular bronchioloalveolar carcinoma: CT patterns and prognostic value. J Comput Assist Tomogr 22:215-219, 1998.
192. Zwirewich CV, Miller RR, Müller NL: Multicentric adenocarcinoma of the lung: CT-pathologic correlation. Radiology 176:185-190, 1990.
193. Adler B, Padley S, Miller RR, et al: High-resolution CT of bronchioloalveolar carcinoma. AJR Am J Roentgenol 159:275-277, 1992.
194. Kuhlman JE, Fishman EK, Kuhajda FP, et al: Solitary bronchioloalveolar carcinoma: CT criteria. Radiology 167:379-382, 1988.
195. Im JG, Han MC, Yu EJ, et al: Lobar bronchioloalveolar carcinoma: "angiogram sign" on CT scans. Radiology 176:749-753, 1990.
196. Aquino SL, Chiles C, Halford P: Distinction of consolidative bronchioloalveolar carcinoma from pneumonia: Do CT criteria work? AJR Am J Roentgenol 171:359-363, 1998.
197. Maldonado RL: The CT angiogram sign. Radiology 210:323-324, 1999.
198. Cohen S, Hossain SA: Primary carcinoma of the lung. A review of 417 histologically proved cases. Dis Chest 49:67-74, 1966.
199. Sahn SA: Pleural effusion in lung cancer. Clin Chest Med 14:189-200, 1993.
200. Heelan RT, Demas BE, Caravelli JF, et al: Superior sulcus tumors: CT and MR imaging. Radiology 170:637-641, 1989.
201. Attar S, Krasna MJ, Sonett JR, et al: Superior sulcus (Pancoast) tumor: Experience with 105 patients. Ann Thorac Surg 66:193-198, 1998.
202. Takasugi JE, Rapoport S, Shaw C: Superior sulcus tumors: The role of imaging. J Thorac Imaging 4:41-48, 1989.
203. Scott IR, Müller NL, Miller RR, et al: Resectable stage III lung cancer: CT, surgical, and pathologic correlation. Radiology 166:75-79, 1988.
204. Pennes DR, Glazer GM, Wimbish KJ, et al: Chest wall invasion by lung cancer: Limitations of CT evaluation. AJR Am J Roentgenol 144:507-511, 1985.
205. Pearlberg JL, Sandler MA, Beute GH, et al: Limitations of CT in evaluation of neoplasms involving chest wall. J Comput Assist Tomogr 11:290-293, 1987.
206. Quint LE, Francis IR: Radiologic staging of lung cancer. J Thorac Imaging 14:235-246, 1999.
207. Webb WR, Gatsonis C, Zerhouni EA, et al: CT and MR imaging in staging non–small cell bronchogenic carcinoma: Report of the Radiologic Diagnostic Oncology Group. Radiology 178:705-713, 1991.
208. Gefter WB: Magnetic resonance imaging in the evaluation of lung cancer. Semin Roentgenol 25:73-84, 1990.
209. Suzuki N, Saitoh T, Kitamura S: Tumor invasion of the chest wall in lung cancer: Diagnosis with US. Radiology 187:39-42, 1993.
210. Pretreatment evaluation of non–small-cell lung cancer. The American Thoracic Society and The European Respiratory Society. Am J Respir Crit Care Med 156:320-332, 1997.
211. Santiago SM, Lehrman S, Williams AJ: Bronchoscopy in patients with haemoptysis and normal chest roentgenograms. Br J Dis Chest 81:186-188, 1987.
212. Marcq M, Galy P: Bronchioloalveolar carcinoma. Clinicopathologic relationships, natural history, and prognosis in 29 cases. Am Rev Respir Dis 107:621-629, 1973.
213. Fraser RS, Viloria JB, Wang NS: Cardiac tamponade as a presentation of extracardiac malignancy. Cancer 45:1697-1704, 1980.
214. Okamoto H, Shinkai T, Yamakido M, et al: Cardiac tamponade caused by primary lung cancer and the management of pericardial effusion. Cancer 71:93-98, 1993.
215. Hirschmann JV, Raugi GJ: Dermatologic features of the superior vena cava syndrome. Arch Dermatol 128:953-956, 1992.
216. Schraufnagel DE, Hill R, Leech JA, et al: Superior vena caval obstruction. Is it a medical emergency? Am J Med 70:1169-1174, 1981.
217. Yellin A, Rosen A, Reichert N, et al: Superior vena cava syndrome. The myth—the facts. Am Rev Respir Dis 141:1114-1118, 1990.
218. Stankey RM, Roshe J, Sogocio RM: Carcinoma of the lung and dysphagia. Dis Chest 55:13-17, 1969.
219. Quint LE, Tummala S, Brisson LJ, et al: Distribution of distant metastases from newly diagnosed non–small cell lung cancer. Ann Thorac Surg 62:246-250, 1996.
220. Bender RA, Hansen H: Hypercalcemia in bronchogenic carcinoma, a prospective study of 200 patients. Ann Intern Med 80:205-208, 1974.
221. Covelli HD, Zaloznik AJ, Shekitka KM: Evaluation of bone pain in carcinoma of the lung. Role of the localized false-negative scan. JAMA 244:2625-2627, 1980.
222. McGuire BM, Cherwitz DL, Rabe KM, et al: Small-cell carcinoma of the lung manifesting as acute hepatic failure. Mayo Clin Proc 72:133-139, 1997.
223. Seidenwurm DJ, Elmer EB, Kaplan LM, et al: Metastases to the adrenal glands and the development of Addison's disease. Cancer 54:552-557, 1984.
224. Antler AS, Ough Y, Pitchumoni CS, et al: Gastrointestinal metastases from malignant tumors of the lung. Cancer 49:170-172, 1982.
225. de la Monte SM, Hutchins GM, Moore GW: Paraneoplastic syndromes and constitutional symptoms in prediction of metastatic behavior of small cell carcinoma of the lung. Am J Med 77:851-857, 1984.
226. Gerber RB, Mazzone P, Arroliga AC: Paraneoplastic syndromes associated with bronchogenic carcinoma. Clin Chest Med 23:257-264, 2002.
227. Patel AM, Davila DG, Peters SG: Paraneoplastic syndromes associated with lung cancer. Mayo Clin Proc 68:278-287, 1993.
228. Small-cell lung cancer. Lancet 345:1285-1289, 1995.
229. Takamori M, Komai K, Iwasa K: Antibodies to calcium channel and synaptotagmin in Lambert-Eaton myasthenic syndrome. Am J Med Sci 319:204-208, 2000.
230. Graus F, Elkon KB, Cordon-Cardo C, et al: Sensory neuronopathy and small cell lung cancer. Antineuronal antibody that also reacts with the tumor. Am J Med 80:45-52, 1986.
231. Rudd AG, Nicholas D, Hodkinson HM: Autonomic neuropathy and hypertrophic myopathy in malignancy. Br J Dis Chest 79:396-399, 1985.
232. Simpson DA, Pawlak AM, Tegmeyer L, et al: Paraneoplastic intestinal pseudo-obstruction, mononeuritis multiplex, and sensory neuropathy/neuronopathy. J Am Osteopath Assoc 96:125-128, 1996.
233. Greenlee JE, Lipton HL: Anticerebellar antibodies in serum and cerebrospinal fluid of a patient with oat cell carcinoma of the lung and paraneoplastic cerebellar degeneration. Ann Neurol 19:82-85, 1986.
234. Morton DL, Itabashi HH, Grimes OF: Nonmetastatic neurological complications of bronchogenic carcinoma: The carcinomatous neuromyopathies. J Thorac Cardiovasc Surg 51:14-29, 1966.
235. Rassam JW, Anderson G: Incidence of paramalignant disorders in bronchogenic carcinoma. Thorax 30:86-90, 1975.
236. Monsieur I, Meysman M, Noppen M, et al: Non–small-cell lung cancer with multiple paraneoplastic syndromes. Eur Respir J 8:1231-1234, 1995.
237. Mazzone PJ, Arroliga AC: Endocrine paraneoplastic syndromes in lung cancer. Curr Opin Pulm Med 9:313-320, 2003.
238. Shepherd FA, Laskey J, Evans WK, et al: Cushing's syndrome associated with ectopic corticotropin production and small-cell lung cancer. J Clin Oncol 10:21-27, 1992.

239. Campbell JH, Ralston S, Boyle IT, et al: Symptomatic hypercalcaemia in lung cancer. Respir Med 85:223-227, 1991.
240. Takai E, Yano T, Iguchi H, et al: Tumor-induced hypercalcemia and parathyroid hormone–related protein in lung carcinoma. Cancer 78:1384-1387, 1996.
241. Coggeshall J, Merrill W, Hande K, et al: Implications of hypercalcemia with respect to diagnosis and treatment of lung cancer. Am J Med 80:325-328, 1986.
242. Segura Dominguez A, Andrade Olivie MA, Rodriguez Sousa T, et al: Plasma parathyroid hormone–related protein levels in patients with cancer, normocalcemic and hypercalcemic. Clin Chim Acta 244:163-172, 1996.
243. Metz SA, Weintraub B, Rosen SW, et al: Ectopic secretion of chorionic gonadotropin by a lung carcinoma. Pituitary gonadotropin and subunit secretion and prolonged chemotherapeutic remission. Am J Med 65:325-333, 1978.
244. Becker KL, Nash DR, Silva OL, et al: Urine calcitonin levels in patients with bronchogenic carcinoma. JAMA 243:670-672, 1980.
245. Byrd RB, Divertie MB, Spittell JA Jr: Bronchogenic carcinoma and thromboembolic disease. JAMA 202:1019-1022, 1967.
246. Ziomek S, Read RC, Tobler HG, et al: Thromboembolism in patients undergoing thoracotomy. Ann Thorac Surg 56:223-226, discussion 227, 1993.
247. Tricerri A, Vangeli M, Errani AR, et al: Plasma thrombin-antithrombin complexes, latent coagulation disorders and metastatic spread in lung cancer: A longitudinal study. Oncology 53:455-460, 1996.
248. Kasuga I, Makino S, Kiyokawa H, et al: Tumor-related leukocytosis is linked with poor prognosis in patients with lung carcinoma. Cancer 92:2399-2405, 2001.
249. Pedersen LM, Milman N: Prognostic significance of thrombocytosis in patients with primary lung cancer. Eur Respir J 9:1826-1830, 1996.
250. Dowlati A, R'Zik S, Fillet G, et al: Anaemia of lung cancer is due to impaired erythroid marrow response to erythropoietin stimulation as well as relative inadequacy of erythropoietin production. Br J Haematol 97:297-299, 1997.
251. Vincent FM: Paraneoplastic CNS and renal syndromes. Simultaneous occurrence in a patient with bronchogenic carcinoma. JAMA 240:862-863, 1978.
252. Singer CR, Boulton-Jones JM: Minimal change nephropathy associated with anaplastic carcinoma of bronchus. Postgrad Med J 62:213-217, 1986.
253. Bocking A, Biesterfeld S, Chatelain R, et al: Diagnosis of bronchial carcinoma on sections of paraffin-embedded sputum. Sensitivity and specificity of an alternative to routine cytology. Acta Cytol 36:37-47, 1992.
254. Naryshkin S, Daniels J, Young NA: Diagnostic correlation of fiberoptic bronchoscopic biopsy and bronchoscopic cytology performed simultaneously. Diagn Cytopathol 8:119-123, 1992.
255. Ng AB, Horak GC: Factors significant in the diagnostic accuracy of lung cytology in bronchial washing and sputum samples. II. Sputum samples. Acta Cytol 27:397-402, 1983.
256. Ng AB, Horak GC: Factors significant in the diagnostic accuracy of lung cytology in bronchial washing and sputum samples. I. Bronchial washings. Acta Cytol 27:391-396, 1983.
257. Pirozynski M: Bronchoalveolar lavage in the diagnosis of peripheral, primary lung cancer. Chest 102:372-374, 1992.
258. Dewald GW, Hicks GA, Dines DE, et al: Cytogenetic diagnosis of malignant pleural effusions: Culture methods to supplement direct preparations in diagnosis. Mayo Clin Proc 57:488-494, 1982.
259. Pastor A, Menendez R, Cremades MJ, et al: Diagnostic value of SCC, CEA and CYFRA 21.1 in lung cancer: A Bayesian analysis. Eur Respir J 10:603-609, 1997.
260. Buccheri G, Ferrigno D: The tissue polypeptide antigen serum test in the preoperative evaluation of non–small-cell lung cancer. Diagnostic yield and comparison with conventional staging methods. Chest 107:471-476, 1995.
261. Paone G, De Angelis G, Munno R, et al: Discriminant analysis on small cell lung cancer and non–small cell lung cancer by means of NSE and CYFRA-21.1. Eur Respir J 8:1136-1140, 1995.
262. Nicholson AG, McCormick CJ, Shimosato Y, et al: The value of PE-10, a monoclonal antibody against pulmonary surfactant, in distinguishing primary and metastatic lung tumours. Histopathology 27:57-60, 1995.
263. Diez M, Torres A, Maestro ML, et al: Prediction of survival and recurrence by serum and cytosolic levels of CEA, CA125 and SCC antigens in resectable non–small-cell lung cancer. Br J Cancer 73:1248-1254, 1996.
264. Graziano SL, Mazid R, Newman N, et al: The use of neuroendocrine immunoperoxidase markers to predict chemotherapy response in patients with non–small-cell lung cancer. J Clin Oncol 7:1398-1406, 1989.
265. Buccheri G, Ferrigno D: Monitoring lung cancer with tissue polypeptide antigen: An ancillary, profitable serum test to evaluate treatment response and posttreatment disease status. Lung Cancer 13:155-168, 1995.
266. Strauss GM, Skarin AT: Use of tumor markers in lung cancer. Hematol Oncol Clin North Am 8:507-532, 1994.
267. Mulshine JL, Zhou J, Treston AM, et al: New approaches to the integrated management of early lung cancer. Hematol Oncol Clin North Am 11:235-252, 1997.
268. Bunn PA Jr: Molecular biology and early diagnosis in lung cancer. Lung Cancer 38:S5-S8, 2002.
269. Huang MS, Jong SB, Tsai MS, et al: Comparison of cytokeratin fragment 19 (CYFRA 21-1), tissue polypeptide antigen (TPA) and carcinoembryonic antigen (CEA) as tumour markers in bronchogenic carcinoma. Respir Med 91:135-142, 1997.
270. Ferrigno D, Buccheri G, Biggi A: Serum tumour markers in lung cancer: History, biology and clinical applications. Eur Respir J 7:186-197, 1994.
271. White CS, Romney BM, Mason AC, et al: Primary carcinoma of the lung overlooked at CT: Analysis of findings in 14 patients. Radiology 199:109-115, 1996.
272. Gurney JW: Missed lung cancer at CT: Imaging findings in nine patients. Radiology 199:117-122, 1996.
273. Boysen PG, Harris JO, Block AJ, et al: Prospective evaluation for pneumonectomy using perfusion scanning: Follow-up beyond one year. Chest 80:163-166, 1981.
274. Chin R Jr, Ward R, Keyes JW, et al: Mediastinal staging of non–small-cell lung cancer with positron emission tomography. Am J Respir Crit Care Med 152:2090-2096, 1995.
275. Erasmus JJ, Patz EF Jr, McAdams HP, et al: Evaluation of adrenal masses in patients with bronchogenic carcinoma using 18F-fluorodeoxyglucose positron emission tomography. AJR Am J Roentgenol 168:1357-1360, 1997.
276. Patz EF Jr, Lowe VJ, Hoffman JM, et al: Persistent or recurrent bronchogenic carcinoma: Detection with PET and 2-[F-18]-2-deoxy-D-glucose. Radiology 191:379-382, 1994.
277. Inoue T, Kim EE, Komaki R, et al: Detecting recurrent or residual lung cancer with FDG-PET. J Nucl Med 36:788-793, 1995.
278. Mountain CF: Revisions in the International System for Staging Lung Cancer. Chest 111:1710-1717, 1997.
279. Mountain CF, Dresler CM: Regional lymph node classification for lung cancer staging. Chest 111:1718-1723, 1997.
280. Abrams J, Doyle LA, Aisner J: Staging, prognostic factors, and special considerations in small cell lung cancer. Semin Oncol 15:261-277, 1988.
281. Gay SB, Black WC, Armstrong P, et al: Chest CT of unresectable lung cancer. Radiographics 8:735-748, 1988.
282. Glazer HS, Kaiser LR, Anderson DJ, et al: Indeterminate mediastinal invasion in bronchogenic carcinoma: CT evaluation. Radiology 173:37-42, 1989.
283. White PG, Adams H, Crane MD, et al: Preoperative staging of carcinoma of the bronchus: Can computed tomographic scanning reliably identify stage III tumours? Thorax 49:951-957, 1994.
284. Mayr B, Lenhard M, Fink U, et al: Preoperative evaluation of bronchogenic carcinoma: Value of MR in T- and N-staging. Eur J Radiol 14:245-251, 1992.
285. Ko JP, Drucker EA, Shepard JA, et al: CT depiction of regional nodal stations for lung cancer staging. AJR Am J Roentgenol 174:775-782, 2000.
286. Quint LE, Glazer GM, Orringer MB, et al: Mediastinal lymph node detection and sizing at CT and autopsy. AJR Am J Roentgenol 147:469-472, 1986.
287. Colice GL: Chest CT for known or suspected lung cancer. Chest 106:1538-1550, 1994.
288. Quint LE, Francis IR, Wahl RL, et al: Preoperative staging of non–small-cell carcinoma of the lung: Imaging methods. AJR Am J Roentgenol 164:1349-1359, 1995.
289. Dales RE, Stark RM, Raman S: Computed tomography to stage lung cancer. Approaching a controversy using meta-analysis. Am Rev Respir Dis 141:1096-1101, 1990.
290. Dwamena BA, Sonnad SS, Angobaldo JO, et al: Metastases from non–small cell lung cancer: Mediastinal staging in the 1990s—meta-analytic comparison of PET and CT. Radiology 213:530-536, 1999.
291. Investigation for mediastinal disease in patients with apparently operable lung cancer. Canadian Lung Oncology Group. Ann Thorac Surg 60:1382-1389, 1995.
292. Poon PY, Bronskill MJ, Henkelman RM, et al: Mediastinal lymph node metastases from bronchogenic carcinoma: Detection with MR imaging and CT. Radiology 162:651-656, 1987.
293. Marom EM, McAdams HP, Erasmus JJ, et al: Staging non–small cell lung cancer with whole-body PET. Radiology 212:803-809, 1999.
294. Cerfolio RJ, Ojha B, Bryant AS, et al: The role of FDG-PET scan in staging patients with nonsmall cell carcinoma. Ann Thorac Surg 76:861-866, 2003.
295. Gould MK, Kuschner WG, Rydzak CE, et al: Test performance of positron emission tomography and computed tomography for mediastinal staging in patients with non–small-cell lung cancer: A meta-analysis. Ann Intern Med 139:879-892, 2003.
296. Falcone F, Fois F, Grosso D: Endobronchial ultrasound. Respiration 70:179-194, 2003.
297. Herth FJ, Becker HD, Ernst A: Ultrasound-guided transbronchial needle aspiration: An experience in 242 patients. Chest 123:604-607, 2003.
298. Fritscher-Ravens A, Bohuslavizki KH, Brandt L, et al: Mediastinal lymph node involvement in potentially resectable lung cancer: Comparison of CT, positron emission tomography, and endoscopic ultrasonography with and without fine-needle aspiration. Chest 123:442-451, 2003.
299. Toloza EM, Harpole L, McCrory DC: Noninvasive staging of non–small cell lung cancer: A review of the current evidence. Chest 123:137S-146S, 2003.
300. Fritscher-Ravens A, Davidson BL, Hauber HP, et al: Endoscopic ultrasound, positron emission tomography, and computerized tomography for lung cancer. Am J Respir Crit Care Med 168:1293-1297, 2003.
301. Ichinose Y, Hara N, Ohta M, et al: Preoperative examination to detect distant metastasis is not advocated for asymptomatic patients with stages 1 and 2 non–small cell lung cancer. Preoperative examination for lung cancer. Chest 96:1104-1109, 1989.
302. Silvestri GA, Littenberg B, Colice GL: The clinical evaluation for detecting metastatic lung cancer. A meta-analysis. Am J Respir Crit Care Med 152:225-230, 1995.
303. Ferrigno D, Buccheri G: Cranial computed tomography as a part of the initial staging procedures for patients with non–small-cell lung cancer. Chest 106:1025-1029, 1994.
304. Webb WR, Golden JA: Imaging strategies in the staging of lung cancer. Clin Chest Med 12:133-150, 1991.
305. Ekholm S, Albrechtsson U, Kugelberg J, et al: Computed tomography in preoperative staging of bronchogenic carcinoma. J Comput Assist Tomogr 4:763-765, 1980.
306. Remer EM, Obuchowski N, Ellis JD, et al: Adrenal mass evaluation in patients with lung carcinoma: A cost-effectiveness analysis. AJR Am J Roentgenol 174:1033-1039, 2000.
307. Heinz-Peer G, Honigschnabl S, Schneider B, et al: Characterization of adrenal masses using MR imaging with histopathologic correlation. AJR Am J Roentgenol 173:15-22, 1999.

308. Maurea S, Mainolfi C, Bazzicalupo L, et al: Imaging of adrenal tumors using FDG PET: Comparison of benign and malignant lesions. AJR Am J Roentgenol 173:25-29, 1999.

309. Ost D, Fein AM, Feinsilver SH: Clinical practice. The solitary pulmonary nodule. N Engl J Med 348:2535-2542, 2003.

310. Siegelman SS, Khouri NF, Scott WW Jr, et al: Pulmonary hamartoma: CT findings. Radiology 160:313-317, 1986.

311. Takashima S, Sone S, Li F, et al: Small solitary pulmonary nodules (< or =1 cm) detected at population-based CT screening for lung cancer: Reliable high-resolution CT features of benign lesions. AJR Am J Roentgenol 180:955-964, 2003.

312. Laking G, Price P: 18-Fluorodeoxyglucose positron emission tomography (FDG-PET) and the staging of early lung cancer. Thorax 56(Suppl 2):ii38-ii44, 2001.

313. Gould MK, Sanders GD, Barnett PG, et al: Cost-effectiveness of alternative management strategies for patients with solitary pulmonary nodules. Ann Intern Med 138:724-735, 2003.

314. Rubins JB, Rubins HB: Temporal trends in the prevalence of malignancy in resected solitary pulmonary lesions. Chest 109:100-103, 1996.

315. Lillington GA: Solitary pulmonary nodules: New wine in old bottles. Curr Opin Pulm Med 7:242-246, 2001.

316. Baaklini WA, Reinoso MA, Gorin AB, et al: Diagnostic yield of fiberoptic bronchoscopy in evaluating solitary pulmonary nodules. Chest 117:1049-1054, 2000.

317. Larscheid RC, Thorpe PE, Scott WJ: Percutaneous transthoracic needle aspiration biopsy: A comprehensive review of its current role in the diagnosis and treatment of lung tumors. Chest 114:704-709, 1998.

318. Takamochi K, Nagai K, Suzuki K, et al: Clinical predictors of N2 disease in non–small cell lung cancer. Chest 117:1577-1582, 2000.

319. Kaplan DK: Mediastinal lymph node metastases in lung cancer: Is size a valid criterion? Thorax 47:332-333, 1992.

320. Pearson M: Is CT scanning essential in the pre-operative assessment of lung cancer? Respir Med 83:93-94, 1989.

321. Gupta NC, Graeber GM, Bishop HA: Comparative efficacy of positron emission tomography with fluorodeoxyglucose in evaluation of small (<1 cm), intermediate (1 to 3 cm), and large (>3 cm) lymph node lesions. Chest 117:773-778, 2000.

322. Kernstine KH, McLaughlin KA, Menda Y, et al: Can FDG-PET reduce the need for mediastinoscopy in potentially resectable nonsmall cell lung cancer? Ann Thorac Surg 73:394-401, discussion 401-402, 2002.

323. Graeter TP, Hellwig D, Hoffmann K, et al: Mediastinal lymph node staging in suspected lung cancer: Comparison of positron emission tomography with F-18-fluorodeoxyglucose and mediastinoscopy. Ann Thorac Surg 75:231-235, discussion 235-236, 2003.

324. Harrow EM, Abi-Saleh W, Blum J, et al: The utility of transbronchial needle aspiration in the staging of bronchogenic carcinoma. Am J Respir Crit Care Med 161:601-607, 2000.

325. Fritscher-Ravens A: Endoscopic ultrasound evaluation in the diagnosis and staging of lung cancer. Lung Cancer 41:259-267, 2003.

326. Wallace MB, Silvestri GA, Sahai AV, et al: Endoscopic ultrasound-guided fine needle aspiration for staging patients with carcinoma of the lung. Ann Thorac Surg 72:1861-1867, 2001.

327. Guidelines for fiberoptic bronchoscopy in adults. American Thoracic Society. Medical Section of the American Lung Association. Am Rev Respir Dis 136:1066, 1987.

328. Flehinger BJ, Melamed MR: Current status of screening for lung cancer. Chest Surg Clin N Am 4:1-15, 1994.

329. Henschke CI, Yankelevitz DF, Libby D, et al: Computed tomography screening for lung cancer. Clin Chest Med 23:49-57, viii, 2002.

330. Bach PB, Kelley MJ, Tate RC, et al: Screening for lung cancer: A review of the current literature. Chest 123:72S-82S, 2003.

331. Saito Y, Takahashi S, Usuda K, et al: [Detection of early cancer by lung cancer screening.] Nippon Rinsho 54:1410-1414, 1996.

332. Strauss GM, Gleason RE, Sugarbaker DJ: Screening for lung cancer. Another look; a different view. Chest 111:754-768, 1997.

333. Patz EF Jr, Goodman PC, Bepler G: Screening for lung cancer. N Engl J Med 343:1627-1633, 2000.

334. Mori K, Tominaga K, Hirose T, et al: Utility of low-dose helical CT as a second step after plain chest radiography for mass screening for lung cancer. J Thorac Imaging 12:173-180, 1997.

335. MacRedmond R, Logan PM, Lee M, et al: Screening for lung cancer using low dose CT scanning. Thorax 59:237-241, 2004.

336. Swensen SJ, Jett JR, Sloan JA, et al: Screening for lung cancer with low-dose spiral computed tomography. Am J Respir Crit Care Med 165:508-513, 2002.

337. Mahadevia PJ, Fleisher LA, Frick KD, et al: Lung cancer screening with helical computed tomography in older adult smokers: A decision and cost-effectiveness analysis. JAMA 289:313-322, 2003.

338. Heffner JE, Silvestri G: CT screening for lung cancer: Is smaller better? Am J Respir Crit Care Med 165:433-434, 2002.

339. Beadsmoore CJ, Screaton NJ: Classification, staging and prognosis of lung cancer. Eur J Radiol 45:8-17, 2003.

340. Shields TW: Surgical therapy for carcinoma of the lung. Clin Chest Med 14:121-147, 1993.

341. Wada H, Tanaka F, Yanagihara K, et al: Time trends and survival after operations for primary lung cancer from 1976 through 1990. J Thorac Cardiovasc Surg 112:349-355, 1996.

342. Roxburgh JC, Thompson J, Goldstraw P: Hospital mortality and long-term survival after pulmonary resection in the elderly. Ann Thorac Surg 51:800-803, 1991.

343. Massard G, Moog R, Wihlm JM, et al: Bronchogenic cancer in the elderly: Operative risk and long-term prognosis. Thorac Cardiovasc Surg 44:40-45, 1996.

344. Antkowiak JG, Regal AM, Takita H: Bronchogenic carcinoma in patients under age 40. Ann Thorac Surg 47:391-393, 1989.

345. Lee-Chiong TL Jr, Matthay RA: Lung cancer in the elderly patient. Clin Chest Med 14:453-478, 1993.

346. Rossing TH, Rossing RG: Survival in lung cancer. An analysis of the effects of age, sex, resectability, and histopathologic type. Am Rev Respir Dis 126:771-777, 1982.

347. Fry WA, Menck HR, Winchester DP: The National Cancer Data Base report on lung cancer. Cancer 77:1947-1955, 1996.

348. Bach PB, Cramer LD, Warren JL, et al: Racial differences in the treatment of early-stage lung cancer. N Engl J Med 341:1198-1205, 1999.

349. Fraire AE, Roggli VL, Vollmer RT, et al: Lung cancer heterogeneity. Prognostic implications. Cancer 60:370-375, 1987.

350. Stanley K, Cox JD, Petrovich Z, et al: Patterns of failure in patients with inoperable carcinoma of the lung. Cancer 47:2725-2729, 1981.

351. Cangemi V, Volpino P, D'Andrea N, et al: Results of surgical treatment of stage IIIA non–small cell lung cancer. Eur J Cardiothorac Surg 9:352-359, 1995.

352. Coen V, Van Lancker M, De Neve W, et al: Prognostic factors in locoregional non–small cell lung cancer treated with radiotherapy. Am J Clin Oncol 18:111-117, 1995.

353. Filderman AE, Silvestri GA, Gatsonis C, et al: Prognostic significance of tumor proliferative fraction and DNA content in stage I non–small cell lung cancer. Am Rev Respir Dis 146:707-710, 1992.

354. Cortese DA, Pairolero PC, Bergstralh EJ, et al: Roentgenographically occult lung cancer. A ten-year experience. J Thorac Cardiovasc Surg 86:373-380, 1983.

355. Martini N, Melamed MR: Occult carcinomas of the lung. Ann Thorac Surg 30:215-223, 1980.

356. Blanke CD, Johnson DH: Treatment of small cell lung cancer. Semin Thorac Cardiovasc Surg 9:101-110, 1997.

357. Skarin AT: Analysis of long-term survivors with small-cell lung cancer. Chest 103:440S-444S, 1993.

358. Johnson BE: Concurrent approaches to combined chemotherapy and chest radiotherapy for the treatment of patients with limited stage small cell lung cancer. Lung Cancer 10(Suppl 1):S281-S287, 1994.

359. Chak LY, Sikic BI, Tucker MA, et al: Increased incidence of acute nonlymphocytic leukemia following therapy in patients with small cell carcinoma of the lung. J Clin Oncol 2:385-390, 1984.

360. Huhti E, Sutinen S, Saloheimo M: Survival among patients with lung cancer. An epidemiologic study. Am Rev Respir Dis 124:13-16, 1981.

361. Gail MH, Eagan RT, Feld R, et al: Prognostic factors in patients with resected stage I non–small cell lung cancer. A report from the Lung Cancer Study Group. Cancer 54:1802-1813, 1984.

362. Liu YY, Chen YM, Huang MH, et al: Prognosis and recurrent patterns in bronchioloalveolar carcinoma. Chest 118:940-947, 2000.

363. Detterbeck FC, Socinski MA: IIB or not IIB: The current question in staging non–small cell lung cancer. Chest 112:229-234, 1997.

364. Patz EF Jr, Rossi S, Harpole DH Jr, et al: Correlation of tumor size and survival in patients with stage IA non–small cell lung cancer. Chest 117:1568-1571, 2000.

365. Feinstein AR, Sosin DM, Wells CK: The Will Rogers phenomenon. Stage migration and new diagnostic techniques as a source of misleading statistics for survival in cancer. N Engl J Med 312:1604-1608, 1985.

366. van Klaveren RJ, Festen J, Otten HJ, et al: Prognosis of unsuspected but completely resectable N2 non–small cell lung cancer. Ann Thorac Surg 56:300-304, 1993.

367. Riquet M, Manac'h D, Saab M, et al: Factors determining survival in resected N2 lung cancer. Eur J Cardiothorac Surg 9:300-304, 1995.

368. Deslauriers J, Brisson J, Cartier R, et al: Carcinoma of the lung. Evaluation of satellite nodules as a factor influencing prognosis after resection. J Thorac Cardiovasc Surg 97:504-512, 1989.

369. Mountain CF: The biological operability of stage III non–small cell lung cancer. Ann Thorac Surg 40:60-64, 1985.

370. van Meerbeeck JP: Staging of non–small cell lung cancer: Consensus, controversies and challenges. Lung Cancer 34(Suppl 2):S95-S107, 2001.

371. Postmus PE, Sleijfer DT, Meinesz AF, et al: No response improvement after sequential chemotherapy for small cell lung cancer. Eur J Respir Dis 68:279-285, 1986.

372. Kochhar R, Frytak S, Shaw EG: Survival of patients with extensive small-cell lung cancer who have only brain metastases at initial diagnosis. Am J Clin Oncol 20:125-127, 1997.

373. Hirsch FR, Hansen HH: Bone marrow involvement in small cell anaplastic carcinoma of the lung: Prognostic and therapeutic aspects. Cancer 46:206-211, 1980.

374. Buccheri G, Ferrigno D: Prognostic factors in lung cancer: Tables and comments. Eur Respir J 7:1350-1364, 1994.

375. Takigawa N, Segawa Y, Okahara M, et al: Prognostic factors for patients with advanced non–small cell lung cancer: Univariate and multivariate analyses including recursive partitioning and amalgamation. Lung Cancer 15:67-77, 1996.

376. Feinstein AR, Wells CK: A clinical-severity staging system for patients with lung cancer. Medicine (Baltimore) 69:1-33, 1990.

377. Mountain CF: New prognostic factors in lung cancer. Biologic prophets of cancer cell aggression. Chest 108:246-254, 1995.

378. Niklinski J, Niklinska W, Laudanski J, et al: Prognostic molecular markers in non–small cell lung cancer. Lung Cancer 34(Suppl 2):S53-S58, 2001.

379. Rosengart TK, Martini N, Ghosn P, et al: Multiple primary lung carcinomas: Prognosis and treatment. Ann Thorac Surg 52:773-778, discussion 778-779, 1991.

380. Antkli T, Schaefer RF, Rutherford JE, et al: Second primary lung cancer. Ann Thorac Surg 59:863-866, discussion 867, 1995.

381. Coffman B, Crum E, Forman WB: Two primary carcinomas of the lung: Adeno-carcinoma and a metachronous squamous cell carcinoma. A case report and review of the literature. Cancer 51:124-126, 1983.

382. Little AG, DeMeester TR, Ferguson MK, et al: Modified stage I (T1N0M0, T2N0M0), nonsmall cell lung cancer: Treatment results, recurrence patterns, and adjuvant immunotherapy. Surgery 100:621-628, 1986.

383. Pommier RF, Vetto JT, Lee JT, et al: Synchronous non–small cell lung cancers. Am J Surg 171:521-524, 1996.

384. Shibuya H, Hisamitsu S, Shioiri S, et al: Multiple primary cancer risk in patients with squamous cell carcinoma of the oral cavity. Cancer 60:3083-3086, 1987.

385. Silvestri F, Bussani R, Cosatti C, et al: High relative risk of a second pulmonary cancer in patients affected by laryngeal cancer: Differences by specific site of occurrence and lung cancer histotype. Laryngoscope 104:222-225, 1994.

386. Engeland A, Bjorge T, Haldorsen T, et al: Use of multiple primary cancers to indicate associations between smoking and cancer incidence: An analysis of 500,000 cancer cases diagnosed in Norway during 1953-93. Int J Cancer 70:401-407, 1997.

387. Salminen E, Pukkala E, Teppo L, et al: Risk of second cancers among lung cancer patients. Acta Oncol 34:165-169, 1995.

388. Bertoldero G, Scribano G, Podda L, et al: Occurrence of second neoplasms in chronic lymphocytic leukemia. Experience at Padua Hospital between 1979 and 1991. Ann Hematol 69:195-198, 1994.

389. van Leeuwen FE, Klokman WJ, Stovall M, et al: Roles of radiotherapy and smoking in lung cancer following Hodgkin's disease. J Natl Cancer Inst 87:1530-1537, 1995.

390. Inskip PD, Stovall M, Flannery JT: Lung cancer risk and radiation dose among women treated for breast cancer. J Natl Cancer Inst 86:983-988, 1994.

391. Paladugu RR, Benfield JR, Pak HY, et al: Bronchopulmonary Kulchitsky cell carcinomas. A new classification scheme for typical and atypical carcinoids. Cancer 55:1303-1311, 1985.

392. Przygodzki RM, Finkelstein SD, Langer JC, et al: Analysis of p53, K-ras-2, and C-raf-1 in pulmonary neuroendocrine tumors. Correlation with histological subtype and clinical outcome. Am J Pathol 148:1531-1541, 1996.

393. Godwin JD 2nd: Carcinoid tumors. An analysis of 2,837 cases. Cancer 36:560-569, 1975.

394. Harpole DH Jr, Feldman JM, Buchanan S, et al: Bronchial carcinoid tumors: A retrospective analysis of 126 patients. Ann Thorac Surg 54:50-54, discussion 54-55, 1992.

395. McCaughan BC, Martini N, Bains MS: Bronchial carcinoids. Review of 124 cases. J Thorac Cardiovasc Surg 89:8-17, 1985.

396. Grote TH, Macon WR, Davis B, et al: Atypical carcinoid of the lung. A distinct clinicopathologic entity. Chest 93:370-375, 1988.

397. Wang LT, Wilkins EW Jr, Bode HH: Bronchial carcinoid tumors in pediatric patients. Chest 103:1426-1428, 1993.

398. Ranchod M, Levine GD: Spindle-cell carcinoid tumors of the lung: A clinicopathologic study of 35 cases. Am J Surg Pathol 4:315-331, 1980.

399. Kinney FJ, Kovarik JL: Bone formation in bronchial adenoma. Am J Clin Pathol 44:52-56, 1965.

400. Al-Kaisi N, Abdul-Karim FW, Mendelsohn G, et al: Bronchial carcinoid tumor with amyloid stroma. Arch Pathol Lab Med 112:211-214, 1988.

401. Martin JM, Maung RT: Differential immunohistochemical reactions of carcinoid tumors. Hum Pathol 18:941-945, 1987.

402. Gould VE, Linnoila RI, Memoli VA, et al: Neuroendocrine cells and neuroendocrine neoplasms of the lung. Pathol Annu 18(Pt 1):287-330, 1983.

403. Addis BJ, Hamid Q, Ibrahim NB, et al: Immunohistochemical markers of small cell carcinoma and related neuroendocrine tumours of the lung. J Pathol 153:137-150, 1987.

404. Hurt R, Bates M: Carcinoid tumours of the bronchus: A 33 year experience. Thorax 39:617-623, 1984.

405. Jordan AG, Predmore L, Sullivan MM, et al: The cytodiagnosis of well-differentiated neuroendocrine carcinoma. A distinct clinicopathologic entity. Acta Cytol 31:464-470, 1987.

406. Arrigoni MG, Woolner LB, Bernatz PE: Atypical carcinoid tumors of the lung. J Thorac Cardiovasc Surg 64:413-421, 1972.

407. Valli M, Fabris GA, Dewar A, et al: Atypical carcinoid tumour of the lung: A study of 33 cases with prognostic features. Histopathology 24:363-369, 1994.

408. Mills SE, Cooper PH, Walker AN, et al: Atypical carcinoid tumor of the lung. A clinicopathologic study of 17 cases. Am J Surg Pathol 6:643-654, 1982.

409. Chaudhuri TK, Shapiro RL, Christie JH: Abnormal lung perfusion in a patient with bronchial adenoma. Chest 62:110-112, 1972.

410. Nessi R, Basso Ricci P, Basso Ricci S, et al: Bronchial carcinoid tumors: Radiologic observations in 49 cases. J Thorac Imaging 6:47-53, 1991.

411. Lawson RM, Ramanathan L, Hurley G, et al: Bronchial adenoma: Review of 18-year experience at the Brompton Hospital. Thorax 31:245-253, 1976.

412. Zwiebel BR, Austin JH, Grimes MM: Bronchial carcinoid tumors: Assessment with CT of location and intratumoral calcification in 31 patients. Radiology 179:483-486, 1991.

413. Magid D, Siegelman SS, Eggleston JC, et al: Pulmonary carcinoid tumors: CT assessment. J Comput Assist Tomogr 13:244-247, 1989.

414. Jeung MY, Gasser B, Gangi A, et al: Bronchial carcinoid tumors of the thorax: Spectrum of radiologic findings. Radiographics 22:351-365, 2002.

415. Kvols LK, Brown ML, O'Connor MK, et al: Evaluation of a radiolabeled somatostatin analog (I-123 octreotide) in the detection and localization of carcinoid and islet cell tumors. Radiology 187:129-133, 1993.

416. Bomanji J, Mather S, Moyes J, et al: A scintigraphic comparison of iodine-123-metaiododobenzylguanidine and an iodine-labeled somatostatin analog (Tyr-3-octreotide) in metastatic carcinoid tumors. J Nucl Med 33:1121-1124, 1992.

417. Gotthardt M, Behe MP, Alfke H, et al: Imaging lung tumors with peptide-based radioligands. Clin Lung Cancer 5:119-124, 2003.

418. Belhocine T, Foidart J, Rigo P, et al: Fluorodeoxyglucose positron emission tomography and somatostatin receptor scintigraphy for diagnosing and staging carcinoid tumours: Correlations with the pathological indexes p53 and Ki-67. Nucl Med Commun 23:727-734, 2002.

419. Sheppard BB, Follette DM, Meyers FJ: Giant carcinoid tumor of the lung. Ann Thorac Surg 63:851-852, 1997.

420. Forster BB, Müller NL, Miller RR, et al: Neuroendocrine carcinomas of the lung: Clinical, radiologic, and pathologic correlation. Radiology 170:441-445, 1989.

421. Rea F, Binda R, Spreafico G, et al: Bronchial carcinoids: A review of 60 patients. Ann Thorac Surg 47:412-414, 1989.

422. Wynn SR, O'Connell EJ, Frigas E, et al: Exercise-induced "asthma" as a presentation of bronchial carcinoid. Ann Allergy 57:139-141, 1986.

423. Johnson LA, Lavin P, Moertel CG, et al: Carcinoids: The association of histologic growth pattern and survival. Cancer 51:882-889, 1983.

424. Oberg K, Norheim I, Wide L: Serum growth hormone in patients with carcinoid tumours; basal levels and response to glucose and thyrotrophin releasing hormone. Acta Endocrinol (Copenh) 109:13-18, 1985.

425. Doppman JL, Nieman L, Miller DL, et al: Ectopic adrenocorticotropic hormone syndrome: Localization studies in 28 patients. Radiology 172:115-124, 1989.

426. Oliaro A, Filosso PL, Casadio C, et al: Bronchial carcinoid associated with Cushing's syndrome. J Cardiovasc Surg (Torino) 36:511-514, 1995.

427. Isawa T, Okubo K, Konno K, et al: Cushing's syndrome caused by recurrent malignant bronchial carcinoid. Case report with 12 years' observation. Am Rev Respir Dis 108:1200-1204, 1973.

428. Johnson NF, Wagner JC, Wills HA: Endocrine cell proliferation in the rat lung following asbestos inhalation. Lung 158:221-228, 1980.

429. Saeed uz Zafar M, Mellinger RC, Fine G, et al: Acromegaly associated with a bronchial carcinoid tumor: Evidence for ectopic production of growth hormone–releasing activity. J Clin Endocrinol Metab 48:66-71, 1979.

430. Bertelsen S, Aasted A, Lund C, et al: Bronchial carcinoid tumours. A clinicopathologic study of 82 cases. Scand J Thorac Cardiovasc Surg 19:105-111, 1985.

431. Cooney T, Benediktsson H, Mukai K: Immunohistochemical evaluation of a complex endocrinopathy. Am J Surg Pathol 4:491-499, 1980.

432. Okike N, Bernatz PE, Woolner LB: Carcinoid tumors of the lung. Ann Thorac Surg 22:270-277, 1976.

433. Collins BT, Cramer HM: Fine needle aspiration cytology of carcinoid tumors. Acta Cytol 40:695-707, 1996.

434. Raff H, Shaker JL, Seifert PE, et al: Intraoperative measurement of adrenocorticotropin (ACTH) during removal of ACTH-secreting bronchial carcinoid tumors. J Clin Endocrinol Metab 80:1036-1039, 1995.

435. Schreurs AJ, Westermann CJ, van den Bosch JM, et al: A twenty-five-year follow-up of ninety-three resected typical carcinoid tumors of the lung. J Thorac Cardiovasc Surg 104:1470-1475, 1992.

436. Ducrocq X, Thomas P, Massard G, et al: Operative risk and prognostic factors of typical bronchial carcinoid tumors. Ann Thorac Surg 65:1410-1414, 1998.

437. Bernstein C, McGoey J, Lertzman M: Recurrent bronchial carcinoid tumor. Chest 95:693-694, 1989.

438. Perkins P, Kemp BL, Putnam JB Jr, et al: Pretreatment characteristics of carcinoid tumors of the lung which predict aggressive behavior. Am J Clin Oncol 20:285-288, 1997.

439. Perkins P, Lee JR, Kemp BL, et al: Carcinoid tumors of the lung and family history of cancer. J Clin Epidemiol 50:705-709, 1997.

440. Shrager JB, Wright CD, Wain JC, et al: Bronchopulmonary carcinoid tumors associated with Cushing's syndrome: A more aggressive variant of typical carcinoid. J Thorac Cardiovasc Surg 114:367-375, 1997.

441. Padberg BC, Woenckhaus J, Hilger G, et al: DNA cytophotometry and prognosis in typical and atypical bronchopulmonary carcinoids. A clinicomorphologic study of 100 neuroendocrine lung tumors. Am J Surg Pathol 20:815-822, 1996.

442. Bohm J, Koch S, Gais P, et al: Prognostic value of MIB-1 in neuroendocrine tumours of the lung. J Pathol 178:402-409, 1996.

443. Marty-Ane CH, Costes V, Pujol JL, et al: Carcinoid tumors of the lung: Do atypical features require aggressive management? Ann Thorac Surg 59:78-83, 1995.

444. DeCaro LF, Paladugu R, Benfield JR, et al: Typical and atypical carcinoids within the pulmonary APUD tumor spectrum. J Thorac Cardiovasc Surg 86:528-536, 1983.

445. el-Naggar AK, Ballance W, Karim FW, et al: Typical and atypical bronchopulmonary carcinoids. A clinicopathologic and flow cytometric study. Am J Clin Pathol 95:828-834, 1991.

446. Lequaglie C, Patriarca C, Cataldo I, et al: Prognosis of resected well-differentiated neuroendocrine carcinoma of the lung. Chest 100:1053-1056, 1991.

447. Miller RR, Müller NL: Neuroendocrine cell hyperplasia and obliterative bronchiolitis in patients with peripheral carcinoid tumors. Am J Surg Pathol 19:653-658, 1995.

448. Cunningham GJ, Nassau E, Walter JB: The frequency of tumour-like formations in bronchiectatic lungs. Thorax 13:64-68, 1958.

449. Churg A, Warnock ML: Pulmonary tumorlet. A form of peripheral carcinoid. Cancer 37:1469-1477, 1976.

450. Bennett GL, Chew FS: Pulmonary carcinoid tumorlets. AJR Am J Roentgenol 162:568, 1994.

451. Brown MJ, English J, Müller NL: Bronchiolitis obliterans due to neuroendocrine hyperplasia: High-resolution CT—pathologic correlation. AJR Am J Roentgenol 168:1561-1562, 1997.

452. Aguayo SM, Miller YE, Waldron JA Jr, et al: Brief report: Idiopathic diffuse hyperplasia of pulmonary neuroendocrine cells and airways disease. N Engl J Med 327:1285-1288, 1992.

453. Rodgers-Sullivan RF, Weiland LH, Palumbo PJ, et al: Pulmonary tumorlets associated with Cushing's syndrome. Am Rev Respir Dis 117:799-806, 1978.

454. Jiang SX, Kameya T, Shoji M, et al: Large cell neuroendocrine carcinoma of the lung: A histologic and immunohistochemical study of 22 cases. Am J Surg Pathol 22:526-537, 1998.

455. Dresler CM, Ritter JH, Patterson GA, et al: Clinical-pathologic analysis of 40 patients with large cell neuroendocrine carcinoma of the lung. Ann Thorac Surg 63:180-185, 1997.

456. Rusch VW, Klimstra DS, Venkatraman ES: Molecular markers help characterize neuroendocrine lung tumors. Ann Thorac Surg 62:798-809, discussion 809-810, 1996.

457. Travis WD, Linnoila RI, Tsokos MG, et al: Neuroendocrine tumors of the lung with proposed criteria for large-cell neuroendocrine carcinoma. An ultrastructural, immunohistochemical, and flow cytometric study of 35 cases. Am J Surg Pathol 15:529-553, 1991.

458. Moran CA: Primary salivary gland–type tumors of the lung. Semin Diagn Pathol 12:106-122, 1995.

459. Gelder CM, Hetzel MR: Primary tracheal tumours: A national survey. Thorax 48:688-692, 1993.

460. Conlan AA, Payne WS, Woolner LB, et al: Adenoid cystic carcinoma (cylindroma) and mucoepidermoid carcinoma of the bronchus. Factors affecting survival. J Thorac Cardiovasc Surg 76:369-377, 1978.

461. Janower ML, Grillo HC, MacMillan AS Jr, et al: The radiological appearance of carcinoma of the trachea. Radiology 96:39-43, 1970.

462. Kwong JS, Adler BD, Padley SP, et al: Diagnosis of diseases of the trachea and main bronchi: Chest radiography vs CT. AJR Am J Roentgenol 161:519-522, 1993.

463. Olmedo G, Rosenberg M, Fonseca R: Primary tumors of the trachea: Clinicopathologic features and surgical results. Chest 81:701, 1982.

464. Moran CA, Suster S, Koss MN: Primary adenoid cystic carcinoma of the lung. A clinicopathologic and immunohistochemical study of 16 cases. Cancer 73:1390-1397, 1994.

465. Maziak DE, Todd TR, Keshavjee SH, et al: Adenoid cystic carcinoma of the airway: Thirty-two-year experience. J Thorac Cardiovasc Surg 112:1522-1531, discussion 1531-1532, 1996.

466. McCarthy MJ, Rosado-de-Christenson ML: Tumors of the trachea. J Thorac Imaging 10:180-198, 1995.

467. Boiselle PM, Reynolds KF, Ernst A: Multiplanar and three-dimensional imaging of the central airways with multidetector CT. AJR Am J Roentgenol 179:301-308, 2002.

468. Finkelstein SE, Schrump DS, Nguyen DM, et al: Comparative evaluation of super high-resolution CT scan and virtual bronchoscopy for the detection of tracheobronchial malignancies. Chest 124:1834-1840, 2003.

469. Kanematsu T, Yohena T, Uehara T, et al: Treatment outcome of resected and non-resected primary adenoid cystic carcinoma of the lung. Ann Thorac Cardiovasc Surg 8:74-77, 2002.

470. Inoue H, Iwashita A, Kanegae H, et al: Peripheral pulmonary adenoid cystic carcinoma with substantial submucosal extension to the proximal bronchus. Thorax 46:147-148, 1991.

471. Yousem SA, Hochholzer L: Mucoepidermoid tumors of the lung. Cancer 60:1346-1352, 1987.

472. Heitmiller RF, Mathisen DJ, Ferry JA, et al: Mucoepidermoid lung tumors. Ann Thorac Surg 47:394-399, 1989.

473. Tsuchiya H, Nagashima K, Ohashi S, et al: Childhood bronchial mucoepidermoid tumors. J Pediatr Surg 32:106-109, 1997.

474. Turnbull AD, Huvos AG, Goodner JT, et al: Mucoepidermoid tumors of bronchial glands. Cancer 28:539-544, 1971.

475. Kim TS, Lee KS, Han J, et al: Mucoepidermoid carcinoma of the tracheobronchial tree: Radiographic and CT findings in 12 patients. Radiology 212:643-648, 1999.

476. Kwong JS, Müller NL, Miller RR: Diseases of the trachea and main-stem bronchi: Correlation of CT with pathologic findings. Radiographics 12:645-657, 1992.

477. Spencer H, Dail DH, Arneaud J: Non-invasive bronchial epithelial papillary tumors. Cancer 45:1486-1497, 1980.

478. Dancey DR, Chamberlain DW, Krajden M, et al: Successful treatment of juvenile laryngeal papillomatosis–related multicystic lung disease with cidofovir: Case report and review of the literature. Chest 118:1210-1214, 2000.

479. Smith J, Gooding CA: Pulmonary involvement in laryngeal papillomatosis. Pediatr Radiol 2:161-166, 1974.

480. Rubel L, Reynolds RE: Cytologic description of squamous cell papilloma of the respiratory tract. Acta Cytol 23:227-231, 1979.

481. Helmuth RA, Strate RW: Squamous carcinoma of the lung in a nonirradiated, non-smoking patient with juvenile laryngotracheal papillomatosis. Am J Surg Pathol 11:643-650, 1987.

482. Kerley SW, Buchon-Zalles C, Moran J, et al: Chronic cavitary respiratory papillomatosis. Arch Pathol Lab Med 113:1166-1169, 1989.

483. Kramer SS, Wehunt WD, Stocker JT, et al: Pulmonary manifestations of juvenile laryngotracheal papillomatosis. AJR Am J Roentgenol 144:687-694, 1985.

484. Takasugi JE, Godwin JD: The airway. Semin Roentgenol 26:175-190, 1991.

485. Laubscher FA: Solitary squamous cell papilloma of bronchial origin. Am J Clin Pathol 52:599-603, 1969.

486. Brach BB, Klein RC, Mathews AJ, et al: Papillomatosis of the respiratory tract. Upper airway obstruction and carcinoma. Arch Otolaryngol 104:413-416, 1978.

487. Drennan JM, Douglas AC: Solitary papilloma of a bronchus. J Clin Pathol 18:401-402, 1965.

488. Wilde E, Duggan MA, Field SK: Bronchogenic squamous cell carcinoma complicating localized recurrent respiratory papillomatosis. Chest 105:1887-1888, 1994.

489. Maxwell RJ, Gibbons JR, O'Hara MD: Solitary squamous papilloma of the bronchus. Thorax 40:68-71, 1985.

490. Zimmermann A, Lang HR, Muhlberger F, et al: Papilloma of the bronchus. Respiration 39:286-290, 1980.

491. Popper HH, el-Shabrawi Y, Wockel W, et al: Prognostic importance of human papilloma virus typing in squamous cell papilloma of the bronchus: Comparison of in situ hybridization and the polymerase chain reaction. Hum Pathol 25:1191-1197, 1994.

492. Dixon AY, Moran JF, Wesselius LJ, et al: Pulmonary mucinous cystic tumor. Case report with review of the literature. Am J Surg Pathol 17:722-728, 1993.

493. Noguchi M, Kodama T, Shimosato Y, et al: Papillary adenoma of type 2 pneumocytes. Am J Surg Pathol 10:134-139, 1986.

494. Yousem SA, Hochholzer L: Alveolar adenoma. Hum Pathol 17:1066-1071, 1986.

495. Koss MN: Pulmonary lymphoid disorders. Semin Diagn Pathol 12:158-171, 1995.

496. Kawahara K, Shiraishi T, Okabayashi K, et al: Nodular lymphoid hyperplasia in the lung. Thorac Cardiovasc Surg 44:210-212, 1996.

497. Bragg DG, Chor PJ, Murray KA, et al: Lymphoproliferative disorders of the lung: Histopathology, clinical manifestations, and imaging features. AJR Am J Roentgenol 163:273-281, 1994.

498. Holland EA, Ghahremani GG, Fry WA, et al: Evolution of pulmonary pseudolymphomas: Clinical and radiologic manifestations. J Thorac Imaging 6:74-80, 1991.

499. Hutchinson WB, Friedenberg MJ, Saltzstein S: Primary pulmonary pseudolymphoma. Radiology 82:48-56, 1964.

500. Koss MN, Hochholzer L, Nichols PW, et al: Primary non-Hodgkin's lymphoma and pseudolymphoma of lung: A study of 161 patients. Hum Pathol 14:1024-1038, 1983.

501. Nicholson AG, Wotherspoon AC, Diss TC, et al: Reactive pulmonary lymphoid disorders. Histopathology 26:405-412, 1995.

502. Turner RR, Colby TV, Doggett RS: Well-differentiated lymphocytic lymphoma. A study of 47 patients with primary manifestation in the lung. Cancer 54:2088-2096, 1984.

503. Kurosu K, Yumoto N, Furukawa M, et al: Third complementarity-determining-region sequence analysis of lymphocytic interstitial pneumonia: Most cases demonstrate a minor monoclonal population hidden among normal lymphocyte clones. Am J Respir Crit Care Med 155:1453-1460, 1997.

504. Herbert A, Walters MT, Cawley MI, et al: Lymphocytic interstitial pneumonia identified as lymphoma of mucosa associated lymphoid tissue. J Pathol 146:129-138, 1985.

505. Deheinzelin D, Capelozzi VL, Kairalla RA, et al: Interstitial lung disease in primary Sjögren's syndrome. Clinical-pathological evaluation and response to treatment. Am J Respir Crit Care Med 154:794-799, 1996.

506. Travis WD, Fox CH, Devaney KO, et al: Lymphoid pneumonitis in 50 adult patients infected with the human immunodeficiency virus: Lymphocytic interstitial pneumonitis versus nonspecific interstitial pneumonitis. Hum Pathol 23:529-541, 1992.

507. DeMartini JC, Brodie SJ, de la Concha-Bermejillo A, et al: Pathogenesis of lymphoid interstitial pneumonia in natural and experimental ovine lentivirus infection. Clin Infect Dis 17(Suppl 1):S236-S242, 1993.

508. Kaan PM, Hegele RG, Hayashi S, et al: Expression of bcl-2 and Epstein-Barr virus LMP1 in lymphocytic interstitial pneumonia. Thorax 52:12-16, 1997.

509. Koss MN, Hochholzer L, Langloss JM, et al: Lymphoid interstitial pneumonia: Clinicopathological and immunopathological findings in 18 cases. Pathology 19:178-185, 1987.

510. Julsrud PR, Brown LR, Li CY, et al: Pulmonary processes of mature-appearing lymphocytes: Pseudolymphoma, well-differentiated lymphocytic lymphoma, and lymphocytic interstitial pneumonitis. Radiology 127:289-296, 1978.

511. Liebow A, Carrington C: The interstitial pneumonias. In Simon M, Potchen E, Le May M (eds): Frontiers of Pulmonary Radiology. New York, Grune & Stratton, 1969, p 102.

512. Ichikawa Y, Kinoshita M, Koga T, et al: Lung cyst formation in lymphocytic interstitial pneumonia: CT features. J Comput Assist Tomogr 18:745-748, 1994.

513. Feigin DS, Siegelman SS, Theros EG, et al: Nonmalignant lymphoid disorders of the chest. AJR Am J Roentgenol 129:221-228, 1977.

514. McGuinness G, Scholes JV, Jagirdar JS, et al: Unusual lymphoproliferative disorders in nine adults with HIV or AIDS: CT and pathologic findings. Radiology 197:59-65, 1995.

515. Johkoh T, Müller NL, Pickford HA, et al: Lymphocytic interstitial pneumonia: Thin-section CT findings in 22 patients. Radiology 212:567-572, 1999.

516. Carignan S, Staples CA, Müller NL: Intrathoracic lymphoproliferative disorders in the immunocompromised patient: CT findings. Radiology 197:53-58, 1995.

517. Saldana M, Mones J: Lymphoid interstitial pneumonia in HIV infected individuals. Prog Surg Pathol 12:181, 1992.

518. Banerjee D, Ahmad D: Malignant lymphoma complicating lymphocytic interstitial pneumonia: A monoclonal B-cell neoplasm arising in a polyclonal lymphoproliferative disorder. Hum Pathol 13:780-782, 1982.

519. Yousem SA, Colby TV, Carrington CB: Follicular bronchitis/bronchiolitis. Hum Pathol 16:700-706, 1985.

520. Howling SJ, Hansell DM, Wells AU, et al: Follicular bronchiolitis: Thin-section CT and histologic findings. Radiology 212:637-642, 1999.

521. Kinoshita M, Higashi T, Tanaka C, et al: Follicular bronchiolitis associated with rheumatoid arthritis. Intern Med 31:674-677, 1992.

522. Fiche M, Caprons F, Berger F, et al: Primary pulmonary non-Hodgkin's lymphomas. Histopathology 26:529-537, 1995.

523. Li G, Hansmann ML, Zwingers T, et al: Primary lymphomas of the lung: Morphological, immunohistochemical and clinical features. Histopathology 16:519-531, 1990.

524. Harris NL: Low-grade B-cell lymphoma of mucosa-associated lymphoid tissue and monocytoid B-cell lymphoma. Related entities that are distinct from other low-grade B-cell lymphomas. Arch Pathol Lab Med 117:771-775, 1993.

525. Koss M, Zeren EH: Low-grade lymphomas of lung and lymphomatoid granulomatosis. Pathology (Phila) 4:125-139, 1996.

526. Nicholson AG, Wotherspoon AC, Diss TC, et al: Pulmonary B-cell non-Hodgkin's lymphomas. The value of immunohistochemistry and gene analysis in diagnosis. Histopathology 26:395-403, 1995.

527. Hytiroglou P, Strauchen JA, Vrettou E, et al: Epstein-Barr virus and primary lung lymphoma: A study utilizing the polymerase chain reaction. Mod Pathol 6:575-580, 1993.

528. Weiss LM, Yousem SA, Warnke RA: Non-Hodgkin's lymphomas of the lung. A study of 19 cases emphasizing the utility of frozen section immunologic studies in differential diagnosis. Am J Surg Pathol 9:480-490, 1985.

529. Subramanian D, Albrecht S, Gonzalez JM, et al: Primary pulmonary lymphoma. Diagnosis by immunoglobulin gene rearrangement study using a novel polymerase chain reaction technique. Am Rev Respir Dis 148:222-226, 1993.

530. Wislez M, Cadranel J, Antoine M, et al: Lymphoma of pulmonary mucosa-associated lymphoid tissue: CT scan findings and pathological correlations. Eur Respir J 14:423-429, 1999.

531. Knisely B, Mastey L, Mergo P, et al: Pulmonary mucosa-associated lymphoid tissue lymphoma: CT and pathologic findings. AJR Am J Roengenol 172:1321, 1999.

532. O'Donnell PG, Jackson SA, Tung KT, et al: Radiological appearances of lymphomas arising from mucosa-associated lymphoid tissue (MALT) in the lung. Clin Radiol 53:258-263, 1998.

533. Cordier JF, Chailleux E, Lauque D, et al: Primary pulmonary lymphomas. A clinical study of 70 cases in nonimmunocompromised patients. Chest 103:201-208, 1993.

534. McCulloch GL, Sinnatamby R, Stewart S, et al: High-resolution computed tomographic appearance of MALToma of the lung. Eur Radiol 8:1669-1673, 1998.

535. Au V, Leung AN: Radiologic manifestations of lymphoma in the thorax. AJR Am J Roentgenol 168:93-98, 1997.

536. Kuruvilla S, Gomathy DV, Shanthi AV, et al: Primary pulmonary lymphoma. Report of a case diagnosed by fine needle aspiration cytology. Acta Cytol 38:601-604, 1994.

537. Keicho N, Oka T, Takeuchi K, et al: Detection of lymphomatous involvement of the lung by bronchoalveolar lavage. Application of immunophenotypic and gene rearrangement analysis. Chest 105:458-462, 1994.

538. L'Hoste RJ Jr, Filippa DA, Lieberman PH, et al: Primary pulmonary lymphomas. A clinicopathologic analysis of 36 cases. Cancer 54:1397-1406, 1984.

539. Tamura A, Komatsu H, Yanai N, et al: Primary pulmonary lymphoma: Relationship between clinical features and pathologic findings in 24 cases. The Japan National Chest Hospital Study Group for Lung Cancer. Jpn J Clin Oncol 25:140-152, 1995.

540. Evans HL: Extranodal small lymphocytic proliferation: A clinicopathologic and immunocytochemical study. Cancer 49:84-96, 1982.

541. Katzenstein AL, Carrington CB, Liebow AA: Lymphomatoid granulomatosis: A clinicopathologic study of 152 cases. Cancer 43:360-373, 1979.

542. Colby TV, Carrington CB: Pulmonary lymphomas simulating lymphomatoid granulomatosis. Am J Surg Pathol 6:19-32, 1982.

543. Myers JL, Kurtin PJ, Katzenstein AL, et al: Lymphomatoid granulomatosis. Evidence of immunophenotypic diversity and relationship to Epstein-Barr virus infection. Am J Surg Pathol 19:1300-1312, 1995.

544. Nicholson AG, Wotherspoon AC, Diss TC, et al: Lymphomatoid granulomatosis: Evidence that some cases represent Epstein-Barr virus-associated B-cell lymphoma. Histopathology 29:317-324, 1996.

545. Prenovault JM, Weisbrod GL, Herman SJ: Lymphomatoid granulomatosis: A review of 12 cases. Can Assoc Radiol J 39:263-266, 1988.

546. Lee JS, Tuder R, Lynch DA: Lymphomatoid granulomatosis: Radiologic features and pathologic correlations. AJR Am J Roentgenol 175:1335-1339, 2000.

547. Wechsler RJ, Steiner RM, Israel HL, et al: Chest radiograph in lymphomatoid granulomatosis: Comparison with Wegener granulomatosis. AJR Am J Roentgenol 142:79-83, 1984.

548. Koss MN, Hochholzer L, Langloss JM, et al: Lymphomatoid granulomatosis: A clinicopathologic study of 42 patients. Pathology 18:283-288, 1986.

549. Liebow AA, Carrington CR, Friedman PJ: Lymphomatoid granulomatosis. Hum Pathol 3:457-558, 1972.

550. Saldana MJ, Patchefsky AS, Israel HI, et al: Pulmonary angiitis and granulomatosis. The relationship between histological features, organ involvement, and response to treatment. Hum Pathol 8:391-409, 1977.

551. Castellino RA, Hilton S, O'Brien JP, et al: Non-Hodgkin lymphoma: Contribution of chest CT in the initial staging evaluation. Radiology 199:129-132, 1996.

552. Mentzer SJ, Reilly JJ, Skarin AT, et al: Patterns of lung involvement by malignant lymphoma. Surgery 113:507-514, 1993.

553. Filly R, Bland N, Castellino RA: Radiographic distribution of intrathoracic disease in previously untreated patients with Hodgkin's disease and non-Hodgkin's lymphoma. Radiology 120:277-281, 1976.

554. Lewis ER, Caskey CI, Fishman EK: Lymphoma of the lung: CT findings in 31 patients. AJR Am J Roentgenol 156:711-714, 1991.

555. Jackson SA, Tung KT, Mead GM: Multiple cavitating pulmonary lesions in non-Hodgkin's lymphoma. Clin Radiol 49:883-885, 1994.

556. Lee KS, Kim Y, Primack SL: Imaging of pulmonary lymphomas. AJR Am J Roentgenol 168:339-345, 1997.

557. Celikoglu F, Teirstein AS, Krellenstein DJ, et al: Pleural effusion in non-Hodgkin's lymphoma. Chest 101:1357-1360, 1992.

558. Leung AN, Müller NL, Miller RR: CT in differential diagnosis of diffuse pleural disease. AJR Am J Roentgenol 154:487-492, 1990.

559. Rees GM: Primary lymphosarcoma of the lung. Thorax 28:429-432, 1973.

560. Colby TV, Hoppe RT, Warnke RA: Hodgkin's disease: A clinicopathologic study of 659 cases. Cancer 49:1848-2858, 1982.

561. Radin AI: Primary pulmonary Hodgkin's disease. Cancer 65:550-563, 1990.

562. Johnson DW, Hoppe RT, Cox RS, et al: Hodgkin's disease limited to intrathoracic sites. Cancer 52:8-13, 1983.

563. Yousem SA, Weiss LM, Colby TV: Primary pulmonary Hodgkin's disease. A clinicopathologic study of 15 cases. Cancer 57:1217-1224, 1986.

564. Castellino RA, Blank N, Hoppe RT, et al: Hodgkin disease: Contributions of chest CT in the initial staging evaluation. Radiology 160:603-605, 1986.

565. Rosenberg SA, Kaplan HS: Evidence for an orderly progression in the spread of Hodgkin's disease. Cancer Res 26:1225-1231, 1966.

566. Fishman EK, Kuhlman JE, Jones RJ: CT of lymphoma: Spectrum of disease. Radiographics 11:647-669, 1991.

567. Brereton HD, Johnson RE: Calcification in mediastinal lymph nodes after radiation therapy of Hodgkin's disease. Radiology 112:705-707, 1974.

568. Wyman SM, Weber AL: Calcification in intrathoracic nodes in Hodgkin's disease. Radiology 93:1021-1024, 1969.

569. Whitcomb ME, Schwarz MI, Keller AR, et al: Hodgkin's disease of the lung. Am Rev Respir Dis 106:79-85, 1972.

570. Press GA, Glazer HS, Wasserman TH, et al: Thoracic wall involvement by Hodgkin disease and non-Hodgkin lymphoma: CT evaluation. Radiology 157:195-198, 1985.

571. Jerusalem G, Beguin Y, Fassotte MF, et al: Whole-body positron emission tomography using ^{18}F-fluorodeoxyglucose compared to standard procedures for staging patients with Hodgkin's disease. Haematologica 86:266-273, 2001.

572. Menzel C, Dobert N, Mitrou P, et al: Positron emission tomography for the staging of Hodgkin's lymphoma—increasing the body of evidence in favor of the method. Acta Oncol 41:430-436, 2002.

573. Wiedmann E, Baican B, Hertel A, et al: Positron emission tomography (PET) for staging and evaluation of response to treatment in patients with Hodgkin's disease. Leuk Lymphoma 34:545-551, 1999.

574. Fisher AM, Kendall B, Van Leuven BD: Hodgkin's disease: A radiological survey. Clin Radiol 13:115-121, 1962.

575. Shuman LS, Libshitz HI: Solid pleural manifestations of lymphoma. AJR Am J Roentgenol 142:269-273, 1984.

576. Cartier Y, Johkoh T, Honda O, et al: Primary pulmonary Hodgkin's disease: CT findings in three patients. Clin Radiol 54:182-184, 1999.

577. Madewell JE, Daroca PJ, Reed JC: Pulmonary parenchymal Hodgkin's disease. RPC from the AFIP. Radiology 117:555-559, 1975.

578. Yellin A, Benfield JR: Pneumothorax associated with lymphoma. Am Rev Respir Dis 134:590-592, 1986.

579. Beachley MC, Lau BP, King ER: Bone involvement in Hodgkin's disease. Am J Roentgenol Radium Ther Nucl Med 114:559-563, 1972.

580. Goldman JM: Parasternal chest wall involvement in Hodgkin's disease. Chest 59:133-137, 1971.

581. North LB, Fuller LM, Sullivan-Halley JA, et al: Regression of mediastinal Hodgkin disease after therapy: Evaluation of time interval. Radiology 164:599-602, 1987.

582. Schuurman HJ, Gooszen HC, Tan IW, et al: Low-grade lymphoma of immature T-cell phenotype in a case of lymphocytic interstitial pneumonia and Sjögren's syndrome. Histopathology 11:1193-1204, 1987.

583. Radford JA, Cowan RA, Flanagan M, et al: The significance of residual mediastinal abnormality on the chest radiograph following treatment for Hodgkin's disease. J Clin Oncol 6:940-946, 1988.

584. Nyman RS, Rehn SM, Glimelius BL, et al: Residual mediastinal masses in Hodgkin disease: Prediction of size with MR imaging. Radiology 170:435-440, 1989.

585. Kramer EL, Divgi CR: Pulmonary applications of nuclear medicine. Clin Chest Med 12:55-75, 1991.

586. Abella-Columna E, Valk PE: Positron emission tomography imaging in melanoma and lymphoma. Semin Roentgenol 37:129-139, 2002.

587. Bar-Shalom R, Yefremov N, Haim N, et al: Camera-based FDG PET and ^{67}Ga SPECT in evaluation of lymphoma: Comparative study. Radiology 227:353-360, 2003.

588. Costello P, Mauch P: Radiographic features of recurrent intrathoracic Hodgkin's disease following radiation therapy. AJR Am J Roentgenol 133:201-206, 1979.

589. Cobby M, Whipp E, Bullimore J, et al: CT appearances of relapse of lymphoma in the lung. Clin Radiol 41:232-238, 1990.

590. Winterbauer RH, Belic N, Moores KD: Clinical interpretation of bilateral hilar adenopathy. Ann Intern Med 78:65-71, 1973.

591. Pinson P, Joos G, Praet M, et al: Primary pulmonary Hodgkin's disease. Respiration 59:314-316, 1992.

592. Arden MJ, Rottino A: Hodgkin's disease complicated by tuberculosis. A twenty-year experience. Am Rev Respir Dis 93:810-815, 1966.

593. Hays DM, Ternberg JL, Chen TT, et al: Postsplenectomy sepsis and other complications following staging laparotomy for Hodgkin's disease in childhood. J Pediatr Surg 21:628-632, 1986.

594. Ragozzino MW, Melton LJ 3rd, Kurland LT, et al: Risk of cancer after herpes zoster: A population-based study. N Engl J Med 307:393-397, 1982.

595. Lund MB, Kongerud J, Nome O, et al: Lung function impairment in long-term survivors of Hodgkin's disease. Ann Oncol 6:495-501, 1995.

596. Horning SJ, Adhikari A, Rizk N, et al: Effect of treatment for Hodgkin's disease on pulmonary function: Results of a prospective study. J Clin Oncol 12:297-305, 1994.

597. Bossi G, Cerveri I, Volpini E, et al: Long-term pulmonary sequelae after treatment of childhood Hodgkin's disease. Ann Oncol 8(Suppl 1):19-24, 1997.

598. Kaldor JM, Day NE, Bell J, et al: Lung cancer following Hodgkin's disease: A case-control study. Int J Cancer 52:677-681, 1992.

599. Waldron JA Jr, Dohring EJ, Farber LR: Primary large cell lymphomas of the mediastinum: An analysis of 20 cases. Semin Diagn Pathol 2:281-295, 1985.

600. Trump DL, Mann RB: Diffuse large cell and undifferentiated lymphomas with prominent mediastinal involvement. Cancer 50:277-282, 1982.

601. Picozzi VJ Jr, Coleman CN: Lymphoblastic lymphoma. Semin Oncol 17:96-103, 1990.

602. Perrone T, Frizzera G, Rosai J: Mediastinal diffuse large-cell lymphoma with sclerosis. A clinicopathologic study of 60 cases. Am J Surg Pathol 10:176-191, 1986.

603. Moller P, Lammler B, Eberlein-Gonska M, et al: Primary mediastinal clear cell lymphoma of B-cell type. Virchows Arch A Pathol Anat Histopathol 409:79-92, 1986.

604. Negendank WG, al-Katib AM, Karanes C, et al: Lymphomas: MR imaging contrast characteristics with clinical-pathologic correlations. Radiology 177:209-216, 1990.

605. Israel O, Front D, Lam M, et al: Gallium 67 imaging in monitoring lymphoma response to treatment. Cancer 61:2439-2443, 1988.

606. Friedberg JW, Chengazi V: PET scans in the staging of lymphoma: Current status. Oncologist 8:438-447, 2003.

607. Elstrom R, Guan L, Baker G, et al: Utility of FDG-PET scanning in lymphoma by WHO classification. Blood 101:3875-3876, 2003.

608. Hoffmann M, Kletter K, Diemling M, et al: Positron emission tomography with fluorine-18-2-fluoro-2-deoxy-D-glucose (F18-FDG) does not visualize extranodal B-cell lymphoma of the mucosa-associated lymphoid tissue (MALT)-type. Ann Oncol 10:1185-1189, 1999.

609. Kintzer JS Jr, Rosenow EC 3rd, Kyle RA: Thoracic and pulmonary abnormalities in multiple myeloma. A review of 958 cases. Arch Intern Med 138:727-730, 1978.

610. Kinare SG, Parulkar GB, Panday SR, et al: Extensive ossification in a pulmonary plasmacytoma. Thorax 20:206-210, 1965.

611. Kwan WC, Lam SC, Klimo P: Kappa light-chain myeloma with pleural involvement. Chest 86:494-496, 1984.

612. Moulopoulos LA, Granfield CA, Dimopoulos MA, et al: Extraosseous multiple myeloma: Imaging features. AJR Am J Roentgenol 161:1083-1087, 1993.

613. Kyle RA: Multiple myeloma: Review of 869 cases. Mayo Clin Proc 50:29-40, 1975.

614. Favis EA, Kerman HD, Schildecker W: Multiple myeloma manifested as a problem in the diagnosis of pulmonary disease. Am J Med 28:323-327, 1960.

615. Badrinas F, Rodriguez-Roisin R, Rives A, et al: Multiple myeloma with pleural involvement. Am Rev Respir Dis 110:82-87, 1974.

616. Wiltshaw E: The natural history of extramedullary plasmacytoma and its relation to solitary myeloma of bone and myelomatosis. Medicine (Baltimore) 55:217-238, 1976.

617. Logan PM, Miller RR, Müller NL: Solitary tracheal plasmacytoma: Computed tomography and pathological findings. Can Assoc Radiol J 46:125-126, 1995.

618. Tenholder MF, Scialla SJ, Weisbaum G: Endobronchial metastatic plasmacytoma. Cancer 49:1465-1468, 1982.

619. Morinaga S, Watanabe H, Gemma A, et al: Plasmacytoma of the lung associated with nodular deposits of immunoglobulin. Am J Surg Pathol 11:989-995, 1987.

620. Wile A, Olinger G, Peter JB, et al: Solitary intraparenchymal pulmonary plasmacytoma associated with production of an M-protein: Report of a case. Cancer 37:2338-2342, 1976.

621. Doran HM, Sheppard MN, Collins PW, et al: Pathology of the lung in leukaemia and lymphoma: A study of 87 autopsies. Histopathology 18:211-219, 1991.

622. Rollins SD, Colby TV: Lung biopsy in chronic lymphocytic leukemia. Arch Pathol Lab Med 112:607-611, 1988.

623. Hildebrand FL Jr, Rosenow EC 3rd, Habermann TM, et al: Pulmonary complications of leukemia. Chest 98:1233-1239, 1990.

624. Maile CW, Moore AV, Ulreich S, et al: Chest radiographic-pathologic correlation in adult leukemia patients. Invest Radiol 18:495-499, 1983.

625. Tenholder MF, Hooper RG: Pulmonary infiltrates in leukemia. Chest 78:468-473, 1980.

626. Callahan M, Wall S, Askin F, et al: Granulocytic sarcoma presenting as pulmonary nodules and lymphadenopathy. Cancer 60:1902-1904, 1987.

627. Genet P, Pulik M, Lionnet F, et al: Leukemic relapse presenting with bronchial obstruction caused by granulocytic sarcoma. Am J Hematol 47:142-143, 1994.

628. McKee LC Jr, Collins RD: Intravascular leukocyte thrombi and aggregates as a cause of morbidity and mortality in leukemia. Medicine (Baltimore) 53:463-478, 1974.

629. Myers TJ, Cole SR, Klatsky AU, et al: Respiratory failure due to pulmonary leukostasis following chemotherapy of acute nonlymphocytic leukemia. Cancer 51:1808-1813, 1983.

630. Vernant JP, Brun B, Mannoni P, et al: Respiratory distress of hyperleukocytic granulocytic leukemias. Cancer 44:264-268, 1979.

631. Takasugi JE, Godwin JD, Marglin SI, et al: Intrathoracic granulocytic sarcomas. J Thorac Imaging 11:223-230, 1996.

632. Sueyoshi E, Uetani M, Hayashi K, et al: Adult T-cell leukemia with multiple pulmonary nodules due to leukemic cell infiltration. AJR Am J Roentgenol 167:540-541, 1996.

633. Kovalski R, Hansen-Flaschen J, Lodato RF, et al: Localized leukemic pulmonary infiltrates. Diagnosis by bronchoscopy and resolution with therapy. Chest 97:674-678, 1990.

634. Jenkins PF, Ward MJ, Davies P, et al: Non-Hodgkin's lymphoma, chronic lymphatic leukaemia and the lung. Br J Dis Chest 75:22-30, 1981.

635. Heyneman LE, Johkoh T, Ward S, et al: Pulmonary leukemic infiltrates: High-resolution CT findings in 10 patients. AJR Am J Roentgenol 174:517-521, 2000.

636. Yamauchi K, Omata T: Leukemic pneumonitis as a poor prognostic factor in chronic myelomonocytic leukemia. Respiration 59:119-121, 1992.

637. Bardales RH, Powers CN, Frierson HF Jr, et al: Exfoliative respiratory cytology in the diagnosis of leukemias and lymphomas in the lung. Diagn Cytopathol 14:108-113, 1996.

638. Janckila AJ, Yam LT, Li CY: Immunocytochemical diagnosis of acute leukemia with pleural involvement. Acta Cytol 29:67-72, 1985.

639. Berkman N, Polliack A, Breuer R, et al: Pulmonary involvement as the major manifestation of chronic lymphocytic leukemia. Leuk Lymphoma 8:495-499, 1992.

640. Tamura K, Yokota T, Mashita R, et al: Pulmonary manifestations in adult T-cell leukemia at the time of diagnosis. Respiration 60:115-119, 1993.

641. Vardiman JW, Variakojis D, Golomb HM: Hairy cell leukemia: An autopsy study. Cancer 43:1339-1349, 1979.

642. Palosaari DE, Colby TV: Bronchiolocentric chronic lymphocytic leukemia. Cancer 58:1695-1698, 1986.

643. Okura T, Tanaka R, Shibata H, et al: Adult T-cell leukemia with a solitary lung mass. Chest 101:1471-1472, 1992.

644. Mainzer F, Taybi H: Thymic enlargement and pleural effusion: An unusual roentgenographic complex in childhood leukemia. Am J Roentgenol Radium Ther Nucl Med 112:35-39, 1971.

645. Nathwani BN, Diamond LW, Winberg CD, et al: Lymphoblastic lymphoma: A clinicopathologic study of 95 patients. Cancer 48:2347-2357, 1981.

646. Rolla G, Bucca C, Chiampo F, et al: Respiratory symptoms, lung function tests, airway responsiveness, and bronchoalveolar lymphocyte subsets in B-chronic lymphocytic leukemia. Lung 171:265-275, 1993.

647. Martini N: Invited commentary. Ann Thorac Surg 58:1155, 1994.

648. Yellin A, Rosenman Y, Lieberman Y: Review of smooth muscle tumours of the lower respiratory tract. Br J Dis Chest 78:337-351, 1984.

649. Suster S: Primary sarcomas of the lung. Semin Diagn Pathol 12:140-157, 1995.

650. Vera-Roman JM, Sobonya RE, Gomez-Garcia JL, et al: Leiomyoma of the lung. Literature review and case report. Cancer 52:936-941, 1983.

651. Guccion JG, Rosen SH: Bronchopulmonary leiomyosarcoma and fibrosarcoma. A study of 32 cases and review of the literature. Cancer 30:836-847, 1972.

652. Gal AA, Brooks JS, Pietra GG: Leiomyomatous neoplasms of the lung: A clinical, histologic, and immunohistochemical study. Mod Pathol 2:209-216, 1989.

653. Martin E: Leiomyomatous lung lesions: A proposed classification. AJR Am J Roentgenol 141:269-272, 1983.

654. Burke AP, Virmani R: Sarcomas of the great vessels. A clinicopathologic study. Cancer 71:1761-1773, 1993.

655. Nonomura A, Kurumaya H, Kono N, et al: Primary pulmonary artery sarcoma. Report of two autopsy cases studied by immunohistochemistry and electron microscopy, and review of 110 cases reported in the literature. Acta Pathol Jpn 38:883-896, 1988.

656. Johansson L, Carlen B: Sarcoma of the pulmonary artery: Report of four cases with electron microscopic and immunohistochemical examinations, and review of the literature. Virchows Arch 424:217-224, 1994.

657. Cox JE, Chiles C, Aquino SL, et al: Pulmonary artery sarcomas: A review of clinical and radiologic features. J Comput Assist Tomogr 21:750-755, 1997.

658. Britton PD: Primary pulmonary artery sarcoma—a report of two cases, with special emphasis on the diagnostic problems. Clin Radiol 41:92-94, 1990.

659. Olsson HE, Spitzer RM, Erston WF: Primary and secondary pulmonary artery neoplasia mimicking acute pulmonary embolism. Radiology 118:49-53, 1976.

660. Lamers RJ, Hochstenbag MM, van Belle AF, et al: Unilateral hilar mass. Chest 108:1444-1446, 1995.

661. Smith WS, Lesar MS, Travis WD, et al: MR and CT findings in pulmonary artery sarcoma. J Comput Assist Tomogr 13:906-909, 1989.

662. Kauczor HU, Schwickert HC, Mayer E, et al: Pulmonary artery sarcoma mimicking chronic thromboembolic disease: Computed tomography and magnetic resonance imaging findings. Cardiovasc Intervent Radiol 17:185-189, 1994.

663. Delany SG, Doyle TC, Bunton RW, et al: Pulmonary artery sarcoma mimicking pulmonary embolism. Chest 103:1631-1633, 1993.

664. Anderson MB, Kriett JM, Kapelanski DP, et al: Primary pulmonary artery sarcoma: A report of six cases. Ann Thorac Surg 59:1487-1490, 1995.

665. Baker PB, Goodwin RA: Pulmonary artery sarcomas. A review and report of a case. Arch Pathol Lab Med 109:35-39, 1985.

666. Yousem SA, Hochholzer L: Primary pulmonary hemangiopericytoma. Cancer 59:549-555, 1987.

667. Halle M, Blum U, Dinkel E, et al: CT and MR features of primary pulmonary hemangiopericytomas. J Comput Assist Tomogr 17:51-55, 1993.

668. Rusch VW, Shuman WP, Schmidt R, et al: Massive pulmonary hemangiopericytoma. An innovative approach to evaluation and treatment. Cancer 64:1928-1936, 1989.

669. Sivit CJ, Schwartz AM, Rockoff SD: Kaposi's sarcoma of the lung in AIDS: Radiologic-pathologic analysis. AJR Am J Roentgenol 148:25-28, 1987.

670. Goodman PC: Kaposi's sarcoma. J Thorac Imaging 6:43-48, 1991.

671. Naidich DP, McGuinness G: Pulmonary manifestations of AIDS. CT and radiographic correlations. Radiol Clin North Am 29:999-1017, 1991.

672. McGuinness G: Changing trends in the pulmonary manifestations of AIDS. Radiol Clin North Am 35:1029-1082, 1997.

673. Wolff SD, Kuhlman JE, Fishman EK: Thoracic Kaposi sarcoma in AIDS: CT findings. J Comput Assist Tomogr 17:60-62, 1993.

674. Khalil AM, Carette MF, Cadranel JL, et al: Intrathoracic Kaposi's sarcoma. CT findings. Chest 108:1622-1626, 1995.

675. Mandel C, Silberstein M, Hennessy O: Case report: Fatal pulmonary Kaposi's sarcoma and Castleman's disease in a renal transplant recipient. Br J Radiol 66:264-265, 1993.

676. Huang L, Schnapp LM, Gruden JF, et al: Presentation of AIDS-related pulmonary Kaposi's sarcoma diagnosed by bronchoscopy. Am J Respir Crit Care Med 153:1385-1390, 1996.

677. Tamm M, Reichenberger F, McGandy CE, et al: Diagnosis of pulmonary Kaposi's sarcoma by detection of human herpes virus 8 in bronchoalveolar lavage. Am J Respir Crit Care Med 157:458-463, 1998.

678. Aboulafia DM: Regression of acquired immunodeficiency syndrome–related pulmonary Kaposi's sarcoma after highly active antiretroviral therapy. Mayo Clin Proc 73:439-443, 1998.

679. Holkova B, Takeshita K, Cheng DM, et al: Effect of highly active antiretroviral therapy on survival of inpatients with AIDS-associated pulmonary Kaposi's sarcoma treated with chemotherapy. J Clin Oncol 19:3848, 2001.

680. Dail DH, Liebow AA, Gmelich JT, et al: Intravascular, bronchiolar, and alveolar tumor of the lung (IVBAT). An analysis of twenty cases of a peculiar sclerosing endothelial tumor. Cancer 51:452-464, 1983.

681. Corrin B, Harrison WJ, Wright DH: The so-called intravascular bronchioloalveolar tumour of lung (low grade sclerosing angiosarcoma): Presentation with extrapulmonary deposits. Diagn Histopathol 6:229-237, 1983.

682. Bollinger BK, Laskin WB, Knight CB: Epithelioid hemangioendothelioma with multiple site involvement. Literature review and observations. Cancer 73:610-615, 1994.

683. Verbeken E, Beyls J, Moerman P, et al: Lung metastasis of malignant epithelioid hemangioendothelioma mimicking a primary intravascular bronchioalveolar tumor. A histologic, ultrastructural, and immunohistochemical study. Cancer 55:1741-1746, 1985.

684. Sherman JL, Rykwalder PJ, Tashkin DP: Intravascular bronchioloalveolar tumor. Am Rev Respir Dis 123:468-470, 1981.

685. Sicilian L, Warson F, Carrington CB, et al: Intravascular bronchioloalveolar tumor (IV-BAT). Respiration 44:387-394, 1983.

686. Luburich P, Ayuso MC, Picado C, et al: CT of pulmonary epithelioid hemangioendothelioma. J Comput Assist Tomogr 18:562-565, 1994.

687. Eggleston JC: The intravascular bronchioloalveolar tumor and the sclerosing hemangioma of the lung: Misnomers of pulmonary neoplasia. Semin Diagn Pathol 2:270-280, 1985.

688. Tomashefski JF Jr: Benign endobronchial mesenchymal tumors: Their relationship to parenchymal pulmonary hamartomas. Am J Surg Pathol 6:531-540, 1982.

689. Carney JA: The triad of gastric epithelioid leiomyosarcoma, functioning extra-adrenal paraganglioma, and pulmonary chondroma. Cancer 43:374-382, 1979.

690. Dajee A, Dajee H, Hinrichs S, et al: Pulmonary chondroma, extra-adrenal paraganglioma, and gastric leiomyosarcoma: Carney's triad. J Thorac Cardiovasc Surg 84:377-381, 1982.

691. Schmutz GR, Fisch-Ponsot C, Sylvestre J: Carney syndrome: Radiologic features. Can Assoc Radiol J 45:148-150, 1994.

692. Lancha C, Diez L, Mitjavila M, et al: A case of complete Carney's syndrome. Clin Nucl Med 19:1008-1010, 1994.

693. Tisell LE, Angervall L, Dahl I, et al: Recurrent and metastasizing gastric leiomyoblastoma (epithelioid leiomyosarcoma) associated with multiple pulmonary chondro-hamartomas: Long survival of a patient treated with repeated operations. Cancer 41:259-265, 1978.

694. Bateson EM: So-called hamartoma of the lung—a true neoplasm of fibrous connective tissue of the bronchi. Cancer 31:1458-1467, 1973.

695. van den Bosch JM, Wagenaar SS, Corrin B, et al: Mesenchymoma of the lung (so called hamartoma): A review of 154 parenchymal and endobronchial cases. Thorax 42:790-793, 1987.

696. Bateson EM, Abbott EK: Mixed tumors of the lung, or hamarto-chondromas. A review of the radiological appearances of cases published in the literature and a report of fifteen new cases. Clin Radiol 11:232-247, 1960.

697. Butler C, Kleinerman J: Pulmonary hamartoma. Arch Pathol 88:584-592, 1969.

698. Hansen CP, Holtveg H, Francis D, et al: Pulmonary hamartoma. J Thorac Cardiovasc Surg 104:674-678, 1992.

699. Incze JS, Lui PS: Morphology of the epithelial component of human lung hamartomas. Hum Pathol 8:411-419, 1977.

700. Fejzo MS, Yoon SJ, Montgomery KT, et al: Identification of a YAC spanning the translocation breakpoints in uterine leiomyomata, pulmonary chondroid hamartoma, and lipoma: Physical mapping of the 12q14-q15 breakpoint region in uterine leiomyomata. Genomics 26:265-271, 1995.

701. Bateson E: Relationship between intrapulmonary and endobronchial cartilage-containing tumors (so-called hamartomata). Thorax 20:447, 1965.

702. Poirier TJ, Van Ordstrand HS: Pulmonary chondromatous hamartomas. Report of seventeen cases and review of the literature. Chest 59:50-55, 1971.

703. Sagel SS, Ablow RC: Hamartoma: On occasion a rapidly growing tumor of the lung. Radiology 91:971-972, 1968.

704. Ahn JM, Im JG, Seo JW, et al: Endobronchial hamartoma: CT findings in three patients. AJR Am J Roentgenol 163:49-50, 1994.

705. Davis WK, Roberts L Jr, Foster WL Jr, et al: Computed tomographic diagnosis of an endobronchial hamartoma. Invest Radiol 23:941-944, 1988.

706. Gjevre JA, Myers JL, Prakash UB: Pulmonary hamartomas. Mayo Clin Proc 71:14-20, 1996.

707. Sharkey RA, Mulloy EM, O'Neill S: Endobronchial hamartoma presenting as massive haemoptysis. Eur Respir J 9:2179-2180, 1996.

708. Dunbar F, Leiman G: The aspiration cytology of pulmonary hamartomas. Diagn Cytopathol 5:174-180, 1989.

709. Roviaro G, Montorsi M, Varoli F, et al: Primary pulmonary tumours of neurogenic origin. Thorax 38:942-945, 1983.

710. Oparah SS, Subramanian VA: Granular cell myoblastoma of the bronchus: Report of 2 cases and review of the literature. Ann Thorac Surg 22:199-202, 1976.

711. Deavers M, Guinee D, Koss MN, et al: Granular cell tumors of the lung. Clinicopathologic study of 20 cases. Am J Surg Pathol 19:627-635, 1995.

712. Korompai FL, Awe RJ, Beall AC, et al: Granular cell myoblastoma of the bronchus: A new case, 12-year followup report, and review of the literature. Chest 66:578-580, 1974.

713. Hirata T, Reshad K, Itoi K, et al: Lipomas of the peripheral lung—a case report and review of the literature. Thorac Cardiovasc Surg 37:385-387, 1989.

714. Eastridge CE, Young JM, Steplock AL: Endobronchial lipoma. South Med J 77:759-761, 1984.

715. Yousem SA, Flynn SD: Intrapulmonary localized fibrous tumor. Intraparenchymal so-called localized fibrous mesothelioma. Am J Clin Pathol 89:365-369, 1988.

716. Halyard MY, Camoriano JK, Culligan JA, et al: Malignant fibrous histiocytoma of the lung. Report of four cases and review of the literature. Cancer 78:2492-2497, 1996.

717. Gal AA, Koss MN, McCarthy WF, et al: Prognostic factors in pulmonary fibrohistiocytic lesions. Cancer 73:1817-1824, 1994.

718. Yousem SA, Hochholzer L: Malignant fibrous histiocytoma of the lung. Cancer 60:2532-2541, 1987.

719. McDonnell T, Kyriakos M, Roper C, et al: Malignant fibrous histiocytoma of the lung. Cancer 61:137-145, 1988.

720. Lee JT, Shelburne JD, Linder J: Primary malignant fibrous histiocytoma of the lung. A clinicopathologic and ultrastructural study of five cases. Cancer 53:1124-1130, 1984.

721. Gaffey MJ, Mills SE, Askin FB, et al: Clear cell tumor of the lung. A clinicopathologic, immunohistochemical, and ultrastructural study of eight cases. Am J Surg Pathol 14:248-259, 1990.

722. Gaffey MJ, Mills SE, Ritter JH: Clear cell tumors of the lower respiratory tract. Semin Diagn Pathol 14:222-232, 1997.

723. Heikkila P, Salminen US: Papillary pneumocytoma of the lung. An immunohistochemical and electron microscopic study. Pathol Res Pract 190:194-200, 1994.

724. Alvarez-Fernandez E, Carretero-Albinana L, Menarguez-Palanca J: Sclerosing hemangioma of the lung. An immunohistochemical study of intermediate filaments and endothelial markers. Arch Pathol Lab Med 113:121-124, 1989.

725. Sugio K, Yokoyama H, Kaneko S, et al: Sclerosing hemangioma of the lung: Radiographic and pathological study. Ann Thorac Surg 53:295-300, 1992.

726. Aihara T, Nakajima T: Sclerosing hemangioma of the lung: Pathological study and enzyme immunoassay for estrogen and progesterone receptors. Acta Pathol Jpn 43:507-515, 1993.

727. Katzenstein AL, Gmelich JT, Carrington CB: Sclerosing hemangioma of the lung: A clinicopathologic study of 51 cases. Am J Surg Pathol 4:343-356, 1980.

728. Nakatani Y, Dickersin GR, Mark EJ: Pulmonary endodermal tumor resembling fetal lung: A clinicopathologic study of five cases with immunohistochemical and ultrastructural characterization. Hum Pathol 21:1097-1107, 1990.

729. Koss MN, Hochholzer L, O'Leary T: Pulmonary blastomas. Cancer 67:2368-2381, 1991.

730. Weisbrod GL, Chamberlain DW, Tao LC: Pulmonary blastoma, report of three cases and a review of the literature. Can Assoc Radiol J 39:130-136, 1988.

731. Senac MO Jr, Wood BP, Isaacs H, et al: Pulmonary blastoma: A rare childhood malignancy. Radiology 179:743-746, 1991.

732. Fung CH, Lo JW, Yonan TN, et al: Pulmonary blastoma: An ultrastructural study with a brief review of literature and a discussion of pathogenesis. Cancer 39:153-163, 1977.

733. Ashley DJ, Danino EA, Davies HD: Bronchial polyps. Thorax 18:45-49, 1963.

734. Greene JG, Tassin L, Saberi A: Endobronchial epithelial papilloma associated with a foreign body. Chest 97:229-230, 1990.

735. Barzo P, Molnar L, Minik K: Bronchial papillomas of various origins. Chest 92:132-136, 1987.

736. Williams DO, Vanecko RM, Glassroth J: Endobronchial polyposis following smoke inhalation. Chest 84:774-776, 1983.

737. Spencer H: The pulmonary plasma cell/histiocytoma complex. Histopathology 8:903-916, 1984.

738. Chen HP, Lee SS, Berardi RS: Inflammatory pseudotumor of the lung. Ultrastructural and light microscopic study of a myxomatous variant. Cancer 54:861-865, 1984.

739. Matsubara O, Tan-Liu NS, Kenney RM, et al: Inflammatory pseudotumors of the lung: Progression from organizing pneumonia to fibrous histiocytoma or to plasma cell granuloma in 32 cases. Hum Pathol 19:807-814, 1988.

740. Pettinato G, Manivel JC, De Rosa N, et al: Inflammatory myofibroblastic tumor (plasma cell granuloma). Clinicopathologic study of 20 cases with immunohistochemical and ultrastructural observations. Am J Clin Pathol 94:538-546, 1990.

741. Wang NS, Morin J: Recurrent endobronchial soft tissue tumors. Chest 85:787-791, 1984.

742. Warter A, Satge D, Roeslin N: Angioinvasive plasma cell granulomas of the lung. Cancer 59:435-443, 1987.

743. Su LD, Atayde-Perez A, Sheldon S, et al: Inflammatory myofibroblastic tumor: Cytogenetic evidence supporting clonal origin. Mod Pathol 11:364-368, 1998.

744. Agrons GA, Rosado-de-Christenson ML, Kirejczyk WM, et al: Pulmonary inflammatory pseudotumor: Radiologic features. Radiology 206:511-518, 1998.

745. McCall IW, Woo-Ming M: The radiological appearances of plasma cell granuloma of the lung. Clin Radiol 29:145-150, 1978.

746. Bahadori M, Liebow AA: Plasma cell granulomas of the lung. Cancer 31:191-208, 1973.
747. Shirakusa T, Kusano T, Motonaga R, et al: Plasma cell granuloma of the lung—resection and steroid therapy. Thorac Cardiovasc Surg 35:185-188, 1987.
748. Jayne D, Bridgewater B, Lawson RA: Endobronchial inflammatory pseudotumour exacerbating asthma. Postgrad Med J 73:98-99, 1997.
749. Mandelbaum I, Brashear RE, Hull MT: Surgical treatment and course of pulmonary pseudotumor (plasma cell granuloma). J Thorac Cardiovasc Surg 82:77-82, 1981.
750. Bando T, Fujimura M, Noda Y, et al: Pulmonary plasma cell granuloma improves with corticosteroid therapy. Chest 105:1574-1575, 1994.
751. Pearl M: Postinflammtory pseudotumor of the lung in children. Radiology 105:391-395, 1972.
752. Engleman P, Liebow AA, Gmelich J, et al: Pulmonary hyalinizing granuloma. Am Rev Respir Dis 115:997-1008, 1977.
753. Yousem SA, Hochholzer L: Pulmonary hyalinizing granuloma. Am J Clin Pathol 87:1-6, 1987.
754. Eschelman DJ, Blickman JG, Lazar HL, et al: Pulmonary hyalinizing granuloma: A rare cause of a solitary pulmonary nodule. J Thorac Imaging 6:54-56, 1991.
755. Dent RG, Godden DJ, Stovin PG, et al: Pulmonary hyalinizing granuloma in association with retroperitoneal fibrosis. Thorax 38:955-956, 1983.
756. Joseph J, Sahn SA: Thoracic endometriosis syndrome: New observations from an analysis of 110 cases. Am J Med 100:164-170, 1996.
757. Foster DC, Stern JL, Buscema J, et al: Pleural and parenchymal pulmonary endometriosis. Obstet Gynecol 58:552-556, 1981.
758. Assor D: Endometriosis of the lung: Report of a case. Am J Clin Pathol 57:311-315, 1972.
759. Hertzanu Y, Heimer D, Hirsch M: Computed tomography of pulmonary endometriosis. Comput Radiol 11:81-84, 1987.
760. Tsumori T, Nakao K, Miyata M, et al: Clinicopathologic study of thyroid carcinoma infiltrating the trachea. Cancer 56:2843-2848, 1985.
761. Wallace A, Chew E-C, Jones D: Arrest and extravasation of cancer cells in the lung. In Weiss L, Gilbert H (eds): Pulmonary Metastasis. Boston, GK Hall, 1978, p 26.
762. Weiss L: Factors leading to the arrest of cancer cells in the lungs. In Weiss L, Gilbert H (eds): Pulmonary Metastasis. Boston, GK Hall, 1978, p 5.
763. Kim U: Pathogenesis of lung matastasis. In Weiss L, Gilbert H (eds): Pulmonary Metastasis. Boston, GK Hall, 1978, p 76.
764. Janower ML, Blennerhassett JB: Lymphangitic spread of metastatic cancer to the lung. A radiologic-pathologic classification. Radiology 101:267-273, 1971.
765. Meyer KK: Direct lymphatic connections from the lower lobes of the lung to the abdomen. J Thorac Surg 35:726-733, 1958.
766. Feldman GB, Knapp RC: Lymphatic drainage of the peritoneal cavity and its significance in ovarian cancer. Am J Obstet Gynecol 119:991-994, 1974.
767. Sampson J: Implantation peritoneal carcinomatosis of ovarian origin. Am J Pathol 7:423, 1931.
768. Crow J, Slavin G, Kreel L: Pulmonary metastasis: A pathologic and radiologic study. Cancer 47:2595-2602, 1981.
769. Hirakata K, Nakata H, Nakagawa T: CT of pulmonary metastases with pathological correlation. Semin Ultrasound CT MR 16:379-394, 1995.
770. Burton RM: A Case of chorion-epithelioma with pulmonary complications. Tubercle 44:487-490, 1963.
771. Peuchot M, Libshitz HI: Pulmonary metastatic disease: Radiologic-surgical correlation. Radiology 164:719-722, 1987.
772. Diederich S, Semik M, Lentschig MG, et al: Helical CT of pulmonary nodules in patients with extrathoracic malignancy: CT-surgical correlation. AJR Am J Roentgenol 172:353-360, 1999.
773. Fischbach F, Knollmann F, Griesshaber V, et al: Detection of pulmonary nodules by multislice computed tomography: Improved detection rate with reduced slice thickness. Eur Radiol 13:2378-2383, 2003.
774. Tillich M, Kammerhuber F, Reittner P, et al: Detection of pulmonary nodules with helical CT: Comparison of cine and film-based viewing. AJR Am J Roentgenol 169:1611-1614, 1997.
775. Chang AE, Schaner EG, Conkle DM, et al: Evaluation of computed tomography in the detection of pulmonary metastases: A prospective study. Cancer 43:913-916, 1979.
776. Brown MS, Goldin JG, Suh RD, et al: Lung micronodules: Automated method for detection at thin-section CT—initial experience. Radiology 226:256-262, 2003.
777. Yokomise H, Mizuno H, Ike O, et al: Importance of intrapulmonary lymph nodes in the differential diagnosis of small pulmonary nodular shadows. Chest 113:703-706, 1998.
778. Edwards SE, Fry IK: Prevalence of lung nodules on computed tomography of patients without known malignant disease. Br J Radiol 55:715-716, 1982.
779. Hirakata K, Nakata H, Haratake J: Appearance of pulmonary metastases on high-resolution CT scans: Comparison with histopathologic findings from autopsy specimens. AJR Am J Roentgenol 161:37-43, 1993.
780. Adkins PC, Wesselhoeft CW Jr, Newman W, et al: Thoracotomy on the patient with previous malignancy: Metastasis or new primary? J Thorac Cardiovasc Surg 56:351-361, 1968.
781. Cahan WG, Castro EB, Hajdu SI: Proceedings: The significance of a solitary lung shadow in patients with colon carcinoma. Cancer 33:414-421, 1974.
782. Askin FB: Something old? Something new? Second primary or pulmonary metastasis in the patient with known extrathoracic carcinoma. Am J Clin Pathol 100:4-5, 1993.
783. Ziskind MM, Weill H, Payzant AR: The recognition and significance of acinus-filling processes of the lungs. Am Rev Respir Dis 87:551-559, 1963.
784. Friedmann G, Bohndorf K, Kruger J: Radiology of pulmonary metastases: Comparison of imaging techniques with operative findings. Thorac Cardiovasc Surg 34(Spec No 2):120-124, 1986.
785. Primack SL, Hartman TE, Lee KS, et al: Pulmonary nodules and the CT halo sign. Radiology 190:513-515, 1994.
786. Shepard JA, Moore EH, Templeton PA, et al: Pulmonary intravascular tumor emboli: Dilated and beaded peripheral pulmonary arteries at CT. Radiology 187:797-801, 1993.
787. Dodd GD, Boyle JJ: Excavating pulmonary metastases. Am J Roentgenol Radium Ther Nucl Med 85:277-293, 1961.
788. Chaudhuri MR: Cavitary pulmonary metastases. Thorax 25:375-381, 1970.
789. Zollikofer C, Castaneda-Zuniga W, Stenlund R, et al: Lung metastases from synovial sarcoma simulating granulomas. AJR Am J Roentgenol 135:161-163, 1980.
790. Cockshott WP, Hendrickse JP: Pulmonary calcification at the site of trophoblastic metastases. Br J Radiol 42:17-20, 1969.
791. Moran CA, Travis WD, Carter D, et al: Metastatic mature teratoma in lung following testicular embryonal carcinoma and teratocarcinoma. Arch Pathol Lab Med 117:641-644, 1993.
792. Dines DE, Cortese DA, Brennan MD, et al: Malignant pulmonary neoplasms predisposing to spontaneous pneumothorax. Mayo Clin Proc 48:541-544, 1973.
793. Smevik B, Klepp O: The risk of spontaneous pneumothorax in patients with osteogenic sarcoma and testicular cancer. Cancer 49:1734-1737, 1982.
794. Fichera G, Hagerstrand I: The small lymph vessels of the lungs in lymphangiosis carcinomatosa. Acta Pathol Microbiol Scand 65:505-513, 1965.
795. Stein MG, Mayo J, Müller N, et al: Pulmonary lymphangitic spread of carcinoma: Appearance on CT scans. Radiology 162:371-375, 1987.
796. Youngberg AS: Unilateral diffuse lung opacity; Differential diagnosis with emphasis on lymphangitic spread of cancer. Radiology 123:277-281, 1977.
797. Munk PL, Müller NL, Miller RR, et al: Pulmonary lymphangitic carcinomatosis: CT and pathologic findings. Radiology 166:705-709, 1988.
798. Ren H, Hruban RH, Kuhlman JE, et al: Computed tomography of inflation-fixed lungs: The beaded septum sign of pulmonary metastases. J Comput Assist Tomogr 13:411-416, 1989.
799. Johkoh T, Ikezoe J, Tomiyama N, et al: CT findings in lymphangitic carcinomatosis of the lung: Correlation with histologic findings and pulmonary function tests. AJR Am J Roentgenol 158:1217-1222, 1992.
800. Kane RD, Hawkins HK, Miller JA, et al: Microscopic pulmonary tumor emboli associated with dyspnea. Cancer 36:1473-1482, 1975.
801. Yutani C, Imakita M, Ishibashi-Ueda H, et al: Pulmonary hypertension due to tumor emboli: A report of three autopsy cases with morphological correlations to radiological findings. Acta Pathol Jpn 43:135-141, 1993.
802. Winterbauer RH, Elfenbein IB, Ball WC Jr: Incidence and clinical significance of tumor embolization to the lungs. Am J Med 45:271-290, 1968.
803. Altemus LR, Lee RE: Carcinomatosis of the lung with pulmonary hypertension. Pathoradiologic spectrum. Arch Intern Med 119:32-38, 1967.
804. Bates SE, Tranum BL: Perfusion lung scan: An aid in detection of lymphangitic carcinomatosis. Cancer 50:232-235, 1982.
805. Goldhaber SZ, Dricker E, Buring JE, et al: Clinical suspicion of autopsy-proven thrombotic and tumor pulmonary embolism in cancer patients. Am Heart J 114:1432-1435, 1987.
806. Albertini RE, Ekberg NL: Endobronchial metastasis in breast cancer. Thorax 35:435-440, 1980.
807. Amer E, Guy J, Vaze B: Endobronchial metastasis from renal adenocarcinoma simulating a foreign body. Thorax 36:183-184, 1981.
808. Sutton FD Jr, Vestal RE, Creagh CE: Varied presentations of metastatic pulmonary melanoma. Chest 65:415-419, 1974.
809. Morency G, Chalaoui J, Samson L, et al: Malignant neoplasms of the trachea. Can Assoc Radiol J 40:198-200, 1989.
810. Braman SS, Whitcomb ME: Endobronchial metastasis. Arch Intern Med 135:543-547, 1975.
811. Meyer PC: Metastatic carcinoma of the pleura. Thorax 21:437-443, 1966.
812. Warren S, Gates O: Lung cancer and metastasis. Arch Pathol 78:467-473, 1964.
812a. Hirsch FR: Histopathologic classification and metastatic pattern of small cell carcinoma of the lung. Copenhagen, Munksgaard, 1983.
813. Katzenstein AL, Purvis R Jr, Gmelich J, et al: Pulmonary resection for metastatic renal adenocarcinoma: Pathologic findings and therapeutic value. Cancer 41:712-723, 1978.
814. McLoud TC, Kalisher L, Stark P, et al: Intrathoracic lymph node metastases from extrathoracic neoplasms. AJR Am J Roentgenol 131:403-407, 1978.
815. Kutty K, Varkey B: Metastatic renal cell carcinoma simulating sarcoidosis. Analysis of 12 patients with bilateral hilar lymphadenopathy. Chest 85:533-536, 1984.
816. Abubakr YA, Chou TH, Redman BG: Spontaneous remission of renal cell carcinoma: A case report and immunological correlates. J Urol 152:156-157, 1994.
817. August DA, Ottow RT, Sugarbaker PH: Clinical perspective of human colorectal cancer metastasis. Cancer Metastasis Rev 3:303-324, 1984.
818. Berg HK, Petrelli NJ, Herrera L, et al: Endobronchial metastasis from colorectal carcinoma. Dis Colon Rectum 27:745-748, 1984.
819. McCormack PM, Burt ME, Bains MS, et al: Lung resection for colorectal metastases. 10-year results. Arch Surg 127:1403-1406, 1992.
820. Sawabe M, Nakamura T, Kanno J, et al: Analysis of morphological factors of hepatocellular carcinoma in 98 autopsy cases with respect to pulmonary metastasis. Acta Pathol Jpn 37:1389-1404, 1987.
821. Papac RJ: Distant metastases from head and neck cancer. Cancer 53:342-345, 1984.

822. Daly BD, Leung SF, Cheung H, et al: Thoracic metastases from carcinoma of the nasopharynx: High frequency of hilar and mediastinal lymphadenopathy. AJR Am J Roentgenol 160:241-244, 1993.

823. Thomas JM, Redding WH, Sloane JP: The spread of breast cancer: Importance of the intrathoracic lymphatic route and its relevance to treatment. Br J Cancer 40:540-547, 1979.

824. Pikoulis E, Varelas PN, Lechago J, et al: Metastatic breast disease 40 years after the initial diagnosis. Chest 114:639-641, 1998.

825. Massin JP, Savoie JC, Garnier H, et al: Pulmonary metastases in differentiated thyroid carcinoma. Study of 58 cases with implications for the primary tumor treatment. Cancer 53:982-992, 1984.

826. Hoie J, Stenwig AE, Kullmann G, et al: Distant metastases in papillary thyroid cancer. A review of 91 patients. Cancer 61:1-6, 1988.

827. Piekarski JD, Schlumberger M, Leclere J, et al: Chest computed tomography (CT) in patients with micronodular lung metastases of differentiated thyroid carcinoma. Int J Radiat Oncol Biol Phys 11:1023-1027, 1985.

828. Bonte FJ, McConnell RW: Pulmonary metastases from differentiated thyroid carcinoma demonstrable only by nuclear imaging. Radiology 107:585-590, 1973.

829. Xiao H, Liu D, Bajorin DF, et al: Medical and surgical management of pulmonary metastases from germ cell tumors. Chest Surg Clin N Am 8:131-143, 1998.

830. Williams MP, Husband JE, Heron CW: Intrathoracic manifestations of metastatic testicular seminoma: A comparison of chest radiographic and CT findings. AJR Am J Roentgenol 149:473-475, 1987.

831. Yousem DM, Scatarige JC, Fishman EK, et al: Low-attenuation thoracic metastases in testicular malignancy. AJR Am J Roentgenol 146:291-293, 1986.

832. Webb WR, Gamsu G: Thoracic metastasis in malignant melanoma. A radiographic survey of 65 patients. Chest 71:176-181, 1977.

833. Ballon S, Donaldson R, Growdon W, et al: Pulmonary metastasis in endometrial carcinoma. In Weiss L, Gilbert H (eds): Pulmonary metastasis. Boston, GK Hall, 1978, p 182.

834. Tellis CJ, Beechler CR: Pulmonary metastasis of carcinoma of the cervix: A retrospective study. Cancer 49:1705-1709, 1982.

835. Imachi M, Tsukamoto N, Matsuyama T, et al: Pulmonary metastasis from carcinoma of the uterine cervix. Gynecol Oncol 33:189-192, 1989.

836. Sostman HD, Matthay RA: Thoracic metastases from cervical carcinoma: Current status. Invest Radiol 15:113-119, 1980.

837. Kerr VE, Cadman E: Pulmonary metastases in ovarian cancer. Analysis of 357 patients. Cancer 56:1209-1213, 1985.

838. Dauplat J, Hacker NF, Nieberg RK, et al: Distant metastases in epithelial ovarian carcinoma. Cancer 60:1561-1566, 1987.

839. Elkin M, Mueller HP: Metastases from cancer of the prostate; autopsy and roentgenological findings. Cancer 7:1246-1248, 1954.

840. Saitoh H, Hida M, Shimbo T, et al: Metastatic patterns of prostatic cancer. Correlation between sites and number of organs involved. Cancer 54:3078-3084, 1984.

841. Apple JS, Paulson DF, Baber C, et al: Advanced prostatic carcinoma: Pulmonary manifestations. Radiology 154:601-604, 1985.

842. Bagshawe KD, Noble MI: Cardio-respiratory aspects of trophoblastic tumours. Q J Med 35:39-54, 1966.

843. Wagner BJ, Woodward PJ, Dickey GE: From the archives of the AFIP. Gestational trophoblastic disease: Radiologic-pathologic correlation. Radiographics 16:131-148, 1996.

844. Levenback C, Rubin SC, McCormack PM, et al: Resection of pulmonary metastases from uterine sarcomas. Gynecol Oncol 45:202-205, 1992.

845. Kayser K, Zink S, Schneider T, et al: Benign metastasizing leiomyoma of the uterus: Documentation of clinical, immunohistochemical and lectin-histochemical data of ten cases. Virchows Arch 437:284-292, 2000.

846. Wolff M, Silva F, Kaye G: Pulmonary metastases (with admixed epithelial elements) from smooth muscle neoplasms. Report of nine cases, including three males. Am J Surg Pathol 3:325-342, 1979.

847. Sargent EN, Barnes RA, Schwinn CP: Multiple pulmonary fibroleiomyomatous hamartomas. Report of a case and review of the literature. Am J Roentgenol Radium Ther Nucl Med 110:694-700, 1970.

848. Maredia R, Snyder BJ, Harvey LA, et al: Benign metastasizing leiomyoma in the lung. Radiographics 18:779-782, 1998.

849. Horstmann JP, Pietra GG, Harman JA, et al: Spontaneous regression of pulmonary leiomyomas during pregnancy. Cancer 39:314-321, 1977.

850. Bachman D, Wolff M: Pulmonary metastases from benign-appearing smooth muscle tumors of the uterus. AJR Am J Roentgenol 127:44144-6, 1976.

851. Vezeridis MP, Moore R, Karakousis CP: Metastatic patterns in soft-tissue sarcomas. Arch Surg 118:915-918, 1983.

852. Kim K, Naylor B, Han IH: Fine needle aspiration cytology of sarcomas metastatic to the lung. Acta Cytol 30:688-694, 1986.

853. Cordier JF, Bailly C, Tabone E, et al: Alveolar soft part sarcoma presenting as asymptomatic pulmonary nodules: Report of a case with ultrastructural diagnosis. Thorax 40:203-204, 1985.

854. Going JJ, Brewin TB, Crompton GK, et al: Soft tissue sarcoma: Two cases of solitary lung metastasis more than 15 years after diagnosis. Clin Radiol 37:579-581, 1986.

855. Huth JF, Eilber FR: Patterns of recurrence after resection of osteosarcoma of the extremity. Strategies for treatment of metastases. Arch Surg 124:122-126, 1989.

856. Poe RH, Ortiz C, Israel RH, et al: Sensitivity, specificity, and predictive values of bronchoscopy in neoplasm metastatic to lung. Chest 88:84-88, 1985.

857. Chuang MT, Padilla ML, Teirstein AS: Flexible fiberoptic bronchoscopy in metastatic cancer to the lungs. Cancer 52:1949-1951, 1983.

858. Mohsenifar Z, Chopra SK, Simmons DH: Diagnostic value of fiberoptic bronchoscopy in metastatic pulmonary tumors. Chest 74:369-371, 1978.

859. Johnston W, Frable W: Other neoplasms of the lung, primary and metastatic. In Baselski V, Wunderink R (eds): Diagnostic Respiratory Cytopathology. Paris, Masson Publishing, 1979.

PULMONARY MANIFESTATIONS OF HIV INFECTION

The impact of the global pandemic of infection by HIV has been enormous. Since illness associated with HIV infection was first reported in 1981, more than 60 million people have been infected.[1] By the end of 2001, an estimated 40 million people were living with it, 20 million having died of AIDS.[2] In the year 2000, an estimated 90.4 million lost healthy years of life were attributed to AIDS, a total exceeding that associated with malaria and tuberculosis combined.[3] In the next 20 years, an estimated 70 million people will die worldwide as a result of the disease.[2]

In the United States, AIDS has developed in over 800,000 people, and nearly 500,000 have died of the disease,[4] a figure exceeding the casualties of both World War I and World War II together. At the end of 2001, approximately 360,000 were living with AIDS.[5] Some have estimated that there may be as many as 400,000 to 500,000 individuals with undiagnosed and/or untreated disease.[6] The advent of highly active antiretroviral therapy (HAART) led to a sharp decline in the incidence of AIDS from 1996 to 1998 and to increasing AIDS prevalence because affected patients lived longer than previously.[7] In 1998 and 1999, this decline began to level, and no change occurred from 1999 to 2001.[7] AIDS develops in more than 40,000 patients annually in the United States. Data for HIV infection in the absence of AIDS are incomplete; however, despite public health measures, significant numbers of individuals continue to be infected with the virus.[5]

The estimated number of cases of HIV infection and AIDS combined is about 2.8 times that of AIDS cases alone.[8] In the absence of effective therapy, AIDS develops about 10 years after the initial HIV infection; as a consequence, focusing on the incidence and prevalence of AIDS alone reflects rates of infection that occurred a decade earlier.[9]

The two most important risk factors for HIV infection are sexual contact with an infected person and intravenous drug use. Among men who have AIDS in the United States, approximately 55% are homosexual and 25% are intravenous drug users; 5% to 10% have both risk factors. About a quarter of all new AIDS cases reported in 2001 were in women. Among them, about 60% were exposed through heterosexual contact and 40% through injection drug use.[5]

In the "developing" world, heterosexual transmission has been the dominant mode of infection and has resulted in a proportionately greater burden of disease among women and children (via transplacental transmission of HIV and breast-feeding) than has been seen in the United States. The highest incidence rates are found in women between the ages of 15 and 25 years.[10] The impact of HIV infection and AIDS in these areas is staggering. For example, more than 2 million Africans died of AIDS in 2001, and 55 million are projected to die of the disease earlier than they would have by 2020.[11] Seven countries in sub-Saharan Africa now have AIDS prevalence rates in excess of 20%, and 11 million African children alive at the end of 2001 had lost one or both parents to AIDS.[11]

The most common and important pulmonary complications of AIDS are infections,[12,13] of which bacteria, *Pneumocystis jiroveci*, *Mycobacterium tuberculosis*, and cytomegalovirus (CMV) are the most frequent causes. Neoplasms—predominantly lymphoma and Kaposi's sarcoma (KS)—are less frequent but also important. Many other relatively uncommon complications are seen in some patients (Table 8–1).

PULMONARY INFECTION

There is a clear association between the degree of immunosuppression, as reflected by the blood CD4+ lymphocyte count, and the risk of development of specific respiratory disorders.[14] Common respiratory tract illnesses such as

TABLE 8–1. Pulmonary Manifestations of AIDS

Infections

Bacteria

Streptococcus pneumoniae
Haemophilus influenzae
Staphylococcus aureus
Legionella species
Pseudomonas aeruginosa
Rhodococcus equi
Nocardia species
Streptococcus agalactiae
Enterobacteriaceae
Moraxella catarrhalis
Treponema pallidum
Pasteurella multocida
Salmonella species
Mycobacterium tuberculosis
Mycobacterium avium–intracellulare complex
Mycobacterium kansasii
Mycobacterium gordonae
Mycobacterium xenopi
Mycobacterium celatum
Mycobacterium haemophilum
Mycobacterium simiae
Mycobacterium fortuitum
Mycobacterium genavense

Fungi

Pneumocystis jiroveci
Cryptococcus species
Histoplasma capsulatum
Coccidioides immitis
Blastomyces dermatitidis
Aspergillus species
Sporothrix schenckii
Paracoccidioides brasiliensis
Mucorales species
Penicillium marneffei

Viruses

Primary HIV pneumonia
Cytomegalovirus
Adenovirus
Varicella
Vaccine-associated measles virus

Parasites

Toxoplasma species
Strongyloides stercoralis
Cryptosporidia
Microsporidia
Platyhelminths

Neoplasms

Kaposi's sarcoma
Non-Hodgkin's lymphoma
Hodgkin's lymphoma
Pulmonary carcinoma
Smooth muscle neoplasms

Miscellaneous Conditions

Nonspecific interstitial pneumonitis
Lymphocytic interstitial pneumonitis
"Primary" pulmonary hypertension
Pulmonary alveolar proteinosis
Diffuse alveolar hemorrhage
Respiratory muscle dysfunction
Cryptogenic organizing pneumonia
Emphysema-like changes
Lymphocytic bronchiolitis
Bronchiectasis
Pulmonary edema secondary to AIDS-related cardiac disease

From Fraser RS, Müller NL, Colman NC, Paré PD: Fraser and Paré's Diagnosis of Diseases of the Chest, 4th ed. Philadelphia, WB Saunders, 1999.

bronchitis, sinusitis, and pharyngitis are seen with all CD4$^+$ T-lymphocyte counts, though at a greater frequency than in a seronegative population.[12] About 80% of cases of bacterial pneumonia and pulmonary tuberculosis are associated with a CD4$^+$ count less than 400 cells/μL. With counts less than 300 cells/μL, bacterial pneumonia is often recurrent, and infection by nontuberculous mycobacteria is seen; counts less than 200 cells/μL are associated with pneumocystis pneumonia (PCP), disseminated tuberculosis, or KS. In patients who have the most severe degree of immunosuppression (counts less than 100 cells/μL), disseminated infection by *Mycobacterium avium-intracellulare*, CMV, and various fungi tends to develop.

Nontuberculous Bacteria

The clinical and radiologic features of bacterial pneumonia are similar in patients with and without HIV infection[15,16]; however, pneumonia in HIV-positive patients tends to progress more rapidly, is more frequently multilobar, and is more often associated with bacteremia.[2,17] Although the risk for development of the complication has been significantly reduced by the use of HAART, increasing risk remains with low CD4$^+$ counts, intravenous drug use, and a history of previous PCP.[18]

Streptococcus pneumoniae is the leading cause of bacterial respiratory disease, with or without bacteremia, in HIV-infected adults[19,20] and may be recurrent.[21] Even with HAART, the risk for infection remains substantially greater than that in the normal population.[18] The incidence of infection is reduced in patients taking trimethoprim-sulfamethoxazole for PCP prophylaxis[22] and in those who have received pneumococcal vaccine after HIV infection and before the development of severe immunosuppression.[23]

Haemophilus influenzae is also a relatively common cause of bacterial pneumonia in HIV-infected individuals.[24] As with other bacterial pneumonias, the risk of infection increases with increasing immunosuppression.[25] Its clinical and radiological manifestations are diverse; subacute disease is seen with worsening degrees of immunosuppression, and bilateral disease on the radiograph is common.[24]

Staphylococcus aureus has been identified uncommonly.[26] However, it should be considered as a cause of pneumonia when illness is severe enough to require hospital admission[20] and in the nosocomial setting.[27] *Legionella* organisms are also infrequent causes of pneumonia,[26,28] in one series accounting for only 1 of 237 cases.[30] Concomitant infection with *P. jiroveci* or mycobacteria is common.[26]

Except at autopsy,[31] *Pseudomonas aeruginosa* is also an uncommon cause of pneumonia.[32] Infection is often indolent[33] and associated with very low CD4$^+$ lymphocyte counts. Radiographically, patchy air space opacification or bronchiectasis may be seen.[22] Relapse after therapy is common.

Rhodococcus equi is an intracellular gram-positive and variably acid-fast bacterium that may be coccoid or have a curved, clubbed shape. More than 100 infections have been described in patients who have AIDS.[34] Infection in other individuals is rare, and identification of the organism should prompt consideration of HIV infection.[28] Risk factors include exposure to farm dust or horses or cohabitation with an infected individual.[35] Histologic findings consist of an infiltrate of neutrophils and macrophages associated with parenchymal destruction.[36] The macrophages typically have abundant vacuolated cytoplasm that contains numerous bacteria.

Radiologic manifestations usually consist of a round opacity or area of consolidation limited to one lobe, most commonly an upper one.[37] Several opacities may coalesce and undergo cavitation associated with a fluid level.[38] Pleural effusion is present in approximately 20% of cases. In most patients, the abnormality persists for more than 1 month despite antibiotic therapy.

Pulmonary disease is usually insidious in onset and characterized by fever, malaise, productive cough, and pleuritic chest pain.[26,39,40] Some patients have evidence of extrathoracic involvement at initial evaluation, most often affecting the eye, subcutaneous tissue, central nervous system (CNS), and lymph nodes. Disease is often chronic and frequently leads to the patient's death.[34]

Bartonella henselae and *Bartonella quintana* are gram-negative bacilli that cause bacillary angiomatosis, a reactive vasoproliferative lesion that occurs almost exclusively in patients who have AIDS.[41,42] The mode of transmission is not known; however, because *B. henselae* is the most common cause of cat-scratch disease,[43] it is likely that it involves animal or insect vectors. The foci of vascular proliferation may affect many tissues, including the skin, bone, brain, and a variety of viscera.[44] Intrathoracic manifestations include polypoid endobronchial lesions, pulmonary parenchymal nodules or masses, mediastinal lymph node enlargement, and pleural effusion.[42,45] Symptoms include fever, chills, night sweats, weight loss, anemia, and (occasionally) hemoptysis or chest pain. Lymph node enlargement is common in the axilla, neck, or groin.[42] Patients usually respond rapidly to appropriate antibiotic therapy; however, if untreated, they may die of overwhelming infection.[42]

The clinical features of lung infection related to *Nocardia asteroides* are similar to those of *R. equi*. The duration of symptoms varies from 1 to 6 months before diagnosis. Although infection is frequently disseminated, the disease is radiographically manifested in the lung as lobar or multilobar areas of air space opacification in more than 50% of patients.[26] The upper lobes are most commonly affected, and areas of cavitation are typical; as such, infection may be confused with tuberculosis.[46] Culture of the organism from sputum or BAL fluid is definitive for the diagnosis; however, the organism may take up to 4 weeks to grow. Identification of typical slender branching filaments on Gram stain of sputum or BAL fluid should suggest the diagnosis.

Mycobacterium tuberculosis

M. tuberculosis is the most important "opportunistic" organism in patients infected with HIV. In fact, such infection is a major factor in the increasing prevalence and incidence of tuberculosis worldwide.[47] Patients who are infected with both HIV and *M. tuberculosis* are at high risk for the development of active tuberculosis. In some HIV-infected groups, such as those in sub-Saharan Africa,[48] the prevalence of tuberculous infection is high; as a result, tuberculosis control measures in many countries are being overwhelmed.[49] Globally, tuberculosis is the most common cause of death in patients who have AIDS[50]; moreover, there is evidence that the infection is

associated with an earlier appearance of AIDS and a worse prognosis once it is established.

Epidemiology

Patients are at risk for the development of both primary and reactivation tuberculosis.[51] There is little doubt that the unexpected increase in the incidence of tuberculosis in the United States that occurred in the mid-1980s to early 1990s can be attributed to the AIDS pandemic.[47] The incidence of tuberculosis in patients who had AIDS at that time was as high as 500 times that in the normal population; in addition, each year tuberculosis developed in as many as 5% to 15% of HIV-infected people who had positive tuberculin skin test results.[47,52] As might be expected, the rates were highest in those who had the most advanced degree of immunosuppression.

Worldwide, a high prevalence of HIV infection has been found in patients who have tuberculosis. In the sub-Saharan region of Africa, more than 50% of patients with tuberculosis are HIV seropositive.[53,54] Although the prevalence of HIV infection in patients who have tuberculosis in "developed" countries is less than that noted in Africa, it is still impressive. For example, in an investigation of 500 patients who had pulmonary tuberculosis in Los Angeles, 25% of the men and 4% of the women who were tested proved to be HIV seropositive[55]; some had no obvious risk factors for HIV infection.

Not unexpectedly, tuberculosis is also a frequent complication of HIV infection, especially in populations in which the prevalence of infection with *M. tuberculosis* is high. In some countries, the risk for development of tuberculosis has been found to be 20-fold higher in HIV-positive individuals than in negative controls.[56,57] This risk persists even after excluding confounding variables such as homelessness and drug addiction.[58] Although most cases of tuberculosis are probably the result of reactivation of latent infection, recently transmitted infection accounts for an important number of cases in some populations.[59]

By fostering reconstitution of the immune response, it is likely that HAART has led to a marked decrease in the incidence of tuberculosis in HIV-infected patients who have been fortunate enough to receive the therapy.[60]

Pathogenesis

HIV infection impairs the cell-mediated immune response to *M. tuberculosis* by interfering with the recruitment and function of both macrophages and CD4[+] T lymphocytes.[61,62] The virus can inhibit macrophage chemotaxis, phagocytosis, and microbicidal activity as well as impair the proper functioning of the macrophage–CD4[+] lymphocyte immune axis. Both the virus and *M. tuberculosis* cause depletion of lymphocytes as well as suppression of their regeneration and maturation. Interference with the association of antigen-presenting cells and antigen-specific lymphocytes, which is part of the normal immune response, also fosters intercellular spread and propagation of HIV. This in turn leads to the selective clonal depletion of mycobacteria-specific CD4[+] lymphocytes.[62]

Functional impairment of CD4[+] lymphocytes occurs even before a significant decline in their number. The T_H2 skewing of lymphocyte response associated with decreased secretion of monocyte-derived T_H1 cytokines (substances that are necessary for effective defense against *M. tuberculosis*) also diminishes effective cell-mediated immunity against the organism. Both HIV replication and infectivity are also enhanced at the site of active mycobacterial infection: in patients who have pulmonary tuberculosis, the HIV-1 load is greater in diseased than in unaffected lung.[63] The net result of all these abnormalities is defective granuloma formation, decreased mycobacterial killing, and an increase in the aggressivity of HIV-1 infection itself.

Radiologic Manifestations

The patterns of abnormality seen in patients who have AIDS differ from those in other patients, the former having a greater likelihood of lymph node enlargement, lower lobe disease, and extensive parenchymal involvement and a lower likelihood of cavitation (Fig. 8–1).[64-66] The prevalence of these abnormalities is influenced by the country of origin of the patient and the degree of immunosuppression. For example, cavitation is seen less commonly in patients from the United States than in those from North and Central Africa.[66,67] In patients who have

relatively normal immune status (>200 CD4+ cells/μL), the appearance is similar to postprimary tuberculosis in a normal host; by contrast, markedly immunosuppressed patients tend to have miliary disease or a pattern similar to primary tuberculosis.[64,65,68] Patients with lower CD4 counts are also more likely to have normal chest radiographs; for example, in an investigation of 48 patients who had fewer than 200 CD4+ cells/μL, 10 (21%) had a normal chest radiograph as opposed to only 1 of 20 (5%) who had a count greater than 200.[68]

Chest radiographs in patients who have AIDS and pulmonary tuberculosis often show transient worsening after antiretroviral therapy.[69] This radiographic deterioration usually occurs 1 to 5 weeks after initiation of the therapy and improves 2 weeks to 3 months later.

The most common abnormality on CT scans consists of enlarged hilar and mediastinal lymph nodes, typically associated with low attenuation (see Fig. 8–1).[70,71] In an investigation of 29 HIV-positive and 47 HIV-negative patients, the most common abnormalities in the former patients were lymph node enlargement (in 22 [76%]), nodules less than 1 cm in diameter (in 20 [69%]), dense consolidation (in

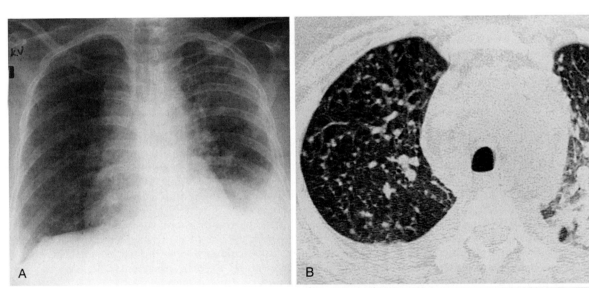

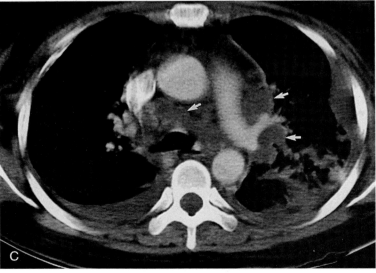

FIGURE 8–1

Pulmonary tuberculosis. An anteroposterior chest radiograph (**A**) in a 43-year-old man who had AIDS shows air space consolidation in the left upper lobe, miliary nodules, mediastinal lymphadenopathy, and bilateral pleural effusions. An HRCT scan (**B**) shows a focal area of consolidation in the left upper lobe and miliary nodules. A scan after the intravenous administration of contrast material (**C**) shows extensive left hilar and mediastinal lymphadenopathy (*arrows*) and small bilateral pleural effusions. The enlarged lymph nodes have low attenuation, a common finding in patients who have AIDS and tuberculosis. (*From Müller NL, Fraser RS, Colman NC, Paré PD: Radiologic Diagnosis of Diseases of the Chest. Philadelphia, WB Saunders, 2001.*)

11 [38%]), and pleural effusion (in 7 [24%])[71]; lymphadenopathy was seen more commonly in HIV-positive than HIV-negative patients (76% versus 55%). Findings seen less commonly in HIV-positive patients included cavitation (24% versus 49%), 1- to 3-cm-diameter nodules (14% versus 47%), and bronchial wall thickening (14% versus 45%). A linear correlation between the CD4[+] cell count and the number of lobes involved ($r = 0.84$) and the number of nodules ($r = 0.97$) was seen in the HIV-positive patients. Patients who had more than 200 CD4[+] cells/μL were more likely to have cavitation than were patients who had lower cell counts (50% versus 13%) and less likely to have lymphadenopathy (33% versus 70%).

The presence of low-attenuation or rim-enhancing hilar or mediastinal lymph nodes in patients with AIDS is most suggestive of tuberculosis or infection with *Mycobacterium avium-intracellulare* complex (MAC). In an investigation of the CT findings in 102 patients, hilar or mediastinal lymph node enlargement was present in 12 of 16 (75%) who had mycobacterial infection, 13 of 26 (50%) who had KS, 4 of 5 (80%) who had lymphoma, and 3 of 5 (60%) who had fungal infection.[72] Low-attenuation lymph nodes with or without rim enhancement were seen only in patients with tuberculosis or MAC infection.

Nodule size and distribution on HRCT are helpful in the differential diagnosis. In an investigation of 43 patients who had opportunistic infection, 36 (84%) had a predominance of nodules smaller than 1 cm in diameter, whereas 14 of 17 (82%) who had KS or lymphoma had a predominance of nodules larger than 1 cm.[73] The nodules had a centrilobular distribution in 65% of patients who had opportunistic infection as opposed to only 1 of 17 (6%) patients with the other two conditions. The most common such infections were caused by bacteria and *M. tuberculosis*; PCP was rare. Nodule size and distribution were not helpful in distinguishing mycobacterial from other bacterial infections.

In HIV-positive patients who have pulmonary tuberculosis and a normal radiograph, CT scan often shows subtle parenchymal abnormalities, including miliary nodules, centrilobular nodules resulting from endobronchial spread, tuberculomas, or lymph node enlargement.[64,74]

Clinical Manifestations

The clinical features of tuberculosis in patients who have AIDS vary with the degree of immunosuppression.[49] When immune function is relatively preserved, the manifestations tend to be the same as those in patients who are not HIV positive.[49] However, in patients in whom CD4 counts are depressed, the likelihood of atypical features is increased. Extrapulmonary tuberculosis is significantly more common in patients who are infected with HIV than in those who are seronegative; in fact, it is seen in more than 50% at some point in the course of the disease and is the sole manifestation of the disease in about 25%.[75] Lymph node involvement, including radiographic evidence of mediastinal node enlargement, is particularly common.[76] As might be expected, disseminated disease is found more often in HIV-positive than HIV-negative individuals.[77] Both it and miliary disease are more likely to be seen when immunosuppression is profound.[78]

Tuberculosis is an uncommon cause of pleural effusion in AIDS patients in North America; however, pleural effusion is still more common as a manifestation of tuberculosis in HIV-infected than in HIV-negative patients.[79] Disease is more often associated with a greater burden of microorganisms, which are thus more likely to be demonstrated in pleural tissue specimens and sputum.[80]

Diagnosis

Significant obstacles hinder a rapid diagnosis of tuberculosis in patients who are HIV positive. The symptoms are nonspecific, the radiographic manifestations are often atypical, and infection is frequently extrapulmonary. Therefore, a high index of suspicion is the first diagnostic step, especially in patients who are at increased risk for the disease.[81,82] Such individuals include intravenous drug abusers, the homeless, prisoners, immigrants from areas where tuberculosis is endemic, patients in whom the tuberculin skin test is positive, and those who have had recent exposure to a person with active disease.

Tuberculin skin testing is of only modest value in diagnosis. Although seropositive purified protein derivative (PPD) reactors are at high risk for the development of tuberculosis, skin test negativity in patients who have an advanced degree of immunosuppression has poor negative predictive value for the presence of infection[83,84]; in fact, only 40% to 55% of HIV-infected patients who have tuberculosis show a positive PPD reaction.[85] Whether a cutaneous induration of 5 mm should be considered positive in patients who are HIV seropositive, as is current practice, is open to question.[86]

The prevalence of positive sputum smears and culture is about the same in HIV-infected and uninfected patients who have pulmonary tuberculosis.[87] Overall, about 60% to 70% of such patients have a positive smear,[87,88] a finding that strongly suggests the presence of tuberculosis, even in the setting of a high prevalence of MAC infection.[89] The use of polymerase chain reaction (PCR) and gene probes permits distinction between the two organisms when the smear is positive and the clinical and radiologic findings are atypical for tuberculosis.[47,51] It may also allow avoidance of invasive procedures for the diagnosis of miliary disease or atypical radiologic findings when sputum smears are negative.[51] Material obtained by a variety of other techniques can also be useful in diagnosis, including sputum induction with aerosolized saline, BAL, transbronchial or bronchial biopsy, and transthoracic needle aspiration.

Prognosis and Natural History

Tuberculosis is an important cause of death in patients who have AIDS.[90] Although most patients in whom the infection is recognized and treated by appropriate drug therapy do well, the disease may progress as a result of noncompliance with therapy or resistance of the organism to drugs.[91] Even though the high mortality rate of patients who have AIDS and tuberculosis is in large part directly related to their degree of immunosuppression,[92] there is evidence that infection with *M. tuberculosis* adversely affects the course of HIV infection; even after consideration of relevant confounders and early death as a result of tuberculosis,[93] the risk of death doubles in affected patients. HIV infection has also been associated with a high prevalence of multidrug-resistant tuberculosis,[91] which is difficult to treat and associated with an extremely high mortality rate.[94]

The immune reconstitution that results from HAART is probably associated with the increased survival of HIV-positive patients who become infected with tuberculosis. However, such therapy may be followed by transient worsening of disease that is not due to failure of therapy or a second new process after its initiation.[95]

Other Mycobacteria

Systemic MAC infection is common in patients who have not received therapy for HIV.[49] However, the incidence of such infection has been strikingly reduced in the United States by the use of HAART and effective prophylactic therapy.[60] The most common radiographic abnormality is mediastinal lymph node enlargement (Fig. 8–2), a finding reflecting the relatively frequent presence of lymph node infection. Radiographically evident pulmonary disease is uncommon[96]; for example, in a study of 48 patients in whom the organism was isolated from respiratory tract specimens, only 2 patients had lung disease attributed to it.[97] The diagnosis of such disease is made by repeated culture of respiratory tract secretions in the setting of a compatible radiographic picture for which no other cause can be demonstrated.

Of the many medically significant mycobacterial species other than *M. avium-intracellulare* or *M. tuberculosis*, more than half have caused disease in HIV-infected patients (see Table 8–1).[98] Both colonization and infection are more common in the HIV-infected population than in uninfected patients. Although some of the organisms also cause systemic illness or focal disease outside the lung, many have been identified only in the lung. The most important are *Mycobacterium kansasii*[99] and *Mycobacterium xenopi*.[100]

Fungi

By far the most important fungus to cause pulmonary disease in patients who are HIV positive is *P. carinii*; however, other organisms account for a significant number of AIDS-defining illnesses,[101] and a variety of additional fungi are occasional causes of infection (see Table 8–1). Despite this rather extensive list, with the exception of PCP, pulmonary fungal infections are uncommon in HIV-infected patients outside the geographic areas in which a given fungus is endemic.[102]

Pneumocystis jiroveci (carinii)

Epidemiology

Since the first descriptions of profound immunodeficiency in previously healthy homosexual men in 1981,[103] the history of AIDS and *P. carinii* (*P. jiroveci*[104]) infection has been closely intertwined. From the early 1980s to the early 1990s, the infection was documented in more than 100,000 Americans, most of whom were also infected with HIV.[105] During this time, PCP occurred in 75% of patients who had AIDS and was the most common AIDS-defining diagnosis and the most common cause of life-threatening illness.[106] Coinciding with the increased use of primary and secondary prophylaxis against *P. jiroveci* and effective antiretroviral therapy in the late 1980s, the incidence of PCP began to decrease,[107] a decline that has accelerated under the influence of HAART.[108] The incidence of PCP in the United States fell by 3.4% per year between 1992 and 1995 and, coincident with the advent of HAART,[109] by 21.5% annually between 1996 and 1998 in a population of AIDS patients who had CD4[+] counts of around 100/μL.

Despite the decrease in its incidence, PCP is still an important infection in the AIDS population. In large part as a result of the unavailability of treatment or nonadherence to therapy,[110] PCP remains the most common AIDS-defining opportunistic infection.[111] Moreover, approximately 50% of individuals who die of AIDS have had PCP at some time during their disease.[111]

The risk for PCP is most pronounced in patients who have CD4[+] lymphocyte counts less than 200 cells/μL; in fact, when counts return to above these levels after the institution of

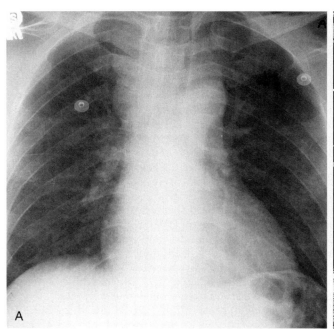
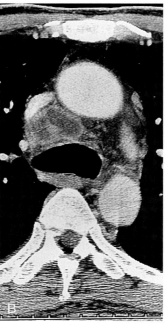

FIGURE 8–2

Mycobacterium avium-intracellulare. An anteroposterior chest radiograph (**A**) in a 47-year-old patient with AIDS demonstrates widening of the right superior mediastinum. A contrast-enhanced CT scan (**B**) demonstrates an enlarged right paratracheal lymph node. The enlarged node has central low attenuation and rim enhancement. The patient had culture-proven disseminated infection with *M. avium-intracellulare* complex. (*From Kang EY, Staples CA, McGuinness G, et al: Detection and differential diagnosis of pulmonary infections and tumors in patients with AIDS: Value of chest radiography versus CT. AJR Am J Roentgenol 166:15, 1996.*)

HAART, PCP prophylaxis can safely be discontinued.[112] The results of molecular typing of *P. jiroveci* isolates have shown that many infections are recently acquired and do not represent activation of latent infection[113]; nevertheless, there is little evidence for person-to-person transmission.[114]

Pathogenesis

The general pathogenetic features of PCP have been discussed previously (see page 278); here, we briefly discuss the mechanisms by which HIV infection alters host defense against the organism. The increased risk for the development of PCP with diminishing CD4 counts is clear evidence for the importance of blood lymphocytes in defense against *P. jiroveci*.[115] As for tuberculosis, there is evidence that the alveolar lymphocytes of patients infected with the organism elaborate greatly increased quantities of HIV when compared with the lymphocytes of HIV-seropositive patients who are not infected with it.[116] In addition, these cells appear to be defective in function and decreased in number.[62] Alveolar macrophages also have an important role in defense[117]; impaired release of tumor necrosis factor-α by infected macrophages is probably key in this regard.[118]

With the relative failure of immune mechanisms to control the infection, an acute inflammatory reaction may be prominent.[119,120] There is also evidence that *P. jiroveci* is toxic to alveolar epithelial cells at points of adherence and that it inhibits their replication,[121] effects that may contribute to the development of alveolar edema and abnormal surfactant function.[122]

Pathologic Characteristics

The type and severity of histologic findings in AIDS-related PCP vary considerably.[123,124] The typical appearance is similar to that seen in immunocompromised individuals who do not have AIDS: alveolar interstitial inflammation, proliferation of type II alveolar epithelial cells, and a finely vacuolated eosinophilic "exudate" within the alveolar air spaces (Fig. 8–3). Unlike disease in individuals not infected with HIV, however, the amount of intra-alveolar exudate is often very large, particularly in patients who die with "active" PCP. In addition, interstitial lymphocytes and plasma cells may be few in number or absent altogether in patients who have very low CD4 counts.

Other histologic findings that may be seen either alone or in association with the typical features include diffuse alveolar damage, granulomatous inflammation (Fig. 8–4A) (in which organisms may be few in number and difficult to identify in BAL fluid),[125] bronchiolitis obliterans with organizing pneumonia,[123] vascular invasion (Fig. 8–4B),[126] parenchymal calcification (usually associated with previous treatment),

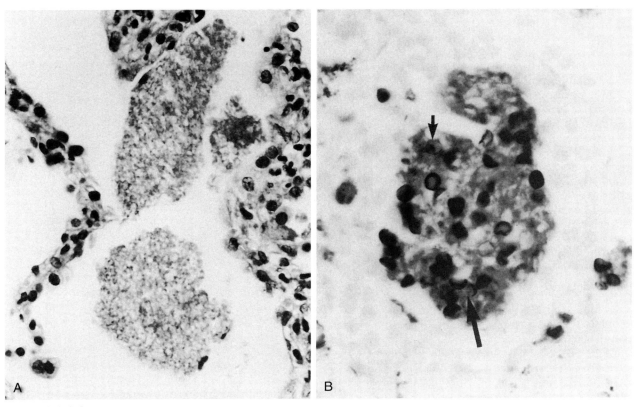

FIGURE 8–3

Pneumocystis pneumonia. A magnified view of a transbronchial biopsy specimen (**A**) from a 42-year-old man with AIDS shows mild interstitial thickening secondary to edema and a mononuclear inflammatory cell infiltrate; two clusters of finely vacuolated proteinaceous material are present within alveolar air spaces. A silver stain of one of these clusters (**B**) shows it to contain multiple round (*short arrow*) or sickle-shaped (*long arrow*) cysts. (**A,** ×440; **B,** Grocott silver methenamine, ×1000.) *(From Fraser RS, Müller NL, Colman NC, Paré PD: Fraser and Paré's Diagnosis of Diseases of the Chest, 4th ed. Philadelphia, WB Saunders, 1999.)*

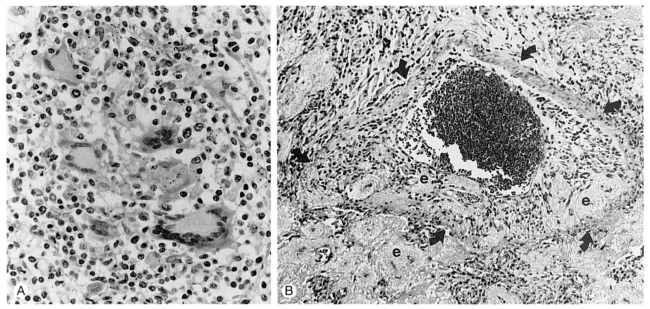

FIGURE 8–4

Pneumocystis pneumonia. A section (**A**) from an autopsy of a patient in whom *P. jiroveci* pneumonia had been diagnosed 2 months before death shows mononuclear cells surround a loosely formed granuloma consisting largely of multinucleated giant cells. A magnified view (**B**) of a pulmonary artery from another patient shows the presence of abundant exudate (e) characteristic of *P. jiroveci* infection. The material is located in the lung parenchyma adjacent to the vessel and in the arterial intima (*arrows* indicate the media, which is partially destroyed in its lower and left portions). (*From Fraser RS, Müller NL, Colman NC, Paré PD: Fraser and Paré's Diagnosis of Diseases of the Chest, 4th ed. Philadelphia, WB Saunders, 1999.*)

necrosis, and cyst formation.[124] The pathologic findings in the last-named complication are variable: some examples consist of blebs and others of parenchymal spaces lined by a thin layer of fibrous tissue or by lung parenchyma consolidated by the foamy exudate of typical *P. jiroveci* infection.[127] There is evidence that the pathogenesis of at least some of the parenchymal cysts is related to tissue invasion by the organisms followed by necrosis.[127] All these atypical pathologic manifestations are more common in patients who have received prophylactic therapy for PCP.

Although organisms often disappear quickly in tissue sections after therapy in patients who have PCP in the absence of AIDS, such clearing is frequently less rapid and may be absent altogether in patients who are HIV positive.[128]

Radiologic Manifestations

The most common radiologic findings in patients with PCP consist of bilateral and symmetrical ground-glass, finely granular, or reticular opacities (Fig. 8–5).[84,129,130] The abnormalities can be diffuse but often have a perihilar, lower lung zone predominance or, less commonly, an upper lung zone predominance. If left untreated, the opacities usually progress to predominantly perihilar or diffuse air space consolidation (Fig. 8–6).[131]

The development of air-filled cysts, or pneumatoceles, has been reported in about 5% to 35% of patients.[131-133] The cysts can be seen anywhere in the lungs, although they are more common in the upper lobes. They range from 1 to 10 cm in diameter and generally have walls 1 mm or less in

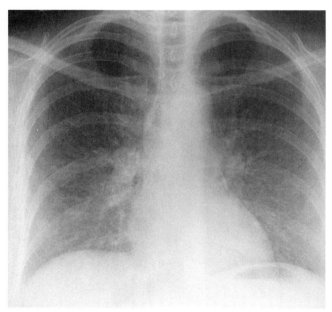

FIGURE 8–5

Pneumocystis pneumonia. A posteroanterior chest radiograph in a 41-year-old woman who had AIDS shows bilateral symmetrical ground-glass opacities involving mainly the middle and lower lung zones. (*From Müller NL, Fraser RS, Colman NC, Paré PD: Radiologic Diagnosis of Diseases of the Chest. Philadelphia, WB Saunders, 2001.*)

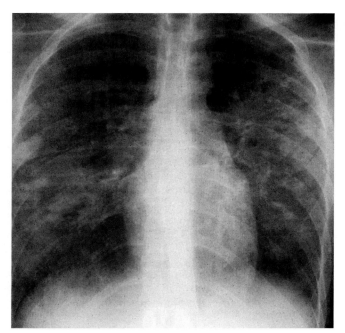

FIGURE 8–6

Pneumocystis pneumonia. A posteroanterior chest radiograph in a 31-year-old patient who had AIDS shows bilateral areas of air space consolidation involving mainly the midlung zones. *(From Müller NL, Fraser RS, Colman NC, Paré PD: Radiologic Diagnosis of Diseases of the Chest. Philadelphia, WB Saunders, 2001.)*

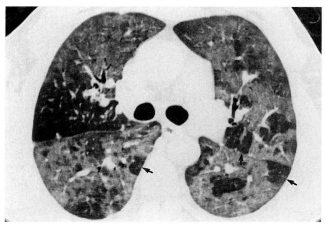

FIGURE 8–7

Pneumocystis pneumonia. An HRCT scan in a 46-year-old man who had AIDS shows bilateral areas of ground-glass attenuation with a mosaic pattern. There is sharp demarcation between normal and abnormal lung parenchyma, with the areas of spared lung parenchyma having a size and configuration that corresponds to that of secondary pulmonary lobules *(arrows). (From Müller NL, Fraser RS, Colman NC, Paré PD: Radiologic Diagnosis of Diseases of the Chest. Philadelphia, WB Saunders, 2001.)*

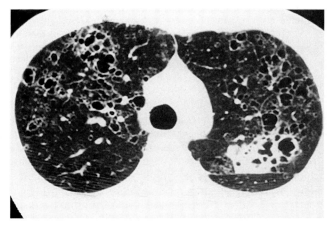

FIGURE 8–8

Pneumocystis pneumonia with cystic change. An HRCT scan through the upper lobes in a 30-year-old patient who had AIDS shows numerous irregularly shaped cysts in a random distribution. Focal areas of ground-glass attenuation and consolidation are evident. *(From Müller NL, Fraser RS, Colman NC, Paré PD: Radiologic Diagnosis of Diseases of the Chest. Philadelphia, WB Saunders, 2001.)*

thickness.[132-134] They are usually spherical. The majority resolve completely over a period of weeks to months.[133]

Pneumothorax occurs in about 5% to 10% of patients.[129,130,135] Factors associated with the complication include the presence of cysts on the chest radiograph,[136,137] a history of cigarette smoking,[138] and the use of aerosolized pentamidine.[135,136] In one investigation, pneumothorax developed in 12 (35%) of the 34 patients who had radiographically evident cysts versus only 2 (7%) patients who did not.[133] The pneumothorax may be unilateral or bilateral and may be recurrent.[139-141] Pneumomediastinum occurs occasionally, either by itself or in association with pneumothorax.[129,142]

Additional radiographic abnormalities seen in a small percentage of patients include focal parenchymal consolidation, single or multiple nodules, miliary nodules, cavitation, hilar or mediastinal lymph node enlargement, lymph node and visceral calcification, and pleural effusion.[129,130,143] Radiographs have been reported to be normal in about 5% to 10% of patients.[144,145]

The characteristic HRCT findings of PCP consist of symmetrical bilateral areas of ground-glass attenuation.[146,147] Similar to findings on radiographs, the abnormalities can be diffuse; however, they often involve mainly the perihilar regions or have a patchy distribution with intervening areas of normal parenchyma that are frequently sharply marginated by the interlobular septa (Fig. 8–7).[146,147] Less common findings include consolidation, cyst formation (Fig. 8–8), small nodules, irregular linear opacities, and interlobular septal thickening.[72,147]

Most patients who have AIDS and PCP have characteristic radiographic findings, thus obviating the need for CT.[148]

However, CT can be helpful in the assessment of patients who have symptoms of pulmonary disease and normal or nonspecific radiographic findings.[149,150] As might be expected, HRCT may show parenchymal abnormalities in patients who have normal radiographs.[149,150] In an investigation of 13 such patients who had a high clinical index of suspicion for PCP, all 4 patients who had patchy areas of ground-glass attenuation on HRCT had *P. jiroveci* identified in BAL fluid specimens[151]; BAL fluid in the 9 patients who had normal HRCT scans was negative. In a second prospective investigation of 51 patients who had a high clinical pretest probability of PCP and normal, equivocal, or nonspecific chest radiograph findings,

HRCT showed parenchymal abnormalities in all 6 patients who had PCP proved by BAL (sensitivity, 100%) and was falsely positive in 5 of 45 patients with negative BAL (specificity, 89%).[150]

HRCT is superior to chest radiography in differentiating PCP from other pulmonary infections and from malignancy in patients who have AIDS.[149] In a review of the radiographs and HRCT scans from 139 HIV-positive patients (including 106 who had proven thoracic complications and 33 who had no evidence of active intrathoracic disease), 96% were identified correctly by two observers as having intrathoracic abnormalities on CT scan as compared with 90% on radiograph.[149] Among the patients who had no pulmonary complications, 73% were identified correctly as such at radiography and 86% at CT. A confident first-choice diagnosis was made in 47% of CT interpretations (correct in 87%) as opposed to 34% on radiograph (correct in 67%). A correct diagnosis of PCP was made in 87% of 19 cases. The diagnosis of PCP in these cases was based on the presence of areas of ground-glass attenuation. The value of this finding was assessed in a study that included 102 patients who had AIDS and proven thoracic complications and 20 HIV-positive patients without active intrathoracic disease.[72] A correct first-choice diagnosis of PCP was made from the HRCT findings in 29 (83%) of 35 patients; the diagnosis was made with a high degree of confidence in 25 patients. Although ground-glass attenuation in patients who have AIDS can be the result of several other abnormalities, such as CMV pneumonia or lymphocytic interstitial pneumonitis (LIP), in most cases it is a manifestation of PCP.

Clinical Manifestations

The clinical features of PCP are nonspecific.[152] Patients commonly complain of fever (temperatures sometimes as high as 39° C to 40° C), nonproductive cough, and progressive dyspnea on exertion.[153] Sputum production has been noted in less than 25% of patients.[154] Less common manifestations include weight loss, chest pain, night sweats, chills, fatigue, and malaise.[115] Wheezing may be evident in patients who have underlying asthma.[155] The constellation of productive cough, shaking chills, and pleuritic chest pain is unusual and should suggest another diagnosis.[156] About 5% of patients do not have symptoms.[157] The rate of progression of the infection varies widely; some patients have fulminant disease with respiratory failure within days of the onset of symptoms, whereas others have relatively insidious disease associated with low-grade symptoms.[106] Recurrence or development of respiratory failure after an initial favorable response to therapy for PCP is sometimes seen when HAART is initiated close to PCP treatment; it is likely that this deterioration is the result of pulmonary damage by an influx of newly immunocompetent lymphocytes (syndrome of "immune reconstitution").[158]

The findings on clinical examination are nonspecific and contribute little to diagnosis[106]; however, the discovery of other abnormalities, such as oral candidiasis or cutaneous KS, may provide an important indicator of underlying HIV infection in patients in whom the diagnosis was not suspected previously.[106] Extrapulmonary disease is well described, but rare.[159]

Biochemical abnormalities are common, but lack specificity. However, the finding of a normal blood lactate dehydrogenase (LDH) level in a *symptomatic* patient should suggest an alternative diagnosis.[160] PCP causes restrictive changes in lung function characterized by a reduction in lung volumes associated with low diffusing capacity, hypoxemia, and deterioration in gas exchange with exercise.[115] After recovery from pneumonia, lung volumes return to normal, and the diffusion capacity improves without returning to normal.[161] Each of these tests has high sensitivity but low specificity for the diagnosis of PCP when applied to patients who have radiologically evident lung disease. However, since both diffusing capacity and arterial oxygen saturation with exercise are decreased in the vast majority of patients, the negative predictive value of normal values is high.[162] Interestingly, recovery from PCP is often associated with persistent abnormalities in lung function that are in keeping with an obstructive pattern.[163]

Diagnosis

Several methods can be used to establish a confident diagnosis of PCP. Induced sputum analysis is a simple procedure that has been widely used.[164] By careful attention to technique, the sensitivity of the procedure has been found to be as high as 92%.[165] However, other investigators have reported less favorable results,[164] and even with the use of monoclonal antibodies[166] or PCR,[167] induced sputum induction is unlikely to be cost-effective when the pretest probability of PCP is low. The unfocused use of PCR for diagnosis is also limited by the test's poor specificity.[168] Overall, the negative predictive value of the test is less than 50%.[166]

Bronchoscopy with BAL remains the procedure of choice for diagnosis. In the absence of previous prolonged empirical therapy,[169] its sensitivity for diagnosis is greater than 95%, a level that effectively negates the need for transbronchial or open lung biopsy in most patients.[170] When the clinical findings suggest a high probability of PCP, some authorities advocate empirical therapy in the absence of a definitive diagnosis to avoid potential complications and decrease cost.[171] There is little doubt that this approach is sound when the prevalence of PCP in the population is high[172]; however, it is likely to lead to a potentially fatal failure to initiate required treatment expeditiously when it is low.

Prognosis and Natural History

Although better results have been described in specific centers,[173,174] the overall 30-day survival rate of patients who have AIDS and PCP in the United States is about 85%.[175] The 12-month survival rate has increased from 40% in 1992-1993 to 63% in 1996-1998.[175] Early death has been associated with a history of previous PCP, low CD4+ count, older age, malnutrition, severity of disease at onset, concurrent infection with CMV, and BAL neutrophilia.[174-177] Improved survival has been associated with the concomitant use of antiretroviral therapy.[175,178]

There is also evidence that PCP is associated with a decrease in long-term survival, possibly by enhancing HIV replication and diminishing the survival of CD4+ cells and macrophages. This adverse effect seems to be independent of the CD4+ cell count and HIV load at the time of PCP.[178] Not surprisingly, skill in care,[179] as well as the use of and access to antiretroviral therapy,[180] also influences both the short- and long-term prognosis. Although early studies of survival in patients who required mechanical ventilation for PCP reported a dismal prognosis,[181] more recent observations have suggested that up to 40% of such individuals survive the hospital admission.[182]

Cryptococcus neoformans

C. neoformans is the most common fungus associated with systemic infection in HIV-infected patients.[101] It is usually seen when the CD4$^+$ count is less than 200 cells/μL.[183] Most cases of pneumonia are discovered serendipitously during the course of investigation of CNS or systemic complaints.[184] Pulmonary signs and symptoms are nonspecific. Exacerbation of cryptococcosis has been described during HAART,[185] including the development of intrathoracic lymphadenopathy, a cavitating lung nodule,[186] and mediastinitis.[187]

The most common radiologic manifestations consist of a reticular or reticulonodular interstitial pattern (seen in about 50% to 60% of patients) or discrete nodules (seen in 30%).[188,189] The latter tend to occur early in the course of AIDS and in patients who have less severe immunosuppression. Less common manifestations include ground-glass opacities, air space consolidation, miliary nodules, lymph node enlargement, and pleural effusions.[70,189]

Culture and smear of expectorated sputum are positive in less than 25% of patients who have cryptococcal pneumonia.[101] Bronchoscopy is usually required to confirm the diagnosis and exclude coexisting disease such as PCP.[190] Culture of *Cryptococcus* species and detection of cryptococcal antigen in BAL fluid obtained by bronchoscopy are sensitive tests.[191] In the absence of immune reconstitution by HAART, the prognosis is poor; less than half these patients survive 1 year despite long-term therapy with antifungal agents.[102]

Histoplasma capsulatum

Overall, histoplasmosis occurs in about 2% of patients who have AIDS in the United States; the prevalence increases to 5% in endemic areas.[70] About 75% of affected patients have disseminated disease and are markedly immunosuppressed, typically having CD4$^+$ counts of less than 100 cells/μL.

More than half of affected individuals have radiographic evidence of pulmonary involvement at the time of diagnosis.[192-194] In a review of 27 patients, the chest radiograph was abnormal in 23 (85%)[195]; findings included diffuse nodular opacities 3 mm or less in diameter in 9 patients (39%), nodules greater than 3 mm in diameter in 1 patient, small linear or irregular opacities in 7 patients (30%), and focal or patchy areas of consolidation in 7 patients (30%). Small pleural effusions were present in five patients, and hilar or paratracheal lymph node enlargement was present in one patient. The radiographic and HRCT findings of miliary histoplasmosis are similar to those of miliary tuberculosis.[195,196]

Fever, weight loss, diarrhea, lymphadenopathy, and hepatosplenomegaly are the most common manifestations.[101] Cough and dyspnea are seen in patients who have lung involvement. Because of the high frequency of concurrent pulmonary infection, the diagnosis of pulmonary histoplasmosis in the setting of disseminated disease should not be assumed in patients who have radiographic abnormalities. Culture of BAL fluid or detection of *Histoplasma* polysaccharide antigen may be used to confirm the diagnosis.[197]

Coccidioides immitis

Coccidioidomycosis is common in HIV-infected patients who live in areas endemic for the infection.[198] An important risk factor is a CD4$^+$ lymphocyte count of less than 250 cells/μL. The majority of patients have pulmonary disease, which may be focal or diffuse.[199] The usual radiologic manifestations consist of focal or diffuse areas of air space consolidation[199]; less common findings include nodules, cavitation, hilar lymph node enlargement, and pleural effusion. Definitive diagnosis requires culture of the organism from tissue or fluid samples or identification of the organism in cytologic or histologic specimens.[184] Sputum, BAL fluid, and bronchial and transbronchial biopsy specimens all have a high diagnostic yield. In the absence of HAART, high mortality rates have been seen in patients who have low CD4$^+$ counts or diffuse lung involvement.[199]

Blastomyces dermatitidis

Blastomycosis has been recognized uncommonly as an opportunistic infection in HIV-infected patients.[200] Almost all affected individuals have a history of residence in an endemic area, CD4$^+$ lymphocyte counts of less than 200 cells/μL, and a history of previous or concomitant opportunistic infection.[200] About half have focal lung disease; the remainder have disseminated infection.[201] Culture of the organism from BAL fluid, skin, or cerebrospinal fluid has provided a definitive diagnosis in most patients; serologic testing has no value. In the absence of immune reconstitution by HAART, about 30% to 35% of patients follow a rapidly fatal course, death occurring within 3 weeks as a result of overwhelming pulmonary disease with or without systemic dissemination.[200]

Aspergillus Species

Invasive pulmonary aspergillosis is uncommon in patients who have AIDS; most have neutropenia and CD4$^+$ counts less than 50 cells/μL and have been treated with glucocorticoids and broad-spectrum antibiotics.[202] The lung is the sole site of infection in somewhat more than half of those who have pulmonary aspergillosis; in the others, systemic spread is evident.[203] The most common pathologic manifestation of pulmonary disease is bronchopneumonia; angioinvasive disease and necrotizing tracheobronchial aspergillosis are seen occasionally.

The radiographic and HRCT manifestations of invasive aspergillosis in patients who have AIDS usually consist of thick-walled cavities measuring 2 to 10 cm in diameter.[204] The cavities can be single or multiple and tend to involve mainly the upper lobes.[204,205] Other common findings include focal areas of consolidation and single or multiple nodules.[202,204] CT may demonstrate nodules and cavitary lesions not apparent on the radiograph.[204]

Symptoms consist of fever, cough, chest pain, and dyspnea[205]; they tend to be insidious in onset and progression. Occasionally, complicating pneumothorax develops; fatal hemoptysis is not uncommon. Concurrent infection, especially by *P. jiroveci* or CMV, is common.[202]

Definitive diagnosis of invasive aspergillosis requires culture of the organism from a normally sterile site or histologic demonstration of tissue invasion, most often by needle aspiration or transbronchial biopsy. Although detection of the organism in BAL fluid is a sensitive test for invasive disease,[206] it lacks specificity.[207] Nonetheless, in the setting of a compatible clinical and radiologic picture and in the absence of identification of another cause for the findings, the possibility of invasive aspergillosis should be seriously considered. Because the infection occurs in the setting of advanced immunosuppression, the long-term survival of patients is usually poor; however, prolonged survival may be seen with improvement in immune function by HAART and the use of antifungal therapy.[208]

Other forms of pulmonary aspergillosis are even less common than invasive disease. Occasionally, all the features of allergic bronchopulmonary aspergillosis are present.[205] Aspergilloma formation has also been described in some patients,[209] sometimes complicated by invasion of adjacent lung parenchyma and life-threatening hemoptysis.

Viruses

The clinical significance of the identification of a viral organism in the lung is often uncertain in HIV-infected patients. Nevertheless, it is clear that a number of viruses can cause pulmonary disease,[210] the most commonly implicated being CMV and HIV itself. Other viruses are recovered from BAL fluid less often. Sometimes they are the only pathogen isolated, thus suggesting that they are truly the cause of the underlying pulmonary disease.[211] The specific virus recovered in the latter cases tends to follow trends in the community and, with few exceptions, is associated with self-limited illness. The major exception is the occurrence of fatal and disseminated adenovirus infection, which has been described in a review of several case reports.[212] Herpesvirus type 1 has also been isolated occasionally.[212]

Pulmonary HIV Infection

HIV can be found in the lungs of patients who are asymptomatic, as well as in those who have pulmonary disease.[213] Asymptomatic patients also frequently have a reduction in diffusing capacity and evidence of lymphocytic alveolitis in the absence of clinical or radiologic findings of pulmonary disease.[214] Since lymphocytic infiltration of pulmonary tissue is the predominant histologic abnormality in LIP and nonspecific interstitial pneumonitis, both of which are seen in patients who have AIDS, it is possible that all these abnormalities represent manifestations of HIV infection.[215]

Cytomegalovirus

CMV can be detected on culture of BAL fluid from many patients infected with HIV.[216] This finding is seldom associated with significant morbidity or mortality, and it is likely that the organism is not pathogenic in most cases. This hypothesis is corroborated by the histologic observation that infected cells may be present in the lung in the absence of evidence of tissue damage or inflammatory reaction. That being said, there is no doubt that CMV can cause pulmonary damage and disseminated infection in some patients.[217] Its clinical findings are similar to those of PCP.[218]

CMV-induced pneumonitis is characterized histologically by a mixed neutrophil and mononuclear inflammatory cell

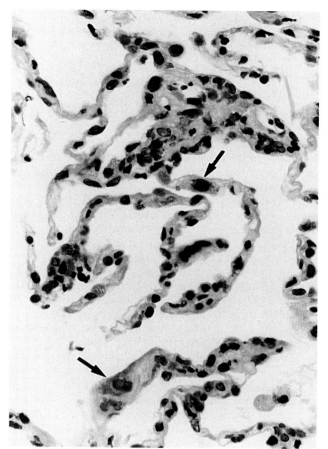

FIGURE 8–9

AIDS—cytomegalovirus (CMV) pneumonitis. A magnified view of a transbronchial biopsy specimen shows mild to moderate alveolar interstitial thickening by lymphocytes and occasional neutrophils. Two enlarged cells with ill-defined nuclear inclusions of CMV are evident (*arrows*). (The presence of the organism was confirmed immunohistochemically.) The intimate association of the virus and inflammatory cells suggests virus-induced tissue damage. (*From Fraser RS, Müller NL, Colman NC, Paré PD: Fraser and Paré's Diagnosis of Diseases of the Chest, 4th ed. Philadelphia, WB Saunders, 1999.*)

infiltrate in alveolar septa and adjacent air spaces (Fig. 8–9). Typical nuclear and cytoplasmic viral inclusions are usually easily identifiable; to be confident of the diagnosis, these inclusions should be seen in cells intimately admixed with the inflamed tissue.

The most common radiologic findings consist of bilateral ground-glass opacities or areas of consolidation (Fig. 8–10).[219,220] Less common manifestations include reticular opacities, discrete nodules or masses, and rarely, miliary nodules.[220] Similar findings have been described on CT scan.[219]

The diagnosis of pulmonary CMV *infection* is made most often by culture or by the identification of viral inclusions in cells in BAL fluid or sputum. The diagnosis of CMV-induced *disease* usually requires the demonstration of tissue damage or an inflammatory reaction in biopsy specimens. The addition of CMV-specific DNA probes and monoclonal antibodies may increase the utility of cytologic examination in this respect; in one study, detection of more than 0.5% positive cells with the

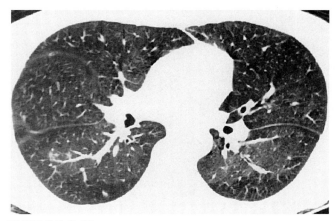

FIGURE 8–10

Cytomegalovirus (CMV) pneumonia. An HRCT scan in a 38-year-old woman with AIDS demonstrates bilateral areas of ground-glass attenuation with relative sparing of the subpleural lung regions. Repeated BAL showed large numbers of CMV organisms and no other organisms. *(From Fraser RS, Müller NL, Colman NC, Paré PD: Fraser and Paré's Diagnosis of Diseases of the Chest, 4th ed. Philadelphia, WB Saunders, 1999.)*

use of monoclonal antibodies correlated with clinical features and histologic evidence of CMV pneumonia.[210] The finding of a negative culture of CMV from BAL fluid has a high negative predictive value for CMV pneumonitis.[221]

Parasites

Although it has been estimated that about half the world's population is infected with *Toxoplasma gondii*, clinically evident disease is uncommon in normal hosts. Even with the profound immunosuppression that accompanies AIDS, pulmonary toxoplasmosis occurs rarely and is usually associated with CNS disease.[222] Signs and symptoms are nonspecific. The principal radiographic manifestation is a fine reticulonodular or ground-glass pattern resembling that seen in patients who have PCP[223]; occasionally, diffuse nodular disease is present. The diagnosis can be established in most cases by the identification of organisms in specimens of BAL fluid stained with methenamine silver.

PULMONARY NEOPLASIA

Three cancers—KS, non-Hodgkin's lymphoma, and cervical squamous cell carcinoma—are indicator conditions for the diagnosis of AIDS.[224] Several other neoplasms, including pulmonary carcinoma and leiomyomas, are also increased in frequency in patients who have HIV infection. These complications are not uncommon: before the availability of HAART, a malignant neoplasm developed in about 25% of patients who had AIDS at some point in the course of the disease.[224] The advent of HAART has resulted in a dramatic decline in the incidence of some of these neoplasms[225]; unfortunately, only a small percentage of patients worldwide receive such therapy, and the prevalence of these neoplasms is increasing. For example, AIDS-related KS is now the most common cancer in parts of sub-Saharan Africa.[226]

Kaposi's Sarcoma

In "developed" countries, KS occurs predominantly in homosexual men. Although its incidence in this group was declining before the use of HAART, this regression has been particularly dramatic after its institution.[225] From a peak of more than 200 cases/100,000 young white men in San Francisco in 1991, the incidence had fallen to 14.7 in 1998.[227] KS has been identified as the cause of pulmonary disease in about a third of patients who have extrapulmonary KS.[228]

Etiology and Pathogenesis

It is now clear that Kaposi's sarcoma–associated herpesvirus (KSHV, human herpesvirus 8) is the primary agent responsible for development of the tumor.[229] Rates of infection with KSHV parallel the incidence of KS, and in advanced lesions, KSHV is latently expressed by nearly all tumor cells. The infection is probably transmitted by anal or genital sex or by oral exposure to infected saliva,[230] although nonsexual contact is probably also important in Africa. Coinfection with HIV exponentially increases the risk for development of KS and increases the tumor's virulence, both by its attendant immunodeficiency and by other mechanisms.

KSHV has tropism for endothelial cells and induces them to produce and become more susceptible to the effects of inflammatory and angiogenesis-inducing cytokines.[231] The virus can produce proteins that are homologous to human oncoproteins, including those that inhibit tumor suppression and apoptosis, as well as chemokines that may activate angiogenesis and help infected cells escape immune surveillance.[226,229] In addition, it transcribes interferon-regulating factor, a protein that prevents interferon from suppressing the c-*myc* oncogene.

In its early stages, KS is more suggestive of a hyperplastic/inflammatory process than a neoplasm. Early lesions consist of scattered spindle cells, blood vessels, and a mixed inflammatory cell infiltrate.[226] These spindle cells are polyclonal and react in tissue culture to the same cytokines that have been identified in the inflammatory cell infiltrate seen in KS lesions.[232] This cytokine milieu, possibly in association with HIV-1 Tat protein, stimulates spindle cell proliferation through autocrine and paracrine loops and promotes increased cell aggressiveness and, eventually, clonal expansion.[226]

Pathologic Characteristics

Grossly, pulmonary involvement is typically most prominent in the pleural, interlobular septal, and bronchovascular interstitium and results in an appearance similar to that of lymphangitic carcinomatosis, except that the affected regions are red or purplish rather than white (Fig. 8–11). Expansion of tumor outside the interstitium may result in nodules or, occasionally, ill-defined areas of parenchymal "consolidation." When present in airway mucosa, the lesions commonly appear as purplish, plaquelike elevations[233]; involvement of lymph nodes is not uncommon and may result in their enlargement. Histologically, the lesions are composed of cytologically atypical spindle cells between which are variable numbers of small, slitlike vascular spaces containing hemosiderin-laden macrophages and red blood cells (see Fig. 8–11).

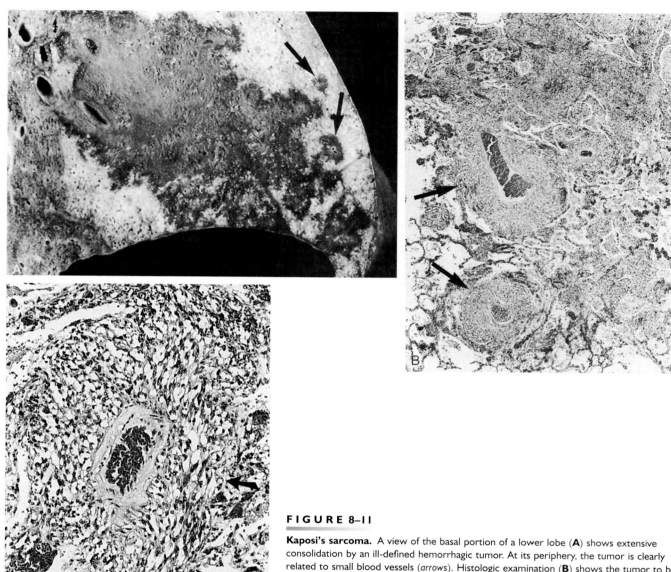

FIGURE 8–11

Kaposi's sarcoma. A view of the basal portion of a lower lobe (**A**) shows extensive consolidation by an ill-defined hemorrhagic tumor. At its periphery, the tumor is clearly related to small blood vessels (*arrows*). Histologic examination (**B**) shows the tumor to be located in perivascular interstitial tissue (*arrows*), as well as the adjacent lung parenchyma. A magnified view (**C**) shows typical spindle-shaped cells at the lower right (*arrows*). The lack of spindle cell appearance elsewhere is the result of the tumor being cut in cross section. (*From Fraser RS, Müller NL, Colman NC, Paré PD· Fraser and Paré's Diagnosis of Diseases of the Chest, 4th ed. Philadelphia, WB Saunders, 1999.*)

Radiologic Manifestations

The characteristic radiographic findings consist of bilateral, symmetrical, poorly defined nodular or linear opacities (Fig. 8–12). Though sometimes diffuse, these opacities often have a predominantly perihilar distribution.[234-236] The nodules measure 0.5 to 3 cm in diameter and tend to coalesce.[235,237] Bronchovascular bundles may show thickening, which often progresses to perihilar consolidation.[236] Other radiographic findings include thickening of interlobular septa (Kerley B lines), pleural effusions (in 30% to 70% of patients),[234,237,238] and hilar or mediastinal lymph node enlargement (in 5% to 15%).[236,239] In 5% to 15% of patients who have pulmonary parenchymal involvement at autopsy or endoscopy, the radiograph is normal.[234,236,237]

The characteristic HRCT findings consist of irregularly shaped, spiculated or poorly defined nodules in a predominantly perihilar and peribronchoarterial distribution (Fig. 8–13).[72,149,240,241] Other common findings include bronchial wall thickening, interlobular septal thickening, focal areas of ground-glass attenuation or air space consolidation, and pleural effusion. The areas of ground-glass attenuation may be the result of hemorrhage,[242] but the finding should raise the possibility of concomitant PCP. Hilar or mediastinal lymph node enlargement is evident on CT scan in 30% to 50% of patients.[72,234,240] Affected nodes usually measure less than 2 cm in diameter.[234] Less common findings include a focal parenchymal mass; cavitation; involvement of the sternum, ribs, or thoracic spine; and pericardial effusion.[72,243]

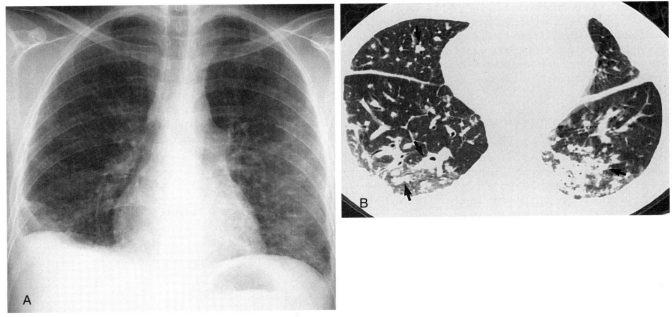

FIGURE 8–12

Kaposi's sarcoma. An anteroposterior chest radiograph (**A**) shows bilateral, symmetrical, poorly defined nodular and linear opacities and small bilateral pleural effusions. HRCT scan (**B**) shows nodular thickening of the bronchoarterial bundles (*arrows*), interlobular septal thickening, and small bilateral pleural effusions. *(From Kang EY, Staples CA, McGuinness G, et al: Detection and differential diagnosis of pulmonary infections and tumors in patients with AIDS: Value of chest radiography versus CT. AJR Am J Roentgenol 166:15, 1996.)*

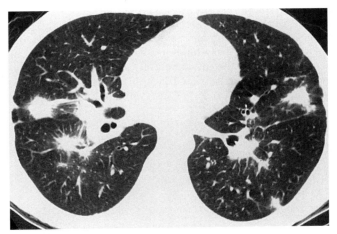

FIGURE 8–13

Kaposi's sarcoma. An HRCT scan in a 34-year-old man who had AIDS shows bilateral nodules with spiculated margins and peribronchial thickening. *(Courtesy of Dr. Andrew Mason, Department of Radiology, St. Paul's Hospital, Vancouver, BC.)*

The characteristic appearance of KS on CT scan allows a confident radiologic diagnosis in most cases. In an investigation of 102 patients who underwent the procedure, a correct first-choice diagnosis of KS was made in 26 (81%) of 32 patients who had the disease.[72] Although CT permits accurate assessment of the presence, pattern, and distribution of parenchymal abnormalities in KS, it is relatively insensitive in the detection of endobronchial lesions.[70] Tumors large enough

to cause atelectasis or stridor may be identified as intraluminal soft tissue lesions,[70,234] but smaller lesions are seldom seen.

Clinical Manifestations

Pulmonary involvement by KS almost invariably follows the development of mucocutaneous lesions. Most patients who have the complication are symptomatic. Dyspnea and cough are reported most commonly[239]; occasionally, blood streaking of sputum, fever, and chest pain are present. These symptoms do not help distinguish KS from opportunistic infection, which commonly accompanies it; however, the presence of blood streaking strongly suggests endobronchial involvement in a patient who has cutaneous KS. Although progression of disease is often relatively indolent, respiratory failure occurring over a period of days has been reported.[244]

The bronchoscopic appearance of the lesions is unique and consists of violaceous or bright red, irregularly shaped, flat or slightly raised plaques, most often located at the carinae of segmental and large subsegmental bronchi. Identification of such lesions is sufficient to make the diagnosis in most cases, and biopsy confirmation is not necessary. The presence of airway tumors is almost always associated with the presence of KS in the more distal portions of the lungs (although the latter can be present by itself).[245] In the absence of endobronchial lesions, the diagnosis is usually based on typical radiologic findings. However, identification of KSHV DNA by PCR in BAL fluid is a sensitive and specific marker for the disease.[246]

The tumor regresses in some patients who have been given intensive antiretroviral therapy,[247] and survival has improved dramatically over that in the pre-HAART era.[248] Nevertheless, the prognosis of untreated or unresponsive patients who have pulmonary KS is poor, the median survival varying between 2 and 10 months. Poor prognostic factors are the presence of pleural effusion, severe breathlessness, a CD4$^+$ lymphocyte count of less than 100 cells/μL, absence of cutaneous KS, previous opportunistic infection, and a low white blood cell count or hemoglobin.[232]

Non-Hodgkin's Lymphoma

Non-Hodgkin's lymphoma develops in about 5% to 10% of HIV-infected patients, an incidence more than 60-fold higher than that expected in the general population.[249] HAART does not seem to have decreased its incidence. Pulmonary involvement has been recognized clinically in about 1% to 15% of affected patients.[250] Thoracic involvement is usually recognized during the staging of lymphoma identified in an extrathoracic site; occasionally, the lung is the initial or sole site of disease.[224]

Tumors are generally high grade, widely disseminated, and extranodal at initial evaluation; about 20% originate in the CNS. Approximately a third are classified histologically as Burkitt-like; most of the remaining are classified as diffuse large B-cell lymphoma.[251] Primary effusion lymphoma is seen in a small number of cases.

The most common radiographic findings consist of single or multiple pulmonary nodules and pleural effusions (Fig. 8–14).[252,253] The nodules are usually well circumscribed and range from 0.5 to 5 cm in diameter.[70,252] On CT scan, they may have smooth or spiculated margins and often contain air bronchograms. Other common manifestations include reticular or reticulonodular opacities and bilateral areas of consolidation.[70,252] The nodules and the masslike areas of consolidation may cavitate.[252,253] Pleural effusions have been reported in 25% to 75% of patients[250,252,253] and are generally seen in association with parenchymal abnormalities; occasionally, they are the only finding.[254,255] The prevalence of lymph node enlargement has ranged from 0%[253,256] to 55%[250] in various studies; a reasonable overall estimate is 30%.[252,254]

Pulmonary signs and symptoms are nonspecific, and comorbid lung disease is common. Most patients have an advanced degree of immunosuppression. An elevated LDH level, high sedimentation rate, hematologic abnormalities, and abnormal gas exchange are present in 90% of patients[250]; however, none of these findings are useful in distinguishing lymphoma from other causes of pulmonary disease. Although pulmonary disease is rarely the direct cause of mortality, the overall prognosis is poor.

Pulmonary Carcinoma

Several epidemiologic studies have shown an increased risk for the development of pulmonary carcinoma in HIV-infected individuals.[257,258] The clinical and radiologic manifestations of the tumors are similar to those in HIV-negative individuals.

MISCELLANEOUS PULMONARY ABNORMALITIES

Nonspecific Interstitial Pneumonitis

Nonspecific interstitial pneumonitis is a relatively common abnormality in HIV-positive patients and is histologically characterized by an infiltrate of lymphocytes and plasma cells in peribronchiolar, perivascular, and interlobular septal interstitial tissue[259]; in contrast to LIP, involvement of the alveolar interstitium is relatively mild or absent altogether. By definition, the cause of the inflammation cannot be detected, and the diagnosis is made after infection and malignancy have been excluded as causes of the radiologic abnormalities.

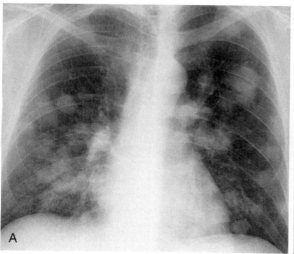
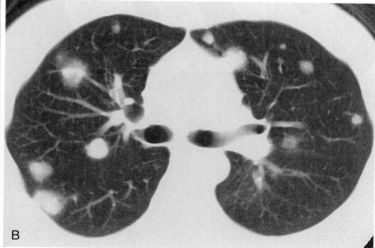

FIGURE 8–14

Non-Hodgkin's lymphoma. A posteroanterior chest radiograph (**A**) in a 41-year-old man who had AIDS shows numerous bilateral nodules of varying size. A CT scan (**B**) shows that the nodules have smooth or slightly irregular margins and are distributed randomly throughout both lungs. There was no evidence of lymphadenopathy on radiograph or CT scan. *(From Müller NL, Fraser RS, Colman NC, Paré PD: Radiologic Diagnosis of Diseases of the Chest. Philadelphia, WB Saunders, 2001.)*

However, as discussed previously, there is evidence that the abnormality is a result of pulmonary HIV infection itself, in at least some individuals.

The radiologic findings resemble those of PCP. In a series of 36 patients in whom pneumonitis was diagnosed by transbronchial or open lung biopsy, 16 (44%) had normal chest radiographs.[260] In general terms, the clinical findings are also indistinguishable from those associated with opportunistic infection.[261] Although subsequent episodes of nonspecific interstitial pneumonitis occur in some patients, resolution or stabilization is the rule, even in the absence of therapy.

Lymphocytic Interstitial Pneumonitis

LIP is a relatively common abnormality in HIV-infected children, in whom it is an AIDS-defining disease; however, it is rare in adults.[262] It is histologically characterized by infiltration of the pulmonary parenchyma by a more or less diffuse infiltrate of mononuclear cells, usually predominantly T lymphocytes (Fig. 8–15).[259] Although involvement of interstitial tissue adjacent to small vessels and airways does occur, the infiltrate is most prominent in the alveolar interstitium. Cytologically, the cells appear mature and show minimal nuclear atypia.

Radiographic findings consist of fine or coarse reticular or reticulonodular opacities, multiple nodules measuring 2 to 5 mm in diameter,[263] or poorly defined hazy (ground-glass) opacities (Fig. 8–16). Occasionally, areas of consolidation are superimposed on a background reticulonodular pattern.[264] HRCT scans show areas of ground-glass attenuation or ill-defined 2- to 4-mm nodules, frequently in a peribronchial distribution.[265] Cysts similar to those seen in PCP have been noted in some patients.[252]

Patients have an insidious onset of dyspnea, usually accompanied by cough and fever. Auscultation may be normal or reveal crackles. The abnormality is often associated with a CD8 lymphocytosis, diffuse hypergammaglobulinemia, a Sjögren syndrome–like disorder, and lymphocytic infiltration of the peripheral lymph nodes, liver, kidneys, bone marrow, and nasopharynx.[262] Pulmonary function studies may reveal restriction and a low diffusing capacity. Gas exchange may be impaired.

Transbronchial biopsy is the procedure of choice for diagnosis[228]; however, open lung biopsy may be required, especially

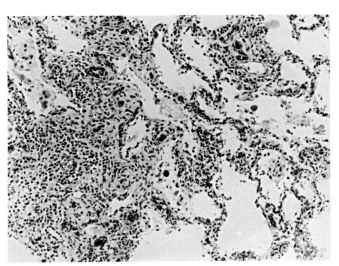

FIGURE 8–15

AIDS—lymphocytic interstitial pneumonitis. The section shows a moderately severe mononuclear inflammatory cell infiltrate composed predominantly of lymphocytes in the peribronchiolar and alveolar interstitium. *(From Fraser RS, Müller NL, Colman NC, Paré PD: Fraser and Paré's Diagnosis of Diseases of the Chest, 4th ed. Philadelphia, WB Saunders, 1999.)*

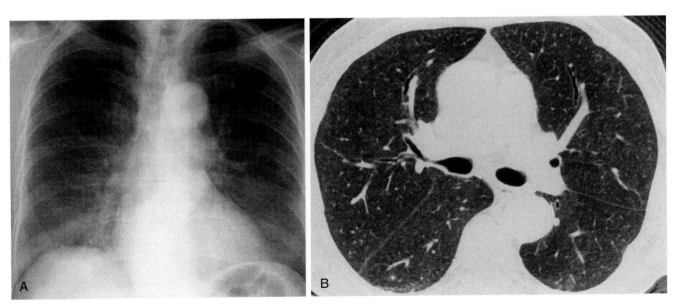

FIGURE 8–16

Lymphocytic interstitial pneumonia. A posteroanterior chest radiograph (**A**) in a 74-year-old man with AIDS demonstrates an extensive bilateral hazy increase in opacity of both lungs. An HRCT scan (**B**) demonstrates diffuse ground-glass attenuation and poorly defined small nodules. *(From Fraser RS, Müller NL, Colman NC, Paré PD: Fraser and Paré's Diagnosis of Diseases of the Chest, 4th ed. Philadelphia, WB Saunders, 1999.)*

when ancillary clinical features of the disease are absent. The finding of lymphocytic alveolitis on analysis of BAL fluid is insufficient for diagnosis because of its lack of specificity. The clinical course is variable. Some patients have very mild disease that resolves spontaneously, whereas respiratory failure develops in others.

Pulmonary Hypertension

Pulmonary hypertension unassociated with a clear-cut cause has been described in more than 100 patients with AIDS.[266] Plexiform arteriopathy is the underlying histologic abnormality in about 85%; recurrent thromboembolism and veno-occlusive disease are seen in most of the remainder. The prognosis is poor: half of reported patients monitored for a median of 8 months died with a median interval of diagnosis to death of 6 months.[266]

REFERENCES

1. Joint United Nations Programme on HIV/AIDS (UNAIDS), World Health Organization (WHO): AIDS Epidemic Update, 2001.
2. Clark S: Experts predict global devastation due to HIV/AIDS. Lancet 360:145, 2002.
3. Thompson D: Charting progress against AIDS, TB and Malaria. Coordinates 2002, prepublication issue. Geneva, World Health Organization, 2002.
4. Sepkowitz KA: AIDS—the first 20 years. N Engl J Med 344:1764-1772, 2001.
5. Department of Health and Human Services, Centers for Disease Control and Prevention. HIV/AIDS surveillance report—U.S. HIV and AIDS cases reported through December 2001. 13:1, 2002.
6. Kates J, Sorian R, Crowley JS, Summers TA: Critical policy challenges in the third decade of the HIV/AIDS epidemic. Am J Public Health 92:1060-1063, 2002.
7. Update: AIDS—United States, 2000. MMWR Morb Mortal Wkly Rep 51(27):592-595, 2002.
8. Diagnosis and reporting of HIV and AIDS in states with HIV/AIDS surveillance—United States 1994-2000. MMWR Morb Mortal Wkly Rep 51(27):595, 2002.
9. Ware J, Antman E: National HIV case reporting for the United States: A defining moment in the history of the epidemic. N Engl J Med 337:1162, 1997.
10. Quinn TC: Global burden of the HIV pandemic. Lancet 348:99-106, 1996.
11. Fact Sheet 2002—Sub-Saharan Africa: UNAIDS, 2002.
12. Rosen MJ: Overview of pulmonary complications. Clin Chest Med 17:621-631, 1996.
13. Wallace JM, Hansen NI, Lavange L, et al: Respiratory disease trends in the Pulmonary Complications of HIV Infection Study cohort. Pulmonary Complications of HIV Infection Study Group. Am J Respir Crit Care Med 155:72-80, 1997.
14. Hanson DL, Chu SY, Farizo KM, Ward JW: Distribution of CD4+ T lymphocytes at diagnosis of acquired immunodeficiency syndrome–defining and other human immunodeficiency virus–related illnesses. The Adult and Adolescent Spectrum of HIV Disease Project Group. Arch Intern Med 155:1537-1542, 1995.
15. Beck JM, Rosen MJ, Peavy HH: Pulmonary complications of HIV infection. Report of the Fourth NHLBI Workshop. Am J Respir Crit Care Med 164:2120-2126, 2001.
16. Amin Z, Miller RF, Shaw PJ: Lobar or segmental consolidation on chest radiographs of patients with HIV infection. Clin Radiol 52:541-545, 1997.
17. Haramati LB, Jenny-Avital ER: Approach to the diagnosis of pulmonary disease in patients infected with the human immunodeficiency virus. J Thorac Imaging 13:247-260, 1998.
18. Sullivan JH, Moore RD, Keruly JC, Chaisson RE: Effect of antiretroviral therapy on the incidence of bacterial pneumonia in patients with advanced HIV infection. Am J Respir Crit Care Med 162:64-67, 2000.
19. Miller RF, Foley NM, Kessel D, Jeffrey AA: Community acquired lobar pneumonia in patients with HIV infection and AIDS. Thorax 49:367-368, 1994.
20. Afessa B, Green B: Bacterial pneumonia in hospitalized patients with HIV infection: The Pulmonary Complications, ICU Support, and Prognostic Factors of Hospitalized Patients with HIV (PIP) Study. Chest 117:1017-1022, 2000.
21. Gilks CF, Ojoo SA, Ojoo JC, et al: Invasive pneumococcal disease in a cohort of predominantly HIV-1 infected female sex-workers in Nairobi, Kenya. Lancet 347:718-723, 1996.
22. Schneider RF: Bacterial pneumonia. Semin Respir Infect 14:327-332, 1999.
23. Dworkin MS, Ward JW, Hanson DL, et al: Pneumococcal disease among human immunodeficiency virus–infected persons: Incidence, risk factors, and impact of vaccination. Clin Infect Dis 32:794-800, 2001.
24. Cordero E, Pachon J, Rivero A, et al: Haemophilus influenzae pneumonia in human immunodeficiency virus–infected patients. The Grupo Andaluz para el Estudio de las Enfermedades Infecciosas. Clin Infect Dis 30:461-465, 2000.
25. Steinhart R, Reingold AL, Taylor F, et al: Invasive Haemophilus influenzae infections in men with HIV infection. JAMA 268:3350-3352, 1992.
26. Daley CL: Bacterial pneumonia in HIV-infected patients. Semin Respir Infect 8:104-115, 1993.
27. Tumbarello M, Tacconelli E, de Gaetano Donati K, et al: Nosocomial bacterial pneumonia in human immunodeficiency virus infected subjects: Incidence, risk factors and outcome. Eur Respir J 17:636-640, 2001.
28. Noskin GA, Glassroth J: Bacterial pneumonia associated with HIV-1 infection. Clin Chest Med 17:713-723, 1996.
29. Blatt SP, Dolan MJ, Hendrix CW, et al: Legionnaire's disease in human immunodeficiency virus infected patients. Clin Infect Dis 18:227, 1994.
30. Hirschtick RE, Glassroth J, Jordan MC, et al: Bacterial pneumonia in persons infected with the human immunodeficiency virus. Pulmonary Complications of HIV Infection Study Group. N Engl J Med 333:845-851, 1995.
31. Afessa B, Green W, Chiao J, Frederick W: Pulmonary complications of HIV infection: Autopsy findings. Chest 113:1225-1229, 1998.
32. Mitchell DM, Miller RF: AIDS and the lung: Update 1995. 2. New developments in the pulmonary diseases affecting HIV infected individuals. Thorax 50:294-302, 1995.
33. Manfredi R, Nanetti A, Ferri M, Chiodo F: Pseudomonas spp. complications in patients with HIV disease: An eight-year clinical and microbiological survey. Eur J Epidemiol 16:111-118, 2000.
34. Verville TD, Huycke MM, Greenfield RA, et al: Rhodococcus equi infections of humans. 12 cases and a review of the literature. Medicine (Baltimore) 73:119-132, 1994.
35. Arlotti M, Zoboli G, Moscatelli GL, et al: Rhodococcus equi infection in HIV-positive subjects: A retrospective analysis of 24 cases. Scand J Infect Dis 28:463-467, 1996.
36. Kwon KY, Colby TV: Rhodococcus equi pneumonia and pulmonary malakoplakia in acquired immunodeficiency syndrome. Pathologic features. Arch Pathol Lab Med 118:744-748, 1994.
37. Scannell KA, Portoni EJ, Finkle HI, Rice M: Pulmonary malacoplakia and Rhodococcus equi infection in a patient with AIDS. Chest 97:1000-1001, 1990.
38. MacGregor JH, Samuelson WM, Sane DC, Godwin JD: Opportunistic lung infection caused by Rhodococcus (Corynebacterium) equi. Radiology 160:83-84, 1986.
39. Scott MA, Graham BS, Verrall R, et al: Rhodococcus equi—an increasingly recognized opportunistic pathogen. Report of 12 cases and review of 65 cases in the literature. Am J Clin Pathol 103:649-655, 1995.
40. Asakura S, Colby TV, Limper AH: Tissue localization of transforming growth factor-β_1 in pulmonary eosinophilic granuloma. Am J Respir Crit Care Med 154:1525-1530, 1996.
41. Slater LN, Welch DF, Hensel D, Coody DW: A newly recognized fastidious gram-negative pathogen as a cause of fever and bacteremia. N Engl J Med 323:1587-1593, 1990.
42. Moore EH, Russell LA, Klein JS, et al: Bacillary angiomatosis in patients with AIDS: Multiorgan imaging findings. Radiology 197:67-72, 1995.
43. Koehler JE, LeBoit PE, Egbert BM, Berger TG: Cutaneous vascular lesions and disseminated cat-scratch disease in patients with the acquired immunodeficiency syndrome (AIDS) and AIDS-related complex. Ann Intern Med 109:449-455, 1988.
44. Adal KA, Cockerell CJ, Petri WA Jr: Cat scratch disease, bacillary angiomatosis, and other infections due to Rochalimaea. N Engl J Med 330:1509-1515, 1994.
45. Foltzer MA, Guiney WB Jr, Wager GC, Alpern HD: Bronchopulmonary bacillary angiomatosis. Chest 104:973-975, 1993.
46. Jones N, Khoosal M, Louw M, Karstaedt A: Nocardial infection as a complication of HIV in South Africa. J Infect 41:232-239, 2000.
47. Perlman DC, El-Helou P, Salomon N: Tuberculosis in patients with human immunodeficiency virus infection. Semin Respir Infect 14:344-352, 1999.
48. Cegielski JP, Chin DP, Espinal MA, et al: The global tuberculosis situation. Progress and problems in the 20th century, prospects for the 21st century. Infect Dis Clin North Am 16:1-58, 2002.
49. Chin DP, Hopewell PC: Mycobacterial complications of HIV infection. Clin Chest Med 17:697-711, 1996.
50. FitzGerald JM, Houston S: Tuberculosis: 8. The disease in association with HIV infection. CMAJ 161:47-51, 1999.
51. Havlir DV, Barnes PF: Tuberculosis in patients with human immunodeficiency virus infection. N Engl J Med 340:367-373, 1999.
52. Selwyn PA, Hartel D, Lewis VA, et al: A prospective study of the risk of tuberculosis among intravenous drug users with human immunodeficiency virus infection. N Engl J Med 320:545-550, 1989.
53. Daley CL, Mugusi F, Chen LL, et al: Pulmonary complications of HIV infection in Dar es Salaam, Tanzania. Role of bronchoscopy and bronchoalveolar lavage. Am J Respir Crit Care Med 154:105-110, 1996.
54. Colvin M, Dawood S, Kleinschmidt I, et al: Prevalence of HIV and HIV-related diseases in the adult medical wards of a tertiary hospital in Durban, South Africa. Int J STD AIDS 12:386-389, 2001.
55. Asch SM, London AS, Barnes PF, Gelberg L: Testing for human immunodeficiency virus infection among tuberculosis patients in Los Angeles. Am J Respir Crit Care Med 155:378-381, 1997.
56. Long R, Scalcini M, Manfreda J, et al: Impact of human immunodeficiency virus type 1 on tuberculosis in rural Haiti. Am Rev Respir Dis 143:69-73, 1991.
57. Seng R, Gustafson P, Gomes VF, et al: Community study of the relative impact of HIV-1 and HIV-2 on intrathoracic tuberculosis. AIDS 16:1059-1066, 2002.
58. Friedman LN, Williams MT, Singh TP, Frieden TR: Tuberculosis, AIDS, and death among substance abusers on welfare in New York City. N Engl J Med 334:828-833, 1996.
59. Moss AR, Hahn JA, Tulsky JP, et al: Tuberculosis in the homeless. A prospective study. Am J Respir Crit Care Med 162:460-464, 2000.

60. Kirk O, Gatell JM, Mocroft A, et al: Infections with *Mycobacterium tuberculosis* and *Mycobacterium avium* among HIV-infected patients after the introduction of highly active antiretroviral therapy. EuroSIDA Study Group JD. Am J Respir Crit Care Med 162:865-872, 2000.

61. Law KF, Jagirdar J, Weiden MD, et al: Tuberculosis in HIV-positive patients: Cellular response and immune activation in the lung. Am J Respir Crit Care Med 153:1377-1384, 1996.

62. Lawn SD, Butera ST, Shinnick TM: Tuberculosis unleashed: The impact of human immunodeficiency virus infection on the host granulomatous response to *Mycobacterium tuberculosis*. Microbes Infect 4:635-646, 2002.

63. Nakata K, Rom WN, Honda Y, et al: *Mycobacterium tuberculosis* enhances human immunodeficiency virus-1 replication in the lung. Am J Respir Crit Care Med 155:996-1003, 1997.

64. Leung AN: Pulmonary tuberculosis: The essentials. Radiology 210:307-322, 1999.

65. Jones BE, Young SM, Antoniskis D, et al: Relationship of the manifestations of tuberculosis to CD4 cell counts in patients with human immunodeficiency virus infection. Am Rev Respir Dis 148:1292-1297, 1993.

66. Long R, Maycher B, Scalcini M, Manfreda J: The chest roentgenogram in pulmonary tuberculosis patients seropositive for human immunodeficiency virus type 1. Chest 99:123-127. 1991

67. Saks AM, Posner R: Tuberculosis in HIV positive patients in South Africa: A comparative radiological study with HIV negative patients. Clin Radiol 46:387-390, 1992.

68. Greenberg SD, Frager D, Suster B, et al: Active pulmonary tuberculosis in patients with AIDS: Spectrum of radiographic findings (including a normal appearance). Radiology 193:115-119, 1994.

69. Fishman JE, Saraf-Lavi E, Narita M, et al: Pulmonary tuberculosis in AIDS patients: Transient chest radiographic worsening after initiation of antiretroviral therapy. AJR Am J Roentgenol 174:43-49, 2000.

70. McGuinness G: Changing trends in the pulmonary manifestations of AIDS. Radiol Clin North Am 35:1029-1082, 1997.

71. Laissy JP, Cadi M, Boudiaf ZE, et al: Pulmonary tuberculosis: Computed tomography and high-resolution computed tomography patterns in patients who are either HIV-negative or HIV-seropositive. J Thorac Imaging 13:58-64, 1998.

72. Hartman TE, Primack SL, Müller NL, Staples CA: Diagnosis of thoracic complications in AIDS: Accuracy of CT. AJR Am J Roentgenol 162:547-553, 1994.

73. Edinburgh KJ, Jasmer RM, Huang L, et al: Multiple pulmonary nodules in AIDS: Usefulness of CT in distinguishing among potential causes. Radiology 214:427-432, 2000.

74. Leung AN, Brauner MW, Gamsu G, et al: Pulmonary tuberculosis: Comparison of CT findings in HIV-seropositive and HIV-seronegative patients. Radiology 198:687-691, 1996.

75. Chaisson RE, Schecter GF, Theuer CP, et al: Tuberculosis in patients with the acquired immunodeficiency syndrome. Clinical features, response to therapy, and survival. Am Rev Respir Dis 136:570-574, 1987.

76. Keiper MD, Beumont M, Elshami A, et al: CD4 T lymphocyte count and the radiographic presentation of pulmonary tuberculosis. A study of the relationship between these factors in patients with human immunodeficiency virus infection. Chest 107:74-80, 1995.

77. Richter C, Perenboom R, Mtoni I, et al: Clinical features of HIV-seropositive and HIV-seronegative patients with tuberculous pleural effusion in Dar es Salaam, Tanzania. Chest 106:1471-1475, 1994.

78. Lee MP, Chan JW, Ng KK, Li PC: Clinical manifestations of tuberculosis in HIV-infected patients. Respirology 5:423-426, 2000.

79. Frye MD, Pozsik CJ, Sahn SA: Tuberculous pleurisy is more common in AIDS than in non-AIDS patients with tuberculosis. Chest 112:393-397, 1997.

80. Relkin F, Aranda CP, Garay SM, et al: Pleural tuberculosis and HIV infection. Chest 105:1338-1341, 1994.

81. Bennett CL, Schwartz DN, Parada JP, et al: Delays in tuberculosis isolation and suspicion among persons hospitalized with HIV-related pneumonia. Chest 117:110-116, 2000.

82. Gold JA, Rom WN, Harkin TJ: Significance of abnormal chest radiograph findings in patients with HIV-1 infection without respiratory symptoms. Chest 121:1472-1477, 2002.

83. Markowitz N, Hansen NI, Wilcosky TC, et al: Tuberculin and anergy testing in HIV-seropositive and HIV-seronegative persons. Pulmonary Complications of HIV Infection Study Group. Ann Intern Med 119:185-193, 1993.

84. Garcia-Garcia ML, Valdespino-Gomez JL, Garcia-Sancho C, et al: Underestimation of *Mycobacterium tuberculosis* infection in HIV-infected subjects using reactivity to tuberculin and anergy panel. Int J Epidemiol 29:369-375, 2000.

85. Ellner JJ: Tuberculosis in the time of AIDS. The facts and the message. Chest 98:1051-1052, 1990.

86. Gourevitch MN, Hartel D, Schoenbaum EE, Klein RS: Lack of association of induration size with HIV infection among drug users reacting to tuberculin. Am J Respir Crit Care Med 154:1029-1033, 1996.

87. Smith RL, Yew K, Berkowitz KA, Aranda CP: Factors affecting the yield of acid-fast sputum smears in patients with HIV and tuberculosis. Chest 106:684-686, 1994.

88. Finch D, Beaty CD: The utility of a single sputum specimen in the diagnosis of tuberculosis. Comparison between HIV-infected and non–HIV-infected patients. Chest 111:1174-1179, 1997.

89. Yajko DM, Nassos PS, Sanders CA, et al: High predictive value of the acid-fast smear for *Mycobacterium tuberculosis* despite the high prevalence of *Mycobacterium avium* complex in respiratory specimens. Clin Infect Dis 19:334-336, 1994.

90. Small PM, Schecter GF, Goodman PC, et al: Treatment of tuberculosis in patients with advanced human immunodeficiency virus infection. N Engl J Med 324:289-294, 1991.

91. Gordin FM, Nelson ET, Matts JP, et al: The impact of human immunodeficiency virus infection on drug-resistant tuberculosis. Am J Respir Crit Care Med 154:1478-1483, 1996.

92. Whalen C, Okwera A, Johnson J, et al: Predictors of survival in human immunodeficiency virus–infected patients with pulmonary tuberculosis. The Makerere University–Case Western Reserve University Research Collaboration. Am J Respir Crit Care Med 153:1977-1981, 1996.

93. Whalen C, Horsburgh CR, Hom D, et al: Accelerated course of human immunodeficiency virus infection after tuberculosis. Am J Respir Crit Care Med 151:129-135, 1995.

94. Fischl MA, Daikos GL, Uttamchandani RB, et al: Clinical presentation and outcome of patients with HIV infection and tuberculosis caused by multiple-drug-resistant bacilli. Ann Intern Med 117:184-190, 1992.

95. Judson MA: Highly active antiretroviral therapy for HIV with tuberculosis: Pardon the granuloma. Chest 122:399-400, 2002.

96. Hocqueloux L, Lesprit P, Herrmann JL, et al: Pulmonary *Mycobacterium avium* complex disease without dissemination in HIV-infected patients. Chest 113:542-548, 1998.

97. Rigsby MO, Curtis AM: Pulmonary disease from nontuberculous mycobacteria in patients with human immunodeficiency virus. Chest 106:913-919, 1994.

98. Benator DA, Gordin FM: Nontuberculous mycobacteria in patients with human immunodeficiency virus infection. Semin Respir Infect 11:285-300, 1996.

99. Bloch KC, Zwerling L, Pletcher MJ, et al: Incidence and clinical implications of isolation of *Mycobacterium kansasii*: Results of a 5-year, population-based study. Ann Intern Med 129:698-704, 1998.

100. El-Solh AA, Nopper J, Abdul-Khoudoud MR, et al: Clinical and radiographic manifestations of uncommon pulmonary nontuberculous mycobacterial disease in AIDS patients. Chest 114:138-145, 1998.

101. Fungal infection in HIV-infected persons. American Thoracic Society. Am J Respir Crit Care Med 152:816-822, 1995.

102. Moore RD, Chaisson RE: Natural history of opportunistic disease in an HIV-infected urban clinical cohort. Ann Intern Med 124:633-642, 1996.

103. Masur H, Michelis MA, Greene JB, et al: An outbreak of community-acquired *Pneumocystis carinii* pneumonia: Initial manifestation of cellular immune dysfunction. N Engl J Med 305:1431-1438, 1981.

104. Stringer JR, Beard CB, Miller RF, Wakefield AE: A new name (*Pneumocystis jiroveci*) for *Pneumocystis* from humans. Emerg Infect Dis 8:891-896, 2002.

105. Safrin S: *Pneumocystis carinii* pneumonia in patients with the acquired immunodeficiency syndrome. Semin Respir Infect 8:96-103, 1993.

106. Murray JF, Mills J: Pulmonary infectious complications of human immunodeficiency virus infection. Part I. Am Rev Respir Dis 141:1356-1372, 1990.

107. Delmas MC, Schwoebel V, Heisterkamp SH, et al: Recent trends in *Pneumocystis carinii* pneumonia as AIDS-defining disease in nine European countries. Coordinators for AIDS Surveillance. J Acquir Immune Defic Syndr Hum Retrovirol 9:74-80, 1995.

108. Wolff AJ, O'Donnell AE: Pulmonary manifestations of HIV infection in the era of highly active antiretroviral therapy. Chest 120:1888-1893, 2001.

109. Kaplan JE, Hanson D, Dworkin MS, et al: Epidemiology of human immunodeficiency virus–associated opportunistic infections in the United States in the era of highly active antiretroviral therapy. Clin Infect Dis 30(Suppl 1):S5-S14, 2000.

110. Lundberg BE, Davidson AJ, Burman WJ: Epidemiology of *Pneumocystis carinii* pneumonia in an era of effective prophylaxis: The relative contribution of non-adherence and drug failure. AIDS 14:2559-2566, 2000.

111. Jones JL, Hanson DL, Dworkin MS, et al: Surveillance for AIDS-defining opportunistic illnesses, 1992-1997. MMWR CDC Surveill Summ 48(2):1-22, 1999.

112. Masur H, Kaplan JE, Holmes KK: Guidelines for preventing opportunistic infections among HIV-infected persons—2002. Recommendations of the U.S. Public Health Service and the Infectious Diseases Society of America. Ann Intern Med 137:435-478, 2002.

113. Kovacs JA, Gill VJ, Meshnick S, Masur H: New insights into transmission, diagnosis, and drug treatment of *Pneumocystis carinii* pneumonia. JAMA 286:2450-2460, 2001.

114. Wohl AR, Simon P, Hu YW, Duchin JS: The role of person-to-person transmission in an epidemiologic study of *Pneumocystis carinii* pneumonia. AIDS 16:1821-1825, 2002.

115. Levine SJ: *Pneumocystis carinii*. Clin Chest Med 17:665-695, 1996.

116. Koziel H, Kim S, Reardon C, et al: Enhanced in vivo human immunodeficiency virus-1 replication in the lungs of human immunodeficiency virus–infected persons with *Pneumocystis carinii* pneumonia. Am J Respir Crit Care Med 160:2048-2055, 1999.

117. Martin WJ 2nd, Pasula R: Role of alveolar macrophages in host defense against *Pneumocystis carinii*. Am J Respir Cell Mol Biol 23:434-435, 2000.

118. Limper AH: Tumor necrosis factor alpha–mediated host defense against *Pneumocystis carinii*. Am J Respir Cell Mol Biol 16:110-111, 1997.

119. Limper AH, Offord KP, Smith TF, Martin WJ 2nd: *Pneumocystis carinii* pneumonia. Differences in lung parasite number and inflammation in patients with and without AIDS. Am Rev Respir Dis 140:1204-1209, 1989.

120. Schliep TC, Yarrish RL: *Pneumocystis carinii* pneumonia. Semin Respir Infect 14:333-343, 1999.

121. Limper AH: Parasitic adherence and host responses in the development of *Pneumocystis carinii* pneumonia. Semin Respir Infect 6:19-26, 1991.

122. Hoffman AG, Lawrence MG, Ognibene FP, et al: Reduction of pulmonary surfactant in patients with human immunodeficiency virus infection and *Pneumocystis carinii* pneumonia. Chest 102:1730-1736, 1992.

123. Foley NM, Griffiths MH, Miller RF: Histologically atypical *Pneumocystis carinii* pneumonia. Thorax 48:996-1001, 1993.

124. Travis WD, Pittaluga S, Lipschik GY, et al: Atypical pathologic manifestations of *Pneumocystis carinii* pneumonia in the acquired immune deficiency syndrome. Review of 123 lung biopsies from 76 patients with emphasis on cysts, vascular invasion, vasculitis, and granulomas. Am J Surg Pathol 14:615-625, 1990.

125. Wakefield AE, Miller RF, Guiver LA, Hopkin JM: Granulomatous *Pneumocystis carinii* pneumonia: DNA amplification studies on bronchoscopic alveolar lavage samples. J Clin Pathol 47:664-666, 1994.

126. Liu YC, Tomashefski JF Jr, Tomford JW, Green H: Necrotizing *Pneumocystis carinii* vasculitis associated with lung necrosis and cavitation in a patient with acquired immunodeficiency syndrome. Arch Pathol Lab Med 113:494-497, 1989.

127. Murry CE, Schmidt RA: Tissue invasion by *Pneumocystis carinii*: A possible cause of cavitary pneumonia and pneumothorax. Hum Pathol 23:1380-1387, 1992.

128. DeLorenzo LJ, Maguire GP, Wormser GP, et al: Persistence of *Pneumocystis carinii* pneumonia in the acquired immunodeficiency syndrome. Evaluation of therapy by follow-up transbronchial lung biopsy. Chest 88:79-83, 1985.

129. DeLorenzo LJ, Huang CT, Maguire GP, Stone DJ: Roentgenographic patterns of *Pneumocystis carinii* pneumonia in 104 patients with AIDS. Chest 91:323-327, 1987.

130. Goodman PC: *Pneumocystis carinii* pneumonia. J Thorac Imaging 6:16-21, 1991.

131. Gamsu G, Hecht ST, Birnberg FA, et al: *Pneumocystis carinii* pneumonia in homosexual men. AJR Am J Roentgenol 139:647-651, 1982.

132. Sandhu JS, Goodman PC: Pulmonary cysts associated with *Pneumocystis carinii* pneumonia in patients with AIDS. Radiology 173:33-35, 1989.

133. Chow C, Templeton PA, White CS: Lung cysts associated with *Pneumocystis carinii* pneumonia: Radiographic characteristics, natural history, and complications. AJR Am J Roentgenol 161:527-531, 1993.

134. Gurney JW, Bates FT: Pulmonary cystic disease: Comparison of *Pneumocystis carinii* pneumatoceles and bullous emphysema due to intravenous drug abuse. Radiology 173:27-31, 1989.

135. Sepkowitz KA, Telzak EE, Gold JW, et al: Pneumothorax in AIDS. Ann Intern Med 114:455-459, 1991.

136. Watts JC, Chandler FW: Evolving concepts of infection by *Pneumocystis carinii*. Pathol Annu 26(Pt 1):93-138, 1991.

137. McClellan MD, Miller SB, Parsons PE, Cohn DL: Pneumothorax with *Pneumocystis carinii* pneumonia in AIDS. Incidence and clinical characteristics. Chest 100:1224-1228, 1991.

138. Metersky ML, Colt HG, Olson LK, Shanks TG: AIDS-related spontaneous pneumothorax. Risk factors and treatment. Chest 108:946-951, 1995.

139. Coker RJ, Moss F, Peters B, et al: Pneumothorax in patients with AIDS. Respir Med 87:43-47, 1993.

140. Alkhuja S, Badhey K, Miller A: Simultaneous bilateral pneumothorax in an HIV-infected men. Chest 112:1417-1418, 1997.

141. Beers MF, Sohn M, Swartz M: Recurrent pneumothorax in AIDS patients with *Pneumocystis* pneumonia. A clinicopathologic report of three cases and review of the literature. Chest 98:266-270, 1990.

142. Takahashi T, Hoshino Y, Nakamura T, Iwamoto A: Mediastinal emphysema with *Pneumocystis carinii* pneumonia in AIDS. AJR Am J Roentgenol 169:1465-1466, 1997.

143. Suster B, Akerman M, Orenstein M, Wax MR: Pulmonary manifestations of AIDS: Review of 106 episodes. Radiology 161:87-93, 1986.

144. Kennedy CA, Goetz MB: Atypical roentgenographic manifestations of *Pneumocystis carinii* pneumonia. Arch Intern Med 152:1390-1398, 1992.

145. Boiselle P, Tocino I, Hooley R, et al: The accuracy of chest radiograph interpretation in the diagnosis of PCP, bacterial pneumonia and TB in HIV positive patients. J Thorac Imaging 12:47, 1997.

146. Bergin CJ, Wirth RL, Berry GJ, Castellino RA: *Pneumocystis carinii* pneumonia: CT and HRCT observations. J Comput Assist Tomogr 14:756-759, 1990.

147. Kuhlman JE, Kavuru M, Fishman EK, Siegelman SS: *Pneumocystis carinii* pneumonia: Spectrum of parenchymal CT findings. Radiology 175:711-714, 1990.

148. Mason AC, Müller NL: The role of computed tomography in the diagnosis and management of human immunodeficiency virus (HIV)-related pulmonary diseases. Semin Ultrasound CT MR 19:154-166, 1998.

149. Kang EY, Staples CA, McGuinness G, et al: Detection and differential diagnosis of pulmonary infections and tumors in patients with AIDS: Value of chest radiography versus CT. AJR Am J Roentgenol 166:15-19, 1996.

150. Gruden JF, Huang L, Turner J, et al: High-resolution CT in the evaluation of clinically suspected *Pneumocystis carinii* pneumonia in AIDS patients with normal, equivocal, or nonspecific radiographic findings. AJR Am J Roentgenol 169:967-975, 1997.

151. Richards PJ, Riddell L, Reznek RH, et al: High resolution computed tomography in HIV patients with suspected *Pneumocystis carinii* pneumonia and a normal chest radiograph. Clin Radiol 51:689-693, 1996.

152. Thomas CF Jr, Limper AH: *Pneumocystis* pneumonia: Clinical presentation and diagnosis in patients with and without acquired immune deficiency syndrome. Semin Respir Infect 13:289-295, 1998.

153. Murray JF, Mills J: Pulmonary infectious complications of human immunodeficiency virus infection. Part II. Am Rev Respir Dis 141:1582-1598, 1990.

154. Kovacs JA, Hiemenz JW, Macher AM, et al: *Pneumocystis carinii* pneumonia: A comparison between patients with the acquired immunodeficiency syndrome and patients with other immunodeficiencies. Ann Intern Med 100:663-671, 1984.

155. Schnipper S, Small CB, Lehach J, et al: *Pneumocystis carinii* pneumonia presenting as asthma: Increased bronchial hyperresponsiveness in *Pneumocystis carinii* pneumonia. Ann Allergy 70:141-146, 1993.

156. Peruzzi WT, Shapiro BA, Noskin GA, et al: Concurrent bacterial lung infection in patients with AIDS, PCP, and respiratory failure. Chest 101:1399-1403, 1992.

157. Balestra DJ, Hennigan SH, Ross GS: Clinical prediction of *Pneumocystis* pneumonia. Arch Intern Med 152:623-624, 1992.

158. Wislez M, Bergot E, Antoine M, et al: Acute respiratory failure following HAART introduction in patients treated for *Pneumocystis carinii* pneumonia. Am J Respir Crit Care Med 164:847-851, 2001.

159. Northfelt DW, Clement MJ, Safrin S: Extrapulmonary pneumocystosis: Clinical features in human immunodeficiency virus infection. Medicine (Baltimore) 69:392-398, 1990.

160. Quist J, Hill AR: Serum lactate dehydrogenase (LDH) in *Pneumocystis carinii* pneumonia, tuberculosis, and bacterial pneumonia. Chest 108:415-418, 1995.

161. Mitchell DM, Fleming J, Pinching AJ, et al: Pulmonary function in human immunodeficiency virus infection. A prospective 18-month study of serial lung function in 474 patients. Am Rev Respir Dis 146:745-751, 1992.

162. Huang L, Stansell J, Osmond D, et al: Performance of an algorithm to detect *Pneumocystis carinii* pneumonia in symptomatic HIV-infected persons. Pulmonary Complications of HIV Infection Study Group. Chest 115:1025-1032, 1999.

163. Morris AM, Huang L, Bacchetti P, et al: Permanent declines in pulmonary function following pneumonia in human immunodeficiency virus–infected persons. The Pulmonary Complications of HIV Infection Study Group. Am J Respir Crit Care Med 162:612-616, 2000.

164. Vander Els NJ, Stover DE: Approach to the patient with pulmonary disease. Clin Chest Med 17:767-785, 1996.

165. Kovacs JA, Ng VL, Masur H, et al: Diagnosis of *Pneumocystis carinii* pneumonia: Improved detection in sputum with use of monoclonal antibodies. N Engl J Med 318:589-593, 1988.

166. Kroe DM, Kirsch CM, Jensen WA: Diagnostic strategies for *Pneumocystis carinii* pneumonia. Semin Respir Infect 12:70-78, 1997.

167. Chouaid C, Roux P, Lavard I, et al: Use of the polymerase chain reaction technique on induced-sputum samples for the diagnosis of *Pneumocystis carinii* pneumonia in HIV-infected patients. A clinical and cost-analysis study. Am J Clin Pathol 104:72-75, 1995.

168. Torres J, Goldman M, Wheat LJ, et al: Diagnosis of *Pneumocystis carinii* pneumonia in human immunodeficiency virus–infected patients with polymerase chain reaction: A blinded comparison to standard methods. Clin Infect Dis 30:141-145, 2000.

169. Gracia JD, Miravitlles M, Mayordomo C, et al: Empiric treatments impair the diagnostic yield of BAL in HIV-positive patients. Chest 111:1180-1186, 1997.

170. Golden JA, Hollander H, Stulbarg MS, Gamsu G: Bronchoalveolar lavage as the exclusive diagnostic modality for *Pneumocystis carinii* pneumonia. A prospective study among patients with acquired immunodeficiency syndrome. Chest 90:18-22, 1986.

171. Tu JV, Biem HJ, Detsky AS: Bronchoscopy versus empirical therapy in HIV-infected patients with presumptive *Pneumocystis carinii* pneumonia. A decision analysis. Am Rev Respir Dis 148:370-377, 1993.

172. Miller RF, Millar AB, Weller IV, Semple SJ: Empirical treatment without bronchoscopy for *Pneumocystis carinii* pneumonia in the acquired immunodeficiency syndrome. Thorax 44:559-564, 1989.

173. Mansharamani NG, Garland R, Delaney D, Koziel H: Management and outcome patterns for adult *Pneumocystis carinii* pneumonia, 1985 to 1995: Comparison of HIV-associated cases to other immunocompromised states. Chest 118:704-711, 2000.

174. Arozullah AM, Yarnold PR, Weinstein RA, et al: A new preadmission staging system for predicting inpatient mortality from HIV-associated *Pneumocystis carinii* pneumonia in the early highly active antiretroviral therapy (HAART) era. Am J Respir Crit Care Med 161:1081-1086, 2000.

175. Dworkin MS, Hanson DL, Navin TR: Survival of patients with AIDS, after diagnosis of *Pneumocystis carinii* pneumonia, in the United States. J Infect Dis 183:1409-1412, 2001.

176. Bang D, Emborg J, Elkjaer J, et al: Independent risk of mechanical ventilation for AIDS-related *Pneumocystis carinii* pneumonia associated with bronchoalveolar lavage neutrophilia. Respir Med 95:661-665, 2001.

177. Benfield TL, Helweg-Larsen J, Bang D, et al: Prognostic markers of short-term mortality in AIDS-associated *Pneumocystis carinii* pneumonia. Chest 119:844-851, 2001.

178. Seage GR 3rd, Losina E, Goldie SJ, et al: The relationship of preventable opportunistic infections, HIV-1 RNA, and CD4 cell counts to chronic mortality. J Acquir Immune Defic Syndr 30:421-428, 2002.

179. Bennett CL, Adams J, Bennett RL, et al: The learning curve for AIDS-related *Pneumocystis carinii* pneumonia: Experience from 3,981 cases in Veterans Affairs Hospitals 1987-1991. J Acquir Immune Defic Syndr Hum Retrovirol 8:373-378, 1995.

180. Laing R, Brettle R, Leen C, Hulks G: Features and outcome of *Pneumocystis carinii* pneumonia according to risk category for HIV infection. Scand J Infect Dis 29:57-61, 1997.

181. Hawley PH, Ronco JJ, Guillemi SA, et al: Decreasing frequency but worsening mortality of acute respiratory failure secondary to AIDS-related *Pneumocystis carinii* pneumonia. Chest 106:1456-1459, 1994.

182. Randall Curtis J, Yarnold PR, Schwartz DN, et al: Improvements in outcomes of acute respiratory failure for patients with human immunodeficiency virus–related *Pneumocystis carinii* pneumonia. Am J Respir Crit Care Med 162:393-398, 2000.

183. Davies SF, Sarosi GA: Fungal pulmonary complications. Clin Chest Med 17:725-744, 1996.

184. Stansell JD: Pulmonary fungal infections in HIV-infected persons. Semin Respir Infect 8:116-123, 1993.

185. Hage CA, Goldman M, Wheat LJ: Mucosal and invasive fungal infections in HIV/AIDS. Eur J Med Res 7:236-241, 2002.

186. Jenny-Avital ER, Abadi M: Immune reconstitution cryptococcosis after initiation of successful highly active antiretroviral therapy. Clin Infect Dis 35:e128-e133, 2002.

187. Trevenzoli M, Cattelan AM, Rea F, et al: Mediastinitis due to cryptococcal infection: A new clinical entity in the HAART era. J Infect 45:173-179, 2002.

188. Sider L, Westcott MA: Pulmonary manifestations of cryptococcosis in patients with AIDS: CT features. J Thorac Imaging 9:78-84, 1994.

189. Friedman EP, Miller RF, Severn A, et al: Cryptococcal pneumonia in patients with the acquired immunodeficiency syndrome. Clin Radiol 50:756-760, 1995.

190. Chuck SL, Sande MA: Infections with *Cryptococcus neoformans* in the acquired immunodeficiency syndrome. N Engl J Med 321:794-799, 1989.

191. Malabonga VM, Basti J, Kamholz SL: Utility of bronchoscopic sampling techniques for cryptococcal disease in AIDS. Chest 99:370-372, 1991.

192. Salzman SH, Smith RL, Aranda CP: Histoplasmosis in patients at risk for the acquired immunodeficiency syndrome in a nonendemic setting. Chest 93:916-921, 1988.

193. Sarosi GA, Johnson PC: Progressive disseminated histoplasmosis in the acquired immunodeficiency syndrome: A model for disseminated disease. Semin Respir Infect 5:146-150, 1990.

194. Johnson PC, Khardori N, Najjar AF, et al: Progressive disseminated histoplasmosis in patients with acquired immunodeficiency syndrome. Am J Med 85:152-158, 1988.

195. Conces DJ Jr, Stockberger SM, Tarver RD, Wheat LJ: Disseminated histoplasmosis in AIDS: Findings on chest radiographs. AJR Am J Roentgenol 160:15-19, 1993.

196. McGuinness G, Naidich DP, Jagirdar J, et al: High resolution CT findings in miliary lung disease. J Comput Assist Tomogr 16:384-390, 1992.

197. Wheat LJ, Connolly-Stringfield PA, Baker RL, et al: Disseminated histoplasmosis in the acquired immune deficiency syndrome: Clinical findings, diagnosis and treatment, and review of the literature. Medicine (Baltimore) 69:361-374, 1990.

198. Ampel NM, Dols CL, Galgiani JN: Coccidioidomycosis during human immunodeficiency virus infection: Results of a prospective study in a coccidioidal endemic area. Am J Med 94:235-240, 1993.

199. Fish DG, Ampel NM, Galgiani JN, et al: Coccidioidomycosis during human immunodeficiency virus infection. A review of 77 patients. Medicine (Baltimore) 69:384-391, 1990.

200. Pappas PG: Blastomycosis in the immunocompromised patient. Semin Respir Infect 12:243-251, 1997.

201. Pappas PG, Pottage JC, Powderly WG, et al: Blastomycosis in patients with the acquired immunodeficiency syndrome. Ann Intern Med 116:847-853, 1992.

202. Mylonakis E, Barlam TF, Flanigan T, Rich JD: Pulmonary aspergillosis and invasive disease in AIDS: Review of 342 cases. Chest 114:251-262, 1998.

203. Minamoto GY, Barlam TF, Vander Els NJ: Invasive aspergillosis in patients with AIDS. Clin Infect Dis 14:66-74, 1992.

204. Staples CA, Kang EY, Wright JL, et al: Invasive pulmonary aspergillosis in AIDS: Radiographic, CT, and pathologic findings. Radiology 196:409-414, 1995.

205. Miller WT Jr, Sais GJ, Frank I, et al: Pulmonary aspergillosis in patients with AIDS. Clinical and radiographic correlations. Chest 105:37-44, 1994.

206. Lortholary O, Meyohas MC, Dupont B, et al: Invasive aspergillosis in patients with acquired immunodeficiency syndrome: Report of 33 cases. French Cooperative Study Group on Aspergillosis in AIDS. Am J Med 95:177-187, 1993.

207. Pursell KJ, Telzak EE, Armstrong D: *Aspergillus* species colonization and invasive disease in patients with AIDS. Clin Infect Dis 14:141-148, 1992.

208. Moreno A, Perez-Elias M, Casado J, et al: Role of antiretroviral therapy in long-term survival of patients with AIDS-related pulmonary aspergillosis. Eur J Clin Microbiol Infect Dis 19:688-693, 2000.

209. Addrizzo-Harris DJ, Harkin TJ, McGuinness G, et al: Pulmonary aspergilloma and AIDS. A comparison of HIV-infected and HIV-negative individuals. Chest 111:612-618, 1997.

210. Wallace JM: Viruses and other miscellaneous organisms. Clin Chest Med 17:745-754, 1996.

211. Connolly MG Jr, Baughman RP, Dohn MN, Linnemann CC Jr: Recovery of viruses other than cytomegalovirus from bronchoalveolar lavage fluid. Chest 105:1775-1781, 1994.

212. King JC Jr: Community respiratory viruses in individuals with human immunodeficiency virus infection. Am J Med 102:19-24, discussion 25-26, 1997.

213. Semenzato G, de Rossi A, Agostini C: Human retroviruses and their aetiological link to pulmonary diseases. Eur Respir J 6:925-929, 1993.

214. Twigg HL, Soliman DM, Day RB, et al: Lymphocytic alveolitis, bronchoalveolar lavage viral load, and outcome in human immunodeficiency virus infection. Am J Respir Crit Care Med 159:1439-1444, 1999.

215. Mayaud CM, Cadranel J: HIV in the lung: Guilty or not guilty? Thorax 48:1191-1195, 1993.

216. Mann M, Shelhamer JH, Masur H, et al: Lack of clinical utility of bronchoalveolar lavage cultures for cytomegalovirus in HIV infection. Am J Respir Crit Care Med 155:1723-1728, 1997.

217. McKenzie R, Travis WD, Dolan SA, et al: The causes of death in patients with human immunodeficiency virus infection: A clinical and pathologic study with emphasis on the role of pulmonary diseases. Medicine (Baltimore) 70:326-343, 1991.

218. Salomon N, Perlman DC: Cytomegalovirus pneumonia. Semin Respir Infect 14:353-358, 1999.

219. Waxman AB, Goldie SJ, Brett-Smith H, Matthay RA: Cytomegalovirus as a primary pulmonary pathogen in AIDS. Chest 111:128-134, 1997.

220. McGuinness G, Scholes JV, Garay SM, et al: Cytomegalovirus pneumonitis: Spectrum of parenchymal CT findings with pathologic correlation in 21 AIDS patients. Radiology 192:451-459, 1994.

221. Uberti-Foppa C, Lillo F, Terreni MR, et al: Cytomegalovirus pneumonia in AIDS patients: Value of cytomegalovirus culture from BAL fluid and correlation with lung disease. Chest 113:919-923, 1998.

222. Campagna AC: Pulmonary toxoplasmosis. Semin Respir Infect 12:98-105, 1997.

223. Rottenberg GT, Miszkiel K, Shaw P, Miller RF: Case report: Fulminant *Toxoplasma gondii* pneumonia in a patient with AIDS. Clin Radiol 52:472-474, 1997.

224. White DA: Pulmonary complications of HIV-associated malignancies. Clin Chest Med 17:755-761, 1996.

225. Eltom MA, Jemal A, Mbulaiteye SM, et al: Trends in Kaposi's sarcoma and non-Hodgkin's lymphoma incidence in the United States from 1973 through 1998. J Natl Cancer Inst 94:1204-1210, 2002.

226. Boshoff C, Weiss R: AIDS-related malignancies. Nat Rev Cancer 2:373-382, 2002.

227. Clarke CA: Changing incidence of Kaposi's sarcoma and non-Hodgkin's lymphoma among young men in San Francisco. AIDS 15:1913-1915, 2001.

228. White DA, Matthay RA: Noninfectious pulmonary complications of infection with the human immunodeficiency virus. Am Rev Respir Dis 140:1763-1787, 1989.

229. Antman K, Chang Y: Kaposi's sarcoma. N Engl J Med 342:1027-1038, 2000.

230. Pauk J, Huang ML, Brodie SJ, et al: Mucosal shedding of human herpesvirus 8 in men. N Engl J Med 343:1369-1377, 2000.

231. Mitsuyasu RT: Update on the pathogenesis and treatment of Kaposi sarcoma. Curr Opin Oncol 12:174-180, 2000.

232. Aboulafia DM: The epidemiologic, pathologic, and clinical features of AIDS-associated pulmonary Kaposi's sarcoma. Chest 117:1128-1145, 2000.

233. Fouret PJ, Touboul JL, Mayaud CM, et al: Pulmonary Kaposi's sarcoma in patients with acquired immune deficiency syndrome: A clinicopathological study. Thorax 42:262-268, 1987.

234. Naidich DP, Tarras M, Garay SM, et al: Kaposi's sarcoma. CT-radiographic correlation. Chest 96:723-728, 1989.

235. Goodman PC: Kaposi's sarcoma. J Thorac Imaging 6:43-48, 1991.

236. Gruden JF, Huang L, Webb WR, et al: AIDS-related Kaposi sarcoma of the lung: Radiographic findings and staging system with bronchoscopic correlation. Radiology 195:545-552, 1995.

237. Davis SD, Henschke CI, Chamides BK, Westcott JL: Intrathoracic Kaposi sarcoma in AIDS patients: Radiographic-pathologic correlation. Radiology 163:495-500, 1987.

238. Sivit CJ, Schwartz AM, Rockoff SD: Kaposi's sarcoma of the lung in AIDS: Radiologic-pathologic analysis. AJR Am J Roentgenol 148:25-28, 1987.

239. Huang L, Schnapp LM, Gruden JF, et al: Presentation of AIDS-related pulmonary Kaposi's sarcoma diagnosed by bronchoscopy. Am J Respir Crit Care Med 153:1385-1390, 1996.

240. Khalil AM, Carette MF, Cadranel JL, et al: Intrathoracic Kaposi's sarcoma. CT findings. Chest 108:1622-1626, 1995.

241. Traill ZC, Miller RF, Shaw PJ: CT appearances of intrathoracic Kaposi's sarcoma in patients with AIDS. Br J Radiol 69:1104-1107, 1996.

242. Primack SL, Hartman TE, Lee KS, Müller NL: Pulmonary nodules and the CT halo sign. Radiology 190:513-515, 1994.

243. Wolff SD, Kuhlman JE, Fishman EK: Thoracic Kaposi sarcoma in AIDS: CT findings. J Comput Assist Tomogr 17:60-62, 1993.

244. Sadaghdar H, Eden E: Pulmonary Kaposi's sarcoma presenting as fulminant respiratory failure. Chest 100:858-860, 1991.

245. Mitchell DM, McCarty M, Fleming J, Moss FM: Bronchopulmonary Kaposi's sarcoma in patients with AIDS. Thorax 47:726-729, 1992.

246. Tamm M, Reichenberger F, McGandy CE, et al: Diagnosis of pulmonary Kaposi's sarcoma by detection of human herpes virus 8 in bronchoalveolar lavage. Am J Respir Crit Care Med 157:458-463, 1998.

247. Aboulafia DM: Regression of acquired immunodeficiency syndrome–related pulmonary Kaposi's sarcoma after highly active antiretroviral therapy. Mayo Clin Proc 73:439-443, 1998.

248. Holkova B, Takeshita K, Cheng DM, et al: Effect of highly active antiretroviral therapy on survival in patients with AIDS-associated pulmonary Kaposi's sarcoma treated with chemotherapy. J Clin Oncol 19:3848-3851, 2001.

249. Lynch JW Jr: AIDS-related non-Hodgkin's lymphoma. Useful techniques for diagnosis. Chest 110:585-587, 1996.

250. Eisner MD, Kaplan LD, Herndier B, Stulbarg MS: The pulmonary manifestations of AIDS-related non-Hodgkin's lymphoma. Chest 110:729-736, 1996.

251. Gabarre J, Raphael M, Lepage E, et al: Human immunodeficiency virus–related lymphoma: Relation between clinical features and histologic subtypes. Am J Med 111:704-711, 2001.

252. Carignan S, Staples CA, Müller NL: Intrathoracic lymphoproliferative disorders in the immunocompromised patient: CT findings. Radiology 197:53-58, 1995.

253. Blunt DM, Padley SP: Radiographic manifestations of AIDS related lymphoma in the thorax. Clin Radiol 50:607-612, 1995.

254. Sider L, Weiss AJ, Smith MD, et al: Varied appearance of AIDS-related lymphoma in the chest. Radiology 171:629-632, 1989.

255. Morassut S, Vaccher E, Balestreri L, et al: HIV-associated human herpesvirus 8–positive primary lymphomatous effusions: Radiologic findings in six patients. Radiology 205:459-463, 1997.

256. Polish LB, Cohn DL, Ryder JW, et al: Pulmonary non-Hodgkin's lymphoma in AIDS. Chest 96:1321-1326, 1989.

257. Parker MS, Leveno DM, Campbell TJ, et al: AIDS-related bronchogenic carcinoma: Fact or fiction? Chest 113:154-161, 1998.

258. Frisch M, Biggar RJ, Engels EA, Goedert JJ: Association of cancer with AIDS-related immunosuppression in adults. JAMA 285:1736-1745, 2001.

259. Travis WD, Fox CH, Devaney KO, et al: Lymphoid pneumonitis in 50 adult patients infected with the human immunodeficiency virus: Lymphocytic interstitial pneumonitis versus nonspecific interstitial pneumonitis. Hum Pathol 23:529-541, 1992.

260. Simmons JT, Suffredini AF, Lack EE, et al: Nonspecific interstitial pneumonitis in patients with AIDS: Radiologic features. AJR Am J Roentgenol 149:265-268, 1987.

261. Sattler F, Nichols L, Hirano L, et al: Nonspecific interstitial pneumonitis mimicking *Pneumocystis carinii* pneumonia. Am J Respir Crit Care Med 156:912-917, 1997.

262. Schneider RF: Lymphocytic interstitial pneumonitis and nonspecific interstitial pneumonitis. Clin Chest Med 17:763-766, 1996.

263. Richards PJ, Armstrong P, Parkin JM, Sharma A: Chest imaging in AIDS. Clin Radiol 53:554-566, 1998.

264. Kramer MR, Saldana MJ, Ramos M, Pitchenik AE: High titers of Epstein-Barr virus antibodies in adult patients with lymphocytic interstitial pneumonitis associated with AIDS. Respir Med 86:49-52, 1992.

265. McGuinness G, Scholes JV, Jagirdar JS, et al: Unusual lymphoproliferative disorders in nine adults with HIV or AIDS: CT and pathologic findings. Radiology 197:59-65, 1995.

266. Mehta NJ, Khan IA, Mehta RN, Sepkowitz DA: HIV-related pulmonary hypertension: Analytic review of 131 cases. Chest 118:1133-1141, 2000.

CHRONIC INTERSTITIAL LUNG DISEASE

SARCOIDOSIS

Sarcoidosis is a relatively common disease of the lungs and other organs that is difficult to characterize precisely. In 1991, members of the World Association of Sarcoidosis and Other Granulomatous Disorders proposed that it should be descriptively defined as follows:

". . . a multisystem disorder of unknown cause(s). It most commonly affects young and middle-aged adults and frequently presents with bilateral hilar lymphadenopathy, pulmonary infiltration, and ocular and skin lesions. Liver, spleen, lymph nodes, salivary glands, heart, nervous system, muscles, bone and other organs may also be involved. The diagnosis is established when clinico-radiological findings are supported by histologic evidence of non-caseating epithelioid cell granulomas. Granulomas of known causes and local sarcoid reactions must be excluded.

Frequently observed immunological features are depression of cutaneous delayed-type hypersensitivity and increased helper cell (CD4)/suppressor cell (CD8) ratio at the site of involvement. Circulating immune complexes along with other signs of B cell hyperactivity may also be detectable. Other markers of the disease include elevated levels of serum angiotensin converting enzyme (ACE), increased uptake of radioactive gallium, abnormal calcium metabolism and abnormal fluorescein angiography. The Kveim-Siltzbach test, when appropriate cell suspensions are available, may be of diagnostic help.

The course and prognosis may correlate with the mode of the onset and the extent of the disease. An acute onset with erythema nodosum or asymptomatic bilateral hilar lymphadenopathy usually heralds a self-limiting course, whereas an insidious onset, especially with multiple extra-pulmonary lesions, may be followed by relentless, progressive fibrosis of the lungs and other organs. Corticosteroids relieve symptoms, suppress the formation of granulomas and normalize the serum ACE levels and the gallium uptake."[1]

Sarcoidosis may occur at any age, but the disease is recognized most commonly in patients between the ages of 20 and 40 years.[2] A second peak in incidence occurs in women older than 50.[3] There is considerable variation in the reported incidence and prevalence in different countries and continents. Disease is particularly common in African Americans, especially women,[4] and particularly rare in Chinese.[5]

Etiology and Pathogenesis

The etiology and pathogenesis of the disease are unclear and undoubtedly complex. The presence of familial clustering[6] and the racial variation in incidence suggest an important genetic contribution. On the other hand, clustering during certain times, in specific regions,[7,8] and in nonconsanguineous relatives[9] and close acquaintances of affected patients,[10] as well as variations in incidence with season,[3] indicates that environmental influences also have an important effect. In fact, the nature of the immunologic disturbances suggests that the disease results from exposure of genetically susceptible individuals to specific environmental agents.[1]

A number of observations suggest that one such agent may be a transmissible microorganism. For example, granulomatous inflammation can be demonstrated in the footpads or viscera of mice after the inoculation of homogenates of human sarcoid tissue,[11] and there is evidence for person-to-person transmission of the disease by bone marrow or cardiac transplantation.[12,13] The most studied potential infectious organisms have been mycobacteria. *Mycobacterium tuberculosis* DNA has been identified in the tissue samples[14] and BAL fluid[15] of some patients, and cell wall–deficient L-forms of the organism have been found in blood.[16] However, these observations have not been consistently reproduced.[17] Moreover, a number of observations argue against mycobacteria as a cause of sarcoidosis, including failure of the disease to progress with the use of corticosteroids and maintenance of the incidence and prevalence of sarcoidosis in the presence of falling rates of infection by *M. tuberculosis*.[18]

A second group of possible causative organisms is *Propionibacterium* species. In a study of 108 lymph node samples taken from Japanese and European patients who had sarcoidosis,[19] *P. acnes* or *P. granulosum* was found in 106, whereas genomes of these organisms were found in 0% to 60% of various groups of control patients and in far fewer numbers. As interesting as these data are, the results require confirmation and elaboration before any particular infectious agent is accepted as being the cause of the disease.

Other observations that touch on the possible etiology include recognition of the strong negative association with smoking[20] and development or relapse in conjunction with the use of interferon-α and interferon-β[21,22] or highly active antiretroviral therapy (HAART).[23,24] Each of these has in common induction or replication (at least in part) of the cytokine milieu associated with the T_H1 immune response that is characteristic of sarcoidosis.

Although the absolute and attributable risk of sarcoidosis in family members of affected individuals is small, there is little doubt that the risk is real, especially in white individuals.[6,25] Even though this increase in risk might be related to common exposure in some cases, evidence suggests that inherited traits that predispose to or protect from the disease are more important.[26,27] The focus of genetic studies has been on the major histocompatibility complex (MHC) region[28,29] and other areas of the genome responsible for immune regulation, T-cell function, and antigen recognition and processing.[30,31] Despite the lack of reproducibility of many of the results among different ethnic groups, the biologic plausibility of the findings suggests that genetic differences between individuals are important in disease expression.[32,33]

The initial reaction in the lung is characterized by the accumulation and proliferation of CD4+ and, to a lesser extent, CD8+ T lymphocytes, both of which are associated with a T_H1 cytokine profile (notably interferon-γ, interleukin-2 [IL-2], and IL-12).[18,34] Several investigators have shown that the T-cell receptor repertoire is restricted, thus indicating oligoclonality in response to a specific antigen.[35] In some patients, particularly those who express the HLA-DR17 allele,[36] there is a strong compartmentalization of activated Va2.3 CD4+ T cells within the lung early in the course of the disease[36]; this finding is associated with a good prognosis and response to therapy and suggests that these lymphocytes may have a protective role.

The mechanisms of T-cell accumulation in the lung are complex and involve interactions with alveolar macrophages, as well as endothelial and epithelial cells. A variety of chemoattractant cytokines, in addition to cytokines that participate in cell adhesion and induce in situ proliferation, contribute to the inflammatory response.[37] It appears that alveolar macrophages both aggregate and proliferate at the site of granuloma formation. They in turn produce a variety of cytokines that activate T cells and induce fibrosis.[18] Dysregulation of T-cell homeostasis may result in excessive granuloma formation and fibrosis in patients who have progressive disease.[37] Some cytokines, such as tumor necrosis factor-α and IL-15, may inhibit T-cell apoptosis, thereby favoring persistent inflammation at disease sites[37]; the same effect may result from overexpression of oncogenes such as *Bcl*-2 by activated T_H1 lymphocytes.

Pathologic Characteristics

The pathologic hallmark of sarcoidosis is the granuloma, which in its early stages is identical to that caused by many other etiologic agents—a well-defined collection of epithelioid histiocytes often containing multinucleated giant cells (Fig. 9–1). Lymphocytes, occasionally plasma cells, and rarely neutrophils and eosinophils can be intermingled. The majority of granulomas are non-necrotizing; however, some contain small foci of necrosis, the presence of which does not exclude the diagnosis.[38] Such necrosis typically occurs in the central portion of the granuloma and appears as amorphous eosinophilic material often associated with degenerated, hyperchromatic nuclei.

Fibroblasts are present in considerable number at the periphery of more "mature" granulomas,[39] and it appears that the fibrosis begins at this site. In this circumstance, concentric lamellae of collagen can be seen to separate the histologically "active" central portion of the granuloma from the adjacent tissue (see Fig. 9–1). With time, the fibrosis proceeds inward until the entire granuloma is converted into a scar. This pattern of peripheral lamellar fibrosis is characteristic of healing sarcoidosis and is itself evidence in favor of the diagnosis.

It should be emphasized that the finding of non-necrotizing granulomas does not in itself constitute absolute evidence of sarcoidosis because such lesions are by no means specific. Local or diffuse non-necrotizing granulomas can be found in the lungs and other organs in association with a wide variety of conditions, including infections (particularly mycobacterial and fungal), extrinsic allergic alveolitis, neoplasms (including pulmonary carcinoma), pneumoconiosis (particularly that caused by beryllium), drugs, and foreign bodies. In some cases, ancillary procedures such as culture or polymerase chain reaction (PCR) analysis of biopsied

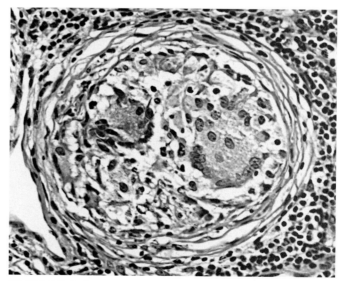

FIGURE 9–1

Sarcoidosis—granuloma. A high-magnification view shows a well-circumscribed collection of epithelioid histiocytes and two multinucleated giant cells. A small amount of lamellated fibrous tissue is evident at the periphery. *(From Fraser RS, Müller NL, Colman NC, Paré PD: Fraser and Paré's Diagnosis of Diseases of the Chest, 4th ed. Philadelphia, WB Saunders, 1999.)*

material, special stains for mycobacteria or fungi, and polarization microscopy may clarify the etiology of the granulomatous process. However, even negative results of these and other investigations do not exclude all specific etiologic agents, and it is necessary to make a careful distinction between the pathologic finding of non-necrotizing granulomatous inflammation and the clinical-radiologic disease known as sarcoidosis.

Pulmonary involvement is characteristically most prominent in the peribronchovascular, interlobular septal, and pleural interstitial tissue (Fig. 9–2; see Color Fig. 9–1). In the early stages, granulomas are discrete and histologically "active"; as the disease progresses, they often become confluent and undergo fibrosis, which results in more or less diffuse interstitial thickening. The parenchymal interstitium may also be affected, though typically much less than in peribronchovascular, septal, and pleural locations. In the early stage of the disease such involvement is manifested by nonspecific pneumonitis[39]; subsequently, typical granulomas develop. These foci of disease are usually microscopic but can conglomerate to form relatively discrete masses several centimeters in diameter, an appearance sometimes referred to as "nodular sarcoidosis."

Possibly because of the prominent peribronchovascular and septal location of the granulomatous inflammation, involvement of pulmonary arteries and veins is common.[40] Although this inflammation can be associated with disruption of the elastic laminae, necrosis does not usually occur. Granulomas are also common in airway mucosa, particularly in small bronchi.[41]

The gross appearance of pulmonary sarcoidosis depends on the stage and severity of disease. In the early, milder forms in which inflammation is most prominent in relation to peribronchovascular, interlobular, and pleural connective tissue, the appearance can resemble lymphangitic carcinomatosis. As disease progresses, involvement of the parenchymal interstitium becomes more evident, and entire lobules can be replaced by granulomas and fibrous tissue. This process is usually most severe in the apical portion of the upper lobes,

where it can take the form of more or less solid areas of fibrous tissue associated with traction bronchiectasis (Fig. 9–3). The latter may be the site of aspergilloma formation.[42]

Lymph node involvement is characterized by more or less diffuse replacement of the node by granulomas (Fig. 9–4), often with a variable histologic appearance.[43] Initially, the granulomas are discrete and appear "active"; as in pulmonary disease, however, they tend to become confluent and undergo progressive fibrosis over time. In advanced disease, this process can result in completely fibrotic nodes in which granulomas are difficult to recognize.

Radiologic Manifestations

Radiographic abnormalities can be usefully classified into four groups or stages for descriptive purposes:[44]

Stage 0: No demonstrable abnormality
Stage 1: Hilar and mediastinal lymph node enlargement unassociated with pulmonary abnormality
Stage 2: Hilar and mediastinal lymph node enlargement associated with pulmonary abnormality
Stage 3: Diffuse pulmonary disease unassociated with lymph node enlargement

The main utility of this staging system is in predicting outcome. In a survey of 3676 patients, 8% were found to have stage 0 disease; 51%, stage 1; 29%, stage 2; and 12%, stage 3.[45] On follow-up, 65% of the patients who had stage 1 disease showed resolution of the radiographic findings as compared with 49% of those who had stage 2 and 20% of those with stage 3.

Lymph Node Enlargement without Pulmonary Abnormality

Lymph node enlargement without parenchymal disease is seen on the initial chest radiograph in approximately 50% of patients.[45,46] The combination of bilateral hilar and right

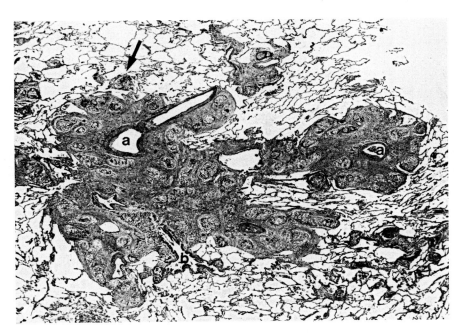

FIGURE 9–2

Pulmonary sarcoidosis. A low-magnification view of lung parenchyma shows numerous granulomas associated with a moderate amount of collagen; both granulomas and fibrous tissue are located predominantly in the interstitium adjacent to pulmonary arteries (a) and bronchioles (b). Only an occasional granuloma appears to be located within the parenchymal interstitium (arrow). (From Fraser RS, Müller NL, Colman NC, Paré PD: Fraser and Paré's Diagnosis of Diseases of the Chest, 4th ed. Philadelphia, WB Saunders, 1999.)

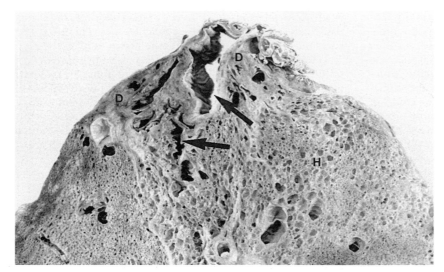

FIGURE 9–3

Sarcoidosis—interstitial fibrosis. A slice of the apical portion of an upper lobe from a patient with long-standing sarcoidosis shows foci of dense fibrosis in which the lung parenchyma is completely destroyed (D); extensive but less severe fibrosis with a "honeycomb" appearance (H) is also present in areas where the parenchyma is evident. Bronchi in the region of severe fibrosis are ectatic (*arrows*). *(From Fraser RS, Müller NL, Colman NC, Paré PD: Fraser and Paré's Diagnosis of Diseases of the Chest, 4th ed. Philadelphia, WB Saunders, 1999.)*

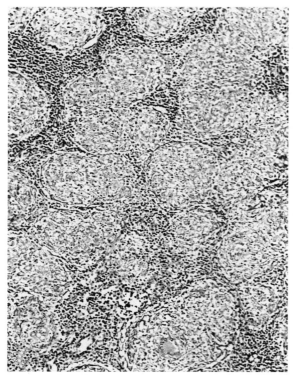

FIGURE 9–4

Sarcoidosis—lymph node involvement. A section of a mediastinal lymph node shows discrete and focally confluent granulomas that are virtually obliterating the normal nodal architecture. There is no necrosis. *(From Fraser RS, Müller NL, Colman NC, Paré PD: Fraser and Paré's Diagnosis of Diseases of the Chest, 4th ed. Philadelphia, WB Saunders, 1999.)*

paratracheal lymph node enlargement is a characteristic and common manifestation (Fig. 9–5).[47] Paratracheal node enlargement seldom occurs without concomitant enlargement of the hilar nodes.[48] Other common sites of lymphadenopathy that are evident include the aortopulmonary window (approximately 50% of cases) and subcarinal region (20% of cases).[47,49] Anterior mediastinal lymph node enlargement is seldom prominent but can be identified on the radiograph in approximately 15% of cases.[49]

Hilar lymph node enlargement is usually bilateral and symmetrical. Unilateral enlargement is uncommon, being reported in only 3% to 5% of proven cases.[50] The bilaterally symmetrical hilar and paratracheal lymph node enlargement contrasts with the node enlargement seen in primary tuberculosis, which tends to be unilateral,[51] and in Hodgkin's lymphoma, which tends to occur predominantly in the anterior mediastinal and paratracheal regions; when the latter involves the hilar nodes, it is predominantly unilateral and asymmetrical. Occasionally, hilar nodal enlargement is sufficient to compress adjacent bronchi and lead to atelectasis (most commonly involving the middle lobe).[52] Calcification of hilar lymph nodes is radiographically apparent in approximately 5% of patients initially[53] and in more than 20% after 10 years of follow-up.[54]

The prevalence of lymph node enlargement and its distribution as described previously refer to findings on the chest radiograph. As might be expected, hilar and mediastinal node enlargement is more commonly evident on CT scans, and the mediastinal disease can be seen to involve more nodal stations,[55] including the internal mammary, axillary, and infradiaphragmatic regions.[56] Calcification of hilar and mediastinal lymph nodes is also more common.[57,58]

As with other interstitial diseases, the lungs can be involved by sarcoidosis in the absence of a demonstrable abnormality on the chest radiograph.[59,60] In fact, the chest radiograph is normal (stage 0) in about 10% of patients who have biopsy-proven pulmonary sarcoidosis.[45,61] Similarly, in a study of 21 consecutive patients with stage 1 disease who underwent open lung biopsy, typical sarcoid granulomas were present in the lung parenchyma in all[60]; however, the extent of granulomatous inflammation and fibrosis was significantly less than that seen in open lung biopsy specimens of patients who had radiographic evidence of diffuse lung involvement. As might be expected, parenchymal abnormalities are seen more commonly on HRCT scans than on radiographs.[55]

Approximately 65% to 80% of patients who have stage 1 disease show complete radiographic resolution.[45,62] Occasionally, enlarged hilar and mediastinal nodes regress to normal

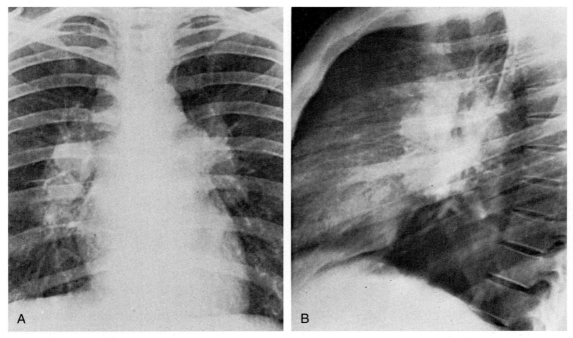

FIGURE 9–5

Sarcoidosis—lymph node involvement alone. Posteroanterior (**A**) and lateral (**B**) radiographs of a 32-year-old asymptomatic woman show marked enlargement of both hila, the lobulated contour being typical of lymph node enlargement. Nodes are also enlarged in the right paratracheal and aortopulmonary regions. The lungs are clear. *(From Müller NL, Fraser RS, Colman NC, Paré PD: Radiologic Diagnosis of Diseases of the Chest. Philadelphia, WB Saunders, 2001.)*

size, only to undergo enlargement again at a later date.[63] On the other hand, node enlargement can persist unchanged for many years.[64]

Diffuse Pulmonary Disease with or without Lymph Node Enlargement

Parenchymal disease is seen on the chest radiograph at initial evaluation in approximately 40% of patients who have sarcoidosis and occurs at some time during the course of the disease in 50% to 65%.[45,62,65] The pulmonary disease is initially found to be associated with lymph node enlargement (stage 2) in approximately 30% of patients; the remaining 10% have no evidence of node enlargement (stage 3).[45,62] In a 15-year follow-up study of 308 patients, 9% who had stage 1 disease at initial examination progressed to stage 2, and an additional 2% progressed to stage 3, apparently without passing through stage 2.[62] In approximately 70% of 128 patients who had stage 2 disease at diagnosis, the radiographic findings returned to normal; in 5% they remained at stage 2, and in 25% they progressed to stage 3.

The parenchymal abnormalities are typically bilateral and symmetrical and involve mainly the upper lung zones in 50% to 80% of patients.[66,67] Occasionally, disease is asymmetrical or unilateral.[64,68] The most frequent patterns are nodular and reticulonodular; less commonly, a reticular pattern, air space consolidation, or ground-glass opacities predominate.[69] Both the pattern and extent of parenchymal abnormalities are depicted better on HRCT scan than on radiographs.[69,70]

Nodular Pattern. A nodular pattern is present on chest radiographs in 30% to 60% of patients (Fig. 9–6).[70,71] The nodules usually have irregular margins and involve mainly the middle and upper lung zones. They range from 1 to 10 mm in diameter, although most measure less than 3 mm.

On HRCT, nodules are seen at initial evaluation in 90% to 100% of patients who have parenchymal abnormalities.[55,72] They are most numerous along the bronchoarterial and pleural interstitium and adjacent to the interlobar fissures (Fig. 9–7). In fact, extensive nodular thickening of the bronchoarterial interstitium involving mainly the middle and upper lung zones is characteristic of the disease.[73] Occasionally, nodules are diffusely distributed throughout the lung and give rise to a miliary pattern.[74] They may also appear as dense, round, sharply marginated opacities greater than 1 cm in diameter, similar to metastatic cancer.[75] Although such nodules are seldom the only finding in pulmonary sarcoidosis, they are seen frequently in association with smaller nodular opacities.[67]

Reticulonodular Pattern. A reticulonodular pattern is present in 25% to 50% of patients who have radiographically evident parenchymal abnormalities (Fig. 9–8).[69,71] The pattern may result from a combination of nodules and thickening of the interlobular septa or a combination of nodules and intralobular linear opacities.

Reticular Pattern. A reticular pattern is seen in 15% to 20% of patients who have radiographically evident parenchymal abnormalities (Fig. 9–9).[69,71] On HRCT, smooth or nodular thickening of the interlobular septa has been described in 20% to 90% of patients, and nonseptal irregular lines have been found in 20% to 70%.[67,69,76] The septal thickening is seldom extensive and, similar to the nodular opacities, tends to involve mainly the central regions of the middle and upper lung

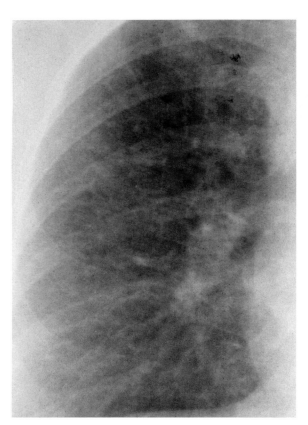

FIGURE 9–6

Sarcoidosis—nodular pattern. A view of the right lung from a posteroanterior chest radiograph shows numerous nodules measuring approximately 3 mm in diameter, most abundant in the middle and upper lung zones. Similar findings were present in the left lung. The patient was a 37-year-old woman. *(From Müller NL, Fraser RS, Colman NC, Paré PD: Radiologic Diagnosis of Diseases of the Chest. Philadelphia, WB Saunders, 2001.)*

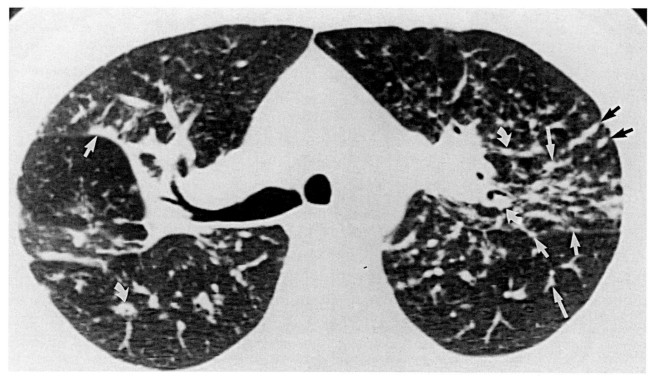

FIGURE 9–7

Sarcoidosis—HRCT appearance. An HRCT scan at the level of the right upper lobe bronchus shows multiple small nodules located mainly along the bronchi *(curved white arrows)*, pulmonary vessels *(long straight white arrows)*, subpleural lung regions, and interlobar fissures *(short straight white arrows)*. Nodular thickening of the interlobular septa is evident *(black arrows)*. The patient was a 37-year-old man. *(From Müller NL, Fraser RS, Colman NC, Paré PD: Radiologic Diagnosis of Diseases of the Chest. Philadelphia, WB Saunders, 2001.)*

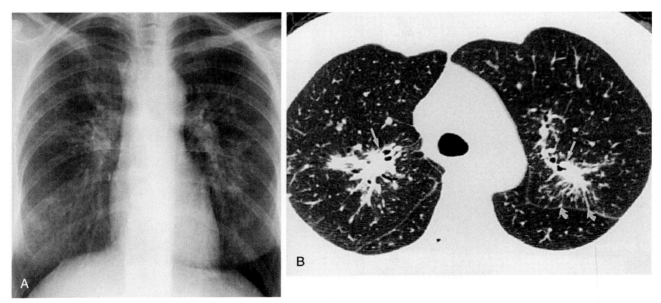

FIGURE 9–8

Sarcoidosis—reticulonodular pattern. A posteroanterior chest radiograph (**A**) shows a coarse reticulonodular pattern involving mainly the perihilar regions of the middle and upper lung zones and evidence of right paratracheal and bilateral hilar lymphadenopathy. An HRCT scan (**B**) shows bilateral nodules with spiculated margins in a predominantly peribronchoarterial distribution (*straight arrows*), as well as thickening of the interlobular septa (*curved arrows*). The patient was a 48-year-old woman. *(From Müller NL, Fraser RS, Colman NC, Paré PD: Radiologic Diagnosis of Diseases of the Chest. Philadelphia, WB Saunders, 2001.)*

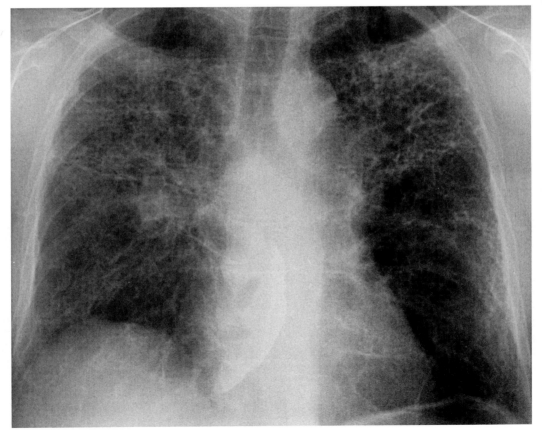

FIGURE 9–9

Sarcoidosis—reticular pattern associated with fibrosis. A posteroanterior chest radiograph in a 67-year-old woman shows a coarse reticular pattern involving mainly the perihilar regions of the middle and upper lung zones. *(From Müller NL, Fraser RS, Colman NC, Paré PD: Radiologic Diagnosis of Diseases of the Chest. Philadelphia, WB Saunders, 2001.)*

zones. Irregular linear opacities are usually associated with distortion of the architecture of the secondary pulmonary lobules, indicative of the presence of fibrosis; however, they are occasionally reversible.[55,70] Fibrosis also leads to dilation and distortion of bronchi (traction bronchiectasis), predominantly in the parahilar regions of the upper lung zones, and to honeycombing.

Air Space Consolidation. Parenchymal consolidation is the predominant finding on the chest radiograph in 10% to 20% of patients who have sarcoidosis with radiographically evident parenchymal disease (Fig. 9–10).[55,65] The consolidation typically has a bilateral and symmetrical distribution involving mainly the middle and upper lung zones. On HRCT scan, the areas of consolidation may be peribronchial (see Fig. 9–10) or, less commonly, peripheral in distribution.[77] Air bronchograms can be seen in most cases.[77]

Ground-Glass Opacities. Hazy areas of increased opacity without obscuration of the vascular markings (ground-glass opacities) are seldom seen on radiography but are commonly present on HRCT (Fig. 9–11).[67,78,79] In most cases, the ground-glass attenuation is a secondary feature seen in association with small nodules.[79,80] Correlation with pathologic findings has shown the pattern to be related to interstitial granulomatous inflammation[79,81]; occasionally, it is the result of microscopic foci of parenchymal fibrosis.[80]

When pulmonary disease and lymph node enlargement coexist, their radiologic appearance is no different from that of separate involvement. The two manifestations may differ greatly, however, in their temporal relationship in different patients. Diffuse pulmonary disease usually appears when hilar node enlargement is present, although the latter may be regressing. Node enlargement may disappear and be replaced by diffuse pulmonary involvement, either concurrently or several years later, or it may remain and diffuse pulmonary involvement may be superimposed on it.

Fibrosis. The fibrosis in sarcoidosis typically involves mainly the upper lung zones.[44,47] It is usually associated with superior retraction of the hila, bulla formation, traction bronchiectasis, and compensatory overinflation of the lower lobes (see Fig. 9–9).[82] When the fibrosis is severe, changes indicative of pulmonary hypertension and cor pulmonale may be seen. On HRCT scan, the fibrosis has a characteristic peribronchovascular distribution radiating from the hila to the upper lobes.[57,72] Additional findings include irregular lines of attenuation with associated architectural distortion, central conglomeration of ectatic bronchi, conglomerate masses, and subpleural honeycombing.[83]

Other Radiologic Manifestations

Pulmonary Disease. Cavitation is a rare manifestation of sarcoidosis and is usually seen in association with other parenchymal abnormalities.[84,85] The cavities may resolve spontaneously or be complicated by superimposed infection or fungus ball formation.[86] The latter complication occurs in approximately 40% of cystic lesions in sarcoidosis; though most often located in foci of bronchiectasis, it may be seen in bullae or cavities of uncertain origin.[76] Atelectasis is also a rare manifestation of the disease.[87] It may be caused by extrinsic compression of bronchi by enlarged lymph nodes, by bronchial mucosal inflammation and fibrosis, or perhaps most commonly, by a combination of the two.[52,88] Evidence of small-airway disease is commonly seen on HRCT.[89,90] Findings include localized areas of decreased attenuation and oligemia on inspiratory scans and air trapping on expiratory scans, both usually having a lobular distribution.[91]

Pleural Disease. Pleural effusion has been documented in about 2% to 7% of patients.[52,92] Affected individuals typically have moderately advanced pulmonary sarcoidosis; nonnecrotizing granulomas are often identified on pleural biopsy. The effusion tends to clear in 4 to 8 weeks but may progress to chronic pleural thickening. Given the rarity with which sarcoidosis causes pleural effusion, its presence should raise the possibility of complicating tuberculosis, coincidental

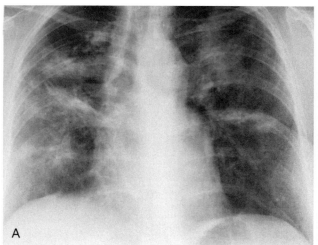
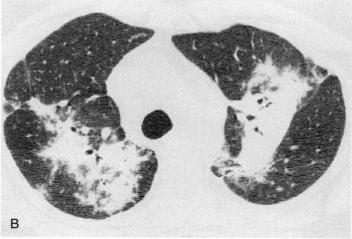

FIGURE 9–10

Sarcoidosis—air space consolidation. A posteroanterior chest radiograph (**A**) in a 39-year-old woman shows patchy bilateral areas of consolidation. Air bronchograms can be seen, particularly on the right side. The consolidation involves mainly the perihilar regions of the middle and upper lung zones. An HRCT scan (**B**) shows a peribronchial distribution of the areas of consolidation and clearly defined air bronchograms. *(From Müller NL, Fraser RS, Colman NC, Paré PD: Radiologic Diagnosis of Diseases of the Chest. Philadelphia, WB Saunders, 2001.)*

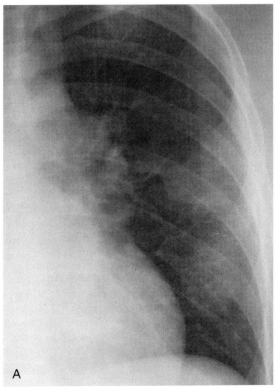

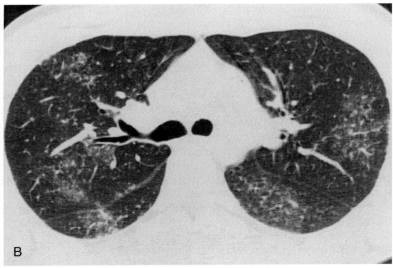

FIGURE 9–11

Sarcoidosis—ground-glass attenuation. A close-up view of the left lung from a posteroanterior chest radiograph (**A**) and an HRCT scan (**B**) show patchy areas of ground-glass attenuation containing a few poorly defined nodules. The patient was a 32-year-old man. *(From Müller NL, Fraser RS, Colman NC, Paré PD: Radiologic Diagnosis of Diseases of the Chest. Philadelphia, WB Saunders, 2001.)*

pneumonia, or heart failure. Focal pleural thickening, or fibrothorax, is not uncommonly identified at thoracotomy or autopsy.[92] It can occur independently of effusion and may be unilateral or bilateral.[93] Spontaneous pneumothorax has been estimated to occur in 1% to 2% of patients.[94]

Cardiovascular Disease. Although abnormalities of the heart, pericardium, and pulmonary vasculature are commonly seen on histologic examination, they are usually of insufficient severity to cause radiographic manifestations. Radiographically evident enlargement of the cardiac silhouette may be the result of cardiomyopathy, valvular disease, pericardial effusion, or left ventricular aneurysm.[95,96] Pulmonary hypertension and cor pulmonale, caused by a combination of obliteration of the pulmonary vascular bed and hypoxic vasoconstriction, tend to occur in the late stage of the disease.

Abdominal Disease. Abdominal lymph node enlargement, hepatomegaly, and splenomegaly are common radiologic findings.[56] Nodules may be seen in the spleen and liver.

Gallium 67 Scanning

Gallium 67 scintigraphy has been used for many years as a marker of disease activity in sarcoidosis. In fact, the results of many (albeit not all[97]) investigations suggest that there is good correlation between the percentage of lymphocytes found in BAL fluid and measurements by gallium 67 scintigraphy.[98,99] The procedure has also been performed to determine the extent and distribution of disease,[100] particularly in patients who have stage 0 or 1 disease.[101,102] Despite these values, the use of gallium 67 has decreased considerably since the advent of HRCT; currently, it is used mainly to assist in the

diagnosis of difficult cases, such as when isolated extrathoracic disease appears to be present.[100]

Clinical Manifestations

The reported prevalence of symptoms in sarcoidosis is variable: patients identified by screening alone are more likely to be asymptomatic, whereas those who have a biopsy-proven diagnosis are almost always symptomatic.[103] It is also likely that the findings at initial examination are related to sex, race, and age.[104]

Symptoms often develop insidiously and are frequently associated with evidence of multisystem involvement, most commonly the lungs, heart, skin, and eyes. Constitutional symptoms are common and include weight loss, fatigue, weakness, and malaise. Fever occurs in 15% to 20% of patients.[2] An acute onset of symptoms, usually with erythema nodosum, is particularly common in Scandinavian, Puerto Rican, and Irish women.[105] The triad of bilateral hilar lymphadenopathy, erythema nodosum, and polyarticular arthritis/arthralgia (Löfgren's syndrome) has also long been recognized as an acute manifestation.[106] Whether coincidental or linked via common susceptibility or exposure, sarcoidosis has been described in association with a variety of connective tissue disorders, including rheumatoid arthritis, ankylosing spondylitis, systemic lupus erythematosus, and progressive systemic sclerosis.[107]

Signs and symptoms of pulmonary involvement develop in about a third of patients[108] and include dry cough and shortness of breath.[109] Hemoptysis is uncommon[110] and is usually attributable to an aspergilloma in an ectatic bronchus or cystic space. Chest pain can be caused by excessive coughing and is rarely pleuritic in type.[111] Symptoms related to pleural involvement (effusion, fibrosis, or pneumothorax) are also rare.[112] Auscultatory signs of pleuropulmonary disease are generally absent in the early stages of the disease, although a few scattered crackles can be heard in some patients; with the development of pulmonary fibrosis, crackles can become more widespread. Rhonchi or wheezes may be audible in patients with endobronchial involvement.[113]

Involvement of the upper respiratory passages is uncommon. The epiglottis is most frequently affected and can be associated with serious obstruction.[114] Laryngeal granulomas have been identified in 1% to 3% of patients.[115] Symptoms include dyspnea, cough, and hoarseness. The latter can also result from extension of the inflammatory process into the recurrent laryngeal nerve from contiguous lymph nodes.[116]

The cardiovascular system can be affected directly or indirectly. Indirect involvement is manifested by pulmonary arterial hypertension and cor pulmonale and can be caused by parenchymal fibrosis and hypoxemia or (rarely) direct compression of the pulmonary arteries[117] or veins[118] by enlarged lymph nodes. Although direct involvement of the myocardium is seen in approximately 25% of cases at autopsy,[119] it is recognized clinically in only a minority. It can be manifested by sudden death, paroxysmal arrhythmias, valvular abnormalities such as mitral insufficiency,[120] angina-like chest pain as a result of small-vessel involvement,[121] left ventricular failure, and ventricular aneurysm. Electrocardiographic abnormalities occur more frequently in patients who have sarcoidosis than in matched controls[122]; in fact, the presence of arrhythmias or unexplained heart failure in a young person should suggest the possibility of myocardial sarcoidosis.

Enlargement of peripheral lymph nodes is said to be clinically evident in about 75% of cases.[2] However, it is probable that nodal involvement occurs at some time in every patient, whether nodes are palpable or not. Palpable lymph nodes are found most frequently in the cervical region, but they may also be felt in the axilla, epitrochlear region, and groin.[123]

The incidence of ocular involvement is probably about 20% to 30%.[124] The characteristic lesion is uveitis[125]; involvement of the conjunctiva, sclera, retina, and lens may also occur and result in cataracts or glaucoma. In general, acute ocular disease is more commonly seen in acute sarcoid syndromes, whereas chronic problems occur in patients who have chronic fibrotic pulmonary and systemic disease.[124]

Cutaneous involvement occurs in 20% to 30% of patients[126] and may be specific (granulomas present pathologically) or nonspecific.[127] The most frequent nonspecific abnormality is erythema nodosum.[128] This inflammatory reaction is a form of panniculitis that most commonly involves the shins and is characterized by the development of crops of transient, nonulcerating nodules that are generally tender, multiple, and bilateral. Lupus pernio ("purple lupus") consists of purplish nodules, usually located on the face, neck, shoulders, and digits and sometimes on the mucous membrane of the nose; it is often associated with involvement of the nasal bones.[129] Large plaques resembling psoriasis may develop over the trunk or extremities. Both lupus pernio and plaques are generally associated with a chronic course and seldom, if ever resolve completely. "Specific" dermal involvement is manifested most often as smooth, soft, red-brown asymptomatic papulonodular lesions; they can be found anywhere on the body and may be solitary or coalescent, deep or superficial. Papules appear in crops and are scattered over the face or grouped closely together at the nape of the neck.[127] Although they tend to occur early in acute disease, like lupus pernio they can be seen in the subacute and chronic phases, during which they tend to coalesce into pebbled, brownish or purplish smooth plaques.[127]

Granulomas can be found in the liver and spleen at autopsy in 60% to 70% of patients; however, palpable enlargement of these organs is seen in only 20%.[130] Most such disease causes no symptoms; however, hepatic involvement can be associated with a variety of histologic and clinical abnormalities that mimic those of other primary liver diseases,[131,132] including primary biliary cirrhosis.[130] Portal hypertension and Budd-Chiari syndrome have been reported rarely.[130] Occasionally, splenomegaly is massive and causes hypersplenism.[133]

Symptomatic involvement of the gastrointestinal tract is very rare.[134] However, markedly increased intestinal permeability (histologically associated with edema and T-cell accumulation) in conjunction with evidence of active, subclinical pulmonary disease in seen in some patients.[135] One study of humoral sensitivity to dietary proteins revealed that about 40% of patients who have sarcoidosis show a specific sensitization to the wheat protein α-gliadin[136]; however, overt celiac disease has been found rarely.[137]

Involvement of minor salivary glands has been noted in almost 60% of random lip biopsies.[138] The combination of parotid gland involvement, uveitis, and pyrexia is called uveoparotid fever; the combination of parotid gland enlargement, uveitis, and facial nerve palsy is known as Heerfordt's syndrome.

Three forms of joint involvement have been described:[139] (1) migratory polyarthritis associated with erythema nodosum, fever, and hilar lymph node enlargement; (2) single or recurrent episodes of polyarticular or monoarticular arthritis; and (3) persistent arthritis. The first of these forms is the most frequent. It is really a polyarthralgia rather than an arthritis and tends to involve the larger joints, particularly the ankles, wrists, elbows, and knees. Symptoms are usually self-limited but occasionally recur or are associated with chronic myalgia and fibromyalgia.[140] Typically, patients are left free of disability. True arthritis is uncommon and is generally seen in patients who have multisystem involvement[141] and chronic pulmonary findings. Syndromes of acute polymyositis or chronic myopathy have been described rarely.[142] Much more commonly, myopathy is due to the use of systemic corticosteroids as therapy.[143] Clubbing is rare and is usually seen in patients who have bronchiectasis or pulmonary fibrosis.[144]

Clinical or functional evidence of renal disease is uncommon[145] despite the fact that granulomas are found in the kidneys in 5% to 20% of autopsied patients.[146] Granulomatous interstitial nephritis is a rare cause of renal failure[147]; when renal insufficiency occurs, it is more commonly due to abnormal calcium metabolism, such as occurs in nephrocalcinosis, urolithiasis, or hypercalcemic renal failure. Given the relative rarity of renal disease, coincidental pathology must be considered in the differential diagnosis.

Involvement of the nervous system is evident in 5% of patients during life[148] and in 15% to 25% at autopsy. Abnormalities may be related to the cranial and peripheral nerves, the brain, the spinal cord, and the meninges.[149] Among patients who have neurologic manifestations, such abnormalities constitute the first clinical evidence of disease in 50% to 75%. Although any cranial nerve can be affected, the second and seventh are most commonly involved, presumably as a result of extension of disease from the underlying meninges[150] or the nose.[151] Unilateral or bilateral facial palsy is sometimes associated with uveoparotid fever. Cerebral lesions can result in grand mal seizures and can simulate metastatic carcinoma.[152] Psychiatric manifestations include delirium, psychosis, personality change, and (possibly) depression.[153,154] Granulomatous inflammation can also affect the hypothalamus and pituitary gland[155]; affected patients often complain of polyuria and polydipsia.

Pulmonary Function Tests

The majority of patients with sarcoidosis and abnormal lung function have restrictive abnormalities[156]; however, many have an obstructive deficit as well.[157] In a small number, the pattern is solely obstructive.[158] Sensitive tests of small-airway dysfunction, such as dynamic compliance, measurement of upstream resistance, and the ratio of closing volume to vital capacity, can be used to demonstrate impairment of small-airway function in asymptomatic nonsmoking patients who have sarcoidosis.[157] Airway hyperresponsiveness has also been reported.[159]

Although attempts have been made in cross-sectional studies to correlate progression of stage with deterioration of lung function,[157] the relationship of function, including diffusing capacity, to radiographic stage is inconstant.[156,160] By contrast, in longitudinal studies, changes in the severity of parenchymal abnormalities on the radiograph correlate well with functional changes over time.[71] Most investigators have shown an increasing prevalence of low DLCO with increasing radiographic stage. Moreover, there is evidence that gas exchange abnormalities on exercise testing correlate better with the radiographic stage than do other measures of lung function.[161]

Reductions in DLCO and alterations in gas exchange can be present on exercise testing even in asymptomatic patients.[162] A reduction in both static and dynamic pulmonary compliance has also been described.[163] Abnormalities in cardiocirculatory function, such as an excessive heart rate and low O_2 pulse, have also been found on exercise testing.[164] These aberrations might be the result of subclinical impairment of right[165] or left[164] ventricular function by cardiac sarcoidosis or, in the case of right-sided disease, the result of changes in lung vasculature secondary to pulmonary disease. Peak inspiratory mouth pressure may also be reduced; in some cases, this decrease has been ascribed to granulomatous inflammation of the respiratory musculature.[166] In one study, the severity of dyspnea on exercise testing correlated better with peak inspiratory and expiratory mouth pressure than it did with other measures of lung function.[167]

Laboratory Findings

A variety of laboratory techniques have been used to support a diagnosis of sarcoidosis, clarify its pathogenesis, assess the likelihood of response to therapy, monitor response to treatment, and estimate prognosis. Attempts have been made to correlate the findings of different tests with each other and with clinical features, radiographic stage, and pulmonary function abnormalities. Such tests include measurement of differential cell counts in BAL fluid, biochemical assay of a variety of substances in BAL fluid and serum (especially serum ACE), and gallium 67 uptake by the lungs. Despite an abundance of information from innumerable published reports, the conclusions of various authors differ in many respects and in some instances are contradictory. The most important variables accounting for these inconsistencies are the methodology used and the variability of the patient population studied.

Analysis of the number, type, and state of activation of inflammatory and immune cells and the presence of cytokines and other mediators of inflammation and fibrosis in BAL fluid has been important in understanding the pathogenesis of the disease, as discussed earlier. However, little evidence has shown that such analysis is useful for either establishing the diagnosis or determining the prognosis (see later). There is evidence that induced sputum can be used to obtain the same information as that from BAL, at least for some substances.[168,169]

Measurement of ACE in serum or BAL fluid has been extensively investigated for its usefulness in diagnosis. High levels of ACE can be found in the BAL fluid of patients who have sarcoidosis, even in the presence of normal serum levels,[170] and elevated levels are found in the serum of many patients who have active disease.[171] Nonetheless, its diagnostic role is limited by lack of specificity[172] and imperfect sensitivity in patients who have early-stage[173] or inactive disease.[174]

Hypercalcemia is seen in about 10% of patients and hypercalciuria in about 30%.[175] The former is said by most investigators to be more evident in the summer months, presumably as a result of increased exposure to sunlight.[150] Aside from the renal effects of hypercalcemia, metastatic calcification can occur in organs and tissues other than the kidney, including the eyes, lungs, stomach, blood vessels, and even ear cartilage.[176]

Hematologic abnormalities are common. In a study of 75 patients who had active pulmonary sarcoidosis, one or more abnormalities were documented in 87%[177]; anemia was present in 21 patients (28%), in 17 of whom bone marrow examination revealed granulomas. Some patients with anemia have evidence of increased hemolysis.[178] Leukopenia and lymphocytopenia are common, with white blood cell counts below 5.0×10^9 per liter observed in approximately 30% of patients. Many patients have a mild degree of peripheral blood eosinophilia.[179] Thrombocytopenia is rare and is associated with a poor prognosis.[180]

Diagnosis

In the appropriate clinical context, a confident diagnosis of sarcoidosis can usually be made on the basis of a combination of clinical, radiographic, and HRCT findings, thus precluding the need for lung biopsy. In a study of 208 patients who had chronic interstitial lung disease, 80 of whom had sarcoidosis, a confident correct diagnosis of sarcoidosis was made on the basis of this combination in 80%.[70] Of the 208 cases, only 1 (berylliosis) was misdiagnosed as sarcoidosis and only 2 cases of sarcoidosis were misdiagnosed (1 as extrinsic allergic alveolitis and the other as silicosis).

In patients in whom the diagnosis cannot be confidently made from these findings, it can usually be established by the identification of non-necrotizing granulomas on biopsy specimens. It should be remembered, however, that other granulomatous diseases, including tuberculosis, brucellosis, fungal infection, and extrinsic allergic alveolitis, can have pathologic and clinical findings similar to those of sarcoidosis. Some of these conditions can be identified by finding microorganisms by special stains, PCR, and/or culture.[181] However, extrinsic allergic alveolitis may be difficult to exclude,[182] particularly with the small biopsy samples obtained by transbronchial biopsy.

When biopsy is required for diagnosis, it is usually obtained bronchoscopically. Biopsy of bronchial mucosa alone yields specimens consistent with sarcoidosis in up to 60% of patients.[183] The yield of transbronchial biopsy is even higher; when multiple biopsy specimens are taken from different sites, granulomas can be identified in almost all patients.[184] Mediastinoscopy with lymph node biopsy is also diagnostic in most cases[185]; however, its use is generally reserved for patients in whom less invasive procedures have not provided a diagnosis or who are suspected to have lymphoma. Fine-needle aspiration biopsy can be useful in patients who have large nodules.[186] Transbronchial needle aspiration of mediastinal nodes performed during bronchoscopy, which may be used in conjunction with endoscopic guidance,[187] has provided a diagnosis in up to 90% of patients.[188] Biopsy of other tissues, such as salivary glands and conjunctiva, is not indicated in most patients because of its relatively low yield.[138,189]

Gallium 67 scanning has a limited role in diagnosis. It can detect disease in the lung parenchyma in stage 0 and stage 1 sarcoidosis,[101] and particular patterns of gallium uptake (*lamda* and *panda*) can suggest the diagnosis when the radiographic pattern is atypical[101]; however, its use in this respect has been largely supplanted by HRCT.

Prognosis and Natural History

The reported prognosis is variable and strongly influenced by referral bias (population versus referral setting), disease severity at initial evaluation, ethnic and genetic factors, and a variety of other clinical features.

The importance of referral bias in estimates of disease mortality is illustrated in a meta-analysis of patients from referral and population-based settings[190]; mortality in the former setting (4.8%) was 10-fold that in the latter (0.5%). Differences in disease stage and ethnicity failed to account for the differences in survival. In the United States, higher mortality has been reported for African American than for white individuals[191]; however, whether this is related to genetically determined differences in disease severity or to confounding factors such as lower socioeconomic status or underinsurance is a matter of debate.[192] Attributable mortality is generally due to progressive respiratory insufficiency[193] or cardiac[194] involvement; occasionally, CNS involvement,[151] disease-related renal failure, or massive hemoptysis as a result of aspergilloma account for death.

Several clinical features have prognostic significance. Löfgren's syndrome generally has a favorable prognosis.[106] On the other hand, persistent skin lesions, bone lesions, hepatosplenomegaly and hypercalcemia,[195] or involvement of the eye, nose, central nervous system, and heart[1] has been associated with a chronic and progressive disease course. As might be expected, higher stage at diagnosis is also linked to a worse prognosis.[196,197] Absence of improvement on the chest radiograph over a 1-year period is a poor prognostic sign, whereas radiographic resolution that lasts for 2 years can be regarded as a cure.[198] Late relapse after disease remission or stabilization is uncommon.[1]

No radiographic criteria allow distinction of reversible from irreversible disease.[47] On HRCT scan, nodules, consolidation, ground-glass attenuation, and interlobular septal thickening may resolve, remain stable, or progress on follow-up.[57,199] Irregular linear opacities are most commonly irreversible but occasionally resolve.[57,199] Irreversible abnormalities indicative of fibrosis on HRCT scan include architectural distortion, traction bronchiectasis, and honeycombing.[57,199] Except for the demonstration of such abnormalities, HRCT is not helpful in predicting outcome because there is no difference in the pattern or extent of parenchymal abnormalities in patients who have persistent or progressive disease and patients who improve on follow-up.[76]

Considerable effort has been directed at identifying markers of "activity" in patients who have sarcoidosis in the hope that such markers will allow identification of those in whom progressive disease is likely to develop. Assessment of these markers includes measurement of an innumerable variety of inflammatory products in BAL fluid[200,201] and blood,[202-205] quantification of serum ACE levels,[206] and determination of delayed cutaneous hypersensitivity[207] and gallium scan activity.[208] Despite the finding that some markers correlate with disease progression,[209] none has been applied to a sufficiently large population of patients in a prospective fashion to allow for intelligent decision making regarding therapy. Moreover, results have been inconsistent in different studies,[210,211] and no test has been demonstrated to be superior to standard clinical evaluation (including lung function testing and chest radiography) in guiding management.

LANGERHANS CELL HISTIOCYTOSIS

Pulmonary Langerhans cell histiocytosis (PLCH) is an uncommon disorder characterized pathologically by infiltration of the lung by Langerhans cells. The latter are antigen-processing and antigen-presenting cells that are normally most prominent in the epidermis but also occur in epithelia elsewhere in the body, including the pulmonary airways. Disease is confined to the lung in more than 85% of affected patients; other sites such as bone and the pituitary gland are occasionally involved.[212] It is a disease of adults and almost inevitably occurs in smokers.[213]

The precise nature of the condition is unclear; however, most evidence suggests that it represents a nonclonal hyperplasia of Langerhans cells that is driven by tobacco smoke. Although occasional clones appear to develop, they do not become neoplastic, and the cellular proliferation seen pathologically often regresses spontaneously.[214] The hyperplastic Langerhans cells have a stimulatory effect on lymphocytes, which, in concert with activated pulmonary alveolar macrophages,[215] are frequently associated with some degree of pulmonary fibrosis.[216] Vasculopathy, sometimes causing pulmonary hypertension that is out of keeping with the calculated functional or gas exchange deficits, can also be seen[217]; its pathogenesis is unclear.

Pathologic Characteristics

In the early stage of disease, the lungs characteristically contain multiple nodules measuring 1 to 10 mm in diameter. With time, these nodules may become confluent and result in irregularly shaped areas of fibrosis containing cysts of variable size. In long-standing disease, the appearance may resemble advanced idiopathic pulmonary fibrosis. The major distinguishing features between the two are that PLCH tends to be more severe in the upper lobes and to affect the peripheral and central regions more evenly.[218]

Early histologic abnormalities are located predominantly in the interstitial connective tissue of small membranous and proximal respiratory bronchioles and consist mainly of a cellular infiltrate composed of variable numbers of Langerhans cells and eosinophils (Fig. 9–12), with lesser numbers of neutrophils, plasma cells, lymphocytes, and multinucleated giant cells.[219] In more advanced disease, the infiltrate extends into the adjacent alveolar interstitium, and the central portion of the lesion undergoes fibrosis, thereby resulting in a characteristic stellate shape (see Color Fig. 9–2). For reasons that are not clear, some affected bronchioles appear to dilate (Fig. 9–13), which results in the cysts that are seen in both gross specimens and radiologic images. It is also possible that some cysts originate by cavitation of the cellular nodules. With progression of disease, individual foci of disease coalesce, fibrous tissue becomes more prominent, and an increasing amount of lung is destroyed.

Alveolar macrophages are commonly increased in number at the periphery of foci of active disease; in some cases they may be so numerous that they simulate desquamative interstitial pneumonitis.

Radiologic Manifestations

Radiographic abnormalities are characteristically bilateral, symmetrical, and diffuse throughout the upper and middle lung zones with sparing of the costophrenic angles.[220] Early in the disease, the appearance consists of a nodular pattern, with individual lesions measuring 1 to 10 mm in diameter. Although cavitated nodules are seen only occasionally during this stage,[221] they can be identified on HRCT scan in approximately 10% of cases.[222,223] In more advanced disease, the pattern often becomes reticulonodular. End-stage disease is characterized by a coarse reticular pattern that often has a cystic appearance, particularly in the upper lung zones (Fig. 9–14). Most cysts are about 1 cm in diameter but may measure 3 cm.

The most common abnormalities on HRCT scan are cysts (present in approximately 80% of patients) and nodules (present in 60% to 80%) (see Fig. 9–14).[222,223] Less common findings include cavitated nodules, reticulation, and areas of ground-glass attenuation. As might be expected, the incidence of these abnormalities depends on the stage of the disease. The predominant abnormality in patients who have recent symptoms consists of small nodules that vary from a few to a myriad and tend to have a centrilobular distribution.[223] Their margins may be smooth or irregular. Occasionally, they disappear after smoking cessation.[224]

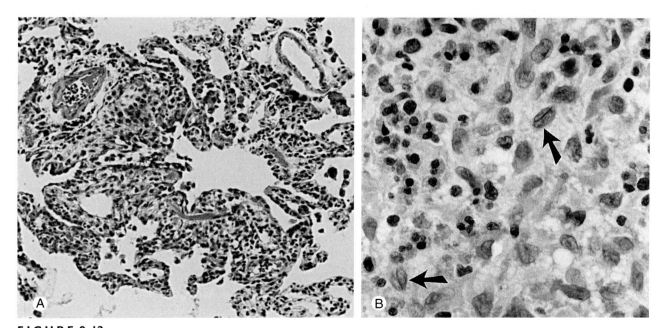

FIGURE 9–12

Langerhans cell histiocytosis—early bronchiolar involvement. The wall of a respiratory bronchiole (**A**) is moderately thickened by a cellular infiltrate; there is no fibrosis. A magnified view (**B**) shows the infiltrate to be composed of scattered bilobed eosinophils and histiocytes with irregularly shaped vesicular nuclei that are focally grooved (*arrows*). (*From Fraser RS, Müller NL, Colman NC, Paré PD: Fraser and Paré's Diagnosis of Diseases of the Chest, 4th ed. Philadelphia, WB Saunders, 1999.*)

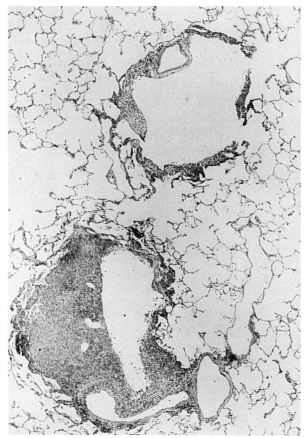

FIGURE 9–13

Langerhans cell histiocytosis—early cystic lesions. Two foci of disease are evident, each centered on a bronchiole. The upper one is mildly dilated and its wall is slightly thickened by a cellular infiltrate; the lower one shows more marked, eccentric thickening as a result of a more pronounced cellular infiltrate. (From Fraser RS, Müller NL, Colman NC, Paré PD: Fraser and Paré's Diagnosis of Diseases of the Chest, 4th ed. Philadelphia, WB Saunders, 1999.)

With progression of disease, cysts become a more prominent feature. In fact, many of the reticular and reticulonodular opacities seen on radiographs represent cysts (see Fig. 9–14).[222] They range from a few millimeters to several centimeters in diameter and may be round, oval, or irregular in shape.[222,225] In many cases, the parenchyma between the cysts is remarkably normal. With progression of disease, however, there is evidence of fibrosis and, eventually, honeycombing.[67] Regardless of the stage of the disease, the abnormalities are most severe in the mid and upper lung zone.[67,226]

The pattern and distribution of abnormalities on HRCT scan are usually characteristic enough to allow a confident diagnosis.[4,83,227] The presence of nodules and cysts throughout the middle and upper lung zones with relative sparing of the lung bases is virtually diagnostic. In patients who have nodules alone, definitive diagnosis is more difficult because the pattern resembles sarcoidosis, tuberculosis, and metastatic cancer. In patients who have only cystic changes, the findings can be easily distinguished from idiopathic pulmonary fibrosis because the latter typically shows the most severe involvement in the subpleural lung regions and the lower lung zones. Cystic

changes similar to those in PLCH may be seen in lymphangioleiomyomatosis and tuberous sclerosis[228]; however, the cysts in these conditions are present diffusely throughout the lungs, without sparing of the lung bases, and nodules are seen rarely.

Spontaneous pneumothorax is a relatively common complication; in two series involving 150 patients, it developed in 18 (12%).[220,229] Hilar and mediastinal node enlargement and pleural effusion are rare in adults,[230,231] although the former is relatively common in children.[231] Concomitant involvement of bones and lungs is uncommon in adults, in one series being evident in only 5 of 100 patients.[229]

Clinical Manifestations

PLCH is seen predominantly in young adults.[213] When it is first discovered, 20% to 25% of patients are asymptomatic,[229] the disease being identified on a screening chest radiograph. About a third of symptomatic patients have only nonspecific constitutional symptoms such as fatigue, weight loss, and fever.[229] Respiratory symptoms are present in the remaining two thirds and usually consist of dry cough and dyspnea. Hemoptysis is uncommon.[229] Chest pain can be caused by pneumothorax or (rarely) an osteolytic rib lesion. Physical findings are of little help in diagnosis; occasionally, crackles or wheezes[232] are heard over the lungs, or there is local tenderness over a bony lesion.[233] Findings of pulmonary hypertension may be present. Finger clubbing is rare.[218] Symptoms caused by the involvement of other organs occur in 5% to 15% of patients.[212] The association of diffuse lung disease with diabetes insipidus should strongly suggest the diagnosis, although this combination occasionally occurs in histoplasmosis and sarcoidosis.

Pulmonary Function Tests and Diagnosis

Even in the presence of radiographic abnormalities, lung function is within the normal predicted range in many patients, in sharp contrast to those who have idiopathic pulmonary fibrosis.[234] The earliest abnormality is a reduction in diffusing capacity.[235] In more advanced disease, both restrictive[236] and obstructive patterns are often present.[229] Exercise impairment is common[236] and probably reflects the consequences of pulmonary vascular changes.

In a young, asymptomatic adult who has the classic radiologic abnormalities, the diagnosis can usually be made with confidence without ancillary studies. When the clinical features are atypical and tissue is required for diagnosis, open lung biopsy is generally required. Transbronchial biopsy is often inadequate for secure diagnosis,[219,237] and the finding of Langerhans cells in BAL fluid[238] lacks specificity unless the proportion of such cells is greater than 5%.[238]

Prognosis and Natural History

Most patients who have disease confined to the lungs experience complete and prolonged remission (as in 74 of 87 patients in one series[213]). Nonetheless, overall survival is shorter than that described in the general population.[239] Respiratory failure accounts for many of the deaths. The prognosis is worse in older patients who have disseminated disease,

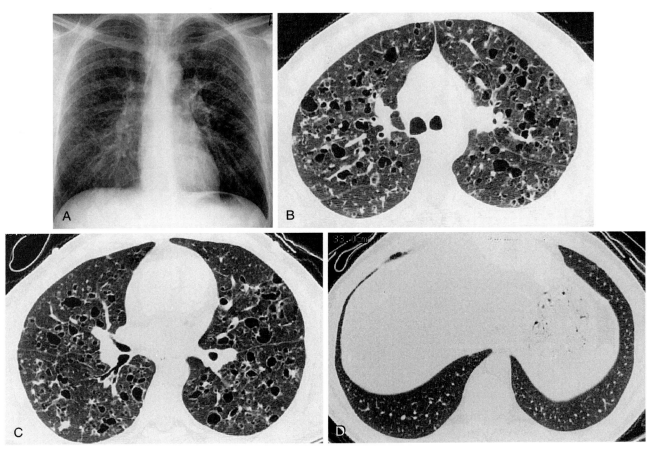

FIGURE 9–14

Langerhans cell histiocytosis. A posteroanterior chest radiograph (**A**) shows a coarse reticular pattern as well as several cysts. Although the abnormalities are relatively diffuse in the upper and middle lung zones, there is sparing of the costophrenic sulci. An HRCT scan at the level of the main bronchi (**B**) shows numerous bilateral cystic lesions of various size. Note the relatively normal intervening lung parenchyma. The apparent reticular opacities on radiograph are shown on CT to be due to cysts, there being little evidence of fibrosis. Bronchi are normal in diameter and do not appear to communicate with the cysts. An HRCT scan at the level of the right middle lobe bronchus (**C**) also shows numerous cysts, as well as a few irregularly marginated small nodules. An HRCT scan through the lung bases (**D**) shows only a few localized cysts. *(From Müller NL, Fraser RS, Colman NC, Paré PD: Radiologic Diagnosis of Diseases of the Chest. Philadelphia, WB Saunders, 2001.)*

in patients who have functional indices of airflow obstruction (lower FEV$_1$/FVC ratio, higher RV/TLC ratio)[239,240] or reduced diffusing capacity,[239] and in patients who have radiographic evidence of honeycombing, especially when associated with repeated episodes of pneumothorax.[218]

An association between PLCH and pulmonary carcinoma has been described by several investigators. Although it may be related to the confounding effect of cigarette smoke,[241] the association of PLCH with a variety of other malignancies, especially Hodgkin's lymphoma,[242] suggests that there may be an underlying pathogenetic relationship. When malignancy is associated with PLCH, it is important to remember that the nodules of PLCH can imitate metastases radiologically.

LYMPHANGIOLEIOMYOMATOSIS

Lymphangioleiomyomatosis (LAM) is a rare pulmonary disease characterized pathologically by cyst formation and an interstitial proliferation of smooth muscle–like cells and clinically by progressive dyspnea and recurrent pneumothorax. It

can occur by itself or in association with tuberous sclerosis complex (TSC).[243] The latter is an inherited autosomal dominant disorder that affects about 1 in 6000 individuals and has various clinical manifestations, including tumors of the brain, heart, and kidney; cognitive defects; and epilepsy.[244] Although the prevalence of LAM in patients who have TSC has traditionally been estimated to be about 2% to 4%, screening by HRCT has found evidence of the disease in as many as a third.[245] Isolated LAM is much less common, with only about 70 cases having been reported by 1997.[246] Whether by itself or associated with TSC, LAM is limited almost entirely to women and is most common during the childbearing years, the average age at the onset of pulmonary symptoms being 30 to 35.[246]

Etiology and Pathogenesis

Tuberous sclerosis is associated with mutations in the *TSC1* and *TSC2* genes. Those involving the latter are common in patients who have LAM, with or without other features of

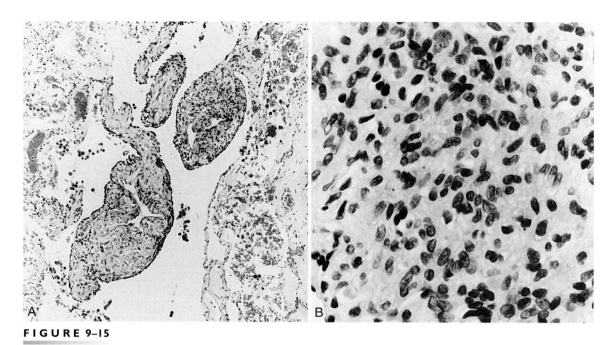

FIGURE 9–15

Lymphangioleiomyomatosis—early lesion. A section of the wall of a small bronchiole (**A**) shows thickening by cellular proliferation, more marked on one side. A magnified view (**B**) shows cells that have oval or round nuclei, somewhat suggestive of smooth muscle. (*From Müller NL, Fraser RS, Colman NC, Paré PD: Radiologic Diagnosis of Diseases of the Chest. Philadelphia, WB Saunders, 2001.*)

TSC, whereas those involving the *TSC1* gene are seen in association with TSC alone.[247] *TSC2* codes for the protein tuberin, which is involved in the regulation of cell growth and may act as a tumor suppressor.[244] An alteration or absence of the protein is associated with localized tumor formation (e.g., renal angiomyolipoma) or with the more diffuse cellular proliferation of smooth muscle–like cells in the lung and lymphatic vessels seen in LAM. In addition to such proliferation, these abnormal muscle cells show increased expression of serum response factor, a substance that indirectly controls the production of several metalloproteinases and their inhibitors. These enzymes include potent elastases and collagenases, and it has been hypothesized that an imbalance in their levels is responsible for development of the cystic spaces characteristic of LAM.[244]

The observation that LAM is almost always seen in women during the reproductive years suggests that altered hormone secretion or tissue response to hormones is also involved in the pathogenesis of the disease. A variety of epidemiologic, clinical, and pathologic evidence supports this hypothesis. For example, receptors for estrogen and progesterone have been identified in the abnormal pulmonary muscle cells.[248,249] More importantly, exacerbations of disease have been documented during pregnancy and after the administration of exogenous estrogens,[250,251] and hormonal therapy has been associated with clinical improvement in some patients.[246] The precise molecular alterations underlying these findings and the mechanism by which they are mediated are unclear.

Pathologic Characteristics

The earliest histologic abnormality in the lung is a proliferation of polygonal or spindle-shaped muscle-like cells in the interstitial tissue of small bronchioles, lymphatic vessels, and the pleura (Fig. 9–15). In more advanced disease, these cells extend into the parenchymal interstitium. Foci of smooth muscle proliferation may also be seen in the thoracic duct and in lymph nodes in the mediastinum and retroperitoneum. Immunohistochemical study shows strong reactivity of the proliferating cells for HMB45 and muscle-specific actin.[252] Slices of lung at autopsy or pneumonectomy typically have innumerable cystic spaces of variable size (usually 0.2 to 2.0 cm in diameter) separated by thickened interstitial tissue.[253] Histologic examination of the cyst walls may show only small foci of abnormal muscle or relatively thick, eccentric or concentric foci of proliferation (Fig. 9–16). Dilated lymphatics (related to lymphatic obstruction by foci of muscle proliferation) and small nodules composed of thickened parenchymal interstitium lined by hyperplastic type II pneumocytes are seen in some cases.[254]

Radiologic Manifestations

The most common radiographic finding is a bilateral reticular pattern (Fig. 9–17).[255-257] In approximately 80% of cases, it involves all lung zones to a similar degree; in the remainder, it is more marked in the lower lung zones. Cysts can be identified on the radiograph in 50% to 60% of cases.[256,257] Evidence of hyperinflation manifested by an increase in the retrosternal air space or flattening of the diaphragm is seen at initial evaluation in many patients. Pneumothorax has been reported in 30% to 40% of cases and unilateral or bilateral pleural effusions in 10% to 20%.[255,257] The pulmonary parenchymal abnormalities may precede, accompany, or follow the pleural manifestations.[255] The chest radiograph has been reported to be normal in 2% to 20% of cases.[255-257]

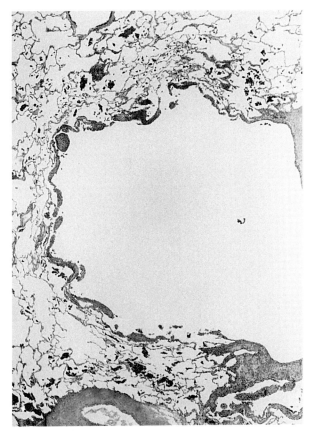

FIGURE 9–16

Lymphangioleiomyomatosis—cystic lesion. A section shows a cystic space with relatively mild wall thickening. *(From Müller NL, Fraser RS, Colman NC, Paré PD: Radiologic Diagnosis of Diseases of the Chest. Philadelphia, WB Saunders, 2001.)*

The characteristic HRCT finding consists of numerous air-filled cysts surrounded by normal lung parenchyma (Fig. 9–18).[255,256] They can be seen in patients who have normal radiographs or radiographs showing only reticular opacities.[255,256] They usually measure between 0.2 and 2 cm in diameter, although they may be as large as 6 cm. The size varies with the severity of disease; most patients who have mild involvement have cysts smaller than 1 cm in diameter. Most cysts are round and have smooth walls ranging from faintly perceptible to 4 mm in thickness. They are distributed diffusely throughout the lungs, without central, peripheral, or lower lung zone predominance. In most cases, the parenchyma between the cysts appears normal; occasionally, there is a slight increase in interstitial markings,[258,259] interlobular septal thickening,[256,259] or patchy areas of ground-glass attenuation.[255]

The cysts can be easily distinguished from the honeycombing associated with idiopathic pulmonary fibrosis by their diffuse distribution and the presence of relatively normal intervening parenchyma.[255,256] The main differential diagnosis on HRCT is with Langerhans cell histiocytosis.[222,255] However, the cysts in this abnormality typically involve the mid and upper lung zones with relative sparing of the lung bases[222]; in addition, most patients who have Langerhans cell histiocytosis have nodules, a finding that is seen rarely in LAM.[223]

Clinical Manifestations

The initial complaint in patients with LAM is usually shortness of breath, most often gradual and occasionally acute, in which case an associated pneumothorax is usually present.[243,246,260] Cough, hemoptysis, and chest pain are uncommon initial symptoms but occur in 35% to 45% of patients at some time in the course of the disease.[260] Chylothorax is also common and may contribute to dyspnea. Extrapulmonary manifestations of disease are generally related to involvement of the thoracic or abdominal lymph nodes and include chyloperitoneum and chylopericardium. When tumors such as renal angiomyolipoma are identified, the possibility of TSC should be considered.

The pulmonary function pattern is generally one of obstruction, with the FEV_1/FVC ratio usually well below the predicted normal value.[260,261] Lung volumes are typically normal or increased, except in patients who have large chylous effusions. DLCO is usually reduced, and hypoxemia is common and may be severe; however, PCO_2 is almost invariably decreased.

Although the classic picture of dyspnea and chylothorax, with or without pneumothorax, in a woman of childbearing age probably suggests the diagnosis to most pulmonary physicians, such a picture appears to be relatively uncommon. In an investigation of 32 patients, the most frequent manifestations were isolated pneumothorax or exertional dyspnea, not uncommonly in association with a normal chest radiograph.[260] Although not all authorities agree,[262] we believe that the diagnosis can be reasonably made in the majority of patients on the basis of a combination of clinical and HRCT findings, thus precluding the need for biopsy.

The prognosis of LAM is generally poor, most patients dying of the disease within 10 years of diagnosis.[246,263] However, as indicated previously, the results of some studies suggest that the prognosis may be better in patients who have been treated with hormonal therapy.[260] Recurrent disease has been seen in some patients who have undergone lung transplantation and is related in at least some cases to migration of residual abnormal muscle cells into the transplanted lung.[264]

NEUROFIBROMATOSIS

Neurofibromatosis (von Recklinghausen's disease) is a relatively common familial disorder with a frequency of about 1 in 3000.[265] The most prominent clinical manifestations are cutaneous café au lait spots and neurofibromas of the cutaneous and subcutaneous peripheral nerves, nerve roots, and viscera. Intrathoracic neurogenic neoplasms can arise in the intercostal nerves (in which case they may be associated with rib destruction and/or a chest wall mass), in the mediastinum, and in the lungs themselves.[266,267] The most common pulmonary manifestations consist of diffuse interstitial fibrosis (histologically characterized by a pattern of nonspecific interstitial pneumonitis) and bullae, either alone or in combination.[268,269]

Radiologically, the interstitial disease is characterized by a reticular pattern that involves both lungs symmetrically with some basal predominance.[269,270] Bullae are usually seen in the upper lobes.[268] Cutaneous neurofibromas appear as nodular opacities on the chest radiograph and may mimic intrapulmonary metastases; in such cases, CT may be helpful

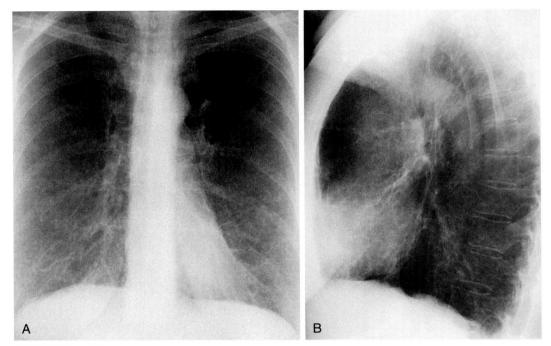

FIGURE 9–17

Lymphangioleiomyomatosis. Posteroanterior (**A**) and lateral (**B**) chest radiographs show a diffuse bilateral reticular pattern. A few small cysts can be identified. Lung volumes are increased. The patient was a 40-year-old woman. *(From Müller NL, Fraser RS, Colman NC, Paré PD: Radiologic Diagnosis of Diseases of the Chest. Philadelphia, WB Saunders, 2001.)*

(Fig. 9–19).[271,272] Plexiform neurofibromas can result in erosion of the inferior or superior margins of one or more ribs.[270] Other abnormalities include scoliosis,[270] scalloping of vertebral bodies,[273] lateral thoracic meningoceles,[274] and "twisted ribbon" deformity of the ribs.[273]

Paraspinal masses may be caused by neural tumors. When the latter arise from the intercostal nerves, they may be seen as extrapleural soft tissue masses running parallel to and occasionally eroding a rib.[274] Tumors of the vagus or phrenic nerves may result in mediastinal masses. The development of a malignant neural tumor should be suspected when a preexisting mass rapidly increases in size or is associated with pain.[270]

Clinically, the diagnosis is usually made readily by the presence of multiple sessile or pedunculated neurofibromas on the skin. Pulmonary disease typically does not become evident until the patient reaches adulthood. Respiratory symptoms are mild, the most common complaint being dyspnea on exertion.[269] Pulmonary function tests generally reveal evidence of obstruction, although a restrictive pattern may be dominant; DLCO is often decreased.

IDIOPATHIC INTERSTITIAL PNEUMONIA

The idiopathic interstitial pneumonias are a heterogeneous group of inflammatory and fibrotic disorders of the lung parenchyma. To resolve the confusion resulting from the use of conflicting classification schemas,[275,276] a multidisciplinary committee of the American Thoracic Society and the European Respiratory Society suggested new guidelines for their categorization in 2002.[277] According to this schema, the clinical-radiologic-pathologic diagnosis of idiopathic interstitial pneumonia is based on the identification of particular histologic patterns. The disorders include idiopathic pulmonary fibrosis (IPF), nonspecific interstitial pneumonitis (NSIP), acute interstitial pneumonia (AIP), respiratory bronchiolitis-associated interstitial lung disease, desquamative interstitial pneumonia (DIP), lymphoid interstitial pneumonia, and cryptogenic organizing pneumonia. The latter two disorders are discussed elsewhere in this text (see pages 377 and 696) since the former is for the most part a lymphoproliferative disorder and the latter has substantial air space disease and is unlikely to be confused clinically, radiologically, or pathologically with the other abnormalities.

A careful clinical history is particularly important in identifying patients who have a specific etiology for interstitial pneumonia. For example, although the histologic pattern of usual interstitial pneumonia (UIP) is generally associated with IPF, it can be seen as well in patients who have connective tissue disease or drug-induced pneumonitis.

Idiopathic Pulmonary Fibrosis

IPF has been defined as "a specific form of chronic fibrosing interstitial pneumonia limited to the lung and associated with the histologic appearance of usual interstitial pneumonia."[278] Like many of the other varieties of interstitial lung disease, it is characterized clinically by dyspnea and radiographically by diffuse reticular opacification.[279] It is the most common cause of idiopathic interstitial lung disease, in one study accounting

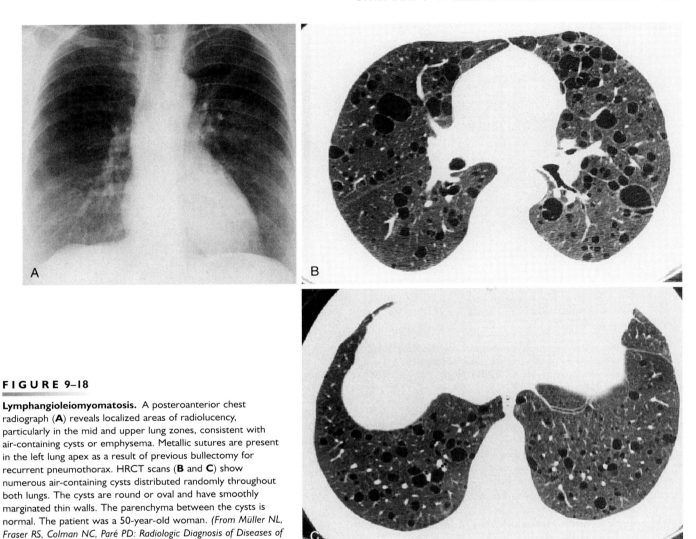

FIGURE 9–18

Lymphangioleiomyomatosis. A posteroanterior chest radiograph (**A**) reveals localized areas of radiolucency, particularly in the mid and upper lung zones, consistent with air-containing cysts or emphysema. Metallic sutures are present in the left lung apex as a result of previous bullectomy for recurrent pneumothorax. HRCT scans (**B** and **C**) show numerous air-containing cysts distributed randomly throughout both lungs. The cysts are round or oval and have smoothly marginated thin walls. The parenchyma between the cysts is normal. The patient was a 50-year-old woman. *(From Müller NL, Fraser RS, Colman NC, Paré PD: Radiologic Diagnosis of Diseases of the Chest. Philadelphia, WB Saunders, 2001.)*

for more than 40% of cases.[280] The calculated prevalence is 20 per 100,000 for males and 13 per 100,000 for females. Both the incidence and the prevalence increase markedly with age; about two thirds of patients are older than 60 when IPF is diagnosed.[278] By using the imperfect tool of death certificate diagnosis, the age-adjusted mortality in 1991 was 5.09 per 100,000 in men and 2.72 per 100,000 in women, rates that seem to have increased since 1979.[281] Disease has been reported worldwide, in both rural and urban settings, with no racial predominance.[278]

Etiology and Pathogenesis

By definition, the etiology of IPF is unknown; however, evidence has accumulated in support of a role for several possible agents. Pathogenetic factors that have been most extensively studied include inherited susceptibility and immunologically mediated inflammation and fibrosis.[282]

Viral Infection. The diagnosis of IPF often coincides with clinical evidence of a viral-type syndrome.[283] In addition, the results of molecular studies suggest that some viruses—especially Epstein-Barr virus—are associated with both the presence of disease[284] and its progression,[285] thus implying that

the organism might be involved in pathogenesis in some patients. Despite these observations, it is rare to identify a specific viral infection that evolves into pathologically proven interstitial fibrosis.[286]

Other Environmental Agents. Although no specific workplace or environmental factor has been clearly linked to the development of IPF,[279] the findings of a number of epidemiologic studies have suggested at least a weak association with solvent[287] or dust[288] exposure. Cigarette smoking has also been associated with an increased risk of disease,[289] although there is little evidence that it is causal.[232]

Gastroesophageal Reflux. Acid reflux has been demonstrated in a substantial number of patients in some series,[290] thus suggesting that it might be a factor in pathogenesis. However, additional investigation is required to confirm this hypothesis.

Genetic Factors. The presence of familial clusters of IPF provides the strongest evidence that genetic factors are involved in development of the disease.[291,292] A mutation in the surfactant protein C gene has been described in some patients with familial disease[293]; although the relationship between this mutation and pathogenesis is unclear, the finding clearly has potential implications for diagnosis and therapy.[294] In patients

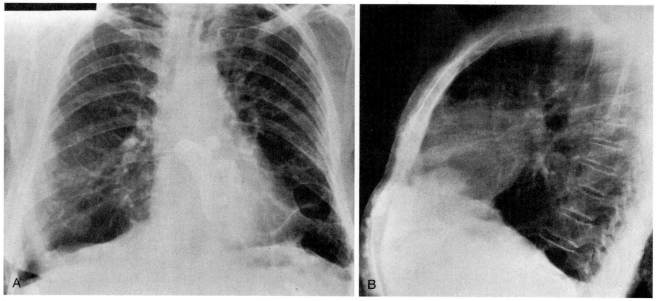

FIGURE 9–19

Neurofibromatosis—pulmonary and cutaneous manifestations. A posteroanterior chest radiograph (**A**) shows numerous bullae in the lower portion of both lungs. Along the anterior and posterior chest walls in lateral projection (**B**) are numerous nodular opacities representing cutaneous neurofibromas. *(From Müller NL, Fraser RS, Colman NC, Paré PD: Radiologic Diagnosis of Diseases of the Chest. Philadelphia, WB Saunders, 2001.)*

who have sporadic disease, specific genetic polymorphisms have been associated with alterations in IL-1 receptor antagonist, tumor necrosis factor-α, IL-6, and ACE[295,296]; mutations in the transforming growth factor-β_1 (TGF-β_1) type I receptor gene have also been described in some patients.[297] Once again, however, the relationship between these abnormalities and disease pathogenesis is unclear.

Immunologic and Inflammatory Influences. Partly because of the identification of lymphocytes and plasma cells in the interstitium on histologic examination, one of the principal hypotheses concerning the pathogenesis of IPF considers inflammation to be the primary pathogenetic process, which in turn induces the production of fibrous tissue.[279] In fact, there is now substantial evidence that this hypothesis is likely to be incorrect.[298] For example, in both human biopsy specimens and tissue derived from experimental animals, the inflammatory cell infiltrate in UIP is usually mild in areas of collagen deposition and is uncommonly seen in otherwise unaltered alveolar septa.[299] Many nonhistologic markers of pulmonary inflammation, including the cellular composition of BAL fluid and gallium 67 lung scan activity, correlate poorly with disease outcome.[299] Moreover, anti-inflammatory therapy has little, if any, effect on disease outcome.[300] On the other hand, a greater extent of fibroblastic foci in biopsy specimens has been found to be associated with decreased survival.[301] Despite these observations, it is possible that transient inflammation early in the course of disease is associated with the production of mediators (such as TGF-β) that result in the more prolonged mesenchymal-epithelial interaction necessary for the development of fibrosis.[302]

A second pathogenetic hypothesis proposes that the foci of fibroblast-myofibroblast proliferation now thought to be characteristic of UIP histologically are the sites of primary damage.[299,303] According to this hypothesis, a complex interaction between epithelial and mesenchymal cells is the basis of the fibrotic reaction. A variety of observations suggest that alveolar epithelial cells are important in pathogenesis. Injury to these cells is associated with secretion of a variety of growth factors, particularly TGF-β_1,[304] that induce migration and proliferation of fibroblasts and their differentiation into myofibroblasts. There is evidence that they also secrete gelatinases that cause disruption of the basement membrane, thereby allowing fibroblast-myofibroblast migration into the adjacent air space.[299] After injury, the process of epithelial cell proliferation and differentiation, which usually allows for restoration of a normal alveolar lining, appears to be slow and incomplete in patients who have IPF, and a deficiency of surfactant and alveolar collapse result.[305] In addition, possibly through the influence of TGF-β_1 and other cytokines, it is likely that epithelial cell apoptosis is increased[306]; in fact, prevention of this process in a murine model of pulmonary fibrosis prevented the development of disease.[307] Finally, epithelial cells have both procoagulant and antithrombolytic activities that could impede the migration of cells necessary for normal repair into the extracellular matrix.[308]

In addition to the abnormalities related to epithelial cells, a variety of processes in the mesenchymal tissue itself are likely to be involved in the development of fibrosis. A defect in synthesis of the antifibrogenic prostaglandin E_2 by interstitial myofibroblasts has been demonstrated in some patients,[309] suggesting that an inherent (possibly genetic) abnormality may be important. The continuing deposition of collagen and other extracellular matrix proteins by myofibroblasts is favored by an imbalance between matrix metalloproteinases in the interstitium and the production of tissue inhibitors of metalloproteinases by the myofibroblasts themselves.[310,311] Myofibroblasts also produce factors such as angiotensinogen that, via angiotensin II, cause alveolar epithelial cell death and fibroblast proliferation, thereby further impairing normal re-epithelialization and increasing fibrosis.[312] A variety of angiogenic factors, such as vascular endothelial growth factor,[299] induce neovascularization in IPF; however, it is not clear whether these factors promote[313] or hinder[299] fibrosis. It is possible that the cytokine profile elicited by the response to injury may also affect the processes of resolution or progression to end-stage fibrosis.[314] For example, predominance of a T_H2 instead of a T_H1 response (which is seen in patients who have IPF) might promote fibrosis.

Pathologic Characteristics

IPF is characterized histologically by a pattern of UIP.[277] Typically, lung biopsy specimens show variably severe disease, with areas of normal and markedly abnormal lung being present in different regions of the same tissue section and, sometimes, in a single lobule (Fig. 9–20). Alveolar septa may be slightly thickened by an infiltrate of inflammatory cells; lymphocytes are usually the most numerous, with plasma cells, histiocytes, eosinophils, and polymorphonuclear leukocytes encountered in lesser numbers. Areas in which interstitial thickening is greater are usually related to the presence of connective tissue, most often mature collagen; however, foci of loose connective tissue indicative of fibrogenesis are common (Fig. 9–21).

In the most severely affected areas, the interstitial thickening is so marked that alveoli are obliterated. This finding is often associated with dilation of transitional airways and represents the histologic counterpart of grossly evident honeycomb lung. Additional abnormalities that can be seen in areas of severe fibrosis include an increase in elastic tissue, smooth muscle hyperplasia, and epithelial metaplasia, the latter usually of squamous or columnar mucus-secreting cells. Dystrophic calcification and osseous metaplasia occur occasionally.

An increased number of macrophages are often seen in the alveolar air spaces; however, in contrast to DIP, they usually vary in number from alveolus to alveolus and are not numerous overall. The adjacent alveolar septa are commonly lined by hyperplastic type II cells. Foci of active-appearing fibrous tissue can also be seen in the alveolar air spaces and lumina of transitional airways; however, such foci are typically patchy and much less prominent than in the interstitium. An air space exudate is absent. The pulmonary arteries generally show some degree of intimal fibrosis and medial muscular hyperplasia, especially in regions of more marked interstitial fibrosis. Although such changes may be related to generalized pulmonary hypertension, in most cases they probably reflect a reaction to local interstitial disease.

Grossly, the early stage of IPF consists of only a slight coarseness of the normal parenchyma, typically most severe in the subpleural parenchyma of the basal and posterior portions of the lower lobes. As disease progresses, clear-cut areas of fibrosis alternating with small cystic spaces 1 to 2 mm in diameter become evident. Eventually, large portions of a lobe can be affected and result in innumerable 5- to 20-mm cystic spaces separated by a variable amount of fibrous tissue (honeycomb lung; see Color Fig. 9–3). Again, these changes are usually most prominent in the lower lobes, particularly the subpleural region; the central portion of the lobes is relatively spared. Traction bronchiectasis is often seen in the more severely affected regions of fibrosis (Fig. 9–22).

Radiologic Manifestations

In patients who have mild disease, the findings usually consist of symmetrical, basal, small to medium-sized irregular linear shadows (reticular pattern, Fig. 9–23).[315,316] Although these opacities may be diffuse throughout both lungs, in 50% to 80% of cases they involve the lower lung zones predominantly or exclusively[317,318]; in 60%, a predominant peripheral distribution is apparent.[70] As the disease progresses, the abnormalities become more diffuse and assume a coarser reticular or reticulonodular pattern associated with progressive loss of volume. Advanced disease is characterized by the presence of

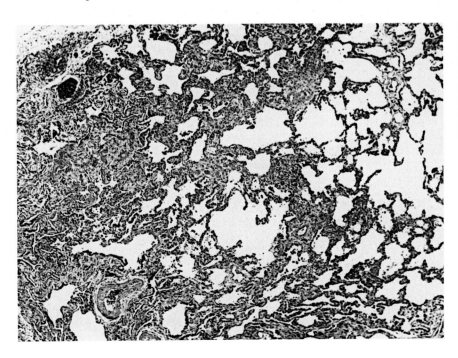

FIGURE 9–20

Usual interstitial pneumonia—variable severity. A low-magnification view of lung parenchyma shows interstitial thickening of variable severity; some alveolar septa are almost normal, whereas others show moderate or marked thickness. (*From Fraser RS, Müller NL, Colman NC, Paré PD: Fraser and Paré's Diagnosis of Diseases of the Chest, 4th ed. Philadelphia, WB Saunders, 1999.*)

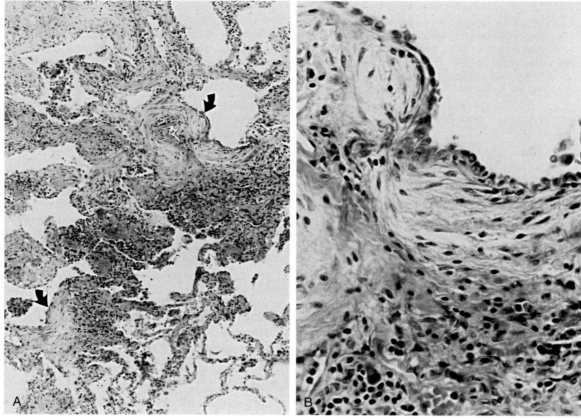

FIGURE 9–21

Usual interstitial pneumonia. Sections show variably severe interstitial thickening by a combination of mononuclear inflammatory cells and collagen. In several areas (*arrows* and magnified view [**B**]), the connective tissue has a loose appearance indicative of active fibrogenesis. *(From Fraser RS, Müller NL, Colman NC, Paré PD: Fraser and Paré's Diagnosis of Diseases of the Chest, 4th ed. Philadelphia, WB Saunders, 1999.)*

cysts measuring 0.5 to 1 cm in diameter (honeycombing).[315,319] Evidence of pleural disease (effusion, pneumothorax, or diffuse thickening) is uncommon.[320]

Decreased lung volumes are radiographically evident at initial evaluation in 50% to 60% of cases.[316,321] We have been impressed by the striking loss of lung volume apparent on serial radiograph studies over a period of several years and believe that a diffuse or predominantly basal reticular pattern accompanied by progressive elevation of the diaphragm strongly suggests the diagnosis of either IPF or progressive systemic sclerosis.[322]

The characteristic finding on HRCT is the presence of irregular intralobular lines of attenuation resulting in a reticular pattern that typically predominantly involves the subpleural lung regions and lower lung zones.[275,323] A patchy distribution consisting of areas that have a reticular pattern intermingled with areas of normal lung is apparent in most patients (Fig. 9–24). The irregular lines are generally associated with irregular pleural, vascular, and bronchial interfaces; evidence of architectural distortion; and dilation of bronchi and bronchioles (traction bronchiectasis and bronchiolectasis).[275,324] Air-containing cysts measuring 2 to 20 mm in diameter (honeycombing) are present in 80% to 90% of patients at diagnosis.[319,325] Serial HRCT scans show an increase in the extent of the reticular pattern and honeycombing in virtually

all cases (Fig. 9–25).[325] Mediastinal lymph node enlargement is evident in 70% to 90% of patients.[326,327]

A confident diagnosis of IPF can be made on CT scan by experienced chest radiologists in about 50% to 70% of cases; such diagnoses are correct about 90% to 100% of the time.[228,328,329] However, the accuracy of interpretation by less experienced observers is substantially lower.[67,79] In one study, the positive predictive value of a confident diagnosis of IPF based on the HRCT findings was 96%.[330] Conditions that can be confused with IPF include progressive systemic sclerosis, rheumatoid arthritis, and asbestosis.[331-333] The latter can usually be distinguished by the presence of pleural plaques. A reticular pattern and honeycombing are also commonly seen in chronic hypersensitivity pneumonitis. However, distinction from IPF can generally be made on HRCT scan by the presence of centrilobular nodules and relative sparing of the lung bases in patients with hypersensitivity pneumonitis.[334]

Clinical Manifestations

Symptoms include progressive dyspnea, nonproductive cough, weight loss, and fatigue.[278] Clubbing is common[335]; its presence can antedate symptoms and other signs of pulmonary disease.[336] Arthralgia and myalgia have been described in patients with early disease.[337] In the early stages, examina-

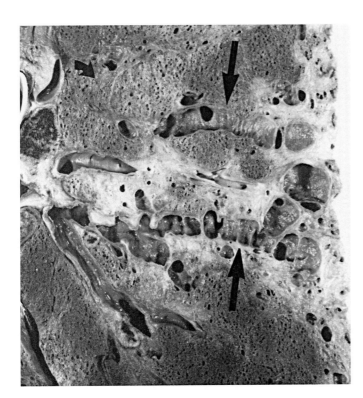

FIGURE 9–22

Idiopathic pulmonary fibrosis—traction bronchiectasis. A magnified view of the midportion of an upper lobe shows patchy fibrosis, most marked in the parenchyma adjacent to the pleura and one bronchus; it is mild elsewhere (*curved arrow*). Two bronchi show a mild to moderate degree of cylindrical bronchiectasis (*straight arrows*). (*From Fraser RS, Müller NL, Colman NC, Paré PD: Fraser and Paré's Diagnosis of Diseases of the Chest, 4th ed. Philadelphia, WB Saunders, 1999.*)

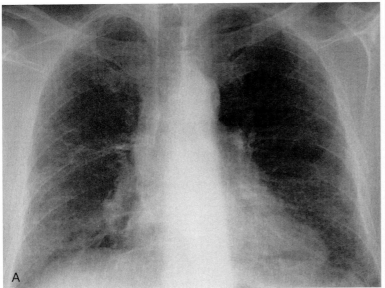

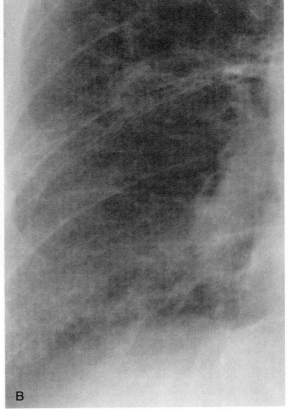

FIGURE 9–23

Idiopathic pulmonary fibrosis. A posteroanterior chest radiograph (**A**) shows irregular linear opacities (reticular pattern) involving predominantly the peripheral regions of the lower lung zones. A magnified view of the right lower lung (**B**) shows the reticular pattern to better advantage. The patient was a 71-year-old man. (*From Müller NL, Fraser RS, Colman NC, Paré PD: Radiologic Diagnosis of Diseases of the Chest. Philadelphia, WB Saunders, 2001.*)

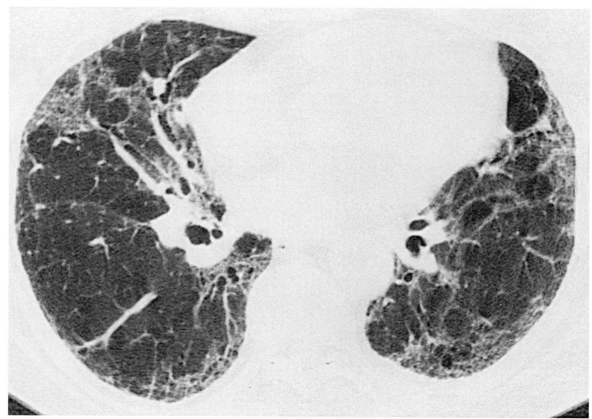

FIGURE 9–24

Idiopathic pulmonary fibrosis. An HRCT scan shows a characteristic variegated pattern consisting of areas with irregular lines, areas with honeycombing, and areas of ground-glass attenuation intermingled with areas of normal lung. The parenchymal abnormalities have a patchy, but predominantly subpleural distribution. The patient was an 80-year-old woman. *(From Müller NL, Fraser RS, Colman NC, Paré PD: Radiologic Diagnosis of Diseases of the Chest. Philadelphia, WB Saunders, 2001.)*

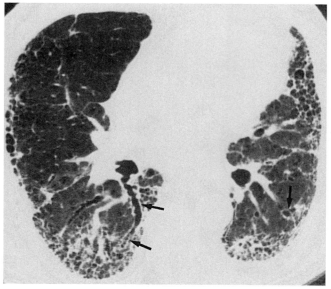

FIGURE 9–25

Idiopathic pulmonary fibrosis: traction bronchiectasis. An HRCT scan shows bilateral honeycombing involving predominantly the subpleural lung regions. Bronchial dilation (traction bronchiectasis) *(arrows)* is evident within the areas of fibrosis, particularly in the right lower lobe. The patient was an 81-year-old man. *(From Müller NL, Fraser RS, Colman NC, Paré PD: Radiologic Diagnosis of Diseases of the Chest. Philadelphia, WB Saunders, 2001.)*

tion of the chest can be within normal limits; however, diffuse crackles, predominantly over the lung bases, are frequently heard as disease becomes more severe.[335] Occasional expiratory crackles may also be heard, particularly when disease is advanced.[338] Cyanosis and signs of pulmonary hypertension and cor pulmonale are late manifestations.

Pulmonary Function Tests

Restrictive derangements in lung function with low diffusing capacity characteristically develop.[339] Most patients have normal or even increased expiratory flow rates when related to absolute lung volume; however, a minority manifest a reduction in the maximum midexpiratory flow rate and FEV_1 relative to the reduction in vital capacity,[340] probably reflecting the effects of cigarette smoking.[341] Indices of airflow obstruction correlate closely with the presence of emphysema as determined by HRCT.[342] Hypoxemia is common at rest and is caused chiefly by $\dot{V}/\dot{Q}$ inequality; however, about 20% of cases can be attributed to a diffusion defect.[343]

A number of abnormalities in tests of exercise performance have been described. Patients typically have a rapid, shallow breathing pattern with total ventilation being excessive for each workload,[344] a finding that is partly related to increased dead space ventilation and partly to hyperventilation. At the same time, maximum ventilatory capacity is reduced.[344] Deterioration in arterial hypoxemia may develop or be present during exercise, largely as a result of diffusion impairment.[343] Although abnormalities in cardiac performance may be evident, exercise limitation is predominantly a result of the respiratory disease.[344] The results of studies examining the relationship between pathologic findings and specific lung function derangements have been inconsistent.[342,345]

Diagnosis

Although the diagnosis if IPF is one of exclusion, careful attention to clinical, functional, and radiologic parameters allows accurate diagnosis in the absence of histologic confirmation in many patients. This is fortunate because the risk of early death after surgical biopsy in such individuals is not insubstantial.[346] By using clinical and HRCT criteria, a diagnosis of IPF can be made in about 75% of patients with a specificity in excess of 90%.[330,347] Open lung biopsy should probably be reserved for patients in whom the radiologic or clinical features of disease are atypical.

Prognosis and Natural History

Deterioration is gradual and inexorable in most patients, with increasing shortness of breath often accompanied by the development of cor pulmonale. Most succumb to respiratory failure, frequently precipitated by infection[348]; about 20% die of cardiac disease.[348] The overall mean survival time is probably less than 5 years.[349,350] A few patients have an acute, severe exacerbation of disease after a period of relative stability[351]; pathologic examination of the lungs of these individuals often shows diffuse alveolar damage. The prognosis in such patients is very poor.[352] Although the pathogenesis of this complication is unclear, the number of cases in which it has been documented suggests that it represents an accelerated phase of IPF rather than an independent process.

When clinical deterioration occurs, progression of IPF must be distinguished from thromboembolism, infection, complications of the disease itself such as pneumothorax and pulmonary carcinoma, and complications of therapy such as steroid-related myopathy, hypokalemia, and uncontrolled diabetes.[353] Given the age of patients usually affected, additional conditions such as ischemic heart disease with left ventricular failure may also explain the increasing breathlessness in some patients.

The incidence of pulmonary carcinoma is increased in patients who have IPF because of the general association between parenchymal scarring of any etiology and pulmonary neoplasia (see page 341). A number of genetic alterations in the epithelial cells of these patients have been described, possibly related to the increased risk.[354,355] The clinical and histologic features of pulmonary carcinoma are similar to those seen in the population at large.[356] Clubbing is an almost invariable finding.[357]

Many attempts have been made to identify specific clinical, functional, laboratory, radiologic, and pathologic features that predict disease progression and mortality. In one well-defined group of patients, survival was significantly worsened in association with increased age at diagnosis, the presence of finger clubbing, absence of cigarette smoking, increased profusion of interstitial opacities, evidence of pulmonary hypertension on the chest radiograph, reduced lung volumes, and gas exchange abnormalities with exercise.[335] The finding of extended survival of current smokers at the time of initial evaluation in compari-

son to never-smokers or ex-smokers was unexpected; although the mechanism of this effect is uncertain, it has been postulated to relate to an inhibitory effect of cigarette smoke on fibroblast function.[335] Although other investigators have shown that severe dyspnea at diagnosis, male sex, and lower diffusion capacity predict poor survival,[301,358] these factors were not found to be independent predictors of survival in this study.

A number of blood and BAL fluid abnormalities have been reported in patients who have IPF; however, none has been shown to have independent prognostic value after considering the clinical, functional, and radiographic findings.[278] A greater extent of fibroblastic foci in biopsy specimens is associated with both decreased survival[331] and a greater decline in lung function at 6 and 12 months.[358] Radiographically and on HRCT, the pattern and extent of parenchymal abnormality and the degree of volume loss correlate with the severity of functional impairment and therefore with the overall prognosis.[359] Reticular changes and honeycombing on HRCT reflect the presence of interstitial fibrosis, whereas areas of ground-glass attenuation usually reflect the presence of inflammation.[360] In the setting of IPF, however, most patients who have ground-glass changes on HRCT progress to frank fibrosis despite treatment with corticosteroids.[361]

Nonspecific Interstitial Pneumonia

NSIP is a form of interstitial lung disease that resembles IPF but is associated with a significantly different course and outcome. Like IPF, it is characterized histologically by a combination of interstitial fibrosis and inflammation (see Color Fig. 9–4); however, the foci of fibroblastic tissue characteristic of UIP are absent, and the overall appearance suggests a single initiating event.[362] Several histologic forms have been described on the basis of the relative proportions of connective tissue and inflammatory cells; the most widely used classification divides the abnormality into two groups: predominantly cellular and predominantly fibrotic.[363] Although the cellular form of NSIP can usually be easily distinguished from UIP histologically, distinction between the fibrotic form and UIP can be difficult, particularly in small biopsy specimens.[364] Even though this difficulty may be the result of sampling error, the observation has given rise to speculation that NSIP is an early stage of UIP, in at least some cases. From a practical point of view, there is evidence that biopsy specimens that show changes of UIP in one lobe and NSIP in another should be regarded as UIP.[365] This is not surprising because this distinction can also be difficult to make histologically.[364,365]

The histologic pattern of NSIP can be seen in a number of clinical contexts, most often connective tissue disease and organic dust exposure (the latter sometimes associated with additional features sufficient to justify a diagnosis of extrinsic allergic alveolitis)[366,367]; occasionally, an infectious cause has been demonstrated.[368] As in the other forms of interstitial pneumonia, an etiology cannot be identified in some patients, and the pneumonia is said to represent idiopathic disease; such a diagnosis must be made after careful exclusion of known causes.

The radiographic manifestations are heterogeneous and range from a predominantly reticular pattern, to mixed reticular and air space patterns, to air space consolidation.[362,369,370] The abnormalities tend to involve the middle and lower lung zones predominantly or exclusively (Fig. 9–26). The most common HRCT manifestation consists of bilateral, symmetrical ground-glass opacities.[371,372] Most scans also show a fine reticular pattern superimposed on the ground-glass opacities, traction bronchiectasis, and architectural distortion (Fig. 9–27).[372,373] Less common findings include areas of consolidation, honeycombing, and centrilobular nodules. The abnormalities may be diffuse, but they involve mainly the lower lung zones in 60% to 90% of cases and predominantly the lung periphery in 50% to 70%.[372,374]

The HRCT manifestations of NSIP can mimic those of UIP, extrinsic allergic alveolitis, and cryptogenic organizing pneumonia.[374] The presence of predominantly ground-glass opacities and absence of honeycombing allow distinction of NSIP from UIP in the majority of cases.[372] However, it may be impossible to distinguish fibrotic NSIP with a predominantly reticular pattern from UIP. Subacute extrinsic allergic alveolitis can usually be distinguished from NSIP by the presence of centrilobular nodules and lobular areas of air trapping.

NSIP accounts for about 5% to 35% of cases in older series of patients considered at the time to have IPF.[375,376] The mean age at onset is about a decade younger than patients who have IPF.[277] Symptoms are the same as those associated with IPF, but they are likely to be less severe and considerably more indolent in progression.

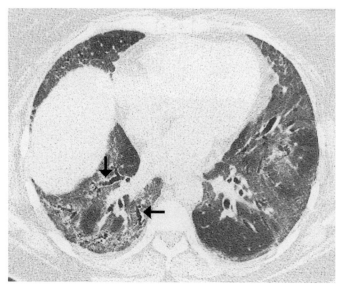

FIGURE 9–27

Nonspecific interstitial pneumonia. An HRCT scan at the level of the right hemidiaphragm shows extensive bilateral ground-glass opacities. Also noted are areas with fine reticulation and traction bronchiectasis (*arrows*), mainly in the right lower lobe. The patient was a 44-year-old woman. (*From Müller NL, Fraser RS, Colman NC, Paré PD: Radiologic Diagnosis of Diseases of the Chest. Philadelphia, WB Saunders, 2001.*)

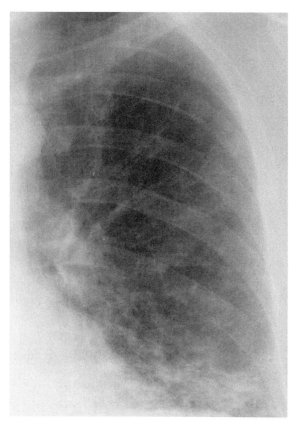

FIGURE 9–26

Nonspecific interstitial pneumonia. A view of the left lung from a posteroanterior chest radiograph shows diffuse ground-glass opacification and focal areas of consolidation as well as irregular linear opacities in the lower lung zone. Similar findings were present in the right lung. (*From Müller NL, Fraser RS, Colman NC, Paré PD: Radiologic Diagnosis of Diseases of the Chest. Philadelphia, WB Saunders, 2001.*)

Patients who have the cellular form of NSIP have an excellent prognosis, but they constitute only a small minority of all patients with the condition.[363,372,377] Patients who have the fibrotic form have a better prognosis than those who have UIP[378,379]; however, their 10-year survival rate is only about 35%.[363,375] In one study, the prognosis of patients whose lung biopsy revealed changes of UIP in one lobe and NSIP in another was that associated with IPF.[377]

Acute Interstitial Pneumonia

In 1935, Hamman and Rich described an acute variety of interstitial lung disease characterized by rapid progression of signs and symptoms leading to death in less than a year.[380] Although this disease was considered for many years to represent a variant of IPF, review of the histologic descriptions of some of Hamman and Rich's patients and more recent studies of patients with similar clinical disease have shown the underlying pathologic abnormality to be diffuse alveolar damage instead of UIP (see Color Fig. 9–5).[381] As a result, the designation "acute interstitial pneumonia (pneumonitis)" has been proposed.[381] As in the other interstitial pneumonias, the histologic pattern of diffuse alveolar damage is associated with a specific etiology in some patients and is idiopathic in others. In addition to these forms of disease, some patients who otherwise have typical IPF clinically and radiologically undergo a phase of rapidly progressive disease whose histologic appearance is that of diffuse alveolar damage.[351] Many of the features of AIP resemble those of acute respiratory distress syndrome (ARDS); however, patients who have AIP have none of the recognized precipitating factors for ARDS and do not develop the multisystem organ failure that is characteristic of it.

The radiologic manifestations are similar to those of ARDS.[381,382] The main abnormality on the chest radiograph is bilateral air space consolidation (Fig. 9–28). HRCT findings consist of extensive bilateral areas of ground-glass attenuation, architectural distortion, traction bronchiectasis, and focal areas of air space consolidation.[382,383] Other common manifestations include intralobular linear opacities, interlobular septal thickening, and thickening of the bronchovascular bundles.[383] An anteroposterior gradient in the ground-glass attenuation or consolidation with a considerable increase in attenuation in the dependent lung regions is present in about 25% of patients.[383]

Patients with AIP have rapidly progressive breathlessness that develops over a period of days to weeks.[384,385] An antecedent viral syndrome is reported by most patients.[384] Cough and dyspnea are frequent, and crackles are common on clinical examination. Neutrophilia and hypoxemia are usually seen.[385] Acute respiratory failure is almost inevitable, and three quarters of affected individuals die,[385] the prognosis being related to the extent of fibrosis on HRCT.[386] Although many survivors do well, persistent interstitial fibrosis or recurrent AIP has been documented in some cases.[385]

Desquamative Interstitial Pneumonia

DIP is a rare disorder that is histologically characterized by relatively uniform parenchymal interstitial fibrosis/inflammation and the presence of numerous cells in the alveolar air spaces (Fig. 9–29). Despite the term "desquamative," it is now recognized that these cells are macrophages rather than sloughed type II cells.[277]

Many authorities consider DIP to be part of a spectrum of smoking-related interstitial lung disease with respiratory bronchiolitis and respiratory bronchiolitis–associated interstitial lung disease, the three differing only in the severity of his-

tologic abnormality.[387,388] However, although the vast majority of cases of DIP occur in cigarette smokers,[277] it should be remembered that the histologic pattern of DIP can be seen rarely in other situations, such as nitrofurantoin therapy[389] and inhalation of particulate matter.[390] The reaction can also be seen focally in association with many other diseases (e.g., Langerhans' cell histiocytosis, carcinoma), and the diagnosis should not be considered definitive by the findings on transbronchial biopsy alone.

The characteristic radiographic pattern consists of symmetrical, bilateral ground-glass opacification, which can be diffuse but usually involves mainly the lower lung zones (Fig. 9–30).[391] In patients who have fibrosis, irregular linear opacities can be seen predominantly in the lower lung zones.[316,392] Radiographs have been reported to be normal in about 5% to 20% of patients who have biopsy-proven disease.[316,392,393]

The predominant abnormality on HRCT scan is the presence of bilateral areas of ground-glass attenuation (see Fig. 9–30).[394,395] These areas can be diffuse but tend to involve mainly the middle and lower lung zones. Irregular lines of attenuation (reticular pattern) suggestive of fibrosis are seen in approximately 50% of cases and mild honeycombing limited to the lung bases in 5% to 30%. Other findings include architectural distortion, traction bronchiectasis, and small cystic changes in areas of ground-glass attenuation.[395]

DIP develops in most patients in the third and fourth decades. Dyspnea on exertion is seen in the majority and cough in about 50%[396]; fever, diaphoresis, weight loss, weakness, myalgia, chest pain, and fatigue occur in a minority. Bibasilar crackles have been described in about 50% of patients; clubbing is somewhat less prevalent. When disease is advanced, cyanosis can be found. Pulmonary function studies may be normal[397] but usually show evidence of a restrictive defect.[396] Associated airflow obstruction may be present,[396] and gas exchange defects are the rule.

Most patients who are treated with corticosteroids have both subjective and objective improvement in the short

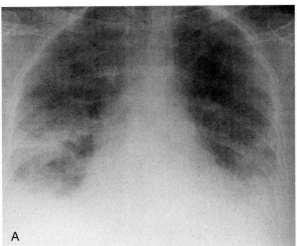
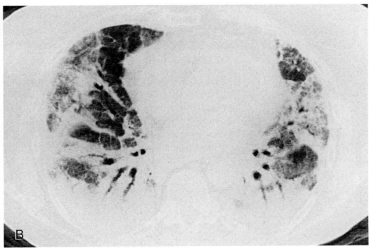

FIGURE 9–28

Acute interstitial pneumonia. A posteroanterior chest radiograph (**A**) shows bilateral areas of consolidation involving predominantly the lower lung zones. A CT scan (**B**) shows areas of consolidation with air bronchograms in the dependent portions of the lower lobes and areas of ground-glass attenuation in the middle lobe and lingula. The patient was an 83-year-old woman. *(From Primack SL, Hartman TE, Ikezoe J, et al: Acute interstitial pneumonia. Radiographic and CT findings in nine patients. Radiology 188:817, 1993.)*

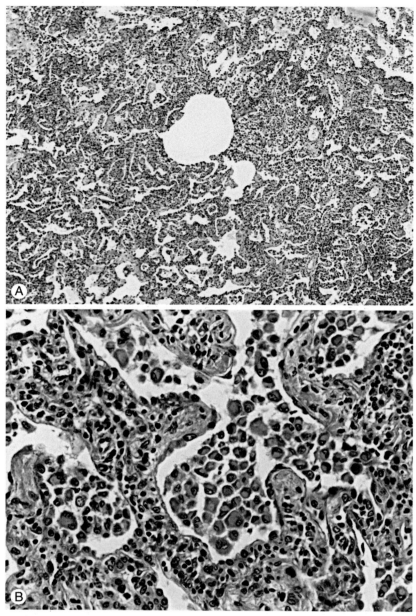

FIGURE 9–29

Desquamative interstitial pneumonitis. A low-magnification view of lung parenchyma
(**A**) shows moderately severe, fairly uniform disease. At higher magnification (**B**),
interstitial thickening can be seen to be caused by a combination of mononuclear
inflammatory cells (predominantly lymphocytes) and a small amount of fibrous tissue; the
adjacent air spaces contain numerous macrophages. *(Courtesy of Dr. Claude Auger, Jean
Talon Hospital, Montreal.)*

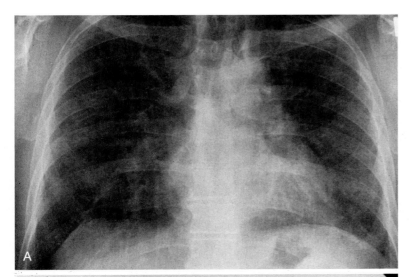

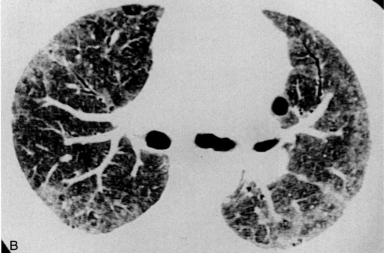

FIGURE 9–30

Desquamative interstitial pneumonia. An anteroposterior chest radiograph (**A**) shows ground-glass opacification throughout all lung zones. An HRCT scan (**B**) shows extensive bilateral ground-glass attenuation most marked in the subpleural lung regions. Incidental note is made of a bulla adjacent to the left heart border. (*From Müller NL, Fraser RS, Colman NC, Paré PD: Radiologic Diagnosis of Diseases of the Chest. Philadelphia, WB Saunders, 2001.*)

term[396]; however, progression of disease despite continued therapy is not uncommon,[361,395,396] and only about half of patients demonstrate persistent improvement 1 year after initiation of therapy.[316] In a study of 40 patients who were monitored for 1 to 22 years, the mortality rate was 28%, and mean survival was 12.2 years.[316]

Respiratory Bronchiolitis–Associated Interstitial Lung Disease

Although the term "respiratory bronchiolitis" has been used to refer to a number of abnormalities histologically, currently it is generally accepted to indicate the accumulation of pigment-laden macrophages in the lumen of first- and second-order respiratory bronchioles and in adjacent alveolar air spaces, accompanied by mild thickening of the airway walls by inflammatory cells and fibrous tissue (see Color Fig. 9–6).[277] The abnormality is invariably associated with cigarette smoke[398] and, in fact, has been considered to be one of the earliest pathologic reactions to this agent. Although most patients with this histologic finding are asymptomatic and have only mild or no evidence of functional airway

obstruction, some have cough, dyspnea, crackles, and a combined restrictive and obstructive pattern on lung function testing. When associated with typical radiologic findings, this condition has been called "respiratory bronchiolitis–associated interstitial lung disease."[398-400] As indicated previously, the abnormality has been considered to represent part of a histologic spectrum of disease that includes DIP.

The radiologic features of respiratory bronchiolitis consist of poorly defined centrilobular nodules or ground-glass opacities (Fig. 9–31).[401] These abnormalities may be diffuse but often involve the upper lobes predominantly or exclusively. The findings in respiratory bronchiolitis–associated interstitial lung disease are similar to those of DIP and consist of ground-glass opacities with or without associated fine reticular or reticulonodular interstitial opacities; in contrast to DIP, however, lung volumes are usually normal.[401] On HRCT, the abnormalities consist of diffuse or patchy areas of ground-glass attenuation or poorly defined centrilobular nodular opacities often superimposed on a background of centrilobular emphysema (Fig. 9–32).[388]

Although the natural history of the condition is uncertain, it improves dramatically with smoking cessation.[232,400]

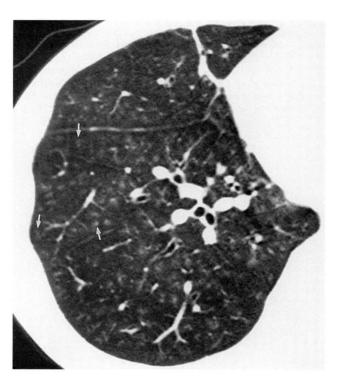

FIGURE 9–31

Respiratory bronchiolitis. A view of the right lower lung from an HRCT scan shows poorly defined centrilobular nodular opacities (*arrows*) and localized areas of ground-glass attenuation. The patient was a 54-year-old heavy smoker who subsequently stopped the habit; a follow-up CT scan performed 5 years later was normal. (*Courtesy of Dr. Takeshi Johkoh, Osaka University Medical School, Osaka, Japan.*)

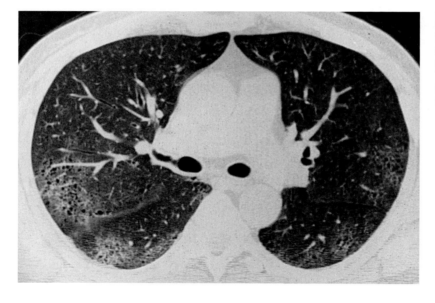

FIGURE 9–32

Respiratory bronchiolitis–associated interstitial lung disease. An HRCT scan shows patchy bilateral areas of ground-glass attenuation and mild centrilobular emphysema. The patient was a heavy smoker. (*Case courtesy of Dr. Kyung Soo Lee, Department of Diagnostic Imaging, Samsung Medical Center, Seoul, South Korea.*)

REFERENCES

1. Yamamoto M, Sharma OP, Hosoda Y: The 1991 descriptive definition of sarcoidosis. Sarcoidosis 9(Suppl):33, 1992.
2. Maycock RL, Bertrand P, Morrison CE, et al: Manifestations of sarcoidosis: Analysis of 145 patients, with a review of nine series selected from the literature. Am J Med 35:67, 1963.
3. Hosoda Y, Sasagawa S, Yasuda Y: Epidemiology of sarcoidosis: New frontiers to explore. Curr Opin Pulm Med 8:424, 2002.
4. Rybicki BA, Maliarik MJ, Popovich J Jr, et al: Epidemiology, demographics and genetics of sarcoidosis. Semin Respir Infect 13:166, 1998.
5. Hsing CT, Han FC, Liu HC, et al: Sarcoidosis among Chinese. Am Rev Respir Dis 89:917, 1964.
6. Rybicki BA, Iannuzzi MC, Frederick MM, et al: Familial aggregation of sarcoidosis. Am J Respir Crit Care Med 164:2085, 2001.
7. Prezant DJ, Dhala A, Goldstein A, et al: The incidence, prevalence, and severity of sarcoidosis in New York City firefighters. Chest 116:1183, 1999.
8. Kajdasz DK, Lackland DT, Mohr LC, Judson MA: A current assessment of rurally linked exposures as potential risk factors for sarcoidosis. Ann Epidemiol 11:111-117, 2001.
9. Edmondstone WM, Wilson AG: Temporal clustering of familial sarcoidosis in nonconsanguineous relatives. Br J Dis Chest 78:184, 1984.
10. Stewart IC, Davidson NM: Clustering of sarcoidosis. Thorax 37:398, 1982.
11. Mitchell DN, Rees RJW: Further observations on the nature and physical characteristics of transmissible agents from human sarcoid and Crohn's disease tissues. In Williams WJ, Davies BH (eds): Eighth International Conference on Sarcoidosis and Other Granulomatous Disease. Cardiff, UK, Omega Publishing, 1978, p 121.
12. Heyll A, Meckenstock G, Aul C, et al: Possible transmission of sarcoidosis via allogenic bone marrow transplantation. Bone Marrow Transplant 14:161, 1994.
13. Burke WM, Keogh A, Maloney PJ, et al: Transmission of sarcoidosis via cardiac transplantation [letter]. Lancet 336:1579, 1990.
14. Grosser M, Lother T, Muller J, et al: Detection of *M. tuberculosis* DNA in sarcoidosis: Correlation with T-cell response. Lab Invest 79:775, 1999.

15. Saboor SA, Johnson NM, McFadden J: Detection of mycobacterial DNA in sarcoidosis and tuberculosis with polymerase chain reaction. Lancet 339:1012-1015, 1992.
16. Almenoff PL, Johnson A, Lesser M, et al: Growth of acid fast L forms in the blood of patients with sarcoidosis. Thorax 51:530, 1996.
17. Vokura M, Lecossier D, du Bois RM, et al: Absence of DNA from mycobacteria of the M. tuberculosis complex in sarcoidosis. Am J Respir Crit Care Med 156:1000, 1997.
18. Conron M, du Bois RM: Immunological mechanisms in sarcoidosis. Clin Exp Allergy 31:543, 2001.
19. Eishi Y, Suga M, Ishige I, et al: Quantitative analysis of mycobacterial and propionibacterial DNA in lymph nodes of Japanese and European patients with sarcoidosis. J Clin Microbiol 40:198, 2002.
20. Valeyre D, Soler P, Clerici C, et al: Smoking and pulmonary sarcoidosis: Effect of cigarette smoking on prevalence, clinical manifestations, alveolitis, and evolution of the disease. Thorax 43:516, 1988.
21. Ravenel JG, McAdams HP, Plankeel JF, et al: Sarcoidosis induced by interferon therapy. AJR Am J Roentgenol 177:199, 2001.
22. Li SD, Yong S, Srinvas D, et al: Reactivation of sarcoidosis during interferon therapy. J Gastroenterol 37:50, 2002.
23. Lenner R, Bregman Z, Teirstein AS, et al: Recurrent pulmonary sarcoidosis in HIV-infected patients receiving highly active antiretroviral therapy. Chest 119:978, 2001.
24. Naccache J-M, Antoine M, Wislez M, et al: Sarcoid-like pulmonary disorder in human immunodeficiency virus–infected patients receiving antiretroviral therapy. Am J Respir Crit Care Med 159:2009, 1999.
25. Rybicki BA, Maliarik MJ, Major M, et al: Genetics of sarcoidosis. Clin Chest Med 18:707, 1997.
26. Rossman M, Thompson B, Frederick M, et al: Sarcoidosis: Association with human leukocyte antigen class II amino acid epitopes and interaction with environmental exposures. Chest 121:14s, 2002.
27. Foley PJ, McGrath DS, Puscinska E, et al: Human leukocyte antigen-DRB1 position 11 residues are a common protective marker for sarcoidosis. Am J Respir Cell Mol Biol 25:272-277, 2001.
28. Schürmann M, Lympany PA, Reichel P, et al: Familial sarcoidosis is linked to the major histocompatibility complex region. Am J Respir Crit Care Med 162:861, 2000.
29. du Bois RM: The genetic predisposition to interstitial lung disease. Chest 121:14s, 2002.
30. Rybicki BA, Maliarik MJ, Malvitgz E, et al: The Influence of T cell receptor and cytokine genes on sarcoidosis susceptibility in African Americans. Hum Immunol 60:867, 1999.
31. Zorzetto M, Bombieri C, Ferraotti I, et al: Complement receptor I gene polymorphisms in sarcoidosis. Am J Respir Cell Mol Biol 27:17, 2002.
32. Yamaguchi E, Itoh A, Hizawa N, et al: The gene polymorphism of tumor necrosis factor-β, but not that of tumor necrosis factor-α, is associated with the prognosis of sarcoidosis. Chest 119:753, 2001.
33. Grutters JC, Sato H, Pantelidis P, et al: increased frequency of the uncommon tumor necrosis factor-857T allele in British and Dutch patients with sarcoidosis. Am J Respir Crit Care Med 165:1119, 2002.
34. Wahlström J, Katchar K, Wigzell H, et al: Analysis of intracellular cytokines in CD4+ and CD8+ lung and blood cells in sarcoidosis. Am J Respir Crit Care Med 163:115, 2001.
35. Zissel G, Bläumer I, Fleischer B, et al: TCR Vβ families in T cell clones from sarcoid lung parenchyma, BAL, and blood. Am J Respir Crit Care Med 156:1593, 1997.
36. Grunewald J, Berlin M, Olerup O, et al: Lung T-helper cells expressing T-cell receptor AV1S3 associate with clinical features of pulmonary sarcoidosis. Am J Respir Crit Care Med 161:814, 2000.
37. Agostini C, Memeghin A, Semenzato G: T-lymphocytes and cytokines in sarcoidosis. Curr Opin Pulm Med 8:435, 2002.
38. Mitchell DN, Scadding JG, Heard BE, et al: Sarcoidosis: Histopathological definition and clinical diagnosis. J Clin Pathol 30:395-408, 1997.
39. Rosen Y, Athanassiades TJ, Moon S, et al: Nongranulomatous interstitial pneumonitis in sarcoidosis. Relationship to development of epithelioid granulomas. Chest 74:122-125, 1978.
40. Rosen Y, Moon S, Huang CT, et al: Granulomatous pulmonary angiitis in sarcoidosis. Arch Pathol Lab Med 101:170-174, 1977.
41. Rossman MD, Daniele RP, Dauber JH: Nodular endobronchial sarcoidosis: A study comparing blood and lung lymphocytes. Chest 79:427-431, 1981.
42. Wollschlager C, Khan F: Aspergillomas complicating sarcoidosis. A prospective study in 100 patients. Chest 86:585-588, 1984.
43. Maarsseveen ACM, Veldhuizen RW, Stan J, et al: A quantitative histomorphologic analysis of lymph node granulomas in sarcoidosis in relation to cardiologic stage I and II. J Pathol 134:441, 1983.
44. De Remee RA: The roentgenographic staging of sarcoidosis: Historic and contemporary perspective. Chest 83:128, 1983.
45. James DG, Neville E, Siltzbach LE, et al: A worldwide review of sarcoidosis. Ann N Y Acad Sci 278:321, 1976.
46. Kirks DR, McCormick VD, Greenspan RH: Pulmonary sarcoidosis: Roentgenologic analysis of 150 patients. AJR Am J Roentgenol 117:77, 1973.
47. Berkmen YM: Radiologic aspects of intrathoracic sarcoidosis. Semin Roentgenol 20:356-375, 1985.
48. Wurm K, Reindell H: [On the differential roentgenological diagnosis of sarcoidosis (Boeck's disease) and lymphogranulomatosis.] Radiologe 2:134-139, 1962.
49. Chiles C, Putman CE: Pulmonary sarcoidosis. Semin Respir Med 13:345, 1992.
50. Spann RW, Rosenow EC 3rd, De Remee RA, et al: Unilateral hilar or paratracheal adenopathy in sarcoidosis: A study of 38 cases. Thorax 26:296, 1971.
51. Wurm K: The stages of pulmonary sarcoidosis. Geriatr Med Monthly 5:386, 1960.
52. Rockoff SD, Rohatgi PK: Unusual manifestations of thoracic sarcoidosis. AJR Am J Roentgenol 144:513, 1985.
53. Rabinowitz JG, Ulreich S, Soriano C: The usual unusual manifestations of sarcoidosis and the "hilar-haze"—a new diagnostic aid. AJR Am J Roentgenol 120:821, 1974.
54. Israel HL, Lenchner G, Steiner RM: Late development of mediastinal calcification in sarcoidosis. Am Rev Respir Dis 124:302, 1981.
55. Müller NL, Kullnig P, Millar RR: The CT findings of pulmonary sarcoidosis: Analysis of 25 patients. AJR Am J Roentgenol 152:1179, 1989.
56. Warshauer DM, Dumbleton SA, Molina PL, et al: Abdominal CT findings in sarcoidosis: Radiologic and clinical correlation. Radiology 192:93, 1994.
57. Murdoch J, Müller NL: Pulmonary sarcoidosis: Changes on follow-up CT examination. AJR Am J Roentgenol 159:473, 1992.
58. Gawne-Cain ML, Hansell DM: The pattern and distribution of calcified mediastinal lymph nodes in sarcoidosis and tuberculosis: A CT study. Clin Radiol 51:263, 1996.
59. Schlossberg O, Sfedu E: Disseminated sarcoidosis. Sarcoidosis 1:149, 1987.
60. Rosen Y, Amorosa JK, Moon S, et al: Occurrence of lung granulomas in patients with stage 1 sarcoidosis. AJR Am J Roentgenol 129:1083, 1977.
61. Epler GR, McLoud TC, Gaensler EA, et al: Normal chest roentgenograms in chronic diffuse infiltrative lung disease. N Engl J Med 298:934, 1978.
62. Hillerdal GN, Nöu E, Osterman K, et al: Sarcoidosis: Epidemiology and prognosis. Am Rev Respir Dis 130:29, 1984.
63. Symmons DPM, Woods KL: Recurrent sarcoidosis. Thorax 35:879, 1980.
64. Stone DJ, Schwartz A: A long-term study of sarcoid and its modification by steroid therapy: Lung function and other factors in prognosis. Am J Med 41:528, 1966.
65. Kirks DR, McCormick VD, Greenspan RH: Pulmonary sarcoidosis: Roentgenologic analysis of 150 patients. AJR Am J Roentgenol 117:777, 1979.
66. Mathieson JR, Mayo JR, Staples CA, et al: Chronic diffuse infiltrative lung disease: Comparison of diagnostic accuracy of CT and chest radiology. Radiology 171:111, 1989.
67. Grenier P, Valeyre D, Cluzel P, et al: Chronic diffuse interstitial lung disease: Diagnostic value of chest radiography and high-resolution CT. Radiology 179:123-132, 1991.
68. Mesbahi SJ, Davies P: Unilateral pulmonary changes in the chest x-ray in sarcoidosis. Clin Radiol 32:283-287, 1981.
69. Müller NL, Mawson JB, Mathieson JR, et al: Sarcoidosis: Correlation of extent of disease at CT with clinical, functional, and radiographic findings. Radiology 171:613-618, 1989.
70. Grenier P, Chevret S, Beigelman C, et al: Chronic diffuse infiltrative lung disease: Determination of the diagnostic value of clinical data, chest radiography, and CT and Bayesian analysis. Radiology 191:383-390, 1994.
71. McLoud TC, Epler GR, Gaensler EA, et al: A radiographic classification for sarcoidosis: Physiologic correlation. Invest Radiol 17:129-138, 1982.
72. Brauner MW, Grenier P, Mompoint D, et al: Pulmonary sarcoidosis: Evaluation with high-resolution CT. Radiology 172:467-471, 1989.
73. Gruden JF, Webb WR: Identification and evaluation of centrilobular opacities on high-resolution CT. Semin Ultrasound CT MR 16:435-449, 1995.
74. Scadding JG: The late stages of pulmonary sarcoidosis. Postgrad Med J 46:530-536, 1970.
75. Rubinstein I, Solomon A, Baum GL, et al: Pulmonary sarcoidosis presenting with unusual roentgenographic manifestations. Eur J Respir Dis 67:335-340, 1985.
76. Remy-Jardin M, Giraud F, Remy J, et al: Pulmonary sarcoidosis: Role of CT in the evaluation of disease activity and functional impairment and in prognosis assessment. Radiology 191:675-680, 1994.
77. Johkoh T, Ikezoe J, Takeuchi N, et al: CT findings in "pseudoalveolar" sarcoidosis. J Comput Assist Tomogr 16:904-907, 1992.
78. Lynch DA, Webb WR, Gamsu G, et al: Computed tomography in pulmonary sarcoidosis. J Comput Assist Tomogr 13:405-410, 1989.
79. Nishimura K, Itoh H, Kitaichi M, et al: Pulmonary sarcoidosis: Correlation of CT and histopathologic findings. Radiology 189:105-109, 1993.
80. Leung AN, Miller RR, Müller NL: Parenchymal opacification in chronic infiltrative lung diseases: CT-pathologic correlation. Radiology 188:209-214, 1993.
81. Nishimura K, Itoh H, Kitaichi M, et al: CT and pathological correlation of pulmonary sarcoidosis. Semin Ultrasound CT MR 16:361-370, 1995.
82. Miller A: The vanishing lung syndrome associated with pulmonary sarcoidosis. Br J Dis Chest 75:209-214, 1981.
83. Primack SL, Hartman TE, Hansell DM, et al: End-stage lung disease: CT findings in 61 patients. Radiology 189:681-686, 1993.
84. Gorske KJ, Fleming RJ: Mycetoma formation in cavitary pulmonary sarcoidosis. Radiology 95:279-285, 1970.
85. Ichikawa Y, Fujimoto K, Shiraishi T, et al: Primary cavitary sarcoidosis: High-resolution CT findings. AJR Am J Roentgenol 163:745, 1994.
86. Biem J, Hoffstein V: Aggressive cavitary pulmonary sarcoidosis. Am Rev Respir Dis 143:428-430, 1991.
87. Freundlich IM, Libshitz HI, Glassman LM, et al: Sarcoidosis. Typical and atypical thoracic manifestations and complications. Clin Radiol 21:376-383, 1970.
88. Dorman RL Jr, Whitman GJ, Chew FS: Thoracic sarcoidosis. AJR Am J Roentgenol 164:1368, 1995.
89. Arakawa H, Niimi H, Kurihara Y, et al: Expiratory high-resolution CT: Diagnostic value in diffuse lung diseases. AJR Am J Roentgenol 175:1537-1543, 2000.

90. Gleeson FV, Traill ZC, Hansell DM: Evidence of expiratory CT scans of small-airway obstruction in sarcoidosis. AJR Am J Roentgenol 166:1052-1054, 1996.
91. Bartz RR, Stern EJ: Airways obstruction in patients with sarcoidosis: Expiratory CT scan findings. J Thorac Imaging 15:285, 2000.
92. Wilen SB, Rabinowitz JG, Ulreich S, et al: Pleural involvement in sarcoidosis. Am J Med 57:200-209, 1974.
93. Lum GH, Poropatich RK: Unilateral pleural thickening. Chest 110:1348-1350, 1996.
94. Gomm SA: An unusual presentation of sarcoidosis—spontaneous haemopneumothorax. Postgrad Med J 60:621-623, 1984.
95. Riedy K, Fisher MR, Belic N, et al: MR imaging of myocardial sarcoidosis. AJR Am J Roentgenol 151:915-916, 1988.
96. Chiles C, Adams GW, Ravin CE: Radiographic manifestations of cardiac sarcoid. AJR Am J Roentgenol 145:711-714, 1985.
97. Myslivecek M, Husak V, Kolek V, et al: Absolute quantitation of gallium-67 citrate accumulation in the lungs and its importance for the evaluation of disease activity in pulmonary sarcoidosis. Eur J Nucl Med 19:1016-1022, 1992.
98. Line BR, Hunninghake GW, Keogh BA, et al: Gallium-67 scanning to stage the alveolitis of sarcoidosis: Correlation with clinical studies, pulmonary function studies, and bronchoalveolar lavage. Am Rev Respir Dis 123:440-446, 1981.
99. Okada M, Takahashi H, Nukiwa T, et al: Correlative analysis of longitudinal changes in bronchoalveolar lavage, ^{67}gallium scanning, serum angiotensin-converting enzyme activity, chest x-ray, and pulmonary function tests in pulmonary sarcoidosis. Jpn J Med 26:360-367, 1987.
100. Tada A: 67 Gallium whole body scintigraphy and single photon emission computed tomography (SPECT) in sarcoidosis. Nippon Rinsho 60:753, 2002.
101. Sulavik SB, Spencer RP, Palestro CJ, et al: Specificity and sensitivity of distinctive chest radiographic and/or ^{67}Ga images in the noninvasive diagnosis of sarcoidosis. Chest 103:403-409, 1993.
102. Klech H, Kohn H, Kummer F, et al: Assessment of activity in sarcoidosis. Sensitivity and specificity of ^{67}gallium scintigraphy, serum ACE levels, chest roentgenography, and blood lymphocyte subpopulations. Chest 82:732-738, 1982.
103. Thrasher DR, Briggs DD Jr: Pulmonary sarcoidosis. Clin Chest Med 3:537-563, 1982.
104. Baughman RP, Teirstein AS, Judson MA, et al: Clinical characteristics of patients in a case control study of sarcoidosis. Am J Respir Crit Care Med 164:1885-1889, 2001.
105. Siltzbach LE, James DG, Neville E, et al: Course and prognosis of sarcoidosis around the world. Am J Med 57:847-852, 1974.
106. Mañá J, Gómez-Vaquero C, Montera A, et al: Löfgren's syndrome revisited: A study of 186 patients. Am J Med 107:240, 1999.
107. Enzenauer RJ, West SG: Sarcoidosis in autoimmune disease. Semin Arthritis Rheum 22:1-17, 1992.
108. Brown JK: Pulmonary sarcoidosis: Clinical manifestations and management. Semin Respir Med 12:215, 1991.
109. Blackmon GM, Raghu G: Pulmonary sarcoidosis: A mimic of respiratory infection. Semin Respir Infect 10:176-186, 1995.
110. Rubinstein I, Baum GL, Hiss Y, et al: Hemoptysis in sarcoidosis. Eur J Respir Dis 66:302-305, 1985.
111. Gardiner IT, Uff JS: Acute pleurisy in sarcoidosis. Thorax 33:124-127, 1978.
112. Soskel NT, Sharma OP: Pleural involvement in sarcoidosis: Case presentation and detailed review of the literature. Semin Respir Med 13:492, 1992.
113. Udwadia ZF, Pilling JR, Jenkins PF, et al: Bronchoscopic and bronchographic findings in 12 patients with sarcoidosis and severe or progressive airways obstruction. Thorax 45:272-275, 1990.
114. Bower JS, Belen JE, Weg JG, et al: Manifestations and treatment of laryngeal sarcoidosis. Am Rev Respir Dis 122:325-332, 1980.
115. Firooznia H, Young R, Lee T: Sarcoidosis of the larynx. Radiology 95:425-428, 1970.
116. Chijimatsu Y, Tajima J, Washizaki M, et al: Hoarseness as an initial manifestation of sarcoidosis. Chest 78:779-781, 1980.
117. Khan MM, Gill DS, McConkey B: Myopathy and external pulmonary artery compression caused by sarcoidosis. Thorax 36:703-704, 1981.
118. Hoffstein V, Ranganathan N, Mullen JB: Sarcoidosis simulating pulmonary veno-occlusive disease. Am Rev Respir Dis 134:809-811, 1986.
119 Sharma OP: Myocardial sarcoidosis. A wolf in sheep's clothing. Chest 106:988-990, 1994.
120. Sharma OP, Maheshwari A, Thaker K: Myocardial sarcoidosis. Chest 103:253-258, 1993.
121. Wait JL, Movahed A: Anginal chest pain in sarcoidosis. Thorax 44:391-395, 1989.
122. Flemming HA: Cardiac sarcoidosis. In James DG (ed): Sarcoidosis and Other Granulomatous Disorders. New York, Marcel Dekker, 1994.
123. Scadding JG: Sarcoidosis. London, Eyre and Spottis Woode, 1967.
124. James DG, Angi MR: Ocular sarcoidosis. In James DG (ed): Sarcoidosis and Other Granulomatous Disorders. New York, Marcel Dekker, 1994.
125. Rothova A: Ocular involvement in sarcoidosis. Br J Ophthalmol 84:110-116, 2000.
126. English JC 3rd, Patel PJ, Greer KE: Sarcoidosis. J Am Acad Dermatol 44:725-743, quiz 744-746, 2001.
127. James DG, Epstein WL: Cutaneous sarcoidosis. In James DG (ed): Sarcoidosis and Other Granulomatous Disorders. New York, Marcel Dekker, 1994.
128. Sheffield EA: Pathology of sarcoidosis. Clin Chest Med 18:741-754, 1997.
129. Spiteri MA, Matthey F, Gordon T, et al: Lupus pernio: A clinico-radiological study of thirty-five cases. Br J Dermatol 112:315-322, 1985.

130. Sherlock S: The liver in sarcoidosis. In James DG (ed): Sarcoidosis and Other Granulomatous Disorders. New York, Marcel Dekker, 1994.
131. Ishak KG: Sarcoidosis of the liver and bile ducts. Mayo Clin Proc 73:467-472, 1998.
132. Devaney K, Goodman ZD, Epstein MS, et al: Hepatic sarcoidosis. Clinicopathologic features in 100 patients. Am J Surg Pathol 17:1272-1280, 1993.
133. Kataria YP, Whitcomb ME: Splenomegaly in sarcoidosis. Arch Intern Med 140:35-37, 1980.
134. James DG: Alimentary tract. In James DG (ed): Sarcoidosis and Other Granulomatous Disorders. New York, Marcel Dekker, 1994.
135. Wallaert B, Colombel JF, Adenis A, et al: Increased intestinal permeability in active pulmonary sarcoidosis. Am Rev Respir Dis 145:1440-1445, 1992.
136. McCormick PA, Feighery C, Dolan C, et al: Altered gastrointestinal immune response in sarcoidosis. Gut 29:1628-1631, 1988.
137. Douglas JG, Gillon J, Logan RF, et al: Sarcoidosis and coeliac disease: An association? Lancet 2:13-15, 1984.
138. Nessan VJ, Jacoway JR: Biopsy of minor salivary glands in the diagnosis of sarcoidosis. N Engl J Med 301:922-924, 1979.
139. Kaplan H: Sarcoid arthritis. A review. Arch Intern Med 112:924-935, 1963.
140. Gran JT, Bohmer E: Acute sarcoid arthritis: A favourable outcome? A retrospective survey of 49 patients with review of the literature. Scand J Rheumatol 25:70-73, 1996.
141. Grigor RR, Hughes GR: Chronic sarcoid arthritis. BMJ 2:1044, 1976.
142. Ost D, Yeldandi A, Cugell D: Acute sarcoid myositis with respiratory muscle involvement. Case report and review of the literature. Chest 107:879-882, 1995.
143. Rizzato G, Montemurro L: The locomotor system. In James DG (ed): Sarcoidosis and Other Granulomatous Disorders. New York, Marcel Dekker, 1994.
144. Shah A, Bhagat R: Digital clubbing in sarcoidosis. Indian J Chest Dis Allied Sci 34:217-218, 1992.
145. Gobel U, Kettritz R, Schneider W, et al: The protean face of renal sarcoidosis. J Am Soc Nephrol 12:616-623, 2001.
146. King BP, Esparza AR, Kahn SI, et al: Sarcoid granulomatous nephritis occurring as isolated renal failure. Arch Intern Med 136:241-245, 1976.
147. Hoffbrand BI: The kidney in sarcoidosis. In James DG (ed): Sarcoidosis and Other Granulomatous Disorders. New York, Marcel Dekker, 1994.
148. Oksanen VE: Neurosarcoidosis. In James DG (ed): Sarcoidosis and Other Granulomatous Disorders. New York, Marcel Dekker, 1994.
149. Sharma OP: Neurosarcoidosis: A personal perspective based on the study of 37 patients. Chest 112:220-228, 1997.
150. Bonnema SJ, Moller J, Marving J, et al: Sarcoidosis causes abnormal seasonal variation in 1,25-dihydroxy-cholecalciferol. J Intern Med 239:393-398, 1996.
151. Delaney P: Neurologic manifestations in sarcoidosis: Review of the literature, with a report of 23 cases. Ann Intern Med 87:336-345, 1977.
152. Karnik AS: Nodular cerebral sarcoidosis simulating metastatic carcinoma. Arch Intern Med 142:385-386, 1982.
153. Chang B, Steimel J, Moller DR, et al: Depression in sarcoidosis. Am J Respir Crit Care Med 163:329-334, 2001.
154. O'Brien GM, Baughman RP, Broderick JP, et al: Paranoid psychosis due to neurosarcoidosis. Sarcoidosis 11:34-36, 1994.
155. Stuart CA, Neelon FA, Lebovitz HE: Disordered control of thirst in hypothalamic-pituitary sarcoidosis. N Engl J Med 303:1078-1082, 1980.
156. Badr AI, Sharma OP: Pulmonary function. In James DG (ed): Sarcoidosis and Other Granulomatous Disorders. New York, Marcel Dekker, 1994.
157. Harrison BD, Shaylor JM, Stokes TC, et al: Airflow limitation in sarcoidosis—a study of pulmonary function in 107 patients with newly diagnosed disease. Respir Med 85:59-64, 1991.
158. Lavergne F, Clerici C, Sadoun D, et al: Airway obstruction in bronchial sarcoidosis: Outcome with treatment. Chest 116:1194-1199, 1999.
159. Shorr AF, Torrington KG, Hnatiuk OW: Endobronchial involvement and airway hyperreactivity in patients with sarcoidosis. Chest 120:881-886, 2001.
160. Winterbauer RH, Hutchinson JF: Use of pulmonary function tests in the management of sarcoidosis. Chest 78:640-647, 1980.
161. Medinger AE, Khouri S, Rohatgi PK: Sarcoidosis: The value of exercise testing. Chest 120:93-101, 2001.
162. Ingram CG, Reid PC, Johnston RN: Exercise testing in pulmonary sarcoidosis. Thorax 37:129-132, 1982.
163. Bradvik I, Wollmer P, Blom-Bulow B, et al: Lung mechanics and gas exchange during exercise in pulmonary sarcoidosis. Chest 99:572-578, 1991.
164. Gibbons WJ, Levy RD, Nava S, et al: Subclinical cardiac dysfunction in sarcoidosis. Chest 100:44-50, 1991.
165. Sietsema KE, Kraft M, Ginzton L, et al: Abnormal oxygen uptake responses to exercise in patients with mild pulmonary sarcoidosis. Chest 102:838-845, 1992.
166. Baydur A, Pandya K, Sharma OP, et al: Control of ventilation, respiratory muscle strength, and granulomatous involvement of skeletal muscle in patients with sarcoidosis. Chest 103:396-402, 1993.
167. Baydur A, Alsalek M, Louie SG, et al: Respiratory muscle strength, lung function, and dyspnea in patients with sarcoidosis. Chest 120:102-108, 2001.
168. Moodley YP, Dorasamy T, Venketasamy S, et al: Correlation of CD4:CD8 ratio and tumour necrosis factor (TNF)alpha levels in induced sputum with bronchoalveolar lavage fluid in pulmonary sarcoidosis. Thorax 55:696-699, 2000.
169. D'Ippolito R, Foresi A, Chetta A, et al: Induced sputum in patients with newly diagnosed sarcoidosis: Comparison with bronchial wash and BAL. Chest 115:1611-1615, 1999.
170. Allen RK, Pierce RJ, Barter CE: Angiotensin-converting enzyme in bronchoalveolar lavage fluid in sarcoidosis. Sarcoidosis 9:54-59, 1992.

171. Brice EA, Friedlander W, Bateman ED, et al: Serum angiotensin-converting enzyme activity, concentration, and specific activity in granulomatous interstitial lung disease, tuberculosis, and COPD. Chest 107:706-710, 1995.

172. Rohatgi PK: Serum angiotensin converting enzyme in pulmonary disease. Lung 160:287-301, 1982.

173. Allen R, Mendelsohn FA, Csicsmann J, et al: A clinical evaluation of serum angiotensin converting enzyme in sarcoidosis. Aust N Z J Med 10:496-501, 1980.

174. Rohrbach MS, DeRemee RA: Pulmonary sarcoidosis and serum angiotensin-converting enzyme. Mayo Clin Proc 57:64-66, 1982.

175. Sharma OP: Vitamin D, calcium, and sarcoidosis. Chest 109:535-539, 1996.

176. Batson JM: Calcification of the ear cartilage associated with the hypercalcemia of sarcoidosis. Report of a case. Nord Hyg Tidskr 265:876-877, 1961.

177. Lower EE, Smith JT, Martelo OJ, et al: The anemia of sarcoidosis. Sarcoidosis 5:51-55, 1988.

178. Kondo H, Sakai S, Sakai Y: Autoimmune haemolytic anaemia, Sjögren's syndrome and idiopathic thrombocytopenic purpura in a patient with sarcoidosis. Acta Haematol 89:209-212, 1993.

179. Renston JP, Goldman ES, Hsu RM, et al: Peripheral blood eosinophilia in association with sarcoidosis. Mayo Clin Proc 75:586-590, 2000.

180. Knodel AR, Beekman JF: Severe thrombocytopenia and sarcoidosis. JAMA 243:258-259, 1980.

181. Hsu RM, Connors AF Jr, Tomashefski JF Jr: Histologic, microbiologic, and clinical correlates of the diagnosis of sarcoidosis by transbronchial biopsy. Arch Pathol Lab Med 120:364-368, 1996.

182. Cohen SH, Fink JN, Garancis JC, et al: Sarcoidosis in hypersensitivity pneumonitis. Chest 72:588-592, 1977.

183. Shorr AF, Torrington KG, Hnatiuk OW: Endobronchial biopsy for sarcoidosis: A prospective study. Chest 120:109-114, 2001.

184. Roethe RA, Fuller PB, Byrd RB, et al: Transbronchoscopic lung biopsy in sarcoidosis. Optimal number and sites for diagnosis. Chest 77:400-402, 1980.

185. Mikhail JR, Mitchell DN, Drury RA, et al: A comparison of the value of mediastinal lymph node biopsy and the Kveim test in sarcoidosis. Am Rev Respir Dis 104:544-550, 1971.

186. Tambouret R, Geisinger KR, Powers CN, et al: The clinical application and cost analysis of fine-needle aspiration biopsy in the diagnosis of mass lesions in sarcoidosis. Chest 117:1004-1011, 2000.

187. Fritscher-Ravens A, Sriram PV, Topalidis T, et al: Diagnosing sarcoidosis using endosonography-guided fine-needle aspiration. Chest 118:928-935, 2000.

188. Cetinkaya E, Yildiz P, Kadakal F, et al: Transbronchial needle aspiration in the diagnosis of intrathoracic lymphadenopathy. Respiration 69:335-338, 2002.

189. Solomon DA, Horn BR, et al: The diagnosis of sarcoidosis by conjunctival biopsy. Chest 74:271-273, 1978.

190. Reich JM: Mortality of intrathoracic sarcoidosis in referral vs population-based settings: Influence of stage, ethnicity, and corticosteroid therapy. Chest 121:32-39, 2002.

191. Gideon NM, Mannino DM: Sarcoidosis mortality in the United States 1979-1991: An analysis of multiple-cause mortality data. Am J Med 100:423-427, 1996.

192. Rabin DL, Richardson MS, Stein SR, et al: Sarcoidosis severity and socioeconomic status. Eur Respir J 18:499-506, 2001.

193. Perry A, Vuitch F: Causes of death in patients with sarcoidosis. A morphologic study of 38 autopsies with clinicopathologic correlations. Arch Pathol Lab Med 119:167-172, 1995.

194. Virmani R, Bures JC, Roberts WC: Cardiac sarcoidosis; a major cause of sudden death in young individuals. Chest 77:423-428, 1980.

195. Neville E, Walker AN, James DG: Prognostic factors predicting the outcome of sarcoidosis: An analysis of 818 patients. Q J Med 52:525-533, 1983.

196. Huhti E, Poukkula A, Lilja M: Prognosis for sarcoidosis in a defined geographical area. Br J Dis Chest 81:381-390, 1987.

197. Viskum K, Vestbo J: Vital prognosis in intrathoracic sarcoidosis with special reference to pulmonary function and radiological stage. Eur Respir J 6:349-353, 1993.

198. Management of pulmonary sarcoidosis. Lancet 1:890-891, 1982.

199. Brauner MW, Lenoir S, Grenier P, et al: Pulmonary sarcoidosis: CT assessment of lesion reversibility. Radiology 182:349-354, 1992.

200. Verstraeten A, Demedts M, Verwilghen J, et al: Predictive value of bronchoalveolar lavage in pulmonary sarcoidosis. Chest 98:560-567, 1990.

201. Laviolette M, La Forge J, Tennina S, et al: Prognostic value of bronchoalveolar lavage lymphocyte count in recently diagnosed pulmonary sarcoidosis. Chest 100:380-384, 1991.

202. Shorr AF, Hnatiuk OW: Circulating D dimer in patients with sarcoidosis. Chest 117:1012-1016, 2000.

203. Kim DS, Paik SH, Lim CM, et al: Value of ICAM-1 expression and soluble ICAM-1 level as a marker of activity in sarcoidosis. Chest 115:1059-1065, 1999.

204. Kobayashi J, Kitamura S: Serum KL-6 for the evaluation of active pneumonitis in pulmonary sarcoidosis. Chest 109:1276-1282, 1996.

205. Hashimoto S, Nakayama T, Gon Y, et al: Correlation of plasma monocyte chemoattractant protein-1 (MCP-1) and monocyte inflammatory protein-1alpha (MIP-1alpha) levels with disease activity and clinical course of sarcoidosis. Clin Exp Immunol 111:604-610, 1998.

206. Selroos O, Gronhagen-Riska C: Angiotensin converting enzyme. III. Changes in serum level as an indicator of disease activity in untreated sarcoidosis. Scand J Respir Dis 60:328-336, 1979.

207. Morell F, Levy G, Orriols R, et al: Delayed cutaneous hypersensitivity tests and lymphopenia as activity markers in sarcoidosis. Chest 121:1239-1244, 2002.

208. Niden AH, Mishkin FS, Salem F, et al: Prognostic significance of gallium lung scans in sarcoidosis. Ann N Y Acad Sci 465:435-443, 1986.

209. Ward K, O'Connor CM, Odlum C, et al: Pulmonary disease progress in sarcoid patients with and without bronchoalveolar lavage collagenase. Am Rev Respir Dis 142:636-641, 1990.

210. Eklund AG, Sigurdardottir O, Ohrn M: Vitronectin and its relationship to other extracellular matrix components in bronchoalveolar lavage fluid in sarcoidosis. Am Rev Respir Dis 145:646-650, 1992.

211. Homolka J, Lorenz J, Zuchold HD, et al: Evaluation of soluble CD 14 and neopterin as serum parameters of the inflammatory activity of pulmonary sarcoidosis. Clin Invest 70:909-916, 1992.

212. Vassallo R, Ryu JH, Colby TV, et al: Pulmonary Langerhans'-cell histiocytosis. N Engl J Med 342:1969-1978, 2000.

213. Howarth DM, Gilchrist GS, Mullan BP, et al: Langerhans cell histiocytosis: Diagnosis, natural history, management, and outcome. Cancer 85:2278-2290, 1999.

214. Yousem SA, Colby TV, Chen YY, et al: Pulmonary Langerhans' cell histiocytosis: Molecular analysis of clonality. Am J Surg Pathol 25:630-636, 2001.

215. Mitchell DN, Rees RJ, Goswami KK: Transmissible agents from human sarcoid and Crohn's disease tissues. Lancet 2:761-765, 1976.

216. Tazi A, Moreau J, Bergeron A, et al: Evidence that Langerhans cells in adult pulmonary Langerhans cell histiocytosis are mature dendritic cells: Importance of the cytokine microenvironment. J Immunol 163:3511-3515, 1999.

217. Fartoukh M, Humbert M, Capron F, et al: Severe pulmonary hypertension in histiocytosis X. Am J Respir Crit Care Med 161:216-223, 2000.

218. Colby TV, Lombard C: Histiocytosis X in the lung. Hum Pathol 14:847-856, 1983.

219. Travis WD, Borok Z, Roum JH, et al: Pulmonary Langerhans cell granulomatosis (histiocytosis X). A clinicopathologic study of 48 cases. Am J Surg Pathol 17:971-986, 1993.

220. Lacronique J, Roth C, Battesti JP, et al: Chest radiological features of pulmonary histiocytosis X: A report based on 50 adult cases. Thorax 37:104-109, 1982.

221. Clark RL, Margulies SI, Mulholland JH: Histiocytosis X. A fatal case with unusual pulmonary manifestations. Radiology 95:631-632, 1970.

222. Moore AD, Godwin JD, Müller NL: Pulmonary histiocytosis X: Comparison of radiographic and CT findings. Radiology 172:249-254, 1989.

223. Brauner MW, Grenier P, Mouelhi MM, et al: Pulmonary histiocytosis X: Evaluation with high-resolution CT. Radiology 172:255-258, 1989.

224. Mogulkoc N, Veral A, Bishop PW, et al: Pulmonary Langerhans' cell histiocytosis: Radiologic resolution following smoking cessation. Chest 115:1452-1455, 1999.

225. Kulwiec EL, Lynch DA, Aguayo SM, et al: Imaging of pulmonary histiocytosis X. Radiographics 12:515-526, 1992.

226. Müller NL, Miller RR: Computed tomography of chronic diffuse infiltrative lung disease. Part 2. Am Rev Respir Dis 142:1440-1448, 1990.

227. Bonelli FS, Hartman TE, Swensen SJ, et al: Accuracy of high-resolution CT in diagnosing lung diseases. AJR Am J Roentgenol 170:1507-1512, 1998.

228. Koyama M, Johkoh T, Honda O, et al: Chronic cystic lung disease: Diagnostic accuracy of high-resolution CT in 92 patients. AJR Am J Roentgenol 180:827, 2003.

229. Friedman PJ, Liebow AA, Sokoloff J: Eosinophilic granuloma of lung. Clinical aspects of primary histiocytosis in the adult. Medicine (Baltimore) 60:385-396, 1981.

230. Tittel PW, Winkler CF: Chronic recurrent pleural effusion in adult histiocytosis-X. Br J Radiol 54:68-69, 1981.

231. Carlson RA, Hattery RR, O'Connell EJ, et al: Pulmonary involvement by histiocytosis X in the pediatric age group. Mayo Clin Proc 51:542-547, 1976.

232. Ryu JH, Colby TV, Hartman TE, et al: Smoking-related interstitial lung diseases: A concise review. Eur Respir J 17:122-132, 2001.

233. Bank A, Christensen C: Unusual manifestation of Langerhans' cell histiocytosis. Acta Med Scand 223:479-480, 1988.

234. Bates DV: Respiratory Function in Disease, 3rd ed. Philadelphia, WB Saunders, 1989.

235. Schonfeld N, Frank W, Wenig S, et al: Clinical and radiologic features, lung function and therapeutic results in pulmonary histiocytosis X. Respiration 60:38-44, 1993.

236. Crausman RS, Jennings CA, Tuder RM, et al: Pulmonary histiocytosis X: Pulmonary function and exercise pathophysiology. Am J Respir Crit Care Med 153:426-435, 1996.

237. Housini I, Tomashefski JF Jr, Cohen A, et al: Transbronchial biopsy in patients with pulmonary eosinophilic granuloma. Comparison with findings on open lung biopsy. Arch Pathol Lab Med 118:523-530, 1994.

238. Auerswald U, Barth J, Magnussen H: Value of CD-1–positive cells in bronchoalveolar lavage fluid for the diagnosis of pulmonary histiocytosis X. Lung 169:305-309, 1991.

239. Vassallo R, Ryu JH, Schroeder DR, et al: Clinical outcomes of pulmonary Langerhans'-cell histiocytosis in adults. N Engl J Med 346:484-490, 2002.

240. Delobbe A, Durieu J, Duhamel A, et al: Determinants of survival in pulmonary Langerhans' cell granulomatosis (histiocytosis X). Groupe d'Etude en Pathologie Interstitielle de la Societe de Pathologie Thoracique du Nord. Eur Respir J 9:2002-2006, 1996.

241. Sadoun D, Vaylet F, Valeyre D, et al: Bronchogenic carcinoma in patients with pulmonary histiocytosis X. Chest 101:1610-1613, 1992.

242. Tomashefski JF, Khiyami A, Kleinerman J: Neoplasms associated with pulmonary eosinophilic granuloma. Arch Pathol Lab Med 115:499-506, 1991.

243. Hancock E, Tomkins S, Sampson J, et al: Lymphangioleiomyomatosis and tuberous sclerosis. Respir Med 96:7-13, 2002.

244. Krymskaya VP, Shipley JM: Lymphangioleiomyomatosis: A complex tale of serum response factor–mediated tissue inhibitor of metalloproteinase-3 regulation. Am J Respir Cell Mol Biol 28:546-550, 2003.

245. Moss J, Avila NA, Barnes PM, et al: Prevalence and clinical characteristics of lymphangioleiomyomatosis (LAM) in patients with tuberous sclerosis complex. Am J Respir Crit Care Med 164:669-671, 2001.
246. Hancock E, Osborne J: Lymphangioleiomyomatosis: A review of the literature. Respir Med 96:1-6, 2002.
247. Pacheco-Rodriguez G, Kristof AS, Stevens LA, et al: Giles F. Filley Lecture. Genetics and gene expression in lymphangioleiomyomatosis. Chest 121:56S-60S, 2002.
248. Brentani MM, Carvalho CR, Saldiva PH, et al: Steroid receptors in pulmonary lymphangiomyomatosis. Chest 85:96-99, 1984.
249. Colley MH, Geppert E, Franklin WA: Immunohistochemical detection of steroid receptors in a case of pulmonary lymphangioleiomyomatosis. Am J Surg Pathol 13:803-807, 1989.
250. Hughes E, Hodder RV: Pulmonary lymphangiomyomatosis complicating pregnancy. A case report. J Reprod Med 32:553-557, 1987.
251. Shen A, Iseman MD, Waldron JA, et al: Exacerbation of pulmonary lymphangioleiomyomatosis by exogenous estrogens. Chest 91:782-785, 1987.
252. Tanaka H, Imada A, Morikawa T, et al: Diagnosis of pulmonary lymphangioleiomyomatosis by HMB45 in surgically treated spontaneous pneumothorax. Eur Respir J 8:1879-1882, 1995.
253. Carrington CB, Cugell DW, Gaensler EA, et al: Lymphangioleiomyomatosis. Physiologic-pathologic-radiologic correlations. Am Rev Respir Dis 116:977-995, 1977.
254. Muir TE, Leslie KO, Popper H, et al: Micronodular pneumocyte hyperplasia. Am J Surg Pathol 22:465-472, 1998.
255. Müller NL, Chiles C, Kullnig P: Pulmonary lymphangiomyomatosis: Correlation of CT with radiographic and functional findings. Radiology 175:335-339, 1990.
256. Lenoir S, Grenier P, Brauner MW, et al: Pulmonary lymphangiomyomatosis and tuberous sclerosis: Comparison of radiographic and thin-section CT findings. Radiology 175:329-334, 1990.
257. Kitaichi M, Nishimura K, Itoh H, et al: Pulmonary lymphangioleiomyomatosis: A report of 46 patients including a clinicopathologic study of prognostic factors. Am J Respir Crit Care Med 151:527-533, 1995.
258. Rappaport DC, Weisbrod GL, Herman SJ, et al: Pulmonary lymphangioleiomyomatosis: High-resolution CT findings in four cases. AJR Am J Roentgenol 152:961-964, 1989.
259. Templeton PA, McLoud TC, Müller NL, et al: Pulmonary lymphangioleiomyomatosis: CT and pathologic findings. J Comput Assist Tomogr 13:54-57, 1989.
260. Taylor JR, Ryu J, Colby TV, et al: Lymphangioleiomyomatosis. Clinical course in 32 patients. N Engl J Med 323:1254-1260, 1990.
261. Crausman RS, Jennings CA, Mortenson RL, et al: Lymphangioleiomyomatosis: The pathophysiology of diminished exercise capacity. Am J Respir Crit Care Med 153:1368-1376, 1996.
262. Kalassian KG, Doyle R, Kao P, et al: Lymphangioleiomyomatosis: New insights. Am J Respir Crit Care Med 155:1183-1186, 1997.
263. Corrin B, Liebow AA, Friedman PJ: Pulmonary lymphangiomyomatosis. A review. Am J Pathol 79:348-382, 1975.
264. Karbowniczek M, Astrinidis A, Balsara BR, et al: Recurrent lymphangiomyomatosis after transplantation: Genetic analyses reveal a metastatic mechanism. Am J Respir Crit Care Med 167:976-982, 2003.
265. Riccardi VM: Von Recklinghausen neurofibromatosis. N Engl J Med 305:1617-1627, 1981.
266. Bourgouin PM, Shepard JO, Moore EH, et al: Plexiform neurofibromatosis of the mediastinum: CT appearance. AJR Am J Roentgenol 151:461-463, 1988.
267. Unger PD, Geller GA, Anderson PJ: Pulmonary lesions in a patient with neurofibromatosis. Arch Pathol Lab Med 108:654-657, 1984.
268. Massaro D, Katz S: Fibrosing alveolitis: Its occurrence, roentgenographic, and pathologic features in von Recklinghausen's neurofibromatosis. Am Rev Respir Dis 93:934-942, 1966.
269. Webb WR, Goodman PC: Fibrosing alveolitis in patients with neurofibromatosis. Radiology 122:289-293, 1977.
270. Rossi SE, Erasmus JJ, McAdams HP, et al: Thoracic manifestations of neurofibromatosis-I. AJR Am J Roentgenol 173:1631-1638, 1999.
271. Patel YD, Morehouse HT: Neurofibrosarcomas in neurofibromatosis: Role of CT scanning and angiography. Clin Radiol 33:555-560, 1982.
272. Schabel SI, Schmidt GE, Vujic I: Overlooked pulmonary malignancy in neurofibromatosis. J Can Assoc Radiol 31:135-136, 1980.
273. Casselman ES, Mandell GA: Vertebral scalloping in neurofibromatosis. Radiology 131:89-94, 1979.
274. Klatte EC, Franken EA, Smith JA: The radiographic spectrum in neurofibromatosis. Semin Roentgenol 11:17-33, 1976.
275. Müller NL, Colby TV: Idiopathic interstitial pneumonias: High-resolution CT and histologic findings. Radiographics 17:1016-1022, 1997.
276. Liebow AA, Carrington CB: The interstitial pneumonias. In Simon M, Potchen EJ, LeMay M (eds): Frontiers of Pulmonary Radiology. New York, Grune & Stratton, 1969, p 102.
277. American Thoracic Society/European Respiratory Society International Multidisciplinary Consensus Classification of the Idiopathic Interstitial Pneumonias. Am J Respir Crit Care Med 165:277, 2002.
278. American Thoracic Society—Idiopathic pulmonary fibrosis: Diagnosis and treatment. Am J Respir Crit Care Med 161:646-664, 2000.
279. Gross TJ, Hunninghake GW: Idiopathic pulmonary fibrosis. N Engl J Med 345:517-525, 2001.
280. Coultas DB, Zumwalt RE, Black WC, et al: The epidemiology of interstitial lung diseases. Am J Respir Crit Care Med 150:967-972, 1994.
281. Mannino DM, Etzel RA, Parrish RG: Pulmonary fibrosis deaths in the United States, 1979-1991. An analysis of multiple-cause mortality data. Am J Respir Crit Care Med 153:1548-1552, 1996.
282. Cherniack RM, Crystal RG, Kalica AR: NHLBI Workshop summary. Current concepts in idiopathic pulmonary fibrosis: A road map for the future. Am Rev Respir Dis 143:680-683, 1991.
283. Geist LJ, Hunninghake GW: Potential role of viruses in the pathogenesis of pulmonary fibrosis. Chest 103:119S-120S, 1993.
284. Kelly BG, Lok SS, Hasleton PS, et al: A rearranged form of Epstein-Barr virus DNA is associated with idiopathic pulmonary fibrosis. Am J Respir Crit Care Med 166:510-513, 2002.
285. Tsukamoto K, Hayakawa H, Sato A, et al: Involvement of Epstein-Barr virus latent membrane protein 1 in disease progression in patients with idiopathic pulmonary fibrosis. Thorax 55:958-961, 2000.
286. Pinsker KL, Schneyer B, Becker N, et al: Usual interstitial pneumonia following Texas A2 influenza infection. Chest 80:123-126, 1981.
287. Iwai K, Mori T, Yamada N, et al: Idiopathic pulmonary fibrosis. Epidemiologic approaches to occupational exposure. Am J Respir Crit Care Med 150:670-675, 1994.
288. Baumgartner KB, Samet JM, Coultas DB, et al: Occupational and environmental risk factors for idiopathic pulmonary fibrosis: A multicenter case-control study. Collaborating Centers. Am J Epidemiol 152:307-315, 2000.
289. Baumgartner KB, Samet JM, Stidley CA, et al: Cigarette smoking: A risk factor for idiopathic pulmonary fibrosis. Am J Respir Crit Care Med 155:242-248, 1997.
290. Tobin RW, Pope CE 2nd, Pellegrini CA, et al: Increased prevalence of gastroesophageal reflux in patients with idiopathic pulmonary fibrosis. Am J Respir Crit Care Med 158:1804-1808, 1998.
291. Hodgson U, Laitinen T, Tukiainen P: Nationwide prevalence of sporadic and familial idiopathic pulmonary fibrosis: Evidence of founder effect among multiplex families in Finland. Thorax 57:338-342, 2002.
292. Wahidi MM, Speer MC, Steele MP, et al: Familial pulmonary fibrosis in the United States. Chest 121:30S, 2002.
293. Thomas AQ, Lane K, Phillips J 3rd, et al: Heterozygosity for a surfactant protein C gene mutation associated with usual interstitial pneumonitis and cellular nonspecific interstitial pneumonitis in one kindred. Am J Respir Crit Care Med 165:1322-1328, 2002.
294. Whitsett JA: Genetic basis of familial interstitial lung disease: Misfolding or function of surfactant protein C? Am J Respir Crit Care Med 165:1201-1202, 2002.
295. Morrison CD, Papp AC, Hejmanowski AQ, et al: Increased D allele frequency of the angiotensin-converting enzyme gene in pulmonary fibrosis. Hum Pathol 32:521-528, 2001.
296. Pantelidis P, Fanning GC, Wells AU, et al: Analysis of tumor necrosis factor-alpha, lymphotoxin-alpha, tumor necrosis factor receptor II, and interleukin-6 polymorphisms in patients with idiopathic pulmonary fibrosis. Am J Respir Crit Care Med 163:1432-1436, 2001.
297. Mori M, Kida H, Morishita H, et al: Microsatellite instability in transforming growth factor-beta 1 type II receptor gene in alveolar lining epithelial cells of idiopathic pulmonary fibrosis. Am J Respir Cell Mol Biol 24:398-404, 2001.
298. Gauldie J: Pro-inflammatory mechanisms are a minor component of the pathogenesis of idiopathic pulmonary fibrosis. Am J Respir Crit Care Med 165:1205-1206, 2002.
299. Selman M, King TE, Pardo A: Idiopathic pulmonary fibrosis: Prevailing and evolving hypotheses about its pathogenesis and implications for therapy. Ann Intern Med 134:136-151, 2001.
300. Douglas WW, Ryu JH, Schroeder DR: Idiopathic pulmonary fibrosis: Impact of oxygen and colchicine, prednisone, or no therapy on survival. Am J Respir Crit Care Med 161:1172-1178, 2000.
301. King TE Jr, Schwarz MI, Brown K, et al: Idiopathic pulmonary fibrosis: Relationship between histopathologic features and mortality. Am J Respir Crit Care Med 164:1025-1032, 2001.
302. Gauldie J, Kolb M, Sime PJ: A new direction in the pathogenesis of idiopathic pulmonary fibrosis? Respir Res 3:1, 2002.
303. Katzenstein AL, Myers JL: Idiopathic pulmonary fibrosis: Clinical relevance of pathologic classification. Am J Respir Crit Care Med 157:1301-1315, 1998.
304. Allen JT, Spiteri MA: Growth factors in idiopathic pulmonary fibrosis: Relative roles. Respir Res 3:13, 2002.
305. Gunther A, Schmidt R, Nix F, et al: Surfactant abnormalities in idiopathic pulmonary fibrosis, hypersensitivity pneumonitis and sarcoidosis. Eur Respir J 14:565-573, 1999.
306. Barbas-Filho JV, Ferreira MA, Sesso A, et al: Evidence of type II pneumocyte apoptosis in the pathogenesis of idiopathic pulmonary fibrosis (IPF)/usual interstitial pneumonia (UIP). J Clin Pathol 54:132-138, 2001.
307. Kuwano K, Hagimoto N, Kawasaki M, et al: Essential roles of the Fas-Fas ligand pathway in the development of pulmonary fibrosis. J Clin Invest 104:13-19, 1999.
308. Fujii M, Hayakawa H, Urano T, et al: Relevance of tissue factor and tissue factor pathway inhibitor for hypercoagulable state in the lungs of patients with idiopathic pulmonary fibrosis. Thromb Res 99:111-117, 2000.
309. Sheppard MN, Harrison NK: New perspectives on basic mechanisms in lung disease. 1. Lung injury, inflammatory mediators, and fibroblast activation in fibrosing alveolitis. Thorax 47:1064-1074, 1992.
310. Kolb M, Bonniaud P, Galt T, et al: Differences in the fibrogenic response after transfer of active transforming growth-beta1 gene to lungs of "fibrosis-prone" and "fibrosis-resistant" mouse strains. Am J Respir Cell Mol Biol 27:141-150, 2002.

311. Crystal RG, Bitterman PB, Mossman B, et al: Future research directions in idiopathic pulmonary fibrosis: Summary of a National Heart, Lung, and Blood Institute working group. Am J Respir Crit Care Med 166:236-246, 2002.
312. Marshall RP, McAnulty RJ, Laurent GJ: Angiotensin II is mitogenic for human lung fibroblasts via activation of the type 1 receptor. Am J Respir Crit Care Med 161:1999-2004, 2000.
313. Keane MP, Belperio JA, Burdick MD, et al: ENA-78 is an important angiogenic factor in idiopathic pulmonary fibrosis. Am J Respir Crit Care Med 164:2239-2242, 2001.
314. Streiter RM: Mechanisms of pulmonary fibrosis—Conference summary. Chest 120:77S, 2001.
315. McAdams HP, Rosado-de-Christenson ML, Wehunt WD, et al: The alphabet soup revisited: The chronic interstitial pneumonias in the 1990s. Radiographics 16:1009-1033, discussion 1033-1034, 1996.
316. Carrington CB, Gaensler EA, Coutu RE, et al: Natural history and treated course of usual and desquamative interstitial pneumonia. N Engl J Med 298:801-809, 1978.
317. Müller NL, Guerry-Force ML, Staples CA, et al: Differential diagnosis of bronchiolitis obliterans with organizing pneumonia and usual interstitial pneumonia: Clinical, functional, and radiologic findings. Radiology 162:151-156, 1987.
318. McLoud TC, Carrington CB, Gaensler EA: Diffuse infiltrative lung disease: A new scheme for description. Radiology 149:353-363, 1983.
319. Staples CA, Müller NL, Vedal S, et al: Usual interstitial pneumonia: Correlation of CT with clinical, functional, and radiologic findings. Radiology 162:377-381, 1987.
320. Picado C, Gomez de Almeida R, Xaubet A, et al: Spontaneous pneumothorax in cryptogenic fibrosing alveolitis. Respiration 48:77-80, 1985.
321. Kawabata H, Nagai S, Hayashi M, et al: Significance of lung shrinkage on CXR as a prognostic factor in patients with idiopathic pulmonary fibrosis. Respirology 8:351-358, 2003.
322. Feigin DS: New perspectives on interstitial lung disease. Radiol Clin North Am 21:683-697, 1983.
323. Müller NL, Miller RR, Webb WR, et al: Fibrosing alveolitis: CT-pathologic correlation. Radiology 160:585-588, 1986.
324. Nishimura K, Kitaichi M, Izumi T, et al: Usual interstitial pneumonia: Histologic correlation with high-resolution CT. Radiology 182:342, 1992.
325. Akira M, Sakatani M, Ueda E: Idiopathic pulmonary fibrosis: Progression of honeycombing at thin-section CT. Radiology 189:687-691, 1993.
326. Bergin C, Castellino RA: Mediastinal lymph node enlargement on CT scans in patients with usual interstitial pneumonitis. AJR Am J Roentgenol 154:251-254, 1990.
327. Niimi H, Kang EY, Kwong JS, et al: CT of chronic infiltrative lung disease: Prevalence of mediastinal lymphadenopathy. J Comput Assist Tomogr 20:305-308, 1996.
328. Mathieson JR, Mayo JR, Staples CA, et al: Chronic diffuse infiltrative lung disease: Comparison of diagnostic accuracy of CT and chest radiography. Radiology 171:111, 1989.
329. Swensen SJ, Aughenbaugh GL, Myers JL: Diffuse lung disease: Diagnostic accuracy of CT in patients undergoing surgical biopsy of the lung. Radiology 205:229, 1997.
330. Hunninghake GW, Zimmerman MB, Schwartz DA, et al: Utility of a lung biopsy for the diagnosis of idiopathic pulmonary fibrosis. Am J Respir Crit Care Med 164:193, 2001.
331. King TE Jr, Costabel U, Cordier J-F, et al: Idiopathic pulmonary fibrosis: Diagnosis and treatment. Consensus statement. Am J Respir Crit Care Med 161:646, 2000.
332. Aberle DR, Gamsu G, Ray CS, et al: Asbestos-related pleural and parenchymal fibrosis: Detection with high-resolution CT. Radiology 166:729-734, 1988.
333. Johkoh T, Ikezoe J, Kohno N, et al: High-resolution CT and pulmonary function tests in collagen vascular disease: Comparison with idiopathic pulmonary fibrosis. Eur J Radiol 18:113-121, 1994.
334. Lynch DA, Newell JD, Logan PM, et al: Can CT distinguish hypersensitivity pneumonitis from idiopathic pulmonary fibrosis? AJR Am J Roentgenol 165:807-811, 1995.
335. King TE Jr, Tooze JA, Schwarz MI, et al: Predicting survival in idiopathic pulmonary fibrosis: Scoring system and survival model. Am J Respir Crit Care Med 164:1171-1181, 2001.
336. Kanematsu T, Kitaichi M, Nishimura K, et al: Clubbing of the fingers and smooth-muscle proliferation in fibrotic changes in the lung in patients with idiopathic pulmonary fibrosis. Chest 105:339-342, 1994.
337. Patchefsky AS, Banner M, Freundlich IM: Desquamative interstitial pneumonia. Significance of intranuclear viral-like inclusion bodies. Ann Intern Med 74:322-327, 1971.
338. Walshaw MJ, Nisar M, Pearson MG, et al: Expiratory lung crackles in patients with fibrosing alveolitis. Chest 97:407-409, 1990.
339. Agusti C, Xaubet A, Agusti AG, et al: Clinical and functional assessment of patients with idiopathic pulmonary fibrosis: Results of a 3 year follow-up. Eur Respir J 7:643-650, 1994.
340. Pande JN: Interrelationship between lung volume, expiratory flow, and lung transfer factor in fibrosing alveolitis. Thorax 36:858-862, 1981.
341. Cherniack RM, Colby TV, Flint A, et al: Correlation of structure and function in idiopathic pulmonary fibrosis. Am J Respir Crit Care Med 151:1180-1188, 1995.
342. Wells AU, King AD, Rubens MB, et al: Lone cryptogenic fibrosing alveolitis: A functional-morphologic correlation based on extent of disease on thin-section computed tomography. Am J Respir Crit Care Med 155:1367-1375, 1997.
343. Agusti AG, Roca J, Gea J, et al: Mechanisms of gas-exchange impairment in idiopathic pulmonary fibrosis. Am Rev Respir Dis 143:219-225, 1991.
344. Marciniuk DD, Watts RE, Gallagher CG: Dead space loading and exercise limitation in patients with interstitial lung disease. Chest 105:183-189, 1994.
345. Chinet T, Jaubert F, Dusser D, et al: Effects of inflammation and fibrosis on pulmonary function in diffuse lung fibrosis. Thorax 45:675-678, 1990.
346. Utz JP, Ryu JH, Douglas WW, et al: High short-term mortality following lung biopsy for usual interstitial pneumonia. Eur Respir J 17:175-179, 2001.
347. Raghu G, Mageto YN, Lockhart D, et al: The accuracy of the clinical diagnosis of new-onset idiopathic pulmonary fibrosis and other interstitial lung disease: A prospective study. Chest 116:1168-1174, 1999.
348. Stack BH, Choo-Kang YF, Heard BE: The prognosis of cryptogenic fibrosing alveolitis. Thorax 27:535-542, 1972.
349. Mapel DW, Hunt WC, Utton R, et al: Idiopathic pulmonary fibrosis: Survival in population based and hospital based cohorts. Thorax 53:469-476, 1998.
350. Hubbard R, Johnston I, Britton J: Survival in patients with cryptogenic fibrosing alveolitis: A population-based cohort study. Chest 113:396-400, 1998.
351. Kondoh Y, Taniguchi H, Kawabata Y, et al: Acute exacerbation in idiopathic pulmonary fibrosis. Analysis of clinical and pathologic findings in three cases. Chest 103:1808-1812, 1993.
352. Stern JB, Mal H, Groussard O, et al: Prognosis of patients with advanced idiopathic pulmonary fibrosis requiring mechanical ventilation for acute respiratory failure. Chest 120:213-219, 2001.
353. Panos RJ, Mortenson RL, Niccoli SA, et al: Clinical deterioration in patients with idiopathic pulmonary fibrosis: Causes and assessment. Am J Med 88:396-404, 1990.
354. Vassilakis DA, Sourvinos G, Spandidos DA, et al: Frequent genetic alterations at the microsatellite level in cytologic sputum samples of patients with idiopathic pulmonary fibrosis. Am J Respir Crit Care Med 162:1115-1119, 2000.
355. Takahashi T, Munakata M, Ohtsuka Y, et al: Expression and alteration of ras and p53 proteins in patients with lung carcinoma accompanied by idiopathic pulmonary fibrosis. Cancer 95:624-633, 2002.
356. Park J, Kim DS, Shim TS, et al: Lung cancer in patients with idiopathic pulmonary fibrosis. Eur Respir J 17:1216-1219, 2001.
357. Turner-Warwick M, Burrows B, Johnson A: Cryptogenic fibrosing alveolitis: Clinical features and their influence on survival. Thorax 35:171-180, 1980.
358. Nicholson AG, Fulford LG, Colby TV, et al: The relationship between individual histologic features and disease progression in idiopathic pulmonary fibrosis. Am J Respir Crit Care Med 166:173-177, 2002.
359. Gay SE, Kazerooni EA, Toews GB, et al: Idiopathic pulmonary fibrosis: Predicting response to therapy and survival. Am J Respir Crit Care Med 157:1063-1072, 1998.
360. Kazerooni EA, Martinez FJ, Flint A, et al: Thin-section CT obtained at 10-mm increments versus limited three-level thin-section CT for idiopathic pulmonary fibrosis: Correlation with pathologic scoring. AJR Am J Roentgenol 169:977-983, 1997.
361. Hartman TE, Primack SL, Kang EY, et al: Disease progression in usual interstitial pneumonia compared with desquamative interstitial pneumonia. Assessment with serial CT. Chest 110:378-382, 1996.
362. Katzenstein AL, Fiorelli RF: Nonspecific interstitial pneumonia/fibrosis. Histologic features and clinical significance. Am J Surg Pathol 18:136-147, 1994.
363. Travis WD, Matsui K, Moss J, et al: Idiopathic nonspecific interstitial pneumonia: Prognostic significance of cellular and fibrosing patterns: Survival comparison with usual interstitial pneumonia and desquamative interstitial pneumonia. Am J Surg Pathol 24:19-33, 2000.
364. Katzenstein A-L, Myers JL: Nonspecific interstitial pneumonia and the other idiopathic interstitial pneumonias: Classification and diagnostic criteria. Am J Surg Pathol 24:1, 2000.
365. Flaherty KR, Travis WD, Colby TV, et al: Histopathologic variability in usual and nonspecific interstitial pneumonias. Am J Respir Crit Care Med 164:1722-1727, 2001.
366. Bouros D, Wells AU, Nicholson AG, et al: Histopathologic subsets of fibrosing alveolitis in patients with systemic sclerosis and their relationship to outcome. Am J Respir Crit Care Med 165:1581-1586, 2002.
367. Vourlekis JS, Schwarz MI, Cool CD, et al: Nonspecific interstitial pneumonitis as the sole histologic expression of hypersensitivity pneumonitis. Am J Med 112:490-493, 2002.
368. Sattler F, Nichols L, Hirano L, et al: Nonspecific interstitial pneumonitis mimicking Pneumocystis carinii pneumonia. Am J Respir Crit Care Med 156:912-917, 1997.
369. Katoh T, Andoh T, Mikawa K, et al: Computed tomographic findings in nonspecific interstitial pneumonia/fibrosis. Respirology 3:69-75, 1998.
370. Park JS, Lee KS, Kim JS, et al: Nonspecific interstitial pneumonia with fibrosis: Radiographic and CT findings in seven patients. Radiology 195:645-648, 1995.
371. Kim TS, Lee KS, Chung MP, et al: Nonspecific interstitial pneumonia with fibrosis: High resolution CT and pathologic findings. AJR Am J Roentgenol 171:1645, 1998.
372. Johkoh T, Müller NL, Colby TV, et al: Nonspecific interstitial pneumonia: Correlation between thin-section CT findings and pathologic subgroups in 55 patients. Radiology 225:199, 2002.
373. MacDonald SL, Rubens MB, Hansell DM, et al: Nonspecific interstitial pneumonia and usual interstitial pneumonia: Comparative appearances at and diagnostic accuracy of thin-section CT. Radiology 221:600, 2001.
374. Hartman TE, Swensen SJ, Hansell DM, et al: Non-specific interstitial pneumonitis: Variable appearance at high resolution chest CT. Radiology 217:701, 2000.

375. Nicholson AG, Colby TV, du Bois RM, et al: The prognostic significance of the histologic pattern of interstitial pneumonia in patients presenting with the clinical entity of cryptogenic fibrosing alveolitis. Am J Respir Crit Care Med 162:2213-2217, 2000.
376. Bjoraker JA, Ryu JH, Edwin MK, et al: Prognostic significance of histopathologic subsets in idiopathic pulmonary fibrosis. Am J Respir Crit Care Med 157:199-203, 1998.
377. Flaherty KR, Travis WD, Colby TV, et al: Histopathologic variability in usual and nonspecific interstitial pneumonia. Am J Respir Crit Care Med 164:1722, 2001.
378. Daniil ZD, Gilchrist FC, Nicholson AG, et al: A histologic pattern of nonspecific interstitial pneumonia is associated with a better prognosis than usual interstitial pneumonia in patients with cryptogenic fibrosing alveolitis. Am J Respir Crit Care Med 160:899-905, 1999.
379. Flaherty KR, Toews GB, Travis WD, et al: Clinical significance of histological classification of idiopathic interstitial pneumonia. Eur Respir J 19:275-283, 2002.
380. Hamman L, Rich AR: Fulminating diffuse interstitial fibrosis of the lungs. Trans Am Climatol Assoc 51:154, 1935.
381. Katzenstein AL, Myers JL, Mazur MT: Acute interstitial pneumonia. A clinicopathologic, ultrastructural, and cell kinetic study. Am J Surg Pathol 10:256-267, 1986.
382. Primack SL, Hartman TE, Ikezoe J, et al: Acute interstitial pneumonia: Radiographic and CT findings in nine patients. Radiology 188:817-820, 1993.
383. Johkoh T, Müller NL, Taniguchi H, et al: Acute interstitial pneumonia: Thin-section CT findings in 36 patients. Radiology 211:859-863, 1999.
384. Bouros D, Nicholson AC, Polychronopoulos V, et al: Acute interstitial pneumonia. Eur Respir J 15:412-418, 2000.
385. Vourlekis JS, Brown KK, Cool CD, et al: Acute interstitial pneumonitis. Case series and review of the literature. Medicine (Baltimore) 79:369-378, 2000.
386. Ichikado K, Suga M, Müller NL, et al: Acute interstitial pneumonia: Comparison of high-resolution computed tomography findings between survivors and nonsurvivors. Am J Respir Crit Care Med 165:1551-1556, 2002.
387. Moon J, du Bois RM, Colby TV, et al: Clinical significance of respiratory bronchiolitis on open lung biopsy and its relationship to smoking related interstitial lung disease. Thorax 54:1009-1014, 1999.
388. Heyneman LE, Ward S, Lynch DA, et al: Respiratory bronchiolitis, respiratory bronchiolitis-associated interstitial lung disease, and desquamative interstitial pneumonia: Different entities or part of the spectrum of the same disease process? AJR Am J Roentgenol 173:1617-1622, 1999.
389. Bone RC, Wolfe J, Sobonya RE, et al: Desquamative interstitial pneumonia following long-term nitrofurantoin therapy. Am J Med 60:697-701, 1976.
390. Lougheed MD, Roos JO, Waddell WR, et al: Desquamative interstitial pneumonitis and diffuse alveolar damage in textile workers. Potential role of mycotoxins. Chest 108:1196-1200, 1995.
391. Gaensler EA, Goff AM, Prowse CM: Desquamative interstitial pneumonia. N Engl J Med 274:113-128, 1966.
392. Feigin DS, Friedman PJ: Chest radiography in desquamative interstitial pneumonitis: A review of 37 patients. AJR Am J Roentgenol 134:91-99, 1980.
393. Padley SP, Hansell DM, Flower CD, et al: Comparative accuracy of high resolution computed tomography and chest radiography in the diagnosis of chronic diffuse infiltrative lung disease. Clin Radiol 44:222-226, 1991.
394. Hartman TE, Primack SL, Swensen SJ, et al: Desquamative interstitial pneumonia: Thin-section CT findings in 22 patients. Radiology 187:787, 1993.
395. Akira M, Yamamoto S, Hara H, et al: Serial computed tomographic evaluation in desquamative interstitial pneumonia. Thorax 52:333, 1997.
396. Tubbs RR, Benjamin SP, Reich NE, et al: Desquamative interstitial pneumonitis. Cellular phase of fibrosing alveolitis. Chest 72:159-165, 1977.
397. Liebow AA, Steer A, Billingsley JG: Desquamative interstitial pneumonia. Am J Med 39:369-404, 1965.
398. Yousem SA, Colby TV, Gaensler EA: Respiratory bronchiolitis-associated interstitial lung disease and its relationship to desquamative interstitial pneumonia. Mayo Clin Proc 64:1373-1380, 1989.
399. Bosi F, Oggionni T, Vaiana E, et al: Respiratory bronchiolitis-associated interstitial lung disease: A case report with bronchoalveolar lavage findings. Monaldi Arch Chest Dis 50:448-450, 1995.
400. King TE Jr: Respiratory bronchiolitis-associated interstitial lung disease. Clin Chest Med 14:693-698, 1993.
401. Müller NL, Miller RR: Diseases of the bronchioles: CT and histopathologic findings. Radiology 196:3-12, 1995.

IMMUNOLOGIC LUNG DISEASE

CONNECTIVE TISSUE DISEASE

The autoimmune connective tissue diseases comprise a group of disorders whose common denominator is damage to components of connective tissue at a variety of sites in the body. At initial evaluation, full clinical expression may be absent, and it may be difficult to place patients in a particular diagnostic category. Ultimately, however, a definitive diagnosis is often possible by considering information derived from laboratory, radiologic, and pathologic studies in concert with the clinical findings. The manifestations of respiratory system involvement vary in type and severity among the different diseases, but in each, such involvement can be a cause of considerable morbidity and, occasionally, mortality.

Systemic Lupus Erythematosus

Systemic lupus erythematosus (SLE) is a multisystem autoimmune disorder characterized by loss of self-tolerance to nuclear autoantigens.[1] The clinical manifestations are varied and probably related to a complex intertwining of genetic,

environmental, hormonal, and immunologic influences.[2-5] Because of this complexity, several diagnostic criteria have been proposed (Table 10–1). The diagnosis can be made confidently when four criteria are met sequentially or simultaneously during any period of observation. However, many patients fail to meet the complete diagnostic criteria[6]; those who have these "lupus-like" disorders tend to have a good prognosis, even with conservative management.

The estimated incidence of SLE is 7.3 per 100,000[7]; estimates of prevalence have been as high as 124 per 100,000 population in the United States.[8] Women are affected 10 times more often than men,[9] and African Americans have an especially high prevalence.[10] Overall, about 50% to 60% of patients have clinically evident pleuropulmonary involvement at some time in the course of the disease.[11]

Pathologic Characteristics

At autopsy, pathologic changes in the lungs and pleura are common in patients who have SLE.[12,13] However, because of the frequent involvement of other organs and tissues, it is not

TABLE 10–1. Clinical Features of Classic Systemic Lupus Erythematosus

Rash	Serositis
Discoid lupus	Renal disorder
Photosensitivity	Neurologic disorder
Oral ulcers	Hematologic disorder
Arthritis	Immunologic disorder

From Panush RS, Greer JM, Morshedian KK: What is lupus? What is not lupus? Rheum Dis Clin North Am 19:223, 1993.

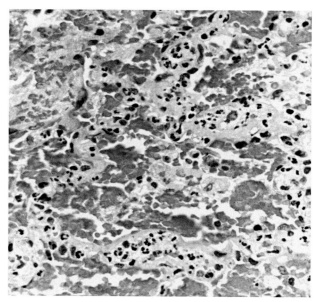

FIGURE 10–1

Systemic lupus erythematosus—capillaritis with pulmonary hemorrhage. A magnified view of lung parenchyma shows several alveolar air spaces filled with red blood cells. The adjacent septa contain a moderate number of neutrophils, some of which appear fragmented (×300). *(From Fraser RS, Müller NL, Colman NC, Paré PD: Fraser and Paré's Diagnosis of Diseases of the Chest, 4th ed. Philadelphia, WB Saunders, 1999.)*

always clear in an individual patient which of these changes is related to a direct effect of SLE and which to an effect of therapy or complicating disease in the lungs or another site. In many instances, it is probably the latter that is important.[12] Pathologic findings that have been proposed as being caused by SLE itself include pleuritis and pleural fibrosis (with or without effusion), interstitial pneumonitis and fibrosis, vasculitis, pulmonary arterial hypertension, lymphocytic interstitial pneumonitis (LIP), and follicular bronchiolitis.[14]

Pleural fibrosis is the most common finding at autopsy and has been reported in as many as 80% to 100% of cases in some series[15]; acute fibrinous pleuritis is seen less frequently. Parenchymal interstitial inflammation and fibrosis are uncommon; in a series of 120 patients, only 5 cases were identified.[12] Pathologic findings in these cases are those of nonspecific interstitial pneumonia or, less commonly, usual interstitial pneumonia.[14]

"Acute lupus pneumonitis" refers to an uncommon manifestation of SLE characterized by fever, dyspnea, hypoxemia, and patchy, diffuse radiographic opacities in the absence of infection. Pathologic features in these patients are variable. Some cases show diffuse alveolar damage (intra-alveolar proteinaceous exudate, hyaline membranes, and an interstitial mononuclear inflammatory infiltrate),[16] whereas others show capillaritis and alveolar hemorrhage (Fig. 10–1).[17]

Pulmonary hypertension in SLE is characterized pathologically by intimal fibrosis, medial hypertrophy, and (sometimes) plexiform lesions (plexogenic arteriopathy).[18] The vessels of some patients who have antiphospholipid syndrome show concentric intimal hyperplasia.[19]

Radiologic Manifestations

Radiologic abnormalities may be seen in the lungs, pleura, and heart, alone or in combination. The most common manifestation is pleural effusion, which occurs in 20% to 35% of patients.[20,21] Pericardial effusion is seen in approximately 20% of patients, and pulmonary involvement in 20%. Pleural effusion is frequently bilateral; though usually small (Fig. 10–2), it may be massive. The effusion may resolve completely or result in mild residual pleural thickening.[22]

Radiologic abnormalities in the lungs consist most commonly of poorly defined patchy areas of parenchymal consolidation involving the lung bases.[23] In most patients, these areas are the result of infection; occasionally, they represent acute lupus pneumonitis,[21] alveolar hemorrhage,[21,23] or cryptogenic organizing pneumonia (COP, BOOP).[24] In patients with severe hemorrhage, radiographs may show extensive bilateral ground-glass opacities or multifocal or confluent areas of consolidation (Fig. 10–3).[25] Radiographic evidence of interstitial

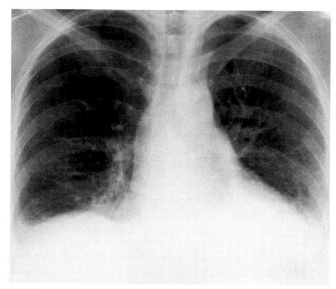

FIGURE 10–2

Systemic lupus erythematosus (SLE). A posteroanterior chest radiograph demonstrates small pleural effusions and decreased lung volumes. Mild enlargement of the cardiopericardial silhouette was shown at echocardiography to be due to pericardial effusion. This constellation of findings is characteristic of SLE. The patient was a 30-year-old woman. *(From Fraser RS, Müller NL, Colman NC, Paré PD: Fraser and Paré's Diagnosis of Diseases of the Chest, 4th ed. Philadelphia, WB Saunders, 1999.)*

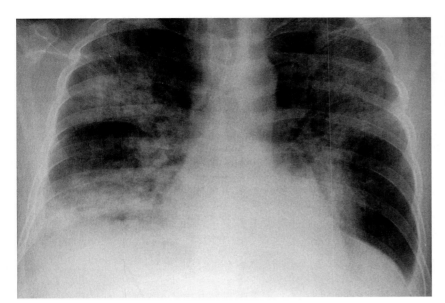

FIGURE 10–3

Diffuse pulmonary hemorrhage in systemic lupus erythematosus (SLE). A posteroanterior chest radiograph demonstrates extensive bilateral areas of consolidation with relative sparing of the peripheral lung regions. Small bilateral pleural effusions are also evident. The patient was a 24-year-old man with SLE who presented with hemoptysis. The parenchymal opacities resolved within 72 hours. *(From Fraser RS, Müller NL, Colman NC, Paré PD: Fraser and Paré's Diagnosis of Diseases of the Chest, 4th ed. Philadelphia, WB Saunders, 1999.)*

fibrosis is seen in 2% to 6% of patients who have SLE.[26,27] Horizontal line shadows are seen relatively commonly in patients with SLE. They are usually present in the lung bases, are sometimes migratory, and are probably attributable to subsegmental atelectasis.

The presence and extent of parenchymal abnormalities are frequently underestimated on the chest radiograph.[28] For example, in a study involving 48 patients, chest radiographs showed evidence of fibrosis in 3 (6%) and no abnormalities in 45 (94%).[27] Seventeen (38%) of the 45 had abnormal findings on HRCT, the most common being interlobular septal thickening (33% of patients), intralobular interstitial thickening (33%), small rounded areas of consolidation (22%), and areas of ground-glass attenuation (13%). As might be expected, the prevalence of parenchymal abnormalities is highest in patients who have long-standing SLE and chronic respiratory symptoms.[28]

Cardiovascular changes frequently occur in association with pulmonary and pleural manifestations. An increase in size of the cardiac silhouette is generally the result of pericardial effusion, which is usually relatively small but may be massive.[29]

Clinical Manifestations

Clinical evidence of *pleural disease* is the most common thoracic manifestation of SLE; it is seen in as many as 70% of patients at some point in the course of the disease and is the first sign in 5% (see page 823).[30]

Acute lupus pneumonitis is uncommon and occurs in only 1% to 4% of patients.[31] The clinical manifestations are similar to those of acute infectious pneumonia and thromboembolic disease; the diagnosis is therefore often one of exclusion. Although *diffuse interstitial pneumonitis and fibrosis* can be appreciated on HRCT in a significant number of patients,[32] clinically evident disease is uncommon and is rarely severe.[33] It may follow acute pneumonitis or appear de novo and has clinical manifestations similar to those of idiopathic pulmonary fibrosis (IPF).

The finding of anemia with a dropping hematocrit in the presence of worsening air space opacification on the chest radiograph suggests *diffuse alveolar hemorrhage*. Associated hemoptysis may be absent, mild, or severe.[34] This complication is rare but when present is usually associated with lupus nephritis.[35]

The presence of high titers of antiphospholipid antibodies in patients with SLE is strongly associated with an elevated risk for pulmonary thromboembolism, deep venous thrombosis, thrombocytopenia, recurrent fetal loss, autoimmune hemolytic anemia, livedo reticularis, and central nervous system (CNS) disease (including stroke) when compared with lupus patients who do not have such titers.[36,37] Nevertheless, the presence of antiphospholipid antibodies has a low predictive value for these conditions in *unselected* patients who have SLE.[38] Microangiopathy and multiorgan failure involving the kidneys, liver, heart, lungs, and brain develop in a small number of patients who have high titers of anticardiolipin antibodies[39]; mortality is high.

Clinically important *pulmonary hypertension* is rare in SLE.[33] Most affected patients demonstrate Raynaud's phenomenon[40] and have disease similar to primary pulmonary hypertension. This complication is strongly associated with anticardiolipin antibodies. However, because there is no relationship between levels of antibody and the severity of hypertension and patients do not usually have any other evidence of antiphospholipid syndrome,[41] their pathogenetic significance is unclear.

Some patients have dyspnea and orthopnea associated with progressive elevation of the hemidiaphragms and plate shadows at the lung bases radiologically, as well as decreased vital capacity on function testing (the "shrinking lung syndrome").[42] The pathogenesis is obscure; when assessed by direct phrenic nerve stimulation, diaphragmatic strength may be conserved.[43,44] Despite the severe abnormalities found in these patients, the clinical course is relatively stable, and some patients improve with therapy.[45,46]

SLE can involve the airways at all levels. Rarely, supraglottic or laryngeal disease causes life-threatening upper airway obstruction.[33] Both obliterative bronchiolitis[47] and COP[24] are well-described pulmonary complications. The former is characterized clinically by progressive dyspnea and the latter by cough, low-grade fever, and dyspnea, usually of several months' duration.

A number of drugs have been associated with the development of a lupus-like syndrome. Systemic manifestations are generally similar to those of idiopathic SLE; however, pulmonary involvement is unusual.[48] Most symptoms resolve with cessation of the offending agent, and rechallenge usually results in recurrence of disease.

Laboratory Findings

The presence of antibodies against specific nuclear and cytoplasmic antigens is one of the diagnostic criteria for SLE. The test most commonly used is a search for antinuclear antibodies (ANAs). The sensitivity of the test is high, with up to 98% of patients being positive. However, a negative test does not completely exclude the diagnosis: rarely, patients who have isolated anti-Ro (anti–SS-A) or anti–single-stranded DNA (anti-ssDNA) have a negative ANA test.[49] Unfortunately, the specificity of the test is poor, with as many as 32% of the general population being positive at low titer.[50] Therefore, it is inadvisable to use the test as a screening tool in patients who have vague complaints or symptoms.[51] Identification of a particular pattern of ANA positivity can be useful in diagnosis; for example, *rim* or *homogeneous* patterns are highly specific for SLE.

Antibodies to double-stranded DNA (dsDNA) are also highly specific for the diagnosis of SLE (95%). However, a negative test does not exclude the diagnosis, because they occur in only 30% of affected individuals.[50] Production of these antibodies is often associated with a reciprocal reduction in serum complement; their level correlates with disease activity in many but not all patients.[52]

Both cytoplasmic (c) and a wide variety of peripheral (p) antineutrophil cytoplasmic antibodies (ANCAs) can be found in SLE,[53,54] the latter in up to 25% of patients.[55] There is no clear association between their presence and disease activity or expression.

Anti-Sm (anti-Smith) antibody, one of a number of antibodies directed against small nuclear ribonucleoproteins (anti-snRNPs), is specific for the diagnosis of SLE; however, it is detected in only 20% to 30% of patients.[49] Although anti–topoisomerase I (anti–Scl-70) has been thought to be relatively specific for progressive systemic sclerosis (PSS),[49] it is found in up to 25% of patients who have SLE.[56] The presence of this antibody has been associated with an increased risk for pulmonary hypertension and nephritis.

Pulmonary Function Tests

The results of lung function studies are frequently abnormal. The most common defect is a reduction in diffusing capacity, which may be evident even in the absence of clinical or radiologic evidence of lung disease.[57] When disease involves the lung parenchyma or chest wall (including the diaphragm), a restrictive pattern of dysfunction consisting of a decrease in lung volumes, diffusing capacity, arterial oxygen saturation, and arterial PCO_2 is seen.[58] Evidence of airflow obstruction unexplained by smoking or asthma should suggest the pres-

ence of obliterative bronchiolitis.[59] Although dyspnea may be secondary to any of these disorders, exercise performance in patients with SLE is often related to peripheral muscle deconditioning.[60,61]

Prognosis and Natural History

SLE typically runs a chronic course, punctuated by acute exacerbations. When medical care is good, the 5-year survival rate exceeds 90%.[62] Death typically occurs after many years from renal failure, CNS involvement, or superimposed infection, the latter often associated with the immunosuppression of therapy.[63,64] Mortality in cases of diffuse alveolar hemorrhage has been reported to exceed 50%[65]; however, early diagnosis and aggressive management may be associated with a more favorable outcome.[66] The prognosis in patients in whom clinically evident pulmonary hypertension develops is guarded, the 2-year mortality exceeding 50%.[31]

Hypocomplementemic Urticarial Vasculitis

The term "hypocomplementemic urticarial vasculitis" refers to a syndrome characterized by persistent urticaria, leukocytoclastic vasculitis, and hypocomplementemia. Although it shares many clinical features with SLE, the paucity of serum autoantibodies as well as the characteristic skin findings suggests that it may be a distinct entity.[67,68] Obstructive lung disease has been described in a number of patients; although many have been smokers, the severity of disease and the age at onset cannot adequately be explained by smoking alone.[68]

Rheumatoid Disease

Rheumatoid arthritis is a common chronic inflammatory and destructive arthropathy; the high prevalence of associated extra-articular manifestations justifies the designation rheumatoid disease (RD). The estimated annual incidence is 54 per 100,000 for women and 24.5 per 100,000 for men in the United States[69]; RD is rare in men younger than 45 years. Many prevalence studies have demonstrated the disease in about 0.5% to 1.0% of the adult population in the United States.[69]

The reported prevalence of lung disease in patients who have RD varies widely, partly as a result of different diagnostic techniques. For example, when based on radiographic findings alone, interstitial lung disease is seen in 1% to 5% of patients[70]; however, the application of more sensitive tests, such as diffusing capacity[71] or HRCT,[72] reveals evidence of pulmonary fibrosis in about 40%. The clinical importance of these early changes remains to be determined by long-term outcome studies.

RD is associated with a variety of pleuropulmonary manifestations (Table 10–2). Most affected patients have arthritis; serum rheumatoid factor, mostly in high titer, can be demonstrated in 70% to 80% of such patients.[73] Occasionally, pleuropulmonary disease precedes the onset of arthritis; in this circumstance, the diagnosis may be suggested by the finding of positive serology.[74]

The pathogenesis of RD is complex. Interestingly, cigarette smoking appears to be an important risk factor for

TABLE 10–2. Pleuropulmonary Manifestations of Rheumatoid Disease

Parenchymal Disease
Interstitial pneumonitis and fibrosis
Upper lobe fibrobullous disease
Rheumatoid nodule
Caplan's syndrome
Pleural Disease
Pleural effusion
Pneumothorax
Airway Disease
Obliterative bronchiolitis
Cryptogenic organizing pneumonia
Follicular bronchiolitis
Bronchiectasis
Upper airway disease
Vascular Disease
Pulmonary hypertension
Pulmonary arteritis
Hyperviscosity syndrome
Secondary Abnormalities
Drug reactions
Infection
Malignancy

From Fraser RS, Müller NL, Colman NC, Paré PD: Fraser and Paré's Diagnosis of Diseases of the Chest, 4th ed. Philadelphia, WB Saunders, 1999.

development of the disease, especially in seropositive men[75]; moreover, its severity may be related to the amount smoked.

Parenchymal Disease

Diffuse Interstitial Pneumonitis and Fibrosis. Interstitial pneumonitis with fibrosis is probably the most common form of pulmonary involvement in RD.[71] The histologic changes are most often those of usual interstitial pneumonia or nonspecific interstitial pneumonia.[76] Nodular aggregates of lymphocytes, sometimes with germinal centers, may be prominent in both the parenchymal interstitium and interstitial tissue adjacent to bronchioles and interlobular septa.[76] With progression of the disease, the inflammatory cellular infiltrate decreases in severity and is replaced by fibrous tissue, which in the advanced stage results in the appearance of a "honeycomb" lung (see Color Fig. 10–1).

The radiographic pattern in the early stage consists of irregular linear opacities causing a fine reticular pattern involving mainly the lower lung zones (Fig. 10–4).[20] With progression of disease, the reticular pattern becomes more coarse and diffuse, and honeycombing may be seen.[20] Similar to the radiograph, the predominant HRCT abnormality consists of a reticular pattern caused by a combination of intralobular linear opacities and irregular thickening of the interlobular septa (see Fig. 10–4).[77,78] Such abnormalities are present mainly in the subpleural region of the lower lung zones.[79] Honeycombing is usually most marked near the diaphragm. The pattern and distribution of fibrosis on the chest radiograph and HRCT scan are indistinguishable from those of IPF.[80]

Interstitial disease is most common in men between the ages of 50 and 60 years.[70] The most frequent symptom is dyspnea on exertion, sometimes associated with cough and pleuritic chest pain. Finger clubbing may be present, albeit at a lower frequency than noted in IPF,[81] and is not uncommonly associated with cor pulmonale. Crackles are generally audible on auscultation of the chest.[82] Anemia and mild lymphocytosis develop in some patients who have advanced disease. Pulmonary function tests typically show a restrictive ventilatory defect.[82] Diffusing capacity is commonly reduced,[82] even in patients who have normal chest radiographs. Although the disease may behave in a more indolent fashion than IPF, it commonly progresses and can lead to death from respiratory insufficiency.[70]

Upper Lobe Fibrobullous Disease. Though rare, the number of reports of fibrosis confined to the upper lobes and associated with bullae or cavities is sufficient to justify inclusion of this form of parenchymal abnormality as a separate manifestation of RD.[83] The pathogenesis of the condition is unknown; searches for acid-fast organisms have proved fruitless. Chest radiographs reveal patchy upper lobe fibrosis and cystic spaces consistent with either cavities or bullae. The pattern closely resembles that observed with advanced ankylosing spondylitis.

Rheumatoid Nodules. A rheumatoid (necrobiotic) nodule is a well-circumscribed focus of connective tissue degeneration found most commonly in the subcutaneous tissue. It is a relatively rare pleuropulmonary manifestation of RD and is typically associated with advanced arthritis and multiple subcutaneous nodules on the elbows or elsewhere.[84] In the lungs, the nodules may be solitary or multiple and are usually situated peripherally in relation to the pleura or interlobular septa.[84] Histologically, they consist of a central portion composed of amorphous necrotic material surrounded by a layer of epithelioid histiocytes; the adjacent tissue shows fibrosis and a variably intense plasma cell and lymphocyte infiltrate.

Radiographically, rheumatoid nodules are visualized as well-circumscribed masses, usually multiple, 5 mm to 7 cm in diameter, and commonly situated in the periphery of the lung next to the pleura (Fig. 10–5).[78] They may be numerous, resembling metastases, and may wax and wane in concert with subcutaneous nodules and in proportion to the activity of the underlying arthritis.[85] Cavitation is common, the walls being thick and having a smooth inner lining. During remission of arthritis, the cavities may become thin walled and disappear gradually, and during exacerbations, they may refill and become opacified.[86]

Patients are usually asymptomatic. Occasionally, the nodules cause hemoptysis or sudden pain and dyspnea when pneumothorax results from rupture into the pleural cavity. Rarely, a nodule develops in the lung before any other manifestation of RD; the possibility of carcinoma must be carefully excluded before accepting this diagnosis for a solitary nodule.[87]

Caplan's Syndrome. This uncommon manifestation of RD is characterized radiologically by the development of one or multiple well-defined spherical opacities in the lungs of individuals exposed to inorganic dust such as silica[88] or coal.[89] Histologically, the central portion of the nodule is composed of necrotic collagen surrounded by layers of macrophages and polymorphonuclear leukocytes, some of which contain dust

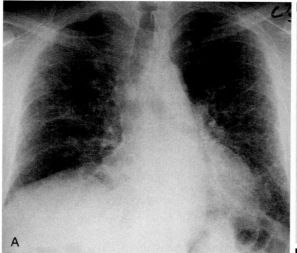

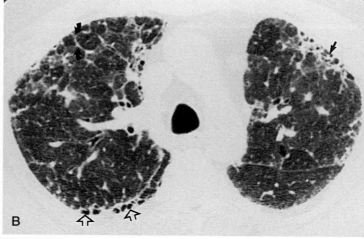

FIGURE 10–4

Rheumatoid disease—interstitial pneumonitis and fibrosis. A posteroanterior chest radiograph (**A**) shows a diffuse reticulonodular pattern associated with a decrease in lung volumes. HRCT scans (**B** and **C**) show a reticular pattern involving mainly the peripheral lung. The reticular pattern is due to a combination of intralobular linear opacities *(straight arrows)* and irregular thickening of interlobular septa *(curved arrows)*. Honeycombing is evident in the right lower lobe *(open arrows)*. No nodules are evident on CT scan. (The nodularity on the radiograph is due to linear opacities seen end-on.) The patient was a 73-year-old man who had long-standing rheumatoid disease. *(From Müller NL, Fraser RS, Colman NC, Paré PD: Radiologic Diagnosis of Diseases of the Chest. Philadelphia, WB Saunders, 2001.)*

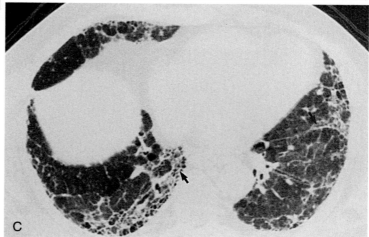

FIGURE 10–5

Rheumatoid nodules. A view of the lower lung zones from a posteroanterior chest radiograph in a 41-year-old man with a 1-year history of rheumatoid arthritis shows two well-circumscribed nodules in the base of the right lung and at least two nodules in the left base *(arrows)*; the more lateral of the two lesions on the right has cavitated. *(From Müller NL, Fraser RS, Colman NC, Paré PD: Radiologic Diagnosis of Diseases of the Chest. Philadelphia, WB Saunders, 2001.)*

particles. It is thought that when these cells die, the dust remains behind and forms the characteristic darkened ring that distinguishes a Caplan nodule from the necrobiotic nodule of uncomplicated RD.[90]

Unlike silicosis, the lesions usually develop rapidly, tend to appear in "crops," and range from 0.5 to 5.0 cm in diameter. They may increase in number, remain unchanged, or calcify. Cavitation may occur and be followed by fibrosis or disappearance of the lesion.[89] The opacities may appear before, coincident with, or after the clinical onset of arthritis, and there is no apparent relationship between the severity of the arthritis and the extent and type of radiographically apparent change in the lungs. Despite the association with inorganic dust, a background of simple pneumoconiosis is slight or absent in many individuals.

Airway Disease

The prevalence of lower respiratory tract airway abnormalities in nonsmoking patients who have RD is high,[91] as determined by both HRCT and lung function testing. Smokers also demonstrate an important interaction between their habit and their disease: the presence of respiratory symptoms and functional abnormalities is much greater in smokers who have rheumatoid arthritis than in control smokers who have osteoarthritis.[92] Specific airway complications of RD include obliterative bronchiolitis, organizing pneumonia (COP), bronchiectasis, and follicular bronchitis/bronchiolitis. Upper airway obstruction, related to ankylosis of the cricoarytenoid and cricothyroid joints, and sleep apnea are additional complications.

Obliterative Bronchiolitis. This abnormality is characterized clinically by the development of rapidly progressive obstructive pulmonary disease.[93,94] An increased risk for the complication has been associated with certain HLA types,[95,96] and obstruction has developed in patients with arthritis who are not taking penicillamine, a drug that is an independent cause of bronchiolitis.[97] Histologically, the abnormality is characterized by a variably intense infiltrate of lymphocytes and plasma cells in and around the bronchiolar wall.[98] Proliferation of fibroblastic tissue between the airway muscle and epithelium ("constrictive" bronchiolitis) results in airway narrowing and, eventually, luminal obliteration (Fig. 10–6). The surrounding parenchyma and pulmonary vasculature are typically unremarkable.

The chest radiograph is usually normal or shows only hyperinflation.[93,99] HRCT typically demonstrates a mosaic perfusion pattern in which some areas of lung have decreased attenuation and vascularity and others have increased attenuation and vascularity.[99,100] Expiratory HRCT images show focal areas of air trapping consistent with small-airway obstruction (Fig. 10–7).[99] Bronchiectasis, mainly at a subsegmental level, may also be seen.[100]

Clinically, patients experience progressive dyspnea, often associated with the development of productive cough; most also have chronic sinusitis.[94] A mid-inspiratory squeak is frequently present on auscultation of the chest.[101] Pulmonary function tests show an obstructive pattern with low diffusing capacity; a few patients have a restrictive or mixed restrictive/obstructive defect.[102]

Organizing Pneumonia (Bronchiolitis Obliterans with Organizing Pneumonia). This condition occasionally occurs in patients who have RD.[103] The pathologic and radiologic findings are identical to those seen in cryptogenic organizing pneumonia (see page 696). Pulmonary function tests reveal a restrictive or mixed obstructive/restrictive pattern.[91] In most cases, a confident diagnosis can be made on the basis of clinical and radiologic (including HRCT) findings.

Follicular Bronchitis/Bronchiolitis. This rare manifestation of pulmonary RD is characterized histologically by the presence of abundant lymphoid tissue, frequently with prominent germinal centers, situated about bronchioles and to a lesser extent bronchi.[104] Despite the name, it is not clear whether it represents active inflammation of the bronchioles (true bronchiolitis) or simply hyperplasia of the lymphoid tissue that normally occurs in this region. The chest radiograph shows a diffuse reticulonodular pattern.[104] HRCT scan typically demonstrates small nodules, mainly in a centrilobular, subpleural, and peribronchial distribution.[94,105] Other findings include bronchial wall thickening, centrilobular branching linear opacities, and ground-glass opacities.[105] The most common clinical finding is progressive shortness of breath; cough, fever, and recurrent pneumonia are occasionally present. Pulmonary function tests reveal evidence of airway obstruction.[106] For unknown reasons, follicular bronchitis/bronchiolitis is more common in adolescents who have clinical features of juvenile rheumatoid arthritis than in adults.

Bronchiectasis/Bronchiolectasis. These relatively common complications of RD are evident on HRCT in almost 30% of unselected patients who have rheumatoid arthritis in the absence of pulmonary fibrosis.[91] There is evidence that the airway abnormalities in some way predispose to the development of arthritis; when recognized clinically, the bronchiectasis precedes a diagnosis of arthritis in almost all patients.[107] The association does not seem to be explained by involvement of the airway with Sjögren's syndrome (SS) or by a common genetic predisposition.[108] The presence of clinically evident bronchiectasis in patients who have RD is associated with a poor 5-year mortality rate.[109]

Vascular Disease

Clinically evident pulmonary hypertension in patients who have RD is usually secondary to interstitial fibrosis[110]; sometimes, it is seen in patients who do not have fibrosis but have Raynaud's phenomenon[111] or (rarely) hyperviscosity syndrome.[112] In one study, echocardiographic evidence of mild pulmonary hypertension was found in 21% of unselected patients who had rheumatoid arthritis and normal lung function[113]; the significance of this finding has not been determined.

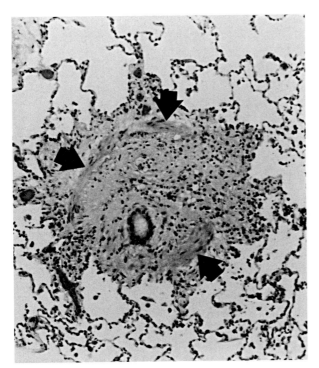

FIGURE 10–6

Rheumatoid disease—obliterative bronchiolitis. A section of a membranous bronchiole shows almost complete luminal obliteration by fibrous tissue with relatively few inflammatory cells (*arrows* indicate the muscularis mucosa). The adjacent lung parenchyma is normal. The patient was a 45-year-old woman who had long-standing rheumatoid disease. *(From Fraser RS, Müller NL, Colman NC, Paré PD: Fraser and Paré's Diagnosis of Diseases of the Chest, 4th ed. Philadelphia, WB Saunders, 1999.)*

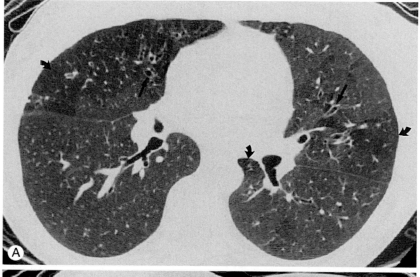

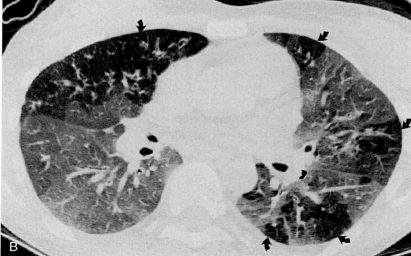

FIGURE 10-7

Rheumatoid disease—obliterative bronchiolitis. An HRCT scan performed at end-inspiration (**A**) shows bronchiectasis in the right middle lobe and lingula (*straight arrows*). Note the areas of decreased attenuation and vascularity in the middle lobe, lingula, and left lower lobe (*curved arrows*), with a slight increase in vascularity in normal lung (mosaic perfusion pattern). Another scan performed at maximal expiration (**B**) shows areas of air trapping (*arrows*). There is a marked decrease in vascularity in the areas of air trapping. The patient was a 30-year-old woman. (*From Müller NL, Fraser RS, Colman NC, Paré PD: Radiologic Diagnosis of Diseases of the Chest. Philadelphia, WB Saunders, 2001.*)

Pleural Disease

Pleural abnormalities are common in patients who have RD.[33] Effusion is unilateral or bilateral in roughly equal proportions and is the sole radiographic abnormality apparent in the thorax in most cases. In fact, it has been suggested that the presence of associated parenchymal disease should suggest a nonrheumatoid etiology.[114] Frequently, the effusion remains relatively unchanged over a period of many months or even years.[114] Pleural thickening without effusion is seen in some cases. The details of its clinical and laboratory features are discussed on page 823.

Though uncommon, pneumothorax may occur as a consequence of rupture of a rheumatoid nodule into the pleural space or as a complication of advanced fibrotic lung disease.[70,115]

Progressive Systemic Sclerosis

PSS (scleroderma) is a systemic autoimmune disease characterized pathologically by microangiopathy and excessive production of collagen with resulting skin and visceral fibrosis.[116]

The major organs affected include the skin, lungs, heart, gastrointestinal tract, and kidneys. There is a strong association with the presence of antibodies to centromeres and to DNA–topoisomerase I.[116] It is an uncommon condition, with an estimated incidence of only 20 cases per million individuals per year and a prevalence of about 1500 per million.[117] PSS occurs more frequently in females than in males at a ratio of 3:1,[118] the majority of cases occurring between the ages of 40 and 60. Severe lung disease and poorer survival are more often seen in black than white patients.[119]

Although pulmonary disease is common in PSS, there is a significant disparity between the clinical, pathologic, radiologic, and functional findings. Even in the absence of clinical or radiographic evidence of fibrotic lung disease, early changes can frequently be found on lung function testing,[120,121] HRCT,[122] or analysis of BAL fluid.[123]

Pathologic Characteristics

At autopsy, some degree of parenchymal interstitial fibrosis is frequent, although in many cases it is only focal.[124] More severely affected lungs show bilateral interstitial thickening that is most marked in the subpleural regions of the lower lobes. Microscopic findings are those of usual interstitial pneumonia or, more commonly, nonspecific interstitial pneumonia.[125] Obliterative bronchiolitis, follicular bronchiolitis, and organizing pneumonia (COP) occur occasionally.[126] Histologic evidence of pulmonary arterial hypertension is seen most often in association with diffuse interstitial fibrosis; occasionally, there is arterial intimal thickening by fibroblastic connective tissue and medial hypertrophy in the absence of interstitial disease.[124] Pleural fibrosis is not uncommon.[127]

Radiologic Manifestations

Evidence of interstitial fibrosis has been reported to be present on chest radiographs in 25% to 65% of patients.[128,129] The initial abnormality may be subtle and typically consists of fine reticulation at the lung bases[128]; as the disease progresses, the reticulation tends to become coarser and easier to detect as it extends from the bases to involve the lower two thirds of the lungs (Fig. 10–8).[128]

HRCT frequently shows evidence of interstitial disease in patients who have normal or questionable radiographic findings.[129,130] Such findings include parenchymal and subpleural micronodules, intralobular linear opacities in a reticular pattern, subpleural lines, areas of ground-glass attenuation,

and honeycombing (see Fig. 10–8). Initial scans usually show ground-glass attenuation with relatively little reticulation and minimal, if any, honeycombing (Fig. 10–9).[131] The abnormalities involve mainly the lower lobes and are located predominantly in the peripheral and posterior regions.[132] Because of this distribution, CT scans should be performed with the patient prone to detect mild abnormalities and avoid confusing early disease with gravity-induced dependent density.[132]

Radiographic evidence of pleural effusion or thickening is less common in PSS than in other connective tissue diseases; such evidence is found in approximately 10% to 15% of patients.[133] Thickening is seen more commonly on CT scan: in a series of 55 patients, it was seen in a third, all of whom had pulmonary abnormalities.[132]

The esophagus is involved clinically and/or radiologically in about 50% of patients.[134] Atrophy and atony can lead to dilation, which may be manifested on plain radiographs as an air esophagogram. The presence of this abnormality in association with typical pulmonary parenchymal changes is virtually pathognomonic of PSS.[135]

Clinical Manifestations

Although pulmonary symptoms are the initial manifestation of disease in less than 1% of patients,[136] more than 60% have

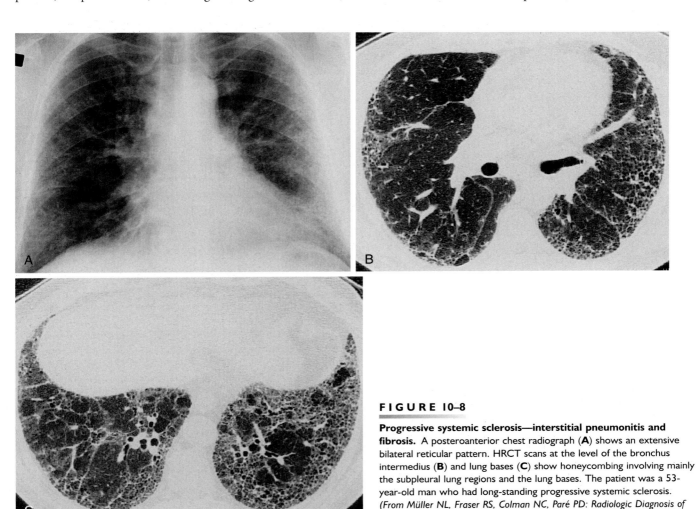

FIGURE 10–8

Progressive systemic sclerosis—interstitial pneumonitis and fibrosis. A posteroanterior chest radiograph (**A**) shows an extensive bilateral reticular pattern. HRCT scans at the level of the bronchus intermedius (**B**) and lung bases (**C**) show honeycombing involving mainly the subpleural lung regions and the lung bases. The patient was a 53-year-old man who had long-standing progressive systemic sclerosis. *(From Müller NL, Fraser RS, Colman NC, Paré PD: Radiologic Diagnosis of Diseases of the Chest. Philadelphia, WB Saunders, 2001.)*

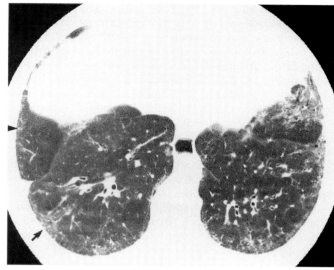

FIGURE 10–9

Progressive systemic sclerosis—nonspecific interstitial pneumonia.
An HRCT scan through the lower lung zones performed with the patient prone shows extensive bilateral ground-glass opacities, a few irregular linear opacities in the peripheral lung regions, and poorly defined subpleural nodules (*arrows*). The esophagus is slightly dilated. The patient was a 47-year-old woman.

dyspnea at some point during the course of disease (usually in the late stages).[137] Basilar crackles are reported to occur in approximately 50% of patients.[138] Patients may have a slightly productive cough or hemoptysis. Massive pulmonary hemorrhage is rare[139]; occasionally, it is part of a lung-renal syndrome.[140] When lung disease is rapidly progressive or the radiologic features are atypical, the diagnosis of COP should be considered.[126]

Patients who have severe esophageal involvement with dysmotility are significantly more likely to have interstitial lung disease than are patients who have lesser degrees of esophageal dysfunction.[141] Although this finding suggests that reflux plays a role in the pathogenesis of the pulmonary fibrosis, it is also possible that both abnormalities are markers of disease severity. Alternatively, since the severity of both abnormalities has been linked to cigarette smoking, the latter could be a confounding variable that explains the apparent association.

Cardiovascular disease is common; it may be primary or secondary to pulmonary or systemic hypertension.[137] Sclerosis of cardiac muscle or PSS-related myocarditis[142] may result in biventricular failure; right ventricular failure alone should suggest the presence of pulmonary vascular disease. Raynaud's phenomenon occurs in the majority of cases of PSS and often antedates the characteristic skin changes of this disease.

Patients who display signs and symptoms of other connective tissue diseases are placed in a category commonly referred to as *overlap syndrome* (see page 494). Another complex that some authorities regard as a variant of PSS is diffuse fasciitis with eosinophilia (eosinophilic fasciitis). Its distinctive features include sparing of the hands and feet, blood eosinophilia, increased serum levels of eosinophilic chemotactic factor, and (sometimes) polyarthritis.[143] Although the lungs are spared, chest wall disease may be

severe enough to cause a restrictive ventilatory defect on lung function testing.

Pulmonary Function Tests

As indicated previously, pulmonary function is often impaired, even when the chest radiograph is normal. A restrictive functional deficit is characteristic of lung fibrosis.[120,144] Airflow obstruction may be present in the absence of a history of cigarette smoking,[145,146] suggesting the presence of bronchiolitis. Both diffusing capacity and lung compliance are often reduced.[121,147]

Prognosis and Natural History

Patients with PSS have statistically higher mortality than the general population; however, the 10-year survival rate is about 70%.[116,117] With the use of multivariate analysis, factors identified at the time of diagnosis that strongly and independently predict PSS-related death include diffuse skin involvement, decreased diffusing capacity, elevated erythrocyte sedimentation rate, anemia, and older age. In one investigation, the observed mortality was 2% in those who had none of these features and 75% in those who had all of them.[116] The prognosis is also worse in men and in patients in whom PSS-associated heart disease or renal impairment develops. There is evidence for an association between pulmonary carcinoma and PSS[148]; most affected patients are women who have pulmonary fibrosis.

CREST Syndrome

CREST syndrome (subcutaneous **c**alcification, **R**aynaud's phenomenon, **e**sophageal dysfunction, **s**clerodactyly, and **t**elangiectasia) possesses certain clinical and laboratory features that differ from those of PSS, and it is generally regarded as a variant of this disorder. The most distinctive serologic abnormality is the presence of anticentromere antibody, which has been found in 50% to 95% of patients judged on clinical grounds to have CREST syndrome, in less than 10% of those who have PSS, and unusually in patients who have other connective tissue diseases.[149,150] However, when all individuals who have this antibody are considered, only a small minority have CREST syndrome.[151] Affected patients have an appreciably lower incidence of arthralgia and arthritis than those with PSS, and their skin involvement is limited to the distal portions of the extremities.[150]

An important feature of CREST syndrome is the occurrence of pulmonary hypertension in the absence of other significant pulmonary disease. In a study of 331 patients, 30 (9%) were so affected[152]; by contrast, none of the 342 patients who had PSS and no CREST features had pulmonary hypertension. When routine echocardiography is performed in patients who have CREST syndrome, a much higher prevalence of pulmonary hypertension can be found.[153] The pathologic and radiographic findings are similar to those reported with primary pulmonary hypertension (Fig. 10–10). The combination of low diffusing capacity and preserved lung volumes should suggest the diagnosis. The prognosis of clinically evident pulmonary hypertension is poor, the 2-year survival rate being only 40%.[152]

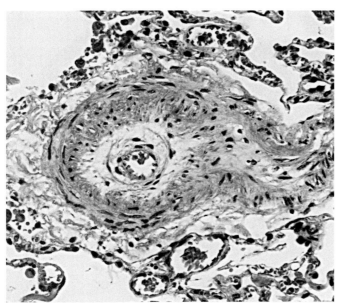

FIGURE 10–10

Overlap syndrome (systemic lupus erythematosus with CREST) and pulmonary arterial hypertension. Clinical evidence of pulmonary hypertension developed in a 26-year-old woman with SLE and CREST syndrome. She died 1 month later. An autopsy showed normal lung parenchyma and extensive narrowing of small pulmonary arteries and arterioles as a result of medial hypertrophy and intimal fibrosis. *(From Fraser RS, Müller NL, Colman NC, Paré PD: Fraser and Paré's Diagnosis of Diseases of the Chest, 4th ed. Philadelphia, WB Saunders, 1999.)*

Dermatomyositis and Polymyositis

The terms "dermatomyositis" and "polymyositis" (DM/PM) refer to a group of disorders characterized by weakness and sometimes pain in the proximal limb muscles and (occasionally) the muscles of the neck. About 50% of patients have a characteristic heliotrope rash, erythema or purpura on the extensor surfaces of the extremity joints, and Gottron's papules (flat-topped violaceous papules on the dorsal aspect of the interphalangeal joints of the hand with central atrophy, hypopigmentation, and telangiectasia), all of which facilitate the distinction of dermatomyositis from polymyositis.[154]

The disease occurs twice as often in women as men. Its incidence has two peaks, the first during the first decade and the second in the fifth and sixth decades.[155] The incidence is approximately 5 to 10 cases per million population.[156]

The respiratory system is commonly affected at some point in the course of the disease, generally in one or more of three forms: (1) hypoventilation and respiratory failure as a result of direct involvement of the respiratory muscles, (2) pulmonary parenchymal disease (most often interstitial pneumonia, organizing pneumonia, or diffuse alveolar damage), and (3) aspiration pneumonia secondary to pharyngeal muscle paresis.

Patients have a high frequency of antibodies to nuclear and cytoplasmic antigens,[157] some of which show strong associations with specific clinical features. In particular, a group of myositis-associated autoantibodies, the antisynthetases, are strongly linked to the development of interstitial lung disease;

about 80% of patients with this complication have these antibodies.[158] They are directed against aminoacyl-tRNA synthetases, cytoplasmic enzymes that catalyze the binding of amino acids to the appropriate tRNA for incorporation into polypeptide chains. A distinct synthetase is present for each amino acid; the most common antibody, anti–Jo-1, is found in about 20% of patients who have DM/PM.[159] These autoantibodies are associated with an "antisynthetase" syndrome, which when compared with disease in patients who have DM/PM unassociated with such antibodies has a high frequency of interstitial lung disease (50% to 100% versus 10%), arthritis, fever during active disease, flaring of disease during treatment withdrawal, and hyperkeratotic lines on the hands with scaling and fissuring ("mechanic's hands").[157] When DM/PM is associated with malignancy, these antibodies are generally absent.[156]

Pathologic Characteristics

Histologic examination of muscle biopsy specimens from patients who have polymyositis reveals both degenerative and regenerative changes, typically associated with phagocytosis of necrotic muscle, a mononuclear inflammatory cell infiltrate, and interstitial fibrosis. Interstitial lung disease may be manifested as usual interstitial pneumonia or nonspecific interstitial pneumonia.[160] COP is seen occasionally.[161]

Radiologic Manifestations

Radiologic evidence of interstitial lung disease occurs in about 5% of patients.[162] The typical finding is a symmetrical, bilateral, predominantly basal, reticular or reticulonodular pattern.[162,163] It can progress slowly and become more or less diffuse and associated with honeycombing.[163] Alternatively, bilateral areas of consolidation superimposed on a reticulonodular pattern develop in some patients over a 2- to 3-week period; this abnormality usually corresponds histologically with diffuse alveolar damage or organizing pneumonia (Fig. 10–11).[161,164] The most common finding on HRCT is ground-glass attenuation, almost invariably seen in association with irregular linear opacities or air space consolidation[165]; small nodules and honeycombing are seen less often.

When polymyositis affects the respiratory muscles, diaphragmatic elevation and small lung volumes may be apparent, often in conjunction with basal linear opacities.[166] Unilateral or bilateral segmental pneumonia may result from aspiration of food and oral secretions in association with pharyngeal muscle involvement; such aspiration pneumonia has been reported in 15% to 20% of patients.[164]

Clinical Manifestations

In patients in whom DM/PM and interstitial lung disease develop, the initial findings are typically either musculoskeletal or pulmonary.[160] Symmetrical weakness of the neck and proximal muscles progressing over a period of weeks or months is characteristic of the former.[167] Rapid destruction of muscle tissue may be associated with profound weakness, pain, tenderness, and swelling of the affected areas.[155] Myositis involving the diaphragm may be severe enough to cause dyspnea, orthopnea, ineffective cough, and respiratory

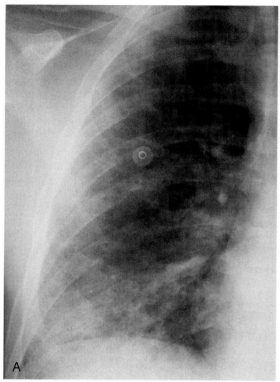

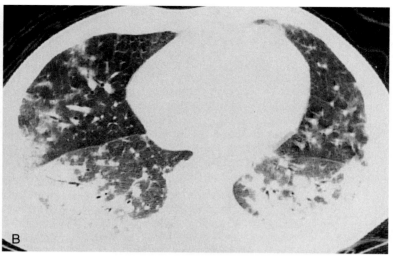

FIGURE 10–11

Polymyositis—cryptogenic organizing pneumonia. A view of the right lung from a posteroanterior chest radiograph (**A**) shows areas of consolidation. Similar findings were present in the left lung. An HRCT scan through the lower lung zones (**B**) shows that the consolidation involves mainly the peripheral lung regions. The patient was a 27-year-old man. (From Müller NL, Fraser RS, Colman NC, Paré PD: Radiologic Diagnosis of Diseases of the Chest. Philadelphia, WB Saunders, 2001.)

insufficiency requiring mechanical ventilation.[160] When pharyngeal weakness is marked, recurrent aspiration and lung infection are common.

Patients with diffuse interstitial lung disease typically have an acute or subacute illness associated with cough and dyspnea. At times the disease is more insidious in onset and may be discovered on a screening chest radiograph.[162] Rare pulmonary complications include diffuse alveolar hemorrhage[168] and acute interstitial pneumonia.[160]

Pulmonary Function Tests

In patients who have interstitial lung disease, lung function abnormalities are identical to those reported in PSS.[160] When the diaphragm is weakened in the absence of other muscle involvement, vital capacity is decreased, flow rates and transdiaphragmatic pressure are reduced, and hypoxemia develops with or without a rise in PCO_2.[166] In some patients who do not have cardiorespiratory symptoms, muscle weakness may mask significant underlying cardiopulmonary disease; in a series of 11 such patients, 7 had echocardiographic evidence of pulmonary hypertension that was associated with abnormalities in exercise performance.[169]

Prognosis and Natural History

When present, pulmonary disease accounts for a significant proportion of the mortality associated with DM/PM.[170] For example, in a study of 58 patients who had the complication, the 5-year survival rate was 60%[160]; of the 11 patients whose cause of death could be determined, progressive interstitial lung disease was responsible in 6 and pneumonia in 4.

Malignancy develops in about 5% to 15% of patients who have DM/PM, a figure that exceeds the expected incidence of cancer in suitable control populations.[171,172] The majority of tumors are identified when DM/PM is diagnosed; the risk for malignancy diminishes with time[173] and approaches that of the general population during the second year of follow-up.[174]

Sjögren's Syndrome

SS is characterized clinically by keratoconjunctivitis sicca, xerostomia, and recurrent swelling of the parotid gland.[175] It occurs as an isolated disorder (primary SS, sicca syndrome) in about 35% to 50% of patients and is associated with other well-defined connective tissue diseases (secondary SS) in the remainder. The most common of the latter is RD; the syndrome has also been described in association with primary biliary cirrhosis, Hashimoto's thyroiditis, pernicious anemia, and primary hypothyroidism and in recipients of bone marrow transplants[176] and individuals infected with HIV.[177] There is a strong female preponderance (90%).[178,179]

Patients with SS frequently have pleuropulmonary abnormalities; some of these abnormalities appear to be a reflection of another underlying connective tissue disease, whereas others are probably specific for the syndrome. The most common of these disorders include LIP, pleuritis with or without effusion, and cough.[180,181]

Pathologic Characteristics

Pathologic findings in the trachea and bronchi include atrophy of the mucous glands associated with a lymphoplasmacytic cellular infiltrate. These abnormalities are believed to be analogous to salivary gland involvement and to be responsible for chronic cough. Fibrosis and mononuclear cell infiltration of the small airways have also been reported in patients who manifest evidence of obstructive airway disease.[182]

Pulmonary parenchymal disease may take several forms, the most common of which is a diffuse, usually bilateral interstitial infiltrate of lymphocytes and plasma cells associated with a variable number of histiocytes and multinucleated giant cells.[183] This infiltrate is generally most dense in relation to bronchioles and their accompanying vessels, but it can extend into the alveolar interstitium itself. Fibrosis may occur and is prominent in some cases.[183] Pathologic differentiation of malignant from benign infiltrates may be difficult (see page 377). Usual interstitial pneumonia or nonspecific interstitial pneumonia is seen in some patients.[184]

Radiologic Manifestations

Pulmonary parenchymal abnormalities are evident on the radiograph in approximately 10% to 15% of patients who have SS.[185,186] The most common finding is a reticulonodular pattern, which usually has a basal predominance.[187]

The characteristic manifestations of LIP on HRCT consist of extensive bilateral ground-glass opacities, poorly defined centrilobular nodules, and scattered thin-walled cysts (Fig. 10–12).[188,189] Other common findings include subpleural nodules, and thickening of the bronchovascular bundles and interlobular septa.[189,190] Nonspecific interstitial pneumonia is manifested by bilateral ground-glass opacities and nonseptal linear opacities resulting in fine reticulation involving mainly the lower lung zones.[190]

Clinical Manifestations

The chief symptoms of SS are grittiness or a burning sensation in the eyes and dryness of the mouth, nose, and skin. Lacrimal or salivary gland enlargement occurs in 25% to 50% of patients.[178] Involvement of the larynx may result in hoarseness and cough.

Clinically evident pulmonary involvement has been reported in approximately 10% to 45% of patients who have primary SS.[183,191] Cough secondary to tracheobronchial inflammation is relatively frequent.[181] Such inflammation may also be associated with atelectasis, bronchitis, bronchiectasis, and recurrent bronchopneumonia.[33] LIP may be associated with dyspnea; in some patients, crackles can be auscultated at the lung bases. Marked infiltration of the airway wall may result in dyspnea associated with hyperinflation and obstructive lung function[192] or airway hyperresponsiveness.[193] Pleuritis is relatively uncommon in primary SS but is seen more often in the secondary form.[181]

Laboratory Findings and Pulmonary Function Tests

Although the diagnosis of SS is usually based on its characteristic clinical manifestations, it may be substantiated by Schirmer's test for the measurement of tear formation and by slit-lamp examination of the eyes for identification of corneal scarring secondary to inadequate lacrimal gland secretion. The diagnosis may also be aided by identification of a panel of autoantibodies that typify this disorder. In more than 90% of patients, primary SS is associated with the presence of autoantibodies to small nuclear/cytoplasmic particles—anti-Ro and anti-La (SS-A and SS-B). Although rheumatoid factor and ANA can be found in individuals who have primary

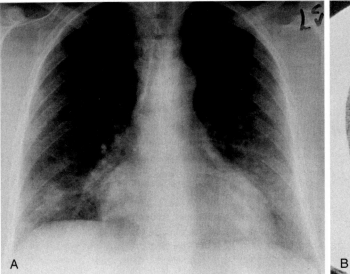
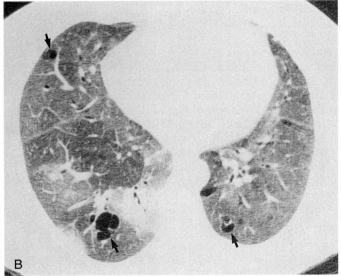

FIGURE 10–12

Sjögren's syndrome—lymphocytic interstitial pneumonia. A posteroanterior chest radiograph (**A**) in a 50-year-old woman with long-standing Sjögren's syndrome shows a poorly defined, hazy increased opacity in both lungs and focal areas of consolidation in the right lower lobe. An HRCT scan (**B**) through the lower lung zones shows extensive areas of ground-glass attenuation in both lungs and a focal area of consolidation in the right lower lobe. Small cystic spaces (*arrows*) are present in both lungs. (*From Müller NL, Fraser RS, Colman NC, Paré PD: Radiologic Diagnosis of Diseases of the Chest. Philadelphia, WB Saunders, 2001.*)

SS, they occur much more commonly in the secondary form.[194]

Significant abnormalities in lung function are found in about 25% of patients who have primary SS.[195] As might be expected of a disease that can involve both the pulmonary interstitium and airways, function testing may show a restrictive, obstructive, or mixed pattern.[179,196,197] Airway hyperresponsiveness is common.[193] Although these abnormalities may appear early in the course of disease and progress over a relatively short time,[195] subsequent stabilization is common.[197]

Overlap Syndromes and Mixed Connective Tissue Disease

Many patients who have connective tissue disease show features of more than one specific entity, in which case they are commonly referred to as having *overlap syndromes* or *unclassified (undifferentiated) connective tissue disease*.[198] These overlap syndromes form a significant proportion of all connective tissue disease; for example, in a series of 73 patients initially thought to have PSS, 20 were noted to have symptoms and signs that overlapped with other autoimmune diseases and to have clinical and radiologic features that differed from PSS and from CREST syndrome alone.[199] By contrast, in another group of 84 patients initially believed to have an overlap syndrome, findings that permitted the diagnosis of a specific connective tissue disease developed in 33 over a 5-year period.[198] There is a strong (9:1) female preponderance among the population of "overlap" patients, and pleuropulmonary disease is common.

One distinctive form of overlap syndrome known as mixed connective tissue disease has clinical features of SLE, PSS, and polymyositis and high serum titers of anti-U1snRNP antibody.[200,201] Though initially thought to be a relatively benign form of connective tissue disease, CNS involvement has been found to develop in 30% to 50% of patients, and pulmonary hypertension is not uncommon.[201] Fatal diffuse interstitial lung disease and diffuse alveolar hemorrhage develop in some patients.[202-204]

As might be expected, the radiologic manifestations of mixed connective tissue disease include those seen in SLE, PSS, and polymyositis. The most common radiographic finding consists of a reticular pattern involving mainly the lung bases.[205,206] With progression of disease, the abnormality gradually extends cephalad; in the late stage, honeycombing may be identified.[205] HRCT corroborates the radiographic findings and shows a predominantly subpleural distribution of fibrosis, similar to that seen in the interstitial fibrosis associated with other connective tissue diseases.[131,205] Other abnormalities include areas of parenchymal consolidation that may be related to aspiration pneumonia or diffuse pulmonary hemorrhage.[207] Pleural effusion has been reported in 5% of patients.[206]

Relapsing Polychondritis

Relapsing polychondritis is characterized principally by inflammation and destruction of cartilage at several sites, including the ribs, tracheobronchial tree, earlobes, nose, and axial and peripheral joints; inflammation of the eye, ear, heart, and systemic vessels is seen occasionally.[208] There may well be a female preponderance[208]; the peak incidence occurs at 40 to 60 years of age. No specific tests can be used to identify this disorder, and the diagnosis is based on clinical grounds alone.[208]

An associated immune disorder is found in 20% to 25% of patients,[209] and anticartilage antibodies have been detected in some individuals.[210] Damage to airway cartilage results in local areas of tracheomalacia and bronchomalacia, which in turn leads to expiratory airway obstruction and an increased risk for pulmonary infection.

Microscopically, affected cartilage shows fragmentation, loss of the normal basophilic staining, and replacement by fibrous tissue. In clinically active disease, an inflammatory infiltrate composed of lymphocytes, plasma cells, and occasional neutrophils is often present at the fibrous-cartilaginous interface.[211]

The most common radiographic manifestation is tracheal stenosis.[212] Less often, narrowing of the major or segmental bronchi is apparent.[213,214] The tracheal narrowing usually measures only a few centimeters in length, although diffuse stenosis may occur.[215] CT demonstrates smooth thickening of the tracheal or bronchial wall, often in association with increased attenuation or calcification, as well as airway stenosis and (during expiration) collapse (Fig. 10–13).[216] Occasionally, bronchiectasis is evident, presumably secondary to recurrent pneumonia.[214]

As the name indicates, the disease is typically relapsing and remitting and usually has a prolonged course. The most common clinical manifestations are swelling, erythema, and pain in the ears and arthralgia[209] that often begin in a precipitous fashion.[208] Nasal chondritis is also frequent and may result in a saddle deformity. The larynx and trachea are involved in about 50% of cases, and in 15%, such involvement is responsible for the initial signs and symptoms.[209] Symptoms of respiratory tract disease include dyspnea, cough, hoarseness, stridor, wheezing, and tenderness over the laryngotracheal cartilage.[217] Airway obstruction can occur as a consequence of encroachment of the airway by inflamed mucosa, by scarring later in the course of disease, or by dynamic collapse of the airway secondary to dissolution of cartilage.[218] Such airway involvement may occur even in the absence of previous nasal or auricular pathology.[33]

The diagnosis is based on the presence of disease in three or more cartilaginous sites.[209] Lesser involvement can also establish the diagnosis if accompanied by histologic corroboration or response to corticosteroid therapy.[218] The prognosis of patients who have airway obstruction is poor, and respiratory complications are responsible for many of the deaths. In a series of 112 patients, the 5- and 10-year survival rates were 74% and 55%, respectively.[219]

Pulmonary function studies in patients who have airway involvement demonstrate signs of intrathoracic or extrathoracic upper airway obstruction on flow-volume curves, the appearance of the curve depending on the site of obstruction.[218]

Pulmonary Involvement in Inflammatory Bowel Disease

Clinically apparent respiratory involvement in patients who have inflammatory bowel disease (IBD, ulcerative colitis,

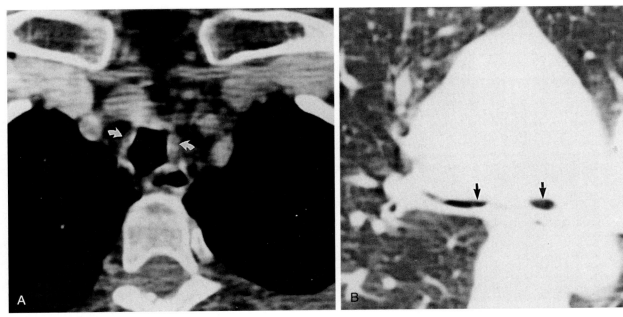

FIGURE 10–13

Relapsing polychondritis. An HRCT scan (**A**) shows mild circumferential thickening of the tracheal wall (*arrows*). A scan at the level of the main bronchi photographed at lung windows (**B**) shows narrowing of the lumen of the right and the left main bronchi (*arrows*). The patient was a 51-year-old woman. *(From Müller NL, Miller RR, Ostrow DN, Pare PD: Diffuse thickening of the tracheal wall. Can Assoc Radiol J 40:213, 1989.)*

Crohn's disease) is rare; in an early report of the association, only 3 examples were identified in a series of 1400 patients monitored for more than 40 years.[220] However, the use of BAL,[222] induced sputum,[223] and lung function testing[224] has revealed abnormalities in up to two thirds of patients in the absence of symptoms or abnormal chest radiographs. A number of specific examples of IBD-related disease that affects the respiratory system from the upper airway to the distal lung parenchyma have been described.[221]

Airway complications are the most common manifestations of pleuropulmonary disease in patients with IBD, especially those who have ulcerative colitis.[225] Chronic bronchitis and bronchiectasis have been seen in a number of such patients in the absence of a smoking history[226]; ulcerative tracheobronchitis,[227] subglottic stenosis, organizing pneumonia,[228] obliterative bronchiolitis, diffuse panbronchiolitis,[229] granulomatous bronchiolitis of uncertain etiology,[230] airway hyperresponsiveness,[224] and eosinophilic bronchitis[231] have also been described. In many patients who have chronic bronchitis and bronchiectasis, the severity of pulmonary symptoms parallels the severity of the bowel disease. For unknown reasons, disease in the lungs may flare dramatically after bowel resection. In contrast to the usual disappointing response to inhaled and systemic corticosteroids in patients who have chronic bronchitis or bronchiectasis, patients who have IBD improve with such therapy.

Apart from organizing pneumonia, parenchymal lung disease is uncommon in patients with IBD. Eosinophilic lung disease has been described most commonly in patients taking sulfasalazine and other anti-inflammatory medications (see page 514); however, some patients do not have this history,[225] which raises the possibility that the reaction may be an intrinsic manifestation of IBD. Granulomatous interstitial lung disease similar to that seen in sarcoidosis has been noted as well, mostly in patients who have Crohn's disease.[232]

The typical radiographic manifestations are bronchial wall thickening and bronchiectasis.[233] The most common findings on HRCT are bronchiectasis, localized areas of decreased attenuation and vascularity adjacent to areas with increased attenuation and vascularity (mosaic perfusion pattern), and air trapping.[233,234] Less common manifestations include thickening of the tracheal or bronchial wall and narrowing of the trachea or major bronchi.[233,235,236]

VASCULITIS

The vasculitides are a diverse group of disorders characterized pathologically by inflammation of blood vessel walls.[236] Clinical manifestations are usually related to ischemic necrosis of tissue supplied by the affected vessel (secondary to stenosis by intraluminal thrombus or by the inflammatory infiltrate itself) or to hemorrhage (as a result of damage to the vessel wall).[237] The current discussion is limited to syndromes in which the inflammatory reaction is directed *primarily* against the vessel wall and is of proved or presumed immunologic origin. The estimated incidence is about 40 per million population.[238] Vasculitis associated with connective tissue diseases, drugs, and infection is discussed elsewhere.

The most widely used classification scheme, based on the size of the vessel affected, is that proposed by the Chapel Hill Consensus Conference on the Nomenclature of Systemic Vasculitis (Table 10–3).[239] It is important to remember that the criteria established at this conference were intended to delineate specific types of vasculitis among patients who *have* vasculitis and not to distinguish patients who have vasculitis from

TABLE 10–3. Names and Definitions of Vasculitides Adopted by the Chapel Hill Consensus Conference on the Nomenclature of Systemic Vasculitis*

Large Vessel Vasculitis	
Giant cell (temporal) arteritis	Granulomatous arteritis of the aorta and its major branches, with a predilection for the extracranial branches of the carotid artery. *Often involves the temporal artery. Usually occurs in patients older than 50 and is often associated with polymyalgia rheumatica*
Takayasu's arteritis	Granulomatous inflammation of the aorta and its major branches. *Usually occurs in patients younger than 50*
Medium-Sized Vessel Vasculitis	
Polyarteritis nodosa[†] (classic polyarteritis nodosa)	Necrotizing inflammation of medium-sized or small arteries without glomerulonephritis or vasculitis in arterioles, capillaries, or venules
Kawasaki's disease	Arteritis involving large, medium-sized, and small arteries associated with mucocutaneous lymph node syndrome. *Coronary arteries are often involved. Aorta and veins may be involved. Usually occurs in children*
Small Vessel Vasculitis	
Wegener's granulomatosis[‡]	Granulomatous inflammation involving the respiratory tract and necrotizing vasculitis affecting small to medium-sized vessels (e.g., capillaries, venules, arterioles, and arteries). *Necrotizing glomerulonephritis is common*
Churg-Strauss syndrome[‡]	Eosinophil-rich and granulomatous inflammation involving the respiratory tract and necrotizing vasculitis affecting small to medium-sized vessels and associated with asthma and eosinophilia
Microscopic polyangiitis[†] (microscopic polyarteritis)[‡]	Necrotizing vasculitis, with few or no immune deposits, affecting small vessels (i.e., capillaries, venules, or arterioles). *Necrotizing arteritis involving small and medium-sized arteries may be present. Necrotizing glomerulonephritis is common. Pulmonary capillaritis often occurs*
Henoch-Schönlein purpura	Vasculitis with IgA-dominant immune deposits affecting small vessels (i.e., capillaries, venules, or arterioles). *Typically involves skin, gut, and glomeruli and is associated with arthralgias or arthritis*
Essential cryoglobulinemic vasculitis	Vasculitis with cryoglobulin immune deposits affecting small vessels (i.e., capillaries, venules, or arterioles) and associated with cryoglobulins in serum. *Skin and glomeruli are often involved*
Cutaneous leukocytoclastic angiitis	Isolated cutaneous leukocytoclastic angiitis without systemic vasculitis or glomerulonephritis

*Large vessel refers to the aorta and the largest branches directed toward major body regions (e.g., to the extremities and the head and neck); *medium-sized vessel* refers to the main visceral arteries (e.g., renal, hepatic, coronary, and mesenteric arteries); *small vessel* refers to venules, capillaries, arterioles, and the intraparenchymal distal arterial radicals that connect with arterioles. Some small and large vessel vasculitides may involve medium-sized arteries, but large and medium-sized vessel vasculitides do not involve vessels smaller than arteries. Essential components are represented by normal type; *italicized type* represents usual but not essential components.
[†]Preferred term.
[‡]Strongly associated with antineutrophil cytoplasmic autoantibodies.
From Jennette C, Falk RJ: Nomenclature of systemic vasculitides: Proposal of an international consensus conference. Arthritis Rheum 37:187, 1994.

those who do not. In fact, in a prospective study of 198 patients in whom vasculitis was suspected but not confirmed, application of the criteria showed them to be a poor diagnostic tool.[236] Even among patients who have vasculitis, difficulties in specific diagnosis also arise because of overlap of the clinical features of the various vasculitides and because features of more than one type of vasculitis develop in some patients.[240]

The clinical and radiologic manifestations of pulmonary vasculitis can be related to the vascular inflammation itself or to the pneumonitis that sometimes accompanies the disorder. During the acute stages, the effects of vasculitis include alveolar hemorrhage and vascular thrombosis, with or without parenchymal necrosis. With more prolonged disease, weakening of the vessel wall can result in aneurysm formation, whereas obliteration of the vessel lumina can cause pulmonary hypertension. Because of the occurrence of concomitant extrapulmonary vasculitis and the common presence of glomerulonephritis, signs and symptoms of extrathoracic disease may overshadow the pulmonary manifestations.

Wegener's Granulomatosis

Wegener's granulomatosis (WG) is a multisystem disease with variable clinical expression that is pathologically characterized by necrotizing granulomatous inflammation of the upper and lower respiratory tracts, glomerulonephritis, and necrotizing vasculitis of the lungs and a variety of other organs and tissues. A classification scheme developed by the American College of Rheumatology in 1990 (before the description of ANCA antibodies) considered four principal criteria in its definition (Table 10–4):[241] (1) nasal and oral inflammation, (2) an abnormal chest radiograph, (3) abnormal urinary sediment, and (4) granulomatous inflammation on a biopsy specimen. In a series of 807 patients *who had vasculitis*, the presence of two or more of these criteria was associated with a diagnostic sensitivity and specificity of 88% and 92%, respectively.[241] The association of c-ANCA with these clinical features greatly strengthens the appropriateness of designating a given vasculitis WG (see Table 10–3).[239] It should be remembered, however, that a number of other disorders can cause lung disease associated with positive c-ANCA,[237,242] including a variety of infections[243] and malignancy.[244]

WG is a rare disease: in the United States the prevalence has been estimated to be about 3 per 100,000.[245] It typically affects adults in their fifth decade, men slightly more often than women.[246]

Two clinical variants of WG have been described in addition to the full-blown systemic disease. The more common is manifested primarily or solely in the respiratory tract and is thus known as *limited (nonrenal) WG*.[247] In many cases, the qualifier "limited" refers chiefly to an absence of clinical evidence of renal or other visceral disease; however, concomitant

TABLE 10–4. Criteria and Definitions Used for the Classification of Wegener's Granulomatosis*

Criterion	Definition
Nasal or oral inflammation	Development of painful or painless oral ulcers or purulent or bloody nasal discharge
Abnormal chest radiograph	Chest radiograph showing the presence of nodules, fixed infiltrates, or cavities
Urinary sediment	Microhematuria (>5 red blood cells per high-power field) or red cell casts in urine sediment
Granulomatous inflammation on biopsy	Histologic changes showing granulomatous inflammation within the wall of an artery or in the perivascular or extravascular area (artery or arteriole)

*For purposes of classification, a patient is said to have Wegener's granulomatosis if at least two of these four criteria are present.
Modified from Leavitt RY, Fauci AS, Bloch DA, et al: The American College of Rheumatology 1990 criteria for the classification of Wegener's granulomatosis. Arthritis Rheum 33:1101, 1990.

involvement of the upper respiratory tract and skin is not uncommon,[248] and a number of patients who apparently have limited disease have been found at autopsy or biopsy to have glomerulonephritis or systemic vasculitis and granulomatous inflammation.[249] Thus, from a pathogenetic point of view, it may be appropriate to consider these cases as part of a spectrum of disease rather than as separate entities. A second, less common clinical variant of WG is characterized by prominent and sometimes prolonged involvement of the mucous membranes of the upper respiratory tract and skin.[250]

Etiology and Pathogenesis

The etiology and pathogenesis of WG are poorly understood. There is experimental evidence that activation of neutrophils leads to the production of proteolytic enzymes and oxidants, which are responsible for the necrosis seen in the lung parenchyma.[251,252] The stimuli that attract and activate the neutrophils are not known. However, the association of disease relapse with bacterial or viral infection[253] and an increased risk of relapse with airway colonization by *Staphylococcus aureus*,[254,255] as well as the beneficial effects of trimethoprim-sulfamethoxazole,[256] suggests that infection initiates the inflammatory cascade in at least some cases.

The results of a number of experimental studies suggest that ANCAs may have a pathogenetic role in WG. These antibodies react with substances in neutrophil azurophilic granules and monocyte lysosomes. Three forms can be identified by indirect immunofluorescence:[257] c-ANCA, which is directed predominantly to proteinase-3 (PR-3); p-ANCA, which reacts predominantly with myeloperoxidase; and atypical ANCA, which is directed to a variety of antigens. c-ANCA is the variant most strongly associated with WG.

It has been demonstrated that mRNA related to PR-3, the target antigen for c-ANCA, is upregulated in the lung tissue of affected patients,[258] especially in type I and II pneumocytes and macrophages. Interaction of these cells with c-ANCA might lead to the production of chemokines or adhesion molecules that are important in inflammation. Furthermore,

cytokine activation of circulating polymorphonuclear cells makes PR-3 accessible for interaction with c-ANCAs on their surface, an interaction that leads to the cell's destruction and release of proteolytic enzymes.[259,260] Pulmonary arterial and capillary endothelial cells may contribute to this injury by increasing their expression of adhesion molecules, which enhance the attachment of activated neutrophils to their surface. c-ANCA has also been shown to have a direct toxic effect on the endothelial cell.[251] Finally, c-ANCA may have an effect on the development of cell-mediated granulomatous inflammation via PR-3–mediated T-cell mitogenesis.[261]

Despite the attractiveness of these hypothetic mechanisms, it is clear that ANCA-mediated injury cannot be the sole factor in the pathogenesis of WG: not all patients have c-ANCA, and the serum level of the antibody does not always correlate with the severity of disease.[262] Moreover, some patients who have c-ANCA do not have the disease.

The frequent presence of granulomatous inflammation in active lesions, both in relation to vessels and in relation to extravascular tissue, implies a cell-mediated component in disease pathogenesis. There is evidence that CD4+ T cells capable of producing interferon-γ and tumor necrosis factor-α (a T_H1 profile) are recruited from the blood of affected patients and promote monocyte accumulation and granuloma formation.[263]

Pathologic Characteristics

The pathologic features of WG are variable but overall are quite characteristic of the disease.[264,265] Grossly, pulmonary involvement typically consists of well-circumscribed nodules or masses ranging in diameter from 1 to 10 cm, often with central necrosis and sometimes with cavity formation. Occasionally, disease is manifested by focal or diffuse hemorrhagic consolidation.[266]

Microscopically, the nodules are composed of variable amounts of inflammatory and necrotic tissue, typically associated with effacement of normal lung architecture. The inflammatory infiltrate is composed predominantly of lymphocytes, plasma cells, and histiocytes, with lesser numbers of eosinophils, multinucleated giant cells, and polymorphonuclear leukocytes (see Color Fig. 10–2). Characteristically, the latter tend to be aggregated in small microabscess-like clusters. As the disease progresses, these clusters become necrotic and delineated by a layer of macrophages or epithelioid histiocytes (granulomatous inflammation). With further progression, individual necrotic areas enlarge, coalesce, and result in a characteristic serpiginous outline. Although inflammation is typically most prominent in the parenchyma, mucosal or submucosal granulomatous inflammation of the airways is also common.[267] The adjacent epithelium may be intact or ulcerated, in which case there may be a polypoid mass of granulation tissue that causes airway obstruction.

Pulmonary arteries and veins of small to medium size show focal or extensive inflammation manifested by one of three patterns (see Color Fig. 10–2): (1) fibrinoid necrosis of the media, (2) infiltration of the vessel wall by an inflammatory cell infiltrate similar to that in the parenchyma, or (3) well-defined granulomas or aggregates of multinucleated giant cells. Thrombosis may or may not be present.

In cases characterized grossly by hemorrhagic consolidation, the histologic appearance is that of microangiitis (capillaritis).[268] In these cases, the underlying lung architecture is maintained, but the alveolar air spaces are filled with red blood cells; hemosiderin-laden macrophages indicative of previous hemorrhage may also be seen. Alveolar septa are thickened by polymorphonuclear leukocytes, some of which may be necrotic (Fig. 10–14). In addition to capillaries, arterioles and venules are also often affected. These findings may be the only histologic manifestation of WG or may be present in association with the classic parenchymal and vascular changes.

Radiologic Manifestations

Pulmonary parenchymal abnormalities are identified on the initial chest radiograph in about 50% of patients and eventually develop in most.[269] The typical abnormality consists of nodules ranging in size from a few millimeters to 10 cm in diameter (Fig. 10–15).[270,271] In most cases, they are fewer than 10, bilateral and widely distributed, with no predilection for any lung zone.[270] With progression of disease, they tend to increase in size and number.[270] Calcification is rare.[272] Cavities develop in approximately 50% of cases.[270,273] They are usually thick walled and tend to have an irregular, shaggy inner lining[270,273]; less commonly, they are thin walled or contain an air-fluid level.

CT may show nodules that are not apparent on radiography and is superior in showing the presence of cavitation[272,274]; in fact, the latter is evident on CT in most nodules that measure more than 2 cm.[275] As on radiography, the nodules tend to have a random distribution[275,276]; occasionally, they are predominantly or exclusively subpleural in location[276] or have a peribronchoarterial distribution.[273,277]

Air space consolidation or ground-glass opacities secondary to diffuse pulmonary hemorrhage may be seen with or without the presence of nodules (Fig. 10–16).[270,273] They are usually bilateral but may be patchy or confluent, or dense and localized.[270,273] The most common manifestation of diffuse hemorrhage on CT scan consists of extensive bilateral ground-glass

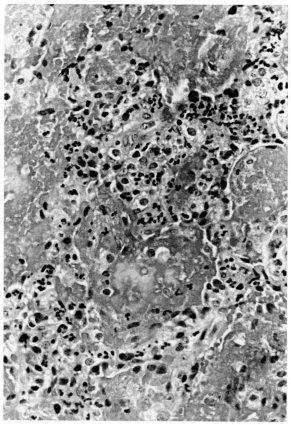

FIGURE 10–14

Wegener's granulomatosis—capillaritis. A section from an open lung biopsy specimen of a patient with bilateral air space disease shows filling of the alveolar air spaces by blood and mild to moderate thickening of the alveolar septa as a result of an infiltrate of polymorphonuclear leukocytes. *(From Fraser RS, Müller NL, Colman NC, Paré PD: Fraser and Paré's Diagnosis of Diseases of the Chest, 4th ed. Philadelphia, WB Saunders, 1999.)*

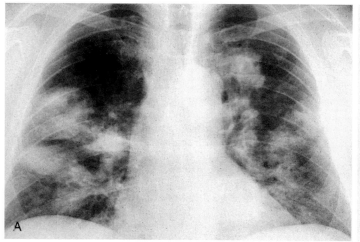
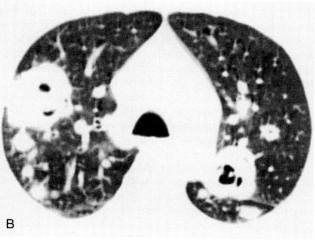

FIGURE 10–15

Wegener's granulomatosis. A posteroanterior chest radiograph (**A**) and a CT scan at the level of the upper lobes (**B**) demonstrate multiple bilateral nodules ranging from a few millimeters to 5 cm in diameter. The larger nodules are cavitated. The patient was a 54-year-old man. *(From Fraser RS, Müller NL, Colman NC, Paré PD: Fraser and Paré's Diagnosis of Diseases of the Chest, 4th ed. Philadelphia, WB Saunders, 1999.)*

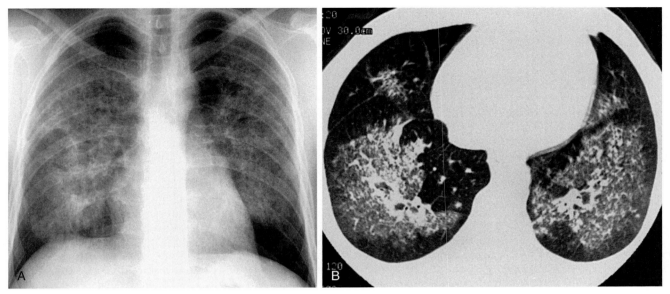

FIGURE 10–16

Wegener's granulomatosis—air space hemorrhage. A posteroanterior chest radiograph (**A**) in a 20-year-old man shows extensive bilateral areas of consolidation with relative sparing of the lung apices and bases. Several irregular linear opacities suggestive of fibrosis are evident. An HRCT scan (**B**) shows bilateral areas of ground-glass attenuation and consolidation with relative sparing of the subpleural lung regions. A few small nodular opacities and irregular linear opacities are evident. *(From Müller NL, Fraser RS, Colman NC, Paré PD: Radiologic Diagnosis of Diseases of the Chest. Philadelphia, WB Saunders, 2001.)*

opacities.[278] Focal areas of consolidation may also be seen in patients without pulmonary hemorrhage. On CT, these areas can have a random distribution, appear as peripheral wedge-shaped lesions abutting the pleura similar to pulmonary infarcts, or have a peribronchoarterial distribution.[277,278]

Tracheal and bronchial disease is seldom visible on the radiograph[271,279] but can usually be detected on CT scans.[276,278,280] The vast majority of tracheal lesions are located in the subglottic region.[281] Common findings include circumferential wall thickening, stenosis, and mucosal irregularity.[281] Pleural effusions occur in about 10% of patients.[270] They may be unilateral or bilateral and small or large. Hilar or mediastinal lymph node enlargement, or both, has been reported on radiography or CT in 2% to 15% of cases[270,273]; hilar involvement may be unilateral or bilateral.

Clinical Manifestations

Although the onset can be acute and its course fulminating, it is more commonly insidious. Initially, the disease may be associated with such nonspecific symptoms as fever, malaise, weight loss, and fatigue; however, the vast majority of patients initially have complaints referable to the nose, paranasal sinuses, or chest.[282] A few have symptoms and signs of widespread disease, including exophthalmos, hematuria, and vesicular and hemorrhagic skin lesions. Although renal manifestations occur in the majority of patients at some time in the course of their disease, only rarely are they the initial clinical feature.

Respiratory symptoms include intractable cough, often associated with hemoptysis, dyspnea, and pleuritic pain. Hemoptysis is occasionally massive, its clinical and radiologic features mimicking those of idiopathic hemorrhage or

Goodpasture's syndrome. Involvement of the larynx and upper part of the trachea can cause hoarseness or frank airway obstruction (the latter usually in the subglottic region).

Virtually any other organ or tissue can be affected. Nasal disease is manifested by rhinitis, sinusitis, and epistaxis; destruction of cartilage and bone may result in nasal deformity. Joint involvement is common and usually takes the form of arthralgia or nondeforming arthritis. Myalgias are also not infrequent. Neurologic manifestations may be central or peripheral, the latter manifested as mononeuritis multiplex or polyneuritis. Cardiac manifestations include conduction abnormalities and pericarditis. CNS and renal involvement is noted more commonly in the elderly than in younger patients.[283]

Laboratory Findings

Laboratory findings include anemia (sometimes hemolytic in type), thrombocytosis, and leukocytosis (occasionally with eosinophilia). As might be expected, markers of endothelial injury and coagulation disturbance such as thrombin–antithrombin III complexes, fibrin D-dimers, von Willebrand's factor, and thrombomodulin are elevated in many patients; their levels may be closely related to disease activity.[284] Rheumatoid factor may be detected in the serum, usually in low titer, and some patients have elevated levels of IgE.[285] Pulmonary function tests may show restrictive or obstructive disease, the latter finding being predominant.[286]

Diagnosis and management of WG have been aided by the ability to measure serum ANCA levels.[287] The presence of c-ANCAs is more specific for WG than p-ANCAs, the latter being seen in a variety of autoimmune disorders and in patients who have IBD.[288] As is true of all laboratory tests, the predictive value of a positive test is a function of the pretest probability of a positive result. Conclusions drawn concerning diagnosis when the test is applied casually may be erroneous.[289]

An important limitation of the test is its relative lack of sensitivity. In a meta-analysis of 15 studies examining the incidence of c-ANCA in WG, there was a pooled sensitivity of 0.66 in all patients who were suspected of having vasculitis. The sensitivity increased to 0.91 in those who had active disease.[290] Therefore, when suspicion of vasculitis is high, a negative test should not discourage further diagnostic testing. Among patients who had vasculitis, the specificity of a positive test was very high (99%). However, in unselected patients, the test may be less useful. For example, in one report of c-ANCA testing over a 10-year period in a single institution, only 32% of positive tests were associated with WG.[291]

The findings of several investigations have indicated that a rise in the titer of blood ANCA or persistence of a high level after therapy can predict relapse of disease before it is clinically apparent.[262,292] However, not all relapses are associated with an increase in titer,[262,292] and relapse is not inevitable when the titer persists in spite of therapy.[262] Therefore, levels of ANCA alone should not be used to dictate treatment regimens.

Bronchoscopy can also be useful in assessing patients who have WG. In a study of 51 individuals who had biopsy-proven disease, 30 (59%) had evidence of tracheobronchial involvement.[279] Biopsy of the affected areas supported the diagnosis in some patients; the diagnosis has also been confirmed occasionally by transbronchial biopsy.[293]

Prognosis

Until the application of immunosuppressive therapy, almost all patients died within 6 months of diagnosis.[294,295] Currently, the estimated median survival after diagnosis is in excess of 20 years,[282] with most deaths being due to either the disease or complications of therapy after a median 5.6 years of observation. Older age, lung involvement, and abnormal renal function at the time of diagnosis adversely affect the prognosis,[282] each being associated with a fourfold to fivefold increase in mortality risk.

Churg-Strauss Syndrome

In 1951, Churg and Strauss described a clinicopathologic syndrome characterized clinically by asthma, fever, and eosinophilia and pathologically by necrotizing vasculitis and extravascular granulomatous inflammation.[296] This condition—which is widely known as Churg-Strauss syndrome (CSS, allergic granulomatosis and angiitis)—has had a somewhat complicated conceptual history. At some times it has been considered to represent a variant of WG[297] and, at others, part of a spectrum of disease that includes polyarteritis nodosa (the term "overlap syndrome" sometimes being used to refer to the latter cases).[240] In addition, some cases of CSS share features with nonvasculitic syndromes such as hypereosinophilic syndrome or eosinophilic pneumonia.[298,299] Despite the fact that it is difficult to precisely classify vasculitic disease with eosinophilia in some patients, maintenance of CSS as a disease entity is generally thought to serve a useful purpose.

The classification system proposed by the American College of Rheumatology in 1990 included the following defining criteria: asthma, peripheral blood eosinophilia greater than 10%, mononeuropathy or polyneuropathy, nonfixed pulmonary "infiltrates," paranasal sinus abnormality, and the presence of extravascular eosinophils[300]; *in patients who have vasculitis*, the presence of four or more of these criteria was found to be diagnostic of CSS with a sensitivity of 85% and a specificity of almost 100%.

The syndrome is rare, the incidence having been estimated to be only 2.4 per million.[301] The mean age at diagnosis in one large series of patients was 48 years (range, 14 to 74 years).[302] There is no sex preponderance.

The cause of CSS is unknown; however, the association with asthma, rhinitis, and an elevated level of IgE, the favorable clinical response to corticosteroids, and the pathologic findings all suggest a hypersensitivity reaction to an unidentified antigen or antigens. Among the possible triggering factors that have been described, a history of desensitization injections is the most frequent.[302] CSS has been reported in patients taking leukotriene receptor antagonists, an observation that raises the possibility that the drug has initiated the disease. However, there is insufficient evidence to validate this hypothesis. On the one hand, the estimated incidence of CSS among these patients is similar to that described in asthmatics before distribution of the drugs[303,304]; on the other, there have been reports of relapse of vasculitis coincident with drug use.[305]

The characteristic histologic findings of CSS in the lungs consist of a combination of vasculitis, necrotizing extravascular granulomatous inflammation, and parenchymal eosinophil infiltration.[306] Vasculitis occurs predominantly in small to medium-sized arteries and veins and is manifested as a transmural infiltrate of lymphocytes, plasma cells, histiocytes, multinucleated giant cells, and a large number of eosinophils. Alveolar interstitial and air space infiltration by eosinophils and macrophages in a pattern similar to eosinophilic pneumonia is common. Histologic changes of chronic asthma (goblet cell metaplasia, basement membrane thickening, and muscle hypertrophy) are frequently evident in bronchioles and small bronchi.

The chest radiograph is abnormal in approximately 70% of patients.[307] In most, the abnormalities consist of transient, patchy nonsegmental areas of consolidation without predilection for any lung zone.[307,308] In 40%, these changes precede the development of clinical evidence of systemic vasculitis. The areas of consolidation may be symmetrical and have a nonsegmental distribution similar to that observed in chronic eosinophilic pneumonia (Fig. 10–17). Occasionally, the abnormalities consist of bilateral small and large nodular opacities that may become confluent; in contrast to WG, cavitation is rare. Unilateral or bilateral pleural effusions occur in approximately 30% of patients.

In a review of the HRCT findings at the time of diagnosis in 17 patients, the most common abnormality (seen in approximately 60%) consisted of areas of ground-glass attenuation or consolidation in a patchy or a predominant peripheral distribution (Fig. 10–18)[309]; other abnormalities seen by themselves or in addition to ground-glass attenuation or consolidation included small centrilobular nodules, cavitated nodules, interlobular septal thickening, bronchial wall thickening or dilation, and small unilateral or bilateral pleural effusions.

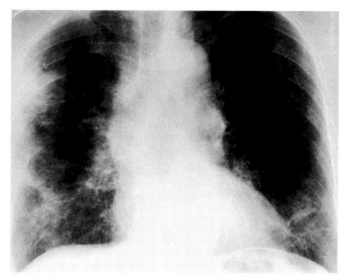

FIGURE 10–17

Churg-Strauss syndrome. A posteroanterior chest radiograph in a 71-year-old woman shows patchy bilateral areas of consolidation in a predominately subpleural distribution. *(From Müller NL, Fraser RS, Colman NC, Paré PD: Radiologic Diagnosis of Diseases of the Chest. Philadelphia, WB Saunders, 2001.)*

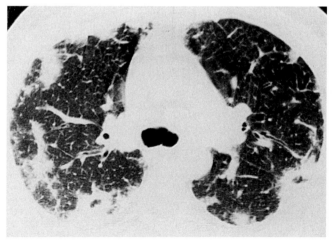

FIGURE 10–18

Churg-Strauss syndrome. An HRCT scan in a 52-year-old man shows bilateral areas of consolidation in a predominantly subpleural distribution. *(From Müller NL, Fraser RS, Colman NC, Paré PD: Radiologic Diagnosis of Diseases of the Chest. Philadelphia, WB Saunders, 2001.)*

CSS is often a triphasic illness.[303] In the prodromal phase, which often begins in adulthood, the patient experiences allergic rhinitis and asthma of variable severity. The second phase is characterized by significant blood eosinophilia and tissue infiltration by eosinophils and the third by life-threatening vasculitis involving multiple organs. Pulmonary manifestations are characterized by cough and, occasionally, hemoptysis. Asthma may precede evidence of vasculitis by as long as 30 years.[310]

Gastrointestinal involvement is common, occurring in 35% to 60% of patients, and is manifested as diarrhea or

bleeding.[311] Neurologic disease most often takes the form of peripheral neuropathy, usually mononeuritis multiplex.[312] Cardiac involvement may be manifested as angina, myocardial infarction, myocarditis, or pericarditis. Skin rash has been reported in up to 70% of patients.[310] Although frank renal failure is uncommon, an active urine sediment or histologic evidence of glomerulonephritis has been described in 30% to 70% of patients.[310]

The white blood cell count is frequently elevated as a result of eosinophilia.[307] BAL eosinophilia has also been described.[313] Hypergammaglobulinemia E is common during the vasculitic phase of illness, and anemia is present in most patients.[307] ANCAs, mostly p-ANCA and, in a smaller number of individuals, c-ANCA, are present in 75% of patients.[314] Their presence does not seem to be related to disease activity.

Clinical remission is achieved with therapy in over 90% of patients,[302] although a substantial minority experience relapse. Severe gastrointestinal or myocardial involvement is associated with a poor outcome.

Polyarteritis Nodosa

Polyarteritis nodosa is characterized by necrotizing vasculitis affecting predominantly small to medium-sized muscular arteries of the systemic circulation; lesions are typically unassociated with granulomatous inflammation, patchy in distribution, and often located at vessel branch points, where they are associated with localized aneurysms. Involvement of the peripheral nervous system, skin, muscle, kidney, and gastrointestinal tract is predominant.[315] An association with hepatitis B virus has been documented in a minority of patients.[237] Involvement of the bronchial artery circulation can occur as part of the systemic vasculitis[316]; however, pulmonary arteritis is rare.[317] The majority of clinical symptoms and radiologic abnormalities related to the lungs are the result of cardiogenic pulmonary edema or infection.

Microscopic Polyangiitis

Microscopic polyangiitis is a necrotizing vasculitis that affects predominantly small vessels (arterioles, venules, capillaries) of the pulmonary and systemic circulations. Although medium-sized vessels may also be affected, involvement of the small vessels by definition excludes a diagnosis of polyarteritis nodosa. Men are affected somewhat more commonly than women; the average age at onset is about 55.[318]

The etiology and pathogenesis are unclear. The association of some cases with the PiZZ phenotype[319] and the recognition that myeloperoxidase promoter polymorphism is linked to certain clinical features of disease[320] suggest that genetic factors play a role in pathogenesis. However, geographic variation in disease incidence[321] and the presence in some patients of apparent initiating events such as drug ingestion[322] or influenza vaccination[323] indicate that environmental factors are likely to be important as well.

ANCAs are present in about 75% of affected individuals, the vast majority being p-ANCA directed to myeloperoxidase.[318] As in WG, these antibodies promote degranulation of neutrophils and release of reactive oxygen species when bound to the cell surface.[324] Changes in antibody-antigen levels have been associated with fatal pulmonary hemorrhage in some patients, thus suggesting an important role in pathogenesis.[324] However, because not all patients with microscopic polyangiitis have p-ANCA and the antibody can be found in association with other diseases, other factors are probably involved in pathogenesis.

Histologically, alveolar air spaces contain fresh blood. In more chronic cases, hemosiderin-laden macrophages and fibroblast proliferation can also be seen.[325] The alveolar walls show capillaritis identical to that seen in WG, specifically, a patchy neutrophil infiltrate associated with edema, necrosis, and (sometimes) fibrin thrombi (see Fig. 10–14). Arterioles and venules may be involved, but larger vessels are unaffected. It is important to remember that the finding of alveolar hemorrhage and capillaritis represents a histologic reaction pattern rather than a specific disease entity.[258] Such a pattern may be seen in a variety of diseases in addition to microscopic polyangiitis, including other vasculitides such as WG,[266] connective tissue diseases (usually SLE),[17] antiphospholipid syndrome,[326] drug hypersensitivity,[325] and so-called pauci-immune pulmonary capillaritis.[327]

The radiographic features consist of patchy, bilateral air space opacities.[328,329] Pleural effusion has been reported in approximately 15% of cases and pulmonary edema in 5%.[329]

The clinical findings are variable. Rapidly progressive glomerulonephritis occurs in 80% to 100% of patients and diffuse alveolar hemorrhage in 10% to 40%.[318] The onset of symptoms may be indolent and precede the diagnosis by a long delay. Arthralgias or hemoptysis may occur for months or even years before acute symptoms bring the patient to medical attention. Other systemic manifestations include weight loss, fever, purpura, arthritis, myositis, hypertension, congestive heart failure, gastrointestinal hemorrhage, peripheral neuropathy (mononeuritis multiplex), and sinusitis.[251,318]

In a group of 85 patients monitored for a mean duration of 70 months, 28 (33%) died as a result of complications of the disease and its therapy.[318] Although therapy induced remission in most patients, relapse was common: 29 patients relapsed after a mean time of 43 months. Both obstructive lung disease and pulmonary fibrosis have been identified as complications of recurrent episodes of bleeding.[318]

Isolated (Pauci-immune) Pulmonary Capillaritis

This rare and relatively recently described abnormality is characterized radiologically by patchy, bilateral air space opacities typical of alveolar hemorrhage and pathologically by capillaritis identical to that seen in microscopic polyangiitis and WG.[327] Unlike the latter conditions, ANCAs and extrapulmonary manifestations of vasculitis are absent. Direct immunofluorescent study of lung biopsy specimens also shows no evidence of immune complex or anti–glomerular basement membrane (GBM) antibody deposition (hence the descriptor "pauci-immune"). It is unclear whether this abnormality is a distinct entity or part of a spectrum of vasculitis that includes pauci-immune disease in other organs such as the kidney.

In an investigation of eight patients who fulfilled the diagnostic criteria for the condition, the mean age at onset was 30 (range, 19 to 37)[327]; initial symptoms included dyspnea,

cough, and hemoptysis. Follow-up found one to have died, five to be in remission, and two to have experienced multiple recurrences of alveolar hemorrhage. In none did evidence of systemic disease develop.

Takayasu's Arteritis

Takayasu's arteritis is an uncommon disease that principally affects the aorta and its major branches; approximately 300 cases had been reported by 1996.[330] According to the American College of Rheumatology vasculitis classification scheme, the presence of three or more of the criteria listed in Table 10–5 is associated with a sensitivity and specificity of diagnosis of approximately 90% and 98% in patients who have vasculitis.[331] Although systemic manifestations of disease are more apparent clinically, pulmonary vascular involvement occurs in the majority of affected individuals.[332-334]

The disease has a marked predilection for women (approximately 90% to 95% of cases)[335] and usually has its onset between 10 and 40 years of age. Most reports have originated from Oriental countries, although it has been suggested that the disease might be underreported in Europe and North America.[336]

The most prominent histologic finding is patchy panarteritis involving the large elastic vessels of the systemic and pulmonary circulations. The adventitia shows fibrosis and a mixed, largely mononuclear inflammatory cell infiltrate resembling that seen in syphilis; fibrous obliteration and a perivascular mononuclear infiltrate of the vasa vasorum occur frequently.[337] The media may show necrotizing or nonnecrotizing granulomatous inflammation or, in older lesions, fibrosis and disruption of the elastic laminae. Intimal fibrosis also occurs frequently.

TABLE 10–5. 1990 Criteria for the Classification of Takayasu's Arteritis*

Criterion	Definition
Age at disease onset ≤40 years	Development of symptoms or findings related to Takayasu's arteritis at age ≤40 years
Claudication of extremities	Development and worsening of fatigue and discomfort in muscles of one or more extremity while in use, especially the upper extremities
Decreased brachial artery pulse	Decreased pulsation of one or both brachial arteries
Blood pressure difference >10 mm Hg	Difference of >10 mm Hg in systolic blood pressure between arms
Bruit over subclavian arteries or aorta	Bruit audible on auscultation over one or both subclavian arteries or abdominal aorta
Arteriogram abnormality	Arteriographic narrowing or occlusion of the entire aorta, its primary branches, or large arteries in the proximal end of the upper or lower extremities, not due to arteriosclerosis, fibromuscular dysplasia, or similar causes; changes usually focal or segmental

*For purposes of classification, a patient is said to have Takayasu's arteritis if at least three of these six criteria are present.
Modified from Arend WP, Michel BA, Bloch DA, et al: The American College of Rheumatology 1990 criteria for the classification of Takayasu arteritis. Arthritis Rheum 33:1131, 1990.

The most common radiographic abnormalities consist of a wavy or scalloped contour of the descending thoracic aorta and ectasia of the aortic arch[333,338]; dilation of the ascending aorta and aneurysm of the descending aorta are seen less frequently. Contrast-enhanced CT shows circumferential thickening of the aortic and, less commonly, the pulmonary artery wall.[339,340] Delayed-phase CT images obtained 20 to 40 minutes after intravenous injection show circumferential enhancement of the vessel wall.[339] Thickening and enhancement of the vessel wall may also be seen on contrast-enhanced MR imaging.[341] Pulmonary artery involvement occurs in 50% to 70% of patients.[342,343] The most common abnormalities consist of stenosis or occlusion of segmental or subsegmental branches, usually in an upper lobe.[343] These abnormalities are associated with localized areas of low attenuation and decreased vascularity on HRCT and perfusion defects on ^{99m}Tc-macroaggregated albumin perfusion scintigraphy.[342]

Constitutional symptoms of fever, myalgias, arthralgias, and weight loss are typically present for months to years before the more specific features of the disease become evident. The latter are usually related to vascular stenosis and include angina pectoris, headache, syncope, impaired vision, and claudication of the upper or lower extremities. A bruit, most commonly heard over the carotid artery, is frequently noted.[335] Localized pain over the affected arteries may be present. Arterial pulses may be diminished or absent altogether; a difference in systolic pressure between the two arms may be appreciated.

Evidence of pulmonary involvement almost always occurs in patients who have systemic findings; rarely, it is the first manifestation of disease.[344] Many patients are asymptomatic despite the presence of clinical signs or radiologic findings of pulmonary disease.[345] Chest pain and hemoptysis occur occasionally.[344]

In a study of 60 patients monitored at the National Institutes of Health over a 6-month to 20-year period, only 2 patients died, apparently of unrelated causes.[335] However, permanent disability as a result of an inability to perform daily functions was found in about 50%, and a further 25% had episodes of temporary disability during periods of active disease.

Giant Cell Arteritis

Giant cell arteritis (temporal arteritis) is a relatively common systemic arteritis that affects predominantly older individuals. Disease is most frequent in the larger arteries of the head and neck; pathologic involvement of both large elastic and medium-sized muscular pulmonary arteries has been documented rarely.[346,347]

Symptoms usually consist of headache, jaw claudication, polymyalgia rheumatica, and loss of vision; tenderness in the region of the temporal artery or scalp is not uncommon. The sedimentation rate is usually high. Upper respiratory tract symptoms and signs, including sore throat, hoarseness, a choking sensation, and tenderness of cervical structures, may be evident as initial findings.[348] Evidence of pleuropulmonary involvement is uncommon but includes findings of pleural effusion,[349] granulomatous interstitial disease,[350] pulmonary infarction,[351] and cough and dyspnea associated with a T4-lymphocytic alveolitis.[352]

Behçet's Disease

Behçet's disease is an uncommon systemic disorder characterized by recurrent aphthous ulcers, skin lesions, genital ulceration, and uveitis. A variety of other organs and tissues may be involved, including the kidneys, joints, CNS, gastrointestinal tract, pericardium, and lung.[353] The age at onset is usually between 20 and 30 years; men are affected slightly more often than women. The disease is most prevalent in the Middle East, especially Turkey, and in eastern Asia.[353]

The etiology and pathogenesis are uncertain. The strong association with HLA-B51 in many ethnic groups[354] and reports of familial clustering of disease unrelated to HLA-B51[353] imply that a genetic influence is important. The observation that oligoclonal T-cell expansion correlates with clinically active disease suggests that an antigen-driven immune response (possibly representing a cross-reaction with an infectious agent) might be important in pathogenesis.[353]

The principal histologic abnormality in the lungs in early disease is transmural vascular inflammation by lymphocytes, plasma cells, and polymorphonuclear leukocytes.[355] The inflammatory process can extend into adjacent airways and cause bronchial or pulmonary artery erosion and hemoptysis. Such active disease is uncommonly seen histologically; more often, microscopic examination shows fibrosis/thinning of muscular and elastic arterial walls, sometimes severe enough to be associated with aneurysm formation. Recent or organized thrombi and parenchymal infarcts may be present and can be related to either local vasculitis and thrombosis or thromboembolism secondary to systemic thrombophlebitis.[356]

Pulmonary artery aneurysms are radiographically visualized as round perihilar opacities or as rapidly developing unilateral hilar enlargement.[357] They may be single or multiple, unilateral or bilateral, and usually measure 1 to 3 cm in diameter.[358,359] Their presence, size, and location can also be better assessed with CT, MR imaging, or angiography (Fig. 10–19)[358-360]; CT and MR imaging may show thrombosed aneurysms, which are not seen at angiography.[358,361] Thrombotic occlusion of the pulmonary vasculature most commonly involves the right interlobar artery and less often the lobar and segmental arteries.[361] It may result in localized areas of consolidation as a result of infarction, areas of oligemia, and areas of atelectasis. Unilateral or bilateral pleural effusions may be seen in association with infarction. Pulmonary hemorrhage as a result of vasculitis or pulmonary artery rupture occasionally results in focal, multifocal, or diffuse air space consolidation.[358,362] Thrombosis of the superior vena cava may be manifested as mediastinal widening on the chest radiograph (see Fig. 10–19).[359]

Behçet's disease follows a waxing and waning course. To establish the diagnosis, patients must have recurrent oral ulceration and two of the following in the absence of other clinical explanations: recurrent genital ulceration, ocular lesions, skin lesions, or a positive pathergy test (development of a papule or pustule after a needle prick to the skin).[353] Pulmonary disease is relatively uncommon and may develop several years after the onset of systemic disease. Pulmonary artery aneurysms, arterial and venous thrombosis, pulmonary infarction, recurrent pneumonia, and pleurisy are the major manifestations.[353] Symptoms typically consist of recurrent hemoptysis, chest pain, dyspnea, and cough. Hemoptysis may

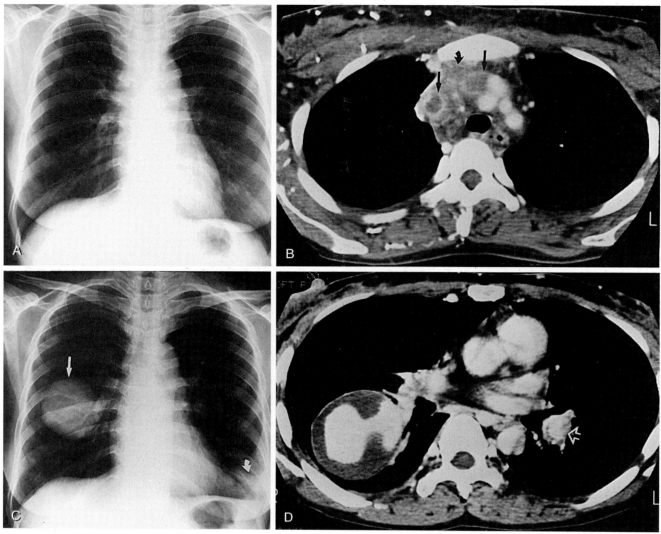

FIGURE 10–19

Behçet's disease. A posteroanterior chest radiograph (**A**) in a 37-year-old woman shows widening of the right upper portion of the mediastinum. A contrast-enhanced CT scan (**B**) shows thrombosis of the right and left brachiocephalic veins (*straight arrows*) and increased attenuation of the mediastinal fat (*curved arrows*), a finding suggestive of edema. Collateral veins are visible in the mediastinum and chest wall. A chest radiograph obtained 6 months later (**C**) shows a round, well-defined mass in the right lower lobe (*straight arrow*) and localized consolidation in the left lower lobe (*curved arrow*). The upper part of the mediastinum appears normal. A contrast-enhanced CT scan (**D**) obtained at the same time as the radiograph demonstrates a thrombus. Note the dilated left descending pulmonary artery (*arrowhead*). (**A** to **D** from Ahn JM, Im JG, Ryoo JW, et al: Thoracic manifestations of Behçet syndrome: Radiographic and CT findings in nine patients. Radiology 194:199-203, 1995. Case courtesy of Dr. Jung-Gi Im, Department of Radiology, Seoul National University Hospital, Seoul, South Korea.)

be massive and is a common cause of death.[363] Obstructive lung function, sometimes responsive to bronchodilator therapy, has been reported[364]; a mild restrictive impairment has also been noted.[363]

Mixed Cryoglobulinemia

Mixed cryoglobulinemia is an uncommon disease characterized by purpura, arthralgia, glomerulonephritis, and the presence in the serum of globulins that precipitate on exposure to cold temperatures (cryoglobulins). These proteins can be present in a wide variety of lymphoproliferative, infectious, and connective tissue diseases; however, the vast majority of

cases are related to hepatitis C virus infection or systemic autoimmune disorders.[365] In a series of 23 patients in whom lung function was studied,[366] radiographic evidence of diffuse interstitial pulmonary disease was present in 18. Symptoms related to the chest were unusual: one patient had hemoptysis, another had pleural pain, and a third had a clinical picture of asthma. Pulmonary function test results indicated small-airway obstruction and abnormal gas exchange.

Henoch-Schönlein Purpura

Henoch-Schönlein purpura, a widespread, necrotizing vasculitis affecting small vessels, is characterized by purpura, abdominal pain, gastrointestinal hemorrhage, arthritis or arthralgia, glomerulonephritis, and tissue deposition of IgA-containing immune complexes. The disease occurs most often in childhood and adolescence.[367] A number of men in whom the disease develops have been found to have underlying malignancy.[368]

The occasional fatal case in which the histologic appearance has been described has shown capillaritis and alveolar hemorrhage.[369,370] Radiographic abnormalities are typically those of bilateral air space disease as a result of intra-alveolar hemorrhage; the pattern is predominantly interstitial in some cases.[371]

Clinically, the disease is characterized by episodes of remission and relapse, typically ending with spontaneous resolution. Evidence of involvement of the respiratory tract is rare; in a review of 77 adults with the condition, only 4 had evidence of pulmonary disease.[367] The principal manifestation is hemoptysis.[369]

Necrotizing Sarcoid Granulomatosis

Necrotizing sarcoid granulomatosis is a rare disorder characterized pathologically by confluent granulomas associated with a variable amount of necrosis and prominent, focally destructive vasculitis.[372] Of the 100 cases reported by 1996, most were in middle-aged adults[373]; there is a strong female preponderance.[374] It is a matter of debate whether the abnormality is a distinct disorder or the histologic counterpart of radiologically evident nodular sarcoidosis.[375]

The radiologic pattern is usually that of multiple 3- to 10-mm-diameter well-defined nodules.[375] On HRCT scan, they have a predominantly peribronchoarterial and subpleural distribution, similar to that of sarcoidosis.[376] Hilar lymph node enlargement was not a feature in the original report of 11 cases,[372] but it was noted in 6 of 12 patients in another series.[377]

Clinically, patients may be asymptomatic or have cough, fever, sweats, malaise, dyspnea, hemoptysis, or pleuritic pain. Infection must be excluded carefully because organisms that cause granulomatous inflammation can produce both the clinical and histologic appearance of the abnormality. The clinical course is typically benign. Radiographic evidence of disease diminishes with corticosteroid therapy or, occasionally, spontaneously; however, relapse has occurred after cessation of therapy.[377]

ORGANIC DUST PULMONARY DISEASE

Extrinsic Allergic Alveolitis

The term "extrinsic allergic alveolitis" (EAA; hypersensitivity pneumonitis) denotes a group of pulmonary diseases characterized by an abnormal immunologic reaction to antigens contained in a wide variety of organic dust. The list of diseases and the antigens associated with them have grown steadily since "farmer's lung" was first described in 1932 (Table 10–6).[378] Regardless of the name of the disease and the specific exposure involved, striking similarities exist among the clinical, pathologic, and radiologic features of all these diseases, thus suggesting that they share a common pathogenesis.

The diagnosis of EAA is hampered by the variability of its clinical expression and by the lack of sensitivity and specificity of its clinical and laboratory features. Although specific diagnostic criteria have been proposed,[379,380] their validity is contingent on the exclusion of other diseases with similar signs and symptoms, which makes strict application difficult.[381] Nonetheless, the diagnosis can usually be considered confirmed if four major and two minor criteria have been fulfilled. Major criteria include the following:

1. A history of symptoms compatible with EAA that appear or worsen within hours after antigen exposure
2. Confirmation of exposure to the offending agent by history, investigation of the environment, serum precipitin test, and/or BAL fluid antibody analysis
3. Compatible changes on chest radiography or HRCT
4. BAL fluid lymphocytosis (however, neutrophilia can also be seen in some settings[382])
5. Compatible histologic changes
6. Positive "natural challenge" (reproduction of symptoms and laboratory abnormalities after exposure to the suspected environment) or positive challenge by controlled inhalation

Minor criteria include the following:

1. Basilar crackles
2. Decreased diffusion capacity
3. Arterial hypoxemia, either at rest or with exercise

Pathogenesis

The development of EAA is dependent on the size, immunogenicity, and number of inhaled organic particles, as well as the duration of exposure and the immune response of the affected individual. A large amount of inhaled antigen is probably necessary to provide a stimulus for the immune response. Investigations of situations known to be associated with EAA have shown such to be the case; for example, it has been estimated that each gram of moldy bagasse has about 500,000,000 potentially antigenic fungal spores.[383]

Details concerning the cellular interactions responsible for pathogenesis of the disease are obscure and undoubtedly complex.[381] There is evidence that immune complex–mediated complement activation and neutrophil chemotaxis are involved in causing tissue injury.[384,385] For example, exposure of patients who have farmer's lung to antigen induces an alveolitis that is characterized in its early stages by the presence of activated neutrophils.[386] In addition, the presence of neutrophils primed to produce collagenase and gelatinase B in the lungs of some patients who have EAA correlates with the development of fibrosis in subacute and chronic disease.[387] There is also evidence from some animal studies that immune complexes play a role both in macrophage-mediated antigen presentation to T cells[384] and in release of proinflammatory cytokines (interleukin-1, tumor necrosis factor-α) involved in the accumulation of lymphocytes[388] and granuloma formation.[389] Despite these observations, it is clear that immune complex–mediated injury is not the only factor in pathogenesis. Affected patients have normal complement levels, the histologic findings are not characteristic of this type of immune response, and abundant evidence has indicated that serum antibodies to an inciting antigen are more a marker of exposure than a marker of disease.[390]

TABLE 10–6. Varieties of Extrinsic Allergic Alveolitis

Disease	Principal Responsible Antigens	Exposure Source	Additional Features
Anhydride-induced lung disease	Trimollitic anhydride (?), phthalic anhydride (?)	Polyester powder paint	Similar to isocyanate-induced lung disease
Bagassosis	*Thermoactinomyces sacchari*	Moldy sugar cane residue (bagasse)	
Bird fancier's (pigeon breeder's) lung	Avian proteins contained in serum, excreta, or feathers	Pigeons, budgerigars, canaries, parakeets, chickens, ducks, turkeys, geese	With farmer's lung, the most common form of EAA
Building-associated EAA	*Thermoactinomyces* species; *Epicoccum nigrum* Various fungi (*Serpula, Paecilomyces, Aspergillus, Leucogyrophana* species)	Decayed wood, damp walls, other materials in human habitations	
Cheese worker's lung	*Penicillium* species	Moldy cheese	
Coffee worker's lung	?	Coffee bean roasting	
Composter's or gardener's lung	?	Yard clippings, poorly ventilated greenhouse	
Detergent worker's lung	*Bacillus subtilis*	Manufacture of proteolytic enzyme by *B. subtilis* for use in detergents	
Farmer's lung	Thermophilic bacteria (*Saccharopolyspora rectivirgula, Micropolyspora faeni, Thermoactinomyces* species, and others)		Affects males aged 40-50 yr; peak incidence during season when stored hay is used for cattle feeding; acute illness in 1/3 of patients, insidious in remainder; prevalence among farmers in different communities 1%-10%; should not be confused with organic dust toxic syndrome.
Fishmeal worker's lung	Fish protein (?)	Preparation of meat	
Herb worker's lung	*Thymus vulgaris*	Threshing of thyme	
Hot tub bather's lung	*Mycobacterium avium–intracellulare* complex		*See also* Humidifier lung
Humidifier lung	Bacteria: *Thermoactinomyces* species Fungi: *Penicillium* species, *Cladosporium* species Amebae: *Sphaeropsidales* species, *Acanthamoeba castellani, Naegleria gruberi*	Air conditioners, humidifiers, damp floors or walls, hot tubs	May be difficult to diagnose because of obscure exposure history; symptoms may develop in the evening of the first day back at work after a long weekend
Isocyanate-induced lung disease	Hexamethylene diisocyanate, diphenylmethane diisocyanate, and others	Electronics industry, autobody shops	Though caused by inorganic material, this abnormality is clinically identical to EAA caused by organic dust
Japanese summer–type allergic alveolitis	*Tricosporum cutaneum*	House dust	Principal form of EAA in Japan; occurs in summer months and subsides in autumn
Laboratory worker's lung	Pauli's reagent, rat serum, and others		
Lycoperdonosis	Mushrooms of genus *Lycoperdon*		
Machine operator's lung	*Pseudomonas fluorescens* (?), *Acinetobacter lwoffi* (?), nontuberculous mycobacteria (?)	Contaminated metalworking fluid	
Malt worker's lung	*Aspergillus clavatus*	Moldy malt	
Maple bark disease	*Cryptostroma corticale*	Tree bark	Affects sawmill workers
Mollusk shell worker's lung		Mollusk shell dust in a button factory	
Mushroom worker's lung	*Micropolyspora faeni, Micromonospora vulgaris, Pleurotus ostreatus, Pholiota namek, Hypsizigus marmoreus*	Compost used for mushroom culture	Steam pasteurization during culture of mushrooms encourages rapid growth of thermophilic actinomycetes
New Guinea lung	*Streptomyces viridis* (?)	Domestic exposure after flooding Thatched roofs	
Orchid grower's lung	*Cryptostroma corticale*		
Peat moss worker's lung	*Monocillium* species (?), *Penicillium* species (?)	Processing plant	
Pituitary snuff taker's lung	Pig or ox pituitary extract	Extract used for treatment of diabetes insipidus	
Polyester powder lung	Phthalic anhydride (?)		
Polyurethane foam injection worker's lung	1,3-*bis* (isocyanatomethyl) cyclohexane prepolymer		
Prawn worker's lung	Shellfish protein (?)	Forced air used to blow meat out of tails	
Salami worker's lung	*Penicillium* species	Salami factory	
Sawmill worker's lung	*Trichoderma konigii*		
Sequoiosis	*Aureobasidium pullulans* (?), *Graphium* species (?)	Moldy redwood sawdust	

TABLE 10–6. Varieties of Extrinsic Allergic Alveolitis—cont'd

Disease	Principal Responsible Antigens	Exposure Source	Additional Features
Soy sauce brewer's lung	*Aspergillus oryzae*		
Starch spray lung	?	Ironing clothes	
Stipatosis	*Aspergillus fumigatus*	Esparto grass	
Suberosis	*Penicillium frequentans*	Moldy cork	Occurs principally in cork workers in Portugal
Swimming pool lung	*Candida albicans*		
Tiger nut lung	*Junia avellaneda*	Tiger nuts	
Tobacco worker's lung	?	Moldy raw tobacco	
Wood pulp worker's disease	*Alternaria* species	Wood pulp	
Wood worker's lung	*Cabreuva* wood dust	Sawing wood	

Modified from Fraser RS, Müller NL, Colman NC, Paré PD: Fraser and Paré's Diagnosis of Diseases of the Chest, 4th ed. Philadelphia, WB Saunders, 1999.

A major feature early in the course of EAA is the development of a lymphocytic alveolitis characterized by the presence of activated CD4+ lymphocytes of the T_H1 phenotype[381] and CD8+ lymphocytes.[391] The presence of these cells appears to be necessary (albeit not sufficient) for the development of subsequent disease.[381] They produce a number of proinflammatory cytokines that activate both macrophages and lymphocytes, eventually resulting in granuloma formation and fibrosis.[381] A number of anti-inflammatory cytokines are also produced by both lymphocytes and alveolar macrophages, and it is likely that expression of disease depends on a balance between proinflammatory and anti-inflammatory processes.[384,392]

Mast cells may also play an immunomodulatory role in EAA. They are increased in number in both tissue sections[393] and samples of BAL fluid (in which they are frequently degranulated).[394] Although their exact role is not understood and their presence in human disease does not appear to correlate with outcome,[395] a model of EAA using mice deficient in mast cells has been characterized by a significant reduction in the inflammatory response.[384]

For obscure reasons, cigarette smoking appears to protect against the development of EAA. A highly significant positive correlation has been observed between lack of cigarette smoking and the development of both active EAA (farmer's and pigeon breeder's lung)[396] and specific serum antibodies.[397] Despite these findings, the results of a study from Japan showed chronic disease, frequent relapse, and poor outcome to be much more prevalent in workers who smoked than in nonsmokers.[398] It is likely that many other individual and environmental factors also influence the development of disease,[399] including HLA haplotype, cytokine polymorphism, and immunomodulation induced by viral infection and by exposure to bacterial lipopolysaccharides and fungal glucan.[400-402]

Pathologic Characteristics

The histologic features of the many different varieties of EAA are strikingly similar. During the acute stage of disease, the histologic appearance consists of a combination of bronchiolitis and alveolitis with granuloma formation.[403,404] The alveolitis is manifested as an interstitial inflammatory infiltrate composed predominantly of lymphocytes with lesser numbers of histiocytes, plasma cells, polymorphonuclear leukocytes,

and eosinophils. The infiltrate is usually patchy in distribution with a tendency to more severe involvement of the peribronchiolar regions (see Color Fig. 10–3). Loosely formed granulomas composed of epithelioid histiocytes, multinucleated giant cells, or both are seen in 65% to 75% of cases (see Color Fig. 10–3); single multinucleated giant cells associated with a lymphocytic infiltrate are also common.[403] Bronchiolitis is frequent as well, the usual pattern being that of an organizing exudate adjacent to a focus of epithelial ulceration or a plug of fibroblastic connective tissue.

Depending on the severity and frequency of individual bouts of lung damage, a variable degree of interstitial fibrosis eventually supervenes. This fibrosis is often most prominent in the peribronchial or periseptal areas; sometimes, it is more diffuse and resembles advanced IPF with honeycombing. If exposure to the inciting antigen is discontinued, the granulomas tend to disappear, although mononuclear inflammatory cells and solitary multinucleated giant cells containing refractile foreign material frequently remain.

Radiologic Manifestations

The radiologic findings vary with the stage of the disease. Early in the course of the acute stage, the chest radiograph may show no abnormality, even in patients who have florid pathologic changes on lung biopsy.[405] Later on, the characteristic finding consists of bilateral areas of consolidation, which may be diffuse or involve primarily the lower lung zones.[406] The radiographic abnormalities in subacute disease usually involve mainly the middle and lower lung zones.[407,408] The most characteristic findings are poorly defined small nodular opacities or a poorly defined hazy increase in lung opacity (ground-glass opacity), or both (Fig. 10–20).[408,409] These abnormalities frequently resolve completely within 10 days to 3 months after exposure if the patient is removed from the environment. If exposure is continued or repeated or if the initial exposure is especially severe, the diffuse nodular or ground-glass pattern is replaced by a reticular pattern characteristic of interstitial fibrosis. Although the fibrosis may be diffuse, there is frequently a zonal predominance, particularly of the middle or lower lung regions (Fig. 10–21).[408,410,411]

As might be expected, HRCT is superior to chest radiography in demonstrating parenchymal abnormalities[406,408]; for example, in a study of 21 patients who had subacute disease and abnormal HRCT scans, 7 (33%) had normal chest

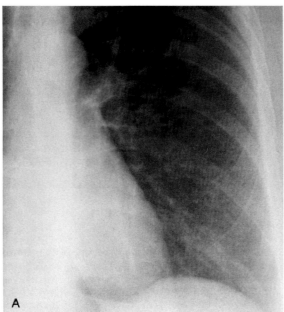
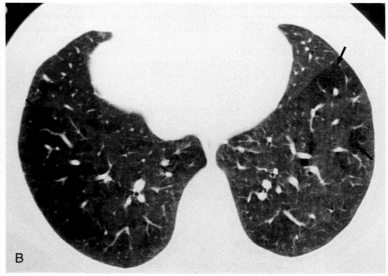

FIGURE 10–20

Subacute hypersensitivity pneumonitis. A 42-year-old woman suffered from progressive shortness of breath over a period of several months. Chest radiographs before admission and at admission were interpreted as normal. Even in retrospect, it is difficult to appreciate the mild, hazy increased opacity on the magnified view of the left lung from the admission chest radiograph (**A**). An HRCT scan (**B**) shows extensive areas of ground-glass attenuation and focal areas of low attenuation and decreased perfusion (*arrows*). *(From Müller NL, Fraser RS, Colman NC, Paré PD: Radiologic Diagnosis of Diseases of the Chest. Philadelphia, WB Saunders, 2001.)*

radiographs.[412] Typical findings in acute disease consist of bilateral areas of consolidation superimposed on small centrilobular nodular opacities.[406,413] The consolidation may be diffuse or involve mainly the lower lung zones. The findings in subacute disease consist of bilateral areas of ground-glass attenuation (see Fig. 10–20), poorly defined centrilobular nodular opacities (Fig. 10–22), or both. Although both abnormalities are usually diffuse, they are often most marked in the middle and lower lung zones.[408] Another frequent finding in patients who have subacute disease is the presence of localized areas of decreased attenuation and vascularity.[414] Such areas usually have a striking lobular distribution and are associated with evidence of air trapping on expiratory HRCT scans (Fig. 10–23). Their extent correlates with an increase in residual volume (RV) and the RV/TLC ratio.

The chronic stage of hypersensitivity pneumonitis is manifested on HRCT by evidence of fibrosis, frequently associated with features of subacute disease (see Fig. 10–21).[406,410,412] In a review of HRCT scans in 16 patients, areas of fibrosis were characterized by the presence of irregular linear opacities and architectural distortion.[410] The irregular lines had a random distribution in the transverse plane in 44% of patients, were predominantly subpleural in 37%, and were peribronchovascular in 19%. Honeycombing was identified in 11 (69%). In 44% of patients, the irregular linear opacities and honeycombing involved mainly the middle lung zones (see Fig. 10–21), and in 38%, they were distributed evenly throughout the three lung zones. Upper lobe predominance was present in only 1 of 16 patients (6%). Extensive areas of ground-glass attenuation and small centrilobular opacities were noted in 15 (94%) and 10 (62%) patients, respectively; these

abnormalities were present mainly in the middle and lower lung zones.

Clinical Manifestations

The clinical findings may be acute, subacute, or chronic. Intermittent exposure of susceptible individuals to a high concentration of antigen is accompanied by recurrent episodes of fever, chills, dry cough, and dyspnea, whereas continuous exposure to a lower concentration characteristically results in gradually progressive dyspnea in the absence of systemic symptoms.[415,416] Episodic symptoms may occur without abnormalities on the chest radiograph,[417] sometimes in patients who have dramatic symptoms.[418] Clearly, the most important first step in diagnosis is to think of the possibility of EAA, thereby avoiding attributing the clinical findings to infection in those who have acute symptoms or to IPF in those whose manifestations are chronic.[419]

Airway disease may also be present in patients who have EAA. In a small number of patients, generally those who have a history of allergy, the findings are confounded by clinical features consistent with asthma.[420] Although chronic cough and sputum production are common in otherwise healthy farmers,[421] there appears to be a strong positive relationship between the syndrome of farmer's lung and chronic bronchitis,[422] thus suggesting that chronic cough and sputum production should be considered features of recurrent or chronic EAA.

No physical findings are specific for the diagnosis of EAA. Auscultatory examination of the chest may at times reveal crackles[423] or a peculiar inspiratory "squawk,"[424] findings that

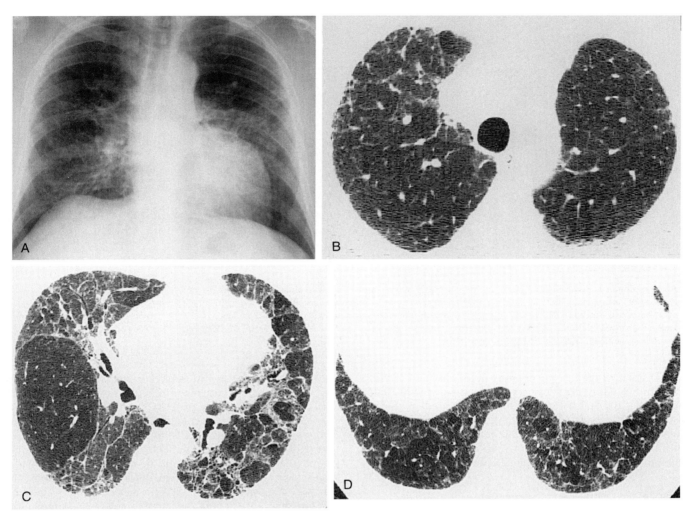

FIGURE 10–21

Chronic hypersensitivity pneumonitis. A posteroanterior chest radiograph (**A**) shows irregular linear opacities involving mainly the middle lung zones. Lung volumes are decreased. An HRCT scan (1-mm collimation) at the level of the aortic arch (**B**) shows mild fibrosis. Much more extensive fibrosis is present at the level of the right middle lobe bronchus (**C**). The fibrosis has a random distribution in the transverse plane and is characterized by the presence of irregular lines of attenuation and distortion of the lung architecture. Mild honeycombing is evident in the posterior basal segments of the lower lobes. An HRCT scan through the lung bases (**D**) shows relative sparing. The distribution of disease is characteristic of chronic hypersensitivity pneumonitis. *(From Müller NL, Fraser RS, Colman NC, Paré PD: Radiologic Diagnosis of Diseases of the Chest. Philadelphia, WB Saunders, 2001.)*

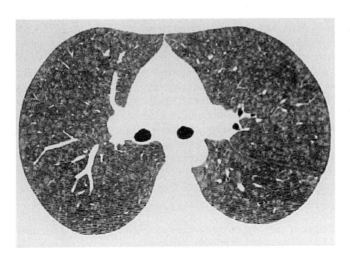

FIGURE 10–22

Subacute hypersensitivity pneumonitis. An HRCT scan (1-mm collimation) shows bilateral, poorly defined, small nodular opacities. These opacities are a few millimeters away from the pleura, including the interlobar fissures, and a few millimeters away from major vessels, a characteristic distribution of centrilobular nodules. The patient had a history of contact with birds. *(From Müller NL, Fraser RS, Colman NC, Paré PD: Radiologic Diagnosis of Diseases of the Chest. Philadelphia, WB Saunders, 2001.)*

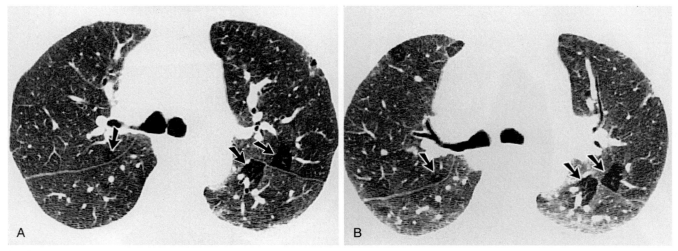

FIGURE 10–23

Air trapping in hypersensitivity pneumonitis. An HRCT scan (1-mm collimation) obtained at end-inspiration (**A**) shows bilateral areas of ground-glass attenuation. Focal areas of low attenuation and decreased vascularity are evident in the right and left lungs (*arrows*). An HRCT scan obtained at end-expiration (**B**) shows the expected loss of volume and increased attenuation of both lungs. The focal areas of decreased attenuation have not changed in volume (*arrows*), a characteristic finding of gas trapping. *(From Müller NL, Fraser RS, Colman NC, Paré PD: Radiologic Diagnosis of Diseases of the Chest. Philadelphia, WB Saunders, 2001.)*

have been attributed to the opening up of airways of various sizes. In one study, crackles persisted in patients who continued to be exposed to antigen but disappeared in those in whom exposure ceased.[425] Clubbing is common in chronic (fibrotic) disease.[415] Although the pathologic manifestations of EAA are confined to the lungs, an association with celiac disease has been noted in some patients.[426]

Laboratory Findings

Generally speaking, laboratory tests are not particularly useful in establishing the diagnosis. Neutrophilia with a shift to the left may be seen in acute disease or after antigen provocation testing; eosinophilia is rare. Although the presence of specific serum precipitins serves as a marker of exposure to an antigen, serologic testing generally lacks sufficient specificity to be of diagnostic value.[379,415] For the same reasons, as well as a lack of reliable commercially available antigen, skin testing is also not useful in diagnosis.[427]

Pulmonary Function Tests

Pulmonary function tests are useful in assessing impairment in naturally occurring disease and in antigen challenge testing. The overall pattern is usually restrictive, with a slight to moderate reduction in FEV_1 that is proportional to the decrease in VC. Both static compliance and diffusing capacity are frequently reduced as a result of the interstitial thickening seen histologically.[428,429] In addition, some patients have evidence of small-airway obstruction as reflected by the finding of air trapping[430] and decreased midexpiratory flow rates.[427]

Although restrictive lung function is the most commonly described long-term outcome in patients who have chronic EAA, airflow obstruction develops in some patients. In fact, in an investigation of 33 nonsmoking farmers who had lung function studies performed 6 years after an initial evaluation, 13 had an obstructive profile, 1 had restrictive changes, 3 had

isolated reductions in diffusing capacity, and 16 had normal tests.[431] Nine of the patients who had airflow obstruction had evidence of emphysema on HRCT. In another study of 88 patients who had farmer's lung and 83 control farmers, emphysema was found in 23% of the former and only 7% of the latter.[432] Among the patients who had farmer's lung, emphysema was seen in 18% of the nonsmokers and 44% of the smokers; corresponding figures for the control individuals were 4% and 20%. These and other studies[433,434] indicate that airflow obstruction and emphysema are common outcomes in patients who have chronic EAA.

Diagnosis

Clinical and radiologic findings often suggest the diagnosis when they develop in the context of exposure to an antigen known to cause EAA. Improvement after avoidance of the offending antigen strengthens the diagnostic presumption. Biopsy may be indicated when the clinical diagnosis is uncertain, especially when other diseases requiring different therapy are serious considerations.[379,415] Transbronchial biopsy specimens may show abnormalities compatible with EAA; in the appropriate context, they can be considered sufficient to confirm the diagnosis.[435] When the results of transbronchial biopsy are nonspecific or when suggestive results are discrepant with other clinical observations, open lung biopsy may be indicated. The latter is usually definitive, although distinction from fungal infection may require a careful search for organisms.[379] Provocation challenge with specific antigens has been useful in confirming the diagnosis of some variants such as bird fancier's lung[436]; however, the sensitivity and specificity are only about 80%.

Prognosis and Natural History

The prognosis is good for patients whose disease is recognized at an early stage and who are removed from exposure to antigen. In the more insidious cases in which the disease is not initially recognized, considerable fibrosis and a variable degree of pulmonary insufficiency can develop before the cause is detected. A better outcome is associated with early detection of disease and avoidance of antigen after diagnosis; chronic symptoms before diagnosis and persistent exposure lead to a progressive decline in lung function.[437,438] In a survey of 86 patients who had farmer's lung and were monitored for a period of 5 years, most of the clinical improvement occurred during the first month and little occurred after 6 months.[439] After 5 years, 65% of patients still had respiratory symptoms, 40% had impaired pulmonary function, and 32% showed persistent diffuse radiographic opacities. With regard to prognosis, it did not appear to make much difference whether patients left or continued working on the farm (presumably while limiting further exposure).

The overall mortality appears to be low. In an investigation of Finnish farmers, only 0.7% died of the disease between 1980 and 1990[440]; most deaths occurred in patients who had chronic symptoms and radiographic abnormalities. On the other hand, mortality in a group of Mexican patients who had chronic pigeon breeder's disease was similar to that of patients who had IPF when correction was made for the degree of fibrosis at initial evaluation.[441] These very different prognoses can be understood by recognizing the differences in findings in the Finnish and Mexican patients: most of the former had episodic EAA, whereas most of the latter had a clinical course of indolently progressive breathlessness associated with radiographic manifestations and functional indices of fibrotic lung disease.

Swine Confinement and the Lung

About 700,000 Americans are exposed to livestock and poultry in confined areas. Although a process of adaptation to this toxic environment clearly takes place in these individuals,[442] nearly 70% regularly have respiratory symptoms related to one or more specific disorders. Workers may be exposed to high concentrations of many organic dusts (including mold, pollen, swine hair, animal food, corn flour, grain mites, and aerosolized fecal matter), endotoxin, hydrogen sulfide, methane, carbon dioxide, carbon monoxide, ammonia, various microorganisms, and a wide variety of volatile compounds produced by anaerobic microorganisms in hog manure pits.[443,444] Which of these substances is responsible for a specific clinical disorder is not always clear. Some investigators have suggested that the total dust or ammonia levels are most closely linked to a decline in lung function,[444] whereas others have postulated that the level of endotoxin or other microbial substances in the bioaerosol is the major determinant.[445,446]

Symptoms of cough, sputum production, throat, nose, and eye irritation, chest tightness, breathlessness, wheezing, and myalgia are each seen in at least 25% of workers[443]; the risk for development of these symptoms escalates with increasing duration and intensity of exposure. Symptoms are also more severe and frequent among cigarette smokers and in patients who are atopic or have preexisting respiratory tract disease.[443] Asthma accounts for symptoms in only a small percentage of workers, most apparently being the result of a nonallergic inflammatory reaction.[447] Swine confinement workers have about a threefold increase in the prevalence of chronic bron-

chitis when compared with nonfarming men.[448] This bronchitis is associated with a small degree of chronic airflow obstruction, a development that has been correlated with the finding of a reduction in lung function over the course of a workshift.[445]

Workers have an excess annual decline in FEV_1 in comparison to nonexposed individuals.[449] Symptomatic patients with[450] and without[451] abnormal baseline lung function are more likely to have airway hyperresponsiveness as assessed by methacholine provocation testing than control individuals are; the hyperresponsiveness worsens with long-term exposure.[452]

Organic Dust Toxic Syndrome

Organic dust toxic syndrome can be defined as a febrile illness after exposure to organic dust in individuals who do not have evidence of EAA.[453] Typically, fever and influenza-like symptoms occur 4 to 8 hours after exposure to organic dust; dry cough, chest tightness, mild dyspnea, and wheezing may also be present.[454] The syndrome encompasses diseases previously described by a variety of names, including humidifier fever (in office and hospital workers), pulmonary mycotoxicosis, grain fever, pig fever, cotton fever, and woodchip fever. The disorder is common, and the characteristic fever develops in up to 10% of exposed farmers[453] and as many as 35% of swine confinement workers.[443] In fact, it has been estimated that the disorder may be 50 times more common than allergic alveolitis in farmers.[455]

The etiology and pathogenesis are unclear; however, the findings in one animal model suggest that they are related to exposure to both fungal organisms and endotoxin.[456] Pulmonary function changes are minimal.[443] The disorder shares some features with EAA: both frequently occur after exposure to moldy vegetable matter and improve rapidly without therapy.[453] However, it is important to distinguish the two because organic dust toxic syndrome causes no permanent impairment of lung function.

EOSINOPHILIC LUNG DISEASE

The term "eosinophilic lung disease" encompasses a group of diverse disorders characterized pathologically by the accumulation of eosinophils in alveolar air spaces and interstitial tissue. Peripheral blood eosinophilia is frequently but not invariably prominent, and the eosinophil is believed to play a major role in the pathogenesis of the resulting disease. The most convenient classification of these disorders divides them into groups with and without established etiologies[457]; those of unknown origin are defined and distinguished from one another largely by their clinical features.

Simple Pulmonary Eosinophilia

Simple pulmonary eosinophilia is an uncommon disorder characterized by local nonsegmental areas of parenchymal consolidation, usually transient, on the chest radiograph and by blood eosinophilia. By definition, the term is confined to cases in which the etiology is unknown; similar illnesses with known causes, such as drugs or parasites, are categorized as specific forms of eosinophilic lung disease.

Documentation of seasonal variation in the prevalence of the disorder, as well as its association with atopy, suggests that unrecognized environmental antigens are responsible in some cases.[457] Because of its benign and transient nature, the pathologic features of the parenchymal consolidation have rarely been documented. In the few cases in which biopsy findings have been reported, there has been interstitial and alveolar edema admixed with a large number of eosinophilic leukocytes.[458]

The radiographic findings characteristically consist of transitory and migratory areas of parenchymal consolidation. These are nonsegmental, may be single or multiple, and usually have ill-defined margins (Fig. 10–24).[457,459] They are often peripheral.[457]

Patients typically have few or no symptoms, the diagnosis often being suspected initially by the finding of characteristic opacities on the chest radiograph. A background of asthma and atopy is often found.[460] A total white blood cell count of more than 20,000/mm[3] is common, an increase in eosinophils being responsible for most of the elevation. When pulmonary parenchymal involvement is extensive, results of function tests usually indicate restrictive impairment, arterial oxygen desaturation, and a decrease in diffusing capacity.[461] Symptoms and signs, if present, usually resolve spontaneously within 1 month.[457]

Acute Eosinophilic Pneumonia

Acute eosinophilic pneumonia is an acute febrile illness associated with hypoxemic respiratory failure, at times so severe that mechanical ventilation is required.[457,462,463] There does not appear to be any sex predominance, and patients of all ages have been affected.[464]

The pathogenesis of the disease is unknown. However, some workers have speculated that it may represent a hypersensitivity reaction to an unrecognized antigen,[465] and indeed, specific exposures seem to have been important in provoking disease in some patients.[466] In many others, an allergic diathesis has been noted.[467] Eosinophils are markedly increased in BAL fluid, but lymphocytes (predominantly CD4[+]) and neutrophils are also increased in number, implying that they may also have a role in disease pathogenesis.[468] There is evidence that interleukin-5 is a key cytokine responsible for accumulation of eosinophils in the lung.[469]

Histologic examination of biopsy specimens from affected patients shows diffuse alveolar damage (either acute or organizing) associated with a large number of interstitial and air space eosinophils.[470]

Radiographically and on CT scan, the findings are similar to those of pulmonary edema. The earliest radiographic manifestation consists of reticular opacities, frequently with Kerley B lines.[457] These opacities progress rapidly over a period of a few hours or days to bilateral interstitial and air space opacities involving mainly the lower lung zones.[467] Small bilateral pleural effusions are seen at some point in the course of the disease in most patients.[471] CT scans show bilateral areas of ground-glass attenuation, smooth interlobular septal thickening, small pleural effusions, and (occasionally) localized areas of consolidation or small nodules.[471] In contrast to chronic eosinophilic pneumonia, a peripheral distribution is seldom seen.[467,472]

Patients typically have breathlessness, myalgias, and pleuritic chest pain at initial evaluation. Physical examination reveals respiratory distress, fever, and bibasilar or diffuse

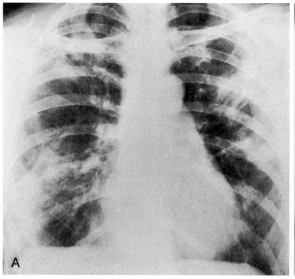 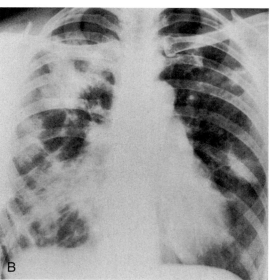

FIGURE 10–24

Simple pulmonary eosinophilia. A posteroanterior chest radiograph (**A**) in a 61-year-old woman shows bilateral areas of consolidation occupying no precise segmental distribution. There is a broad shadow of increased density along the lower axillary zone of the right lung. At this time her total white blood cell count was 11,000/mL with 1700 (15%) eosinophils. One week later (**B**), the anatomic distribution of the areas of consolidation had changed considerably; they were more extensive in the right upper and both lower lobes and less extensive in the left upper lobe. The total white blood cell count was 14,000/mL with 20% eosinophils. A diagnosis of simple pulmonary eosinophilia was made; treatment resulted in prompt remission of symptoms and complete resolution of the radiographic abnormalities. (*From Müller NL, Fraser RS, Colman NC, Paré PD: Radiologic Diagnosis of Diseases of the Chest. Philadelphia, WB Saunders, 2001.*)

crackles on auscultation.[457] Wheezing has been noted in patients with an associated bronchiolitis.[473] Peripheral eosinophilia is usually absent, although a marked elevation in BAL eosinophils—up to 80% in some patients—is characteristic and important in establishing the diagnosis.[463] Pulmonary function studies in patients who have eosinophilic infiltration of small airways show a low diffusing capacity and evidence of small-airway dysfunction.[473]

Typically, the response to corticosteroid therapy is rapid, although some patients improve spontaneously. Unlike with chronic eosinophilic pneumonia, relapse is not a feature. It is important to distinguish the disease from drug reactions and fungal or parasitic infection, which can have similar clinical and laboratory manifestations. It is also important to keep in mind that patients who have fulminant respiratory failure may have an easily reversible cause of their disease.

Chronic Eosinophilic Pneumonia

This uncommon pulmonary disorder has a more protracted clinical and radiographic course than either acute eosinophilic pneumonia or simple pulmonary eosinophilia. As in the latter condition, an atopic background (particularly asthma) is common. Females are affected more than twice as often as males; about half the cases occur between 30 and 50 years of age.

The etiology is usually unknown. The frequent association with atopy and the presence of high levels of circulating IgE during peak disease activity and their return to normal during remission suggest that a reagin-mediated hypersensitivity response to an unidentified antigen is involved in pathogenesis.[474]

The predominant histologic finding is filling of alveolar air spaces by an inflammatory infiltrate containing a high proportion of eosinophils (see Color Fig. 10–4).[475] Although necrosis of lung parenchyma is unusual, aggregates of necrotic eosinophils surrounded by a rim of palisaded histiocytes ("eosinophilic microabscesses") are often present. Airway epithelium may be ulcerated and associated with obliterative bronchiolitis,[475] a finding probably related to the development of obstructive airway disease in some patients.

The characteristic radiographic pattern consists of bilateral, nonsegmental consolidation involving predominately or exclusively the outer two thirds of the lungs (Fig. 10–25).[476] This peripheral distribution, typically involving mainly the upper lobes, is apparent in approximately 60% of patients on radiographs[476,477] and can be identified in virtually all cases on CT scans.[472,477] When compared with the transitory and migratory character of the areas of consolidation in simple pulmonary eosinophilia, the lesions tend to persist unchanged for many days or weeks unless corticosteroid therapy is instituted.

Atopy is present in about 50% of patients, asthma being the most common manifestation.[467] In our experience and that of others,[478] there appears to be an unusual association with therapeutic desensitization to a variety of antigens. Disease may develop insidiously and is generally characterized by high fever, malaise, weight loss, cough, and dyspnea[457]; hemoptysis, chest pain, and myalgia occur rarely.

Laboratory investigation reveals blood eosinophilia in most patients, although its absence does not exclude the

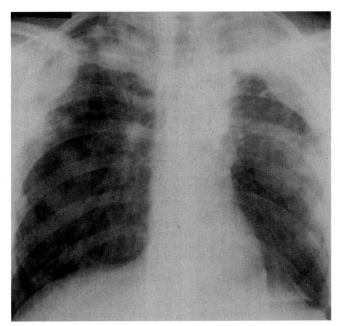

FIGURE 10–25

Chronic eosinophilic pneumonia. A posteroanterior chest radiograph reveals bilateral air space consolidation, predominantly upper lobe in distribution; the peripheral (cortical) distribution is highly characteristic of the disease. *(From Müller NL, Fraser RS, Colman NC, Paré PD: Radiologic Diagnosis of Diseases of the Chest. Philadelphia, WB Saunders, 2001.)*

diagnosis.[476] Pulmonary function tests usually show a restrictive pattern with reduced diffusing capacity and impaired gas exchange, accompanied in some cases by severe hypoxemia during the acute phase.[475] After remission, an obstructive ventilatory defect is a common finding.[479] The diagnosis can almost always be made on clinical and radiologic grounds alone without resorting to invasive procedures before the institution of therapy. Although it can be confirmed histologically, the presence of numerous eosinophils in BAL fluid also supports the diagnosis.[480]

The response to corticosteroid therapy is characteristically dramatic, with rapid radiographic resolution and clear-cut clinical improvement within 24 hours.[478] Most patients are completely well within 2 weeks,[476] although residual pulmonary fibrosis has been described.[481] Many patients require therapy for months or even years because exacerbations are common when corticosteroid therapy is reduced or stopped.[482]

Hypereosinophilic Syndrome

Hypereosinophilic syndrome (HES) is an uncommon condition characterized by prolonged blood eosinophilia and multiple organ dysfunction.[483] The etiology is usually unknown (idiopathic HES) and is probably multifactorial. In a series of 50 patients, 35 (70%) experienced the onset of disease between the ages of 20 and 50 years (mean, 33 years).[483] Although the incidence by sex was not revealed in this series, other authors have noted a male preponderance.[484]

Three criteria have been established for the diagnosis of idiopathic HES:[483] (1) persistent eosinophilia of 1500/mm³ for at least 6 months or death before 6 months in individuals with appropriate signs and symptoms; (2) lack of evidence for a parasitic, allergic, or other recognized cause of eosinophilia; and (3) signs and symptoms of organ involvement, either directly related to eosinophilia or unexplained in the given clinical setting.

The principal organs affected in HES are the heart (valvular fibrosis with regurgitation) and the nervous system (meningitis, peripheral neuropathies, and behavioral or cognitive abnormalities). Direct involvement of the respiratory system is relatively uncommon but can take several forms, including vascular infiltration by eosinophils and interstitial fibrosis.

Chest radiographs may reveal transient air space opacities that can resolve spontaneously and are sometimes associated with clinical evidence of bronchospasm. An interstitial pattern has also been described, usually in association with involvement of other organs and presumably caused by perivascular eosinophilic infiltration or fibrosis.[457] Cardiac decompensation is manifested by cardiomegaly, pulmonary edema, and pleural effusion.

The initial symptoms are nonspecific, and the diagnosis is often considered only when leukocytosis and eosinophilia are detected. Cough and dyspnea may reflect either pulmonary or cardiac involvement (or both).

Eosinophilic Lung Disease of Specific Etiology

Drugs. Drugs are an important cause of eosinophilic lung disease.[457] It is important to consider the reaction in any patient who has pulmonary opacities on the radiograph, blood or BAL eosinophilia, and a history of drug exposure by any route. Reactions range from those similar to simple pulmonary eosinophilia to those resembling acute eosinophilic pneumonia. Implicated drugs include antibiotics, nonsteroidal anti-inflammatory agents, drugs used for IBD, and inhaled agents such as cocaine[485] or heroin.[486]

Parasitic Infestation. Parasitic infestation is a common cause of eosinophilic lung infiltration and peripheral blood eosinophilia in "developing" countries. However, with increasing immigration to industrialized countries from these areas and with ever-increasing foreign travel, physicians should be familiar with the manifestations of these infections. All infestations are caused by metazoans, the majority from roundworms. Most patients initially have signs and symptoms similar to those of simple pulmonary eosinophilia. Among the more commonly implicated organisms are *Ascaris lumbricoides, Strongyloides stercoralis, Ancylostoma duodenale, Wuchereria bancrofti, Toxocara canis* and *cati,* and *Schistosoma* species.

PULMONARY HEMORRHAGE

Goodpasture's Syndrome and Idiopathic Pulmonary Hemorrhage

Both of these diseases are characterized by repeated episodes of pulmonary hemorrhage, iron deficiency anemia, and in long-standing cases, pulmonary insufficiency. Goodpasture's syndrome (GPS) also includes glomerulonephritis and the presence of anti-GBM antibodies. Idiopathic pulmonary hemorrhage (IPH) occurs most commonly in children, usually those younger than 10 years, and shows no sex predominance; by contrast, GPS is a disease of young adults and has a male preponderance.[487]

Since hemorrhage is the primary abnormality in IPH and hemosiderosis is only part of the pathologic consequence of the disease (and sometimes only a very minor part), we prefer the term *idiopathic pulmonary hemorrhage* to the more traditional "hemosiderosis."

Etiology and Pathogenesis

Although most cases of GPS occur sporadically, the strong association of disease with the HLA-DR15 and HLA-DR4 alleles[488] and the under-representation of HLA-DR7 and HLA-DR1[489,490] suggest an important genetic link in pathogenesis.

The presence of anti-GBM antibody is clearly pathogenetic: a positive correlation has been found between disease severity and antibody titer in some cases,[491] and the disease does not recur in renal transplant patients in the absence of antibody. The basement membrane autoantigen is located at the amino terminus of the α3 chain of type IV collagen—α3(IV)NC1 (noncollagenous domain).[492] T lymphocytes reactive to the same antigen have also been identified in some patients,[493] thus suggesting a role in disease beyond their enhancement of B-cell function and antibody production.

Why only alveolar hemorrhage or glomerulonephritis instead of the more usual combination of the two develop in some patients who have anti-GBM antibody is not clear. This finding may be related to structural differences between alveoli and glomeruli that could allow antibodies increased access to the basement membrane.[487] Increased capillary permeability could also be necessary for the antibody to gain access to the alveolar basement membrane. This hypothesis is supported by data from experimental animal studies[487] and by the clinical observations that recurrent pulmonary hemorrhage may develop after infection,[494] fluid overload, cigarette smoking,[495] and exposure to a variety of toxins.[487]

The precise pathogenesis of the pulmonary hemorrhage in GPS is also uncertain. In the kidney, complement activation and inflammatory cell enzymes are responsible for glomerular damage. Because capillaritis has been seen in human biopsy material[268] and because an early influx of neutrophils into alveolar septa has been documented in experimental animals,[496] it is possible that similar mechanisms are involved in the lung. The results of an experimental animal model of disease suggest that expression of CD44 by endothelial cells may contribute to leukocyte recruitment and subsequent alveolar septal injury.[497]

The etiology and pathogenesis of IPH are also unknown. Although the clinical and pathologic similarities to GPS suggest an autoimmune disease, serologic evidence is lacking in most cases. In addition, immunologic and ultrastructural studies of lung tissue have failed to reveal evidence of deposition of immunoglobulin or complement components.[498] On the other hand, both circulating[499] and tissue[500] immune complexes have been identified in some patients, and the abnormality has been found in association with a number of well-recognized immune disorders, including celiac disease[501] in approximately 25% of patients.

Pathologic Characteristics

The histologic features of the lung in GPS and IPH are virtually identical. Hemorrhage is confined largely to the alveolar air spaces and smaller airways (see Color Fig. 10–5); in fact, massive blood loss into the lungs can occur without associated hemoptysis, and the trachea and major bronchi may contain little or no blood. Other histologic changes depend on the duration and severity of the disease at the time of examination, but they usually include the presence of hemosiderin-laden macrophages in the alveolar air spaces and interstitial tissue, mild to moderate interstitial fibrosis, and type II cell hyperplasia. Focal or (less commonly) diffuse acute interstitial inflammation can also be seen.[502] This inflammation is manifested as capillaritis identical to that of microscopic polyangiitis and appears as a neutrophil infiltrate intimately associated with alveolar septa with or without fibrin thrombi and necrosis.

Immunofluorescence studies of fresh lung tissue obtained from patients who have GPS typically show diffuse linear staining along the alveolar wall.[503] IgG is the usual antibody detected, although IgA and IgM are occasionally present as well; C3 is variably present. In distinct contrast to the positive immunofluorescent studies in GPS, the results in IPH are almost always negative.

Radiologic Manifestations

The radiologic manifestations of GPS and IPH are identical. In early disease, the radiographic pattern is one of patchy areas of air space consolidation scattered fairly evenly throughout the lungs (Fig. 10–26). An air bronchogram is often identifiable in areas of major consolidation. Opacities are usually widespread but may be more prominent in the perihilar areas and the mid and lower lung zones. The apices and costophrenic angles are almost invariably spared.[504] Although parenchymal involvement is usually bilateral, it is commonly asymmetrical and occasionally unilateral.[505] The CT manifestations consist of areas of ground-glass attenuation or consolidation; they may also be patchy or diffuse[207,506] but tend to involve mainly the dependent lung regions.[507]

Serial radiographs obtained over the several days after an acute episode of hemorrhage often reveal a characteristic progressive change in pattern (see Fig. 10–26): the areas of air space consolidation resolve in 2 to 3 days and are replaced by a reticulonodular pattern whose distribution is identical to that of the air space disease.[508] This reticular pattern diminishes gradually during the next several days, and the chest radiograph usually returns to normal about 10 to 12 days after the original episode.[207] With repeated episodes of hemorrhage, the chest radiograph generally shows only partial clearing after each episode, with persistence of a fine reticulonodular pattern indicative of the irreversible interstitial disease (fibrosis and accumulation of hemosiderin-laden macrophages).[509,510]

Clinical Manifestations

The onset of IPH may be insidious, with anemia, pallor, weakness, lethargy, and dry cough. In other cases, the onset is acute, with fever and hemoptysis. Finger clubbing, hepatosplenomegaly, and jaundice may develop with progression of disease.[501,511] Physical examination during the acute stage of pulmonary hemorrhage may reveal fine crackles and dullness to percussion over the affected areas of lung; the liver, spleen, and lymph nodes are palpably enlarged in 20% to 25% of patients.[512] Iron deficiency anemia develops in most patients.[501] When associated with celiac disease, steatorrhea may be present.[513] Occasionally, a discrepancy between the degree of hemoptysis and the severity of the anemia can be explained by unrecognized malabsorption caused by celiac disease.[514] Peripheral eosinophilia was present in 12% of patients in one series, and cold agglutinins were detected in 10 of the 20 patients tested.[512]

Hemoptysis, the most common initial symptom in patients with GPS, occurs in about 80% to 95%.[487] Although it may be life-threatening, it is seldom as copious as in IPH. It may occur late in the course of the disease or be absent altogether, and it typically precedes the clinical manifestations of renal disease by several months.[487] The latter observation is helpful in distinguishing GPS from hemoptysis associated with chronic renal failure of other etiology. Other initial symptoms include dyspnea, fatigue, weakness, lassitude, pallor, cough, and (occasionally) frank hematuria.[515] Acute hemorrhage may be associated with chills, fever, and diaphoresis.[487] Chest pain, often worsened by cough, is not uncommon. Physical findings are similar to those of IPH. Although results of the initial urinalysis may be normal, proteinuria, hematuria, and cellular and granular casts almost invariably develop at some stage. Repeated and careful urine analysis is mandatory. Occasionally, urinary sediment findings are normal, and the presence of renal involvement is established by biopsy.[516] Of 51 cases in one review, anemia was present in all and leukocytosis (with a shift to the left) in half.[515]

Only a few reports have described pulmonary function in patients who have either IPH or GPS. Some patients tested during remission have had a predominantly restrictive pattern, with decreased diffusing capacity and sometimes a fall in resting PaO_2.[517] Such a pattern has been said to persist in both diseases after the chest radiograph has returned to normal.[518] A greater than normal uptake of carbon monoxide is a useful sign that the air space opacities observed radiographically are caused by hemorrhage.[519]

Diagnosis

The diagnosis of GPS should be suspected when a patient in the late second or third decade of life has hemoptysis and radiologic evidence of air space hemorrhage, particularly when manifestations of renal disease are also present. Confirmation is obtained by demonstration of circulating or tissue-bound anti-GBM antibodies by enzyme-linked immunosorbent assay or immunofluorescent examination.[520] Most other disorders characterized by hemoptysis and renal dysfunction can be recognized by associated clinical and laboratory manifestations of vasculitis or by the observation of immunoglobulin and complement deposition in a granular pattern on immunofluorescent examination of a kidney biopsy specimen.[521] The diagnosis can be confirmed by examination of a transbronchial biopsy specimen[503]; however, a negative result does not exclude the diagnosis since anti-GBM antibody may not be identified in alveolar septa and yet still be present in glomeruli.[522]

When all patients who have glomerulonephritis and pulmonary hemorrhage are considered, about 20% are found to have GPS[521,523] and 50% some form of systemic vasculitis[523]; most of the remainder have diffuse alveolar hemorrhage in

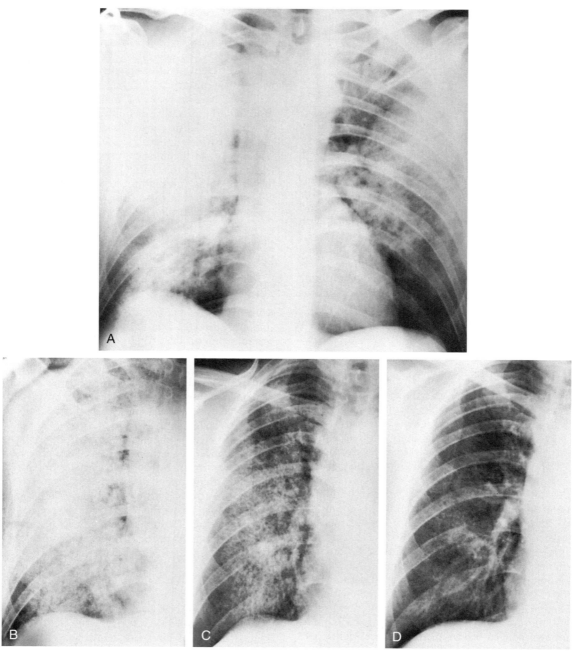

FIGURE 10–26

Goodpasture's syndrome. A posteroanterior radiograph (**A**) of a 49-year-old man reveals extensive consolidation of both lungs. A well-defined air bronchogram is evident. Three days later (**B**), the pattern was somewhat more granular, and 10 days after the initial episode (**C**) the pattern has become distinctly reticular. Six days later (**D**), only a fine reticular pattern remains in an anatomic distribution identical to the original involvement. The sequence of changes illustrated is typical of massive pulmonary hemorrhage. *(From Müller NL, Fraser RS, Colman NC, Paré PD: Radiologic Diagnosis of Diseases of the Chest. Philadelphia, WB Saunders, 2001.)*

association with other forms of glomerulonephritis.[523] Because renal involvement in GPS may not be apparent initially,[524] the diagnosis must still be considered in any patient who has radiologic and clinical findings consistent with diffuse alveolar hemorrhage and no evidence of kidney disease. The differential diagnosis in this situation is large and includes (1) aspirated blood after vascular disruption,[525] (2)

connective tissue disease or systemic vasculitis,[140,526] and (3) certain metastatic neoplasms such as choriocarcinoma.[527]

Prognosis

The prognosis in patients with IPH varies considerably. In one early report, the average interval from the onset of symptoms until death was only 2.5 years[512]; however, in recent pediatric evaluations, prolonged survival is the rule,[501,511] probably because of the current use of corticosteroids and immunosuppressive agents in management. The prognosis in adults also seems relatively favorable. Of seven adults reported in one series (four of whom had associated celiac disease), five survived for 10 to 40 years.[528]

With current therapy (including corticosteroids, immunosuppressive agents, and plasmapheresis), the outlook for patients who have GPS has also improved substantially.[529] Overall, more than 50% of patients are long-term survivors, although some are dependent on dialysis.[487] The prognosis is closely associated with the degree of initial renal impairment[530]; preservation of renal function is favored by early diagnosis. Rarely, GPS can recur years later in patients whose disease remits spontaneously or as a result of therapy.[531]

REFERENCES

1. Shlomchik MJ, Craft JE, Mamula MJ: From T to B and back again: Positive feedback in systemic autoimmune disease. Nat Rev Immunol 1:147-153, 2001.
2. Robson MG, Walport MJ: Pathogenesis of systemic lupus erythematosus (SLE). Clin Exp Allergy 31:678-685, 2001.
3. Rao S, Olson JM, Moser KL, et al: Linkage analysis of human systemic lupus erythematosus–related traits: A principal component approach. Arthritis Rheum 44:2807-2818, 2001.
4. Salmon M, Gordon C: The role of apoptosis in systemic lupus erythematosus. Rheumatology (Oxford) 38:1177-1183, 1999.
5. Dean GS, Tyrrell-Price J, Crawley E, Isenberg DA: Cytokines and systemic lupus erythematosus. Ann Rheum Dis 59:243-251, 2000.
6. Panush RS, Greer JM, Morshedian KK: What is lupus? What is not lupus? Rheum Dis Clin North Am 19:223-234, 1993.
7. Jacobson DL, Gange SJ, Rose NR, Graham NM: Epidemiology and estimated population burden of selected autoimmune diseases in the United States. Clin Immunol Immunopathol 84:223-243, 1997.
8. Hochberg MC, Perlmutter DL, Medsger TA, et al: Prevalence of self-reported physician-diagnosed systemic lupus erythematosus in the USA. Lupus 4:454-456, 1995.
9. Hopkinson ND, Doherty M, Powell RJ: Clinical features and race-specific incidence/prevalence rates of systemic lupus erythematosus in a geographically complete cohort of patients. Ann Rheum Dis 53:675-680, 1994.
10. Fessel WJ: Systemic lupus erythematosus in the community. Incidence, prevalence, outcome, and first symptoms; the high prevalence in black women. Arch Intern Med 134:1027-1035, 1974.
11. Quismorio F: Clinical and pathologic features of lung involvement in systemic lupus erythematosus. Semin Respir Med 9:297, 1988.
12. Haupt HM, Moore GW, Hutchins GM: The lung in systemic lupus erythematosus. Analysis of the pathologic changes in 120 patients. Am J Med 71:791-798, 1981.
13. Pertschuk LP, Moccia LF, Rosen Y, et al: Acute pulmonary complications in systemic lupus erythematosus. Immunofluorescence and light microscopic study. Am J Clin Pathol 68:553-557, 1977.
14. Colby TV: Pulmonary pathology in patients with systemic autoimmune diseases. Clin Chest Med 19:587-612, 1998.
15. Miller LR, Greenberg SD, McLarty JW: Lupus lung. Chest 88:265-269, 1985.
16. Matthay RA, Schwarz MI, Petty TL, et al: Pulmonary manifestations of systemic lupus erythematosus: Review of twelve cases of acute lupus pneumonitis. Medicine (Baltimore) 54:397-409, 1975.
17. Myers JL, Katzenstein AA: Microangiitis in lupus-induced pulmonary hemorrhage. Am J Clin Pathol 85:552-556, 1986.
18. Nair SS, Askari AD, Popelka CG, Kleinerman JF: Pulmonary hypertension and systemic lupus erythematosus. Arch Intern Med 140:109-111, 1980.
19. Hughson MD, McCarty GA, Brumback RA: Spectrum of vascular pathology affecting patients with the antiphospholipid syndrome. Hum Pathol 26:716-724, 1995.
20. Primack SL, Müller NL: Radiologic manifestations of the systemic autoimmune diseases. Clin Chest Med 19:573-586, 1998.
21. Kim JS, Lee KS, Koh EM, et al: Thoracic involvement of systemic lupus erythematosus: Clinical, pathologic, and radiologic findings. J Comput Assist Tomogr 24:9-18, 2000.
22. Gamsu G: Radiographic manifestations of thoracic involvement by collagen vascular diseases. J Thorac Imaging 7:1-12, 1992.
23. Wiedemann HP, Matthay RA: Pulmonary manifestations of systemic lupus erythematosus. J Thorac Imaging 7:711-718, 1992.
24. Gammon RB, Bridges TA, al-Nezir H, et al: Bronchiolitis obliterans organizing pneumonia associated with systemic lupus erythematosus. Chest 102:1171-1174, 1992.
25. Onomura K, Nakata H, Tanaka Y, Tsuda T: Pulmonary hemorrhage in patients with systemic lupus erythematosus. J Thorac Imaging 6:57-61, 1991.
26. Gross M, Esterly JR, Earle RH: Pulmonary alterations in systemic lupus erythematosus. Am Rev Respir Dis 105:572-577, 1972.
27. Bankier AA, Kiener HP, Wiesmayr MN, et al: Discrete lung involvement in systemic lupus erythematosus: CT assessment. Radiology 196:835-840, 1995.
28. Ooi GC, Ngan H, Peh WC, et al: Systemic lupus erythematosus patients with respiratory symptoms: The value of HRCT. Clin Radiol 52:775-781, 1997.
29. Bulgrin JG, Dubois EL, Jacobson G: Chest roentgenographic changes in systemic lupus erythematosus. Radiology 74:42-49, 1960.
30. Joseph J, Sahn SA: Connective tissue diseases and the pleura. Chest 104:262-270, 1993.
31. Orens JB, Martinez FJ, Lynch JP 3rd: Pleuropulmonary manifestations of systemic lupus erythematosus. Rheum Dis Clin North Am 20:159-193, 1994.
32. Fenlon HM, Doran M, Sant SM, Breatnach E: High-resolution chest CT in systemic lupus erythematosus. AJR Am J Roentgenol 166:301-307, 1996.
33. Wiedemann HP, Matthay RA: Pulmonary manifestations of the collagen vascular diseases. Clin Chest Med 10:677-722, 1989.
34. Eagen JW, Memoli VA, Roberts JL, et al: Pulmonary hemorrhage in systemic lupus erythematosus. Medicine (Baltimore) 57:545-560, 1978.
35. Santos-Ocampo AS, Mandell BF, Fessler BJ: Alveolar hemorrhage in systemic lupus erythematosus: Presentation and management. Chest 118:1083-1090, 2000.
36. Alarcon-Segovia D, Deleze M, Oria CV, et al: Antiphospholipid antibodies and the antiphospholipid syndrome in systemic lupus erythematosus. A prospective analysis of 500 consecutive patients. Medicine (Baltimore) 68:353-365, 1989.
37. Gomez-Pacheco L, Villa AR, Drenkard C, et al: Serum anti-beta2-glycoprotein-I and anticardiolipin antibodies during thrombosis in systemic lupus erythematosus patients. Am J Med 106:417-423, 1999.
38. Merkel PA, Chang Y, Pierangeli SS, et al: The prevalence and clinical associations of anticardiolipin antibodies in a large inception cohort of patients with connective tissue diseases. Am J Med 101:576-583, 1996.
39. Asherson RA, Cervera R, Piette JC, et al: Catastrophic antiphospholipid syndrome. Clinical and laboratory features of 50 patients. Medicine (Baltimore) 77:195-207, 1998.
40. Quismorio FP Jr, Sharma O, Koss M, et al: Immunopathologic and clinical studies in pulmonary hypertension associated with systemic lupus erythematosus. Semin Arthritis Rheum 13:349-359, 1984.
41. Miyata M, Suzuki K, Sakuma F, et al: Anticardiolipin antibodies are associated with pulmonary hypertension in patients with mixed connective tissue disease or systemic lupus erythematosus. Int Arch Allergy Immunol 100:351-354, 1993.
42. Thompson PJ, Dhillon DP, Ledingham J, Turner-Warwick M: Shrinking lungs, diaphragmatic dysfunction, and systemic lupus erythematosus. Am Rev Respir Dis 132:926-928, 1985.
43. Laroche CM, Mulvey DA, Hawkins PN, et al: Diaphragm strength in the shrinking lung syndrome of systemic lupus erythematosus. Q J Med 71:429-439, 1989.
44. Hawkins P, Davison AG, Dasgupta B, Moxham J: Diaphragm strength in acute systemic lupus erythematosus in a patient with paradoxical abdominal motion and reduced lung volumes. Thorax 56:329-330, 2001.
45. Martens J, Demedts M, Vanmeenen MT, Dequeker J: Respiratory muscle dysfunction in systemic lupus erythematosus. Chest 84:170-175, 1983.
46. Walz-Leblanc BA, Urowitz MB, Gladman DD, Hanly PJ: The "shrinking lungs syndrome" in systemic lupus erythematosus—improvement with corticosteroid therapy. J Rheumatol 19:1970-1972, 1992.
47. Kinney WW, Angelillo VA: Bronchiolitis in systemic lupus erythematosus. Chest 82:646-649, 1982.
48. Skaer TL: Medication-induced systemic lupus erythematosus. Clin Ther 14:496-506, discussion 495, 1992.
49. Lane SK, Gravel JW Jr: Clinical utility of common serum rheumatologic tests. Am Fam Physician 65:1073-1080, 2002.
50. Shojania K: Rheumatology: 2. What laboratory tests are needed? CMAJ 162:1157-1163, 2000.
51. Thomas C, Robinson JA: The antinuclear antibody test. When is a positive result clinically relevant? Postgrad Med 94:55-58, 63, 66, 1993.
52. Vlachoyiannopoulos PG, Karassa FB, Karakostas KX, et al: Systemic lupus erythematosus in Greece. Clinical features, evolution and outcome: A descriptive analysis of 292 patients. Lupus 2:303-312, 1993.
53. Merkel PA, Polisson RP, Chang Y, et al: Prevalence of antineutrophil cytoplasmic antibodies in a large inception cohort of patients with connective tissue disease. Ann Intern Med 126:866-873, 1997.
54. Manolova I, Dancheva M, Halacheva K: Antineutrophil cytoplasmic antibodies in patients with systemic lupus erythematosus: Prevalence, antigen specificity, and clinical associations. Rheumatol Int 20:197-204, 2001.
55. Pauzner R, Urowitz M, Gladman D, Gough J: Antineutrophil cytoplasmic antibodies in systemic lupus erythematosus. J Rheumatol 21:1670-1673, 1994.
56. Gussin HA, Ignat GP, Varga J, Teodorescu M: Anti–topoisomerase I (anti-Scl-70) antibodies in patients with systemic lupus erythematosus. Arthritis Rheum 44:376-383, 2001.
57. Nakano M, Hasegawa H, Takada T, et al: Pulmonary diffusion capacity in patients with systemic lupus erythematosus. Respirology 7:45-49, 2002.
58. Huang CT, Lyons HA: Comparison of pulmonary function in patients with systemic lupus erythematosus, scleroderma, and rheumatoid arthritis. Am Rev Respir Dis 93:865-875, 1966.
59. Eichacker PQ, Pinsker K, Epstein A, et al: Serial pulmonary function testing in patients with systemic lupus erythematosus. Chest 94:129-132, 1988.
60. Forte S, Carlone S, Vaccaro F, et al: Pulmonary gas exchange and exercise capacity in patients with systemic lupus erythematosus. J Rheumatol 26:2591-2594, 1999.

61. Tenca C, Bentley D, Vleck V, et al: Aerobic fitness, fatigue, and physical disability in systemic lupus erythematosus. J Rheumatol 29:474-481, 2002.
62. Ruiz-Irastorza G, Khamashta MA, Castellino G, Hughes GR: Systemic lupus erythematosus. Lancet 357:1027-1032, 2001.
63. Hellmann DB, Petri M, Whiting-O'Keefe Q: Fatal infections in systemic lupus erythematosus: The role of opportunistic organisms. Medicine (Baltimore) 66:341-348, 1987.
64. Bellomio V, Spindler A, Lucero E, et al: Systemic lupus erythematosus: Mortality and survival in Argentina. A multicenter study. Lupus 9:377-381, 2000.
65. Zamora MR, Warner ML, Tuder R, Schwarz MI: Diffuse alveolar hemorrhage and systemic lupus erythematosus. Clinical presentation, histology, survival, and outcome. Medicine (Baltimore) 76:192-202, 1997.
66. Schwab EP, Schumacher HR Jr, Freundlich B, Callegari PE: Pulmonary alveolar hemorrhage in systemic lupus erythematosus. Semin Arthritis Rheum 23:8-15, 1993.
67. Zeiss CR, Burch FX, Marder RJ, et al: A hypocomplementemic vasculitic urticarial syndrome. Report of four new cases and definition of the disease. Am J Med 68:867-875, 1980.
68. Schwartz HR, McDuffie FC, Black LF, et al: Hypocomplementemic urticarial vasculitis: Association with chronic obstructive pulmonary disease. Mayo Clin Proc 57:231-238, 1982.
69. Gabriel SE: The epidemiology of rheumatoid arthritis. Rheum Dis Clin North Am 27:269-281, 2001.
70. Anaya JM, Diethelm L, Ortiz LA, et al: Pulmonary involvement in rheumatoid arthritis. Semin Arthritis Rheum 24:242-254, 1995.
71. Roschmann RA, Rothenberg RJ: Pulmonary fibrosis in rheumatoid arthritis: A review of clinical features and therapy. Semin Arthritis Rheum 16:174-185, 1987.
72. Gabbay E, Tarala R, Will R, et al: Interstitial lung disease in recent onset rheumatoid arthritis. Am J Respir Crit Care Med 156:528-535, 1997.
73. Kohler PF, Vaughan J: The autoimmune diseases. JAMA 248:2646-2657, 1982.
74. Nusslein HG, Rodl W, Giedel J, et al: Multiple peripheral pulmonary nodules preceding rheumatoid arthritis. Rheumatol Int 7:89-91, 1987.
75. Albano SA, Santana-Sahagun E, Weisman MH: Cigarette smoking and rheumatoid arthritis. Semin Arthritis Rheum 31:146-159, 2001.
76. Yousem SA, Colby TV, Carrington CB: Lung biopsy in rheumatoid arthritis. Am Rev Respir Dis 131:770-777, 1985.
77. Staples CA, Müller NL, Vedal S, et al: Usual interstitial pneumonia: Correlation of CT with clinical, functional, and radiologic findings. Radiology 162:377-381, 1987.
78. Remy-Jardin M, Remy J, Cortet B, et al: Lung changes in rheumatoid arthritis: CT findings. Radiology 193:375-382, 1994.
79. McCann BG, Hart GJ, Stokes TC, Harrison BD: Obliterative bronchiolitis and upper-zone pulmonary consolidation in rheumatoid arthritis. Thorax 38:73-74, 1983.
80. Akira M, Sakatani M, Hara H: Thin-section CT findings in rheumatoid arthritis–associated lung disease: CT patterns and their courses. J Comput Assist Tomogr 23:941-948, 1999.
81. Rajasekaran BA, Shovlin D, Lord P, Kelly CA: Interstitial lung disease in patients with rheumatoid arthritis: A comparison with cryptogenic fibrosing alveolitis. Rheumatology (Oxford) 40:1022-1025, 2001.
82. Dawson JK, Fewins HE, Desmond J, et al: Fibrosing alveolitis in patients with rheumatoid arthritis as assessed by high resolution computed tomography, chest radiography, and pulmonary function tests. Thorax 56:622-627, 2001.
83. Petrie GR, Bloomfield P, Grant IW, Crompton GK: Upper lobe fibrosis and cavitation in rheumatoid disease. Br J Dis Chest 74:263-267, 1980.
84. Walters MN, Ojeda VJ: Pleuropulmonary necrobiotic rheumatoid nodules. A review and clinicopathological study of six patients. Med J Aust 144:648-651, 1986.
85. Morgan WK, Wolfel DA: The lungs and pleura in rheumatoid arthritis. Am J Roentgenol Radium Ther Nucl Med 98:334-342, 1966.
86. Burrows FG: Pulmonary nodules in rheumatoid disease: A report of two cases. Br J Radiol 40:256-261, 1967.
87. Jolles H, Moseley PL, Peterson MW: Nodular pulmonary opacities in patients with rheumatoid arthritis. A diagnostic dilemma. Chest 96:1022-1025, 1989.
88. Caplan A, Cowen ED, Gough J: Rheumatoid pneumoconiosis in a foundry worker. Thorax 13:181-184, 1958.
89. Caplan A: Certain unusual radiological appearances in the chest of coal-miners suffering from rheumatoid arthritis. Thorax 8:29-37, 1953.
90. Gough J, Rivers D, Seal RM: Pathological studies of modified pneumoconiosis in coal-miners with rheumatoid arthritis; Caplan's syndrome. Thorax 10:9-18, 1955.
91. Perez T, Remy-Jardin M, Cortet B: Airways involvement in rheumatoid arthritis: Clinical, functional, and HRCT findings. Am J Respir Crit Care Med 157:1658-1665, 1998.
92. Hassan WU, Keaney NP, Holland CD, Kelly CA: Bronchial reactivity and airflow obstruction in rheumatoid arthritis. Ann Rheum Dis 53:511-514, 1994.
93. Geddes DM, Corrin B, Brewerton DA, et al: Progressive airway obliteration in adults and its association with rheumatoid disease. Q J Med 46:427-444, 1977.
94. Hayakawa H, Sato A, Imokawa S, et al: Bronchiolar disease in rheumatoid arthritis. Am J Respir Crit Care Med 154:1531-1536, 1996.
95. Scott TE, Wise RA, Hochberg MC, Wigley FM: HLA-DR4 and pulmonary dysfunction in rheumatoid arthritis. Am J Med 82:765-771, 1987.
96. Sweatman MC, Markwick JR, Charles PJ, et al: Histocompatibility antigens in adult obliterative bronchiolitis with or without rheumatoid arthritis. Dis Markers 4:19-26, 1986.
97. Epler GR, Snider GL, Gaensler EA, et al: Bronchiolitis and bronchitis in connective tissue disease. A possible relationship to the use of penicillamine. JAMA 242:528-532, 1979.
98. Begin R, Masse S, Cantin A, et al: Airway disease in a subset of nonsmoking rheumatoid patients. Characterization of the disease and evidence for an autoimmune pathogenesis. Am J Med 72:743-750, 1982.
99. Aquino SL, Webb WR, Golden J: Bronchiolitis obliterans associated with rheumatoid arthritis: Findings on HRCT and dynamic expiratory CT. J Comput Assist Tomogr 18:555-558, 1994.
100. Padley SP, Adler BD, Hansell DM, Müller NL: Bronchiolitis obliterans: High resolution CT findings and correlation with pulmonary function tests. Clin Radiol 47:236-240, 1993.
101. Herzog CA, Miller RR, Hoidal JR: Bronchiolitis and rheumatoid arthritis. Am Rev Respir Dis 124:636-639, 1981.
102. Wells AU, du Bois RM: Bronchiolitis in association with connective tissue disorders. Clin Chest Med 14:655-666, 1993.
103. Ippolito JA, Palmer L, Spector S, et al: Bronchiolitis obliterans organizing pneumonia and rheumatoid arthritis. Semin Arthritis Rheum 23:70-78, 1993.
104. Yousem SA, Colby TV, Carrington CB: Follicular bronchitis/bronchiolitis. Hum Pathol 16:700-706, 1985.
105. Howling SJ, Hansell DM, Wells AU, et al: Follicular bronchiolitis: Thin-section CT and histologic findings. Radiology 212:637-642, 1999.
106. Fortoul TI, Cano-Valle F, Oliva E, Barrios R: Follicular bronchiolitis in association with connective tissue diseases. Lung 163:305-314, 1985.
107. McMahon MJ, Swinson DR, Shettar S, et al: Bronchiectasis and rheumatoid arthritis: A clinical study. Ann Rheum Dis 52:776-779, 1993.
108. Cohen M, Sahn SA: Bronchiectasis in systemic diseases. Chest 116:1063-1074, 1999.
109. Swinson DR, Symmons D, Suresh U, et al: Decreased survival in patients with co-existent rheumatoid arthritis and bronchiectasis. Br J Rheumatol 36:689-691, 1997.
110. Heath D, Gillund TD, Kay JM, Hawkins CF: Pulmonary vascular disease in honeycomb lung. J Pathol Bacteriol 95:423-430, 1968.
111. Gardner DL, Duthie JJ, Macleod J, Allan WS: Pulmonary hypertension in rheumatoid arthritis: Report of a case with intimal sclerosis of the pulmonary and digital arteries. Scott Med J 2:183-188, 1957.
112. Eaton AM, Serota H, Kernodle GW Jr, et al: Pulmonary hypertension secondary to serum hyperviscosity in a patient with rheumatoid arthritis. Am J Med 82:1039-1045, 1987.
113. Dawson JK, Goodson NG, Graham DR, Lynch MP: Raised pulmonary artery pressures measured with Doppler echocardiography in rheumatoid arthritis patients. Rheumatology (Oxford) 39:1320-1325, 2000.
114. Carr DT, Mayne JG: Pleurisy with effusion in rheumatoid arthritis, with reference to the low concentration of glucose in pleural fluid. Am Rev Respir Dis 85:345-350, 1962.
115. Adelman HM, Dupont EL, Flannery MT, Wallach PM: Case report: Recurrent pneumothorax in a patient with rheumatoid arthritis. Am J Med Sci 308:171-172, 1994.
116. Scussel-Lonzetti L, Joyal F, Raynauld JP, et al: Predicting mortality in systemic sclerosis: Analysis of a cohort of 309 French Canadian patients with emphasis on features at diagnosis as predictive factors for survival. Medicine (Baltimore) 81:154-167, 2002.
117. Ferri C, Valentini G, Cozzi F, et al: Systemic sclerosis: Demographic, clinical, and serologic features and survival in 1,012 Italian patients. Medicine (Baltimore) 81:139-153, 2002.
118. Medsger TA Jr, Masi AT: Epidemiology of systemic sclerosis (scleroderma). Ann Intern Med 74:714-721, 1971.
119. Kuwana M, Kaburaki J, Arnett FC, et al: Influence of ethnic background on clinical and serologic features in patients with systemic sclerosis and anti-DNA topoisomerase I antibody. Arthritis Rheum 42:465-474, 1999.
120. Steen VD, Conte C, Owens GR, Medsger TA Jr: Severe restrictive lung disease in systemic sclerosis. Arthritis Rheum 37:1283-1289, 1994.
121. Sud A, Gupta D, Wanchu A, et al: Static lung compliance as an index of early pulmonary disease in systemic sclerosis. Clin Rheumatol 20:177-180, 2001.
122. Dellafiore L, Colombo B, Del Sante M, et al: [Pulmonary involvement in scleroderma assessed with high-resolution computerized tomography and functional tests.] Radiol Med (Torino) 87:608-613, 1994.
123. Witt C, Borges AC, John M, et al: Pulmonary involvement in diffuse cutaneous systemic sclerosis: Bronchioalveolar fluid granulocytosis predicts progression of fibrosing alveolitis. Ann Rheum Dis 58:635-640, 1999.
124. Young RH, Mark GJ: Pulmonary vascular changes in scleroderma. Am J Med 64:998-1004, 1978.
125. Bouros D, Wells AU, Nicholson AG, et al: Histopathologic subsets of fibrosing alveolitis in patients with systemic sclerosis and their relationship to outcome. Am J Respir Crit Care Med 165:1581-1586, 2002.
126. Bridges AJ, Hsu KC, Dias-Arias AA, Chechani V: Bronchiolitis obliterans organizing pneumonia and scleroderma. J Rheumatol 19:1136-1140, 1992.
127. D'Angelo WA, Fries JF, Masi AT, Shulman LE: Pathologic observations in systemic sclerosis (scleroderma). A study of fifty-eight autopsy cases and fifty-eight matched controls. Am J Med 46:428-440, 1969.
128. Minai OA, Dweik RA, Arroliga AC: Manifestations of scleroderma pulmonary disease. Clin Chest Med 19:713-731, 1998.
129. Schurawitzki H, Stiglbauer R, Graninger W, et al: Interstitial lung disease in progressive systemic sclerosis: High-resolution CT versus radiography. Radiology 176:755-759, 1990.
130. Harrison NK, Glanville AR, Strickland B, et al: Pulmonary involvement in systemic sclerosis: The detection of early changes by thin section CT scan, bronchoalveolar lavage and ^{99m}Tc-DTPA clearance. Respir Med 83:403-414, 1989.

131. Kim EA, Johkoh T, Lee KS, et al: Interstitial pneumonia in progressive systemic sclerosis: Serial high-resolution CT findings with functional correlation. J Comput Assist Tomogr 25:757-763, 2001.
132. Remy-Jardin M, Remy J, Wallaert B, et al: Pulmonary involvement in progressive systemic sclerosis: Sequential evaluation with CT, pulmonary function tests, and bronchoalveolar lavage. Radiology 188:499-506, 1993.
133. McCarthy DS, Baragar FD, Dhingra S, et al: The lungs in systemic sclerosis (scleroderma): A review and new information. Semin Arthritis Rheum 17:271-283, 1988.
134. Farmer RG, Gifford RW Jr, Hines EA Jr: Prognostic significance of Raynaud's phenomenon and other clinical characteristics of systemic scleroderma. A study of 271 cases. Circulation 21:1088-1095, 1960.
135. Dinsmore RE, Goodman D, Dreyfuss JR: The air esophagram: A sign of scleroderma involving the esophagus. Radiology 87:348-349, 1966.
136. Bettmann MA, Kantrowitz F: Rapid onset of lung involvement in progressive systemic sclerosis. Chest 75:509-510, 1979.
137. Owens GR, Follansbee WP: Cardiopulmonary manifestations of systemic sclerosis. Chest 91:118-127, 1987.
138. Weaver AL, Divertie MB, Titus JL: Pulmonary scleroderma. Dis Chest 54:490-498, 1968.
139. Kallenbach J, Prinsloo I, Zwi S: Progressive systemic sclerosis complicated by diffuse pulmonary haemorrhage. Thorax 32:767-770, 1977.
140. Bar J, Ehrenfeld M, Rozenman J, et al: Pulmonary-renal syndrome in systemic sclerosis. Semin Arthritis Rheum 30:403-410, 2001.
141. Marie I, Dominique S, Levesque H, et al: Esophageal involvement and pulmonary manifestations in systemic sclerosis. Arthritis Rheum 45:346-354, 2001.
142. Clemson BS, Miller WR, Luck JC, Feriss JA: Acute myocarditis in fulminant systemic sclerosis. Chest 101:872-874, 1992.
143. Kent LT, Cramer SF, Moskowitz RW:. Eosinophilic fasciitis: Clinical, laboratory, and microscopic considerations. Arthritis Rheum 24:677-683, 1981.
144. Jacobsen S, Halberg P, Ullman S, et al: A longitudinal study of pulmonary function in Danish patients with systemic sclerosis. Clin Rheumatol 16:384-390, 1997.
145. Blom-Bulow B, Jonson B, Brauer K: Lung function in progressive systemic sclerosis is dominated by poorly compliant lungs and stiff airways. Eur J Respir Dis 66:1-8, 1985.
146. Guttadauria M, Ellman H, Emmanuel G, et al: Pulmonary function in scleroderma. Arthritis Rheum 20:1071-1079, 1977.
147. Diot E, Boissinot E, Asquier E, et al: Relationship between abnormalities on high-resolution CT and pulmonary function in systemic sclerosis. Chest 114:1623-1629, 1998.
148. Yang Y, Fujita J, Tokuda M, et al: Lung cancer associated with several connective tissue diseases: With a review of literature. Rheumatol Int 21:106-111, 2001.
149. Spencer-Green G, Alter D, Welch HG: Test performance in systemic sclerosis: Anticentromere and anti–Scl-70 antibodies. Am J Med 103:242-248, 1997.
150. Steen VD, Ziegler GL, Rodnan GP, Medsger TA Jr: Clinical and laboratory associations of anticentromere antibody in patients with progressive systemic sclerosis. Arthritis Rheum 27:125-131, 1984.
151. Zuber M, Gotzen R, Filler I: Clinical correlation of anticentromere antibodies. Clin Rheumatol 13:427-432, 1994.
152. Stupi AM, Steen VD, Owens GR, et al: Pulmonary hypertension in the CREST syndrome variant of systemic sclerosis. Arthritis Rheum 29:515-524, 1986.
153. Battle RW, Davitt MA, Cooper SM, et al: Prevalence of pulmonary hypertension in limited and diffuse scleroderma. Chest 110:1515-1519, 1996.
154. Tanimoto K, Nakano K, Kano S, et al: Classification criteria for polymyositis and dermatomyositis. J Rheumatol 22:668-674, 1995.
155. Bohan A, Peter JB: Polymyositis and dermatomyositis (first of two parts). N Engl J Med 292:344-347, 1975.
156. Plotz PH, Rider LG, Targoff IN, et al: NIH conference. Myositis: Immunologic contributions to understanding cause, pathogenesis, and therapy. Ann Intern Med 122:715-724, 1995.
157. Targoff IN: Immune manifestations of inflammatory muscle disease. Rheum Dis Clin North Am 20:857-880, 1994.
158. Schmidt WA, Wetzel W, Friedlander R, et al: Clinical and serological aspects of patients with anti–Jo-1 antibodies—an evolving spectrum of disease manifestations. Clin Rheumatol 19:371-377, 2000.
159. Wasicek CA, Reichlin M, Montes M, Raghu G: Polymyositis and interstitial lung disease in a patient with anti-Jo1 prototype. Am J Med 76:538-544, 1984.
160. Douglas WW, Tazelaar HD, Hartman TE, et al: Polymyositis-dermatomyositis–associated interstitial lung disease. Am J Respir Crit Care Med 164:1182-1185, 2001.
161. Tazelaar HD, Viggiano RW, Pickersgill J, Colby TV: Interstitial lung disease in polymyositis and dermatomyositis. Clinical features and prognosis as correlated with histologic findings. Am Rev Respir Dis 141:727-733, 1990.
162. Frazier AR, Miller RD: Interstitial pneumonitis in association with polymyositis and dermatomyositis. Chest 65:403-407, 1974.
163. Schwarz MI, Matthay RA, Sahn SA, et al: Interstitial lung disease in polymyositis and dermatomyositis: Analysis of six cases and review of the literature. Medicine (Baltimore) 55:89-104, 1976.
164. Schwarz MI: Pulmonary and cardiac manifestations of polymyositis-dermatomyositis. J Thorac Imaging 7:46-54, 1992.
165. Ikezoe J, Johkoh T, Kohno N, et al: High-resolution CT findings of lung disease in patients with polymyositis and dermatomyositis. J Thorac Imaging 11:250-259, 1996.
166. Schiavi EA, Roncoroni AJ, Puy RJ: Isolated bilateral diaphragmatic paresis with interstitial lung disease. An unusual presentation of dermatomyositis. Am Rev Respir Dis 129:337-339, 1984.
167. Ogle S: Retrospective study of polymyositis in Auckland over 10 years. N Z Med J 92:433-435, 1980.
168. Schwarz MI, Sutarik JM, Nick JA, et al: Pulmonary capillaritis and diffuse alveolar hemorrhage. A primary manifestation of polymyositis. Am J Respir Crit Care Med 151:2037-2040, 1995.
169. Hebert CA, Byrnes TJ, Baethge BA, et al: Exercise limitation in patients with polymyositis. Chest 98:352-357, 1990.
170. Marie I, Dominique S, Remy-Jardin M, et al: [Interstitial lung diseases in polymyositis and dermatomyositis.] Rev Med Interne 22:1083-1096, 2001.
171. Callen JP: Relationship of cancer to inflammatory muscle diseases. Dermatomyositis, polymyositis, and inclusion body myositis. Rheum Dis Clin North Am 20:943-953, 1994.
172. Stockton D, Doherty VR, Brewster DH: Risk of cancer in patients with dermatomyositis or polymyositis, and follow-up implications: A Scottish population-based cohort study. Br J Cancer 85:41-45, 2001.
173. Buchbinder R, Forbes A, Hall S, et al: Incidence of malignant disease in biopsy-proven inflammatory myopathy. A population-based cohort study. Ann Intern Med 134:1087-1095, 2001.
174. Chow WH, Gridley G, Mellemkjaer L, et al: Cancer risk following polymyositis and dermatomyositis: A nationwide cohort study in Denmark. Cancer Causes Control 6:9-13, 1995.
175. Sjögren H: Zur Kenntnis der Keratoconjunctivitis sicca (Keratitis filiformis bei Hypofunktion der Tranendrusen). [Keratoconjunctivitis sicca (keratitis filiformis with hypofunction of the lacrimal glands).] Acta Ophthalmol 2(Suppl):1, 1933.
176. Gratwhol AA, Moutsopoulos HM, Chused TM, et al: Sjögren-type syndrome after allogeneic bone-marrow transplantation. Ann Intern Med 87:703-706, 1977.
177. Itescu S, Brancato LJ, Buxbaum J, et al: A diffuse infiltrative CD8 lymphocytosis syndrome in human immunodeficiency virus (HIV) infection: A host immune response associated with HLA-DR5. Ann Intern Med 112:3-10, 1990.
178. Shearn MA: Sjögren's syndrome. Med Clin North Am 61:271-282, 1977.
179. Papiris SA, Maniati M, Constantopoulos SH, et al: Lung involvement in primary Sjögren's syndrome is mainly related to the small airway disease. Ann Rheum Dis 58:61-64, 1999.
180. Fairfax AJ, Haslam PL, Pavia D, et al: Pulmonary disorders associated with Sjögren's syndrome. Q J Med 50:279-295, 1981.
181. Constantopoulos SH, Tsianos EV, Moutsopoulos HM: Pulmonary and gastrointestinal manifestations of Sjögren's syndrome. Rheum Dis Clin North Am 18:617-635, 1992.
182. Newball HH, Brahim SA: Chronic obstructive airway disease in patients with Sjögren's syndrome. Am Rev Respir Dis 115:295-304, 1977.
183. Deheinzelin D, Capelozzi VL, Kairalla RA, et al: Interstitial lung disease in primary Sjögren's syndrome. Clinical-pathological evaluation and response to treatment. Am J Respir Crit Care Med 154:794-799, 1996.
184. Kadota J, Kusano S, Kawakami K, et al: Usual interstitial pneumonia associated with primary Sjögren's syndrome. Chest 108:1756-1758, 1995.
185. Strimlan CV, Rosenow EC 3rd, Divertie MB, Harrison EG Jr: Pulmonary manifestations of Sjögren's syndrome. Chest 70:354-361, 1976.
186. Franquet T, Gimenez A, Monill JM, et al: Primary Sjögren's syndrome and associated lung disease: CT findings in 50 patients. AJR Am J Roentgenol 169:655-658, 1997.
187. Tanoue LT: Pulmonary involvement in collagen vascular disease: A review of the pulmonary manifestations of the Marfan syndrome, ankylosing spondylitis, Sjögren's syndrome, and relapsing polychondritis. J Thorac Imaging 7:62-77, 1992.
188. Carignan S, Staples CA, Müller NL: Intrathoracic lymphoproliferative disorders in the immunocompromised patient: CT findings. Radiology 197:53-58, 1995.
189. Johkoh T, Müller NL, Pickford HA, et al: Lymphocytic interstitial pneumonia: Thin-section CT findings in 22 patients. Radiology 212:567-572, 1999.
190. Koyama M, Johkoh T, Honda O, et al: Pulmonary involvement in primary Sjögren's syndrome: Spectrum of pulmonary abnormalities and computed tomography findings in 60 patients. J Thorac Imaging 16:290-296, 2001.
191. Salaffi F, Manganelli P, Carotti M, et al: A longitudinal study of pulmonary involvement in primary Sjögren's syndrome: Relationship between alveolitis and subsequent lung changes on high-resolution computed tomography. Br J Rheumatol 37:263-269, 1998.
192. Lahdensuo A, Korpela M: Pulmonary findings in patients with primary Sjögren's syndrome. Chest 108:316-319, 1995.
193. Gudbjornsson B, Hedenstrom H, Stalenheim G, Hallgren R: Bronchial hyperresponsiveness to methacholine in patients with primary Sjögren's syndrome. Ann Rheum Dis 50:36-40, 1991.
194. Moutsopoulos HM, Chused TM, Mann DL, et al: Sjögren's syndrome (sicca syndrome): Current issues. Ann Intern Med 92:212-226, 1980.
195. Kelly C, Gardiner P, Pal B, Griffiths I: Lung function in primary Sjögren's syndrome: A cross sectional and longitudinal study. Thorax 46:180-183, 1991.
196. Papathanasiou MP, Constantopoulos SH, Tsampoulas C, et al: Reappraisal of respiratory abnormalities in primary and secondary Sjögren's syndrome. A controlled study. Chest 90:370-374, 1986.
197. Davidson BK, Kelly CA, Griffiths ID: Ten year follow up of pulmonary function in patients with primary Sjögren's syndrome. Ann Rheum Dis 59:709-712, 2000.
198. Danieli MG, Fraticelli P, Salvi A, et al: Undifferentiated connective tissue disease: Natural history and evolution into definite CTD assessed in 84 patients initially diagnosed as early UCTD. Clin Rheumatol 17:195-201, 1998.

199. Lazaro MA, Maldonado Cocco JA, et al: Clinical and serologic characteristics of patients with overlap syndrome: Is mixed connective tissue disease a distinct clinical entity? Medicine (Baltimore) 68:58-65, 1989.

200. Sullivan WD, Hurst DJ, Harmon CE, et al: A prospective evaluation emphasizing pulmonary involvement in patients with mixed connective tissue disease. Medicine (Baltimore) 63:92-107, 1984.

201. Kasukawa R: Mixed connective tissue disease. Intern Med 38:386-393, 1999.

202. Schwarz MI, Zamora MR, Hodges TN, et al: Isolated pulmonary capillaritis and diffuse alveolar hemorrhage in rheumatoid arthritis and mixed connective tissue disease. Chest 113:1609-1615, 1998.

203. Wiener-Kronish JP, Solinger AM, Warnock ML, et al: Severe pulmonary involvement in mixed connective tissue disease. Am Rev Respir Dis 124:499-503, 1981.

204. Horiki T, Fuyuno G, Ishii M, et al: Fatal alveolar hemorrhage in a patient with mixed connective tissue disease presenting polymyositis features. Intern Med 37:554-560, 1998.

205. Prakash UB: Lungs in mixed connective tissue disease. J Thorac Imaging 7:55-61, 1992.

206. Prakash UB, Luthra HS, Divertie MB: Intrathoracic manifestations in mixed connective tissue disease. Mayo Clin Proc 60:813-821, 1985.

207. Müller NL, Miller RR: Diffuse pulmonary hemorrhage. Radiol Clin North Am 29:965-971, 1991.

208. Trentham DE, Le CH: Relapsing polychondritis. Ann Intern Med 129:114-122, 1998.

209. McAdam LP, O'Hanlan MA, Bluestone R, Pearson CM: Relapsing polychondritis: Prospective study of 23 patients and a review of the literature. Medicine (Baltimore) 55:193-215, 1976.

210. Yang CL, Brinckmann J, Rui HF, et al: Autoantibodies to cartilage collagens in relapsing polychondritis. Arch Dermatol Res 285:245-249, 1993.

211. Valenzuela R, Cooperrider PA, Gogate P, et al: Relapsing polychondritis. Immunomicroscopic findings in cartilage of ear biopsy specimens. Hum Pathol 11:19-22, 1980.

212. Dolan DL, Lemmon GB Jr, Teitelbaum SL: Relapsing polychondritis. Analytical literature review and studies on pathogenesis. Am J Med 41:285-299, 1966.

213. Crockford MP, Kerr IH: Relapsing polychondritis. Clin Radiol 39:386-390, 1988.

214. Davis SD, Berkmen YM, King T: Peripheral bronchial involvement in relapsing polychondritis: Demonstration by thin-section CT. AJR Am J Roentgenol 153:953-954, 1989.

215. Choplin RH, Wehunt WD, Theros EG: Diffuse lesions of the trachea. Semin Roentgenol 18:38-50, 1983.

216. Tillie-Leblond I, Wallaert B, Leblond D, et al: Respiratory involvement in relapsing polychondritis. Clinical, functional, endoscopic, and radiographic evaluations. Medicine (Baltimore) 77:168-176, 1998.

217. Eng J, Sabanathan S: Airway complications in relapsing polychondritis. Ann Thorac Surg 51:686-692, 1991.

218. Sarodia BD, Dasgupta A, Mehta AC: Management of airway manifestations of relapsing polychondritis: Case reports and review of literature. Chest 116:1669-1675, 1999.

219. Michet CJ Jr, McKenna CH, Luthra HS, O'Fallon WM: Relapsing polychondritis. Survival and predictive role of early disease manifestations. Ann Intern Med 104:74-78, 1986.

220. Kraft SC, Earle RH, Roesler M, Esterly JR: Unexplained bronchopulmonary disease with inflammatory bowel disease. Arch Intern Med 136:454-459, 1976.

221. Camus P, Colby TV: The lung in inflammatory bowel disease. Eur Respir J 15:5-10, 2000.

222. Karadag F, Ozhan MH, Akcicek E, et al: Is it possible to detect ulcerative colitis–related respiratory syndrome early? Respirology 6:341-346, 2001.

223. Fireman Z, Osipov A, Kivity S, et al: The use of induced sputum in the assessment of pulmonary involvement in Crohn's disease. Am J Gastroenterol 95:730-734, 2000.

224. Mansi A, Cucchiara S, Greco L, et al: Bronchial hyperresponsiveness in children and adolescents with Crohn's disease. Am J Respir Crit Care Med 161:1051-1054, 2000.

225. Camus P, Piard F, Ashcroft T, et al: The lung in inflammatory bowel disease. Medicine (Baltimore) 72:151-183, 1993.

226. Eaton TE, Lambie N, Wells AU: Bronchiectasis following colectomy for Crohn's disease. Thorax 53:529-531, 1998.

227. Vasishta S, Wood DB, McGinty F: Ulcerative tracheobronchitis years after colectomy for ulcerative colitis. Chest 106:1279-1281, 1994.

228. Swinburn CR, Jackson GJ, Cobden I, et al: Bronchiolitis obliterans organising pneumonia in a patient with ulcerative colitis. Thorax 43:735-736, 1988.

229. Desai SJ, Gephardt GN, Stoller JK: Diffuse panbronchiolitis preceding ulcerative colitis. Chest 95:1342-1344, 1989.

230. Vandenplas O, Casel S, Delos M, et al: Granulomatous bronchiolitis associated with Crohn's disease. Am J Respir Crit Care Med 158:1676-1679, 1998.

231. Louis E, Louis R, Shute J, et al: Bronchial eosinophilic infiltration in Crohn's disease in the absence of pulmonary disease. Clin Exp Allergy 29:660-666, 1999.

232. Storch I, Rosoff L, Katz S: Sarcoidosis and inflammatory bowel disease. J Clin Gastroenterol 33:345, 2001.

233. Garg K, Lynch DA, Newell JD: Inflammatory airways disease in ulcerative colitis: CT and high-resolution CT features. J Thorac Imaging 8:159-163, 1993.

234. Mahadeva R, Walsh G, Flower CD, Shneerson JM: Clinical and radiological characteristics of lung disease in inflammatory bowel disease. Eur Respir J 15:41-48, 2000.

235. Wilcox P, Miller R, Miller G, et al: Airway involvement in ulcerative colitis. Chest 92:18-22, 1987.

236. Rao JK, Allen NB, Pincus T: Limitations of the 1990 American College of Rheumatology classification criteria in the diagnosis of vasculitis. Ann Intern Med 129:345-352, 1998.

237. Hunder G: Vasculitis: Diagnosis and therapy. Am J Med 100:37S-45S, 1996.

238. Luqmani RA: Is it possible to offer evidence-based treatment for systemic vasculitis? Scand J Rheumatol 29:211-215, 2000.

239. Jennette JC, Falk RJ, Andrassy K, et al: Nomenclature of systemic vasculitides. Proposal of an international consensus conference. Arthritis Rheum 37:187-192, 1994.

240. Leavitt RY, Fauci AS: Pulmonary vasculitis. Am Rev Respir Dis 134:149-166, 1986.

241. Leavitt RY, Fauci AS, Bloch DA, et al: The American College of Rheumatology 1990 criteria for the classification of Wegener's granulomatosis. Arthritis Rheum 33:1101-1107, 1990.

242. Gal AA, Velasquez A: Antineutrophil cytoplasmic autoantibody in the absence of Wegener's granulomatosis or microscopic polyangiitis: Implications for the surgical pathologist. Mod Pathol 15:197-204, 2002.

243. Choi HK, Lamprecht P, Niles JL, et al: Subacute bacterial endocarditis with positive cytoplasmic antineutrophil cytoplasmic antibodies and anti–proteinase 3 antibodies. Arthritis Rheum 43:226-231, 2000.

244. Miyahara N, Eda R, Umemori Y, et al: Pulmonary lymphoma of large B-cell type mimicking Wegener's granulomatosis. Intern Med 40:786-790, 2001.

245. Cotch MF, Hoffman GS, Yerg DE, et al: The epidemiology of Wegener's granulomatosis. Estimates of the five-year period prevalence, annual mortality, and geographic disease distribution from population-based data sources. Arthritis Rheum 39:87-92, 1996.

246. Littlejohn GO, Ryan PJ, Holdsworth SR: Wegener's granulomatosis: Clinical features and outcome in seventeen patients. Aust N Z J Med 15:241-245, 1985.

247. Luqmani RA, Bacon PA, Beaman M, et al: Classical versus non-renal Wegener's granulomatosis. Q J Med 87:161-167, 1994.

248. Cassan SM, Coles DT, Harrison EG Jr: The concept of limited forms of Wegener's granulomatosis. Am J Med 49:366-379, 1970.

249. Wolff SM, Fauci AS, Horn RG, Dale DC: Wegener's granulomatosis. Ann Intern Med 81:513-525, 1974.

250. Kihiczak D, Nychay SG, Schwartz RA, et al: Protracted superficial Wegener's granulomatosis. J Am Acad Dermatol 30:863-866, 1994.

251. Schwarz MI, Brown KK: Small vessel vasculitis of the lung. Thorax 55:502-510, 2000.

252. Schnabel A, Csernok E, Braun J, Gross WL: Activation of neutrophils, eosinophils, and lymphocytes in the lower respiratory tract in Wegener's granulomatosis. Am J Respir Crit Care Med 161:399-405, 2000.

253. Pinching AJ, Rees AJ, Pussell BA, et al: Relapses in Wegener's granulomatosis: The role of infection. BMJ 281:836-838, 1980.

254. Stegeman CA, Tervaert JW, Sluiter WJ, et al: Association of chronic nasal carriage of Staphylococcus aureus and higher relapse rates in Wegener granulomatosis. Ann Intern Med 120:12-17, 1994.

255. van Putten JW, van Haren EH, Lammers JW: Association between Wegener's granulomatosis and Staphylococcus aureus infection? Eur Respir J 9:1955-1957, 1996.

256. Reinhold-Keller E, De Groot K, Rudert H, et al: Response to trimethoprim/sulfamethoxazole in Wegener's granulomatosis depends on the phase of disease. QJM 89:15-23, 1996.

257. Savige JA, Davies DJ, Gatenby PA: Anti-neutrophil cytoplasmic antibodies (ANCA): Their detection and significance: Report from workshops. Pathology 26:186-193, 1994.

258. Brockmann H, Schwarting A, Kriegsmann J, et al: Proteinase-3 as the major autoantigen of c-ANCA is strongly expressed in lung tissue of patients with Wegener's granulomatosis. Arthritis Res 4:220-225, 2002.

259. Falk RJ, Terrell RS, Charles LA, Jennette JC: Anti-neutrophil cytoplasmic autoantibodies induce neutrophils to degranulate and produce oxygen radicals in vitro. Proc Natl Acad Sci U S A 87:4115-4119, 1990.

260. Grimminger F, Hattar K, Papavassilis C, et al: Neutrophil activation by anti–proteinase 3 antibodies in Wegener's granulomatosis: Role of exogenous arachidonic acid and leukotriene B$_4$ generation. J Exp Med 184:1567-1572, 1996.

261. Brouwer E, Stegeman CA, Huitema MG, et al: T cell reactivity to proteinase 3 and myeloperoxidase in patients with Wegener's granulomatosis (WG). Clin Exp Immunol 98:448-453, 1994.

262. Girard T, Mahr A, Noel LH, et al: Are antineutrophil cytoplasmic antibodies a marker predictive of relapse in Wegener's granulomatosis? A prospective study. Rheumatology (Oxford) 40:147-151, 2001.

263. Komocsi A, Lamprecht P, Csernok E, et al: Peripheral blood and granuloma CD4(+)CD28(–) T cells are a major source of interferon-gamma and tumor necrosis factor-alpha in Wegener's granulomatosis. Am J Pathol 160:1717-1724, 2002.

264. Travis WD, Hoffman GS, Leavitt RY, et al: Surgical pathology of the lung in Wegener's granulomatosis. Review of 87 open lung biopsies from 67 patients. Am J Surg Pathol 15:315-333, 1991.

265. Mark EJ, Matsubara O, Tan-Liu NS, Fienberg R: The pulmonary biopsy in the early diagnosis of Wegener's (pathergic) granulomatosis: A study based on 35 open lung biopsies. Hum Pathol 19:1065-1071, 1988.

266. Yoshikawa Y, Watanabe T: Pulmonary lesions in Wegener's granulomatosis: A clinicopathologic study of 22 autopsy cases. Hum Pathol 17:401-410, 1986.

267. Yousem SA: Bronchocentric injury in Wegener's granulomatosis: A report of five cases. Hum Pathol 22:535-540, 1991.

268. Travis WD, Colby TV, Lombard C, Carpenter HA: A clinicopathologic study of 34 cases of diffuse pulmonary hemorrhage with lung biopsy confirmation. Am J Surg Pathol 14:1112-1125, 1990.

269. Hoffman GS, Kerr GS, Leavitt RY, et al: Wegener granulomatosis: An analysis of 158 patients. Ann Intern Med 116:488-498, 1992.

270. Cordier JF, Valeyre D, Guillevin L, et al: Pulmonary Wegener's granulomatosis. A clinical and imaging study of 77 cases. Chest 97:906-912, 1990.
271. Aberle DR, Gamsu G, Lynch D: Thoracic manifestations of Wegener granulomatosis: Diagnosis and course. Radiology 174:703-709, 1990.
272. Frazier AA, Rosado-de-Christenson ML, Galvin JR, Fleming MV: Pulmonary angiitis and granulomatosis: Radiologic-pathologic correlation. Radiographics 18:687-710, quiz 727, 1998.
273. Papiris SA, Manoussakis MN, Drosos AA, et al: Imaging of thoracic Wegener's granulomatosis: The computed tomographic appearance. Am J Med 93:529-536, 1992.
274. Reuter M, Schnabel A, Wesner F, et al: Pulmonary Wegener's granulomatosis: Correlation between high-resolution CT findings and clinical scoring of disease activity. Chest 114:500-506, 1998.
275. Weir IH, Müller NL, Chiles C, et al: Wegener's granulomatosis: Findings from computed tomography of the chest in 10 patients. Can Assoc Radiol J 43:31-34, 1992.
276. Maskell GF, Lockwood CM, Flower CD: Computed tomography of the lung in Wegener's granulomatosis. Clin Radiol 48:377-380, 1993.
277. Kuhlman JE, Hruban RH, Fishman EK: Wegener granulomatosis: CT features of parenchymal lung disease. J Comput Assist Tomogr 15:948-952, 1991.
278. Sheehan RE, Flint JD, Müller NL: Computed tomography features of the thoracic manifestations of Wegener granulomatosis. J Thorac Imaging 18:34-41, 2003.
279. Daum TE, Specks U, Colby TV, et al: Tracheobronchial involvement in Wegener's granulomatosis. Am J Respir Crit Care Med 151:522-526, 1995.
280. Gohel VK, Dalinka MK, Israel HL, Libshitz HI: The radiological manifestations of Wegener's granulomatosis. Br J Radiol 46:427-432, 1973.
281. Screaton NJ, Sivasothy P, Flower CD, Lockwood CM: Tracheal involvement in Wegener's granulomatosis: Evaluation using spiral CT. Clin Radiol 53:809-815, 1998.
282. Reinhold-Keller E, Beuge N, Latza U, et al: An interdisciplinary approach to the care of patients with Wegener's granulomatosis: Long-term outcome in 155 patients. Arthritis Rheum 43:1021-1032, 2000.
283. Krafcik SS, Covin RB, Lynch JP 3rd, Sitrin RG: Wegener's granulomatosis in the elderly. Chest 109:430-437, 1996.
284. Hergesell O, Andrassy K, Nawroth P: Elevated levels of markers of endothelial cell damage and markers of activated coagulation in patients with systemic necrotizing vasculitis. Thromb Haemost 75:892-898, 1996.
285. Davenport A, Goodfellow J, Goel S, et al: Aortic valve disease in patients with Wegener's granulomatosis. Am J Kidney Dis 24:205-208, 1994.
286. Chung MP, Rhee CH: Airway obstruction in interstitial lung disease. Curr Opin Pulm Med 3:332-335, 1997.
287. Sorensen SF, Slot O, Tvede N, Petersen J: A prospective study of vasculitis patients collected in a five year period: Evaluation of the Chapel Hill nomenclature. Ann Rheum Dis 59:478-482, 2000.
288. Gross WL, Trabandt A, Reinhold-Keller E: Diagnosis and evaluation of vasculitis. Rheumatology (Oxford) 39:245-252, 2000.
289. Byrd VM, Fogo A: The double-edged sword of ANCA: A useful but limited test for screening of pauci-immune vasculitides. Am J Kidney Dis 32:344-349, 1998.
290. Rao JK, Weinberger M, Oddone EZ, et al: The role of antineutrophil cytoplasmic antibody (c-ANCA) testing in the diagnosis of Wegener granulomatosis. A literature review and meta-analysis. Ann Intern Med 123:925-932, 1995.
291. Perroux-Goumy L, Carrere F, Boivinet R: The spectrum of diseases with antineutrophil cytoplasmic antibodies (ANCA) in 189 patients [abstract]. Arthritis Rheum 40:S68, 1997.
292. De'Oliviera J, Gaskin G, Dash A, et al: Relationship between disease activity and anti-neutrophil cytoplasmic antibody concentration in long-term management of systemic vasculitis. Am J Kidney Dis 25:380-389, 1995.
293. Givens CD Jr, Newman JH, McCurley TL: Diagnosis of Wegener's granulomatosis by transbronchial biopsy. Chest 88:794-796, 1985.
294. Fauci AS, Wolff SM: Wegener's granulomatosis: Studies in eighteen patients and a review of the literature. Medicine (Baltimore) 52:535-561, 1973.
295. Burns A: Pulmonary vasculitis. Thorax 53:220-227, 1998.
296. Churg J, Strauss L: Allergic granulomatosis, allergic angiitis, and periarteritis nodosa. Am J Pathol 27:277, 1951.
297. Fienberg R: Allergic granulomatosis. Am J Surg Pathol 6:189-190, 1982.
298. Steinfeld S, Golstein M, De Vuyst P: Chronic eosinophilic pneumonia (CEP) as a presenting feature of Churg-Strauss syndrome (CSS). Eur Respir J 7:2098, 1994.
299. Hueto-Perez-de-Heredia JJ, Dominguez-del-Valle FJ, Garcia E, et al: Chronic eosinophilic pneumonia as a presenting feature of Churg-Strauss syndrome. Eur Respir J 7:1006-1008, 1994.
300. Masi AT, Hunder GG, Lie JT, et al: The American College of Rheumatology 1990 criteria for the classification of Churg-Strauss syndrome (allergic granulomatosis and angiitis). Arthritis Rheum 33:1094-1100, 1990.
301. Watts RA, Carruthers DM, Scott DG: Epidemiology of systemic vasculitis: Changing incidence or definition? Semin Arthritis Rheum 25:28-34, 1995.
302. Guillevin L, Cohen P, Gayraud M, et al: Churg-Strauss syndrome. Clinical study and long-term follow-up of 96 patients. Medicine (Baltimore) 78:26-37, 1999.
303. Weller PF, Plaut M, Taggart V, Trontell A: The relationship of asthma therapy and Churg-Strauss syndrome: NIH workshop summary report. J Allergy Clin Immunol 108:175-183, 2001.
304. Loughlin JE, Cole JA, Rothman KJ, Johnson ES: Prevalence of serious eosinophilia and incidence of Churg-Strauss syndrome in a cohort of asthma patients. Ann Allergy Asthma Immunol 88:319-325, 2002.
305. Solans R, Bosch JA, Selva A, et al: Montelukast and Churg-Strauss syndrome. Thorax 57:183-185, 2002.
306. Koss MN, Antonovych T, Hochholzer L: Allergic granulomatosis (Churg-Strauss syndrome): Pulmonary and renal morphologic findings. Am J Surg Pathol 5:21-28, 1981.
307. Lanham JG, Elkon KB, Pusey CD, Hughes GR: Systemic vasculitis with asthma and eosinophilia: A clinical approach to the Churg-Strauss syndrome. Medicine (Baltimore) 63:65-81, 1984.
308. Chumbley LC, Harrison EG Jr, DeRemee RA: Allergic granulomatosis and angiitis (Churg-Strauss syndrome). Report and analysis of 30 cases. Mayo Clin Proc 52:477-484, 1977.
309. Worthy SA, Müller NL, Hansell DM, Flower CD: Churg-Strauss syndrome: The spectrum of pulmonary CT findings in 17 patients. AJR Am J Roentgenol 170:297-300, 1998.
310. Ramakrishna G, Midthun DE: Churg-Strauss syndrome. Ann Allergy Asthma Immunol 86:603-613, quiz 613, 2001.
311. Lhote F, Guillevin L: Polyarteritis nodosa, microscopic polyangiitis, and Churg-Strauss syndrome. Clinical aspects and treatment. Rheum Dis Clin North Am 21:911-947, 1995.
312. Sehgal M, Swanson JW, DeRemee RA, Colby TV: Neurologic manifestations of Churg-Strauss syndrome. Mayo Clin Proc 70:337-341, 1995.
313. Wallaert B, Gosset P, Prin L, et al: Bronchoalveolar lavage in allergic granulomatosis and angiitis. Eur Respir J 6:413-417, 1993.
314. Tervaert JW, Goldschmeding R, Elema JD, et al: Antimyeloperoxidase antibodies in the Churg-Strauss syndrome. Thorax 46:70-71, 1991.
315. Mouthon L, Le Toumelin P, Andre MH, et al: Polyarteritis nodosa and Churg-Strauss angiitis: Characteristics and outcome in 38 patients over 65 years. Medicine (Baltimore) 81:27-40, 2002.
316. Matsumoto T, Homma S, Okada M, et al: The lung in polyarteritis nodosa: A pathologic study of 10 cases. Hum Pathol 24:717-724, 1993.
317. Nick J, Tuder R, May R, Fisher J: Polyarteritis nodosa with pulmonary vasculitis. Am J Respir Crit Care Med 153:450-453, 1996.
318. Guillevin L, Durand-Gasselin B, Cevallos R, et al: Microscopic polyangiitis: Clinical and laboratory findings in eighty-five patients. Arthritis Rheum 42:421-430, 1999.
319. Mazodier P, Elzouki AN, Segelmark M, Eriksson S: Systemic necrotizing vasculitides in severe α_1-antitrypsin deficiency. QJM 89:599-611, 1996.
320. Reynolds WF, Stegeman CA, Tervaert JW: -463 G/A myeloperoxidase promoter polymorphism is associated with clinical manifestations and the course of disease in MPO-ANCA-associated vasculitis. Clin Immunol 103:154-160, 2002.
321. Watts RA, Gonzalez-Gay MA, Lane SE, et al: Geoepidemiology of systemic vasculitis: Comparison of the incidence in two regions of Europe. Ann Rheum Dis 60:170-172, 2001.
322. Ohtsuka M, Yamashita Y, Doi M, Hasegawa S: Propylthiouracil-induced alveolar haemorrhage associated with antineutrophil cytoplasmic antibody. Eur Respir J 10:1045-1047, 1997.
323. Kelsall JT, Chalmers A, Sherlock CH, et al: Microscopic polyangiitis after influenza vaccination. J Rheumatol 24:1198-1202, 1997.
324. Minota S, Horie S, Yamada A, et al: Circulating myeloperoxidase and anti-myeloperoxidase antibody in patients with vasculitis. Scand J Rheumatol 28:94-99, 1999.
325. Mark EJ, Ramirez JF: Pulmonary capillaritis and hemorrhage in patients with systemic vasculitis. Arch Pathol Lab Med 109:413-418, 1985.
326. Gertner E, Lie JT: Pulmonary capillaritis, alveolar hemorrhage, and recurrent microvascular thrombosis in primary antiphospholipid syndrome. J Rheumatol 20:1224-1228, 1993.
327. Jennings CA, King TE Jr, Tuder R, et al: Diffuse alveolar hemorrhage with underlying isolated, pauciimmune pulmonary capillaritis. Am J Respir Crit Care Med 155:1101-1109, 1997.
328. Lewis EJ, Schur PH, Busch GJ, et al: Immunopathologic features of a patient with glomerulonephritis and pulmonary hemorrhage. Am J Med 54:507-513, 1973.
329. Haworth SJ, Savage CO, Carr D, et al: Pulmonary haemorrhage complicating Wegener's granulomatosis and microscopic polyarteritis. Br Med J (Clin Res Ed) 290:1775-1778, 1985.
330. Dabague J, Reyes PA: Takayasu arteritis in Mexico: A 38-year clinical perspective through literature review. Int J Cardiol 54(Suppl):S103-S109, 1996.
331. Arend WP, Michel BA, Bloch DA, et al: The American College of Rheumatology 1990 criteria for the classification of Takayasu arteritis. Arthritis Rheum 33:1129-1134, 1990.
332. Sharma S, Kamalakar T, Rajani M, et al: The incidence and patterns of pulmonary artery involvement in Takayasu's arteritis. Clin Radiol 42:177-181, 1990.
333. Yamato M, Lecky JW, Hiramatsu K, Kohda E: Takayasu arteritis: Radiographic and angiographic findings in 59 patients. Radiology 161:329-334, 1986.
334. Vanoli M, Castellani M, Bacchiani G, et al: Non-invasive assessment of pulmonary artery involvement in Takayasu's arteritis. Clin Exp Rheumatol 17:215-218, 1999.
335. Kerr GS, Hallahan CW, Giordano J, et al: Takayasu arteritis. Ann Intern Med 120:919-929, 1994.
336. Sharma BK, Siveski-Iliskovic N, Singal PK: Takayasu arteritis may be underdiagnosed in North America. Can J Cardiol 11:311-316, 1995.
337. Saito Y, Hirota K, Ito I, et al: Clinical and pathological studies of five autopsied cases of aortitis syndrome. I. Findings of the aorta and its branches, peripheral arteries and pulmonary arteries. Jpn Heart J 13:20-33, 1972.
338. Hachiya J: Current concept of Takayasu's arteritis. Semin Roentgenol 5:245, 1970.
339. Park JH, Chung JW, Im JG, et al: Takayasu arteritis: Evaluation of mural changes in the aorta and pulmonary artery with CT angiography. Radiology 196:89-93, 1995.

340. Matsunaga N, Hayashi K, Sakamoto I, et al: Takayasu arteritis: Protean radiologic manifestations and diagnosis. Radiographics 17:579-594, 1997.
341. Choe YH, Han BK, Koh EM, et al: Takayasu's arteritis: Assessment of disease activity with contrast-enhanced MR imaging. AJR Am J Roentgenol 175:505-511, 2000.
342. Takahashi K, Honda M, Furuse M, et al: CT findings of pulmonary parenchyma in Takayasu arteritis. J Comput Assist Tomogr 20:742-748, 1996.
343. Yamada I, Numano F, Suzuki S: Takayasu arteritis: Evaluation with MR imaging. Radiology 188:89-94, 1993.
344. Nakabayashi K, Kurata N, Nangi N, et al: Pulmonary artery involvement as first manifestation in three cases of Takayasu arteritis. Int J Cardiol 54(Suppl):S177-S183, 1996.
345. Lupi E, Sanchez G, Horwitz S, Gutierrez E: Pulmonary artery involvement in Takayasu's arteritis. Chest 67:69-74, 1975.
346. Ladanyi M, Fraser RS: Pulmonary involvement in giant cell arteritis. Arch Pathol Lab Med 111:1178-1180, 1987.
347. Schott G, Winkler S, Hollenstein U, et al: Obstruction of the pulmonary artery by granulomatous vasculitis: A clinical, morphological, and immunological analysis. Ann Rheum Dis 61:463-467, 2002.
348. Larson TS, Hall S, Hepper NG, Hunder GG: Respiratory tract symptoms as a clue to giant cell arteritis. Ann Intern Med 101:594-597, 1984.
349. Gur H, Rapman E, Ehrenfeld M, Sidi Y: Clinical manifestations of temporal arteritis: A report from Israel. J Rheumatol 23:1927-1931, 1996.
350. Karam GH, Fulmer JD: Giant cell arteritis presenting as interstitial lung disease. Chest 82:781-784, 1982.
351. de Heide LJ, Pieterman H, Hennemann G: Pulmonary infarction caused by giant-cell arteritis of the pulmonary artery. Neth J Med 46:36-40, 1995.
352. Blockmans D, Knockaert D, Bobbaers H: Giant cell arteritis can be associated with T4-lymphocytic alveolitis. Clin Rheumatol 18:330-333, 1999.
353. Erkan F, Gul A, Tasali E: Pulmonary manifestations of Behçet's disease. Thorax 56:572-578, 2001.
354. Mizuki N, Inoko H, Ohno S: Pathogenic gene responsible for the predisposition of Behçet's disease. Int Rev Immunol 14:33-48, 1997.
355. Slavin RE, de Groot WJ: Pathology of the lung in Behçet's disease. Case report and review of the literature. Am J Surg Pathol 5:779-788, 1981.
356. Efthimiou J, Johnston C, Spiro SG, Turner-Warwick M: Pulmonary disease in Behçet's syndrome. Q J Med 58:259-280, 1986.
357. Ko GY, Byun JY, Choi BG, Cho SH: The vascular manifestations of Behçet's disease: Angiographic and CT findings. Br J Radiol 73:1270-1274, 2000.
358. Tunaci A, Berkmen YM, Gokmen E: Thoracic involvement in Behçet's disease: Pathologic, clinical, and imaging features. AJR Am J Roentgenol 164:51-56, 1995.
359. Ahn JM, Im JG, Ryoo JW, et al: Thoracic manifestations of Behçet syndrome: Radiographic and CT findings in nine patients. Radiology 194:199-203, 1995.
360. Puckette TC, Jolles H, Proto AV: Magnetic resonance imaging confirmation of pulmonary artery aneurysm in Behçet's disease. J Thorac Imaging 9:172-175, 1994.
361. Numan F, Islak C, Berkmen T, et al: Behçet disease: Pulmonary arterial involvement in 15 cases. Radiology 192:465-468, 1994.
362. Erkan F, Cavdar T: Pulmonary vasculitis in Behçet's disease. Am Rev Respir Dis 146:232-239, 1992.
363. Raz I, Okon E, Chajek-Shaul T: Pulmonary manifestations in Behçet's syndrome. Chest 95:585-589, 1989.
364. Ahonen AV, Stenius-Aarniala BS, Viljanen BC, et al: Obstructive lung disease in Behçet's syndrome. Scand J Respir Dis 59:44-50, 1978.
365. Rieu V, Cohen P, Andre MH, et al: Characteristics and outcome of 49 patients with symptomatic cryoglobulinaemia. Rheumatology (Oxford) 41:290-300, 2002.
366. Bombardieri S, Paoletti P, Ferri C, et al: Lung involvement in essential mixed cryoglobulinemia. Am J Med 66:748-756, 1979.
367. Cream JJ, Gumpel JM, Peachey RD: Schönlein-Henoch purpura in the adult. A study of 77 adults with anaphylactoid or Schönlein-Henoch purpura. Q J Med 39:461-484, 1970.
368. Pertuiset E, Liote F, Launay-Russ E, et al: Adult Henoch-Schönlein purpura associated with malignancy. Semin Arthritis Rheum 29:360-367, 2000.
369. Kathuria S, Cheifec G: Fatal pulmonary Henoch-Schönlein syndrome. Chest 82:654-656, 1982.
370. Wright WK, Krous HF, Griswold WR, et al: Pulmonary vasculitis with hemorrhage in anaphylactoid purpura. Pediatr Pulmonol 17:269-271, 1994.
371. Fulmer JD, Kaltreider HB: The pulmonary vasculitides. Chest 82:615-624, 1982.
372. Liebow AA: The J. Burns Amberson lecture—pulmonary angiitis and granulomatosis. Am Rev Respir Dis 108:1-18, 1973.
373. Le Gall F, Loeuillet L, Delaval P, et al: Necrotizing sarcoid granulomatosis with and without extrapulmonary involvement. Pathol Res Pract 192:306-313, discussion 314, 1996.
374. Chittock DR, Joseph MG, Paterson NA, McFadden RG: Necrotizing sarcoid granulomatosis with pleural involvement. Clinical and radiographic features. Chest 106:672-676, 1994.
375. Churg A, Carrington CB, Gupta R: Necrotizing sarcoid granulomatosis. Chest 76:406-413, 1979.
376. Niimi H, Hartman TE, Müller NL: Necrotizing sarcoid granulomatosis: Computed tomography and pathologic findings. J Comput Assist Tomogr 19:920-923, 1995.
377. Koss MN, Hochholzer L, Feigin DS, et al: Necrotizing sarcoid-like granulomatosis: Clinical, pathologic, and immunopathologic findings. Hum Pathol 11:510-519, 1980.
378. Campbell J: Acute symptoms following work with hay. BMJ 2:1143, 1932.
379. Richerson HB, Bernstein IL, Fink JN, et al: Guidelines for the clinical evaluation of hypersensitivity pneumonitis. Report of the Subcommittee on Hypersensitivity Pneumonitis. J Allergy Clin Immunol 84:839-844, 1989.
380. Schuyler M, Cormier Y: The diagnosis of hypersensitivity pneumonitis. Chest 111:534-536, 1997.
381. Patel AM, Ryu JH, Reed CE: Hypersensitivity pneumonitis: Current concepts and future questions. J Allergy Clin Immunol 108:661-670, 2001.
382. Ohtani Y, Kojima K, Sumi Y, et al: Inhalation provocation tests in chronic bird fancier's lung. Chest 118:1382-1389, 2000.
383. Salvaggio JE: Hypersensitivity pneumonitis: "Pandora's box." N Engl J Med 283:314-315, 1970.
384. Salvaggio JE, Millhollon BW: Allergic alveolitis: New insights into old mysteries. Respir Med 87:495-501, 1993.
385. Chouchakova N, Skokowa J, Baumann U, et al: Fc gamma RIII–mediated production of TNF-alpha induces immune complex alveolitis independently of CXC chemokine generation. J Immunol 166:5193-5200, 2001.
386. Tremblay GM, Sallenave JM, Israel-Assayag E, et al: Elafin/elastase-specific inhibitor in bronchoalveolar lavage of normal subjects and farmer's lung. Am J Respir Crit Care Med 154:1092-1098, 1996.
387. Pardo A, Barrios R, Gaxiola M, et al: Increase of lung neutrophils in hypersensitivity pneumonitis is associated with lung fibrosis. Am J Respir Crit Care Med 161:1698-1704, 2000.
388. Dakhama A, Israel-Assayag E, Cormier Y: Altered immunosuppressive activity of alveolar macrophages in farmer's lung disease. Eur Respir J 9:1456-1462, 1996.
389. Denis M, Bedard M, Laviolette M, Cormier Y: A study of monokine release and natural killer activity in the bronchoalveolar lavage of subjects with farmer's lung. Am Rev Respir Dis 147:934-939, 1993.
390. Rodriguez de Castro F, Carrillo T, Castillo R, et al: Relationships between characteristics of exposure to pigeon antigens. Clinical manifestations and humoral immune response. Chest 103:1059-1063, 1993.
391. Trentin L, Zambello R, Facco M, et al: Selection of T lymphocytes bearing limited TCR-Vβ regions in the lung of hypersensitivity pneumonitis and sarcoidosis. Am J Respir Crit Care Med 155:587-596, 1997.
392. Denis M: Mouse hypersensitivity pneumonitis: Depletion of NK cells abrogates the spontaneous regression phase and leads to massive fibrosis. Exp Lung Res 18:761-773, 1992.
393. Pesci A, Bertorelli G, Olivieri D: Mast cells in bronchoalveolar lavage fluid and in transbronchial biopsy specimens of patients with farmer's lung disease. Chest 100:1197-1202, 1991.
394. Miadonna A, Pesci A, Tedeschi A, et al: Mast cell and histamine involvement in farmer's lung disease. Chest 105:1184-1189, 1994.
395. Laviolette M, Cormier Y, Loiseau A, et al: Bronchoalveolar mast cells in normal farmers and subjects with farmer's lung. Diagnostic, prognostic, and physiologic significance. Am Rev Respir Dis 144:855-860, 1991.
396. Warren CP: Extrinsic allergic alveolitis: A disease commoner in non-smokers. Thorax 32:567-569, 1977.
397. Baldwin CI, Todd A, Bourke S, et al: Pigeon fanciers' lung: Effects of smoking on serum and salivary antibody responses to pigeon antigens. Clin Exp Immunol 113:166-172, 1998.
398. Ohtsuka Y, Munakata M, Tanimura K, et al: Smoking promotes insidious and chronic farmer's lung disease, and deteriorates the clinical outcome. Intern Med 34:966-971, 1995.
399. McSharry C, Anderson K, Bourke SJ, Boyd G: Takes your breath away—the immunology of allergic alveolitis. Clin Exp Immunol 128:3-9, 2002.
400. Camarena A, Juarez A, Mejia M, et al: Major histocompatibility complex and tumor necrosis factor-alpha polymorphisms in pigeon breeder's disease. Am J Respir Crit Care Med 163:1528-1533, 2001.
401. Israel-Assayag E, Dakhama A, Lavigne S, et al: Expression of costimulatory molecules on alveolar macrophages in hypersensitivity pneumonitis. Am J Respir Crit Care Med 159:1830-1834, 1999.
402. Dakhama A, Hegele RG, Laflamme G, et al: Common respiratory viruses in lower airways of patients with acute hypersensitivity pneumonitis. Am J Respir Crit Care Med 159:1316-1322, 1999.
403. Reyes CN, Wenzel FJ, Lawton BR, Emanuel DA: The pulmonary pathology of farmer's lung disease. Chest 81:142-146, 1982.
404. Hogg JC: The histologic appearance of farmer's lung. Chest 81:133-134, 1982.
405. Hargreave F, Hinson KF, Reid L, et al: The radiological appearances of allergic alveolitis due to bird sensitivity (bird fancier's lung). Clin Radiol 23:1-10, 1972.
406. Silver SF, Müller NL, Miller RR, Lefcoe MS: Hypersensitivity pneumonitis: Evaluation with CT. Radiology 173:441-445, 1989.
407. Cook PG, Wells IP, McGavin CR: The distribution of pulmonary shadowing in farmer's lung. Clin Radiol 39:21-27, 1988.
408. Hansell DM, Moskovic E: High-resolution computed tomography in extrinsic allergic alveolitis. Clin Radiol 43:8-12, 1991.
409. Monkare S, Ikonen M, Haahtela T: Radiologic findings in farmer's lung. Prognosis and correlation to lung function. Chest 87:460-466, 1985.
410. Adler BD, Padley SP, Müller NL, et al: Chronic hypersensitivity pneumonitis: High-resolution CT and radiographic features in 16 patients. Radiology 185:91-95, 1992.
411. Lynch DA, Newell JD, Logan PM, et al: Can CT distinguish hypersensitivity pneumonitis from idiopathic pulmonary fibrosis? AJR Am J Roentgenol 165:807-811, 1995.
412. Remy-Jardin M, Remy J, Wallaert B, Müller NL: Subacute and chronic bird breeder hypersensitivity pneumonitis: Sequential evaluation with CT and correlation with lung function tests and bronchoalveolar lavage. Radiology 189:111-118, 1993.
413. Akira M, Kita N, Higashihara T, et al: Summer-type hypersensitivity pneumonitis: Comparison of high-resolution CT and plain radiographic findings. AJR Am J Roentgenol 158:1223-1228, 1992.

414. Hansell DM, Wells AU, Padley SP, Müller NL: Hypersensitivity pneumonitis: Correlation of individual CT patterns with functional abnormalities. Radiology 199:123-128, 1996.
415. Selman M, Chapela R, Raghu G: Hypersensitivity pneumonitis: Clinical manifestations, pathogenesis, diagnosis and therapeutic strategies. Semin Respir Med 14:353, 1993.
416. Respiratory health hazards in agriculture. Am J Respir Crit Care Med 158:S1-S76, 1998.
417. Cormier Y, Laviolette M: Farmer's lung. Semin Respir Med 14:31, 1993.
418. Arshad M, Braun SR, Sunderrajan EV: Severe hypoxemia in farmer's lung disease with normal findings on chest roentgenogram. Chest 91:274-275, 1987.
419. Yoshizawa Y, Ohtani Y, Hayakawa H, et al: Chronic hypersensitivity pneumonitis in Japan: A nationwide epidemiologic survey. J Allergy Clin Immunol 103:315-320, 1999.
420. Pepys J, Jenkins PA: Precipitin (F.L.H.) test in farmer's lung. Thorax 20:21-35, 1965.
421. Dalphin JC, Dubiez A, Monnet E, et al: Prevalence of asthma and respiratory symptoms in dairy farmers in the French province of the Doubs. Am J Respir Crit Care Med 158:1493-1498, 1998.
422. Dalphin JC, Debieuvre D, Pernet D, et al: Prevalence and risk factors for chronic bronchitis and farmer's lung in French dairy farmers. Br J Ind Med 50:941-944, 1993.
423. Davies D: Bird fancier's disease. Br Med J (Clin Res Ed) 287:1239-1240, 1983.
424. Earis JE, Marsh K, Pearson MG, Ogilvie CM: The inspiratory "squawk" in extrinsic allergic alveolitis and other pulmonary fibroses. Thorax 37:923-926, 1982.
425. Leblanc P, Belanger J, Laviolette M, Cormier Y: Relationship among antigen contact, alveolitis, and clinical status in farmer's lung disease. Arch Intern Med 146:153-157, 1986.
426. A national survey of bird fanciers' lung: Including its possible association with jejunal villous atrophy. (A report to the Research Committee of the British Thoracic Society.) Br J Dis Chest 78:75-88, 1984.
427. Sharma OP, Fujimura N: Hypersensitivity pneumonitis: A noninfectious granulomatosis. Semin Respir Infect 10:96-106, 1995.
428. Monkare S: Clinical aspects of farmer's lung: Airway reactivity, treatment and prognosis. Eur J Respir Dis Suppl 137:1-68, 1984.
429. Warren CP, Tse KS, Cherniack RM: Mechanical properties of the lung in extrinsic allergic alveolitis. Thorax 33:315-321, 1978.
430. Sovijarvi AR, Kuusisto P, Muittari A, Kauppinen-Walin K: Trapped air in extrinsic allergic alveolitis. Respiration 40:57-64, 1980.
431. Lalancette M, Carrier G, Laviolette M, et al: Farmer's lung. Long-term outcome and lack of predictive value of bronchoalveolar lavage fibrosing factors. Am Rev Respir Dis 148:216-221, 1993.
432. Erkinjuntti-Pekkanen R, Rytkonen H, Kokkarinen JI, et al: Long-term risk of emphysema in patients with farmer's lung and matched control farmers. Am J Respir Crit Care Med 158:662-665, 1998.
433. de Gracia J, Morell F, Bofill JM, et al: Time of exposure as a prognostic factor in avian hypersensitivity pneumonitis. Respir Med 83:139-143, 1989.
434. Zacharisen MC, Schlueter DP, Kurup VP, Fink JN: The long-term outcome in acute, subacute, and chronic forms of pigeon breeder's disease hypersensitivity pneumonitis. Ann Allergy Asthma Immunol 88:175-182, 2002.
435. Lacasse Y, Fraser RS, Fournier M, Cormier Y: Diagnostic accuracy of transbronchial biopsy in acute farmer's lung disease. Chest 112:1459-1465, 1997.
436. Ramirez-Venegas A, Sansores RH, Perez-Padilla R, et al: Utility of a provocation test for diagnosis of chronic pigeon breeder's disease. Am J Respir Crit Care Med 158:862-869, 1998.
437. Schmidt CD, Jensen RL, Christensen LT, et al: Longitudinal pulmonary function changes in pigeon breeders. Chest 93:359-363, 1988.
438. Cormier Y, Belanger J: Long-term physiologic outcome after acute farmer's lung. Chest 87:796-800, 1985.
439. Monkare S, Haahtela T: Farmer's lung—a 5-year follow-up of eighty-six patients. Clin Allergy 17:143-151, 1987.
440. Kokkarinen J, Tukiainen H, Terho EO: Mortality due to farmer's lung in Finland. Chest 106:509-512, 1994.
441. Perez-Padilla R, Salas J, Chapela R, et al: Mortality in Mexican patients with chronic pigeon breeder's lung compared with those with usual interstitial pneumonia. Am Rev Respir Dis 148:49-53, 1993.
442. Israel-Assayag E, Cormier Y: Adaptation to organic dust exposure: A potential role of L-selectin shedding? Eur Respir J 19:833-837, 2002.
443. Donham K: Respiratory disease hazards to workers in livestock and poultry confinement structures. Semin Respir Med 14:49, 1993.
444. Donham KJ, Reynolds SJ, Whitten P, et al: Respiratory dysfunction in swine production facility workers: Dose-response relationships of environmental exposures and pulmonary function. Am J Ind Med 27:405-418, 1995.
445. Schwartz DA, Donham KJ, Olenchock SA, et al: Determinants of longitudinal changes in spirometric function among swine confinement operators and farmers. Am J Respir Crit Care Med 151:47-53, 1995.
446. Zhiping W, Malmberg P, Larsson BM, et al: Exposure to bacteria in swine-house dust and acute inflammatory reactions in humans. Am J Respir Crit Care Med 154:1261-1266, 1996.
447. Zuskin E, Kanceljak B, Schachter EN, et al: Immunological and respiratory findings in swine farmers. Environ Res 56:120-130, 1991.
448. Zejda JE, Hurst TS, Rhodes CS, et al: Respiratory health of swine producers. Focus on young workers. Chest 103:702-709, 1993.
449. Iversen M, Dahl R: Working in swine-confinement buildings causes an accelerated decline in FEV₁: A 7-yr follow-up of Danish farmers. Eur Respir J 16:404-408, 2000.
450. Bessette L, Boulet LP, Tremblay G, Cormier Y: Bronchial responsiveness to methacholine in swine confinement building workers. Arch Environ Health 48:73-77, 1993.
451. Carvalheiro MF, Peterson Y, Rubenowitz E, Rylander R: Bronchial reactivity and work-related symptoms in farmers. Am J Ind Med 27:65-74, 1995.
452. Vogelzang PF, van der Gulden JW, Folgering H, et al: Longitudinal changes in bronchial responsiveness associated with swine confinement dust exposure. Chest 117:1488-1495, 2000.
453. Rask-Andersen A: Organic dust toxic syndrome among farmers. Br J Ind Med 46:233-238, 1989.
454. do Pico GA: Hazardous exposure and lung disease among farm workers. Clin Chest Med 13:311-328, 1992.
455. Wright JL: Inhalational lung injury causing bronchiolitis. Clin Chest Med 14:635-644, 1993.
456. Shahan TA, Sorenson WG, Lewis DM: Superoxide anion production in response to bacterial lipopolysaccharide and fungal spores implicated in organic dust toxic syndrome. Environ Res 67:98-107, 1994.
457. Allen JN, Davis WB: Eosinophilic lung diseases. Am J Respir Crit Care Med 150:1423-1438, 1994.
458. Baggenstoss A, Bayley E, Lindberg D: Löffler's syndrome. Report of a case with pathologic examination of the lungs. Proc Mayo Clin 21:457, 1946.
459. Citro LA, Gordon ME, Miller WT: Eosinophilic lung disease (or how to slice P.I.E.). Am J Roentgenol Radium Ther Nucl Med 117:787-797, 1973.
460. Chapman BJ, Capewell S, Gibson R, et al: Pulmonary eosinophilia with and without allergic bronchopulmonary aspergillosis. Thorax 44:919-924, 1989.
461. Morrissey JF, Gibbs GM: Pulmonary infiltration with eosinophilia occurring postpartum. Arch Intern Med 107:95-99, 1961.
462. Pope-Harman AL, Davis WB, Allen ED, et al: Acute eosinophilic pneumonia. A summary of 15 cases and review of the literature. Medicine (Baltimore) 75:334-342, 1996.
463. Allen JN, Pacht ER, Gadek JE, Davis WB: Acute eosinophilic pneumonia as a reversible cause of noninfectious respiratory failure. N Engl J Med 321:569-574, 1989.
464. Buchheit J, Eid N, Rodgers G Jr, et al: Acute eosinophilic pneumonia with respiratory failure: A new syndrome? Am Rev Respir Dis 145:716-718, 1992.
465. Badesch DB, King TE Jr, Schwarz MI: Acute eosinophilic pneumonia: A hypersensitivity phenomenon? Am Rev Respir Dis 139:249-252, 1989.
466. Hirai K, Yamazaki Y, Okada K, et al: Acute eosinophilic pneumonia associated with smoke from fireworks. Intern Med 39:401-403, 2000.
467. Hayakawa H, Sato A, Toyoshima M, et al: A clinical study of idiopathic eosinophilic pneumonia. Chest 105:1462-1466, 1994.
468. Fujimura M, Yasui M, Shinagawa S, et al: Bronchoalveolar lavage cell findings in three types of eosinophilic pneumonia: Acute, chronic and drug-induced eosinophilic pneumonia. Respir Med 92:743-749, 1998.
469. Nakahara Y, Hayashi S, Fukuno Y, et al: Increased interleukin-5 levels in bronchoalveolar lavage fluid is a major factor for eosinophil accumulation in acute eosinophilic pneumonia. Respiration 68:389-395, 2001.
470. Tazelaar HD, Linz LJ, Colby TV, et al: Acute eosinophilic pneumonia: Histopathologic findings in nine patients. Am J Respir Crit Care Med 155:296-302, 1997.
471. Cheon JE, Lee KS, Jung GS, et al: Acute eosinophilic pneumonia: Radiographic and CT findings in six patients. AJR Am J Roentgenol 167:1195-1199, 1996.
472. Johkoh T, Müller NL, Akira M, et al: Eosinophilic lung diseases: Diagnostic accuracy of thin-section CT in 111 patients. Radiology 216:773-780, 2000.
473. Ogawa H, Fujimura M, Matsuda T, et al: Transient wheeze. Eosinophilic bronchobronchiolitis in acute eosinophilic pneumonia. Chest 104:493-496, 1993.
474. Turner-Warwick M, Assem ES, Lockwood M: Cryptogenic pulmonary eosinophilia. Clin Allergy 6:135-145, 1976.
475. Fox B, Seed WA: Chronic eosinophilic pneumonia. Thorax 35:570-580, 1980.
476. Jederlinic PJ, Sicilian L, Gaensler EA: Chronic eosinophilic pneumonia. A report of 19 cases and a review of the literature. Medicine (Baltimore) 67:154-162, 1988.
477. Mayo JR, Müller NL, Road J, et al: Chronic eosinophilic pneumonia: CT findings in six cases. AJR Am J Roentgenol 153:727-730, 1989.
478. Carrington CB, Addington WW, Goff AM, et al: Chronic eosinophilic pneumonia. N Engl J Med 280:787-798, 1969.
479. Durieu J, Wallaert B, Tonnel AB: Long-term follow-up of pulmonary function in chronic eosinophilic pneumonia. Groupe d'Etude en Pathologie Interstitielle de la Societe de Pathologie Thoracique du Nord. Eur Respir J 10:286-291, 1997.
480. Lieske TR, Sunderrajan EV, Passamonte PM: Bronchoalveolar lavage and technetium-99m glucoheptonate imaging in chronic eosinophilic pneumonia. Chest 85:282-284, 1984.
481. Yoshida K, Shijubo N, Koba H, et al: Chronic eosinophilic pneumonia progressing to lung fibrosis. Eur Respir J 7:1541-1544, 1994.
482. Naughton M, Fahy J, FitzGerald MX: Chronic eosinophilic pneumonia. A long-term follow-up of 12 patients. Chest 103:162-165, 1993.
483. Fauci AS, Harley JB, Roberts WC, et al: NIH conference. The idiopathic hypereosinophilic syndrome. Clinical, pathophysiologic, and therapeutic considerations. Ann Intern Med 97:78-92, 1982.
484. Clinicopathologic conference: Hypereosinophilic syndrome with pulmonary hypertension. Am J Med 60:239-247, 1976.
485. Nadeem S, Nasir N, Israel RH: Löffler's syndrome secondary to crack cocaine. Chest 105:1599-1600, 1994.
486. Brander PE, Tukiainen P: Acute eosinophilic pneumonia in a heroin smoker. Eur Respir J 6:750-752, 1993.
487. Kelly PT, Haponik EF: Goodpasture syndrome: Molecular and clinical advances. Medicine (Baltimore) 73:171-185, 1994.

488. Burns AP, Fisher M, Li P, et al: Molecular analysis of HLA class II genes in Goodpasture's disease. QJM 88:93-100, 1995.

489. Fisher M, Pusey CD, Vaughan RW, Rees AJ: Susceptibility to anti–glomerular basement membrane disease is strongly associated with HLA-DRB1 genes. Kidney Int 51:222-229, 1997.

490. Phelps RG, Jones V, Turner AN, Rees AJ: Properties of HLA class II molecules divergently associated with Goodpasture's disease. Int Immunol 12:1135-1143, 2000.

491. Levy JB, Lachmann RH, Pusey CD: Recurrent Goodpasture's disease. Am J Kidney Dis 27:573-578, 1996.

492. Borza DB, Bondar O, Todd P, et al: Quaternary organization of the Goodpasture autoantigen, the alpha 3(IV) collagen chain. Sequestration of two cryptic autoepitopes by intrapromoter interactions with the alpha4 and alpha5 NC1 domains. J Biol Chem 277:40075-40083, 2002.

493. Salama AD, Chaudhry AN, Ryan JJ, et al: In Goodpasture's disease, CD4(+) T cells escape thymic deletion and are reactive with the autoantigen alpha3(IV)NC1. J Am Soc Nephrol 12:1908-1915, 2001.

494. Lucas Guillen E, Martinez Ruiz A, Alegria Fernandez M, Martinez Losa A: [Goodpasture syndrome: Re-exacerbations associated with intercurrent infections.] Rev Clin Esp 195:761-764, 1995.

495. Donaghy M, Rees AJ: Cigarette smoking and lung haemorrhage in glomerulonephritis caused by autoantibodies to glomerular basement membrane. Lancet 2:1390-1393, 1983.

496. Lan HY, Paterson DJ, Hutchinson P, Atkins RC: Leukocyte involvement in the pathogenesis of pulmonary injury in experimental Goodpasture's syndrome. Lab Invest 64:330-338, 1991.

497. Hill PA, Lan HY, Atkins RC, Nikolic-Paterson DJ: Ultrastructural localisation of CD44 in the rat lung in experimental Goodpasture's syndrome. Pathology 29:380-384, 1997.

498. Corrin B, Jagusch M, Dewar A, et al: Fine structural changes in idiopathic pulmonary haemosiderosis. J Pathol 153:249-256, 1987.

499. Louie S, Russell LA, Richeson RB 3rd, Cross CE: Circulating immune complexes with pulmonary hemorrhage during pregnancy in idiopathic pulmonary hemosiderosis. Chest 104:1907-1909, 1993.

500. van der Ent CK, Walenkamp MJ, Donckerwolcke RA, et al: Pulmonary hemosiderosis and immune complex glomerulonephritis. Clin Nephrol 43:339-341, 1995.

501. Le Clainche L, Le Bourgeois M, Fauroux B, et al: Long-term outcome of idiopathic pulmonary hemosiderosis in children. Medicine (Baltimore) 79:318-326, 2000.

502. Lombard CM, Colby TV, Elliott CG: Surgical pathology of the lung in anti–basement membrane antibody–associated Goodpasture's syndrome. Hum Pathol 20:445-451, 1989.

503. Beechler CR, Enquist RW, Hunt KK, et al: Immunofluorescence of transbronchial biopsies in Goodpasture's syndrome. Am Rev Respir Dis 121:869-872, 1980.

504. Slonim L: Goodpasture's syndrome and its radiological features. Australas Radiol 13:164-172, 1969.

505. Bowley NB, Steiner RE, Chin WS: The chest x-ray in antiglomerular basement membrane antibody disease (Goodpasture's syndrome). Clin Radiol 30:419-429, 1979.

506. Cheah FK, Sheppard MN, Hansell DM: Computed tomography of diffuse pulmonary haemorrhage with pathological correlation. Clin Radiol 48:89-93, 1993.

507. Niimi A, Amitani R, Kurasawa T, et al: [Two cases of idiopathic pulmonary hemosiderosis: Analysis of chest CT findings.] Nihon Kyobu Shikkan Gakkai Zasshi 30:1749-1755, 1992.

508. Theros EG, Reeder MM, Eckert JF: An exercise in radiologic-pathologic correlation. Radiology 90:784-791, 1968.

509. Bruwer AJ, Kennedy RL, Edwards JE: Recurrent pulmonary hemorrhage with hemosiderosis: So-called idiopathic pulmonary hemosiderosis. Am J Roentgenol Radium Ther Nucl Med 76:98-107, 1956.

510. Sybers RG, Sybers JL, Dickie HA, Paul LW: Roentgenographic aspects of hemorrhagic pulmonary-renal disease (Goodpasture's syndrome). Am J Roentgenol Radium Ther Nucl Med 94:674-680, 1965.

511. Saeed MM, Woo MS, MacLaughlin EF, et al: Prognosis in pediatric idiopathic pulmonary hemosiderosis. Chest 116:721-725, 1999.

512. Soergel H, Sommers S: Idiopathic pulmonary hemosiderosis and related syndromes. Am J Med 32:499, 1962.

513. Wright PH, Menzies IS, Pounder RE, Keeling PW: Adult idiopathic pulmonary haemosiderosis and coeliac disease. Q J Med 50:95-102, 1981.

514. Lane DJ, Hamilton WS: Idiopathic steatorrhoea and idiopathic pulmonary haemosiderosis. BMJ 2:89-90, 1971.

515. Proskey AJ, Weatherbee L, Easterling RE, et al: Goodpasture's syndrome. A report of five cases and review of the literature. Am J Med 48:162-173, 1970.

516. Mathew TH, Hobbs JB, Kalowski S, et al: Goodpasture's syndrome: Normal renal diagnostic findings. Ann Intern Med 82:215-218, 1975.

517. Allue X, Wise MB, Beaudry PH: Pulmonary function studies in idiopathic pulmonary hemosiderosis in children. Am Rev Respir Dis 107:410-415, 1973.

518. Donald KJ, Edwards RL, McEvoy JD: Alveolar capillary basement membrane lesions in Goodpasture's syndrome and idiopathic pulmonary hemosiderosis. Am J Med 59:642-649, 1975.

519. Addleman M, Logan AS, Grossman RF: Monitoring intrapulmonary hemorrhage in Goodpasture's syndrome. Chest 87:119-120, 1985.

520. Salama AD, Dougan T, Levy JB, et al: Goodpasture's disease in the absence of circulating anti–glomerular basement membrane antibodies as detected by standard techniques. Am J Kidney Dis 39:1162-1167, 2002.

521. Leatherman JW: Immune alveolar hemorrhage. Chest 91:891-897, 1987.

522. Kurki P, Helve T, von Bonsdorff M, et al: Transformation of membranous glomerulonephritis into crescentic glomerulonephritis with glomerular basement membrane antibodies. Serial determinations of anti-GBM before the transformation. Nephron 38:134-137, 1984.

523. Boyce NW, Holdsworth SR: Pulmonary manifestations of the clinical syndrome of acute glomerulonephritis and lung hemorrhage. Am J Kidney Dis 8:31-36, 1986.

524. Tobler A, Schurch E, Altermatt HJ, Im Hof V: Anti–basement membrane antibody disease with severe pulmonary haemorrhage and normal renal function. Thorax 46:68-70, 1991.

525. Favre JP, Gournier JP, Adham M, et al: Aortobronchial fistula: Report of three cases and review of the literature. Surgery 115:264-270, 1994.

526. Hughson MD, He Z, Henegar J, McMurray R: Alveolar hemorrhage and renal microangiopathy in systemic lupus erythematosus. Arch Pathol Lab Med 125:475-483, 2001.

527. Benditt JO, Farber HW, Wright J, Karnad AB: Pulmonary hemorrhage with diffuse alveolar infiltrates in men with high-volume choriocarcinoma. Ann Intern Med 109:674-675, 1988.

528. Wright PH, Buxton-Thomas M, Keeling PW, Kreel L: Adult idiopathic pulmonary haemosiderosis: A comparison of lung function changes and the distribution of pulmonary disease in patients with and without coeliac disease. Br J Dis Chest 77:282-292, 1983.

529. Merkel F, Pullig O, Marx M, et al: Course and prognosis of anti–basement membrane antibody (anti-BM-Ab)-mediated disease: Report of 35 cases. Nephrol Dial Transplant 9:372-376, 1994.

530. Levy JB, Turner AN, Rees AJ, Pusey CD: Long-term outcome of anti–glomerular basement membrane antibody disease treated with plasma exchange and immunosuppression. Ann Intern Med 134:1033-1042, 2001.

531. Klasa RJ, Abboud RT, Ballon HS, Grossman L: Goodpasture's syndrome: Recurrence after a five-year remission. Case report and review of the literature. Am J Med 84:751-755, 1988.

TRANSPLANTATION

Largely as a result of an increased understanding of the immunologic mechanisms of organ rejection and the development of powerful immunosuppressive drugs, transplantation has become an important form of therapy for many diseases. These procedures have resulted in improved quality and length of life in many patients; however, they are frequently accompanied by profound side effects. As might be expected, the necessity of preventing graft rejection by chemotherapeutic immunosuppression is associated with a significant risk of infection, often severe and caused by opportunistic organisms. In addition, a variety of noninfectious pulmonary complications are seen in many patients, particularly those undergoing lung, heart-lung, or bone marrow transplantation.

LUNG AND HEART-LUNG TRANSPLANTATION

Since the mid-1980s, lung and heart-lung transplantation has passed from the status of experimental procedure to standard therapy for a variety of otherwise fatal pulmonary conditions, the most common being idiopathic pulmonary fibrosis, cystic fibrosis, COPD (including α_1-antiprotease–associated emphysema), and primary pulmonary hypertension. Between 1995 and 2001, almost 9000 single or bilateral lung transplantations were reported to the registry of the International Society for Heart and Lung Transplantation.[1] The number of heart-lung transplantations is much lower and has actually declined, with less than 100 procedures now being performed annually. Unfortunately, the number of available organs for donation is limited, and both the waiting time for transplantation and the number of patients who die while awaiting transplantation have increased.[2]

Technique and Patient Selection

Operative Procedures

Four major surgical approaches may be used for lung transplantation: single-lung transplantation, bilateral sequential transplantation, heart-lung transplantation, and transplantation of lobes from living donors.[2] Single-lung transplantation is suitable for most patients and is preferable to bilateral transplantation since it is technically easier and allows for a greater number of procedures overall. It has been used successfully in patients who have primary pulmonary hypertension, even in the presence of right ventricular failure,[3] and in advanced emphysema.[4] Bilateral lung transplantation is required for patients who have septic lung disease[5] and is preferred in some centers for younger patients who have COPD.[6] Heart-lung transplantation is required in patients who have Eisenmenger's complex without correctable cardiac defects, pulmonary disease with unrelated heart disease, and chronic thromboembolic pulmonary hypertension when thromboendarterectomy is not feasible.[7] There is limited, albeit favorable, experience with the use of living related donor, bilateral lobar transplantation in patients who have cystic fibrosis.[8]

Patient Selection

General recommendations for patient selection are outlined in Table 11–1. The timing for referral of a patient to a transplant clinic is difficult; provision must be made for the 1- to 2-year delay that the patient is likely to experience while on a waiting list. The expectation that transplantation will prolong life implies that estimations of survival have been established for specific diseases. In reality, such approximations are in evolution and imperfect.[9,10] Ultimately, the decision to refer a

TABLE 11–1. Selection Criteria for Lung Transplant Recipients

1. Age younger than 65 years for single-lung transplantation and 60 years for double-lung transplantation
2. End-stage lung disease with life expectancy of less than 12 to 18 months
3. Absence of other significant medical disease (including HIV seropositivity)
4. Acceptable nutritional status (both marked obesity and marked malnutrition are relative contraindications)
5. Ambulatory with rehabilitation potential
6. Good psychological profile and demonstrated compliance with medical regimens, abstinence from cigarette smoking or other drug abuse for at least 6 months, and good emotional and logistic support system
7. Absence of multiresistant organisms on sputum culture
8. Absence of previous major thoracic surgery
9. Adequate financial resources for both transplantation and postoperative care

From Fraser RS, Müller NL, Colman NC, Paré PD: Fraser and Paré's Diagnosis of Diseases of the Chest, 4th ed. Philadelphia, WB Saunders, 1999.

patient may have as much to do with the patient's perception of quality of life as with the physician's estimate of its duration.[11] The ability to participate in a preoperative rehabilitation program is mandatory; such participation may help optimize the patient's condition before transplantation and shorten postoperative recovery, and it serves as an indicator of motivation and compliance with post-transplant medical regimens. General medical conditions that have an impact on eligibility and disease-specific guidelines for transplantation have been published.[12]

Ischemia-Reperfusion Injury

The lung injury caused by ischemia-reperfusion during the transplant procedure (the "pulmonary reimplantation response") is a result of alveolar epithelial/endothelial damage and is characterized clinically by pulmonary edema and hypoxemia occurring within 72 hours of lung transplantation.[13] It usually begins in the first 24 hours and progresses to reach a peak in 4 to 7 days.[14] So-called primary graft failure, which occurs in about 15% of patients and frequently leads to death or the need for prolonged mechanical ventilation, is considered to be its most severe form. The reimplantation response has also been associated with an increased risk for the development and progression of bronchiolitis obliterans and late graft failure.[15] The diagnosis of ischemia-reperfusion–induced lung injury should be considered after the exclusion of other causes of air space disease, such as volume overload, acute rejection, infection, left heart failure, or pulmonary venous obstruction.[16]

Pulmonary injury during the transplantation procedure is mediated primarily by activated neutrophils, which damage alveolar capillary endothelium and result in fluid accumulation in the adjacent air spaces.[17] The severity of endothelial injury is related to FIO_2, temperature, and the degree of lung inflation during transport and the use of cardiopulmonary bypass during surgery[14]; it does not appear to be influenced by ischemia time under current conditions of storage and reperfusion.[18] Biophysical factors such as maintenance of vascular distention during the ischemic time[19] and reperfusion

pressure[20] may also influence the severity of injury. The pathogenesis of endothelial injury is related to a variety of processes, including enhanced neutrophil adhesion and activation, the formation of reactive oxygen species, and the elaboration of proinflammatory cytokines (especially interleukin-8[21]), which may be of donor origin.[22] Decreased surfactant production secondary to alveolar epithelial injury may also impair gas exchange.[23]

Mild cases of reperfusion injury are manifested histologically by air space and alveolar septal edema and congestion[24]; in severe cases, the appearance is that of diffuse alveolar damage. Plugs of fibroblastic tissue may be identified in the air spaces several weeks after transplantation and represent organization of the exudate.[25]

The radiologic findings are nonspecific and similar to those seen in patients who have left ventricular failure, fluid overload, and acute rejection.[26,27] They range from a subtle perihilar haze to patchy or confluent air space consolidation involving mainly the middle and lower lung zones. Other common findings include peribronchial and perivascular thickening and a reticular pattern. Abnormalities are typically first evident on the chest radiograph within 24 hours after transplantation, reach a peak by day 3 or 4, and usually resolve between days 5 and 14.

Hyperacute Rejection

Hyperacute rejection typically occurs within minutes of re-establishment of pulmonary perfusion and is caused by pre-formed alloantibodies that bind to the donor organ and activate complement.[28] The abnormality has been described rarely in lung transplant recipients. It is manifested histologically by diffuse alveolar damage, a neutrophil infiltrate, and IgG fluorescence in the alveolar spaces and septa.[29-31] Screening of recipient blood for anti-HLA antibodies formed as a result of previous exposure to alloantigens and ensuring ABO compatibility have virtually eliminated this complication as a cause of early graft dysfunction.

Acute Rejection

Acute rejection is an almost invariable complication of lung transplantation and an important cause of morbidity.[32] Although the reaction can be seen as early as 3 days after transplantation, it is usually first manifested after 1 to 2 weeks. Sixty percent of cases occur during the first 3 postoperative months; rejection after 4 years is uncommon.[33] The minority of patients in whom clinical evidence of rejection does not develop during the first 4 months after transplantation generally continue to be free of the complication.[34]

Pathogenesis

Acute rejection is predominantly a cell-mediated immune response that results from the activation and proliferation of effector T cells directed against the HLA complex (major histocompatibility complex [MHC]) of donor cells.[35] More specifically, recipient CD8$^+$ T lymphocytes recognize donor class I MHC molecules and, after differentiation under the influence of cytokines secreted from T-helper lymphocytes, directly lyse graft endothelial and epithelial cells.[28] As might be expected, the risk for development of the complication has been strongly associated with mismatches at HLA loci.[36,37]

Pathologic Characteristics

Although the histologic features of acute lung rejection overlap somewhat with those seen in other conditions (e.g., infection),[38] they are sufficiently characteristic to enable confident diagnosis in most cases.[39] As might be expected, the abnormalities vary with the severity of rejection, and grading systems reflecting such variation have been devised (Table 11–2).[39] Minimal and mild rejection is seen most often; severe rejection is rare.

The principal abnormality is a mononuclear cell infiltrate that in the lower grades is located predominantly in the interstitial tissue surrounding venules, arterioles, and small veins and arteries. Vessels are usually affected in a patchy fashion, and it is recommended that a minimum of five transbronchial biopsy fragments be obtained for adequate assessment.[40] In more severe disease, the inflammatory infiltrate extends through the vessel wall to involve the endothelium ("endotheliitis") and into the adjacent alveolar interstitium (Fig. 11–1). Air spaces are usually unaffected except in severe disease, in which case alveolar septal necrosis may be accompanied by hemorrhage, a proteinaceous exudate, hyaline membranes, and a neutrophil infiltrate.

Radiologic Manifestations

Radiographic abnormalities include a fine reticular interstitial pattern, septal lines, ground-glass opacities, patchy or confluent air space consolidation, and new or increasing pleural effusions (Fig. 11–2).[41] The parenchymal abnormalities tend to involve mainly the mid and lower lung zones.[42] They are more likely to be seen when rejection occurs early in the postoperative course than when it occurs later.[43] The most common HRCT manifestations are localized, patchy, or widespread areas of ground-glass attenuation, septal lines, and pleural effusion.[27,44] HRCT may be normal, particularly in patients who have mild degrees of rejection.[44,45]

TABLE 11–2. Working Formulation for Classification and Grading of Lung Allograft Rejection

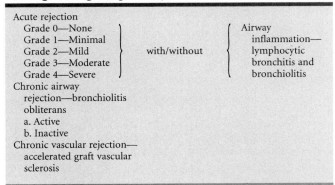

Acute rejection
  Grade 0—None
  Grade 1—Minimal
  Grade 2—Mild   } with/without { Airway inflammation—lymphocytic bronchitis and bronchiolitis
  Grade 3—Moderate
  Grade 4—Severe
Chronic airway rejection—bronchiolitis obliterans
  a. Active
  b. Inactive
Chronic vascular rejection—accelerated graft vascular sclerosis

Adapted from Yousem S: A perspective on the revised working formulation for the grading of lung allograft rejection. Transplant Proc 28:477, 1996. Reprinted by permission of Appleton & Lange, Inc.

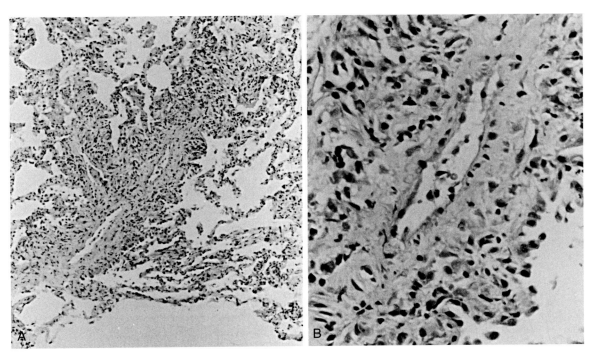

FIGURE 11–1

Pulmonary transplantation: acute rejection. The wall of a small pulmonary artery (**A**) shows moderate thickening by edema and an infiltrate of inflammatory cells, some of which extend into the adjacent alveolar septa. A magnified view (**B**) shows some of the inflammatory cells to have enlarged, somewhat irregularly shaped nuclei ("transformed lymphocytes"); occasional cells are intimately associated with the endothelium ("endotheliitis"). *(From Fraser RS, Müller NL, Colman NC, Paré PD: Fraser and Paré's Diagnosis of Diseases of the Chest, 4th ed. Philadelphia, WB Saunders, 1999.)*

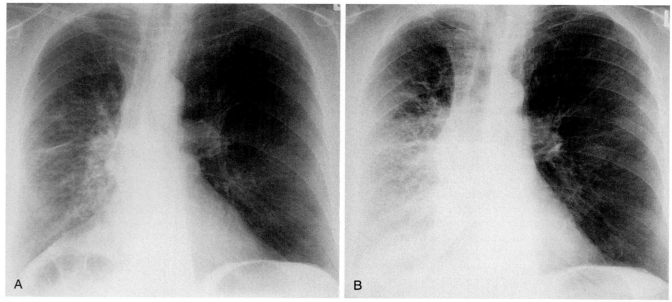

FIGURE 11–2

Pulmonary transplantation: acute rejection. A 62-year-old woman underwent right lung transplantation for emphysema. A posteroanterior chest radiograph performed 6 days later (**A**) shows mild interstitial thickening involving mainly the right perihilar region and right lower lobe. A radiograph 2 days later (**B**) shows an increase in the parenchymal abnormalities associated with the development of septal lines, ground-glass opacities throughout the right middle and lower lung zones, and focal areas of consolidation. The diagnosis of acute rejection was confirmed by transbronchial biopsy. *(From Müller NL, Fraser RS, Colman NC, Paré PD: Radiologic Diagnosis of Diseases of the Chest. Philadelphia, WB Saunders, 2001.)*

The radiographic and HRCT findings of acute rejection are nonspecific and similar to those of reperfusion injury, left heart failure, and infection.[44,45] However, findings suggestive of acute rejection include new or worsening opacities 1 to 2 weeks after transplantation, new or increasing pleural effusions, and septal lines without other signs of left heart failure.[27,46]

Clinical Manifestations

Acute pulmonary rejection is characterized by a nonspecific clinical picture of cough, dyspnea, fever, tachypnea, and crackles on auscultation[7]; consequently, transbronchial biopsy is often required for diagnosis. Although the use of surveillance transbronchial biopsy (procedures performed in the absence of abnormal clinical, functional, or radiologic findings) has clearly demonstrated that some episodes of rejection are clinically silent,[47] there is little evidence that management based on the results of surveillance biopsies improves the prognosis and outcome.[48]

Pulmonary Function Tests

Persistent declines in FEV_1 and FVC of greater than 10% usually signal the development of a complication of transplantation. The specificity of such findings is obviously limited; the sensitivity for acute rejection has been found to vary from about 40% to 85%[49] in single-lung transplant recipients. The best results have been found for small changes in FVC in patients who have underlying pulmonary fibrosis, whereas the worst have been associated with small changes in FEV_1 in patients who have COPD.

Obliterative Bronchiolitis

Progressive airflow obstruction as a result of bronchiolitis has been reported in up to 70% of patients who have undergone lung transplantation.[50] As many as 55% of affected individuals die as a result of the complication, thus making it the major cause of late graft failure.[51]

Pathogenesis

Although the precise pathogenesis of obliterative bronchiolitis (OB) is uncertain, the bulk of evidence points to immunologically mediated airway injury as the underlying mechanism. In fact, most authorities use the terms "post-transplantation obliterative bronchiolitis" or "obliterative bronchiolitis syndrome" (BOS, the latter referring to pulmonary dysfunction in the absence of histologic evidence of OB and other apparent reasons for airflow obstruction) interchangeably with chronic rejection.[52] Numerous clinical and experimental observations support this hypothesis, including the following:

1. There is a strong (albeit not inevitable) association between the frequency, severity, and persistence of acute rejection and the development of OB.[53]
2. Identical pathologic changes are seen in the lungs of bone marrow transplant recipients who have graft-versus-host disease and patients who have immunologically mediated connective tissue disease such as rheumatoid disease.
3. The prevalence of OB has been reduced by augmented immunosuppression in the post-transplantation period,[54] and established OB sometimes improves

with increased immunosuppression.[55] Medication noncompliance, by contrast, is a risk factor for BOS.[3]

4. Patients with OB have higher numbers of T and B lymphocytes in the peribronchiolar tissue and bronchiolar lumen than controls do[56]; in addition, there is evidence that the presence of lymphocytic bronchitis/bronchiolitis, in the absence of infection, is both a manifestation of acute rejection and a risk factor for the development of OB.[57]

5. Analysis of lymphocytes in peripheral blood[58] and BAL fluid[59] from some patients who have OB has revealed clonal or oligoclonal populations, suggesting that their expansion has been the result of a response to a limited number of alloantigens.

6. In a number of other assays, lymphocytes obtained by both BAL[60] and bronchial biopsy[61] have shown donor antigen–specific reactivity in patients who have OB.

7. The bronchial epithelium of patients with OB has upregulated expression of class II MHC antigens when compared with patients who have normal airways,[62] thereby providing both an inducement and a target for an immunologic response. This response is augmented by upregulated expression of the costimulatory molecules B7-1 and B7-2 on antigen-presenting cells.[63]

8. BAL fluid lymphocytes from patients who have BOS are reactive to donor-specific class I HLA antigens,[64] and their presence correlates with progression of OB.[65]

9. The presence of serum anti-HLA antibodies has been associated with a higher risk for the development of OB, thus suggesting a role for humoral immunity.[66]

10. OB has failed to develop in some patients who have lymphocytic hyporeactivity to donor antigens.[67]

The precise pathway by which these immunologic reactions result in OB is unclear. It is likely, however, that they stimulate an inflammatory response,[68,69] which in turn triggers excessive airway fibrosis, presumably mediated by cytokines such as transforming growth factor-β.[70-73]

Several additional mechanisms may contribute to airway injury and subsequent OB.[52] There is evidence that cytomegalovirus (CMV) pneumonitis/bronchiolitis may increase the risk for OB by increasing graft immunogenicity.[74] There is also a significant correlation between ischemia-reperfusion injury and the development of BOS[15]; although the mechanism for this correlation is uncertain, it has been speculated that the inflammatory reaction to the tissue injury may contribute to increased expression of HLA antigens.

Pathologic Characteristics

Histologically, OB is manifested by an eccentric or, more often, concentric increase in connective tissue between the muscularis mucosa and the epithelium of membranous and proximal respiratory bronchioles (Fig. 11–3).[75] In early disease, the connective tissue appears to be active and is composed of fibroblasts separated by a loose-appearing stroma. In more advanced disease, the fibrous tissue is typically mature in appearance and may completely occlude the airway lumen. Although a mononuclear inflammatory cell infiltrate is often present in both peribronchiolar interstitial tissue and the fibroblastic tissue itself, it is typically mild in severity. The airway epithelium may be normal but is frequently flattened or shows squamous metaplasia.

Radiologic Manifestations

The chest radiograph is often normal. When present, radiographic manifestations include decreased peripheral vascular markings, a slight decrease in lung volumes, and

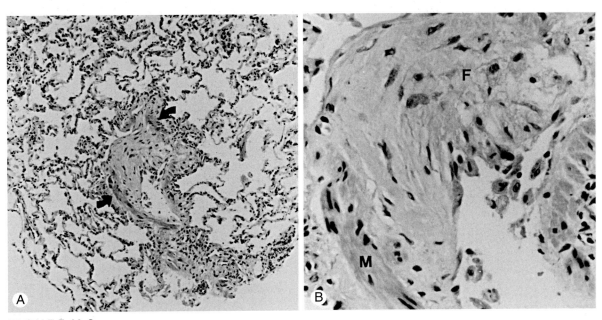

FIGURE 11–3

Post-transplantation obliterative bronchiolitis. A portion of a transbronchial biopsy specimen (**A**) shows mild interstitial pneumonitis and partial occlusion of a small bronchiole by fibrous tissue situated between the muscularis mucosae (*arrows*) and the epithelium. A magnified view (**B**) shows the fibrous tissue (F) to contain active-appearing fibroblasts. M, muscle. (*From Fraser RS, Müller NL, Colman NC, Paré PD: Fraser and Paré's Diagnosis of Diseases of the Chest, 4th ed. Philadelphia, WB Saunders, 1999.*)

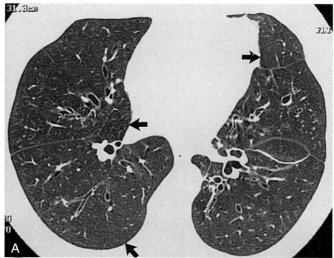

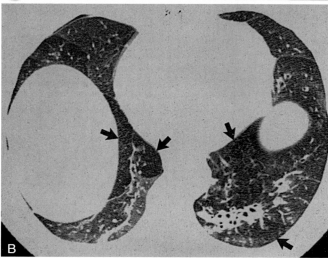

FIGURE 11–4

Pulmonary transplantation—obliterative bronchiolitis. An inspiratory HRCT scan (**A**) shows marked bronchial dilatation and areas of reduced attenuation and vascularity (*arrows*). An expiratory scan (**B**) at the level of the diaphragmatic domes shows air trapping (*arrows*). The patient was a 60-year-old woman who had undergone transplantation 2 years previously. *(From Müller NL, Fraser RS, Colman NC, Paré PD: Radiologic Diagnosis of Diseases of the Chest. Philadelphia, WB Saunders, 2001.)*

occasionally, bronchial dilation.[76,77] HRCT findings include areas of decreased attenuation and vascularity, bronchial dilation, bronchial wall thickening, and air trapping (Fig. 11–4).[78,79] The most sensitive and accurate radiologic indicator of BOS is the presence of air trapping on HRCT scans performed after maximal expiration.[80,81] For example, in a study of 38 heart-lung transplant recipients, air trapping involving more than 32% of the lung parenchyma had a sensitivity of 83% and a specificity of 89% in distinguishing patients with and without the syndrome.[80] However, other groups of investigators have found lower diagnostic accuracy, and the role of

HRCT in early detection of the complication and in monitoring patients who have it is controversial.[82-84]

Clinical Manifestations

The mean time between transplantation and recognition of OB is 6 to 12 months.[28] The clinical course is variable: in some patients, the disease has an insidious onset with indolent progression, whereas in others, both the onset and course are rapid.[85] Some patients are asymptomatic, the disease being detected after surveillance lung function testing and biopsy. Symptoms are nonspecific and include malaise, dry cough, and shortness of breath on exertion. As pulmonary function deteriorates, dyspnea worsens. Wheezing and chest tightness are common; both symptoms respond poorly to bronchodilator medication.[86] Sputum production is typically absent; however, chronic colonization of the airway by *Pseudomonas aeruginosa* may be associated with recurrent purulent tracheobronchitis.[2]

Few physical signs are present in early OB. Late inspiratory wheezes and bibasilar crackles have been noted in some patients. With advanced disease, diminished breath sounds, prolonged expiration, cyanosis, and signs of cor pulmonale may develop.[87]

Diagnosis

The diagnosis of OB is usually based on a combination of clinical, radiologic, and functional findings. Although the reported sensitivity of bronchoscopy and transbronchial biopsy is variable (ranging from 15%[88] to 70%[50]), the procedures are often useful by excluding abnormalities that may be confused with OB clinically, such as anastomotic stenosis, infection, disease recurrence, and acute rejection. In addition, some abnormalities in BAL fluid are sensitive (albeit nonspecific) markers for BOS.[89,90]

The most characteristic functional abnormality of OB is a decline in FEV_1. A working formulation for clinical staging of graft dysfunction based on the ratio of the current FEV_1 to the average of the two highest post-transplant values obtained at least 3 weeks apart has generally been adopted.[91] A potential BOS stage, "BOS 0-p," refers to possible early disease that warrants careful surveillance; it has been defined as a 10% to 19% decline in FEV_1 from baseline and/or a 25% or greater decline in forced expiratory flow, midexpiratory phase ($FEF_{25\%-75\%}$). Methacholine hyperresponsiveness,[92] bronchodilator response at low lung volumes,[93] and an alteration in ventilation distribution[94] are also indicators of an increased risk for BOS. "BOS 1" is defined as an FEV_1 that is 66% to 80% of baseline and "BOS 3" as an FEV_1 50% or less of baseline. When another abnormality, such as pleural effusion, causes new restriction, the "diagnostic" FEV_1 should be reset to a lower value.[91]

Cryptogenic Organizing Pneumonia

This abnormality is most often associated with mild acute rejection or infection, usually CMV pneumonia[95]; rarely, it occurs as an isolated finding. It has both followed and preceded the development of OB. The pathologic, radiologic, and clinical features of the disease are similar to those reported in the nontransplant population.

Post-transplantation Lymphoproliferative Disorder

The term "post-transplantation lymphoproliferative disorder" (PTLD) refers to a localized proliferation of abnormal lymphoid cells that develops after transplantation.[96] Specific lesions may be histologically and biologically benign (plasmacytic hyperplasia) to frankly malignant with clonal chromosomal abnormalities (lymphoma).[97] Incidence rates in patients who have undergone lung transplantation range from about 5% to 10%. Most tumors are found in the lung itself,[98] especially in patients whose disease develops in the first year after transplantation.[99]

The abnormality is strongly associated with Epstein-Barr virus (EBV)-infected B cells,[100] and it is likely that such infection is an essential step in the development of most lesions. The complication is much more likely to develop in patients who are seronegative before transplantation than in those who are EBV positive,[101] a risk that can be reduced by the use of antiviral prophylaxis.[102] Although EBV infection thus appears to be important in the development of PTLD, it is clear that therapeutic immunosuppression is also essential. The precise mechanism of the interaction between these two factors is uncertain; however, it is likely to be a combination of events, including EBV-induced B-cell proliferation, drug-related inhibition of cytotoxic T cells, cyclosporine- and EBV-associated inhibition of apoptosis, and activation of oncogenes or inactivation of tumor suppressor genes.[97]

The most common radiographic and HRCT manifestations consist of single or multiple pulmonary nodules and hilar or mediastinal lymph node enlargement (Fig. 11–5).[27,103] Less common findings include interlobular septal thickening, ground-glass opacities, consolidation, pleural effusion, and pericardial effusion. The nodules may have smooth or irregular margins and are often surrounded by a halo of ground-glass attenuation.[104] Pathologic correlation has shown that the halo is related to infiltration of the adjacent lung by a less dense infiltrate of lymphoid cells.[105]

Diagnosis may be possible on a specimen obtained by fine-needle aspiration[106]; however, core needle or open lung biopsy

specimens are often necessary. Regression of disease may follow a reduction in the intensity of maintenance immunosuppression; death may be the result of subsequent chronic rejection or progressive lymphoma.[107] The overall 1- and 2-year actuarial survival rates are about 50% and 20%, respectively[107]; patients with a solitary pulmonary nodule as the initial manifestation of disease have a relatively favorable prognosis.[108]

Infection

Pulmonary infection is the most common cause of morbidity and mortality in lung transplant recipients[107]; it accounts for about half the deaths occurring during the initial hospitalization and up to three quarters of those thereafter.[109] In addition to the effect of immunosuppressive therapy necessary to prevent rejection, patients are prone to pulmonary infection because of impaired mucociliary clearance,[110] impaired lymphatic drainage, and depression of the cough reflex as a result of lung denervation.[107] Handling, ischemia, preservation, and reimplantation of the donor lung also probably impair its defense against infection in the immediate post-transplant period.[111] The development of anastomotic stenosis or dehiscence is a risk factor later on.[112]

Although infection is most often caused by organisms first contacted in the post-transplantation period, it is occasionally transmitted from the donor organ[113] or originates in the proximal airways or sinuses of the recipient that became colonized before transplantation.[114] As might be expected, the spectrum of organisms responsible for infection includes a variety of bacteria, viruses, fungi, and *Mycoplasma* species.

The radiologic manifestations of the various infections in lung transplant recipients are nonspecific. One group of investigators reviewed the CT findings of 39 patients who had 45 documented pneumonias,[115] most frequently caused by CMV, *Pseudomonas* species, and *Aspergillus* species. The most common CT findings consisted of consolidation (seen in 37 episodes), ground-glass opacities (in 34), septal thickening (in 33), pleural effusion (in 33), and multiple nodules (in 25).

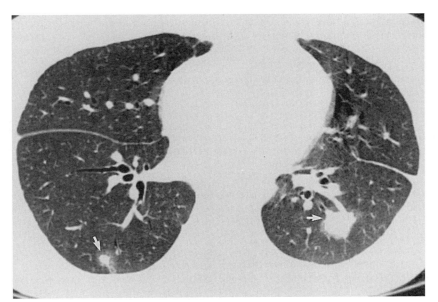

FIGURE 11–5

Post-transplantation lymphoproliferative disorder. An HRCT scan shows bilateral lung nodules (*arrows*) surrounded by a poorly defined halo of ground-glass attenuation. Thickening of the left interlobar fissure as a result of a small pleural effusion is also evident. The patient was a 52-year-old woman who had undergone double-lung transplantation 3 months previously. (*From Müller NL, Fraser RS, Colman NC, Paré PD: Radiologic Diagnosis of Diseases of the Chest. Philadelphia, WB Saunders, 2001.*)

Identification of specific abnormalities was not helpful in distinguishing the different causes of the pneumonia. Of 25 pneumonias in patients who had a single transplanted lung, parenchymal abnormalities involved both lungs in 12 (48%), only the transplanted lung in 11 (44%), and only the native lung in 2 (8%).

Bacteria

Bacteria are the most common cause of infection in heart-lung and lung transplant recipients.[16] Pneumonia occurs in a bimodal fashion; it is common in the early period after transplantation, whereas tracheobronchitis is seen in association with the bronchiectasis that accompanies late OB.[2] Gram-negative organisms, especially *P. aeruginosa*, are the most common agents.[116] Although the overall incidence of bacterial pneumonia in patients who have cystic fibrosis is not higher than that in other lung transplant recipients, previous infection with multiresistant organisms such as *Burkholderia cepacia* is a particularly important and often fatal complication.[117] Gram-positive species, including methicillin-resistant *Staphylococcus aureus*, are next in importance.[118] Other organisms, such as *Actinomyces* and *Mycobacterium* species, are identified less often.[119] Tuberculosis may develop as a primary infection, as reactivation of latent disease,[120] or by transmission from the donor.[121]

It is important to remember that the clinical features of bacterial pneumonia may be atypical in the setting of lung transplantation. Cough may be decreased and tachypnea may not be as prominent as a result of lung denervation, and fever may be suppressed and the leukocyte response blunted by the use of immunosuppressive agents. Although infection by bacterial organisms is associated with significant morbidity, mortality is low.[116]

Viruses

Cytomegalovirus. CMV is the second most common cause of infection in lung transplant recipients[122]; pneumonia is its most common manifestation. The organism can be transmitted by a lung harvested from a CMV-seropositive donor or from the transfusion of blood products from a CMV-seropositive individual; disease may likewise result from reactivation of latent infection in a seropositive recipient. Asymptomatic active infection has also been discovered in recipients who are receiving immunosuppressive agents before transplantation.[123]

Because CMV is so common in the general population, it is necessary to make a careful distinction between infection and disease. The former can be defined as identification of the organism in material obtained from any body site by culture, cytologic examination, or immunohistochemical or molecular techniques in the absence of symptoms and histologic changes indicative of tissue injury.[124] CMV disease can be considered to be present if the organism is identified by these means in the presence of histologic evidence of tissue damage.

The risk and consequences of CMV infection and disease are dependent on the serologic status of both the recipient and the donor. As might be expected, the risk of infection is lowest in seronegative recipients who have received organs from seronegative donors. When seropositive blood products are also avoided in such patients, infection occurs in only about 15%. However, in these and other patients in whom *primary*

infection develops, clinical disease occurs in most and is associated with a high fatality rate (about 20% to 25%). By contrast, despite the high prevalence of infection in patients who are donor positive and recipient positive or donor negative and recipient positive, disease develops in less than a third, and the fatality rate is lower.[107]

The pathologic features of CMV infection in biopsy specimens taken from patients who have undergone lung transplantation are similar to those from other immunosuppressed patients. It is worth noting, however, that the use of antiviral agents such as ganciclovir can result in smaller, apparently degenerated nuclear inclusions that can be overlooked unless there is a high index of suspicion, examination of several tissue levels, and/or use of immunohistochemistry.

Nonspecific signs and symptoms such as fever, malaise, myalgia, arthralgia, anorexia, and fatigue are common and may occur without evident involvement of a specific organ. Pulmonary signs and symptoms are similar to those of acute rejection. Hepatitis, colitis, retinitis, lymphopenia, thrombocytopenia, and gastroenteritis are other manifestations; their presence may provide a clue to the diagnosis of pulmonary disease.[125]

A *presumptive* diagnosis of CMV pneumonia can be made if a culture of BAL fluid is positive for CMV, the clinical and radiologic findings are compatible with the infection, and other causes of disease have been reasonably excluded.[107] CMV infection is usually documented by the shell-vial assay technique, which allows identification of the organism in 24 to 48 hours. The sensitivity and negative predictive value of the technique are extremely high; however, its specificity for the diagnosis of pneumonia is low.[126] Detection of CMV antigenemia by polymerase chain reaction has also been used to identify infection; there is evidence that quantification of viral load by this technique can be useful in identifying disease.[127] Cytologic examination of cells in BAL fluid for viral inclusions has low sensitivity (about 20%) but high specificity (98%) for the diagnosis of pneumonia.[119] When tissue is required, transbronchial biopsy is the procedure of choice; open lung biopsy is seldom required.

Miscellaneous Viruses. A variety of other viruses, including herpes simplex virus, adenovirus, influenza virus, the paramyxoviruses, respiratory syncytial virus, and parainfluenza virus, also cause pneumonia in lung transplant recipients, albeit less commonly than CMV.[128] Most are community acquired and occur months after transplantation. They are important causes of morbidity and mortality; adenovirus, in particular, carries a grave prognosis.[129]

Fungi

In the absence of appropriate prophylaxis, invasive fungal disease accounts for about 10% to 15% of pulmonary infections after lung transplantation.[130] Most cases occur between 10 and 60 days after transplantation. Disease may result from reactivation of latent infection or from recent exposure to a new environmental source, including the donor lung itself.[131] *Aspergillus* is the most common organism. Its presence in specimens obtained prospectively from the lung usually represents colonization; however, in about 3% of colonized individuals, pneumonia or disseminated disease eventually develops.[132]

Pulmonary disease caused by *Aspergillus* species may have any of the patterns seen in nontransplanted patients, including tracheobronchitis, bronchopneumonia, angioinvasive disease, allergic bronchopulmonary aspergillosis, fungus ball, and empyema.[133] The site of lung disease is usually the allograft; however, the native lung has been involved in some single-lung recipients. In some cases, the infection begins by colonization of necrotic tissue at the bronchial anastomosis. Although colonies that develop in this way may remain localized to the necrotic bronchial wall, they may also extend through it into the mediastinum or pleural space or distally along the airways, where they may cause pseudomembranous bronchitis or bronchopneumonia.[134] Definitive diagnosis of invasive disease requires biopsy; however, a presumptive diagnosis can be made when the organism is identified in BAL fluid and the clinical picture is consistent.

Recurrence of the Primary Disease

The frequency of recurrence of the pulmonary disease underlying the need for transplantation is about 1%.[135] Sarcoidosis is the most common; however, such recurrence has also been described in a variety of other conditions, including lymphangioleiomyomatosis, Langerhans cell histiocytosis, talc granulomatosis, diffuse panbronchiolitis, pulmonary alveolar proteinosis, bronchioloalveolar carcinoma,[136] desquamative interstitial pneumonitis,[137] and giant cell pneumonitis.[138]

Pleural Complications

Pleural effusion is virtually inevitable after lung transplantation.[139] Effusions are generally small to moderate in size but may be massive.[140] Their pathogenesis is probably related to a combination of surgical trauma and disruption of lymphatic flow in the allograft; postoperative positive fluid balance may also be a factor in some patients. New or increasing pleural fluid may be a sign of acute rejection; in one investigation, the presence of these radiographic findings and septal lines predicted the complication with a sensitivity of 68% and a specificity of 90%.[140]

Other causes of pleural effusion in the post-transplantation period include parapneumonic effusion and empyema. In a series of 392 patients, empyema developed in 3.6%.[141] It was not related to the type of operation or to previous septic lung disease. Other investigators have reported an increased risk for empyema in patients with cystic fibrosis who are infected with *B. cepacia* or other antibiotic-resistant organisms.[142] Additional unusual causes of pleural effusion include chylothorax and hemothorax.

Persistent or recurrent pneumothorax has been reported in about 10% of patients who have received a lung transplant. Although iatrogenic causes account for most episodes, the complication can be related to invasive fungal infection or the primary disease in the residual native lung.[140,142] After heart-lung transplantation or sequential bilateral lung transplantation, pneumothorax can be bilateral as a result of direct communication between the right and left pleural spaces.[143]

Bronchial Complications

The two main complications related to the anastomosis are dehiscence and stenosis. The former usually occurs in the first few months after transplantation; with current surgical and management techniques, however, it is rare.[144] Anastomotic stenosis has been described in about 5% to 20% of patients[145]; it occurs most often in association with saprophytic fungal infection or excessive granulation tissue at the anastomotic site or with localized airway wall necrosis/fibrosis as a result of ischemia.

Chest radiographs are of limited value in diagnosis, but both stenosis and dehiscence can usually be recognized on CT (Fig. 11–6).[146-148] The procedure is not 100% accurate, however, and bronchoscopy is required for definitive diagnosis.[149] The size of the bronchial defects on CT ranges from 0.1 to 1.5 cm, with most measuring 0.5 cm or less.[146] Optimal assessment of bronchial caliber requires thin-section spiral CT and multiplanar reconstruction.[150]

Wheezing, breathlessness, or stridor typically develops in patients who have anastomotic stenosis; most show progressive deterioration in lung function.[151] Flow-volume loops may be useful in monitoring the patency of the anastomosis and in evaluating the functional response to stent insertion.[152] The diagnosis has been confirmed an average of about 60 days after transplantation (range, 3 to 245 days). Although most stenoses can be managed successfully with stent insertion, fatal pulmonary infection originating in the stenotic area occasionally ensues.

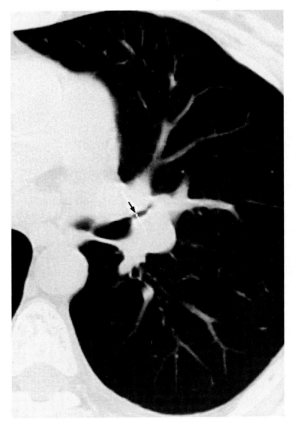

FIGURE 11–6

Bronchial stenosis. A CT scan shows severe stenosis of the left upper lobe bronchus (*arrow*). The patient was a 31-year-old woman who had undergone double-lung transplantation for cystic fibrosis 4 months earlier. (*Case courtesy of Dr. Ann Leung, Stanford University School of Medicine, Stanford, CA.*)

Pulmonary Vascular Complications

Postoperative pulmonary arterial or venous obstruction at the anastomotic site occurs infrequently.[153] Nonanastomotic pulmonary vascular abnormalities are much more common than those related to the anastomoses. They tend to be associated with the development of OB and may represent a vascular component of chronic rejection.[154] Histologic abnormalities consist of patchy intimal thickening by loose connective tissue containing myofibroblast-like cells[75]; the large elastic and muscular arteries, arterioles, and small veins are the most affected. Although the clinical effects of such thickening are generally absent or minimal, there is evidence that the complication occurs earlier and is associated with a bad prognosis in younger patients.[155]

As in other postoperative patients, deep venous thrombosis and pulmonary thromboembolism may develop in lung transplant recipients; these complications were documented in 14 (12%) of 116 patients in one series and were thought to contribute to death in 3 of them.[156]

Pulmonary Function Post-transplantation

Pulmonary function improves markedly in patients after lung transplantation.[107] As might be expected, double-lung recipients have significantly better function than single-lung recipients do; in fact, they are able to attain nearly normal function. After single-lung transplantation, maximal ventilatory function is usually reached within 3 months. In patients who have COPD, FEV_1 increases to about 50% to 60% of the predicted value, but an obstructive pattern persists; in those with underlying pulmonary fibrosis, a mild restrictive pattern remains.[2]

When single-lung transplantation is performed for the treatment of COPD, the transplanted lung is significantly restricted and contributes only about a third of TLC.[157] The mechanism of this restriction is thought to be low transpulmonary pressure generation related to an abnormal configuration of the recipient's chest wall[158]; this problem results in the persistent hyperinflation and air trapping noted in these patients after bilateral lung transplantation.[159] Diffusion capacity is about 75% of predicted after double-lung transplantation and 60% of predicted after a single-lung procedure.[160] Oxygenation returns to normal in most patients; in previously hypercapnic patients, the average time to normalization of arterial P_{CO_2} after transplantation is about 15 days.[111]

Although most patients report no limitation in activity 1 year after transplantation,[2] formal assessment of exercise performance reveals a reduction in most. Most investigators have reported maximal oxygen uptake to be about half normal and the anaerobic threshold to be reduced in both single and bilateral transplant patients.[161] These limitations are probably the result of impaired oxygen utilization by skeletal muscles,[162] possibly as a result of cyclosporine-induced changes in muscle mitochondrial respiration and deconditioning.[2] Despite these observations, some authors have reported that exercise capacity after bilateral lung transplantation is better than that after single-lung transplantation[6]; this finding might be explained by flow limitation during exercise (as described in some patients who have received single lungs for COPD[163]) or by the younger age of bilateral lung transplant recipients.

Despite the pulmonary denervation necessitated by the transplantation procedure, control of breathing is not significantly altered.[107] The breathing pattern is slow and deep, a finding consistent with the absence of vagally mediated inhibition of inflation.[164] The prevalence of airway hyperresponsiveness to methacholine or histamine is increased[92]; such hyperresponsiveness has been attributed to denervation hypersensitivity of muscarinic receptors and to changes in the small airways as a result of incipient BOS.[165]

Prognosis

Two phases of survival can be seen on analysis of registry data—an early decline followed by slow attrition.[1] Both early and late survival of patients older than 50 years is somewhat less than that of younger patients.[1] Bilateral lung transplant recipients tend to live longer than those who have received only one lung, the "half-life" (50% survival) of the former being 4.9 years and the latter, 3.7 years. The "conditional half-life" (survival after the first year) is 7.9 years for bilateral lung recipients and 5.9 years for single. These differences are largely applicable to patients who have COPD, there being no significant differences between those who have underlying idiopathic pulmonary fibrosis or primary pulmonary hypertension.[1] However, higher perioperative mortality has been found in patients with idiopathic pulmonary fibrosis, primary pulmonary hypertension, or sarcoidosis than in patients with COPD.[1] Patients who are undergoing retransplantation or who are receiving mechanical ventilation or require transplantation for congenital heart disease also have a higher perioperative mortality rate.[1] Infection and graft failure are the major causes of perioperative mortality, whereas infection and OB are primarily responsible for late death.

Although some patients remain ill as a result of transplant-related complications, prospective evaluation of the quality of life has revealed a highly significant improvement in physical, social, and emotional health in some cohorts.[166] Nonetheless, only about 40% of transplant survivors report feeling able to return to work,[167] and only about 10% actually return to full-time employment.[168]

BONE MARROW TRANSPLANTATION

Bone marrow transplantation (BMT) or transplantation of stem cells harvested from umbilical cord blood or peripheral blood is now standard therapy for aplastic anemia, acute and chronic leukemia, and some forms of lymphoma. It has also been used in patients who have hemoglobinopathies, immunodeficiency disorders, myelodysplastic syndrome, multiple myeloma, and some solid tumors.[169] More than 50,000 procedures were performed in 1998, the majority of which were autologous.[170]

Pulmonary disease accounts for a substantial proportion of the morbidity and mortality associated with the procedure: more than 30% of transplantation-related deaths are caused by respiratory disorders, and pulmonary complications occur in 40% to 60% of recipients.[169,171] These complications are classified as early or late according to whether they occur during or after the first 100 days of transplantation.[171] Specific complications are related to the type and duration of immunologic defects produced by the underlying disease and the therapy, the nature of the conditioning regimens used in the pretransplantation period, and the development of graft-versus-host disease (GVHD).[169] Although recipients of syngeneic (identical twin) and autologous transplants are subject to fewer complications than recipients of allogeneic grafts, the incidence of disease is nevertheless significant.

Pulmonary Edema

Pulmonary edema develops in as many as 50% of patients after both allogeneic and autologous BMT.[172] When accompanied by multiorgan dysfunction, it suggests that the edema is one manifestation of a systemic process that has been called the "engraftment syndrome."[172,173] In fact, the pathogenesis is probably multifactorial. Hydrostatic forces related to fluid overload or to the cardiotoxicity of immunosuppressive agents such as doxorubicin favor the development of edema.[169] Increased capillary permeability may also occur secondary to sepsis or to toxicity from the conditioning regimen, which may include total-body irradiation and high-dose cyclophosphamide.[171]

The onset of edema is rapid and usually occurs in the second or third week after transplantation.[169] Clinical manifestations include dyspnea, weight gain, and crackles on physical examination. Radiographic findings are similar to those of pulmonary edema associated with fluid overload.[174] HRCT frequently demonstrates areas of ground-glass attenuation involving mainly the dependent lung regions. A variable degree of hypoxemia may be present.

Diffuse Alveolar Hemorrhage

Diffuse alveolar hemorrhage has been reported in up to 21% of patients who have undergone autologous or allogeneic transplantation.[170] Risk factors include age older than 40 years, high fever, severe mucositis, white blood cell recovery, pretransplant BAL neutrophilia, and renal insufficiency.[170,175] Although air space hemorrhage is seen histologically, a pattern of diffuse alveolar damage is also commonly found at autopsy.[176]

The characteristic radiographic and HRCT findings consist of bilateral or, less commonly, unilateral ground-glass opacities and patchy or confluent air space consolidation (Fig. 11–7).[174,177] These abnormalities tend to involve mainly the perihilar region and lower lung zones.[177]

The condition is clinically characterized by progressive dyspnea, cough, fever, and hypoxemia; hemoptysis is rare.[169] Symptoms develop about 12 days after transplantation (range, 7 to 40 days). Although some investigators have found successive aliquots of BAL fluid to contain increasing amounts of blood,[178] this finding is neither sensitive nor specific for the diagnosis.[176] Most patients require admission to an intensive care unit and mechanical ventilation; half of affected individuals die.[179] Systemic corticosteroids probably moderate the effects of the hemorrhage and appear to improve survival[180,181]; clearly, excluding infection and aspiration of blood from a focal process is mandatory.

Graft-versus-Host Disease

GVHD results when the recipient's tissue is recognized as foreign by donor T lymphocytes. It may be acute or chronic, the former occurring in about two thirds of patients. A variety

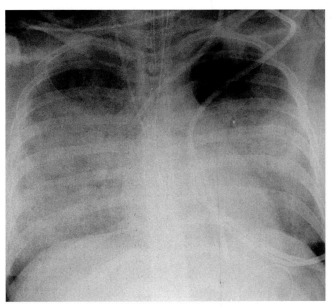

FIGURE 11–7

Bone marrow transplantation—diffuse alveolar hemorrhage. An anteroposterior chest radiograph shows extensive bilateral consolidation with air bronchograms. The patient was a 27-year-old woman in whom diffuse alveolar hemorrhage developed 2 weeks after bone marrow transplantation. *(From Müller NL, Fraser RS, Colman NC, Paré PD: Radiologic Diagnosis of Diseases of the Chest. Philadelphia, WB Saunders, 2001.)*

of pulmonary disorders are seen in patients who have GVHD, and it is possible that the condition is pathogenetically associated with one or more of them. Such disorders include idiopathic pneumonia syndrome, lymphocytic bronchiolitis, bronchiolitis obliterans, and (rarely) cryptogenic organizing pneumonia (bronchiolitis obliterans with organizing pneumonia).[182] Patients with chronic GVHD frequently have concomitant pulmonary infection by bacteria and opportunistic organisms. A sicca syndrome accompanied by chronic bronchitis may also develop.[169]

Idiopathic Pneumonia Syndrome

Idiopathic pneumonia syndrome has been defined as diffuse lung injury occurring after BMT for which an infectious etiology is not identified.[169] The complication develops in about 10% of patients who have undergone BMT.[183] An early peak occurs in the first 14 days after transplantation and is followed by a lower but consistent incidence in the following 80 days. Most cases of pneumonia occurring in the first 28 days after transplantation are idiopathic; after this period, the rate of idiopathic pneumonia syndrome is about 20%.[183]

Risk factors for idiopathic pneumonia syndrome include poor performance status before transplantation, transplantation for a malignancy other than leukemia, longer interval from diagnosis to transplantation, high-dose total-body irradiation, older age, the use of high-dose BCNU (carmustine) or methotrexate before transplantation, positive donor CMV serology, and GVHD.[169,182] Its etiology is probably varied, and its pathogenesis is poorly defined. One hypothesis is that chemotherapy results in the generation of proinflammatory cytokines and oxidants by pulmonary epithelial cells and macrophages.[184] A second injury, such as that caused by conditioning irradiation or GVHD, may also be necessary for development of the syndrome.[185]

The radiologic findings are nonspecific and consist of bilateral interstitial thickening occasionally associated with ground-glass opacities and poorly defined small nodular opacities.[174,183] The clinical manifestations are varied: radiographic changes may be associated with a complete lack of symptoms in the early stages or with acute and severe respiratory distress.[183] The diagnosis is one of exclusion, particularly of infection. The mortality rate is high, in some series approaching 80%.[171] However, less than a third of patients die of progressive respiratory failure as a direct result of idiopathic pneumonia syndrome,[186] complicating infection being a more common cause of death.

Delayed Pulmonary Toxicity Syndrome

This uncommon complication of autologous BMT has features that overlap those of idiopathic pneumonia syndrome. It is characterized by the development of interstitial pneumonitis and fibrosis months to years after transplantation in patients who have received high-dose chemotherapy for breast cancer.[182] Its timing, low mortality, and good response to corticosteroids help distinguish the complication from idiopathic pneumonia syndrome.

Obliterative Bronchiolitis

Obstructive airway disease caused by OB is an uncommon complication of BMT.[187] With few exceptions, it follows allogeneic transplantation. The median interval between the procedure and diagnosis is about 260 days. The histologic features are identical to those of OB after lung transplantation and most often consist of mild bronchiolitis and a proliferation of fibroblastic tissue between the epithelium and muscularis mucosa. Parenchymal interstitial disease is typically absent or minimal.

The chest radiograph may be normal or may show evidence of hyperinflation and attenuation of the peripheral vascular markings. Characteristic HRCT findings consist of dilation of the segmental and subsegmental bronchi and localized areas of decreased attenuation and perfusion.[174,188] HRCT scans performed at end-expiration show air trapping.[174] Recurrent pneumothorax and pneumomediastinum have been described in several patients.[189]

Symptoms include cough, which is progressively productive, as well as wheeze and exertional dyspnea.[187] In some patients, the abnormality is discovered because of deterioration in lung function in the absence of symptoms.[169] Findings of chronic GVHD are almost always present.[182] Pulmonary function studies usually show an obstructive pattern; diffusing capacity may be normal or reduced. The rate of progression of these functional abnormalities is variable.[190]

Lymphocytic Bronchitis

A lymphocytic infiltrate in the bronchial epithelium and submucosa associated with focal epithelial necrosis is not uncommon in patients who have undergone allogeneic BMT.[191] Clinical findings include a dry, nonproductive cough. Frequently, associated GVHD is present in skin, liver, and intestine; however, similar findings can be seen in the airways of patients who do not have GVHD and in autografted dogs,[192] thus making a pathogenetic relationship with GVHD uncertain.

Infection

Specific infections in patients who undergo BMT tend to occur at particular times corresponding to specific defects in host defense.[193] The conditioning regimen virtually eliminates all preexisting immunity. The pattern of immune reconstitution varies with the nature of the underlying disorder, the source of stem cells used for transplantation, and the presence of GVHD.[194] Patients who have the latter complication are particularly at risk for infection by encapsulated bacteria and opportunistic organisms.[193] From the point of view of the differential diagnosis, it is useful to remember that most diffuse disease is noninfectious in origin whereas focal disease is frequently the result of bacterial or fungal infection.

The pre-engraftment period is characterized by neutropenia. Unless prolonged, bacterial pneumonia is the major respiratory complication and occurs in 20% to 50% of patients in the first 2 weeks[194] after transplantation. Gram-negative organisms are the most common agents; gram-positive organisms such as *Streptococcus pneumoniae* and *S. aureus* are occasionally identified.[195] After immune reconstitution, bacterial pneumonia is predominantly caused by gram-positive organisms, especially *S. pneumoniae*.[196] The presence of GVHD increases the risk for pneumonia caused by encapsulated bacteria and *P. aeruginosa*.[197]

Aspergillus is the most common fungus associated with pneumonia after BMT and has been identified as the cause of up to 36% of all nosocomial pneumonias in this setting.[193] Most cases have occurred within 30 days of transplantation and have been associated with granulocytopenia and the use of broad-spectrum antibiotics and corticosteroids.[169] The use of growth factors and air filtration diminishes the risk. After engraftment, such infections are often associated with GVHD and its therapy.[194] The mortality rate is very high, approaching 85%.[169]

CMV pneumonia has been identified in 10% to 40% of allogeneic BMT recipients[169] and in about 2% of those receiving autologous transplants.[198] Most cases develop 6 to 12 weeks after the procedure. The complication accounts for about half of all episodes of diffuse interstitial pneumonia in patients who have allogeneic transplants. Pneumonia occurs in about a third of patients infected with the virus; the risk is increased by the presence of severe GVHD, the treatment of GVHD, older age, total-body irradiation during the conditioning regimen, and the transfusion of CMV-positive blood products to CMV-negative recipients.[194,199] Although aggressive prophylaxis reduces the risk substantially,[197] mortality is high in patients in whom pneumonia develops.[194]

The radiologic manifestations of pneumonia in BMT recipients are the same as those in otherwise healthy individuals.[200] CT can provide information that establishes the pattern and extent of pulmonary disease more clearly than radiography (Fig. 11–8).[201,202] For example, in a study of 87

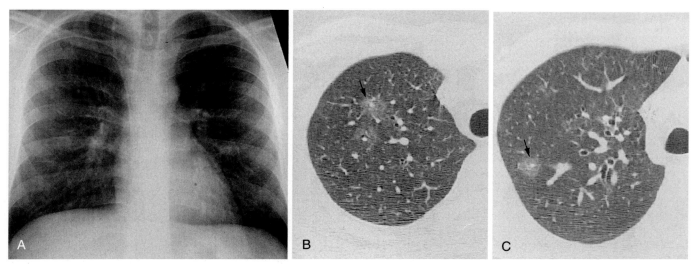

FIGURE 11–8

Bone marrow transplantation—angioinvasive aspergillosis. An anteroposterior chest radiograph (**A**) in a 19-year-old man 3 weeks after bone marrow transplantation shows questionable parenchymal opacities. HRCT scan images of the right upper lobe (**B** and **C**) show small nodules with surrounding halos of ground-glass attenuation (*arrows*). These findings are most suggestive of angioinvasive aspergillosis. The diagnosis was confirmed by open lung biopsy. *(From Müller NL, Fraser RS, Colman NC, Paré PD: Radiologic Diagnosis of Diseases of the Chest. Philadelphia, WB Saunders, 2001.)*

neutropenic patients who had 146 episodes of fever that persisted for more than 2 days despite empirical antibiotic therapy, chest radiographs were normal and HRCT scans were abnormal in 70 (48%) episodes.[202] Microorganisms were detected in 30 (43%) of the 70 cases; in 22 (31%) of them, abnormalities became apparent on the radiograph later. The median interval (delay) until abnormalities were evident was 5 days (range, 1 to 22 days).

Miscellaneous Complications

Pleural effusion is usually seen in well-defined clinical settings, such as pulmonary edema, fluid overload, infection, noninfectious pneumonia, recurrence of neoplasm, or veno-occlusive disease.[203] The latter should be suggested by the triad of pulmonary edema, pulmonary hypertension, and normal left ventricular function.[204]

Because of the use of immunosuppressive agents, patients have a substantially increased risk for the development of secondary malignancies,[205] a risk that increases with time. Such malignancies include nonhematologic malignancies as well as new hematologic malignancies, especially EBV-related lymphoma (PTLD).[206]

Pulmonary Function Tests

Restrictive lung function with deterioration in diffusing capacity develops in a significant number of patients.[207] In the absence of an obvious cause for these changes, they are usually transient.[208] The pathogenesis of this abnormality is unclear; toxicity as a result of the pretransplantation conditioning regimen, muscle weakness, and sequelae of intercurrent infection have been hypothesized.[169]

Somewhat surprisingly, alterations in both preoperative and postoperative lung function have been found to have prognostic significance.[207,209] Although respiratory failure is more common in patients who have pulmonary function abnormalities before transplantation, this finding does not entirely account for the described increase in mortality. On the other hand, when lung function is abnormal in the postoperative period, the risk for death from respiratory causes explains the increased mortality.[207]

LIVER TRANSPLANTATION

The lungs are frequently abnormal in patients who have severe liver disease, as well as in those who have undergone liver transplantation.[210] The respiratory complications of liver disease, the complications of abdominal surgery, and the infections that follow immunosuppressive medication are discussed in the appropriate areas of this text. However, several complications of liver transplantation and concerns unique to the procedure are briefly discussed here.

Pulmonary Calcification

When the relatively insensitive tool of chest radiography is used, metastatic calcification of the lung has been noted in 5% of patients who have undergone liver transplantation.[211] The importance of the abnormality is related principally to the ease with which it can be confused radiographically with other complications such as edema or infection. The pathogenesis is unclear but is probably related to complicating renal failure, acid-base disturbances, and the administration of exogenous calcium and citrate. Patients do not usually have symptoms; however, dyspnea and nonproductive cough occur occasionally, and respiratory failure has been described.[212] The diagnosis can be confirmed by the use of technetium 99m phosphate scans, which show increased uptake in the lungs, and by CT scanning.

Pulmonary Thrombosis

Massive pulmonary platelet aggregation is an important cause of early death in patients who have undergone liver transplantation.[213] An elevation in pulmonary artery pressure before death should suggest the diagnosis.[214]

Hypoxemia

Hypoxemia is common in patients who have cirrhosis.[215] In many cases it appears to be related to the presence of intrapulmonary shunts caused by dilatation of small pulmonary arteries (the hepatopulmonary syndrome).[216,217] The observation that liver transplantation can reverse even severe preoperative hypoxemia confirms the functional nature of the disorder.[218] However, a preoperative PaO_2 value of 50 mm Hg or less alone or in combination with a shunt fraction of 20% or greater is a strong predictor of postoperative mortality.[218,219]

REFERENCES

1. Hertz MI, Taylor DO, Trulock EP, et al: The registry of the International Society for Heart and Lung Transplantation: Nineteenth official report—2002. J Heart Lung Transplant 21:950-970, 2002.
2. Arcasoy SM, Kotloff RM: Lung transplantation. N Engl J Med 340:1081-1091, 1999.
3. Gammie JS, Keenan RJ, Pham SM, et al: Single- versus double-lung transplantation for pulmonary hypertension. J Thorac Cardiovasc Surg 115:397-402, discussion 402-403, 1998.
4. Weill D, Keshavjee S: Lung transplantation for emphysema: Two lungs or one. J Heart Lung Transplant 20:739-742, 2001.
5. Rao JN, Forty J, Hasan A, et al: Bilateral lung transplant: The procedure of choice for end-stage septic lung disease. Transplant Proc 33:1622-1623, 2001.
6. Pochettino A, Kotloff RM, Rosengard BR, et al: Bilateral versus single lung transplantation for chronic obstructive pulmonary disease: Intermediate-term results. Ann Thorac Surg 70:1813-1818, discussion 1818-1819, 2000.
7. Jenkinson SG, Levine SM: Lung transplantation. Dis Mon 40:1-38, 1994.
8. Cohen RG, Starnes VA: Living donor lung transplantation. World J Surg 25:244-250, 2001.
9. Mayer-Hamblett N, Rosenfeld M, Emerson J, et al: Developing cystic fibrosis lung transplant referral criteria using predictors of 2-year mortality. Am J Respir Crit Care Med 166:1550-1555, 2002.
10. Mogulkoc N, Brutsche MH, Bishop PW, et al: Pulmonary function in idiopathic pulmonary fibrosis and referral for lung transplantation. Am J Respir Crit Care Med 164:103, 2002.
11. Hosenpud JD, Bennett LE, Keck BM, et al: Effect of diagnosis on survival benefit of lung transplantation for end-stage lung disease. Lancet 351:24-27, 1998.
12. International guidelines for the selection of lung transplant candidates. The American Society for Transplant Physicians (ASTP)/American Thoracic Society (ATS)/European Respiratory Society (ERS)/International Society for Heart and Lung Transplantation (ISHLT). Am J Respir Crit Care Med 158:335-339, 1998.
13. de Perrot M, Liu M, Waddell TK, Keshavjee S: Ischemia-reperfusion–induced lung injury. Am J Respir Crit Care Med 167:490-511, 2003.
14. Khan SU, Salloum J, O'Donovan PB, et al: Acute pulmonary edema after lung transplantation: The pulmonary reimplantation response. Chest 116:187-194, 1999.
15. Fiser SM, Tribble CG, Long SM, et al: Ischemia-reperfusion injury after lung transplantation increases risk of late bronchiolitis obliterans syndrome. Ann Thorac Surg 73:1041-1047, discussion 1047-1048, 2002.
16. DeMeo DL, Ginns LC: Clinical status of lung transplantation. Transplantation 72:1713-1724, 2001.
17. Stewart KC, Patterson GA: Current trends in lung transplantation. Am J Transplant 1:204-210, 2001.
18. Fiser SM, Kron IL, Long SM, et al: Influence of graft ischemic time on outcomes following lung transplantation. J Heart Lung Transplant 20:1291-1296, 2001.
19. Schutte H, Hermle G, Seeger W, Grimminger F: Vascular distension and continued ventilation are protective in lung ischemia/reperfusion. Am J Respir Crit Care Med 157:171-177, 1998.
20. Halldorsson AO, Kronon MT, Allen BS, et al: Lowering reperfusion pressure reduces the injury after pulmonary ischemia. Ann Thorac Surg 69:198-203, discussion 204, 2000.
21. De Perrot M, Sekine Y, Fischer S, et al: Interleukin-8 release during early reperfusion predicts graft function in human lung transplantation. Am J Respir Crit Care Med 165:211-215, 2002.
22. Fisher AJ, Donnelly SC, Hirani N, et al: Elevated levels of interleukin-8 in donor lungs is associated with early graft failure after lung transplantation. Am J Respir Crit Care Med 163:259-265, 2001.
23. Hohlfeld JM, Tiryaki E, Hamm H, et al: Pulmonary surfactant activity is impaired in lung transplant recipients. Am J Respir Crit Care Med 158:706-712, 1998.
24. Zenati M, Yousem SA, Dowling RD, et al: Primary graft failure following pulmonary transplantation. Transplantation 50:165-167, 1990.
25. Yousem SA, Duncan SR, Griffith BP: Interstitial and airspace granulation tissue reactions in lung transplant recipients. Am J Surg Pathol 16:877-884, 1992.
26. Ward S, Müller NL: Pulmonary complications following lung transplantation. Clin Radiol 55:332-339, 2000.
27. Collins J: Imaging of the chest after lung transplantation. J Thorac Imaging 17:102-112, 2002.
28. Trulock EP: Management of lung transplant rejection. Chest 103:1566-1576, 1993.
29. Frost AE, Jammal CT, Cagle PT: Hyperacute rejection following lung transplantation. Chest 110:559-562, 1996.
30. Choi JK, Kearns J, Palevsky HI, et al: Hyperacute rejection of a pulmonary allograft. Immediate clinical and pathologic findings. Am J Respir Crit Care Med 160:1015-1018, 1999.
31. Bittner HB, Dunitz J, Hertz M, et al: Hyperacute rejection in single lung transplantation—case report of successful management by means of plasmapheresis and antithymocyte globulin treatment. Transplantation 71:649-651, 2001.
32. Keenan RJ, Zeevi A: Immunologic consequences of transplantation. Chest Surg Clin N Am 5:107-120, 1995.
33. Kesten S, Chamberlain D, Maurer J: Yield of surveillance transbronchial biopsies performed beyond two years after lung transplantation. J Heart Lung Transplant 15:384-388, 1996.
34. Baz MA, Layish DT, Govert JA, et al: Diagnostic yield of bronchoscopies after isolated lung transplantation. Chest 110:84-88, 1996.
35. Sayegh MH, Turka LA: The role of T-cell costimulatory activation pathways in transplant rejection. N Engl J Med 338:1813-1821, 1998.
36. Schulman LL, Weinberg AD, McGregor C, et al: Mismatches at the HLA-DR and HLA-B loci are risk factors for acute rejection after lung transplantation. Am J Respir Crit Care Med 157:1833-1837, 1998.
37. Quantz MA, Bennett LE, Meyer DM, Novick RJ: Does human leukocyte antigen matching influence the outcome of lung transplantation? An analysis of 3,549 lung transplantations. J Heart Lung Transplant 19:473-479, 2000.
38. Nakhleh RE, Bolman RM 3rd, Henke CA, Hertz MI: Lung transplant pathology. A comparative study of pulmonary acute rejection and cytomegaloviral infection. Am J Surg Pathol 15:1197-1201, 1991.
39. Yousem SA, Berry GJ, Cagle PT, et al: Revision of the 1990 working formulation for the classification of pulmonary allograft rejection: Lung Rejection Study Group. J Heart Lung Transplant 15:1-15, 1996.
40. Berry GJ, Brunt EM, Chamberlain D, et al: A working formulation for the standardization of nomenclature in the diagnosis of heart and lung rejection: Lung Rejection Study Group. The International Society for Heart Transplantation. J Heart Transplant 9:593-601, 1990.
41. Erasmus JJ, McAdams HP, Tapson VF, et al: Radiologic issues in lung transplantation for end-stage pulmonary disease. AJR Am J Roentgenol 169:69-78, 1997.
42. Kundu S, Herman SJ, Larhs A, et al: Correlation of chest radiographic findings with biopsy-proven acute lung rejection. J Thorac Imaging 14:178-184, 1999.
43. Millet B, Higenbottam TW, Flower CD, et al: The radiographic appearances of infection and acute rejection of the lung after heart-lung transplantation. Am Rev Respir Dis 140:62-67, 1989.
44. Loubeyre P, Revel D, Delignette A, et al: High-resolution computed tomographic findings associated with histologically diagnosed acute lung rejection in heart-lung transplant recipients. Chest 107:132-138, 1995.
45. Gotway MB, Dawn SK, Sellami D, et al: Acute rejection following lung transplantation: Limitations in accuracy of thin-section CT for diagnosis. Radiology 221:207-212, 2001.
46. Bergin CJ, Castellino RA, Blank N, et al: Acute lung rejection after heart-lung transplantation: Correlation of findings on chest radiographs with lung biopsy results. AJR Am J Roentgenol 155:23-27, 1990.
47. Hopkins PM, Aboyoun CL, Chhajed PN, et al: Prospective analysis of 1,235 transbronchial lung biopsies in lung transplant recipients. J Heart Lung Transplant 21:1062-1067, 2002.
48. Valentine VG, Taylor DE, Dhillon GS, et al: Success of lung transplantation without surveillance bronchoscopy. J Heart Lung Transplant 21:319-326, 2002.
49. Becker FS, Martinez FJ, Brunsting LA, et al: Limitations of spirometry in detecting rejection after single-lung transplantation. Am J Respir Crit Care Med 150:159-166, 1994.
50. Reichenspurner H, Girgis RE, Robbins RC, et al: Stanford experience with obliterative bronchiolitis after lung and heart-lung transplantation. Ann Thorac Surg 62:1467-1472, discussion 1472-1473, 1996.
51. Boehler A, Kesten S, Weder W, Speich R: Bronchiolitis obliterans after lung transplantation: A review. Chest 114:1411-1426, 1998.
52. Estenne M, Hertz MI: Bronchiolitis obliterans after human lung transplantation. Am J Respir Crit Care Med 166:440-444, 2002.
53. Bando K, Paradis IL, Similo S, et al: Obliterative bronchiolitis after lung and heart-lung transplantation. An analysis of risk factors and management. J Thorac Cardiovasc Surg 110:4-13, discussion 13-14, 1995.
54. Ross DJ, Jordan SC, Nathan SD, et al: Delayed development of obliterative bronchiolitis syndrome with OKT3 after unilateral lung transplantation. A plea for multicenter immunosuppressive trials. Chest 109:870-873, 1996.
55. Ross DJ, Lewis MI, Kramer M, et al: FK 506 'rescue' immunosuppression for obliterative bronchiolitis after lung transplantation. Chest 112:1175-1179, 1997.

56. Ohori NP, Iacono AT, Grgurich WF, Yousem SA: Significance of acute bronchi-tis/bronchiolitis in the lung transplant recipient. Am J Surg Pathol 18:1192-1204, 1994.

57. Husain AN, Siddiqui MT, Holmes EW, et al: Analysis of risk factors for the development of bronchiolitis obliterans syndrome. Am J Respir Crit Care Med 159:829-833, 1999.

58. Duncan SR, Leonard C, Theodore J, et al: Oligoclonal CD4(+) T cell expansions in lung transplant recipients with obliterative bronchiolitis. Am J Respir Crit Care Med 165:1439-1444, 2002.

59. DeBruyne LA, Lynch JP 3rd, Baker LA, et al: Restricted V beta usage by T cells infiltrating rejecting human lung allografts. J Immunol 156:3493-3500, 1996.

60. Reinsmoen NL, Bolman RM, Savik K, et al: Differentiation of class I– and class II–directed donor-specific alloreactivity in bronchoalveolar lavage lymphocytes from lung transplant recipients. Transplantation 53:181-189, 1992.

61. Schulman LL, Ho EK, Reed EF, et al: Immunologic monitoring in lung allograft recipients. Transplantation 61:252-257, 1996.

62. Hasegawa S, Ockner DM, Patterson GA, et al: Expression of class II major histocompatibility complex antigens and lymphocyte subset immunotyping in chronic pulmonary transplant rejection. Transplant Proc 27:1290-1292, 1995.

63. Elssner A, Jaumann F, Wolf WP, et al: Bronchial epithelial cell B7-1 and B7-2 mRNA expression after lung transplantation: A role in allograft rejection? Eur Respir J 20:165-169, 2002.

64. Jaramillo A, Smith MA, Phelan D, et al: Development of ELISA-detected anti-HLA antibodies precedes the development of bronchiolitis obliterans syndrome and correlates with progressive decline in pulmonary function after lung transplantation. Transplantation 67:1155-1161, 1999.

65. Reinsmoen NL, Bolman RM, Savik K, et al: Are multiple immunopathogenetic events occurring during the development of obliterative bronchiolitis and acute rejection? Transplantation 55:1040-1044, 1993.

66. Palmer SM, Davis RD, Hadjiliadis D, et al: Development of an antibody specific to major histocompatibility antigens detectable by flow cytometry after lung transplant is associated with bronchiolitis obliterans syndrome. Transplantation 74:799-804, 2002.

67. Reinsmoen NL, Bolman RM, Savik K, et al: Improved long-term graft outcome in lung transplant recipients who have donor antigen-specific hyporeactivity. J Heart Lung Transplant 13:30-36, discussion 36-37, 1994.

68. Riise GC, Andersson BA, Kjellstrom C, et al: Persistent high BAL fluid granulocyte activation marker levels as early indicators of bronchiolitis obliterans after lung transplant. Eur Respir J 14:1123-1130, 1999.

69. Behr J, Maier K, Braun B, et al: Evidence for oxidative stress in bronchiolitis obliterans syndrome after lung and heart-lung transplantation. The Munich Lung Transplant Group. Transplantation 69:1856-1860, 2000.

70. El-Gamel A, Sim E, Hasleton P, et al: Transforming growth factor beta (TGF-beta) and obliterative bronchiolitis following pulmonary transplantation. J Heart Lung Transplant 17:828-837, 1998.

71. Liu M, Suga M, Maclean AA, et al: Soluble transforming growth factor-beta type III receptor gene transfection inhibits fibrous airway obliteration in a rat model of bronchiolitis obliterans. Am J Respir Crit Care Med 165:419-423, 2002.

72. Charpin JM, Stern M, Grenet D, Israel-Biet D: Insulinlike growth factor-1 in lung transplants with obliterative bronchiolitis. Am J Respir Crit Care Med 161:1991-1998, 2000.

73. Elssner A, Jaumann F, Dobmann S, et al: Elevated levels of interleukin-8 and transforming growth factor-beta in bronchoalveolar lavage fluid from patients with bronchiolitis obliterans syndrome: Proinflammatory role of bronchial epithelial cells. Munich Lung Transplant Group. Transplantation 70:362-367, 2000.

74. Duncan SR, Paradis IL, Yousem SA, et al: Sequelae of cytomegalovirus pulmonary infections in lung allograft recipients. Am Rev Respir Dis 146:1419-1425, 1992.

75. Tazelaar HD, Yousem SA: The pathology of combined heart-lung transplantation: An autopsy study. Hum Pathol 19:1403-1416, 1988.

76. Skeens JL, Fuhrman CR, Yousem SA: Bronchiolitis obliterans in heart-lung transplantation patients: Radiologic findings in 11 patients. AJR Am J Roentgenol 153:253-256, 1989.

77. Morrish WF, Herman SJ, Weisbrod GL, Chamberlain DW: Bronchiolitis obliterans after lung transplantation: Findings at chest radiography and high-resolution CT: The Toronto Lung Transplant Group. Radiology 179:487-490, 1991.

78. Lentz D, Bergin CJ, Berry GJ, et al: Diagnosis of bronchiolitis obliterans in heart-lung transplantation patients: Importance of bronchial dilatation on CT. AJR Am J Roentgenol 159:463-467, 1992.

79. Leung AN, Fisher K, Valentine V, et al: Bronchiolitis obliterans after lung transplantation: Detection using expiratory HRCT. Chest 113:365-370, 1998.

80. Bankier AA, Van Muylem A, Knoop C, et al: Bronchiolitis obliterans syndrome in heart-lung transplant recipients: Diagnosis with expiratory CT. Radiology 218:533-539, 2001.

81. Siegel MJ, Bhalla S, Gutierrez FR, et al: Post-lung transplantation bronchiolitis obliterans syndrome: Usefulness of expiratory thin-section CT for diagnosis. Radiology 220:455-462, 2001.

82. Lee ES, Gotway MB, Reddy GP, et al: Early bronchiolitis obliterans following lung transplantation: Accuracy of expiratory thin-section CT for diagnosis. Radiology 216:472-477, 2000.

83. Choi YW, Rossi SE, Palmer SM, et al: Bronchiolitis obliterans syndrome in lung transplant recipients: Correlation of computed tomography findings with bronchiolitis obliterans syndrome stage. J Thorac Imaging 18:72-79, 2003.

84. Cook RC, Fradet G, Müller NL, et al: Noninvasive investigations for the early detection of chronic airways dysfunction following lung transplantation. Can Respir J 10:76-83, 2003.

85. Nathan SD, Ross DJ, Belman MJ, et al: Bronchiolitis obliterans in single-lung transplant recipients. Chest 107:967-972, 1995.

86. Kramer MR: Bronchiolitis obliterans following heart-lung and lung transplantation. Respir Med 88:9-15, 1994.

87. Reichenspurner H, Girgis RE, Robbins RC, et al: Obliterative bronchiolitis after lung and heart-lung transplantation. Ann Thorac Surg 60:1845-1853, 1995.

88. Kramer MR, Stoehr C, Whang JL, et al: The diagnosis of obliterative bronchiolitis after heart-lung and lung transplantation: Low yield of transbronchial lung biopsy. J Heart Lung Transplant 12:675-681, 1993.

89. Ward C, Snell GI, Zheng L, et al: Endobronchial biopsy and bronchoalveolar lavage in stable lung transplant recipients and chronic rejection. Am J Respir Crit Care Med 158:84-91, 1998.

90. Reynaud-Gaubert M, Thomas P, Badier M, et al: Early detection of airway involvement in obliterative bronchiolitis after lung transplantation. Functional and bronchoalveolar lavage cell findings. Am J Respir Crit Care Med 161:1924-1929, 2000.

91. Estenne M, Maurer JR, Boehler A, et al: Bronchiolitis obliterans syndrome 2001: An update of the diagnostic criteria. J Heart Lung Transplant 21:297-310, 2002.

92. Stanbrook MB, Kesten S: Bronchial hyperreactivity after lung transplantation predicts early bronchiolitis obliterans. Am J Respir Crit Care Med 160:2034-2039, 1999.

93. Rajagopalan N, Maurer J, Kesten S: Bronchodilator response at low lung volumes predicts bronchiolitis obliterans in lung transplant recipients. Chest 109:405-407, 1996.

94. Estenne M, Van Muylem A, Knoop C, Antoine M: Detection of obliterative bronchiolitis after lung transplantation by indexes of ventilation distribution. Am J Respir Crit Care Med 162:1047-1051, 2000.

95. Chaparro C, Chamberlain D, Maurer J, et al: Bronchiolitis obliterans organizing pneumonia (BOOP) in lung transplant recipients. Chest 110:1150-1154, 1996.

96. Wigle DA, Chaparro C, Humar A, et al: Epstein-Barr virus serology and posttransplant lymphoproliferative disease in lung transplantation. Transplantation 72:1783-1786, 2001.

97. Chadburn A, Cesarman E, Knowles DM: Molecular pathology of posttransplantation lymphoproliferative disorders. Semin Diagn Pathol 14:15-26, 1997.

98. Ramalingam P, Rybicki L, Smith MD, et al: Posttransplant lymphoproliferative disorders in lung transplant patients: The Cleveland Clinic experience. Mod Pathol 15:647-656, 2002.

99. Paranjothi S, Yusen RD, Kraus MD, et al: Lymphoproliferative disease after lung transplantation: Comparison of presentation and outcome of early and late cases. J Heart Lung Transplant 20:1054-1063, 2001.

100. Schenkein DP, Schwartz RS: Neoplasms and transplantation—trading swords for plowshares. N Engl J Med 336:949-950, 1997.

101. Aris RM, Maia DM, Neuringer IP, et al: Post-transplantation lymphoproliferative disorder in the Epstein-Barr virus–naive lung transplant recipient. Am J Respir Crit Care Med 154:1712-1717, 1996.

102. Malouf MA, Chhajed PN, Hopkins P, et al: Anti-viral prophylaxis reduces the incidence of lymphoproliferative disease in lung transplant recipients. J Heart Lung Transplant 21:547-554, 2002.

103. Dodd GD 3rd, Ledesma-Medina J, Baron RL, Fuhrman CR: Posttransplant lymphoproliferative disorder: Intrathoracic manifestations. Radiology 184:65-69, 1992.

104. Carignan S, Staples CA, Müller NL: Intrathoracic lymphoproliferative disorders in the immunocompromised patient: CT findings. Radiology 197:53-58, 1995.

105. Brown MJ, Miller RR, Müller NL: Acute lung disease in the immunocompromised host: CT and pathologic examination findings. Radiology 190:247-254, 1994.

106. Gattuso P, Castelli MJ, Peng Y, Reddy VB: Posttransplant lymphoproliferative disorders: A fine-needle aspiration biopsy study. Diagn Cytopathol 16:392-395, 1997.

107. Trulock EP: Lung transplantation. Am J Respir Crit Care Med 155:789-818, 1997.

108. Pickhardt PJ, Siegel MJ, Anderson DC, et al: Chest radiography as a predictor of outcome in posttransplantation lymphoproliferative disorder in lung allograft recipients. AJR Am J Roentgenol 171:375-382, 1998.

109. Husain AN, Siddiqui MT, Reddy VB, et al: Postmortem findings in lung transplant recipients. Mod Pathol 9:752-761, 1996.

110. Herve P, Silbert D, Cerrina J, et al: Impairment of bronchial mucociliary clearance in long-term survivors of heart/lung and double-lung transplantation. The Paris-Sud Lung Transplant Group. Chest 103:59-63, 1993.

111. Ettinger NA, Trulock EP: Pulmonary considerations of organ transplantation. Part 3. Am Rev Respir Dis 144:433-451, 1991.

112. Horvath J, Dummer S, Loyd J, et al: Infection in the transplanted and native lung after single lung transplantation. Chest 104:681-685, 1993.

113. Low DE, Kaiser LR, Haydock DA, et al: The donor lung: Infectious and pathologic factors affecting outcome in lung transplantation. J Thorac Cardiovasc Surg 106:614-621, 1993.

114. Maurer JR, Tullis DE, Grossman RF, et al: Infectious complications following isolated lung transplantation. Chest 101:1056-1059, 1992.

115. Collins J, Müller NL, Kazerooni EA, Paciocco G: CT findings of pneumonia after lung transplantation. AJR Am J Roentgenol 175:811-818, 2000.

116. Deusch E, End A, Grimm M, et al: Early bacterial infections in lung transplant recipients. Chest 104:1412-1416, 1993.

117. Flume PA, Egan TM, Paradowski LJ, et al: Infectious complications of lung transplantation. Impact of cystic fibrosis. Am J Respir Crit Care Med 149:1601-1607, 1994.

118. Kramer MR, Marshall SE, Starnes VA, et al: Infectious complications in heart-lung transplantation. Analysis of 200 episodes. Arch Intern Med 153:2010-2016, 1993.

119. Malouf MA, Glanville AR: The spectrum of mycobacterial infection after lung transplantation. Am J Respir Crit Care Med 160:1611-1616, 1999.

120. Dromer C, Nashef SA, Velly JF, et al: Tuberculosis in transplanted lungs. J Heart Lung Transplant 12:924-927, 1993.

121. Schulman LL, Scully B, McGregor CC, Austin JH: Pulmonary tuberculosis after lung transplantation. Chest 111:1459-1462, 1997.

122. Shreeniwas R, Schulman LL, Berkmen YM, et al: Opportunistic bronchopulmonary infections after lung transplantation: Clinical and radiographic findings. Radiology 200:349-356, 1996.

123. Milstone AP, Brumble LM, Loyd JE, et al: Active CMV infection before lung transplantation: Risk factors and clinical implications. J Heart Lung Transplant 19:744-750, 2000.

124. Paradis IL, Williams P: Infection after lung transplantation. Semin Respir Infect 8:207-215, 1993.

125. Anderson DJ, Jordan MC: Viral pneumonia in recipients of solid organ transplants. Semin Respir Infect 5:38-49, 1990.

126. Solans EP, Garrity ER Jr, McCabe M, et al: Early diagnosis of cytomegalovirus pneumonitis in lung transplant patients. Arch Pathol Lab Med 119:33-35, 1995.

127. Sanchez JL, Kruger RM, Paranjothi S, et al: Relationship of cytomegalovirus viral load in blood to pneumonitis in lung transplant recipients. Transplantation 72:733-735, 2001.

128. Palmer SM Jr, Henshaw NG, Howell DN, et al: Community respiratory viral infection in adult lung transplant recipients. Chest 113:944-950, 1998.

129. Matar LD, McAdams HP, Palmer SM, et al: Respiratory viral infections in lung transplant recipients: Radiologic findings with clinical correlation. Radiology 213:735-742, 1999.

130. Minari A, Husni R, Avery RK, et al: The incidence of invasive aspergillosis among solid organ transplant recipients and implications for prophylaxis in lung transplants. Transpl Infect Dis 4:195-200, 2002.

131. Kanj SS, Welty-Wolf K, Madden J, et al: Fungal infections in lung and heart-lung transplant recipients. Report of 9 cases and review of the literature. Medicine (Baltimore) 75:142-156, 1996.

132. Mehrad B, Paciocco G, Martinez FJ, et al: Spectrum of *Aspergillus* infection in lung transplant recipients: Case series and review of the literature. Chest 119:169-175, 2001.

133. Westney GE, Kesten S, De Hoyos A, et al: *Aspergillus* infection in single and double lung transplant recipients. Transplantation 61:915-919, 1996.

134. Kramer MR, Denning DW, Marshall SE, et al: Ulcerative tracheobronchitis after lung transplantation. A new form of invasive aspergillosis. Am Rev Respir Dis 144:552-556, 1991.

135. Collins J, Hartman MJ, Warner TF, et al: Frequency and CT findings of recurrent disease after lung transplantation. Radiology 219:503-509, 2001.

136. Garver RI Jr, Zorn GL, Wu X, et al: Recurrence of bronchioloalveolar carcinoma in transplanted lungs. N Engl J Med 340:1071-1074, 1999.

137. King MB, Jessurun J, Hertz MI: Recurrence of desquamative interstitial pneumonia after lung transplantation. Am J Respir Crit Care Med 156:2003-2005, 1997.

138. Frost AE, Keller CA, Brown RW, et al: Giant cell interstitial pneumonitis. Disease recurrence in the transplanted lung. Am Rev Respir Dis 148:1401-1404, 1993.

139. Judson MA, Handy JR, Sahn SA: Pleural effusions following lung transplantation. Time course, characteristics, and clinical implications. Chest 109:1190-1194, 1996.

140. Judson MA, Sahn SA: The pleural space and organ transplantation. Am J Respir Crit Care Med 153:1153-1165, 1996.

141. Nunley DR, Grgurich WF, Keenan RJ, Dauber JH: Empyema complicating successful lung transplantation. Chest 115:1312-1315, 1999.

142. Herridge MS, de Hoyos AL, Chaparro C, et al: Pleural complications in lung transplant recipients. J Thorac Cardiovasc Surg 110:22-26, 1995.

143. Paranjpe DV, Wittich GR, Hamid LW, Bergin CJ: Frequency and management of pneumothoraces in heart-lung transplant recipients. Radiology 190:255-256, 1994.

144. Alvarez A, Algar J, Santos F, et al: Airway complications after lung transplantation: A review of 151 anastomoses. Eur J Cardiothorac Surg 19:381-387, 2001.

145. Herrera JM, McNeil KD, Higgins RS, et al: Airway complications after lung transplantation: Treatment and long-term outcome. Ann Thorac Surg 71:989-993, discussion 993-994, 2001.

146. Semenkovich JW, Glazer HS, Anderson DC, et al: Bronchial dehiscence in lung transplantation: CT evaluation. Radiology 194:205-208, 1995.

147. Herman SJ, Rappaport DC, Weisbrod GL, et al: Single-lung transplantation: Imaging features. Radiology 170:89-93, 1989.

148. Herman SJ: Radiologic assessment after lung transplantation. Radiol Clin North Am 32:663-678, 1994.

149. McAdams HP, Palmer SM, Erasmus JJ, et al: Bronchial anastomotic complications in lung transplant recipients: Virtual bronchoscopy for noninvasive assessment. Radiology 209:689-695, 1998.

150. Quint LE, Whyte RI, Kazerooni EA, et al: Stenosis of the central airways: Evaluation by using helical CT with multiplanar reconstructions. Radiology 194:871-877, 1995.

151. Higgins R, McNeil K, Dennis C, et al: Airway stenoses after lung transplantation: Management with expanding metal stents. J Heart Lung Transplant 13:774-778, 1994.

152. Anzueto A, Levine SM, Tillis WP, et al: Use of the flow-volume loop in the diagnosis of bronchial stenosis after single lung transplantation. Chest 105:934-936, 1994.

153. Clark SC, Levine AJ, Hasan A, et al: Vascular complications of lung transplantation. Ann Thorac Surg 61:1079-1082, 1996.

154. Yousem SA, Paradis IL, Dauber JH, et al: Pulmonary arteriosclerosis in long-term human heart-lung transplant recipients. Transplantation 47:564-569, 1989.

155. Badizadegan K, Perez-Atayde AR: Pathology of lung allografts in children and young adults. Hum Pathol 28:704-713, 1997.

156. Kroshus TJ, Kshettry VR, Hertz MI, Bolman RM 3rd: Deep venous thrombosis and pulmonary embolism after lung transplantation. J Thorac Cardiovasc Surg 110:540-544, 1995.

157. Cheriyan AF, Garrity ER Jr, Pifarre R, et al: Reduced transplant lung volumes after single lung transplantation for chronic obstructive pulmonary disease. Am J Respir Crit Care Med 151:851-853, 1995.

158. Loring SH, Leith DE, Connolly MJ, et al: Model of functional restriction in chronic obstructive pulmonary disease, transplantation, and lung reduction surgery. Am J Respir Crit Care Med 160:821-828, 1999.

159. Pinet C, Estenne M: Effect of preoperative hyperinflation on static lung volumes after lung transplantation. Eur Respir J 16:482-485, 2000.

160. Davis RD Jr, Pasque MK: Pulmonary transplantation. Ann Surg 221:14-28, 1995.

161. Orens JB, Becker FS, Lynch JP 3rd, et al: Cardiopulmonary exercise testing following allogeneic lung transplantation for different underlying disease states. Chest 107:144-149, 1995.

162. Lands LC, Smountas AA, Mesiano G, et al: Maximal exercise capacity and peripheral skeletal muscle function following lung transplantation. J Heart Lung Transplant 18:113-120, 1999.

163. Murciano D, Ferretti A, Boczkowski J, et al: Flow limitation and dynamic hyperinflation during exercise in COPD patients after single lung transplantation. Chest 118:1248-1254, 2000.

164. Mattila IP, Sovijarvi A, Malmberg P, et al: Altered regulation of breathing after bilateral lung transplantation. Eur J Cardiothorac Surg 9:237-241, 1995.

165. Higenbottam T, Jackson M, Rashdi T, et al: Lung rejection and bronchial hyperresponsiveness to methacholine and ultrasonically nebulized distilled water in heart-lung transplantation patients. Am Rev Respir Dis 140:52-57, 1989.

166. TenVergert EM, Essink-Bot ML, Geertsma A, et al: The effect of lung transplantation on health-related quality of life: A longitudinal study. Chest 113:358-364, 1998.

167. Paris W, Diercks M, Bright J, et al: Return to work after lung transplantation. J Heart Lung Transplant 17:430-436, 1998.

168. Schulman LL: Quality of life after lung transplantation. Chest 108:1489-1490, 1995.

169. Soubani AO, Miller KB, Hassoun PM: Pulmonary complications of bone marrow transplantation. Chest 109:1066-1077, 1996.

170. Afessa B, Tefferi A, Litzow MR, et al: Diffuse alveolar hemorrhage in hematopoietic stem cell transplant recipients. Am J Respir Crit Care Med 166:641-645, 2002.

171. Breuer R, Lossos IS, Berkman N, Or R: Pulmonary complications of bone marrow transplantation. Respir Med 87:571-579, 1993.

172. Cahill RA, Spitzer TR, Mazumder A: Marrow engraftment and clinical manifestations of capillary leak syndrome. Bone Marrow Transplant 18:177-184, 1996.

173. Ravenel JG, Scalzetti EM, Zamkoff KW: Chest radiographic features of engraftment syndrome. J Thorac Imaging 15:56-60, 2000.

174. Worthy SA, Flint JD, Müller NL: Pulmonary complications after bone marrow transplantation: High-resolution CT and pathologic findings. Radiographics 17:1359-1371, 1997.

175. Robbins RA, Linder J, Stahl MG, et al: Diffuse alveolar hemorrhage in autologous bone marrow transplant recipients. Am J Med 87:511-518, 1989.

176. Agusti C, Ramirez J, Picado C, et al: Diffuse alveolar hemorrhage in allogeneic bone marrow transplantation. A postmortem study. Am J Respir Crit Care Med 151:1006-1010, 1995.

177. Witte RJ, Gurney JW, Robbins RA, et al: Diffuse pulmonary alveolar hemorrhage after bone marrow transplantation: Radiographic findings in 39 patients. AJR Am J Roentgenol 157:461-464, 1991.

178. Corso S, Vukelja SJ, Wiener D, Baker WJ: Diffuse alveolar hemorrhage following autologous bone marrow infusion. Bone Marrow Transplant 12:301-303, 1993.

179. Afessa B, Tefferi A, Litzow MR, Peters SG: Outcome of diffuse alveolar hemorrhage in hematopoietic stem cell transplant recipients. Am J Respir Crit Care Med 166:1364-1368, 2002.

180. Metcalf JP, Rennard SI, Reed EC, et al: Corticosteroids as adjunctive therapy for diffuse alveolar hemorrhage associated with bone marrow transplantation. University of Nebraska Medical Center Bone Marrow Transplant Group. Am J Med 96:327-334, 1994.

181. Chao NJ, Duncan SR, Long GD, et al: Corticosteroid therapy for diffuse alveolar hemorrhage in autologous bone marrow transplant recipients. Ann Intern Med 114:145-146, 1991.

182. Afessa B, Litzow MR, Tefferi A: Bronchiolitis obliterans and other late onset non-infectious pulmonary complications in hematopoietic stem cell transplantation. Bone Marrow Transplant 28:425-434, 2001.

183. Clark JG, Hansen JA, Hertz MI, et al: NHLBI workshop summary. Idiopathic pneumonia syndrome after bone marrow transplantation. Am Rev Respir Dis 147:1601-1606, 1993.

184. Haddad IY: Idiopathic pneumonia after marrow transplantation: When are antioxidants effective? Am J Respir Crit Care Med 166:1532-1534, 2002.

185. Shankar G, Scott Bryson J, Darrell Jennings C, et al: Idiopathic pneumonia syndrome after allogeneic bone marrow transplantation in mice. Role of pretransplant radiation conditioning. Am J Respir Cell Mol Biol 20:1116-1124, 1999.

186. Crawford SW, Hackman RC: Clinical course of idiopathic pneumonia after bone marrow transplantation. Am Rev Respir Dis 147:1393-1400, 1993.

187. Philit F, Wiesendanger T, Archimbaud E, et al: Post-transplant obstructive lung disease ("bronchiolitis obliterans"): A clinical comparative study of bone marrow and lung transplant patients. Eur Respir J 8:551-558, 1995.

188. Padley SP, Adler BD, Hansell DM, Müller NL: Bronchiolitis obliterans: High resolution CT findings and correlation with pulmonary function tests. Clin Radiol 47:236-240, 1993.

189. Krowka MJ, Rosenow EC 3rd, Hoagland HC: Pulmonary complications of bone marrow transplantation. Chest 87:237-246, 1985.
190. Clark JG, Crawford SW, Madtes DK, Sullivan KM: Obstructive lung disease after allogeneic marrow transplantation. Clinical presentation and course. Ann Intern Med 111:368-376, 1989.
191. Beschorner WE, Saral R, Hutchins GM, et al: Lymphocytic bronchitis associated with graft-versus-host disease in recipients of bone-marrow transplants. N Engl J Med 299:1030-1036, 1978.
192. O'Brien KD, Hackman RC, Sale GE, et al: Lymphocytic bronchitis unrelated to acute graft-versus-host disease in canine marrow graft recipients. Transplantation 37:233-238, 1984.
193. Crawford SW: Bone-marrow transplantation and related infections. Semin Respir Infect 8:183-190, 1993.
194. Matulis M, High KP: Immune reconstitution after hematopoietic stem-cell transplantation and its influence on respiratory infections. Semin Respir Infect 17:130-139, 2002.
195. Ettinger NA, Trulock EP: Pulmonary considerations of organ transplantation. Part 2. Am Rev Respir Dis 144:213-223, 1991.
196. Hoyle C, Goldman JM: Life-threatening infections occurring more than 3 months after BMT: 18 UK Bone Marrow Transplant Teams. Bone Marrow Transplant 14:247-252, 1994.
197. Gosselin MV, Adams RH: Pulmonary complications in bone marrow transplantation. J Thorac Imaging 17:132-144, 2002.
198. Konoplev S, Champlin RE, Giralt S, et al: Cytomegalovirus pneumonia in adult autologous blood and marrow transplant recipients. Bone Marrow Transplant 27:877-881, 2001.
199. Horak DA, Schmidt GM, Zaia JA, et al: Pretransplant pulmonary function predicts cytomegalovirus-associated interstitial pneumonia following bone marrow transplantation. Chest 102:1484-1490, 1992.
200. Barloon TJ, Galvin JR, Mori M, et al: High-resolution ultrafast chest CT in the clinical management of febrile bone marrow transplant patients with normal or nonspecific chest roentgenograms. Chest 99:928-933, 1991.
201. Graham NJ, Müller NL, Miller RR, Shepherd JD: Intrathoracic complications following allogeneic bone marrow transplantation: CT findings. Radiology 181:153-156, 1991.
202. Heussel CP, Kauczor HU, Heussel G, et al: Early detection of pneumonia in febrile neutropenic patients: Use of thin-section CT. AJR Am J Roentgenol 169:1347-1353, 1997.
203. Seber A, Khan SP, Kersey JH: Unexplained effusions: Association with allogeneic bone marrow transplantation and acute or chronic graft-versus-host disease. Bone Marrow Transplant 17:207-211, 1996.
204. Williams LM, Fussell S, Veith RW, et al: Pulmonary veno-occlusive disease in an adult following bone marrow transplantation. Case report and review of the literature. Chest 109:1388-1391, 1996.
205. Kolb HJ, Socie G, Duell T, et al: Malignant neoplasms in long-term survivors of bone marrow transplantation. Late Effects Working Party of the European Cooperative Group for Blood and Marrow Transplantation and the European Late Effect Project Group. Ann Intern Med 131:738-744, 1999.
206. Bhatia S, Ramsay NK, Steinbuch M, et al: Malignant neoplasms following bone marrow transplantation. Blood 87:3633-3639, 1996.
207. Crawford SW, Pepe M, Lin D, et al: Abnormalities of pulmonary function tests after marrow transplantation predict nonrelapse mortality. Am J Respir Crit Care Med 152:690-695, 1995.
208. Carlson K, Backlund L, Smedmyr B, et al: Pulmonary function and complications subsequent to autologous bone marrow transplantation. Bone Marrow Transplant 14:805-811, 1994.
209. Crawford SW, Fisher L: Predictive value of pulmonary function tests before marrow transplantation. Chest 101:1257-1264, 1992.
210. Torbenson M, Wang J, Nichols L, et al: Causes of death in autopsied liver transplantation patients. Mod Pathol 11:37-46, 1998.
211. Chan ED, Morales DV, Welsh CH, et al: Calcium deposition with or without bone formation in the lung. Am J Respir Crit Care Med 165:1654-1669, 2002.
212. O'Brien JD, Ettinger NA: Pulmonary complications of liver transplantation. Clin Chest Med 17:99-114, 1996.
213. Sankey EA, Crow J, Mallett SV, et al: Pulmonary platelet aggregates: Possible cause of sudden peroperative death in adults undergoing liver transplantation. J Clin Pathol 46:222-227, 1993.
214. Gosseye S, van Obbergh L, Weynand B, et al: Platelet aggregates in small lung vessels and death during liver transplantation. Lancet 338:532-534, 1991.
215. Agusti AG, Roca J, Rodriguez-Roisin R: Mechanisms of gas exchange impairment in patients with liver cirrhosis. Clin Chest Med 17:49-66, 1996.
216. Martinez GP, Barbera JA, Visa J, et al: Hepatopulmonary syndrome in candidates for liver transplantation. J Hepatol 34:651-657, 2001.
217. Herve P, Lebrec D, Brenot F, et al: Pulmonary vascular disorders in portal hypertension. Eur Respir J 11:1153-1166, 1998.
218. Krowka MJ, Porayko MK, Plevak DJ, et al: Hepatopulmonary syndrome with progressive hypoxemia as an indication for liver transplantation: Case reports and literature review. Mayo Clin Proc 72:44-53, 1997.
219. Arguedas MR, Abrams GA, Krowka MJ, Fallon MB: Prospective evaluation of outcomes and predictors of mortality in patients with hepatopulmonary syndrome undergoing liver transplantation. Hepatology 37:192-197, 2003.

CHAPTER TWELVE

EMBOLIC AND THROMBOTIC DISEASES OF THE LUNGS

PULMONARY THROMBOSIS

Although embolization is undoubtedly the most frequent mechanism invoked to explain the presence of intrapulmonary thrombus, in situ thrombosis of pulmonary vessels is probably more common than is generally appreciated. The pathogenesis and the effects of such thrombosis are related to a large extent to the particular vessels affected.

Pulmonary Arteries

The most common cause of in situ arterial thrombosis is probably infectious pneumonia; the vascular damage in this situation occurs adjacent to an abscess or a focus of granulomatous inflammation. Thrombosis related to a primary or metastatic neoplasm is also frequent as a result of invasion of the vessel by the neoplasm or vascular compression by expanding tumor. Less common causes include immune-mediated vasculitis,[1] aneurysm,[2] use of an intravascular catheter,[3] and sickle cell trait or disease.[4] It is also likely that propagation of thrombus proximal to peripheral

thromboemboli is responsible for some cases of chronic thrombosis of major pulmonary arteries.[5]

Pathologically, in situ arterial thrombosis should be suspected if there is adjacent parenchymal disease or an associated vascular abnormality known to cause thrombosis (e.g., vasculitis or carcinoma). Despite these diagnostic clues, the distinction between in situ thrombosis and embolism can be difficult and, in some cases, impossible.

Since thrombosis occurs most often in arteries supplying lung that is already involved by disease, the role of the thrombus in determining radiologic or clinical manifestations is probably limited in most cases. An exception is the necrosis and cavitation that develop in some cases of pneumonia (lung "gangrene") or vasculitis, the pathogenesis being related at least in part to the thrombosis and resulting ischemia. Thrombosis has also been implicated as a cause of sudden death in patients who have sickle cell disease.[6]

Pulmonary Arterioles and Capillaries

Thrombosis of small pulmonary vessels occurs frequently in immune-mediated capillaritis (microangiitis); in this situation, it is usually associated with other evidence of vascular damage, particularly parenchymal hemorrhage. In addition, fibrin thrombi can be found in the small vessels of patients who have disseminated intravascular coagulation (DIC) related to such conditions as septicemia and amniotic fluid embolism.[7,8] Pulmonary microvascular thrombosis (sometimes associated with DIC) is also frequent in the early stage of acute respiratory distress syndrome (ARDS) and, in fact, has been implicated in its pathogenesis. In situ thrombosis of small pulmonary vessels can occur in sickle cell disease as well and may be responsible for some cases of acute chest syndrome in patents with this condition.[4]

Pulmonary Veins

As in the arterial circulation, pulmonary venous thrombosis commonly develops secondary to a focus of infectious pneumonia or a neoplasm. Other related conditions include those in which there is decreased blood flow (e.g., tetralogy of Fallot),[9] fibrosing mediastinitis (occasionally associated with pulmonary infarction),[10] and veno-occlusive disease; in fact, venous thrombosis has been thought to be intimately involved in the pathogenesis of veno-occlusive disease.

PULMONARY THROMBOEMBOLISM

Emboli of fragments of thrombus to the pulmonary vasculature are common and range from minute fibrin-platelet aggregates unassociated with clinical, radiologic, or functional consequences to massive clots that completely occlude the pulmonary trunk and cause sudden death. Because pulmonary thromboembolism (PTE) by definition implies the formation of thrombi elsewhere than the lungs, the two processes are frequently discussed together under the term *venous thromboembolic disease* (VTED). The term *deep venous thrombosis* (DVT) usually implies thrombosis of the deep veins of the leg, the most common site of clinically significant thrombosis.

Epidemiology

The precise incidence of VTED and its relationship to patient morbidity and mortality are difficult to determine for several reasons. Up to 80% of patients who have PTE are asymptomatic[11]; moreover, when signs and symptoms are present, they lack sensitivity and specificity.[12] Both these features are associated with underdiagnosis. Another factor that has the same effect is the failure of many physicians to appreciate the poor sensitivity of clinical examination to detect DVT[13]; as a result, the possibility of PTE may not be considered in patients who do not have clinical signs of DVT and appropriate diagnostic testing is not performed. Finally, even when PTE is included as part of the differential diagnosis, diagnostic criteria are uneven.[14]

With these caveats in mind, the reported incidence of DVT depends largely on the specific risk factors of the population studied and whether the diagnosis is made during screening or at the onset of symptoms. As an example, DVT develops in the vast majority of patients who have undergone hip replacement in the absence of anticoagulation prophylaxis,[15] when

assessed prospectively; by contrast, DVT was appreciated in only 1.9% of 1162 patients who had this procedure when diagnostic testing was confined to those who were symptomatic.[16] In a recent review and meta-analysis of studies addressing the overall incidence of DVT in the general population, the incidence of initial episodes of DVT per 10,000 population was found to be 5.04.[17] As indicated earlier, however, the risk within specific populations can be much greater. For example, hospitalization was associated with an 8-fold increase in the risk for DVT or PTE; this figure increased to 22-fold when surgery had been performed. The presence of cancer was associated with a fivefold increase in risk. In fact, the risk for DVT increases in proportion to the number of risk factors present.[18] Symptomatic PTE occurs in about 30% of patients who have proximal (thigh) DVT.[19]

The risk for PTE also increases with age.[20] However, it is not clear whether this increase in risk is independent of the conditions that commonly accompany aging, such as heart failure, cancer, and surgical immobilization. Ethnicity may also be a factor in the risk for VTED; for example, there is evidence that Asians have a very low risk for DVT/PTE in comparison to white individuals.[21,22] For unknown reasons, there seems to be a significant seasonal variation in hospital admissions for DVT and PTE, both occurring more commonly in the winter months.[23]

An accurate determination of the frequency of PTE as the sole or significant contributory cause of death is difficult to establish because of the subjectivity involved in such estimation. Although autopsy studies indicate that PTE is a common finding in patients dying in the hospital, it is likely that the majority of emboli have not contributed to death.[24] Reflecting this difficulty, some have concluded that PTE is the sole cause of death in as many as 7% of hospitalized patients and a major contributing cause in an additional 7% to 10%,[25] whereas others have found a figure of only 1%.[26] Nevertheless, the condition is clearly important: it is estimated that more than 200,000 new cases of VTED occur annually in the United States and result in excess of 50,000 deaths[19]; in the vast majority of these cases, the diagnosis is not suspected before death.[27,28] Fortunately, mortality from PTE in the Unites States appears to be declining,[29,30] probably because of improvements in prevention, diagnosis, and treatment.

Etiology and Pathogenesis

The pathogenesis of PTE can be conveniently considered under two headings: (1) factors determining the development of thrombus and (2) consequences to the lungs of the thromboemboli that follow.

Factors Determining the Development of Thrombus

More than 90% of PTEs identified during life originate in the lower extremity.[13] Those confined to the calf generally do not embolize to the lung, whereas those that extend to or arise from the popliteal veins or higher are at risk to do so.[31] Other sites, such as the pelvic veins (including the periprostatic veins in men), the inferior vena cava, and the right atrium, are seen occasionally. Although the arms have been estimated to be the site of thrombus in less than 2% of all cases of DVT,[32] complicating PTE occurs in up to a third of affected patients.[33] As might be expected, thrombus originating in this site is often associated with the use of a central venous catheter.[33] It should be emphasized that the source of thrombus is not found during life in as many as 50% of cases of fatal embolism and may not be identifiable even at autopsy.

The eponymous Virchow's triad of venous stasis, intimal injury, and alteration in coagulation remains the basis of our understanding of the mechanisms of venous thrombosis. Most instances of venous thrombosis and PTE, particularly those that are acute and massive, are associated with medical, surgical, or obstetric conditions that have well-defined risk factors for one or more of these three abnormalities.[34]

Altered Blood Flow. The velocity of blood flow through the systemic veins to the heart depends on cardiac output; resistance to venous flow; the milking action of the local musculature; and, in veins in which they are present, intraluminal valves. Many of the clinical conditions associated with venous thrombosis, particularly in the legs, are related to an abnormality in one or more of these factors.[18,27,35] Such conditions include left-sided heart failure and shock (decreased cardiac output, immobilization); obesity, pregnancy, intra-abdominal tumors, right-sided heart failure, and external pressure from leg casts or bandages (increased resistance to flow); the postsurgical or paraplegic state (immobility with loss or decrease of muscle activity); and varicose veins (valve incompetence). Immobilization, usually as a result of surgery, was the most common risk factor for PTE in the Prospective Investigation of Pulmonary Embolism Diagnosis (PIOPED) study.[36] It also seems likely that prolonged air and other travel constitutes a small but real risk for PTE.[37] An alteration in blood flow resulting in localized areas of turbulence may also be related to the formation of thrombus associated with a variety of indwelling venous catheters.[38,39]

Endothelial Injury. Venous thrombosis secondary to injury or inflammation of the vessel wall (thrombophlebitis) is probably uncommon in patients who have DVT. However, endothelial injury can be a significant factor in some situations in which localized venous trauma occurs, such as hip replacement.[40] It is also likely to be important in the thrombosis associated with bacterial endocarditis, immunologically mediated vasculitis, and trauma related to intravenous devices. Ironically, the contrast medium used to detect venous thrombosis can itself initiate thrombosis, possibly as a result of endothelial damage.[41]

Coagulation Abnormalities. *Thrombophilia* describes a tendency to undergo thrombosis as a result of inherited or acquired disorders of blood coagulation or fibrinolysis.[42] Such disorders frequently interact, and it is thus useful to view the thrombosis as being the result of gene-gene and gene-environment interactions.[42-44] Inherited abnormalities of coagulation have been identified in up to a third of unselected patients who have VTED.[45] They should be particularly suspected in patients in whom VTED develops at a young age or in those who have recurrent thrombosis, thrombosis at an unusual site, recurrent unexplained pregnancy loss, any episode of VTED unassociated with a known risk factor, or a family history of thrombotic disorders.[46,47]

Inherited Thrombophilia. Inherited thrombophilia can be conveniently divided into two groups.[43,45] The first encompasses abnormalities associated with reduced levels of the inhibitors of the coagulation cascade, such as protein C deficiency, protein S deficiency, and antithrombin deficiency. The second group consists of thrombophilia associated with an increased effect of coagulation factors, including factor V Leiden and activated protein C resistance, prothrombin regulatory sequence mutation, and other disorders. Although these abnormalities are more common than those in the first group, the risk for thrombosis is less. In fact, most such patients will not have had a thrombotic event by the age of 60. Moreover, even though the abnormalities are associated with an increased risk for a single thrombotic event, there is evidence that they are not associated with an increased risk for recurrent episodes.[48,49]

Abnormalities causing reduced levels of inhibitors of the coagulation cascade were the first of the inherited thrombophilias to be described. Antithrombin III is an α_2-globulin that inactivates thrombin as well as other procoagulants such as factors XIIa, IXa, XIa, and Xa.[50] Up to 90% of patients who have a deficiency of the substance will have an episode of venous thrombosis before the age of 60 years.[50] The deficiency is rare and occurs in only 0.2% of the general population and 0.5% to 7.5% of patients who have VTED.[43]

Protein C is activated by thrombin complexed to thrombomodulin. In this state, it is a potent anticoagulant that inactivates factors Va and VIIIa, a process requiring its cofactor protein S.[43] A deficiency is found in 0.2% of the normal population and 2.5% to 6.0% of patients who have VTED. Most patients will have a thrombotic event by the age of 60.[50]

Protein S is a vitamin K–dependent protein that serves as a cofactor for activated protein C. Deficiency of protein S can be identified in 1.3% to 5% of patients who have venous thrombosis; its frequency in the general population is unknown.[43] As for protein C deficiency, more than half of the initial thrombotic events are spontaneous; most patients will have an episode of thrombosis by 60 years of age.[50]

Resistance to the anticoagulant effects of activated protein C was first demonstrated when some patients who had thrombotic disorders failed to increase their activated partial thromboplastin time when activated protein C was added to their plasma.[43] About 90% of such individuals have a factor V allele, *factor V Leiden*, that is associated with a single amino acid change at one of the sites on the factor V molecule where it is normally cleaved by activated protein C.[51] It is a common finding and is present in 5% of healthy individuals of North European ancestry, 10% of patients who have venous thrombosis, and 30% to 50% of patients investigated for thrombophilia.[43,45] Despite a 5- to 10-fold increase in risk for DVT in heterozygote carriers and an 80-fold increase in risk in homozygotes, the absolute increase in risk for thrombotic events in patients who have factor V Leiden is relatively low,[52] with most events occurring during high-risk periods such as postoperatively or in association with another thrombophilic disorder.[53]

The prothrombin gene mutation (*G20210A*) occurs in about 4% of the population, in about 5% to 10% of patients who have venous thrombosis, and in about 15% of patients who are investigated for thrombophilia.[43] The mutation is associated with increased basal levels of functionally normal prothrombin. The risk for thrombosis is low, and most patients will not have a thrombotic event before the age of 50. The increase in risk is expressed in the presence of other risk factors and older age.[54]

Increases in the levels of factors VIII, IX, and XI and fibrinogen have been found more commonly in patients who have VTED than in healthy individuals.[55-58] The mechanisms for the increases in their levels have not been elucidated; however, the finding of elevated levels of factor VIII in family members of similarly affected patients suggests a genetic basis in at least some cases. The magnitude of risk seems to be small, similar to that caused by factor V Leiden.

Hyperhomocysteinemia can be congenital or acquired. Although high levels of homocysteine are associated with venous thrombosis,[59] no causal role has yet been established.[60] Some studies, however, have suggested that hyperhomocysteinemia can be synergistic with other defects in promoting VTED, such as factor V Leiden.[61]

Acquired Thrombophilia. A variety of acquired thrombophilias are also important in the pathogenesis of VTED. Their association with malignancy and oral contraceptives is particularly important. The role of antiphospholipid antibodies is discussed in Chapter 10 (see page 483).

Thromboembolic disease affects 10% to 15% of patients who have cancer and is the second most common cause of death in these patients.[62] Mucin-secreting adenocarcinomas of the lung, gastrointestinal tract, and pancreas are particularly associated with the complication; affected patients have an approximately fourfold increased incidence of VTED.[63] Although no particular anomaly is predictive of thrombosis in an individual patient, a number of procoagulant abnormalities have been described, including acquired activated protein C resistance,[64] tissue factor expression and induction by tumor-infiltrating macrophages, cancer cell procoagulant production, alterations in platelet aggregation,[65] macrophage cytokine-induced production of fibrinogen and factor VIII, and suppression of fibrinolytic activity.[66,67] With extensive evaluation, occult cancer has been found in up to 13% of patients who have "idiopathic" DVT[50,63,66]; whether early detection favors improved survival remains to be determined.[68]

Since the 1960s there have been many reports of an increased risk for VTED in women taking oral contraceptives.[69-71] With current agents, the absolute risk is low, the baseline risk of less than 1 per 10,000 person-years being increased to 3 to 4 per 10,000 person-years.[72] The risk is dose related. The major culpable agent is thought to be estrogen,[62] which both augments clotting and impairs fibrinolysis. Higher risk has also been associated with current third-generation progestogens than with earlier agents.[72] An inherited thrombophilic trait significantly increases the risk; for example, women who have the factor V Leiden mutation and use oral contraceptives have a 35-fold increase in VTED risk when compared with factor V Leiden–negative nonusers.[62] Not surprisingly, an increase in risk for VTED is also associated with pregnancy and the puerperium, an increase that worsens in the presence of inherited thrombophilias.[73]

Testing. The optimal time to test for a hypercoagulable state is 6 months after a thrombotic event.[74] Earlier testing is not desirable because of alterations in coagulation factors caused by the thrombosis itself. Most testing can be done while the patient is receiving warfarin. Therapy with low-molecular-weight heparin for a 2-week period allows for subsequent accurate assessment of levels of protein C activity and free protein S antigen. It is important to exclude acquired conditions that could account for abnormal test results, such as liver disease, before accepting a diagnosis of an inherited coagulation disorder.[74]

Consequences to the Lungs of Thromboemboli

A fragment of embolized thrombus lodged within a pulmonary artery has two immediate consequences—an increase in pressure proximal to the thrombus and a decrease or cessation of flow distal to it. Although the effects of thromboemboli are largely a result of these two consequences, the final clinical, radiologic, and pathologic manifestations are modified by a number of factors, including the size of the embolus, the presence of bacteria within the thrombus (septic embolism, see page 564), the presence and extent of underlying lung disease (including previous thromboemboli), and the presence of extrapulmonary disease, particularly of the heart. These manifestations can be discussed under five headings: (1) hemorrhage and infarction, (2) bronchoconstriction and atelectasis, (3) acute pulmonary hypertension, (4) chronic pulmonary hypertension, and (5) edema. The contribution of these abnormalities to the gas exchange derangements that follow PTE is discussed at the end of this section.

Hemorrhage and Infarction. Excluding septic embolism, parenchymal consolidation secondary to occlusion of a pulmonary artery is due to either hemorrhage alone or to hemorrhage with necrosis of lung parenchyma (infarction). Because clinical and radiographic findings seldom permit reliable differentiation between the two, at least in their early stages, they are usually referred to by the single term "infarction." Apart from pathologic examination, the true nature of the abnormality can be determined only by observing its radiologic evolution: should follow-up examinations show rapid clearing, it is reasonable to consider a lesion to be caused by hemorrhage alone; should the opacity clear slowly over a period of several weeks, the inference can be made that the vascular insult resulted in tissue death.

Although the precise pathogenesis of pulmonary hemorrhage after thromboembolism has not been clearly established, the probable mechanism is ischemic damage to endothelial and alveolar epithelial cells and subsequent passage of red blood cells and edema into the air spaces. The hemorrhage has been thought to be derived from the bronchial arteries via bronchopulmonary anastomoses,[75] but it may also come from the pulmonary artery itself when the vessel is only partly occluded or after fibrinolysis has partly reopened the vessel.

It is unclear why some thromboemboli have no effect on the lung parenchyma or result in hemorrhage alone whereas others cause infarction. However, it is known that pulmonary vascular occlusion usually results in no permanent tissue damage unless other factors coexist[76]; in fact, the results of some autopsy reviews suggest that the frequency of infarction is as low as 10% to 15% of all cases of thromboemboli.[77] The most common underlying condition that predisposes to infarction is congestive heart failure, an association believed to be explained by increased pulmonary venous pressure and the resulting decreased bronchial artery blood flow. Other conditions associated with an increased likelihood of infarction include shock, malignancy, multiple emboli, and the presence of peripheral (as opposed to central) emboli.[78,79]

Bronchoconstriction and Atelectasis. The pathophysiologic consequences of sudden occlusion of a pulmonary vessel include a local decrease in compliance and ventilation caused at least partly by bronchoconstriction. This may result from decreased PCO_2 within the airways supplying the occluded segment[80] or from the release of vasoactive and bronchoconstrictive substances such as serotonin, prostaglandins, and histamine. Although such bronchoconstriction may in part be a cause of loss of lung volume, it is likely that it is attributable mostly to surfactant depletion. This manifestation of PTE is a common radiographic finding and is usually more striking when accompanied by infarction.[81] Although physiologic evidence of bronchoconstriction is common in patients who have PTE, wheezing is uncommon and more likely to be evident in patients who have asthma.[82]

Acute Pulmonary Hypertension. Information regarding the precise hemodynamic changes in humans after PTE is of necessity imprecise. The measurements that have been obtained are from a survivor population, and premorbid data regarding baseline hemodynamics in affected patients are not usually available for comparison with postembolic findings.[83] Nevertheless, certain observations concerning hemodynamic changes can be made.

In patients who do not have underlying cardiopulmonary disease, PTE increases pulmonary arterial pressure, the rise depending on both mechanical blockage and the increase in venous return as a result of hypoxemia-induced increase in sympathetic tone.[84] However, these factors alone cannot explain the importance of the increase in pressure that has been observed,[85] and it is likely that neural or humoral mechanisms, or both, are implicated.[86,87] In previously healthy individuals, the severity of pulmonary hypertension correlates with the severity of vascular occlusion; however, mean pulmonary artery pressures greater than 40 mm Hg are rarely seen in the absence of pre-embolic cardiopulmonary disease or a history of otherwise unrecognized recurrent PTE.[88]

Although patients with small PTE may have no symptoms or signs, occlusion of a major portion of the pulmonary arterial system almost invariably results in acute pulmonary hypertension and right-sided heart failure. However, pulmonary hypertension is not sustained in patients who do not have previous cardiopulmonary disease until at least 50% of the pulmonary vascular tree is occluded.[89] When an increase in pulmonary artery pressure is discovered in patients with recent PTE, it is usually necessary to exclude previous embolic occlusions or underlying disease. In patients who have COPD, measurement of FEV_1 as an indicator of the severity of disease may be useful in assessing its contribution to the elevation in pulmonary artery pressure.[90] In practical terms, a large thromboembolus in a patient who has normal cardiopulmonary reserve may have the same hemodynamic and clinical outcome as a smaller embolus in a patient who has impaired cardiopulmonary reserve.[91]

Chronic Pulmonary Hypertension. It has been estimated that chronic hypertension will develop in up to 1% of patients who have PTE (see page 596).[92] Although classically this has been attributed to recurrent emboli[93] and failure of clot to resolve,[94] clinical and pathologic observations and findings at surgery suggest that it is more often the result of propagation of clot in situ and secondary structural changes in the pulmonary vasculature not directly affected by thrombus.[95] It is likely that vasoconstriction is also important, since the hypertension is partially reversible after the administration of vasodilating agents in some patients.[96] Systemic procoagulant states are identified in less than 10% of patients.[97] Through mechanisms of ventricular interdependence, left ventricular systolic and diastolic performance is impaired in patients who have chronic thromboembolic pulmonary hypertension; these effects are reversible after thromboendarterectomy and only rarely result in clinical evidence of pulmonary edema.[98]

Edema. Diffuse pulmonary edema is sometimes seen in patients who have PTE.[99] In many, this edema is the result of independent heart failure at the time of the embolic episode. In others, it is possible that the systemic hypotension that results from right ventricular failure impairs coronary perfusion and causes acute myocardial ischemia.[91] However, increased permeability edema has also been reported in some patients,[100] and data from animal experiments suggest that obstruction of the pulmonary vasculature can precipitate edema via humoral mechanisms.[101]

Gas Exchange Abnormalities. Hypoxemia and hypocapnia are common in patients who have PTE; however, it cannot be overemphasized that evaluation of gas exchange neither permits nor excludes the diagnosis.[102,103] Obstruction of the vascular bed leads to an increase in dead space ventilation, the magnitude of which may correlate with the degree of vascular obstruction.[104] In some hands, measurement of alveolar dead space, in combination with other tests such as D-dimer assessment, has proved useful in excluding the diagnosis of VTED in a noninvasive manner.[103,105]

Areas of low ventilation-perfusion ($\dot{V}/\dot{Q}$) account for most of the hypoxemia seen in patients who have PTE. Although mechanical diversion of blood to unobstructed vessels explains part of this phenomenon,[106] reflex and humorally mediated bronchoconstriction is probably more significant. Shunt may become important as a cause of hypoxemia when there is perfusion of atelectatic areas or when pulmonary hypertension is associated with opening of the foramen ovale.[107] When the cardiac index falls, a low mixed venous oxygen tension can augment the hypoxemia caused by areas of shunt and $\dot{V}/\dot{Q}$ mismatch.[108] Though not contributing to hypoxemia, a substantial bronchial artery–pulmonary venous shunt develops in chronic thromboembolic pulmonary hypertension.[109]

Pathologic Characteristics

Lung Parenchyma

In the majority of instances, lung parenchyma distal to a pulmonary thromboembolus is either normal or shows only mild atelectasis and minimal intra-alveolar hemorrhage or edema. When changes are more marked, they consist of either hemorrhage alone or a combination of hemorrhage and necrosis.

Parenchymal hemorrhage is grossly similar to infarction in its early stage and consists of a more or less wedge-shaped area of red, consolidated lung. In the absence of tissue death, the blood usually disappears fairly rapidly, and its residue may not be grossly detectable if the lung is examined a week or more after the embolic episode. In the early stages, histologic examination shows only intra-alveolar hemorrhage and edema with intact alveolar walls. Later on, hemosiderin-laden macrophages or interstitial pigment is usually the only evidence of previous damage.

Within 1 or 2 days of thromboembolism, an infarct becomes easily recognizable as a firm, more or less wedge-shaped area of hemorrhagic consolidation typically abutting

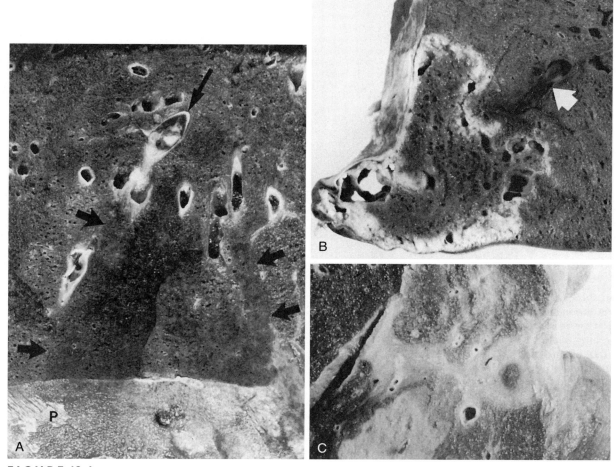

FIGURE 12–1

Pulmonary infarcts: gross appearance. Recent (**A**), organizing (**B**), and remote (**C**) infarcts are illustrated. In **A,** a relatively ill-defined, but roughly triangular focus of hemorrhagic and necrotic lung parenchyma can be seen adjacent to the pleura (*small arrows*). Note the thrombus in the feeding pulmonary artery (*large arrow*) and the fibrinous pleuritis (P). The basal aspect of a lower lobe (**B**) shows a distinct zone of white tissue at the junction of necrotic and viable parenchyma that represents an acute inflammatory reaction to the presence of necrotic tissue; focal cavitation is also evident. Note again the pulmonary artery thrombus (*arrow*) and the residual pleuritis. Such an appearance suggests an interval of several weeks since the original thromboembolic episode. In **C,** an organized infarct in a superior segment of a lower lobe is manifested by a roughly linear band of fibrous tissue associated with pleural puckering. (*A and B from Fraser RS, Müller NL, Colman NC, Paré PD: Fraser and Paré's Diagnosis of Diseases of the Chest, 4th ed. Philadelphia, WB Saunders, 1999. C from Fraser RS: Pathologic characteristics of venous thromboembolism. In Leclerc JR [ed]: Venous Thromboembolic Disorders. Philadelphia, Lea & Febiger, 1991.)*

the pleura (Fig. 12–1 and Color Fig. 12–1). Although it is usually well demarcated, patchy areas of parenchymal hemorrhage may be present adjacent to it (a feature that accounts for the poor definition of infarcts radiographically). Overlying fibrinous pleuritis is often present (see Fig. 12–1). Infarction is usually seen in association with occlusion of segmental or subsegmental arteries.[78]

With time, the necrotic parenchyma becomes clearly demarcated from adjacent lung by a zone of organization tissue that may be red in appearance (reflecting its pronounced vascularity) or distinctly white (as a result of the influx of polymorphonuclear leukocytes (see Fig. 12–1). Cavitation within the infarct usually indicates the presence of superimposed infection (see Color Fig. 12–2). It is typically associated with a prominent leukocytic infiltrate, the enzymes from these cells

presumably causing liquefaction of necrotic tissue as a precursor to drainage and cavity formation. Eventually, the infarcted parenchyma is completely replaced by fibrous tissue, which results in a contracted, somewhat elongated scar frequently associated with pleural puckering (see Fig. 12–1).

Histologically, infarcted lung is manifested by coagulative necrosis of alveolar septa associated with air space hemorrhage and edema. Organization by granulation tissue is identifiable at the periphery after several days (Fig. 12–2). Reactive epithelial changes, particularly of type II pneumocytes, may be seen at the margin of the infarct; when expectorated, these cells occasionally give rise to a false-positive cytologic diagnosis of malignancy.[110] Long-standing infarcts show dense parenchymal fibrosis in which the underlying lung architecture can often still be recognized.

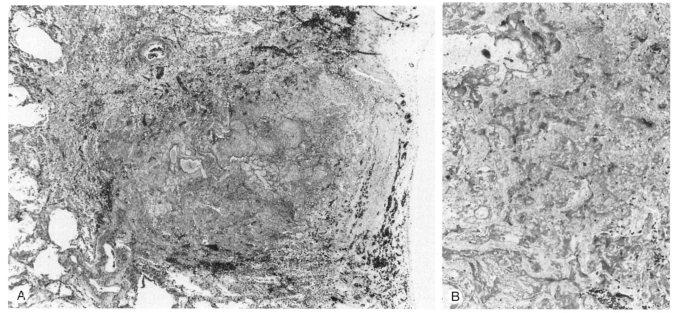

FIGURE 12–2

Organizing pulmonary infarct. A histologic section at low power (**A**) reveals a fairly well demarcated focus of necrotic lung parenchyma surrounded by granulation tissue. A magnified view (**B**) shows coagulative necrosis of lung tissue. *(From Fraser RS, Müller NL, Colman NC, Paré PD: Fraser and Paré's Diagnosis of Diseases of the Chest, 4th ed. Philadelphia, WB Saunders, 1999.)*

Thromboemboli and Pulmonary Vessels

The fate of pulmonary thromboemboli depends on multiple factors, including the status of the patient's fibrinolytic system, the degree of organization of the thrombus before its embolization, and the amount of new thrombus added in situ. Although emboli occasionally change little in size, thereby causing chronic vascular obstruction, the majority are largely degraded by one or more of three mechanisms—lysis, fragmentation and peripheral embolization, and organization and recanalization.

The results of radiologic and perfusion scanning studies in both animals[111] and humans[112,113] have shown that in many cases the flow through obstructed arteries returns relatively rapidly in the first few days after embolization, thus suggesting the presence of fibrinolysis. This process may also be important in preventing additional formation of thrombus in situ. Despite the angiographic evidence of dissolution in many cases, some recent thromboemboli remain intact and can be recognized grossly at autopsy by one or more of three characteristics: (1) the presence of distinct laminations (Fig. 12–3A and B) corresponding to alternating bands of red blood cells and platelet-fibrin aggregates formed during the initial stage of venous thrombosis; (2) adherence to the vessel wall (see Fig 12–3C); and (3) in larger vessels, the presence of a coiled appearance as a result of an imperfect fit and folding of the thrombus as it lodges in the artery (see Fig. 12–3D). Older (organized) thromboemboli may be identified grossly as foci of mural thickening or as fibrous bands or webs traversing the lumen (Fig. 12–4).

In some experimental studies, clots have been observed to fragment into small pieces that embolize farther toward the periphery of the lung.[111] The pathogenesis of this fragmentation may be related to splitting of the thrombus into smaller and smaller pieces as a result of ingrowth of endothelial cells and macrophages from the vessel wall.[114] Similar growth of myofibroblasts, macrophages, and endothelial cells from the vessel wall into the peripheral portion of a thrombus can result in its organization and eventual incorporation into the wall as a fibrous plaque, typically in an eccentric location (Fig. 12–5). Alternatively, some thrombi undergo lysis and organization in their central portion at the same time that they undergo peripheral organization, thereby resulting in the formation of multiple small vascular channels within the original lumen (recanalization) (Fig. 12–6). Although the lumina of such embolized vessels are inevitably diminished in cross-sectional area, these processes undoubtedly result in much greater flow than would have been possible without organization.

Radiographic Manifestations

Most episodes of PTE produce no detectable changes on the chest radiograph. Even if the diagnosis is suspected clinically and confirmed angiographically, no abnormalities are seen in approximately 10% to 15% of cases.[115] Moreover, even when abnormalities are evident, the chest radiograph is of limited value in diagnosis: although the specificity of some abnormalities, such as oligemia, is good, the sensitivity is poor. For example, in a study of 152 patients suspected of having PTE, a predictive index that reflected the overall accuracy of diagnosis was only 0.40.[116] The major value of radiography lies in excluding other disease processes that can mimic PTE, such as pneumonia and pneumothorax, and in providing correlation with $\dot{V}/\dot{Q}$ lung scans.[115-117]

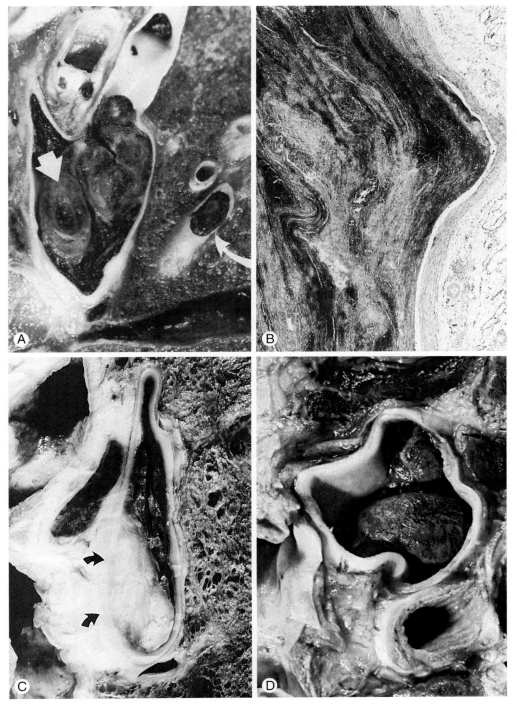

FIGURE 12–3

Thromboemboli: variable appearance. The illustration shows three gross features characteristic of thromboemboli. In **A**, a recent embolus has a laminated appearance (*arrow*) corresponding to alternating layers of red blood cells and fibrin platelet aggregates (also seen in a corresponding histologic section in **B**). Occlusion of a small segmental artery is also apparent (*curved arrow*). In **C**, a remote thromboembolus is largely organized, as evidenced by its fibrous (white) appearance and the indistinct junction between the thrombus and adjacent vessel wall (*arrows*). In **D**, the right interlobar artery is completely occluded by a smooth-surfaced, coiled thrombus. (**B**, ×25.) (*D from Fraser RS: Pathologic characteristics of venous thromboembolism. In Leclerc JR [ed]: Venous Thromboembolic Disorders. Philadelphia, Lea & Febiger, 1991.*)

Thromboembolism without Hemorrhage or Infarction

Changes related to thromboembolism without hemorrhage or infarction include oligemia, change in vessel size, loss of lung volume, and alteration in size and configuration of the heart.
Oligemia. Oligemia is an uncommon manifestation of acute PTE; in a review of the radiographic findings in 123 patients, it was present in only 7 (5%).[118] It may be focal (Westermark's sign), in which case it is usually seen in the periphery of the

lung and is associated with occlusion of a lobar or segmental pulmonary artery (Fig. 12–7). Occasionally, it is generalized as a result of widespread small-vessel occlusion.[81,119] In a study of 1063 patients, the finding had a sensitivity of 14% and a specificity of 92% for the diagnosis.[115]
Changes in the Pulmonary Arteries. Enlargement of a major pulmonary artery (Fleischner's sign) is a helpful sign in diagnosis, particularly when serial radiographs reveal a progressive increase in size of the affected vessel (see Fig. 12–7).[81] Of equal diagnostic importance is abrupt tapering of the

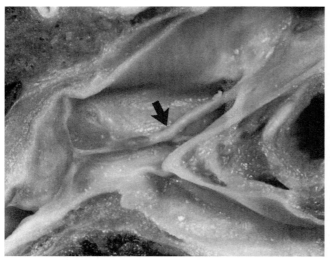

FIGURE 12–4

Remote thromboembolus: intraluminal fibrous bands. A gross specimen of a lobar pulmonary artery and its proximal branches shows a cordlike fibrous band traversing the vessel lumen (*arrow*). This appearance is diagnostic of organized thrombus, most often caused by embolism. (*From Fraser RS, Müller NL, Colman NC, Paré PD: Fraser and Paré's Diagnosis of Diseases of the Chest, 4th ed. Philadelphia, WB Saunders, 1999.*)

occluded vessel distally, in some cases so marked that the so-called knuckle sign is created (see Fig. 12–7).[120] As with oligemia, enlargement of a hilar pulmonary artery is usually seen in patients who have large emboli, and the sign has relatively low sensitivity in diagnosis. In the investigation referred to earlier, a prominent central pulmonary artery was found to have a diagnostic specificity of 80% but a sensitivity of only 20%.[115]

Volume Loss. Loss of volume of a lower lobe associated with PTE may be manifested radiographically by elevation of the hemidiaphragm, downward displacement of the major fissure, or both. In a review of 1063 patients, elevation of the hemidiaphragm had a diagnostic sensitivity and specificity of 20% and 85%, respectively.[115] Another relatively common abnormality is the presence of line shadows representing linear atelectasis, as found in 22% of cases in one study.[121] These shadows are roughly horizontal, usually occur in the lower lung zones, are 1 to 3 mm thick and several centimeters long, and abut the pleural surface.

Cardiac Changes. Radiographic findings suggestive of acute pulmonary artery hypertension are seen in about 10% of patients.[118,122] They occur most often with widespread small emboli. The signs are those of cardiac enlargement as a result of dilation of the right ventricle, an increase in size of the main

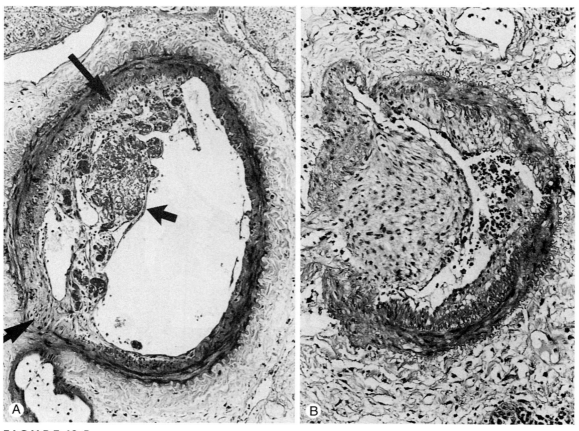

FIGURE 12–5

Pulmonary thromboemboli: organization. A histologic section of a muscular artery of medium size (**A**) shows a small amount of thrombus (*short arrow*) covered by endothelial cells; the thrombus has been partly replaced by fibrous tissue (*long arrows*), which is continuous with the intima. A section of another vessel (**B**) shows a more advanced stage of organization, the thrombus being completely replaced by an eccentric plaque of fibrous tissue. (*From Fraser RS, Müller NL, Colman NC, Paré PD: Fraser and Paré's Diagnosis of Diseases of the Chest, 4th ed. Philadelphia, WB Saunders, 1999.*)

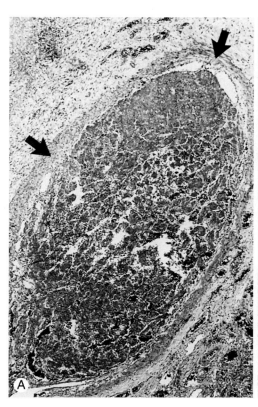
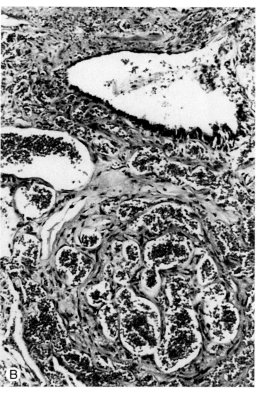

FIGURE 12–6

Pulmonary thromboemboli: recanalization. The photomicrograph on the left (**A**) shows a large muscular pulmonary artery that is almost completely occluded by thrombus. Adherence of the thrombus to the vessel wall as a result of fibroblastic ingrowth is evident at several places (*arrows*). The central portion of the thrombus is partly subdivided into numerous small fragments secondary to lysis and organization; the end result of such processes is often multiple small intraluminal channels (as illustrated in a small muscular artery in **B**). (**A,** ×40; **B,** ×150.) *(From Fraser RS, Müller NL, Colman NC, Paré PD: Fraser and Paré's Diagnosis of Diseases of the Chest, 4th ed. Philadelphia, WB Saunders, 1999.)*

pulmonary artery, and usually, an increase in size and rapidity of tapering of the hilar pulmonary vessels.[123,124]

Thromboembolism with Hemorrhage or Infarction

The radiographic changes in PTE with hemorrhage or infarction consist of segmental areas of consolidation associated with volume loss. Their relative frequency is influenced by the time interval between the onset of symptoms and performance of radiography. In a study of 50 patients who had angiographically documented acute PTE, loss of lung volume as evidenced by elevation of a hemidiaphragm was observed in 50% within 24 hours of the onset of symptoms and in only 15% when symptoms had been present longer.[125] By contrast, pulmonary opacities were found in 37% of patients within 24 hours and 57% thereafter.

In the early stages of infarction, parenchymal opacities are ill defined. They are most common in the base of the right lower lobe, often nestled in the costophrenic sulcus. Most parenchymal opacities involve no more than one or two segments and thus affect a relatively small volume of lung parenchyma; however, the major portion of the lobe is occasionally affected.[126,127] The interval between the embolic episode and the development of an opacity ranges from about 10 hours to several days[128,129]; in one series, the opacity developed within 24 hours in half the patients.[121]

The typical appearance of a pulmonary infarct consists of a homogeneous wedge-shaped area of consolidation in the lung periphery, with its base contiguous to a visceral pleural surface and its rounded, convex apex directed toward the hilum (Fig. 12–8), a configuration known as *Hampton's hump*.[117,128] The consolidated area is usually 3 to 5 cm in diameter but may be as large as 10 cm.[128] Cavitation is rare and generally indicates the presence of a septic embolus.[130]

Pleural Disease

Pleural effusion is seen in 35% to 55% of patients who have documented acute PTE.[115,118] It occurs most commonly in patients who have infarction but may be present in patients who do not have parenchymal consolidation.[115] The amount of fluid is usually small but may be abundant. It is more often unilateral.[128]

Special Radiologic Techniques

Although it is well recognized that pulmonary angiography is the definitive method of establishing a diagnosis of PTE and showing the extent of embolism, the procedure is expensive and time-consuming and may lead to significant morbidity. As a result, V̇/Q̇ scintigraphy has been widely used as an initial screening procedure. More recently, contrast-enhanced CT using a spiral or electron beam technique has become the method of choice in several centers. Other techniques that have a role in the diagnosis of PTE and/or DVT are MR imaging, venography, and ultrasonography.

Scintigraphy

The radiopharmaceuticals of choice for perfusion lung scanning are technetium 99m–labeled human albumin microsphere (^{99m}Tc-HAM) particles or macroaggregated albumin

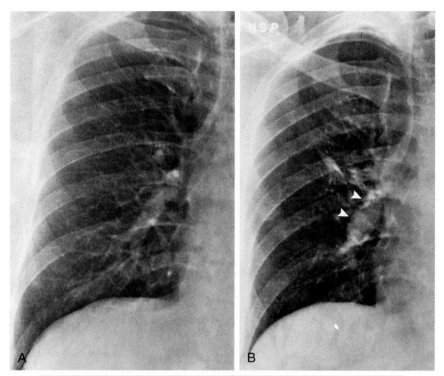

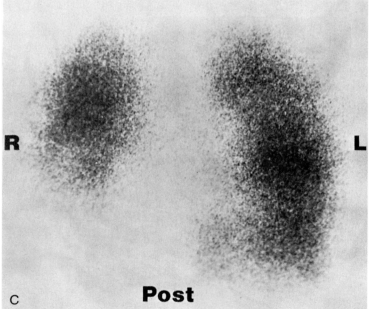

FIGURE 12–7

Pulmonary thromboembolism without infarction. On admission of a 52-year-old man to the hospital, a posteroanterior radiograph (**A**) revealed no significant abnormalities. Several days after abdominal surgery, he experienced an abrupt onset of right chest pain and dyspnea. A radiograph at this time (**B**) showed an obvious increase in diameter and a change in configuration of the right interlobar artery (*arrowheads*); in addition, the distal end of this artery appeared *knuckled* and the vessels peripheral to it diminutive. The right lower zone showed increased radiolucency indicating diminished perfusion (Westermark's sign). A lung scan (**C**) revealed absence of perfusion of the lower half of the right lung. *(From Müller NL, Fraser RS, Colman NC, Paré PD: Radiologic Diagnosis of Diseases of the Chest. Philadelphia, WB Saunders, 2001.)*

(^{99m}Tc-MAA) particles.[131,132] These particles lodge within precapillary pulmonary arterioles; their distribution is proportional to regional pulmonary blood flow at the time of injection. It has been estimated that the particles cause transient blocks in approximately 0.1% of precapillary pulmonary arterioles,[133] thereby providing a static image of regional flow. For diagnostic purposes, at least six views of the lungs should be obtained, including anterior, posterior, right and left lateral, and right and left posterior oblique views. Additional right and left anterior oblique views may be helpful in selected cases.[131,132]

Perfusion scintigraphy is a sensitive but nonspecific technique for identifying pulmonary disease: virtually all parenchymal and airway diseases can cause decreased pulmonary artery blood flow within the affected lung. Because thromboemboli characteristically cause abnormal perfusion with preserved ventilation (mismatched defects) (Fig. 12–9) whereas parenchymal lung disease most often causes ventilation and perfusion abnormalities in the same lung region (matched defects), combined $\dot{V}/\dot{Q}$ scintigraphy is performed routinely in most centers to improve diagnostic specificity. Most experience with ventilation imaging has been with xenon 133.[117]

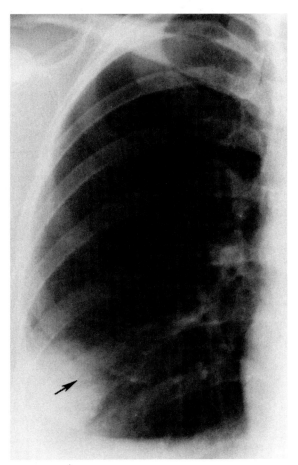

FIGURE 12–8

Pulmonary infarction—Hampton's hump. A view of the right lung from a posteroanterior chest radiograph reveals a homogeneous opacity in the right costophrenic angle with a convex contour *(arrow)* toward the hilum. This appearance constitutes the typical features of Hampton's hump and is highly suggestive of a pulmonary infarct. The patient was a young man who had a history of acute chest pain associated with thrombophlebitis of the right leg. *(From Müller NL, Fraser RS, Colman NC, Paré PD: Radiologic Diagnosis of Diseases of the Chest. Philadelphia, WB Saunders, 2001.)*

With xenon 133, ventilation imaging is generally performed before perfusion imaging.[117] An initial posterior wash-in or first-breath image is acquired; equilibrium images are then obtained while the patient rebreathes the gas within a closed system. The wash-in or breath-hold images show regional lung ventilation. Regions of the lungs that appear as defects on the wash-in images may normalize on the equilibrium image because of collateral ventilation. Finally, serial wash-out images acquired while the patient breathes ambient air allow regional air trapping to be detected as focal areas of retained activity.

Diagnostic Criteria. As indicated, the diagnosis of PTE by scintigraphy is based on the presence of $\dot{V}/\dot{Q}$ mismatch, that is, the presence of ventilation in the absence of perfusion distal to obstructing emboli. The findings are classified in terms of probability of embolism, the most commonly used reporting terms being normal, near-normal, low, intermediate, and high.

TABLE 12–1. Revised PIOPED Criteria for Interpretation of Ventilation-Perfusion Images

Probability of Pulmonary Embolism	Diagnostic Criteria
High probability (≥80%)	Two or more large mismatched segmental perfusion defects or the arithmetic equivalent in moderate or large and moderate defects, i.e., one large plus two or more moderate defects or four or more moderate mismatches
Intermediate probability (20%-79%)	One moderate plus one large mismatched segmental perfusion defect or the arithmetic equivalent in moderate defects
	One matched ventilation-perfusion defect with a normal chest radiograph. Difficult to categorize as low or high or not described as low or high
Low probability (≤19%)	Nonsegmental perfusion defects (e.g., cardiomegaly, enlarged aorta, enlarged hila, elevated diaphragm). Any perfusion defect with a substantially larger abnormality at chest radiography
	Perfusion defects matched by ventilation abnormality provided that there are (1) normal chest radiographs and (2) some areas of normal perfusion in the lungs
	Any number of small perfusion defects with a normal chest radiograph
Normal	No perfusion defects or perfusion defects that outline exactly the shape of the lungs seen on the chest radiograph (hilar and aortic impressions may be seen, and the chest radiograph and/or ventilation scan may be abnormal)

Modified from Gottschalk A, Sostman HD, Coleman RE, et al: Ventilation-perfusion scintigraphy in the PIOPED study. Part II. Evaluation of the scintigraphic criteria and interpretations. J Nucl Med 34:1119-1126, 1993; and Sostman HD, Coleman RE, DeLong DM, et al: Evaluation of revised criteria for ventilation-perfusion scintigraphy in patients with suspected pulmonary embolism. Radiology 193:103-107, 1994.

Several diagnostic criteria have been suggested for interpretation of $\dot{V}/\dot{Q}$ lung scans,[134,135] many of which criteria were assessed in the PIOPED study.[36] In an investigation comparing various diagnostic algorithms, the original PIOPED criteria had the highest likelihood ratio for predicting the presence of emboli on pulmonary angiography.[136] Use of these criteria was associated with the highest proportion of $\dot{V}/\dot{Q}$ scans being interpreted as intermediate probability, however. Several amendments to the original PIOPED criteria have been made (Table 12–1).[131,135] By using the revised criteria, it is possible to decrease the number of intermediate-probability interpretations and classify them correctly as low probability.

Several criteria have been identified that have a positive predictive value (PPV) of less than 10% for PTE,[137] including nonsegmental perfusion abnormalities (PPV = 8%), matched $\dot{V}/\dot{Q}$ abnormalities in two or three zones of a single lung (PPV = 3%), and one to three perfusion defects involving less than 25% of a segment (PPV = 1%). These abnormalities constitute criteria for a very-low-probability interpretation and increase the utility of $\dot{V}/\dot{Q}$ scintigraphy in the assessment of patients who have suspected acute PTE. Use of the revised PIOPED criteria has been shown in clinical studies to provide a more accurate assessment of angiographically proven PTE than has use of the original criteria.[131,138]

Diagnostic Accuracy. In a random sample of 931 patients who underwent scintigraphy in the PIOPED study, 13% had high-probability scans, 39% had intermediate-probability

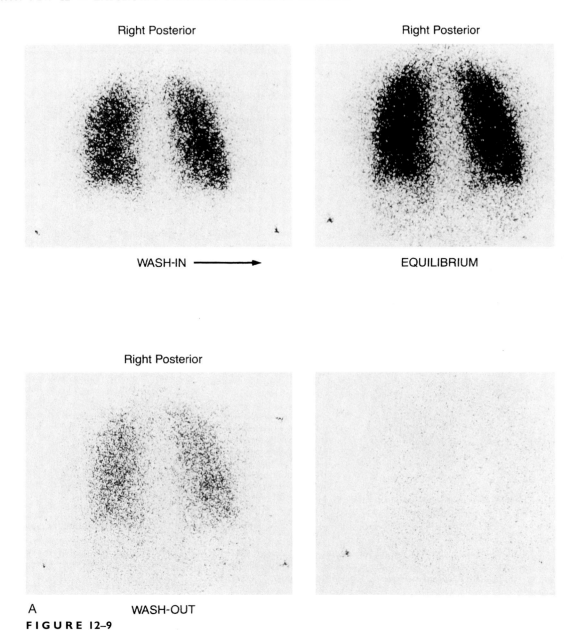

FIGURE 12–9

Value of ventilation-perfusion lung scans in the diagnosis of thromboembolism. A xenon 133 posterior inhalation lung scan (**A**) shows normal ventilation parameters during the wash-in, equilibrium, and wash-out phases.

scans, 34% had low-probability scans, and 14% had normal or near-normal scans.[36] There was good agreement for classifying $\dot{V}/\dot{Q}$ scans as high probability (95%) or as normal (94%); however, there was 25% to 75% disagreement in interpreting intermediate-probability and low-probability scans.[36] Of the 931 patients, 755 underwent pulmonary angiography. Of those who had high-probability scans and a definitive diagnosis at angiography, 88% had emboli as compared with 33% of patients who had intermediate-probability scans, 16% who had low-probability scans, and 9% who had near-normal or normal scans. The sensitivity, specificity, and PPV of $\dot{V}/\dot{Q}$ scanning for detecting acute PTE in this study are presented in Table 12–2. The diagnostic value was not significantly different between men and women, patients of different ages, or

patients who had preexisting cardiac or pulmonary disease when compared with patients who had no such disease.[139,140] In a subset of patients who had COPD, the sensitivity of a high-probability scan was significantly lower than that in patients who had no preexisting cardiopulmonary disease[141]; however, the PPV of a high-probability scan was 100%, and the negative predictive value of a low-probability or very-low-probability scan was 94%.

Although clinical assessment of patients who have suspected PTE does not lead to a definitive diagnosis in most instances, the results from the PIOPED study emphasize the importance of incorporating the pretest clinical likelihood of PTE into the overall diagnostic evaluation (Table 12–3). In patients who have low-probability or very-low-probability

Anterior

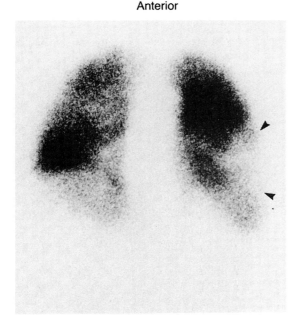

Posterior

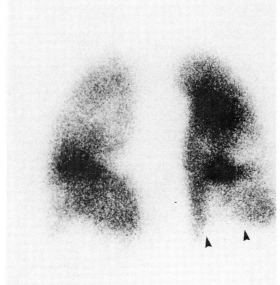

Right Posterior Oblique

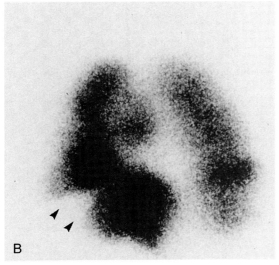

Left Posterior Oblique

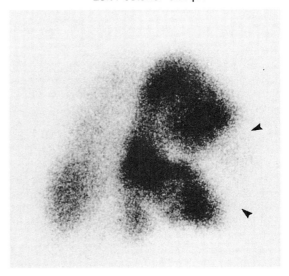

FIGURE 12–9—cont'd

Corresponding technetium 99m MAA perfusion lung scans (**B**) in the anterior, posterior, and right and left posterior oblique projections identify multiple segmental filling defects throughout both lungs (*arrowheads*). These findings, in concert with the ventilation study, are virtually diagnostic (high probability) of pulmonary thromboembolism. The patient was a 65-year-old man with acute dyspnea. (*From Müller NL, Fraser RS, Colman NC, Paré PD: Radiologic Diagnosis of Diseases of the Chest. Philadelphia, WB Saunders, 2001.*)

$\dot{V}/\dot{Q}$ scans and no history of immobilization, recent surgery, trauma to the lower extremities, or central venous instrumentation, the prevalence of PTE was only 4.5%.[142] By contrast, in patients who had low-probability or very-low-probability scan interpretations and one risk factor, the prevalence was 12%, whereas in patients who had two or more risk factors, the prevalence was 21%. In the PIOPED study, however, most patients had intermediate-probability or low-probability $\dot{V}/\dot{Q}$ scans and an intermediate clinical likelihood of PTE; for these patients, the combination of clinical assessment and $\dot{V}/\dot{Q}$ scans does not provide adequate information to direct patient management accurately.

Patients with COPD have a greater likelihood of having intermediate-probability $\dot{V}/\dot{Q}$ scans. In an investigation of

TABLE 12–2. Sensitivity, Specificity, and Positive Predictive Value of Ventilation-Perfusion Lung Scanning for Detecting Acute Pulmonary Embolism Using the Original PIOPED Interpretation Criteria

$\dot{V}/\dot{Q}$ Scan Interpretation	Sensitivity (%)	Specificity (%)	PPV (%)
High	40	98	87
High, intermediate	82	64	49
High, intermediate, low	98	12	32

PPV, positive predictive value; $\dot{V}/\dot{Q}$, ventilation-perfusion.
Results based on the study by Worsley DF, Palevsky HI, Alavi A: A detailed evaluation of patients with acute pulmonary embolism and low- or very-low-probability lung scan interpretations. Arch Intern Med 154:2737-2741, 1994.

TABLE 12–3. Effect of Selected Risk Factors on the Prevalence of Pulmonary Embolism

$\dot{V}/\dot{Q}$ Scan Interpretation	0 Risk Factor*	1 Risk Factor*	≥2 Risk Factors*
High	63/77 (82%)	41/49 (84%)	56/58 (97%)
Intermediate	52/207 (25%)	40/107 (37%)	77/173 (45%)
Low/very low	14/315 (4%)	19/155 (12%)	37/179 (21%)

*Risk factors include immobilization, trauma to the lower extremities, surgery, or central venous instrumentation within 3 months of enrollment.
Results based on the study by Worsley DF, Palevsky HI, Alavi A: A detailed evaluation of patients with acute pulmonary embolism and low- or very-low-probability lung scan interpretations. Arch Intern Med 154:2737-2741, 1994.

108 patients who had COPD and who were suspected of having PTE (21 of whom had the diagnosis confirmed by angiography), high-probability, intermediate-probability, low-probability, and normal-probability scan results were present in 5%, 60%, 30%, and 5%, respectively.[141] The frequency of PTE in these categories was 100%, 22%, 2%, and 0%, respectively.

One group of investigators assessed the accuracy of chest radiography in predicting the extent of airway disease in patients who had suspected PTE.[143] The investigators found that $\dot{V}/\dot{Q}$ scans were indeterminate in all 21 patients who had radiographic evidence of widespread COPD, in 35% of patients who had focal obstructive disease, and in only 18% of patients whose chest radiographs revealed no evidence of COPD.[143] They concluded that ventilation imaging is probably not warranted in patients who have radiographic evidence of widespread COPD.

In summary, approximately 15% of patients with PTE have high-probability $\dot{V}/\dot{Q}$ scans, 40% have intermediate-probability scans, 30% have low-probability scans, and 15% have normal or near-normal scan results.[36] Approximately 90% of those with high-probability scans have PTE versus 30% of patients who have intermediate-probability scans, 15% who have low-probability scans, and 10% who have normal or near-normal scans.[36,144] The diagnostic accuracy can be improved by combining the results of $\dot{V}/\dot{Q}$ scanning with the clinical impression.[36] However, even under optimal circumstances of excellent clinical assessment and expert interpretation of lung scans, further investigation is often required.

Computed Tomography

The introduction of spiral CT and ultrafast electron beam CT technology in the late 1980s has made it possible to image the entire chest in a short time, often during a single breath-hold. When used with intravenous contrast material, these techniques (CT angiography) have high sensitivity and specificity for the detection of emboli in the main, lobar, and segmental pulmonary arteries.[145-147] Imaging of the chest with single-detector spiral CT scanners was typically performed with the use of relatively thick sections (3- to 5-mm collimation). Assessment of the pulmonary vessels has been improved considerably with the introduction of multidetector row (4, 8, and since 2002, 16 rows) CT scanners and greater rotation speeds.[148,149] These scanners allow imaging of the entire chest with 1- to 1.5-mm sections within a short breath-hold (10 seconds or less). The improved spatial resolution provided by the thin sections allows accurate analysis of pulmonary arteries down to the fifth order[150] and thus results in improved accuracy in the identification of segmental and, in many cases, even subsegmental emboli.[151,152]

Vascular Findings

Acute Thromboembolism. The diagnosis of acute PTE on contrast-enhanced CT scan is based on the presence of partial or complete intravascular filling defects.[145,146] The former is defined as a central or marginal area of low attenuation surrounded by a variable amount of contrast material (Fig. 12–10); the latter is defined as an area of low attenuation that occupies the entire arterial section (i.e., by the abrupt absence of contrast material in a clearly evident vessel) (Fig. 12–11).[145,153] The most reliable sign of an acute embolus is a filling defect that forms an acute angle with the vessel wall outlined by contrast material. Although a defect that forms a smooth, obtuse angle with the vessel wall or a complete cutoff of contrast opacification may be related to an acute embolus, these findings may also be seen with chronic emboli.

The accuracy of CT angiography in the diagnosis of acute PTE has been assessed in several prospective studies. Despite some controversy,[153,154] most investigators have shown an overall sensitivity of 80% to 90% and a specificity of 80% to 95% with the use of single-detector spiral CT.[147,155,156] Similar results have been reported with ultrafast electron beam CT.[146,157] Preliminary studies have shown an improvement in sensitivity and specificity with the use of thin sections (1- to 1.5-mm collimation) and multidetector CT.[151,152] It has also been shown experimentally that spiral CT performed with 1-mm collimation is comparable to angiography in the detection of segmental and subsegmental emboli.[158]

Several groups of investigators have shown that CT angiography is superior to $\dot{V}/\dot{Q}$ scintigraphy in the diagnosis of acute PTE.[155,159,160] In a prospective comparison of spiral CT angiography and $\dot{V}/\dot{Q}$ scintigraphy in 142 patients, the results of both procedures were assessed independently by two experienced observers.[155] The combination of a high-probability $\dot{V}/\dot{Q}$ scan plus a spiral CT finding of PTE was considered diagnostic, and no further imaging studies were performed. The combination of a normal, very-low-probability, or low-probability $\dot{V}/\dot{Q}$ scan and a negative spiral CT scan in a patient who had a low clinical suspicion of PTE was considered sufficient to exclude the disease. All other patients underwent pulmonary angiography.

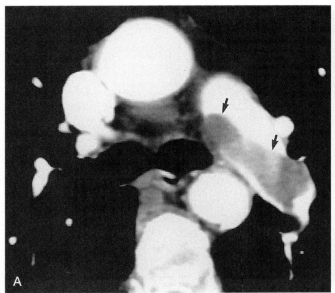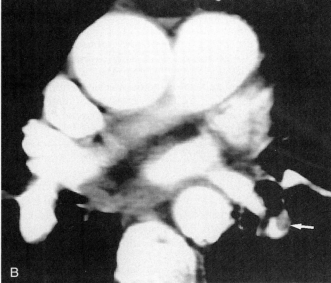

FIGURE 12–10

Acute pulmonary thromboembolism. A contrast-enhanced spiral CT scan at the level of the left pulmonary artery (**A**) in an 84-year-old woman shows a large intraluminal filling defect (*arrows*). Contrast material is present around and distal to the embolus, indicative of partial occlusion of the artery. A scan at a more caudal level (**B**) shows embolus (*arrow*) within the left lower lobe pulmonary artery. *(From Müller NL, Fraser RS, Colman NC, Paré PD: Radiologic Diagnosis of Diseases of the Chest. Philadelphia, WB Saunders, 2001.)*

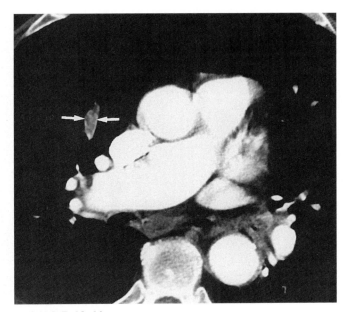

FIGURE 12–11

Acute pulmonary thromboembolism. A contrast-enhanced spiral CT scan in an 83-year-old man shows an abrupt absence of contrast material within the medial segmental artery of the right middle lobe (*arrows*) consistent with complete occlusion of the artery by an embolus. Increased diameter of the occluded vessel is apparent. *(From Müller NL, Fraser RS, Colman NC, Paré PD: Radiologic Diagnosis of Diseases of the Chest. Philadelphia, WB Saunders, 2001.)*

Twelve patients had discordant spiral CT and $\dot{V}/\dot{Q}$ scans; when angiographic results were used as the gold standard, the spiral CT interpretation was correct in 11 patients and the $\dot{V}/\dot{Q}$ scan in 1 patient. Overall, CT angiography had a sensitivity of 87% and a specificity of 98% versus a sensitivity of 65% and a specificity of 94% for a high-probability $\dot{V}/\dot{Q}$ scan. There was also better interobserver agreement in interpretation of the spiral CT scans than the $\dot{V}/\dot{Q}$ scans.

CT angiography also has an advantage over nuclear scanning by allowing assessment of the mediastinum and pulmonary parenchyma and evaluation of vascular abnormalities associated with nonembolic disease, such as may be seen with carcinoma and emphysema.[156] In a prospective randomized trial of 78 patients who had suspected PTE, spiral CT or $\dot{V}/\dot{Q}$ scans were performed as part of the initial investigation.[159] A confident diagnosis was made in 35 of 39 patients (90%) who underwent spiral CT, versus 21 of 39 patients (54%) who underwent scintigraphy first. The main reason for this difference was the ability of CT to show abnormalities other than emboli that were considered to be responsible for symptoms in 13 of 39 (33%) patients. Potential pitfalls in the diagnosis of PTE by CT include confusion of emboli with hilar lymph nodes, poor opacification of the pulmonary arteries, increased image noise in large patients, and obscuration of vessels by surrounding parenchymal opacification.[155,161,162]

The clinical validity of a negative CT angiography examination and the implications for patient outcome have been assessed by a number of investigators.[163-166] One group of investigators reviewed 1512 consecutive patients who were referred for CT with clinically suspected acute PTE[165]; 993 of these patients received no anticoagulation and had CT scans interpreted as negative for embolism. The 3-month probability of development of venous thrombosis or PTE was 0.8% (8 of 993 patients). By comparison, in a study of 380 patients who had suspected PTE and normal pulmonary angiograms, PTE developed in 6 (1.6%) within 1 year of follow-up.[166]

Analysis of a decision model based on published data has shown that the use of spiral CT is likely to improve cost-effectiveness in the workup of PTE and to be associated with decreased mortality.[167] Investigators assessed a number of diagnostic algorithms that included various combinations of V̇/Q̇ scintigraphy, ultrasound, D-dimer assay, spiral CT, and conventional angiography; for all realistic values of the pretest probability of PTE and coexisting DVT and the diagnostic accuracy of spiral CT, all of the best diagnostic strategies included CT angiography.[167]

Although there is little doubt that CT angiography can be helpful in the assessment of patients who have suspected PTE, there is considerable controversy about the specific indications for its use.[168-170] Some investigators recommend that the procedure be performed in patients who have indeterminate or low-probability V̇/Q̇ scans and a high clinical index of suspicion for PTE.[147,155,145] Others have suggested that it should be performed instead of scintigraphy in patients who have underlying cardiopulmonary disease and an abnormal chest radiograph.[159,170] It has also been proposed that spiral CT should replace scintigraphy in the assessment of all patients whose symptoms are suggestive of acute PTE and who have no symptoms or signs of DVT (lower extremity ultrasonography being recognized as the primary imaging modality in the assessment of patients who have suspected DVT).[148,171,172]

We and others believe that CT angiography is the modality of choice for the diagnosis of acute PTE in centers that have multidetector spiral CT scanners.[148,149,165] In centers with only single-detector CT scanners, we recommend the use of CT angiography in patients who have symptoms that are suggestive of acute PTE and who have intermediate-probability V̇/Q̇ scans, as well as in patients who have low-probability or normal scans and a high clinical index of suspicion. We also believe that the procedure is the initial imaging modality of choice and should replace V̇/Q̇ scintigraphy in patients who have severe COPD or extensive parenchymal abnormalities on their chest radiograph. Although both single-detector CT and multidetector CT have high accuracy in the diagnosis of acute PTE in patients with extensive parenchymal disease, multidetector CT results in better image quality.[173]

Occasionally, clinically unsuspected emboli are found incidentally on CT scans performed during the assessment of patients who have a history of trauma, thoracic tumors, aortic disease, or pulmonary abnormalities.[174-176] Not surprisingly, such patients generally have at least one risk factor for PTE.

Chronic Thromboembolism. Although most patients treated for acute PTE improve, chronic disease related either to the initial thromboembolic episode or to recurrent embolism develops in a small number. In a study of 62 patients, spiral CT scans were performed 1 to 53 months (median, 8 months) after the initial diagnosis of PTE.[177] All patients had been treated with anticoagulants, and 31 had received fibrinolytic therapy. On the follow-up spiral CT scan, emboli were considered acute if they partially or completely occluded the arterial lumen and the arterial diameter was not reduced. They were considered chronic if at least two of the following were present: (1) an eccentric location contiguous to the vessel wall (Fig. 12–12), (2) evidence of recanalization within the intraluminal filling defect, (3) arterial stenosis or

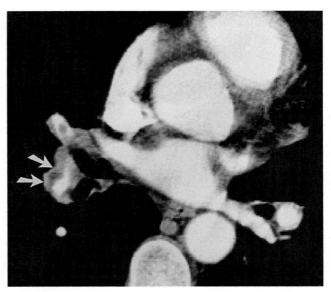

FIGURE 12–12

Chronic pulmonary thromboembolism. A contrast-enhanced spiral CT scan shows an eccentric filling defect along the lateral margin of the right lower lobe pulmonary artery (*arrows*). A small intraluminal filling defect is present in the middle lobe pulmonary artery. The patient was a 53-year-old man with recurrent pulmonary embolism. (*From Müller NL, Fraser RS, Colman NC, Paré PD: Radiologic Diagnosis of Diseases of the Chest. Philadelphia, WB Saunders, 2001.*)

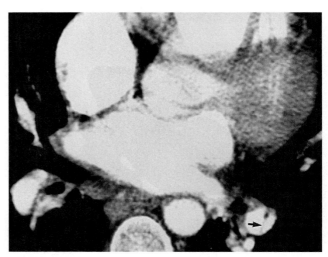

FIGURE 12–13

Chronic pulmonary thromboembolism. A contrast-enhanced spiral CT scan shows a linear filling defect (web) (*arrow*) in the left lower lobe pulmonary artery. The patient was a 39-year-old woman with pulmonary arterial hypertension secondary to chronic pulmonary thromboembolism. (*From Müller NL, Fraser RS, Colman NC, Paré PD: Radiologic Diagnosis of Diseases of the Chest. Philadelphia, WB Saunders, 2001.*)

webs (Fig. 12–13), (4) reduction of more than 50% of the arterial diameter, and (5) complete occlusion at the level of the stenosed artery. Thirty of 62 patients (48%) had complete resolution of the initial embolus on the follow-up CT scan and 24 (39%) had partial resolution; 8 (13%) patients had features of chronic embolism. The clinical features, risk factors at diagnosis, and treatment did not differ among the patients who had or did not have complete resolution; however, the patients who showed residual abnormalities or chronic emboli had more extensive embolization at initial diagnosis.

As in acute PTE, contrast-enhanced spiral CT allows a confident diagnosis of chronic emboli in most patients.[178,179] In a study of 75 patients who had this abnormality, CT showed thrombi in the pulmonary trunk, right and left main arteries, or lobar arteries in 53 patients[179]; thromboendarterectomy performed in 48 of these patients confirmed the CT findings of surgically resectable central chronic embolism. Organized thrombi were also excised at surgery in 14 of the 22 patients whose scans failed to show central emboli. CT had 78% sensitivity and 100% specificity in the diagnosis of surgically resectable chronic PTE.

Parenchymal Findings

Acute Thromboembolism. Parenchymal manifestations of acute PTE on CT are similar to those on chest radiography and include oligemia, loss of lung volume, and wedge-shaped pleural-based opacities.[180,181] Localized areas of decreased attenuation secondary to oligemia are uncommon except in patients who have massive emboli. In fact, this finding is an unreliable sign of embolization since it is seen in approximately the same number of patients who have and do not have emboli.[181]

As a manifestation of PTE, a wedge-shaped pulmonary opacity abutting the pleural surface is seen more commonly on a CT scan than on a chest radiograph.[182] The opacities may have the configuration of a full triangle or a truncated cone with a concave or convex apex (Fig. 12–14). However, though characteristic of infarction, such opacities may be seen in other conditions, including hemorrhage, pneumonia, neoplasm, and edema.[183]

Chronic Thromboembolism. Although parenchymal findings on CT are of limited value in the diagnosis of acute PTE,

they are characteristic enough to suggest the diagnosis of chronic embolism in many cases.[179,184] The most common abnormality consists of localized areas of decreased attenuation and vascularity that are sharply marginated from adjacent areas with increased or normal attenuation and vessel size, a pattern known as *mosaic perfusion*.[185] Although this pattern can also be seen with airway disease, particularly obliterative bronchiolitis and asthma, when associated with enlarged central pulmonary arteries or asymmetry in size of the central or segmental pulmonary arteries, it is suggestive of pulmonary hypertension secondary to chronic PTE (Fig. 12–15).[185,186]

Chronic PTE is sometimes associated with bronchiectasis.[187] In a study of 52 patients, this abnormality was seen on HRCT in 21 of 33 patients (64%) who had chronic PTE but in only 2 of 19 (11%) who had acute embolism.[187] Since the abnormal bronchi were located next to pulmonary arteries completely obstructed by emboli, it was postulated that the pathogenesis may be one of traction by fibrous tissue located in the vessel lumen similar to the mechanism of bronchiectasis seen in interstitial pulmonary fibrosis.

Magnetic Resonance Imaging

MR imaging also allows direct visualization of thromboemboli (Fig. 12–16). It has the additional advantage of not requiring radiation or the use of iodinated intravenous contrast material; however, it is more expensive and less readily available and may be associated with cardiac and respiratory motion artifacts and complex pulmonary blood flow patterns that mimic embolism. These problems have been minimized with the development of gradient-recalled echo (GRE) imaging techniques obtained during a single breath-hold. The combination of these techniques with gadolinium enhancement generally results in good-quality MR angiographic images of the pulmonary arteries.[188,189] Sensitivities of 75% to 100% and a specificity of about 95% have been found in studies using conventional or digital subtraction angiography as the gold standard.[188,189]

Pulmonary Angiography

Pulmonary arteriography is the most definitive technique for diagnosing PTE (Fig. 12–17).[36,190,191] Best results are obtained if the contrast medium is injected through a catheter whose tip is placed in the right or left pulmonary artery, a procedure that permits not only a clear view of the ipsilateral arterial tree but also measurement of pulmonary artery pressure. Although the procedure is valuable in identifying occlusion of lobar or segmental vessels, it is considerably less useful in showing obstruction of subsegmental ones.[192,193] The last-named vessels are seen inadequately for several reasons, including dilution of contrast medium during cardiac systole, obscuration of vascular detail because of overlap of opacified vessels, and diversion of blood flow away from embolized vessels. This difficulty can result in significant interobserver disagreement. For example, in a study in which three angiographers independently reviewed the arteriograms of 60 patients, the interobserver agreement was 100% for emboli involving the main, lobar, and segmental arteries but only 13% for those affecting subsegmental vessels.[194]

Although pulmonary angiography is considered to be the gold standard for the diagnosis of PTE, the procedure is

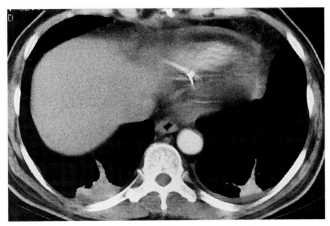

FIGURE 12–14

Pulmonary infarcts on CT scan. A contrast-enhanced spiral CT scan in a 57-year-old patient with acute pulmonary embolism shows pleura-based, wedge-shaped opacities in both lower lobes. The triangular opacity in the right lower lobe did not enhance with intravenous contrast material. A small left pleural effusion is evident. (*From Müller NL, Fraser RS, Colman NC, Paré PD: Radiologic Diagnosis of Diseases of the Chest. Philadelphia, WB Saunders, 2001.*)

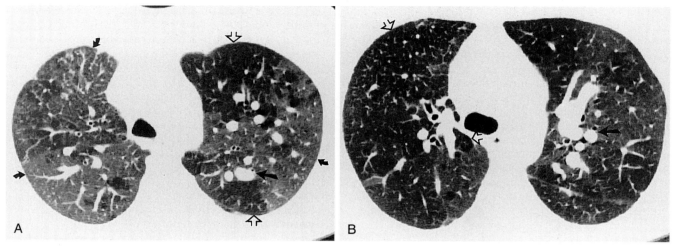

FIGURE 12–15

Chronic pulmonary embolism: mosaic perfusion. HRCT scans (**A** and **B**) show localized areas of decreased attenuation (*open arrows*) and vascularity and areas with increased attenuation and vascularity (*curved arrows*), a pattern known as *mosaic perfusion*. Markedly increased pulmonary artery–to–bronchus diameter ratios are visible (*straight arrows*), particularly in the left upper lobe. The patient was a 43-year-old woman with pulmonary arterial hypertension as a result of chronic pulmonary thromboembolism. *(From Müller NL, Fraser RS, Colman NC, Paré PD: Radiologic Diagnosis of Diseases of the Chest. Philadelphia, WB Saunders, 2001.)*

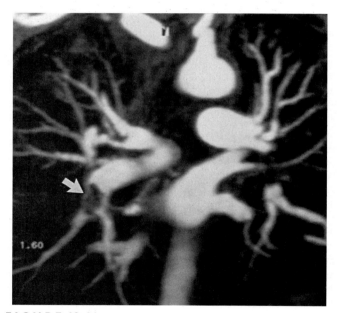

FIGURE 12–16

MR imaging of acute pulmonary thromboembolism. A coronal MR image shows a filling defect (*arrow*) in the right interlobar pulmonary artery. *(Case courtesy of Dr. Jaime Fernández-Cuadrado, Hospital La Paz, Madrid, Spain.)*

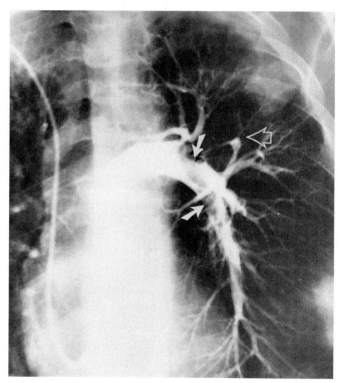

FIGURE 12–17

Pulmonary thromboembolism: arteriography. A selective left pulmonary arteriogram in the left anterior oblique projection shows multiple central intraluminal filling defects (*arrows*). A segmental artery is amputated (*open arrow*). *(From Müller NL, Fraser RS, Colman NC, Paré PD: Radiologic Diagnosis of Diseases of the Chest. Philadelphia, WB Saunders, 2001.)*

requested in only a small percentage of patients who have clinically suspected emboli.[195,196] The reluctance to request it stems to some extent from concern over the perceived risks.[195,197] However, when modern techniques are used, including nonosmotic contrast media and pigtail or flow-directed catheters, significant complications are rare.[197]

The angiographic criteria for the diagnosis of acute PTE include primary and secondary signs.[198] The only primary sign is a filling defect, which may be manifested as a persistent intraluminal radiolucency without complete obstruction of blood flow or as a trailing edge of an intraluminal radiolucency when there is complete obstruction of distal blood flow. Secondary signs include abrupt occlusion (*cutoff*) of a pulmonary artery without visualization of an intraluminal filling defect and perfusion defects. The latter may be manifested as areas of oligemia or avascularity or as abruptly tapering peripheral vessels with a paucity of branching vessels (*pruning*).[198] Although these findings reflect nothing more than diminished pulmonary arterial perfusion, as may be seen with several pulmonary and cardiac diseases from which PTE must be differentiated,[199] they may be useful by directing attention to areas in which manifestations of embolism may be subtle; in such cases, segmental arteriography, especially with magnification, may reveal intraluminal defects in smaller vessels.

The angiographic findings of chronic PTE include abrupt vascular narrowing, complete vascular obstruction, webs or bands, intimal irregularities, and "pouching" defects.[200] The last-named finding is defined as the presence of obstructing or partially occlusive emboli that have organized in a concave configuration toward the lumen of the artery. Tapering of vessels usually connotes circumferential organization and recanalization. Abrupt narrowing of a large artery is also a characteristic finding of chronic PTE, the normal gentle tapering of the vessel being replaced by an abrupt decrease in diameter of the opacified lumen.[200,201] Pulmonary artery webs or bands are lines of low opacity that traverse the vessel lumen; they are often associated with narrowing and post-stenotic dilation and have been shown in follow-up angiographic studies to be located at the sites of previously identified filling defects.[202] Another common finding of chronic PTE is the presence of a scalloped appearance of the pulmonary arterial wall, an abnormality that has been shown to be related to irregularly organized thrombus.[200]

Diagnosis of Deep Vein Thrombosis

Conventional Venography

Conventional contrast venography is used to outline the deep veins extending from the calf to the inferior vena cava and has been considered the gold standard imaging modality in the diagnosis of DVT.[203] In one prospective study, 70% of patients who had PTE proved by angiography showed evidence of thrombosis of the deep veins of the legs[204]; it must be assumed that the remaining 30% had other sources for embolism (e.g., the deep pelvic veins) or that all or most of the thrombi in the legs had embolized. Usually, the veins are opacified by injecting contrast medium into a foot vein; the iliac veins can be visualized by femoral vein injection.

Despite these observations, venography has several disadvantages: (1) it can be painful, (2) it *induces* thrombosis in 3%

to 4% of patients when ionic contrast medium is used, (3) inadequate examinations as a result of incomplete venous filling and other technical problems occur in 5% of cases, and (4) there is an approximately 10% interobserver disagreement in assessment of the presence of thrombus.[205,206] Although the incidence of complications can be decreased with the use of nonionic contrast medium,[205,207] venography has been largely replaced by other imaging techniques, particularly ultrasound, in the initial investigation of patients who have suspected DVT.

Ultrasonography

Studies of the use of ultrasound in the diagnosis of DVT in the 1980s were based on the observation that the normal vein lumen is obliterated after compression by the ultrasound probe whereas a vein containing thrombus remains distended, the thrombus often being seen as an echogenic area within the normal nonechoic vein lumen.[203] Such studies had a sensitivity of approximately 90% and a specificity of 97% to 100% for the diagnosis of popliteal and femoral vein thrombosis in patients who had symptoms or signs suggestive of DVT.[208,209] Assessment of DVT by ultrasound improved with the advent of color flow technology in the late 1980s.[203] In a normal vein, color-coded flow fills the lumen completely. Thrombosis results in the absence of flow or the presence of isoechoic or echogenic thrombus within the lumen and the absence or persistent underfilling of color-coded flow.[203] Color Doppler ultrasound has a sensitivity greater than 95% and a specificity greater than 98% in the diagnosis of popliteal and femoral vein thrombosis.[210,211] The procedure has similar sensitivity and specificity in the diagnosis of calf vein thrombosis.[212,213] However, the clinical value of such diagnosis is controversial,[203,214] and the results of most investigations suggest that thrombosis localized to this site is not associated with an increased risk for PTE.[215,216]

Because of its ready accessibility, low cost, and high diagnostic accuracy, ultrasonography has become the imaging modality of choice in the diagnosis of DVT in most centers. In patients who have symptoms of acute PTE and DVT, the procedure has been recommended as the initial imaging modality.[168,169,217] A positive examination in this clinical setting allows a confident diagnosis of PTE with no need for further investigation.[168,169] By contrast, lower extremity Doppler ultrasound has a limited role in the assessment of patients who do not have symptoms or signs of DVT; several groups have shown poor sensitivity in the detection of venous thrombi in this setting, including those that develop in the postoperative period.[203,218]

Computed Tomography

Contrast-enhanced spiral CT assessment of the leg veins can be performed with direct or indirect techniques. Direct CT venography is performed by placing a 22-gauge intravenous cannula in the dorsal vein of each foot and a tourniquet around each ankle. Diluted intravenous contrast material is injected simultaneously into both legs. After a 35-second delay, spiral CT is performed from the ankle to the inferior vena. The diagnosis of DVT is based on visualization of a filling defect in an opacified vein or a nonopacified venous segment interposed between a proximally and distally opacified vein.[219] Although this technique has been found to have high sensitivity and specificity for the diagnosis, it is seldom performed in clinical practice.[219,220]

Indirect CT venography is performed by injecting contrast material into an arm vein.[221,222] Its main advantage is that it can be performed after CT angiography of the pulmonary vasculature without the need for another venipuncture or additional intravenous contrast material. Several groups of investigators have shown that the procedure has high sensitivity (90% to 100%) and specificity (70% to 100%) in the diagnosis of DVT.[221,223,224] The procedure is particularly useful in patients clinically suspected of having PTE who have a negative spiral CT scan of the chest.[225] In an investigation of 96 patients who had suspected PTE, 29 (30%) had embolism confirmed on CT and 10 (10%) had positive CT venography[226]; only 5 of the 10 patients who had DVT had evidence of PTE.

Combining CT venography with CT angiography simplifies and shortens the assessment of patients suspected of having VTED and increases confidence in withholding treatment when both examinations are negative.[227] The main disadvantage is increased radiation[228]; consequently, particularly as it applies to the ovaries and testicles, we recommend CT venography only in patients who have negative CT angiography (as assessed during the course of the procedure) and are older than 50 years.

Magnetic Resonance Imaging

Several groups have shown that MR imaging is comparable or superior to conventional venography or ultrasound in the diagnosis of DVT.[229,230] The diagnosis is based on the presence of an intravascular filling defect with low signal intensity surrounded by high signal intensity resulting from flowing blood or on the presence of occlusion of an enlarged vein with a clot that has decreased or absent signal intensity. Because of its high diagnostic accuracy,[231] the procedure is recommended in patients who have suspected DVT and a nondiagnostic ultrasound examination or suspected pelvic vein thrombosis.

Summary

On the basis of published observations and our own experience, the following imaging algorithm is recommended for the evaluation of patients suspected of having acute PTE:

1. All patients should have a chest radiograph to exclude abnormalities that may mimic PTE clinically, such as pneumonia.
2. Patients who have symptoms or signs of DVT should undergo evaluation of the leg veins, preferably by Doppler ultrasound. If the result of this investigation is positive, the patient can be considered to have PTE and will not usually require further investigation.
3. Patients who have no signs or symptoms of DVT should undergo spiral CT pulmonary angiography. Those who have a contraindication to use of the iodinated contrast material necessitated by this procedure should undergo ventilation-perfusion scintigraphy.
4. Patients who are deemed to have a high clinical index of suspicion for acute PTE and who have suboptimal or negative CT scans should undergo pulmonary angiography.

Clinical Manifestations

The clinical manifestations of PTE are variable and the diagnosis can be difficult to make. Analysis of autopsy studies and the finding of objective evidence for PTE in patients who have DVT and no chest symptoms have established that many emboli cause no symptoms.[11] When symptoms occur, they are nonspecific and are often attributed to underlying comorbid conditions such as COPD and congestive heart failure.[232] Nevertheless, the history and clinical examination are important components of algorithms that identify the relative prevalence of PTE in populations of patients requiring evaluation and are therefore crucial in the interpretation of abnormal test results.[233,234]

Dyspnea is the most common symptom of angiographically proven PTE and occurs in more than 80% of patients. Its onset is usually abrupt; rarely, it is sporadic and associated with wheezing, similar to asthma.[235] In about 50% of patients, close questioning will elicit a history of one or more transitory episodes of dyspnea, harbingers of later, more distressing embolism.[236]

Pulmonary infarction is the most common clinically identified complication after PTE.[237] Typically, the patient complains of dyspnea of acute onset, pain on breathing, and (sometimes) hemoptysis. Occasionally, the chest pain is unaccompanied by dyspnea and tachypnea. Tachycardia[238] and fever,[239] usually low grade, may accompany the pain. High fever persisting longer than 6 days should suggest a diagnosis other than PTE.[240] Physical findings in patients who have pulmonary infarction include locally decreased breath sounds, crackles, rhonchi, friction rub, and signs of pleural effusion.[241] The differential diagnosis of such findings includes pneumonia and atelectasis or pleural effusion of other etiology. Embolism may be especially difficult to differentiate from atelectasis secondary to bronchial mucus plugging since both are common postoperative complications. The pleural effusion that develops in the context of pulmonary infarction is usually grossly bloody.

Massive PTE results when thrombus acutely obstructs at least 50% of the pulmonary vascular bed. It is an uncommon event that was observed in less than 10% of patients in the PIOPED study.[242] Characteristically, patients complain of severe dyspnea and retrosternal pain. Tachycardia, tachypnea, and at times, cyanosis are evident on examination. The jugular veins are distended, a gallop rhythm may be audible, and there may be a diffuse systolic lift at the left sternal border with accentuation of the pulmonic component of the second heart sound. If the right ventricle fails acutely—a finding often associated with severe systemic hypotension and, on occasion, with accompanying right ventricular infarction[243]—signs of pulmonary hypertension may be absent. Massive pulmonary embolism must be distinguished from left ventricular infarction[244] and, when neurologic manifestations predominate,[245] from a cerebrovascular accident.

Patients who have chronic thromboembolic pulmonary hypertension may complain of episodic transient dyspnea, possibly as a result of intermittent microembolism; others have a history of progressive breathlessness with or without clear-cut evidence of previous acute thromboembolic events.[246] Substernal chest pain and syncope occur late in the course of disease.[246] The finding of bruits over the lung fields as a result of turbulent flow in partially obstructed pulmonary arteries may help distinguish this disorder from primary pulmonary hypertension.[246]

The presence of signs and symptoms of DVT, particularly in the legs, is supportive evidence for the diagnosis of PTE. Localized pain or tenderness in the calf, popliteal fossa, or thigh, especially if associated with a discrepancy in the diameter of the legs, suggests venous thrombosis. In some cases, pain may be elicited by dorsiflexion of the foot (Homans' sign). However, although these findings are helpful when present, their absence does not in any way militate against a diagnosis of PTE: approximately 50% of patients who suffer a fatal embolism show no clinical evidence of DVT.[247]

Even though the clinical manifestations of PTE and infarction are chiefly respiratory, cardiac, or both,[238] they can also mimic acute abdominal or cerebral disease.[248] Diaphragmatic pleuritis, paralytic ileus, and a rise in serum bilirubin may suggest a diagnosis of acute cholecystitis. Neurologic signs include restlessness, apprehension, syncope, seizures, irrational behavior, hemiparesis or monoparesis, confusion, and coma.[249,250] They appear mainly in elderly, bedridden, or cardiac patients and are usually caused by a combination of previous cerebrovascular disease, hypoxemia, and diminished cerebral oxygen delivery as a result of decreased cardiac output or cerebral vasospasm secondary to hypocapnia. Occasionally, paradoxical embolism through a patent foramen ovale is demonstrated.[251]

Laboratory Findings

Biochemical tests lack both sensitivity and specificity for PTE and are of little value in the diagnosis.[125,213] Assays of several markers of coagulation and fibrinolysis are more useful. The most promising of these assays is the measurement of plasma D-dimers, which are circulating cross-linked fibrin degradation products that are specific markers for plasmin activity. The finding of an elevated D-dimer level lacks specificity for the diagnosis of PTE[252,253]; however, there is evidence that it has high sensitivity,[254,255] such that a negative test has a sufficiently high negative predictive value that invasive testing can be avoided in the appropriate circumstance. Variability in assay sensitivity, the heterogeneity of subjects tested, and the inconsistency of diagnostic criteria have provided the foundation for debate about the validity of this statement.[256-258] However, it appears reasonable to conclude that a negative D-dimer test result safely excludes the diagnosis when the probability of VTED is low. In addition, the negative predictive value for the combined use of D-dimer testing and clinical assessment in patients evaluated in the emergency department for VTED is as high as 100%.[233,259] Similarly, in patients who have a low to moderate probability of VTED and a nondiagnostic ventilation-perfusion scan, a negative D-dimer result safely excludes the diagnosis.[260,261]

In patients who have DVT, the platelet count often falls with the onset of PTE[262]; however, a decrease may also be seen with pneumonia or as a side effect of antibiotic therapy.[12] The leukocyte count seldom exceeds 15,000/mm[3]; in a study of 386 patients who had a diagnosis of acute PTE, the white blood cell count never exceeded 20,000.[263]

Pleural fluid is grossly bloody in approximately two thirds of patients who have PTE and effusion.[264] In other cases, the effusion is a serous exudate; when transudate is present, it is probably secondary to associated heart failure.[265] Polymorphonuclear leukocytosis and mesothelial cell hyperplasia are common; pleural fluid eosinophilia greater than 10% has been described in almost 20% of patients.[266]

Pulmonary function studies may reveal restrictive disease: resting lung volume is decreased, airway resistance is increased, and lung compliance and diffusing capacity are reduced.

Electrocardiographic changes are common.[267] Nonspecific ST-segment or T-wave changes are the most frequent and supraventricular arrhythmias are not uncommon. Changes that are considered typical for PTE include (1) an S_1Q_3 or $S_1Q_3T_3$ pattern, (2) a rightward shift of the QRS axis, (3) transient complete or incomplete right bundle branch block, and (4) T-wave inversion in the right precordial leads. These findings correlate with the presence of pulmonary hypertension and massive PTE.[268,269]

Prognosis and Natural History

As discussed previously, most thromboembolic episodes are unrecognized clinically: careful search of the pulmonary vascular tree at autopsy has revealed recent or organized thrombi in more than 50% of unselected patients, most of whom had neither a clinical history suggestive of PTE nor pathologic evidence that the emboli had caused morbidity or mortality.[77] In most of these cases, the emboli are small and lodged in subsegmental or segmental vessels.

The short-term outcome of patients who have *clinically evident* PTE depends on a number of factors, including the size and number of emboli, the age of the patient, and the presence or absence of hemodynamic instability, right heart dysfunction (as assessed echocardiographically), and underlying disease (especially cancer and disease of the heart and lungs).[270-272] Many fatal pulmonary emboli are massive and occur without warning, with inadequate time for initiation of investigation or therapy. Overall, in treated patients, death occurs in 1.5% to 7.5% of affected individuals within 3 months of the initial event[271,272]; most patients who die do so as a result of associated comorbid conditions. Patients who have massive PTE and shock and who survive long enough for confirmation of the diagnosis have a poor prognosis, death occurring in more than a third.

In nearly all patients who survive the acute event, clinical and hemodynamic resolution is complete within 4 to 6 weeks[273]; however, radiologic resolution may take somewhat longer. Most patients show improvement in the perfusion lung scan within 2 weeks of initiation of therapy[274]; however, patients who have large emboli or associated cardiopulmonary disease may never achieve complete recovery.[275] In the absence of prolonged anticoagulation, it is important to recognize that patients whose risk for VTED is transient are at substantially less risk of having recurrent events than those who have a persisting risk such as cancer or neurologic disease.[276,277]

The prognosis of patients who have chronic thromboembolic pulmonary hypertension, whether treated or untreated, is poor.[92] Although the majority of patients meeting selection criteria for surgery improve significantly, the mortality rate of attempted surgical embolectomy has varied from 5% to 24%.[246] Furthermore, only a small percentage of patients meet selection criteria for surgery.

SEPTIC THROMBOEMBOLISM

Septic embolism occurs when fragments of thrombus contain organisms, usually bacteria and occasionally fungi or parasites. The pulmonary manifestations of such emboli may be the only indication of serious underlying infection; because the radiologic changes are often distinctive, recognition of such changes early in the disease should permit diagnosis and prompt institution of therapy. Although most cases of pulmonary infection associated with thromboembolism are the result of the presence of organisms within the thrombus itself (true septic emboli), it should be appreciated that secondary bacterial infection of initially sterile infarcts occasionally results in a similar pathologic and radiographic appearance.

Septic pulmonary embolism occurs most often in young adults.[278] The organism most often grown on blood cultures is coagulase-positive *Staphylococcus aureus*. A predisposing factor is nearly always present, most often drug addiction, alcoholism, immunologic deficiency (particularly lymphoma), congenital heart disease, and skin infection.[279,280]

Most emboli originate from the heart (in association with endocarditis of the tricuspid valve or a ventricular septal defect[281]) or the peripheral veins (septic thrombophlebitis). Occasionally, they arise in the pharynx when infection extends to the parapharyngeal space and internal jugular venous system and result in a clinical condition referred to as Lemierre's syndrome, or postanginal sepsis.[282] The oral anaerobes, particularly *Bacteroides* and *Fusobacterium* species, are the most common pathogens associated with this syndrome. A wide variety of other sites have served as sources occasionally, including the bones (staphylococcal osteomyelitis),[283] the arm veins in patients who have a history of intravenous drug abuse, veins near infected indwelling catheters, the oral cavity (periodontal infection[284]), and arteriovenous shunts such as those used for hemodialysis.[285]

The radiographic manifestations consist of multiple, ill-defined, round or wedge-shaped peripheral opacities (Fig. 12–18). They may be uniform in size or vary widely as a result of recurrent showers of emboli. The opacities are usually bilateral, although they may be asymmetrical and are occasionally unilateral.[286] They may be migratory, first appearing in one area and then in another as older lesions resolve and new ones appear.[278] Cavitation is frequent and may occur rapidly; the cavities are generally thin walled, and many have no fluid level. Hilar and mediastinal lymph node enlargement may be present and is occasionally massive.[287]

The diagnosis can be confirmed in questionable cases by CT.[288] The characteristic findings consist of multiple nodules in various stages of cavitation (Fig. 12–19). Most vary from 0.5 to 3.5 cm in diameter and involve the peripheral lung regions. Wedge-shaped pleura-based areas of consolidation that frequently contain central areas of heterogeneous lucency or frank cavitation are also often seen. Pleural effusions are evident in approximately 60% of patients and hilar or mediastinal lymph node enlargement in 25%.

Fever, cough (with or without expectoration of purulent material), and hemoptysis (occasionally massive)[289] are the most common symptoms. Although infection originating in a right-sided heart valve may give rise to a murmur, in many cases it is soft and atypically located.[290]

PULMONARY MANIFESTATIONS OF SICKLE CELL DISEASE

Sickle cell lung disease occurs in all of the more common sickle hemoglobinopathies, including homozygous hemoglobin SS and the compound heterozygous states of hemoglobin S/C and hemoglobin S/β-thalassemia.[291] Approximately 85% of affected individuals survive into the second decade of life and therefore

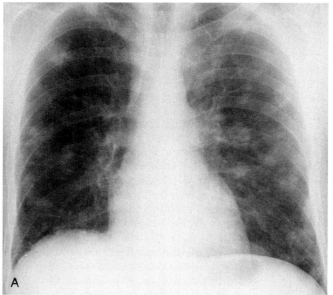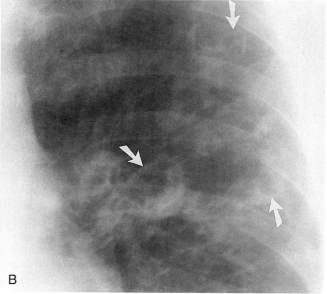

FIGURE 12–18

Septic embolism. A view of a posteroanterior chest radiograph (**A**) in a 28-year-old man with fever shows poorly defined bilateral nodular opacities. Blood cultures grew *Staphylococcus aureus*. A view of the left lung (**B**) from a chest radiograph performed 1 week later shows multiple thin-walled cavities *(arrows)*. *(From Müller NL, Fraser RS, Colman NC, Paré PD: Radiologic Diagnosis of Diseases of the Chest. Philadelphia, WB Saunders, 2001.)*

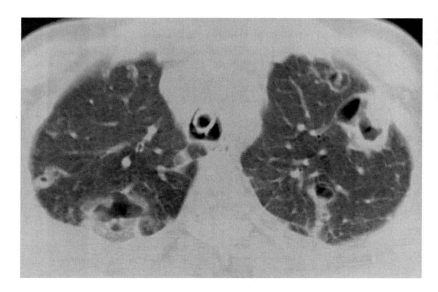

FIGURE 12–19

Septic embolism. A CT scan shows cavitating nodules in both upper lobes. Blood cultures grew enterococci. The patient was a 20-year-old drug addict. *(From Müller NL, Fraser RS, Colman NC, Paré PD: Radiologic Diagnosis of Diseases of the Chest. Philadelphia, WB Saunders, 2001.)*

come to the attention of chest physicians and internists treating adults.[291] The sickle cell gene is carried by 8% of African Americans, so the disease is relatively common in the United States.[292]

Several pulmonary complications can occur. The most common, termed *acute chest syndrome*, is characterized by fever, pleuritic chest pain, dyspnea, leukocytosis, and new lung opacities on radiographs. The abnormality occurs in up to 50% of patients who have sickle cell disease and is frequently recurrent.[291,292] It is second only to pain as a cause for hospitalization and is responsible for 25% of all deaths in sickle cell disease.[292] The pathogenesis of the syndrome is multifactorial.[293] Infection,[294] fat embolization,[295,296] iatrogenic fluid overload, hypoxemia and atelectasis as a result of splinting from painful bone infarcts, and sickling and endothelial adhesion of red blood cells resulting in pulmonary vascular obstruction and lung infarction[297] have all been implicated.

Abnormalities in lung function develop in most patients who have sickle cell anemia. Changes may be restrictive or obstructive (in part reversible), or both, and may be associated with abnormal gas exchange and hypoxemia.[293] Clinically evident pulmonary hypertension can develop and is associated with early mortality.[293] Less severe elevations in pulmonary artery pressure can be detected echocardiographically in a substantial minority of patients.[293]

The radiographic findings in acute chest syndrome consist of bilateral patchy areas of consolidation, which have been attributed to edema and infarction.[298] In addition to consolidation, HRCT demonstrates areas of vascular attenuation attributed to hypoperfusion.[299] In patients who have repeated pulmonary infections and episodes of acute chest syndrome, focal or, rarely, diffuse interstitial fibrosis may develop and be manifested by interlobular septal thickening, parenchymal bands of attenuation, and pleural tags with associated architectural distortion.[300]

EMBOLI OF EXTRAVASCULAR TISSUE AND SECRETIONS

Theoretically, fragments of virtually any organ, tissue, or body secretion can gain access to the systemic circulation and be transported to the lungs. Some, such as megakaryocytes, do so with such frequency that the process can be considered a normal phenomenon. Others are found only in pathologic conditions, in which circumstance tissue disruption with vascular laceration is a necessary precondition; thus, the underlying pathogenesis is usually trauma, most often associated with labor, accidental or battlefield injuries, or medical procedures such as venipuncture or surgery. With the exception of amniotic fluid and fat, clinicopathologic and radiologic effects of such emboli are almost invariably absent.

In addition to normal body tissues, abnormal tissue can also embolize to the pulmonary circulation. Perhaps the most common of such substances are neoplastic cells, which, because of their inherent invasive properties, can gain access to the circulation without the aid of trauma; although such emboli are usually microscopic and of no direct vascular consequence, large fragments or numerous small ones occasionally cause significant pulmonary arterial obstruction. Similar obstruction can occur with embolized parasites, either as eggs in the microvasculature (as in schistosomiasis) or as whole or fragmented adult worms in large arteries (as in dirofilariasis).

Fat Embolism

Although intact fragments of adipose tissue (usually with admixed hematopoietic cells) are often found in the pulmonary arteries after severe trauma, the term *fat embolism* traditionally refers to the presence of globules of free fat within the vasculature.[301,302] Exogenous fatty material, such as ethiodized oil used as radiographic contrast media and vegetable oil, is also usually excluded from the definition and is discussed separately (see page 573).

Epidemiology

The precise incidence of pulmonary fat embolism is difficult to ascertain, partly because diagnostic criteria are variable and partly because the majority of cases result in no clinical manifestations. It is likely, however, that asymptomatic emboli are very common; autopsy studies of patients who have experienced severe trauma reveal them in the vast majority of cases,[303] and measurement of fat globules in the venous circulation shows that they occur almost invariably during insertion of orthopedic prostheses.[302] The incidence of clinically significant disease in patients who have simple tibial or femoral fractures is generally believed to be about 1% to 3%.[301] In individuals who have more severe trauma, the incidence of clinically evident embolism is probably in the range of 10% to 20%.[301,302]

In addition to these forms of trauma, a wide variety of surgical procedures and medical conditions that disrupt the marrow occasionally cause fat emboli (Table 12–4). One of the more important of these conditions is sickle cell disease, in which fat emboli have been hypothesized to be the cause of some cases of acute chest syndrome seen in this condition (see page 564).[304]

Pathogenesis

The fat in fat embolism syndrome has two possible origins. The first and probably much more common is bone marrow, with embolism developing after entry of disrupted fat into lacerated medullary veins. A wide variety of clinical and experimental observations support this hypothesis.[305] Although intuitively one might expect an increase in intramedullary pressure to accompany the entry of fat into torn veins, experimental evidence suggests that this may not be necessary.[306] It has also been postulated that embolized fat can be derived from altered blood lipoproteins or chylomicrons or from stress-induced lipemia.[305,307] According to this hypothesis, a substance in the blood—the most likely being C-reactive protein—causes agglutination of plasma lipid into particles sufficient in size to obstruct pulmonary capillaries.

Two pathogenetic mechanisms have been implicated in the development of pulmonary abnormalities after fat embolism. The first is mechanical vascular obstruction, predominantly by fat globules themselves and possibly enhanced in some cases by platelet or red blood cell aggregates.[308] Evidence suggesting the importance of this effect includes the histologic

identification of fat within small pulmonary vessels (Fig. 12–20) and the observation that pulmonary arterial pressure rises transiently in experimental animals soon after embolization.[309] A second potential mechanism involves conversion of neutral triglycerides (the form in which fat appears to be transported to the lungs) into free fatty acids by endothelial lipases. These substances can damage the alveolar wall and

TABLE 12–4. Pulmonary Fat Embolism

External Trauma

Major accident/battlefield trauma
Isolated long bone fracture
External cardiac massage

Surgery or Medical Procedures

Orthopedic procedures (e.g., intramedullary prosthesis insertion, arthroplasty)
Intraosseous venography
Liposuction
Bone marrow transplantation and harvesting
Venous hyperalimentation
Lung transplantation (e.g., after trauma-related embolism in the donor lung)
Drug therapy (e.g., cyclosporine, cisplatin)

Underlying Disease

Pancreatitis
Diabetes mellitus
Acute osteomyelitis
Osteoporosis (compression fracture)
Sickle cell disease
Thalassemia
Hepatic steatosis (secondary to drugs [e.g., steroids], poisons [e.g., carbon tetrachloride], or alcohol)
Epilepsy
Burns
Decompression sickness

Modified from Fraser RS, Müller NL, Colman NC, Paré PD: Fraser and Paré's Diagnosis of Diseases of the Chest, 4th ed. Philadelphia, WB Saunders, 1999.

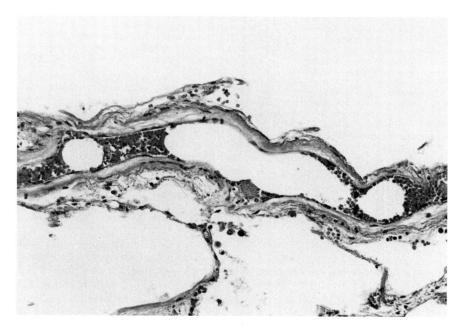

FIGURE 12–20

Fat embolus. The lumen of this pulmonary arteriole shows one elongated and two circular spaces that are devoid of blood cells. Such an appearance is suggestive of fat and was confirmed by lipid stains. This histologic section is from a young man who died several hours after a motor vehicle accident; there was no clinical or pathologic evidence of acute lung damage. (×190.) (From Fraser RS, Müller NL, Colman NC, Paré PD: Fraser and Paré's Diagnosis of Diseases of the Chest, 4th ed. Philadelphia, WB Saunders, 1999.)

lead to activation of complement or release of inflammatory mediators, thereby further exaggerating the injury. Supporting this hypothesis are experimental investigations in which severe pulmonary edema and hemorrhage have resulted from the injection of free fatty acids into the pulmonary arteries.[310,311] However, in other experimental studies in which neutral fat has been injected into the systemic veins, evidence for conversion to free fatty acids has not been found.[310]

Although the results of animal experiments and the presence of radiologic changes and clinical signs and symptoms shortly after trauma have understandably led to the belief that intravascular fat is responsible for the pulmonary disease that develops in patients who have fat embolism, there is evidence that this conclusion may not be correct in all cases. For example, in some autopsy[312] and clinical investigations,[313] poor correlation has been found between the presence of intravascular fat and clinical manifestations. In addition, some investigators have found that pelvic or long bone fractures unaccompanied by sepsis or by severe injuries to the brain, chest, or abdomen are associated with relatively mild pulmonary disease and quick clinical recovery.[314] As a result of these observations, the significance of pulmonary fat emboli in previously healthy individuals has been questioned, and it has been hypothesized that the clinical findings associated with the emboli may be the result of a concomitant disease process.[313]

Pathologic Characteristics

The presence of fat within pulmonary arterioles and capillaries can be suspected on hematoxylin and eosin–stained sections when there are round to oval spaces, 20 to 40 μm in diameter, apparently compressing red blood cells to one side (see Fig. 12–20). Definitive diagnosis requires the use of fat-soluble dyes on unfixed (frozen) tissue or other special techniques.

Radiologic Manifestations

Most patients have a normal chest radiograph.[315] When present, the radiographic manifestations consist of bilateral areas of air space consolidation involving predominantly the peripheral lung regions and lung bases.[316,317] Pleural effusions are typically absent. The time lapse between trauma and radiographic signs is usually 1 to 2 days.[316,318] This delay differentiates fat embolism from traumatic lung contusion, in which the radiographic opacity invariably appears immediately after injury. In addition, although the latter opacity usually clears rapidly (in about 24 hours), resolution of fat embolism generally takes 7 to 10 days and occasionally as long as 4 weeks.[319] Further differentiation lies in the extent of lung involvement, contusion seldom affecting both lungs diffusely and symmetrically.

In an investigation of nine patients who had normal radiographs, all were found to have abnormal HRCT scans: seven had ground-glass opacities and two had small nodular opacities.[320] The ground-glass opacities had a patchy or predominately peripheral distribution. The nodular opacities tended to be located in the centrilobular regions, along the interlobular septa, and along the interlobar fissures. Smooth or nodular septal thickening was present in five of the nine patients.

Clinical Manifestations

Although symptoms may appear almost immediately after the event causing embolization,[321] in most cases there is a delay of 12 to 24 hours. The most common pulmonary symptom is dyspnea; cough, hemoptysis, and pleural pain occur occasionally. Signs include pyrexia, tachypnea, tachycardia, fine inspiratory crackles, and (occasionally) rhonchi and friction rub.[322] Acute cor pulmonale with cardiac failure, cyanosis, and circulatory shock may occur.

Symptoms of systemic fat embolism are seen in up to 85% of patients who have pulmonary disease.[301] They are chiefly related to the central nervous system and include confusion, restlessness, stupor, delirium, seizures, and coma. A petechial rash often develops 2 to 3 days after embolization,[322] particularly along the anterior axillary folds and in the conjunctiva and retina.

Laboratory Findings and Diagnosis

Hypocalcemia may develop because of the affinity of calcium ions for free fatty acids released by the hydrolysis of embolized fat.[322] Thrombocytopenia is frequently present and may be associated with DIC. Lipiduria is not uncommon,[322] and hematuria and proteinuria are seen occasionally.[301] Pulmonary function tests reveal decreased compliance and an increased A-a O_2 gradient as a result of $\dot{V}/\dot{Q}$ inequality.[322,323] Severe hypoxemia may persist despite inhalation of 100% oxygen.

The diagnosis can be difficult to make, partly because of the relative nonspecificity of signs and symptoms and partly because clinical abnormalities may be related more directly to the cause of the emboli (e.g., trauma-associated shock). Some investigators have advocated the use of BAL and analysis of harvested macrophages for the presence of fat.[324,325] However, patients who do not have fat embolism syndrome may also have lipid-laden macrophages in their BAL fluid, and the definitive diagnostic threshold is unclear, some investigators proposing a value as low as 5%[324] and others one as high as 30%.[325]

Analysis of blood aspirated from a wedged pulmonary artery catheter has also been used to identify fat.[326] Again, however, serum fat globules are probably present in the majority of patients who have had skeletal trauma, regardless of whether they have fat embolism syndrome, and the number of such globules required for diagnosis is uncertain.[302] Transesophageal echocardiography has been used by some investigators to detect emboli during bone marrow reaming.[327]

In current practice, the diagnosis is probably best based on the presence of a combination of clinical and laboratory findings.[328,329]

Prognosis and Natural History

It has been estimated that approximately 10% of patients who have pulmonary symptoms of fat embolism syndrome progress to respiratory failure.[330] As might be expected, those in whom features of ARDS develop are the most likely to die.[322] Follow-up of survivors generally shows a return to normal pulmonary function.[331]

Amniotic Fluid Embolism

Amniotic fluid embolism is a rare but highly lethal complication of pregnancy.[332,333] Its precise incidence is uncertain. It has been estimated that it is associated with a maternal mortality rate of about 5 to 15 per 100,000 deliveries and accounts for about 5% to 10% of maternal deaths in "developed" countries.[333] However, because of the difficulty in confirming the diagnosis, both during life and at autopsy, and because of the existence of nonlethal disease in an unspecified number of women,[334] the overall incidence is almost certainly higher than these figures suggest.

Pathogenesis

It is likely that little, if any, amniotic fluid enters the maternal circulation during normal labor and that significant embolism occurs only when there is disruption of the uterine wall in association with rupture of the placental membranes.[335] Such disruption can occur at several sites, the most common probably being the endocervix or lower uterine segment. Traumatic tears in the small veins in these regions can occur during normal labor but are of no significance if they are covered by fetal membranes; however, if such veins have separated from the fetal membranes, uterine contractions against a head impacted in the birth canal can repeatedly "pump" amniotic fluid into the maternal venous circulation. Amniotic fluid can also enter the maternal circulation at the placental site—usually in cases of uterine rupture, placenta previa, or cesarean section when the incision involves the site—and rarely elsewhere in the uterine wall in association with myometrial trauma.

The pathophysiologic consequences of intravascular amniotic fluid are complex and probably related to several processes,[332] including (1) pulmonary vascular obstruction by amniotic fluid particulates such as meconium,[336] (2) left ventricular dysfunction (possibly as a result of ischemia secondary to pulmonary hypertension and right ventricular dysfunction or direct myocardial injury by a substance in the embolized amniotic fluid such as endothelin[332,337]), (3) pulmonary edema (related to the left ventricular dysfunction just described or to damage to the vascular endothelium by some constituent of amniotic fluid[338,339]), (4) an immunologic reaction pathogenetically similar to anaphylaxis,[340] (5) infection and septic shock, and (6) coagulation disturbances.

Pathologic Characteristics

The most striking histologic abnormality is the presence of squames, mucin, and bile derived from meconium within small pulmonary vessels. Although much of this material can be recognized with hematoxylin and eosin stain, its presence is more reliably demonstrated by special histochemical techniques or immunohistochemistry,[335,341] which should be performed before excluding a diagnosis of amniotic fluid embolism pathologically.

Radiologic Manifestations

The principal radiographic finding is air space edema indistinguishable from acute pulmonary edema of other cause.[342,343] Whether cardiac enlargement accompanies the edema depends on the severity of pulmonary arterial hypertension and consequent cor pulmonale with or without left ventricular failure. The consolidation may persist or resolve within a few days.[343] Because the predominant radiographic manifestation is widespread air space consolidation, the chief differential diagnoses are massive pulmonary hemorrhage and aspiration of liquid gastric contents.

Clinical Manifestations

The vast majority of patients are in the 35th to 42nd week of pregnancy at the time of embolization. The clinical manifestations are typically abrupt in onset and rapid in progression. Respiratory distress is the initial symptom in about 50% of patients; unexplained hypotension, cyanosis, or seizures may also be evident.[332] Although these abnormalities begin during spontaneous labor in most patients, they occur after delivery in about 30% (10% spontaneous and 20% after cesarean section).[340] Clinical evidence of coagulopathy (DIC) is present in many patients and is the initial feature in 10% to 15%.[344] There appears to be no significant predisposing risk factors.[340]

Laboratory Findings and Diagnosis

Fibrinogen levels are low in many patients, even in the absence of clinical features of DIC. A decreased platelet count as well as increased prothrombin and partial thromboplastin times may be evident.

Because of the frequently rapid and lethal course, the possibility of amniotic fluid embolism should be considered seriously on the basis of the appropriate clinical findings alone. It is supported by identifying squames (particularly when associated with neutrophils), mucin, or hair fragments in samples of pulmonary capillary blood aspirated via a Swan-Ganz catheter.[334] Other potential but as yet unvalidated techniques for diagnosis involve measurement of substances in maternal blood, such as sialyl Tn antigen,[345] zinc coproporphyrin I[346] (both components of amniotic fluid), or tryptase.[333]

Prognosis

The mortality rate of clinically recognized cases varies from 60% to 85%[340]; 25% to 50% of patients die within the first hour of the disease and most of the rest within 12 hours. Serious neurologic sequelae are common in survivors.[340]

Embolic Manifestations of Parasitic Infestation

Immature forms of many human metazoan parasites travel through the systemic circulation to the lungs, where they lodge within pulmonary arterioles and capillaries. Though strictly speaking this represents embolization, in most cases the clinical and pathologic effects are not related to vascular obstruction or damage; instead, pulmonary disease typically occurs in the adjacent lung parenchyma and represents a host reaction to the migrating organism during part of its life cycle. Examples of parasites that cause this form of disease include *Ascaris lumbricoides*, *Strongyloides stercoralis*, *Ancylostoma duodenale*, *Necator americanus*, *Toxocara canis* and *cati*, *Paragonimus* species, and probably *Wuchereria bancrofti* and *Brugia malayi*.

In some instances, however, parasites cause disease that is related directly to pulmonary vascular obstruction. Undoubtedly, the most important of these organisms are *Schistosoma* species, whose eggs, when released into the systemic or portal venous circulation, lodge within pulmonary arteries and arterioles and cause endarteritis obliterans and pulmonary arterial hypertension. Occasionally, whole mature organisms are transported to the lung and become lodged within larger pulmonary vessels; the most common of these organisms is *Dirofilaria immitis*, which is typically associated with adjacent parenchymal necrosis that is manifested radiologically as a solitary pulmonary nodule. A more thorough discussion of these parasites and the diseases that they cause is presented in Chapter 6 (see page 312).

Embolism of Neoplastic Tissue

Because all cases of hematogenous pulmonary metastases must be derived from tumor fragments lodged within pulmonary vessels, it is evident that these are one of the most common forms of emboli. Because of the small size of most tumor fragments, however, effects related to vascular obstruction are seldom apparent. However, when tumor emboli are of sufficient size or number, the clinical, pathologic, and radiographic manifestations are identical to those of thromboemboli and include pulmonary infarction, acute cor pulmonale and sudden death, and a slowly progressive syndrome of dyspnea and pulmonary hypertension.[347] Although the diagnosis is rarely made on conventional radiography,[348] it may be suspected on CT by the presence of multifocal nodular opacities in the distribution of peripheral pulmonary arteries leading to a beaded appearance of these vessels.[349] The subject is considered in greater detail on page 406.

EMBOLI OF FOREIGN MATERIAL

Foreign particulate material can enter the venous side of the systemic circulation and embolize to the lungs. In some situations, this material is introduced by the patient directly into the vasculature (as in intravenous talcosis); in most cases, however, material gains access to the circulation as the result of a medical procedure. The vast majority of these emboli are discovered incidentally at autopsy and are of little or no clinical or radiologic importance.

Air Embolism

As with thrombi and other solid material, embolism of air* within the circulation can have important consequences, including cerebral infarction, cardiovascular collapse, and death.[349a] Although such emboli are uncommonly recognized clinically, it is likely that subclinical emboli occur much more frequently than generally appreciated.[350,351]

---

*Although air itself is frequently the substance that enters the vasculature, in some cases the causative agent is gas, either altered air from the lungs or pure gas such as carbon dioxide, oxygen, or helium.[352,353] Though strictly speaking the appropriate term for the abnormality is thus *gas embolism*, because of conventional use we retain the designation *air embolism* in this text.

Pathogenesis

Air emboli may have their origin in either the greater or the lesser circulation, the predisposing situations and pathophysiologic effects differing significantly between the two sites.[349a] In *systemic (arterial)* air embolism, air typically enters the pulmonary venous circulation and passes to the left side of the heart and then to the systemic arteries; the effects are therefore manifested chiefly in the heart, the spinal cord, and the brain. By contrast, in *pulmonary (venous)* air embolism, air usually enters the systemic venous circulation and passes to the right side of the heart and then to the lungs; clinical and functional manifestations are thus related to obstruction of the pulmonary circulation and are felt predominantly by the lungs.

Systemic Air Embolism. The most frequent site of entry of air into the systemic circulation is the pulmonary veins. This occurs when the wall of a vessel exposed to air is disrupted and the pressure of the air exceeds the pressure in the vessel. These two criteria are met in a variety of circumstances (Table 12–5), the most common of which is probably penetrating thoracic trauma, either iatrogenic or accidental.

Embolism can also occur in several situations in which the thorax is intact. One of the most common is scuba diving, in which the pathogenesis may be related to poor ventilation of a bulla or cyst because of partial or complete obstruction of its feeding airway.[354] Identical barotrauma of ascent can occur in

TABLE 12–5. Systemic (Arterial) Air Embolism

Etiology	Comment
Cardiac Surgery	
Open heart	Most common; residual air in pulmonary veins released into circulation after cross-clamping terminated
Coronary artery bypass	
Iatrogenic fistula	Between lung and left atrium
Penetrating Thoracic Trauma	
Transthoracic needle aspiration	
Thoracentesis	
YAG laser bronchial surgery	Laser-related bronchovascular fistula
Accidents	
Intrinsic Lung Disease	
Asthma	
Neonatal respiratory distress syndrome	
Pulmonary abscess	Fistula between pulmonary vessel and bronchus
Barotrauma	
Positive pressure ventilation	
Compressed air diving	
Air travel	
Miscellaneous	
Hydrogen peroxide ingestion	
Prosthetic aortic valves	

From Fraser RS, Müller NL, Colman NC, Paré PD: Fraser and Paré's Diagnosis of Diseases of the Chest, 4th ed. Philadelphia, WB Saunders, 1999.

airplane passengers.[355] In both these situations, tissue disruption is related to the increase in air pressure in an enclosed space as a result of a decrease in ambient pressure. Most commonly, the resulting pulmonary overpressurization syndrome is related to the presence of mediastinal or subcutaneous air and is characterized by chest pain, hoarseness, and/or neck fullness; more serious consequences develop if air also disseminates into the systemic circulation. Air embolism after decompression can likewise develop as a result of nitrogen coming out of solution directly in the systemic vessels (see later).

Systemic air embolization can also occur in a variety of situations in which there is underlying lung disease, such as severe asthma,[356] and during assisted positive pressure ventilation, particularly in neonates but also in adults.[357,358] In these situations, the sequence of events probably consists of alveolar rupture, interstitial emphysema, and pneumomediastinum and/or pneumothorax; as air dissects through the perivenous interstitial tissue, it also extends into the vein wall and lumen. Air that enters the systemic veins can gain access to the systemic arteries via a patent foramen ovale (paradoxical embolism) or, when abundant, by "spillover" from the pulmonary arterioles/capillaries.

Pulmonary Air Embolism. This abnormality occurs in a wide variety of circumstances (Table 12–6).[359] Iatrogenic causes are by far the most common and include surgery, insertion and maintenance of intravenous apparatus, and diagnostic and therapeutic air insufflation procedures. Venous air embolism has been reported to occur in more than half of all cesarean sections.[360]

As with systemic embolism, pulmonary air embolism requires both vascular disruption and a pressure gradient between the source of extravascular gas and the vascular lumen. This gradient can occur by two mechanisms: (1) positive pressure forcing gas into the veins, as seen in such situations as pressurized infusion of CT contrast material or CO_2 insufflation of the peritoneal cavity before laparoscopy,[361,362] and (2) movement of gas into the veins as a result of a pressure gradient between the site of entry and the pulmonary vessels, a situation best exemplified by head and neck surgery in the sitting position, in which the incidence of emboli may be as high as 40%.[363]

The physiologic effects of embolized air in the pulmonary circulation depend on its quantity and rate of entry.[301] Rapid injection of a large amount of air may result in the formation of an air block in the outflow tract of the right ventricle that prevents pulmonary arterial blood flow. Smaller amounts infused slowly appear to exert an effect at the level of the distal pulmonary arteries and arterioles. Some of this effect is probably related to vascular obstruction by air bubbles themselves; however, reflex vasoconstriction[364] and the formation of fibrin emboli as blood and air are whipped together in the right heart chambers[365] may also be important. The overall effect of these processes is a transient increase in pulmonary vascular resistance and arterial pressure.[366] Both clinical[367] and experimental observations[368] indicate that pulmonary edema complicates some cases of pulmonary air embolism, probably as a result of increased microvascular permeability. The edema results in decreased lung compliance, ventilation-perfusion mismatching, and alterations in gas exchange.[369]

Another cause of pulmonary air embolism is related to the air that reaches the pulmonary vasculature as part of the decompression syndrome. When a diver spends a prolonged

TABLE 12–6. Pulmonary (Venous) Air Embolism

Etiology	Comment
Surgery	
Central nervous system	Paticularly in the sitting (Fowler's) position, in which the incidence is as high as 40%
Uterus	Curettage, hysterectomy, cesarean section, laser ablation
Lung	After bronchus/azygous vein fistula
Bone and joint	Dental implantation, intramedullary nailing, arthroscopic knee surgery, laminectomy
Prostate	Transurethral resection, radical prostatectomy
Kidney	Percutaneous nephrostomy
Diagnostic/Therapeutic Air Injection	
Laparoscopic intra-abdominal surgery	Related to pneumoperitoneum; particularly cholecystectomy
Arthrography	
Pneumoperitoneum	Historical therapy for tuberculosis
Pulsatile saline wound irrigation	
Intravenous Devices	
Cardiac pacemaker	
Central venous catheters for hyperalimentation/ chemotherapy	
Pressurized infusion of intravenous fluids	For example, CT contrast material, blood
Hemodialysis catheters	
Vena cava filters	
Miscellaneous	
Vaginal inflation	Most common in pregnant women after orogenital sex; rarely manual sex or vaginal cocaine insufflation
Penis/scrotal inflation	
Hydrogen peroxide ingestion/ irrigation	After accidental ingestion of H_2O_2 (with gastric catabolism producing excessive oxygen) or wound irrigation
Positive pressure ventilation	
Head trauma	
Air-turbine dental drilling	
Recovery and readministration of blood products	
Decompression syndrome	Rapid ascent after diving or loss of cockpit pressure at high altitude

From Fraser RS, Müller NL, Colman NC, Paré PD: Fraser and Paré's Diagnosis of Diseases of the Chest, 4th ed. Philadelphia, WB Saunders, 1999.

period breathing gas at greater than atmospheric pressure, excess air dissolves in the blood and tissue fluids. With too rapid an ascent and return of partial pressures to lower values, air comes out of solution and forms small bubbles that can be carried in the systemic veins to the right side of the heart and pulmonary vasculature. Oxygen coming out of solution can be disposed of easily by metabolic consumption, but the inert nitrogen is much slower to be cleared. The bubbles cause lung microvascular damage and noncardiac pulmonary edema in the same manner as discussed earlier. This form of pulmonary decompression sickness, which has been called "the chokes," is a relatively uncommon form of decompression illness that is sometimes fatal.[370]

Pathologic Characteristics

In patients who die of pulmonary air embolism, bloody froth formed by the whipping action of the right atrium and ventricle may be seen to partly fill these chambers and extend into the proximal branches of the pulmonary artery. The pulmonary veins are virtually empty of blood, as are the left atrium and left ventricle, which are typically contracted.

Radiologic Manifestations

The principal sign of air embolism is the presence of gas in cardiac chambers or pulmonary or systemic vessels.[371,372] In pulmonary air embolism, the gas is present in the right heart chambers, central pulmonary arteries, and (sometimes) the hepatic veins[373]; in systemic air embolism, it can be identified in the left heart chambers, aorta, or more peripheral branches of the systemic arterial tree such as the neck, shoulder girdles, or upper part of the abdomen. Other manifestations of pulmonary air embolism include pulmonary edema, focal oligemia, enlarged central pulmonary arteries, and atelectasis.[372] The radiographic findings associated with air embolism in a study of 31 scuba divers included pneumomediastinum (in 8), subcutaneous emphysema (3), pneumocardium (2), and pneumothorax and pneumoperitoneum (1 each).[374]

Pulmonary air embolism is seen particularly well on CT. In a study of 100 patients who received intravenous contrast material that was injected by hand and followed by a drip infusion, asymptomatic venous air embolism was documented in 23.[362] The most common site was the main pulmonary artery. In another series of 677 patients who underwent contrast-enhanced CT, air emboli were detected in 79 (12%)[375]; they were located in the main pulmonary artery in 54 (8%), the superior vena cava in 12 (1.8%), the right ventricle in 10 (1.5%), the subclavian or brachiocephalic vein in 6 (0.9%), and the right atrium in 5 (0.7%). Seven patients (1%) had emboli at more than one site.

Clinical Manifestations

The vast majority of patients with pulmonary air embolism are asymptomatic. However, when the amount of air entering the lung is considerable, particularly if the entry is rapid, clinical manifestations may ensue. Symptoms are nonspecific and include faintness, lightheadedness, and dyspnea; chest pain occurs occasionally. One group of investigators has described a "gasp" reflex consisting of a cough followed by a short expiration and several seconds of inspiration.[376]

Physical findings include tachycardia, tachypnea, and systemic hypotension. A precordial murmur resembling the sound of a "mill wheel" has been described in some patients.[377] Signs of pulmonary edema may also be evident. Migration of air into systemic vessels supplying the brain or heart may result in convulsions, coma, or chest pain. Bubbles can be visualized in the retinal vessels in some patients.[302] Similar findings are evident in "primary" systemic air embolism.

Laboratory Findings and Diagnosis

Laboratory findings are nonspecific. Elevated levels of lactate dehydrogenase and transaminases have been found in some patients who have had arterial air embolism after underwater diving.[378] If coronary vessels are obstructed, electrocardiographic changes may indicate myocardial ischemia or ventricular dysrhythmia. Arterial blood gas analysis may show hypoxemia and hypercapnia.

The most commonly used techniques for confirming the diagnosis are precordial Doppler ultrasonography and transesophageal echocardiography. The former is probably the more sensitive; it is able to detect air bubbles as small as 0.1 mL because of the high echogenic interface between air and blood.[301]

Prognosis

Pulmonary air embolism is usually a benign event unrecognized by the patient or physician.[379] Systemic air embolism is probably also often unnoticed; however, because of the serious consequences potentially associated with occlusion of cardiac or cerebral arteries, only a small amount of embolized air may be lethal. The precise incidence of this outcome is uncertain because of difficulty in diagnosis, both during life and after death.

Embolism of Talc, Starch, and Cellulose

Emboli of talc, starch, and cellulose are seen almost invariably in individuals who have engaged in intravenous drug abuse over a long period.[380] In most instances, the complication occurs with medications intended solely for oral use; pills are crushed in a spoon or bottle top, water is added, and the mixture is drawn into a syringe and injected. The habit is usually the result of a shortage of available heroin, although some addicts use the drugs in this manner to counteract the sedative effect of the narcotic drugs themselves. Oral medications misused in this way include amphetamines and closely related drugs such as methylphenidate hydrochloride (Ritalin) and tripelennamine, methadone hydrochloride, hydromorphone hydrochloride (Dilaudid), phenyltoloxamine, propoxyphene (Darvon), secobarbital, pentazocine (Talwin), meperidine, and propylhexedrine.

All these medications have in common the addition of an insoluble filler to bind the medicinal particles together and act as a lubricant to prevent the tablets from sticking to punches and dies during manufacture. The most widely used filler is talc; cornstarch and microcrystalline cellulose are used occasionally. As might be predicted, the severity of radiographic and pulmonary function abnormalities is related to the quantity of drug injected.[381]

Pathogenesis

When injected intravenously, the fillers become trapped within pulmonary arterioles and capillaries and cause vascular occlusion, sometimes associated with thrombosis. Transient pulmonary hypertension has been reported after the intravenous injection of pentazocine, possibly related to this mechanism.[382] In time, the foreign particles migrate through the vessel wall and come to lie in the adjacent perivascular and parenchymal interstitial tissue, where they engender a foreign body giant cell reaction and fibrosis. Chronic pulmonary hypertension typically develops at this stage if the quantity of foreign material is sufficient. Although such hypertension is undoubtedly related to vascular alterations directly caused by the emboli, it is possible that parenchymal fibrosis and emphysema are also involved. The pathogenesis of the emphysema is unclear.

Pathologic Characteristics

In early disease, the lungs show variable numbers of more or less discrete parenchymal nodules measuring up to 1 mm in diameter (Fig. 12–21). In long-standing disease, the nodules tend to become confluent, especially in the upper lobes, and produce large areas of consolidation resembling the progressive massive fibrosis seen in the pneumoconioses (see Color Fig. 12–3). Panacinar emphysema, sometimes with bulla formation, is often evident.[380,383]

Histologically, the small nodules consist of loosely formed granulomas containing many large multinucleated giant cells (see Fig. 12–21). Sections of the large foci of upper lobe consolidation seen in long-standing disease show sheets of multinucleated giant cells, usually not organized in discrete granulomas; a variable degree of fibrosis is also present. Foreign material is readily identifiable within the giant cells and is particularly well seen in polarized light.

Radiologic Manifestations

The earliest radiologic manifestation is widespread nodules ranging from barely visible to about 1 mm in diameter (Fig. 12–22). They are distinct and "pinpoint" in character, similar to alveolar microlithiasis. Although some authors have described a midzonal predominance of these nodules,[384] the distribution that we have observed has been diffuse and uniform throughout the lungs.[385]

In more advanced disease, the upper lobe nodules may coalesce to form an almost homogeneous opacity that resembles the progressive massive fibrosis of silicosis or coal workers' pneumoconiosis, except for the frequent presence of an air bronchogram.[380,386] Pulmonary arterial hypertension and cor pulmonale may develop.[384,387] In the late stages of the disease, increasing disability and deteriorating function are associated with radiographic evidence of emphysema and bullae.[380] HRCT findings consist of diffuse ground-glass attenuation, a diffuse micronodular pattern, and perihilar upper lobe conglomerate areas of fibrosis.[385,388] Localized areas of high attenuation consistent with talc deposition can be seen within the conglomerate masses (Fig. 12–23).

The radiographic and CT findings of intravenous abuse of methylphenidate (crushed Ritalin tablets) differ somewhat from those of other types of intravenous drug abuse,[385,389] the main abnormality characteristically consisting of bilateral, symmetrical emphysema involving mainly the lower lung zones and unassociated with bulla formation.

Clinical Manifestations

Most addicts are asymptomatic, granulomas being found incidentally at autopsy in those who die of other causes.[390]

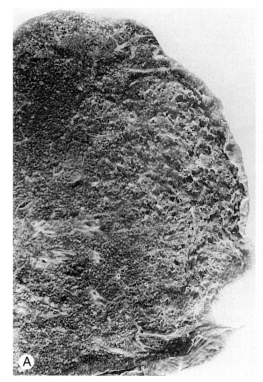
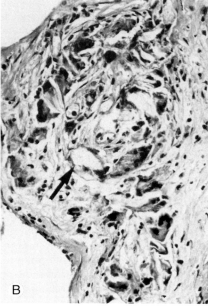
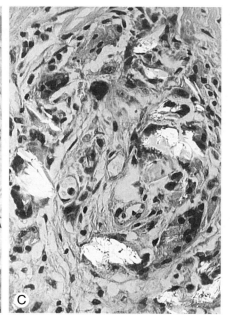

FIGURE 12–21

Intravenous talcosis. A slice of an upper lobe (**A**) shows severe panacinar emphysema in its anterior portion and a fine nodularity in the remaining parenchyma. A histologic view (**B**) reveals aggregates of multinucleated giant cells containing talc crystals (*arrow*). A photomicrograph taken with polarized light (**C**) shows the refractile talc to better advantage. *(From Fraser RS, Müller NL, Colman NC, Paré PD: Fraser and Paré's Diagnosis of Diseases of the Chest, 4th ed. Philadelphia, WB Saunders, 1999.)*

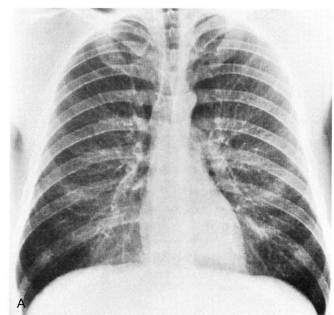

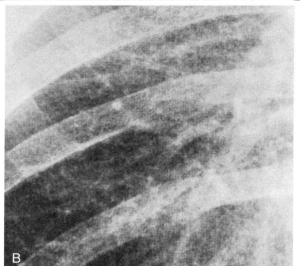

FIGURE 12-22

Pulmonary talcosis in intravenous drug abuse. This asymptomatic 22-year-old man had been shooting heroin and methadone for 4 years at the time that these radiographs were obtained. There is widespread involvement of both lungs by tiny micronodular opacities (**A**), seen to better advantage on a magnified image (2:1) of the right lower zone (**B**). There is no anatomic predominance. The pattern is similar to the discrete opacities of alveolar microlithiasis. (*From Müller NL, Fraser RS, Colman NC, Paré PD: Radiologic Diagnosis of Diseases of the Chest. Philadelphia, WB Saunders, 2001.*)

Typically, symptoms develop only in very heavy users (not infrequently with a history of injection of thousands of pills) and consist of slowly progressive dyspnea and (occasionally) persistent cough. Cor pulmonale may be evident as a result of extensive disease. As in silicosis, disease may progress and disability may increase after cessation of exposure.[381] Organized thrombi and scars are visible on the forearms of nearly all addicts who inject drugs intravenously. Glistening particles can be seen in the fundi, principally at the posterior pole sur-

rounding the foveal area, and may be the earliest clue to the drug use.[381,391]

Pulmonary Function Studies

Studies of addicts who admit intravenous abuse of oral medications have found significant impairment of gas transfer[392] accompanied by a combination of obstructive and restrictive defects but little or no hyperinflation or air trapping, at least in the early stages.[381] In more advanced disease, a severe reduction in flow rates and diffusion accompanied by hyperinflation and air trapping may become evident.[380]

Iodized Oil Embolism

Pulmonary oil embolism is usually a complication of lymphangiography with ethiodized poppy seed oil (Ethiodol). It is probably common; both postmortem studies shortly after the procedure[393] and photoscans of sputum after lymphangiography with ^{131}I-labeled oil[394] have shown that a considerable quantity of oil may be present in the lungs, even without any radiographically demonstrable abnormality.

In an investigation of 80 patients, radiographic evidence of oil embolism was found in 44 (55%), most of whom had pelvic or abdominal lymphatic obstruction.[395] It has been postulated that such obstruction permits uptake of the contrast medium by systemic veins, so the oil arrives in the lungs earlier and in greater concentration than it would otherwise. The findings usually consist of a fine reticular pattern, which may persist for 1 to 2 weeks (Fig. 12–24).[395] In addition, small peripheral vessels may be so filled with contrast material that they have an arborizing pattern similar to that seen on pulmonary arteriography.[393]

Few patients have symptoms. Mild fever may develop within 48 hours after lymphangiography; rarely, cough, chills, dyspnea, cyanosis, hemoptysis, or hypotension is present.[395,396] Decreased diffusing capacity is not uncommon, the abnormality being most marked at 24 to 48 hours.[397] Additional abnormalities include a reduction in lung compliance and arterial PO_2, particularly after a high dose of a contrast agent.[398]

Miscellaneous Foreign Body Embolism

Metallic Mercury Embolism. Pulmonary embolization of mercury may be accidental or intentional—the former after injury from a broken thermometer and the latter as a result of injection by drug abusers or patients attempting suicide.[399] The radiographic appearance is distinctive because of the very high density of mercury and takes the form of small spherules or short tubular structures representing mercury-filled arterial segments.[400] The distribution is generally bilateral and fairly symmetrical. A local collection of mercury may be apparent in the heart, usually near the apex of the right ventricle. Pulmonary, cardiac, and systemic localization of mercury droplets has also been described on CT.[401] Clinically, toxicity is manifested by a metallic taste, excessive salivation, gingivitis, stomatitis, diarrhea, nephrosis, tremor (hatter's shakes), and irritability.[402] Pulmonary symptoms and function abnormalities are very mild or absent.[403]

Liquid Acrylate. Liquid acrylate glues—most commonly isobutyl-2-cyanoacrylate and *n*-butyl-2-cyanoacrylate—are

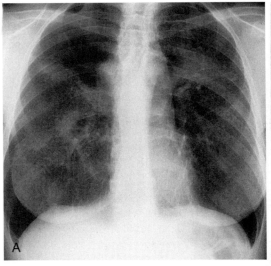

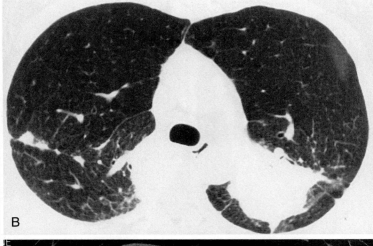

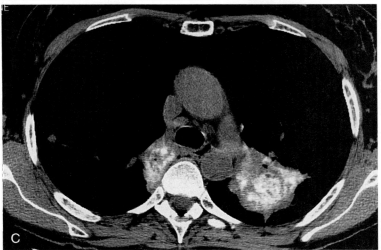

FIGURE 12–23

Talcosis: progressive massive fibrosis. A posteroanterior chest radiograph (**A**) shows bilateral large opacities in the middle and upper lung zones. Note the dense large opacity adjacent to the right tracheobronchial angle and the right upper lobe emphysema. An HRCT scan (**B**) shows dense large opacities with associated distortion of the lung architecture. Soft tissue windows (**C**) reveal areas of increased attenuation with the opacities consistent with talc deposition. The patient was a 54-year-old woman with exercise-induced dyspnea. Although she had a 12-year history of intravenous drug abuse (heroin and methadone), she emphatically stated that she had stopped using any intravenous drugs 23 years previously. *(From Müller NL, Fraser RS, Colman NC, Paré PD: Radiologic Diagnosis of Diseases of the Chest. Philadelphia, WB Saunders, 2001.)*

FIGURE 12–24

Lipiodol emboli. A magnified view of the apex of the left upper lobe approximately $1\frac{1}{2}$ hours after the injection of 7 mL of Lipiodol into the lymphatics of each leg reveals a fine network of shadows of high density. This network is caused by the presence of contrast medium in the microvascular circulation of the lung. The thoracic duct can be identified on the left *(arrows)*. *(From Fraser RS, Müller NL, Colman NC, Paré PD: Fraser and Paré's Diagnosis of Diseases of the Chest, 4th ed. Philadelphia, WB Saunders, 1999.)*

frequently used in embolization therapy for vascular malformations.[404] Asymptomatic pulmonary embolism associated with the procedure is probably more frequent than generally appreciated[404,405]; however, symptomatic embolization is uncommon. Radiographic findings consist of subsegmental areas of consolidation.[404] CT scans have shown subsegmental, predominantly pleural-based wedge-shaped areas of consolidation consistent with infarction. Because the acrylate glue is mixed with radiopaque substances to allow accurate localization during embolization therapy, CT also shows punctate radiodensities within pulmonary arteries. Patients may complain of pleuritic chest pain with or without associated cough and bloody sputum.

Bullets and Shrapnel. Uncommonly, these agents enter the extrathoracic systemic veins or the right side of the heart, are carried to the lungs, and then lodge within pulmonary arteries.[406] Both clinical observations and experimental studies have shown that such foreign bodies can remain within the pulmonary vasculature for prolonged periods without untoward effects.[407]

Radiopaque Foreign Bodies. A variety of devices such as wire loops and balloons filled with contrast medium have been used therapeutically in both the pulmonary and systemic circulations to obliterate arteriovenous malformations or to control intractable hemorrhage. Escape of such material into the systemic veins can result in opacities of metallic density within the lungs.[408]

Plastic Intravenous Catheters. These devices, either whole or in fragments, usually embolize to the lungs when cut by the sharp bevel of the needle housing them[409]; occasionally, they are detached from their connector or fracture spontaneously.[410]

Silicone. Silicone fluid (polydimethylsiloxane) embolism has been reported in some patients in whom the substance has been injected subcutaneously for breast augmentation.[411] Radiographs have shown a combination of interstitial and air space disease, which in severe cases progresses to a pattern of ARDS.

REFERENCES

1. Slavin RE, de Groot WJ: Pathology of the lung in Behçet's disease. Case report and review of the literature. Am J Surg Pathol 5:779-788, 1981.
2. Chiu B, Magil A: Idiopathic pulmonary arterial trunk aneurysm presenting as cor pulmonale: Report of a case. Hum Pathol 16:947-949, 1985.
3. Connors AF Jr, Castele RJ, Farhat NZ, Tomashefski JF Jr: Complications of right heart catheterization. A prospective autopsy study. Chest 88:567-572, 1985.
4. Haupt HM, Moore GW, Bauer TW, Hutchins GM: The lung in sickle cell disease. Chest 81:332-337, 1982.
5. Presti B, Berthrong M, Sherwin RM: Chronic thrombosis of major pulmonary arteries. Hum Pathol 21:601-606, 1990.
6. Heath D, Thompson IM: Bronchopulmonary anastomoses in sickle-cell anaemia. Thorax 24:232-238, 1969.
7. Robboy SJ, Major MC, Colman RW, Minna JD: Pathology of disseminated intravascular coagulation (DIC). Analysis of 26 cases. Hum Pathol 3:327-343, 1972.
8. Cramer SF, Tomkiewicz ZM: Septic pulmonary thrombosis in streptococcal toxic shock syndrome. Hum Pathol 26:1157-1160, 1995.
9. Ferencz C: The pulmonary vascular bed in tetralogy of Fallot. II. Changes following a systemic-pulmonary arterial anastomosis. Bull Johns Hopkins Hosp 106:100-118, 1960.
10. Berry DF, Buccigrossi D, Peabody J, et al: Pulmonary vascular occlusion and fibrosing mediastinitis. Chest 89:296-301, 1986.
11. Huisman MV, Buller HR, ten Cate JW, et al: Unexpected high prevalence of silent pulmonary embolism in patients with deep venous thrombosis. Chest 95:498-502, 1989.
12. Hampson NB: Pulmonary embolism: Difficulties in the clinical diagnosis. Semin Respir Infect 10:123-130, 1995.
13. Moser KM: Venous thromboembolism. Am Rev Respir Dis 141:235-249, 1990.
14. Goldhaber SZ, Morpurgo M: Diagnosis, treatment, and prevention of pulmonary embolism. Report of the WHO/International Society and Federation of Cardiology Task Force. JAMA 268:1727-1733, 1992.
15. Kalodiki E, Domjan J, Nicolaides AN, et al: V/Q defects and deep venous thrombosis following total hip replacement. Clin Radiol 50:400-403, 1995.
16. Warwick D, Williams MH, Bannister GC: Death and thromboembolic disease after total hip replacement. A series of 1162 cases with no routine chemical prophylaxis. J Bone Joint Surg Br 77:6-10, 1995.
17. Fowkes FJ, Price JF, Fowkes FG: Incidence of diagnosed deep vein thrombosis in the general population: Systematic review. Eur J Vasc Endovasc Surg 25:1-5, 2003.
18. Samama MM: An epidemiologic study of risk factors for deep vein thrombosis in medical outpatients: The Sirius study. Arch Intern Med 160:3415-3420, 2000.
19. Hyers TM: Venous thromboembolism. Am J Respir Crit Care Med 159:1-14, 1999.
20. Silverstein MD, Heit JA, Mohr DN, et al: Trends in the incidence of deep vein thrombosis and pulmonary embolism: A 25-year population-based study. Arch Intern Med 158:585-593, 1998.
21. White RH, Zhou H, Romano PS: Incidence of idiopathic deep venous thrombosis and secondary thromboembolism among ethnic groups in California. Ann Intern Med 128:737-740, 1998.
22. Klatsky AL, Armstrong MA, Poggi J: Risk of pulmonary embolism and/or deep venous thrombosis in Asian-Americans. Am J Cardiol 85:1334-1337, 2000.
23. Boulay F, Berthier F, Schoukroun G, et al: Seasonal variations in hospital admission for deep vein thrombosis and pulmonary embolism: Analysis of discharge data. BMJ 323:601-602, 2001.
24. Morrell MT, Dunnill MS: The post-mortem incidence of pulmonary embolism in a hospital population. Br J Surg 55:347-352, 1968.
25. Dalen JE, Alpert JS: Natural history of pulmonary embolism. Prog Cardiovasc Dis 17:259-270, 1975.
26. Lau G: Pulmonary thromboembolism is not uncommon—results and implications of a five-year study of 116 necropsies. Ann Acad Med Singapore 24:356-365, 1995.
27. Kim V, Spandorfer J: Epidemiology of venous thromboembolic disease. Emerg Med Clin North Am 19:839-859, 2001.
28. Dalen JE: Pulmonary embolism: What have we learned since Virchow? Natural history, pathophysiology, and diagnosis. Chest 122:1440-1456, 2002.
29. Lilienfeld DE: Decreasing mortality from pulmonary embolism in the United States, 1979-1996. Int J Epidemiol 29:465-469, 2000.
30. Janke RM, McGovern PG, Folsom AR: Mortality, hospital discharges, and case fatality for pulmonary embolism in the Twin Cities: 1980-1995. J Clin Epidemiol 53:103-109, 2000.
31. Kakkar VV, Howe CT, Flanc C, Clarke MB: Natural history of postoperative deep-vein thrombosis. Lancet 2:230-232, 1969.
32. Coon WW, Willis PW 3rd: Thrombosis of axillary and subclavian veins. Arch Surg 94:657-663, 1967.
33. Joffe HV, Goldhaber SZ: Upper-extremity deep vein thrombosis. Circulation 106:1874-1880, 2002.
34. Anderson FA Jr, Wheeler HB, Goldberg RJ, et al: The prevalence of risk factors for venous thromboembolism among hospital patients. Arch Intern Med 152:1660-1664, 1992.
35. Heit JA, Silverstein MD, Mohr DN, et al: Risk factors for deep vein thrombosis and pulmonary embolism: A population-based case-control study. Arch Intern Med 160:809-815, 2000.
36. The PIOPED Investigators: Value of the ventilation/perfusion scan in acute pulmonary embolism. Results of the Prospective Investigation of Pulmonary Embolism Diagnosis (PIOPED). JAMA 263:2753-2759, 1990.
37. Ferrari E, Chevallier T, Chapelier A, Baudouy M: Travel as a risk factor for venous thromboembolic disease: A case-control study. Chest 115:440-444, 1999.
38. Joynt GM, Kew J, Gomersall CD, et al: Deep venous thrombosis caused by femoral venous catheters in critically ill adult patients. Chest 117:178-183, 2000.
39. Otten TR, Stein PD, Patel KC, et al: Thromboembolic disease involving the superior vena cava and brachiocephalic veins. Chest 123:809-812, 2003.
40. Stamatakis JD, Kakkar VV, Sagar S, et al: Femoral vein thrombosis and total hip replacement. BMJ 2:223-225, 1977.
41. Hull R, Hirsh J, Sackett DL, Stoddart G: Cost effectiveness of clinical diagnosis, venography, and noninvasive testing in patients with symptomatic deep-vein thrombosis. N Engl J Med 304:1561-1567, 1981.
42. De Stefano V, Rossi E, Paciaroni K, Leone G: Screening for inherited thrombophilia: Indications and therapeutic implications. Haematologica 87:1095-1108, 2002.
43. Crowther MA, Kelton JG: Congenital thrombophilic states associated with venous thrombosis: A qualitative overview and proposed classification system. Ann Intern Med 138:128-134, 2003.
44. Franco RF, Reitsma PH: Genetic risk factors of venous thrombosis. Hum Genet 109:369-384, 2001.
45. Murin S, Marelich GP, Arroliga AC, Matthay RA: Hereditary thrombophilia and venous thromboembolism. Am J Respir Crit Care Med 158:1369-1373, 1998.
46. McGlennen RC, Key NS: Clinical and laboratory management of the prothrombin G20210A mutation. Arch Pathol Lab Med 126:1319-1325, 2002.
47. Joffe HV, Goldhaber SZ: Laboratory thrombophilias and venous thromboembolism. Vasc Med 7:93-102, 2002.
48. Eichinger S, Weltermann A, Mannhalter C, et al: The risk of recurrent venous thromboembolism in heterozygous carriers of factor V Leiden and a first spontaneous venous thromboembolism. Arch Intern Med 162:2357-2360, 2002.
49. De Stefano V, Martinelli I, Mannucci PM, et al: The risk of recurrent venous thromboembolism among heterozygous carriers of the G20210A prothrombin gene mutation. Br J Haematol 113:630-635, 2001.
50. Perry SL, Ortel TL: Clinical and laboratory evaluation of thrombophilia. Clin Chest Med 24:153-170, 2003.
51. De Stefano V, Leone G: Resistance to activated protein C due to mutated factor V as a novel cause of inherited thrombophilia. Haematologica 80:344-356, 1995.
52. Middeldorp S, Meinardi JR, Koopman MM, et al: A prospective study of asymptomatic carriers of the factor V Leiden mutation to determine the incidence of venous thromboembolism. Ann Intern Med 135:322-327, 2001.
53. Meinardi JR, Middeldorp S, de Kam PJ, et al: The incidence of recurrent venous thromboembolism in carriers of factor V Leiden is related to concomitant thrombophilic disorders. Br J Haematol 116:625-631, 2002.
54. De Stefano V, Rossi E, Paciaroni K, et al: Different circumstances of the first venous thromboembolism among younger or older heterozygous carriers of the G20210A polymorphism in the prothrombin gene. Haematologica 88:61-66, 2003.
55. Kraaijenhagen RA, in't Anker PS, Koopman MM, et al: High plasma concentration of factor VIIIc is a major risk factor for venous thromboembolism. Thromb Haemost 83:5-9, 2000.
56. van Hylckama Vlieg A, van der Linden IK, Bertina RM, Rosendaal FR: High levels of factor IX increase the risk of venous thrombosis. Blood 95:3678-3682, 2000.
57. Meijers JC, Tekelenburg WL, Bouma BN, et al: High levels of coagulation factor XI as a risk factor for venous thrombosis. N Engl J Med 342:696-701, 2000.

58. Koster T, Rosendaal FR, Reitsma PH, et al: Factor VII and fibrinogen levels as risk factors for venous thrombosis. A case-control study of plasma levels and DNA polymorphisms—the Leiden Thrombophilia Study (LETS). Thromb Haemost 71:719-722, 1994.

59. den Heijer M, Koster T, Blom HJ, et al: Hyperhomocysteinemia as a risk factor for deep-vein thrombosis. N Engl J Med 334:759-762, 1996.

60. Key NS, McGlennen RC: Hyperhomocyst(e)inemia and thrombophilia. Arch Pathol Lab Med 126:1367-1375, 2002.

61. De Stefano V, Casorelli I, Rossi E, et al: Interaction between hyperhomocysteinemia and inherited thrombophilic factors in venous thromboembolism. Semin Thromb Hemost 26:305-311, 2000.

62. Matei D, Brenner B, Marder VJ: Acquired thrombophilic syndromes. Blood Rev 15:31-48, 2001.

63. Prandoni P: Cancer and thromboembolic disease: How important is the risk of thrombosis? Cancer Treat Rev 28:133-136, 2002.

64. Haim N, Lanir N, Hoffman R, et al: Acquired activated protein C resistance is common in cancer patients and is associated with venous thromboembolism. Am J Med 110:91-96, 2001.

65. Patterson WP, Ringenberg QS: The pathophysiology of thrombosis in cancer. Semin Oncol 17:140-146, 1990.

66. Sutherland DE, Weitz IC, Liebman HA: Thromboembolic complications of cancer: Epidemiology, pathogenesis, diagnosis, and treatment. Am J Hematol 72:43-52, 2003.

67. Lee AY: Cancer and thromboembolic disease: Pathogenic mechanisms. Cancer Treat Rev 28:137-140, 2002.

68. Fennerty T: Screening for cancer in venous thromboembolic disease. BMJ 323:704-705, 2001.

69. Oral contraception and thrombo-embolic disease. J R Coll Gen Pract 13:267-279, 1967.

70. Grady D, Sawaya G: Postmenopausal hormone therapy increases risk of deep vein thrombosis and pulmonary embolism. Am J Med 105:41-43, 1998.

71. Venous thromboembolic disease and combined oral contraceptives: Results of international multicentre case-control study. World Health Organization Collaborative Study of Cardiovascular Disease and Steroid Hormone Contraception. Lancet 346:1575-1582, 1995.

72. Vandenbroucke JP, Rosing J, Bloemenkamp KW, et al: Oral contraceptives and the risk of venous thrombosis. N Engl J Med 344:1527-1535, 2001.

73. Gerhardt A, Scharf RE, Beckmann MW, et al: Prothrombin and factor V mutations in women with a history of thrombosis during pregnancy and the puerperium. N Engl J Med 342:374-380, 2000.

74. Seligsohn U, Lubetsky A: Genetic susceptibility to venous thrombosis. N Engl J Med 344:1222-1231, 2001.

75. Dalen JE, Haffajee CI, Alpert JS 3rd, et al: Pulmonary embolism, pulmonary hemorrhage and pulmonary infarction. N Engl J Med 296:1431-1435, 1977.

76. Parker B, Smith J: Pulmonary embolism and infarction. A review of the physiologic consequences of pulmonary arterial obstruction. Am J Med 24:402, 1958.

77. Lindblad B, Sternby NH, Bergqvist D: Incidence of venous thromboembolism verified by necropsy over 30 years. BMJ 302:709-711, 1991.

78. Tsao MS, Schraufnagel D, Wang NS: Pathogenesis of pulmonary infarction. Am J Med 72:599-606, 1982.

79. Schraufnagel DE, Tsao MS, Yao YT, Wang NS: Factors associated with pulmonary infarction. A discriminant analysis study. Am J Clin Pathol 84:15-18, 1985.

80. Newhouse MT, Becklake MR, Macklem PT, McGregor M: Effect of alterations in end-tidal CO_2 tension on flow resistance. J Appl Physiol 19:745-749, 1964.

81. Kerr IH, Simon G, Sutton GC: The value of the plain radiograph in acute massive pulmonary embolism. Br J Radiol 44:751-757, 1971.

82. Windebank WJ, Boyd G, Moran F: Pulmonary thrombo-embolism presenting as cardiac emergencies. Scott Med J 19:221-228, 1974.

83. Colman NC: Pathophysiology of pulmonary embolism. In Leclerc JR (ed): Venous Thromboembolic Disorders. Philadelphia, Lea & Febiger, 1991, p 65.

84. Soloff LA, Rodman T: Acute pulmonary embolism. 1. Review. Am Heart J 74:710-724, 1967.

85. McIntyre KM, Sasahara AA: The hemodynamic response to pulmonary embolism in patients without prior cardiopulmonary disease. Am J Cardiol 28:288-294, 1971.

86. Sofia M, Faraone S, Alifano M, et al: Endothelin abnormalities in patients with pulmonary embolism. Chest 111:544-549, 1997.

87. Egermayer P, Town GI, Peacock AJ: Role of serotonin in the pathogenesis of acute and chronic pulmonary hypertension. Thorax 54:161-168, 1999.

88. Sasahara AA: The clinical and hemodynamic features of acute pulmonary embolism. In Simmons DH (ed): Current Pulmonology. Chicago, Mosby Year Book, 1988.

89. Wiener SN, Edelstein J, Charms BL: Observations on pulmonary embolism and the pulmonary angiogram. Am J Roentgenol Radium Ther Nucl Med 98:859-873, 1966.

90. Fanta CH, Wright TC, McFadden ER Jr: Differentiation of recurrent pulmonary emboli from chronic obstructive lung disease as a cause of cor pulmonale. Chest 79:92-95, 1981.

91. Wood KE: Major pulmonary embolism: Review of a pathophysiologic approach to the golden hour of hemodynamically significant pulmonary embolism. Chest 121:877-905, 2002.

92. Moser KM, Auger WR, Fedullo PF, Jamieson SW: Chronic thromboembolic pulmonary hypertension: Clinical picture and surgical treatment. Eur Respir J 5:334-342, 1992.

93. Benotti JR, Dalen JE: The natural history of pulmonary embolism. Clin Chest Med 5:403-410, 1984.

94. Fedullo PF, Auger WR, Channick RN, et al: Chronic thromboembolic pulmonary hypertension. Clin Chest Med 22:561-581, 2001.

95. Kimura H, Okada O, Tanabe N, et al: Plasma monocyte chemoattractant protein-1 and pulmonary vascular resistance in chronic thromboembolic pulmonary hypertension. Am J Respir Crit Care Med 164:319-324, 2001.

96. Dantzker DR, Bower JS: Partial reversibility of chronic pulmonary hypertension caused by pulmonary thromboembolic disease. Am Rev Respir Dis 124:129-131, 1981.

97. Fedullo PF, Auger WR, Channick RN, et al: Chronic thromboembolic pulmonary hypertension. Clin Chest Med 16:353-374, 1995.

98. Menzel T, Wagner S, Kramm T, et al: Pathophysiology of impaired right and left ventricular function in chronic embolic pulmonary hypertension: Changes after pulmonary thromboendarterectomy. Chest 118:897-903, 2000.

99. Dombert MC, Rouby JJ, Smiejan JM, et al: Pulmonary oedema during pulmonary embolism. Br J Dis Chest 81:407-410, 1987.

100. tenHoopen DJ, Sherer DM, Abramowicz JS, Papadakos PJ: Extensive pulmonary embolism presenting as severe adult respiratory distress syndrome after surgical resection of a cornual pregnancy. Am J Obstet Gynecol 165:41-42, 1991.

101. Perlman MB, Johnson A, Jubiz W, Malik AB: Lipoxygenase products induce neutrophil activation and increase endothelial permeability after thrombin-induced pulmonary microembolism. Circ Res 64:62-73, 1989.

102. Rodger MA, Carrier M, Jones GN, et al: Diagnostic value of arterial blood gas measurement in suspected pulmonary embolism. Am J Respir Crit Care Med 162:2105-2108, 2000.

103. Kline JA, Johns KL, Colucciello SA, Israel EG: New diagnostic tests for pulmonary embolism. Ann Emerg Med 35:168-180, 2000.

104. Kline JA, Kubin AK, Patel MM, et al: Alveolar dead space as a predictor of severity of pulmonary embolism. Acad Emerg Med 7:611-617, 2000.

105. Rodger MA, Jones G, Rasuli P, et al: Steady-state end-tidal alveolar dead space fraction and D-dimer: Bedside tests to exclude pulmonary embolism. Chest 120:115-119, 2001.

106. Santolicandro A, Prediletto R, Fornai E, et al: Mechanisms of hypoxemia and hypocapnia in pulmonary embolism. Am J Respir Crit Care Med 152:336-347, 1995.

107. Elliott CG: Pulmonary physiology during pulmonary embolism. Chest 101:163S-171S, 1992.

108. Manier G, Castaing Y: Influence of cardiac output on oxygen exchange in acute pulmonary embolism. Am Rev Respir Dis 145:130-136, 1992.

109. Ley S, Kreitner KF, Morgenstern I, et al: Bronchopulmonary shunts in patients with chronic thromboembolic pulmonary hypertension: Evaluation with helical CT and MR imaging. AJR Am J Roentgenol 179:1209-1215, 2002.

110. Bewtra C, Dewan N, O'Donahue WJ Jr: Exfoliative sputum cytology in pulmonary embolism. Acta Cytol 27:489-496, 1983.

111. Austin HM, Wilner GD, Dominguez C: Natural history of pulmonary thromboemboli in dogs. Serial radiographic observation of clots labeled with powdered tantalum. Radiology 116:519-525, 1975.

112. Dalen JE, Banas JS Jr, Brooks HL, et al: Resolution rate of acute pulmonary embolism in man. N Engl J Med 280:1194-1199, 1969.

113. Walker RH, Goodwin J, Jackson JA: Resolution of pulmonary embolism. BMJ 4:135-139, 1970.

114. Sevitt S: Organic fragmentation in pulmonary thrombo-emboli. J Pathol 122:95-103, 1977.

115. Worsley DF, Alavi A, Aronchick JM, et al: Chest radiographic findings in patients with acute pulmonary embolism: Observations from the PIOPED Study. Radiology 189:133-136, 1993.

116. Greenspan RH, Ravin CE, Polansky SM, McLoud TC: Accuracy of the chest radiograph in diagnosis of pulmonary embolism. Invest Radiol 17:539-543, 1982.

117. Alderson PO, Martin EC: Pulmonary embolism: Diagnosis with multiple imaging modalities. Radiology 164:297-312, 1987.

118. Stein PD, Athanasoulis C, Greenspan RH, Henry JW: Relation of plain chest radiographic findings to pulmonary arterial pressure and arterial blood oxygen levels in patients with acute pulmonary embolism. Am J Cardiol 69:394-396, 1992.

119. Westermark N: On the roentgen diagnosis of lung embolism. Acta Radiol 19:357, 1938.

120. Llamas R, Swenson EW: Diagnostic clues in pulmonary thrombo-embolism evaluated by angiographic and ventilation-blood flow studies. Thorax 20:327-336, 1965.

121. Stein GN, Chen JT, Goldstein F, et al: The importance of chest roentgenography in the diagnosis of pulmonary embolism. Am J Roentgenol Radium Ther Nucl Med 81:255-263, 1959.

122. Laur A: Roentgen diagnosis of pulmonary embolism and its differentiation from myocardial infarction. Am J Roentgenol Radium Ther Nucl Med 90:632-637, 1963.

123. Fleischner FG: Pulmonary embolism. Clin Radiol 13:169-182, 1962.

124. Williams JR, Wilcox WC: Pulmonary embolism. Roentgenographic and angiographic considerations. Am J Roentgenol Radium Ther Nucl Med 89:333-342, 1963.

125. Szucs MM Jr, Brooks HL, Grossman W, et al: Diagnostic sensitivity of laboratory findings in acute pulmonary embolism. Ann Intern Med 74:161-166, 1971.

126. Talbot S, Worthington BS, Roebuck EJ: Radiographic signs of pulmonary embolism and pulmonary infarction. Thorax 28:198-203, 1973.

127. Jacoby CG, Mindell HJ: Lobar consolidation in pulmonary embolism. Radiology 118:287-290, 1976.

128. Fleischner FG: Roentgenology of the pulmonary infarct. Semin Roentgenol 2:61, 1967.

129. Beilin D, Fink J, Leslie L: Correlation of postmortem pathological observations with chest roentgenograms. Radiology 57:361, 1951.

130. Redline S, Tomashefski JF Jr, Altose MD: Cavitating lung infarction after bland pulmonary thromboembolism in patients with the adult respiratory distress syndrome. Thorax 40:915-919, 1985.

131. Sostman HD, Coleman RE, DeLong DM, et al: Evaluation of revised criteria for ventilation-perfusion scintigraphy in patients with suspected pulmonary embolism. Radiology 193:103-107, 1994.

132. Miniati M, Pistolesi M, Marini C, et al: Value of perfusion lung scan in the diagnosis of pulmonary embolism: Results of the Prospective Investigative Study of Acute Pulmonary Embolism Diagnosis (PISA-PED). Am J Respir Crit Care Med 154:1387-1393, 1996.

133. Heck L, Duley J: Statistical considerations in lung scanning with Tc-99m albumin particles. Radiology 113:675, 1975.

134. Sostman HD, Rapoport S, Gottschalk A, Greenspan RH: Imaging of pulmonary embolism. Invest Radiol 21:443-454, 1986.

135. Gottschalk A, Sostman HD, Coleman RE, et al: Ventilation-perfusion scintigraphy in the PIOPED study. Part II. Evaluation of the scintigraphic criteria and interpretations. J Nucl Med 34:1119-1126, 1993.

136. Webber MM, Gomes AS, Roe D, et al: Comparison of Biello, McNeil, and PIOPED criteria for the diagnosis of pulmonary emboli on lung scans. AJR Am J Roentgenol 154:975-981, 1990.

137. Stein PD, Gottschalk A: Review of criteria appropriate for a very low probability of pulmonary embolism on ventilation-perfusion lung scans: A position paper. Radiographics 20:99-105, 2000.

138. Freitas JE, Sarosi MG, Nagle CC, et al: Modified PIOPED criteria used in clinical practice. J Nucl Med 36:1573-1578, 1995.

139. Quinn DA, Thompson BT, Terrin ML, et al: A prospective investigation of pulmonary embolism in women and men. JAMA 268:1689-1696, 1992.

140. Worsley DF, Alavi A, Palevsky HI, Kundel HL: Comparison of diagnostic performance with ventilation-perfusion lung imaging in different patient populations. Radiology 199:481-483, 1996.

141. Lesser BA, Leeper KV Jr, Stein PD, et al: The diagnosis of acute pulmonary embolism in patients with chronic obstructive pulmonary disease. Chest 102:17-22, 1992.

142. Worsley DF, Palevsky HI, Alavi A: A detailed evaluation of patients with acute pulmonary embolism and low- or very-low-probability lung scan interpretations. Arch Intern Med 154:2737-2741, 1994.

143. Smith R, Ellis K, Alderson PO: Role of chest radiography in predicting the extent of airway disease in patients with suspected pulmonary embolism. Radiology 159:391-394, 1986.

144. Ralph DD: Pulmonary embolism. The implications of Prospective Investigation of Pulmonary Embolism Diagnosis. Radiol Clin North Am 32:679-687, 1994.

145. Remy-Jardin M, Remy J, Wattinne L, Giraud F: Central pulmonary thromboembolism: Diagnosis with spiral volumetric CT with the single-breath-hold technique—comparison with pulmonary angiography. Radiology 185:381-387, 1992.

146. Teigen CL, Maus TP, Sheedy PF 2nd, et al: Pulmonary embolism: Diagnosis with electron-beam CT: Radiology 188:839-845, 1993.

147. van Rossum AB, Pattynama PM, Ton ER: Pulmonary embolism: Validation of spiral CT angiography in 149 patients. Radiology 201:467-470, 1996.

148. Powell T, Müller NL: Imaging of acute pulmonary thromboembolism: Should spiral computed tomography replace the ventilation-perfusion scan? Clin Chest Med 24:29-38, 2003.

149. Schoepf UJ, Costello P: Multidetector-row CT imaging of pulmonary embolism. Semin Roentgenol 38:106-114, 2003.

150. Ghaye B, Szapiro D, Mastora I, et al: Peripheral pulmonary arteries: How far in the lung does multi-detector row spiral CT allow analysis? Radiology 219:629-636, 2001.

151. Schoepf UJ, Holzknecht N, Helmberger TK, et al: Subsegmental pulmonary emboli: Improved detection with thin-collimation multi-detector row spiral CT: Radiology 222:483-490, 2002.

152. Patel S, Kazerooni EA, Cascade PN: Pulmonary embolism: Optimization of small pulmonary artery visualization at multi-detector row CT. Radiology 227:455-460, 2003.

153. Goodman LR, Curtin JJ, Mewissen MW, et al: Detection of pulmonary embolism in patients with unresolved clinical and scintigraphic diagnosis: Helical CT versus angiography. AJR Am J Roentgenol 164:1369-1374, 1995.

154. Drucker EA, Rivitz SM, Shepard JA, et al: Acute pulmonary embolism: Assessment of helical CT for diagnosis. Radiology 209:235-241, 1998.

155. Mayo JR, Remy-Jardin M, Müller NL, et al: Pulmonary embolism: Prospective comparison of spiral CT with ventilation-perfusion scintigraphy. Radiology 205:447-452, 1997.

156. Kim KI, Müller NL, Mayo JR: Clinically suspected pulmonary embolism: Utility of spiral CT. Radiology 210:693-697, 1999.

157. Teigen CL, Maus TP, Sheedy PF 2nd, et al: Pulmonary embolism: Diagnosis with contrast-enhanced electron-beam CT and comparison with pulmonary angiography. Radiology 194:313-319, 1995.

158. Baile EM, King GG, Müller NL, et al: Spiral computed tomography is comparable to angiography for the diagnosis of pulmonary embolism. Am J Respir Crit Care Med 161:1010-1015, 2000.

159. Cross JJ, Kemp PM, Walsh CG, et al: A randomized trial of spiral CT and ventilation perfusion scintigraphy for the diagnosis of pulmonary embolism. Clin Radiol 53:177-182, 1998.

160. Blachere H, Latrabe V, Montaudon M, et al: Pulmonary embolism revealed on helical CT angiography: Comparison with ventilation-perfusion radionuclide lung scanning. AJR Am J Roentgenol 174:1041-1047, 2000.

161. Remy-Jardin M, Remy J, Artaud D, et al: Spiral CT of pulmonary embolism: Technical considerations and interpretive pitfalls. J Thorac Imaging 12:103-117, 1997.

162. Gefter WB, Hatabu H, Holland GA, et al: Pulmonary thromboembolism: Recent developments in diagnosis with CT and MR imaging. Radiology 197:561-574, 1995.

163. Garg K, Sieler H, Welsh CH, et al: Clinical validity of helical CT being interpreted as negative for pulmonary embolism: Implications for patient treatment. AJR Am J Roentgenol 172:1627-1631, 1999.

164. Goodman LR, Lipchik RJ, Kuzo RS, et al: Subsequent pulmonary embolism: Risk after a negative helical CT pulmonary angiogram—prospective comparison with scintigraphy. Radiology 215:535-542, 2000.

165. Swensen SJ, Sheedy PF 2nd, Ryu JH, et al: Outcomes after withholding anticoagulation from patients with suspected acute pulmonary embolism and negative computed tomographic findings: A cohort study. Mayo Clin Proc 77:130-138, 2002.

166. Henry JW, Relyea B, Stein PD: Continuing risk of thromboemboli among patients with normal pulmonary angiograms. Chest 107:1375-1378, 1995.

167. van Erkel AR, van Rossum AB, Bloem JL, et al: Spiral CT angiography for suspected pulmonary embolism: A cost-effectiveness analysis. Radiology 201:29-36, 1996.

168. Goodman LR, Lipchik RJ, Kuzo RS: Acute pulmonary embolism: The role of computed tomographic imaging. J Thorac Imaging 12:83-86, discussion 86-102, 1997.

169. Sostman HD: Opinion response to acute pulmonary embolism: The role of computed tomographic imaging. J Thorac Imaging 12:89, 1997.

170. Gefter WB, Palevsky HI: Opinion response to acute pulmonary embolism: The role of computed tomographic imaging. J Thorac Imaging 12:97, 1997.

171. Garg K, Welsh CH, Feyerabend AJ, et al: Pulmonary embolism: Diagnosis with spiral CT and ventilation-perfusion scanning—correlation with pulmonary angiographic results or clinical outcome. Radiology 208:201-208, 1998.

172. van Rossum AB, Pattynama PM, Mallens WM, et al: Can helical CT replace scintigraphy in the diagnostic process in suspected pulmonary embolism? A retrospective-prospective cohort study focusing on total diagnostic yield. Eur Radiol 8:90-96, 1998.

173. Remy-Jardin M, Tillie-Leblond I, Szapiro D, et al: CT angiography of pulmonary embolism in patients with underlying respiratory disease: Impact of multislice CT on image quality and negative predictive value. Eur Radiol 12:1971-1978, 2002.

174. Romano WM, Cascade PN, Korobkin MT, et al: Implications of unsuspected pulmonary embolism detected by computed tomography. Can Assoc Radiol J 46:363-367, 1995.

175. Winston CB, Wechsler RJ, Salazar AM, et al: Incidental pulmonary emboli detected at helical CT: Effect on patient care. Radiology 201:23-27, 1996.

176. Gosselin MV, Rubin GD, Leung AN, et al: Unsuspected pulmonary embolism: Prospective detection on routine helical CT scans. Radiology 208:209-215, 1998.

177. Remy-Jardin M, Louvegny S, Remy J, et al: Acute central thromboembolic disease: Posttherapeutic follow-up with spiral CT angiography. Radiology 203:173-180, 1997.

178. Tardivon AA, Musset D, Maitre S, et al: Role of CT in chronic pulmonary embolism: Comparison with pulmonary angiography. J Comput Assist Tomogr 17:345-351, 1993.

179. Schwickert HC, Schweden F, Schild HH, et al: Pulmonary arteries and lung parenchyma in chronic pulmonary embolism: Preoperative and postoperative CT findings. Radiology 191:351-357, 1994.

180. Greaves SM, Hart EM, Brown K, et al: Pulmonary thromboembolism: Spectrum of findings on CT: AJR Am J Roentgenol 165:1359-1363, 1995.

181. Coche EE, Müller NL, Kim KI, et al: Acute pulmonary embolism: Ancillary findings at spiral CT. Radiology 207:753-758, 1998.

182. Sinner WN: Computed tomographic patterns of pulmonary thromboembolism and infarction. J Comput Assist Tomogr 2:395-399, 1978.

183. Ren H, Kuhlman JE, Hruban RH, et al: CT of inflation-fixed lungs: Wedge-shaped density and vascular sign in the diagnosis of infarction. J Comput Assist Tomogr 14:82-86, 1990.

184. King MA, Bergin CJ, Yeung DW, et al: Chronic pulmonary thromboembolism: Detection of regional hypoperfusion with CT. Radiology 191:359-363, 1994.

185. Austin JH, Müller NL, Friedman PJ, et al: Glossary of terms for CT of the lungs: Recommendations of the Nomenclature Committee of the Fleischner Society. Radiology 200:327-331, 1996.

186. King MA, Ysrael M, Bergin CJ: Chronic thromboembolic pulmonary hypertension: CT findings. AJR Am J Roentgenol 170:955-960, 1998.

187. Remy-Jardin M, Remy J, Louvegny S, et al: Airway changes in chronic pulmonary embolism: CT findings in 33 patients. Radiology 203:355-360, 1997.

188. Meaney JF, Weg JG, Chenevert TL, et al: Diagnosis of pulmonary embolism with magnetic resonance angiography. N Engl J Med 336:1422-1427, 1997.

189. Gupta A, Frazer CK, Ferguson JM, et al: Acute pulmonary embolism: Diagnosis with MR angiography. Radiology 210:353-359, 1999.

190. Stein PD, Hull RD, Saltzman HA, Pineo G: Strategy for diagnosis of patients with suspected acute pulmonary embolism. Chest 103:1553-1559, 1993.

191. Oudkerk M, van Beek EJ, van Putten WL, Buller HR: Cost-effectiveness analysis of various strategies in the diagnostic management of pulmonary embolism. Arch Intern Med 153:947-954, 1993.

192. Weidner W, Swanson L, Wilson G: Roentgen techniques in the diagnosis of pulmonary thromboembolism. Am J Roentgenol Radium Ther Nucl Med 100:397-407, 1967.

193. Ormond RS, Gale HH, Drake EH, Gahagan T: Pulmonary angiography and pulmonary embolism. Radiology 86:658-662, 1966.

194. Quinn MF, Lundell CJ, Klotz TA, et al: Reliability of selective pulmonary arteriography in the diagnosis of pulmonary embolism. AJR Am J Roentgenol 149:469-471, 1987.

195. Schlager N, Henschke C, King T, et al: Diagnosis of pulmonary embolism at a large teaching hospital. J Thorac Imaging 9:180-184, 1994.

196. Cooper TJ, Hayward MW, Hartog M: Survey on the use of pulmonary scintigraphy and angiography for suspected pulmonary thromboembolism in the UK. Clin Radiol 43:243-245, 1991.

197. Hudson ER, Smith TP, McDermott VG, et al: Pulmonary angiography performed with iopamidol: Complications in 1,434 patients. Radiology 198:61-65, 1996.

198. Sagel SS, Greenspan RH: Nonuniform pulmonary arterial perfusion. Pulmonary embolism? Radiology 99:541-548, 1971.

199. Goldhaber SZ, Hennekens CH, Evans DA, et al: Factors associated with correct antemortem diagnosis of major pulmonary embolism. Am J Med 73:822-826, 1982.

200. Auger WR, Fedullo PF, Moser KM, et al: Chronic major-vessel thromboembolic pulmonary artery obstruction: Appearance at angiography. Radiology 182:393-398, 1992.

201. Moser KM, Bloor CM: Pulmonary vascular lesions occurring in patients with chronic major vessel thromboembolic pulmonary hypertension. Chest 103:685-692, 1993.

202. Peterson KL, Fred HL, Alexander JK: Pulmonary arterial webs. A new angiographic sign of previous thromboembolism. N Engl J Med 277:33-35, 1967.

203. Baxter GM: The role of ultrasound in deep venous thrombosis. Clin Radiol 52:1-3, 1997.

204. Hull RD, Hirsh J, Carter CJ, et al: Pulmonary angiography, ventilation lung scanning, and venography for clinically suspected pulmonary embolism with abnormal perfusion lung scan. Ann Intern Med 98:891-899, 1983.

205. Lensing AW, Prandoni P, Buller HR, et al: Lower extremity venography with iohexol: Results and complications. Radiology 177:503-505, 1990.

206. McLachlan MS, Thomson JG, Taylor DW, et al: Observer variation in the interpretation of lower limb venograms. AJR Am J Roentgenol 132:227-229, 1979.

207. Bettmann MA, Robbins A, Braun SD, et al: Contrast venography of the leg: Diagnostic efficacy, tolerance, and complication rates with ionic and nonionic contrast media. Radiology 165:113-116, 1987.

208. Aitken AG, Godden DJ: Real-time ultrasound diagnosis of deep vein thrombosis: A comparison with venography. Clin Radiol 38:309-313, 1987.

209. Cronan JJ, Dorfman GS, Scola FH, et al: Deep venous thrombosis: US assessment using vein compression. Radiology 162:191-194, 1987.

210. Rose SC, Zwiebel WJ, Nelson BD, et al: Symptomatic lower extremity deep venous thrombosis: Accuracy, limitations, and role of color duplex flow imaging in diagnosis. Radiology 175:639-644, 1990.

211. Lewis BD, James EM, Welch TJ, et al: Diagnosis of acute deep venous thrombosis of the lower extremities: Prospective evaluation of color Doppler flow imaging versus venography. Radiology 192:651-655, 1994.

212. Baxter GM, Duffy P, Partridge E: Colour flow imaging of calf vein thrombosis. Clin Radiol 46:198-201, 1992.

213. Atri M, Herba MS, Reinhold C, et al: Accuracy of sonography in the evaluation of calf deep vein thrombosis in both postoperative surveillance and symptomatic patients. Am J Roentgenol 166:1361, 1996.

214. Fraser JD, Anderson DR: Deep venous thrombosis: Recent advances and optimal investigation with US. Radiology 211:9-24, 1999.

215. Gottlieb RH, Widjaja J, Mehra S, Robinette WB: Clinically important pulmonary emboli: Does calf vein US alter outcomes? Radiology 211:25-29, 1999.

216. Vaccaro JP, Cronan JJ, Dorfman GS: Outcome analysis of patients with normal compression US examinations. Radiology 175:645-649, 1990.

217. Sheiman RG, McArdle CR: Clinically suspected pulmonary embolism: Use of bilateral lower extremity US as the initial examination—a prospective study. Radiology 212:75-78, 1999.

218. Ginsberg JS, Caco CC, Brill-Edwards PA, et al: Venous thrombosis in patients who have undergone major hip or knee surgery: Detection with compression US and impedance plethysmography. Radiology 181:651-654, 1991.

219. Baldt MM, Zontsich T, Stumpflen A, et al: Deep venous thrombosis of the lower extremity: Efficacy of spiral CT venography compared with conventional venography in diagnosis. Radiology 200:423-428, 1996.

220. Lomas DJ, Britton PD: CT demonstration of acute and chronic iliofemoral thrombosis. J Comput Assist Tomogr 15:861-862, 1991.

221. Loud PA, Katz DS, Klippenstein DL, et al: Combined CT venography and pulmonary angiography in suspected thromboembolic disease: Diagnostic accuracy for deep venous evaluation. AJR Am J Roentgenol 174:61-65, 2000.

222. Yankelevitz DF, Gamsu G, Shah A, et al: Optimization of combined CT pulmonary angiography with lower extremity CT venography. AJR Am J Roentgenol 174:67-69, 2000.

223. Garg K, Kemp JL, Wojcik D, et al: Thromboembolic disease: Comparison of combined CT pulmonary angiography and venography with bilateral leg sonography in 70 patients. AJR Am J Roentgenol 175:997-1001, 2000.

224. Duwe KM, Shiau M, Budorick NE, et al: Evaluation of the lower extremity veins in patients with suspected pulmonary embolism: A retrospective comparison of helical CT venography and sonography. 2000 ARRS Executive Council Award I. American Roentgen Ray Society. AJR Am J Roentgenol 175:1525-1531, 2000.

225. Cham MD, Yankelevitz DF, Shaham D, et al: Deep venous thrombosis: Detection by using indirect CT venography. The Pulmonary Angiography–Indirect CT Venography Cooperative Group. Radiology 216:744-751, 2000.

226. Walsh G, Redmond S: Does addition of CT pelvic venography to CT pulmonary angiography protocols contribute to the diagnosis of thromboembolic disease? Clin Radiol 57:462-465, 2002.

227. Ciccotosto C, Goodman LR, Washington L, Quiroz FA: Indirect CT venography following CT pulmonary angiography: Spectrum of CT findings. J Thorac Imaging 17:18-27, 2002.

228. Rademaker J, Griesshaber V, Hidajat N, et al: Combined CT pulmonary angiography and venography for diagnosis of pulmonary embolism and deep vein thrombosis: Radiation dose. J Thorac Imaging 16:297-299, 2001.

229. Spritzer CE, Sussman SK, Blinder RA, et al: Deep venous thrombosis evaluation with limited-flip-angle, gradient-refocused MR imaging: Preliminary experience. Radiology 166:371-375, 1988.

230. Spritzer CE, Norconk JJ Jr, Sostman HD, Coleman RE: Detection of deep venous thrombosis by magnetic resonance imaging. Chest 104:54-60, 1993.

231. Evans AJ, Sostman HD, Knelson MH, et al: 1992 ARRS Executive Council Award. Detection of deep venous thrombosis: Prospective comparison of MR imaging with contrast venography. AJR Am J Roentgenol 161:131-139, 1993.

232. Pineda LA, Hathwar VS, Grant BJ: Clinical suspicion of fatal pulmonary embolism. Chest 120:791-795, 2001.

233. Wells PS, Anderson DR, Rodger M, et al: Excluding pulmonary embolism at the bedside without diagnostic imaging: Management of patients with suspected pulmonary embolism presenting to the emergency department by using a simple clinical model and d-dimer. Ann Intern Med 135:98-107, 2001.

234. Perrier A, Miron MJ, Desmarais S, et al: Using clinical evaluation and lung scan to rule out suspected pulmonary embolism: Is it a valid option in patients with normal results of lower-limb venous compression ultrasonography? Arch Intern Med 160:512-516, 2000.

235. Windebank WJ, Boyd G, Moran F: Pulmonary thromboembolism presenting as asthma. BMJ 1:90, 1973.

236. Goodwin JF: The clinical diagnosis of pulmonary thromboembolism. In Sasahara AA, Stein M (eds): Pulmonary Embolic Disease. New York, Grune & Stratton, 1965, pp 239-255.

237. Stein PD, Henry JW: Clinical characteristics of patients with acute pulmonary embolism stratified according to their presenting syndromes. Chest 112:974-979, 1997.

238. Miniati M, Prediletto R, Formichi B, et al: Accuracy of clinical assessment in the diagnosis of pulmonary embolism. Am J Respir Crit Care Med 159:864-871, 1999.

239. Stein PD, Afzal A, Henry JW, Villareal CG: Fever in acute pulmonary embolism. Chest 117:39-42, 2000.

240. Murray HW, Ellis GC, Blumenthal DS, Sos TA: Fever and pulmonary thromboembolism. Am J Med 67:232-235, 1979.

241. Manganelli D, Palla A, Donnamaria V, Giuntini C: Clinical features of pulmonary embolism. Doubts and certainties. Chest 107:25S-32S, 1995.

242. Stein PD, Terrin ML, Hales CA, et al: Clinical, laboratory, roentgenographic, and electrocardiographic findings in patients with acute pulmonary embolism and no pre-existing cardiac or pulmonary disease. Chest 100:598-603, 1991.

243. Coma-Canella I, Gamallo C, Martinez Onsurbe P, Lopez-Sendon J: Acute right ventricular infarction secondary to massive pulmonary embolism. Eur Heart J 9:534-540, 1988.

244. Shaw RA, Schonfeld SA, Whitcomb ME: Pulmonary embolism presenting as coronary insufficiency. Arch Intern Med 141:651, 1981.

245. Fred HL, Willerson JT, Alexander JK: Neurological manifestations of pulmonary thromboembolism. Arch Intern Med 120:33-37, 1967.

246. Fedullo PF, Auger WR, Kerr KM, Rubin LJ: Chronic thromboembolic pulmonary hypertension. N Engl J Med 345:1465-1472, 2001.

247. Stein PD, Henry JW, Gopalakrishnan D, Relyea B: Asymmetry of the calves in the assessment of patients with suspected acute pulmonary embolism. Chest 107:936-939, 1995.

248. Israel H, Goldstein F: The varied clinical manifestations of pulmonary embolism. Ann Intern Med 47:202, 1957.

249. Wolfe TR, Allen TL: Syncope as an emergency department presentation of pulmonary embolism. J Emerg Med 16:27-31, 1998.

250. Marine JE, Goldhaber SZ: Pulmonary embolism presenting as seizures. Chest 112:840-842, 1997.

251. Ward R, Jones D, Haponik EF: Paradoxical embolism. An underrecognized problem. Chest 108:549-558, 1995.

252. Perrier A, Desmarais S, Goehring C, et al: D-dimer testing for suspected pulmonary embolism in outpatients. Am J Respir Crit Care Med 156:492-496, 1997.

253. Brotman DJ, Segal JB, Jani JT, et al: Limitations of D-dimer testing in unselected inpatients with suspected venous thromboembolism. Am J Med 114:276-282, 2003.

254. Kearon C: Diagnosis of pulmonary embolism. CMAJ 168:183-194, 2003.

255. Brown MD, Rowe BH, Reeves MJ, et al: The accuracy of the enzyme-linked immunosorbent assay D-dimer test in the diagnosis of pulmonary embolism: A meta-analysis. Ann Emerg Med 40:133-144, 2002.

256. Sijens PE, Oudkerk M: Exclusion of pulmonary embolism using quantitative plasma D-dimer assays. Clin Lab 47:321-326, 2001.

257. Kelly J, Rudd A, Lewis RR, Hunt BJ: Plasma D-dimers in the diagnosis of venous thromboembolism. Arch Intern Med 162:747-756, 2002.

258. De Monye W, Sanson BJ, MacGillavry MR, et al: Embolus location affects the sensitivity of a rapid quantitative D-dimer assay in the diagnosis of pulmonary embolism. Am J Respir Crit Care Med 165:345-348, 2002.

259. Kruip MJ, Slob MJ, Schijen JH, et al: Use of a clinical decision rule in combination with D-dimer concentration in diagnostic workup of patients with suspected pulmonary embolism: A prospective management study. Arch Intern Med 162:1631-1635, 2002.

260. Dalsey WC, Jagoda AS, Decker WW, et al: Clinical policy: Critical issues in the evaluation and management of adult patients presenting with suspected pulmonary embolism. Ann Emerg Med 41:257-270, 2003.

261. Perrier A, Bounameaux H, Morabia A, et al: Diagnosis of pulmonary embolism by a decision analysis-based strategy including clinical probability, D-dimer levels, and ultrasonography: A management study. Arch Intern Med 156:531-536, 1996.

262. Monreal M, Lafoz E, Casals A, et al: Platelet count and venous thromboembolism. A useful test for suspected pulmonary embolism. Chest 100:1493-1496, 1991.

263. Afzal A, Noor HA, Gill SA, et al: Leukocytosis in acute pulmonary embolism. Chest 115:1329-1332, 1999.

264. Bynum LJ, Wilson JE 3rd: Characteristics of pleural effusions associated with pulmonary embolism. Arch Intern Med 136:159-162, 1976.

265. Griner PF: Bloody pleural fluid following pulmonary infarction. JAMA 202:947-949, 1967.

266. Romero Candeira S, Hernandez Blasco L, Soler MJ, et al: Biochemical and cytologic characteristics of pleural effusions secondary to pulmonary embolism. Chest 121:465-469, 2002.

267. Falterman TJ, Martinez JA, Daberkow D, Weiss LD: Pulmonary embolism with ST segment elevation in leads V1 to V4: Case report and review of the literature regarding electrocardiographic changes in acute pulmonary embolism. J Emerg Med 21:255-261, 2001.

268. Ferrari E, Imbert A, Chevalier T, et al: The ECG in pulmonary embolism. Predictive value of negative T waves in precordial leads—80 case reports. Chest 111:537-543, 1997.

269. Daniel KR, Courtney DM, Kline JA: Assessment of cardiac stress from massive pulmonary embolism with 12-lead ECG. Chest 120:474-481, 2001.

270. Becattini C, Agnelli G: Risk factors for adverse short-term outcome in patients with pulmonary embolism. Thromb Res 103:V239-V244, 2001.

271. Goldhaber SZ, Visani L, De Rosa M: Acute pulmonary embolism: Clinical outcomes in the International Cooperative Pulmonary Embolism Registry (ICOPER). Lancet 353:1386-1389, 1999.

272. Grifoni S, Olivotto I, Cecchini P, et al: Short-term clinical outcome of patients with acute pulmonary embolism, normal blood pressure, and echocardiographic right ventricular dysfunction. Circulation 101:2817-2822, 2000.

273. Donnamaria V, Palla A, Petruzzelli S, et al: Early and late follow-up of pulmonary embolism. Respiration 60:15-20, 1993.

274. Alderson PO, Dzebolo NN, Biello DR, et al: Serial lung scintigraphy: Utility in diagnosis of pulmonary embolism. Radiology 149:797-802, 1983.

275. Menendez R, Nauffal D, Cremades MJ: Prognostic factors in restoration of pulmonary flow after submassive pulmonary embolism: A multiple regression analysis. Eur Respir J 11:560-564, 1998.

276. Colp CR, Williams MH Jr: Pulmonary function following pulmonary embolization. Am Rev Respir Dis 85:799-807, 1962.

277. Heit JA, Mohr DN, Silverstein MD, et al: Predictors of recurrence after deep vein thrombosis and pulmonary embolism: A population-based cohort study. Arch Intern Med 160:761-768, 2000.

278. Jaffe RB, Koschmann EB: Septic pulmonary emboli. Radiology 96:527-532, 1970.

279. Wong KS, Lin TY, Huang YC, et al: Clinical and radiographic spectrum of septic pulmonary embolism. Arch Dis Child 87:312-315, 2002.

280. Thomson EC, Lynn WA: Clinical picture—septic thrombophlebitis with multiple pulmonary embolism. Lancet Infect Dis 3:86, 2003.

281. Iwama T, Shigematsu S, Asami K, et al: Tricuspid valve endocarditis with large vegetations in a non–drug addict without underlying cardiac disease. Intern Med 35:203-206, 1996.

282. Weesner CL, Cisek JE: Lemierre syndrome: The forgotten disease. Ann Emerg Med 22:256-258, 1993.

283. Felman AH, Shulman ST: Staphylococcal osteomyelitis, sepsis, and pulmonary disease. Observations of 10 patients with combined osseous and pulmonary infections. Radiology 117:649-655, 1975.

284. Shiota Y, Arikita H, Horita N, et al: Septic pulmonary embolism associated with periodontal disease: Reports of two cases and review of the literature. Chest 121:652-654, 2002.

285. Goodwin NJ, Castronuovo JJ, Friedman EA: Recurrent septic pulmonary embolism complicating maintenance hemodialysis. Ann Intern Med 71:29-38, 1969.

286. Huang RM, Naidich DP, Lubat E, et al: Septic pulmonary emboli: CT-radiographic correlation. AJR Am J Roentgenol 153:41-45, 1989.

287. Gumbs RV, McCauley DI: Hilar and mediastinal adenopathy in septic pulmonary embolic disease. Radiology 142:313-315, 1982.

288. Kuhlman JE, Fishman EK, Teigen C: Pulmonary septic emboli: Diagnosis with CT. Radiology 174:211-213, 1990.

289. Webb DW, Thadepalli H: Hemoptysis in patients with septic pulmonary infarcts from tricuspid endocarditis. Chest 76:99-100, 1979.

290. Roberts WC, Buchbinder NA: Right-sided infective endocarditis. A clinicopathologic study of twelve necropsy patients. Am J Med 53:7-19, 1972.

291. Dreyer ZE: Chest infections and syndromes in sickle cell disease of childhood. Semin Respir Infect 11:163-172, 1996.

292. Verdegem T, Yee S: Lung disease in sickle cell anemia: A tropical disease with a twist. Sem Respir Med 12:107, 1991.

293. Minter KR, Gladwin MT: Pulmonary complications of sickle cell anemia. A need for increased recognition, treatment, and research. Am J Respir Crit Care Med 164:2016-2019, 2001.

294. Vichinsky EP, Neumayr LD, Earles AN, et al: Causes and outcomes of the acute chest syndrome in sickle cell disease. National Acute Chest Syndrome Study Group. N Engl J Med 342:1855-1865, 2000.

295. Gladwin MT, Rodgers GP: Pathogenesis and treatment of acute chest syndrome of sickle-cell anaemia. Lancet 355:1476-1478, 2000.

296. Maitre B, Habibi A, Roudot-Thoraval F, et al: Acute chest syndrome in adults with sickle cell disease. Chest 117:1386-1392, 2000.

297. Stuart MJ, Setty BN: Acute chest syndrome of sickle cell disease: New light on an old problem. Curr Opin Hematol 8:111-122, 2001.

298. Cockshott WP: Rib infarcts in sickling disease. Eur J Radiol 14:63-66, 1992.

299. Bhalla M, Abboud MR, McLoud TC, et al: Acute chest syndrome in sickle cell disease: CT evidence of microvascular occlusion. Radiology 187:45-49, 1993.

300. Aquino SL, Gamsu G, Fahy JV, et al: Chronic pulmonary disorders in sickle cell disease: Findings at thin-section CT. Radiology 193:807-811, 1994.

301. Dudney TM, Elliott CG: Pulmonary embolism from amniotic fluid, fat, and air. Prog Cardiovasc Dis 36:447-474, 1994.

302. King MB, Harmon KR: Unusual forms of pulmonary embolism. Clin Chest Med 15:561-580, 1994.

303. Palmovic V, McCarroll JR: Fat embolism in trauma. Arch Pathol 80:630-635, 1965.

304. Vichinsky E, Williams R, Das M, et al: Pulmonary fat embolism: A distinct cause of severe acute chest syndrome in sickle cell anemia. Blood 83:3107-3112, 1994.

305. Sevitt S: Fat Embolism. London, Butterworths, 1962.

306. Wozasek GE, Simon P, Redl H, Schlag G: Intramedullary pressure changes and fat intravasation during intramedullary nailing: An experimental study in sheep. J Trauma 36:202-207, 1994.

307. Hulman G: The pathogenesis of fat embolism. J Pathol 176:3-9, 1995.

308. Thompson PL, Williams KE, Walters MN: Fat embolism in the microcirculation: An in-vivo study. J Pathol 97:23-28, 1969.

309. Schemitsch EH, Jain R, Turchin DC, et al: Pulmonary effects of fixation of a fracture with a plate compared with intramedullary nailing. A canine model of fat embolism and fracture fixation. J Bone Joint Surg Am 79:984-996, 1997.

310. Jones JG, Minty BD, Beeley JM, et al: Pulmonary epithelial permeability is immediately increased after embolisation with oleic acid but not with neutral fat. Thorax 37:169-174, 1982.

311. Syrbu S, Thrall RS, Smilowitz HM: Sequential appearance of inflammatory mediators in rat bronchoalveolar lavage fluid after oleic acid–induced lung injury. Exp Lung Res 22:33-49, 1996.

312. Dines DE, Burgher LW, Okazaki H: The clinical and pathologic correlation of fat embolism syndrome. Mayo Clin Proc 50:407-411, 1975.

313. Gitin TA, Seidel T, Cera PJ, et al: Pulmonary microvascular fat: The significance? Crit Care Med 21:673-677, 1993.

314. Modig J, Hedstrand U, Wegenius G: Determinants of early adult respiratory distress syndrome. A retrospective study of 220 patients with major fractures. Acta Chir Scand 151:413-418, 1985.

315. Glas WW, Grekin TD, Musselman MM: Fat embolism. Am J Surg 85:363-369, 1953.

316. Berrigan TJ Jr, Carsky EW, Heitzman ER: Fat embolism. Roentgenographic pathologic correlation in 3 cases. Am J Roentgenol Radium Ther Nucl Med 96:967-971, 1966.

317. Heitzman ER: The Lung: Radiologic-Pathologic Correlations. St Louis, CV Mosby, 1973.

318. Maruyama Y, Little JB: Roentgen manifestations of traumatic pulmonary fat embolism. Radiology 79:945-952, 1962.

319. Williams JR, Bonte FJ: Pulmonary damage in nonpenetrating chest injuries. Radiol Clin North Am 1:439, 1963.

320. Malagari K, Economopoulos N, Stoupis C, et al: High-resolution CT findings in mild pulmonary fat embolism. Chest 123:1196-1201, 2003.

321. Peter RE, Schopfer A, Le Coultre B, Hoffmeyer P: Fat embolism and death during prophylactic osteosynthesis of a metastatic femur using an unreamed femoral nail. J Orthop Trauma 11:233-234, 1997.

322. Burgher LW, Dines DE, Linscheid RL, Didier EP: Fat embolism and the adult respiratory distress syndrome. Mayo Clin Proc 49:107-109, 1974.

323. Wiener L, Forsyth D: Pulmonary pathophysiology of fat embolism. Am Rev Respir Dis 92:113, 1965.

324. Chastre J, Fagon JY, Soler P, et al: Bronchoalveolar lavage for rapid diagnosis of the fat embolism syndrome in trauma patients. Ann Intern Med 113:583-588, 1990.

325. Mimoz O, Edouard A, Beydon L, et al: Contribution of bronchoalveolar lavage to the diagnosis of posttraumatic pulmonary fat embolism. Intensive Care Med 21:973-980, 1995.

326. Castella X, Valles J, Cabezuelo MA, et al: Fat embolism syndrome and pulmonary microvascular cytology. Chest 101:1710-1711, 1992.

327. Pell AC, Christie J, Keating JF, Sutherland GR: The detection of fat embolism by transoesophageal echocardiography during reamed intramedullary nailing. A study of 24 patients with femoral and tibial fractures. J Bone Joint Surg Br 75:921-925, 1993.

328. Schonfeld SA, Ploysongsang Y, DiLisio R, et al: Fat embolism prophylaxis with corticosteroids. A prospective study in high-risk patients. Ann Intern Med 99:438-443, 1983.

329. Vedrinne JM, Guillaume C, Gagnieu MC, et al: Bronchoalveolar lavage in trauma patients for diagnosis of fat embolism syndrome. Chest 102:1323-1327, 1992.

330. Guenter CA, Braun TE: Fat embolism syndrome. Changing prognosis. Chest 79:143-145, 1981.

331. Benatar SR, Ferguson AD, Goldschmidt RB: Fat embolism—some clinical observations and a review of controversial aspects. Q J Med 41:85-98, 1972.

332. Davies S: Amniotic fluid embolus: A review of the literature. Can J Anaesth 48:88-98, 2001.

333. Tuffnell DJ: Amniotic fluid embolism. Curr Opin Obstet Gynecol 15:119-122, 2003.

334. Karetzky M, Ramirez M: Acute respiratory failure in pregnancy. An analysis of 19 cases. Medicine (Baltimore) 77:41-49, 1998.

335. Roche WD Jr, Norris HJ: Detection and significance of maternal pulmonary amniotic fluid embolism. Obstet Gynecol 43:729-731, 1974.

336. Attwood HD: Amniotic fluid embolism. Pathol Annu 7:145-172, 1972.

337. Dib N, Bajwa T: Amniotic fluid embolism causing severe left ventricular dysfunction and death: Case report and review of the literature. Cathet Cardiovasc Diagn 39:177-180, 1996.

338. Romero R, Emamian M, Wan M, et al: Increased concentrations of arachidonic acid lipoxygenase metabolites in amniotic fluid during parturition. Obstet Gynecol 70:849, 1987.
339. Masson RG, Ruggieri J, Siddiqui MM: Amniotic fluid embolism: Definitive diagnosis in a survivor. Am Rev Respir Dis 120:187-192, 1979.
340. Clark SL, Hankins GD, Dudley DA, et al: Amniotic fluid embolism: Analysis of the national registry. Am J Obstet Gynecol 172:1158-1167, discussion 1167-1169, 1995.
341. Kobayashi H, Ooi H, Hayakawa H, et al: Histological diagnosis of amniotic fluid embolism by monoclonal antibody TKH-2 that recognizes NeuAc alpha 2-6GalNAc epitope. Hum Pathol 28:428-433, 1997.
342. Lumley J, Owen R, Morgan M: Amniotic fluid embolism. A report of three cases. Anaesthesia 34:33-36, 1979.
343. Fidler JL, Patz EF Jr, Ravin CE: Cardiopulmonary complications of pregnancy: Radiographic findings. AJR Am J Roentgenol 161:937-942, 1993.
344. Morgan M: Amniotic fluid embolism. Anaesthesia 34:20-32, 1979.
345. Kobayashi H, Ohi H, Terao T: A simple, noninvasive, sensitive method for diagnosis of amniotic fluid embolism by monoclonal antibody TKH-2 that recognizes NeuAc alpha 2-6GalNAc. Am J Obstet Gynecol 168:848-953, 1993.
346. Kanayama N, Yamazaki T, Naruse H, et al: Determining zinc coproporphyrin in maternal plasma—a new method for diagnosing amniotic fluid embolism. Clin Chem 38:526-529, 1992.
347. Schriner RW, Ryu JH, Edwards WD: Microscopic pulmonary tumor embolism causing subacute cor pulmonale: A difficult antemortem diagnosis. Mayo Clin Proc 66:143-148, 1991.
348. Chan CK, Hutcheon MA, Hyland RH, et al: Pulmonary tumor embolism: A critical review of clinical, imaging, and hemodynamic features. J Thorac Imaging 2:4-14, 1987.
349. Shepard JA, Moore EH, Templeton PA, McLoud TC: Pulmonary intravascular tumor emboli: Dilated and beaded peripheral pulmonary arteries at CT. Radiology 187:797-801, 1993.
349a. Muth CM, Shank ES: Gas embolism. N Engl J Med 342:476-482, 2000.
350. Tingleff J, Joyce FS, Pettersson G: Intraoperative echocardiographic study of air embolism during cardiac operations. Ann Thorac Surg 60:673-677, 1995.
351. Lew TW, Tay DH, Thomas E: Venous air embolism during cesarean section: More common than previously thought. Anesth Analg 77:448-452, 1993.
352. Despond O, Fiset P: Oxygen venous embolism after the use of hydrogen peroxide during lumbar discectomy. Can J Anaesth 44:410-413, 1997.
353. Pao BS, Hayden SR: Cerebral gas embolism resulting from inhalation of pressurized helium. Ann Emerg Med 28:363-366, 1996.
354. Moon RE, Vann RD, Bennett PB: The physiology of decompression illness. Sci Am 273:70-77, 1995.
355. Zaugg M, Kaplan V, Widmer U, et al: Fatal air embolism in an airplane passenger with a giant intrapulmonary bronchogenic cyst. Am J Respir Crit Care Med 157:1686-1689, 1998.
356. Segal AJ, Wasserman M: Arterial air embolism: A cause of sudden death in status asthmaticus. Radiology 99:271-272, 1971.
357. Kogutt MS: Systemic air embolism secondary to respiratory therapy in the neonate: Six cases including one survivor. AJR Am J Roentgenol 131:425-429, 1978.
358. Weaver LK, Morris A: Venous and arterial gas embolism associated with positive pressure ventilation. Chest 113:1132-1134, 1998.
359. Palmon SC, Moore LE, Lundberg J, Toung T: Venous air embolism: A review. J Clin Anesth 9:251-257, 1997.
360. Lowenwirt IP, Chi DS, Handwerker SM: Nonfatal venous air embolism during cesarean section: A case report and review of the literature. Obstet Gynecol Surv 49:72-76, 1994.
361. Lantz PE, Smith JD: Fatal carbon dioxide embolism complicating attempted laparoscopic cholecystectomy—case report and literature review. J Forensic Sci 39:1468-1480, 1994.
362. Woodring JH, Fried AM: Nonfatal venous air embolism after contrast-enhanced CT. Radiology 167:405-407, 1988.
363. Matjasko J, Petrozza P, Cohen M, Steinberg P: Anesthesia and surgery in the seated position: Analysis of 554 cases. Neurosurgery 17:695-702, 1985.
364. O'Quin RJ, Lakshminarayan S: Venous air embolism. Arch Intern Med 142:2173-2176, 1982.
365. Warren BA, Philp RB, Inwood MJ: The ultrastructural morphology of air embolism: Platelet adhesion to the interface and endothelial damage. Br J Exp Pathol 54:163-172, 1973.
366. Butler BD, Hills BA: Transpulmonary passage of venous air emboli. J Appl Physiol 59:543-547, 1985.
367. Clark MC, Flick MR: Permeability pulmonary edema caused by venous air embolism. Am Rev Respir Dis 129:633-635, 1984.
368. Pou NA, Roselli RJ, Parker RE, Clanton JC: Effects of air embolism on sheep lung fluid volumes. J Appl Physiol 75:986-993, 1993.
369. Hlastala MP, Robertson HT, Ross BK: Gas exchange abnormalities produced by venous gas emboli. Respir Physiol 36:1-17, 1979.
370. Kizer KW: Diving medicine. Emerg Med Clin North Am 2:513-530, 1984.
371. Cholankeril JV, Joshi RR, Cenizal JS, et al: Massive air embolism from the pulmonary artery. Radiology 142:33-44, 1982.
372. Kizer KW, Goodman PC: Radiographic manifestations of venous air embolism. Radiology 144:35-39, 1982.
373. Vinstein AL, Gresham EL, Lim MO, Franken EA Jr: Pulmonary venous air embolism in hyaline membrane disease. Radiology 105:627-630, 1972.
374. Harker CP, Neuman TS, Olson LK, et al: The roentgenographic findings associated with air embolism in sport scuba divers. J Emerg Med 11:443-449, 1993.

375. Groell R, Schaffler GJ, Rienmueller R, Kern R: Vascular air embolism: Location, frequency, and cause on electron-beam CT studies of the chest. Radiology 202:459-462, 1997.
376. Adornato DC, Gildenberg PL, Ferrario CM, et al: Pathophysiology of intravenous air embolism in dogs. Anesthesiology 49:120-127, 1978.
377. Ericsson JA, Gottlieb JD, Sweet RB: Closed-chest cardiac massage in the treatment of venous air embolism. N Engl J Med 270:1353-1354, 1964.
378. Smith RM, Neuman TS: Abnormal serum biochemistries in association with arterial gas embolism. J Emerg Med 15:285-289, 1997.
379. Young M, Smith D, Murtaugh F: Comparison of surgical and anesthetic complications in neurosurgical patients experiencing venous air embolism in the sitting position. Neurosurgery 18:157, 1986.
380. Paré JP, Cote G, Fraser RS: Long-term follow-up of drug abusers with intravenous talcosis. Am Rev Respir Dis 139:233-241, 1989.
381. Paré JA, Fraser RG, Hogg JC, et al: Pulmonary 'mainline' granulomatosis: Talcosis of intravenous methadone abuse. Medicine (Baltimore) 58:229-239, 1979.
382. Farber HW, Falls R, Glauser FL: Transient pulmonary hypertension from the intravenous injection of crushed, suspended pentazocine tablets. Chest 80:178-182, 1981.
383. Schmidt RA, Glenny RW, Godwin JD, et al: Panlobular emphysema in young intravenous Ritalin abusers. Am Rev Respir Dis 143:649-656, 1991.
384. Genereux GP, Emson HE: Talc granulomatosis and angiothrombotic pulmonary hypertension in drug addicts. J Can Assoc Radiol 25:87-93, 1974.
385. Ward S, Heyneman LE, Reittner P, et al: Talcosis associated with IV abuse of oral medications: CT findings. AJR Am J Roentgenol 174:789-793, 2000.
386. Feigin DS: Talc: Understanding its manifestations in the chest. AJR Am J Roentgenol 146:295-301, 1986.
387. Robertson CH Jr, Reynolds RC, Wilson JE 3rd: Pulmonary hypertension and foreign body granulomas in intravenous drug abusers. Documentation by cardiac catheterization and lung biopsy. Am J Med 61:657-664, 1976.
388. Demeter S, Raymond GS, Puttagunta L, et al: Intravenous pulmonary talcosis with complicating massive fibrosis. Can Assoc Radiol J 50:413, 1999.
389. Stern EJ, Frank MS, Schmutz JF, et al: Panlobular pulmonary emphysema caused by i.v. injection of methylphenidate (Ritalin): Findings on chest radiographs and CT scans. AJR Am J Roentgenol 162:555-560, 1994.
390. Siegel H, Bloustein P: Continuing studies in the diagnosis and pathology of death from intravenous narcotism. J Forensic Sci 15:179-184, 1970.
391. Murphy SB, Jackson WB, Paré JA: Talc retinopathy. Can J Ophthalmol 13:152-156, 1978.
392. Itkonen J, Schnoll S, Daghestani A, Glassroth J: Accelerated development of pulmonary complications due to illicit intravenous use of pentazocine and tripelennamine. Am J Med 76:617-622, 1984.
393. Takahashi M, Abrams HL: Arborizing pulmonary embolization following lymphangiography. Report of three cases and an experimental study. Radiology 89:633-638, 1967.
394. Richardson P, Crosby EH, Bean HA, Dexter D: Pulmonary oil deposition in patients subjected to lymphography: Detection by thoracic photoscan and sputum examination. Can Med Assoc J 94:1086-1091, 1966.
395. Bron KM, Baum S, Abrams HL: Oil embolism in lymphangiography. Incidence, manifestations, and mechanism. Radiology 80:194-202, 1963.
396. Chung JW, Park JH, Im JG, et al: Pulmonary oil embolism after transcatheter oily chemoembolization of hepatocellular carcinoma. Radiology 187:689-693, 1993.
397. Fallat RJ, Powell MR, Youker JE, Nadel JA: Pulmonary deposition and clearance of 131-I–labeled oil after lymphography in man. Correlation with lung function. Radiology 97:511-520, 1970.
398. LaMonte CS, Lacher MJ: Lymphangiography in patients with pulmonary dysfunction. Arch Intern Med 132:365-367, 1973.
399. Hill DM: Self-administration of mercury by subcutaneous injection. BMJ 1:342, 1967.
400. Cowan NC, Kane P, Karani J: Case report: Metallic mercury embolism—deliberate self-injection. Clin Radiol 46:357-358, 1992.
401. Maniatis V, Zois G, Stringaris K: I.V. mercury self-injection: CT imaging. AJR Am J Roentgenol 169:1197-1198, 1997.
402. Naidich TP, Bartelt D, Wheeler PS, Stern WZ: Metallic mercury emboli. Am J Roentgenol Radium Ther Nucl Med 117:886-891, 1973.
403. Torres-Alanis O, Garza-Ocanas L, Pineyro-Lopez A: Intravenous self-administration of metallic mercury: Report of a case with a 5-year follow-up. J Toxicol Clin Toxicol 35:83-87, 1997.
404. Pelz DM, Lownie SP, Fox AJ, Hutton LC: Symptomatic pulmonary complications from liquid acrylate embolization of brain arteriovenous malformations. AJNR Am J Neuroradiol 16:19-26, 1995.
405. Takasugi JE, Shaw C: Inadvertent bucrylate pulmonary embolization: A case report. J Thorac Imaging 4:71-73, 1989.
406. Hafez A, Darteville P, Lafont D, et al: Pulmonary arterial embolus by an unusual wandering bullet. Thorac Cardiovasc Surg 31:392-394, 1983.
407. Brewer LL, Bai A, King E, et al: The pathologic effects of metallic foreign bodies in the pulmonary circulation. J Thorac Cardiovasc Surg 38:670, 1959.
408. Terry PB, Barth KH, Kaufman SL, White RI Jr: Balloon embolization for treatment of pulmonary arteriovenous fistulas. N Engl J Med 302:1189-1190, 1980.
409. Ross AM: Polyethylene emboli: How many more? Chest 57:307-308, 1970.
410. Prager D, Hertzberg RW: Spontaneous intravenous catheter fracture and embolization from an implanted venous access port and analysis by scanning electron microscopy. Cancer 60:270-273, 1987.
411. Chen YM, Lu CC, Perng RP: Silicone fluid–induced pulmonary embolism. Am Rev Respir Dis 147:1299-1302, 1993.

PULMONARY HYPERTENSION

Pulmonary arterial hypertension can be defined as an increase in systolic pressure to 30 mm Hg or higher or an increase in mean pressure to 18 mm Hg or higher.[1] Pulmonary venous hypertension is present when the pressure in the pulmonary veins measured indirectly by a catheter wedged in a pulmonary artery exceeds 12 mm Hg. Both forms can be classified in a number of ways. The classification scheme followed here is adopted from the one derived at the World Symposium on Primary Pulmonary Hypertension in 1998 (Table 13–1).[2]

Before discussing the features of the specific conditions listed in this classification, it is useful to briefly review some features characteristic to all forms.

GENERAL FEATURES OF PULMONARY HYPERTENSION

Anatomic and Physiologic Considerations

The normal anatomy and physiology of the pulmonary circulation are outlined in Chapter 1, and only a few points relevant to an understanding of altered pulmonary hemodynamics are reviewed here. Unlike the tracheobronchial tree, in which most of the resistance to airflow occurs in the large airways, most of the resistance in the pulmonary arterial tree is in the smaller blood vessels (muscular arteries and arterioles). As illustrated in Figure 13–1,[3] although the conducting airways and pulmonary arterial system begin with similar-sized "trunks," the total cross-sectional area of the airways greatly exceeds that of the vessels in the lung periphery. The vessels in this location also contain the majority of vascular smooth muscle, and it is modulation of their caliber that causes the best match of ventilation and perfusion.

The pulmonary vascular circuit is a low-pressure system, with mean arterial pressure being only about a sixth of systemic arterial pressure. It has a remarkable capacity to compensate for a large physiologic increase in blood flow (e.g., during exercise) without a corresponding increase in pressure. This reduction in vascular resistance is achieved mainly by "recruiting" pulmonary vessels that are not perfused at rest. This ability is reflected in the pulmonary vascular pressure-flow curve (Fig. 13–2). When cardiac output is low (A), pulmonary vascular resistance is given by the slope A-X, or

$$10.5 \text{ mm Hg}/5 \text{ L/min} = 2.1 \text{ mm Hg/L/min}$$

If cardiac output is increased to 15 L/min (B), pulmonary artery pressure increases only slightly, to 12 mm Hg, and now pulmonary vascular resistance is given by the slope B-X, or

$$12 \text{ mm Hg}/15 \text{ L/min} = 0.8 \text{ mm Hg/L/min}$$

This substantial decrease in resistance occurs simply because of vascular recruitment and *not* because of relaxation of pulmonary vascular smooth muscle.

Pulmonary vascular resistance is calculated by dividing driving pressure by cardiac output:

$$PVR = \frac{Ppa - Pla}{\dot{Q}}$$

where PVR is pulmonary vascular resistance, Ppa is pulmonary artery pressure, Pla is left atrial pressure, and $\dot{Q}$ is cardiac output. The driving pressure is the difference between mean pulmonary arterial and mean left atrial pressure. In practice, pulmonary wedge pressure provides a reliable estimate of left atrial pressure in the absence of large-vein obstruction.

The pressure across any vascular bed is directly related to the blood flow through that particular bed and the blood

TABLE 13–1. Classification of Pulmonary Hypertension

Pulmonary Arterial Hypertension

Primary pulmonary hypertension
    Sporadic disorders
    Familial disorders
Related conditions
    Collagen vascular disease
    Congenital systemic-to-pulmonary shunt
    Portal hypertension
    HIV infection
    Drugs and toxins
       Anorectic agents
       Others
Persistent pulmonary hypertension of the newborn

Pulmonary Venous Hypertension

Left-sided atrial or ventricular heart disease
Left-sided valvular disease
Congenital stenosis of the pulmonary veins
Extrinsic compression of central pulmonary veins
    Fibrosing mediastinitis
    Adenopathy and/or tumors
Pulmonary veno-occlusive disease

Pulmonary Hypertension Caused by Diseases of the Respiratory System and/or Hypoxemia

COPD, cystic fibrosis, bronchiectasis
Interstitial lung disease
Sleep-disordered breathing
Chest wall deformity (kyphoscoliosis, thoracoplasty)
Pleural disease (fibrothorax)
Alveolar hypoventilation disorders (neuromuscular disease, Ondine's curse)
Chronic exposure to high altitude
Neonatal lung disease
Alveolar-capillary dysplasia

Pulmonary Hypertension Caused by Chronic Thrombotic and/or Embolic Disease

Thomboembolic obstruction of proximal pulmonary arteries
Obstruction of distal pulmonary arteries
    Pulmonary embolism (thrombus, tumor, ova and/or parasites, foreign material)
    In situ thrombosis
    Sickle cell disease
    Tumor emboli
    Miscellaneous (talc, fat, amnionic fluid)

Pulmonary Hypertension Caused by Disorders Directly Affecting the Pulmonary Vasculature

Inflammatory conditions
    Schistosomiasis
    Sarcoidosis
Pulmonary capillary hemangiomatoisis

Modified from Executive Summary from the World Symposium on Primary Pulmonary Hypertension 1998, Evian, France, September 6-10, 1998.

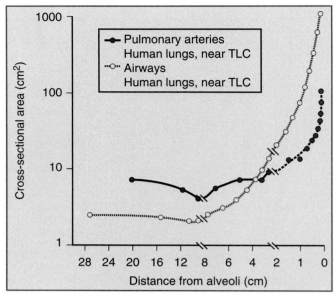

FIGURE 13–1

Pulmonary arterial and airway cross-sectional area. The total cross-sectional area of the tracheobronchial tree and the pulmonary vascular tree increases greatly as they branch toward the gas-exchanging portion of the lung. These data show that the total area occupied by small airways exceeds that occupied by small pulmonary vessels. (*From Culver BH, Butler J: Mechanical influences on the pulmonary microcirculation. Annu Rev Physiol 40:187, 1980.*)

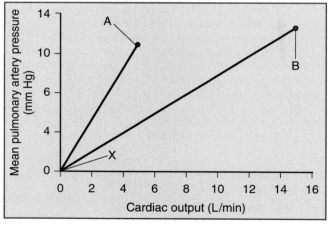

FIGURE 13–2

Pulmonary vascular pressure-flow curves. Mean pulmonary arterial pressure is plotted against cardiac output. The slope of the line is pulmonary vascular resistance. A large increase in cardiac output is associated with only a slight increase in mean pulmonary vascular pressure.

viscosity within it; an increase in either will cause an increase in pressure for any given vascular geometry. The pressure across the vascular bed is also inversely related to the number and radii of its vessels. The total cross-sectional area of the vascular tree can decrease because of a loss of pulmonary vessels, intraluminal occlusion of a proportion of the vessels, or a decrease in vascular radius as a result of smooth muscle contraction or vascular wall thickening and remodeling. Finally, pulmonary arterial pressure can be increased as a result of an increase in the downstream or venous pressure.

Pulmonary artery vasoconstriction can be produced by hypoxemia or acidosis, either metabolic or respiratory in origin, and may thus be reversed, at least partly, by the administration of oxygen or by raising the pH of the blood.[4] Vasoconstriction can also be caused by a variety of mediators of inflammation, including serotonin, histamine, angiotensin, catecholamines, prostaglandins, and leukotrienes.[5] The release of such mediators partly explains the acute pulmonary hypertension that develops in thromboembolic disease. The increase in pressure in the pulmonary arteries resulting from postcapillary hypertension is also initially vasospastic in origin, probably mediated through a vasovagal reflex originating from a rise in left atrial and pulmonary venous pressure.[6] The pulmonary vascular endothelium plays an important role in control of the pulmonary circulation; it produces a variety of substances, including prostacyclin, endothelin, and nitric oxide, that affect tone in the underlying vascular smooth muscle cells.[7]

Pathologic Characteristics

The pathologic abnormalities seen in the pulmonary vasculature differ somewhat depending on the etiology of the hypertension.[8] However, partly because of the limited response that can occur in the pulmonary vessels and partly because some of the abnormalities are secondary to the hypertension, some findings are common to all causes. This is particularly true for changes in the large muscular and elastic arteries in patients who have hypertension of many etiologies and in the smaller arteries in patients who have primary (idiopathic) pulmonary hypertension or hypertension related to congenital cardiovascular disease, hepatic disease, AIDS, connective tissue disease, and some drugs—conditions that are characterized by a group of vascular changes collectively known as *plexogenic pulmonary arteriopathy.*

In pulmonary arterial hypertension of significant degree, the large elastic arteries, especially the main pulmonary artery, are often dilated and are sometimes larger in diameter than the aorta; the dilation may be so severe that localized aneurysm formation is the result. Pulmonary arterial atherosclerosis, usually mild and predominantly affecting the large elastic vessels, is a relatively common finding in older individuals; however, in the presence of pulmonary hypertension, atherosclerotic foci tend to be larger and to involve more distal branches.[9] Intimal fibrosis of elastic and large muscular arteries is also frequent in pulmonary hypertension of any cause and may be so severe that it virtually obliterates the vascular lumen (Fig. 13–3). Thickening of the media of small muscular arteries is a characteristic feature of many forms of pulmonary hypertension. It is most often caused by a combination of muscle hypertrophy and hyperplasia and an increase in interstitial connective tissue.[10] Muscle hypertrophy

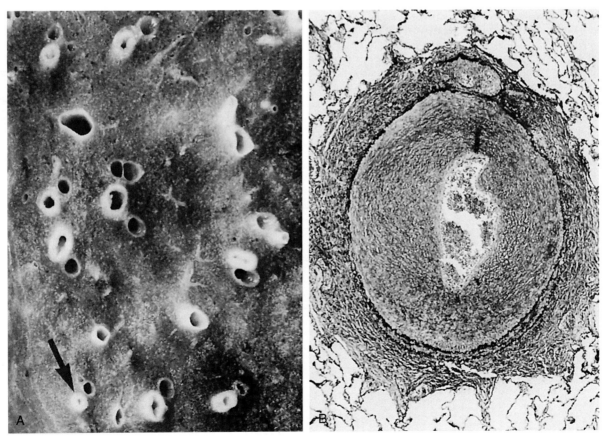

FIGURE 13–3

Pulmonary hypertension: intimal fibrosis. A magnified view of an autopsy specimen of the lung (**A**) of a 25-year-old woman who had systemic lupus erythematosus shows marked thickening of the walls of many muscular arteries; in some (*arrow*), the lumen is almost obliterated. A corresponding histologic section (**B**) demonstrates the thickening to be caused predominantly by intimal fibrosis; marked medial atrophy is also evident. (*From Fraser RS, Müller NL, Colman NC, Paré PD: Fraser and Paré's Diagnosis of Diseases of the Chest, 4th ed. Philadelphia, WB Saunders, 1999.*)

also occurs in pulmonary arterioles. In some cases, it is caused by an increase in the size and number of muscle fibers already present in the arteriolar wall; in others, it represents extension of muscle into vessels that formerly contained none ("arterialization" of pulmonary arterioles).[11]

In addition to muscle hypertrophy-hyperplasia, several abnormalities are often present in small to medium-sized muscular arteries that together characterize plexogenic pulmonary arteriopathy.[12] These abnormalities include cellular intimal proliferation and fibrosis, plexiform lesions, fibrinoid "necrosis," and vasculitis. In the early stages, intimal thickening is characterized by the presence of loose connective tissue containing cells that are often elongated and arranged in more or less concentric layers encompassing the entire vascular lumen, thereby resulting in a distinctive "onion skin" appearance (Fig. 13–4).[13] With time, the connective tissue component—particularly collagen and sometimes elastin—becomes prominent. The term *fibrinoid necrosis* is used to describe the presence of homogeneous eosinophilic material in the walls of small arteries and arterioles. Although luminal thrombosis may occur adjacent to the site of "necrosis," there is usually no inflammation of the vessel wall and the lesion most likely represents an accumulation of fibrin and other proteins within the media as a result of endothelial damage.

Plexiform lesions are seen in small supernumerary arteries a short distance beyond their origin from the parent vessel.[14] The lesion consists of a localized focus of vascular dilation associated with an intraluminal plexus of slitlike vascular channels (Fig. 13–5); the latter are separated by a small amount of connective tissue and a variable number of plump endothelium-like cells. The plexus itself often continues distally into a thin-walled, somewhat tortuous and dilated vascular channel. The pathogenesis of plexiform lesions is uncertain; however, one group of investigators found that the proliferating endothelial cells are a monoclonal expansion. This observation suggests that acquired genetic abnormalities, such as occur in malignancy, may be causative.[15]

Radiologic Manifestations

The characteristic radiologic features of pulmonary hypertension, regardless of etiology, consist of enlargement of the central pulmonary arteries and rapid tapering of the vessels as they extend to the periphery of the lungs (Fig. 13–6).[16] The heart may be normal in size or enlarged. Enlargement of the hilar arteries can be assessed by measuring the diameter of the interlobar arteries.[17] The main pulmonary artery can be identified and measured with CT and MR imaging; it is considered enlarged if it measures 29 mm or more in diameter.[18,19] The cross-sectional area of the main and left pulmonary arteries normalized for body surface area shows good correlation with mean pulmonary arterial pressure. It has also been suggested that a segmental artery–to–bronchus diameter ratio greater than 1 in three or more lobes is helpful in predicting the presence of hypertension.[19]

The most accurate noninvasive method of assessing the presence of pulmonary arterial hypertension is echocardiography. A number of variables derived from continuous wave or pulsed Doppler echocardiography can be used to determine right ventricular peak systolic pressure, which is used as an estimate of pulmonary artery pressure.[20] Echocardiographic assessment of pulmonary hemodynamics can be carried out during exercise,[21] and transesophageal echocardiography can detect the presence and site of intracardiac shunts.[22]

MR imaging is particularly useful in assessment and has been shown to accurately predict right heart hemodynamics in patients who have primary pulmonary hypertension (PPH).[23] The procedure can be used to define the direction and velocity of blood flow within the cardiac chambers and great vessels, assess cardiovascular structure (Fig. 13–7), make measurements of end-systolic and end-diastolic right ventricular volume, and calculate ejection volume and fraction.[24,25]

Ventilation-perfusion scintigraphy is used mainly to distinguish PPH from hypertension associated with chronic thromboembolism, a normal or low-probability scan virtually

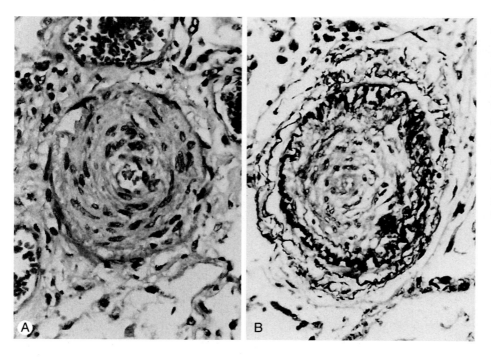

FIGURE 13–4

Pulmonary hypertension: cellular intimal fibrosis. A section of a small pulmonary artery (**A**) from a young man with an atrial septal defect shows almost complete obliteration of the lumen by fibrous tissue. The cell nuclei are somewhat elongated and arranged in roughly concentric layers, the result being a somewhat whorled appearance. A section of the same vessel stained for elastic tissue (**B**) shows the cellular proliferation to be entirely within the intima. *(From Fraser RS, Müller NL, Colman NC, Paré PD: Fraser and Paré's Diagnosis of Diseases of the Chest, 4th ed. Philadelphia, WB Saunders, 1999.)*

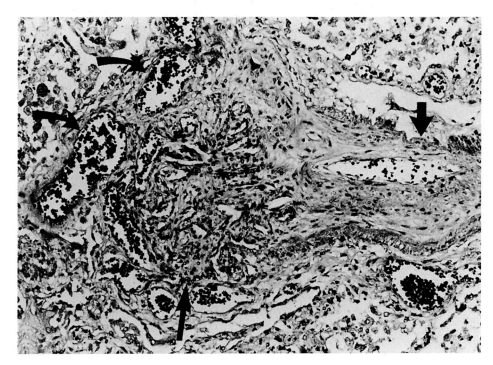

Pulmonary hypertension: plexiform lesion. A section of a medium-sized pulmonary artery from a young patient who had cirrhosis and portal hypertension reveals moderate intimal fibrosis (*short arrow*) continuous with a plexus of small, irregularly shaped vascular channels. These channels are separated by fibrous tissue containing many plump cells resembling fibroblasts (*long arrow*). The plexus itself is continuous with a dilated, relatively thin-walled vascular channel (*curved arrows*). *(From Fraser RS, Müller NL, Colman NC, Paré PD: Fraser and Paré's Diagnosis of Diseases of the Chest, 4th ed. Philadelphia, WB Saunders, 1999.)*

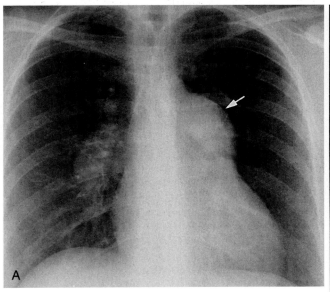
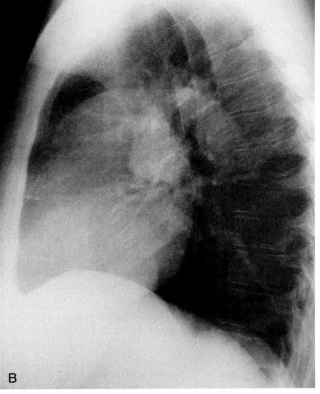

FIGURE 13–6

Pulmonary arterial hypertension. Posteroanterior (**A**) and lateral (**B**) chest radiographs demonstrate enlargement of the central pulmonary arteries with rapid tapering of the vessels. On the posteroanterior view, marked enlargement of the main pulmonary artery results in a focal convexity (*arrow*) immediately below the level of the aortic arch. On the lateral view, right ventricular enlargement and dilation of the pulmonary outflow tract result in filling of the lower retrosternal air space. The patient was a 36-year-old woman who had primary pulmonary hypertension. *(From Fraser RS, Müller NL, Colman NC, Paré PD: Fraser and Paré's Diagnosis of Diseases of the Chest, 4th ed. Philadelphia, WB Saunders, 1999.)*

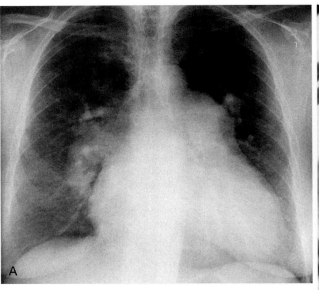

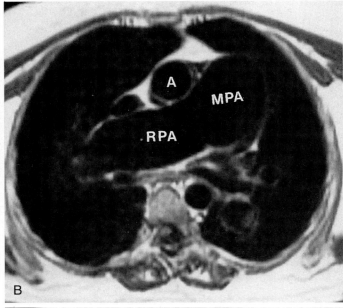

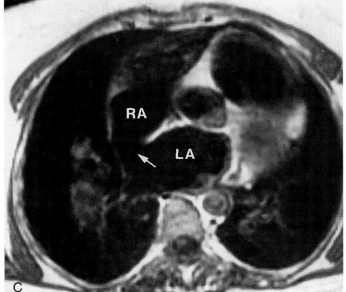

FIGURE 13–7

Pulmonary arterial hypertension—atrial septal defect. A posteroanterior chest radiograph (**A**) shows cardiomegaly and marked enlargement of the central pulmonary arteries. Although there is rapid tapering, increased vascularity is still present in the lung periphery, particularly on the right side. A cardiac-gated spin-echo MR image (**B**) shows enlargement of the main (MPA) and right (RPA) pulmonary arteries. The diameter of the main pulmonary artery is considerably larger than that of the aorta (A). An MR image at the level of the right (RA) and left (LA) atria (**C**) demonstrates an atrial septal defect (*arrow*). The patient was a 61-year-old woman. (*From Fraser RS, Müller NL, Colman NC, Paré PD: Fraser and Paré's Diagnosis of Diseases of the Chest, 4th ed. Philadelphia, WB Saunders, 1999.*)

excluding the latter process. In patients who have intermediate- or high-probability scans, the diagnosis of chronic thromboembolic disease can usually be confirmed with contrast-enhanced spiral CT (Fig. 13–8)[26]; however, angiography may be required for definitive diagnosis in some patients.

Cor Pulmonale

The presence of pulmonary hypertension does not necessarily imply cor pulmonale, but it does indicate that there is a strain on the right ventricle that, if prolonged, will inevitably lead to the abnormality. Although the term "cor pulmonale" was originally restricted to instances in which an abnormality in lung structure or function results in right ventricular hypertrophy, it is increasingly being used to describe right heart failure secondary to pulmonary hypertension caused by pulmonary vascular obstruction. Approximately 80% of cases result from COPD.[27]

Radiographically, cardiac enlargement is not always apparent, even when right ventricular hypertrophy is evident at postmortem examination.[28] This is particularly likely to occur in the presence of pulmonary emphysema, when only serial radiographs may reveal evidence of increased heart size. Clinically, right ventricular thrust, usually felt along the left sternal border, may also be obscured by pulmonary overinflation in emphysema. As right-sided heart failure develops, a systolic murmur that is louder during inspiration may become audible along the left sternal border. It may be associated with a palpable pulse in the (enlarged) liver, a systolic venous pulse in the neck, and in many cases, peripheral edema and ascites. The electrocardiogram (ECG) may be normal, even in cases of known severe right ventricular hypertrophy.[29]

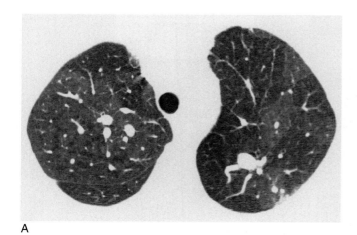

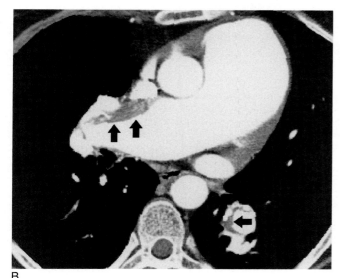

FIGURE 13–8

Thromboembolic pulmonary arterial hypertension. An HRCT image (**A**) shows localized areas of increased and decreased attenuation and vascularity (mosaic perfusion pattern). Contrast-enhanced CT (**B**) demonstrates enlargement of the main pulmonary artery and filling defects contiguous with the wall of the right interlobar and left lower lobar pulmonary arteries (*arrows*). This eccentric location of the filling defects is characteristic of chronic pulmonary thromboembolism. The patient was a 54-year-old woman.

The term *acute cor pulmonale* has been used to describe the syndrome of acute right ventricular pressure overload and failure, which occurs in a variety of clinical settings, including massive pulmonary embolism, severe asthma, and episodes of primary lactic acidosis, as well as infrequently during the course of acute respiratory distress syndrome.[30]

PULMONARY ARTERIAL HYPERTENSION

Primary Pulmonary Hypertension

PPH is a rare abnormality, with an incidence of only about 1 per million population.[31,32] The mean age of patients in the

National Institutes of Health (NIH) Pulmonary Hypertension Registry in 1987 was 36 ± 15 years with a female-to-male preponderance of 1.7:1.[31] Although the majority of cases appear to be sporadic, about 5% of the patients in the NIH registry have a family history (familial primary pulmonary hypertension [FPPH]). The inheritance most closely conforms to an autosomal dominant pattern. However, FPPH also shows an incomplete pattern of penetrance, with overt disease actually developing in only 10% to 20% of family members, which suggests that additional environmental and/or genetic events are required for its complete expression.

A gene on chromosome 2 that codes for bone morphogenic protein receptor (BMPR-2) has been closely associated with PPH.[33,34] In fact, abnormalities in BMPR-2 are seen in more than half the cases of familial disease and may be involved in many cases of sporadic PPH, as well as other forms of hypertension such as that induced by anorexigens.[35] BMPR-2 is a member of the transforming growth factor-β receptor family and has been implicated in various developmental processes. At least 46 germline mutations in the BMPR-2 gene have been described in FPPH and sporadic PPH; it remains unclear how such mutations lead to PPH.[36] It is also uncertain why mutations in such an important gene, which is expressed in multiple tissues, lead to abnormalities in only specific regions of the pulmonary vascular system.

A potential role for immunologically mediated processes in the pathogenesis of PPH is suggested by the observation that pulmonary hypertension occurs as a complication of several connective tissue diseases, particularly systemic lupus erythematosus (SLE) and progressive systemic sclerosis (PSS).[37,38] Moreover, the incidence of Raynaud's phenomenon in patients who have PPH is higher than would be expected by chance. It is believed that the early stages of PPH are characterized by constriction of pulmonary vascular smooth muscle; with prolonged vasoconstriction, vascular remodeling and the changes of plexogenic pulmonary arteriopathy eventually ensue. There is also evidence that in situ thrombosis contributes to progression of disease in many cases.[39]

The pathologic findings in PPH are those of plexogenic arteriopathy, although not all histologic manifestations of this complex of abnormalities are identified in every case.[40] The radiographic findings consist of enlargement of the central pulmonary arteries, rapid tapering, and peripheral oligemia (Fig. 13–9). Overinflation does not occur, thus permitting ready differentiation from the diffuse pulmonary oligemia associated with emphysema. Ventilation-perfusion scans may be normal or show patchy nonsegmental perfusion defects.[41]

The main symptom is dyspnea on exertion, which is often insidious in onset.[42] Less frequent manifestations include Raynaud's phenomenon, syncope, easy fatigability, chest pain, and cough. The mean interval from the onset of symptoms to diagnosis averages about 2 years. Signs of cor pulmonale and cardiac failure may be present, including giant jugular A waves, right atrial gallop, a loud pulmonary ejection click, an accentuated pulmonic sound, a palpable lift along the left sternal border, and in some cases, murmurs caused by pulmonic and tricuspid insufficiency.[43]

Catheterization of the right side of the heart reveals increased pulmonary artery pressure, normal pulmonary wedge pressure, high pulmonary vascular resistance, and in patients who have right ventricular failure, low cardiac output.[31] Although pulmonary function may be normal,

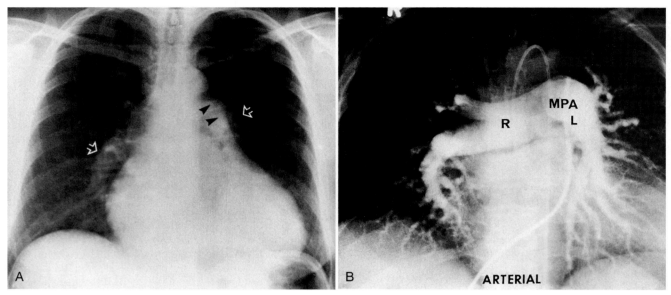

FIGURE 13-9

Primary pulmonary hypertension. A posteroanterior chest radiograph (**A**) shows enlargement of the right ventricle, dilation of the main (*arrowheads*) and hilar (*open arrows*) pulmonary arteries, and increased rapidity of tapering of pulmonary arteries as they proceed distally. These findings are confirmed on a pulmonary angiogram during the arterial (**B**) phase (main pulmonary artery [MPA], right [R] and left [L] pulmonary arteries); the middle and distal pulmonary arteries taper rapidly and display a sinuous ("corkscrew") appearance. *(From Fraser RS, Müller NL, Colman NC, Paré PD: Fraser and Paré's Diagnosis of Diseases of the Chest, 4th ed. Philadelphia, WB Saunders, 1999.)*

arterial oxygen saturation and diffusing capacity are often decreased.[44,45] The finding of a marked decrease in arterial oxygen saturation during exercise, related in part to a decrease in cardiac output, is a useful diagnostic finding.[46]

The majority of patients who have PPH experience progressive dyspnea, cor pulmonale, and death within a few years.[47] In a retrospective study of 61 patients, 2-, 5-, and 10-year survival rates were 48%, 32%, and 12%, respectively.[48] In the NIH study, a reduced FVC and cardiac index and increased right atrial pressure were significant risk factors for decreased survival after diagnosis.[49] A reduced cardiac index and symptoms that reflect decreased cardiac output, such as syncope, have been also found to be indicators of a poor prognosis.[50]

Related Conditions

Connective Tissue Disease

As indicated, pulmonary arterial hypertension unaccompanied by parenchymal lung disease and manifested pathologically by plexogenic arteriopathy occurs occasionally in a number of connective tissue disorders, particularly PSS, mixed connective tissue disease, and SLE (Fig. 13–10).[51] Pulmonary hypertension can also occur in patients who have interstitial fibrosis complicating rheumatoid disease and PSS; in these cases, the pathogenesis as well as the radiologic and pathologic features are identical to those associated with chronic interstitial lung disease of other etiologies. Rarely, hypertension is a complication of pulmonary vasculitis, most often Takayasu's or Behçet's disease; in these cases, the pathogenesis of the hypertension is probably related to in situ arterial thrombosis.

Congenital Systemic-to-Pulmonary Shunt

Included in this category are the congenital heart defects with left-to-right shunt, atrial septal and ventricular septal defects, patent ductus arteriosus, aorticopulmonary window, transposition of the great vessels, and partial anomalous pulmonary venous drainage. The pathogenetic feature common to all these conditions is increased blood flow in the pulmonary circulation. A similar mechanism may be responsible for the pulmonary hypertension occasionally seen in thyrotoxicosis[52] and chronic renal failure[53] and after extensive lung resection.[54]

Pulmonary arterial flow may be greatly increased for a long time before increased resistance results in hypertension. Ultimately, left-to-right shunting can lead to the development of severe irreversible pulmonary arterial hypertension with dilation of the central pulmonary arteries and reversal of the left-to-right shunt at the atrial, ventricular, or aortopulmonary level (Eisenmenger's syndrome).[55,56] The pathologic features of pulmonary hypertension associated with increased flow are those of plexogenic arteriopathy.

The main radiographic sign in all these conditions is an increase in caliber of the pulmonary arteries throughout the lungs (Fig. 13–11). The diagnosis of a left-to-right shunt can be made readily with echocardiography or MR imaging (see Fig. 13–7);[57] however, cardiac catheterization, with or without angiocardiography, is often required to define the abnormality and determine the severity of pulmonary arterial hypertension.

Many patients who have left-to-right shunts are asymptomatic. If the shunt is large, the patient may complain of fatigue, palpitations, and dyspnea on exertion and may exhibit signs of right-sided cardiac failure. Examination of the heart and systemic vessels may provide valuable clues

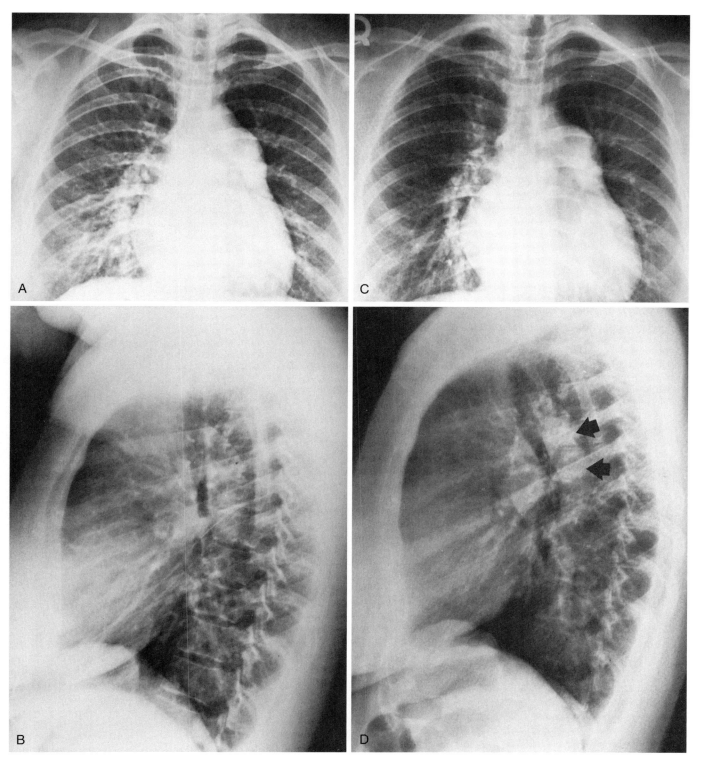

FIGURE 13–10

Pulmonary arterial hypertension—systemic lupus erythematosus. The first chest radiographs in posteroanterior (**A**) and lateral (**B**) projection in this 32-year-old reveal prominence of the main pulmonary artery and mild to moderate cardiomegaly consistent with right ventricular enlargement. The pulmonary vasculature looks plethoric, but the lungs are otherwise unremarkable. Eight months later, repeat chest radiographs (**C** and **D**) show an increase in size of the heart and greater prominence of the main and hilar pulmonary arteries; note the markedly dilated left interlobar artery in **D** (*arrows*). However, a more remarkable change has occurred in the pulmonary vasculature, which now displays diffuse oligemia. (*From Fraser RS, Müller NL, Colman NC, Paré PD: Fraser and Paré's Diagnosis of Diseases of the Chest, 4th ed. Philadelphia, WB Saunders, 1999.*)

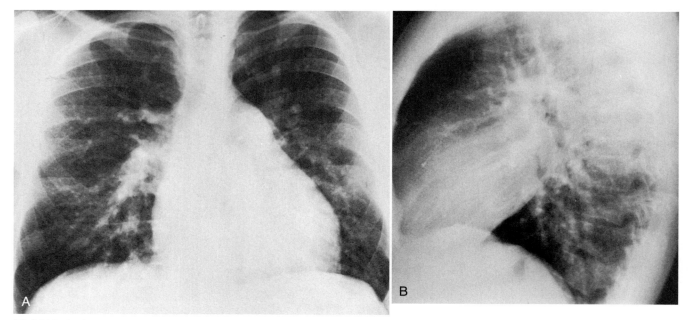

FIGURE 13–11

Pulmonary pleonemia—atrial septal defect. Posteroanterior (**A**) and lateral (**B**) radiographs of an asymptomatic 19-year-old man with an atrial septal defect reveal an increase in caliber of the pulmonary arteries and veins throughout both lungs; the vessels taper normally. The heart is moderately enlarged and has a contour consistent with enlargement of the right atrium and right ventricle. *(From Fraser RS, Müller NL, Colman NC, Paré PD: Fraser and Paré's Diagnosis of Diseases of the Chest, 4th ed. Philadelphia, WB Saunders, 1999.)*

regarding the nature of the shunt. Atrial septal defects, ventricular septal defects, and patent ductus arteriosus lead to characteristic murmurs and other cardiac signs indicative of right ventricular strain and hypertrophy. The development of pulmonary hypertension in patients with left-to-right shunt gives rise to changes in the physical findings. In atrial septal defect, atrial fibrillation is a frequent occurrence and may be followed by tricuspid regurgitation and heart failure; the fixed splitting of the second heart sound becomes much narrower, and the systolic murmur may become fainter. In ventricular septal defect, the systolic murmur decreases in length, and an ejection systolic murmur and click may appear.

A number of additional symptoms and signs are related to cor pulmonale and right heart failure, including retrosternal pain identical to angina pectoris, parasternal thrust, a murmur of tricuspid insufficiency, and liver and neck pulsations. Pulmonary hypertension may also cause accentuation of the second pulmonic sound and an early diastolic murmur along the left sternal border as a result of pulmonary valvular insufficiency. A variety of additional manifestations, such as cyanosis, clubbing, and cachexia, may also be seen.

The hemodynamic consequences and clinical outcome in patients who have severe pulmonary hypertension as a result of Eisenmenger's syndrome appear to be better than those in patients who have PPH of similar magnitude.[58]

Portal Hypertension

Pulmonary hypertension is a well-recognized complication of chronic liver disease, particularly (but not invariably[59]) when accompanied by portal hypertension.[60] The prevalence of pulmonary hypertension in all patients who have cirrhosis is low (0.61% to 0.73%)[61]; however, it is much higher in those being considered for liver transplantation.[62] Slow but steady improvement in pulmonary hemodynamics has been reported after successful liver transplantation.[63]

The pathogenesis of pulmonary hypertension in liver disease may be related to vasoactive or vasotoxic substances that are normally produced in the gut and metabolized by the liver, the increased pressure in the portal veins enabling these substances to reach the pulmonary circulation via a porto-systemic shunt.[64] Pulmonary thromboemboli originating in a congested portal circulation and reaching the lung via varices is another potential, albeit less likely, contributing mechanism.[65]

The radiologic manifestations range from normal to the characteristic findings of pulmonary arterial hypertension (Fig. 13–12).[66] Symptoms and signs are similar to those in patients who have pulmonary hypertension of other cause, although they may be masked by the inactivity caused by the underlying liver disease.

HIV Infection

An association between pulmonary hypertension and HIV infection has been clearly established.[67,68] However, there is no evidence of a direct effect of the virus on the pulmonary vasculature, which has led to the speculation that the hypertension is the result of an immunologic response.[69] In most cases, the pathologic appearance is that of plexogenic pulmonary hypertension[70]; nonetheless, cases of thrombus-associated hypertension and veno-occlusive disease have also been reported.[71,72]

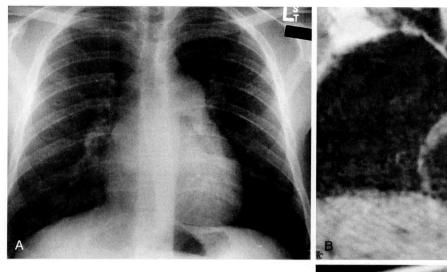

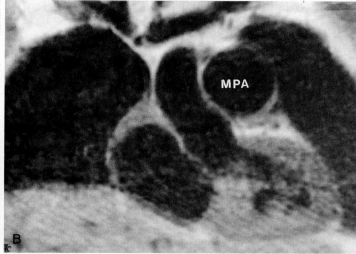

FIGURE 13–12

Pulmonary arterial hypertension related to cirrhosis. A posteroanterior chest radiograph (**A**) in a 17-year-old man demonstrates cardiomegaly and enlargement of the central pulmonary arteries. A coronal spin-echo MR image (**B**) shows marked enlargement of the main pulmonary artery (MPA). A transverse MR image (**C**) shows enlargement of the MPA, which has a greater diameter than that of the aorta (A). Increased signal is evident within the right and left pulmonary arteries (*arrows*) as a result of slow blood flow because of hypertension. (*From Fraser RS, Müller NL, Colman NC, Paré PD: Fraser and Paré's Diagnosis of Diseases of the Chest, 4th ed. Philadelphia, WB Saunders, 1999.*)

The clinical manifestations are identical to those of PPH, except that the age at onset is younger.[73] In most cases, the hypertension develops in the absence of other manifestations of HIV infection. The CD4 count is usually greater than 200/μL. The natural history of the pulmonary hypertension is one of rapid deterioration.[73]

Toxins and Drugs

A variety of toxins and drugs have been implicated in the pathogenesis of pulmonary hypertension. For example, in the exposure to contaminated rapeseed oil that occurred in Spain in 1981, hypertension was the principal pulmonary manifestation during the later stages of disease (see page 781).[74] Eosinophilia-myalgia syndrome, a condition similar to rapeseed oil toxicity, may also be accompanied by pulmonary hypertension and has been reported after the ingestion of medicinal preparations containing large amounts of the amino acid L-tryptophan.[75] In addition, pulmonary hypertension has been associated with the ingestion or inhalation of cocaine,[76] amphetamines,[77] and phenformin.[78]

A significant increase in incidence of "PPH" was noted in certain European countries after use of the anorectic drug aminorex fumarate in the 1960s.[79] In the 1970s, use of another class of appetite suppressors, the fenfluramine derivatives, was again followed by sporadic reports and small series of cases of pulmonary hypertension[80]; a multicenter case-control study showed an odds ratio of 6.5 for the development of "PPH" with these drugs (mainly fenfluramine and dexfenfluramine).[81] The mechanism by which the drugs cause pulmonary hypertension is unknown; however, they are all substrates for serotonin uptake transporters, and it is possible that some alteration in processing or metabolism of this substance is involved.[82]

The pathologic features of toxin- or drug-related pulmonary hypertension are those of plexogenic arteriopathy. Radiologic and clinical manifestations are identical to those of primary disease.

Persistent Pulmonary Hypertension of the Newborn

Persistent pulmonary hypertension of the newborn (persistent fetal circulation syndrome) is a pathophysiologic syndrome that results when pulmonary vascular resistance fails to decrease after birth despite normal lung expansion and ventilation. The increased pulmonary vascular pressure results in continuation of blood flow through the foramen ovale and ductus arteriosus and causes systemic hypoxemia.

The pathogenesis of the hypertension is not known. Possible mechanisms include intrauterine hypoxia causing pulmonary vascular remodeling,[83] hypoplasia of the pulmonary vascular tree, dysregulation of vasoactive mediators,[84] and microthrombus formation.[85] The syndrome occurs in term or post-term infants who have tachypnea, respiratory distress, and cyanosis. The chest radiograph is characteristically normal; the diagnosis can be confirmed by echocardiography.

PULMONARY VENOUS HYPERTENSION

Pulmonary venous hypertension (postcapillary pulmonary hypertension) results from conditions that increase pulmonary venous pressure above a critical level. The most common of these conditions are diseases of the left side of the heart, usually those that cause left ventricular failure, such as systemic hypertension and coronary artery disease. Less common causes include mitral stenosis, congenital cardiac anomalies such as cor triatriatum, chronic sclerosing mediastinitis, atrial myxoma, total anomalous venous drainage, and pulmonary veno-occlusive disease.

Left-Sided Heart Disease

The increase in pulmonary arterial pressure that follows pulmonary venous hypertension is initially the result of arterial vasoconstriction[86]; however, when postcapillary hypertension is severe and long-standing, it induces structural changes within the arteries that perpetuate the increased resistance. These changes are typically manifested as medial hypertrophy and intimal fibrosis[87]; muscularization of arterioles is also common. Findings of plexogenic arteriopathy are not seen. Medial hypertrophy and intimal fibrosis also occur in the pulmonary veins.[88]

The pulmonary parenchyma itself is usually abnormal, probably because of chronic leakage of fluid and red blood cells from alveolar capillaries. Parenchymal interstitial fibrosis, type II cell hyperplasia, and foci of air space hemorrhage are often evident (Fig. 13–13)[88]; remote episodes of hemorrhage are manifested by the presence of hemosiderin-laden macrophages within alveolar air spaces. Organization of intra-alveolar edema may be responsible for the presence of mature bone within alveolar air spaces or the lumen of alveolar ducts, a finding that is particularly common in mitral stenosis.

Pulmonary venous hypertension of any cause is characterized radiographically by narrowing of pulmonary vessels in the lower lobes and distention of those in the upper lobes.[89] This pattern is most striking in the setting of chronic rather than acute venous hypertension.[90] The exact mechanism for the change in vascular volume (and presumably blood flow) is unclear. Hypotheses include reflex vasoconstriction in the dependent lung,[91] hypoxic vasoconstriction caused by the presence of interstitial edema,[92] and interstitial fibrosis in the lower lung zones. Regardless of the mechanism, there is no doubt that a disparity between the caliber of upper and lower lobe vessels is one of the most useful radiographic signs of pulmonary venous hypertension (Fig. 13–14). In fact, the radiographic sign may be apparent

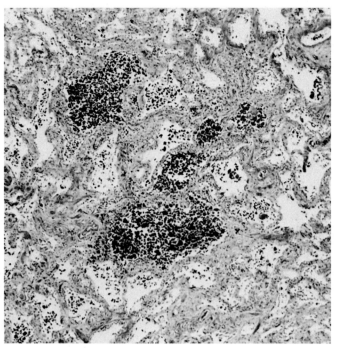

FIGURE 13–13

Postcapillary hypertension in mitral stenosis. A section of lung parenchyma from a 68-year-old woman with long-standing mitral stenosis shows several intra-alveolar aggregates of hemosiderin-laden macrophages (black cells) and a moderate degree of interstitial fibrosis. *(From Fraser RS, Müller NL, Colman NC, Paré PD: Fraser and Paré's Diagnosis of Diseases of the Chest, 4th ed. Philadelphia, WB Saunders, 1999.)*

without clinical evidence of left ventricular decompensation. Additional radiographic abnormalities seen with venous hypertension include loss of the normal sharp margins of the pulmonary vessels, perihilar haze, and Kerley A and B lines (Fig. 13–15).[93]

The symptoms associated with postcapillary hypertension are usually readily differentiated from those of precapillary origin. In left ventricular failure, which is the most common cause, the symptoms and signs are predominantly those arising from acute or subacute pulmonary edema and include dyspnea, orthopnea, and paroxysmal nocturnal dyspnea. Mitral stenosis can be diagnosed on auscultation of the heart by the loud opening snap and rumbling diastolic murmur. When pulmonary venous hypertension develops as a result of a myxoma or thrombus blocking the mitral valve orifice, the clinical course is usually punctuated by episodes of pulmonary edema or positional syncope.

The ECG findings reflect the cause of the hypertension and the rapidity of increase in pressure. In pure mitral stenosis, the changes may be identical to those of primary arterial hypertension with right ventricular hypertrophy. In mitral insufficiency, the ECG usually shows left ventricular hypertrophy, with or without evidence of right ventricular hypertrophy.

In the early stages of mitral stenosis, the diffusing capacity for carbon monoxide may be increased, presumably as a result of an increase in pulmonary capillary blood volume; however, in patients who have moderate or severe disease, it is reduced significantly.[94] Pulmonary function studies in patients who

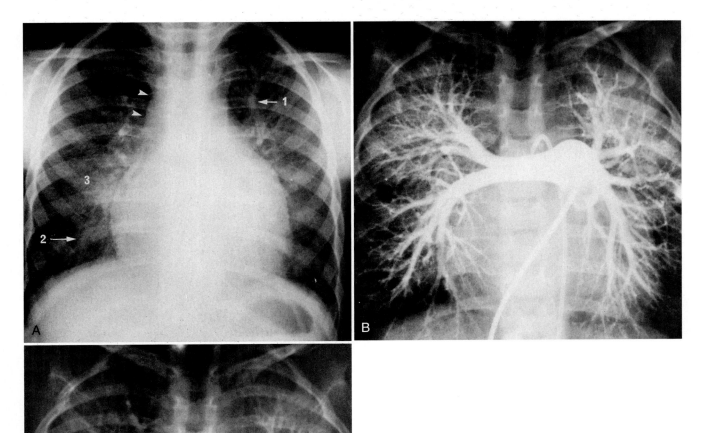

FIGURE 13–14

Severe postcapillary pulmonary hypertension and edema—mitral valve prolapse. A posteroanterior chest radiograph (**A**) shows dilated upper lobe vessels (1), ill-defined lower lobe vessels (2), and diffuse interstitial edema (3). Cardiac size is increased in a nonspecific fashion. The vascular pedicle is increased in width as a result of distention of the superior vena cava (*arrowheads*), indicative of systemic venous hypertension. Anteroposterior views of the thorax from a selective main pulmonary angiogram during the arterial (**B**) and venous (**C**) phases reveal increased blood flow to the upper lobes (compare the degree of contrast filling of the upper lobe arteries with the relatively branchless lower lobe arterial vasculature). The mid and upper zones show a "background blush"; the lower lobes do not. Note the persistence of the lower lobe arterial pattern, the well-distended upper lobe veins (V1), and the poorly filled lower lobe veins (V2) during the venous phase. *(From Fraser RS, Müller NL, Colman NC, Paré PD: Fraser and Paré's Diagnosis of Diseases of the Chest, 4th ed. Philadelphia, WB Saunders, 1999.)*

have mitral valve disease show a progressive decrease in vital capacity and diffusing capacity and, with advanced disease, in expiratory flow rates.[95]

Pulmonary Veno-occlusive Disease

Pulmonary veno-occlusive disease is a rare abnormality characterized pathologically by intimal thickening and evidence of repeated thrombosis of pulmonary veins and clinically by pulmonary arterial hypertension, pulmonary edema, or both.[96] In most of the cases reported before 1990, the diagnosis was made at autopsy[97]; however, as a result of the more widespread

recognition of the variable manifestations of the disease and the availability of HRCT, the diagnosis is now being made more frequently antemortem. The condition can occur at any age but is most common during childhood and adolescence. In adolescent patients, the sex incidence is approximately equal; however, in older individuals, there appears to be a slight male preponderance.[98]

The pathogenesis is unclear and may be related to more than one mechanism. Familial clusters of the disease suggest a genetic predisposition.[99] The disorder has been reported in association with a variety of diseases known to have an autoimmune basis, including chronic active hepatitis, celiac disease, Raynaud's disease, and SLE,[100-102] and it is possible that

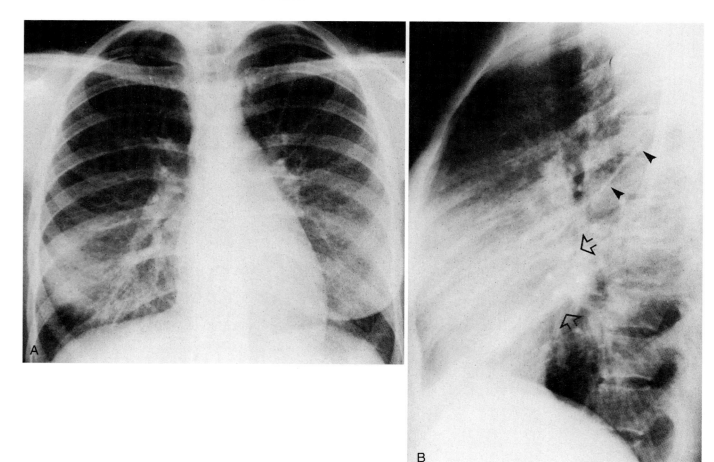

FIGURE 13–15

Postcapillary hypertension—left atrial myxoma. Posteroanterior (**A**) and lateral (**B**) chest radiographs show a perihilar and lower lobe parenchymal haze, ill-defined lower lobe bronchovascular bundles, and thickening of interlobar fissures as a result of pleural edema (*arrowheads*). On the posteroanterior projection, the heart does not appear enlarged; however, on the lateral view, there is a suggestion of left atrial (*open arrows*) and right ventricular enlargement. The findings are consistent with obstruction at or proximal to the mitral valve. (*From Fraser RS, Müller NL, Colman NC, Paré PD: Fraser and Paré's Diagnosis of Diseases of the Chest, 4th ed. Philadelphia, WB Saunders, 1999.*)

an abnormality in immune function is involved in some cases. It appears to be a complication of several drugs, including bleomycin,[103] mitomycin,[104] and oral contraceptives[105]; the mechanism underlying oral contraceptives may be related to pulmonary vascular prostaglandin balance. The abnormality has also been reported after bone marrow transplantation and radiation therapy involving the thorax.[106,107]

Pathologically, the most prominent feature is stenosis or obliteration of the lumina of small pulmonary veins and venules by intimal fibrous tissue, sometimes resembling organized thrombus (Fig. 13–16).[100] Occasionally, an inflammatory infiltrate can be identified in the adjacent wall[108]; however, recent or organizing thrombus is uncommon. Histologic evidence of pulmonary arterial hypertension is usually present, but changes of plexogenic arteriopathy are absent.[109] The lung parenchyma may show evidence of hemorrhage (interstitial and air space hemosiderin-laden macrophages); some degree of interstitial fibrosis and chronic inflammation are also often evident.[110]

Radiographic findings are identical to those associated with PPH, with the important addition of signs of postcapillary

hypertension, chiefly pulmonary edema.[111] HRCT demonstrates smooth thickening of the interlobular septa and interlobar fissures and areas of ground-glass attenuation consistent with interstitial pulmonary edema (Fig. 13–17).[112] Small pleural effusions are present in most patients.[112]

Patients typically have slowly progressive dyspnea and orthopnea punctuated by attacks of acute pulmonary edema; hemoptysis may occur. Crackles can be heard over the lung bases, and the second pulmonic sound is accentuated in most cases. As the condition progresses, a right ventricular heave develops, together with murmurs indicative of pulmonic and tricuspid insufficiency.

Pulmonary function tests reveal arterial oxygen desaturation and a reduction in diffusing capacity and lung compliance.[113] Pulmonary arterial wedge pressure is usually normal or low,[111] a finding best explained by the fact that the wedged pulmonary artery catheter measures the pressure not in the small pulmonary veins (which are narrowed by the obliterative process) but in the large pulmonary veins (which are usually distal to the site of obstruction); the wedge pressure therefore reflects the pressure in the

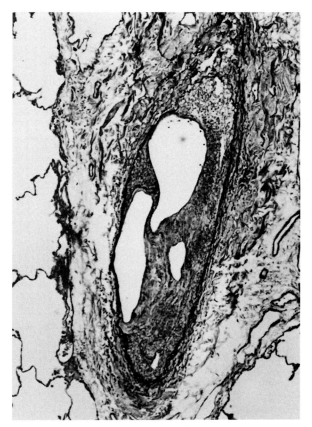

FIGURE 13–16

Veno-occlusive disease. A section of a medium-sized pulmonary vein shows intraluminal fibrosis and multiple variable-sized spaces suggesting recanalized thrombus. *(From Fraser RS, Müller NL, Colman NC, Paré PD: Fraser and Paré's Diagnosis of Diseases of the Chest, 4th ed. Philadelphia, WB Saunders, 1999.)*

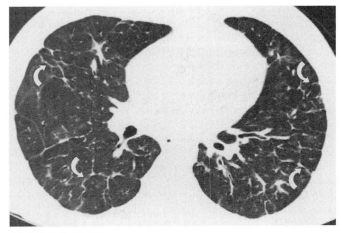

FIGURE 13–17

Primary veno-occlusive disease. An HRCT image shows thickening of the interlobular septa *(arrows)*, localized ground-glass opacities, and areas of decreased attenuation and vascularity. The patient was a 19-year-old man.

large pulmonary veins and left atrium, which is normal, and not the pressure in the pulmonary capillaries, which is elevated.[114]

Most patients die within 2 years of the onset of symptoms.[97]

PULMONARY HYPERTENSION CAUSED BY DISEASES OF THE RESPIRATORY SYSTEM AND/OR HYPOXEMIA

A wide variety of primary diseases of the lungs, pleura, chest wall, and respiratory control center can cause pulmonary hypertension (see Table 13–1); however, pulmonary arterial pressures seldom reach the levels attained in cases of primary vascular disease, and the arterial and arteriolar narrowing as a result of intimal thickening and medial hypertrophy is less.[115] The main cause of hypertension in this group of conditions is hypoxemia, with or without respiratory acidosis.

Chronic Obstructive Pulmonary Disease

Pulmonary hypertension in patients who have COPD is related to a combination of hypoxemia and destruction of the microvasculature.[116] Acute and reversible worsening of pulmonary hypertension can occur during exacerbations of respiratory insufficiency[117] and contribute to exercise impairment independent of the degree of ventilatory impairment.[118] The radiographic manifestations of pulmonary hypertension in emphysema are identical to those of primary vascular disease; however, the invariable presence of overinflation permits ready differentiation (Fig. 13–18).

Diffuse Interstitial or Air Space Disease

In most conditions associated with diffuse interstitial or air space disease, elevation of pulmonary artery pressure is probably related to hypoxemia and the limited distensibility of the pulmonary vascular tree; as a result, hypertension becomes particularly evident during exercise-induced increases in cardiac output. The radiologic changes are dominated by the underlying pulmonary disease, and in many cases, the peripheral vascular markings are obscured. Usually, symptoms are attributable to the underlying parenchymal disease, and the presence of pulmonary hypertension may not be clinically detectable until cor pulmonale and cardiac failure develop.

Alveolar Hypoventilation Syndromes

Underventilation of normal lungs, with consequently decreased arterial blood PO_2 and increased PCO_2, may result in pulmonary hypertension. This syndrome may be primary in origin (Ondine's curse) or related to obesity-hypoventilation syndrome, obstructive sleep apnea, loss of altitude acclimatization, or continuous depression of the respiratory center by drugs.[119,120] In obstructive sleep apnea, hemodynamically significant pulmonary hypertension is more often seen in patients who have more severe daytime hypoxemia, a higher body mass index, and worse lung function.[121]

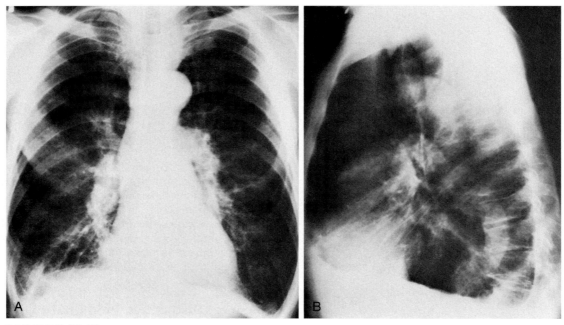

FIGURE 13–18

Pulmonary arterial hypertension secondary to emphysema. Posteroanterior (**A**) and lateral (**B**) radiographs reveal marked overinflation of both lungs, with a low flat position of the diaphragm and an increase in depth of the retrosternal air space. The lungs are diffusely oligemic, the peripheral vessels being narrow and attenuated. A discrepancy in size of the central and peripheral pulmonary vessels is caused not only by a decrease in caliber peripherally but also by an increase in size centrally; the latter constitutes convincing evidence of pulmonary arterial hypertension. *(From Fraser RS, Müller NL, Colman NC, Paré PD: Fraser and Paré's Diagnosis of Diseases of the Chest, 4th ed. Philadelphia, WB Saunders, 1999.)*

Miscellaneous Conditions

Pathologic and physiologic evidence of hypertension can be found several years after pneumonectomy and lung reduction surgery[122]; the complication may result from intimal/medial fibrosis secondary to increased blood flow.[123] Severe degrees of kyphoscoliosis and thoracoplasty may lead to hypertension on the basis of ventilation-perfusion imbalance and hypoventilation. Chronic pleural thickening is rarely associated with pulmonary arterial hypertension.

PULMONARY HYPERTENSION CAUSED BY CHRONIC THROMBOTIC AND/OR EMBOLIC DISEASE

It is inevitable that hypertension will develop if a sufficient portion of the pulmonary arterial system is occluded by thrombus. Such occlusion may be caused by several mechanisms, including (1) multiple recurrent embolic episodes involving small thrombi and occurring over a number of months or years, (2) one or a few embolic episodes involving a large thrombus that occludes a significant proportion of the proximal pulmonary vasculature either directly or by propagation of clot in situ,[124] and (3) in situ thrombosis of small or large pulmonary arteries unassociated with emboli. The last two are the most frequent.[125]

As discussed previously (see page 548), the most common natural history of a pulmonary thromboembolic episode is resolution with restoration of normal pulmonary hemodynamics, gas exchange, and exercise tolerance[126]; occasionally, however, thrombi lodged in proximal arteries fail to undergo significant recanalization or dissolution and thereby cause chronic pulmonary hypertension (Fig. 13–19). This condition, which has been called *chronic thromboembolic pulmonary hypertension* (CTEPH), is important to distinguish from hypertension associated with predominantly peripheral pulmonary vascular disease because surgical removal of the central thrombi is possible with reasonably low surgical mortality.[127] It is unclear why some patients eventually progress to CTEPH rather than recanalize or lyse their thrombi. The abnormality is uncommon; it has been estimated that CTEPH ultimately develops in only about 0.1% to 0.5% of patients who have an acute thromboembolic episode.[127]

Pathologically, cases hypothesized to represent in situ thrombosis of small pulmonary vessels demonstrate foci of eccentric intimal fibrosis and transluminal fibrous bands (colander or cribriform pattern) (Fig. 13–20).[128,129] Thrombus itself is relatively sparse but can often be identified focally. Examination of tissue removed from large pulmonary arteries by endarterectomy shows thrombi in various stages of organization[130]; histologic evidence of recurrent (in situ) thrombosis adjacent to partially organized emboli may be seen. The small pulmonary vessels may also be abnormal in patients who have CTEPH,[124] the most common features being medial hypertrophy and intimal fibrosis (which may be eccentric, concentric, or in a colander pattern consistent with recanalized thrombus).

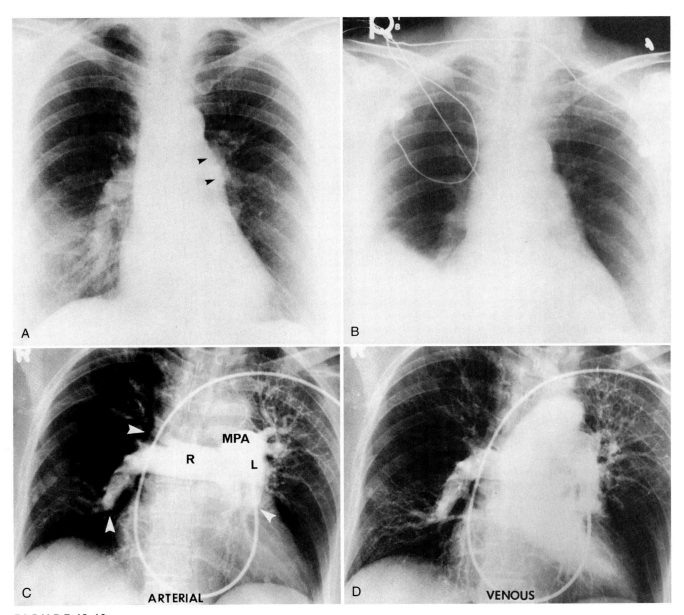

FIGURE 13-19

Precapillary pulmonary hypertension—massive pulmonary thromboembolism. A posteroanterior chest radiograph (**A**) shows moderate enlargement of the main pulmonary artery (*arrowheads*), dilation of the hilar pulmonary arteries, and slight enlargement of the heart. There is a suggestion of oligemia in the right upper lobe. The patient was a middle-aged woman who had experienced vague chest discomfort several days before this examination. Approximately 6 weeks later, after the sudden onset of severe chest pain and circulatory collapse, a chest radiograph (**B**) discloses an increase in size of the heart, diffuse oligemia of the right lung, and elevation of the right hemidiaphragm. These features are consistent with acute cor pulmonale caused by thromboembolism. Four and a half months later, arterial (**C**) and venous (**D**) phases of a pulmonary arteriogram reveal multiple amputated arteries (*arrowheads*) in the lower lobes and right upper lobe. The main pulmonary artery (MPA) and its right (R) and left (L) branches are dilated. During the venous phase, note the oligemia in the right mid and upper lung zones and the left lower lobe. The arterial vasculature is tortuous and sinuous. *(From Fraser RS, Müller NL, Colman NC, Paré PD: Fraser and Paré's Diagnosis of Diseases of the Chest, 4th ed. Philadelphia, WB Saunders, 1999.)*

Characteristic radiographic findings include right ventricular enlargement, prominence of the central pulmonary arteries, rapid tapering of smaller vessels, and areas of decreased vascularity.[131] When either thrombosis or embolism occurs in the major hilar pulmonary arteries, the combination of bulging hilar pulmonary arteries, severe peripheral oligemia, and cor pulmonale constitutes a virtually pathognomonic triad.

A variety of additional procedures can be used for assessment. Ventilation-perfusion scintigraphy is a safe and highly sensitive test to evaluate patients suspected of having the disease (Fig. 13–21).[41,132] The diagnosis can also be suggested

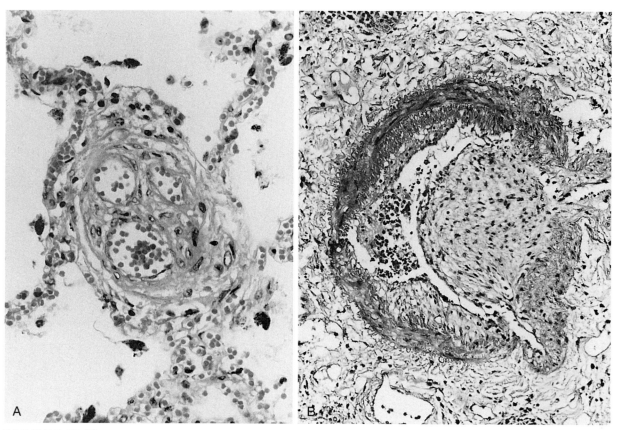

FIGURE 13–20

Pulmonary hypertension: organized thromboemboli. Two lesions consistent with organized thromboemboli are illustrated. In **A,** a small artery is subdivided by fibrous bands into three small channels (colander lesion). In **B,** a somewhat nodular focus of loose fibroblastic tissue is present on one side of the vessel wall (eccentric fibrosis). *(From Fraser RS, Müller NL, Colman NC, Paré PD: Fraser and Paré's Diagnosis of Diseases of the Chest, 4th ed. Philadelphia, WB Saunders, 1999.)*

on the basis of a mosaic perfusion pattern on HRCT (see Fig. 13–8, page 587).[133] Contrast-enhanced spiral CT is the imaging modality of choice for the evaluation of patients who have pulmonary arterial hypertension and suspected chronic thromboembolism based on a combination of radiographic and scintigraphic findings or HRCT (Fig. 13–22).[134,135] Pulmonary angiography is recommended when there is a discrepancy between the CT and clinical findings and when assessing selected patients in whom thromboendarterectomy is being considered.[136] Pulsed Doppler echocardiography permits assessment of right ventricular size and systolic function in patients who have recent or chronic emboli; thromboemboli within the heart or pulmonary artery may also be detected.[137]

The symptoms and signs of pulmonary thromboemboli are described in Chapter 12 (see page 562). Pulmonary function changes include an increase in physiologic dead space and the arterial-alveolar gradient,[138] reduced diffusing capacity[138a] and (sometimes) evidence of lung restriction.[139]

The prognosis is related to the site in which the thrombi occur. In specialized centers, surgical removal of thrombi from large pulmonary arteries can lead to significant clinical improvement; although surgical mortality has been reported to be about 10%, the rate has been decreasing.[127] The prognosis of patients who have histologic features of small-vessel

thrombosis or thromboembolism in the absence of proximal vessel disease is poor; the average survival in one investigation was only about 3 years.[128]

PULMONARY HYPERTENSION CAUSED BY DISORDERS DIRECTLY AFFECTING THE PULMONARY VASCULATURE

Pulmonary Capillary Hemangiomatosis

Pulmonary capillary hemangiomatosis is a rare form of pulmonary hypertension. Although the etiology and pathogenesis are uncertain, the infiltrative nature of the vessels on histologic examination has suggested to some that it may represent a low-grade, locally aggressive neoplasm of the pulmonary endothelial cell.[140] A familial association has been documented in some cases.[141] Pathologically, the most striking feature is a patchy interstitial proliferation of thin-walled blood vessels the size of capillaries.[142] The vessels appear to invade the walls of pulmonary veins and to a lesser extent the pulmonary arteries. The venular infiltration is often accompanied by intimal fibrosis, which may lead to significant stenosis.

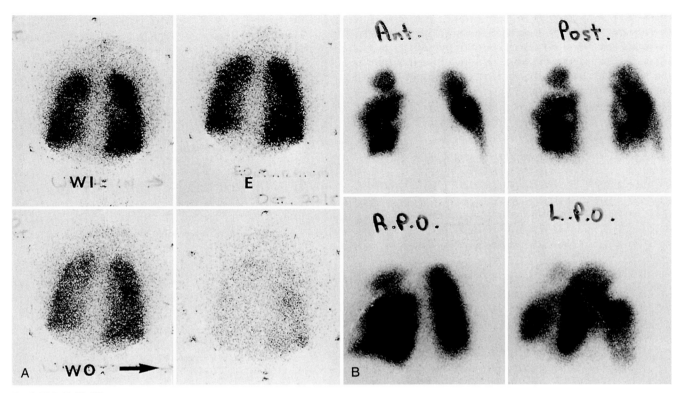

FIGURE 13–21

Pulmonary hypertension—perfusion pattern on scintigraphy in chronic thromboembolism without infarction. Ventilation (**A**) and perfusion (**B**) lung scintigrams reveal features that are considered "high probability" for thromboembolism. WI, E, and WO represent the wash-in, equilibrium, and wash-out phases, respectively, of the ventilation study. The patient was a 64-year-old man. *(From Fraser RS, Müller NL, Colman NC, Paré PD: Fraser and Paré's Diagnosis of Diseases of the Chest, 4th ed. Philadelphia, WB Saunders, 1999.)*

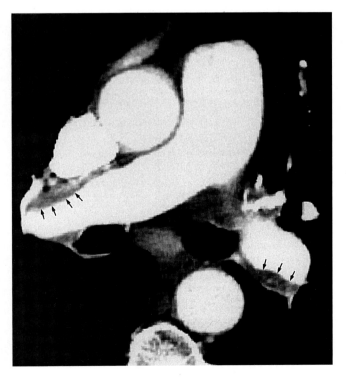

FIGURE 13–22

Chronic thromboembolism. A contrast-enhanced spiral CT scan in a 56-year-old woman demonstrates filling defects adjacent to the wall of the right and left interlobar pulmonary arteries (*arrows*). This eccentric location is characteristic of chronic thromboembolism. *(From Fraser RS, Müller NL, Colman NC, Paré PD: Fraser and Paré's Diagnosis of Diseases of the Chest, 4th ed. Philadelphia, WB Saunders, 1999.)*

The chest radiograph may demonstrate a predominantly reticulonodular or micronodular pattern, or the appearance may be normal except for the evidence of pulmonary hypertension.[140] HRCT demonstrates thickening of the interlobular septa, poorly defined centrilobular nodular opacities, and areas of ground-glass attenuation.[143] Patients are generally young adults and have a clinical picture of pulmonary hypertension; the course is one of slow progression.

REFERENCES

1. Fowler NO, Westcott RN, Scott RC: Normal pressure in the right heart and pulmonary artery. Am Heart J 46:264-267, 1953.
2. Chatterjee K, De Marco T, Alpert JS: Pulmonary hypertension: Hemodynamic diagnosis and management. Arch Intern Med 162:1925-1933, 2002.
3. Culver BH, Butler J: Mechanical influences on the pulmonary microcirculation. Annu Rev Physiol 42:187-198, 1980.
4. Harvey RM, Enson Y, Ferrer MI: A reconsideration of the origins of pulmonary hypertension. Chest 59:82-94, 1971.
5. Rounds S, Hill NS: Pulmonary hypertensive diseases. Chest 85:397, 1984.
6. Harris P, Heath D: The Human Pulmonary Circulation: Its Form and Function in Health and Disease. Baltimore, Williams & Wilkins, 1962.
7. Higenbottam T: Pathophysiology of pulmonary hypertension. A role for endothelial dysfunction. Chest 105:7S-12S, 1994.
8. Pietra G: The pathology of primary pulmonary hypertension. In Rubin L, Rich S (eds): Primary Pulmonary Hypertension. New York, Marcel Dekker, 1997.
9. Moore GW, Smith RR, Hutchins GM: Pulmonary artery atherosclerosis: Correlation with systemic atherosclerosis and hypertensive pulmonary vascular disease. Arch Pathol Lab Med 106:378-380, 1982.
10. Hall SM, Haworth SG: Onset and evolution of pulmonary vascular disease in young children: Abnormal postnatal remodelling studied in lung biopsies. J Pathol 166:183-193, 1992.
11. Heath D, Williams D, Rios-Dalenz J, et al: Small pulmonary arterial vessels of Aymara Indians from the Bolivian Andes. Histopathology 16:565-571, 1990.
12. Wagenvoort CA: Plexogenic arteriopathy. Thorax 49(Suppl):S39-S45, 1994.
13. Jones PL, Cowan KN, Rabinovitch M: Tenascin-C, proliferation and subendothelial fibronectin in progressive pulmonary vascular disease. Am J Pathol 150:1349-1360, 1997.
14. Yaginuma G, Mohri H, Takahashi T: Distribution of arterial lesions and collateral pathways in the pulmonary hypertension of congenital heart disease: A computer aided reconstruction study. Thorax 45:586-590, 1990.
15. Lee SD, Shroyer KR, Markham NE, et al: Monoclonal endothelial cell proliferation is present in primary but not secondary pulmonary hypertension. J Clin Invest 101:927-934, 1998.
16. Randall PA, Heitzman ER, Bull MJ, et al: Pulmonary arterial hypertension: A contemporary review. Radiographics 9:905-927, 1989.
17. Chang CH: The normal roentgenographic measurement of the right descending pulmonary artery in 1,085 cases. Am J Roentgenol Radium Ther Nucl Med 87:929-935, 1962.
18. Kuriyama K, Gamsu G, Stern RG, et al: CT-determined pulmonary artery diameters in predicting pulmonary hypertension. Invest Radiol 19:16-22, 1984.
19. Tan RT, Kuzo R, Goodman LR, et al: Utility of CT scan evaluation for predicting pulmonary hypertension in patients with parenchymal lung disease. Medical College of Wisconsin Lung Transplant Group. Chest 113:1250-1256, 1998.
20. Burghuber OC, Brunner CH, Schenk P, et al: Pulsed Doppler echocardiography to assess pulmonary artery hypertension in chronic obstructive pulmonary disease. Monaldi Arch Chest Dis 48:121-125, 1993.
21. Bach DS: Stress echocardiography for evaluation of hemodynamics: Valvular heart disease, prosthetic valve function, and pulmonary hypertension. Prog Cardiovasc Dis 39:543-554, 1997.
22. Chen WJ, Chen JJ, Lin SC, et al: Detection of cardiovascular shunts by transesophageal echocardiography in patients with pulmonary hypertension of unexplained cause. Chest 107:8-13, 1995.
23. Tardivon AA, Mousseaux E, Brenot F, et al: Quantification of hemodynamics in primary pulmonary hypertension with magnetic resonance imaging. Am J Respir Crit Care Med 150:1075-1080, 1994.
24. Boxt LM, Katz J: Magnetic resonance imaging for quantitation of right ventricular volume in patients with pulmonary hypertension. J Thorac Imaging 8:92-97, 1993.
25. Frank H, Globits S, Glogar D, et al: Detection and quantification of pulmonary artery hypertension with MR imaging: Results in 23 patients. AJR Am J Roentgenol 161:27-31, 1993.
26. Bergin CJ, Sirlin CB, Hauschildt JP, et al: Chronic thromboembolism: Diagnosis with helical CT and MR imaging with angiographic and surgical correlation. Radiology 204:695-702, 1997.
27. Stevens PM, Terplan M, Knowles JH: Prognosis of cor pulmonale. N Engl J Med 269:1289-1291, 1963.
28. Chronic cor pulmonale: Report of an expert committee (Reprinted from World Health Organization Technical Report Series No. 213). Circulation 27:594, 1963.
29. Sepulveda G, Rios E, Leon J, et al: Clinico-pathologic correlation in chronic cor pulmonale. Dis Chest 52:205-212, 1967.
30. Jardin F, Dubourg O, Bourdarias JP: Echocardiographic pattern of acute cor pulmonale. Chest 111:209-217, 1997.
31. Rich S, Dantzker DR, Ayres SM, et al: Primary pulmonary hypertension. A national prospective study. Ann Intern Med 107:216-223, 1987.
32. D'Alonzo G, Dantzker D: Diagnosing primary pulmonary hypertension. In Rubin L, Rich S (eds): Primary Pulmonary Hypertension, vol 99. In Lenfant C (executive ed): Lung Biology and Disease. New York, Marcel Dekker, 1997.
33. Thomson JR, Machado RD, Pauciulo MW, et al: Sporadic primary pulmonary hypertension is associated with germline mutations of the gene encoding BMPR-II, a receptor member of the TGF-beta family. J Med Genet 37:741-745, 2000.
34. Morse JH, Jones AC, Barst RJ, et al: Familial primary pulmonary hypertension locus mapped to chromosome 2q31-q32. Chest 114:57S-58S, 1998.
35. Humbert M, Deng Z, Simonneau G, et al: BMPR2 germline mutations in pulmonary hypertension associated with fenfluramine derivatives. Eur Respir J 20:518-523, 2002.
36. Machado RD, Pauciulo MW, Thomson JR, et al: BMPR2 haploinsufficiency as the inherited molecular mechanism for primary pulmonary hypertension. Am J Hum Genet 68:92-102, 2001.
37. Perez HD, Kramer N: Pulmonary hypertension in systemic lupus erythematosus: Report of four cases and review of the literature. Semin Arthritis Rheum 11:177-181, 1981.
38. Salerni R, Rodnan GP, Leon DF, et al: Pulmonary hypertension in the CREST syndrome variant of progressive systemic sclerosis (scleroderma). Ann Intern Med 86:394-399, 1977.
39. Chaouat A, Weitzenblum E, Higenbottam T: The role of thrombosis in severe pulmonary hypertension. Eur Respir J 9:356-363, 1996.
40. Chazova I, Loyd JE, Zhdanov VS, et al: Pulmonary artery adventitial changes and venous involvement in primary pulmonary hypertension. Am J Pathol 146:389-397, 1995.
41. Worsley DF, Palevsky HI, Alavi A: Ventilation-perfusion lung scanning in the evaluation of pulmonary hypertension. J Nucl Med 35:793-796, 1994.
42. Selby C: Living with primary pulmonary hypertension. In Rubin L, Rich S (eds): Primary Pulmonary Hypertension, vol 99. In Lenfant C (executive ed): Lung Biology in Health and Disease. New York, Marcel Dekker, 1997, pp 319-325.
43. Walcott G, Burchell HB, Brown AL Jr: Primary pulmonary hypertension. Am J Med 49:70-79, 1970.
44. Sleeper JC, Orgain ES, Mc IH: Primary pulmonary hypertension. Review of clinical features and pathologic physiology with a report of pulmonary hemodynamics derived from repeated catheterization. Circulation 26:1358-1369, 1962.
45. Romano AM, Tomaselli S, Gualtieri G, et al: Respiratory function in precapillary pulmonary hypertension. Monaldi Arch Chest Dis 48:201-204, 1993.
46. Dantzker DR, D'Alonzo GE, Bower JS, et al: Pulmonary gas exchange during exercise in patients with chronic obliterative pulmonary hypertension. Am Rev Respir Dis 130:412-416, 1984.
47. Hughes JD, Rubin LJ: Primary pulmonary hypertension. An analysis of 28 cases and a review of the literature. Medicine (Baltimore) 65:56-72, 1986.
48. Rajasekhar D, Balakrishnan KG, Venkitachalam CG, et al: Primary pulmonary hypertension: Natural history and prognostic factors. Indian Heart J 46:165-170, 1994.
49. Sandoval J, Bauerle O, Palomar A, et al: Survival in primary pulmonary hypertension. Validation of a prognostic equation. Circulation 89:1733-1744, 1994.
50. Rich S, Levy PS: Characteristics of surviving and nonsurviving patients with primary pulmonary hypertension. Am J Med 76:573-578, 1984.
51. Hoeper MM: Pulmonary hypertension in collagen vascular disease. Eur Respir J 19:571-576, 2002.
52. Nakchbandi IA, Wirth JA, Inzucchi SE: Pulmonary hypertension caused by Graves' thyrotoxicosis: Normal pulmonary hemodynamics restored by 131I treatment. Chest 116:1483-1485, 1999.
53. Amin M, Fawzy A, Hamid MA, et al: Pulmonary hypertension in patients with chronic renal failure: Role of parathyroid hormone and pulmonary artery calcifications. Chest 124:2093-2097, 2003.
54. Cachecho R, Isik FF, Hirsch EF: Pathologic consequences of bilateral pulmonary lower lobectomies: Case report. J Trauma 32:268-270, 1992.
55. Hopkins WE: Severe pulmonary hypertension in congenital heart disease: A review of Eisenmenger syndrome. Curr Opin Cardiol 10:517-523, 1995.
56. Granton JT, Rabinovitch M: Pulmonary arterial hypertension in congenital heart disease. Cardiol Clin 20:441-457, 2002.
57. Rebergen SA, Niezen RA, Helbing WA, et al: Cine gradient-echo MR imaging and MR velocity mapping in the evaluation of congenital heart disease. Radiographics 16:467-481, 1996.
58. Hopkins WE, Ochoa LL, Richardson GW, et al: Comparison of the hemodynamics and survival of adults with severe primary pulmonary hypertension or Eisenmenger syndrome. J Heart Lung Transplant 15:100-105, 1996.
59. Yoshida EM, Erb SR, Ostrow DN, et al: Pulmonary hypertension associated with primary biliary cirrhosis in the absence of portal hypertension: A case report. Gut 35:280-282, 1994.
60. Budhiraja R, Hassoun PM: Portopulmonary hypertension: A tale of two circulations. Chest 123:562-576, 2003.
61. McDonnell PJ, Toye PA, Hutchins GM: Primary pulmonary hypertension and cirrhosis: Are they related? Am Rev Respir Dis 127:437-441, 1983.
62. Kuo P: Pulmonary hypertension: Considerations in the liver transplant candidate. Transpl Int 9:141-150, 1996.

63. Levy MT, Torzillo P, Bookallil M, et al: Case report: Delayed resolution of severe pulmonary hypertension after isolated liver transplantation in a patient with cirrhosis. J Gastroenterol Hepatol 11:734-737, 1996.
64. Kibria G, Smith P, Heath D, et al: Observations on the rare association between portal and pulmonary hypertension. Thorax 35:945-949, 1980.
65. King PD, Rumbaut R, Sanchez C: Pulmonary manifestations of chronic liver disease. Dig Dis 14:73-82, 1996.
66. Chan T, Palevsky HI, Miller WT: Pulmonary hypertension complicating portal hypertension: Findings on chest radiographs. AJR Am J Roentgenol 151:909-914, 1988.
67. Mesa RA, Edell ES, Dunn WF, et al: Human immunodeficiency virus infection and pulmonary hypertension: Two new cases and a review of 86 reported cases. Mayo Clin Proc 73:37-45, 1998.
68. Burkart KM, Farber HW: HIV-associated pulmonary hypertension: Diagnosis and treatment. Adv Cardiol 40:197-207, 2003.
69. Mette SA, Palevsky HI, Pietra GG, et al: Primary pulmonary hypertension in association with human immunodeficiency virus infection. A possible viral etiology for some forms of hypertensive pulmonary arteriopathy. Am Rev Respir Dis 145:1196-1200, 1992.
70. Cool CD, Kennedy D, Voelkel NF, et al: Pathogenesis and evolution of plexiform lesions in pulmonary hypertension associated with scleroderma and human immunodeficiency virus infection. Hum Pathol 28:434-442, 1997.
71. Heron E, Laaban JP, Capron F, et al: Thrombotic primary pulmonary hypertension in an HIV+ patient. Eur Heart J 15:394-396, 1994.
72. Escamilla R, Hermant C, Berjaud J, et al: Pulmonary veno-occlusive disease in a HIV-infected intravenous drug abuser. Eur Respir J 8:1982-1984, 1995.
73. Petitpretz P, Brenot F, Azarian R, et al: Pulmonary hypertension in patients with human immunodeficiency virus infection. Comparison with primary pulmonary hypertension. Circulation 89:2722-2727, 1994.
74. Kilbourne EM, Posada de la Paz M, Abaitua Borda I, et al: Toxic oil syndrome: A current clinical and epidemiologic summary, including comparisons with the eosinophilia-myalgia syndrome. J Am Coll Cardiol 18:711-717, 1991.
75. Yakovlevitch M, Siegel M, Hoch DH, et al: Pulmonary hypertension in a patient with tryptophan-induced eosinophilia-myalgia syndrome. Am J Med 90:272-273, 1991.
76. Albertson TE, Walby WF, Derlet RW: Stimulant-induced pulmonary toxicity. Chest 108:1140-1149, 1995.
77. Schaiberger PH, Kennedy TC, Miller FC, et al: Pulmonary hypertension associated with long-term inhalation of "crank" methamphetamine. Chest 104:614-616, 1993.
78. Fahlen M, Bergman H, Helder G, et al: Phenformin and pulmonary hypertension. Br Heart J 35:824-828, 1973.
79. Follath F, Burkart F, Schweizer W: Drug-induced pulmonary hypertension? BMJ 1:265-266, 1971.
80. Thomas SH, Butt AY, Corris PA, et al: Appetite suppressants and primary pulmonary hypertension in the United Kingdom. Br Heart J 74:660-663, 1995.
81. Abenhaim L, Moride Y, Brenot F, et al: Appetite-suppressant drugs and the risk of primary pulmonary hypertension. International Primary Pulmonary Hypertension Study Group. N Engl J Med 335:609-616, 1996.
82. Rothman RB, Ayestas MA, Dersch CM, et al: Aminorex, fenfluramine, and chlorphentermine are serotonin transporter substrates. Implications for primary pulmonary hypertension. Circulation 100:869-875, 1999.
83. Geggel RL, Reid LM: The structural basis of PPHN. Clin Perinatol 11:525-549, 1984.
84. Steinhorn RH, Millard SL, Morin FC 3rd: Persistent pulmonary hypertension of the newborn. Role of nitric oxide and endothelin in pathophysiology and treatment. Clin Perinatol 22:405-428, 1995.
85. Levin DL, Weinberg AG, Perkin RM: Pulmonary microthrombi syndrome in newborn infants with unresponsive persistent pulmonary hypertension. J Pediatr 102:299-303, 1983.
86. Cody RJ: The potential role of endothelin as a vasoconstrictor substance in congestive heart failure. Eur Heart J 13:1573-1578, 1992.
87. Wagenvoort C: Pathology of congested pulmonary hypertension. Prog Respir Res 9:195, 1975.
88. Wagenvoort CA: Morphologic changes in intrapulmonary veins. Hum Pathol 1:205-213, 1970.
89. Simon M: The pulmonary veins in mitral stenosis. J Fac Radiol 9:25, 1958.
90. Ravin CE: Pulmonary vascularity: Radiographic considerations. J Thorac Imaging 3:1-13, 1988.
91. West JB, Dollery CT, Heard BE: Increased pulmonary vascular resistance in the dependent zone of the isolated dog lung caused by perivascular edema. Circ Res 17:191-206, 1965.
92. Hughes JM, Glazier JB, Maloney JE, et al: Effect of interstitial pressure on pulmonary blood-flow. Lancet 1:192-193, 1967.
93. McHugh TJ, Forrester JS, Adler L, et al: Pulmonary vascular congestion in acute myocardial infarction: Hemodynamic and radiologic correlations. Ann Intern Med 76:29-33, 1972.
94. Rhodes KM, Evemy K, Nariman S, et al: Effects of mitral valve surgery on static lung function and exercise performance. Thorax 40:107-112, 1985.
95. Palmer WH, Gee JB, Bates DV: Disturbances of pulmonary function in mitral valve disease. Can Med Assoc J 89:744-750, 1963.
96. Mandel J, Mark EJ, Hales CA: Pulmonary veno-occlusive disease. Am J Respir Crit Care Med 162:1964-1973, 2000.
97. Shackelford GD, Sacks EJ, Mullins JD, et al: Pulmonary venoocclusive disease: Case report and review of the literature. AJR Am J Roentgenol 128:643-648, 1977.
98. Wagenvoort CA, Wagenvoort N, Takahashi T: Pulmonary veno-occlusive disease: Involvement of pulmonary arteries and review of the literature. Hum Pathol 16:1033-1041, 1985.
99. Voordes CG, Kuipers JR, Elema JD: Familial pulmonary veno-occlusive disease: A case report. Thorax 32:763-736, 1977.
100. Hasleton PS, Ironside JW, Whittaker JS, et al: Pulmonary veno-occlusive disease. A report of four cases. Histopathology 10:933-944, 1986.
101. Leinonen H, Pohjola-Sintonen S, Krogerus L: Pulmonary veno-occlusive disease. Acta Med Scand 221:307-310, 1987.
102. Kishida Y, Kanai Y, Kuramochi S, et al: Pulmonary venoocclusive disease in a patient with systemic lupus erythematosus. J Rheumatol 20:2161-2162, 1993.
103. Lombard CM, Churg A, Winokur S: Pulmonary veno-occlusive disease following therapy for malignant neoplasms. Chest 92:871-876, 1987.
104. Waldhorn RE, Tsou E, Smith FP, et al: Pulmonary veno-occlusive disease associated with microangiopathic hemolytic anemia and chemotherapy of gastric adenocarcinoma. Med Pediatr Oncol 12:394-396, 1984.
105. Townend JN, Roberts DH, Jones EL, et al: Fatal pulmonary venoocclusive disease after use of oral contraceptives. Am Heart J 124:1643-1644, 1992.
106. Williams LM, Fussell S, Veith RW, et al: Pulmonary veno-occlusive disease in an adult following bone marrow transplantation. Case report and review of the literature. Chest 109:1388-1391, 1996.
107. Kramer MR, Estenne M, Berkman N, et al: Radiation-induced pulmonary veno-occlusive disease. Chest 104:1282-1284, 1993.
108. McDonnell PJ, Summer WR, Hutchins GM: Pulmonary veno-occlusive disease. Morphological changes suggesting a viral cause. JAMA 246:667-671, 1981.
109. Case records of the Massachusetts General Hospital. Weekly clinicopathological exercises. Case 14-1983. A 67-year-old woman with pulmonary hypertension. N Engl J Med 308:823-834, 1983.
110. Wagenvoort CA, Wagenvoort N: The pathology of pulmonary veno-occlusive disease. Virchows Arch A Pathol Anat Histol 364:69-79, 1974.
111. Rambihar VS, Fallen EL, Cairns JA: Pulmonary veno-occlusive disease: Antemortem diagnosis from roentgenographic and hemodynamic findings. Can Med Assoc J 120:1519-1522, 1979.
112. Swensen SJ, Tashjian JH, Myers JL, et al: Pulmonary venoocclusive disease: CT findings in eight patients. AJR Am J Roentgenol 167:937-940, 1996.
113. Stovin PGI, Mitchinson MJ: Pulmonary hypertension due to obstruction of intrapulmonary veins. Thorax 20:106, 1965.
114. Wiedemann HP: Wedge pressure in pulmonary veno-occlusive disease. N Engl J Med 315:1233, 1986.
115. Wright JL, Petty T, Thurlbeck WM: Analysis of the structure of the muscular pulmonary arteries in patients with pulmonary hypertension and COPD: National Institutes of Health nocturnal oxygen therapy trial. Lung 170:109-124, 1992.
116. MacNee W: Pathophysiology of cor pulmonale in chronic obstructive pulmonary disease. Part One. Am J Respir Crit Care Med 150:833-852, 1994.
117. Weitzenblum E: The pulmonary circulation and the heart in chronic lung disease. Monaldi Arch Chest Dis 49:231-234, 1994.
118. Fujii T, Kurihara N, Fujimoto S, et al: Role of pulmonary vascular disorder in determining exercise capacity in patients with severe chronic obstructive pulmonary disease. Clin Physiol 16:521-533, 1996.
119. Penaloza D, Sime F: Chronic cor pulmonale due to loss of altitude acclimatization (chronic mountain sickness). Am J Med 50:728-743, 1971.
120. Marks CE Jr, Goldring RM: Chronic hypercapnia during methadone maintenance. Am Rev Respir Dis 108:1088-1093, 1973.
121. Sajkov D, Cowie RJ, Thornton AT, et al: Pulmonary hypertension and hypoxemia in obstructive sleep apnea syndrome. Am J Respir Crit Care Med 149:416-422, 1994.
122. Weg IL, Rossoff L, McKeon LM, et al: Development of pulmonary hypertension after lung volume reduction surgery. Am J Respir Crit Care Med 159:552–556, 1999.
123. Fry WA, Archer FA, Adams WE: Long-term clinical-pathologic study of the pneumonectomy patient. Dis Chest 52:720-726, 1967.
124. Moser KM, Bloor CM: Pulmonary vascular lesions occurring in patients with chronic major vessel thromboembolic pulmonary hypertension. Chest 103:685-692, 1993.
125. Rich S, Levitsky S, Brundage BH: Pulmonary hypertension from chronic pulmonary thromboembolism. Ann Intern Med 108:425-434, 1988.
126. Benotti JR, Dalen JE: The natural history of pulmonary embolism. Clin Chest Med 5:403-410, 1984.
127. Fedullo PF, Auger WR, Channick RN, et al: Chronic thromboembolic pulmonary hypertension. Clin Chest Med 16:353-374, 1995.
128. Palevsky HI, Schloo BL, Pietra GG, et al: Primary pulmonary hypertension. Vascular structure, morphometry, and responsiveness to vasodilator agents. Circulation 80:1207-1221, 1989.
129. Pietra GG, Ruttner JR: Specificity of pulmonary vascular lesions in primary pulmonary hypertension. A reappraisal. Respiration 52:81-85, 1987.
130. Presti B, Berthrong M, Sherwin RM: Chronic thrombosis of major pulmonary arteries. Hum Pathol 21:601-606, 1990.
131. Chitwood WR Jr, Sabiston DC Jr, Wechsler AS: Surgical treatment of chronic unresolved pulmonary embolism. Clin Chest Med 5:507-536, 1984.
132. Powe JE, Palevsky HI, McCarthy KE: Pulmonary arterial hypertension: Value of perfusion scintigraphy. Radiology 164:727, 1987.
133. Bergin CJ, Rios G, King MA, et al: Accuracy of high-resolution CT in identifying chronic pulmonary thromboembolic disease. AJR Am J Roentgenol 166:1371-1377, 1996.
134. Remy-Jardin M, Louvegny S, Remy J, et al: Acute central thromboembolic disease: Posttherapeutic follow-up with spiral CT angiography. Radiology 203:173-180, 1997.

135. Bergin CJ, Sirlin C, Deutsch R, et al: Predictors of patient response to pulmonary thromboendarterectomy. AJR Am J Roentgenol 174:509-515, 2000.

136. Oikonomou A, Dennie CJ, Müller NL, et al: Chronic thromboembolic pulmonary arterial hypertension: Correlation of postoperative results of thromboendarterectomy with preoperative helical contrast-enhanced computed tomography. J Thorac Imaging 19:67-73, 2004.

137. Come PC: Echocardiographic evaluation of pulmonary embolism and its response to therapeutic interventions. Chest 101:151S-162S, 1992.

138. Nadel JA, Gold WM, Burgess JH: Early diagnosis of chronic pulmonary vascular obstruction. Value of pulmonary function tests. Am J Med 44:16-25, 1968.

138a. Bernstein RJ, Ford RL, Clausen JL, et al: Membrane diffusion and capillary blood volume in chronic thromboembolic pulmonary hypertension. Chest 110:1430-1436, 1996.

139. Morris TA, Auger WR, Ysrael MZ, et al: Parenchymal scarring is associated with restrictive spirometric defects in patients with chronic thromboembolic pulmonary hypertension. Chest 110:399-403, 1996.

140. Eltorky MA, Headley AS, Winer-Muram H, et al: Pulmonary capillary hemangiomatosis: A clinicopathologic review. Ann Thorac Surg 57:772-726, 1994.

141. Langleben D, Heneghan JM, Batten AP, et al: Familial pulmonary capillary hemangiomatosis resulting in primary pulmonary hypertension. Ann Intern Med 109:106-109, 1988.

142. Faber CN, Yousem SA, Dauber JH, et al: Pulmonary capillary hemangiomatosis. A report of three cases and a review of the literature. Am Rev Respir Dis 140:808-813, 1989.

143. Hansell DM: Small-vessel diseases of the lung: CT-pathologic correlates. Radiology 225:639-653, 2002.

PULMONARY EDEMA

GENERAL PATHOGENETIC FEATURES

Although the absolute amount of fluid within the pulmonary interstitium and alveolar air spaces is more or less constant, there is considerable transport of water between different tissue compartments within the lung. Normally, an ultrafiltrate of plasma moves from the pulmonary microvessels through the endothelium into the interstitial tissue. Fluid is removed from this space by the pulmonary lymphatics, evaporative water loss from the alveolar surface, resorption into the pulmonary and bronchial microvasculature, and transport into the pleural space. The volume of water and protein movement is dependent on the balance of pressure across the pulmonary microvasculature (determined by the relationship between microvascular and perimicrovascular hydrostatic pressure and between plasma and perimicrovascular osmotic pressure) and on the permeability of the microvascular membrane. A disturbance of sufficient magnitude in one or both of these factors will result in an increase in the transudation or exudation of fluid from the microvessels into interstitial tissue. Sufficient accumulation of fluid in this compartment constitutes interstitial edema; when the storage capacity of the interstitial space is exceeded, edema develops in the alveolar air spaces.[1,2]

Anatomic Considerations

The large surface area available for gas exchange (approximately 70 m^2 in the average adult[3]) is also potentially available for fluid exchange. Although most of this exchange occurs in relation to pulmonary capillaries, precapillary and postcapillary vessels also take part; as a result, the most appropriate term for the process is *microvascular fluid exchange*.[4]

The microvasculature can be considered to comprise two functional compartments based on the response to an increase in alveolar pressure: (1) *alveolar vessels*, which are affected directly by an increase in pressure that compresses them and narrows their lumen, and (2) *extra-alveolar vessels*, which are affected indirectly in that they expand during pulmonary distention as a result of the development of a more negative interstitial pressure.

As discussed elsewhere (see page 10), the alveolar septa have thin and thick sides, the former for gas exchange and the latter for structural support and fluid exchange.[5] On the thin side, the membrane measures about 0.5 μm in thickness and consists of type I epithelial and endothelial cells that have a common basement membrane without intervening interstitial tissue. On the thick side, the basement membranes of the endothelium and epithelium are separated by an interstitial compartment consisting of collagen and elastic fibers, interstitial cells, and connective tissue matrix. When excess water and protein accumulate in the septa, as in interstitial pulmonary edema, they do so exclusively or predominantly on the thick side (Fig. 14–1).[6]

The exact pathway for fluid and solute transport across the pulmonary microvasculature is uncertain. It is reasonable to assume that lipid-soluble substances can traverse the capillary endothelium by passing directly through cell membranes. However, water-soluble substances must be transported by pinocytosis or pass through the "paracellular pathway" (intercellular "pores"). Selective sieving of protein molecules according to their molecular size suggests that the latter mechanism is the more important. Small molecules traverse the pulmonary capillary endothelium with ease, whereas larger molecules are excluded in direct proportion to their molecular size; in fact, very large molecules do not reach the pulmonary interstitium at all in normal circumstances.

The anatomic counterpart of the physiologic "pores" is uncertain but may be discontinuities in the tight junctions that join the endothelial cells.[7] It has been hypothesized that

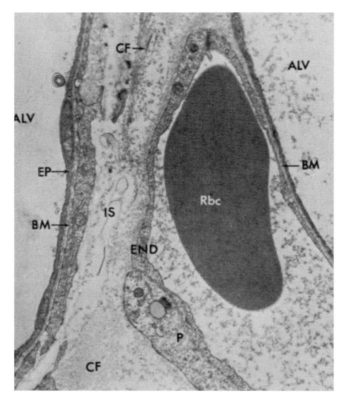

FIGURE 14–1

Interstitial pulmonary edema. The interstitial space of the thick portion of the alveolar septum has been considerably widened by edema fluid during hydrostatic pulmonary edema, whereas the opposite thin part, which contains the fused basement membranes (BM), remains unchanged in thickness. ALV, alveolar space; CF, collagen fibers; END, capillary endothelium; EP, alveolar epithelium; IS, interstitial space; Rbc, red blood cell. Transmission electron microscope (TEM) section stained with uranil acetate and lead citrate (×12,000). *(Reprinted from Fishman A: Circulation 46:389, 1972. With permission of the author and The American Heart Association, Inc.)*

an increase in pulmonary microvascular pressure increases the size of these discontinuities, which in turn increases protein permeability (the stretched-pore theory). Support for this theory is provided by the results of experimental studies that have shown a correlation between the number of junctional strands and the permeability of a cellular membrane.[8] Although it is probable that endothelial permeability is not directly affected by moderately elevated microvascular pressure,[9] when it exceeds a critical value of about 30 cm H_2O, stress failure leads to the development of edema.[10] It should be appreciated that the "pores" through which this fluid movement occurs represent a minute fraction of the total capillary surface area[11]; as a result, doubling or tripling of the surface area occupied by pores might not be detected by conventional microscopic techniques, whereas it would markedly enhance fluid and solute transport.

Although the surface area of the epithelial side of the alveolocapillary membrane is approximately equal to that of the capillary endothelial surface, it is much less permeable. This is reflected in physiologic tracer studies in which it has been

shown that the epithelium is restrictive to all but small molecules such as urea, sucrose, and sodium.[12] In fact, the "pore" size of the epithelium has been calculated to average 3 to 4 nm,[12] whereas "pores" as large as 100 nm are postulated to be present in the capillary endothelium.[13] As a result, excess fluid that leaks from the alveolar capillaries accumulates first in the interstitium instead of flowing into the adjacent air space.

The interstitial connective tissue is a gel that contains fibers and cells. The gel itself is composed of a matrix of highly polymerized mucopolysaccharides that, in combination with proteins, form proteoglycans (glycosaminoglycans). In the lung, the principal mucopolysaccharides are chondroitin sulfate and hyaluronic acid. The proteoglycan complexes are extremely hydrophilic and can bind large amounts of water; 40% of the extravascular water is in the interstitial space. During the development of pulmonary edema, this volume can more than double before alveolar flooding occurs. The fluid storage capacity of the interstitial space increases with lung volume.[14] In fact, when positive end-expiratory pressure (PEEP) is used to increase lung volume, fluid can shift from the alveolar air space to the interstitial space, where it has a less detrimental effect on gas exchange.[15]

The pulmonary interstitium itself can be divided into two compartments—an alveolar septal (parenchymal) compartment and a peribronchovascular and interlobular septal (axial) compartment. Although the former constitutes a large percentage of the total interstitial space, its relatively low compliance means that fluid tends to accumulate to a much lesser extent within it than in the peribronchovascular and interlobular septal connective tissue (see Color Fig. 14–1).[16] Fluid within the interlobular septa can be appreciated in lung slices as a somewhat gelatinous-appearing thickening of the connective tissue between secondary lobules (see Color Fig. 14–2).

Pulmonary lymphatic drainage is one of the important mechanisms by which interstitial fluid is removed from the lung. As discussed previously (see page 63), the lymphatics begin as blind-ended vessels in the region of the alveolar ducts and respiratory bronchioles and course in the interstitial connective tissue of the bronchovascular bundles and interlobular septa (see Color Fig. 14–1). Fluid that enters the lymphatics is pumped toward the hila by the passive action of respiratory motion and by active contraction of the lymphatic vessels, which in large lymphatics can generate pressures as high as 60 cm H_2O.

Physiologic Considerations

The Starling Equation

The factors that govern the formation and removal of extravascular water within the lungs are described by the fluid transport equation originally proposed by Starling (Fig. 14–2):[17]

$$f = Kf[(Pmv - Ppmv) - \sigma(\pi mv - \pi pmv)]$$

where f = net transvascular fluid flow; Kf = the filtration coefficient, a measure of fluid conductance of the microvascular endothelium; Pmv = hydrostatic pressure in the lumen of the fluid-exchanging microvessels; Ppmv = hydrostatic pressure in

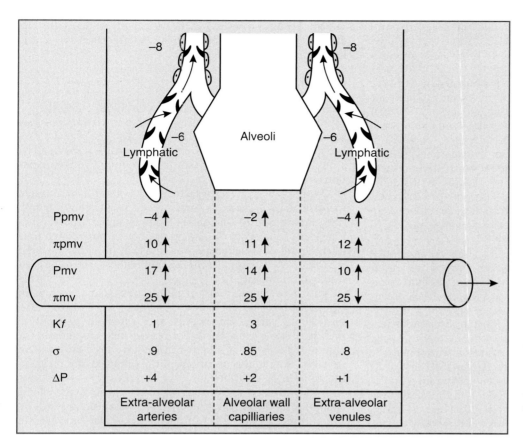

FIGURE 14–2

A three-compartment model of Starling's forces. The values for microvascular and perimicrovascular hydrostatic and osmotic pressure represent rough estimates and have been chosen to illustrate the longitudinal variation in net driving pressure (ΔP) within the exchanging vessels. The arbitrary values for Kf illustrate the relative importance of the different compartments to overall lung fluid exchange, and the values for the reflection coefficient (σ) are indicative of the morphometric complexity of endothelial intercellular junctions on the arterial and venous side of the microcirculation. A value of 1.0 for σ would represent a membrane that was freely permeable to water but completely impermeable to protein. The driving pressure is greatest in the precapillary vessels and least in the postcapillary venules. There is a gradient in interstitial pressure that drives fluid from the pericapillary interstitial space toward the hilum. *(Modified from Staub NC: Pathophysiology of pulmonary edema. In Staub NC, Taylor AE [eds]: Edema. New York, Raven Press, 1984, p. 719.)*

the interstitial tissue surrounding the fluid-exchanging microvessels; σ = the osmotic reflection coefficient (i.e., a number between 0 and 1 that describes the effectiveness of the membrane in preventing the flow of protein versus the flow of water); πmv = protein osmotic pressure in the microvascular lumen; and πpmv = protein osmotic pressure in the interstitial fluid surrounding the microvessels.

Movement of protein across the endothelium occurs by diffusion and is related to the concentration difference between the capillary lumen and the interstitial space and to the size of the protein molecules relative to the size of the endothelial "pores." Since the permeability is different for protein molecules of different size, their net flux is inversely related to molecular weight. When pulmonary microvascular permeability and pressure are normal, the ratios of interstitial to plasma protein concentrations for albumin, globulin, and fibrinogen are approximately 0.8, 0.5, and 0.2, respectively.[18]

Under normal steady-state conditions, there is continual flow of fluid and protein from the pulmonary microvasculature to the interstitium; these substances are then returned to the bloodstream by the lymphatics. When this balance is disrupted, edema results. Although an increase in capillary hydrostatic pressure (Pmv) or an increase in endothelial permeability (Kf) is the most common cause of such imbalance, each of the factors in the Starling equation can have an effect. **Microvascular Hydrostatic Pressure (Pmv).** The hydrostatic pressure in the fluid-exchanging vessels of the lung must be somewhere between the mean pulmonary arterial pressure (about 20 cm H_2O) and the mean left atrial pressure (about 5 cm H_2O). The actual value is dependent on the relative

resistance of the vessels upstream and downstream from the fluid-exchanging vessels and can be calculated as

$$Pmv = PLa + RV(PPa - PLa)/RA + RV$$

where Pmv = microvascular pressure; PLa = left atrial pressure; RV and RA = venous and arterial resistance, respectively; and PPa = pulmonary arterial pressure.[19] If arterial resistance is high relative to venous resistance, microvascular pressure will be close to venous pressure. Conversely, if venous resistance is high relative to arterial resistance, pulmonary microvascular pressure will approach arterial pressure.

Normally, arterial resistance is slightly higher than venous resistance, which results in an average capillary pressure of approximately 10 cm H_2O.[19] Microvascular pressure differs between the arterial and the venous ends of the fluid-exchanging vessels as a result of capillary resistance; there may also be fluid filtration at the arterial end of the capillaries and reabsorption at the venous end.[18] Although it is usual to talk of a single microvascular pressure within the pulmonary vasculature, pulmonary arterial pressure and venous pressure decrease or increase by 1 cm H_2O for each centimeter that the vessel in question is above or below the left atrium. Since there is as much lung above as below this level, the integrated microvascular pressure over the height of the lung is not much different from what would be calculated from the average Ppa and PLa at the level of the left atrium.[18] **Perimicrovascular Interstitial Hydrostatic Pressure (Ppmv).** Just as there is no unique value for microvascular pressure, there is also no single value for the interstitial pressure of the lung. For example, the pressure in close proximity to the alveolar septa is about −3 cm H_2O,[20] whereas that in the perihilar connective tissue is −5 cm H_2O (a value that becomes about −12 cm H_2O when the lung is inflated to TLC).[21] As indicated previously, there is a gradient in pressure that drives fluid from the pericapillary to the perihilar (axial) interstitial space (see Fig. 14–2).[18] There is also a vertical gradient in interstitial pressure from the top to the bottom of the lung, the pressure being more negative at the apex of the lung.

Plasma Protein Osmotic Pressure (πmv). The pressure exerted by plasma proteins is dependent on their concentration and on the permeability of the endothelium to them. The term πmv represents the maximal osmotic pressure that would be produced by that concentration of plasma protein acting across a membrane that is completely impermeable to protein.

Interstitial Protein Osmotic Pressure (πpmv). Interstitial osmotic pressure is also related to the concentration of protein within it. This concentration decreases as fluid filtration increases, an effect that protects against the development of pulmonary edema.

The Filtration Coefficient (Kf). The filtration coefficient (expressed as milliliters per minute per cm H_2O per unit lung weight) is a measure of endothelial permeability to water. The more permeable the endothelium, the larger the value of Kf (i.e., the greater the fluid flux for a given driving pressure). It is impossible to measure Kf in vivo, and even in excised lung preparations the reported values represent the best estimates. However, it is clear that in many forms of pulmonary edema, an increase in Kf—rather than an imbalance in hydrostatic and osmotic pressure—is responsible for edema formation.

The Osmotic Reflection Coefficient (σ). The reflection coefficient is a numerical estimate of the permeability of the membrane to a solute and is therefore also an estimate of the effectiveness with which a given concentration of solute can exert osmotic pressure. A reflection coefficient of 1 means that the membrane is completely impermeable to the solute and that the osmotic pressure exerted by that solute will be equal to that measured in an osmometer. When the reflection coefficient is 0, the membrane is completely permeable to the solute, and the solute exerts no osmotic pressure.[22] A coefficient of 0.5 means that one half of the potentially available osmotic pressure is exerted by the solute. In the presence of noncardiogenic pulmonary edema, the capillary endothelial permeability for water (Kf) and protein (σ) ia altered; when the endothelium is severely damaged, the reflection coefficient approaches 0. In this case, plasma proteins exert no effective pressure across the endothelium, and the most powerful force preventing the formation of edema is lost.

Fluid Transport across the Alveolar Epithelium

The principles that govern fluid and solute transport across the epithelium are the same as those that operate across the endothelium; however, the overall fluid conductivity is at least one order of magnitude lower. The epithelium can restrict the movement of electrolytes so that they can exert an osmotic pressure, and their concentration can be altered by active transport.[23] The surface tension at the interface between alveolar liquid and gas exerts a pressure that tends to suck fluid from the interstitium into the air spaces. Because surfactant lowers surface tension, this pressure is normally small (about 15 cm H_2O); however, when surfactant is deficient, the increase in surface tension can play an important role in the formation of alveolar edema.[24]

Safety Factors

Normally, the alveolar air spaces remain ideally moist despite substantial changes in microvascular and interstitial pressure related to posture, gravity, variations in the state of hydration, and changes in lung volume. This homeostasis is provided by a number of safety factors that tend to minimize accumulation of fluid in the lung.[18]

Lymph flow is one such factor. In the presence of an acute increase in microvascular pressure or permeability, lymph flow can increase 10-fold before a significant accumulation of interstitial fluid occurs.[19] The precise rate of lung lymph flow during pulmonary edema is unknown in humans; however, maximal flow rates of 200 mL/hr are predicted on the basis of results of animal studies.[25]

With repeated episodes of pulmonary edema, such as in chronic left ventricular failure, lymphatic vessels proliferate, increase in caliber, and result in a threefold to fourfold increase in flow capacity.[26,27] For reasons that are unclear, the ability of the lymphatic system to remove fluid and protein from the lung is also enhanced in the presence of damage to the pulmonary endothelium.[28]

A second safety factor that operates in hydrostatic edema is dilution of interstitial protein. This mechanism depends on the relative impermeability of the microvascular endothelium to protein. As transvascular fluid movement increases as a result of elevated microvascular hydrostatic pressure, water transport outstrips protein transport. The resulting dilution of interstitial protein decreases interstitial osmotic pressure.[29]

The increase in tissue pressure that accompanies the accumulation of edema fluid within the alveolar interstitium also acts as a safety factor. As fluid accumulates in this space, the tightly compacted gel resists deformation and pressure increases. Since the peribronchovascular interstitium appears to be more compliant than that of the alveolar septa, fluid flows proximally and accumulates first around the airways and vessels, where it has a significantly less detrimental effect on gas exchange.[16] When the fluid storage capacity of the peribronchovascular interstitium is exceeded, alveolar interstitial pressure increases and results in disruption of the alveolar epithelium and alveolar flooding.[30]

Active transport of solute and water from the alveolar surface into the interstitium is another mechanism that serves to keep the alveolar air spaces free of excessive fluid.[31] Distal airway epithelial cells and alveolar type II cells have amiloride-sensitive Na^+ channels on their apical (luminal) surface and ouabain-sensitive Na^+ and K^+-ATPase pumps on their basal (abluminal) surfaces. These ion channels can be stimulated to remove Na^+ from the alveolar and airway lumen; water follows passively through specialized channels ("aquaporins"), which are made up of channel-forming integral membrane proteins.[32]

Development and Classification of Pulmonary Edema

The sequence of events that occur during the development of pulmonary edema is similar for both hydrostatic and

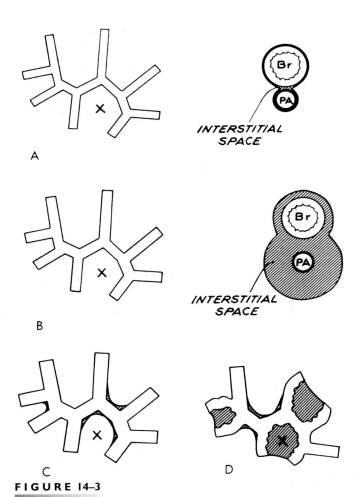

FIGURE 14–3

Schematic representation of the sequence of fluid accumulation in acute pulmonary edema. A, Normal lung (alveolar wall and alveoli on the *left*, bronchovascular bundle on the *right*); **B,** interstitial edema in which fluid has accumulated preferentially in the interstitial space around the conducting blood vessels and airways without affecting the alveolar walls; **C,** early alveolar edema showing the interstitial spaces filled and fluid present in the alveoli, preferentially at the corners at which the curvature is greatest; **D,** alveolar flooding in which individual alveoli have reached a critical configuration at which existing inflation pressure can no longer maintain stability and the alveolar gas volume rapidly passes to a new configuration with much reduced curvature. X, alveolar air space. *(Slightly modified from Staub NC, Nagano H, Pearce ML: Pulmonary edema in dogs, especially the sequence of fluid accumulation in lungs. J Appl Physiol 22:227-240, 1967.)*

permeability edema (Fig. 14–3).[16] The earliest manifestation observed through the light microscope is widening of the peribronchovascular interstitial space and interlobular septa accompanied by lymphatic distention. Fluid appears within this tissue before there is evidence of alveolar flooding and when measurements of alveolar wall thickness are virtually normal.

As the amount of fluid increases, there is a progressive increase in alveolar wall thickness as fluid accumulates in the thick side of the alveolocapillary membrane. Small amounts of fluid may also accumulate within the air spaces confined to the alveolar "corners." When the fluid storage capacity of the interstitium is exceeded, alveolar flooding tends to occur in an all-or-nothing manner, individual alveoli being either liquid

TABLE 14–1. Classification of Pulmonary Edema

Hydrostatic Pulmonary Edema

Cardiogenic
    Left ventricular failure
    Mitral valve disease
    Left atrial myxoma or thrombus
    Cor triatriatum
Disease of the pulmonary veins
    Primary (idiopathic) veno-occlusive disease
    Fibrosing mediastinitis
Neurogenic (combined hydrostatic and permeability pulmonary edema)
    Head trauma
    Increased intracranial pressure
    Postictal
Decreased capillary osmotic pressure
    Renal disease
    Fluid overload
    Cirrhosis

Increased Permeability Pulmonary Edema (ARDS)

Systemic sepsis
Pulmonary infection
Trauma
Inhalation of noxious fumes and gases
Aspiration of noxious fluids
Ingestion or injection of drugs or poisons

filled or air filled.[6] In both hydrostatic and permeability edema, the protein content of the fluid in the flooded alveolar air spaces is the same as that in the interstitium,[33] suggesting that during alveolar flooding the epithelium loses all ability to sieve and therefore permits the outpouring of pure interstitial fluid.

Despite some overlap,[34] it is convenient to classify the causes of pulmonary edema into two major categories on the basis of the underlying pathogenetic abnormality: an increase in pulmonary microvascular pressure (hydrostatic edema) or an increase in microvascular permeability (Table 14–1). Left ventricular decompensation (cardiogenic edema) is the most important cause of hydrostatic edema; others include stenosis of pulmonary veins (e.g., veno-occlusive disease), neurogenic edema, and conditions associated with decreased plasma oncotic pressure (such as cirrhosis and glomerulopathy). Although many specific insults can cause permeability pulmonary edema, the resulting constellation of clinical and radiologic findings is remarkably similar and commonly referred to as acute respiratory distress syndrome (ARDS).[35] A combination of permeability and hydrostatic edema is common and is particularly devastating because many of the safety factors that normally impede the accumulation of excess extravascular fluid are lost when the endothelium loses its selectivity for solutes.

PULMONARY EDEMA ASSOCIATED WITH ELEVATED MICROVASCULAR PRESSURE

Cardiogenic Pulmonary Edema

The most common cause of pulmonary edema is a rise in pulmonary venous pressure secondary to disease of the left side of the heart. Increased pressure within the left atrium is transmitted to the pulmonary veins as a result of backpressure, most often from a failing left ventricle or obstruction to left atrial outflow. Rarely, venous hypertension is caused by stenosis of the pulmonary veins themselves, such as occurs in congenital or acquired veno-occlusive disease or fibrosing mediastinitis; the manifestations of pulmonary edema in such cases are usually indistinguishable from those of pulmonary venous hypertension from cardiac causes, except for the presence of a normal size heart.

Hydrostatic edema results in two principal radiologic patterns related to whether the fluid remains localized in the interstitial space or whether it also occupies the air spaces.

Radiologic Manifestations

Predominantly Interstitial Edema

Transudation of fluid into the interstitial space of the lung necessarily constitutes the first stage of pulmonary edema. As discussed previously, however, the first radiographic sign of cardiac decompensation or pulmonary venous hypertension may be a redistribution of blood "flow" from the lower to the upper lung zones (Fig. 14–4).[36]

When pulmonary venous hypertension is moderate in degree (17 to 20 mm Hg or higher), fluid accumulates within the perivascular interstitial tissue and interlobular septa.[37] As a result of this localization, edema fluid produces a characteristic radiographic pattern of loss of the normal sharp definition of pulmonary vascular markings and thickening of the interlobular septa (Kerley A and B lines) (Fig. 14–5). Although the presence of septal lines can be of value in confirming the diagnosis when other signs are equivocal, in our experience the frequency with which they can be identified is low in comparison to the loss of definition of vessel markings; thus, their absence should not be construed as evidence against the diagnosis.

In circumstances in which edema fluid accumulates in the parenchymal interstitial tissue before the development of overt air space edema, the accumulation is usually invisible or only faintly discernible radiographically as a "haze," which tends to be predominantly lower zonal or perihilar in distribution. Although the severity of radiographic abnormalities correlates with pulmonary wedge pressure,[38] there is often a phase lag between the elevation in wedge pressure and radiographic signs of pulmonary edema, possibly because of the time required for transudation of fluid into the extravascular space.[39] The heart is generally enlarged; however, it may be normal in size when the cause of the edema is recent myocardial infarction, coronary insufficiency, or restrictive cardiomyopathy.[40]

Evidence for interstitial pulmonary edema is also provided by an increase in the thickness of the walls of bronchi seen

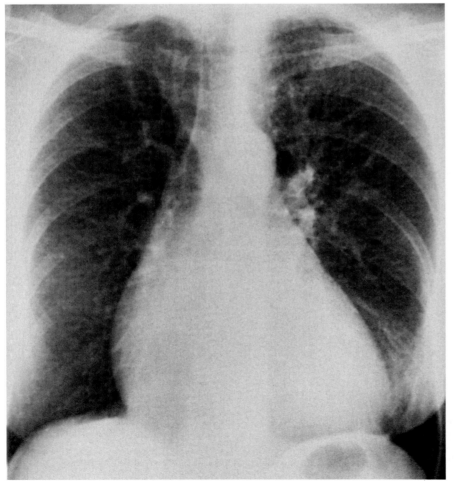

FIGURE 14–4

Redistribution of blood flow to the upper lung zones caused by pulmonary venous hypertension. A posteroanterior radiograph reveals unusually prominent vascular markings in the upper zones and rather sparse markings in the lower zones. The patient was a 42-year-old woman who had recurrent episodes of left ventricular decompensation as a result of cardiomyopathy.

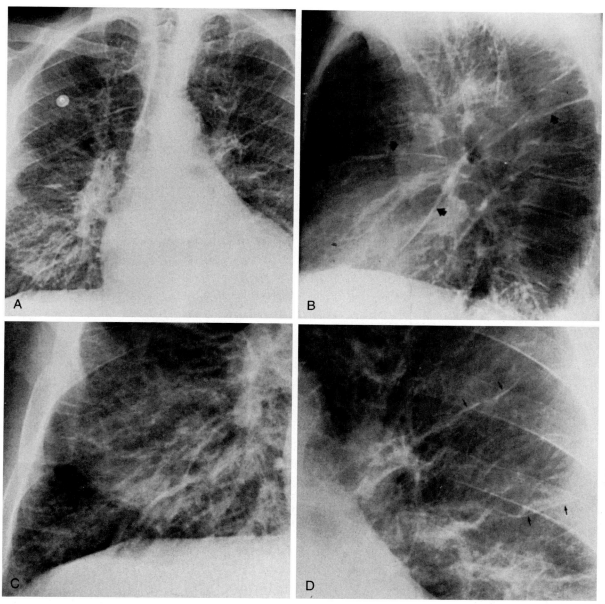

FIGURE 14–5

Interstitial pulmonary edema. Posteroanterior (**A**) and lateral (**B**) radiographs show multiple linear opacities throughout both lungs that are seen to better advantage in a magnified view of the right lower (**C**) and left upper (**D**) lungs. These lines consist of a combination of long septal lines (Kerley A), predominantly in the midlung zones (*arrows* in **D**), and shorter peripheral septal lines (Kerley B). In lateral projection (**B**), the interlobar fissures are prominent (*arrows*), representing pleural edema.

end-on in the perihilar zones. In the absence of chronic airway disease such as COPD or asthma, these structures measure less than 1 mm in thickness. When fluid accumulates in the interstitial tissue surrounding them, their shadow thickens and loses its sharp definition (Fig. 14–6). Another sign of interstitial edema is thickening of the interlobar fissures (see Fig. 14–5).[36] After adequate treatment of edema, all these radiologic signs may disappear within a matter of hours.

Although a diagnosis of hydrostatic pulmonary edema is usually based on clinical information and findings on conventional chest radiography, it is important to recognize its appearance on CT and HRCT, both because it can mimic other diseases and because it is seen occasionally in patients not suspected clinically to have edema.[41] Findings include a disproportionate enlargement of nondependent pulmonary arteries and veins and smooth thickening of the interlobular septa, subpleural connective tissue, and peribronchovascular connective tissue (Fig. 14–7).[42] Areas of ground-glass attenuation can result from either interstitial or air space edema, whereas consolidation specifically reflects the presence of air space edema.

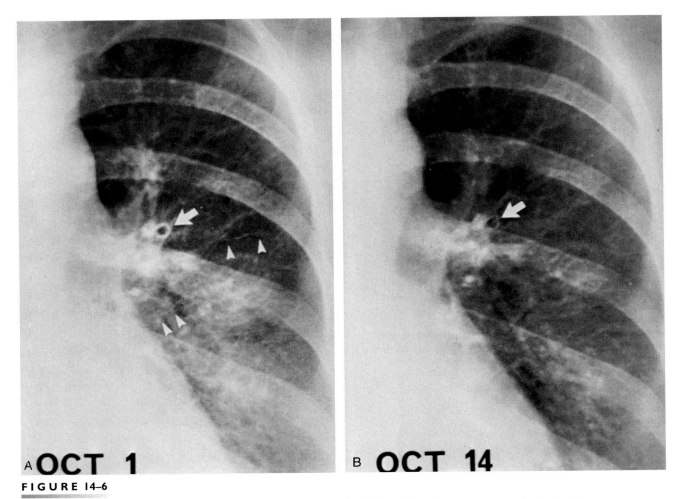

FIGURE 14–6

Peribronchial cuffing in pulmonary edema. A detail view of the upper half of the left lung from a posteroanterior chest radiograph
(**A**) reveals distended upper lobe vessels, perihilar haze, septal A lines (*arrowheads*), and a thickened bronchial wall viewed end-on (*arrow*).
A few days later, after diuretic therapy (**B**), signs of pulmonary edema had resolved. Note the decreased thickness of the bronchial wall (*arrow*).
The patient was a middle-aged woman with renal failure.

Air Space Edema

Although interstitial edema usually precedes air space edema
(Fig. 14–8), the chest radiograph may show evidence of both
simultaneously.[43] The characteristic radiographic abnormality
is the presence of patchy or confluent bilateral areas of consolidation that tend to be symmetrical and to involve mainly
the perihilar regions and the lower lung zones. Air bronchograms can be seen.[43] In the majority of cases, the shadows
are confluent and create irregular, rather poorly defined
patchy opacities of unit density scattered randomly throughout the lungs; in the medial third of the lungs particularly,
coalescence of areas of consolidation is common. The distribution varies from patient to patient but may be surprisingly similar during different episodes in the same individual.
Patchy air space consolidation sometimes extends to the subpleural zone or "cortex" of the lung (Fig. 14–9); however, the
cortex may be completely spared, thus creating the "bat's
wing" or "butterfly" pattern (Fig. 14–10).

Edema secondary to cardiac disease is generally bilateral
and fairly symmetrical. Occasionally, it is predominantly unilateral or occupies zones of one or both lungs out of keeping

with the "expected" distribution of disease arising from a
central influence (Fig. 14–11).[44] Unilateral pulmonary edema
can occur in a wide variety of conditions in which the pathogenetic mechanism exists either on the same side as the edema
(ipsilateral edema) or on the opposite side (contralateral
edema).[45] In patients who have cardiac decompensation, unilateral edema is probably related primarily to dependency.[46]

Like hydrostatic interstitial pulmonary edema, air space
edema usually clears fairly rapidly in response to adequate
treatment of the underlying condition, and resolution appears
to be radiographically complete in less than 3 days in most
cases.

Clinical Manifestations

The clinical manifestations of cardiogenic pulmonary edema
depend on whether the onset of edema is acute or insidious.
When severe, the acute form is dramatic, with dyspnea developing over a period of minutes to hours. The patient characteristically sits bolt upright in obvious respiratory distress and
uses the accessory muscles of respiration. Peripheral and

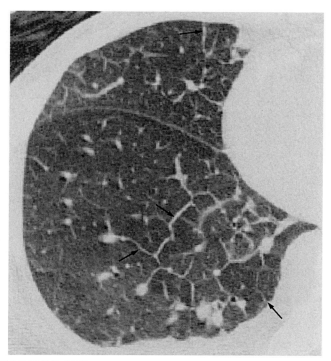

FIGURE 14–7

Interstitial pulmonary edema. A view of the right lung from an HRCT scan demonstrates increased diameter of the pulmonary vessels, smooth thickening of the interlobular septa (*arrows*), and localized areas of ground-glass attenuation in the dependent lung regions. A small pleural effusion is also present. The patient was a 49-year-old woman with interstitial pulmonary edema as a result of fluid overload.

central cyanosis, tachycardia, pallor, cool sweaty skin, anxiety, and elevated blood pressure are often present as a result of sympathetic stimulation. In the most severe cases, the patient may expectorate frothy, blood-tinged fluid. "Air hunger" may be sufficient to interfere with normal speech.

Physical examination may reveal elevated jugular venous pressure; however, in severe edema the jugular veins may be difficult to evaluate because of the patient's use of the cervical accessory muscles of respiration and the considerable swings in pleural pressure transmitted to the cervical veins. Other signs of congestive failure may be present, such as hepatosplenomegaly and peripheral edema. Auscultation of the thorax reveals widespread crackles. Findings suggestive of airway narrowing such as expiratory wheezes are frequent, probably because of airway compression by distended vessels and expanded peribronchovascular interstitial tissue.[47] In the terminal stages, the patient's level of consciousness decreases and circulatory collapse ensues.

In patients in whom pulmonary edema develops less precipitously, the onset of symptoms may be insidious and there may be few physical findings. Dyspnea in such patients may occur only during exertion; a history of orthopnea and paroxysmal nocturnal dyspnea is a helpful diagnostic feature in these individuals, although these symptoms, accompanied by cough, are also common in patients who have asthma or COPD. Occasionally, the clinical manifestations of "butterfly" edema are almost as unimpressive as the radiographic appearance is dramatic.

When the edema is confined to the interstitial space, auscultatory findings may be absent, although expiratory wheezing is present in some patients at this stage. The quieter chest allows more careful auscultation of the heart, which may reveal a gallop rhythm or a murmur caused by valvular dysfunction. An estimate of right-sided heart filling pressure can be obtained by examining the jugular veins, and the increase in jugular venous pressure caused by compression of the abdomen (hepatojugular [abdominojugular] reflux) can be assessed by performing a standardized maneuver.[48]

Acute cardiogenic pulmonary edema is not a static condition, and there is usually improvement or worsening during a relatively short time course. The differential diagnosis includes fulminant pneumonia, an exacerbation of COPD or asthma, pulmonary hemorrhage, and upper airway obstruction.

Pulmonary Function and Other Tests

The abnormalities in lung function that occur in pulmonary edema are caused by the effects of pulmonary vascular engorgement, interstitial fluid accumulation, and alveolar flooding. Pulmonary vascular congestion and interstitial edema stiffen the lung and contribute to a decrease in VC and TLC.[49] These respiratory parameters are further decreased by alveolar flooding as a result of replacement of alveolar gas by fluid and disruption of the surfactant-air interface.[50]

The distribution of ventilation and perfusion is usually altered and results in $\dot{V}/\dot{Q}$ mismatching and arterial hypoxemia. When edema is confined to the interstitium, it is usually mild; when air spaces are involved, true shunting of pulmonary blood combines with the $\dot{V}/\dot{Q}$ mismatching to cause more severe hypoxemia. In patients who have interstitial and mild to moderate air space edema, arterial PCO_2 is normal or low because of an overall increase in alveolar ventilation. Although most patients who have acute pulmonary edema are hypocapnic or eucapnic, many are acidemic as a result of hypoperfusion of peripheral tissues and the development of lactic acidosis.[51] Approximately 10% of patients are hypercapnic; almost invariably, this respiratory acidosis is accompanied by metabolic acidosis.

Occasionally, it is necessary to use a pulmonary artery catheter and measure pulmonary arterial wedge pressure to establish that the cause of pulmonary edema is an increase in pulmonary venous pressure. However, echocardiographic techniques such as transesophageal echo and pulsed Doppler can be used to assess ventricular function and provide a fairly accurate estimate of pulmonary capillary wedge pressure.[52] Blood levels of atrial and brain natriuretic peptide are increased in dyspneic patients who are in mild heart failure but not in similarly dyspneic patients whose symptoms are secondary to primary lung disease.[53]

Pulmonary Edema Associated with Renal Disease, Hypervolemia, or Hypoproteinemia

Both acute and chronic renal disease—with or without uremia—can be associated with acute pulmonary edema.[54] A major contributing cause in these cases is left ventricular failure; however, it is likely that decreased protein osmotic pressure, hypervolemia, and increased capillary permeability

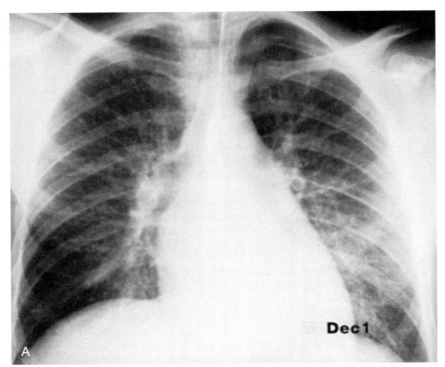

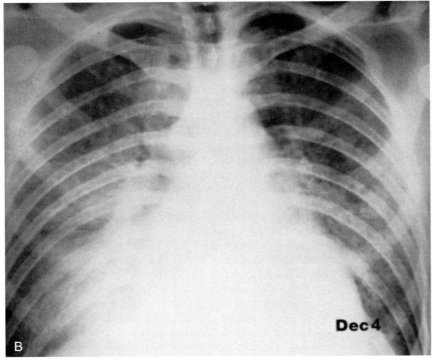

FIGURE 14–8

Interstitial edema progressing to air space edema in association with severe valvular disease and bacterial endocarditis. The initial posteroanterior radiograph of this 22-year-old man (**A**) reveals diffuse interstitial edema manifested by loss of definition of the vascular markings throughout both lungs and by septal lines in both costophrenic recesses. Three days later (**B**), the lungs had become massively consolidated by air space edema. Heart size had increased considerably in this interval. The patient had clinical evidence of both aortic and mitral insufficiency.

also have a role.[55] Factors contributing to hydrostatic pulmonary edema in uremic patients include a constant high cardiac output secondary to anemia and arteriovenous fistula (in patients maintained on chronic hemodialysis), coronary artery disease, fluid overload, and left ventricular hypertrophy.[56] In fact, patients undergoing dialysis often have subclinical interstitial pulmonary edema that can be detected by indicator dilution methods[57]; the abnormality is corrected during dialysis.

Administration of large volumes of intravenous fluids has been shown to cause pulmonary edema in patients who do not have underlying heart disease,[58] particularly during the postoperative period and in the elderly. As might be expected, the effects of volume overload are amplified in patients who are on the verge of cardiac or renal failure. Pulmonary edema occurs with increased frequency in patients who have hepatic disease and have undergone liver transplantation.[59] It also frequently accompanies the development of acute hepatic

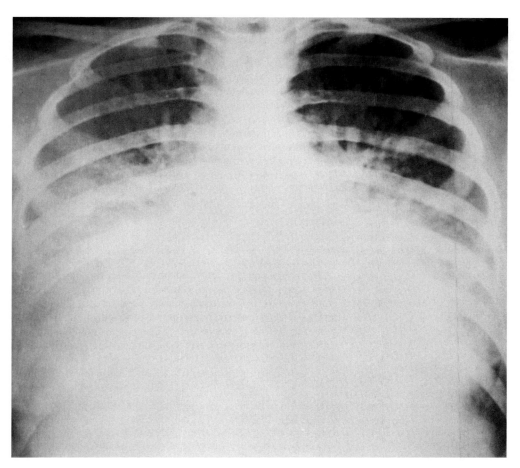

FIGURE 14–9

Acute pulmonary edema secondary to left ventricular failure. A posteroanterior radiograph reveals extensive consolidation of both lungs extending to the visceral pleural surfaces. The heart is moderately enlarged. Six hours before this radiograph was taken, the patient had an abrupt onset of severe dyspnea, pleuritic pain, and cough productive of copious frothy sputum. Both the clinical and radiographic pictures are typical of acute pulmonary edema secondary to left ventricular failure.

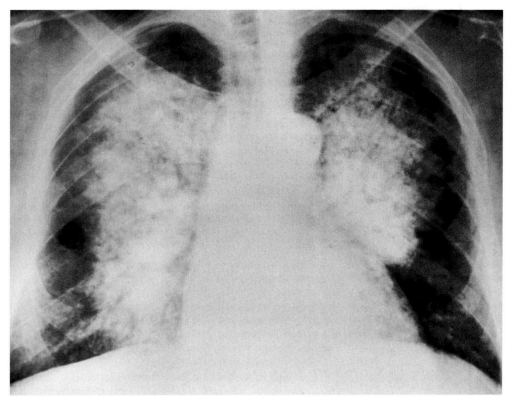

FIGURE 14–10

Pulmonary edema—"bat's wing" pattern. A posteroanterior radiograph demonstrates consolidation of the parahilar and "medullary" portions of both lungs, a combination that creates a bat's wing or "butterfly" appearance; the "cortex" of both lungs is relatively unaffected. The margins of the edematous lung are rather sharply defined. The consolidation is fairly homogeneous and associated with well-defined air bronchograms on both sides. This 59-year-old man had suffered a massive myocardial infarct 48 hours previously.

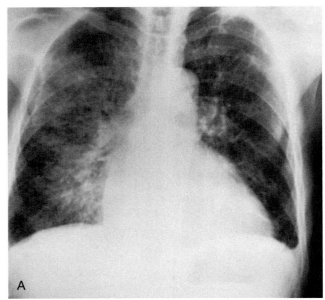

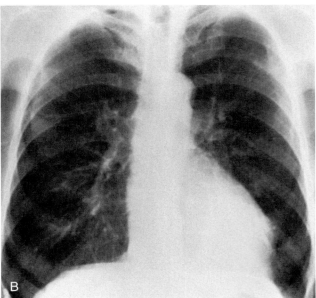

FIGURE 14–11

Predominantly unilateral pulmonary edema. A posteroanterior radiograph (**A**) of a 70-year-old man admitted with an acute myocardial infarct reveals patchy air space consolidation occupying the medial two thirds of the right lung characteristic of acute pulmonary edema. The left lung is relatively unaffected and there is a small left pleural effusion. The heart is moderately enlarged. A visit to the patient's bedside revealed the fact that he lay on his right side most of the time since other positions seemed to intensify his shortness of breath. A radiograph after resolution of the edema (**B**) shows a marked increase in volume of both lungs characteristic of diffuse pulmonary emphysema. The unilaterality of the edema was clearly related to the influence of gravity. It cannot be explained on the basis of emphysema because this disease is bilateral and symmetrical.

failure.[60] It is unclear whether increased capillary pressure, increased endothelial permeability, or decreased plasma osmotic pressure is the major contributor to the development of edema in these patients; it is likely that a combination of factors is responsible.

Neurogenic and Postictal Pulmonary Edema

Acute pulmonary edema is a well-described but infrequent complication of raised intracranial pressure, head trauma, and seizures. Although its mechanism is poorly understood, experimental studies have shown transient, massive sympathetic discharge from the central nervous system, which results in generalized vasoconstriction, a shift of blood volume into the pulmonary vascular compartment, and elevation of pulmonary microvascular pressure.[61,62] A number of investigators have reported normal microvascular pressure and protein-rich edema fluid in patients who have neurogenic pulmonary edema,[63,64] suggesting that an alteration in microvascular permeability also occurs. The combination of increased pressure and increased permeability have led to the hypothesis that an acute increase in intracranial pressure causes a generalized sympathetic discharge that results in a massive increase in pulmonary vascular pressure, barotrauma to the endothelium, and consequent increased permeability; by the time microvascular pressure is measured, it may have returned to control levels, thereby leaving barotrauma-induced changes in permeability as the major culprit.[65] There is also evidence that a direct negative inotropic effect on the heart may contribute to pathogenesis of the edema.[66]

The radiographic distribution of neurogenic pulmonary edema is usually generalized.[64] Characteristically, the edema disappears within several days after surgical relief of increased intracranial pressure. Most patients are comatose and experience frequent periods of apnea when pulmonary edema develops. Thus, they are likely to aspirate gastric secretions and suffer prolonged hypoxemia. In fact, it is possible that aspiration is the cause of the edema in some cases.

Head trauma is one of the most frequent causes of neurogenic edema; although it is often severe, it may be relatively mild.[67] In nontraumatized patients in whom edema develops as a consequence of raised intracranial pressure, the rise in pressure may or may not be abrupt. Postictal pulmonary edema can develop immediately after an epileptic seizure or can be delayed for several hours.

PULMONARY EDEMA ASSOCIATED WITH NORMAL MICROVASCULAR PRESSURE

After a variety of direct or indirect pulmonary insults (Table 14–2), a number of patients suffer progressive respiratory distress characterized by tachypnea, dyspnea, cough, and the physical findings of air space consolidation. The chest radiograph reveals diffuse air space disease; blood gas analysis demonstrates severe arterial desaturation that is resistant to high concentrations of inhaled oxygen; the lungs become stiff and difficult to ventilate; pulmonary vascular pressure and resistance increase; and it becomes necessary to institute prolonged oxygen therapy and ventilatory support. Despite the varying inciting events, the histologic changes are similar and consist of diffuse alveolar damage (interstitial and air space edema, hyaline membrane formation in transitional airways, and in later stages, fibrosis).[68]

Although a number of terms have been used to describe this disease,[69,70] the term *acute* (or *adult*) *respiratory distress*

TABLE 14–2. Causes of Increased Permeability Pulmonary Edema

Direct Pulmonary Insults
Inhalation or Aspiration
Smoke
Toxic gases (e.g., nitrogen dioxide [silo filler's disease], sulfur dioxide, ammonia, oxygen)
Gastric acid
Water (near-drowning)
Cocaine inhalation
Drugs
Heroin and morphine
Cocaine and amphetamines
Methadone
Salicylates
Bleomycin
Amiodarone
Ethylene glycol
Lithium
Ketamine (possibly a hydrostatic component)
Propoxyphene
Paclitaxel (possibly a hydrostatic component)
Gemcitabine
Hydrochlorothiazide
Tocolytic therapy (e.g., terbutaline infused to prevent the onset of labor)
Ergometrine (possibly a hydrostatic component)
Tricyclic antidepressants (possibly a hydrostatic component)
Triazolam
Interleukin-2 (combined hydrostatic and permeability edema)
Chemicals and Poisons
Carbamate and organophosphate
Paraquat
Polyethylene glycol
Fish or insect venom (e.g., scorpion or stonefish)
Infection
Viruses, bacteria, and fungi
Mycobacteria
Miscellaneous Causes
Fat emboli
Amniotic fluid emboli
Air emboli
Decompression sickness
Pulmonary contusion
Radiologic contrast media
Thoracic irradiation
Indirect Pulmonary Insults
Sepsis
Anaphylaxis
Multisystem trauma
Multiple transfusions
Antilymphocyte globulin therapy
Disseminated intravascular coagulation
Pancreatitis
Pheochromocytoma
Diabetic ketoacidosis
Cardiopulmonary bypass
High altitude
Rapid lung re-expansion
Neurogenic
Sickle cell crisis
Hyperthermia
Hypothermia
Hyponatremic encephalopathy
Eclampsia
Extreme physical exertion

syndrome (ARDS) is now in general usage. A second relatively common designation is *permeability edema*; although *increased permeability edema* is more appropriate, the abbreviated nomenclature serves to distinguish this form of edema from that resulting primarily from increased microvascular pressure. When increased permeability edema is of lesser severity, it is sometimes designated "acute lung injury."[71] Because of their familiarity and brevity, "permeability edema" and "ARDS" are used throughout this text.

In the United States, the incidence of ARDS is about 1.5 cases per 100,000 people per year.[72] Conditions often associated with it include sepsis, aspiration of liquid gastric contents, severe trauma (including long-bone and pelvic fractures and pulmonary contusion), multiple blood transfusions, near-drowning, pancreatitis, prolonged hypotension, overwhelming pneumonia, and disseminated intravascular coagulation (DIC) (often associated with sepsis).[73] Less common risk factors are drug overdose, major burns,[74] and coronary artery bypass surgery.[73]

Pathogenesis

ARDS is the end result of the effects of a number of cellular and molecular reactions that are initiated by a variety of local or systemic insults.[75] Even though ARDS is often regarded as a manifestation of increased microvascular permeability localized to the lungs, there is abundant evidence that it is really a specific feature of a generalized inflammatory disorder termed the *systemic inflammatory response syndrome* (SIRS).[76] Although an increase in microvascular permeability and the development of interstitial and air space edema are initially the major clinical consequences of this inflammatory process, the injury also involves damage to endothelial cells in other organs, especially in the setting of sepsis and trauma. Initially, this generalized endothelial injury is often clinically silent; however, if the patient survives the consequences of pulmonary edema, manifestations of renal, cardiac, gastrointestinal, and/or cerebral dysfunction soon appear. In fact, patients who die of ARDS after 72 hours almost invariably have evidence of a syndrome termed *multiple system organ failure* (MSOF) (or *multiple organ dysfunction syndrome* [MODS]).[76,77]

The pathogenesis of this syndrome involves a complex series of inflammatory events and includes the participation of cytokines and chemokines, preformed plasma-derived inflammatory mediators, and newly generated arachidonic acid mediators from both the cyclooxygenase and lipoxygenase pathways.[78] Activation of the complement and blood-clotting systems is also involved. These biochemical substances, as well as integrins and selectins on endothelial cells and epithelial cells, mediate the recruitment of a variety of inflammatory cells to affected tissues. There is no unifying theory that ties together the actions of these intricate inflammatory cascades and cytokine networks, and we present only a brief summary of the various pathways and mechanisms that are thought to be important.

Pulmonary Endothelial and Epithelial Cells. The major targets for agents that precipitate ARDS are the endothelial and epithelial cells that line the alveolar walls. The same cells also have an important role in orchestrating the inflammatory response by secreting a number of cytokines and expressing a variety of surface glycoproteins (selectins and integrins).

Cultured pulmonary endothelial cells are sensitive to the effects of bacterial endotoxin, as well as to many of the constituents of the cytokine "soup" that is generated by inflammatory and tissue cells during acute lung injury.[79,80] In such models, endothelial injury is first manifested by cell retraction, which causes a reduction in barrier function, release of intracellular enzymes, and ultimately, cell death. Endothelial cells exposed to endotoxin can produce a variety of inflammatory cytokines (e.g., interleukin-1 [IL-1], IL-6, and IL-8), as well as factors such as granulocyte–macrophage colony-stimulating factor (GM-CSF), that can influence the bone marrow to increase the production of inflammatory cells.[81] The stimulated endothelial cells also express surface molecules that cause circulating inflammatory cells to adhere to them and migrate through their intercellular junctions.[82]

Although alveolar epithelial cells are more resistant to injury than endothelial cells are, they are invariably damaged in the course of ARDS and may also have an active role in mediating the inflammatory response. For example, they are capable of expressing a variety of cytokines and surface-active molecules; such expression is associated with attraction of leukocytes as well as adherence to and migration across the epithelium.[83]

Alveolar Macrophages. Alveolar macrophages also have an important role in modulating the inflammatory reaction in ARDS. After exposure to endotoxin, they release tumor necrosis factor (TNF) and IL-1, both of which are powerful proinflammatory mediators that can initiate and perpetuate the inflammatory cascade directly and by secondary induction of additional cytokines.[80]

Polymorphonuclear Leukocytes. Considerable evidence from both experimental and clinical studies has shown that polymorphonuclear leukocytes are important in the pathogenesis of ARDS. A large pool of marginated neutrophils normally reside within the pulmonary microvessels. These cells, as well as circulating neutrophils, respond to a gradient mediated by a variety of chemotaxins and chemokines that causes them to migrate toward a site of injury.[84] Leukocyte–endothelial cell adherence is mediated by surface molecules on neutrophils such as L-selectin, which is responsible for loose adherence (rolling), and the β_2-integrins, which cause firm adherence and are necessary for migration into the pulmonary interstitium and air spaces.[85,86] These leukocyte-specific molecules interact with intercellular adhesion molecule type 1 (ICAM-1) and ICAM-2 on both endothelial and epithelial cell surfaces. Activation of neutrophils is associated with the production of several species of oxygen radicals that damage the endothelial and epithelial cells. In addition to oxygen radicals, neutrophils can also release prostaglandins, leukotrienes, and enzymes that are designed for bacterial digestion but are also capable of degrading the extracellular matrix.[87]

Surfactant. In the respiratory distress syndrome of newborns, a deficiency of surfactant production is believed to be the primary cause of pulmonary injury. By contrast, the abnormalities in surfactant function and synthesis that occur in adults who have ARDS are more the result than the cause of the injury. This has been well illustrated by the lack of a substantial clinical benefit of exogenous surfactant replacement.[88] Nonetheless, disruption of the surfactant layer and the resultant increase in surface tension undoubtedly contribute to both the development and perpetuation of alveolar edema in ARDS.[24]

Both qualitative and quantitative abnormalities of surfactant have been demonstrated in fluid obtained by BAL.[89] These abnormalities may have several causes, including dilution of the normal amount of surface-active phospholipid by exudate within the alveoli, deficiency in phospholipid production as a result of epithelial injury, and inactivation of surfactant by oxygen radicals or other substances.[90] A number of the cytokines and mediators implicated in the pathogenesis of ARDS also have an effect on surfactant function or synthesis.[91,92]

Complement. Activation of the complement system can occur in a variety of conditions, including trauma, infection, extracorporeal circulation during hemodialysis, and cardiopulmonary bypass for coronary artery grafting.[93,94] Complement components derived from such activation can have a direct toxic effect on certain cells; neutrophil activation can then cause a release of enzymes and oxygen radicals that can secondarily damage other cells and tissues.[95] Despite these observations, the importance of complement activation in the pathogenesis of ARDS has been questioned,[96] since levels of complement fragments can be elevated in severely injured patients regardless of whether they eventually experience ARDS or MSOF.[97]

The Clotting System. Abnormalities of the clotting system ranging from activation of the clotting cascade and inhibition of fibrinolysis to full-blown DIC are common in ARDS and have been implicated in its pathogenesis.[98] Exposure of collagen after pulmonary microvascular injury can activate the intrinsic system that initiates clotting, whereas tissue thromboplastin generated from damaged lung can activate the extrinsic system. Such activation results in the production of thrombin and fibrin, both of which can induce endothelial cell damage and increase pulmonary vascular permeability. Fibrin monomers and fibrin split products can also cause microvascular endothelial injury and stimulate pulmonary vasoconstriction.[99]

The results of experimental studies suggest the following sequence of events in the pathogenesis of vascular injury after the initiation of coagulation: (1) fibrin is generated from fibrinogen and activates the fibrinolytic system, which results in the formation of plasmin from plasminogen; (2) plasmin breaks down fibrin and causes cleavage of complement proteins and formation of the chemotactic peptides C3a and C5a; (3) complement fragments cause sequestration of neutrophils within the lung; and (4) neutrophil activation results in vascular injury and pulmonary edema.

Oxygen Radicals. Short-lived unstable species of oxygen molecules (oxygen free radicals) such as the superoxide radical ($O_2^{\cdot-}$), hydrogen peroxide (H_2O_2), hydroxyl radical ($OH^{\star}$), and singlet oxygen ($O_2^{\star}$) are generated by enzymes such as xanthine oxidase and as a byproduct of normal mitochondrial energy transfer reactions. Under normal conditions, these radicals are inactivated by antioxidant defense mechanisms that include specific enzymes such as superoxide dismutase (which catalyzes the conversion of $O_2^{\cdot-}$ to hydrogen peroxide), catalase (which catalyzes the conversion of hydrogen peroxide to oxygen and water), and glutathione peroxidase (which converts peroxide radicals to nontoxic lipids). Several nonspecific "free radical scavengers," such as ascorbic acid, β-carotene, and glutathione, can also neutralize the radicals.

Pulmonary sources of oxygen radicals include activated neutrophils, macrophages, and even endothelial cells. Many proinflammatory stimuli such as endotoxin, TNF, platelet-activating factor, and complement fragments can facilitate or directly stimulate these cells to produce oxygen radicals.[100] The results of a number of experimental studies suggest that the damage that they induce on other cells and tissue may be the final common pathway in a variety of acute lung injuries, including ARDS.[101,102]

Enzymes and Mediators. Both mediators of inflammation and a number of enzymes play important roles in initiating and modifying lung injury in ARDS. Among the most important of such mediators are the cytokines, a diverse group of proteins and peptides that act as soluble signals between cells.[84,103] TNF and IL-1 generated by alveolar and tissue macrophages are the first cytokines that can be detected. They have the ability to alter hemodynamics and lung oxygenation, induce fever, and activate neutrophils and the coagulation cascade. They also induce the upregulation of endothelial and epithelial adhesion molecules and cause secretion of the powerful neutrophil chemoattractant IL-8[104]; the level of this mediator is particularly increased in patients whose ARDS is related to sepsis.[105] TNF and IL-1 also stimulate the liver to synthesize and secrete IL-6 and acute phase proteins and decrease the synthesis of albumin.[106,107] In addition, cytokines cause the generation and secretion of arachidonic acid metabolites (prostaglandins, thromboxanes, and leukotrienes), which can either cause or protect against lung injury.[108]

Shock. Episodes of hypotension, either brief or prolonged and caused by hypovolemia, impaired cardiac output, and/or a decrease in systemic vascular smooth muscle tone, are frequent precursors of ARDS. Although this relationship suggests a pathogenetic role, it is difficult to cause lung damage by shock alone,[109] and it is probable that other factors are involved to produce the complete syndrome in most instances.

Pathologic Characteristics

The pathologic changes in the lungs of patients who have ARDS are virtually the same regardless of etiology and are described by the term *diffuse alveolar damage*. Although a continuum of histologic abnormalities exists, for purposes of discussion the changes can conveniently be described in three phases: exudative, proliferative, and fibrotic.[68,110]

The exudative phase is manifested histologically by interstitial edema and vascular congestion, and air space filling is manifested by a proteinaceous exudate and a variable number of red blood cells (see Color Fig. 14–3A). Fibrin thrombi may be present in capillaries and small arterioles and venules. After several days, the exudate that is present in alveolar ducts and respiratory bronchioles appears more compact and becomes flattened against the airway wall, resulting in hyaline membranes. Soon after the initial injury, type II alveolar epithelial cells begin to proliferate, which eventually results in relining of the alveolar surfaces.

The proliferative phase is seen from 7 to 28 days after the initial pulmonary insult and is characterized by a proliferation of myofibroblasts, predominantly within the alveolar air spaces but also in the parenchymal interstitium (see Color Fig. 14–3B).[111] The cellular proliferation is accompanied by synthesis and deposition of proteoglycans in the interstitium[112];

in time, collagen may be laid down within this provisional matrix. Mononuclear inflammatory cells, predominantly lymphocytes, may be apparent. In patients who have less severe disease, much of the fibroblastic proliferation resolves without residual fibrosis; in others, significant mature fibrous tissue remains.

Pulmonary vascular abnormalities are also commonly seen during all stages of ARDS and are sometimes extensive.[113] They probably result from several causes, including microvascular thrombosis initiated by the initial pulmonary insult and thromboembolism.

Radiologic Manifestations

Typically, a delay of up to 12 hours elapses from the clinical onset of respiratory failure to the appearance of abnormalities on the chest radiograph. The earliest findings consist of patchy, ill-defined opacities throughout both lungs.[114] The appearance is similar to air space edema of cardiac origin, except that the heart size is usually normal and the edema tends to show a more peripheral distribution. The patchy zones of consolidation rapidly coalesce to the point of massive air space consolidation (Fig. 14–12). Characteristically, involvement is diffuse and affects all lung zones from the apex to the base and to the extreme periphery of each lung; in our experience, this widespread distribution can be of considerable value in distinguishing ARDS from cardiogenic pulmonary edema, whose distribution is seldom as extensive. Also in contrast to cardiogenic edema, an air bronchogram is frequently visible. Pleural effusion is characteristically inapparent on supine radiographs; its presence should strongly suggest concomitant hydrostatic pulmonary edema or complicating acute pneumonia or pulmonary infarction. Institution of PEEP can result in a dramatic decrease in the radiographic abnormality within minutes of application.[115]

After approximately 1 week the lungs remain diffusely abnormal, but the pattern tends to become reticular or "bubbly."[116] It is likely that this pattern represents interstitial and air space fibrosis characteristic of the proliferative phase seen pathologically (Fig. 14–13). In the vast majority of patients who survive, the radiograph shows improvement within the first 10 to 14 days.

Findings on CT and HRCT also depend on the stage. In early disease, most patients show diffuse, non–gravity-dependent patchy consolidation or mixed air space and ground-glass opacification.[117] Air bronchograms and small pleural effusions are common. Later in the exudative phase, the consolidation becomes more homogeneous and gravity dependent (Fig. 14–14). During the organizing phase, there is often a decrease in overall lung density and the appearance of reticulation.[42] Examination at this stage often shows evidence of complications of ARDS and its treatment, such as interstitial emphysema, pneumomediastinum, pneumothorax, and subpleural bullae or cysts (Fig. 14–15).[34,118] As with the radiograph, the CT features of ARDS are altered when the patient's lungs are inflated by the application of PEEP.[119]

Clinical Manifestations

Risk factors for the development of ARDS include the "sepsis syndrome," documented aspiration of gastric contents,

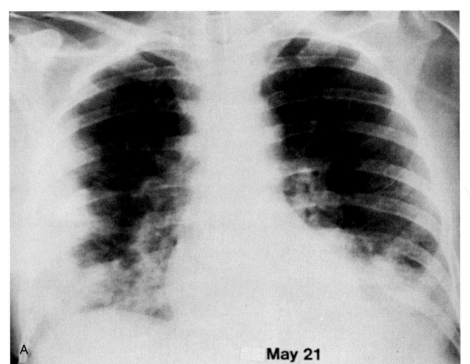

May 21

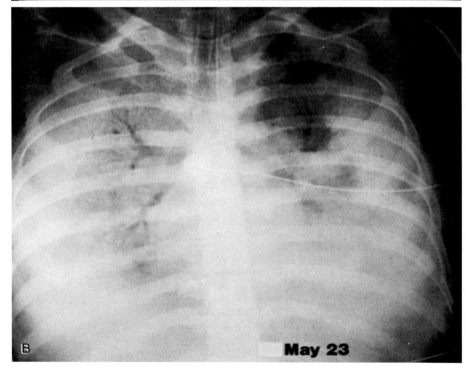

May 23

FIGURE 14–12

Acute respiratory distress syndrome. This 18-year-old girl was admitted to the intensive care unit in severe shock after a motor vehicle accident. A radiograph the day after admission (**A**) revealed homogeneous consolidation of the left lower lobe and the axillary portion of the right lung. Two days later (**B**), both lungs were massively consolidated; note the prominent air bronchogram.

near-drowning, pulmonary contusion, multiple long-bone fractures, multiple transfusions (more than 10 U of blood over a 6-hour period), and hypotension (systolic blood pressure less than 90 mm Hg for more than 2 hours).[77] Detailed formulas for calculating a patient's degree of illness or injury, such as the APACHE II score (Acute Physiology and Chronic Health Evaluation) or the Injury Severity Score, are modestly predictive of the likelihood of the development of ARDS.[120,121]

The clinical manifestations of ARDS can develop either insidiously, hours or days after the initiating event (e.g., sepsis or fat emboli), or acutely, coincident with the event (e.g., aspiration of liquid gastric contents). Typical symptoms are dyspnea, tachypnea, dry cough, retrosternal discomfort, and agitation; cyanosis may be present. Expectoration of copious blood-tinged fluid signifies the presence of the full-blown syndrome. Examination of the chest reveals coarse crackles and bronchial breath sounds.

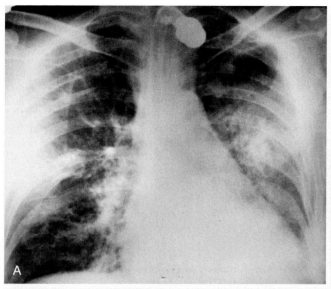

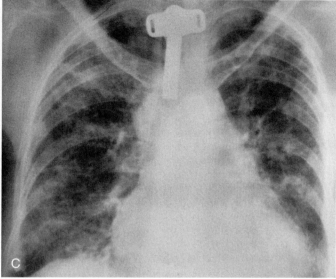

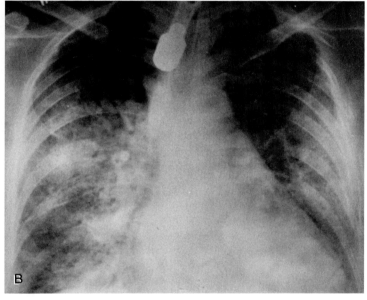

FIGURE 14-13

Acute respiratory distress syndrome—prolonged course and partial resolution. Twenty-four hours after admission of a young woman with multiple bone fractures sustained in a motor vehicle accident, a radiograph of the chest in anteroposterior projection, supine position (**A**), shows a mixture of reticular and air space opacities asymmetrically distributed throughout the lungs. An endotracheal tube is evident. Four days later, a repeat radiograph (**B**) demonstrates worsening of the air space consolidation. Approximately 2 months later, a predischarge radiograph (**C**) shows that most of the air space component has resolved; however, there is persistent coarse reticulation that represents residual parenchymal fibrosis. Follow-up films over the ensuing months demonstrated only modest improvement.

Pulmonary Function and Cardiovascular Tests

The most important pathophysiologic effect of lung edema in ARDS is on gas exchange; in fact, profound hypoxemia rather than ventilatory failure is the major indication for intubation and mechanical ventilation. The hypoxemia is difficult or impossible to correct, even with the use of very high concentrations of inspired oxygen. Its pathogenesis is related predominantly to the development of a shunt rather than to other forms of $\dot{V}/\dot{Q}$ mismatching.[122] Prone positioning improves gas exchange, an effect that is related to a more even distribution of blood flow.[123] Though not routinely measured, diffusing capacity and FRC are decreased and pulmonary resistance is increased.[124,125] There is also evidence that peripheral oxygen uptake is impaired.[126] Although the mechanism is incompletely understood, it is presumably a reflection of the generalized abnormality in microvascular function seen in patients who have MSOF.

ARDS is often accompanied by pulmonary arterial hypertension, and the resultant increase in right ventricular afterload usually causes right ventricular dysfunction.[127] There is also evidence that right ventricular dysfunction can result in left ventricular dysfunction, most likely related to a shift in the shared interventricular septum.[128] In the late stages of ARDS, the lung becomes progressively noncompliant, and although gas exchange may improve somewhat, it is harder to maintain a normal $PaCO_2$.[118]

Although the radiographic features can often distinguish cardiogenic from increased permeability pulmonary edema, measurement of pulmonary vascular pressure with a balloon-tipped, flow-directed (Swan-Ganz) catheter is often required for definitive diagnosis. Wedge pressure provides an accurate estimate of the filling pressure of the left ventricle and is therefore a reflection of left ventricular preload. A normal or low pulmonary arterial wedge pressure measurement provides strong, indirect evidence that endothelial damage and increased permeability are the cause of the pulmonary edema.

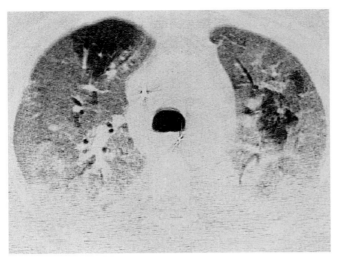

FIGURE 14–14

Acute respiratory distress syndrome. An HRCT scan demonstrates extensive bilateral areas of ground-glass attenuation, air bronchograms, areas of consolidation in the dependent lung regions, and focal areas of relatively normal lung. The patient was a 45-year-old woman with ARDS secondary to a cytotoxic drug reaction.

Central venous pressure measurement does not provide similar information because the right and left ventricles often differ considerably in their performance characteristics and filling pressure.[129]

In addition to giving an accurate estimate of left atrial filling pressure, pulmonary wedge pressure provides information concerning pulmonary microvascular pressure. Its measurement thus serves as an effective management tool in testing the effectiveness of agents and therapies designed to lower intravascular pressure. In the presence of increased microvascular permeability, a transient or prolonged elevation in microvascular pressure can significantly increase the amount of edema fluid (Fig. 14–16).[130] However, despite the theoretical benefit of monitoring wedge pressure, clinical studies have shown no survival benefit of measuring wedge pressure in critically ill patients at risk for ARDS.[131,132]

Natural History and Prognosis

Regardless of the availability of modern diagnostic techniques and therapies, ARDS has a mortality rate of greater than 50%.[133] Patients who die of pulmonary insufficiency usually show a progressive decrease in lung compliance and

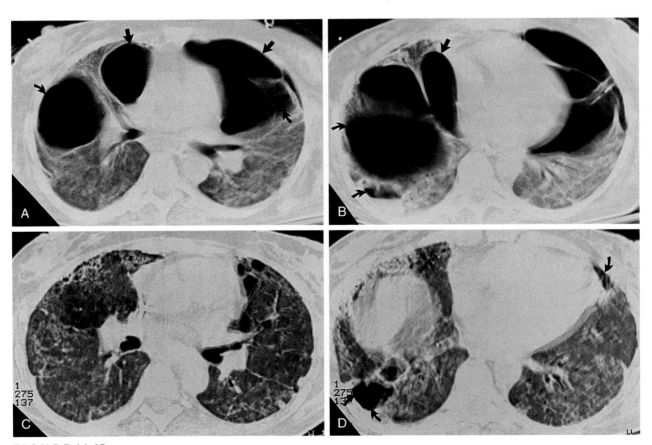

FIGURE 14–15

Cystic changes in ARDS. Sepsis and ARDS developed in a 30-year-old woman after cesarean section. HRCT scans 1 week later (**A** and **B**) demonstrate bilateral loculated pneumothoraces (*straight arrows*) and cystic changes (*curved arrows*) in both lungs. HRCT scans 1 month later (**C** and **D**) demonstrate bilateral areas of ground-glass attenuation, irregular linear opacities, and residual cystic changes (*curved arrows*). (*Courtesy of Dr. Maura Brown, Surrey Memorial Hospital, Surrey, British Columbia.*)

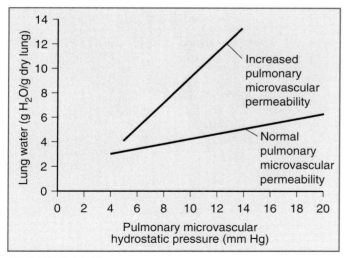

FIGURE 14–16

Lung water versus pulmonary microvascular pressure. Lung water, expressed as grams of water per gram of dry lung, is plotted against mean pulmonary microvascular pressure. When pulmonary microvascular permeability is normal, increased microvascular pressure causes a modest increase in lung water (hydrostatic edema); when microvascular permeability is increased, the same changes in pressure cause a marked accumulation of lung water.

worsening gas exchange; in the terminal stages, barotrauma and hypercapnia may develop even in the presence of enormous minute ventilation. Despite these observations, the development of multiple organ failure rather than the severity of pulmonary dysfunction appears to be a better predictor of survival.[134] For example, in one study only 40% of those who had pulmonary insufficiency alone died, whereas patients who had clinical evidence of two, three, four, or five organs affected had mortality rates of 54%, 72%, 84%, or 100%, respectively.[135] Renal failure is a particularly important complication in this regard.[136] In addition to being the most common initiator of ARDS, sepsis is also a common fatal complication; infection is most often caused by gram-negative organisms, and the most frequent sources are the lung and abdominal cavity.[137]

Patients who survive ARDS have surprisingly little long-term impairment in lung function.[138] Some have a mild restrictive impairment and gas exchange deficit,[139] whereas others have partly reversible airway obstruction.[140] Most of these abnormalities improve in the first year after ARDS; however, if deficits persist at 1 year, further improvement is unlikely.[141]

Specific Forms of Permeability Edema

High-Altitude Pulmonary Edema

In some individuals, a symptom complex known as high-altitude pulmonary edema (HAPE) can develop while at high altitude.[142] The illness may develop after both acute and prolonged exposure to an altitude of 3500 to 4000 m (11,500 to 13,000 ft).[143,144] Usually, the move from sea level to high altitude is abrupt.[145] Affected individuals are characteristically

young and otherwise healthy. The condition appears to show a predilection for former residents who are returning to high altitude after being at sea level for a few days to several weeks.[146] Other risk factors include a previous episode of HAPE, a lower than average ventilatory response to hypoxia, and higher resting pulmonary artery pressure at sea level. Physical exertion and cold weather are precipitating factors in some cases.[147]

Although the pathogenesis is uncertain, the fact that the edema usually occurs in individuals in whom an inordinate degree of pulmonary arterial hypertension develops after exposure to normally tolerable levels of hypoxia suggests that increased intravascular pressure is important.[148] On the other hand, the results of numerous studies have clearly demonstrated that increased capillary permeability is a contributing factor.[149] It is possible that hypoxia secondary to the low FIO_2 causes intense but inhomogeneous constriction of a large proportion of the pulmonary arteries, thereby forcing blood at high pressure through the remaining patent vessels. Thus, in regions where arterial constriction is deficient, there will be high flow and transmission of the increased pulmonary arterial pressure directly to the capillary bed. The high capillary pressure along with the shear stress caused by the high flow in the unconstricted areas results in pulmonary microvascular endothelial damage and permeability edema.[150]

According to this hypothesis, the inflammatory reaction, which can be seen by examination of BAL fluid,[149] represents a response to the injury caused by high pressure and flow. Some patients who die of HAPE have been found at autopsy to have thrombi in small pulmonary arteries in addition to diffuse pulmonary edema.[151] This observation, coupled with the finding of increased circulating levels of fibrinopeptide A in severe cases, raises the possibility that activation of the clotting system also plays a role in pathogenesis. However, similar to the inflammation seen on BAL, these abnormalities are more likely secondary to endothelial damage.[150]

This "mechanical" hypothesis for pulmonary capillary endothelial damage in HAPE has been strengthened by development of the concept of "stress failure" in the pulmonary capillaries.[152] The thin alveolocapillary membrane can be disrupted by capillary pressures above 30 cm H_2O.[153] When blood flow is increased, as occurs at altitude, capillary pressure becomes closer to arterial pressure,[154] and stress-related disruption of the vessels can occur. A similar mechanism has been postulated to explain the capillary damage seen in neurogenic pulmonary edema and the occasional instance of exercise-induced pulmonary hemorrhage in elite athletes.[152]

The radiographic appearances are those of acute pulmonary edema of any etiology. The consolidation tends to be most severe in the lower lobes and most commonly involves both central and peripheral lung regions.[155] On CT, the edema is patchy and predominantly peripheral in distribution.[156] Although the central pulmonary vessels may be prominent as a result of acute pulmonary hypertension, cardiac enlargement is not seen. The edema usually resolves within 1 to 2 days,[157] but it may be present for as long as 10 days.[158]

Clinical features include symptoms of "mountain sickness" (headache, giddiness, dizziness, tiredness, weakness, body aches, anorexia, nausea, vomiting, abdominal pain, insomnia, and restlessness) in addition to cough, dyspnea on exertion, and fever.[159] Cyanosis and tachycardia are common; crackles may be heard throughout the lungs. Papilledema and retinal hemorrhages indicate accompanying cerebral edema.[160] Fever occurs in about a third of patients and leukocytosis is common, ranging from 13,000/mm^3 to as high as 30,000/mm^3.[161] Symptoms develop within 12 hours to 3 days after arrival at high altitude and characteristically disappear on descent to sea level.[145]

Postpneumonectomy Pulmonary Edema

Acute pulmonary edema is an uncommon complication of lung resection, especially pneumonectomy.[162] In a study of 197 patients who underwent the procedure, it was diagnosed in 2.5%.[163] Risk factors include the use of fresh frozen plasma, high mechanical ventilation pressure, low preoperative diffusing capacity, and right pneumonectomy.[163-165]

Although fluid overload was formerly believed to be the major contributing factor, it is now clear that the edema is related to increased pulmonary capillary permeability.[166] It is possible that the mechanism is the result of stress failure of the pulmonary capillaries, as has been suggested to occur in HAPE and neurogenic pulmonary edema.[152] The combination of surgical reduction in the cross-sectional area of the pulmonary capillary bed to one half of normal, ventilation of one lung with high pressure, administration of fluid and inotropic agents, and preexisting emphysema and/or pulmonary vascular disease could interact to cause transient elevations in capillary pressure to very high levels.

Clinical and radiologic manifestations are similar to those of other forms of increased permeability edema. The complication has a very high mortality rate, in most series exceeding 80%.[163,165]

Pulmonary Edema after Lung Re-expansion

Unilateral pulmonary edema can develop after rapid removal of air or liquid from the pleural space in the presence of pneumothorax or hydrothorax.[167] Three features are common to most cases:[168] (1) the pneumothorax or hydrothorax is moderate or large in size (amounting to at least 50% of the affected hemithorax), (2) the pulmonary edema is strictly localized to the ipsilateral lung, and (3) the pneumothorax or hydrothorax has been present for a considerable period, usually several days, before rapid re-expansion.

The pathogenesis is unclear; however, increased capillary permeability appears to be involved since the condition is associated with elevated protein content of the edema fluid.[169] Possible mechanisms include (1) a sudden increase in negative intrapleural pressure transmitted to the interstitial space,[170] (2) a deficit in venous or lymphatic return caused by stasis in the pulmonary venules and lymphatics during prolonged collapse,[171] (3) an increase in alveolar surface tension after prolonged relaxation atelectasis causing a more negative interstitial pressure,[172] and (4) reperfusion injury to the pulmonary endothelium caused by the local production of toxic oxygen free radicals.

The radiographic manifestations consist of unilateral air space consolidation.[173] Although it usually affects the entire re-expanded lung, occasionally it involves only one lobe.[173] CT shows a patchy distribution of the areas of consolidation (Fig. 14-17). Resolution occurs after 5 to 7 days.

The edema usually develops immediately or within 1 hour of re-expansion and always within 24 hours.[167] The

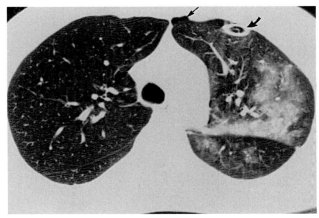

FIGURE 14–17

Re-expansion pulmonary edema. An HRCT scan in a 23-year-old man shows patchy areas of consolidation involving the left lung. Also noted are a small residual left pneumothorax (*straight arrow*) and a left chest tube (*curved arrow*) in place. Edema developed after chest tube drainage of a large left pneumothorax.

development of edema is often preceded by a feeling of tightness in the chest and by spasmodic coughing; when such symptoms develop, thoracentesis should be discontinued. Although the complication is unassociated with significant clinical consequences in most instances, severe respiratory disability can occur and fatalities have been reported.[174] It can be prevented by slow withdrawal of gas or liquid by underwater drainage.

Pulmonary Edema Associated with Severe Upper Airway Obstruction

This complication occurs exclusively in lesions affecting the extrathoracic airway from the nasopharynx to the thoracic inlet (Fig. 14–18).[175] It is often precipitated by laryngospasm, which develops especially after surgery on or near the upper airway.[176] Its pathogenesis is probably multifactorial. When significant upper airway obstruction is present, the effort to inspire is associated with an increase in negative intrathoracic pressure—in effect, a sustained Müller maneuver. This may in turn cause transudation of fluid from capillaries into the interstitium and air spaces. Cardiac "dysfunction" almost certainly contributes to development of the edema: an inspiratory effort against a severely narrowed or occluded upper airway can generate pressures of −140 cm H_2O or greater[177]; for the left side of the heart, this is analogous to adding an afterload of approximately 100 mm Hg (i.e., an increase in mean aortic pressure from 90 to 190 mm Hg). Clinical manifestations are the same as in other forms of edema. Vigorous treatment usually results in prompt resolution.[177]

Miscellaneous Causes of Permeability Edema

As indicated previously (see Table 14–2), many direct and indirect pulmonary insults have been associated with the development of ARDS.

Transfusion. The pulmonary edema that occasionally develops after blood transfusion is due to increased pulmonary vascular permeability as a result of leukoagglutinins and/or

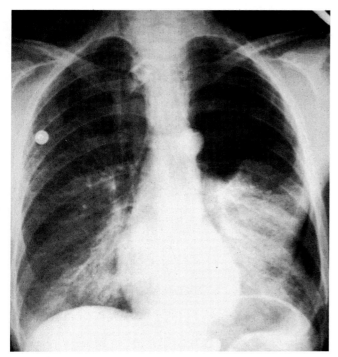

FIGURE 14–18

Acute pulmonary edema related to excessive negative intra-alveolar pressure. A 52-year-old woman was brought to the emergency department in severe respiratory distress and was found to have a huge mass (subsequently proved to be a primary carcinoma) almost completely obstructing the larynx. An emergency tracheostomy was performed. A radiograph taken shortly thereafter shows diffuse interstitial and air space pulmonary edema and a moderate-sized left pneumothorax; cardiac size and configuration are within normal limits. It is assumed that the edema resulted from prolonged, sustained negative intrathoracic pressure occasioned by the patient's attempts to inspire beyond the laryngeal obstruction—in essence a sustained Müller maneuver. The edema disappeared in less than 24 hours after tracheostomy.

human leukocyte antigen incompatibility.[178] Patients have an abrupt onset of chills, fever, tachycardia, nonproductive cough, and dyspnea; blood eosinophilia is sometimes evident. The differential diagnosis should include hemolytic transfusion reactions, anaphylaxis caused by IgA antibodies in the recipient reacting with IgA in the donor's blood (a reaction seen in patients who have IgA deficiency), hypervolemia, and bacterial sepsis.[179]

Pancreatitis. ARDS develops in a small but significant number of patients who have acute pancreatitis unassociated with other precipitating causes such as sepsis or aspiration.[180] The mechanism by which the disease causes pulmonary edema is unclear; however, it has been proposed that the pancreatic enzymes in blood may cause activation of the coagulation pathway or complement system or the generation of kinins.[181,182] It should be remembered that secondary pancreatic injury may also develop in patients who have ARDS.[183]

Fat Embolism. ARDS frequently occurs after major trauma, particularly in the presence of multiple pelvic and long-bone fractures. The contribution of fat embolism to development of the complication is often difficult to assess since patients who have such trauma are frequently hypotensive, have had

transfusions, or have sepsis, each of which is a risk factor for the development of ARDS.

Parenteral Contrast Media. Pulmonary edema has been described after parenteral administration of the oil-based medium used for lymphangiography and the water-based media used in urography, angiography, and contrast-enhanced CT.[184,185] The pathogenesis is unclear; however, it is possible that the oil microemboli are acted on by esterases in the lung, which causes a breakdown of the esterified compounds to free fatty acids and resultant pulmonary capillary damage. The onset of the edema is characteristically acute, occurring minutes to hours after the injection, and is associated with systemic hypotension.

REFERENCES

1. Taylor A, Khimenko P, Moore T, et al: Fluid balance. In Crystal R, West J (eds): The Lung: Scientific Foundations, ed 2. Philadelphia, Lippincott-Raven, 1997.
2. Matthay MA, Folkesson HG, Verkman AS: Salt and water transport across alveolar and distal airway epithelia in the adult lung. Am J Physiol 270:L487-L503, 1996.
3. Weibel ER: Morphological basis of alveolar-capillary gas exchange. Physiol Rev 53:419-495, 1973.
4. Albert R: Sites of leakage in pulmonary edema. In Said S (ed): The Pulmonary Circulation and Acute Lung Injury. New York, Futura, 1985, p 189.
5. Fishman AP: Pulmonary edema. The water-exchanging function of the lung. Circulation 46:390-408, 1972.
6. Cottrell TS, Levine OR, Senior RM, et al: Electron microscopic alterations at the alveolar level in pulmonary edema. Circ Res 21:783-797, 1967.
7. Schneeburger E: Barrier function of intercellular junctions in adult and foetal lungs. In Fishman A, Renkin E (eds): Pulmonary Edema. Baltimore, Williams & Wilkins, 1979.
8. Claude P, Goodenough DA: Fracture faces of zonulae occludentes from "tight" and "leaky" epithelia. J Cell Biol 58:390-400, 1973.
9. Brigham K: Lung edema due to increased vascular permeability. In Staub N (ed): Lung Water and Solute Exchange. New York, Marcel Dekker, 1978.
10. Bhattacharya J: Pressure-induced capillary stress failure: Is it regulated? Am J Physiol Lung Cell Mol Physiol 284:L701-L702, 2003.
11. Todd TR, Baile E, Hogg JC: Pulmonary capillary and permeability during hemorrhagic shock. J Appl Physiol 45:298-306, 1978.
12. Egan E: Effects of lung inflation on alveolar permeability to solutes. In Lung Liquids. Ciba Symposium (New Series) 38. New York, Excerpta Medica, 1976.
13. Harris TR, Roselli RJ: A theoretical model of protein, fluid, and small molecule transport in the lung. J Appl Physiol 50:1-14, 1981.
14. Gee MH, Williams DO: Effect of lung inflation on perivascular cuff fluid volume in isolated dog lung lobes. Microvasc Res 17:192-201, 1979.
15. Malo J, Ali J, Duke K, et al: Effects of PEEP on lung liquid distribution and pulmonary shunt in canine oleic acid pulmonary edema. Clin Res 28:703, 1980.
16. Staub NC, Nagano H, Pearce ML: Pulmonary edema in dogs, especially the sequence of fluid accumulation in lungs. J Appl Physiol 22:227-240, 1967.
17. Starling E: On the absorption of fluids from the connective tissue spaces. J Physiol (Lond) 19:312, 1896.
18. Staub N: Pathophysiology of pulmonary edema. In Staub N, Taylor A (eds): Edema. New York, Raven Press, 1984, p 719.
19. Staub NC: Pulmonary edema. Physiol Rev 54:678-811, 1974.
20. Bhattacharya J, Staub NC: Direct measurement of microvascular pressures in the isolated perfused dog lung. Science 210:327-328, 1980.
21. Lai-Fook SJ: Perivascular interstitial fluid pressure measured by micropipettes in isolated dog lung. J Appl Physiol 52:9-15, 1982.
22. Pritchard J: Edema of the Lung. Springfield, IL, Charles C Thomas, 1982.
23. Olver R: Ion transport and water flow in the mammalian lung. In Lung Liquids. Ciba Symposium (New Series) 38. New York, Excerpta Medica, 1976.
24. Albert RK, Lakshminarayan S, Hildebrandt J, et al: Increased surface tension favors pulmonary edema formation in anesthetized dogs' lungs. J Clin Invest 63:1015-1018, 1979.
25. Brigham KL, Woolverton WC, Staub NC: Reversible increase in pulmonary vascular permeability after *Pseudomonas aeruginosa* bacteremia in unanesthetized sheep. Chest 65(Suppl):51S-54S, 1974.
26. Sampson JJ, Leeds SE, Uhley HN, et al: Studies of lymph flow and changes in pulmonary structures as indexes of circulatory changes in experimental pulmonary edema. Isr J Med Sci 5:826-830, 1969.
27. Leeds SE, Uhley HN, Sampson JJ, et al: Significance of changes in the pulmonary lymph flow in acute and chronic experimental pulmonary edema. Am J Surg 114:254-258, 1967.
28. Casley-Smith JR: Increased initial lymphatic uptake in high-flow high-protein oedema: An additional safety factor against tissue oedema. Lymphology 24:2-6, 1991.
29. Erdmann AJ 3rd, Vaughan TR Jr, Brigham KL, et al: Effect of increased vascular pressure on lung fluid balance in unanesthetized sheep. Circ Res 37:271-284, 1975.

30. Montaner JS, Tsang J, Evans KG, et al: Alveolar epithelial damage. A critical difference between high pressure and oleic acid–induced low pressure pulmonary edema. J Clin Invest 77:1786-1796, 1986.
31. Matthay MA, Clerici C, Saumon G: Invited review: Active fluid clearance from the distal air spaces of the lung. J Appl Physiol 93:1533-1541, 2002.
32. Matthay MA: Function of the alveolar epithelial barrier under pathologic conditions. Chest 105:67S-74S, 1994.
33. Vreim CE, Snashall PD, Staub NC: Protein composition of lung fluids in anesthetized dogs with acute cardiogenic edema. Am J Physiol 231:1466-1469, 1976.
34. Ketai LH, Godwin JD: A new view of pulmonary edema and acute respiratory distress syndrome. J Thorac Imaging 13:147-171, 1998.
35. Petty TL, Ashbaugh DG: The adult respiratory distress syndrome. Clinical features, factors influencing prognosis and principles of management. Chest 60:233-239, 1971.
36. Morgan PW, Goodman LR: Pulmonary edema and adult respiratory distress syndrome. Radiol Clin North Am 29:943-963, 1991.
37. Milne E: Physiologic interpretation of the plain radiograph in mitral stenosis, including a review of the criteria for the radiologic estimation of pulmonary arterial and venous pressure. Br J Radiol 36:902, 1963.
38. McHugh TJ, Forrester JS, Adler L, et al: Pulmonary vascular congestion in acute myocardial infarction: Hemodynamic and radiologic correlations. Ann Intern Med 76:29-33, 1972.
39. Slutsky RA, Higgins CB: Intravascular and extravascular pulmonary fluid volumes II. Response to rapid increases in left atrial pressure and the theoretical implications for pulmonary radiographic and radionuclide imaging. Invest Radiol 18:33-39, 1983.
40. Dodek A, Kassebaum DG, Bristow D: Pulmonary edema in coronary-artery disease without cardiomegaly. Paradox of the stiff heart. N Engl J Med 286:1347-1350, 1972.
41. Primack SL, Remy-Jardin M, Remy J, et al: High-resolution CT of the lung: Pitfalls in the diagnosis of infiltrative lung disease. AJR Am J Roentgenol 167:413-418, 1996.
42. Goodman LR: Congestive heart failure and adult respiratory distress syndrome. New insights using computed tomography. Radiol Clin North Am 34:33-46, 1996.
43. Milne EN: Hydrostatic versus increased permeability pulmonary edema. Radiology 170:891-894, 1989.
44. Richman SM, Godar TJ: Unilateral pulmonary edema. N Engl J Med 264:1148-1149, 1961.
45. Calenoff L, Kruglik GD, Woodruff A: Unilateral pulmonary edema. Radiology 126:19-24, 1978.
46. Leeming BW: Gravitational edema of the lungs observed during assisted respiration. Chest 64:719-722, 1973.
47. Hogg JC, Agarawal JB, Gardiner AJ, et al: Distribution of airway resistance with developing pulmonary edema in dogs. J Appl Physiol 32:20-24, 1972.
48. Ewy GA: The abdominojugular test: Technique and hemodynamic correlates. Ann Intern Med 109:456-460, 1988.
49. Cooke C, Mead J, Schreiner G, et al: Pulmonary mechanics during induced pulmonary edema in anesthetized dogs. J Appl Physiol 14:17, 1964.
50. Said SI, Longacher JW Jr, Davis RK, et al: Pulmonary gas exchange during induction of pulmonary edema in anesthetized dogs. J Appl Physiol 19:403-407, 1964.
51. Fulop M, Horowitz M, Aberman A, et al: Lactic acidosis in pulmonary edema due to left ventricular failure. Ann Intern Med 79:180-186, 1973.
52. Berger M, Bach M, Hecht SR, et al: Estimation of pulmonary arterial wedge pressure by pulsed Doppler echocardiography and phonocardiography. Am J Cardiol 69:562-564, 1992.
53. de Denus S, Pharand C, Williamson DR: Brain natriuretic peptide in the management of heart failure: The versatile neurohormone. Chest 125:652-668, 2004.
54. Macpherson RI, Banerjee AK: Acute glomerulonephritis: A chest film diagnosis? J Can Assoc Radiol 25:58-64, 1974.
55. Gibson DG: Haemodynamic factors in the development of acute pulmonary oedema in renal failure. Lancet 2:1217-1220, 1966.
56. Kooman JP, Leunissen KM: Cardiovascular aspects in renal disease. Curr Opin Nephrol Hypertens 2:791-797 1993.
57. Wallin CJ, Jacobson SH, Leksell LG: Subclinical pulmonary oedema and intermittent haemodialysis. Nephrol Dial Transplant 11:2269-2275, 1996.
58. Stein L, Beraud JJ, Cavanilles J, et al: Pulmonary edema during fluid infusion in the absence of heart failure. JAMA 229:65-68, 1974.
59. O'Brien JD, Ettinger NA: Pulmonary complications of liver transplantation. Clin Chest Med 17:99-114, 1996.
60. Trewby PN, Warren R, Contini S, et al: Incidence and pathophysiology of pulmonary edema in fulminant hepatic failure. Gastroenterology 74:859-865, 1978.
61. Benowitz NL, Simon RP, Copeland JR: Status epilepticus: Divergence of sympathetic activity and cardiovascular response. Ann Neurol 19:197-199, 1986.
62. Johnston SC, Darragh TM, Simon RP: Postictal pulmonary edema requires pulmonary vascular pressure increases. Epilepsia 37:428-432, 1996.
63. Melon E, Bonnet F, Lepresle E, et al: Altered capillary permeability in neurogenic pulmonary oedema. Intensive Care Med 11:323-325, 1985.
64. Ducker TB: Increased intracranial pressure and pulmonary edema. 1. Clinical study of 11 patients. J Neurosurg 28:112-117, 1968.
65. Theodore J, Robin ED: Speculations on neurogenic pulmonary edema (NPE). Am Rev Respir Dis 113:405-411 1976.
66. Samuels MA: Neurally induced cardiac damage. Definition of the problem. Neurol Clin 11:273-292, 1993.
67. Felman AH: Neurogenic pulmonary edema. Observations in 6 patients. Am J Roentgenol Radium Ther Nucl Med 112:393-396, 1971.
68. Blennerhassett JB: Shock lung and diffuse alveolar damage; pathological and pathogenetic considerations. Pathology 17:239-247, 1985.
69. The pulmonary edema of heroin toxicity—an example of the stiff lung syndrome. Chest 62:199-205, 1972.
70. Briscoe WA, Smith JP, Bergofsky E, et al: Catastrophic pulmonary failure. Am J Med 60:248-258, 1976.
71. Bernard GR, Artigas A, Brigham KL, et al: The American-European Consensus Conference on ARDS. Definitions, mechanisms, relevant outcomes, and clinical trial coordination. Am J Respir Crit Care Med 149:818-824, 1994.
72. Villar J, Slutsky AS: The incidence of the adult respiratory distress syndrome. Am Rev Respir Dis 140:814-816, 1989.
73. Connelly KG, Repine JE: Markers for predicting the development of acute respiratory distress syndrome. Annu Rev Med 48:429-445, 1997.
74. Wittram C, Kenny JB: The admission chest radiograph after acute inhalation injury and burns. Br J Radiol 67:751-754, 1994.
75. Downey GP, Granton JT: Mechanisms of acute lung injury. Curr Opin Pulm Med 3:234-241, 1997.
76. Bone RC, Balk RA, Cerra FB, et al: Definitions for sepsis and organ failure and guidelines for the use of innovative therapies in sepsis. The ACCP/SCCM Consensus Conference Committee. American College of Chest Physicians/Society of Critical Care Medicine. Chest 101:1644-1655, 1992.
77. Montgomery AB, Stager MA, Carrico CJ, et al: Causes of mortality in patients with the adult respiratory distress syndrome. Am Rev Respir Dis 132:485-489, 1985.
78. Bone R: Toward a theory regarding the pathogenesis of the systemic inflammatory response syndrome: What we do and do not know about cytokine regulation. Crit Care Med 24:163, 1996.
79. Meyrick B, Berry LC Jr, Christman BW: Response of cultured human pulmonary artery endothelial cells to endotoxin. Am J Physiol 268:L239-244, 1995.
80. Canonico A, Brigham K: Biology of acute injury. In Crystal R, West J (eds): The Lung. Philadelphia, Lippincott-Raven, 1997, pp 2475-2498.
81. Clinton SK, Underwood R, Hayes L, et al: Macrophage colony-stimulating factor gene expression in vascular cells and in experimental and human atherosclerosis. Am J Pathol 140:301-316, 1992.
82. Springer TA: Adhesion receptors of the immune system. Nature 346:425-434, 1990.
83. Tosi MF, Stark JM, Smith CW, et al: Induction of ICAM-1 expression on human airway epithelial cells by inflammatory cytokines: Effects on neutrophil-epithelial cell adhesion. Am J Respir Cell Mol Biol 7:214-221, 1992.
84. Nicod LP: Cytokines. 1. Overview. Thorax 48:660-667, 1993.
85. Larson RS, Springer TA: Structure and function of leukocyte integrins. Immunol Rev 114:181-217, 1990.
86. Springer TA: Traffic signals for lymphocyte recirculation and leukocyte emigration: The multistep paradigm. Cell 76:301-314, 1994.
87. Tenholder MF, Rajagopal KR, Phillips YY, et al: Urinary desmosine excretion as a marker of lung injury in the adult respiratory distress syndrome. Chest 100:1385-1390, 1991.
88. Poynter SE, LeVine AM: Surfactant biology and clinical application. Crit Care Clin 19:459-472, 2003.
89. Hallman M, Spragg R, Harrell JH, et al: Evidence of lung surfactant abnormality in respiratory failure. Study of bronchoalveolar lavage phospholipids, surface activity, phospholipase activity, and plasma myoinositol. J Clin Invest 70:673-683, 1982.
90. Lewis JF, Jobe AH: Surfactant and the adult respiratory distress syndrome. Am Rev Respir Dis 147:218-233, 1993.
91. Arias-Diaz J, Vara E, Garcia C, et al: Tumor necrosis factor-alpha–induced inhibition of phosphatidylcholine synthesis by human type II pneumocytes is partially mediated by prostaglandins. J Clin Invest 94:244-250, 1994.
92. Pison U, Tam EK, Caughey GH, et al: Proteolytic inactivation of dog lung surfactant-associated proteins by neutrophil elastase. Biochim Biophys Acta 992:251-257, 1989.
93. Knudsen F, Nielsen AH, Pedersen JO, et al: Adult respiratory distress–like syndrome during hemodialysis: Relationship between activation of complement, leukopenia, and release of granulocyte elastase. Int J Artif Organs 8:187-194, 1985.
94. Lew PD, Forster A, Perrin LH, et al: Complement activation in the adult respiratory distress syndrome following cardiopulmonary bypass. Bull Eur Physiopathol Respir 21:231-235, 1985.
95. Till G, Ward P: Complement-induced lung injury. In Said S (ed): The Pulmonary Circulation and Acute Lung Injury. Mount Kisco, NY, Futura, 1985.
96. Rinaldo JE, Rogers RM: Adult respiratory distress syndrome. N Engl J Med 315:578-580, 1986.
97. Donnelly TJ, Meade P, Jagels M, et al: Cytokine, complement, and endotoxin profiles associated with the development of the adult respiratory distress syndrome after severe injury. Crit Care Med 22:768-776, 1994.
98. Idell S: Coagulation, fibrinolysis, and fibrin deposition in acute lung injury. Crit Care Med 31:S213-S220, 2003.
99. Carlson RW, Schaeffer RC Jr, Carpio M, et al: Edema fluid and coagulation changes during fulminant pulmonary edema. Chest 79:43-49, 1981.
100. Nakae H, Endo S, Inada K, et al: Significance of alpha-tocopherol and interleukin 8 in septic adult respiratory distress syndrome. Res Commun Chem Pathol Pharmacol 84:197-202, 1994.
101. Taylor A, Martin D, Townsley M: Oxygen radicals and pulmonary edema. In Said S (ed): The Pulmonary Circulation and Acute Injury. Mount Kisco, NY, Futura, 1985, p 307.
102. Mathru M, Rooney MW, Dries DJ, et al: Urine hydrogen peroxide during adult respiratory distress syndrome in patients with and without sepsis. Chest 105:232-236, 1994.

103. White C, Kumuda C: Role of cytokines in acute lung injury. In Crystal R (ed): The Lung, ed 2. Philadelphia, Lippincott-Raven, 1997, pp 2451-2464.
104. Sica A, Matsushima K, Van Damme J, et al: IL-1 transcriptionally activates the neutrophil chemotactic factor/IL-8 gene in endothelial cells. Immunology 69:548-553, 1990.
105. Miller EJ, Cohen AB, Matthay MA: Increased interleukin-8 concentrations in the pulmonary edema fluid of patients with acute respiratory distress syndrome from sepsis. Crit Care Med 24:1448-1454, 1996.
106. Dinarello CA: Interleukin-1 and its biologically related cytokines. Adv Immunol 44:153-205, 1989.
107. Gauldie J, Richards C, Harnish D, et al: Interferon beta 2/B-cell stimulatory factor type 2 shares identity with monocyte-derived hepatocyte-stimulating factor and regulates the major acute phase protein response in liver cells. Proc Natl Acad Sci U S A 84:7251-7255, 1987.
108. Seeger W, Grimminger F, Barden M, et al: Omega-oxidized leukotriene B₄ detected in the broncho-alveolar lavage fluid of patients with non-cardiogenic pulmonary edema, but not in those with cardiogenic edema. Intensive Care Med 17:1-6, 1991.
109. Blaisdell FW, Schlobohm RM: The respiratory distress syndrome: A review. Surgery 74:251-262, 1973.
110. Hasleton PS: Adult respiratory distress syndrome—a review. Histopathology 7:307-332, 1983.
111. Fukuda Y, Ishizaki M, Masuda Y, et al: The role of intraalveolar fibrosis in the process of pulmonary structural remodeling in patients with diffuse alveolar damage. Am J Pathol 126:171-182, 1987.
112. Bensadoun ES, Burke AK, Hogg JC, et al: Proteoglycan deposition in pulmonary fibrosis. Am J Respir Crit Care Med 154:1819-1828, 1996.
113. Tomashefski JF Jr, Davies P, Boggis C, et al: The pulmonary vascular lesions of the adult respiratory distress syndrome. Am J Pathol 112:112-126, 1983.
114. Ostendorf P, Birzle H, Vogel W, et al: Pulmonary radiographic abnormalities in shock. Roentgen-clinical-pathological correlation. Radiology 115:257-263, 1975.
115. Zimmerman JE, Goodman LR, Shahvari MB: Effect of mechanical ventilation and positive end-expiratory pressure (PEEP) on chest radiograph. AJR Am J Roentgenol 133:811-815, 1979.
116. Dyck DR, Zylak CJ: Acute respiratory distress in adults. Radiology 106:497-501, 1973.
117. Tagliabue M, Casella TC, Zincone GE, et al: CT and chest radiography in the evaluation of adult respiratory distress syndrome. Acta Radiol 35:230-234, 1994.
118. Gattinoni L, Bombino M, Pelosi P, et al: Lung structure and function in different stages of severe adult respiratory distress syndrome. JAMA 271:1772-1779, 1994.
119. Gattinoni L, D'Andrea L, Pelosi P, et al: Regional effects and mechanism of positive end-expiratory pressure in early adult respiratory distress syndrome. JAMA 269:2122-2127, 1993.
120. Hudson LD, Milberg JA, Anardi D, et al: Clinical risks for development of the acute respiratory distress syndrome. Am J Respir Crit Care Med 151:293-301, 1995.
121. Roumen RM, Redl H, Schlag G, et al: Scoring systems and blood lactate concentrations in relation to the development of adult respiratory distress syndrome and multiple organ failure in severely traumatized patients. J Trauma 35:349-355, 1993.
122. Ralph DD, Robertson HT, Weaver LJ, et al: Distribution of ventilation and perfusion during positive end-expiratory pressure in the adult respiratory distress syndrome. Am Rev Respir Dis 131:54-60, 1985.
123. Wiener CM, Kirk W, Albert RK: Prone position reverses gravitational distribution of perfusion in dog lungs with oleic acid–induced injury. J Appl Physiol 68:1386-1392, 1990.
124. Macnaughton PD, Evans TW: Measurement of lung volume and DLCO in acute respiratory failure. Am J Respir Crit Care Med 150:770-775, 1994.
125. Pesenti A, Pelosi P, Rossi N, et al: Respiratory mechanics and bronchodilator responsiveness in patients with the adult respiratory distress syndrome. Crit Care Med 21:78-83, 1993.
126. Kariman K, Burns SR: Regulation of tissue oxygen extraction is disturbed in adult respiratory distress syndrome. Am Rev Respir Dis 132:109-114, 1985.
127. Zapol WM, Snider MT: Pulmonary hypertension in severe acute respiratory failure. N Engl J Med 296:476-480, 1977.
128. Sibbald WJ, Driedger AA, Cunningham DG, et al: Right and left ventricular performance in acute hypoxemic respiratory failure. Crit Care Med 14:852-857, 1986.
129. Toussaint GP, Burgess JH, Hampson LG: Central venous pressure and pulmonary wedge pressure in critical surgical illness. A comparison. Arch Surg 109:265-269, 1974.
130. Cope DK, Grimbert F, Downey JM, et al: Pulmonary capillary pressure: A review. Crit Care Med 20:1043-1056, 1992.
131. Sandham JD, Hull RD, Brant RF, et al: A randomized, controlled trial of the use of pulmonary-artery catheters in high-risk surgical patients. N Engl J Med 348:5-14, 2003.
132. Connors AF Jr, Speroff T, Dawson NV, et al: The effectiveness of right heart catheterization in the initial care of critically ill patients. SUPPORT Investigators. JAMA 276:889-897, 1996.
133. Lee J, Turner JS, Morgan CJ, et al: Adult respiratory distress syndrome: Has there been a change in outcome predictive measures? Thorax 49:596-597, 1994.
134. Fowler AA, Hamman RF, Good JT, et al: Adult respiratory distress syndrome: Risk with common predispositions. Ann Intern Med 98:593-597, 1983.
135. Bartlett RH, Morris AH, Fairley HB, et al: A prospective study of acute hypoxic respiratory failure. Chest 89:684-689, 1986.
136. Gillespie DJ, Marsh HM, Divertie MB, et al: Clinical outcome of respiratory failure in patients requiring prolonged (greater than 24 hours) mechanical ventilation. Chest 90:364-369, 1986.
137. Seidenfeld JJ, Pohl DF, Bell RC, et al: Incidence, site, and outcome of infections in patients with the adult respiratory distress syndrome. Am Rev Respir Dis 134:12-16, 1986.
138. Towne BH, Lott IT, Hicks DA, et al: Long-term follow-up of infants and children treated with extracorporeal membrane oxygenation (ECMO): A preliminary report. J Pediatr Surg 20:410-414, 1985.
139. Elliott CG, Morris AH, Cengiz M: Pulmonary function and exercise gas exchange in survivors of adult respiratory distress syndrome. Am Rev Respir Dis 123:492-495, 1981.
140. Simpson DL, Goodman M, Spector SL, et al: Long-term follow-up and bronchial reactivity testing in survivors of the adult respiratory distress syndrome. Am Rev Respir Dis 117:449-454, 1978.
141. Hert R, Albert RK: Sequelae of the adult respiratory distress syndrome. Thorax 49:8-13, 1994.
142. Wilson R: Acute high-altitude illness in mountaineers and problems of rescue. Ann Intern Med 78:421-428, 1973.
143. Kamat SR, Banerji BC: Study of cardiopulmonary function on exposure to high altitude. I. Acute acclimatization to an altitude of 3,500 to 4,000 meters in relation to altitude sickness and cardiopulmonary function. Am Rev Respir Dis 106:404-413, 1972.
144. Kamat SR, Rao TL, Sarma BS, et al: Study of cardiopulmonary function on exposure to high altitude. II. Effects of prolonged stay at 3,500 to 4,000 meters and reversal on return to sea level. Am Rev Respir Dis 106:414-431, 1972.
145. Menon ND: High-altitude pulmonary edema: A clinical study. N Engl J Med 273:66-73, 1965.
146. Viswanathan R, Jain SK, Subramanian S, et al: Pulmonary edema of high altitude. II. Clinical, aerohemodynamic, and biochemical studies in a group with history of pulmonary edema of high altitude. Am Rev Respir Dis 100:334-341, 1969.
147. Singh I, Kapila CC, Khanna PK, et al: High-altitude pulmonary oedema. Lancet 191:229-234, 1965.
148. Hackett PH, Roach RC, Schoene RB, et al: Abnormal control of ventilation in high-altitude pulmonary edema. J Appl Physiol 64:1268-1272, 1988.
149. Hultgren HN: High-altitude pulmonary edema: Current concepts. Ann Rev Med 47:267-284, 1996.
150. Hultgren HN: High altitude pulmonary edema: Hemodynamic aspects. Int J Sports Med 18:20-25, 1997.
151. Hultgren H, Spickard W, Lopez C: Further studies of high altitude pulmonary oedema. Br Heart J 24:95-102, 1962.
152. West J, Mathieu-Costello O: Stress failure of pulmonary capillaries. In Crystal R, West J (eds): The Lung. Philadelphia, Lippincott-Raven, 1997, pp 1493-1501.
153. Costello ML, Mathieu-Costello O, West JB: Stress failure of alveolar epithelial cells studied by scanning electron microscopy. Am Rev Respir Dis 145:1446-1455, 1992.
154. Younes M, Bshouty Z, Ali J: Longitudinal distribution of pulmonary vascular resistance with very high pulmonary blood flow. J Appl Physiol 62:344-358, 1987.
155. Vock P, Brutsche MH, Nanzer A, et al: Variable radiomorphologic data of high altitude pulmonary edema. Features from 60 patients. Chest 100:1306-1311, 1991.
156. Bartsch P: High altitude pulmonary edema. Respiration 64:435-443, 1997.
157. Colice GL, Matthay MA, Bass E, et al: Neurogenic pulmonary edema. Am Rev Respir Dis 130:941-948, 1984.
158. Im JG, Yu YJ, Ahn JM, et al: Hydrostatic versus oleic acid–induced pulmonary edema: High-resolution computed tomography findings in the pig lung. Acad Radiol 1:364-372, 1994.
159. Maggiorini M, Bartsch P, Oelz O: Association between raised body temperature and acute mountain sickness: Cross sectional study. BMJ 315:403-404, 1997.
160. Kobayashi T, Koyama S, Kubo K, et al: Clinical features of patients with high-altitude pulmonary edema in Japan. Chest 92:814-821, 1987.
161. Kleiner JP, Nelson WP: High altitude pulmonary edema. A rare disease? JAMA 234:491-495, 1975.
162. Kopec SE, Irwin RS, Umali-Torres CB, et al: The postpneumonectomy state. Chest 114:1158-1184, 1998.
163. van der Werff YD, van der Houwen HK, Heijmans PJ, et al: Postpneumonectomy pulmonary edema. A retrospective analysis of incidence and possible risk factors. Chest 111:1278-1284, 1997.
164. Dong S, Paré P: Postpneumonectomy pulmonary edema and cardiac dysrhythmias are the major cause of postoperative mortality and morbidity. Am J Respir Crit Care Med 147:A740, 1993.
165. Turnage WS, Lunn JJ: Postpneumonectomy pulmonary edema. A retrospective analysis of associated variables. Chest 103:1646-1650, 1993.
166. Williams EA, Evans TW, Goldstraw P: Acute lung injury following lung resection: Is one lung anaesthesia to blame? Thorax 51:114-116, 1996.
167. Mahfood S, Hix WR, Aaron BL, et al: Reexpansion pulmonary edema. Ann Thorac Surg 45:340-345, 1988.
168. Waqaruddin M, Bernstein A: Re-expansion pulmonary oedema. Thorax 30:54-60, 1975.
169. Buczko GB, Grossman RF, Goldberg M: Re-expansion pulmonary edema: Evidence for increased capillary permeability. Can Med Assoc J 125:460-461, 1981.
170. Humphreys RL, Berne AS: Rapid re-expansion of pneumothorax. A cause of unilateral pulmonary edema. Radiology 96:509-512, 1970.
171. Rigler L: Pulmonary edema. Semin Roentgenol 2:33, 1967.
172. Ratliff JL, Chavez CM, Jamchuk A, et al: Re-expansion pulmonary edema. Chest 64:654-656, 1973.
173. Tarver RD, Broderick LS, Conces DJ Jr: Reexpansion pulmonary edema. J Thorac Imaging 11:198-209, 1996.
174. Olcott EW: Fatal reexpansion pulmonary edema following pleural catheter placement. J Vasc Interv Radiol 5:176-178, 1994.

175. Pacley SP, Downes MO: Case report: Pulmonary oedema secondary to laryngospasm following general anaesthesia. Br J Radiol 67:654-655, 1994.
176. Ingrams D, Burton M, Goodwin A, et al: Acute pulmonary oedema complicating laryngospasm. J Laryngol Otol 111:482-484, 1997.
177. Goldenberg JD, Portugal LG, Wenig BL, et al: Negative-pressure pulmonary edema in the otolaryngology patient. Otolaryngol Head Neck Surg 117:62-66, 1997.
178. Jeter EK, Spivey MA: Noninfectious complications of blood transfusion. Hematol Oncol Clin North Am 9:187-204, 1995.
179. Virchis AE, Patel RK, Contreras M, et al: Lesson of the week. Acute non-cardiogenic lung oedema after platelet transfusion. BMJ 314:880-882, 1997.
180. Renner IG, Savage WT 3rd, Pantoja JL, et al: Death due to acute pancreatitis. A retrospective analysis of 405 autopsy cases. Dig Dis Sci 30:1005-1018, 1985.
181. Satake K, Rozmanith JS, Appert H, et al: Hemodynamic change and bradykinin levels in plasma and lymph during experimental acute pancreatitis in dogs. Ann Surg 178:659-662, 1973.
182. Minta JO, Man D, Movat HZ: Kinetic studies on the fragmentation of the third component of complement (C3) by trypsin. J Immunol 118:2192-2198, 1977.
183. Nicod L, Leuenberger P, Seydoux C, et al: Evidence for pancreas injury in adult respiratory distress syndrome. Am Rev Respir Dis 131:696-699, 1985.
184. Boden WE: Anaphylactoid pulmonary edema ("shock lung") and hypotension after radiologic contrast media injection. Chest 81:759-761, 1982.
185. Bouachour G, Varache N, Szapiro N, et al: Noncardiogenic pulmonary edema resulting from intravascular administration of contrast material. AJR Am J Roentgenol 157:255-256, 1991.

DISEASE OF THE AIRWAYS

This chapter is concerned with a variety of lung diseases that are grouped together because of their common characteristic of obstruction of the airways. Such obstruction may be acute or chronic, and acute episodes may be isolated or recurrent; obstruction can occur in either the upper or the lower airways, and in the latter site it may be local or diffuse.

The designation "chronic obstructive pulmonary disease" is frequently used in association with patients who have persistent diffuse lower airway obstruction. In its broadest sense, this term is applied to those who have chronic bronchitis with airway narrowing, intractable asthma, emphysema, bronchiectasis, cystic fibrosis, or a combination of these disorders. However, COPD is also frequently used in a narrower sense to refer to irreversible obstruction to expiratory flow predominantly attributable to cigarette smoking. This obstruction is related to a combination of loss of lung elasticity and narrowing of the membranous and respiratory bronchioles. For the most part, use of the term COPD in this chapter refers to this more restrictive definition.

OBSTRUCTIVE DISEASE OF THE UPPER AIRWAYS

The upper airway extends from the external nares (during nose breathing) or the lips (during mouth breathing) to the tracheal carina. Although the clinical manifestations of obstruction of this passage are usually sufficiently distinctive to permit prompt and accurate recognition, an appreciable number of cases are misdiagnosed.

The most important considerations in diagnosis are a high index of suspicion and the appropriate application of specific physiologic, bronchoscopic, and radiologic tests.[1]

General Considerations

Physiologic Findings

An excellent method of portraying how physiologic determinants of flow can be affected by various obstructing lesions of the conducting system is the flow-volume loop, which combines maximal expiratory and inspiratory curves from total lung capacity (TLC) and residual volume (RV), respectively (Fig. 15–1). In normal individuals, the maximal, or peak, expiratory flow rate (PEFR) occurs early in forced expiration, and the flow ratio between expiratory and inspiratory limbs at mid–vital capacity (50% VC) is approximately 1.[2] In asthma, COPD, and other conditions that cause diffuse lower airway obstruction, peak expiratory flow is decreased less than flow at lower lung volumes, and expiratory flow is decreased much more than inspiratory flow, so the mid-VC expiratory-inspiratory ratio is usually less than 0.5 (see Fig. 15–1). By contrast, in upper airway obstruction, flow is decreased to approximately the same extent throughout the forced VC (FVC), and there tends to be a plateau in one or both segments of the flow-volume curve.

The dynamic effects of lesions of the upper airway depend in part on the extent to which the obstruction is "fixed" or "variable." In "fixed" obstruction, the airway is unable to change cross-sectional area in response to transmural pressure differences. By contrast, in "variable" obstruction—a situation that occurs most often with neoplasms that arise from the airway wall and create a crescentic lumen—the airway is able to respond to transmural pressure, thus permitting a variable cross-sectional area throughout the forced ventilatory maneuver. Characteristic flow-volume loop patterns are produced by fixed and variable lesions (see Fig. 15–1). Since fixed upper airway obstruction, either intrathoracic or extrathoracic, is not influenced by transmural pressure gradients, both inspiratory flow and expiratory flow are proportionately lowered.

When a lesion is variable, however, its location within or outside the thorax becomes important. During *inspiration*, the extrathoracic airway has a transmural pressure favoring narrowing because intraluminal pressure is subatmospheric while extraluminal pressure is approximately atmospheric. During *expiration*, intraluminal pressure is positive relative to extraluminal pressure, thus tending to dilate the airway and obscure the presence of the lesion. Consequently, a variable extrathoracic lesion tends to cause a predominant decrease in maximal inspiratory flow and has relatively little effect on maximal expiratory flow.[3]

This situation is reversed when a variable lesion is intrathoracic in location. During *inspiration*, extraluminal pressure (equivalent to pleural pressure) is negative relative to intraluminal pressure, so transmural pressure favors airway dilation. By contrast, during *expiration*, extraluminal pressure is positive relative to intraluminal pressure, so airway narrowing occurs. Thus, a variable intrathoracic lesion results in a predominant reduction in maximal expiratory flow with relative preservation of maximal inspiratory flow (see Fig. 15–1).[3]

In addition to flow-volume curve abnormalities, periodic flow oscillations caused by fluttering of upper airway structures, either passively or as a result of periodic muscle contraction, may be an important indicator of an abnormality in control of upper airway caliber in neuromuscular disease.[4] Such oscillations are also seen in some patients who have obstructive sleep apnea.[5]

A comparison of FEV_1 and midexpiratory phase flow ($FEF_{25\%-75\%}$) may be useful in detecting upper airway obstruction when flow-volume loops are not available. In the absence of airflow obstruction, the numerical values of FEV_1 and $FEF_{25\%-75\%}$ are roughly comparable; however, as lower airway obstruction develops (e.g., in asthma or COPD), $FEF_{25\%-75\%}$ becomes disproportionately lowered. In upper airway obstruction, FEV_1 is decreased to the same extent as $FEF_{25\%-75\%}$.[6] Despite considerable obstruction, patients with upper airway lesions often have normal diffusing capacity and no response to bronchodilators.[7]

Radiologic Manifestations

Plain radiography plays a limited role in the assessment of patients who have pharyngeal or laryngeal abnormalities. The main exception is the use of lateral radiographs of the soft tissues of the neck in the evaluation of patients suspected of having acute epiglottitis, retropharyngeal abscess, or foreign body obstruction. Imaging of intrinsic abnormalities of the pharynx and larynx is better performed with CT or MR imaging.[8,9]

The initial radiologic examination in patients suspected of having a tracheal abnormality usually consists of standard frontal and lateral chest radiographs.[10] Adequate visualization of the trachea, mediastinum, and lungs requires the use of high (120 to 150) kilovolts (peak). Unfortunately, the trachea

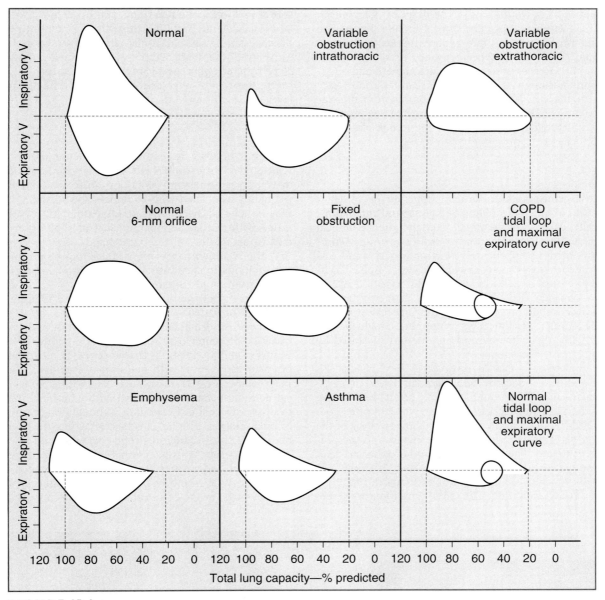

FIGURE 15-1

Flow-volume loops of various obstructive conditions. Volume is given as a percentage of predicted TLC. The bottom two curves on the *right* show a tidal flow-volume loop and a complete maximal expiratory flow-volume curve in a patient with COPD and a normal subject. There is considerable reserve for increased expiratory flow in the normal person; however, in the patient with COPD, the tidal loop is superimposed on the maximal expiratory curve. *(Modified from Miller RD, Hyatt RE: Obstructing lesions of the larynx and trachea: Clinical and physiologic characteristics. Mayo Clin Proc 44:145-161, 1969.)*

is all too often a "blind spot" for the radiologist, a deficiency that can be corrected only by paying particular attention to this region. CT, especially spiral CT, allows assessment of the location and extent of tracheal obstruction, as well as the presence of mediastinal involvement. The use of volume-rendered three-dimensional images improves recognition of early tracheal abnormalities not readily apparent on conventional cross-sectional images.[11]

Clinical Manifestations

The symptoms and signs of upper airway obstruction vary with the nature of the underlying lesion, its location, and to

some extent the age of the patient. As might be expected, the major complaint is dyspnea, either during exercise or at rest, depending on the severity of obstruction. Stridor may also be noted either at rest or during exercise, and its timing may be inspiratory, expiratory, or both. Nonproductive cough is common.

Acute Upper Airway Obstruction

Because of the small intraluminal caliber and greater compliance of their upper airways, disorders that cause acute upper airway obstruction occur most commonly in infants and young children. The sudden onset of dyspnea, hoarseness, and stridor is the most frequent clinical manifestation. The cause of the obstruction is often apparent from the history. For example, fever and cough are usually present with infections and previous episodes of obstruction with angioneurotic edema. Although the radiologic manifestations vary according to the specific etiology, the combination of relatively small lung volumes and dilation of the airway proximal to the site of obstruction should alert the radiologist to the diagnosis.[12]

Infection

A variety of organisms can cause acute upper airway obstruction as a result of mucosal swelling by edema fluid and inflammatory cells or an intraluminal exudate after epithelial ulceration. Acute pharyngitis and tonsillitis are most commonly associated with β-hemolytic streptococci[13] and less often with adenoviruses and coxsackieviruses.[14,15] Acute laryngotracheitis (croup) is caused most often by parainfluenza or respiratory syncytial virus and results in a characteristic narrowing of the subglottic trachea; staphylococcal tracheitis can closely simulate it clinically.[16] Whooping cough may be associated with upper airway obstruction and is caused by *Bordetella pertussis* and adenovirus.[17]

Acute epiglottitis is caused most often by *Haemophilus influenzae* and occasionally by *Staphylococcus aureus* or *Streptococcus pneumoniae*.[18] Although it usually affects infants and young children, it also occurs in adults, in whom it often goes unrecognized.[19] Radiographic findings include swelling of the epiglottis, aryepiglottic folds, arytenoids, uvula, and the prevertebral soft tissues. The hypopharynx and oropharynx tend to be ballooned and the valleculae obliterated. Narrowing of the subglottic trachea, simulating croup, occurs in roughly a quarter of affected children.[20] The initial symptoms are severe

sore throat, difficulty breathing, and hoarseness; stridor may be present. Acute bacterial tracheitis is a rare but potentially life-threatening cause of upper airway obstruction.[21]

Many of the abnormalities just described can be complicated by a retropharyngeal abscess, which in turn can result in severe upper airway obstruction in both infants and adults (Fig. 15–2).

Edema

As a cause of acute upper airway obstruction, non–infection-related edema most often affects the larynx. It can be caused by trauma or inhalation of irritant noxious gases but is most frequently associated with angioneurotic edema.[22] The latter may be allergic, hereditary, or idiopathic and is often associated with pruritic, nonpainful foci of swelling in the subcutaneous tissues of the face, hands, feet, and genitalia; urticaria is sometimes seen. An attack may be precipitated by certain foods, inhaled substances, bee stings, or drugs (including aspirin and angiotensin-converting enzyme [ACE] inhibitors)[23]; however, the precise etiology is identified in less than 20% of patients. The hereditary form is associated with absence or abnormal function of an inhibitor of the first component of complement (C1 esterase inhibitor). It usually begins in childhood and is characterized by recurrent attacks, often in association with abdominal cramps.[24] The attacks may follow local trauma, such as tonsillectomy or tooth extraction, or may be associated with emotional upsets. The disorder can be life-threatening, although long-term prophylactic measures can be effective[24]; the prognosis for non-hereditary chronic angioneurotic edema is good.[25]

Edema resulting from thermal injury to the upper airway is common and responsible for many fire-related deaths.[26] Singed nasal hairs and hoarseness provide clues to the diagnosis, which can be confirmed with inspiratory and expira-

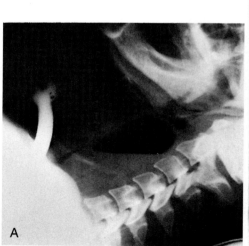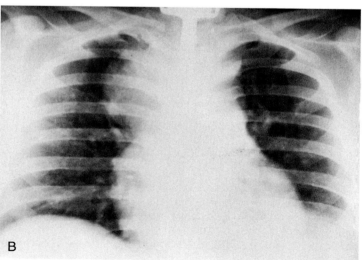

FIGURE 15–2

Acute retropharyngeal and mediastinal abscess. A 29-year-old woman was admitted to the hospital with an 8-day history of increasing dyspnea, difficulty swallowing, and loss of voice. An emergency tracheostomy was performed. A lateral radiograph of the soft tissues of the neck with a horizontal x-ray beam (**A**) reveals a large accumulation of gas and fluid in the retropharyngeal space associated with complete obliteration of the air space of the hypopharynx and anterior displacement of the cervical trachea. An anteroposterior (**B**) radiograph shows a large mediastinal mass projecting predominantly to the right of midline. (*From Fraser RS, Müller NL, Colman NC, Paré PD: Fraser and Paré's Diagnosis of Diseases of the Chest, 4th ed. Philadelphia, WB Saunders, 1999.*)

tory flow-volume curves and fiberoptic laryngoscopy[27]; tracheal stenosis as a result of mucosal fibrosis may also occur months after the initial injury.[28]

Retropharyngeal Hemorrhage

Acute upper airway obstruction from hemorrhage into the retropharyngeal space can be associated with a variety of causes, including neck surgery, external trauma, carotid angiography, transbrachial retrograde catheterization, and erosion of an artery secondary to infection or rupture of an aneurysm.[29,30] Hemorrhage can also occur spontaneously in patients who have hematologic disorders, such as hemophilia or acute leukemia, or in those receiving anticoagulant therapy.[31,32]

Foreign Body Aspiration

Airway obstruction by foreign bodies occurs most frequently in infants and young children and tends to affect the major bronchi much more commonly than the upper airway (see page 744). The objects most frequently aspirated are food particles such as peanuts. In adults, larger bodies such as partially masticated pieces of meat may obstruct the larynx ("café coronary" syndrome) and cause death rapidly (Fig. 15–3). Large foreign bodies within the esophagus can also cause acute obstruction by pressure on the adjacent airway.[33]

Faulty Placement of an Endotracheal Tube

This problem occurs most commonly in the right main bronchus.[34] The radiographic findings are typical and consist of visualization of the tube in a main bronchus and atelecta-sis of the contralateral lung as a result of complete obstruction of its main bronchus. Clinically, the examining physician should not be misled by hearing breath sounds transmitted from the normal or overinflated contralateral lung through the collapsed lung.

Chronic Upper Airway Obstruction

In contrast to acute upper airway obstruction, in which the cause is often apparent, chronic obstructive disease is frequently misdiagnosed as asthma or COPD. Dyspnea is the usual initial complaint, although an insidious onset of cor pulmonale or sleep disturbance can occur. A great variety of conditions are responsible (Table 15–1).

Hypertrophy of the Tonsils and Adenoids

Hypertrophy of the palatine tonsils sufficient to cause airway obstruction occurs chiefly in children.[35] Though uncommon, alveolar hypoventilation with resultant hypoxia, hypercapnia, and pulmonary arterial hypertension and cor pulmonale may be seen.[36] The characteristic radiographic appearance is that of a smooth, well-defined, elliptical soft tissue mass extending downward from the soft palate into the hypopharynx; hypertrophy of the nasopharyngeal adenoids is commonly associated.

Thyroid Disease

Goiter is a relatively common cause of upper airway obstruction and can be diagnosed by using flow-volume curves, CT,

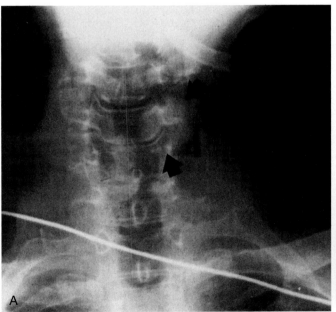
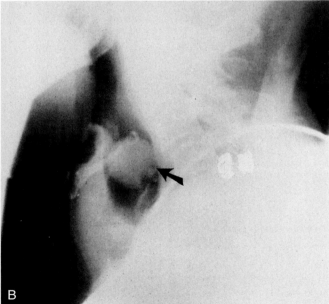

FIGURE 15–3

Acute upper airway obstruction caused by a foreign body. A radiograph of the neck in anteroposterior projection (**A**) reveals a grape-sized opacity (*arrows*) situated in the region of the left piriform sinus immediately above the false vocal cords. The object can be seen with greater clarity (*arrow*) on a detail lateral view of the soft tissues of the neck (**B**). This 71-year-old woman presented in acute respiratory distress; she was cyanotic and stuporous. Direct laryngoscopy revealed a grape, removal of which resulted in prompt improvement. (*Courtesy of Dr. John Fleetham, University of British Columbia, Vancouver.*)

TABLE 15–1. Selected Causes of Chronic Upper Airway Obstruction

Infection
Chronic granulomatous infection with *Klebsiella rhinoscleromatis* Laryngotracheal papillomatosis
Ectopic Tissue
Endotracheal thymus or thyroid Lingual thyroid
Neoplasms
Primary Neoplasms
Tracheobronchial squamous cell carcinoma Tracheobronchial gland neoplasms Plasmacytoma Lymphoma Kaposi's sarcoma
Metastatic Carcinoma
Direct Extension of Neoplasm
Thyroid carcinoma Esophageal carcinoma
Cysts
Thyroglossal duct cyst Mediastinal bronchogenic cyst Laryngoceles
Musculoskeletal Abnormalities
Ankylosis of the cricoarytenoid joint in rheumatoid arthritis Temporomandibular joint ankylosis Cervical osteophytes Ankylosing spondylitis of the cervical spine
Metabolic Abnormalities
Acromegaly (macroglossia and pharyngeal soft tissue hypertrophy) Amyloidosis Mucopolysaccharidosis
Immunologic Abnormalities
Wegener's granulomatosis Ulcerative colitis Relapsing polychondritis
Vascular Abnormalities
Right-sided aortic arch Aberrant subclavian, innominate, or common carotid artery Pulmonary artery sling Aortic aneurysm
Trauma
Postintubation tracheal fibrosis

MR imaging, or ultrasound.[37-39] Riedel's thyroiditis, thyroid cancer, and ectopic intratracheal thyroid tissue are additional uncommon causes.[40,41]

Laryngeal Dysfunction

Laryngeal dysfunction, caused by either decreased activity of dilating muscle groups or increased activity of constricting ones, can result in either acute or chronic airway obstruction.[42]

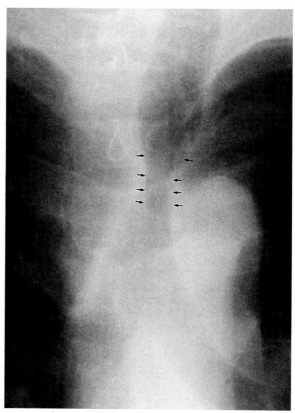

FIGURE 15–4

Tracheal stenosis after intubation. A view of the trachea from a posteroanterior chest radiograph demonstrates focal circumferential tracheal narrowing (*arrows*). (*From Fraser RS, Müller NL, Colman NC, Paré PD: Fraser and Paré's Diagnosis of Diseases of the Chest, 4th ed. Philadelphia, WB Saunders, 1999.*)

Specific causes include neuromuscular disease, such as Parkinson's disease and myasthenia gravis,[43,44] and inadvertent surgical interruption of the laryngeal nerves.[45] Vocal cord paralysis predominantly affects inspiratory flow. Paradoxical expiratory glottic narrowing and episodic psychogenic stridor caused by adduction of the vocal cords during inspiration can be confused with organic obstruction.[46,47]

Tracheal Stenosis

One of the most common causes of chronic upper airway obstruction is tracheal stenosis after intubation or tracheostomy.[48] It occurs most often at the site of the stoma or the inflatable cuff. The mechanism in the latter situation is compression of the tracheal mucosa between the cuff's balloon and the underlying cartilage and subsequent mucosal necrosis and eventual fibrosis and/or destruction of the cartilaginous support.[49] The radiographic appearance includes circumferential narrowing of the tracheal lumen (Fig. 15–4) or a thin membrane or thickened, eccentric opacity within its lumen.[50] Optimal assessment requires the use of spiral CT (Fig. 15–5).[51]

Clinically, most patients are symptom free for a variable period after removal of the tracheostomy tube. Eventually, there is increasing difficulty in raising secretions and shortness of breath on exertion. These symptoms may progress to stridor and marked dyspnea on minimal exertion.[50]

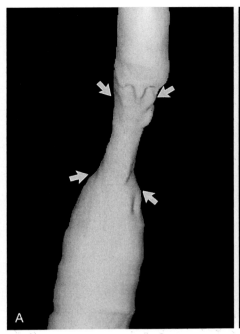
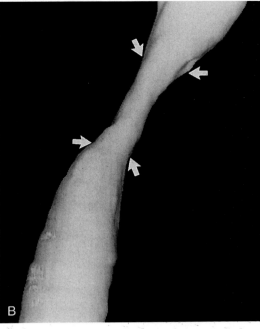

FIGURE 15–5

Post-tracheotomy tracheal stenosis. Three-dimensional reconstructions from spiral CT in anteroposterior (**A**) and lateral (**B**) projections demonstrate tracheal stenosis (between *arrows*). The reconstructions were performed with a surface-shading technique. *(Courtesy of Dr. Martine Remy-Jardin, Centre Hospitalier Regional et Universitaire de Lille, Lille, France.)*

Tracheal Neoplasms

The trachea is a rare site of primary cancer. Squamous cell carcinoma and adenocystic carcinoma account for the vast majority (see page 371). The tumors are usually manifested radiologically as an intraluminal nodule with smooth, irregular, or lobulated margins or as an eccentric or circumferential thickening of the tracheal wall associated with narrowing of its lumen.[52] Spiral CT and MR imaging are helpful in assessing their extent.[53,54] Patients often give a history of treatment of asthma for a considerable period before the correct diagnosis is made. Dyspnea, hoarseness, cough, and wheeze are common; hemoptysis may also occur. A characteristic wheeze (stridor) may be heard with or without a stethoscope placed over the trachea. The timing of the stridor is characteristically inspiratory with extrathoracic lesions and expiratory with intrathoracic lesions.

"Saber Sheath" Trachea

The coronal and sagittal diameters of the tracheal air column are usually roughly equal. A "saber sheath" trachea is characterized by a markedly reduced coronal diameter and an increased sagittal diameter confined to the intrathoracic portion (Fig. 15–6).[55] The majority of affected patients are smokers with COPD[56] and physiologic evidence of lower rather than upper airway obstruction. It remains unclear whether the abnormality is a result or a cause of airflow obstruction.[57]

Relapsing Polychondritis

This uncommon disease affects cartilage in many sites throughout the body, including the ribs, ear lobes, nose, central and peripheral joints, and tracheobronchial tree (see page 494).[58] Obstructive effects on the major airways may be fixed or variable.[59] Variable effects are caused by increased compliance as a result of cartilage destruction and lead to airway collapse on expiration. Involvement of the airway can be rapidly progressive and severe and is the most common cause of death.[60] Because a beneficial effect of corticosteroid therapy has been reported, prompt recognition and institution of therapy are important.[61] The typical radiographic finding consists of diffuse circumferential narrowing of the trachea and main bronchi[62]; CT also demonstrates mild circumferential thickening of their walls (Fig. 15–7).[63,64]

Tracheobronchopathia Osteochondroplastica

Tracheobronchopathia osteochondroplastica is a rare condition characterized by nodules of cartilage and bone in the mucosa of the trachea and bronchi.[65] In most cases, it is identified as an incidental finding at autopsy or during bronchoscopy.[66,67] The cause is uncertain; however, it has been speculated to be an end stage of amyloidosis or to represent enchondroses arising from the tracheobronchial cartilage rings.[68,69] The nodules appear as numerous sessile polyps that give the trachea and bronchi a beaded appearance at both autopsy and bronchoscopy.

The typical radiographic manifestation is nodular or irregular thickening of the tracheal and bronchial walls (Fig. 15–8).[70] CT also shows nodular thickening resulting in undulating narrowing of the airway lumen (Fig. 15–9).[71] Most patients do not have symptoms because the degree of osteochondromatous proliferation is insufficient to cause clinically significant airway narrowing. Occasionally, there is dyspnea, hoarseness, cough, expectoration, wheezing, or hemoptysis.[72] The diagnosis can be made at bronchoscopy, the spicule-like formations of bone and cartilage producing a grating sensation as the instrument is passed.

Tracheomalacia

Tracheomalacia is characterized by a weakness of the tracheal wall and supporting cartilage with resultant easy collapsibility.[73] It may be accompanied by tracheomegaly. Causes

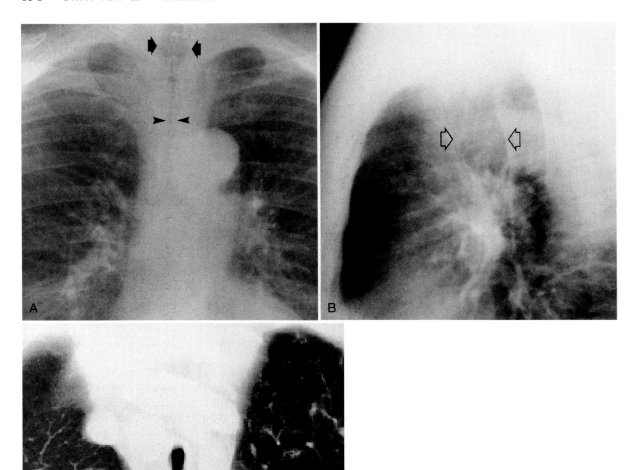

FIGURE 15–6

Saber sheath trachea. Views of posteroanterior (**A**) and lateral (**B**) chest radiographs reveal severe narrowing of the intrathoracic trachea in the coronal plane (*arrowheads*) and widening in the sagittal plane (*open arrows*). Note that the extrathoracic trachea (*arrows*) is normal, the narrowing beginning at the thoracic inlet. **C,** A CT scan from another patient demonstrates narrowing of the coronal diameter and an increase in sagittal diameter of the trachea. Emphysema and a 2-cm-diameter left upper lobe nodule (subsequently shown to be pulmonary carcinoma) are also evident. (*From Fraser RS, Müller NL, Colman NC, Paré PD: Fraser and Paré's Diagnosis of Diseases of the Chest, 4th ed. Philadelphia, WB Saunders, 1999.*)

include necrosis of cartilage following intubation, congenital abnormality of cartilage rings, thyroid enlargement, vascular malformations, trauma, chronic or recurrent infection, radiation therapy, and relapsing polychondritis.[74] The abnormal flaccidity is associated with inefficiency of the cough mechanism and thus results in retention of mucus, recurrent pneumonitis, and bronchiectasis. Symptoms include stridor and shortness of breath. In both tracheomalacia and tracheobronchomegaly, radiologic studies reveal dilation of the conducting airways during inspiration and their premature collapse during expiration.[73] Expiratory CT is the imaging modality of choice for definitive assessment.[75]

Tracheobronchomegaly

Tracheobronchomegaly (Mounier-Kuhn syndrome) is characterized by dilation of the tracheobronchial tree that may extend all the way from the larynx to the periphery of the lung.[76] Although the etiology is unclear, its association with connective tissue disorders such as Ehlers-Danlos syndrome[77] and Marfan's syndrome[78] suggests an underlying defect in elastic tissue. Pathologically, both the cartilaginous and membranous portions of the trachea and bronchi are affected, each having thin atrophied muscular and elastic tissue.[79]

Radiographically (Fig. 15–10), the caliber of the trachea and major bronchi is increased, and the air columns have an irregular, corrugated appearance caused by the protrusion of mucosal and submucosal tissue between the cartilaginous rings ("tracheal diverticulosis"). Both CT and MR imaging can be used to identify the dilation (see Fig. 15–10)[80]; dynamic CT demonstrates collapse of the airways on expiration.[81] In contrast to bronchiectasis, the dilated bronchi of patients who have tracheobronchomegaly typically have thin walls.

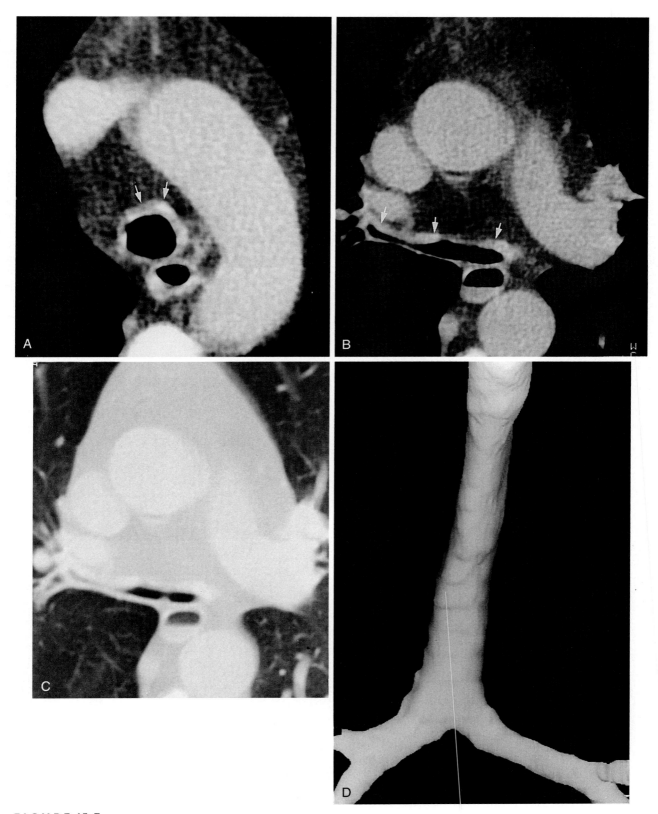

FIGURE 15–7

Relapsing polychondritis. Spiral CT scans demonstrate mild thickening and calcification of the walls of the trachea (*arrows*) (**A**) and main and right upper lobe bronchi (**B**) (*arrows*). Lung windows (**C**) demonstrate narrowing of the bronchial lumen. A three-dimensional reconstruction using the surface-shading technique (**D**) demonstrates relatively mild, but extensive narrowing of the trachea and main bronchi, particularly the left. (*Courtesy of Dr. Martine Remy-Jardin, Centre Hospitalier Regional et Universitaire de Lille, Lille, France.*)

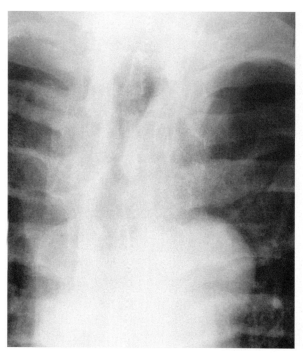

FIGURE 15–8

Tracheobronchopathia osteochondroplastica. A view of the trachea from a posteroanterior chest radiograph in a 69-year-old man demonstrates irregular narrowing of the trachea. The wall has a nodular appearance; no definite calcification is evident. *(From Fraser RS, Müller NL, Colman NC, Paré PD: Fraser and Paré's Diagnosis of Diseases of the Chest, 4th ed. Philadelphia, WB Saunders, 1999.)*

As in tracheomalacia, tracheobronchomegaly is associated with an inefficient cough mechanism and recurrent pneumonia.[82] The presence of prolonged cough and a loud, harsh, rasping sound on auscultation in a patient who complains of an inability to expectorate secretions should arouse suspicion of the diagnosis.[81]

OBSTRUCTIVE SLEEP APNEA

Obstructive apnea can be defined as complete closure of the upper airway despite continued respiratory efforts lasting at least 10 seconds.[83] *Central* apnea is the absence of both airflow and respiratory effort for at least 10 seconds. *Mixed* apnea begins with a cessation of respiratory effort but continues during increasing respiratory effort against a closed airway. *Hypopnea* is a transient reduction in breathing that may be central or obstructive. Obstructive and mixed apneas characterize patients who have the obstructive sleep apnea-hypopnea (OSA) syndrome, which is described in this chapter. Pure central apnea is related to abnormalities of the respiratory control centers in the pons and medulla and is discussed in Chapter 23 (see page 914).

Physiologic Characteristics of Normal Sleep

Sleep has profound effects on respiratory system mechanics, the control of breathing, metabolism, and hemodynamics. During the initial two stages of non–rapid eye movement (NREM) sleep, breathing is unsteady and irregular; the average minute ventilation ($\dot{V}E$) decreases, and alveolar and arterial PCO_2 increase slightly. Periods of relative hyperpnea

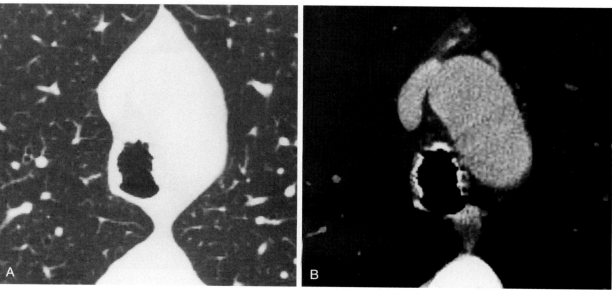

FIGURE 15–9

Tracheobronchopathia osteochondroplastica. A CT scan (**A**) in a 64-year-old man demonstrates nodular thickening of the tracheal wall. Soft tissue windows (**B**) show extensive calcification of the submucosal nodules. Note the lack of involvement of the posterior membranous portion of the trachea, a characteristic finding of tracheobronchopathia osteochondroplastica. *(From Fraser RS, Müller NL, Colman NC, Paré PD: Fraser and Paré's Diagnosis of Diseases of the Chest, 4th ed. Philadelphia, WB Saunders, 1999.)*

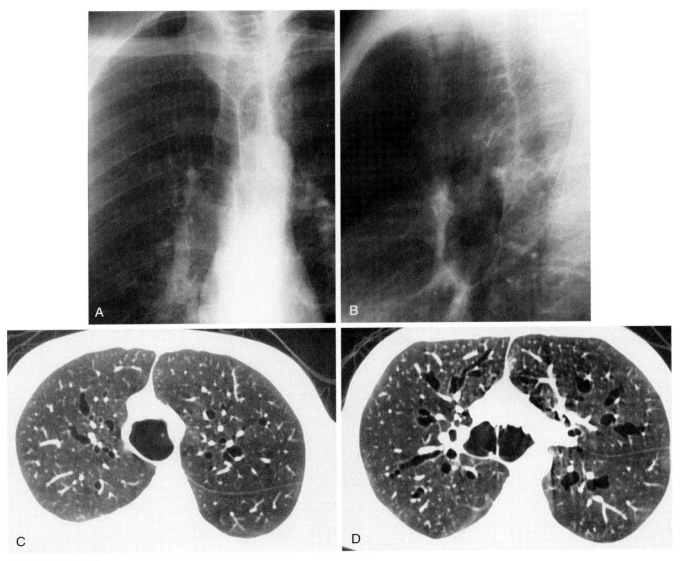

FIGURE 15–10

Tracheobronchomegaly. Views from posteroanterior (**A**) and lateral (**B**) chest radiographs demonstrate marked dilation of the trachea and main bronchi. HRCT scans through the trachea (**C**) and main bronchi (**D**) show diffuse dilation of the trachea, both main bronchi, and the intraparenchymal bronchi. Note that the bronchi have thin walls. The trachea measured 3.3 cm in diameter and the right and left main bronchi 3.0 and 3.4 cm, respectively. The patient was a 21-year-old man. *(From Kwong JS, Müller NL, Miller RR: Diseases of the trachea and main-stem bronchi: Correlation of CT with pathologic findings. Radiographics 12:645, 1992.)*

may be followed by brief central apnea. During stages 3 and 4 (slow-wave sleep), breathing becomes remarkably regular, and there are further decreases in $\dot{V}_E$ ranging from 5% to 30% of awake $\dot{V}_E$, with a 2– to 7–mm Hg rise in $PaCO_2$.[84,85] The decreased $\dot{V}_E$ is the result of increased airway resistance rather than decreased respiratory drive.[86] Breathing becomes irregular again with the onset of rapid eye movement (REM) sleep, and there is a decrease in intercostal electromyographic activation and in the contribution of rib cage expansion to V_T. There is a further overall decrease in $\dot{V}_E$ with considerable fluctuation in breath-by-breath alveolar ventilation.[84]

Ventilatory chemosensitivity to hypoxia and hypercapnia decreases during all stages of sleep.[87] The depression in chemosensitivity is more pronounced during REM than during NREM sleep. The normal rapid adjustment to

external resistive loads is diminished,[87] and there is a decrease in the rate of mucociliary clearance and a depression in the cough threshold.

The ultimate safeguard is arousal, which results in a rapid decrease in upper airway resistance and an increase in sensitivity of the chemical and mechanical responses.[88] There is considerable individual variation in the threshold for such arousal in response to changes in blood gases; a high threshold may be an important risk factor for OSA.[89]

Epidemiology

The estimated prevalence of OSA in the general population is dependent on the diagnostic threshold selected.[90] For example, in one study in which the diagnosis was based on the presence of habitual snoring, breathing pauses during sleep, and daytime drowsiness as reported in telephone interviews, 3.5% of men and 1.5% of women were found to be affected.[91] However, in another in which the condition was defined by more than five episodes of apnea per hour of sleep, OSA was identified in approximately 11% of men and 6% of women.[92]

A useful measure of severity is the apnea-hypopnea index (AHI), defined as the number of apneic or hypopneic episodes that cause a decrease in SaO_2 of 4% or greater per hour.[93] An AHI greater than 10 is often used as the cutoff for the definition of OSA. With this definition, estimates of prevalence have been 2.7% in a study of 1510 Italian men[94] and 10% in men and 7% in women in an investigation of 400 Australian adults.[95] In the Wisconsin Sleep Cohort Study, in which a random sample of approximately 600 men and women aged 30 to 60 years was assessed, 4% of men and 2% of women had OSA.[96] The prevalence of OSA is higher during early childhood and old age and in African Americans and Hispanics.[97,98]

A great variety of conditions predispose to OSA (Table 15–2), the most important of which is obesity. Although OSA can be seen in individuals of normal weight, 60% to 90% of cases are diagnosed in those who are obese (defined as a body mass index [BMI] greater than 28 kg/m²).[90] Moreover, the severity of the disorder increases with increasing BMI, and weight loss can be associated with dramatic improvement.[99] Even more powerful than BMI as a predictor of OSA are measures of central and visceral obesity, such as a higher waist-to-hip ratio and greater neck circumference.[100]

Although approximately 85% to 90% of clinically diagnosed patients are male,[101] some data suggest that this striking gender imbalance may be due to diagnostic bias.[102] In women, the condition usually occurs in the postmenopausal period. Pregnancy may also be associated with its development.[103] Additional risk factors for OSA include a family history of the condition, lower VC, and the use of tobacco, alcohol, and medications such as sedatives.

Etiology and Pathogenesis

OSA is caused by loss of upper airway muscle tone during sleep superimposed on a degree of upper airway narrowing.[104] The episodes of obstruction and apnea occur during all stages of sleep but especially during stage 2 of NREM sleep and during REM sleep, when the apneas tend to be the longest and the resultant arterial desaturation most severe.[105] Factors implicated in pathogenesis include an intrinsically (anatomically) narrowed airway, an abnormally collapsible airway, decreased neural drive, and uncoordinated activation of the upper airway muscles (Fig. 15–11).[106]

Genetic Factors

There is compelling evidence that OSA is partly determined by genetic factors. In fact, it has been estimated that about 40% of the variance in AHI can be explained by this influence.[107] Although the basis for the genetic contribution is unclear, it is likely that genes associated with craniofacial structure, body fat distribution, ventilatory control, and neural control of the upper airway muscles are involved.[107]

TABLE 15–2. Conditions Associated with Obstructive Sleep Apnea

Neurologic
Alzheimer's disease
Parkinson's disease
Syringomyelia
Arnold-Chiari malformation
Poliomyelitis
Autonomic neuropathies
Normal-pressure hydrocephalus
Diabetic neuropathy
Shy-Drager syndrome
Acid maltase deficiency
Mucopolysaccharidosis
Alpert's syndrome
Myasthenia gravis
Möbius' syndrome
Fragile X syndrome
Klippel-Feil sequence
Myotonic dystrophy
Duchenne's muscular dystrophy
Tourette's syndrome
Quadriplegia
Rubinstein-Taybi syndrome
Metabolic
Obesity
Hypothyroidism
Acromegaly
Diabetes
Growth hormone therapy
Testosterone treatment
Cushing's disease
Musculoskeletal
Kyphoscoliosis
Pectus excavatum
Achondroplasia
Fibromyalgia
Ollier's disease (skeletal chondromatosis)
Miscellaneous
Chronic renal failure
Hemodialysis
Marfan's syndrome
Pregnancy
Chronic fatigue syndrome
Tracheobronchomalacia and laryngomalacia
Carcinoid syndrome
Obstructing upper airway tumor
Floppy eyelid syndrome
Sarcoidosis
Repaired cleft palate

Familial aggregation of OSA has been documented in both obese and nonobese individuals,[108] and snoring has been shown to have a hereditary component. In one radiographic study, measurements of craniofacial structure in monozygotic and dizygotic twins showed high heritability,[109] and disproportionate craniofacial anatomy is common in relatives of patients who have OSA.[110] Down's syndrome is the most common congenital disease associated with OSA,[111] and the apnea is usually secondary to tonsillar hypertrophy. The results of twin studies suggest that approximately 70% of the variance in obesity is genetic[112]; in addition, genes also contribute to the intersubject variability in body fat

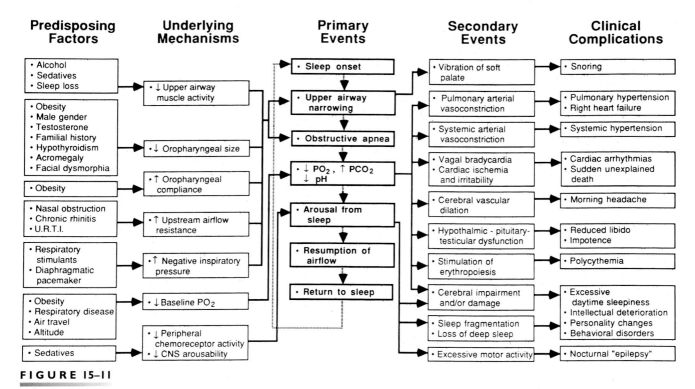

Predisposing Factors	Underlying Mechanisms	Primary Events	Secondary Events	Clinical Complications
• Alcohol • Sedatives • Sleep loss	• ↓ Upper airway muscle activity	• Sleep onset	• Vibration of soft palate	• Snoring
• Obesity • Male gender • Testosterone • Familial history • Hypothyroidism • Acromegaly • Facial dysmorphia	• ↓ Oropharyngeal size	• Upper airway narrowing	• Pulmonary arterial vasoconstriction	• Pulmonary hypertension • Right heart failure
• Obesity	• ↑ Oropharyngeal compliance	• Obstructive apnea	• Systemic arterial vasoconstriction	• Systemic hypertension
• Nasal obstruction • Chronic rhinitis • U.R.T.I.	• ↑ Upstream airflow resistance	• ↓ PO_2, ↑ PCO_2 ↓ pH	• Vagal bradycardia • Cardiac ischemia and irritability	• Cardiac arrhythmias • Sudden unexplained death
• Respiratory stimulants • Diaphragmatic pacemaker	• ↑ Negative inspiratory pressure	• Arousal from sleep	• Cerebral vascular dilation	• Morning headache
			• Hypothalmic - pituitary-testicular dysfunction	• Reduced libido • Impotence
• Obesity • Respiratory disease • Air travel • Altitude	• ↓ Baseline PO_2	• Resumption of airflow	• Stimulation of erythropoiesis	• Polycythemia
• Sedatives	• ↓ Peripheral chemoreceptor activity • ↓ CNS arousability	• Return to sleep	• Cerebral impairment and/or damage	• Excessive daytime sleepiness • Intellectual deterioration • Personality changes • Behavioral disorders
			• Sleep fragmentation • Loss of deep sleep	
			• Excessive motor activity	• Nocturnal "epilepsy"

FIGURE 15–11

Pathogenesis of obstructive sleep apnea. CNS, central nervous system; U.R.T.I., upper respiratory tract infection. *(Modified from a table constructed by Dr. John Fleetham, Vancouver General Hospital, University of British Columbia, Vancouver.)*

distribution.[113] Family members of patients with OSA have decreased ventilatory responses to hypoxemia and a greater increase in airway impedance in response to inspiratory loading than do age- and gender-matched control subjects.[114]

In a linkage analysis study of 66 pedigrees in whom a proband had OSA, weak evidence of linkage for both AHI and BMI was found on several chromosomes[115]; except for the locus on 19p, evidence for linkage to AHI disappeared after adjustment for BMI, thus suggesting that both shared and unshared genetic factors underlie the susceptibility to OSA and obesity. In fact, there could be a common causal pathway involving one or more genes regulating both AHI and BMI.

Endocrine Factors

As indicated previously, OSA predominantly affects men. Moreover, women with the disorder have elevated androgen levels, and administration of androgens can induce the abnormal state in previously unaffected men and women.[116] These observations, together with the known ventilatory stimulant effect of medroxyprogesterone, have led to the hypothesis that the male predominance in OSA is related to a detrimental effect of testosterone and the lack of a protective effect of progesterone.[117]

Structural Narrowing

Structural narrowing of the upper airway is a major risk factor in the vast majority of patients who have clinically significant OSA.[118] An example of its importance is given by the results of a study of 300 consecutive patients in which a prediction

model based on BMI, neck circumference, and oral cavity measurements was found to be 98% sensitive and 100% specific in detecting OSA.[119]

Only a minority of the implicated structural abnormalities are grossly evident.[120] The airway obstruction that develops during sleep apnea usually occurs in the oropharynx.[121] Although nasopharyngeal obstruction does not cause apnea by itself, it can precipitate it by virtue of the more negative downstream inspiratory pressures that must be generated.[122] Breathing through the mouth may also increase the risk for OSA, since opening the mouth tends to displace the tongue posteriorly and encourages airway closure.[123]

Cephalometry (lateral radiography of the head and neck with the use of soft tissue technique) has demonstrated a variety of abnormalities in craniofacial and upper airway soft tissue anatomy that may predispose patients to upper airway obstruction during sleep and affect the severity of OSA.[124] Many patients have been shown to have a small posteriorly placed mandible, a narrow posterior airway space, an enlarged tongue and soft palate, an inferiorly placed hyoid bone, or a combination of these abnormalities. Differences in cephalometric parameters have also been identified in some racial groups, a finding that could be relevant to the ethnic variation in the prevalence of OSA mentioned previously.[125]

An important cause of upper airway narrowing is deposition of adipose tissue in the soft tissues surrounding the pharynx. Neck circumference is a simple clinical measurement that reflects obesity in the region of the upper airway and correlates with several soft tissue variables measured from cephalometry.[126,127] It also predicts apnea severity better than BMI does.[128] These findings suggest that obesity mediates its effect in OSA through fat deposition in the neck.[128]

It is also possible that some of the pharyngeal narrowing seen in patients with OSA occurs as a *result* of the obstruction rather than its cause. Many patients have swollen pharyngeal walls and soft palate, as well as a pendulous uvula,[106] and it has been suggested that chronic obstruction and snoring cause edema of these structures.

Increased Compliance

Increased compliance of the upper airway is an additional important factor implicated in the pathogenesis of OSA.[129] It can be measured during sleep or anesthesia by applying negative pressure at the airway opening and determining the pressure that will result in airway closure. In normal individuals, negative pressures of -25 cm H_2O or lower can be applied before closure occurs; however, in patients who have OSA, closure occurs with pressures as high as -0.5 cm H_2O. Closing pressure is less negative in the supine than in the lateral decubitus position,[130] and opening of the mouth increases the collapsibility.[131] Once the airway closes, the pressure necessary to re-establish patency increases as a result of surface adhesive forces. Closure can also be demonstrated dynamically with digital fluoroscopy.[132]

Neuromuscular Dysfunction

A variety of neurologic disorders are associated with an increased prevalence of obstructive as well as central sleep apnea.[133,134] The dilating muscles of the upper airway display tonic and phasic respiratory electromyographic activity: contraction of these muscles stiffens the walls of the oropharynx, thereby counteracting the tendency of the airway to narrow in response to the negative intraluminal pressure that develops during inspiration. This protective mechanism is depressed during sleep, as well as by alcohol and sedative drugs. REM sleep is associated with the greatest decrease in activation and maximal vulnerability for airway closure.[135] The sleep deprivation and hypoxia that result from OSA can cause further depression of phasic respiratory activity in the upper airway muscles and can lead to worsening obstruction and more fragmented sleep.[136]

Radiologic Manifestations

Although imaging of the upper airway has led to an understanding of the mechanisms involved in OSA, it plays a limited role in assessment of individual patients.[137] Nonetheless, cephalometry (Fig. 15–12), CT, or a combination of the two has been used to characterize the abnormalities of soft tissue and bony structures in patients who have proven OSA and may aid in planning of the most appropriate therapy.[138] Some investigators have also found that cephalometry allows separation of snorers who do or do not have OSA with a precision of approximately 80%[139]; however, others have not reproduced this result.[140]

The dimensions of the upper airway can be assessed with three-dimensional CT reconstruction and cine CT.[141] The narrowest cross-sectional area of the upper airway is at the level of the oropharynx (0.52 ± 0.18 cm^2) in the majority of individuals and is significantly narrower in those who have OSA (Fig. 15–13). Additional findings on CT may include an increase in fat or nonfatty tissues in the pharyngeal wall,

thickening of the mucosa of the nasopharnyx and oropharynx, and enlargement of lymphoid tissue, the tongue, or the soft palate.[142] Upper airway dimensions and increased pharyngeal fat can also be assessed with MR imaging.[143] Ultrafast MR imaging in particular generates dynamic three-dimensional images and allows demonstration of the site of airway narrowing or closure.[144]

Clinical Manifestations

The principal signs and symptoms of OSA are snoring, apneas witnessed by a bed partner, and excessive daytime sleepiness.[145] Snoring is almost invariable and often precedes the diagnosis of OSA, sometimes by many years.[146] However, the symptom is by no means specific for OSA. For example, almost 40% of men and 30% of women were found in one investigation to be occasional or habitual snorers, a prevalence much higher than that seen in OSA.[147] Descriptions of the sleep and snoring patterns from a spouse or bed partner may be helpful in diagnosis. The snoring of individuals who have OSA tends to be loud, irregular, and interrupted by frequent periods of apnea. The apneic periods are typically terminated by loud snorting and motor activity associated with arousal, and the cycle then repeats itself.

Another characteristic symptom of OSA is excessive daytime sleepiness. Its severity correlates with the intensity of nocturnal apnea and sleep deprivation and can be estimated by taking a careful history and applying questionnaires that have been designed to test for daytime sleepiness, such as the Stanford Sleepiness Scale,[148] the Rotterdam Daytime Sleepiness Scale,[149] and the Epworth Sleepiness Scale.[150]

Three clinical levels of increasing severity have been described.[151] In category 1, or mild sleepiness, the individual falls asleep only when reading, watching television, or listening to lectures; although the sleepiness is more severe when the person is overtired, it does not completely disappear despite a "good" night's sleep. The patient and family members do not view the sleepiness as a problem, and it does not interfere with the patient's work. Category 2, or moderate sleepiness, is characterized by unequivocal hypersomnolence; the patient falls asleep not only while relaxing but also while engaged in activities such as driving. The patient and family members are aware that excessive sleepiness is a problem and is interfering with the individual's work. Category 3, or severe sleepiness, implies extreme hypersomnolence; patients may fall asleep while talking, eating, or relating their medical history and are unable to work or drive a car.

OSA is associated with an increased prevalence of systemic hypertension, coronary artery disease and its various complications, and stroke.[152-154] Hypertension is present in more than 50% of patients and is independent of age and obesity.[155] Its pathogenesis is contributed to by vascular smooth muscle contraction related to hypoxemia and respiratory acidosis, increased sympathetic nervous system activity, and/or increased secretion of catecholamines.[156,157] Electrocardiographic monitoring shows that episodes of apnea are frequently associated with myocardial ischemia.[158] Patients with OSA also have a high incidence of left and right ventricular hypertrophy as assessed by echocardiography.[159] OSA may exacerbate heart failure by virtue of the negative intrathoracic pressure that develops during periods of apnea. This negative

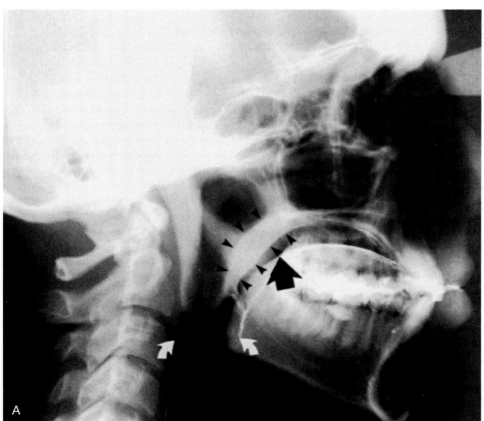

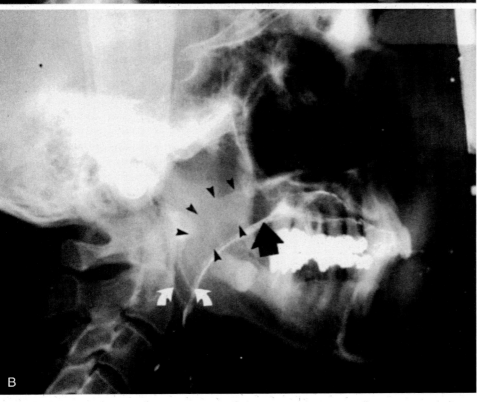

FIGURE 15–12

Radiography of the upper airway in a normal subject and a patient with obstructive sleep apnea. A lateral radiograph of the face and neck (**A**) of a normal individual after the ingestion of barium paste to outline the top of the tongue (*large arrow*) reveals a widely patent oropharynx, normal uvula (*arrowheads*), and normal hypopharynx (*curved arrow*). A similar view in a patient who has obstructive sleep apnea (**B**) shows a markedly narrowed oropharynx (*large arrow*) and hypopharynx (*curved arrows*) and a very large uvula (*arrowheads*). (*From Fraser RS, Müller NL, Colman NC, Paré PD: Fraser and Paré's Diagnosis of Diseases of the Chest, 4th ed. Philadelphia, WB Saunders, 1999.*)

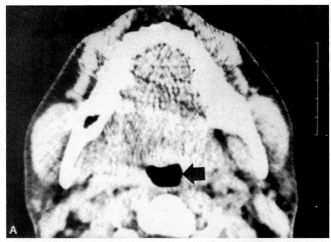

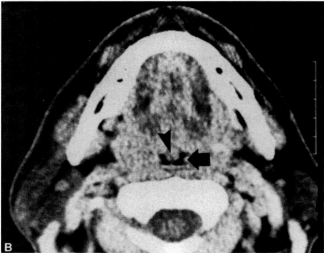

FIGURE 15–13

Computed tomography of the upper airway in a normal subject and a patient with obstructive sleep apnea. A CT scan at the level of the oropharynx in a normal subject (**A**) reveals a widely patent oropharynx (*arrow*). In a patient who has obstructive sleep apnea, a CT image at approximately the same level (**B**) shows a markedly reduced cross-sectional area of the airway (*arrow*) and a prominent uvula (*arrowhead*). *(From Fraser RS, Müller NL, Colman NC, Paré PD: Fraser and Paré's Diagnosis of Diseases of the Chest, 4th ed. Philadelphia, WB Saunders, 1999.)*

pressure is transmitted to the chambers of the heart and acts as an increased afterload in the same way that an increase in arterial blood pressure would.[160]

The arterial oxygen desaturation associated with apneic episodes causes pulmonary arterial hypertension and an increase in right ventricular afterload.[161] Persistent pulmonary hypertension develops in approximately 15% to 20% of patients who have OSA,[162] most often in association with concomitant COPD.[163] If significant hypoxemia precedes the apneic episodes, as it may in individuals with intrinsic pulmonary disease, a similar duration of apnea will cause more profound desaturation.[164]

In addition to an increased incidence of cerebrovascular accidents and pronounced sleepiness,[165] patients who have OSA may manifest cognitive impairment, depression, and personality changes.[166] It should also be remembered that OSA may subsequently develop in patients who have had cerebrovascular accidents.[167] Headache, especially on awakening, is significantly more common in snorers and patients who have OSA than in appropriate control subjects.[168]

A subset of patients with OSA have the pickwickian syndrome (or as it is more often called, the obesity-hypoventilation syndrome). Such patients tend to be morbidly obese and experience not only severe arterial oxygen desaturation at night but also arterial oxygen desaturation and hypercapnia during the day[169]; ultimately, cor pulmonale develops. It has been suggested that the chronic sleep deprivation combined with nocturnal hypoxia and hypercapnia in these individuals leads to a disruption of normal central ventilatory control.[170]

Diagnosis

Although OSA can be suspected on the basis of the clinical history, definitive diagnosis requires a study of breathing during sleep. A complete polysomnographic investigation includes sleep staging and measurement of respiratory effort, airflow, and arterial blood gas tensions (Fig. 15–14).[101] Staging is done by recording the electroencephalogram, the electro-oculogram, and the electromyogram of a skeletal muscle (usually the submental). The frequency and amplitude of the brain waves are the most important signals. The onset of REM sleep is signaled by low-amplitude, rapid-frequency electroencephalographic waves and by rapid eye movements detected by electro-oculography. Approximately 20% to 25% of sleep is spent in REM sleep. Stages vary throughout sleep, and on average about 40 changes occur between stages during a sleep of 7.5 hours' duration. Respiratory effort can be determined by using devices that measure rib cage and/or abdominal movement or changes in intrathoracic pressure. Respiratory airflow can be measured with a thermistor, a microphone, a pneumotachograph, or a device that measures fluctuations in expired CO_2.[171]

Changes in arterial oxygen saturation can be monitored noninvasively with a pulse-type or transmittance-type ear oximeter. The final measurements are an electrocardiogram to record cardiac dysrhythmias and an audio signal to detect snoring.

Since a complete overnight sleep study is expensive and time-consuming, a number of simpler methods have been investigated for the detection of clinically significant OSA, including anthropometric analysis, questionnaires,[172] abbreviated sleep studies,[173] overnight home monitoring,[174] and video recording[175]; a combination of methods has also been proposed.[176] The British Thoracic Society has suggested that if baseline arterial saturation is greater than 90% by pulse oximetry, the presence of more than 15 episodes of 4% oxygen desaturation per hour of sleep is indicative of OSA.[177] As with other diagnostic tests, the positive predictive value of overnight oximetry increases when the pretest probability for OSA is judged to be high on the basis of the clinical history and physical examination.[177]

Sophisticated portable monitoring devices are now available that allow in-home detection of the sleep state, electro-oculography, electromyography, arterial saturation, airflow, and respiratory effort with an accuracy comparable to that of

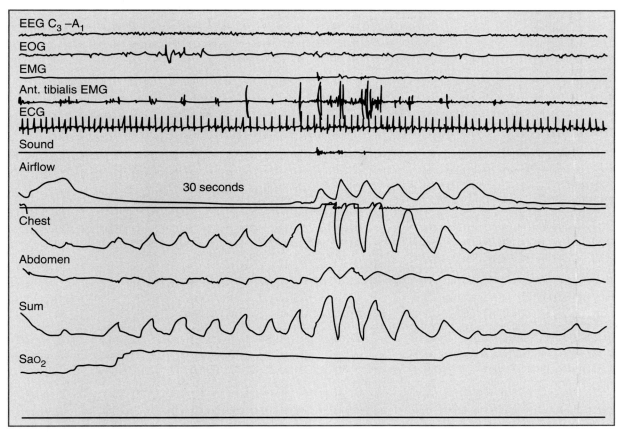

FIGURE 15–14

Polysomnographic record—obstructive sleep apnea. The rows, from top to bottom, show an electroencephalogram (EEG), an electro-oculogram (EOG), an electromyogram (EMG) of the anterior tibialis muscle, an electrocardiogram (ECG), a sound recording to detect snoring (Sound), a tracing of airflow at the mouth (Airflow), Respitrace recordings of the chest and abdominal movement and their sum (Sum), and a pulse oximeter tracing of arterial saturation (SaO_2). Airflow ceases shortly after the start of the record and remains zero for approximately 30 seconds, indicative of prolonged apnea. The evidence that this condition is obstructive apnea is continued movement of the chest wall and abdomen despite the absence of airflow. At the termination of the apnea there is resumption of airflow, accompanied by snoring and leg movements (tibialis EMG) suggesting arousal; however, after six unobstructed breaths another period of apnea begins. The apparently paradoxical increase in oxygen saturation during apnea is due to the time lag of this recording; the rise reflects the previous short burst of unobstructed breathing. Repeated apnea and brief arousal are characteristic of severe obstructive sleep apnea. *(Courtesy of Dr. John Fleetham, University of British Columbia.)*

polysomnography in the diagnosis of OSA.[178] A useful two-stage approach is to conduct portable monitoring of oxygen saturation, snoring, and body position in patients selected on the basis of neck circumference, blood pressure, habitual snoring, and witnessed nocturnal choking and gasping.[176]

Prognosis

Although OSA is associated with increased mortality, its direct contribution to this increase is unclear, in part because of variation in the experimental design of studies addressing this issue and in part because of the confounding influences of comorbid disease such as obesity and hypertension.[179] Early studies of mortality in OSA focused on severely affected patients referred to clinics and were associated with quite alarming statistics, especially in men younger than 50 years (10% mortality over a period of 8 years).[180,181] However, in more recent studies, the contribution of OSA to excess mortality has been shown to be lower, especially in older individuals.[182]

ASTHMA

According to the Global Initiative for Asthma, asthma can be defined as

> *A chronic inflammatory disorder of the airways in which many cells play a role, in particular mast cells, eosinophils, and T lymphocytes. In susceptible individuals this inflammation causes recurrent episodes of wheezing, breathlessness, chest tightness, and cough, particularly at night and/or in the early morning. These symptoms are usually associated with widespread but variable airflow limitation that is at least partly reversible either spontaneously or with treatment. The inflammation also causes an associated increase in airway responsiveness to a variety of stimuli.*[183]

Because airway inflammation and hyperresponsiveness are seen in other diseases and because information concerning the cellular inflammation is most often not available, this comprehensive definition is of limited value in routine clinical practice.[184] Nevertheless, elements of the definition are used by clinicians, epidemiologists, and basic scientists. For clinicians, symptoms and evidence of variable, partly reversible airflow obstruction usually suffice. For epidemiologic studies, symptom questionnaires are probably the most valid approach.[185]

The airway narrowing that occurs in asthma is intermittent and variable; complete remission can occur between attacks, although some abnormality in function is often detectable with sensitive tests.[186] During attacks, generalized narrowing of the bronchi and bronchioles results in diffuse wheezing often associated with dyspnea, even at rest. Although the reversibility may be suspected from the clinical history, it should always be evaluated objectively by measurement of airway function after the administration of a bronchodilator or after a course of anti-inflammatory therapy.[187] Asthma should be a diagnosis of exclusion; several diseases can be associated with a clinical picture that simulates it, including acute bronchitis and bronchiolitis, COPD, bronchiectasis, lymphangitic carcinomatosis, left-sided heart failure, and anatomic or functional upper airway obstruction.[188]

Despite some overlap, asthma can be considered in two major categories: extrinsic and intrinsic.

Extrinsic Asthma. This form occurs in patients who are atopic, a term used to refer to the genetic predisposition to respond to antigenic challenge with excessive IgE production. The inheritance is complex but usually incomplete, and evidence of it is much greater if both parents are atopic. The prevalence increases until approximately 20 years of age, at which point it gradually declines. Peak IgE levels occur at 14 years of age; in infants and young children, atopy and asthma are twice as common in males.[189] Although patients with extrinsic asthma are invariably atopic, it is important to realize that atopy itself is not synonymous with asthma. The former occurs in more than 30% of the population, whereas the incidence of asthma is generally less than 5%. In addition, although atopy invariably develops in both identical twins if one is affected, the development of asthmatic symptoms and nonspecific bronchial hyperresponsiveness is often discordant.[190]

In addition to atopy and elevated blood levels of IgE, extrinsic asthma is characterized by (1) a high incidence of eczema and rhinitis, (2) onset during the first 3 decades of life, (3) seasonal symptoms, (4) positive skin and bronchial challenge tests to specific allergens, and (5) a tendency for remission in later life.[191]

Intrinsic Asthma. Intrinsic asthma occurs in patients in whom atopy or specific external triggers of bronchoconstriction cannot be identified and may be a distinct immunopathologic entity.[192] Affected patients are characterized by (1) being older than patients with extrinsic disease, (2) having no or a less convincing family history of asthma or atopy, (3) an absence of elevated blood levels of IgE or positive skin or bronchial response to allergen challenge, (4) increased numbers of blood and sputum eosinophils, (5) an increased incidence of autoimmune disease and autoantibodies to smooth muscle, (6) decreased responsiveness to therapy, (7) a greater risk of being aspirin sensitive, and (8) a tendency to persistent and progressive disease resulting in fixed airflow obstruction.[191]

Epidemiology

Asthma is a very common disease, and there is good evidence that its prevalence as well as the prevalence of other allergic

disorders is increasing worldwide.[193] The reasons for this increase are unclear[194]; the most persistent theory is the "hygiene hypothesis," which holds that a high prevalence of respiratory infection, parasitic infestation, and/or "poor hygiene" in some way protects against the development of atopic disease.[195] Whatever the protective mechanism, it appears that migration from rural to urban areas is associated with an increase in asthma prevalence.[196]

Estimates of prevalence vary by definition, geography, ethnicity, and age. When the diagnosis of asthma is based on the presence of wheeze in the previous 12 months, the range has varied from 2% to 5% in China and Hong Kong; to 10% to 15% in Canada, the United States, and the United Kingdom; and to 20% to 27% in Fiji, Australia, and Chile.[197] These differences are probably related to environmental rather than genetic factors.[198] For example, the lower incidence of asthma in some tropical countries may be related to a protective effect of high serum IgE levels induced by parasitic infestation.[199]

The most important risk factors for the development of asthma are atopy, passive cigarette smoke exposure, and childhood bronchiolitis.[200-202] The risk appears to be especially high in those with allergic sensitivity to certain allergens such as house dust mites or fungi (such as *Alternaria* species).[203] The prevalence of asthma is highest in childhood and decreases during adolescence and adulthood. However, diagnosing the condition in infants and young children is difficult: about 20% of infants wheeze during viral infections in their first 3 years of life but do not ultimately develop asthma. A second group of young children (10% of the population) who also wheeze during viral infections show evidence of atopy (high serum IgE levels, family history of allergy) and develop persistent or recurrent asthma.[204] The prevalence of asthma before the age of 10 is higher in boys than girls[205]; after that, it is higher in females. Females are also more likely to visit the emergency room and be admitted for acute severe asthma.[206]

Genetic Considerations

Despite abundant evidence that heredity has an important role in the pathogenesis of asthma and allergic diseases,[207] the inheritance does not conform to a classic mendelian pattern such as recessive or dominant. Asthma and allergy are complex genetic disorders in which more than one abnormal gene is required in an affected person (i.e., inheritance is polygenic) and different combinations of genes produce the disease in different individuals (i.e., genetic heterogeneity). Moreover, environmental factors are also necessary for expression of the disease phenotype.

The phenotype in genetic studies of allergic disorders can be symptoms, exaggerated IgE production (positive skin prick tests or serum levels), or bronchial hyperresponsiveness. Evidence for a genetic contribution to these traits includes the observation of greater concordance in monozygotic than dizygotic twins[208]; this is true for both asthma symptoms and measures of excessive IgE and is seen even when twins are reared apart. There is also an increased prevalence of disease in the first-degree relatives of affected individuals[209]; for asthma, the prevalence in the general population is about 5%, whereas in first-degree relatives of asthmatics it is approximately 20%. In addition, there is evidence that airway hyperresponsiveness is heritable, although it is also a consequence of allergic airway inflammation.[210,211]

Numerous chromosomal locations have been linked to asthma and allergy phenotypes.[212,213] At some of these loci, function-altering polymorphisms have been identified in candidate genes implicated in the pathogenesis of allergy and asthma. Examples include the interleukin-4 and interleukin-9 genes, the high-affinity IgE receptor, and the β-adrenergic receptor. At other loci, novel genes not previously known have been localized. Examples include the *ADAM33* gene on chromosome 20, which has both integrin and metalloproteinase activities,[214] and a unique peptidase on chromosome 2q that may activate chemokines.[215] In addition to imparting risk for allergy and asthma, polymorphisms in certain genes may influence the severity of asthma and the efficacy of specific asthma therapy, such as β-adrenergic agonists and antileukotriene medications.[216,217]

Pathologic Characteristics

At autopsy, the lungs of patients who die of asthma are distended and the bronchi and bronchioles are plugged with viscid mucus that contains proteinaceous material and ciliated epithelial and inflammatory cells, most of which are eosinophils.[218] Histologic changes in the bronchial and bronchiolar walls involve the epithelium, lamina propria, muscularis mucosae, and submucosa.[219] The constellation of abnormalities is referred to as *airway wall remodeling* and consists of changes in the composition, quantity, and organization of the cellular and molecular constituents of the airway wall as a consequence of chronic injury and repair.[220]

Epithelial abnormalities include goblet cell hyperplasia and detachment of ciliated cells such that only a layer of basal cells is left[221] (see Color Fig. 15–1). The subepithelial layer of connective tissue, the lamina reticularis, is typically thickened ("basement membrane" thickening) as a result of the deposition of collagen and fibronectin.[222] There may be edema, vascular congestion and proliferation, and inflammatory cell infiltration of the lamina propria, submucosa, and adventitia.[223] The collagen deposition in the subepithelial layer, as well as in the adventitia, may underlie the decreased airway distensibility that may be seen in asthmatic patients.[224] An increase in smooth muscle is also a characteristic feature; it is the result of both hyperplasia and hypertrophy and is most pronounced in subjects who die of the disease.[225,226] Eosinophils are the most characteristic and numerous inflammatory cells in the airway wall (see Color Fig. 15–1); however, there may also be increases in lymphocytes, macrophages, neutrophils, and mast cells.[227]

Pathogenesis

Cellular Mechanisms

The basic pathophysiologic abnormality that determines the functional and symptomatic status of an asthmatic patient is airway narrowing, which can occur by four mechanisms: (1) airway smooth muscle contraction, (2) edema and congestion of the airway wall, (3) plugging of the airway lumen by mucus and inflammatory exudate, and (4) airway wall remodeling. For the most part, it is difficult if not impossible to determine in a given patient at a given time what proportion of airway obstruction is caused by each of these mechanisms. However, it may reasonably be concluded that when obstruction is rapidly reversible after the inhalation of smooth muscle relaxants, the pathogenesis is smooth muscle contraction. On the other hand, when obstruction responds over a period of days to steroids and other therapeutic interventions, it is probably caused predominantly by edema and mucus plugging. Reversal of airway remodeling may take many months.[228]

The symptoms of asthma, including wheeze, cough, and breathlessness, are caused both directly and indirectly by acute and chronic inflammation in the airways. An allergic response to inhaled allergens is the most frequent cause of the inflammation.[229] The first interaction is with intraepithelial dendritic cells, which process antigens and present them to local T lymphocytes.[230] CD4+ T lymphocytes then differentiate into distinct subsets: T_H1 cells, which secrete interferon-γ (INF-γ) and tumor necrosis factor-β (TNF-β), and T_H2 cells, which secrete several interleukins. These T_H2 cytokines stimulate IgE production against the antigen. The latter binds to IgE receptors on mast cells, basophils, and other inflammatory cells and triggers an allergic immune response when next exposed to the specific allergen. Which subset of T lymphocytes predominates is genetically determined and modified by the intensity, timing, and mode of exposure to allergens and other environmental factors.

T_H2 cytokines perpetuate the inflammatory response by initiating chemotaxis and migration of circulating inflammatory cells, particularly eosinophils, and by activating resident cells to express and secrete molecules that enhance inflammation. The cytokines also cause an upregulation of expression of adhesion molecules, such as vascular cell adhesion molecule-1 (VCAM-1) and intercellular adhesion molecule-1 (ICAM-1), on the surface of endothelial and epithelial cells; these surface molecules interact with complementary ligands on inflammatory cells to enhance their adherence and migration. Other environmental agents, such as viruses and tobacco smoke, can be inhaled in addition to the pathogenic allergens; in genetically predisposed individuals, these agents can aggravate the airway obstruction produced by the allergic inflammatory reaction.

The long list of mediators, cytokines, chemokines, and proteases involved in the inflammatory response includes histamine, prostaglandins, leukotrienes, platelet-activating factor, tryptase, chymase, eotaxin, RANTES, and eosinophil-derived toxic cationic proteins such as major basic protein and eosinophil cationic protein.[231] They have a variety of effects, including increased vascular permeability, mucus hypersecretion, inflammatory cell chemotaxis and migration, and smooth muscle contraction. The endothelium and airway epithelium are also involved in the reaction via the production of nitric oxide and endothelin.[232] Tachykinins such as substance P and the neurokinins are released from afferent nerve endings and initiate neurogenic inflammation. Resident tissue cells, including fibroblasts, smooth muscle cells, and epithelial cells, can produce chemotactic cytokines as well as growth factors such as platelet-derived growth factor (PDGF) and transforming growth factor-β (TGF-β), which can drive tissue remodeling.[233]

Nonspecific Bronchial Hyperresponsiveness

One of the important consequences of chronic airway inflammation is a structural and functional alteration that renders the airways hyperresponsive to a variety of nonspecific (nonallergic) irritants. Because such alterations are relatively irreversible, airway hyperresponsiveness and symptoms can persist despite removal of the inciting allergens. Such nonspecific bronchial hyperresponsiveness (NSBH) (bronchial hyperreactivity, bronchial hyperexcitability) is often defined in practice as a lower than normal dose or concentration—PD_{20} or PC_{20}, respectively—of inhaled methacholine or histamine that causes a 20% decline in FEV_1.[234]

Although all the stimuli used to demonstrate NSBH result in some degree of airway narrowing in normal individuals, it is the excessive narrowing at very much lower doses or concentrations that characterizes NSBH. There is considerable interest in the mechanisms behind this reaction because many of the symptoms of asthma are related to its presence. In fact, asthmatic patients respond excessively to a wide variety of pharmacologic agonists and mediators and experience excessive airway narrowing after the inhalation of atmospheric pollutants, dust, and cold and dry air and after certain respiratory maneuvers such as a deep inspiration or forced expiration to RV[235]; as a result, NSBH has been considered to be a sine qua non of the disease.[236]

Measurement. The various methods that have been used to quantify NSBH are described in Chapter 4 (see page 183). Asthmatics show exaggerated airway narrowing with whatever test is used; however, better differentiation between asthmatic patients and normal individuals can be achieved by using a test that includes a maximal inspiratory maneuver (FEV_1, PEFR, or maximal expiratory flow rather than airway or pulmonary resistance) because in addition to exhibiting exaggerated narrowing, the airways of asthmatic patients show less bronchodilation after a big breath.[237]

Pathogenesis. The various links between airway smooth muscle stimulation, airway narrowing, and an increase in airway resistance are shown diagrammatically in Figure 15–15. Abnormalities at any level of this cascade can theoretically produce an exaggeration of airway narrowing in asthmatic patients. Possible mechanisms include the following:

1. Because of the nonlinear relationship between airway radius and resistance, factors that narrow the airways, such as airway edema and mucus plugging, will exaggerate the effect of subsequent smooth muscle contraction.[238]
2. Deposition of aerosolized particles of the size used for testing airway responsiveness is dependent on impaction; more central deposition because of the turbulent airflow pattern in the already narrowed airways of asthmatics could contribute to hyperresponsiveness.[239]
3. The amount of drug that reaches smooth muscle is dependent on the balance between penetration of the mucosa and its removal by the bronchial vasculature, lymphatics, and enzymatic degradation; since the respiratory epithelium is characteristically damaged in patients who have asthma, a greater proportion of inhaled agonist might reach smooth muscle.[240]
4. Because airway smooth muscle is innervated by the autonomic nervous system, an exaggerated excitatory or deficient inhibitory neural control could contribute

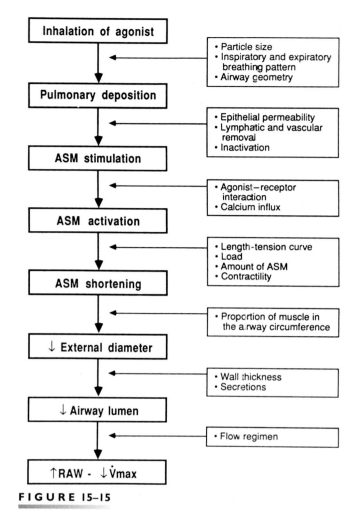

FIGURE 15–15

Airway responsiveness cascade. ASM, airway smooth muscle. (*From Fraser RS, Müller NL, Colman NC, Paré PD: Fraser and Paré's Diagnosis of Diseases of the Chest, 4th ed. Philadelphia, WB Saunders, 1999.*)

to NSBH[241]; possible mechanisms include an imbalance between the M_3 (excitatory) and M_2 (inhibitory) cholinergic receptors, decreased responsiveness to β-adrenergic agonists,[242] or defective nonadrenergic noncholinergic inhibition of bronchoconstriction.[243]
5. The increase in the amount of airway smooth muscle may be an important determinant of NSBH if its contractile capacity is maintained[244]; in fact, some evidence suggests that the smooth muscle is more contractile than normal.[245] Similarly, a decrease in load on the muscle as a result of remodeling or edema could facilitate excessive shortening.[246]

Clinical Usefulness. NSBH is so characteristic of asthma that it is questionable whether the diagnosis can be made in its absence.[236] Rare patients who have occupational asthma do not show NSBH at the time of diagnosis; this lack of NSBH occurs most often when exposure to the offending agent has been remote. However, increased responsiveness often develops with prolonged exposure.[247] There are also patients in whom a clinical history of asthma may not be clear and who have normal spirometric values at the time of examination,

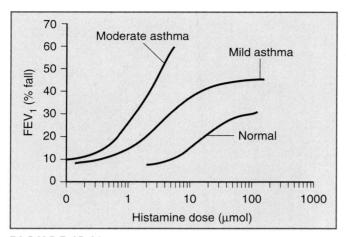

FIGURE 15–16

Histamine dose-response curves. The percent fall in FEV₁ is plotted against the dose of inhaled histamine for a normal subject and patients with mild and moderate asthma. In normal subjects and patients with mild asthma, a plateau is often reached on the dose-response curve. In patients with moderate asthma, there is no plateau despite a 60% decrease in FEV₁. Asthma is characterized by a shift of the dose-response curve to the left and an increase in the maximal response. *(Modified from Woolcock AJ, Salome CM, Yan K: The shape of the dose-response curve to histamine in asthmatic and normal subjects. Am Rev Respir Dis 130:71, 1984.)*

thus precluding assessment of bronchodilator response; in these individuals, measurement of NSBH is a useful adjunct to diagnosis (Fig. 15–16).[248] Such measurement is particularly helpful in patients who complain only of chronic cough, in whom the demonstration of increased NSBH aids in predicting whether the patient will respond symptomatically to asthma therapy.[249] Tests of NSBH are less useful in patients who are already obstructed, in which case the history and response to bronchodilators are usually diagnostic.[250] Because NSBH can be altered by treatment, it can also be used as an indicator of the effectiveness of therapy and the need for more or less intensive administration.[251]

Despite being a very sensitive indicator of asthma, NSBH is far from being specific; it may be seen in patients who have sarcoidosis,[252] extrinsic allergic alveolitis,[253] or COPD.[254] Moreover, in surveys of airway responsiveness, the incidence of NSBH is higher than that of clinically diagnosed asthma.[255]

Mucus and Mucociliary Clearance

Although mucus plugging plays an important role in the airway obstruction of asthma, there are no specific abnormalities in the biochemical composition or viscoelastic properties of airway mucus in asthmatic subjects.[256,257] However, many putative mediators of asthma are known to increase mucus secretion, including histamine, prostaglandins, and lipoxygenase products of arachidonic acid metabolism.[258,259]

Radioaerosol techniques reveal impaired mucociliary clearance rates in patients who have stable asthma[260] and further impairment during acute attacks.[261] The depressed clearance is most likely related to the excessive mucus production because the mediators actually stimulate increased ciliary beat frequency.[262] Nonetheless, some asthmatic patients have been found to have a ciliary inhibitory compound in

their sputum.[263] Prolonged therapy with corticosteroids has been shown to result in improved mucociliary clearance.[264]

Provoking Factors

Although asthma is a chronic disease, a variety of insults can induce exacerbations and result in acute episodes of dyspnea and wheezing. Some of these provoking factors contribute to the ongoing inflammatory process, as well as cause acute airway narrowing (i.e., inducers). Other factors simply stimulate airway narrowing because of NSBH (i.e., inciters).[265]

Allergens

Specific antigens can provoke asthmatic attacks in sensitized persons. These individuals frequently suffer from other allergic manifestations, such as hay fever and eczema, and usually have positive prick or intradermal skin test results to a variety of allergens. Such hypersensitivity is common and appears to be increasing in prevalence.[266] Surveys of the population at large by skin tests indicate that approximately 30% of individuals have a positive reaction to at least one allergen.[267] Many such individuals are asymptomatic, and some suffer only from rhinitis. Besides skin tests, specific allergy to individual antigens can be proved by using an inhalation challenge test or an assay of the specific IgE blood levels for various antigens—the radioallergosorbent test (RAST).

Potential antigens in our environment are innumerable. Although grass and tree pollen cause positive skin reactions and a response to inhalation challenge in many allergic asthmatic patients, they are not common causes of asthmatic attacks. Whole ragweed pollen grains are too large to be inspired into the lower respiratory tract; however, fragmented particles are a common cause of hay fever and asthma.[268] Fungal spores are a major source of airborne allergens, usually outnumbering pollen by as much as 1000:1. The most commonly recognized forms are the imperfect fungi, which include *Alternaria, Aspergillus, Cladosporium, Mucor,* and *Penicillium* species.[269]

There is substantial evidence that indoor allergens are the most important cause of chronic allergic asthma.[270] Animal dander from a variety of household pets, including the gerbil and guinea pig, in addition to the more ubiquitous cat and dog, may cause ocular and nasal symptoms, as well as asthma. Proteins derived from a variety of insects are also an important source of aeroallergens; the most potent and ubiquitous is that derived from the house dust mite, *Dermatophagoides pteronyssinus.* This organism thrives in house dust, especially in damp environments, and is an important cause of asthma, particularly in children.[271,272] Another indoor insect that appears to be important is the cockroach; in fact, it has been hypothesized that exposure to high levels of cockroach allergen may explain the high frequency of asthma-related health problems in inner-city children.[273]

Although latex allergy is primarily an occupational risk (see later), the prevalence of such allergy is increasing in nonoccupational settings; affected persons often have cross-reacting hypersensitivity to foods such as avocado, banana, kiwi fruit, and chestnuts.[274] In addition to aeroallergens, a variety of protein antigens in foods, particularly eggs, fish, nuts, spices, and chocolate, can cause allergy and asthma, again especially in children. Although asthmatic patients associate symptoms with the ingestion of specific foods in about 20% of attacks, objective evidence incriminating them is obtained only rarely.[275] From a clinical point of view, it is relatively rare that wheeze is the sole manifestation of food allergy; the majority of affected persons also have atopic eczema, gastrointestinal symptoms, and/or angioedema or urticaria.[276]

The pathogenesis of allergen-mediated asthma is related to binding of IgE to tissue mast cells and blood basophils. As indicated previously, when a specific allergen is inhaled or ingested and comes in contact with antibody in the airway, it induces the synthesis and release of inflammatory mediators. The latter results in contraction of airway smooth muscle, increased bronchial vascular and airway epithelial permeability, increased airway mucus secretion, and attraction of inflammatory cells to the airway, as well as activation of these cells. Clinically, patients have an immediate or early response characterized by bronchoconstriction that reaches a maximum in 15 to 30 minutes and is followed by a return toward normal lung function, even without treatment.[277] The severity of bronchoconstriction is related to the degree of allergy and nonspecific bronchial responsiveness.[278] The former can be determined by performing quantitative skin tests[278] or RAST[279] and relates to the amounts of specific IgE and mediator released for a given antigen dose. The severity of NSBH determines the degree of bronchial narrowing that will occur when a given amount of mediator is released.

In some patients, the early response is followed by a late or delayed response that develops between 3 and 10 hours after the initial challenge and may persist for 48 hours (Fig. 15–17). This late response may be related to the presence of inflammatory cells attracted by chemotactic factors released during the early response. In some patients, a single-antigen inhalation challenge is followed by recurrent nocturnal episodes of asthma.[280] Occasionally, only a delayed response to inhaled antigen develops. Although it was initially believed that the late response might be mediated by IgG antibody, it is now accepted that it is a delayed result of the immediate IgE–mast cell interaction.

Besides being more prolonged, the late asthmatic response differs from the immediate response with respect to modulation by pharmacologic interventions. β-Adrenergic agonists in sufficient concentration effectively block the immediate response, but they are much less effective against the delayed one; on the other hand, corticosteroids do not influence the immediate response but attenuate the late response, and sodium cromoglycate and antileukotrienes block both the immediate and the late response.[281,282] The similarity of the pathology of the late phase response to that of chronic asthma suggests that chronic asthma may be the link between immediate hypersensitivity reactions and the subacute or chronic airway disease that characterizes the majority of patients who have asthma. A similar common final pathway of airway inflammation may explain the similarity of airway function and pathology in asthmatic patients in whom asthma is triggered by nonallergic mechanisms.[283]

When IgE antibody and antigen interaction occurs on mast cells throughout the body, anaphylaxis develops. Airway narrowing as a result of the local release of mediators in the airways is only a component of this generalized response; hypotension and upper airway obstruction caused by edema may play a more striking role. Anaphylaxis may occur after the oral or parenteral administration of drugs, of which penicillin

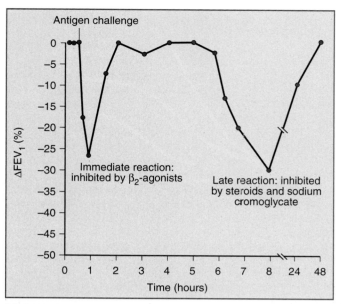

FIGURE 15–17

Immediate and late allergic airway response. This graph reveals the response when asthmatic patients are challenged with a specific antigen to which they are allergic: immediate bronchoconstriction can develop that generally wanes by 1 hour, followed by a late reaction that begins 3 to 10 hours after challenge and can last as long as 24 hours. β-Adrenergic agonists effectively inhibit the immediate allergic reaction but have less effect on alleviating the late response. Both the immediate and late responses can be inhibited by sodium cromoglycate, whereas steroid therapy attenuates the late response but has no influence on the immediate response.

is the most frequent culprit. Other causes include bee and wasp stings and parenteral administration of iodinated contrast agents. The condition can be rapidly fatal, most often as a result of asphyxia secondary to laryngeal edema or acute bronchoconstriction.

Exercise

Exercise-induced asthma (EIA) can be considered to be present when airway narrowing accompanies moderate or vigorous exercise.[284] It can be specifically defined as a decrease in FEV_1 or PEFR greater than 10% or a decrease in specific airway conductance (SGaw), $FEF_{25\%-75\%}$, or $Vmax_{50}$ greater than 35%. Rather than being a separate form of asthma, EIA should be considered a trigger for airway narrowing in patients *who have asthma.* In fact, it occurs in 70% to 80% of patients with asthma who exercise at 80% to 90% of their maximal workload for 6 to 8 minutes.[285] The bronchoconstriction usually peaks 5 to 12 minutes after the cessation of exercise and spontaneously remits within 30 to 60 minutes. The majority of patients are refractory to the induction of a second episode of EIA for approximately 2 hours.

A major advance in the understanding of EIA came with the observation that airway narrowing can be completely abolished if the inspired air during exercise is warmed to body temperature and saturated with water vapor (37° C and a water content of about 46 mg/L).[286] In fact, the degree of airway obstruction after identical exercise challenges can be modified by altering the inspired air conditions: the colder and drier the air breathed during exercise, the greater the subsequent response.[287] Moreover, exercise is not even necessary to produce "EIA," the airway response being reproducible by the isocapnic hyperventilation of unconditioned air.[288] With identical inspired air conditions, there is a dose-response relationship between ventilation and the severity of bronchoconstriction in patients with asthma, regardless of whether the bronchoconstriction is associated with exercise or with isocapnic hyperventilation (hyperventilation-induced bronchoconstriction). Similar refractoriness to subsequent challenge can be produced by matched levels of isocapnic hyperventilation.[289] In individual patients, the degree of bronchoconstriction in response to either exercise or isocapnic hyperventilation depends on the level of nonspecific bronchial responsiveness.[290]

These observations have led to the conclusion that EIA is related to an exaggerated response to cooling and/or drying of the airways. When the temperature and water content of inspired air are less than 37° C and 100% relative humidity, heat and water are lost from the respiratory tract. During resting levels of ventilation, especially during nose breathing, the inspired air is warmed and humidified before it reaches the glottis, and any cooling or drying is confined to the upper airway. During exercise or isocapnic hyperventilation, however, unconditioned air can reach the lung and cool and dry the tracheobronchial tree. It is still unclear whether it is the cooling of the lower airway or the drying of the surface liquid that triggers EIA and hyperventilation-induced bronchoconstriction.[291] However, when the temperature and water content of inspired air are varied so that a range of total respiratory heat and water loss is produced, the magnitude of bronchoconstriction correlates more closely with calculated water loss than with heat loss.[292] The hypothesis that drying, with consequent hyperosmolarity of the surface liquid, is the important stimulus has been strengthened by studies that have shown that inhalation of hyperosmolar aerosols elicits bronchoconstriction in patients with EIA.[293]

The bronchoconstriction that occurs in asthmatic patients in response to ventilation of unconditioned air appears to result not from a defect in inspired air conditioning but rather from an abnormal response to a normal stimulus. Normal individuals do not seem to have more efficient air conditioning because equivalent airway cooling develops at matched levels of ventilation and inspired air conditions.[294] With identical levels of ventilation and inspired air conditions, nasal breathing results in much less airway cooling and bronchoconstriction than oral breathing.[295]

The precise mechanism by which airway cooling or drying results in airway narrowing is uncertain. Possibilities include the release of mediators such as histamine and neutrophil chemotactic factor of anaphylaxis from mast cells or other sources,[296] stimulation of afferent receptors,[297] a direct effect on smooth muscle,[298] and mucosal vascular dilation and edema.[299]

From 50% to 80% of asthmatic patients in whom EIA develops show a refractory period after challenge; during this period, similar levels of exercise produce no response or an attenuated response.[300] The degree of attenuation of the second response depends on the intensity of the initial exercise and on time. Thirty minutes after an initial episode, EIA is considerably less; by 4 hours, however, the protective effect has completely disappeared.[301] The exact explanation for the refractory period is unknown; however, some evidence suggests a relative depletion or attenuated release of mast cell mediators,[302] as well as the release of bronchodilating prostaglandins during the postexercise period.

Exercise and isocapnic hyperventilation of cold and/or dry air causes cough as well as bronchoconstriction. The time course of the cough is similar to that of bronchoconstriction, with a peak 5 minutes after exercise or hypoventilation and a duration of approximately 30 minutes. It correlates better with respiratory water loss than with heat loss and occurs in both normal and asthmatic subjects. Cough also occurs in response to inhaled hypertonic aerosols, suggesting that the stimulus is the change in airway fluid osmolarity as a result of evaporative water loss.

Infection

Viral infection of the respiratory tract can have important consequences for airway function. In otherwise normal adults, small but measurable transient changes in flow rates and pharmacologic responsiveness can result from infection with respiratory syncytial virus (RSV) or influenza A virus or vaccination with live attenuated virus.[303] In asthmatic patients, heat-killed and live attenuated influenza vaccination, as well as naturally occurring infection with RSV, rhinovirus, and influenza A virus, has been found to cause increased NSBH.[304] More severe "cold" symptoms develop in allergic individuals in response to an experimental rhinoviral infection than in nonallergic controls, suggesting synergy between viral- and allergen-induced inflammation.[305]

The effect of viruses in provoking bronchoconstriction appears to be more pronounced in children than in adults; in some studies, for example, viral infections have been associated with exacerbations of asthma in as many as 70% of episodes in children[306] but only 10% of episodes in adults.[307] The mechanism by which infection precipitates these attacks is not clear. Interaction with cholinergic or sensory nerves, epithelial damage, and stimulation of cytokine synthesis have been suggested.[308] It is possible that airway wall edema and increased secretions within the airway lumina further diminish the caliber of already narrowed airways. It is also conceivable that the mucosal inflammation associated with the infection results in airway smooth muscle contraction secondary to release of mediators from inflammatory cells.

In addition to inducing attacks in individuals known to have asthma, there is evidence that viral infection predisposes to development of the disease. Recurrent wheezing and asthma develop in as many as 50% of children who have an episode of RSV bronchiolitis during infancy[309]; moreover, the more severe the initial episode of bronchiolitis, the higher the subsequent risk.[310] The mechanisms by which such infection might lead to subsequent asthma are unclear. In some instances, the attack of bronchiolitis may be the first attack of asthma in a genetically susceptible child.[311] Alternatively, the bronchiolitis could alter the subsequent immune response to aeroallergens, or the viral genome could persist or become latent within the airways, thereby establishing a potentially persistent inflammatory stimulus.[312]

Our understanding of the relationship between respiratory infection and asthma has become more complicated with the rise to prominence of the hygiene hypothesis, which supports a role for early and frequent respiratory infections in *preventing* subsequent allergic asthma.[313] It is possible that infection protects against the development of allergic asthma but precipitates exacerbations in patients who have established disease.[266]

Analgesics

Acetylsalicylic acid (ASA) and several other nonsteroidal analgesics and anti-inflammatory drugs (NSAIDs) such as indomethacin are capable of provoking attacks in about 5% to 30% of patients who have asthma.[314,315] The typical ASA-sensitive patient is a nonatopic woman older than 20 years with a long history of perennial rhinitis and nasal polyps.[316] Long-standing asthma and rhinitis usually precede development of the sensitivity, and the intolerance increases with age, being six times more common after the age of 50 than before the age of 20.[317] Peripheral eosinophilia is observed in more than 50% of patients, although serum IgE levels are usually normal and specific IgE directed toward ASA is not detectable.[315]

Symptoms and signs develop 20 minutes to 3 hours after ingestion. Two forms of response can occur: a predominantly respiratory form and an urticarial-angioedema form. Rarely, both occur in the same individual.[315] The respiratory response is dominated by bronchoconstriction and can be severe and life-threatening; it is usually associated with rhinitis and conjunctivitis. The diagnosis can be confirmed by challenging the patient, preferentially via the oral route.[318]

The most likely mechanism by which the drugs cause bronchoconstriction is by blocking the metabolism of arachidonic acid via the cyclooxygenase pathway (COX-1).[319] Supporting this hypothesis is the observation that the degree of bronchoconstriction that the drugs induce in vivo is proportional to their ability to retard prostaglandin synthesis in vitro.[320] On the other hand, acetaminophen, sodium salicylate, and trisalicylates have little anti-COX activity and can be safely used in most ASA-sensitive patients.[321] The new COX-2 inhibitors also appear to be safe in ASA-sensitive individuals.[322] Although it has been postulated that NSAIDs produce their effect by causing an acute decrease in the synthesis of bronchodilating prostanoids,[323] a more likely explanation is that blockade of the COX-1 enzyme diverts more arachidonic acid toward the lipoxygenase metabolic pathway and thereby results in excessive production of bronchoconstricting leukotrienes.[324]

Gastroesophageal Reflux

The association of asthma and gastroesophageal reflux (GER) is common, various investigators having estimated the concordance to be from 30% to over 80%.[325] There is evidence that GER can induce asthma and that asthma can cause a worsening of GER. It is possible that GER triggers airway narrowing in susceptible persons by reflex bronchoconstriction secondary to stimulation of afferent nerves in the esophagus or pharynx and/or by direct aspiration of a small amount of esophageal contents.[326] When acid is instilled into the esophagus of asthmatic patients, bronchoconstriction occurs primarily in those in whom symptoms of esophagitis develop.[327] It has been suggested that GER contributes to the nocturnal worsening of asthma because recumbency and decreased tone in the lower esophageal sphincter during sleep enhance reflux.[328] Although the results are inconsistent,[329] antireflux therapy has been reported to reduce the respiratory symptoms caused by GER,[330] and some data indicate long-term improvement in respiratory function after antireflux therapy.[331] There is also a strong association of cough and GER in patients who have asthma; however, GER is associated with cough in nonasthmatics as well.[325]

Emotion

It is difficult to evaluate the influence of psychological factors as provocative triggers of asthmatic attacks.[332] Although some asthmatic patients are emotionally unstable and dependent, this is almost certainly a result of their disease rather than a factor predisposing to its development. Mild bronchoconstriction and bronchodilation can be produced by suggestion, presumably as a result of changes in cholinergic vagal activity.[333] Hyperventilation provoked by anxiety is common in asthmatic patients. In fact, a vicious cycle can be established because the hyperventilation itself can cause bronchoconstriction as a result of hypocapnia and airway drying, thus tending to increase the anxiety.[334] Despite evidence for neural effects on the immune response, resistance to infection, and endocrine function, all of which could also have an influence on the development of asthma,[335] there is no direct evidence that psychoneural interaction plays a role in the basic pathophysiologic processes that cause the asthmatic state.

Environment

It is clear that low levels of atmospheric chemical pollutants can cause functional abnormalities in patients who have hyperresponsive airways.[336] In fact, epidemiologic studies in industrial areas have shown that asthma symptoms and admissions to the hospital are increased during periods of heavy pollution,[337] which may be seasonal.[338] The major respirable atmospheric chemicals that affect lung function are ozone and the oxides of sulfur and nitrogen.

In normal subjects, inhalation of sulfur dioxide (SO_2) in concentrations of 0.5 to 1.0 ppm causes mild, transient, asymptomatic bronchoconstriction, albeit only when the subjects exercise during the exposure, thereby increasing the dose of SO_2 reaching the airways.[339] As might be expected, patients who have asthma are more sensitive than normal subjects. A concentration as low as 0.25 ppm can cause detectable obstruction during mild exercise,[340] and 5 minutes of heavy exercise in 0.4 or 0.5 ppm SO_2 can cause transient symptomatic exacerbation (followed by recovery within 24 hours).[341]

In both normal and asthmatic subjects and at a concentration as low as 0.12 ppm, ozone causes a dose-dependent decrease in expiratory flow rates and volumes, as well as TLC, thus making it the most potent irritant gas.[342] As with SO_2, its effects are enhanced with exercise. Even brief ozone exposure increases subsequent nonspecific airway responsiveness in normal subjects[343]; the results of some animal and human studies suggest that this effect is mediated by airway inflammation.[344] At a population level, the prevalence of airway hyperresponsiveness is related to the level of pollution.[345]

The oxides of nitrogen are another component of smog and industrial pollution that in low concentration can precipitate symptomatic episodes in hyperresponsive individuals.

A transient increase in the nitrogen oxide level to more than 500 parts per billion was blamed for an acute outbreak of asthma in Barcelona, Spain, in which 44 patients were admitted to the hospital over a 2- to 3-hour period.[346] Inhalation of nitrogen dioxide (0.3 ppm) increases the severity of exercise-induced bronchoconstriction in asthmatic patients.[347] In most studies, low-level NO_2 exposure (0.1 ppm for 1 hour or 910 $\mu g/m^3$ for 20 minutes) enhances nonspecific airway responsiveness in asthmatic subjects but does not do so in normal individuals.[348]

Although there is little evidence to suggest that environmental pollution has contributed to the increased prevalence of asthma,[349] certain pollutants may alter the immunologic response to inhaled allergen and thus foster an increase in allergic airway disease.[350] "Domestic air pollution" from wood stoves, fireplaces, and gas stoves may also be associated with increased morbidity.[351]

Deep Inspiration

Normal subjects show a transient decrease in airway resistance after a deep inspiration, a reaction believed to be caused by relaxation of airway smooth muscle.[352] By contrast, asthmatic subjects often show paradoxical airway narrowing.[353] The difference between asthmatic subjects and normal individuals is also evident after pharmacologically induced bronchoconstriction: a deep inspiration in these circumstances has a profound bronchodilating effect in normal subjects that is absent or deficient in asthmatic subjects.[354] The effectiveness of deep inspiration in asthmatics correlates with severity and is modified by treatment.[355] The reason for the abnormal response to a big breath in asthmatic subjects is not known. It is possible that the stretch on the airways stimulates irritant receptors and initiates reflex bronchoconstriction or causes a myogenic contraction of the muscle.[356] Alternatively, the stretch may not be adequately transmitted to the muscle because of airway remodeling, or the hypertrophied airway smooth muscle layer may show a deficient or abnormal response to stretch.[357,358]

In addition to a deficient bronchodilating effect of deep inspiration, asthmatic subjects have a deficient "bronchoprotective" effect. When normal subjects take a few deep inspirations before the administration of a bronchoconstricting stimulus, subsequent airway narrowing is attenuated[359]; this effect is absent or markedly attenuated in asthmatic subjects.[360]

Miscellaneous Provoking Factors

Alcohol-containing beverages have been reported to precipitate attacks of bronchoconstriction in some patients who have asthma.[361] Although in certain cases this effect is caused by the preservative metabisulfite (see later), in others ethanol alone seems to be responsible.[362] A rapid onset of flushing, nasal congestion, and wheeze develops; the response is attenuated by histamine H_1 and COX blockers but not by atropine.[363] Asians, who have a very high incidence of acetylaldehyde dehydrogenase deficiency and who have a tendency to manifest vasomotor responsiveness to ethanol, may be particularly sensitive to its bronchoconstricting effects.[363]

In addition to food itself, several artificial additives to food can provoke airway narrowing in sensitive individuals. Metabisulfite salts are used as preservatives in a wide variety of foods and beverages and cause bronchoconstriction in approximately 4% of asthmatic subjects[364]; sensitivity can be documented by careful oral challenge with capsules containing increasing amounts of metabisulfite. Monosodium glutamate and the food-coloring additive tartrazine can also cause attacks.[365]

β-Adrenergic blocking agents can cause acute attacks of asthma in as many as 50% of asthmatic patients, even when used topically in the eye.[321] Although ACE inhibitors can cause cough and angioedema, they do not seem to cause these complications more often in asthmatic patients than in nonasthmatics,[366] although asthma may deteriorate during ACE therapy.

A large number of asthmatic patients report a worsening of symptoms in the presence of certain odors, of which perfume and cologne are the most frequently mentioned sources.[367] Environmental cigarette smoke exposure can also cause symptoms and airflow obstruction in asthmatic individuals.[368] As many as 30% of women with asthma complain of increased symptoms and demonstrate decreased maximal flow rates during the premenstrual period[369]; though presumably related to a hormonal effect, the precise pathogenesis is unclear.

Occupational Asthma

Occupational asthma is a particularly important form of the disease to recognize because it is becoming more frequent[370] and it is potentially completely reversible if recognized early. More than 250 chemicals have been implicated as causative agents, and it is estimated that up 20% of cases of asthma may be occupationally related.[371] Bronchial obstruction in the workplace can be induced by reflex, inflammatory, pharmacologic, or immunologic mechanisms. In this discussion we limit the term occupational asthma to the immunologic category in which the patient's asthma is caused by exposure to a specific sensitizing agent in the workplace. We do not include worsening of preexisting asthma as a result of nonspecific bronchoconstriction in response to irritants in the workplace (reflex), nor do we include variable airway obstruction caused by a single exposure to a toxic substance (reactive airways dysfunction syndrome [RADS]) or chronic exposure to a nonimmunologic irritant (e.g., byssinosis). These entities are discussed separately. The "immunologic" category can itself be subdivided into exposures with proven allergic pathophysiology—in which high-molecular-weight substances can be implicated—and those in which an immunologic mechanism is likely but unproven—in which low-molecular-weight substances are the offending agents.

Proven Allergic Bronchoconstriction

For the most part, the antigens implicated in this form of asthma are high-molecular-weight proteins, polysaccharides, or glycoproteins derived from plants or animals. Sensitivity develops predominantly in workers with an atopic predisposition, and positive immediate skin test or specific IgE responses (RAST) can be demonstrated. Smokers have a substantial increase in risk for this form of occupational asthma.[372]

Symptoms develop in up to 30% of workers chronically exposed to proteins from the fur or urine of rats, mice, guinea pigs, or rabbits.[373] Seafood exposure has emerged as an important cause of occupational asthma.[374] Exposed workers include fishers, processing plant personnel, and cooks; recreational anglers exposed to live baitfish are also at risk. IgE-mediated acute and delayed airway responses to specific antigens such as grain mites and weevils and to the grains themselves develop in a small percentage of atopic grain workers.[370] Symptoms of allergy (rhinitis and asthma) eventually develop in 7% to 20% of bakers.[375] There has been a substantial increase in the prevalence of allergic skin and airway sensitivity to latex in workers involved in the manufacture and inspection of latex products and in health care workers and patients who use latex gloves or are exposed to latex products.[376]

Possible Allergic Bronchoconstriction

An ever-increasing number of low-molecular-weight substances (<1000 daltons) have been shown to induce asthma in exposed workers. Although the mechanism of sensitization to these substances is uncertain, some features are suggestive of an allergic origin: (1) sensitivity develops in only about 5% of exposed individuals, (2) there is a latent period between exposure and the onset of bronchoconstriction, (3) increasing exposure increases the incidence of sensitivity, and (4) exposure to minute quantities of the substances causes acute bronchoconstriction followed by a delayed response. On the other hand, classic skin test sensitivity is usually absent, and sensitivity is not more likely to develop in atopic individuals. Strangely, sensitivity is less likely to develop in cigarette smokers, the exact opposite of allergic bronchoconstriction associated with high-molecular-weight allergens.[377]

The best-studied agent in this category is plicatic acid, which is a component of red cedar saw dust.[378] Sensitivity to this substance develops in approximately 4% of exposed workers over an exposure period ranging from months to years. Nonatopic individuals are equally as prone as atopic individuals to the development of sensitization, and no clinical or historical characteristics permit a prediction of which workers will be affected. Specific IgE antibody to plicatic acid–human serum albumin conjugate is found in approximately 40% of patients tested. Cough and dyspnea can be insidious in onset and predominantly nocturnal, presumably as a result of the delayed response; these characteristics make diagnosis difficult. Symptoms and pulmonary function abnormalities increase with the duration and intensity of exposure.[379] Approximately 60% of sensitive individuals have persistent symptoms for 4 years after cessation of exposure; those whose symptoms are of longer duration before diagnosis and whose pulmonary function is worse at diagnosis are less likely to recover completely.[380]

Isocyanates are used as hardeners in paint, varnish, molds, and plastics, and exposure to them, particularly toluene diisocyanate (TDI), is the most common cause of occupational asthma. Airway sensitivity develops in as many as 20% of exposed workers.[381] TDI hypersensitivity can cause prolonged asthma despite removal from occupational exposure.[382] The clinical, epidemiologic, and pathophysiologic features are similar to those of plicatic acid sensitivity, although nonspecific irritant and allergic alveolitis–type syndromes have also been reported.[383,384]

Diagnosis

The diagnosis of occupational asthma is aided by a high index of suspicion and requires a demonstration that the patient's symptoms are caused by asthma and are related to the work environment. It is established by a combination of clinical history, pulmonary function tests, bronchodilator response, and tests of nonspecific and specific bronchial responsiveness. A carefully taken occupational history should be obtained from all patients with adult-onset asthma. It is especially helpful if symptoms develop during or immediately after exposure to a specific agent; however, symptoms can begin after working hours or can be solely nocturnal. Patients should be questioned concerning remission of their symptoms during weekends and holidays and exacerbation on return to work. It should be remembered that asthma may begin as long as 10 years after first exposure.[385] Positive results of skin tests or RAST to known occupational allergens are supportive of the diagnosis.

Patients with occupational asthma frequently have normal lung function at initial evaluation, and it may be necessary to document functional impairment related to work exposure.[386] Because of the potential for delayed responses, 24-hour records of PEFR with mini–peak flowmeters may be particularly helpful in establishing the diagnosis.[387] Serial tests of NSBH can also help document that the asthma is work related.[388] An increase in NSBH during a period of exposure and a decrease during absence from work provide strong evidence for occupational sensitivity.[389] In addition, tests of NSBH help predict the severity of the response to a challenge with a specific sensitizing agent.[390]

Bronchial provocation testing with suspected occupational agents should not be undertaken lightly and should be performed only by experienced personnel in a hospital setting where resuscitation facilities are available.[370] However, a significant airway response to a specific challenge remains the most definitive means of establishing a causative relationship, provided that a nonspecific irritant response can be ruled out.

Miscellaneous Occupational Airway Disorders

Patients who have asthma that is unrelated to a specific occupational exposure can suffer episodic exacerbation of their symptoms when exposed to a variety of irritants in the workplace.

Acute exposure to a high concentration of certain gases, vapors, and smoke can produce severe bronchial and bronchiolar injury that causes narrowing and hyperresponsiveness of airways in an exposed worker.[384] This condition, which has been called *reactive airways dysfunction syndrome*, develops after a single exposure to a high concentration of gases (such as hydrogen sulfide, ammonia, diethylene diamine, and chlorine), fumes from plastics, and smoke from a variety of materials.[391] Airway obstruction develops within 24 hours of exposure, and some degree of obstruction and exaggerated nonspecific airway responsiveness can persist for months, usually followed by slow resolution.

Some occupations involve exposure to substances that are thought to cause a direct, nonidiosyncratic airway effect in a dose-dependent fashion in all or most exposed workers.[370] The most common substances implicated in this type of reaction are cotton dust (byssinosis), grain dust (grain fever), and the noxious aerosols generated in livestock confinement buildings.[392] These disorders are referred to collectively as *organic dust toxic syndrome* (see page 511).[393] Certain organophosphate insecticides have anticholinesterase activity and can produce vagally mediated airway narrowing.[370]

Radiologic Manifestations

The most common radiographic abnormalities in patients who have asthma are hyperinflation and bronchial wall thickening; less frequent manifestations include peripheral oligemia, increased central lung markings, and prominence of the hila.[394] The prevalence of these abnormalities is influenced by several factors, including the age at onset and severity of asthma and the presence of other diseases or complications of asthma.[395]

In the presence of acute severe asthma or during a prolonged, intractable attack, the most characteristic radiographic signs are pulmonary hyperinflation and expiratory air trapping (Fig. 15–18).[396] The former is manifested as an increase in the depth of the retrosternal space, an increase in lung height, and flattening of the diaphragm. Thickening of the airways occurs in both segmental and subsegmental bronchi and can be seen either as ring shadows when viewed end-on or as "tramline" opacities when viewed en face. Prominence of the main pulmonary artery and its hilar branches with rapid tapering is indicative of transient precapillary pulmonary arterial hypertension secondary to hypoxia (Fig. 15–19).[397] Additional vascular findings include diffuse narrowing and blood flow redistribution into the upper lobes (the latter in the absence of other signs of postcapillary hypertension) and a paucity of vessels in the outer 2 to 4 cm of the lungs (Fig. 15–20).

Despite the observations just outlined, the chest radiograph has a limited role in the diagnosis of asthma. It is often normal, even during an acute attack; moreover, when it is abnormal, the findings are nonspecific.[398] In fact, the two main indications for chest radiography are to exclude other conditions that cause wheezing throughout the chest (particularly emphysema, congestive heart failure, and obstruction of the trachea or major bronchi) and to identify complications such as pneumothorax.[399]

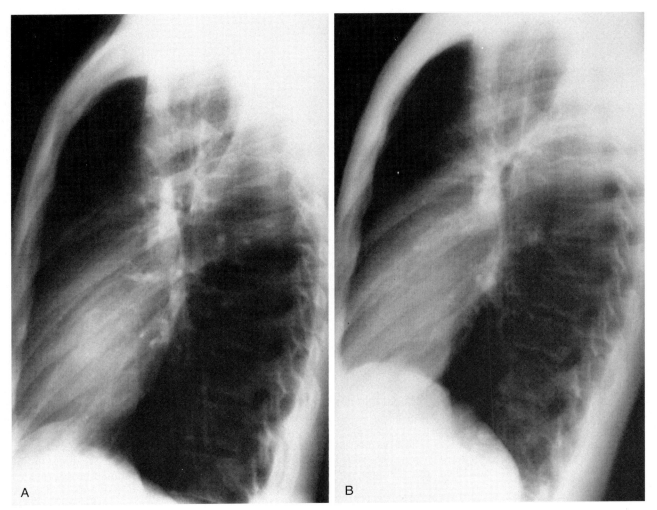

FIGURE 15–18

Asthma—reversible pulmonary overinflation (adult). A lateral chest radiograph (**A**) of an adult asthmatic patient during an attack of severe bronchospasm reveals a low position and flat configuration of the diaphragm, indicative of severe pulmonary overinflation. Approximately 1 year later during a remission (**B**), lung volume had returned to normal. Note that the curvature of the sternum and thoracic spine did not change because these structures do not participate in acute hyperinflation in an adult. *(From Fraser RS, Müller NL, Colman NC, Paré PD: Fraser and Paré's Diagnosis of Diseases of the Chest, 4th ed. Philadelphia, WB Saunders, 1999.)*

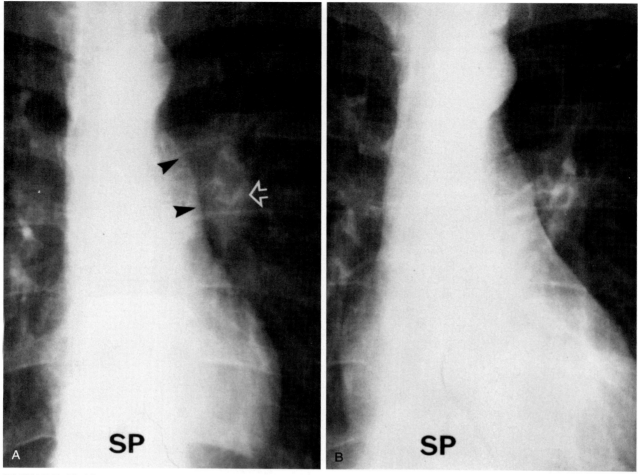

FIGURE 15–19

Asthma—reversible precapillary pulmonary hypertension. A detail view of the heart and left hilum from a posteroanterior radiograph (**A**) reveals enlargement of the main pulmonary artery (*arrowheads*) and left interlobar artery (*open arrow*), consistent with the presence of pulmonary arterial hypertension. At the time of this study, the patient, a young man, was experiencing a severe attack of acute bronchospasm. Approximately 2 years later during a period of remission, a repeat radiograph (**B**) demonstrates a return to normal configuration of the main and interlobar arteries. Note that the heart has increased in size during this interval, reflecting a decrease in the high transpulmonary pressure that existed during the acute attack and the consequent reduction in venous return. *(From Fraser RS, Müller NL, Colman NC, Paré PD: Fraser and Paré's Diagnosis of Diseases of the Chest, 4th ed. Philadelphia, WB Saunders, 1999.)*

HRCT allows visualization of the airways and parenchyma in asthmatic patients in much greater detail than plain radiography does (Fig. 15–21).[220,400] The thickening and narrowing of the airways can be quantified and have been shown to increase with increasing severity of disease.[401,402] Additional findings include bronchial dilation, gas trapping, and patchy areas of decreased attenuation and vascularity (Fig. 15–22). The latter result from abnormalities in ventilation-perfusion distribution; they may be seen even during clinically stable periods and have been well described by scintigraphy (Fig. 15–23).[403]

Clinical Manifestations

The diagnosis of asthma is based largely on a history of periodic paroxysms of dyspnea, when the individual is at rest as well as exercising, alternating with intervals of complete or nearly complete remission. Some patients have a more chronic form of the disease, but periodic exacerbation and remission occur in all cases. Cough can be a prominent symptom, and nonsmoking patients who have asthma can fulfill the diagnostic criteria for chronic bronchitis.[404] The diagnosis is strengthened by a history of eczema or hay fever or by a family history of allergies.

Meticulous inquiry into the circumstances that initiate attacks, though time-consuming, is a particularly important diagnostic procedure. Questioning should be directed toward the possible association with ingestion of a specific food (particularly in children) or the season of the year (suggesting either pollen or insect sensitivity). Careful inquiry should be made into possible antigens in the home, especially those from domestic pets, feather pillows, cockroaches, and bedding or carpets, which can harbor dust mites. The patient may also have recognized an association between the onset of symptoms and exposure to the work environment.

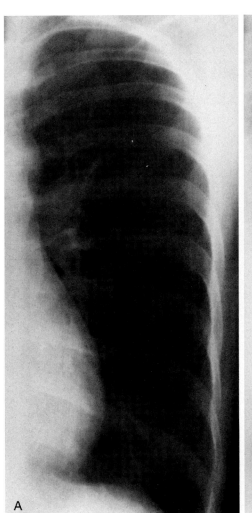
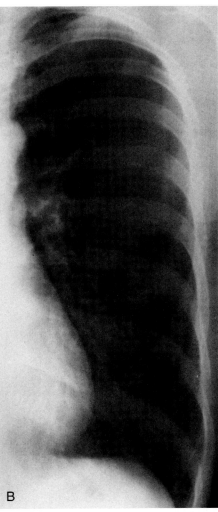

FIGURE 15-20

Asthma—peripheral oligemia. A detail view of the left lung from a posteroanterior chest radiograph (**A**) of a young man during an episode of acute bronchospasm reveals moderate hyperinflation. The vasculature in the outer 2 to 3 cm of lung is inconspicuous and barely visible, thus creating a subpleural shell of oligemic lung. A repeat study 1 year later during remission (**B**) shows less hyperinflation; the pulmonary vessels now taper normally, and most are visible well into the lung periphery. (*From Fraser RS, Müller NL, Colman NC, Paré PD: Fraser and Paré's Diagnosis of Diseases of the Chest, 4th ed. Philadelphia, WB Saunders, 1999.*)

A history of drug intake should always be sought, particularly with respect to β-blockers, NSAIDs, and ACE inhibitors. The patient should be questioned about whether there is an association between the onset of asthmatic attacks and infections of the upper or lower respiratory tract, with particular emphasis on the occurrence of symptoms suggestive of sinusitis, such as postnasal drip and facial pain. An attempt should be made to correlate the onset of attacks with emotional disturbance; if the patient is a child, interview of the parents should be included. Additional historical features of importance include a previous history of rhinitis, eczema, or anaphylaxis and symptoms suggestive of GER. Finally, the patient should be questioned regarding the relationship between the onset of attacks and exercise; exposure to cold air, irritating dust, fumes, or odors; and changes in temperature and humidity. When a history of exercise-induced attacks is elicited, it should be determined whether the prior ingestion of any particular food precipitates the attacks.[405]

In both atopic and nonatopic patients, particularly those who are elderly, the original asthmatic episode is commonly termed *acute bronchitis*, regardless of whether concomitant fever or symptoms of upper respiratory tract disease are present.[406,407] In such patients, wheezing and paroxysmal nocturnal dyspnea are often attributed to COPD or left ventricular failure.[408] In fact, nocturnal breathlessness is a common symptom of asthma, and careful history taking may be necessary to distinguish the disease from paroxysmal nocturnal dyspnea of cardiac origin.

In the majority of patients, the onset of an attack is heralded by a nonproductive cough and wheeze. The onset of dyspnea is usually gradual and seldom abrupt. Paroxysms occur most commonly at night; when they are severe, the patient may feel obliged to sit on the edge of the bed or open the window in the vain hope of relieving breathlessness. The lowest values for expiratory flow are recorded in the early hours of the morning (2 to 4 AM) (a phenomenon known as "morning dipping").[409] The mechanisms of nocturnal asthma are unclear. Asthmatic patients show a circadian rhythm in airway responsiveness, plasma epinephrine, cortisol, cyclic adenosine monophosphate (cAMP), and histamine, each of which may have an effect.[410] Sleep itself is not a necessary factor because the obstruction develops, albeit somewhat less severely, even when nocturnal sleep is prevented.[411]

Cough (with normal pulmonary function) is the sole initial symptom in some patients, in which case measurement of NSBH may be helpful in diagnosis.[412] Patients in whom asthma is the underlying cause of cough usually have an increase in nonspecific airway responsiveness, and the cough

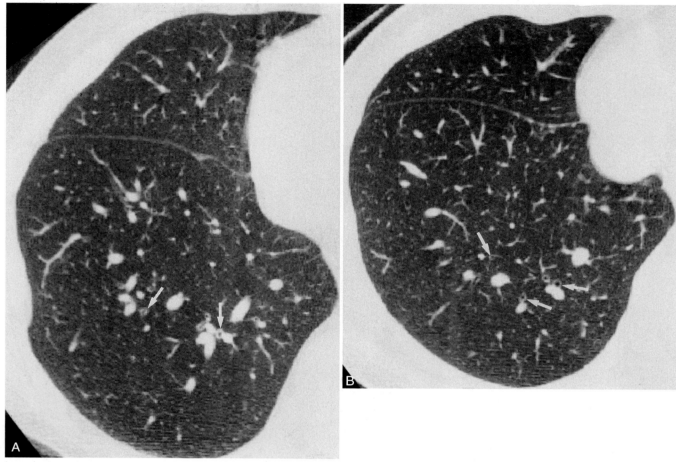

FIGURE 15–21

Asthma—bronchial wall thickening. An HRCT scan in a patient who has chronic asthma (**A**) demonstrates thickening of the walls of several bronchi (*arrows*) and a decreased diameter of their lumen (compare with the image from a healthy individual in **B**). *(From Fraser RS, Müller NL, Colman NC, Paré PD: Fraser and Paré's Diagnosis of Diseases of the Chest, 4th ed. Philadelphia, WB Saunders, 1999.)*

is alleviated by treatment of the asthma. Measurement of the total eosinophil count may be a useful screening technique to select patients for this test.[413]

Although some patients have attacks of asthma that develop over a period of hours, most have had progressive symptoms over days to weeks, often with more rapid deterioration during the previous 24 hours. Younger atopic subjects are more likely to have exacerbations of rapid onset.[414] Occasionally, the onset of asthma is so insidious that the diagnosis is not considered, particularly in elderly smokers, who usually are labeled as having COPD; intensive therapy in such patients may result in a dramatic reversal of obstruction.[415] The sudden onset of chest pain should arouse suspicion of pneumomediastinum or pneumothorax.

Physical findings in asthma include hyperventilation, hyper-resonance on percussion, inspiratory and expiratory rhonchi and wheezes, decreased breath sounds, and prolonged expiration. In very severe attacks, wheezing may not be apparent, the clinical picture being one of air hunger. In this situation there is evidence of the use of accessory muscles of respiration, diminished breath sounds without rhonchi, and often cyanosis.[416] A precordial "click" or "crunch" synchronous

with the heartbeat (Hamman's sign) may be present in association with pneumomediastinum or pneumothorax.

Patients who have acute severe asthma may be too dyspneic or exhausted to speak or may be stuporous or even comatose as a result of hypoxemia and hypercapnia; in these situations, they commonly have tachycardia and pulsus paradoxus. In fact, measurement of the pulsus paradoxus can provide an index of the severity of the bronchoconstriction.[417] On inspiration, the systolic arterial pressure of normal individuals decreases by as much as 5 mm Hg, whereas in patients with asthma it may drop by 10 mm Hg or more. This greater decrease is probably the result of increased negative intrathoracic pressure secondary to airway obstruction and may be related to two mechanisms:[418] (1) the increased right ventricular volume caused by the negative pressure may result in a leftward shift of the interventricular septum and interfere with left ventricular diastolic filling, and (2) because there is communication between the ventricle and the great vessels outside the thorax that are not exposed to the negative pressure, the negative intrathoracic pressure may act as an afterload on the left ventricle.[419]

A number of algorithms have been designed in an attempt to assess asthma severity in order to provide prognostic

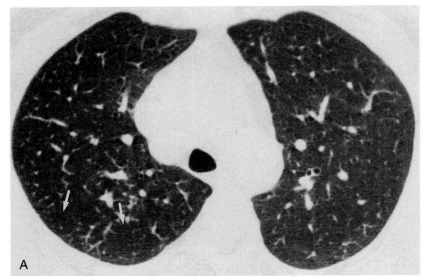

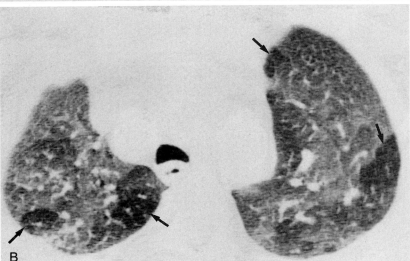

FIGURE 15–22

Asthma—air trapping. An HRCT scan performed at end-inspiration (**A**) shows subtle localized areas of decreased attenuation and vascularity (*arrows*). HRCT performed at the end of maximal expiration (**B**) shows several bilateral areas of air trapping (*arrows*). The patient was a 45-year-old lifelong nonsmoker who had chronic asthma. (*From Fraser RS, Müller NL, Colman NC, Paré PD: Fraser and Paré's Diagnosis of Diseases of the Chest, 4th ed. Philadelphia, WB Saunders, 1999.*)

information and guide therapy.[420] When present, pulsus paradoxus and the use of accessory muscles of inspiration suggest more severe obstruction, but overall neither symptoms nor physical sign can be used to reliably judge severity.[421] Appropriate assessment requires objective measurement of maximal expiratory flow.[422] Another index of asthma severity is the intensity of therapy required for its control. This has led to inclusion of the intensity of therapy in estimates of severity and separation of the concept of asthma "control" from asthma "severity"[423] (e.g., a patient may have severe asthma but it can be well controlled because of intensive therapy; alternatively, a relatively mild asthmatic may have significant symptoms if not taking any medication). In a small subset of patients who have very severe asthma, the disease appears to be refractory to intensive therapy.[424] It should be remembered, however, that such "refractory asthma" must be distinguished from other conditions in which symptoms and signs of airflow obstruction are not reversible with anti-inflammatory and bronchodilator therapy, including COPD, laryngeal dyskinesia, vocal cord dysfunction, airway obstruction by neoplasm, bronchiectasis, and bronchiolitis. Additional causes of "refractory asthma" are lack of compliance with medications, poor technique in the administration of inhaled medications, and persistent exposure to allergens.

Laboratory Findings

Cytologic and chemical alterations in sputum have been systematically explored as means of assessing the severity of airway inflammation, and rigorous standards of analysis have been proposed.[425] The combination of sputum eosinophil count and a measure of the level of eosinophil cationic protein has been shown to be a more sensitive and specific means of distinguishing between asthmatic patients and normal individuals than are measurement of these parameters in peripheral blood.[426] Blood eosinophils do not usually exceed 10% of the total white cell count, but they may account for up to 35%. Skin tests may be useful in identifying specific food or aeroallergens to which patients are sensitive, and confirmation of specific sensitivity may be obtained by RAST. It is important to remember, however, that skin application of the

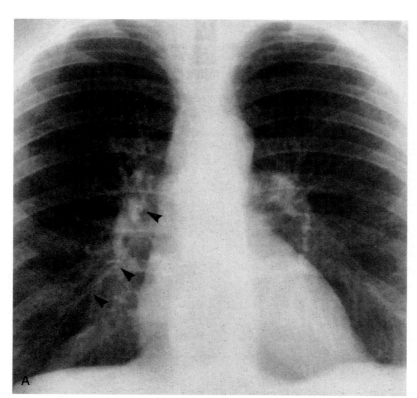

FIGURE 15–23

Asthma—ventilation-perfusion abnormalities. A posteroanterior chest radiograph (**A**) is normal except for mild overinflation and bronchial wall thickening (*arrowheads*). A ventilation lung scintigram (**B**) reveals unequal deposition of radioisotope in the central parenchyma on the initial breath (IB), with relative sparing peripherally; equilibration (EQ) was eventually achieved centrally and peripherally, although air trapping occurred in both areas during the washout (WO) phase. A perfusion scan (**C**) in anterior (A), posterior (P), right lateral (RL), and left lateral (LL) positions demonstrates deficits in the perfusion pattern in the lower lobes and posterior portions of the upper lobes. Note the rim of maintained perfusion in the cortex (1) that alternates with adjacent regions of cortical hypoperfusion (2); in both instances, the proximal medulla (3) is focally underperfused. The presence of maintained perfusion adjacent to contiguous medullary hypoperfusion on a scintigram is designated the "stripe sign," identification of which effectively excludes thromboembolic disease as the cause of the oligemia. (*From Fraser RS, Müller NL, Colman NC, Paré PD: Fraser and Paré's Diagnosis of Diseases of the Chest, 4th ed. Philadelphia, WB Saunders, 1999.*)

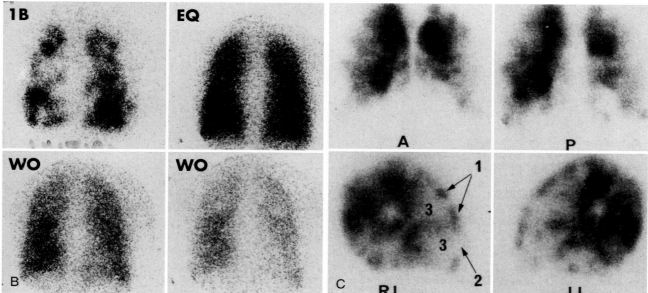

recommended dilutions of individual allergens may precipitate an attack. The patient must be watched carefully for reactions, and countermeasures should be at hand.[427]

Although inhalation challenge is a more reliable method of identifying specific allergens, it is rarely indicated in clinical practice because profound immediate and delayed bronchoconstriction may occur. It should be reserved for research studies in carefully controlled settings and for incriminating a specific antigen in occupational asthma.[428] Nonspecific inhalation challenge with methacholine is an important diagnostic technique in some patients and may have value in monitoring the response to long-term therapy.

A variety of electrocardiographic changes may occur during severe episodes of asthma.[429] Sinus tachycardia is almost always present; in addition, there may be right axis deviation, clockwise rotation of the heart, right ventricular hypertrophy, right atrial P waves, and ST-segment or T-wave abnormalities.

Pulmonary Function Tests

As might be expected, abnormalities in pulmonary function in patients with asthma vary, depending largely on whether the disease is in remission or exacerbation and, if the latter, on the severity of the attack. Many patients whose asthma is in remission have normal routine pulmonary function,[430] although "sensitive" tests of small-airway function may demonstrate abnormalities.[431] Even when maximal expiratory flow and volume are within the normal predicted range, inhalation of a bronchodilator may result in greater than a 15% increase in FEV_1 or FVC. The relationship between symptoms and function depends on the patient's ability to detect airway obstruction and is quite variable; some patients are unable to sense the presence of severe airway obstruction (FEV_1 less than 50% of predicted).[432]

Diffuse airway narrowing is the basic functional abnormality of symptomatic asthma; the resulting increase in resistance leads to decreased flow, hyperinflation, gas trapping, and ultimately, an increase in the work of breathing. It is most easily detected and quantified by measurements of maximal expiratory flow derived from either volume-time or flow-volume plots.[433] The increase in airway resistance is also associated with hyperinflation, as manifested by an increase in FRC and, to a lesser extent, TLC.[396] The latter is significantly higher and lung elastic recoil lower in asthmatic individuals whose disease began in childhood than in those who have the adult-onset type.[434] The hyperinflation has both advantages and disadvantages.[435] By dilating the intraparenchymal airways, it improves the distribution of ventilation and prevents limitation of expiratory flow during tidal breathing.[435] On the negative side, it increases the elastic work of breathing and places inspiratory muscles on an inefficient portion of their length-tension curve.

As an asthmatic episode resolves, there is improvement in expiratory flow and VC and a decrease in FRC and RV. A decrease in symptoms may accompany the return of lung volumes to normal before changes in FEV_1 are observed, presumably because of the reversal of hyperinflation and gas trapping.[436] Flow rates measured at low lung volumes ($FEF_{25\%-75\%}$, $\dot{V}_{50}$, $\dot{V}_{25}$) may take longer to improve or may never return to normal predicted values.[437]

The single-breath diffusing capacity is often elevated in both stable and acute asthma.[438] The most plausible explanation for this apparent paradox is the transient increase in pulmonary capillary blood volume that occurs as a result of the more negative inspiratory intrathoracic pressure secondary to obstruction of the airways.

Most patients experiencing an acute attack have some degree of hypoxemia as a result of $\dot{V}/\dot{Q}$ mismatch.[302] Inhalation of a β-adrenergic bronchodilator increases the perfusion to low $\dot{V}/\dot{Q}$ regions and lowers arterial PO_2, suggesting pharmacologic reversal of hypoxic vasoconstriction in these regions.[439] Respiratory alkalosis is the only acid-base disturbance seen during mild asthmatic attacks, but metabolic and mixed acidosis can occur during severe exacerbations.[440]

There is not a close relationship between measures of airway obstruction and gas exchange in asthma.[441] However, in severe acute attacks, PaO_2 generally drops to below 60 mm Hg, FEV_1 is less than 1 L, and peak flow is less than 60 L/min.[442] As the severity and duration of obstruction increase, patients become exhausted, their respiratory muscles fatigue, and values of $PaCO_2$ rise into the hypercapnic range.[443] In asthma, unlike COPD, hypercapnia is *never* a steady-state situation. PCO_2 can rise steeply within minutes or hours, and patients should be under constant surveillance.

Prognosis and Natural History

Complications of asthma are much more common in children than adults and consist of pneumonia, atelectasis, mucoid impaction, pneumomediastinum, and rarely, arterial air embolism. Radiographic examination of large groups of children who have acute asthma demonstrates one of these complications in about 5% to 25% of individuals,[444,445] whereas similar studies in adults have shown them in as few as 1%.[446]

Atelectasis is the result of mucus plugging of small or large airways.[444] Although it is uncommonly identified radiologically in adults, it is probable that mucus plugging of smaller bronchi and bronchioles occurs much more frequently than recognized, atelectasis being prevented by collateral ventilation of obstructed regions.

Pneumomediastinum is also an uncommon complication that is most often identified in males. Infants in particular have a tendency for the additional development of pneumothorax.[447] Should the pneumothorax fail to respond to chest tube drainage and the ipsilateral lung undergo progressive loss of volume, obstruction of central airways by impacted mucus should be suspected. In asthmatic patients who require mechanical ventilation during an acute attack, systemic hypotension and barotrauma can occur secondary to dynamic hyperinflation.[448] In addition to complications that result directly from an asthmatic attack, lower respiratory tract infection occurs more frequently in patients who have asthma than in the population at large, and the clinical severity of viral infections tends to be worse in asthmatic individuals.[449] The reason for these effects is unclear.

Three issues need to be considered when determining the prognosis of patients with asthma: the determinants of recovery from an individual acute episode, the likelihood of achieving complete remission, and the chance of dying of the disease.

Recovery from an Acute Asthmatic Episode. Features that have been associated with a need for hospitalization and a prolonged symptomatic and functional recovery from acute asthma include (1) age older than 40 years, (2) absence of atopy, (3) a longer duration of symptoms before admission, (4) poor long-term control of symptoms, and (5) the use of maintenance steroids.[450] The rapidity with which flow rates improve during the first 6 hours also predicts a patient's recovery time.[451] In one retrospective study, a scoring system based on pulse rate, respiratory rate, pulsus paradoxus, PEFR, the use of accessory muscles, and the severity of dyspnea and wheeze was 90% effective in predicting the need for hospitalization and the relapse rate after discharge from the emergency room.[452] The mortality among asthmatic patients who require mechanical ventilation during an acute attack is about 10% to 15%.[453]

Remission. Determination of the ultimate long-term prognosis requires a long period of follow-up. The likelihood of remission is much greater in childhood-onset asthma. Almost 60% of children who "wheeze" before the age of 3 years are asymptomatic by the age of 6.[454] Fifty percent to 70% of patients whose onset of disease is before 16 years of age experience remission in early adult life.[455] A number of factors are associated with a poor prognosis in this respect, including early onset of symptoms, multiple attacks in the initial year, clinical and physiologic evidence of persistent airway obstruction, hyperinflation, chest deformity, and growth impairment.[456] In an 8-year follow-up study of 2289 children who were 6 to 8 years of age when first seen, active and passive cigarette smoking, lower socioeconomic status, number of children and furry pets in the household, and the use of gas cookers were associated with persistent symptoms.[457] The prognosis in patients whose asthmatic attacks are intermittent and who show evidence of lability is considerably better than in those whose symptoms are continuous and whose obstruction is relatively fixed.[458]

The remissions experienced by adolescents and young adults may or may not be permanent. In a 14-year follow-up of 441 children, the cumulative prevalence of asthma increased until the age of 7 years and then progressively decreased until the age of 17 to 18 years, at which time 70% were "cured" (no symptoms or treatment for 1 year).[459] Subsequent "relapses" occurred, however, and at an average age of 26 years, only 57% were still "cured." Additional relapses tend to occur with increasing age.

Although a characteristic feature of asthma is some degree of reversibility of the airflow obstruction, it is clear that long-standing disease can lead to a relatively fixed narrowing and accelerated decline in lung function,[460] despite prolonged and aggressive therapy with bronchodilators and corticosteroids.[461]

Mortality. Death from asthma is rare and occurs predominantly in adults between the ages of 40 and 60 years and in children younger than 2 years.[462] Racial and ethnic differences in asthma mortality rates have been well documented; for example, in the United States, age-adjusted mortality in African Americans and Hispanics is higher than that in whites.[463]

In 1980, death rates from asthma in patients aged 5 to 34 years ranged from 0.2 per 100,000 in the United States to 3 per 100,000 in New Zealand.[199] Since that time, the death rate in New Zealand has fallen dramatically (to about 0.5 per 100,000 in 1994), whereas it has increased slowly and steadily in most other countries.[464] Two largely unexplained and transient increases in asthma mortality occurred between 1959 and 1966 in the United Kingdom, New Zealand, and Australia[262] and, more recently, in New Zealand again.[465] Although excessive use of β-adrenergic bronchodilators has been suggested as a possible cause of these "epidemics," the authors of a meta-analysis of β-agonist use and death from asthma concluded that although there was a significant relationship, the effect was very small and potentially confounded.[466]

Case-control studies have identified several factors that are linked to near-fatal or fatal asthma, including (1) a history of previous mechanical ventilation or admission to an intensive care unit, (2) increased asthma symptoms in the week preceding death, (3) a decrease in corticosteroid dosage, (4) inadequate steroid and bronchodilator administration, (5) excessive theophylline dosage, (6) over-reliance on home nebulized bronchodilators, and (7) failure to institute artificial ventilation.[260,467] Patient education is also an important factor in preventing death. Patients who are considered to be at risk of dying should be admitted to the hospital promptly when their clinical and physiologic findings indicate a severe attack.[468]

CHRONIC OBSTRUCTIVE PULMONARY DISEASE

The Global Initiative on Obstructive Lung Disease (GOLD) has proposed a definition of COPD that is based on evidence of airflow obstruction. Accordingly, it is defined as *a disease*

TABLE 15–3. GOLD Classification of Severity*

Stage	Characteristics
0	At risk. Normal spirometry Chronic symptoms (cough, sputum production)
1	Mild COPD. $FEV_1/FVC < 70\%$ $FEV_1 > 80\%$ of predicted With or without chronic symptoms (cough, sputum production)
2	Moderate COPD. $FEV_1/FVC < 70\%$ FEV_1 between 50% and 80% of predicted With or without chronic symptoms (cough, sputum production)
3	Severe COPD. $FEV_1/FVC < 70\%$ FEV_1 between 30% and 50% of predicted With or without chronic symptoms (cough, sputum production)
4	Very severe COPD. $FEV_1/FVC < 70\%$ $FEV_1 < 30\%$ of predicted or $FEV_1 < 50\%$ of predicted plus chronic respiratory failure[†]

*Classification based on postbronchodilator FEV_1.
[†]Respiratory failure: Pao_2 less than 60 mm Hg with or without $Paco_2$ greater than 50 mm Hg while breathing air at sea level.
GOLD, Global Initiative on Obstructive Lung Disease.

state characterized by airflow limitation that is not fully reversible. The airflow limitation is usually both progressive and associated with an abnormal inflammatory response of the lungs to noxious particles or gases.[469] A classification based on severity of disease has also been proposed (Table 15–3). The cutoff for the presence of disease (stage 1) is a postbronchodilator FEV_1/FVC ratio less than 70%. Synonyms for COPD include chronic obstructive lung disease, chronic airflow obstruction, and chronic airflow limitation. Although the first two are acceptable, chronic airflow limitation is misleading because it suggests that airflow limitation is unique to this entity. In fact, everyone has maximal expiratory airflow limitation; it is the severity of the limitation that is abnormal in COPD. We use the GOLD definition of COPD in this text along with the following definitions of chronic bronchitis and emphysema.[470]

Chronic bronchitis refers to a clinical condition diagnosed on the basis of a history of excessive mucus expectoration on most days during at least 3 consecutive months for not less than 2 consecutive years.[471] All other causes of chronic coughing and expectoration must be eliminated before the diagnosis is accepted. In some cases, it may be difficult to differentiate chronic bronchitis from asthma, and the term *asthmatic bronchitis* has been used to describe patients who fulfill the diagnostic criteria for both conditions.

The relationship between chronic bronchitis and airway obstruction is unclear.[472] In an investigation of 2718 male smokers monitored for 20 years, coughing and sputum production were found not to be related to a decline in lung function[473]; the initial value of FEV_1 as percent predicted and persistent smoking were the most important determinants of eventual symptomatic airflow obstruction. In another 10-year follow-up study of 13,756 men and women, the importance of baseline FEV_1 was confirmed[474]; however, mucus hypersecretion was also a significant predictor of the rate of decline in lung function, as well as risk for hospitalization and death from COPD.[475] Despite these findings, it is clear that cough and sputum production can develop in smokers in the absence of airway obstruction and that obstruction can occur in the absence of mucus hypersecretion. This discordance means that it is misleading to equate chronic bronchitis with COPD.

Emphysema is defined as abnormal permanent enlargement of air spaces distal to the terminal bronchioles, accompanied by destruction of their walls, without obvious fibrosis.[476] Strictly speaking, the condition can be diagnosed only pathologically; however, certain clinical, pulmonary function, and CT features allow an in vivo estimation of its presence and severity. Although emphysema is generally accompanied by loss of lung elastic recoil—which in turn is thought to cause airflow obstruction, hyperinflation, and gas trapping—loss of recoil can occur without the development of emphysema and vice versa.

The term *small-airway disease* has been used to describe not only the pathologic abnormalities seen in the small airways of patients with COPD but also a variant of the clinical findings in a small number of patients with COPD.[259] We believe that use of the term in the latter context should be abandoned because it only leads to confusion; disease of the small airways is one of the abnormalities that leads to airway obstruction in COPD, not a disease in its own right.

Epidemiology

Whichever terms one accepts, it is clear that these conditions have an important impact on health throughout the world. Mortality rates for COPD in the United States increased steeply between 1930 and 1980 and have continued to rise.[261] According to projections from the World Health Organization, rates of morbidity and mortality from COPD will increase over the next 20 years and make COPD the 3rd leading cause of death (currently 4th) and 5th leading cause of disability (currently 12th) worldwide.[477,478] In addition, there is good evidence that chronic respiratory disease is a very important cause of work incapacity and restricted activity in both Europe and North America.[479,480] The worldwide prevalence of COPD in 1990 was estimated to be 9.3/1000 in men and 7.3/1000 in women.[481] The exponential increase in cigarette smoking in some "developing" countries promises a continued increase in global prevalence.[482]

Although it has been proposed that men are more susceptible to the effects of cigarette smoke,[483] there is in fact evidence that gender differences are related to differences in cigarette consumption or that women are more susceptible than men for the same smoke exposure.[484,485] There may also be a gender bias in the diagnosis; women who have clinical and physiologic findings characteristic of COPD are more likely to have asthma diagnosed than are men who have the same findings.[486] COPD is generally more severe in white than in nonwhite cigarette smokers, a difference that cannot be explained by the amount, mechanism, or duration of cigarette smoking.[487]

Etiology

Cigarette smoking is clearly the most important factor in the development of COPD. The condition is rare in those who do not smoke.[488] However, since COPD develops in only a relatively small percentage of chronic smokers,[489] other factors must be important. Possible modifiers and amplifiers of the response to cigarette smoke include air pollution, infection (especially during childhood), climate, heredity, socioeconomic status, atopy, nonspecific airway hyperresponsiveness, diet, and nutrition.[490]

Tobacco Smoke

Cigarette smoking is overwhelmingly the most important etiologic agent in the development of COPD.[491] Healthy people who are nonsmokers show a yearly decline in FEV_1 that is largely secondary to the age-related decrease in lung elastic recoil; smokers, however, show an exaggerated decline, the rate increasing with the intensity of cigarette smoking (Fig. 15–24).[492] Cigarette smoking also retards the normal increase in expiratory flow that occurs during growth in childhood or adolescence.[493] The duration and intensity of smoking are of equal importance in determining these effects. Smoking cessation is associated with a small improvement in lung function, a decrease in coughing and sputum expectoration, and normalization of the rate of annual decline in lung function.[494,495]

It is not known which of the components of tobacco smoke are responsible for the development of COPD; however, the tar content, the use of filters, and the development of allergy to cigarette smoke components do not appear to be important. The pattern of inhalation may influence the site and intensity of lung exposure to the various particulates and gases and could be a factor leading to the variable response between individuals.[496]

Although personal cigarette smoking is certainly the most important risk factor in the development of COPD, passive or sidestream (i.e., environmental tobacco smoke) exposure may

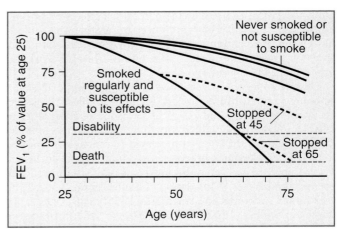

FIGURE 15–24

Changes in FEV_1 with aging. The graph shows the percent change in FEV_1 versus age for smokers and nonsmokers. Nonsmokers show a gradual decline in FEV_1 with age, and smokers who are not susceptible to the effects of cigarette smoke show a similar, though somewhat accelerated decline. Individuals who are susceptible to cigarette smoke and who smoke regularly demonstrate an accelerated decline in FEV_1, which increases in rapidity with increasing age ("horse race effect"). Smoking cessation returns the rate of decline to that observed in the nonsmoking or nonsusceptible population. *(Modified from Peto R, Speizer FE, Cochrane AL, et al: The relevance in adults of air-flow obstruction, but not of mucus hypersecretion, to mortality from chronic lung disease. Results from 20 years of prospective observation. Am Rev Respir Dis 128:491-500, 1983.)*

also be harmful, especially in infants and children.[491] Such individuals who live in the same household as parents or siblings who smoke have an increased incidence of respiratory illness, functional impairment, and a less than expected increase in lung function during growth.[497]

Air Pollution

Air pollution may be domestic, urban, or occupational. Although the effects are usually minor when compared with the influence of cigarette smoking, in heavily polluted regions and with certain industrial exposures they may be significant.

Domestic exposure to pollutants is often overlooked, but it is likely to be an important factor in certain situations. For example, the use of natural gas in home cooking has been shown to be associated with an increased incidence of childhood respiratory illness and pulmonary dysfunction that is independent of the effects of parental smoking.[498] Cooking fires are a major cause of domestic pollution worldwide, and in rural communities in "developing" countries, prolonged exposure can lead to obstructive lung disease and cor pulmonale.[499]

Although a sudden increase in the degree of air pollution—such as occurs with smog—can result in increased morbidity and mortality in patients with established COPD,[500] there is less evidence that urban air pollution per se causes obstructive pulmonary disease in adult nonsmokers.[501] However, it does appear to have an effect additive to that of cigarette smoke and may be partly responsible for progression of disability in patients already affected.[502] There are also significant relationships between hospital admission and emergency room visit rates for COPD and atmospheric levels of SO_2 and O_3 and the atmospheric concentration of particulate particles less than 10 μm in diameter (PM_{10}).[503] Children with growing lungs may be particularly vulnerable to the effects of air pollution. The incidence of acute lower respiratory tract infections is higher in children who live in environments with high levels of air pollution[504]; such infection increases the risk for impairment in lung function.

Despite some controversy over the relative importance of smoking and exposure to dust in the workplace, in some occupations there is unequivocal evidence of a significant effect of inhaled dust on lung function.[505] An increased annual rate of decline in FEV_1 or an increased prevalence of emphysema has been seen in workers exposed to inorganic dust such as coal, in hard rock miners, and in those in the metal and chemical industries.[506] Inhalation of cotton, grain, wood dust, and fumes generated in slaughterhouses and livestock confinement buildings has also been shown to contribute to chronic airway obstruction.[507]

Infection

There is evidence that lower respiratory tract infection in children is a significant risk factor for the subsequent development of COPD during adulthood.[508] Childhood "bronchitis" and pneumonia, especially in children younger than 2 years, are associated with persistently abnormal lung function[509]; moreover, this impairment appears to predispose to accelerated deterioration. The precise mechanism of this effect is uncertain, but it may reflect an alteration in growth or pulmonary defense. Alternatively, these associations could be due to the fact that children predisposed to the later development of COPD have an increased susceptibility to infection.[510] It has also been speculated that chronic latent adenovirus infection of airway epithelium may be a factor.[511]

Respiratory infection in patients who have established COPD may accelerate subsequent functional deterioration and can lead to an irreversible deficit[512]; of particular importance in this regard is the possibility that established COPD itself may increase the incidence and severity of respiratory infection. However, despite a severe decline in pulmonary function during respiratory infections, most patients who have COPD improve to their pre-exacerbation status after resolution of the infection.

Viral infection is responsible for the majority of clinical exacerbations in patients with COPD.[513] The rhinoviruses and myxoviruses—the latter particularly during epidemics—appear to be the most common etiologic agents.[514] H. influenzae, M. pneumoniae, and Chlamydia pneumoniae may also precipitate exacerbations.[515]

Climate

Patients who have COPD often relate exacerbations of their disease to climatic factors, particularly extreme variations in humidity and temperature. There are also seasonal variations in morbidity from obstructive lung disease that are incompletely explained by known risk factors.[516] In patients who have established COPD, both inhalation and exposure of facial skin to cold dry air cause bronchoconstriction.[517]

Socioeconomic Factors, Diet, and Nutrition

An increased risk for the development of COPD is seen in individuals of lower socioeconomic status. Although the precise mechanism is unclear, it has been shown to be independent of factors such as smoking habit, industrial exposure, passive smoking, diet, and childhood infection.[518]

Nutritional status as judged by BMI is a predictor of survival in patients who have established COPD; however, it is unclear whether this represents a causal relationship.[519] Specific associations between vitamin C levels and chronic bronchitis and between polyunsaturated fatty acid consumption and COPD have been reported.[520,521]

Heredity

First-degree relatives of patients with COPD have a likelihood of developing the disease that is 1.2 to 3 times that of the general population.[522] The observation that concordance for indices of airway obstruction is greater between first-degree relatives than between spouses and greater between monozygotic than dizygotic twins supports the influence of a genetic predisposition rather than the effects of a shared environment.[523] The results of twin studies suggest that the proportion of the variability in lung function that is due to genetic factors (i.e., the heritability) ranges from 0.5 to 0.8.[523a]

One of the most important hereditary abnormalities associated with COPD is α_1-antiprotease inhibitor (α_1-PI) deficiency. The relative risk for the development of symptomatic COPD imparted by the presence of homozygous deficiency (Pi^{ZZ}) is approximately 30. However, such deficiency accounts for less than 1% of cases of COPD because the frequency of the genetic defect is only 1 in 2000 to 1 in 4000 in white populations.[524] α_1-PI is an acute phase reactant that is synthesized in the liver and released into the blood. Normal values for serum concentrations are between 0.93 and 1.77 g/L, and values less than 0.30 g/L represent severe deficiency; values can also be expressed as micromoles per liter, the lower limit of normal being about 11 µmol/L.[525] Heterozygous deficiency (Pi^{MZ}) is much more common than the homozygous form (1 in 100 to 4 in 100) and is associated with serum α_1-antiprotease levels that are approximately 60% of normal. However, because of the well-documented overlap of serum concentrations of α_1-PI, particularly between normal individuals and patients in the intermediate range, identification of protease inhibitor protein (Pi) by electrophoresis or genotyping is necessary for the recognition of heterozygotes.[525]

More than 25 different α_1-PI isoforms have been described; approximately 90% of the population is homozygous for M (Pi^{MM}).[526] The gene Pi^Z in the homozygous state (ZZ) is associated with the lowest serum concentration of α_1-PI ($\approx$20% of normal).[527] The Z isoform of the antiprotease has a lysine molecule substituted for glutamic acid at position 342.[528] In the normal molecule, the latter is the site of attachment of sialic acid; the lack of this substance results in intracellular polymerization, defective secretion, and accumulation of α_1-PI in hepatocytes.[529] In a small percentage of Pi^{ZZ} individuals, liver disease (cholestasis, hepatitis, and cirrhosis) develops as a result of intrahepatic retention of the protein.[530]

Cigarette smoking plays an important role in the production of emphysema in patients who have α_1-PI deficiency. The symptom of dyspnea and other evidence of airflow obstruction bring smokers with α_1-PI deficiency to medical attention in the third and fourth decades of life, whereas nonsmokers may not become symptomatic until the sixth or seventh decade.[531] In fact, respiratory symptoms may never develop in PI^{ZZ} individuals who do not smoke. A family history of COPD is an additional risk factor for the development of obstruction with or without smoking.[525]

Occasionally, emphysema is described in patients who have Pi variants other than Pi^{ZZ}. The heterozygous Pi^{SZ} phenotype has been associated with α_1-PI levels as low as those seen in Pi^{ZZ} patients and is associated with a modest increase in risk for COPD.[525] Despite some controversy, the bulk of the evidence suggests that the heterozygous Pi^{MZ} phenotype increases the risk approximately twofold in those who smoke.[532] There is also evidence of an increased risk for the development of bronchiectasis in patients who have severe α_1-PI deficiency.[533]

After recognition of the association between emphysema and α_1-PI deficiency, it was hypothesized that other inherited forms of COPD would be discovered to explain the genetic tendency for the development of COPD. Linkage analysis of severe early-onset COPD has revealed a number of promising loci,[534] and many genes and gene products have been tested for potential involvement in pathogenesis (Table 15–4).[535] The relative risk imparted by the mutant forms of these genes is generally small in comparison to homozygous α_1-PI deficiency.

Nonspecific Bronchial Hyperresponsiveness (the "Dutch Hypothesis")

This hypothesis proposes that patients who are atopic and have increased nonspecific bronchial responsiveness have an increased risk for irreversible airflow obstruction.[536] It is not

TABLE 15–4. Candidate Genes in COPD

Gene Class	Gene
Protease and antiprotease genes	α_1-Antitrypsin
	Tissue inhibitors of metalloproteinases (TIMPs)
	α_1-Antichymotrypsin
	Matrix metalloproteinases (MMPs 1, 2, 9, and 12)
	α_2-Macroglobulin
Antioxidant and xenobiotic metabolizing enzyme genes	Heme oxygenase-1
	Microsomal epoxide hydrolase
	Glutathione-S-transferases
	Cytochrome P-450 1A1
Inflammatory mediator genes	Tumor necrosis factor-α
	Vitamin D–binding protein
	Interleukin-1α, interleukin-1β
	Interleukin-1 receptor, type 1
	Interleukin-1 receptor, type 2
	Interleukin-13
	Interleukin-1 receptor antagonist
Genes involved in airway defense	Human leukocyte antigens
	Cystic fibrosis transmembrane conductance regulator
	Defensins (α-defensin-1, -2)
	Surfactant proteins

clear exactly how these conditions might be involved in the pathogenesis of COPD. However, in individuals with hyperresponsive airways, it is possible that repeated episodes of acute bronchoconstriction related to smoke inhalation might by themselves cause fixed narrowing. Alternatively, an exaggerated inflammatory response to smoke in atopic individuals could be responsible.[537]

In the 5-year follow-up study of nearly 6000 smokers in the U.S. Lung Health Study, airway reactivity to methacholine was shown to be an important predictor of progression of airway obstruction independent of the baseline level of obstruction.[538] Additional support for the Dutch hypothesis derives from population studies that have shown a positive relationship between decreased FEV_1 levels and skin test responses to allergens, blood eosinophilia, and elevated serum IgE levels.[539,540] In a study of 1533 individuals monitored for 20 years, an elevated total serum IgE level was predictive of the development of airflow obstruction, even after correction for asthma and cigarette smoking.[541]

Pathogenesis

COPD is caused by two fundamental processes, each of which is based on exaggerated inflammation; one affects the airways and results in fibrosis and narrowing, and the other affects the parenchyma and results in emphysema. The latter process is caused by enzymatic destruction of the elastic and collagen framework of the lung.[542] Although the most important enzyme in this regard is elastase derived from polymorphonuclear leukocytes, evidence is increasing that the matrix metalloproteinases (MMPs) and other proteolytic enzymes are involved.[543,544] For example, both alveolar and interstitial macrophages, which contain a variety of MMPs that have elastase and collagenase activity, are significantly increased in number in smokers. In addition, in mice in whom the

MMP-12 gene has been "knocked out," emphysema does not develop after smoke exposure.[545]

The lung is normally protected against excessive elastolytic damage by antiproteases, including α_1-PI, α_1-macroglobulin, low-molecular-weight antiproteases present in airway mucus (e.g., secretory leukocyte proteinase inhibitor), and the tissue inhibitors of metalloproteinases.[546,547] The balance between proteolytic and antiproteolytic forces and the factors that influence them (Fig. 15–25) are of fundamental importance in the pathogenesis of emphysema.

The effect of cigarette smoke may be explained by its action on both proteolytic and antiproteolytic factors. It decreases the level of lysyl oxidase, an enzyme involved in the repair of damaged elastin and collagen[542]; increases the number of circulating and pulmonary neutrophils and alveolar macrophages[548]; enhances neutrophil adhesion to the endothelium[549]; delays the transit of neutrophils through the pulmonary circulation[550]; causes the release of elastase from neutrophils; and may enhance the chemotaxis of neutrophils from the vasculature to the lung interstitium.[551] The peripheral neutrophils of smokers also show a higher than normal content of myeloperoxidase—an enzyme that can oxidatively inactivate α_1-PI—and neutrophil elastase.[552]

An oxidant/antioxidant imbalance is also an important mechanism in the pathogenesis of COPD. The gas phase of cigarette smoke is a rich source of oxidizing agents, one puff of cigarette smoke having been estimated to contain more than 10^{14} free radicals.[553] Nitric oxide is also present in cigarette smoke at concentrations of 500 to 1000 ppm, and it can form damaging radicals.[554] Reactive oxygen species are released from activated leukocytes, and cigarette smoke decreases antioxidant defenses.[555] Oxidants can inactivate antiproteinases, cause air space epithelial injury, increase sequestration of neutrophils in the pulmonary microvasculature, and increase the expression of proinflammatory mediators.

The mechanisms underlying the airway inflammation, scarring, and narrowing, which constitute the second important pathophysiologic mechanism in COPD, are less well understood. Oxidant damage to the epithelium, secondary inflammatory cell infiltration, and mucus hypersecretion all contribute. Although there is evidence of activation of the innate immune response, the presence of lymphocytes and lymphoid aggregates also suggests activation of the adaptive immune system, perhaps in response to microbial antigens.[556] Cigarette smoking is associated with an increased amount of serum protein in airway mucus,[557] alterations in the viscoelastic properties of mucus,[558] and decreased clearance of particulate matter from the airways[559]; however, patients may have significant impairment in airflow without alterations in mucociliary clearance and vice versa.[560] In fact, only mild

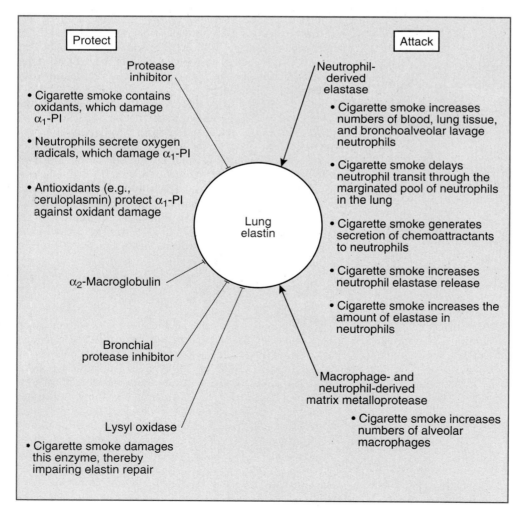

FIGURE 15–25

Pathogenesis of emphysema. Cigarette smoke acts to disrupt the proteolysis-antiproteolysis balance at a number of sites. The overall effect is to promote increased breakdown of elastin and interfere with repair. α_1-PI, α_1-protease inhibitor.

Protect

Protease inhibitor

• Cigarette smoke contains oxidants, which damage α_1-PI

• Neutrophils secrete oxygen radicals, which damage α_1-PI

• Antioxidants (e.g., ceruloplasmin) protect α_1-PI against oxidant damage

α_2-Macroglobulin

Bronchial protease inhibitor

Lysyl oxidase
• Cigarette smoke damages this enzyme, thereby impairing elastin repair

Lung elastin

Attack

Neutrophil-derived elastase

• Cigarette smoke increases numbers of blood, lung tissue, and bronchoalveolar lavage neutrophils

• Cigarette smoke delays neutrophil transit through the marginated pool of neutrophils in the lung

• Cigarette smoke generates secretion of chemoattractants to neutrophils

• Cigarette smoke increases neutrophil elastase release

• Cigarette smoke increases the amount of elastase in neutrophils

Macrophage- and neutrophil-derived matrix metalloprotease

• Cigarette smoke increases numbers of alveolar macrophages

airflow obstruction develops in nonsmoking individuals who have primary ciliary dyskinesia and virtual absence of particulate clearance from the lung.[561] Anatomic factors are probably involved: patients with chronic bronchitis have an increased number of ultrastructurally abnormal cilia,[562] as well as replacement of ciliated cells by goblet cells and metaplastic squamous cells.

Pathologic Characteristics

The majority of patients with COPD have pathologic abnormalities in the large airways, small airways, and lung parenchyma, although the changes in an individual patient may be located predominantly in one of these sites.[563]

Large Airways

Hyperplasia of the tracheobronchial glands is common and partly explains the increase in mucus production seen in chronic bronchitis. However, measurements of gland hyperplasia generally do not correlate with the severity of airway obstruction.[564] The tracheobronchial epithelium often shows foci of goblet and basal cell hyperplasia and squamous metaplasia, sometimes associated with dysplasia. Other bronchial wall abnormalities include an increase in total wall thickness and smooth muscle,[565] chronic inflammation,[557] and decreased cartilage and elastic tissue.[566]

Small Airways

Airways smaller than 2 to 3 mm in internal diameter are the major site of increased resistance to airflow in the lungs of patients with COPD.[567] The principal histologic abnormalities underlying this increased airflow resistance are seen in the membranous and respiratory bronchioles and include (1) thickening of the walls by a chronic inflammatory cell infiltrate and fibrous tissue (see Color Fig. 15–2) and (2) goblet cell metaplasia associated with partial or complete plugging of the lumina by mucus.[568] An increase in alveolar macrophages in airway lumina and adjacent alveolar air spaces is common. Disruption of the surrounding alveolar walls, which normally provide structural support to the airways, may also be evident.[569]

The severity of these abnormalities and the accompanying airway narrowing can be assessed by using a semiquantitative microscopic scoring system based on a comparison of the airways to be measured to a set of standard photomicrographs that show different degrees of cellular infiltration and fibrosis.[570] These and other more quantitative measurements correlate with decreased maximal expiratory flow and increased total airway resistance.[571] Patients who have normal expiratory flow but abnormal tests of small-airway function—such as the closing volume or the slope of phase III of the single-breath nitrogen washout test—are also more likely to have pathologic abnormalities of their small airways.[572]

Lung Parenchyma

The basic pathologic abnormality of the lung parenchyma is destruction of alveolar walls and the formation of enlarged air spaces (i.e., emphysema). Four morphologic types of emphysema have been described, depending on the localization of disease within the acinus. Selective or predominant involvement of the respiratory bronchioles is termed *centrilobular emphysema*, whereas diffuse and more selective terminal acinar destruction are termed *panacinar emphysema* and *distal acinar emphysema*, respectively. The fourth form shows no specific localization and is termed *irregular emphysema*.

Although the pathologic diagnosis of emphysema is usually made on gross examination, microscopic estimation of its severity can be performed by measuring the average distance between alveolar walls, measuring the alveolar wall surface area per unit volume, or using a semiquantitative index of lung destruction.[573]

Centrilobular Emphysema. Centrilobular is the most common form of emphysema that has clinical and functional significance; it is found predominantly in cigarette smokers. The earliest lesions are seen in the region of the proximal respiratory bronchioles (Fig. 15–26). Although the term *centrilobular* is frequently used to refer to this region, the fact that each lobule contains multiple acini means that instead of disease being found precisely in the center of the lobule, it is characteristically distributed in a multifocal fashion within it (Fig. 15–27).

The histologic appearance of early disease and the reasons for its proximal acinar predilection have not been well established. The earliest abnormality may be fenestrae, or holes, which can be seen in the alveolar walls adjacent to small airways (Fig. 15–28).[574] Theoretically, these fenestrae coalesce as they increase in size and number, so eventually the alveolar wall disappears. Morphometric studies have shown that the number of alveolar walls attached to the small airways decreases in emphysema, thus supporting this concept.[575] These early morphologic abnormalities are associated with loss of lung elasticity and decreased maximal expiratory flow and can occur in the absence of gross pathologic changes.

As disease progresses, respiratory bronchioles dilate and the adjacent parenchymal tissue is lost, thereby resulting in abnormal foci clearly identifiable both microscopically and

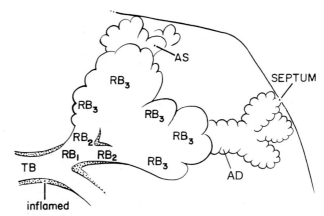

FIGURE 15–26

Centrilobular emphysema. In centrilobular (proximal acinar) emphysema, respiratory bronchioles (RB) are predominantly involved. AD, alveolar duct; AS, alveolar sac; TB, terminal bronchiole. *(Modified from Thurlbeck WM: Chronic Airflow Obstruction in Lung Disease. Philadelphia, WB Saunders, 1976, p 15.)*

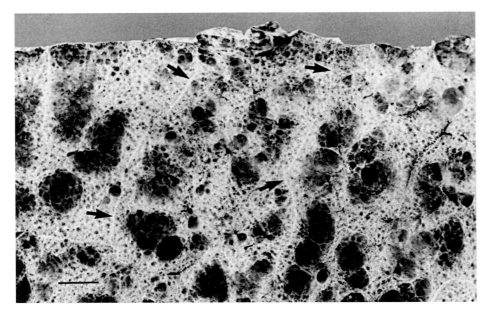

FIGURE 15–27

Centrilobular emphysema—anatomic location within the lobule. A highly magnified view of lung parenchyma shows multiple foci of emphysema distributed in a patchy fashion; most appear black as a result of deposition of carbon in residual tissue. The parenchyma adjacent to the interlobular septa *(arrows)* is essentially normal. The location of the emphysematous spaces corresponds approximately to that of the proximal respiratory bronchioles. (The specimen was inflated with polyethylene glycol and air-dried.) *(From Fraser RS, Müller NL, Colman NC, Paré PD: Fraser and Paré's Diagnosis of Diseases of the Chest, 4th ed. Philadelphia, WB Saunders, 1999.)*

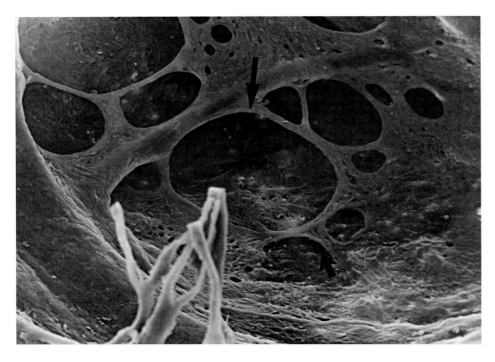

FIGURE 15–28

Alveolar wall fenestrae. A scanning electron micrograph of an alveolar wall shows multiple small *(short arrow)* and large *(long arrow)* fenestrae. *(From Fraser RS, Müller NL, Colman NC, Paré PD: Fraser and Paré's Diagnosis of Diseases of the Chest, 4th ed. Philadelphia, WB Saunders, 1999.)*

grossly. The usually prominent deposition of carbonaceous pigment derived from tobacco smoke in the emphysematous foci results in a distinctive "checkerboard" appearance (see Fig. 15–27). With further progression, the relatively discrete foci of early disease become confluent, and eventually an entire lobule or whole segments of lung can be destroyed (see Color Fig. 15–3).

Centrilobular emphysema has an upper zone predominance in which the apical and posterior segments of the upper lobes and the superior segments of the lower lobes are particularly affected (see Color Fig. 15–3).[576] The precise reasons for this predominance are unclear but may be related to differences in zonal deposition or clearance of inhaled tobacco smoke, differences in perfusion between the upper and lower lobes (leukocyte transit time being prolonged and antielastases being less available in the relatively underperfused upper zones), or differences in pleural pressure (the more negative pressure and resultant hyperinflation of nondependent lung regions resulting in relatively greater mechanical stress on the alveolar walls in these regions).

Panacinar Emphysema. Panacinar (panlobular) emphysema is characteristic of disease in patients with α_1-antiprotease deficiency; however, it can also be seen in smokers and (rarely) nonsmokers without protease deficiency.[577] As with centrilobular emphysema, the early morphologic changes have been poorly documented. However, examination of thick sections of lung reveals fenestrations in alveolar walls similar to those seen in centrilobular emphysema,[578] and it is possible that these fenestrations represent the initial abnormality. As the name implies, the disease affects tissue more or less uniformly throughout the acinus (Fig. 15–29).

In severe disease, affected parenchyma consists of no more than large air spaces through which strands of tissue and blood vessels pass like struts—so-called cotton candy lung. Histologic examination shows dilated air spaces with virtually no alveolar septa. Panacinar emphysema characteristically shows a predilection for the lower and anterior lung zones.

Distal Acinar Emphysema. Distal acinar (paraseptal) emphysema is usually focal and consists of a row of more or less continuous, variably sized spaces located in the periphery of the lung adjacent to the pleura or along interlobular septa (Fig. 15–30). Bullae may develop in these regions and are usually multiple; in fact, paraseptal emphysema may represent an early form of bullous lung disease. In the vast majority of cases, the abnormal spaces are limited in extent and, with the exception of the occasional occurrence of spontaneous pneumothorax, result in no clinical disease.

Irregular Emphysema. This form is always associated with fibrosis and, according to the definition given previously, should not even be classified as emphysema.[579] The association with fibrosis suggests a relationship with inflammation. In some instances—such as remote granulomas—this

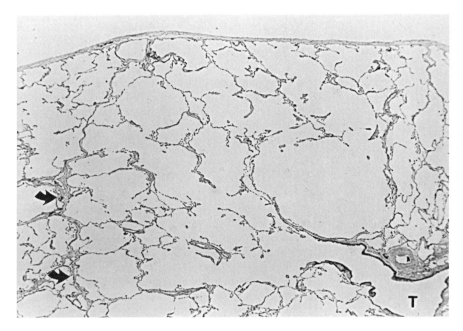

FIGURE 15–29

Panacinar emphysema. This section from a 52-year-old man who had α_1-antiprotease inhibitor deficiency shows more or less diffuse air space enlargement and loss of alveolar septa involving all the tissue between the pleura, interlobular septum (*arrows*), and terminal bronchiole (T). *(From Fraser RS, Müller NL, Colman NC, Paré PD: Fraser and Paré's Diagnosis of Diseases of the Chest, 4th ed. Philadelphia, WB Saunders, 1999.)*

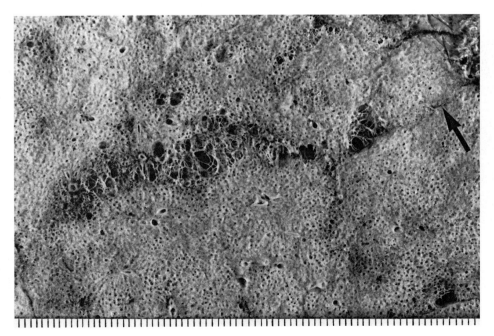

FIGURE 15–30

Paraseptal emphysema. A magnified view of an upper lobe lung slice reveals a well-delimited zone of emphysema in a linear pattern contiguous with an interlobular septum (*arrow*) immediately under the pleura. The adjacent lung parenchyma is normal. The linearity and proximity to the septum indicate the paraseptal nature of the emphysema. *(From Fraser RS, Müller NL, Colman NC, Paré PD: Fraser and Paré's Diagnosis of Diseases of the Chest, 4th ed. Philadelphia, WB Saunders, 1999.)*

association is clearly evident (Fig. 15–31); in many others, on the other hand, it can only be assumed. Typically, however, the tissue affected is limited in extent, and functional or clinical abnormalities are not apparent.

Radiologic Manifestations

As discussed previously, chronic bronchitis is defined clinically, emphysema is defined pathologically, and COPD is

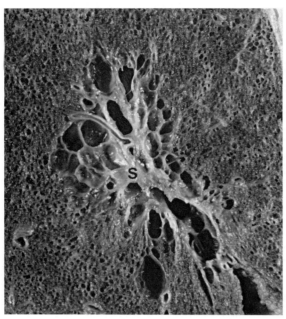

FIGURE 15–31

Irregular emphysema. A magnified slice of lung parenchyma reveals a small scar (S) surrounded by irregularly shaped emphysematous spaces. The cause of the disease was not determined. *(From Fraser RS, Müller NL, Colman NC, Paré PD: Fraser and Paré's Diagnosis of Diseases of the Chest, 4th ed. Philadelphia, WB Saunders, 1999.)*

defined functionally. As a diagnostic tool that predominantly reveals morphologic abnormalities, the chest radiograph can demonstrate changes attributable to chronic bronchitis or emphysema but can disclose variations caused by COPD only by inference.

Chronic Bronchitis

It should be remembered that chronic bronchitis is not a radiologic diagnosis. Although changes suggesting that bronchitis is present may be observed, it is inappropriate for the radiologist to do other than indicate that the findings are compatible with that diagnosis. The principal abnormalities are bronchial wall thickening and an increase in lung markings.[580] The latter (sometimes termed "dirty chest" or simply "prominent lung markings") refers to a general accentuation of linear markings throughout the lungs associated with loss of definition of the vascular margins.[581] Bronchial wall thickening may be manifested as ring shadows end-on or as tubular shadows en face ("tram tracks") (Fig. 15–32).[582] Objective measurements of these abnormalities have been made on both plain chest radiographs and HRCT scans.[583] With HRCT, the thickness of the right apical segmental bronchus has been found to correlate with measures of expiratory flow limitation in smokers that are independent of the degree of emphysema.[584]

Emphysema

Radiography. The radiographic abnormalities in emphysema reflect the presence of lung destruction, secondary alterations in the vascular pattern, and increased lung volume. Direct signs of emphysema such as bullae can be seen on the chest radiograph in some patients (Fig. 15–33).[581] Vascular abnormalities include local avascular areas, distortion of the vessels, increased branching angles and loss of the normal sinuosity of vessels, decrease in peripheral vascular markings, and enlargement of the main pulmonary arteries (Fig. 15–34).[585] The most reliable sign of overinflation is flattening of the diaphragmatic domes (see Fig. 15–33).[586] Other helpful signs

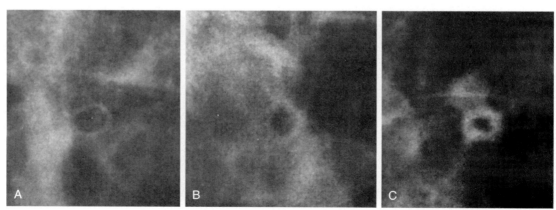

FIGURE 15–32

Bronchial wall thickening as assessed from parahilar bronchi viewed end-on. Views of the left parahilar zone from posteroanterior chest radiographs from three different patients show a normal bronchus (**A**), a bronchus with moderate wall thickening (**B**), and a bronchus with marked wall thickening (**C**). *(From Fraser RG, Fraser RS, Renner JW, et al: The roentgenologic diagnosis of chronic bronchitis: A reassessment with emphasis on parahilar bronchi seen end-on. Radiology 120:1-9, 1976.)*

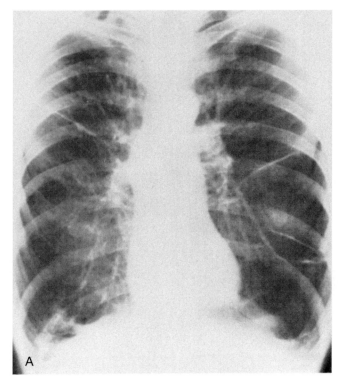

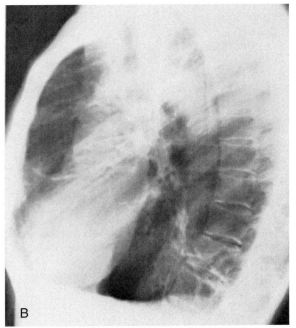

FIGURE 15-33

Emphysema associated with bullae. Posteroanterior (**A**) and lateral (**B**) chest radiographs from a 43-year-old woman reveal severe overinflation of both lungs. The diaphragm is low and its superior surface concave. Note the prominent costophrenic muscle slips. The retrosternal air space is deepened. Numerous bullae are present in both lower lung zones, particularly the left. The peripheral vasculature of the lungs is severely diminished, but there is no evidence of pulmonary arterial hypertension. *(From Fraser RS, Müller NL, Colman NC, Paré PD: Fraser and Paré's Diagnosis of Diseases of the Chest, 4th ed. Philadelphia, WB Saunders, 1999.)*

of overinflation include an increase in the retrosternal air space, an increase in lung height, and a low position (depression) of the diaphragm. When the configuration of the diaphragm is concave superiorly, the presence of emphysema is virtually certain in adults. The greatest diagnostic accuracy on the radiograph is obtained by using a combination of findings.[587]

Computed Tomography. On CT scans, emphysema is detected by the presence of areas of abnormally low attenuation, usually without visible walls (Fig. 15–35).[588] Centrilobular emphysema is characterized by the presence of multiple localized small areas of low attenuation, which often measure less than 1 cm in diameter and typically involve mainly the upper lobes. Panacinar emphysema involves mainly the lower lobes and is characterized by more diffuse areas of low attenuation and a paucity of vessels (Fig. 15–36).[589] Paraseptal (distal acinar) emphysema is characterized by the presence of areas of low attenuation in the subpleural lung regions separated by intact interlobular septa (Fig. 15–37). Because centrilobular emphysema and paraseptal emphysema produce localized areas of low attenuation, they are easier to recognize on CT scans than panacinar disease.[587] Severe centrilobular emphysema may be indistinguishable from panacinar emphysema on HRCT (compare Figs. 15–34C and 15–36B). Mild emphysema can be missed on standard CT scans[590]; visualization of such disease can be improved by the use of spiral scans and narrow window widths.

Semiquantitative scoring of CT findings correlates closely with the presence and severity of pathologically detected emphysema.[591] However, the extent of emphysema can be assessed objectively and more accurately by CT with the use of computer programs that quantify the volume of lung that has abnormally low attenuation values.[592] Lung density measured by this technique is affected by many variables, including patient size, location of the emphysema, depth of inspiration, type of CT scanner, collimation, kilovoltage, and reconstruction algorithm. Despite these limitations, correlation between the mean density mask score and the pathologic score for emphysema is excellent, especially when a Hounsfield unit (HU) cutoff of −910 is used.[593]

Spiral CT allows rapid quantification of the volume of lung affected by emphysema. The use of predetermined threshold attenuation values with this technique enables display of the distribution of emphysema in multiple planes and in three dimensions (Fig. 15–38).[594] CT also allows measurement of overall lung volumes and regional changes in lung volume after lung volume reduction surgery or bullectomy.[595] The introduction of multislice CT scanners now makes it feasible to reconstruct contiguous thin 1- to 2-mm sections through the entire lung volume.[596]

Clinical Manifestations

Respiratory Manifestations

Patients may complain of cough, expectoration, and/or dyspnea. The majority of patients with cough and expectoration have mucoid sputum, only periodically yellow or green. Cough can precede the onset of dyspnea by many years.[597] Hemoptysis is very uncommon, and its presence should stimulate a careful search for other causes, such as superimposed infectious bronchitis or carcinoma. Most patients are heavy

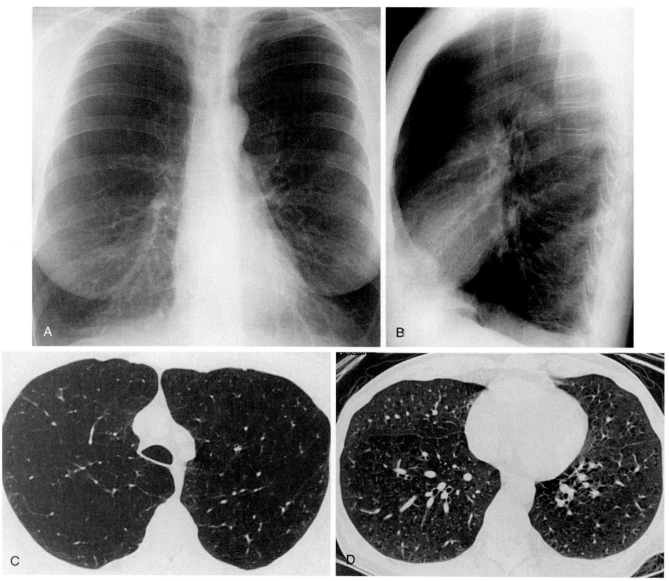

FIGURE 15-34

Centrilobular emphysema. Posteroanterior (**A**) and lateral (**B**) chest radiographs demonstrate increased lucency and decreased vascularity in the upper lobes, marked overinflation with flattening of the diaphragm, and an increase in the retrosternal air space. An HRCT scan through the upper lobes (**C**) reveals severe emphysema; a scan at a more caudal level (**D**) demonstrates relatively mild centrilobular emphysema. The patient was a 49-year-old smoker. (*From Fraser RS, Müller NL, Colman NC, Paré PD: Fraser and Paré's Diagnosis of Diseases of the Chest, 4th ed. Philadelphia, WB Saunders, 1999.*)

smokers; however, in individual patients the number of years of smoking may not correlate with the amount and duration of coughing and expectoration or the degree of pulmonary dysfunction.[598]

When COPD is mild or moderate in severity, dyspnea occurs only on exertion. As the disease worsens, it is precipitated by less and less effort and in advanced disease is present at rest. Airflow obstruction does not usually become symptomatic until after 20 or 30 years of smoking. In patients who have severe disease, dyspnea may be influenced by posture, being worse when they are in the erect, sitting, or standing position than when they are supine (platypnea) or sitting while leaning forward[599]; other patients have orthopnea. In

temperate climates, the frequency of respiratory infections is increased during the winter; such episodes cause an exacerbation of symptoms, including an increase in the severity of dyspnea.

Dyspnea is not closely related to abnormalities in arterial blood gases, a dissociation that is highlighted by the clinical differentiation of patients into "pink puffers" and "blue bloaters."[600] A typical "pink puffer," or type A patient, complains of severe dyspnea but has a relatively good blood oxygen level and does not have hypercapnia. Such patients tend to be thin and do not have cor pulmonale or right heart failure. On the other hand, a typical "blue bloater," or type B patient, has peripheral edema caused by right heart failure and

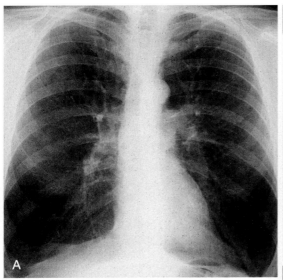

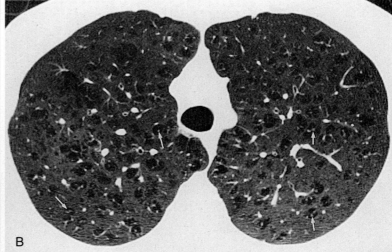

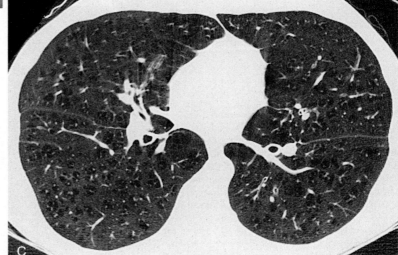

FIGURE 15–35

Centrilobular emphysema. A posteroanterior chest radiograph (**A**) demonstrates overinflation and attenuation of the peripheral vascular markings. An HRCT scan through the upper lobes (**B**) reveals localized areas of low attenuation characteristic of centrilobular emphysema. Persistent vessels (*arrows*) can be seen in the center of several of the areas of low attenuation; this feature is characteristic of emphysema and helpful in the distinction from cystic lung disease. An HRCT scan obtained at a more caudal level (**C**) demonstrates slightly less severe emphysema. The patient was a 49-year-old man. (*From Fraser RS, Müller NL, Colman NC, Paré PD: Fraser and Paré's Diagnosis of Diseases of the Chest, 4th ed. Philadelphia, WB Saunders, 1999.*)

has more severe hypoxemia and hypercapnia and less dyspnea. Although the great majority of patients with COPD cannot be placed precisely into one of these categories, the concept that there is a spectrum of clinical manifestations is a valuable one.

The physiologic and clinical responses to a given degree of airflow narrowing differ between individual patients, part of the variation probably being the result of differences in the responsiveness of the respiratory center to hypoxia and hypercapnia. It is likely that in individuals who have a well-developed ventilatory response, blood gases will be preserved at the expense of increased respiratory effort. Conversely, those who have relatively blunted respiratory center responsiveness may hypoventilate, thus allowing PO_2 to fall further and PCO_2 to rise higher. Genetic differences contribute to this variation in respiratory drive.[601] The other major determinant of dyspnea on exertion is the degree of hyperinflation: dynamic hyperinflation occurs during exercise, increasing the work of breathing and decreasing the effectiveness of the inspiratory muscles.[602]

In many patients with chronic cough and expectoration and mild airflow obstruction, physical examination of the chest reveals no abnormalities, at least during quiet breathing.

Wheezing is often audible during forced expiration, but it does not relate closely to the degree of obstruction.[603] During quiet expiration, however, it is a more reliable indicator in this regard, and symptomatic patients usually have diffuse inspiratory and expiratory wheezing. Signs associated with more severe disease include decreased intensity of breath sounds, prolonged expiration, and increased resonance of the percussion note.[604]

When lung volumes are markedly increased and the thoracic cage is fixed in an inspiratory position, the chest becomes barrel shaped, kyphosis is increased, the shoulders are raised, and the chest tends to move en bloc, often with contraction of the accessory muscles of respiration in the neck.[605] Depression of the diaphragm is believed to be responsible for a paradoxical movement of the lower thoracic costal margins during inspiration; known as Hoover's sign, it consists of an inward pulling of the costal cartilage from the flattened diaphragm.[606] Paradoxical abdominal motion at rest is a sign of inspiratory muscle fatigue or recruitment of expiratory muscles and is seen with particularly severe disease.

When a low BMI develops in patients with advanced COPD,[607] it is due to a complex interaction of nutritional

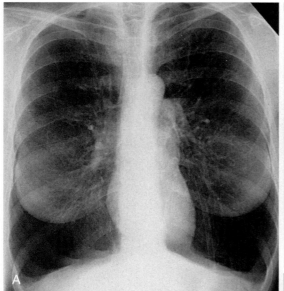

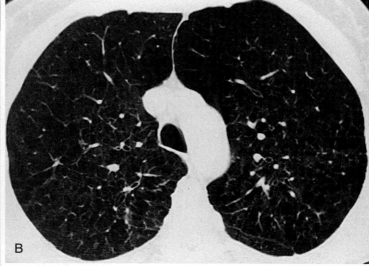

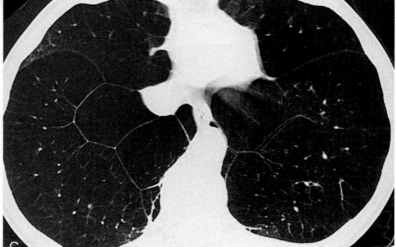

FIGURE 15–36

Panlobular emphysema. A posteroanterior chest radiograph (**A**) demonstrates overinflation, increased height of the lungs, and flattening of the diaphragm. Decreased vascularity in the peripheral lung regions is also apparent. A high-resolution CT scan at the level of the aortic arch (**B**) reveals moderately severe emphysema; a scan at the lung bases (**C**) demonstrates severe emphysema. Note the presence of blood flow redistribution (decreased size of the lower lobe vessels in comparison to the upper lobe vessels). The patient was a 47-year-old woman who had α_1-protease inhibitor deficiency. *(From Fraser RS, Müller NL, Colman NC, Paré PD: Fraser and Paré's Diagnosis of Diseases of the Chest, 4th ed. Philadelphia, WB Saunders, 1999.)*

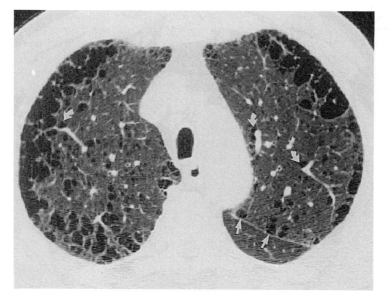

FIGURE 15–37

Paraseptal emphysema. An HRCT scan demonstrates emphysema, predominantly in a subpleural distribution and focally along the interlobar fissure (*straight arrow*) and vessels (*curved arrows*). *(From Fraser RS, Müller NL, Colman NC, Paré PD: Fraser and Paré's Diagnosis of Diseases of the Chest, 4th ed. Philadelphia, WB Saunders, 1999.)*

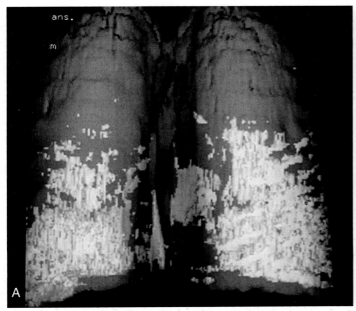

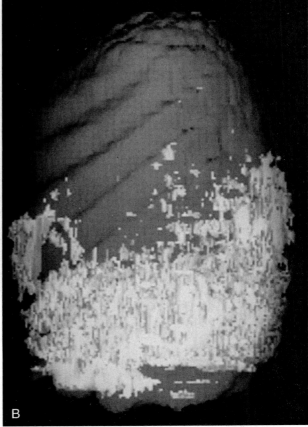

FIGURE 15–38

Objective quantification of panacinar emphysema. Posterior (**A**) and left lateral (**B**) three-dimensional reconstruction images from a spiral CT study show the areas of emphysema highlighted in white and normal lung tissue as areas of gray. The emphysema involves almost exclusively the lower lung zones. The areas that are highlighted have attenuation values equal or less than –910 HU. *(Courtesy Dr. Ella Kazerooni, University of Michigan Medical Center, Ann Arbor.)*

deficiency, chronic inflammation, hypoxia, hypercapnia, and energy deprivation.[608] Decreased muscle mass may contribute, along with mechanical disadvantage and chronic fatigue,[609] to the decreased inspiratory muscle strength of patients who have advanced disease.[610]

Cardiovascular Manifestations

COPD is associated with several complications, the most serious of which are pulmonary arterial hypertension, right ventricular hypertrophy (cor pulmonale), and right ventricular failure.[611,612] Pulmonary hypertension is caused by a combination of hypoxic vasoconstriction of the muscular pulmonary arteries, a loss of pulmonary capillary bed, and a decrease in pulmonary vascular compliance associated with arterial intimal and medial hypertrophy. With mild to moderate grades of COPD (FEV_1 40% to 80% of predicted), pulmonary artery pressure (Ppa) is usually normal at rest but increases with moderate exercise or exposure to cold.[613] In the presence of severe COPD (FEV_1 < 40% of predicted), hypertension is usually present at rest (mean Ppa > 20 mm Hg), and pulmonary arterial pressure undergoes a disproportionate increase with mild exercise[614]; its severity correlates with the degree of arterial desaturation and arterial P_{CO_2}.[615]

Exacerbations of COPD are associated with acute worsening of pulmonary hypertension, although Ppa usually returns to pre-exacerbation levels with treatment.[615] Ppa can also increase acutely during episodes of hypoxemia that occur during sleep, and it has been suggested that recurrent

nocturnal pulmonary hypertension can eventually lead to "fixed" hypertension as a result of structural changes in the arterial wall.[616] In the absence of therapy, the hypertension progresses slowly but inexorably.[617]

Although left ventricular function is normal in most patients who have COPD, it may deteriorate when cor pulmonale and right ventricular failure develop because of right ventricular dilation, septal shift, and decreased left ventricular compliance.[618] Chronic cor pulmonale is associated with a high incidence of cardiac arrhythmias, particularly supraventricular arrhythmia.[619]

The electrocardiogram may be normal. As airway obstruction becomes more severe, however, signs of right axis deviation develop, with large S waves and biphasic T waves over the left precordium beyond the V_2 position. These changes correlate best with total pulmonary vascular resistance.[620] With decreasing FEV_1/FVC ratios, there is an increased frequency of P waves greater than 2.0 mm, P axis greater than +75 degrees, S waves greater than 5 mm in V_5 and V_6, and QRS axis greater than +75 degrees.[621] The most reliable indicators of right ventricular hypertrophy are an S_1Q_3 pattern, right axis deviation (>110), an $S_1S_2S_3$ pattern, and an RS ratio in V_6 greater than 1.0.[622]

Pulmonary Function Tests

The most important applications of pulmonary function tests lie in detecting the presence of disease (preferably at an early stage) and in monitoring its progression. Because COPD follows an insidiously progressive course for years before clinical manifestation,[623] affected individuals can be identified long before the development of symptoms. Smoking cessation in such individuals results in some functional improvement but, more importantly, causes a normalization in the rate of age-related decline in lung function.[495] A number of tests specifically aimed at detecting small-airway obstruction have been proposed as sensitive screens for early COPD; the available evidence suggests that carefully performed spirometry is the most valuable one.

Spirometry

A decrease in maximal expiratory flow is the diagnostic functional hallmark of COPD and occurs as a result of increased airway resistance and loss of lung elastic recoil.[624] Expiratory flow can be measured as peak flow (PEFR), flow in the first second of an FVC maneuver (FEV$_1$), average flow over the middle half of the forced expired volume (FEF$_{25\%-75\%}$ or maximal midexpiratory flow rate [MMEF]), or instantaneous flow rates at different percentages of FVC ($\dot{V}max_{50}$, $\dot{V}max_{25}$). All these measures decrease with the development of COPD. FEV$_1$ has the advantage of being the most reproducible in a given individual, and there is little evidence that FEF$_{25\%-75\%}$, $\dot{V}max_{50}$, or $\dot{V}max_{25}$ is more sensitive in detecting the early stages of the disease.[625] Despite a wide range of values within the normal population for these tests, the range can be narrowed by expressing forced expiratory flow as a percentage of FVC (FEV$_1$/FVC percent). Forced expiratory flow decreases over the entire VC range, and the effort-independent portion of the curve (from 80% TLC to RV) becomes more curvilinear than normal and is convex (lower toward the volume axis) (Fig. 15–39).[626]

Patients with COPD can show a substantial increase in forced expiratory flow after the inhalation of a bronchodilator, 30% of patients achieving greater than 20% improvement in FEV$_1$. Therefore, distinction of patients who have asthma from those who have COPD cannot be established by their response to bronchodilators.[627] Some patients with COPD also have substantial improvement in function after a course of oral or inhaled corticosteroid therapy and, like asthmatic patients, can show substantial diurnal variation in expiratory

flow.[628,629] It is possible that such patients have a combination of asthma and COPD; the term *asthmatic bronchitis* has been used to describe them. Irrespective of mechanism, distinction between the conditions can be difficult. Bronchodilators and steroid therapy can also cause a reduction in the dynamic hyperinflation that characterizes COPD.[630] This parameter can be measured as an increase in inspiratory capacity and may correlate more closely with alleviation of symptoms than does an increase in maximal flow.[631]

As indicated previously, smoking cessation results in a sustained increase in maximal expiratory flow[632] and normalization in the rate of decline in lung function.[495] The improvement begins as early as 1 week after cessation and continues for 6 to 8 months.[633]

Lung Volumes

The initial alteration in lung volumes is an increase in RV.[634] This change is probably related to premature airway closure at the lung bases, as has been demonstrated in asymptomatic young smokers.[635] As RV increases further, FRC and TLC also increase, and VC decreases. VC can decrease further when patients assume the supine posture (about 10% on average).[636] The increase in FRC is caused by loss of lung elastic recoil, which allows the chest wall to expand, and by dynamic hyperinflation caused by the development of "auto-PEEP" (positive end-expiratory pressure). The latter occurs when a patient inspires before a reduction in alveolar pressure to zero[637]; the resulting increased intrathoracic pressure can adversely affect venous return to the right side of the heart. Moreover, the hyperinflation puts the inspiratory muscles at a mechanical disadvantage and at a shorter length on their length-tension curve.[638] On the positive side, the hyperinflation dilates the intraparenchymal airways and decreases the resistive work of breathing.

The increase in TLC is related to a combination of loss in lung elasticity and, possibly, adaptive shortening of the inspiratory muscles.[639] The magnitude of the increase in TLC is controversial. Both the helium dilution technique and the body plethysmograph are subject to errors in patients who have airway obstruction. With helium, there is a tendency to underestimate TLC,[640] whereas with plethysmography, thoracic gas volume may be overestimated.[641]

The changes in lung distensibility that occur in COPD are also reflected by an alteration in the pulmonary pressure-volume curve. The maximal elastic recoil pressure at TLC and recoil pressures at various percentages of TLC normally decrease with increasing age; however, this decrease is accelerated in smokers.[642] The entire pressure-volume curve can be described by an exponential equation in which the constant k indicates the shape (see page 180); increased k indicates loss of recoil and correlates with the presence of emphysema in smokers.[643]

Arterial Blood Gases

Arterial blood gas tensions are commonly abnormal; as a rule, the more severe the disease, the more frequent the hypoxemia and hypercapnia.[644] Arterial hypoxemia is the result of alveolar hypoventilation and ventilation-perfusion mismatching. In COPD of mild to moderate severity, hypoxemia exists without hypercapnia. Although the $\dot{V}/\dot{Q}$ inequality impairs

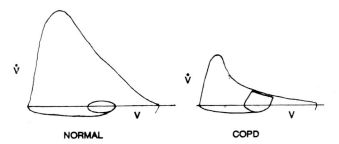

FIGURE 15–39

Flow-volume curve in a normal individual and a patient with severe COPD. A normal tidal flow-volume ($\dot{V}$-V) loop and a complete maximal expiratory flow-volume curve show that during tidal breathing, a patient with COPD achieves maximal expiratory flow. There is considerable reserve for increased expiratory flow in a normal person. *(From Fraser RS, Müller NL, Colman NC, Paré PD: Fraser and Paré's Diagnosis of Diseases of the Chest, 4th ed. Philadelphia, WB Saunders, 1999.)*

both the uptake of O_2 and the elimination of CO_2, the tendency for elevation of $PaCO_2$ is overcome by an increase in alveolar ventilation to well-perfused units. However, the increase in ventilation cannot correct the hypoxemia because of the nonlinear shape of the oxygen dissociation curve. When COPD becomes severe, carbon dioxide retention eventually occurs as total alveolar ventilation decreases. An increase in arterial $PaCO_2$ does not generally occur until FEV_1 is less than approximately 1.2 L, and the presence of hypercapnia in a patient with an FEV_1 greater than 1.5 L should raise the possibility of central hypoventilation or OSA.

The hypoxemia of COPD is easily corrected by increasing the concentration of inspired oxygen; however, such an increase also causes a variable increase in arterial PCO_2, especially during episodes of acute ventilatory respiratory failure.[645] The administration of supplemental oxygen causes a decrease in minute ventilation ($\dot{V}E$) and a worsening of ventilation-perfusion matching, the latter as a result of the increased alveolar oxygen's attenuating hypoxic vasoconstriction.[646]

During exacerbations of COPD, blood gas tensions deteriorate.[647] Such exacerbations are frequently associated with right-sided heart failure and fluid overload, which by themselves may impair arterial blood gas tensions.[648] Cardiac output can also influence arterial blood gases by changing the mixed venous tensions of oxygen and carbon dioxide. Given a certain disturbance in $\dot{V}/\dot{Q}$ matching and metabolic rate, mixed venous PO_2 will fall and mixed venous PCO_2 will rise as cardiac output decreases, changes that are reflected in arterial gas tensions.[649]

COPD is not associated with an increase in the incidence of obstructive apnea, but because both are relatively common chronic disorders, their simultaneous occurrence is not infrequent.[650] Even without obstructive apnea, sleep has profound effects on ventilatory control and arterial blood gases in patients with COPD and is frequently associated with a worsening of hypoxemia and hypercapnia.[651] Since PaO_2 values may fall onto the steep portion of the oxygen dissociation curve, the decrease in arterial saturation may be considerable. Despite the lack of frank apneas, patients with COPD may experience episodic arterial desaturation during sleep, episodes of decreased saturation being more severe in patients categorized as blue bloaters than as pink puffers.[652] The desaturation is also more severe during REM sleep than during slow-wave sleep[653] and appears to be related to periods of hypoventilation or "hypopnea" that are in part due to the phasic inhibition of intercostal inspiratory muscle tone that is characteristic of REM sleep. Episodes of nocturnal desaturation are associated with a worsening of pulmonary hypertension; although nocturnal oxygen administration does not prevent hypopnea, it does block the pulmonary vascular response by preventing the nocturnal hypoxemia.[654]

Exercise can also influence arterial blood gas tensions; in some patients, it induces pronounced arterial desaturation and hypercapnia, whereas in others, gas exchange is improved.[655] Patients in whom desaturation occurs tend to have significantly worse airflow obstruction, a lower diffusing capacity, a higher dead space–tidal volume ratio (VD/VT), and a lower VT.[656,657] Even during maximal exercise, normal individuals do not achieve the level of ventilation of which they are capable, and considerable ventilatory reserve remains. By contrast, patients who have COPD usually stop exercising when they reach their maximal achievable ventilation; this

level can be estimated from combined measurements of FEV_1 and inspiratory muscle strength.[658]

Secondary polycythemia develops in some hypoxemic patients, especially those with severe nocturnal desaturation.[659] Increased carboxyhemoglobin levels can also contribute to the development of polycythemia.[660] Air travel can be associated with significant arterial oxygen desaturation.[661]

Measurement of arterial pH, hydrogen ion concentration, and bicarbonate levels provides important information about the acid-base status of patients who have COPD. When an excess of carbon dioxide is compensated for by an increase in bicarbonate, it is a clear indication that the respiratory failure is not of "acute" onset. An arterial pH above the normal range in uncomplicated respiratory acidosis suggests the possibility of concomitant metabolic alkalosis, often secondary to the use of diuretics. An elevated $PaCO_2$ associated with a normal or only slightly raised bicarbonate level may indicate that the hypoventilation and respiratory acidosis are of recent onset. However, this conclusion is not justified if there is coexisting metabolic acidosis that has depressed the bicarbonate level. Measurement of the anion gap is useful in making this distinction.

Diffusing Capacity

The single-breath diffusing capacity ($DLCOSB$) of individuals who smoke cigarettes is lower than that of age-matched non-smoking individuals, even in the absence of other evidence of lung dysfunction.[662] Part of this decrease is caused by elevated blood carboxyhemoglobin levels; however, even after correction for the backpressure of carbon monoxide, smoking subjects have lower values of $DLCOSB$.[663] $DLCOSB$ decreases significantly during active smoking[664] but returns toward normal within a week of smoking cessation.[665] Some of these changes may be a result of decreased pulmonary vascular volume in smokers.

In the presence of established COPD, there is a further reduction in diffusing capacity that is related to the extent of emphysema. This reduction is generally considered to be caused by both a decrease in the membrane component and $\dot{V}/\dot{Q}$ mismatch. It is probable, however, that there are other contributing factors, including a reduction in capillary volume and perhaps limitation of gas-phase diffusion within large emphysematous spaces.[666]

Prognosis and Natural History

Over a period of years, most patients with COPD experience slow but inexorable worsening of symptoms and progressive impairment in pulmonary function.[495] When the impairment results in dyspnea, progression to severe disability can be expected within 6 to 10 years.[623]

The course of the disease is frequently punctuated with periodic exacerbations that have been defined as *"a sustained worsening of the patient's condition, from the stable state and beyond normal day-to-day variations that is acute in onset and may warrant additional treatment."*[667] Exacerbations can be precipitated by viral or bacterial infection, superimposed heart failure, or exposure to atmospheric pollution. They vary widely in severity but account for a substantial proportion of health care use by COPD patients.[668] In advanced disease, severe exacerbations with "acute-on-chronic" respiratory failure may occur. Although most patients survive such crises,[669] the subsequent mortality rate is high. For example, in one study, the in-hospital mortality was only 11%; however, the 6-month, 1-year, and 2-year mortality was 33%, 43%, and 49%, respectively.[670] Predictors of a favorable outcome include younger age, better premorbid quality of life, higher mental status and blood pressure, and lower heart rate, creatinine, white blood cell count, and plasma glucose.[671] Nutritional status as reflected in the percentage of ideal body weight also influences the prognosis.[672] The prognosis is improved by smoking cessation and by participation in comprehensive pulmonary rehabilitation programs.[672]

The prognosis is also significantly related to the pulmonary hemodynamic and right ventricular consequences of COPD.[673] Patients who have a pulmonary artery pressure of less than 20 mm Hg have an average 5-year survival rate of about 70% as compared with less than 50% in those whose pressure exceeds 20 mm Hg. However, the prognosis is equally well predicted by measurements of arterial PCO_2 or FEV_1.[674,675]

Long-term supplemental oxygen increases the survival of patients with advanced COPD,[676] but the exact mechanism by which this occurs is not clear. In one study, lung function did not improve and pulmonary artery pressure did not decrease significantly in the patients who received oxygen, although the increase in pulmonary artery pressure was less than would have been expected without oxygen.[677] Prevention of severe oxygen desaturation during sleep may decrease cardiac irritability, a possible contributing factor to the beneficial effects of oxygen.[678]

Despite the foregoing, the use of *uncontrolled oxygen therapy* for respiratory failure in patients with severe COPD can cause serious complications, a high concentration of inspired alveolar oxygen causing worsening of hypercapnia by interfering with hypoxic vasoconstriction, increasing "physiologic" dead space, and depressing minute ventilation.[679] In fact, an abrupt rise in $PaCO_2$ can result in marked deterioration leading to coma and death.[680]

CYSTIC FIBROSIS

Cystic fibrosis (CF) is a hereditary disease of mendelian recessive transmission. The fundamental abnormality consists of the production of abnormal secretions from exocrine glands, such as the salivary and sweat glands, as well as the pancreas, large bowel, and tracheobronchial tree. The major clinical manifestations are obstructive pulmonary disease, which is found in varying degrees of severity in almost all patients, and pancreatic insufficiency (present in 80% to 90%).[681] The condition is the most common lethal genetically transmitted disease in white persons, the estimated incidence being about 1 per 2000 to 3500 live births.[682] It is uncommon in nonwhites; the incidence is 1 in 17,000 among African Americans and 1 in 90,000 among North American Indians and Asians.[683] There is no sex preponderance. The diagnosis is made before the age of 5 years in about 80% of individuals and during adolescence in 10%[684]; occasionally, it is identified in adulthood.[685]

Etiology and Pathogenesis

The gene responsible is located on the long arm of chromosome 7.[686] Its protein product, the cystic fibrosis transmembrane

regulator (CFTR), contains 1480 amino acids and has two transmembrane-spanning domains and two intracellular nucleotide-binding domains. It is part of a cAMP-regulated channel located in the apical membrane of airway and tracheobronchial gland epithelial cells and is involved in chloride and water transport from these cells into the airway lumen.[687]

The most common mutation associated with gene dysfunction is a three–base pair deletion, which causes loss of the amino acid phenylalanine at position 508 of the protein. This mutation, termed ΔF508, accounts for about 70% of the mutant alleles on the CFTR gene; however, more than 1000 additional mutations have been identified that can result in the CF phenotype. About 1 in 20 to 25 whites is heterozygous for one of the abnormal CF genes. No clinical characteristics that identify these individuals have been demonstrated. Prenatal screening is possible by genotyping DNA in cells obtained by amniocentesis or chorionic villus aspiration.[688]

All the mutations that cause CF affect the function of CFTR, although the manner in which they do so is different for different mutations. They have been classified into five categories:[689] class 1 mutations, in which no protein is produced; class 2, in which most of the protein does not reach the cell membrane (e.g., ΔF508); class 3, in which the protein fails to respond to cAMP; class 4, associated with the production of a protein that has a reduced response to cAMP; and class 5, in which there is decreased production of a normally functioning chloride channel. Patients who have class 4 and 5 mutations are less likely to have pancreatic deficiency; however, there is no close correlation between mutation class and the severity of airway disease.[690]

CFTR has a major influence on airway ion and water transport.[691,692] In addition to defective chloride secretion, the mutations indirectly cause excessive sodium absorption and a decrease in volume of the periciliary liquid layer. This in turn decreases the effectiveness of mucociliary clearance, causes adherence of mucus to epithelial cells, and impairs antimicrobial defense.[693] Respiratory infection by bacteria such as *S. aureus*, *Pseudomonas aeruginosa*, and *Burkholderia cepacia* plays a major role in the pathogenesis of pulmonary disease in CF. Chronic airway "colonization" by mucoid, alginate-producing variants of *P. aeruginosa* is particularly important as a cause of clinical deterioration.[694,695] The presence of *B. cepacia* has also been associated with an accelerated course. In addition to its direct effects on the airway wall, this organism is especially important because (1) it is often resistant to antimicrobial agents[696]; (2) it can result in a fulminating, potentially fatal pneumonia[697]; and (3) it appears to be particularly prone to person-to-person transmission through nosocomial or social contacts.[698]

The inflammatory reaction to airway colonization by *P. aeruginosa* and *B. cepacia* is characterized by an influx of polymorphonuclear leukocytes; these cells release proteolytic enzymes such as elastase and collagenase, which contribute to airway epithelial ulceration and, eventually, bronchiectasis.[699,700] Aggregates of mucus and neutrophils within the airway lumen partially or completely occlude the lumina, thereby leading to productive cough and functional obstruction characteristic of the condition. Part of these effects is related to increased sputum viscosity as a result of neutrophil death, increased sputum DNA content, and intertwining of the long DNA molecules with mucus glycoproteins, which increases the rigidity of the gel.[701]

Pathologic Characteristics

Most pathologic studies of neonates or infants who have died of CF have shown essentially normal lungs.[702] The lungs of older patients who die of the disease or who undergo lung transplantation usually show airway plugging by mucopurulent debris, bronchiectasis (typically more severe in the upper lobes), and acute and organizing pneumonia (often with abscess formation) (see Color Fig. 15–4).[703] Focal emphysema, bullae, and blebs can also be seen.[704,705] Histologic examination typically reveals chronic inflammation and fibrosis of the bronchial wall, partial or complete luminal occlusion by purulent material, focal epithelial ulceration, and cartilage destruction (see Color Fig. 15–4).[706] Membranous bronchioles may have similar inflammatory changes or may show narrowing or obliteration as a result of fibrosis.

Radiologic Manifestations

The earliest manifestations of CF on the chest radiograph consist of round or poorly defined linear opacities measuring 3 to 5 mm in diameter and located within 2 to 3 cm of the pleura[707]; thickened bronchial walls without bronchial dilation (usually seen as ring shadows), mild hyperinflation, and hilar lymph node enlargement are seen less commonly.[707] Progression of disease is characterized by increases in bronchial diameter, bronchial wall thickness, lung volume, and the number and size of peripheral nodular opacities and by the development of mucoid impaction and focal areas of consolidation (Fig. 15–40).[707] Bronchiectasis, bronchial wall thickening, and mucus plugging are particularly frequent and in fact are evident in almost all adult patients.[708]

Recurrent foci of consolidation occur in most patients and lobar or segmental atelectasis in many.[709] Hilar enlargement may be due to lymph node enlargement or dilation of the central pulmonary arteries secondary to pulmonary arterial hypertension.[710] The chest radiographic abnormalities have been incorporated into a number of semiquantitative scoring schemes that are believed to be of value in predicting prognosis and directing therapy.[710,711]

HRCT is clearly more sensitive than radiography in detecting mild disease in CF (Fig. 15–41)[712]; moreover, there is evidence that incorporating the results of serial HRCT scans into a semiquantitative scoring system can show evidence of progressive structural damage that is not reflected in pulmonary function abnormalities.[713] Typical findings include widespread, predominantly upper lobe bronchiectasis and small nodular opacities in the center of secondary lobules (Fig. 15–42).[714] The presence of gas trapping can be appreciated on images obtained after expiration to RV.[715]

Clinical Manifestations

Involvement of the lungs is clinically manifested by recurrent chest infections associated with wheezing, dyspnea, and productive cough. Malnutrition and protein depletion are

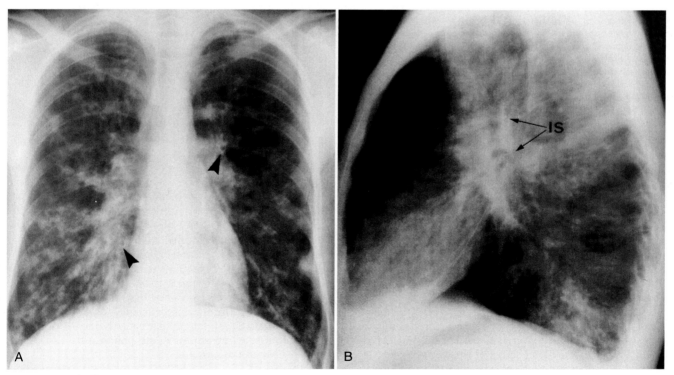

FIGURE 15–40

Cystic fibrosis. Posteroanterior (**A**) and lateral (**B**) chest radiographs demonstrate diffuse bronchial wall thickening (*arrowheads*), peribronchial thickening, diffuse small patchy opacities, and areas of inhomogeneous air space consolidation. Note the remarkable thickening of the posterior wall of the bronchus intermedius (IS). The lungs are moderately overinflated. Both hila are enlarged, almost certainly as a result of lymph node enlargement rather than pulmonary arterial hypertension. The patient was a 24-year-old man. (*From Fraser RS, Müller NL, Colman NC, Paré PD: Fraser and Paré's Diagnosis of Diseases of the Chest, 4th ed. Philadelphia, WB Saunders, 1999.*)

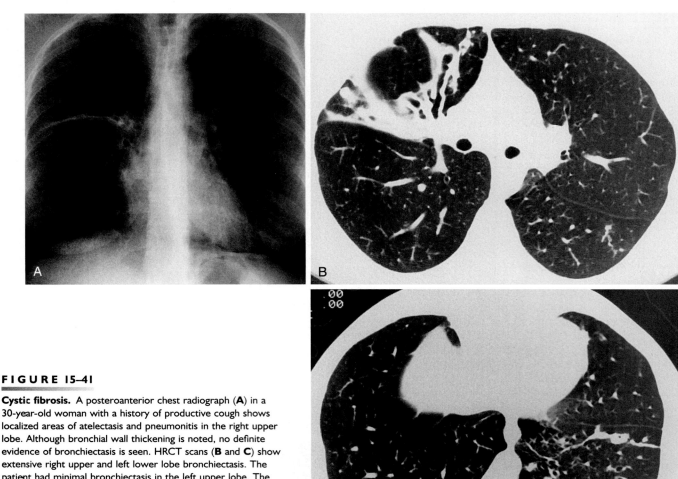

FIGURE 15–41

Cystic fibrosis. A posteroanterior chest radiograph (**A**) in a 30-year-old woman with a history of productive cough shows localized areas of atelectasis and pneumonitis in the right upper lobe. Although bronchial wall thickening is noted, no definite evidence of bronchiectasis is seen. HRCT scans (**B** and **C**) show extensive right upper and left lower lobe bronchiectasis. The patient had minimal bronchiectasis in the left upper lobe. The diagnosis of cystic fibrosis was made after the CT findings. The markedly asymmetrical distribution of the bronchiectasis seen in this patient is a relatively uncommon manifestation of the disease. *(From Fraser RS, Müller NL, Colman NC, Paré PD: Fraser and Paré's Diagnosis of Diseases of the Chest, 4th ed. Philadelphia, WB Saunders, 1999.)*

consequences of such infection and can in turn accelerate the course of pulmonary disease.[716] The infection is predominantly caused by bacteria such as *P. aeruginosa*, *S. aureus*, and *H. influenzae*, although viruses, mycoplasmas, and fungi are occasionally responsible. The presence of *B. cepacia* is usually associated with advanced disease. Hemoptysis and pneumothorax are common complications[717]; the latter is frequently recurrent.[718] Patients with CF have a higher incidence of atopy and asthma than that in the general population.[719] Allergic bronchopulmonary aspergillosis occurs in 5% to 10% of patients and can be associated with an accelerated decline in lung function.[720,721] Respiratory insufficiency accompanied by persistent pulmonary arterial hypertension and cor pulmonale develops in the later stages of the disease.

Physical findings are those of bronchiectasis and obstructive airway disease. Coarse crackles may be localized but are often diffuse; generalized wheezing should suggest the possibility of asthma. Finger clubbing is an almost invariable sign in patients who have advanced disease.

Additional clinical manifestations relate to the genitourinary and gastrointestinal tracts. Reproductive failure is common in males and usually occurs as a result of the absence of the vas deferens.[722] Women with CF are also relatively infertile, the probable cause being abnormal cervical mucus. Intestinal obstruction as a result of meconium ileus develops in about 10% to 15% of neonates who have CF; surgical therapy is sometimes required. *Meconium ileus equivalent* and *distal intestinal obstruction syndrome* are terms used to describe intestinal obstruction that occurs after the neonatal period. Hepatic involvement is manifested by steatosis and focal biliary cirrhosis. Pancreatic dysfunction occurs in about 90% of patients; the enzyme deficiency results in poor digestion, particularly of fat, so patients characteristically have bulky, foul-smelling stools. Acute pancreatitis and diabetes mellitus can also occur.

Diagnosis and Laboratory Findings

Although the diagnosis of CF may be suggested by a positive family history, persistent respiratory disease, or clinical evidence of pancreatic insufficiency, confirmation requires a

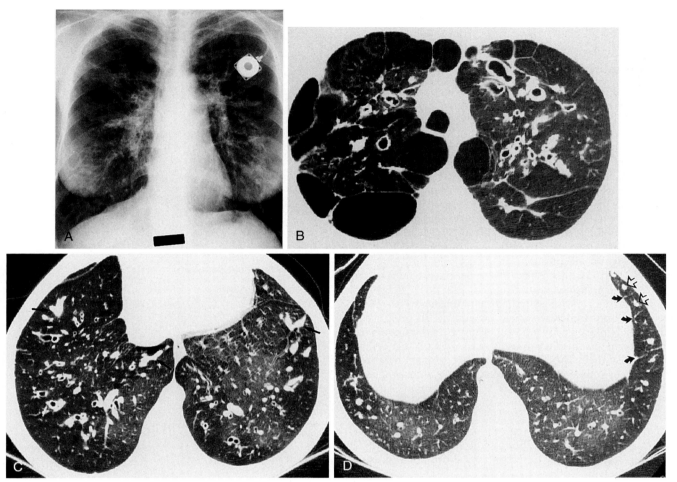

FIGURE 15–42

Cystic fibrosis. A posteroanterior chest radiograph (**A**) in a 39-year-old woman shows evidence of extensive bronchiectasis and several large bullae, particularly in the right upper lobe. An HRCT scan at the level of the upper lobes (**B**) also demonstrates bullae, more severe on the right, and widespread bronchiectasis. A scan at the level of the lower lung zones (**C**) demonstrates less severe bronchiectasis, branching opacities representing mucoid impaction (*straight arrows*), and areas of decreased attenuation and vascularity, particularly in the dependent lung regions and in the medial segment of the right lower lobe. A third scan at a more caudal level (**D**) demonstrates centrilobular nodular opacities (*open arrows*) measuring 3 to 5 mm in diameter and representing dilated bronchioles. Decreased attenuation and vascularity within the secondary lobules demarcated by interlobular septa (*curved arrows*) can also be identified. *(From Fraser RS, Müller NL, Colman NC, Paré PD: Fraser and Paré's Diagnosis of Diseases of the Chest, 4th ed. Philadelphia, WB Saunders, 1999.)*

positive sweat test or identification of two abnormal copies of the CFTR gene. However, the large number of uncommon mutations that can lead to CF makes it difficult to provide a routine screen that is comprehensive enough to rival the sensitivity of sweat testing. On the other hand, sweat electrolyte testing is not reliable in newborn infants, and certain class 4 and 5 mutations that cause lesser degrees of CFTR dysfunction may be associated with sweat chloride values in the normal range.[689] In children, a chloride concentration of 60 mEq/L or higher indicates the presence of CF. Values for sodium and chloride concentrations in sweat increase with advancing age.[723]

Incorporation of molecular biologic techniques into rapid, cost-efficient, and specific diagnostic tests for most CF genotypes is now possible by using the multiplex polymerase chain reaction.[724] This development has allowed the implementation of prenatal,[725] neonatal,[726] and population-based screening for CFTR mutations.[727] However, the exact role of these screening tests is still not clear.

Pulmonary Function Tests

Tests of pulmonary function can be performed on infants who have CF by using the technique of thoracic squeeze and measurement of expiratory flow. With this method, abnormal function has been found in affected infants even before the development of signs and symptoms.[728] As disease progresses, FEV_1 and VC decrease and RV increases.[729] The bronchodilator response is less than in asthma. Dynamic hyperinflation and arterial desaturation occur during exercise in severely obstructed patients.[730] Exercise capacity is typically reduced as a result of both pulmonary and nutritional factors.[731]

Hypoxemia is present in some patients, and hypercapnia in a minority. Episodes of arterial desaturation occur during sleep, the largest decrease occurring during REM sleep.[732] The rate of change in lung function is highly variable and to some extent dependent on CFTR phenotype,[733] as well as environmental factors such as compliance with therapy and exposure to secondhand cigarette smoke.[734]

Prognosis and Natural History

As a result of improved medical care, chiefly antibiotic therapy, life expectancy has increased dramatically during the latter part of the 20th century.[735] In fact, an important part of the variability in prognosis seen in different countries is related to the availability of centralized specialist centers and government-funded health insurance.[736] The predicted mean life expectancy has been estimated to be 40 years for infants born in "developed" countries today.[737] With the development of programs for lung transplantation, the survival in advanced CF is being extended even longer; the survival rate after transplantation is about 85% at 1 year and up to 70% at 2 years.[738]

The prognosis has also been related to a number of specific features. Age at diagnosis is an important indicator, with patients detected earlier as part of a screening program having a better outcome than those detected clinically.[739] Scoring of abnormalities on the chest radiograph (Brasfield system) has been used both to define patient groups and to predict survival.[740] Maximal exercise test results have been found to be no more informative in predicting survival over a 5-year follow-up than FEV_1 is.[741] The development of pulmonary hypertension and cor pulmonale is associated with a poor prognosis; most patients die within 2 years of the appearance of right heart failure.[742] Nutritional status and *B. cepacia* colonization have also been identified as negative prognostic indicators.[743] By contrast, the CFTR genotype has relatively little influence; in fact, patients and even siblings who have the same CFTR mutations can have very different clinical courses, suggesting that there may be "modifier genes."[744]

BRONCHIECTASIS

General Features

Bronchiectasis is best defined as irreversible dilation of a portion of the bronchial tree. As such, it is a relatively common pathologic or HRCT finding that occurs in association with many conditions (Table 15–5).[745] Although it has decreased in importance as a clinically significant disease since the advent of antibiotic therapy,[746] it has engendered increased interest because of (1) prolonged survival in patients who have diseases associated with it, such as CF, ciliary dyskinetic syndromes, and some immune deficiency syndromes; (2) its association with HIV infection[747]; (3) its emergence as a complication of heart, lung, and bone marrow transplantation[748,749]; and (4) advances in radiologic imaging that have improved the recognition of relatively minor degrees of airway dilation in a number of conditions, such as rheumatoid disease.[750]

Etiology and Pathogenesis

The most important processes contributing to bronchiectasis are infection, obstruction, or immunologically mediated injury to the airway itself or fibrosis of the adjacent parenchyma. A number of respiratory infections (e.g., measles

TABLE 15–5. Causes of Bronchiectasis

Inherited Cellular or Molecular Defects

Cystic fibrosis
Dyskinetic cilia syndromes

Inherited or Acquired Deficiency in Host Defense

X-linked agammaglobulinemia
Selective immunoglobulin deficiency
Common variable immunodeficiency
Chronic granulomatous disease of childhood
HIV infection

Congenital Abnormalities of Bronchial or Vascular Structure

Absent or defective cartilage (Williams-Campbell syndrome)
Intraluminal webs
Mounier-Kuhn syndrome
Bronchial atresia
Unilateral pulmonary artery agenesis

Acquired Bronchial Obstruction

Intraluminal obstruction
   Neoplasms
   Aspirated foreign body
   Broncholithiasis
   Papillomatosis
External compression
   Lymph node enlargement
   Pulmonary artery band migration

Infection

Mycobacterium tuberculosis
Mycobacterium avium-intracellulare
Bordetella species
Viruses (usually following childhood infection)
Allergic bronchopulmonary aspergillosis

Toxins and Poisons

Toxic gas inhalation
Smoke inhalation
Gastric acid aspiration
Paraquat ingestion

Parenchymal Fibrosis

Chronic tuberculosis
Sarcoidosis
Idiopathic pulmonary fibrosis

Immunologic Disease

Lung allograft rejection
Graft-versus-host disease after bone marrow transplantation
Rheumatoid disease
Sjögren's syndrome
Inflammatory bowel disease

Miscellaneous

Yellow nail syndrome
Young's syndrome

and pertussis) are associated with an inflammatory response and the release of proteolytic enzymes, such as collagenase and elastase,[751,752] that result in damage to the airway wall sufficient to cause dilation.[753] This in turn is associated with impairment of bacterial clearance and an increased susceptibility to colonization by organisms such as *H. influenzae*, *P. aeruginosa*, and

Branhamella catarrhalis.[754] These bacteria perpetuate the inflammatory reaction and lead to a vicious cycle of progressive bronchial wall damage and increasing dilation.[755] The impaired mucociliary clearance that occurs in CF and primary ciliary dyskinesia and the increased susceptibility to infection associated with immunologic deficiency states predispose to the development of bronchiectasis by similar mechanisms.[756] The bronchiectasis that develops after the inhalation of various fumes or gases such as ammonia or smoke is probably caused by a similar mechanism of airway damage and chronic bacterial colonization.[757,758]

Airway obstruction is typically followed by retention of mucus in distal airway lumina and atelectasis of the surrounding parenchyma; both the increased luminal pressure and retraction of the adjacent parenchyma favor airway dilation. Secondary bacterial infection, usually localized to the airway wall, may also ensue and contribute to airway injury and dilation.[759] These mechanisms are the probable ones seen in association with endobronchial neoplasms and in some cases of right middle lobe syndrome in which the middle lobe bronchus is compressed by enlarged peribronchial lymph nodes.

Peribronchial fibrosis contributes to the development of bronchiectasis in patients who have tuberculosis, interstitial lung diseases such as sarcoidosis and idiopathic pulmonary fibrosis,[760] and pneumonitis secondary to the ingestion of poisons such as paraquat.[761] In all these conditions, the parenchyma is the primary site of disease, with contraction of interstitial fibrous tissue resulting in secondary bronchial dilation (*traction bronchiectasis*).

The bronchiectasis that develops in allergic bronchopulmonary aspergillosis, lung allograft rejection, and graft-versus-host reaction after bone marrow transplantation appears to be a consequence of immunologically mediated airway damage. A similar process may also be responsible for the bronchiectasis associated with diseases such as rheumatoid disease,[762] ulcerative colitis,[763] Felty's syndrome, and Sjögren's syndrome.[764]

The relative importance of the various causes of bronchiectasis undoubtedly varies in different areas of the world, as well as in specific populations in such areas. In a study of 193 patients referred to Papworth Hospital, England, for investigation of known or suspected bronchiectasis, 150 had confirmation of the disease by HRCT.[754] One or more presumed causes were identified in 47%, including early childhood pneumonia, pertussis or measles (in 44 patients), immune defects other than hypogammaglobulinemia (in 12 patients), allergic bronchopulmonary aspergillosis (11), aspiration (6), Young's syndrome (5), CF (4), rheumatoid disease (4), and ciliary dysfunction (3).

Pathologic Characteristics

The pathologic findings vary according to the severity of bronchial dilation and the degree of distal bronchial and bronchiolar obliteration. In mild disease (cylindrical bronchiectasis), the bronchi are of fairly regular outline, their diameter remaining constant or increasing only slightly as they extend distally (Fig. 15–43). The number of subdivisions of the bronchial tree from the main bronchus to the periphery is within normal limits. In more severe disease (varicose bronchiectasis), the degree of dilation is greater, and local constrictions cause an irregularity in outline of the bronchial wall that resembles varicose veins. The lumina of smaller bronchi and bronchioles distal to those that are dilated may be obliterated by granulation or fibrous tissue. In the most severe cases (saccular [cystic] bronchiectasis), bronchial dilatation increases progressively toward the periphery and results in cystic spaces measuring up to several centimeters in diameter (see Fig. 15–43). The maximal number of bronchial subdivisions that can be counted may be no more than five, and bronchioles may be entirely absent.

The intervening pulmonary parenchyma may be normal but often shows foci of organizing or organized pneumonia as a result of the frequent bouts of infection experienced by these patients. The bronchial arterial circulation is typically markedly increased and is probably the source of hemoptysis in most cases.[765]

Localization of bronchiectasis within the lungs depends to some extent on the underlying cause. For example, it tends to involve the basal segments of the lower lobes after viral childhood infection,[766] is likely to be localized to the posterior segment of an upper lobe after tuberculosis, and tends to occur in the large (central) bronchi in allergic bronchopulmonary aspergillosis.

Radiologic Manifestations

A number of radiographic features are seen in bronchiectasis.[767] Those that involve the airways include parallel line opacities (*tram tracks*), which represent thickened bronchial walls (Fig. 15–44); tubular opacities, which represent mucus-filled bronchi; and ring opacities or cystic spaces, which measure up to 2 cm in diameter and sometimes contain air-fluid levels (Fig. 15–45). An increase in size and loss of definition of the pulmonary markings in specific segmental areas of the lungs are also common. Vascular abnormalities include crowding of the pulmonary vascular markings, a finding indicative of the almost invariable loss of volume associated with the condition (Fig. 15–46), and evidence of oligemia as a result of a reduction in pulmonary artery perfusion, a finding usually noted in more severe disease. Signs of compensatory overinflation may be apparent in the remainder of the lung (see Fig. 15–46).

Despite the list of abnormalities just presented, the chest radiograph is often normal when CT reveals significant bronchiectasis,[767] and it is now generally accepted that HRCT is the imaging modality of choice to establish the presence of bronchiectasis and determine its precise extent.[768] Characteristic findings include an internal bronchial diameter greater than that of the adjacent pulmonary artery (Fig. 15–47), lack of bronchial tapering (defined as a bronchus that has the same diameter as its parent branch for a distance of more than 2 cm) (Fig. 15–48), visualization of bronchi within 1 cm of the costal pleura or abutting the mediastinal pleura (Fig. 15–49), and bronchial wall thickening.[768-770]

The HRCT appearance of ectatic bronchi varies depending on the type of bronchiectasis and the orientation of the airways relative to the plane of the HRCT scan. For example, in cylindrical bronchiectasis, bronchi coursing horizontally are visualized as parallel lines ("tram tracks") (see Fig. 15–48), whereas vertically oriented bronchi appear as circular lucencies larger than the diameter of the adjacent pulmonary artery

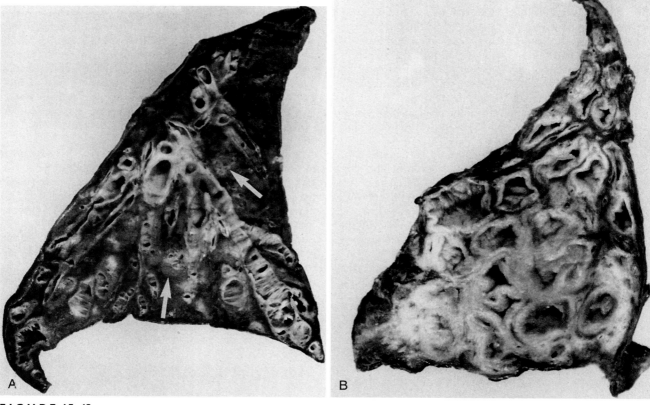

FIGURE 15–43

Bronchiectasis. Slices of lower lobes from two patients who had bronchiectasis are illustrated. The slice in **A** shows mild ("cylindrical") bronchiectasis and the slice in **B**, severe ("saccular" or "cystic") disease. Although much of the parenchyma in **A** is normal, focal areas of organizing pneumonia are apparent (*arrows*). This process is advanced in **B**, there being almost no evidence of residual normal parenchyma. (*From Fraser RS, Müller NL, Colman NC, Paré PD: Fraser and Paré's Diagnosis of Diseases of the Chest, 4th ed. Philadelphia, WB Saunders, 1999.*)

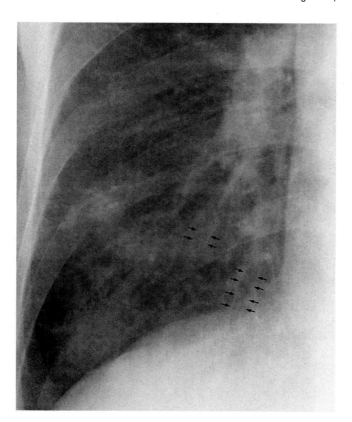

FIGURE 15–44

Bronchiectasis—"tram tracks." A view of the right lower portion of the chest from a posteroanterior radiograph demonstrates opacities in a parallel line ("tram tracks") (*arrows*) as a result of thickened dilated bronchi. The diagnosis of bronchiectasis was confirmed on HRCT. The patient was a 46-year-old man who had chronic productive cough. (*From Fraser RS, Müller NL, Colman NC, Paré PD: Fraser and Paré's Diagnosis of Diseases of the Chest, 4th ed. Philadelphia, WB Saunders, 1999.*)

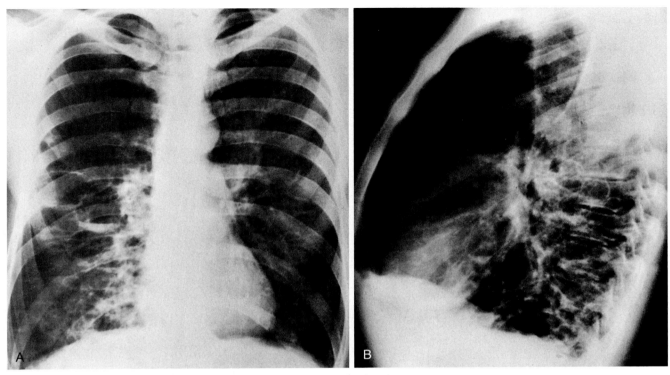

FIGURE 15–45

Cystic bronchiectasis. Posteroanterior (**A**) and lateral (**B**) radiographs in a 46-year-old man who had chronic productive cough demonstrate extensive replacement of the right lower lobe by multiple thin-walled cysts, many of which contain air-fluid levels. The left lung is normal; the right upper and middle lobes show severe oligemia. *(From Fraser RS, Müller NL, Colman NC, Paré PD: Fraser and Paré's Diagnosis of Diseases of the Chest, 4th ed. Philadelphia, WB Saunders, 1999.)*

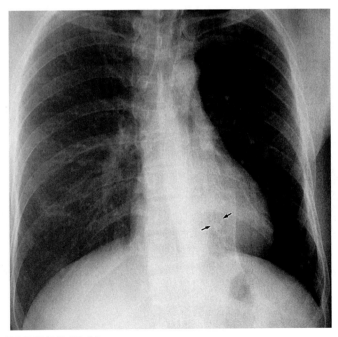

FIGURE 15–46

Bronchiectasis with left lower lobe atelectasis. A posteroanterior chest radiograph demonstrates left lower lobe atelectasis. Ectatic thick-walled bronchi *(arrows)* can be seen within the atelectatic lobe. Note the compensatory overinflation of the left upper lobe. *(From Fraser RS, Müller NL, Colman NC, Paré PD: Fraser and Paré's Diagnosis of Diseases of the Chest, 4th ed. Philadelphia, WB Saunders, 1999.)*

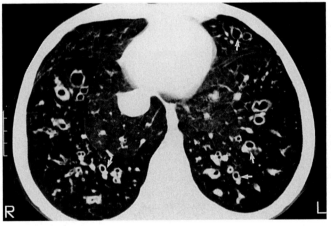

FIGURE 15–47

Bronchiectasis with the signet ring sign. An HRCT scan demonstrates numerous bronchi with an internal diameter greater than that of the adjacent pulmonary artery (signet ring sign) in the lower lobes and lingula *(arrows)*. The patient was a 15-year-old boy who had cystic fibrosis. *(From Fraser RS, Müller NL, Colman NC, Paré PD: Fraser and Paré's Diagnosis of Diseases of the Chest, 4th ed. Philadelphia, WB Saunders, 1999.)*

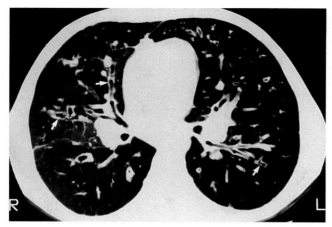

FIGURE 15–48

Bronchiectasis with lack of bronchial tapering. An HRCT scan demonstrates lack of tapering (*arrows*) and thickening of the walls of bronchi in the right middle and left lower lobes. Ectatic bronchi are also evident in cross section (signet ring sign). The patient was a 15-year-old boy with cystic fibrosis. (*From Fraser RS, Müller NL, Colman NC, Paré PD: Fraser and Paré's Diagnosis of Diseases of the Chest, 4th ed. Philadelphia, WB Saunders, 1999.*)

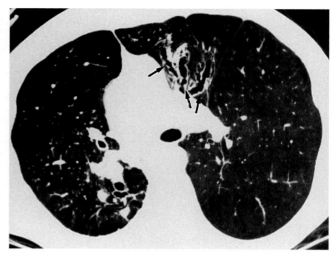

FIGURE 15–50

Varicose bronchiectasis. An HRCT scan demonstrates ectatic bronchi that have an undulating wall (*arrows*) characteristic of varicose bronchiectasis. Bronchiectasis is also evident in the right lung. The patient was a 46-year-old man who had long-standing central bronchiectasis as a result of allergic bronchopulmonary aspergillosis. (*From Fraser RS, Müller NL, Colman NC, Paré PD: Fraser and Paré's Diagnosis of Diseases of the Chest, 4th ed. Philadelphia, WB Saunders, 1999.*)

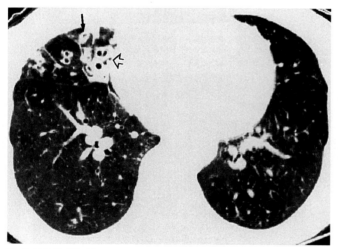

FIGURE 15–49

Bronchiectasis. An HRCT scan in a 50-year-old woman who had bronchiectasis demonstrates bronchi within 1 cm of the costal pleura (*straight arrow*) and abutting the mediastinal pleura (*open arrow*). The bronchiectasis was presumed to be the result of previous tuberculosis. (*From Fraser RS, Müller NL, Colman NC, Paré PD: Fraser and Paré's Diagnosis of Diseases of the Chest, 4th ed. Philadelphia, WB Saunders, 1999.*)

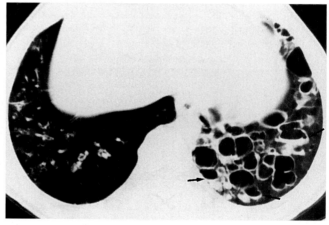

FIGURE 15–51

Cystic bronchiectasis. An HRCT scan demonstrates thin-walled cystic spaces throughout the left lower lobe and lingula; several have air-fluid levels (*arrows*). Mild bronchiectasis is present in the right lower lobe. The patient was a 32-year-old man who had bronchiectasis after childhood viral infection. (*From Fraser RS, Müller NL, Colman NC, Paré PD: Fraser and Paré's Diagnosis of Diseases of the Chest, 4th ed. Philadelphia, WB Saunders, 1999.*)

("signet ring" appearance) (see Fig. 15–47).[771,772] Varicose bronchiectasis is characterized by the presence of nonuniform bronchial dilation (Fig. 15–50), whereas cystic bronchiectasis results in a cluster of thin-walled cystic spaces often containing air-fluid levels (Fig. 15–51). Although bronchial wall thickening on HRCT is fairly common in bronchiectasis, it should be remembered that it is a nonspecific finding that may also be seen in asthmatic patients and asymptomatic smokers.[583,769]

Other abnormalities that are seen with increased frequency in patients who have bronchiectasis include areas of decreased lung attenuation and perfusion, tracheomegaly, and mediastinal lymph node enlargement.[773,774]

Clinical Manifestations

Many patients have no symptoms referable to the bronchiectasis itself. When present, the main symptoms are cough and expectoration of purulent sputum; hemoptysis, recurrent fever, and chest pain are less common. Some patients become aware of purulent expectoration only after respiratory infections (which tend to be frequent). In patients who have postinfective bronchiectasis, symptoms commonly originate in early childhood, and there may be a history of "pneumonia" developing as a complication of measles or some other contagious childhood infection.[775] Hemoptysis occurs in about 50% of older patients. If the disease is widespread, the patient may complain of shortness of breath.

Persistent crackles localized to the area of major involvement are detectable in about 70% of cases.[775] If the bronchiectasis is associated with significant airway obstruction, diffuse or localized wheezing may be audible. The most common extrathoracic manifestation is finger clubbing, seen in about a third of cases.[766] Occasional patients show evidence of a systemic inflammatory response, as evidenced by decreased body weight and serum albumin and increased total serum globulin, α_1-antitrypsin, and white blood cell count.[776]

Pulmonary Function Studies

Bronchiectasis is not associated with any specific pattern of pulmonary function abnormality, although a combination of obstruction and restriction is characteristic. Patients who have localized disease suffer little or no functional impairment. In the presence of appreciable atelectasis, the abnormality in function may be restrictive, with a decrease in VC, FRC, and TLC. In more diffuse disease, the pattern is obstructive, with a proportionally greater decrease in FEV_1 and, in many cases, an increase in FRC and a reduction in diffusing capacity.[777] Lung function tends to be worse and its rate of decline faster in patients who are chronically infected with *P. aeruginosa* as opposed to other organisms.[778]

Prognosis and Natural History

Before 1940, 70% of patients died before the age of 40 years, about 90% as a direct result of the disease.[779] With the advent of antibiotics, the prognosis has improved significantly.[780] In a 1981 review of 116 patients, the reported mortality rate was 19% during a 14-year follow-up period, the mean age at death being 54 years.[781] After pulmonary resection for localized bronchiectasis, the disease commonly affects segments previously shown to be normal.[782] Brain abscess, amyloidosis, and neuropathy are occasional complications. It is emphasized that these survival statistics and complications relate predominantly to patients who have radiographic and clinical features of bronchiectasis; patients whose disease is identified by HRCT alone undoubtedly have a much better outcome.

Specific Causes of Bronchiectasis

Dyskinetic Cilia Syndrome

The syndrome of situs inversus, paranasal sinusitis, and bronchiectasis was first reported in 1904 but acquired its eponym somewhat later after Kartagener described it in detail.[783] Although the descriptive term *immotile cilia syndrome* was suggested to replace the eponymous name, it has become apparent that even structurally abnormal cilia move, albeit in an ineffective, uncoordinated fashion.[784] As a result, the terms now accepted for these disorders are *dyskinetic cilia*

syndrome or *primary ciliary dyskinesia*. The incidence of the syndrome in white persons is estimated to be between 1 in 12,500 and 1 in 40,000[785,786]; a higher prevalence has been reported in Japan.[787]

The abnormality has a strong familial association, with the results of most studies suggesting an autosomal recessive pattern of inheritance[788]; however, the variety of ultrastructural defects associated with the clinical syndrome suggests considerable genetic heterogeneity.[789] In addition, patients have been described with classic Kartagener's syndrome and abnormal airway ciliary ultrastructure but with normal spermatozoa, indicating that discordance in phenotypic manifestations can occur.[790]

Ultrastructural abnormalities in each of the components of the cilium have been identified (Fig. 15–52) and include a lack of outer dynein arms, absent or short radial spokes, absent or defective inner dynein arms, absent or disoriented central microtubules, and transposition of peripheral microtubules[791,792]; the most common is a lack of dynein arms. A combination of structural defects is often present.[793]

The radiographic manifestations of dyskinetic cilia syndrome are similar to those of CF, although they tend to be less severe and less progressive. Findings include bronchial wall thickening, hyperinflation, segmental atelectasis or consolidation, and bronchiectasis.[794] Although the bronchiectasis can be widespread on HRCT, it involves the lower lobes predominantly or exclusively in approximately 50% of patients.[795] In addition to these abnormalities, evidence of otitis, sinusitis, and situs inversus is found in about 50% of patients (Fig. 15–53).

Individuals who have full-blown dyskinetic cilia syndrome have symptoms of chronic rhinitis, sinusitis, and otitis. Recurrent infections of the lower respiratory tract, sterility (in males), corneal abnormalities, and a poor sense of smell are also evident in many. To make the diagnosis, patients should have signs of chronic bronchial infection and rhinitis from early childhood, combined with one or more of the following features: (1) situs inversus or dextrocardia in the patient or a sibling, (2) living but immotile spermatozoa of normal appearance, (3) tracheobronchial clearance that is absent or nearly so, and (4) a nasal or bronchial biopsy specimen that has ultrastructural ciliary defects characteristic of the syndrome.[796]

Mild to moderate airflow obstruction develops in many patients.[561] The decrease in mucociliary clearance is profound and greater than that seen in advanced CF, postinfective bronchiectasis, COPD, or asthma.[797]

Young's Syndrome

Young's syndrome (obstructive azoospermia) is characterized by infertility related to mechanical obstruction of the genital tract accompanied by sinusitis and bronchiectasis.[798] The combination of infertility and sinopulmonary infections may suggest a diagnosis of CF or dyskinetic cilia syndrome. Although some mutations in the CFTR gene are associated with congenital bilateral absence of the vas deferens,[799] the available evidence suggests that Young's syndrome is unrelated to CFTR.[800] Although patients with Young's syndrome have reduced mucociliary clearance, the mechanism is unclear.[801]

It has been suggested that in some cases the condition is acquired as a result of exposure to mercury-containing compounds.[802]

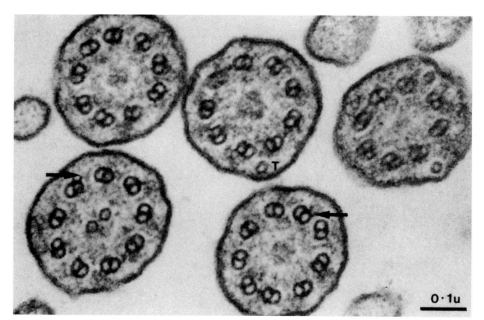

FIGURE 15-52

Ciliary abnormalities in dyskinetic cilia syndrome. A cross section of a group of cilia and microvilli shows that most of the outer ciliary doublets lack dynein arms; some partially developed arms are present (*arrows*). The central tubules are also absent in four of the cilia; supernumerary single tubules (T) are present. (*From Wakefield St J, Waite D: Mucociliary transport and ultrastructural abnormalities in Polynesian bronchiectasis. Am Rev Respir Dis 121:1003, 1980.*)

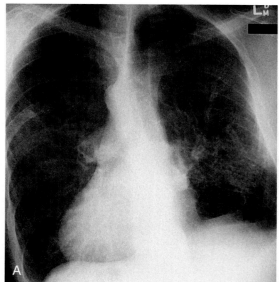

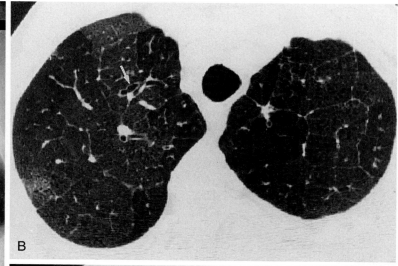

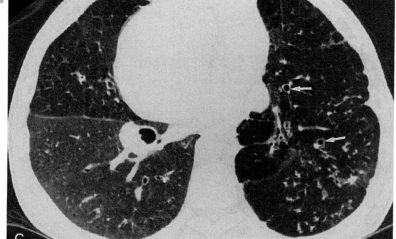

FIGURE 15-53

Kartagener's syndrome. A posteroanterior chest radiograph (**A**) demonstrates dextrocardia and situs inversus. Ectatic, thick-walled bronchi are seen, particularly on the left side. Hyperlucency and oligemia of the left lung are also evident. HRCT scans (**B** and **C**) demonstrate bilateral bronchiectasis (*arrows*), more severe in the left lung. The areas of bronchiectasis are associated with decreased attenuation and vascularity, suggesting the presence of obliterative bronchiolitis. Note the relative sparing of the right lower lobe. (*From Fraser RS, Müller NL, Colman NC, Paré PD: Fraser and Paré's Diagnosis of Diseases of the Chest, 4th ed. Philadelphia, WB Saunders, 1999.*)

Syndrome of Yellow Nails, Lymphedema, Pleural Effusion, and Bronchiectasis

A syndrome of yellow nails and lymphedema was first described in 1964[803]; pleural effusion and bronchiectasis are frequent concomitant features. The pleural fluid is characteristically an exudate and may be chylous.[804] Typically, the nails grow slowly, are yellowish green, and are thickened and excessively curved from side to side; they have a tendency to become infected. The pathogenesis of the bronchiectasis is unknown.

Williams-Campbell Syndrome

Williams-Campbell syndrome is a congenital form of bronchiectasis that is believed to be caused by a deficiency in the amount of airway cartilage.[805] The condition shows familial clustering and may be associated with other congenital abnormalities.[806] HRCT findings consist of cystic bronchiectasis limited to the fourth-, fifth-, and sixth-generation bronchi associated with collapse of the bronchi and distal air trapping on expiratory scans.[807] Affected individuals are usually identified in infancy because of repeated chest infections and evidence of bronchiectasis.

"Lady Windermere Syndrome"

Bronchiectasis associated with *Mycobacterium avium-intracellulare* infection is an increasingly common cause of airway disease, particularly in elderly women.[808] The name of the syndrome derives from the suggestion that voluntary suppression of coughing is the basis for the susceptibility.[809] The dependent portions of the lung and the middle lobe and lingula tend to be involved.

BRONCHOLITHIASIS

The term *broncholithiasis* is used to denote the presence of calcified or ossified material within the lumen of the tracheobronchial tree. Although this material can be in situ calcification of aspirated foreign material, calcification and extrusion of bronchial cartilage plates, or migration of calcified material to a bronchus from a distant site such as a pleural plaque,[810] the most common cause is erosion and extrusion of calcified necrotic material from a bronchopulmonary lymph node affected by long-standing necrotizing granulomatous lymphadenitis. Broncholiths can cause cough, hemoptysis, distal bronchiectasis, and obstructive pneumonitis or may be expectorated (lithoptysis).

Radiographic manifestations of broncholithiasis include a change of position or disappearance of a calcific focus on serial radiographs or the development of airway obstruction resulting in lobar or segmental atelectasis, mucoid impaction, or expiratory air trapping.[811] Although a specific diagnosis can seldom be made on the plain chest radiograph, broncholiths can usually be readily identified on CT (Fig. 15–54).[812]

BRONCHIAL FISTULAS

Bronchial fistulas can be established with many structures, both within the thorax and outside it. The principal underlying causes are infection and carcinoma[813]; either may originate in the lung or in the organ with which the fistula is associated. Bronchopleural fistulas may be radiographically manifested as persistent pneumothorax, tension pneumothorax, or hydropneumothorax.[814] CT often allows direct visualization and localization of the fistula, as well as assessment of the underlying cause.[815]

BRONCHIOLITIS

Classification and Pathologic Characteristics

A variety of pulmonary diseases are characterized predominantly by inflammation of the membranous and respiratory bronchioles.[816] Such bronchiolitis can be classified in several ways, including (1) by its proved or presumed etiology or the pulmonary or systemic diseases with which it is often associated (Table 15–6) and (2) by its histologic features (Table 15–7). Although an etiologic classification is useful for reminding the physician when to suspect the presence of bronchiolitis, a scheme based on histologic characteristics is more valuable for two reasons: (1) the histologic patterns of bronchiolitis generally show better correlation with the clinical and radiologic manifestations of disease than the various etiologies do, and (2) the histologic classification shows better correlation with the natural history of the disease and the response to therapy.

The classification scheme presented in Table 15–7 is based on a consideration of two pathologic processes: inflammation and fibrosis. The first is related simply to the traditional separation of inflammation into acute and chronic reactions, the former characterized by an exudate of fluid and neutrophils and, frequently, by tissue necrosis (see Color Fig. 15–5) and the latter by tissue infiltration by mononuclear cells (see Color Fig. 15–2). From this perspective, bronchiolitis can be

TABLE 15–6. Etiologic Agents and Clinical Conditions Associated with Bronchiolitis

Inhalation of gases, fumes, and dust
  Toxic fumes
  Cigarette smoke
  Irritant gases (NO_2, SO_2, ammonia, chlorine, phosgene, HCl)
  Mineral dust fumes (e.g., from welding)
  Mineral dust particles (e.g., asbestos, silica)
  Grain dust
Infection
  Viruses
  Aspergillus species
  Bordetella pertussis
  Mycoplasma pneumoniae
  Chlamydia species
Drugs and chemicals
Immunologic disease
  Organ transplantation
  Rheumatoid disease
  Systemic lupus erythematosus
  Dermatomyositis
  Sjögren's syndrome
  Progressive systemic sclerosis
  Extrinsic allergic alveolitis
  Ulcerative colitis
Aspiration

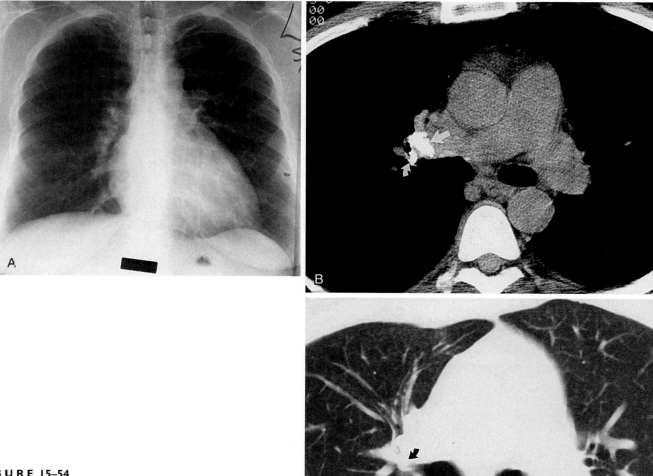

FIGURE 15–54

Broncholithiasis. A posteroanterior chest radiograph (**A**) demonstrates calcified right hilar nodes. Five-millimeter-collimation CT scans (**B** and **C**) show the calcification (*straight arrow*) and a broncholith within the right upper lobe bronchus (*curved arrow*). The patient was a 45-year-old woman who had a history of hemoptysis and lithoptysis. (*From Fraser RS, Müller NL, Colman NC, Paré PD: Fraser and Paré's Diagnosis of Diseases of the Chest, 4th ed. Philadelphia, WB Saunders, 1999.*)

subdivided into acute and chronic forms. The first of these forms is typically associated with processes that cause bronchiolar injury over a short time frame, such as viral infection or the inhalation of toxic gases. The second form is typically associated with more prolonged injury and may itself have a variety of pathologic patterns. Some of these patterns are histologically distinctive and have thus been described by specific terms, such as *respiratory bronchiolitis*, *follicular bronchiolitis*, and *diffuse panbronchiolitis*. The histologic categorization of these conditions clearly depends on the availability of tissue; however, the clinical and radiologic features associated with specific histologic patterns are often sufficiently characteristic to permit a strong presumptive diagnosis.

In addition to these relatively distinctive patterns of chronic bronchiolitis, nonspecific chronic bronchiolitis characterized by infiltration of the bronchiolar wall by lymphocytes, plasma cells, and histiocytes, accompanied by a variable degree of fibrosis, can be encountered in a variety of situations, including COPD,[817] bronchiectasis (Fig. 15–55), lung transplantation (in which it has sometimes been designated *lymphocytic bronchiolitis*),[818] aspiration of oral or gastric secretions,[819] and chronic inhalation of organic and inorganic dust.[820]

Despite some degree of overlap, bronchiolitis can also be subdivided histologically into two forms on the basis of the pattern of fibrosis (Fig. 15–56). The first, which we prefer to call *obliterative bronchiolitis* but which has also been termed *constrictive bronchiolitis*, is characterized by a proliferation of fibrous tissue predominantly between the epithelium and the muscularis mucosae; the proliferation results in more or less concentric narrowing of the airway lumen, which in its most extreme form results in complete obliteration. The epithelium overlying the abnormal fibrous tissue may be flattened or metaplastic but is usually intact (i.e., without evidence of ulceration). By contrast, the epithelium in the second form of bronchiolitis is invariably absent, at least focally. Granulation

TABLE 15–7. Bronchiolitis: Pathologic Classification with Corresponding Clinical, Functional, and Radiologic Features

Forms of Bronchiolitis	Histologic Characteristics	Clinical Features	Functional Features	Radiographic Features	HRCT Features
Acute bronchiolitis	Predominantly acute but also chronic inflammation associated with epithelial necrosis and a variable degree of inflammation in the adjacent lung parenchyma	Characteristic of infection (particularly viruses and *Mycoplasma pneumoniae*). Also seen as an early reaction after the inhalation of toxic fumes or gases	Obstruction and hyperinflation	Reticulonodular opacities	Centrilobular nodules and branching lines; patchy or diffuse distribution
Chronic bronchiolitis	Chronic inflammation (variable number of lymphocytes, plasma cells, and histiocytes) and fibrosis. The epithelium may be metaplastic (goblet cells), and there may be increased smooth muscle. Several relatively specific clinicopathologic variants can be seen	This pattern is the major pathologic finding in the membranous bronchioles of cigarette smokers. It can also be seen after chronic irritation of the airways caused by a variety of inhaled substances (e.g., grain dust and some minerals) and in bronchiectasis and extrinsic allergic alveolitis	Along with loss of lung elastic recoil, this is the cause of airflow obstruction in COPD	Reticulonodular opacities	Centrilobular nodules
Respiratory bronchiolitis	Accumulation of macrophages within membranous and respiratory bronchioles accompanied by a variable degree of lymphocyte infiltration and fibrosis in the bronchiolar wall and peribronchiolar interstitium	This is the earliest lesion seen in cigarette smokers. Patients are usually young and asymptomatic. When dyspnea is associated with radiographic abnormalities and restrictive lung function, the abnormality has been termed *respiratory bronchiolitis–associated interstitial pneumonia* (possibly representing an early manifestation of desquamative interstitial pneumonitis)	May be associated with a mild obstructive pattern or, in some patients, restrictive changes	Ground-glass opacities	Ground-glass attenuation and poorly defined centrilobular nodular opacities; upper lobe predominance
Follicular bronchiolitis	Abundant lymphoid tissue, frequently with prominent germinal centers, situated in the walls of bronchioles and, to some extent, bronchi	Most often described in association with rheumatoid arthritis but may be seen in immunodeficiency syndromes and hypersensitivity reactions	Restrictive or obstructive functional abnormality	Reticulonodular opacities	Centrilobular nodules and branching lines
Diffuse panbronchiolitis	Mural and intraluminal infiltrates of acute and chronic inflammatory cells. The lesions are centered predominantly on respiratory bronchioles and are associated with a striking accumulation of foamy macrophages within the airway wall and adjacent parenchyma	Typically seen in patients from Japan and Southeast Asia	Associated with progressive development of an obstructive ventilatory defect	Reticulonodular opacities	Centrilobular nodules and branching lines; bronchiolectasis, bronchiectasis, diffuse distribution
Obliterative bronchiolitis	Fibrous tissue predominantly between the muscularis mucosa and epithelium of membranous bronchioles resulting in more or less concentric airway narrowing. An inflammatory cell infiltrate and fibrosis in the submucosa are variable in intensity but often mild	Characteristically seen in bone marrow and lung transplant recipients and in some connective tissue diseases (particularly rheumatoid disease)	Progressive airflow obstruction, hyperinflation, and ventilatory respiratory failure	Hyperinflation and peripheral areas of vascular attenuation	Low attenuation and mosaic attenuation; air trapping on expiratory HRCT

Continued

TABLE 15–7. Bronchiolitis: Pathologic Classification with Corresponding Clinical, Functional, and Radiologic Features—cont'd

Forms of Bronchiolitis	Histologic Characteristics	Clinical Features	Functional Features	Radiographic Features	HRCT Features
Cryptogenic organizing pneumonia	Focal necrosis of the respiratory bronchiolar and alveolar duct epithelium associated with partial or complete air space occlusion by fibroblast (myofibroblast) proliferation. Mild to moderate interstitial pneumonitis and air space fibrosis in adjacent parenchyma	The lesion is most often of unknown etiology but may occur in association with many causes, including connective tissue diseases, viral and bacterial pneumonia, drugs, and aspiration	Restrictive pattern	Patchy, usually bilateral air space consolidation	Multifocal consolidation, often predominantly peribronchial or subpleural; ground-glass opacities

From Fraser RS, Müller NL, Colman NC, Paré PD: Fraser and Paré's Diagnosis of Diseases of the Chest, 4th ed. Philadelphia, WB Saunders, 1999.

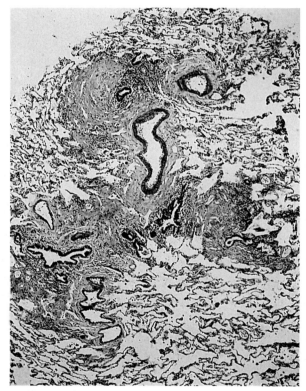

FIGURE 15–55

Chronic bronchiolitis—cystic fibrosis. A section of lung parenchyma from a 22-year-old patient with cystic fibrosis shows marked fibrosis and patchy chronic inflammation of the walls of several membranous bronchioles. *(From Fraser RS, Müller NL, Colman NC, Paré PD: Fraser and Paré's Diagnosis of Diseases of the Chest, 4th ed. Philadelphia, WB Saunders, 1999.)*

tissue or plugs of fibroblastic tissue extend from these areas of epithelial damage into the airway lumen and result in partial or, occasionally, complete obstruction. Although this histologic pattern may be the only abnormality seen in the lung, in the vast majority of cases it is associated with similar epithelial injury and fibroblastic reaction in the adjacent parenchyma. As a result, the terms *bronchiolitis obliterans with*

organizing pneumonia (BOOP) or *cryptogenic organizing pneumonia (COP)* are frequently used to describe this form of disease.[821,822]

Radiologic Manifestations

The radiographic features of bronchiolitis are highly variable and related to a number of factors, including the extent of airway involvement, the chronicity of the disorder, and the presence or absence of underlying parenchymal abnormality. Nonetheless, they are essentially limited to two patterns: hyperinflation and peripheral attenuation of vascular markings (Fig. 15–57) (associated with obliterative bronchiolitis) and air space consolidation (Fig. 15–58) (in COP).[823,824] There is considerable interobserver and intraobserver variability in interpretation of these abnormalities and poor correlation between the clinical severity of disease and the degree of radiologic change.[825,826]

The anatomic detail that can be revealed with HRCT allows better assessment of the presence and extent of abnormalities; in fact, the results of several radiologic and pathologic correlative studies show that HRCT can suggest the predominant histologic pattern of bronchiolitis in some cases.[827-829] Because of this ability, HRCT is clearly the radiologic method of choice for investigating a patient suspected on clinical or radiographic grounds of having bronchiolitis. A number of patterns can be seen, including centrilobular nodules and branching lines, areas of decreased attenuation, air space consolidation, and ground-glass attenuation. Fibrosis/inflammation of the bronchiolar wall or filling of dilated bronchioles with granulation tissue, mucus, or pus results in a pattern of small centrilobular nodules and branching lines (tree-in-bud pattern [Fig. 15–59]). This pattern is characteristic of acute infectious bronchiolitis, including that seen with endobronchial spread of tuberculosis; in some cases, it is accompanied by scattered areas of ground-glass attenuation or consolidation.[828] A tree-in-bud pattern can also be seen in diffuse panbronchiolitis and in association with large-airway disease, such as bronchiectasis.[830,831]

A heterogeneous pattern of attenuation consisting of areas of decreased density and vascularity (mosaic perfusion) is characteristic of obliterative bronchiolitis (Fig. 15–60).[832,833] The variation in attenuation of individual lobules is

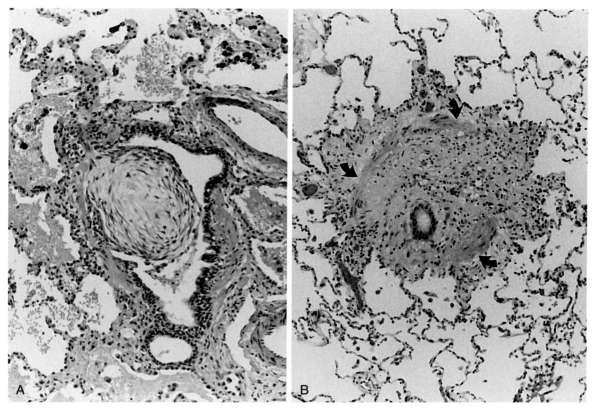

FIGURE 15–56

Bronchiolitis with fibrosis. Sections of membranous bronchioles from two patients show two major histologic patterns of bronchiolar fibrosis. In **A,** a plug of fibroblastic tissue partially occludes the airway lumen. The epithelium is absent where the fibrous tissue is in contact with the airway wall, suggesting that the latter represents organization of an exudate secondary to epithelial ulceration. The patient had experienced an episode of presumed bacterial pneumonia about 1 month before death. This pattern of fibrosis is usually seen in association with similar plugs of fibroblastic tissue in transitional airways and alveolar air spaces, in which case the abnormality is termed *cryptogenic organizing pneumonia (bronchiolitis obliterans with organizing pneumonia).* In **B,** the airway lumen is markedly narrowed by fibrous tissue that more or less completely surrounds intact epithelium (residual muscularis mucosae is indicated by *arrows*), a pattern sometimes referred to as *constrictive bronchiolitis.* The patient had long-standing rheumatoid disease and had suffered progressive dyspnea associated with obstructive lung function. *(From Fraser RS, Müller NL, Colman NC, Paré PD: Fraser and Paré's Diagnosis of Diseases of the Chest, 4th ed. Philadelphia, WB Saunders, 1999.)*

accentuated when images are obtained after the patient exhales to RV.[834] The areas of decreased attenuation are the result of airway closure (causing air trapping) and local hypoxemia (causing pulmonary arterial vasoconstriction). The increased attenuation is due to redistribution of blood flow to the relatively normal lung. It should be remembered that small, focal areas of low attenuation, as well as small areas of air trapping, can also be seen in healthy individuals.[835] Although these findings can affect one or several lobules at various sites, they are most commonly seen in the superior segments of the lower lobes and near the tip of the lingula and usually involve less than 25% of the cross-sectional area of one lung at one scan level.[835] Mosaic perfusion and air trapping can be considered abnormal when they affect a volume of lung equal to or greater than a pulmonary segment and are not limited to the superior segment of the lower lobe or the lingula tip.[833] Mosaic perfusion can also be seen in patients who have pulmonary vascular abnormalities (particularly hypertension secondary to chronic thromboembolism),[836] extrinsic allergic alveolitis,[837] asthma,[838] and bronchiectasis.[839]

Unilateral or bilateral areas of consolidation are characteristic of COP (Fig. 15–61). The consolidation is often patchy; although it may have a random distribution, it affects mainly the peribronchial or subpleural lung regions in about 60% of cases.[840] Centrilobular nodular opacities may reflect the presence of intrabronchiolar fibroblastic tissue or peribronchiolar consolidation. Focal areas of consolidation can also be seen in association with centrilobular nodular and branching linear opacities in infectious bronchiolitis and bronchopneumonia.

Ground-glass attenuation can occur in association with isolated respiratory bronchiolitis, respiratory bronchiolitis with interstitial lung disease, and COP.[828,840] Occasionally, particularly in immunocompromised patients who have COP, ground-glass attenuation is the only abnormality evident on HRCT.[840] Extrinsic allergic alveolitis is characterized on HRCT by the presence of poorly defined centrilobular opacities and extensive bilateral areas of ground-glass attenuation. Localized areas of low attenuation are also observed frequently (Fig. 15–62)[841]; these areas have been confirmed to represent air

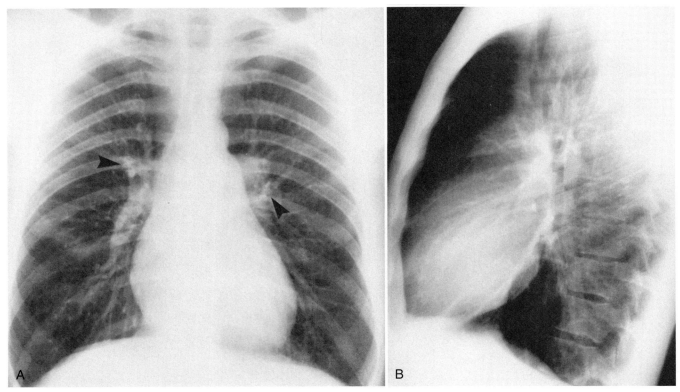

FIGURE 15–57

Obliterative bronchiolitis of unknown etiology. Posteroanterior (**A**) and lateral (**B**) chest radiographs demonstrate pulmonary overinflation. The vasculature in the lower lung zones appears somewhat attenuated and that in the upper lung zones more prominent than normal, indicative of recruitment. When these changes are considered in conjunction with prominence of the main pulmonary artery and probable right ventricular enlargement, the findings are consistent with pulmonary arterial hypertension. The bronchial walls are thickened (*arrowheads*). Histologic examination of the lungs at autopsy showed typical changes of obliterative bronchiolitis and pulmonary artery hypertension. The patient was a young man with progressive dyspnea and right-sided heart failure. *(From Fraser RS, Müller NL, Colman NC, Paré PD: Fraser and Paré's Diagnosis of Diseases of the Chest, 4th ed. Philadelphia, WB Saunders, 1999.)*

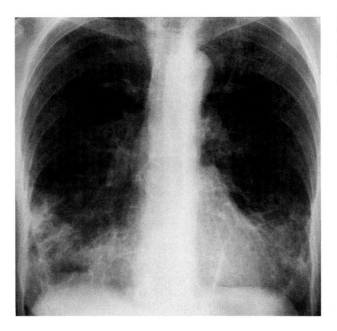

FIGURE 15–58

Cryptogenic organizing pneumonia. A posteroanterior chest radiograph in a 64-year-old woman demonstrates bilateral areas of consolidation involving the lower lung zones. *(From Fraser RS, Müller NL, Colman NC, Paré PD: Fraser and Paré's Diagnosis of Diseases of the Chest, 4th ed. Philadelphia, WB Saunders, 1999.)*

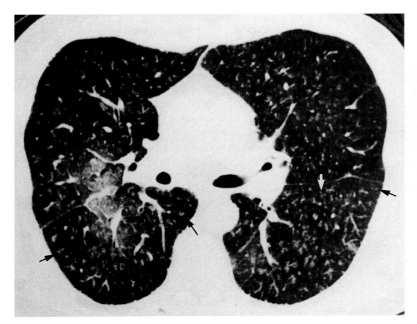

FIGURE 15–59

Bronchiolitis related to *Aspergillus* species. An HRCT scan demonstrates bilateral centrilobular nodular and branching opacities (*arrows*). Also noted is a focal area of ground-glass attenuation in the right lung. The diagnosis of *Aspergillus* bronchiolitis and early bronchopneumonia was confirmed by open lung biopsy. The patient was a 52-year-old man with leukemia. (*From Fraser RS, Müller NL, Colman NC, Paré PD: Fraser and Paré's Diagnosis of Diseases of the Chest, 4th ed. Philadelphia, WB Saunders, 1999.*)

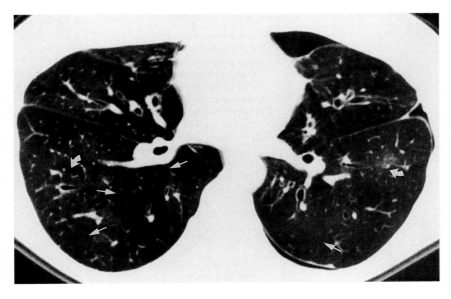

FIGURE 15–60

Obliterative bronchiolitis. An HRCT scan demonstrates localized areas of decreased attenuation (*straight arrows*) and areas of slightly increased attenuation (*curved arrows*), a pattern known as *mosaic attenuation*. Note the greater number and size of vessels within the areas that have increased attenuation. The patient was a 29-year-old woman with bronchiolitis as a result of chronic graft-versus-host disease. Incidental note is made of a small left pneumothorax. (*From Fraser RS, Müller NL, Colman NC, Paré PD: Fraser and Paré's Diagnosis of Diseases of the Chest, 4th ed. Philadelphia, WB Saunders, 1999.*)

trapping on expiratory CT scan and are presumed to be secondary to bronchiolitis.[837,841]

Specific Clinicopathologic Forms of Bronchiolitis

Acute Infectious Bronchiolitis

Acute infectious bronchiolitis is characteristically the result of infection by viruses, *Mycoplasma pneumonia*, and *Chlamydia* species. Symptomatic viral infection is most common and severe in children, in whom the incidence has been found to be as high as 10 per 100 children per year in the first year of life in the United States.[842] The most common agents are RSV, the adenoviruses, and parainfluenza virus (especially type 3).

The clinical manifestations typically begin with symptoms of an upper respiratory tract infection, followed 2 to 3 days later by the abrupt onset of dyspnea, tachypnea, and fever; cyanosis and prostration may be seen in severe cases. In previously healthy infants, the usual course of the disease consists of 2 or 3 days of severe symptoms followed by progressive recovery. Adults are probably infected with respiratory tract viruses as often as infants; however, the severity and consequences of infection in otherwise healthy individuals are usually much less, probably because their small airways contribute less to total pulmonary resistance.[843] Nonetheless, severe and sometimes fatal disease can occur.[844]

Bronchiolitis Related to Toxic Gases, Fumes, and Dust

A variety of inorganic and organic agents can cause acute inhalational lung injury (see page 754); bronchiolitis may be the major manifestation or a minor component of such

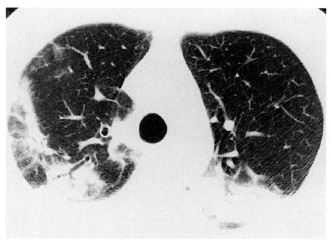

FIGURE 15–61

Cryptogenic organizing pneumonia. An HRCT scan at the level of the aortic arch shows bilateral areas of consolidation in a predominantly subpleural and peribronchial distribution. The patient was a 46-year-old man. *(From Worthy SL, Müller NL: Small airways disease. Radiol Clin North Am 36:163, 1998.)*

injury.[845] Acute exposure to smoke and the oxides of nitrogen, sulfur, and a variety of other gases and fumes can cause bronchiolitis that is associated with severe airflow obstruction. Symptoms of cough and dyspnea appear minutes or hours after exposure and may be accompanied by the development of pulmonary edema within 4 to 24 hours. If patients survive this acute disease, a delayed second phase characterized by fever, chills, cough, dyspnea, and cyanosis may occur within 2 to 5 weeks[846]; corresponding pathologic findings are predominantly those of obliterative bronchiolitis.[847] When concentrations of gas or fume are not so high, acute symptoms may be minimal, and there can be a symptom-free period before the second phase begins.

As indicated previously, bronchiolitis is a prominent component of extrinsic allergic alveolitis and is also the probable cause of the obstructive ventilatory defect seen in workers chronically exposed to grain dust.[848,849] Exposure to a variety of organic substances containing microorganisms may also result in organic dust toxic syndrome,[850] which is characterized histologically by a mononuclear inflammatory infiltrate within the walls of respiratory bronchioles. Although the

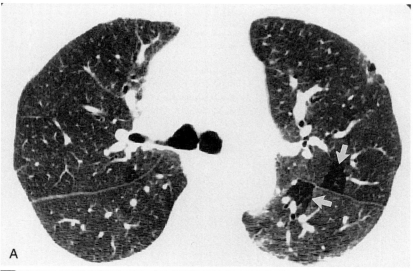

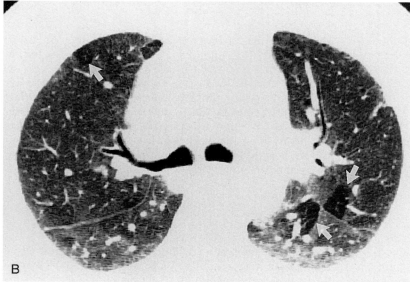

FIGURE 15–62

Extrinsic allergic alveolitis. An HRCT scan obtained at end-inspiration (**A**) shows bilateral areas of ground-glass attenuation and focal areas of decreased attenuation and decreased vascularity (*arrows*). The areas of decreased attenuation have a configuration and size that correspond to a secondary pulmonary lobule. A scan obtained at end-expiration (**B**) shows air trapping (*arrows*). The latter is presumably related to bronchiolitis, whereas the areas of ground-glass attenuation reflect the presence of alveolitis. *(From Fraser RS, Müller NL, Colman NC, Paré PD: Fraser and Paré's Diagnosis of Diseases of the Chest, 4th ed. Philadelphia, WB Saunders, 1999.)*

pathogenesis is not known, it has been hypothesized that it is caused by high concentrations of endotoxin in the dust; a similar mechanism may underlie the obstructive lung function abnormalities and bronchiolitis experienced by workers in the poultry and swine confinement industries (see page 511).

Bronchiolitis Associated with Connective Tissue Disease

Bronchiolitis is an occasional complication of a number of connective tissue diseases, particularly rheumatoid disease.[851] In the latter condition, it may take a variety of forms, including obliterative bronchiolitis, follicular bronchiolitis, and COP; nonspecific chronic bronchiolitis may also be seen in association with bronchiectasis. The obliterative form of disease may be more frequent in patients who have been treated with penicillamine or gold.[852,853] Lymphocytic bronchiolitis and follicular bronchiolitis are the most frequently encountered histologic forms of bronchiolitis in patients who have Sjögren's syndrome; either may be part of a more generalized process of lymphocytic interstitial pneumonitis.

Obliterative Bronchiolitis Associated with Organ Transplantation

Obliterative bronchiolitis is an important complication of bone marrow, lung, and heart-lung transplantation (see pages 528 and 536).[854] It is a relatively uncommon complication of bone marrow transplantation and is seen in 5% or less of patients who receive allogeneic transplants[855]; however, it has been reported in up to 70% of lung transplant recipients and has been the cause of death of more than half of affected individuals.[856,857] Most patients have a history of cough and progressive breathlessness. Lung function testing reveals progressive airflow obstruction.

Swyer-James Syndrome

Swyer-James syndrome (Macleod's syndrome, unilateral or lobar emphysema, unilateral hyperlucent lung) is an uncommon abnormality that is characterized radiographically by a hyperlucent lobe or lung and functionally by normal or reduced volume during inspiration and air trapping during expiration. As some of its names suggest, the abnormality has been considered by some to represent a variant of emphysema. However, since the hyperlucency is primarily the result of decreased pulmonary blood volume secondary to bronchiolar obliteration rather than destruction of pulmonary parenchyma, we prefer to regard it as a disease of the airways.

Substantial evidence indicates that the syndrome is initiated by viral bronchiolitis. In many cases, the disease is recognized (or at least suspected) in childhood when chest radiography is carried out for investigation of repeated respiratory infections. In others, it does not become apparent until adulthood when it is recognized on the basis of a screening chest radiograph of an asymptomatic patient; inquiry in these cases often reveals a history of acute lower respiratory tract infection, generally during childhood.[858] Most cases of Swyer-James syndrome therefore probably begin as an acute bronchiolitis that progresses to fibrous obliteration of the airway lumen; the peripheral parenchyma is largely unaffected and

remains inflated because of collateral ventilation with resulting air trapping. However, destructive changes characteristic of emphysema also supervene in some cases.[859]

The radiographic manifestations are usually easily recognized and are virtually pathognomonic. A posteroanterior radiograph exposed at TLC reveals a remarkable difference in radiolucency of the two lungs (or the affected and unaffected lobes) (Fig. 15–63) caused not by a relative increase in air in the affected lung but by decreased perfusion. The peripheral pulmonary markings are diminutive as a result of vascular narrowing and attenuation. The ipsilateral hilum is also diminutive but is present, a feature of value in the differentiation from proximal interruption of a pulmonary artery (pulmonary artery agenesis). In radiographs exposed at TLC, the volume of the affected lung (or lobe) either is comparable to that of the normal contralateral lung or is reduced; it is seldom, if ever, increased.

One of the characteristic radiologic features of Swyer-James syndrome—in fact, a sine qua non for diagnosis—is the presence of air trapping during expiration (see Fig. 15–63). This finding is a reflection of airway obstruction and is extremely valuable in differentiating the syndrome from other conditions that may give rise to unilateral or lobar hyperlucency. Because the contralateral lung is normal, expiration causes the mediastinum to shift toward the normal lung; in addition, excursion of the hemidiaphragms is markedly asymmetrical because it is severely diminished on the affected side. Radiographs exposed at RV also accentuate the disparity in radiolucency of the two lungs, the density of the normal lung being much greater. This disparity is related to the fact that the normal lung contains less air and, perhaps more important, its blood flow is virtually the total output of the right ventricle.

The diagnosis can be confirmed readily with HRCT or spiral CT angiography.[860] The characteristic CT findings are decreased size, decreased attenuation and vascularity of the involved lung, and air trapping on expiration (see Fig. 15–63). Bronchiectasis is seen in the vast majority of cases. In some patients, areas of normal attenuation are found within the hyperlucent lung and focal areas of decreased attenuation and vascularity in the contralateral lung.[861]

Although a number of conditions can have a radiographic appearance similar to that of Swyer-James syndrome, in only one is there a serious potential difficulty. A partly obstructing lesion situated within a main bronchus can create a triad of radiographic signs that are indistinguishable from Swyer-James syndrome—a smaller than normal lung volume, air trapping on expiration, and diffuse oligemia as a result of hypoxic vasoconstriction. As a consequence, in any patient with these signs, the presence of a lesion within the ipsilateral main bronchus must be excluded before a diagnosis of the syndrome is accepted; the easiest way to accomplish such exclusion is by bronchoscopy or spiral CT.

The clinical findings are highly variable. Some patients have no symptoms; others complain of dyspnea on exertion or a history of repeated lower respiratory tract infections.[862] Physical examination reveals restriction of chest expansion on the affected side in association with diminished breath sounds, relative hyper-resonance, and (sometimes) scattered crackles. In cases in which an entire lung is involved, VC and expiratory flow are reduced. Diffusing capacity measured by the steady-state method is usually reduced; however, it may be normal with the single-breath method because

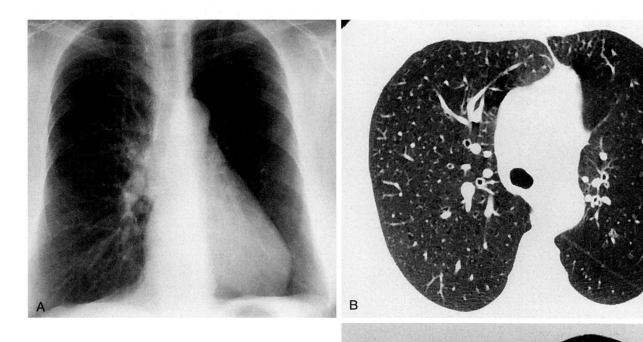

FIGURE 15–63

Swyer-James syndrome. A posteroanterior chest radiograph (**A**) shows increased radiolucency and decreased vascularity and size of the left lung. An HRCT scan (**B**) at end-inspiration confirms the radiographic findings. The left lung is decreased in volume in association with a shift of the mediastinum and the anterior junction line to the left. A scan performed at end-expiration (**C**) reveals air trapping in the left lung associated with a shift of the mediastinum and the junction line to the midline. The patient was a 61-year-old woman. *(From Fraser RS, Müller NL, Colman NC, Paré PD: Fraser and Paré's Diagnosis of Diseases of the Chest, 4th ed. Philadelphia, WB Saunders, 1999.)*

breath-holding permits time for more uniform gas distribution. Blood gas concentrations are generally normal but may decrease during exercise.

Cryptogenic Organizing Pneumonia (Bronchiolitis Obliterans with Organizing Pneumonia)

Although *organizing pneumonia* has been used as a descriptive term histologically in a variety of conditions for a long time, the idea that it could represent a distinct clinicopathologic entity was first recognized only in 1982.[863]

Because no causative agent was identified in the patients described in this report, the authors suggested that it could be referred to as *cryptogenic organizing pneumonia*, an appellation that has now been accepted by a classification committee of the American Thoracic Society and European Respiratory Society.[822] In 1985, another group described an identical

clinicopathologic disorder that they termed *bronchiolitis obliterans organizing pneumonia* to emphasize its two characteristic histologic features; the acronym derived therefrom (BOOP) is also widely used to refer to the abnormality.[821]

It is important to remember that the histologic reaction pattern of COP can be seen in association with a number of etiologies, including connective tissue diseases, drugs, infection, and aspiration; the following discussion refers mainly to cases in which an etiology is not identified ("idiopathic" COP). It is also important to note that the radiographic appearance occasionally suggests interstitial disease and that pulmonary function studies reveal a restrictive rather than an obstructive derangement, in which situation COP can be confused with idiopathic pulmonary fibrosis or other forms of interstitial lung disease.

COP is typically distributed in a patchy fashion throughout the lung, both grossly and microscopically within secondary lobules. Characteristically, plugs of fibroblastic connective tissue can be identified within respiratory bronchioles and alveolar ducts (Fig. 15–64). The parenchyma adjacent to the affected bronchioles shows filling of alveolar air spaces by similar fibroblastic tissue; occasionally, a proteinaceous exudate can be identified in the central portion of the fibroblastic tissue that represents a more direct manifestation of previous epithelial or endothelial injury. A variable degree of nonspecific chronic inflammation and interstitial fibrosis is also evident.

COP has four distinctive radiographic and CT patterns: (1) multiple, usually bilateral, symmetrical, patchy air space opacities; (2) bilateral interstitial opacities, which may be reticular, nodular, or reticulonodular; (3) focal consolidation; and (4) multiple large nodules or masses.[864,865] A mixed pattern of combined air space and interstitial opacities has also been described.

Patchy air space consolidation is the most characteristic and the most common of these patterns (Fig. 15–65). The opacities are most often peripheral and pleural based. They may decrease in size in one area and appear in previously unaffected regions.[866] The size of the individual opacities ranges from about 3 cm to nearly complete lobar consolidation. The margins of the individual opacities are indistinct,

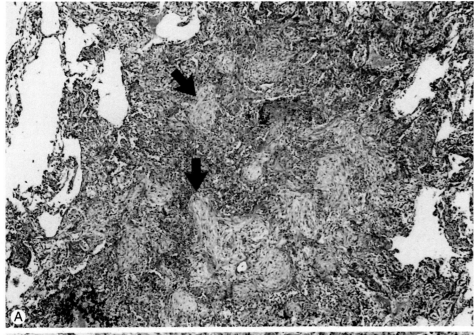

FIGURE 15–64

Cryptogenic organizing pneumonia. A section of lung parenchyma (**A**) shows a poorly defined focus of chronic inflammation associated with numerous small foci of loose connective tissue (*arrows*). A magnified view of similar disease from another area (**B**) shows branching of the connective tissue plugs, which implies that they are present in the lumina of alveolar ducts and respiratory bronchioles. The interstitial nature of the chronic inflammatory infiltrate is apparent at the junction with normal lung (*arrows*). (*From Fraser RS, Müller NL, Colman NC, Paré PD: Fraser and Paré's Diagnosis of Diseases of the Chest, 4th ed. Philadelphia, WB Saunders, 1999.*)

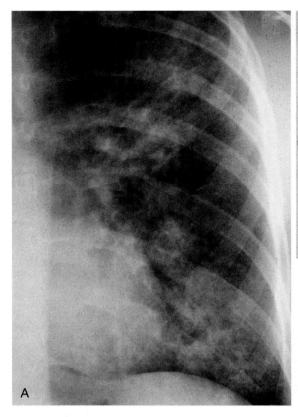

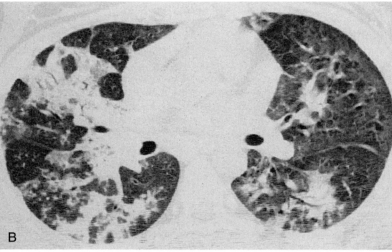

FIGURE 15–65

Cryptogenic organizing pneumonia. A view of the left lung from a posteroanterior chest radiograph (**A**) in a 20-year-old woman demonstrates patchy areas of consolidation. An HRCT scan (**B**) shows a predominantly peribronchial and subpleural distribution of the consolidation. Air bronchograms, focal areas of ground-glass attenuation, and a few centrilobular nodules are also evident. (*From Fraser RS, Müller NL, Colman NC, Paré PD: Fraser and Paré's Diagnosis of Diseases of the Chest, 4th ed. Philadelphia, WB Saunders, 1999.*)

and they may contain air bronchograms. Lung volume may appear preserved or decreased. Concomitant small pleural effusions are seen in 20% to 30% of patients.[867,868] Although this consolidation pattern is characteristic of COP, it is by no means specific, and the differential diagnosis includes chronic eosinophilic pneumonia, bronchioalveolar carcinoma, lymphoma, pulmonary alveolar proteinosis, and alveolar hemorrhage.[864]

A pattern of reticular or reticulonodular opacities may be seen in association with air space opacities or, occasionally, as an isolated finding.[867,868] A focal area of consolidation is a relatively uncommon manifestation; the differential diagnosis includes pulmonary carcinoma, a suspicion that may be enhanced by the presence of fever, weight loss, and hemoptysis.[859] The last and least common manifestation of COP is multiple large nodules or masses, which may simulate metastatic disease.[865]

On HRCT, most patients show areas of air space consolidation, small nodules, or both[870,871]; peripheral reticular areas of increased attenuation and ground-glass opacities are seen less often.[871] Occasionally, patients have a pattern of small centrilobular nodules and branching shadows that is more characteristic of acute infectious bronchiolitis or diffuse panbronchiolitis.[828]

COP is usually manifested as a subacute illness whose duration of symptoms before diagnosis varies from 2 to 6 months.[872] The most common symptoms are cough (often productive), dyspnea, fever, malaise, and weight loss. Crackles are audible on auscultation in 75% of cases. Clubbing is not observed. Most patients have restrictive disease and gas exchange impairment.[873,874] Organizing pneumonia that is manifested as an asymptomatic focal opacity is most often

detected on a chest radiograph and diagnosed on lung biopsy performed because of a suspicion of carcinoma.

In many patients, the clinical and radiographic signs of disease remit completely after systemic corticosteroid therapy.[872,875] However, a minority have disease that pursues a rapid course and has a worse prognosis; although some of these patients are still found to have idiopathic disease after careful investigation,[876] such rapid progression is more likely to be associated with an underlying condition such as connective tissue disease or drug therapy.[877] Patients with focal COP usually have no relapse or respiratory-related deaths.[878]

Respiratory Bronchiolitis

The term *respiratory bronchiolitis* has been used to describe a variety of histologic abnormalities, including accumulation of pigment-laden macrophages in the respiratory bronchioles and adjacent alveoli and thickening of the respiratory bronchiolar walls by inflammatory cells and fibrous tissue (see Color Fig. 9–6).[879,880] The abnormality is invariably associated with cigarette smoking and, in fact, has been considered to be one of the earliest pathologic reactions to this agent.[881]

In its mildest form, respiratory bronchiolitis is associated with few, if any, symptoms and minimal abnormalities in lung function. In this situation, it is typically discovered as an incidental finding on histologic examination of lungs removed at autopsy or for transplantation. Rarely, a patient presents with cough, dyspnea, crackles, and a combined restrictive and obstructive pattern on lung function testing. When associated with typical radiologic and pathologic findings (see later), this clinicopathologic syndrome has been called *respiratory bronchiolitis–associated interstitial lung disease*.[882] Patients with this syndrome may constitute no more than a subset of individuals who have a more severe form of cigarette smoke–induced respiratory bronchiolitis. However, the lesion has also been thought to represent part of a histologic spectrum of disease that includes desquamative interstitial pneumonitis (see page 471).[883]

The radiologic features consist of poorly defined centrilobular nodules or ground-glass opacities (Fig. 15–66).[828,884] These abnormalities may be diffuse but often involve the upper lobes predominantly or exclusively. The findings in respiratory bronchiolitis–associated interstitial lung disease are similar to those of desquamative interstitial pneumonia and consist of ground-glass opacities with or without associated fine reticular or reticulonodular interstitial opacities; in contrast to desquamative interstitial pneumonia, lung volumes are usually normal.[828,882] On HRCT, the abnormalities consist of diffuse or patchy areas of ground-glass attenuation and/or poorly defined centrilobular nodular opacities often superimposed on a background of emphysema.[885]

Although the natural history of the condition is uncertain, it responds dramatically to smoking cessation and corticosteroid therapy.[882]

Follicular Bronchiolitis

This form of bronchiolar disease is characterized histologically by the presence of abundant lymphoid tissue, frequently with prominent germinal centers, situated in the walls of

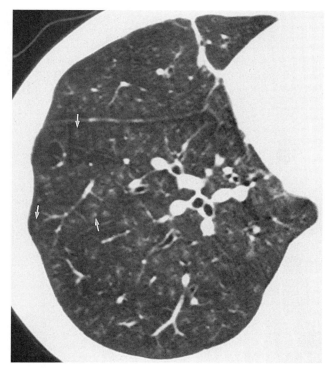

FIGURE 15–66

Respiratory bronchiolitis. A view of the right lower lung from an HRCT scan demonstrates poorly defined centrilobular nodular opacities (*arrows*) and localized areas of ground-glass attenuation. The patient was a 54-year-old heavy smoker who subsequently stopped the habit; a follow-up CT scan performed 5 years later was normal. (*Courtesy of Dr. Takeshi Johkoh, Osaka University Medical School, Osaka, Japan.*)

bronchioles and, to some extent, bronchi (see page 378).[886] Although the alveolar interstitium may contain a similar lymphocytic infiltrate, it is typically minimal. The most common clinical finding is progressive shortness of breath[887]; cough, fever, and recurrent pneumonia are occasionally present. Pulmonary function studies reveal evidence of airway obstruction, restriction, or both.

The abnormality can be found in association with connective tissue diseases (particularly rheumatoid disease and Sjögren's syndrome), immunodeficiency diseases, systemic hypersensitivity reactions, and infection by *M. pneumoniae* or viruses.[886,887] The chest radiograph characteristically shows a diffuse reticulonodular pattern.[886,887] The most common HRCT finding consists of small bilateral centrilobular nodules.[888] Less common manifestations include small subpleural nodules, bronchial wall thickening, peribronchial nodular opacities (Fig. 15–67), and patchy ground-glass opacities.

Diffuse Panbronchiolitis

Diffuse panbronchiolitis is a disease of unknown etiology and pathogenesis associated with chronic inflammation of the paranasal sinuses and respiratory bronchioles, the latter characterized histologically by a striking accumulation of foamy macrophages.[889,890] It has been recognized almost exclusively in Asia, particularly Japan. The average age at onset is about 40 years[890]; the male-to-female ratio is about 2:1.[891]

Investigation for a causative organism has not yielded consistent results. Although patients are frequently infected with *P. aeruginosa* and *H. influenzae*, this is thought to represent opportunistic infection in damaged airways rather than a cause of the disorder.[892] The condition has a strong association with specific HLA antigens, suggesting the possibility of a hereditary factor.[890] Although some patients have been reported to have a history of rheumatoid arthritis or adult T-cell leukemia,[893,894] evidence of abnormal immune function has not been found in most patients.

Histologically, the condition is characterized by an accumulation of mononuclear inflammatory cells (predominantly lymphocytes, plasma cells, and foamy histiocytes) in the walls of respiratory bronchioles, alveolar ducts, and to a lesser extent, adjacent alveoli.[895] Mucus and aggregates of neutrophils may be seen within the airway lumen.[896] The distal lung parenchyma may be normal or may show features of airway obstruction (such as an increase in alveolar macrophages and a mild degree of interstitial inflammation).

Radiographic abnormalities consist of diffuse nodules smaller than 5 mm in diameter and mild to moderate hyperinflation.[897] Findings on HRCT include small centrilobular nodules and branching linear opacities, bronchiolectasis, bronchiectasis, and mosaic areas of decreased parenchymal attenuation and vascularity (Fig. 15–68).[830] The presence of these findings is related to the stage of the disease:[898] the earliest manifestation consists of centrilobular nodular opacities, followed by branching linear opacities that connect to the nodules, followed by bronchiolectasis and, eventually, bronchiectasis. Large cystic spaces or bullae may be seen in the late stage.

The chief clinical manifestations are dyspnea on exertion and cough, often with sputum production. Features of chronic sinusitis are also typical.[891] Elevated cold agglutinin levels are

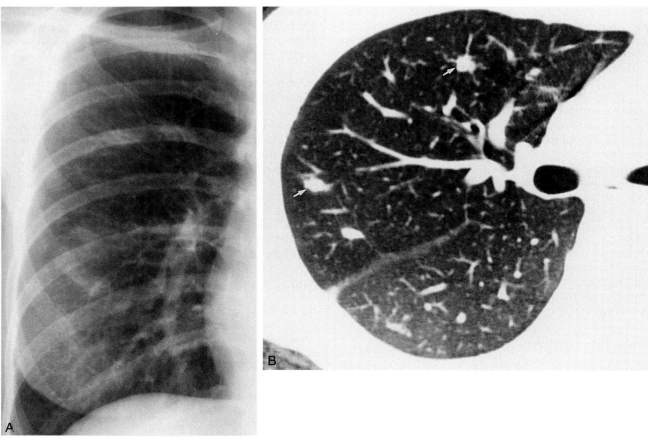

FIGURE 15–67

Follicular bronchiolitis. A view of the right lung from a posteroanterior chest radiograph (**A**) shows ill-defined nodular opacities; a similar pattern was present in the left lung. HRCT targeted to the right lung (**B**) demonstrates sharply defined peribronchovascular nodular opacities in the right upper lobe (*arrows*). The patient was a 24-year-old woman with rheumatoid disease. *(From Fraser RS, Müller NL, Colman NC, Paré PD: Fraser and Paré's Diagnosis of Diseases of the Chest, 4th ed. Philadelphia, WB Saunders, 1999.)*

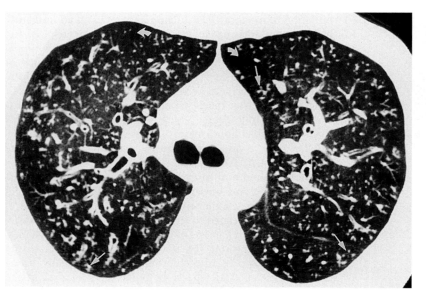

FIGURE 15–68

Diffuse panbronchiolitis. An HRCT scan in a 32-year-old man demonstrates centrilobular nodules (*straight arrows*), marked bronchial wall thickening, bronchiectasis, and localized areas of decreased attenuation and perfusion (*curved arrows*). *(Courtesy of Dr. Kyung Soo Lee, Samsung Medical Center, Seoul, South Korea.)*

frequently seen.[816] Pulmonary function tests show marked obstructive and mild restrictive impairment. Progressive disease is the rule in untreated patients and may be accompanied by respiratory failure. Colonization with *P. aeruginosa* frequently complicates the late stage of the disease and appears to be associated with a worse prognosis; in one study, the 10-year survival rate for those infected with the organism was only 12% as compared with 73% for those who remained uninfected.[892] The beneficial effect of macrolide therapy has been well established and is hypothesized to be related to inhibition of inflammatory cytokine production rather than a direct antibacterial effect[899]; the 10-year survival rate of patients receiving such treatment is over 90% in some studies.[890]

REFERENCES

1. Aboussouan LS, Stoller JK: Diagnosis and management of upper airway obstruction. Clin Chest Med 15:35-53, 1994.
2. Bass H: The flow volume loop: Normal standards and abnormalities in chronic obstructive pulmonary disease. Chest 63:171-176, 1973.
3. Miller RD, Hyatt RE: Obstructing lesions of the larynx and trachea: Clinical and physiologic characteristics. Mayo Clin Proc 44:145-161, 1969.
4. Vincken W, Dollfuss RE, Cosio MG: Upper airway dysfunction detected by respiratory flow oscillations. Eur J Respir Dis 68:50-57, 1986.
5. Katz I, Zamel N, Slutsky AS, et al: An evaluation of flow-volume curves as a screening test for obstructive sleep apnea. Chest 98:337-340, 1990.
6. Paré PD, Donevan RE, Nelems JM: Clues to unrecognized upper airway obstruction. Can Med Assoc J 127:39-41, 1982.
7. Sackner MA: Physiologic features of upper airway obstruction. Chest 62:414-417, 1972.
8. Keberle M, Kenn W, Hahn D: Current concepts in imaging of laryngeal and hypopharyngeal cancer. Eur Radiol 12:1672-1683, 2002.
9. Hasegawa K, Nishimura T, Yagisawa M, et al: Dynamic MRI diagnosis of sleep-disordered breathing. Acta Otolaryngol Suppl 550:29-31, 2003.
10. Kwong JS, Adler BD, Padley SP, et al: Diagnosis of diseases of the trachea and main bronchi: Chest radiography vs CT. AJR Am J Roentgenol 161:519-522, 1993.
11. Remy-Jardin M, Remy J, Artaud D, et al: Volume rendering of the tracheobronchial tree: Clinical evaluation of bronchographic images. Radiology 208:761-770, 1998.
12. Capitanio MA, Kirkpatrick JA: Obstructions of the upper airway in children as reflected on the chest radiograph. Radiology 107:159-161, 1973.
13. Evans AS: Clinical syndromes in adults caused by respiratory infection. Med Clin North Am 51:803-818, 1967.
14. Hobson D: Acute respiratory virus infections. BMJ 2:229-231, 1973.
15. Hawley HB, Morin DP, Geraghty ME, et al: Coxsackievirus B epidemic at a boy's summer camp. Isolation of virus from swimming water. JAMA 226:33-36, 1973.
16. Kasian GF, Bingham WT, Steinberg J, et al: Bacterial tracheitis in children. CMAJ 140:46-50, 1989.
17. Connor JD: Evidence for an etiologic role of adenoviral infection in pertussis syndrome. N Engl J Med 283:390-394, 1970.
18. Bass JW, Steele RW, Wiebe RA: Acute epiglottitis. A surgical emergency. JAMA 229:671-675, 1974.
19. Ossoff RH, Wolff AP: Acute epiglottitis in adults. JAMA 244:2639-2640, 1980.
20. Shackelford GD, Siegel MJ, McAlister WH: Subglottic edema in acute epiglottitis in children. AJR Am J Roentgenol 131:603-605, 1978.
21. Valor RR, Polnitsky CA, Tanis DJ, et al: Bacterial tracheitis with upper airway obstruction in a patient with the acquired immunodeficiency syndrome. Am Rev Respir Dis 146:1598-1599, 1992.
22. Frigas E, Nzeako UC: Angioedema. Pathogenesis, differential diagnosis, and treatment. Clin Rev Allergy Immunol 23:217-231, 2002.
23. Gabb GM, Ryan P, Wing LM, et al: Epidemiological study of angioedema and ACE inhibitors. Aust N Z J Med 26:777-782, 1996.
24. Frank MM, Gelfand JA, Atkinson JP: Hereditary angioedema: The clinical syndrome and its management. Ann Intern Med 84:580-593, 1976.
25. van der Valk PG, Moret G, Kiemeney LA: The natural history of chronic urticaria and angioedema in patients visiting a tertiary referral centre. Br J Dermatol 146:110-113, 2002.
26. Cahalane M, Demling RH: Early respiratory abnormalities from smoke inhalation. JAMA 251:771-773, 1984
27. Haponik EF, Munster AM, Wise RA, et al: Upper airway function in burn patients. Correlation of flow-volume curves and nasopharyngoscopy. Am Rev Respir Dis 129:251-257, 1984.
28. Colice GL, Munster AM, Haponik EF: Tracheal stenosis complicating cutaneous burns: An underestimated problem. Am Rev Respir Dis 134:1315-1318, 1986.
29. Eshaghy B, Loeb HS, Miller SE, et al: Mediastinal and retropharyngeal hemorrhage. A complication of cardiac catheterization. JAMA 226:427-431, 1973.
30. Primack SL, Mayo JR, Fradet G: Perforated atherosclerotic ulcer of the aorta presenting with upper airway obstruction. Can Assoc Radiol J 46:209-211, 1995.
31. O'Leary TG, Kotecha B, Rothera MP: Upper airway obstruction secondary to anticoagulant induced haemorrhage necessitating a tracheostomy. Ir Med J 83:151, 1990.
32. Joynt GM, Wickham NW, Young RJ, et al: Upper airway obstruction caused by acquired inhibitor to factor VIII. Anaesthesia 51:689-691, 1996.
33. Handler SD, Beaugard ME, Canalis RF, et al: Unsuspected esophageal foreign bodies in adults with upper airway obstruction. Chest 80:234-237, 1981.
34. Feller-Kopman D: Acute complications of artificial airways. Clin Chest Med 24:445-455, 2003.
35. Messner AH: Treating pediatric patients with obstructive sleep disorders: An update. Otolaryngol Clin North Am 36:519-530, 2003.
36. Djalilian M, Kern EB, Brown HA, et al: Hypoventilation secondary to chronic upper airway obstruction in childhood. Mayo Clin Proc 50:11-14, 1975.
37. Miller MR, Pincock AC, Oates GD, et al: Upper airway obstruction due to goitre: Detection, prevalence and results of surgical management. Q J Med 74:177-188, 1990.
38. Weber AL, Randolph G, Aksoy FG: The thyroid and parathyroid glands. CT and MR imaging and correlation with pathology and clinical findings. Radiol Clin North Am 38:1105-1129, 2000.
39. Nygaard B, Nygaard T, Court-Payen M, et al: Thyroid volume measured by ultrasonography and CT. Acta Radiol 43:269-274, 2002.
40. Som PM, Sacher M, Lanzieri CF, et al: Two benign CT presentations of thyroid-related papillary adenocarcinoma. J Comput Assist Tomogr 9:162-166, 1985.
41. Muysoms F, Boedts M, Claeys D: Intratracheal ectopic thyroid tissue mass. Chest 112:1684-1685, 1997.
42. Rothe TB, Karrer W: Functional upper airway obstruction and chronic irritation of the larynx. Eur Respir J 11:498-500, 1998.
43. Vincken WG, Gauthier SG, Dollfuss RE, et al: Involvement of upper-airway muscles in extrapyramidal disorders. A cause of airflow limitation. N Engl J Med 311:438-442, 1984.
44. Putman MT, Wise RA: Myasthenia gravis and upper airway obstruction. Chest 109:400-404, 1996.
45. Bogaard JM, Pauw KH, Stam H, et al: Interpretation of changes in spirographic and flow-volume variables after operative treatment in bilateral vocal cord paralysis. Bull Eur Physiopathol Respir 21:131-135, 1985.
46. Rodenstein DO, Francis C, Stanescu DC: Emotional laryngeal wheezing: A new syndrome. Am Rev Respir Dis 127:354-356, 1983.
47. Nahmias J, Tansey M, Karetzky MS: Asthmatic extrathoracic upper airway obstruction: Laryngeal dyskinesis. N J Med 91:616-620, 1994.
48. Sue RD, Susanto I: Long-term complications of artificial airways. Clin Chest Med 24:457-471, 2003.
49. Messahel BF: Total tracheal obliteration after intubation with a low-pressure cuffed tracheal tube. Br J Anaesth 73:697-699, 1994.
50. James AE Jr, Macmillan AS Jr, Eaton SB, et al: Roentgenology of tracheal stenosis resulting from cuffed tracheostomy tubes. Am J Roentgenol Radium Ther Nucl Med 109:455-466, 1970.
51. Whyte RI, Quint LE, Kazerooni EA, et al: Helical computed tomography for the evaluation of tracheal stenosis. Ann Thorac Surg 60:27-30, discussion 30-31, 1995.
52. McCarthy MJ, Rosado-de-Christenson ML: Tumors of the trachea. J Thorac Imaging 10:180-198, 1995.
53. Shepard JO, McLoud TC: Imaging the airways. Computed tomography and magnetic resonance imaging. Clin Chest Med 12:151-168, 1991.
54. Lawler LP, Corl FM, Haponik EF, et al: Multidetector row computed tomography and 3-dimensional volume rendering for adult airway imaging. Curr Probl Diagn Radiol 31:115-133, 2002.
55. Greene R, Lechner GL: "Saber-sheath" trachea: A clinical and functional study of marked coronal narrowing of the intrathoracic trachea. Radiology 115:265-268, 1975.
56. Greene R: "Saber-sheath" trachea: Relation to chronic obstructive pulmonary disease. AJR Am J Roentgenol 130:441-445, 1978.
57. Trigaux JP, Hermes G, Dubois P, et al: CT of saber-sheath trachea. Correlation with clinical, chest radiographic and functional findings. Acta Radiol 35:247-250, 1994.
58. Letko E, Zafirakis P, Baltatzis S, et al: Relapsing polychondritis: A clinical review. Semin Arthritis Rheum 31:384-395, 2002.
59. Gibson GJ, Davis P: Respiratory complications of relapsing polychondritis. Thorax 29:726-731, 1974.
60. Tillie-Leblond I, Wallaert B, Leblond D, et al: Respiratory involvement in relapsing polychondritis. Clinical, functional, endoscopic, and radiographic evaluations. Medicine (Baltimore) 77:168-176, 1998.
61. Neilly JB, Winter JH, Stevenson RD: Progressive tracheobronchial polychondritis: Need for early diagnosis. Thorax 40:78-79, 1985.
62. Dolan DL, Lemmon GB Jr, Teitelbaum SL: Relapsing polychondritis. Analytical literature review and studies on pathogenesis. Am J Med 41:285-299, 1966.
63. Prince JS, Duhamel DR, Levin DL, et al: Nonneoplastic lesions of the tracheobronchial wall: Radiologic findings with bronchoscopic correlation. Radiographics 22(Spec No):S215-S230, 2002.
64. Behar JV, Choi YW, Hartman TA, et al: Relapsing polychondritis affecting the lower respiratory tract. AJR Am J Roentgenol 178:173-177, 2002.
65. van Nierop MA, Wagenaar SS, van den Bosch JM, et al: Tracheobronchopathia osteochondroplastica. Report of four cases. Eur J Respir Dis 64:129-133, 1983.
66. Baird RB, Macartney JN: Tracheopathia osteoplastica. Thorax 21:321-324, 1966.
67. Coetmeur D, Bovyn G, Leroux P, et al: Tracheobronchopathia osteochondroplastica presenting at the time of a difficult intubation. Respir Med 91:496-498, 1997.
68. Alroy GG, Lichtig C, Kaftori JK: Tracheobronchopathia osteoplastica: End stage of primary lung amyloidosis? Chest 61:465-468, 1972.

69. Pounder DJ, Pieterse AS: Tracheopathia osteoplastica: Report of four cases. Pathology 14:429-433, 1982.
70. Dernie CJ, Coblentz CL: The trachea: Pathologic conditions and trauma. Can Assoc Radiol J 44:157-167, 1993.
71. Zack JR, Rozenshtein A: Tracheobronchopathia osteochondroplastica: Report of three cases. J Comput Assist Tomogr 26:33-36, 2002.
72. Park SS, Shin DH, Lee DH, et al: Tracheopathia osteoplastica simulating asthmatic symptoms. Diagnosis by bronchoscopy and computerized tomography. Respiration 62:43-45, 1995.
73. Aquino SL, Shepard JA, Ginns LC, et al: Acquired tracheomalacia: Detection by expiratory CT scan. J Comput Assist Tomogr 25:394-399, 2001.
74. Feist JH, Johnson TH, Wilson RJ: Acquired tracheomalacia, etiology and differential diagnosis. Chest 68:340-345, 1975.
75. Wright CD: Tracheomalacia. Chest Surg Clin N Am 13:349-357, viii, 2003.
76. Mounier-Kuhn P: Dilatation de la trachée: Constations radiographiques et bronchoscopiques. (Tracheal dilation: Roentgenographic and bronchographic findings.) Lyon Med 150:106, 1932.
77. Ayres J, Rees J, Cochrane GM: Haemoptysis and non-organic upper airways obstruction in a patient with previously undiagnosed Ehlers-Danlos syndrome. Br J Dis Chest 75:309-310, 1981.
78. Shivaram U, Shivaram I, Cash M: Acquired tracheobronchomegaly resulting in severe respiratory failure. Chest 98:491-492, 1990.
79. el-Mallah Z, Quantock OP: Tracheobronchomegaly. Thorax 23:320-324, 1968.
80. Doyle AJ: Demonstration on computed tomography of tracheomalacia in tracheobronchomegaly (Mounier-Kuhn syndrome). Br J Radiol 62:176-177, 1989.
81. Goh RH, Dobranowski J, Kanaha L, et al: Dynamic computed tomography evaluation of tracheobronchomegaly. Can Assoc Radiol J 46:212-215, 1995.
82. Smith DL, Withers N, Holloway B, et al: Tracheobronchomegaly: An unusual presentation of a rare condition. Thorax 49:840-841, 1994.
83. Stradling JR, Davies RJ: Sleep. 1: Obstructive sleep apnoea/hypopnoea syndrome: Definitions, epidemiology, and natural history. Thorax 59:73-78, 2004.
84. Krieger J: Breathing during sleep in normal subjects. Clin Chest Med 6:577-594, 1985.
85. Gothe B, Altose MD, Goldman MD, et al: Effect of quiet sleep on resting and CO_2-stimulated breathing in humans. J Appl Physiol 50:724-730, 1981.
86. Hudgel DW, Martin RJ, Johnson B, et al: Mechanics of the respiratory system and breathing pattern during sleep in normal humans. J Appl Physiol 56:133-137, 1984.
87. Douglas NJ: Control of ventilation during sleep. Clin Chest Med 6:563-575, 1985.
88. Phillipson EA, Sullivan CE: Arousal: The forgotten response to respiratory stimuli. Am Rev Respir Dis 118:807-809, 1978.
89. Berthon-Jones M, Sullivan CE: Ventilatory and arousal responses to hypoxia in sleeping humans. Am Rev Respir Dis 125:632-639, 1982.
90. Strohl KP, Redline S: Recognition of obstructive sleep apnea. Am J Respir Crit Care Med 154:279-289, 1996.
91. Ohayon MM, Guilleminault C, Priest RG, et al: Snoring and breathing pauses during sleep: Telephone interview survey of a United Kingdom population sample. BMJ 314:860-863, 1997.
92. Jennum P, Sjol A: Epidemiology of snoring and obstructive sleep apnoea in a Danish population, age 30-60. J Sleep Res 1:240-244, 1992.
93. Wiegand L, Zwillich CW: Obstructive sleep apnea. Dis Mon 40:197-252, 1994.
94. Cirignotta F, D'Alessandro R, Partinen M, et al: Prevalence of every night snoring and obstructive sleep apnoeas among 30-69-year-old men in Bologna, Italy. Acta Neurol Scand 79:366-372, 1989.
95. Bearpark H, Elliott L, Grunstein R, et al: Snoring and sleep apnea. A population study in Australian men. Am J Respir Crit Care Med 151:1459-1465, 1995.
96. Young T, Palta M, Dempsey J, et al: The occurrence of sleep-disordered breathing among middle-aged adults. N Engl J Med 328:1230-1235, 1993.
97. Redline S, Tishler PV, Hans MG, et al: Racial differences in sleep-disordered breathing in African-Americans and Caucasians. Am J Respir Crit Care Med 155:186-192, 1997.
98. Standards and indications for cardiopulmonary sleep studies in children. American Thoracic Society. Am J Respir Crit Care Med 153:866-878, 1996.
99. Suratt PM, McTier RF, Findley LJ, et al: Changes in breathing and the pharynx after weight loss in obstructive sleep apnea. Chest 92:631-637, 1987.
100. Grunstein R, Wilcox I, Yang TS, et al: Snoring and sleep apnoea in men: Association with central obesity and hypertension. Int J Obes Relat Metab Disord 17:533-540, 1993.
101. Fletcher E: History, techniques and definitions in sleep-related respiratory disorders. In Fletcher E (ed): Abnormalities of Respiration During Sleep. Orlando, FL, Grune & Stratton, 1986, p 1.
102. Redline S, Kump K, Tishler PV, et al: Gender differences in sleep disordered breathing in a community-based sample. Am J Respir Crit Care Med 149:722-726, 1994.
103. Lefcourt LA, Rodis JF: Obstructive sleep apnea in pregnancy. Obstet Gynecol Surv 51:503-506, 1996.
104. White DP: Sleep-related breathing disorder.2. Pathophysiology of obstructive sleep apnoea. Thorax 50:797-804, 1995.
105. Findley LJ, Wilhoit SC, Suratt PM: Apnea duration and hypoxemia during REM sleep in patients with obstructive sleep apnea. Chest 87:432-436, 1985.
106. Sullivan CE, Issa FG: Obstructive sleep apnea. Clin Chest Med 6:633-650, 1985.
107. Redline S, Tishler PV: The genetics of sleep apnea. Sleep Med Rev 4:583-602, 2000.
108. el Bayadi S, Millman RP, Tishler PV, et al: A family study of sleep apnea. Anatomic and physiologic interactions. Chest 98:554-559, 1990.
109. Nance W, Nakata M, Paul T, et al: Congenital defects. In Janerich D, Skalko R, Porter I (eds): New Directions in Research. New York, Academic Press, 1974, pp 23-49.
110. Guilleminault C, Partinen M, Hollman K, et al: Familial aggregates in obstructive sleep apnea syndrome. Chest 107:1545-1551, 1995.
111. Ferri R, Curzi-Dascalova L, Del Gracco S, et al: Respiratory patterns during sleep in Down's syndrome: Importance of central apnoeas. J Sleep Res 6:134-141, 1997.
112. Stunkard AJ, Harris JR, Pedersen NL, et al: The body-mass index of twins who have been reared apart. N Engl J Med 322:1483-1487, 1990.
113. Bouchard C: Genetic factors in obesity. Med Clin North Am 73:67-81, 1989.
114. Redline S, Leitner J, Arnold J, et al: Ventilatory-control abnormalities in familial sleep apnea. Am J Respir Crit Care Med 156:155-160, 1997.
115. Palmer LJ, Buxbaum SG, Larkin E, et al: A whole-genome scan for obstructive sleep apnea and obesity. Am J Hum Genet 72:340-350, 2003.
116. Matsumoto AM, Sandblom RE, Schoene RB, et al: Testosterone replacement in hypogonadal men: Effects on obstructive sleep apnoea, respiratory drives, and sleep. Clin Endocrinol (Oxf) 22:713-721, 1985.
117. Robinson RW, Zwillich CW: The effect of drugs on breathing during sleep. Clin Chest Med 6:603-614, 1985.
118. Ayappa I, Rapoport DM: The upper airway in sleep: Physiology of the pharynx. Sleep Med Rev 7:9-33, 2003.
119. Kushida CA, Efron B, Guilleminault C: A predictive morphometric model for the obstructive sleep apnea syndrome. Ann Intern Med 127:581-587, 1997.
120. Spier S, Rivlin J, Rowe RD, et al: Sleep in Pierre Robin syndrome. Chest 90:711-715, 1986.
121. Rama AN, Tekwani SH, Kushida CA: Sites of obstruction in obstructive sleep apnea. Chest 122:1139-1147, 2002.
122. Papsidero MJ: The role of nasal obstruction in obstructive sleep apnea syndrome. Ear Nose Throat J 72:82-84, 1993.
123. Masumi S, Nishigawa K, Williams AJ, et al: Effect of jaw position and posture on forced inspiratory airflow in normal subjects and patients with obstructive sleep apnea. Chest 109:1484-1489, 1996.
124. Nelson S, Hans M: Contribution of craniofacial risk factors in increasing apneic activity among obese and nonobese habitual snorers. Chest 111:154-162, 1997.
125. Lee JJ, Ramirez SG, Will MJ: Gender and racial variations in cephalometric analysis. Otolaryngol Head Neck Surg 117:326-329, 1997.
126. Hoffstein V, Mateika S: Differences in abdominal and neck circumferences in patients with and without obstructive sleep apnoea. Eur Respir J 5:377-381, 1992.
127. Davies RJ, Stradling JR: The relationship between neck circumference, radiographic pharyngeal anatomy, and the obstructive sleep apnoea syndrome. Eur Respir J 3:509-514, 1990.
128. Davies RJ, Ali NJ, Stradling JR: Neck circumference and other clinical features in the diagnosis of the obstructive sleep apnoea syndrome. Thorax 47:101-105, 1992.
129. Isono S, Remmers JE, Tanaka A, et al: Static properties of the passive pharynx in sleep apnea. Sleep 19:S175-S177, 1996.
130. Issa FG, Sullivan CE: Upper airway closing pressures in obstructive sleep apnea. J Appl Physiol 57:520-527, 1984.
131. Meurice JC, Marc I, Carrier G, et al: Effects of mouth opening on upper airway collapsibility in normal sleeping subjects. Am J Respir Crit Care Med 153:255-259, 1996.
132. Tsushima Y, Antila J, Svedstrom E, et al: Upper airway size and collapsibility in snorers: Evaluation with digital fluoroscopy. Eur Respir J 9:1611-1618, 1996.
133. Younes M: Contributions of upper airway mechanics and control mechanisms to severity of obstructive apnea. Am J Respir Crit Care Med 168:645-658, 2003.
134. Horner RL: Motor control of the pharyngeal musculature and implications for the pathogenesis of obstructive sleep apnea. Sleep 19:827-853, 1996.
135. Berry DT, Webb WB, Block AJ, et al: Sleep-disordered breathing and its concomitants in a subclinical population. Sleep 9:478-483, 1986.
136. Leiter JC, Knuth SL, Bartlett D Jr: The effect of sleep deprivation on activity of the genioglossus muscle. Am Rev Respir Dis 132:1242-1245, 1985.
137. Faber CE, Grymer L: Available techniques for objective assessment of upper airway narrowing in snoring and sleep apnea. Sleep Breath 7:77-86, 2003.
138. Lowe AA, Fleetham JA, Adachi S, et al: Cephalometric and computed tomographic predictors of obstructive sleep apnea severity. Am J Orthod Dentofacial Orthop 107:589-595, 1995.
139. Pracharktam N, Nelson S, Hans MG, et al: Cephalometric assessment in obstructive sleep apnea. Am J Orthod Dentofacial Orthop 109:410-419, 1996.
140. Frohberg U, Naples RJ, Jones DL: Cephalometric comparison of characteristics in chronically snoring patients with and without sleep apnea syndrome. Oral Surg Oral Med Oral Pathol Oral Radiol Endod 80:28-33, 1995.
141. Schwab RJ, Gefter WB, Hoffman EA, et al: Dynamic upper airway imaging during awake respiration in normal subjects and patients with sleep disordered breathing. Am Rev Respir Dis 148:1385-1400, 1993.
142. Lowe AA, Gionhaku N, Takeuchi K, et al: Three-dimensional CT reconstructions of tongue and airway in adult subjects with obstructive sleep apnea. Am J Orthod Dentofacial Orthop 90:364-374, 1986.
143. Shelton KE, Woodson H, Gay SB, et al: Adipose tissue deposition in sleep apnea. Sleep 16:S103, discussion S103-S105, 1993.
144. Abbott MB, Dardzinski BJ, Donnelly LF: Using volume segmentation of cine MR data to evaluate dynamic motion of the airway in pediatric patients. AJR Am J Roentgenol 181:857-859, 2003.
145. McNamara SG, Grunstein RR, Sullivan CE: Obstructive sleep apnoea. Thorax 48:754-764, 1993.
146. Redline S, Young T: Epidemiology and natural history of obstructive sleep apnea. Ear Nose Throat J 72:20-21, 24-26, 1993.
147. Lugaresi E, Cirignotta F, Coccagna G, et al: Some epidemiological data on snoring and cardiocirculatory disturbances. Sleep 3:221-224, 1980.

148. Hoddes E, Zarcone V, Smythe H, et al: Quantification of sleepiness: A new approach. Psychophysiology 10:431-436, 1973.
149. van Knippenberg FC, Passchier J, Heysteck D, et al: The Rotterdam Daytime Sleepiness Scale: A new daytime sleepiness scale. Psychol Rep 76:83-87, 1995.
150. Johns MW: A new method for measuring daytime sleepiness: The Epworth sleepiness scale. Sleep 14:540-45, 1991.
151. Sleep-related breathing disorders in adults: Recommendations for syndrome definition and measurement techniques in clinical research. The Report of an American Academy of Sleep Medicine Task Force. Sleep 22:667-689, 1999.
152. Hung J, Whitford EG, Parsons RW, et al: Association of sleep apnoea with myocardial infarction in men. Lancet 336:261-264, 1990.
153. Guilleminault C, Connolly SJ, Winkle RA: Cardiac arrhythmia and conduction disturbances during sleep in 400 patients with sleep apnea syndrome. Am J Cardiol 52:490-494, 1983.
154. Shamsuzzaman AS, Gersh BJ, Somers VK: Obstructive sleep apnea: Implications for cardiac and vascular disease. JAMA 290:1906-1914, 2003.
155. Young T, Peppard P, Palta M, et al: Population-based study of sleep-disordered breathing as a risk factor for hypertension. Arch Intern Med 157:1746-1752, 1997.
156. Ziegler MG, Nelesen R, Mills P, et al: Sleep apnea, norepinephrine-release rate, and daytime hypertension. Sleep 20:224-231, 1997.
157. Narkiewicz K, Somers VK: Sympathetic nerve activity in obstructive sleep apnoea. Acta Physiol Scand 177:385-390, 2003.
158. Schafer H, Koehler U, Ploch T, et al: Sleep-related myocardial ischemia and sleep structure in patients with obstructive sleep apnea and coronary heart disease. Chest 111:387-393, 1997.
159. Noda A, Okada T, Yasuma F, et al: Cardiac hypertrophy in obstructive sleep apnea syndrome. Chest 107:1538-1544, 1995.
160. Malone S, Liu PP, Holloway R, et al: Obstructive sleep apnoea in patients with dilated cardiomyopathy: Effects of continuous positive airway pressure. Lancet 338:1480-1484, 1991.
161. Marrone O, Bonsignore MR: Pulmonary haemodynamics in obstructive sleep apnoea. Sleep Med Rev 6:175-193, 2002.
162. Kessler R, Chaouat A, Weitzenblum E, et al: Pulmonary hypertension in the obstructive sleep apnoea syndrome: Prevalence, causes and therapeutic consequences. Eur Respir J 9:787-794, 1996.
163. Chaouat A, Weitzenblum E, Krieger J, et al: Pulmonary hemodynamics in the obstructive sleep apnea syndrome. Results in 220 consecutive patients. Chest 109:380-386, 1996.
164. Bradley TD, Martinez D, Rutherford R, et al: Physiological determinants of nocturnal arterial oxygenation in patients with obstructive sleep apnea. J Appl Physiol 59:1364-1368, 1985.
165. Yaggi H, Mohsenin V: Sleep-disordered breathing and stroke. Clin Chest Med 24:223-237, 2003.
166. Beebe DW, Groesz L, Wells C, et al: The neuropsychological effects of obstructive sleep apnea: A meta-analysis of norm-referenced and case-controlled data. Sleep 26:298-307, 2003.
167. Bassetti C, Aldrich MS, Quint D: Sleep-disordered breathing in patients with acute supra- and infratentorial strokes. A prospective study of 39 patients. Stroke 28:1765-1772, 1997.
168. Ulfberg J, Carter N, Talback M, et al: Headache, snoring and sleep apnoea. J Neurol 243:621-625, 1996.
169. Javaheri S, Colangelo G, Lacey W, et al: Chronic hypercapnia in obstructive sleep apnea—hypopnea syndrome. Sleep 17:416-423, 1994.
170. Chin K, Hirai M, Kuriyama T, et al: Changes in the arterial PCO_2 during a single night's sleep in patients with obstructive sleep apnea. Intern Med 36:454-460, 1997.
171. Cummiskey J, Williams TC, Krumpe PE, et al: The detection and quantification of sleep apnea by tracheal sound recordings. Am Rev Respir Dis 126:221-224, 1982.
172. Flemons WW, Whitelaw WA, Brant R, et al: Likelihood ratios for a sleep apnea clinical prediction rule. Am J Respir Crit Care Med 150:1279-1285, 1994.
173. Ruhle KH, Schlenker E, Randerath W: Upper airway resistance syndrome. Respiration 64(Suppl 1):29-34, 1997.
174. Broughton R, Fleming J, Fleetham J: Home assessment of sleep disorders by portable monitoring. J Clin Neurophysiol 13:272-284, 1996.
175. Sivan Y, Kornecki A, Schonfeld T: Screening obstructive sleep apnoea syndrome by home videotape recording in children. Eur Respir J 9:2127-2131, 1996.
176. Flemons WW, Remmers JE: The diagnosis of sleep apnea: Questionnaires and home studies. Sleep 19:S243-S247, 1996.
177. Gyulay S, Olson LG, Hensley MJ, et al: A comparison of clinical assessment and home oximetry in the diagnosis of obstructive sleep apnea. Am Rev Respir Dis 147:50-53, 1993.
178. Douglas NJ: Home diagnosis of the obstructive sleep apnoea/hypopnoea syndrome. Sleep Med Rev 7:53-59, 2003.
179. Baltzan M, Suissa S: Mortality in sleep apnea patients: A multivariate analysis of risk factors—a response to Lavie and collaborators. Sleep 20:377-380, 1997.
180. He J, Kryger MH, Zorick FJ, et al: Mortality and apnea index in obstructive sleep apnea. Experience in 385 male patients. Chest 94:9-14, 1988.
181. Partinen M, Jamieson A, Guilleminault C: Long-term outcome for obstructive sleep apnea syndrome patients. Mortality. Chest 94:1200-1204, 1988.
182. Ancoli-Israel S, Kripke DF, Klauber MR, et al: Morbidity, mortality and sleep-disordered breathing in community dwelling elderly. Sleep 19:277-282, 1996.
183. Global Initiative for Asthma: Global Strategy for Asthma Management and Prevention. NHLBI/WHO Workshop Report. Bethseda, MD, National Institutes of Health, National Heart, Lung, and Blood Institute, 1995.
184. Scadding JG: Asthma and bronchial reactivity. Br Med J (Clin Res Ed) 294:1115-1116, 1987.
185. Pekkanen J, Pearce N: Defining asthma in epidemiological studies. Eur Respir J 14:951-957, 1999.
186. Mok JY, Simpson H: Pulmonary function in severe chronic asthma in children during apparent clinical remission. Eur J Respir Dis 64:487-493, 1983.
187. Criteria for the assessment of reversibility in airways obstruction. Report of the Committee on Emphysema American, College of Chest Physicians. Chest 65:552-553, 1974.
188. Stirling RG, Chung KF: Severe asthma: Definition and mechanisms. Allergy 56:825-840, 2001.
189. Marsh DG, Meyers DA, Bias WB: The epidemiology and genetics of atopic allergy. N Engl J Med 305:1551-1559, 1981.
190. Hopp RJ, Bewtra AK, Watt GD, et al: Genetic analysis of allergic disease in twins. J Allergy Clin Immunol 73:265-270, 1984.
191. Scadding J: Definition and the clinical categories of asthma. In Clark T, Godfrey S (eds): Asthma, ed 2. London, Chapman & Hall, 1983, pp 1-11.
192. Kroegel C, Jager L, Walker C: Is there a place for intrinsic asthma as a distinct immunopathological entity? Eur Respir J 10:513-515, 1997.
193. Woolcock AJ, Peat JK: Evidence for the increase in asthma worldwide. Ciba Found Symp 206:122-134, discussion 134-139, 157-159, 1997.
194. Ciba Foundation Symposium 206. The Rising Trends in Asthma. Chichester, John Wiley & Sons, 1997.
195. Woolcock AJ, Peat JK, Trevillion LM: Is the increase in asthma prevalence linked to increase in allergen load? Allergy 50:935-940, 1995.
196. Becklake MR, Ernst P: Environmental factors. Lancet 350(Suppl 2):SII10-SII13, 1997.
197. Salome C, Woolcock A: Ethnic differences. In Barnes P, Grunstein M, Leff A, et al (eds): Asthma. Philadelphia, Lippincott-Raven, 1997, p 63.
198. Wichmann HE: Possible explanation for the different trends of asthma and allergy in East and West Germany. Clin Exp Allergy 26:621-623, 1996.
199. Woolcock AJ: Worldwide differences in asthma prevalence and mortality. Why is asthma mortality so low in the USA? Chest 90:40S-45S, 1986.
200. Landau LI: Bronchiolitis and asthma: Are they related? Thorax 49:293-296, 1994.
201. Sears MR, Burrows B, Flannery EM, et al: Atopy in childhood. I. Gender and allergen related risks for development of hay fever and asthma. Clin Exp Allergy 23:941-948, 1993.
202. Cook DG, Strachan DP: Health effects of passive smoking. 3. Parental smoking and prevalence of respiratory symptoms and asthma in school age children. Thorax 52:1081-1094, 1997.
203. Gergen PJ, Turkeltaub PC: The association of individual allergen reactivity with respiratory disease in a national sample: Data from the second National Health and Nutrition Examination Survey, 1976-80 (NHANES II). J Allergy Clin Immunol 90:579-588, 1992.
204. Martinez FD: Definition of pediatric asthma and associated risk factors. Pediatr Pulmonol Suppl 15:9-12, 1997.
205. Zannolli R, Morgese G: Does puberty interfere with asthma? Med Hypotheses 48:27-32, 1997.
206. Skobeloff EM, Spivey WH, St Clair SS, et al: The influence of age and sex on asthma admissions. JAMA 268:3437-3440, 1992.
207. Sandford A, Weir T, Paré P: The genetics of asthma. Am J Respir Crit Care Med 153:1749-1765, 1996.
208. Hanson B, McGue M, Roitman-Johnson B, et al: Atopic disease and immunoglobulin E in twins reared apart and together. Am J Hum Genet 48:873-879, 1991.
209. Dold S, Wjst M, von Mutius E, et al: Genetic risk for asthma, allergic rhinitis, and atopic dermatitis. Arch Dis Child 67:1018-1022, 1992.
210. Longo G, Strinati R, Poli F, et al: Genetic factors in nonspecific bronchial hyperreactivity. An epidemiologic study. Am J Dis Child 141:331-334, 1987.
211. Ericsson CH, Svartengren M, Mossberg B, et al: Bronchial reactivity and allergy-promoting factors in monozygotic twins discordant for allergic rhinitis. Ann Allergy 67:53-59, 1991.
212. Cookson W: A new gene for asthma: Would you ADAM and Eve it? Trends Genet 19:169-172, 2003.
213. Zhang Y, Leaves NI, Anderson GG, et al: Positional cloning of a quantitative trait locus on chromosome 13q14 that influences immunoglobulin E levels and asthma. Nat Genet 34:181-186, 2003.
214. Van Eerdewegh P, Little RD, Dupuis J, et al: Association of the ADAM33 gene with asthma and bronchial hyperresponsiveness. Nature 418:426-430, 2002.
215. Allen M, Heinzmann A, Noguchi E, et al: Positional cloning of a novel gene influencing asthma from chromosome 2q14. Nat Genet 35:258-263, 2003.
216. Weir TD, Mallek N, Sandford AJ, et al: β_2-Adrenergic receptor haplotypes in mild, moderate and fatal/near fatal asthma. Am J Respir Crit Care Med 158:787-791, 1998.
217. Palmer LJ, Silverman ES, Weiss ST, et al: Pharmacogenetics of asthma. Am J Respir Crit Care Med 165:861-866, 2002.
218. Dunnill MS: The pathology of asthma, with special reference to changes in the bronchial mucosa. J Clin Pathol 13:27-33, 1960.
219. Jeffery PK: Remodeling in asthma and chronic obstructive lung disease. Am J Respir Crit Care Med 164:S28-S38, 2001.
220. Nakano Y, Müller NL, King GG, et al: Quantitative assessment of airway remodeling using high-resolution CT. Chest 122:271S-275S, 2002.
221. Montefort S, Roberts JA, Beasley R, et al: The site of disruption of the bronchial epithelium in asthmatic and non-asthmatic subjects. Thorax 47:499-503, 1992.
222. Roche WR, Beasley R, Williams JH, et al: Subepithelial fibrosis in the bronchi of asthmatics. Lancet 1:520-524, 1989.
223. Wilson J: The bronchial microcirculation in asthma. Clin Exp Allergy 30(Suppl 1):51-53, 2000.

224. Wilson JW, Li X, Pain MC: The lack of distensibility of asthmatic airways. Am Rev Respir Dis 148:806-809, 1993.
225. Carroll N, Elliot J, Morton A, et al: The structure of large and small airways in non-fatal and fatal asthma. Am Rev Respir Dis 147:405-410, 1993.
226. Ebina M, Takahashi T, Chiba T, et al: Cellular hypertrophy and hyperplasia of airway smooth muscles underlying bronchial asthma. A 3-D morphometric study. Am Rev Respir Dis 148:720-726, 1993.
227. Saetta M, Di Stefano A, Rosina C, et al: Quantitative structural analysis of peripheral airways and arteries in sudden fatal asthma. Am Rev Respir Dis 143:138-143, 1991.
228. Jeffery PK, Godfrey RW, Adelroth E, et al: Effects of treatment on airway inflammation and thickening of basement membrane reticular collagen in asthma. A quantitative light and electron microscopic study. Am Rev Respir Dis 145:890-899, 1992.
229. Neurath MF, Finotto S, Glimcher LH: The role of Th1/Th2 polarization in mucosal immunity. Nat Med 8:567-573, 2002.
230. Stumbles PA, Upham JW, Holt PG: Airway dendritic cells: Co-ordinators of immunological homeostasis and immunity in the respiratory tract. APMIS 111:741-755, 2003.
231. Ayars GH, Altman LC, Gleich GJ, et al: Eosinophil- and eosinophil granule-mediated pneumocyte injury. J Allergy Clin Immunol 76:595-604, 1985.
232. Gossett P, Jeannin P, Lassalle P, et al: The role of the endothelial cells in asthma. Asthma 1:507, 1997.
233. Sine J, Tremblay G, Xing Z, et al: Interstitial and bronchial fibroblasts. Asthma 1:475, 1997.
234. Woodstock A: Definitions and clinical classification. In Barnes P, Grunstein M, Leff A, et al (eds): Asthma. Philadelphia, Lippincott-Raven, 1997, p 27.
235. Boushey HA, Holtzman MJ, Sheller JR, et al: Bronchial hyperreactivity. Am Rev Respir Dis 121:389-413, 1980.
236. Orehek J: Asthma without airway hyperreactivity: Fact or artifact? Eur J Respir Dis 63:1-4, 1982.
237. Fish JE, Ankin MG, Kelly JF, et al: Regulation of bronchomotor tone by lung inflation in asthmatic and nonasthmatic subjects. J Appl Physiol 50:1079-1086, 1981.
238. Moreno RH, Hogg JC, Paré PD: Mechanics of airway narrowing. Am Rev Respir Dis 133:1171-1180, 1986.
239. Ruffin RE, Dolovich MB, Wolff RK, et al: The effects of preferential deposition of histamine in the human airway. Am Rev Respir Dis 117:485-492, 1978.
240. Hogg JC: Bronchial mucosal permeability and its relationship to airways hyperreactivity. J Allergy Clin Immunol 67:421-425, 1981.
241. Widdicombe JG: Overview of neural pathways in allergy and asthma. Pulm Pharmacol Ther 16:23-30, 2003.
242. Shore SA, Drazen JM: Beta-agonists and asthma: Too much of a good thing? J Clin Invest 112:495-497, 2003.
243. Joos GF, Germonpre PR, Pauwels RA: Neural mechanisms in asthma. Clin Exp Allergy 30(Suppl):60-65, 2000.
244. Lambert RK, Wiggs BR, Kuwano K, et al: Functional significance of increased airway smooth muscle in asthma and COPD. J Appl Physiol 74:2771-2781, 1993.
245. Schellenberg RR, Paré PD, Hards J, et al: Smooth muscle mechanics: Implications for airway hyperresponsiveness. Int Arch Allergy Appl Immunol 94:291-292, 1991.
246. Macklem PT: A theoretical analysis of the effect of airway smooth muscle load on airway narrowing. Am J Respir Crit Care Med 153:83-89, 1996.
247. Giffon E, Orehek J, Vervloet D, et al: Asthma without airway hyperresponsiveness to carbachol. Eur J Respir Dis 70:229-233, 1987.
248. Hargreave F, Ramsdale H, Dolovich J: Measurement of airway responsiveness in clinical practice. In Hargreave F, Woolcock A (eds): Airway Responsiveness: Measurement and Interpretation. Mississauga, Ontario, Canada, 1985, p 122.
249. Morice AH, Kastelik JA: Cough. 1: Chronic cough in adults. Thorax 58:901-907, 2003.
250. Woolcock A: Test of airway responsiveness in epidemiology. In Hargeave F, Woolcock A (eds): Airway responsiveness: Measurement and Interpretation. Mississauga, Ontario, Canada, 1985, p 136.
251. Sont JK, Willems LN, Bel EH, et al: Clinical control and histopathologic outcome of asthma when using airway hyperresponsiveness as an additional guide to long-term treatment. The AMPUL Study Group. Am J Respir Crit Care Med 159:1043-1051, 1999.
252. Olafsson M, Simonsson BG, Hansson SB: Bronchial reactivity in patients with recent pulmonary sarcoidosis. Thorax 40:51-53, 1985.
253. Monkare S: Clinical aspects of farmer's lung: Airway reactivity, treatment and prognosis. Eur J Respir Dis Suppl 137:1-68, 1984.
254. Bahous J, Cartier A, Ouimet G, et al: Nonallergic bronchial hyperexcitability in chronic bronchitis. Am Rev Respir Dis 129:216-220, 1984.
255. Mortagy AK, Howell JB, Waters WE: Respiratory symptoms and bronchial reactivity: Identification of a syndrome and its relation to asthma. Br Med J (Clin Res Ed) 293:525-529, 1986.
256. Del Donno M, Bittesnich D, Chetta A, et al: The effect of inflammation on mucociliary clearance in asthma: An overview. Chest 118:1142-1149, 2000.
257. Wanner A, Salathe M, O'Riordan TG: Mucociliary clearance in the airways. Am J Respir Crit Care Med 154:1868-1902, 1996.
258. Shelhamer JH, Kaliner MA: Respiratory mucus production in asthma. Bull Eur Physiopathol Respir 21:301-307, 1985.
259. Pavia D, Bateman JR, Sheahan NF, et al: Tracheobronchial mucociliary clearance in asthma: Impairment during remission. Thorax 40:171-175, 1985.
260. O'Riordan TG, Zwang J, Smaldone GC: Mucociliary clearance in adult asthma. Am Rev Respir Dis 146:598-603, 1992.
261. Messina MS, O'Riordan TG, Smaldone GC: Changes in mucociliary clearance during acute exacerbations of asthma. Am Rev Respir Dis 143:993-997, 1991.
262. Maurer DR, Sielczak M, Oliver W Jr., et al: Role of ciliary motility in acute allergic mucociliary dysfunction. J Appl Physiol 52:1018-1023, 1982.
263. Dulfano MJ, Luk CK: Sputum and ciliary inhibition in asthma. Thorax 37:646-651, 1982.
264. Agnew JE, Bateman JR, Sheahan NF, et al: Effect of oral corticosteroids on mucus clearance by cough and mucociliary transport in stable asthma. Bull Eur Physiopathol Respir 19:37-41, 1983.
265. Dolovich J, Hargreave F: The asthma syndrome: Inciters, inducers, and host characteristics. Thorax 36:641-643, 1981.
266. Martinez FD: The coming-of-age of the hygiene hypothesis. Respir Res 2:129-132, 2001.
267. Barbee RA, Lebowitz MD, Thompson HC, et al: Immediate skin-test reactivity in a general population sample. Ann Intern Med 84:129-133, 1976.
268. Rosenberg GL, Rosenthal RR, Norman PS: Inhalation challenge with ragweed pollen in ragweed-sensitive asthmatics. J Allergy Clin Immunol 71:302-310, 1983.
269. Salvaggio J, Aukrust L: Postgraduate course presentations. Mold-induced asthma. J Allergy Clin Immunol 68:327-346, 1981.
270. Platt-Mills TA, Sporik RB, Chapman MD, et al: The role of indoor allergens in asthma. Allergy 50:5-12, 1995.
271. Blythe ME, Al Ubaydi F, Williams JD, et al: Study of dust mites in three Birmingham hospitals. BMJ 1:62-64, 1975.
272. Squillace SP, Sporik RB, Rakes G, et al: Sensitization to dust mites as a dominant risk factor for asthma among adolescents living in central Virginia. Multiple regression analysis of a population-based study. Am J Respir Crit Care Med 156:1760-1764, 1997.
273. Rosenstreich DL, Eggleston P, Kattan M, et al: The role of cockroach allergy and exposure to cockroach allergen in causing morbidity among inner-city children with asthma. N Engl J Med 336:1356-1363, 1997.
274. Wooding LG, Teuber SS, Gershwin ME: Latex allergy. Compr Ther 22:384-392, 1996.
275. Warner JO: Food intolerance and asthma. Clin Exp Allergy 25(Suppl 1):29-30, 1995.
276. Bock SA, Sampson HA: Food allergy in infancy. Pediatr Clin North Am 41:1047-1067, 1994.
277. Wanner A, Russi E, Brodnan JM, et al: Prolonged bronchial obstruction after a single antigen challenge in ragweed asthma. J Allergy Clin Immunol 76:177-181, 1985.
278. Cockcroft DW, Ruffin RE, Frith PA, et al: Determinants of allergen-induced asthma: Dose of allergen, circulating IgE antibody concentration, and bronchial responsiveness to inhaled histamine. Am Rev Respir Dis 120:1053-1058, 1979.
279. Valenti S, Crimi E, Brusasco V: Bronchial provocation tests with RAST-standardized allergens and dosimetric technique. Respiration 48:97-102, 1985.
280. Cockcroft DW, Hoeppner VH, Werner GD: Recurrent nocturnal asthma after bronchoprovocation with western red cedar sawdust: Association with acute increase in non-allergic bronchial responsiveness. Clin Allergy 14:61-68, 1984.
281. Kalinen M: Hypotheses on the contribution of late-phase allergic responses to the understanding and treatment of allergic diseases. J Allergy Clin Immunol 73:311-315, 1984.
282. O'Byrne PM, Israel E, Drazen JM: Antileukotrienes in the treatment of asthma. Ann Intern Med 127:472-480, 1997.
283. Hogg JC: The pathology of asthma. Clin Chest Med 5:567-571, 1984.
284. McFadden ER Jr: Exercise-induced airway obstruction. Clin Chest Med 16:671-682, 1995.
285. Custovic A, Arifhodzic N, Robinson A, et al: Exercise testing revisited. The response to exercise in normal and atopic children. Chest 105:1127-1132, 1994.
286. Strauss RH, McFadden ER Jr, Ingram RH Jr, et al: Enhancement of exercise-induced asthma by cold air. N Engl J Med 297:743-747, 1977.
287. Deal EC Jr, McFadden ER Jr, Ingram RH Jr, et al: Role of respiratory heat exchange in production of exercise-induced asthma. J Appl Physiol 46:467-475, 1979.
288. Deal EC Jr, McFadden ER Jr, Ingram RH Jr, et al: Hyperpnea and heat flux: Initial reaction sequence in exercise-induced asthma. J Appl Physiol 46:476-483, 1979.
289. Nowak D, Kuziek G, Jorres R, et al: Comparison of refractoriness after exercise- and hyperventilation-induced asthma. Lung 169:57-67, 1991.
290. Neijens HJ, Wesselius T, Kerrebijn KF: Exercise-induced bronchoconstriction as an expression of bronchial hyperreactivity: A study of its mechanisms in children. Thorax 36:517-522, 1981.
291. Anderson SD, Daviskas E: The mechanism of exercise-induced asthma is. J Allergy Clin Immunol 106:453-459, 2000.
292. Argyros GJ, Phillips YY, Rayburn DB, et al: Water loss without heat flux in exercise-induced bronchospasm. Am Rev Respir Dis 147:1419-1424, 1993.
293. Anderson SD, Brannan JD: Methods for "indirect" challenge tests including exercise, eucapnic voluntary hyperpnea, and hypertonic aerosols. Clin Rev Allergy Immunol 24:27-54, 2003.
294. Deal EC Jr, McFadden ER Jr, Ingram RH Jr, et al: Esophageal temperature during exercise in asthmatic and nonasthmatic subjects. J Appl Physiol 46:484-490, 1979.
295. Griffin MP, McFadden ER Jr, Ingram RH Jr: Airway cooling in asthmatic and nonasthmatic subjects during nasal and oral breathing. J Allergy Clin Immunol 69:354-359, 1982.
296. Lee TH, Nagakura T, Cromwell O, et al: Neutrophil chemotactic activity and histamine in atopic and nonatopic subjects after exercise-induced asthma. Am Rev Respir Dis 129:409-412, 1984.
297. O'Byrne PM, Thomson NC, Morris M, et al: The protective effect of inhaled chlorpheniramine and atropine on bronchoconstriction stimulated by airway cooling. Am Rev Respir Dis 128:611-617, 1983.

298. Black JL, Armour CL, Shaw J: The effect of alteration in temperature on contractile responses in human airways in vitro. Respir Physiol 57:269-277, 1984.
299. McFadden ER Jr, Lenner KA, Strohl KP: Postexertional airway rewarming and thermally induced asthma. New insights into pathophysiology and possible pathogenesis. J Clin Invest 78:18-25, 1986.
300. Lee TH, Anderson SD: Heterogeneity of mechanisms in exercise induced asthma. Thorax 40:481-487, 1985.
301. Edmunds AT, Tooley M, Godfrey S: The refractory period after exercise-induced asthma: Its duration and relation to the severity of exercise. Am Rev Respir Dis 117:247-254, 1978.
302. Wasserman SI: Mast cells and airway inflammation in asthma. Am J Respir Crit Care Med 150:S39-41, 1994.
303. Laitinen LA, Elkin RB, Empey DW, et al: Bronchial hyperresponsiveness in normal subjects during attenuated influenza virus infection. Am Rev Respir Dis 143:358-361, 1991.
304. Sterk PJ: Virus-induced airway hyperresponsiveness in man. Eur Respir J 6:894-902, 1993.
305. Bardin PG, Fraenkel DJ, Sanderson G, et al: Amplified rhinovirus colds in atopic subjects. Clin Exp Allergy 24:457-464, 1994.
306. Minor TE, Dick EC, DeMeo AN, et al: Viruses as precipitants of asthmatic attacks in children. JAMA 227:292-298, 1974.
307. Clarke CW: Relationship of bacterial and viral infections to exacerbations of asthma. Thorax 34:344-347, 1979.
308. Corne JM, Holgate ST: Mechanisms of virus induced exacerbations of asthma. Thorax 52:380-389, 1997.
309. Korppi M, Reijonen T, Poysa L, et al: A 2- to 3-year outcome after bronchiolitis. Am J Dis Child 147:628-631, 1993.
310. Priftis K, Everard M, Milner AD: Outcome of severe acute bronchiolitis needing mechanical ventilation. Lancet 335:607, 1990.
311. Welliver RC: RSV and chronic asthma. Lancet 346:789-790, 1995.
312. Vitalis TZ, Keicho N, Itabashi S, et al: A model of latent adenovirus 5 infection in the guinea pig (Cavia porcellus). Am J Respir Cell Mol Biol 14:225-231, 1996.
313. Strachan DP: Hay fever, hygiene, and household size. BMJ 299:1259-1260, 1989.
314. Namazy JA, Simon RA: Sensitivity to nonsteroidal anti-inflammatory drugs. Ann Allergy Asthma Immunol 89:542-550, quiz 550, 605, 2002.
315. Slepian IK, Mathews KP, McLean JA: Aspirin-sensitive asthma. Chest 87:386-391, 1985.
316. Ogino S, Harada T, Okawachi I, et al: Aspirin-induced asthma and nasal polyps. Acta Otolaryngol Suppl 430:21-27, 1986.
317. Settipane GA, Chafee FH, Klein DE: Aspirin intolerance. II. A prospective study in an atopic and normal population. J Allergy Clin Immunol 53:200-204, 1974.
318. Grzelewska-Rzymowska I, Bogucki A, Szmidt M, et al: Migraine in aspirin-sensitive asthmatics. Allergol Immunopathol (Madr) 13:13-16, 1985.
319. Bianco S, Robuschi M, Petrigni G, et al: Efficacy and tolerability of nimesulide in asthmatic patients intolerant to aspirin. Drugs 46(Suppl 1):115-120, 1993.
320. Szczeklik A, Gryglewski RJ, Czerniawska-Mysik G: Relationship of inhibition of prostaglandin biosynthesis by analgesics to asthma attacks in aspirin-sensitive patients. BMJ 1:67-69, 1975.
321. Craig T, Richerson HB, Moeckli J: Problem drugs for the patient with asthma. Compr Ther 22:339-344, 1996.
322. Zembowicz A, Mastalerz L, Setkowicz M, et al: Safety of cyclooxygenase 2 inhibitors and increased leukotriene synthesis in chronic idiopathic urticaria with sensitivity to nonsteroidal anti-inflammatory drugs. Arch Dermatol 139:1577-1582, 2003.
323. Parker C: Aspirin-sensitive asthma. In Lichtenstein L, Austen K (eds): Asthma: Physiology, Immunopharmacology and Treatment. New York, Academic Press, 1977, p 301.
324. Szczeklik A, Nizankowska E, Sanak M, et al: Aspirin-induced rhinitis and asthma. Curr Opin Allergy Clin Immunol 1:27-33, 2001.
325. Ayres JG, Miles JF: Oesophageal reflux and asthma. Eur Respir J 9:1073-1078, 1996.
326. Boyle JT, Tuchman DN, Altschuler SM, et al: Mechanisms for the association of gastroesophageal reflux and bronchospasm. Am Rev Respir Dis 131:S16-S20, 1985.
327. Schan CA, Harding SM, Haile JM, et al: Gastroesophageal reflux–induced bronchoconstriction. An intraesophageal acid infusion study using state-of-the-art technology. Chest 106:731-737, 1994.
328. Cibella F, Cuttitta G: Nocturnal asthma and gastroesophageal reflux. Am J Med 111(Suppl 8A):31S-36S, 2001.
329. Gibson PG, Henry RL, Coughlan JL: Gastro-oesophageal reflux treatment for asthma in adults and children. Cochrane Database Syst Rev CD001496, 2003.
330. Kiljander TO: The role of proton pump inhibitors in the management of gastroesophageal reflux disease–related asthma and chronic cough. Am J Med 115(Suppl 3A):65S-71S, 2003.
331. Simpson WG: Gastroesophageal reflux disease and asthma. Diagnosis and management. Arch Intern Med 155:798-803, 1995.
332. Sandberg S, Paton JY, Ahola S, et al: The role of acute and chronic stress in asthma attacks in children. Lancet 356:982-987, 2000.
333. Horton DJ, Suda WL, Kinsman RA, et al: Bronchoconstrictive suggestion in asthma: A role for airways hyperreactivity and emotions. Am Rev Respir Dis 117:1029-1038, 1978.
334. Demeter SL, Cordasco EM: Hyperventilation syndrome and asthma. Am J Med 81:989-994, 1986.
335. Busse WW, Kiecolt-Glaser JK, Coe C, et al: NHLBI Workshop summary. Stress and asthma. Am J Respir Crit Care Med 151:249-252, 1995.
336. Etzel RA: How environmental exposures influence the development and exacerbation of asthma. Pediatrics 112:233-239, 2003.
337. Bates DV: The effects of air pollution on children. Environ Health Perspect 103(Suppl 6):49-53, 1995.
338. Bates DV, Baker-Anderson M, Sizto R: Asthma attack periodicity: A study of hospital emergency visits in Vancouver. Environ Res 51:51-70, 1990.
339. Folinsbee LJ, Bedi JF, Horvath SM: Pulmonary response to threshold levels of sulfur dioxide (1.0 ppm) and ozone (0.3 ppm). J Appl Physiol 58:1783-1787, 1985.
340. Roger LJ, Kehrl HR, Hazucha M, et al: Bronchoconstriction in asthmatics exposed to sulfur dioxide during repeated exercise. J Appl Physiol 59:784-791, 1985.
341. Linn WS, Venet TG, Shamoo DA, et al: Respiratory effects of sulfur dioxide in heavily exercising asthmatics. A dose-response study. Am Rev Respir Dis 127:278-283, 1983.
342. Kulle TJ, Sauder LR, Hebel JR, et al: Ozone response relationships in healthy nonsmokers. Am Rev Respir Dis 132:36-41, 1985.
343. Holtzman MJ, Cunningham JH, Sheller JR, et al: Effect of ozone on bronchial reactivity in atopic and nonatopic subjects. Am Rev Respir Dis 120:1059-1067, 1979.
344. McBride DE, Koenig JQ, Luchtel DL, et al: Inflammatory effects of ozone in the upper airways of subjects with asthma. Am J Respir Crit Care Med 149:1192-1197, 1994.
345. Forastiere F, Corbo GM, Pistelli R, et al: Bronchial responsiveness in children living in areas with different air pollution levels. Arch Environ Health 49:111-118, 1994.
346. Ussetti P, Roca J, Agusti AG, et al: Another asthma outbreak in Barcelona: Role of oxides of nitrogen. Lancet 1:156, 1984.
347. Bauer MA, Utell MJ, Morrow PE, et al: Inhalation of 0.30 ppm nitrogen dioxide potentiates exercise-induced bronchospasm in asthmatics. Am Rev Respir Dis 134:1203-1208, 1986.
348. Bylin G, Lindvall T, Rehn T, et al: Effects of short-term exposure to ambient nitrogen dioxide concentrations on human bronchial reactivity and lung function. Eur J Respir Dis 66:205-217, 1985.
349. Newman-Taylor A: Environmental determinants of asthma. Lancet 345:296-299, 1995.
350. Casillas AM, Nel AE: An update on the immunopathogenesis of asthma as an inflammatory disease enhanced by environmental pollutants. Allergy Asthma Proc 18:227-233, 1997.
351. Ostro BD, Lipsett MJ, Mann JK, et al: Indoor air pollution and asthma. Results from a panel study. Am J Respir Crit Care Med 149:1400-1406, 1994.
352. Parham WM, Shepard RH, Norman PS, et al: Analysis of time course and magnitude of lung inflation effects on airway tone: Relation to airway reactivity. Am Rev Respir Dis 128:240-245, 1983.
353. Ingram RH Jr: Relationships among airway-parenchymal interactions, lung responsiveness, and inflammation in asthma. Giles F. Filley Lecture. Chest 107:148S-152S, 1995.
354. Beaupre A, Badier M, Delpierre S, et al: Airway response of asthmatics to carbachol and to deep inspiration. Eur J Respir Dis 64:108-112, 1983.
355. Lim TK, Ang SM, Rossing TH, et al: The effects of deep inhalation on maximal expiratory flow during intensive treatment of spontaneous asthmatic episodes. Am Rev Respir Dis 140:340-343, 1989.
356. Mitchell RW, Rabe KF, Magnussen H, et al: Passive sensitization of human airways induces myogenic contractile responses in vitro. J Appl Physiol 83:1276-1281, 1997.
357. Wang L, Paré PD: Deep inspiration and airway smooth muscle adaptation to length change. Respir Physiol Neurobiol 137:169-178, 2003.
358. Burns CB, Taylor WR, Ingram RH Jr: Effects of deep inhalation in asthma: Relative airway and parenchymal hysteresis. J Appl Physiol 59:1590-1596, 1985.
359. Malmberg P, Larsson K, Sundblad BM, et al: Importance of the time interval between FEV₁ measurements in a methacholine provocation test. Eur Respir J 6:680-686, 1993.
360. Kapsali T, Permutt S, Laube B, et al: Potent bronchoprotective effect of deep inspiration and its absence in asthma. J Appl Physiol 89:711-720, 2000.
361. Ayres JG, Clark TJ: Alcoholic drinks and asthma: A survey. Br J Dis Chest 77:370-375, 1983.
362. Shimoda T, Kohno S, Takao A, et al: Investigation of the mechanism of alcohol-induced bronchial asthma. J Allergy Clin Immunol 97:74-84, 1996.
363. Gong H Jr, Tashkin DP, Calvarese BM: Alcohol-induced bronchospasm in an asthmatic patient: Pharmacologic evaluation of the mechanism. Chest 80:167-173, 1981.
364. Bush RK, Taylor SL, Holden K, et al: Prevalence of sensitivity to sulfiting agents in asthmatic patients. Am J Med 81:816-820, 1986.
365. Genton C, Frei PC, Pecoud A: Value of oral provocation tests to aspirin and food additives in the routine investigation of asthma and chronic urticaria. J Allergy Clin Immunol 76:40-45, 1985.
366. Kaufman J, Schmitt S, Barnard J, et al: Angiotensin-converting enzyme inhibitors in patients with bronchial responsiveness and asthma. Chest 101:922-925, 1992.
367. Millqvist E, Lowhagen O: Placebo-controlled challenges with perfume in patients with asthma-like symptoms. Allergy 51:434-439, 1996.
368. Dahms TE, Bolin JF, Slavin RG: Passive smoking. Effects on bronchial asthma. Chest 80:530-534, 1981.
369. Eliasson O, Scherzer HH, DeGraff AC Jr: Morbidity in asthma in relation to the menstrual cycle. J Allergy Clin Immunol 77:87-94, 1986.
370. Chan-Yeung M, Lam S: Occupational asthma. Am Rev Respir Dis 133:686-703, 1986.
371. Venables KM, Chan-Yeung M: Occupational asthma. Lancet 349:1465-1469, 1997.
372. McSharry C, Anderson K, McKay IC, et al: The IgE and IgG antibody responses to aerosols of Nephrops norvegicus (prawn) antigens: The association with clinical hypersensitivity and with cigarette smoking. Clin Exp Immunol 97:499-504, 1994.
373. Agrup G, Belin L, Sjostedt L, et al: Allergy to laboratory animals in laboratory technicians and animal keepers. Br J Ind Med 43:192-198, 1986.

374. Malo JL, Cartier A: Occupational reactions in the seafood industry. Clin Rev Allergy 11:223-240, 1993.
375. Thiel H, Ulmer WT: Bakers' asthma: Development and possibility for treatment. Chest 78:400-405, 1980.
376. Fish JE: Occupational asthma and rhinoconjunctivitis induced by natural rubber latex exposure. J Allergy Clin Immunol 110:S75-S81, 2002.
377. Chan-Yeung M: Occupational asthma. Chest 98:148S-161S, 1990.
378. Chan-Yeung M, Vedal S, Kus J, et al: Symptoms, pulmonary function, and bronchial hyperreactivity in western red cedar workers compared with those in office workers. Am Rev Respir Dis 130:1038-1041, 1984.
379. Vedal S, Chan-Yeung M, Enarson D, et al: Symptoms and pulmonary function in western red cedar workers related to duration of employment and dust exposure. Arch Environ Health 41:179-183, 1986.
380. Chan-Yeung M, MacLean L, Paggiaro PL: Follow-up study of 232 patients with occupational asthma caused by western red cedar (Thuja plicata). J Allergy Clin Immunol 79:792-796, 1987.
381. Bernstein JA: Overview of diisocyanate occupational asthma. Toxicology 111:181-189, 1996.
382. Moller DR, McKay RT, Bernstein IL, et al: Persistent airways disease caused by toluene diisocyanate. Am Rev Respir Dis 134:175-186, 1986.
383. Vandenplas O, Malo JL, Saetta M, et al: Occupational asthma and extrinsic alveolitis due to isocyanates: Current status and perspectives, Br J Ind Med 50:213-228, 1993.
384. Lemiere C, Malo JL, Gautrin D: Nonsensitizing causes of occupational asthma. Med Clin North Am 80:749-774, 1996.
385. Chan-Yeung M, Malo JL: Occupational asthma. N Engl J Med 333:107-112, 1995.
386. Burge PS, O'Brien IM, Harries MG: Peak flow rate records in the diagnosis of occupational asthma due to isocyanates. Thorax 34:317-323, 1979.
387. Burge PS, O'Brien IM, Harries MG: Peak flow rate records in the diagnosis of occupational asthma due to colophony. Thorax 34:308-316, 1979.
388. Vandenplas O, Delwiche JP, Jamart J, et al: Increase in non-specific bronchial hyperresponsiveness as an early marker of bronchial response to occupational agents during specific inhalation challenges. Thorax 51:472-478, 1996.
389. Chan-Yeung M, Lam S, Tse K: Measurement of airway responsiveness in occupational asthma. In Hargreave F, Woolcock A (eds): Airway Responsiveness: Measurement and Interpretation. Mississauga, Ontario, Canada, 1985, p 129.
390. Lam S, Tan F, Chan H, et al: Relationship between types of asthmatic reaction, non-specific bronchial reactivity, and specific IgE antibodies in patients with red cedar asthma. J Allergy Clin Immunol 72:134-139, 1983.
391. Tarlo SM: Workplace irritant exposures: Do they produce true occupational asthma? Ann Allergy Asthma Immunol 90:19-23, 2003.
392. Choudat D, Goehen M, Korobaeff M, et al: Respiratory symptoms and bronchial reactivity among pig and dairy farmers. Scand J Work Environ Health 20:48-54, 1994.
393. Seifert SA, Von Essen S, Jacobitz K, et al: Organic dust toxic syndrome: A review. J Toxicol Clin Toxicol 41:185-193, 2003.
394. Lynch DA: Imaging of asthma and allergic bronchopulmonary mycosis. Radiol Clin North Am 36:129-142, 1998.
395. Paganin F, Trussard V, Seneterre E, et al: Chest radiography and high resolution computed tomography of the lungs in asthma. Am Rev Respir Dis 146:1084-1087, 1992.
396. Blackie SP, al-Majed S, Staples CA, et al: Changes in total lung capacity during acute spontaneous asthma. Am Rev Respir Dis 142:79-83, 1990.
397. Genereux G: Radiology and pulmonary immunopathologic lung disease. In Steiner R (ed): Recent Advances in Radiology and Medical Imaging. New York, Churchill Livingstone, 1983, pp 213-240.
398. Zieverink SE, Harper AP, Holden RW, et al: Emergency room radiography of asthma: An efficacy study. Radiology 145:27-29, 1982.
399. Rossi OV, Lahde S, Laitinen J, et al: Contribution of chest and paranasal sinus radiographs to the management of acute asthma. Int Arch Allergy Immunol 105:96-100, 1994.
400. Grenier PA, Beigelman-Aubry C, Fetita C, et al: New frontiers in CT imaging of airway disease. Eur Radiol 12:1022-1044, 2002.
401. Niimi A, Matsumoto H, Amitani R, et al: Airway wall thickness in asthma assessed by computed tomography. Relation to clinical indices. Am J Respir Crit Care Med 162:1518-1523, 2000
402. Awadh N, Müller NL, Park CS, et al: Airway wall thickness in patients with near fatal asthma and control groups: Assessment with high resolution computed tomographic scanning. Thorax 53:248-253, 1998.
403. King GG, Eberl S, Salome CM, et al: Differences in airway closure between normal and asthmatic subjects measured with single-photon emission computed tomography and technegas. Am J Respir Crit Care Med 158:1900-1906, 1998.
404. Simonsson BG: Chronic cough and expectoration in patients with asthma and in patients with α_1-antitrypsin deficiency. Eur J Respir Dis Suppl 118:123-128, 1982.
405. Wade JP, Liang MH, Sheffer AL: Exercise-induced anaphylaxis: Epidemiologic observations. Prog Clin Biol Res 297:175-182, 1989.
406. Lee HY, Stretton TB: Asthma in the elderly. BMJ 4:93-95, 1972.
407. Jack CI, Lye M: Asthma in the elderly patient. Gerontology 42:61-68, 1996.
408. McFadden ER Jr: Exertional dyspnea and cough as preludes to acute attacks of bronchial asthma. N Engl J Med 292:555-559, 1975.
409. Turner-Warwick M: On observing patterns of airflow obstruction in chronic asthma. Br J Dis Chest 71:73-86, 1977.
410. Oosterhoff Y, Koeter GH, De Monchy JG, et al: Circadian variation in airway responsiveness to methacholine, propranolol, and AMP in atopic asthmatic subjects. Am Rev Respir Dis 147:512-517, 1993.
411. Catterall JR, Rhind GB, Stewart IC, et al: Effect of sleep deprivation on overnight bronchoconstriction in nocturnal asthma. Thorax 41:676-680, 1986.
412. Puolijoki H, Lahdensuo A: Chronic cough as a risk indicator of bronchopulmonary disease. Eur J Respir Dis 71:77-85, 1987.
413. Cohen RM, Grant W, Lieberman P, et al: The use of methacholine inhalation, methacholine skin testing, distilled water inhalation challenge and eosinophil counts in the evaluation of patients presenting with cough and/or nonwheezing dyspnea. Ann Allergy 56:308-312, 1986.
414. Arnold AG, Lane DJ, Zapata E: The speed of onset and severity of acute severe asthma. Br J Dis Chest 76:157-163, 1982.
415. Stellman JL, Spicer JE, Cayton RM: Morbidity from chronic asthma. Thorax 37:218-221, 1982.
416. McFadden ER Jr, Kiser R, DeGroot WJ: Acute bronchial asthma. Relations between clinical and physiologic manifestations. N Engl J Med 288:221-225, 1973.
417. Knowles GK, Clark TJ: Pulsus paradoxus as a valuable sign indicating severity of asthma. Lancet 2:1356-1359, 1973.
418. Galant SP, Groncy CE, Shaw KC: The value of pulsus paradoxus in assessing the child with status asthmaticus. Pediatrics 61:46-51, 1978.
419. McGregor M: Current concepts: Pulsus paradoxus. N Engl J Med 301:480-482, 1979.
420. Woolcock A: Assessment of asthma severity. In Barnes P, Grunstein M, Leff A, et al (eds): Asthma. Philadelphia, Lippincott-Raven, 1997, pp 1499-1503.
421. O'Connor GT, Weiss ST: Clinical and symptom measures. Am J Respir Crit Care Med 149:S21-S28; discussion S29-S30, 1994.
422. Li JT, O'Connell EJ: Clinical evaluation of asthma. Ann Allergy Asthma Immunol 76:1-13, quiz 13-15, 1996.
423. Cockcroft DW, Swystun VA: Asthma control versus asthma severity. J Allergy Clin Immunol 98:1016-1018, 1996.
424. Szefler SJ, Leung DY: Glucocorticoid-resistant asthma: Pathogenesis and clinical implications for management. Eur Respir J 10:1640-1647, 1997.
425. Pavord ID, Pizzichini MM, Pizzichini E, et al: The use of induced sputum to investigate airway inflammation. Thorax 52:498-501, 1997.
426. Pizzichini E, Pizzichini MM, Efthimiadis A, et al: Measuring airway inflammation in asthma: Eosinophils and eosinophilic cationic protein in induced sputum compared with peripheral blood. J Allergy Clin Immunol 99:539-544, 1997.
427. Beers R: Skin tests. In Samter M, Alexander H (eds): Immunologic Disorders. Boston, Little, Brown, 1965, p 539.
428. Pepys J: New tests to assess lung function. Inhalation challenge tests in asthma. N Engl J Med 293:758-759, 1975.
429. Ahonen A: Analysis of the changes in ECG during status asthmaticus. Respiration 37:85-90, 1979.
430. Orzalesi MM, Cook CD, Hart MC: pulmonary function in symptom-free asthmatic patients. Acta Paediatr 53:401-407, 1964.
431. McCarthy D, Milic-Emili J: Closing volume in asymptomatic asthma. Am Rev Respir Dis 107:559-570, 1973.
432. Rubinfeld AR, Pain MC: Perception of asthma. Lancet 1:882-884, 1976.
433. Olive JT Jr, Hyatt RE: Maximal expiratory flow and total respiratory resistance during induced bronchoconstriction in asthmatic subjects. Am Rev Respir Dis 106:366-376, 1972.
434. Greaves IA, Colebatch HJ: Large lungs after childhood asthma: A consequence of enlarged airspaces. Aust N Z J Med 15:427-434, 1985.
435. Macklem PT: Hyperinflation. Am Rev Respir Dis 129:1-2, 1984.
436. Woolcock AJ, Read J: Improvement in bronchial asthma not reflected in forced expiratory volume. Lancet 2:1323-1325, 1965..
437. Wang T-R, Levison H: Pulmonary function in children with asthma at acute attack and symptom-free status. Am Rev Respir Dis 99:719, 1969.
438. Collard P, Njinou B, Nejadnik B, et al: Single breath diffusing capacity for carbon monoxide in stable asthma. Chest 105:1426-1429, 1994.
439. Wagner PD, Dantzker DR, Iacovoni VE, et al: Ventilation-perfusion inequality in asymptomatic asthma. Am Rev Respir Dis 118:511-524, 1978.
440. Alberts WM, Williams JH, Ramsdell JW: Metabolic acidosis as a presenting feature in acute asthma. Ann Allergy 57:107-109, 1986.
441. Wagner PD, Hedenstierna G, Rodriguez-Roisin R: Gas exchange, expiratory flow obstruction and the clinical spectrum of asthma. Eur Respir J 9:1278-1282, 1996.
442. Banner AS, Shah RS, Addington WW: Rapid prediction of need for hospitalization in acute asthma. JAMA 235:1337-1338, 1976.
443. Palmer KN, Diament ML: Dynamic and static lung volumes and blood-gas tensions in bronchial asthma. Lancet 1:591-593, 1969.
444. Eggleston PA, Ward BH, Pierson WE, et al: Radiographic abnormalities in acute asthma in children. Pediatrics 54:442-449, 1974.
445. Gershel JC, Goldman HS, Stein RE, et al: The usefulness of chest radiographs in first asthma attacks. N Engl J Med 309:336-339, 1983.
446. Findley LJ, Sahn SA: The value of chest roentgenograms in acute asthma in adults. Chest 80:535-536, 1981.
447. Bierman CW: Pneumomediastinum and pneumothorax complicating asthma in children. Am J Dis Child 114:42-50, 1967.
448. Leatherman J: Life-threatening asthma. Clin Chest Med 15:453-479, 1994.
449. Bendkowski B: Asian influenza (1957) in allergic patients. BMJ 5108:1314-1315, 1958.
450. Jenkins PF, Benfield GF, Smith AP: Predicting recovery from acute severe asthma. Thorax 36:835-841, 1981.
451. Benfield GF, Smith AP: Predicting rapid and slow response to treatment in acute severe asthma. Br J Dis Chest 77:249-254, 1983.

452. Fischl MA, Pitchenik A, Gardner LB: An index predicting relapse and need for hospitalization in patients with acute bronchial asthma. N Engl J Med 305:783-789, 1981.

453. Williams TJ, Tuxen DV, Scheinkestel CD, et al: Risk factors for morbidity in mechanically ventilated patients with acute severe asthma. Am Rev Respir Dis 146:607-615, 1992.

454. Martinez FD, Wright AL, Taussig LM, et al: Asthma and wheezing in the first six years of life. The Group Health Medical Associates. N Engl J Med 332:133-138, 1995.

455. Rackemann FM, Edwards MC: A follow-up study of 688 patients after an interval of twenty years. N Engl J Med 246:815-823, contd, 1952.

456. Roorda RJ: Prognostic factors for the outcome of childhood asthma in adolescence. Thorax 51(Suppl 1):S7-S12, 1996.

457. Withers NJ, Low L, Holgate ST, et al: The natural history of respiratory symptoms in a cohort of adolescents. Am J Respir Crit Care Med 158:352-357, 1998.

458. Blackhall MI: Effect of age on fixed and labile components of airways resistance in asthma. Thorax 26:325-330, 1971.

459. Cserhati E, Mezei G, Kelemen J: Late prognosis of bronchial asthma in children. Respiration 46:160-165, 1984.

460. Ulrik CS, Lange P: Decline of lung function in adults with bronchial asthma. Am J Respir Crit Care Med 150:629-634, 1994.

461. Brown PJ, Greville HW, Finucane KE: Asthma and irreversible airflow obstruction. Thorax 39:131-136, 1984.

462. Alexander HL: A historical account of death from asthma. J Allergy Clin Immunol 34:305-322, 1963.

463. Sly RM, O'Donnell R: Stabilization of asthma mortality. Ann Allergy Asthma Immunol 78:347-354, 1997.

464. Beasley R, Pearce N, Crane J: International trends in asthma mortality. Ciba Found Symp 206:140-150, discussion 150-156, 157-159, 1997.

465. Sears MR, Rea HH, Beaglehole R, et al: Asthma mortality in New Zealand: A two year national study. N Z Med J 98:271-275, 1985.

466. Mullen M, Mullen B, Carey M: The association between beta-agonist use and death from asthma. A meta-analytic integration of case-control studies. JAMA 270:1842-1845, 1993.

467. Sears MR, Rea HH, Fenwick J, et al: 75 deaths in asthmatics prescribed home nebulisers. Br Med J (Clin Res Ed) 294:477-480, 1987.

468. Turner MO, Noertjojo K, Vedal S, et al: Risk factors for near-fatal asthma. A case-control study in hospitalized patients with asthma. Am J Respir Crit Care Med 157:1804-1809, 1998.

469. WWW: http://www.hereditaryangioedema.com.

470. Standards for the diagnosis and care of patients with chronic obstructive pulmonary disease. American Thoracic Society. Am J Respir Crit Care Med 152(5 Pt 2):S77-S121, 1995.

471. American Thoracic Society (Statement by Committee on Diagnostic Standards for Nontuberculous Respiratory Diseases): Definitions and classification of chronic bronchitis, asthma, and pulmonary emphysema. Am Rev Respir Dis 85:762, 1962.

472. Snider GL: What's in a name? Names, definitions, descriptions, and diagnostic criteria of diseases, with emphasis on chronic obstructive pulmonary disease. Respiration 62:297-301, 1995.

473. Peto R, Speizer FE, Cochrane AL, et al: The relevance in adults of air-flow obstruction, but not of mucus hypersecretion, to mortality from chronic lung disease. Results from 20 years of prospective observation. Am Rev Respir Dis 128:491-500, 1983.

474. Vestbo J, Prescott E, Lange P: Association of chronic mucus hypersecretion with FEV_1 decline and chronic obstructive pulmonary disease morbidity. Copenhagen City Heart Study Group. Am J Respir Crit Care Med 153:1530-1535, 1996.

475. Prescott E, Lange P, Vestbo J: Chronic mucus hypersecretion in COPD and death from pulmonary infection. Eur Respir J 8:1333-1338, 1995.

476. The definition of emphysema. Report of a National Heart, Lung, and Blood Institute, Division of Lung Diseases workshop. Am Rev Respir Dis 132:182-185, 1985.

477. Murray CJ, Lopez AD: Global mortality, disability, and the contribution of risk factors: Global Burden of Disease Study. Lancet 349:1436-1442, 1997.

478. Murray CJ, Lopez AD: Regional patterns of disability-free life expectancy and disability-adjusted life expectancy: Global Burden of Disease Study. Lancet 349:1347-1352, 1997.

479. Sin DD, Stafinski T, Ng YC, et al: The impact of chronic obstructive pulmonary disease on work loss in the United States. Am J Respir Crit Care Med 165:704-707, 2002.

480. Dahl R, Lofdahl CG: The economic impact of COPD in North America and Europe. Analysis of the Confronting COPD survey. Introduction. Respir Med 97(Suppl C):S1-S2, 2003.

481. Murray CJ, Lopez AD: Evidence-based health policy—lessons from the Global Burden of Disease Study. Science 274:740-743, 1996.

482. Zhang H, Cai B: The impact of tobacco on lung health in China. Respirology 8:17-21, 2003.

483. Sherrill DL, Lebowitz MD, Burrows B: Epidemiology of chronic obstructive pulmonary disease. Clin Chest Med 11:375-387, 1990.

484. Marang-van de Mheen PJ, Smith GD, Hart CL, et al: Are women more sensitive to smoking than men? Findings from the Renfrew and Paisley study. Int J Epidemiol 30:787-792, 2001.

485. Silverman EK, Weiss ST, Drazen JM, et al: Gender-related differences in severe, early-onset chronic obstructive pulmonary disease. Am J Respir Crit Care Med 162:2152-2158, 2000.

486. Chapman KR, Tashkin DP, Pye DJ: Gender bias in the diagnosis of COPD. Chest 119:1691-1695, 2001.

487. Gillum RF: Chronic obstructive pulmonary disease in blacks and whites: Mortality and morbidity. J Natl Med Assoc 82:417-428, 1990.

488. Whittemore AS, Perlin SA, DiCiccio Y: Chronic obstructive pulmonary disease in lifelong nonsmokers: Results from NHANES. Am J Public Health 85:702-706, 1995.

489. Bascom R: Differential susceptibility to tobacco smoke: Possible mechanisms. Pharmacogenetics 1:102-106, 1991.

490. Silverman EK, Speizer FE: Risk factors for the development of chronic obstructive pulmonary disease. Med Clin North Am 80:501-522, 1996.

491. Cigarette smoking and health. American Thoracic Society. Am J Respir Crit Care Med 153:861-865, 1996.

492. Clement J, Van de Woestijne KP: Rapidly decreasing forced expiratory volume in one second or vital capacity and development of chronic airflow obstruction. Am Rev Respir Dis 125:553-558, 1982.

493. Tager IB, Munoz A, Rosner B, et al: Effect of cigarette smoking on the pulmonary function of children and adolescents. Am Rev Respir Dis 131:752-759, 1985.

494. Pauwels RA, Lofdahl CG, Laitinen LA, et al: Long-term treatment with inhaled budesonide in persons with mild chronic obstructive pulmonary disease who continue smoking. European Respiratory Society Study on Chronic Obstructive Pulmonary Disease. N Engl J Med 340:1948-1953, 1999.

495. Anthonisen NR, Connett JE, Kiley JP, et al: Effects of smoking intervention and the use of an inhaled anticholinergic bronchodilator on the rate of decline of FEV_1. The Lung Health Study. JAMA 272:1497-1505, 1994.

496. Taylor DR, Reid WD, Paré PD, et al: Cigarette smoke inhalation patterns and bronchial reactivity. Thorax 43:65-70, 1988.

497. Stick S: Pediatric origins of adult lung disease. 1. The contribution of airway development to paediatric and adult lung disease. Thorax 55:587-594, 2000.

498. Ware JH, Dockery DW, Spiro A 3rd, et al: Passive smoking, gas cooking, and respiratory health of children living in six cities. Am Rev Respir Dis 129:366-374, 1984.

499. Perez-Padilla R, Regalado J, Vedal S, et al: Exposure to biomass smoke and chronic airway disease in Mexican women. A case-control study. Am J Respir Crit Care Med 154:701-706, 1996.

500. Vedal S: Update on the health effects of outdoor air pollution. Clin Chest Med 23:763-775, 2002.

501. Cohen CA, Hudson AR, Clausen JL, et al: Respiratory symptoms, spirometry, and oxidant air pollution in nonsmoking adults. Am Rev Respir Dis 105:251-261, 1972.

502. Tashkin DP, Detels R, Simmons M, et al: The UCLA population studies of chronic obstructive respiratory disease: XI. Impact of air pollution and smoking on annual change in forced expiratory volume in one second. Am J Respir Crit Care Med 149:1209-1217, 1994.

503. Anderson HR, Spix C, Medina S, et al: Air pollution and daily admissions for chronic obstructive pulmonary disease in 6 European cities: Results from the APHEA project. Eur Respir J 10:1064-1071, 1997.

504. Lunn JE, Knowelden J, Handyside AJ: Patterns of respiratory illness in Sheffield infant schoolchildren. Br J Prev Soc Med 21:7-16, 1967.

505. Balmes J, Becklake M, Blanc P, et al: American Thoracic Society Statement: Occupational contribution to the burden of airway disease. Am J Respir Crit Care Med 167:787-797, 2003.

506. Oxman AD, Muir DC, Shannon HS, et al: Occupational dust exposure and chronic obstructive pulmonary disease. A systematic overview of the evidence. Am Rev Respir Dis 148:38-48, 1993.

507. Respiratory health hazards in agriculture. Am J Respir Crit Care Med 158:S1-S76, 1998.

508. Britton J, Martinez FD: The relationship of childhood respiratory infection to growth and decline in lung function. Am J Respir Crit Care Med 154:S240-S245, 1996.

509. Shaheen SO, Barker DJ, Holgate ST: Do lower respiratory tract infections in early childhood cause chronic obstructive pulmonary disease? Am J Respir Crit Care Med 151:1649-1651, discussion 1651-1652, 1995.

510. Martinez FD, Morgan WJ, Wright AL, et al: Diminished lung function as a predisposing factor for wheezing respiratory illness in infants. N Engl J Med 319:1112-1117, 1988.

511. Ogawa E, Elliott WM, Hughes F, et al: Latent adenoviral infection induces production of growth factors relevant to airway remodeling in COPD. Am J Physiol Lung Cell Mol Physiol 286:L189-L197, 2004.

512. Sethi S, Murphy TF: Bacterial infection in chronic obstructive pulmonary disease in 2000: A state-of-the-art review. Clin Microbiol Rev 14:336-363, 2001.

513. Gump DW, Phillips CA, Forsyth BR, et al: Role of infection in chronic bronchitis. Am Rev Respir Dis 113:465-474, 1976.

514. Wedzicha JA, Donaldson GC: Exacerbations of chronic obstructive pulmonary disease. Respir Care 48:1204-1215, 2003.

515. Von Hertzen L, Alakarppa H, Koskinen R, et al: *Chlamydia pneumoniae* infection in patients with chronic obstructive pulmonary disease. Epidemiol Infect 118:155-164, 1997.

516. Osborne ML, Vollmer WM, Buist AS: Periodicity of asthma, emphysema, and chronic bronchitis in a northwest health maintenance organization. Chest 110:1458-1462, 1996.

517. Koskela HO, Koskela AK, Tukiainen HO: Bronchoconstriction due to cold weather in COPD. The roles of direct airway effects and cutaneous reflex mechanisms. Chest 110:632-636, 1996.

518. Strachan D: Epidemiology: A British prospective. In Calverley PM, Pride NB (eds): Chronic Obstructive Pulmonary Disease. London, Chapman & Hall, 1995, pp 47-68.

519. Gray-Donald K, Gibbons L, Shapiro SH, et al: Nutritional status and mortality in chronic obstructive pulmonary disease. Am J Respir Crit Care Med 153:961-966, 1996.

520. Britton J: Dietary fish oil and airways obstruction. Thorax 50(Suppl 1):S11-S15, 1995.

521. Schwartz J, Weiss ST: Dietary factors and their relation to respiratory symptoms. The Second National Health and Nutrition Examination Survey. Am J Epidemiol 132:67-76, 1990.

522. Tockman M, Khoury M, Cohen B: The epidemiology of COPD. In Petty T (ed): Chronic Obstructive Disease. New York, Marcel Dekker, 1985, p 43.

523. Sandford AJ, Weir TD, Paré PD: Genetic risk factors for chronic obstructive pulmonary disease. Eur Respir J 10:1380-1391, 1997.

523a. Redline S, Tishler PV, Lewitter FI, et al: Assessment of genetic and nongenetic influences on pulmonary function. A twin study. Am Rev Respir Dis 135:217-222, 1987.

524. Lilienfeld A, Lilienfeld D: Foundations of Epidemiology, ed 2. New York, Oxford University Press, 1980.

525. American Thoracic Society/European Respiratory Society Statement: Standards for the diagnosis and management of individuals with alpha-1 antitrypsin deficiency. Am J Respir Crit Care Med 168:818-900, 2003.

526. Talamo RC, Thurlbeck WM: Alpha-antitrypsin Pi types in postmortem blood. Am Rev Respir Dis 112:201-207, 1975.

527. Falk GA, Briscoe WA: Alpha-1-antitrypsin deficiency in chronic obstructive pulmonary disease. Ann Intern Med 72:427-429, 1970.

528. Jeppsson JO, Larsson C, Eriksson S: Characterization of alpha1-antitrypsin in the inclusion bodies from the liver in alpha 1-antitrypsin deficiency. N Engl J Med 293:576-579, 1975.

529. Carrell RW, Lomas DA: Alpha1-antitrypsin deficiency—a model for conformational diseases. N Engl J Med 346:45-53, 2002.

530. Perlmutter DH: Alpha-1-antitrypsin deficiency: Biochemistry and clinical manifestations. Ann Med 28:385-394, 1996.

531. Black LF, Kueppers F: α_1-Antitrypsin deficiency in nonsmokers. Am Rev Respir Dis 117:421-428, 1978.

532. Sandford AJ, Chagani T, Weir TD, et al: Susceptibility genes for rapid decline of lung function in the lung health study. Am J Respir Crit Care Med 163:469-473, 2001.

533. King MA, Stone JA, Diaz PT, et al: Alpha 1-antitrypsin deficiency: Evaluation of bronchiectasis with CT. Radiology 199:137-141, 1996.

534. Silverman EK, Palmer LJ, Mosley JD, et al: Genomewide linkage analysis of quantitative spirometric phenotypes in severe early-onset chronic obstructive pulmonary disease. Am J Hum Genet 70:1229-1239, 2002.

535. Sandford AJ, Joos L, Paré PD: Genetic risk factors for chronic obstructive pulmonary disease. Curr Opin Pulm Med 8:87-94, 2002.

536. Sluiter HJ, Koeter GH, de Monchy JG, et al: The Dutch hypothesis (chronic nonspecific lung disease) revisited. Eur Respir J 4:479-489, 1991.

537. de Jong JW, Koeter GH, Postma DS: The significance of airway responsiveness in the onset and evolution of chronic obstructive pulmonary disease. Clin Exp Allergy 27:1114-1119, 1997.

538. Tashkin DP, Altose MD, Connett JE, et al: Methacholine reactivity predicts changes in lung function over time in smokers with early chronic obstructive pulmonary disease. The Lung Health Study Research Group. Am J Respir Crit Care Med 153:1802-1811, 1996.

539. Taylor RG, Gross E, Joyce H, et al: Smoking, allergy, and the differential white blood cell count. Thorax 40:17-22, 1985.

540. Frette C, Annesi I, Korobaeff M, et al: Blood eosinophilia and FEV_1. Cross-sectional and longitudinal analyses. Am Rev Respir Dis 143:987-992, 1991.

541. Sherrill DL, Lebowitz MD, Halonen M, et al: Longitudinal evaluation of the association between pulmonary function and total serum IgE. Am J Respir Crit Care Med 152:98-102, 1995.

542. Janoff A: Elastases and emphysema. Current assessment of the protease-antiprotease hypothesis. Am Rev Respir Dis 132:417-433, 1985.

543. Shapiro SD: Proteinases in chronic obstructive pulmonary disease. Biochem Soc Trans 30:98-102, 2002.

544. Belvisi MG, Bottomley KM: The role of matrix metalloproteinases (MMPs) in the pathophysiology of chronic obstructive pulmonary disease (COPD): A therapeutic role for inhibitors of MMPs? Inflamm Res 52:95-100, 2003.

545. Hautamaki RD, Kobayashi DK, Senior RM, et al: Requirement for macrophage elastase for cigarette smoke-induced emphysema in mice. Science 277:2002-2004, 1997.

546. Cawston T, Carrere S, Catterall J, et al: Matrix metalloproteinases and TIMPs: Properties and implications for the treatment of chronic obstructive pulmonary disease. Novartis Found Symp 234:205-218, discussion 218-228, 2001.

547. Sallenave JM: The role of secretory leukocyte proteinase inhibitor and elafin (elastase-specific inhibitor/skin-derived antileukoprotease) as alarm antiproteinases in inflammatory lung disease. Respir Res 1:87-92, 2000.

548. Selby C, Drost E, Gillooly M, et al: Neutrophil sequestration in lungs removed at surgery. The effect of microscopic emphysema. Am J Respir Crit Care Med 149:1526-1533, 1994.

549. Klut ME, Doerschuk CM, Van Eeden SF, et al: Activation of neutrophils within pulmonary microvessels of rabbits exposed to cigarette smoke. Am J Respir Cell Mol Biol 9:82-89, 1993.

550. MacNee W, Martin B, Tanco S, et al: Cigarette smoking delays polymorphonuclear leukocyte (PMN) transit through the pulmonary circulation. Am Rev Respir Dis 135:A146, 1987.

551. Shoji S, Ertl RF, Koyama S, et al: Cigarette smoke stimulates release of neutrophil chemotactic activity from cultured bovine bronchial epithelial cells. Clin Sci (Lond) 88:337-344, 1995.

552. Kramps JA, Bakker W, Dijkman JH: A matched-pair study of the leukocyte elastase-like activity in normal persons and in emphysematous patients with and without alpha 1-antitrypsin deficiency. Am Rev Respir Dis 121:253-261, 1980.

553. Pryor WA, Stone K: Oxidants in cigarette smoke. Radicals, hydrogen peroxide, peroxynitrate, and peroxynitrite. Ann N Y Acad Sci 686:12-27, discussion 27-28, 1993.

554. Padmaja S, Huie RE: The reaction of nitric oxide with organic peroxyl radicals. Biochem Biophys Res Commun 195:539-544, 1993.

555. MacNee W: Oxidants/antioxidants and COPD. Chest 117:303S-317S, 2000.

556. Hogg JC: Chronic obstructive pulmonary disease: An overview of pathology and pathogenesis. Novartis Found Symp 234:4-19, discussion 19-26, 2001.

557. Saetta M, Turato G, Maestrelli P, et al: Cellular and structural bases of chronic obstructive pulmonary disease. Am J Respir Crit Care Med 163:1304-1309, 2001.

558. Puchelle E, Zahm JM, Aug F: Viscoelasticity, protein content and ciliary transport rate of sputum in patients with recurrent and chronic bronchitis. Biorheology 18:659-666, 1981.

559. Foster WM, Langenback EG, Bergofsky EH: Disassociation in the mucociliary function of central and peripheral airways of asymptomatic smokers. Am Rev Respir Dis 132:633-639, 1985.

560. Matthys H, Vastag E, Kohler D, et al: Mucociliary clearance in patients with chronic bronchitis and bronchial carcinoma. Respiration 44:329-337, 1983.

561. Mossberg B, Camner P: Impaired mucociliary transport as a pathogenetic factor in obstructive pulmonary diseases. Chest 77:265-266, 1980.

562. Verra F, Escudier E, Lebargy F, et al: Ciliary abnormalities in bronchial epithelium of smokers, ex-smokers, and nonsmokers. Am J Respir Crit Care Med 151:630-634, 1995.

563. Jeffery PK: Structural and inflammatory changes in COPD: A comparison with asthma. Thorax 53:129-136, 1998.

564. Jamal K, Cooney TP, Fleetham JA, et al: Chronic bronchitis. Correlation of morphologic findings to sputum production and flow rates. Am Rev Respir Dis 129:719-722, 1984.

565. Opazo Saez AM, Seow CY, Paré PD: Peripheral airway smooth muscle mechanics in obstructive airways disease. Am J Respir Crit Care Med 161:910-917, 2000.

566. Nagai A, West WW, Paul JL, et al: The National Institutes of Health Intermittent Positive-Pressure Breathing trial: Pathology studies. I. Interrelationship between morphologic lesions. Am Rev Respir Dis 132:937-945, 1985.

567. Yanai M, Sekizawa K, Ohrui T, et al: Site of airway obstruction in pulmonary disease: Direct measurement of intrabronchial pressure. J Appl Physiol 72:1016-1023, 1992.

568. Kuwano K, Bosken CH, Paré PD, et al: Small airways dimensions in asthma and in chronic obstructive pulmonary disease. Am Rev Respir Dis 148:1220-1225, 1993.

569. Hogg JC: Airway pathology of functional significance in chronic bronchitis and chronic obstructive airway disease. Agents Actions Suppl 30:11-20, 1990.

570. Wright JL, Cosio M, Wiggs B, et al: A morphologic grading scheme for membranous and respiratory bronchioles. Arch Pathol Lab Med 109:163-185, 1985.

571. Niewoehner DE, Kleinerman J: Morphologic basis of pulmonary resistance in the human lung and effects of aging. J Appl Physiol 36:412-418, 1974.

572. Wright JL, Lawson LM, Paré PD, et al: The detection of small airways disease. Am Rev Respir Dis 129:989-994, 1984.

573. Eidelman DH, Ghezzo H, Kim WD, et al: The destructive index and early lung destruction in smokers. Am Rev Respir Dis 144:156-159, 1991.

574. Cosio MG, Shiner RJ, Saetta M, et al: Alveolar fenestrae in smokers. Relationship with light microscopic and functional abnormalities. Am Rev Respir Dis 133:126-131, 1986.

575. Nagai A, Yamawaki I, Takizawa T, et al: Alveolar attachments in emphysema of human lungs. Am Rev Respir Dis 144:888-891, 1991.

576. Anderson AE Jr, Foraker AG: Centrilobular emphysema and panlobular emphysema: Two different diseases. Thorax 28:547-550, 1973.

577. Anderson AE Jr, Furlaneto JA, Foraker AG: Bronchopulmonary derangements in nonsmokers. Am Rev Respir Dis 101:518-527, 1970.

578. Boren HG: Alveolar fenestrae. Relationship to the pathology and pathogenesis of pulmonary emphysema. Am Rev Respir Dis 85:328-344, 1962.

579. Standards for the diagnosis and care of patients with chronic obstructive pulmonary disease. American Thoracic Society. Am J Respir Crit Care Med 152:S77-S121, 1995.

580. Webb WR: Radiology of obstructive pulmonary disease. AJR Am J Roentgenol 169:637-647, 1997.

581. Takasugi JE, Godwin JD: Radiology of chronic obstructive pulmonary disease. Radiol Clin North Am 36:29-55, 1998.

582. Fraser RG, Fraser RS, Renner JW, et al: The roentgenologic diagnosis of chronic bronchitis: A reassessment with emphasis on parahilar bronchi seen end-on. Radiology 120:1-9, 1976.

583. Remy-Jardin M, Remy J, Boulenguez C, et al: Morphologic effects of cigarette smoking on airways and pulmonary parenchyma in healthy adult volunteers: CT evaluation and correlation with pulmonary function tests. Radiology 186:107-115, 1993.

584. Nakano Y, Muro S, Sakai H, et al: Computed tomographic measurements of airway dimensions and emphysema in smokers. Correlation with lung function. Am J Respir Crit Care Med 162:1102-1108, 2000.

585. Miniati M, Filippi E, Falaschi F, et al: Radiologic evaluation of emphysema in patients with chronic obstructive pulmonary disease. Chest radiography versus high resolution computed tomography. Am J Respir Crit Care Med 151:1359-1367, 1995.

586. Pratt PC: Role of conventional chest radiography in diagnosis and exclusion of emphysema. Am J Med 82:998-1006, 1987.

587. Thurlbeck WM, Müller NL: Emphysema: Definition, imaging, and quantification. AJR Am J Roentgenol 163:1017-1025, 1994.

588. Austin JH, Müller NL, Friedman PJ, et al: Glossary of terms for CT of the lungs: Recommendations of the Nomenclature Committee of the Fleischner Society. Radiology 200:327-331, 1996.

589. Spouge D, Mayo JR, Cardoso W, et al: Panacinar emphysema: CT and pathologic findings. J Comput Assist Tomogr 17:710-713, 1993.
590. Miller RR, Müller NL, Vedal S, et al: Limitations of computed tomography in the assessment of emphysema. Am Rev Respir Dis 139:980-983, 1989.
591. Gevenois PA, de Maertelaer V, De Vuyst P, et al: Comparison of computed density and macroscopic morphometry in pulmonary emphysema. Am J Respir Crit Care Med 152:653-657, 1995.
592. Sakai N, Mishima M, Nishimura K, et al: An automated method to assess the distribution of low attenuation areas on chest CT scans in chronic pulmonary emphysema patients. Chest 106:1319-1325, 1994.
593. Müller NL, Staples CA, Miller RR, et al: "Density mask." An objective method to quantitate emphysema using computed tomography. Chest 94:782-787, 1988.
594. Mergo PJ, Williams WF, Gonzalez-Rothi R, et al: Three-dimensional volumetric assessment of abnormally low attenuation of the lung from routine helical CT: Inspiratory and expiratory quantification. AJR Am J Roentgenol 170:1355-1360, 1998.
595. Bae KT, Slone RM, Gierada DS, et al: Patients with emphysema: Quantitative CT analysis before and after lung volume reduction surgery. Work in progress. Radiology 203:705-714, 1997.
596. Müller NL, Coxson H: Chronic obstructive pulmonary disease. 4: Imaging the lungs in patients with chronic obstructive pulmonary disease. Thorax 57:982-985, 2002.
597. Burrows B, Niden AH, Barclay WR, et al: Chronic obstructive lung disease. II. Relationship of clinical and physiologic findings to the severity of airways obstruction. Am Rev Respir Dis 91:665-678, 1965.
598. Kass I, O'Brien LE, Zamel N, et al: Lack of correlation between clinical background and pulmonary function tests in patients with chronic obstructive pulmonary diseases. A retrospective study of 140 cases. Am Rev Respir Dis 107:64-69, 1973.
599. Seward JB, Hayes DL, Smith HC, et al: Platypnea-orthodeoxia: Clinical profile, diagnostic workup, management, and report of seven cases. Mayo Clin Proc 59:221-231, 1984.
600. Burrows B, Fletcher CM, Heard BE, et al: The emphysematous and bronchial types of chronic airways obstruction. A clinicopathological study of patients in London and Chicago. Lancet 1:830-835, 1966.
601. Kawakami Y, Irie T, Shida A, et al: Familial factors affecting arterial blood gas values and respiratory chemosensitivity in chronic obstructive pulmonary disease. Am Rev Respir Dis 125:420-425, 1982.
602. O'Donnell DE, D'Arsigny C, Fitzpatrick M, et al: Exercise hypercapnia in advanced chronic obstructive pulmonary disease: The role of lung hyperinflation. Am J Respir Crit Care Med 166:663-668, 2002.
603. Marini JJ, Pierson DJ, Hudson LD, et al: The significance of wheezing in chronic airflow obstruction. Am Rev Respir Dis 120:1069-1072, 1979.
604. Campbell EJ: Physical signs of diffuse airways obstruction and lung distension. Thorax 24:1-3, 1969.
605. Christe R: Emphysema of the lungs. BMJ 1:105, 1944.
606. Gilmartin JJ, Gibson GJ: Mechanisms of paradoxical rib cage motion in patients with chronic obstructive pulmonary disease. Am Rev Respir Dis 134:683-687, 1986.
607. Openbrier DR, Irwin MM, Rogers RM, et al: Nutritional status and lung function in patients with emphysema and chronic bronchitis. Chest 83:17-22, 1983.
608. Wouters EF: Nutrition and metabolism in COPD. Chest 117:274S-280S, 2000.
609. De Troyer A: Effect of hyperinflation on the diaphragm. Eur Respir J 10:708-713, 1997.
610. Polkey MI, Kyroussis D, Hamnegard CH, et al: Diaphragm strength in chronic obstructive pulmonary disease. Am J Respir Crit Care Med 154:1310-1317, 1996.
611. MacNee W: Pathophysiology of cor pulmonale in chronic obstructive pulmonary disease. Part One. Am J Respir Crit Care Med 150:833-852, 1994.
612. MacNee W: Pathophysiology of cor pulmonale in chronic obstructive pulmonary disease. Part two. Am J Respir Crit Care Med 150:1158-1168, 1994.
613. Oswald-Mammosser M, Apprill M, Bachez P, et al: Pulmonary hemodynamics in chronic obstructive pulmonary disease of the emphysematous type. Respiration 58:304-310, 1991.
614. Albert RK, Muramoto A, Caldwell J, et al: Increases in intrathoracic pressure do not explain the rise in left ventricular end-diastolic pressure that occurs during exercise in patients with chronic obstructive pulmonary disease. Am Rev Respir Dis 132:623-627, 1985.
615. Weitzenblum E, Hirth C, Parini JP, et al: Clinical, functional and pulmonary hemodynamic course of patients with chronic obstructive pulmonary disease followed-up over 3 years. Respiration 36:1-9, 1978.
616. Midgren B, White T, Petersson K, et al: Nocturnal hypoxaemia and cor pulmonale in severe chronic lung disease. Bull Eur Physiopathol Respir 21:527-533, 1985.
617. Weitzenblum E, Jezek V: Evolution of pulmonary hypertension in chronic respiratory diseases. Bull Eur Physiopathol Respir 20:73-81, 1984.
618. Vonk Noordegraaf A, Marcus JT, Roseboom B, et al: The effect of right ventricular hypertrophy on left ventricular ejection fraction in pulmonary emphysema. Chest 112:640-645, 1997.
619. Holford FD, Mithoefer JC: Cardiac arrhythmias in hospitalized patients with chronic obstructive pulmonary disease. Am Rev Respir Dis 108:879-885, 1973.
620. Thompson HK Jr, North LD, Aboumrad MH: The electrocardiogram in chronic obstructive pulmonary disease. Am Rev Respir Dis 107:1067-1070, 1973.
621. Tandon MK: Correlations of electrocardiographic features with airway obstruction in chronic bronchitis. Chest 63:146-148, 1973.
622. Murphy ML, Hutcheson F: The electrocardiographic diagnosis of right ventricular hypertrophy in chronic obstructive pulmonary disease. Chest 65:622-627, 1974.
623. Burrows B, Earle RH: Course and prognosis of chronic obstructive lung disease. A prospective study of 200 patients. N Engl J Med 280:397-404, 1969.
624. Paré P: Lung structure-function relationships. In Calverley PM, Pride NB (eds): Chronic Obstructive Pulmonary Disease. London, Chapman & Hall, 1995, p 33.
625. Marrero O, Beck GJ, Schachter EN: Discriminating power of measurements from maximum expiratory flow-volume curves. Respiration 49:263-273, 1986.
626. Hyatt R, Rodarte J: Changes in lung mechanics. In Macklem P, Permutt S (eds): The Lung in the Transition between Health and Disease. New York, Marcel Dekker, 1979, p 73.
627. Anthonisen NR, Wright EC: Bronchodilator response in chronic obstructive pulmonary disease. Am Rev Respir Dis 133:814-819, 1986.
628. Kerstjens HA, Brand PL, Quanjer PH, et al: Variability of bronchodilator response and effects of inhaled corticosteroid treatment in obstructive airways disease. Dutch CNSLD Study Group. Thorax 48:722-729, 1993.
629. Ramsdale EH, Morris MM, Hargreave FE: Interpretation of the variability of peak flow rates in chronic bronchitis. Thorax 41:771-776, 1986.
630. Pellegrino R, Brusasco V: Lung hyperinflation and flow limitation in chronic airway obstruction. Eur Respir J 10:543-549, 1997.
631. O'Donnell DE: Assessment of bronchodilator efficacy in symptomatic COPD: Is spirometry useful? Chest 117:42S-47S, 2000.
632. Buist AS, Nagy JM, Sexton GJ: The effect of smoking cessation on pulmonary function: A 30-month follow-up of two smoking cessation clinics. Am Rev Respir Dis 120:953-957, 1979.
633. Simonsson BG, Rolf C: Bronchial reactivity to methacholine in ten non-obstructive heavy smokers before and up to one year after cessation of smoking. Eur J Respir Dis 63:526-534, 1982.
634. Hogg JC, Wright JL, Paré PD: Airways disease: Evolution, pathology, and recognition. Med J Aust 142:605-607, 1985.
635. York EL, Jones RL: Effects of smoking on regional residual volume in young adults. Chest 79:12-15, 1981.
636. Dawkins KD, Muers MF: Diurnal variation in airflow obstruction in chronic bronchitis. Thorax 36:618-621, 1981.
637. Purro A, Appendini L, Patessio A, et al: Static intrinsic PEEP in COPD patients during spontaneous breathing. Am J Respir Crit Care Med 157:1044-1050, 1998.
638. O'Donnell DE: Ventilatory limitations in chronic obstructive pulmonary disease. Med Sci Sports Exerc 33:S647-S655, 2001.
639. Farkas GA, Roussos C: Adaptability of the hamster diaphragm to exercise and/or emphysema. J Appl Physiol 53:1263-1272, 1982.
640. Paré PD, Wiggs BJ, Coppin CA: Errors in the measurement of total lung capacity in chronic obstructive lung disease. Thorax 38:468-471, 1983.
641. Piquet J, Harf A, Lorino H, et al: Lung volume measurements by plethysmography in chronic obstructive pulmonary disease: Influence of the panting pattern. Bull Eur Physiopathol Respir 20:31, 1985.
642. Colebatch HJ, Greaves IA, Ng CK: Pulmonary distensibility and ventilatory function in smokers. Bull Eur Physiopathol Respir 21:439-447, 1985.
643. Paré PD, Brooks LA, Bates J, et al: Exponential analysis of the lung pressure-volume curve as a predictor of pulmonary emphysema. Am Rev Respir Dis 126:54-61, 1982.
644. Soguel Schenkel N, Burdet L, de Muralt B, et al: Oxygen saturation during daily activities in chronic obstructive pulmonary disease. Eur Respir J 9:2584-2589, 1996.
645. Aubier M, Murciano D, Fournier M, et al: Central respiratory drive in acute respiratory failure of patients with chronic obstructive pulmonary disease. Am Rev Respir Dis 122:191-199, 1980.
646. Guenard H, Verhas M, Todd-Prokopek A, et al: Effects of oxygen breathing on regional distribution of ventilation and perfusion in hypoxemic patients with chronic lung disease. Am Rev Respir Dis 125:12-17, 1982.
647. MacNee W: Acute exacerbations of COPD. Swiss Med Wkly 133:247-257, 2003.
648. Paré PD, Brooks LA, Baile EM: Effect of systemic venous hypertension on pulmonary function and lung water. J Appl Physiol 51:592-597, 1981.
649. Mithoefer JC, Ramirez C, Cook W: The effect of mixed venous oxygenation on arterial blood in chronic obstructive pulmonary disease: The basis for a classification. Am Rev Respir Dis 117:259-264, 1978.
650. Weitzenblum E, Chaouat A, Charpentier C, et al: Sleep-related hypoxaemia in chronic obstructive pulmonary disease: Causes, consequences and treatment. Respiration 64:187-193, 1997.
651. Flick MR, Block AJ: Continuous in-vivo monitoring of arterial oxygenation in chronic obstructive lung disease. Ann Intern Med 86:725-730, 1977.
652. Guilleminault C, Cummiskey J, Motta J: Chronic obstructive airflow disease and sleep studies. Am Rev Respir Dis 122:397-406, 1980.
653. Douglas NJ, Calverley PM, Leggett RJ, et al: Transient hypoxaemia during sleep in chronic bronchitis and emphysema. Lancet 1:1-4, 1979.
654. Boysen PG, Block AJ, Wynne JW, et al: Nocturnal pulmonary hypertension in patients with chronic obstructive pulmonary disease. Chest 76:536-542, 1979.
655. Stewart RI, Lewis CM: Arterial oxygenation and oxygen transport during exercise in patients with chronic obstructive pulmonary disease. Respiration 49:161-169, 1986.
656. Owens GR, Rogers RM, Pennock BE, et al: The diffusing capacity as a predictor of arterial oxygen desaturation during exercise in patients with chronic obstructive pulmonary disease. N Engl J Med 310:1218-1221, 1984.
657. Gimenez M, Servera E, Candina R, et al: Hypercapnia during maximal exercise in patients with chronic airflow obstruction. Bull Eur Physiopathol Respir 20:113-119, 1984.
658. Montes de Oca M, Rassulo J, Celli BR: Respiratory muscle and cardiopulmonary function during exercise in very severe COPD. Am J Respir Crit Care Med 154:1284-1289, 1996.
659. Wedzicha JA, Cotes PM, Empey DW, et al: Serum immunoreactive erythropoietin in hypoxic lung disease with and without polycythaemia. Clin Sci (Lond) 69:413-422, 1985.

660. Calverley PM, Leggett RJ, McElderry L, et al: Cigarette smoking and secondary poly-cythemia in hypoxic cor pulmonale. Am Rev Respir Dis 125:507-510, 1982.

661. Schwartz JS, Bencowitz HZ, Moser KM: Air travel hypoxemia with chronic obstructive pulmonary disease. Ann Intern Med 100:473-477, 1984.

662. Knudson RJ, Kaltenborn WT, Burrows B: Single breath carbon monoxide transfer factor in different forms of chronic airflow obstruction in a general population sample. Thorax 45:514-519, 1990.

663. Miller A, Thornton JC, Warshaw R, et al: Single breath diffusing capacity in a representative sample of the population of Michigan, a large industrial state. Predicted values, lower limits of normal, and frequencies of abnormality by smoking history. Am Rev Respir Dis 127:270-277, 1983.

664. Sansores RH, Paré PD, Abboud RT: Acute effect of cigarette smoking on the carbon monoxide diffusing capacity of the lung. Am Rev Respir Dis 146:951-958, 1992.

665. Sansores RH, Paré P, Abboud RT: Effect of smoking cessation on pulmonary carbon monoxide diffusing capacity and capillary blood volume. Am Rev Respir Dis 146:959-964, 1992.

666. Williams MH Jr, Park SS: Diffusion of gases within the lungs of patients with chronic obstructive pulmonary disease. Am Rev Respir Dis 98:210-216, 1968.

667. Burge S, Wedzicha JA: COPD exacerbations: Definitions and classifications. Eur Respir J Suppl 41:46s-53s, 2003.

668. Miravitlles M, Murio C, Guerrero T, et al: Costs of chronic bronchitis and COPD: A 1-year follow-up study. Chest 123:784-791, 2003.

669. Moser KM, Shibel EM, Beamon AJ: Acute respiratory failure in obstructive lung disease. Long-term survival after treatment in an intensive care unit. JAMA 225:705-707, 1973.

670. Connors AF Jr, Dawson NV, Thomas C, et al: Outcomes following acute exacerbation of severe chronic obstructive lung disease. The SUPPORT investigators (Study to Understand Prognoses and Preferences for Outcomes and Risks of Treatments). Am J Respir Crit Care Med 154:959-967, 1996.

671. Sun X, Muir J-F, Kakim R, et al: Prognosis of acute respiratory failure in patients with chronic obstructive pulmonary disease. In Enfant C (ed): Lung Biology in Health and Disease. Acute Respiratory Failure in Chronic Obstructive Pulmonary Disease. New York, Marcel Dekker, 1996.

672. Hodgkin JE: Prognosis in chronic obstructive pulmonary disease. Clin Chest Med 11:555-569, 1990.

673. Bishop JM, Cross KW: Physiological variables and mortality in patients with various categories of chronic respiratory disease. Bull Eur Physiopathol Respir 20:495-500, 1984.

674. Weitzenblum E, Hirth C, Ducolone A, et al: Prognostic value of pulmonary artery pressure in chronic obstructive pulmonary disease. Thorax 36:752-758, 1981.

675. Strom K: Survival of patients with chronic obstructive pulmonary disease receiving long-term domiciliary oxygen therapy. Am Rev Respir Dis 147:585-591, 1993.

676. Long term domiciliary oxygen therapy in chronic hypoxic cor pulmonale complicating chronic bronchitis and emphysema. Report of the Medical Research Council Working Party. Lancet 1:681-686, 1981.

677. Timms RM, Khaja FU, Williams GW: Hemodynamic response to oxygen therapy in chronic obstructive pulmonary disease. Ann Intern Med 102:29-36, 1985.

678. Flick MR, Block AJ: Nocturnal vs diurnal cardiac arrhythmias in patients with chronic obstructive pulmonary disease. Chest 75:8-11, 1979.

679. Sassoon CS, Hassell KT, Mahutte CK: Hyperoxic-induced hypercapnia in stable chronic obstructive pulmonary disease. Am Rev Respir Dis 135:907-911, 1987.

680. McNicol MW, Campbell EJ: Severity of respiratory failure. Arterial blood-gases in untreated patients. Lancet 13:336-338, 1965.

681. Wood RE, Boat TF, Doershuk CF: Cystic fibrosis. Am Rev Respir Dis 113:833-878, 1976.

682. Bye MR, Ewig JM, Quittell LM: Cystic fibrosis. Lung 172:251-270, 1994.

683. Rosenstein BJ, Langbaum TS, Metz SJ: Cystic fibrosis: Diagnostic considerations. Johns Hopkins Med J 150:113-120, 1982.

684. Fitzpatrick SB, Rosenstein BJ, Langbaum TS: Diagnosis of cystic fibrosis during adolescence. J Adolesc Health Care 7:38-43, 1986.

685. Hunt B, Geddes DM: Newly diagnosed cystic fibrosis in middle and later life. Thorax 40:23-26, 1985.

686. Zielenski J, Rozmahel R, Bozon D, et al: Genomic DNA sequence of the cystic fibrosis transmembrane conductance regulator (CFTR) gene. Genomics 10:214-228, 1991.

687. Engelhardt JF, Yankaskas JR, Ernst SA, et al: Submucosal glands are the predominant site of CFTR expression in the human bronchus. Nat Genet 2:240-248, 1992.

688. Findlay I, Atkinson G, Chambers M, et al: Rapid genetic diagnosis at 7-9 weeks gestation: Diagnosis of sex, single gene defects and DNA fingerprint from coelomic samples. Hum Reprod 11:2548-2553, 1996.

689. Wilschanski M, Zielenski J, Markiewicz D, et al: Correlation of sweat chloride concentration with classes of the cystic fibrosis transmembrane conductance regulator gene mutations. J Pediatr 127:705-710, 1995.

690. Kulczycki LL, Kostuch M, Bellanti JA: A clinical perspective of cystic fibrosis and new genetic findings: Relationship of CFTR mutations to genotype-phenotype manifestations. Am J Med Genet 116A:262-267, 2003.

691. Boucher RC: Human airway ion transport. Part one. Am J Respir Crit Care Med 150:271-281, 1994.

692. Boucher RC: Human airway ion transport. Part two. Am J Respir Crit Care Med 150:581-593, 1994.

693. Boucher RC: Regulation of airway surface liquid volume by human airway epithelia. Pflugers Arch 445:495-498, 2003.

694. Govan JR, Deretic V: Microbial pathogenesis in cystic fibrosis: Mucoid *Pseudomonas aeruginosa* and *Burkholderia cepacia*. Microbiol Rev 60:539-574, 1996.

695. Govan JR, Nelson JW: Microbiology of lung infection in cystic fibrosis. Br Med Bull 48:912-930, 1992.

696. Taylor RF, Gaya H, Hodson ME: *Pseudomonas cepacia*: Pulmonary infection in patients with cystic fibrosis. Respir Med 87:187-192, 1993.

697. Govan JR, Hughes JE, Vandamme P: *Burkholderia cepacia*: Medical, taxonomic and ecological issues. J Med Microbiol 45:395-407, 1996.

698. Mahenthiralingam E, Campbell ME, Henry DA, et al: Epidemiology of *Burkholderia cepacia* infection in patients with cystic fibrosis: Analysis by randomly amplified polymorphic DNA fingerprinting. J Clin Microbiol 34:2914-2920, 1996.

699. Doring G: The role of neutrophil elastase in chronic inflammation. Am J Respir Crit Care Med 150:S114-S117, 1994.

700. Elborn JS, Shale DJ: Cystic fibrosis. 2. Lung injury in cystic fibrosis. Thorax 45:970-973, 1990.

701. Fuchs HJ, Borowitz DS, Christiansen DH, et al: Effect of aerosolized recombinant human DNase on exacerbations of respiratory symptoms and on pulmonary function in patients with cystic fibrosis. The Pulmozyme Study Group. N Engl J Med 331:637-642, 1994.

702. Ogrinc G, Kampalath B, Tomashefski JF Jr: Destruction and loss of bronchial cartilage in cystic fibrosis. Hum Pathol 29:65-73, 1998.

703. Vawter G, Shwachman H: Cystic fibrosis in adults: An autopsy study. In Sommers S, Rosen P (eds): Pathology Annual. Part 2. New York, Appleton-Century-Crofts, 1979, p 357.

704. Sobonya RE, Taussig LM: Quantitative aspects of lung pathology in cystic fibrosis. Am Rev Respir Dis 134:290-295, 1986.

705. Tomashefski JF Jr, Konstan MW, Bruce MC, et al: The pathologic characteristics of interstitial pneumonia in cystic fibrosis. A retrospective autopsy study. Am J Clin Pathol 91:522-530, 1989.

706. Tiddens HA, Koopman LP, Lambert RK, et al: Cartilaginous airway wall dimensions and airway resistance in cystic fibrosis lungs. Eur Respir J 15:735-742, 2000.

707. Friedman PJ, Harwood IR, Ellenbogen PH: Pulmonary cystic fibrosis in the adult: Early and late radiologic findings with pathologic correlations. AJR Am J Roentgenol 136:1131-1144, 1981.

708. Grum CM, Lynch JP 3rd: Chest radiographic findings in cystic fibrosis. Semin Respir Infect 7:193-209, 1992.

709. Friedman PJ: Chest radiographic findings in the adult with cystic fibrosis. Semin Roentgenol 22:114-124, 1987.

710. Shale DJ: Chest radiology in cystic fibrosis: Is scoring useful? Thorax 49:847, 1994.

711. Conway SP, Pond MN, Bowler I, et al: The chest radiograph in cystic fibrosis: A new scoring system compared with the Chrispin-Norman and Brasfield scores. Thorax 49:860-862, 1994.

712. Santis G, Hodson ME, Strickland B: High resolution computed tomography in adult cystic fibrosis patients with mild lung disease. Clin Radiol 44:20-22, 1991.

713. de Jong PA, Nakano Y, Lequin MH, et al: Progressive damage on high resolution computed tomography despite stable lung function in cystic fibrosis. Eur Respir J 23:93-97, 2004.

714. Wood BP: Cystic fibrosis: 1997. Radiology 204:1-10, 1997.

715. Stern E, Frank M: Small airway diseases of the lung: Findings at expiration. AJR Am J Roentgenol 147:670, 1986.

716. Shepherd RW, Holt TL, Thomas BJ, et al: Nutritional rehabilitation in cystic fibrosis: Controlled studies of effects on nutritional growth retardation, body protein turnover, and course of pulmonary disease. J Pediatr 109:788-794, 1986.

717. Cipolli M, Perini S, Valletta EA, et al: Bronchial artery embolization in the management of hemoptysis in cystic fibrosis. Pediatr Pulmonol 19:344-347, 1995.

718. McLaughlin FJ, Matthews WJ Jr, Strieder DJ, et al: Pneumothorax in cystic fibrosis: Management and outcome. J Pediatr 100:863-869, 1982.

719. Wonne R, Hofmann D, Posselt HG, et al: Bronchial allergy in cystic fibrosis. Clin Allergy 15:455-463, 1985.

720. Knutsen A, Slavin RG: Allergic bronchopulmonary mycosis complicating cystic fibrosis. Semin Respir Infect 7:179-192, 1992.

721. Laufer P, Fink JN, Bruns WT, et al: Allergic bronchopulmonary aspergillosis in cystic fibrosis. J Allerg Clin Immunol 73:44-48, 1984.

722. Kaplan E, Shwachman H, Perlmutter AD, et al: Reproductive failure in males with cystic fibrosis. N Engl J Med 279:65-69, 1968.

723. Jones JD, Steige H, Logan GB: Variations of sweat sodium values in children and adults with cystic fibrosis and other diseases. Mayo Clin Proc 45:768-773, 1970.

724. Kant JA, Mifflin TE, McGlennen R, et al: Molecular diagnosis of cystic fibrosis. Clin Lab Med 15:877-898, 1995.

725. Farrell PM, Fost N: Prenatal screening for cystic fibrosis: Where are we now? J Pediatr 141:758-763, 2002.

726. Farrell MH, Farrell PM: Newborn screening for cystic fibrosis: Ensuring more good than harm. J Pediatr 143:707-712, 2003.

727. Khoury MJ, McCabe LL, McCabe ER: Population screening in the age of genomic medicine. N Engl J Med 348:50-58, 2003.

728. Tepper RS, Montgomery GL, Ackerman V, et al: Longitudinal evaluation of pulmonary function in infants and very young children with cystic fibrosis. Pediatr Pulmonol 16:96-100, 1993.

729. Featherby EA, Weng TR, Crozier DN, et al: Dynamic and static lung volumes, blood gas tensions, and diffusing capacity in patients with cystic fibrosis. Am Rev Respir Dis 102:737-749, 1970.

730. Lebecque P, Lapierre JG, Lamarre A, et al: Diffusion capacity and oxygen desaturation effects on exercise in patients with cystic fibrosis. Chest 91:693-697, 1987.

731. Lands LC, Heigenhauser GJ, Jones NL: Analysis of factors limiting maximal exercise performance in cystic fibrosis. Clin Sci (Lond) 83:391-397, 1992.

732. Tepper RS, Skatrud JB, Dempsey JA: Ventilation and oxygenation changes during sleep in cystic fibrosis. Chest 84:388-393, 1983.

733. Corey M, Edwards L, Levison H, et al: Longitudinal analysis of pulmonary function decline in patients with cystic fibrosis. J Pediatr 131:809-814, 1997.

734. Smyth A, O'Hea U, Williams G, et al: Passive smoking and impaired lung function in cystic fibrosis. Arch Dis Child 71:353-354, 1994.

735. Dodge JA, Morison S, Lewis PA, et al: Incidence, population, and survival of cystic fibrosis in the UK, 1968-95. UK Cystic Fibrosis Survey Management Committee. Arch Dis Child 77:493-496, 1997.

736. Phelan P, Hey E: Cystic fibrosis mortality in England and Wales and in Victoria, Australia 1976-80. Arch Dis Child 59:71-73, 1984.

737. Elborn JS, Shale DJ, Britton JR: Cystic fibrosis: Current survival and population estimates to the year 2000. Thorax 46:881-885, 1991.

738. Mendeloff EN, Huddleston CB, Mallory GB, et al: Pediatric and adult lung transplantation for cystic fibrosis. J Thorac Cardiovasc Surg 115:404-413, discussion 413-414, 1998.

739. Dankert-Roelse JE, te Meerman GJ: Long term prognosis of patients with cystic fibrosis in relation to early detection by neonatal screening and treatment in a cystic fibrosis centre. Thorax 50:712-718, 1995.

740. Doershuk CF, Matthews LW, Tucker AS, et al: Evaluation of a prophylactic and therapeutic program for patients with cystic fibrosis. Pediatrics 36:675-688, 1965.

741. Moorcroft AJ, Dodd ME, Webb AK: Exercise testing and prognosis in adult cystic fibrosis. Thorax 52:291-293, 1997.

742. Penketh AR, Wise A, Mearns MB, et al: Cystic fibrosis in adolescents and adults. Thorax 42:526-532, 1987.

743. Lewin LO, Byard PJ, Davis PB: Effect of Pseudomonas cepacia colonization on survival and pulmonary function of cystic fibrosis patients. J Clin Epidemiol 43:125-131, 1990.

744. Salvatore F, Scudiero O, Castaldo G: Genotype-phenotype correlation in cystic fibrosis: The role of modifier genes. Am J Med Genet 111:88-95, 2002.

745. Barker AF: Bronchiectasis. Semin Thorac Cardiovasc Surg 7:112-118, 1995.

746. Sanderson JM, Kennedy MC, Johnson MF, et al: Bronchiectasis: Results of surgical and conservative management. A review of 393 cases. Thorax 29:407-416, 1974.

747. Bard M, Couderc LJ, Saimot AG, et al: Accelerated obstructive pulmonary disease in HIV infected patients with bronchiectasis. Eur Respir J 11:771-775, 1998.

748. Loubeyre P, Revel D, Delignette A, et al: Bronchiectasis detected with thin-section CT as a predictor of chronic lung allograft rejection. Radiology 194:213-216, 1995.

749. Morehead RS: Bronchiectasis in bone marrow transplantation. Thorax 52:392-393, 1997.

750. Smith IE, Flower CD: Review article: Imaging in bronchiectasis. Br J Radiol 69:589-593, 1996.

751. Sepper R, Konttinen YT, Ding Y, et al: Human neutrophil collagenase (MMP-8), identified in bronchiectasis BAL fluid, correlates with severity of disease. Chest 107:1641-1647, 1995.

752. Lloberes P, Montserrat E, Montserrat JM, et al: Sputum sol phase proteins and elastase activity in patients with clinically stable bronchiectasis. Thorax 47:88-92, 1992.

753. Eller J, Lapa e Silva JR, Poulter LW, et al: Cells and cytokines in chronic bronchial infection. Ann N Y Acad Sci 725:331-345, 1994.

754. Pasteur MC, Helliwell SM, Houghton SJ, et al: An investigation into causative factors in patients with bronchiectasis. Am J Respir Crit Care Med 162:1277-1284, 2000.

755. Klingman KL, Pye A, Murphy TF, et al: Dynamics of respiratory tract colonization by Branhamella catarrhalis in bronchiectasis. Am J Respir Crit Care Med 152:1072-1078, 1995.

756. Verghese A, al-Samman M, Nabhan D, et al: Bacterial bronchitis and bronchiectasis in human immunodeficiency virus infection. Arch Intern Med 154:2086-2091, 1994.

757. Hoeffler HB, Schweppe HI, Greenberg SD: Bronchiectasis following pulmonary ammonia burn. Arch Pathol Lab Med 106:686-687, 1982.

758. Tasaka S, Kanazawa M, Mori M, et al: Long-term course of bronchiectasis and bronchiolitis obliterans as late complication of smoke inhalation. Respiration 62:40-42, 1995.

759. Croxatto OC, Lanari A: Pathogenesis of bronchiectasis; experimental study and anatomic findings. J Thorac Surg 27:514-528, 1954.

760. Udwadia ZF, Pilling JR, Jenkins PF, et al: Bronchoscopic and bronchographic findings in 12 patients with sarcoidosis and severe or progressive airways obstruction. Thorax 45:272-275, 1990.

761. Lee SH, Lee KS, Ahn JM, et al: Paraquat poisoning of the lung: Thin-section CT findings. Radiology 195:271-274, 1995.

762. Takanami I, Imamuma T, Yamamoto Y, et al: Bronchiectasis complicating rheumatoid arthritis. Respir Med 89:453-454, 1995.

763. Garg K, Lynch DA, Newell JD: Inflammatory airways disease in ulcerative colitis: CT and high-resolution CT features. J Thorac Imaging 8:159-163, 1993.

764. Robinson DA, Meyer CF: Primary Sjögren's syndrome associated with recurrent sinopulmonary infections and bronchiectasis. J Allergy Clin Immunol 94:263-264, 1994.

765. Cudkowicz L: Bronchiectasis and bronchial artery circulation. In Moser KM (ed): Pulmonary Vascular Diseases. Lung Biology in Health and Diseases. New York, Marcel Dekker, 1979, p 165.

766. Clark NS: Bronchiectasis in childhood. BMJ 5323:80-88, 1963.

767. van der Bruggen-Bogaarts BA, van der Bruggen HM, van Waes PF, et al: Screening for bronchiectasis. A comparative study between chest radiography and high-resolution CT. Chest 109:608-611, 1996.

768. Kim JS, Müller NL, Park CS, et al: Cylindrical bronchiectasis: Diagnostic findings on thin-section CT. AJR Am J Roentgenol 168:751-754, 1997.

769. Park CS, Müller NL, Worthy SA, et al: Airway obstruction in asthmatic and healthy individuals: Inspiratory and expiratory thin-section CT findings. Radiology 203:361-367, 1997.

770. Kang EY, Miller RR, Müller NL: Bronchiectasis: Comparison of preoperative thin-section CT and pathologic findings in resected specimens. Radiology 195:649-654, 1995.

771. McGuinness G, Naidich DP, Leitman BS, et al: Bronchiectasis: CT evaluation. AJR Am J Roentgenol 160:253-259, 1993.

772. Naidich DP, McCauley DI, Khouri NF, et al: Computed tomography of bronchiectasis. J Comput Assist Tomogr 6:437-444, 1982.

773. Hansell DM, Wells AU, Rubens MB, et al: Bronchiectasis: Functional significance of areas of decreased attenuation at expiratory CT. Radiology 193:369-374, 1994.

774. Thomas RD, Blaquiere RM: Reactive mediastinal lymphadenopathy in bronchiectasis assessed by CT. Acta Radiol 34:489-491, 1993.

775. Nicotra MB, Rivera M, Dale AM, et al: Clinical, pathophysiologic, and microbiologic characterization of bronchiectasis in an aging cohort. Chest 108:955-961, 1995.

776. Tanaka E, Tada K, Amitani R, et al: Systemic hypersensitivity vasculitis associated with bronchiectasis. Chest 102:647-649, 1992.

777. Cherniack N, Vosti KL, Saxton GA, et al: Pulmonary function tests in fifty patients with bronchiectasis. J Lab Clin Med 53:693-707, 1959.

778. Evans SA, Turner SM, Bosch BJ, et al: Lung function in bronchiectasis: The influence of Pseudomonas aeruginosa. Eur Respir J 9:1601-1604, 1996.

779. Perry K, King D: Bronchiectasis: A study of prognosis based on a follow-up of 400 patients. Am Rev Respir Dis 41:531, 1940.

780. Evans DJ, Greenstone M: Long-term antibiotics in the management of non-CF bronchiectasis—do they improve outcome? Respir Med 97:851-8.58, 2003.

781. Ellis DA, Thornley PE, Wightman AJ, et al: Present outlook in bronchiectasis: Clinical and social study and review of factors influencing prognosis. Thorax 36:659-664, 1981.

782. Helm WH, Thompson VC: The long-term results of resection for bronchiectasis. Q J Med 27:353-367, 1958.

783. Kartagener M: Zur Pathogenese der Bronchiektasien: Bronchiektasien bei Situs viscerum inversum. Beitr Klin Tuberk 83:489, 1933.

784. Rossman CM, Forrest JB, Lee RM, et al: The dyskinetic cilia syndrome; abnormal ciliary motility in association with abnormal ciliary ultrastructure. Chest 80:860-865, 1981.

785. Holmes LB, Blennerhassett JB, Austen KF: A reappraisal of Kartagener's syndrome. Am J Med Sci 255:13-28, 1968.

786. Kroon AA, Heij JM, Kuijper WA, et al: Function and morphology of respiratory cilia in situs inversus. Clin Otolaryngol 16:294-297, 1991.

787. Katsuhara K, Kawamoto S, Wakabayashi T, et al: Situs inversus totalis and Kartagener's syndrome in a Japanese population. Chest 61:56-61, 1972.

788. Rott HD: Genetics of Kartagener's syndrome. Eur J Respir Dis Suppl 127:1-4, 1983.

789. Chao J, Turner JA, Sturgess JM: Genetic heterogeneity of dynein-deficiency in cilia from patients with respiratory disease. Am Rev Respir Dis 126:302-305, 1982.

790. Matwijiw I, Thliveris JA, Faiman C: Aplasia of nasal cilia with situs inversus, azoospermia and normal sperm flagella: A unique variant of the immotile cilia syndrome. J Urol 137:522-524, 1987.

791. Sturgess JM, Chao J, Wong J, et al: Cilia with defective radial spokes: A cause of human respiratory disease. N Engl J Med 300:53-56, 1979.

792. Wilton LJ, Teichtahl H, Temple-Smith PD, et al: Kartagener's syndrome with motile cilia and immotile spermatozoa: Axonemal ultrastructure and function. Am Rev Respir Dis 134:1233-1236, 1986.

793. Min YG, Shin JS, Choi SH, et al: Primary ciliary dyskinesia: Ultrastructural defects and clinical features. Rhinology 33:189-193, 1995.

794. Nadel HR, Stringer DA, Levison H, et al: The immotile cilia syndrome: Radiological manifestations. Radiology 154:651-655, 1985.

795. Reiff DB, Wells AU, Carr DH, et al: CT findings in bronchiectasis: Limited value in distinguishing between idiopathic and specific types. AJR Am J Roentgenol 165:261-267, 1995.

796. Newhouse MT: "Immotile-cilia" syndrome and ciliary abnormalities induced by infection and injury. Am Rev Respir Dis 125:371, 1982.

797. Kollberg H, Mossberg B, Afzelius BA, et al: Cystic fibrosis compared with the immotile-cilia syndrome. A study of mucociliary clearance, ciliary ultrastructure, clinical picture and ventilatory function. Scand J Respir Dis 59:297-306, 1978.

798. Le Lannou D, Jezequel P, Blayau M, et al: Obstructive azoospermia with agenesis of vas deferens or with bronchiectasia (Young's syndrome): A genetic approach. Hum Reprod 10:338-341, 1995.

799. Oates RD, Amos JA: The genetic basis of congenital bilateral absence of the vas deferens and cystic fibrosis. J Androl 15:1-8, 1994.

800. Lissens W, Mercier B, Tournaye H, et al: Cystic fibrosis and infertility caused by congenital bilateral absence of the vas deferens and related clinical entities. Hum Reprod 11(Suppl 4):55-78, discussion 79-80, 1996.

801. de Iongh R, Ing A, Rutland J: Mucociliary function, ciliary ultrastructure, and ciliary orientation in Young's syndrome. Thorax 47:184-187, 1992.

802. Hendry WF, A'Hern RP, Cole PJ: Was Young's syndrome caused by exposure to mercury in childhood? BMJ 307:1579-1582, 1993.

803. Hershko A, Hirshberg B, Nahir M, et al: Yellow nail syndrome. Postgrad Med J 73:466-468, 1997.

804. Morandi U, Golinelli M, Brandi L, et al: "Yellow nail syndrome" associated with chronic recurrent pericardial and pleural effusions. Eur J Cardiothorac Surg 9:42-44, 1995.

805. Palmer SM Jr, Layish DT, Kussin PS, et al: Lung transplantation for Williams-Campbell syndrome. Chest 113:534-537, 1998.

806. Lee P, Bush A, Warner JO: Left bronchial isomerism associated with bronchomalacia, presenting with intractable wheeze. Thorax 46:459-461, 1991.

807. Kaneko K, Kudo S, Tashiro M, et al: Case report: Computed tomography findings in Williams-Campbell syndrome. J Thorac Imaging 6:11-13, 1991.

808. Chalermskulrat W, Gilbey JG, Donohue JF: Nontuberculous mycobacteria in women, young and old. Clin Chest Med 23:675-686, 2002.

809. Reich JM, Johnson RE: *Mycobacterium avium* complex pulmonary disease presenting as an isolated lingular or middle lobe pattern. The Lady Windermere syndrome. Chest 101:1605-1609, 1992.

810. Uragoda CG: Broncholithiasis secondary to intrapleural calcification. BMJ 2:1635-1636, 1966.

811. Vix VA: Radiographic manifestations of broncholithiasis. Radiology 128:295-299, 1978.

812. Conces DJ Jr, Tarver RD, Vix VA: Broncholithiasis: CT features in 15 patients. AJR Am J Roentgenol 157:249-253, 1991.

813. Hollaus PH, Lax F, el-Nashef BB, et al: Natural history of bronchopleural fistula after pneumonectomy: A review of 96 cases. Ann Thorac Surg 63:1391-1396, discussion 1397, 1997.

814. Powner DJ, Bierman MI: Thoracic and extrathoracic bronchial fistulas. Chest 100:480-486, 1991.

815. Stern EJ, Sun H, Haramati LB: Peripheral bronchopleural fistulas: CT imaging features. AJR Am J Roentgenol 167:117-120, 1996.

816. Ryu JH, Myers JL, Swensen SJ: Bronchiolar disorders. Am J Respir Crit Care Med 168:1277-1292, 2003.

817. Adesina AM, Vallyathan V, McQuillen EN, et al: Bronchiolar inflammation and fibrosis associated with smoking. A morphologic cross-sectional population analysis. Am Rev Respir Dis 143:144-149, 1991.

818. Yousem SA: Lymphocytic bronchitis/bronchiolitis in lung allograft recipients. Am J Surg Pathol 17:491-496, 1993.

819. Matsuse T, Oka T, Kida K, et al: Importance of diffuse aspiration bronchiolitis caused by chronic occult aspiration in the elderly. Chest 110:1289-1293, 1996.

820. Wright JL, Churg A: Morphology of small-airway lesions in patients with asbestos exposure. Hum Pathol 15:68-74, 1984.

821. Epler GR, Colby TV, McLoud TC, et al: Bronchiolitis obliterans organizing pneumonia. N Engl J Med 312:152-158, 1985.

822. American Thoracic Society/European Respiratory Society International Multidisciplinary Consensus Classification of the Idiopathic Interstitial Pneumonias. This joint statement of the American Thoracic Society (ATS), and the European Respiratory Society (ERS) was adopted by the ATS board of directors, June 2001 and by the ERS Executive Committee, June 2001. Am J Respir Crit Care Med 165:277-304, 2002.

823. McLoud TC, Epler GR, Colby TV, et al: Bronchiolitis obliterans. Radiology 159:1-8, 1986.

824. Sweatman MC, Millar AB, Strickland B, et al: Computed tomography in adult obliterative bronchiolitis. Clin Radiol 41:116-119, 1990.

825. Davies HD, Wang EE, Manson D, et al: Reliability of the chest radiograph in the diagnosis of lower respiratory infections in young children. Pediatr Infect Dis J 15:600-604, 1996.

826. Dawson KP, Long A, Kennedy J, et al: The chest radiograph in acute bronchiolitis. J Paediatr Child Health 26:209-211, 1990.

827. Lynch DA: Imaging of small airways diseases. Clin Chest Med 14:623-634, 1993.

828. Müller NL, Miller RR: Diseases of the bronchioles: CT and histopathologic findings. Radiology 196:3-12, 1995.

829. Worthy SA, Flint JD, Müller NL: Pulmonary complications after bone marrow transplantation: High-resolution CT and pathologic findings. Radiographics 17:1359-1371, 1997.

830. Nishimura K, Kitaichi M, Izumi T, et al: Diffuse panbronchiolitis: Correlation of high-resolution CT and pathologic findings. Radiology 184:779-785, 1992.

831. Gruden JF, Webb WR, Warnock M: Centrilobular opacities in the lung on high-resolution CT: Diagnostic considerations and pathologic correlation. AJR Am J Roentgenol 162:569-574, 1994.

832. Padley SP, Adler BD, Hansell DM, et al: Bronchiolitis obliterans: High resolution CT findings and correlation with pulmonary function tests. Clin Radiol 47:236-240, 1993.

833. Worthy SA, Park CS, Kim JS, et al: Bronchiolitis obliterans after lung transplantation: High-resolution CT findings in 15 patients. AJR Am J Roentgenol 169:673-677, 1997.

834. Desai SR, Hansell DM: Small airways disease: Expiratory computed tomography comes of age. Clin Radiol 52:332-337, 1997.

835. Webb WR, Stern EJ, Kanth N, et al: Dynamic pulmonary CT: Findings in healthy adult men. Radiology 186:117-124, 1993.

836. Worthy SA, Müller NL, Hartman TE, et al: Mosaic attenuation pattern on thin-section CT scans of the lung: Differentiation among infiltrative lung, airway, and vascular diseases as a cause. Radiology 205:465-470, 1997.

837. Hansell DM, Wells AU, Padley SP, et al: Hypersensitivity pneumonitis: Correlation of individual CT patterns with functional abnormalities. Radiology 199:123-128, 1996.

838. Lynch DA, Newell JD, Tschomper BA, et al: Uncomplicated asthma in adults: Comparison of CT appearance of the lungs in asthmatic and healthy subjects. Radiology 188:829-833, 1993.

839. Arakawa H, Webb WR, McCowin M, et al: Inhomogeneous lung attenuation at thin-section CT: Diagnostic value of expiratory scans. Radiology 206:89-94, 1998.

840. Lee KS, Kullnig P, Hartman TE, et al: Cryptogenic organizing pneumonia: CT findings in 43 patients. AJR Am J Roentgenol 162:543-546, 1994.

841. Small JH, Flower CD, Traill ZC, et al: Air-trapping in extrinsic allergic alveolitis on computed tomography. Clin Radiol 51:684-688, 1996.

842. Welliver JR, Welliver RC: Bronchiolitis. Pediatr Rev 14:134-139, 1993.

843. Hogg JC, Williams J, Richardson JB, et al: Age as a factor in the distribution of lower-airway conductance and in the pathologic anatomy of obstructive lung disease. N Engl J Med 282:1283-1287, 1970.

844. Chan ED, Kalayanamit T, Lynch DA, et al: *Mycoplasma pneumoniae*–associated bronchiolitis causing severe restrictive lung disease in adults: Report of three cases and literature review. Chest 115:1188-1194, 1999.

845. Wright JL: Inhalational lung injury causing bronchiolitis. Clin Chest Med 14:635-644, 1993.

846. Tse RL, Bockman AA: Nitrogen dioxide toxicity. Report of four cases in firemen. JAMA 212:1341-1344, 1970.

847. Wright JL, Cagle P, Churg A, et al: Diseases of the small airways. Am Rev Respir Dis 146:240-262, 1992.

848. Selman-Lama M, Perez-Padilla R: Airflow obstruction and airway lesions in hypersensitivity pneumonitis. Clin Chest Med 14:699-714, 1993.

849. Moira CY, Enarson DA, Kennedy SM: The impact of grain dust on respiratory health. Am Rev Respir Dis 145:476-487, 1992.

850. Malmberg P, Rask-Andersen A, Hoglund S, et al: Incidence of organic dust toxic syndrome and allergic alveolitis in Swedish farmers. Int Arch Allergy Appl Immunol 87:47-54, 1988.

851. Wells AU, du Bois RM: Bronchiolitis in association with connective tissue disorders. Clin Chest Med 14:655-666, 1993.

852. Wolfe F, Schurle DR, Lin JJ, et al: Upper and lower airway disease in penicillamine treated patients with rheumatoid arthritis. J Rheumatol 10:406-410, 1983.

853. Tomioka R, King TE Jr: Gold-induced pulmonary disease: Clinical features, outcome, and differentiation from rheumatoid lung disease. Am J Respir Crit Care Med 155:1011-1020, 1997.

854. Reichenspurner H, Girgis RE, Robbins RC, et al: Stanford experience with obliterative bronchiolitis after lung and heart-lung transplantation. Ann Thorac Surg 62:1467-1472, discussion 1472-1473, 1996.

855. Philit F, Wiesendanger T, Archimbaud E, et al: Post-transplant obstructive lung disease ("bronchiolitis obliterans"): A clinical comparative study of bone marrow and lung transplant patients. Eur Respir J 8:551-558, 1995.

856. Dauber JH: Posttransplant bronchiolitis obliterans syndrome. Where have we been and where are we going? Chest 109:857-859, 1996.

857. Sundaresan S, Trulock EP, Mohanakumar T, et al: Prevalence and outcome of bronchiolitis obliterans syndrome after lung transplantation. Washington University Lung Transplant Group. Ann Thorac Surg 60:1341-1346, discussion 1346-1347, 1995.

858. Houk VN, Kent DC, Fosburg RG: Unilateral hyperlucent lung: A study in pathophysiology and etiology. Am J Med Sci 253:406-416, 1967.

859. Reid L, Simon G: Unilateral lung transradiancy. Thorax 17:230-239, 1962.

860. Ghossain MA, Achkar A, Buy JN, et al: Swyer-James syndrome documented by spiral CT angiography and high resolution inspiratory and expiratory CT: An accurate single modality exploration. J Comput Assist Tomogr 21:616-618, 1997.

861. Moore AD, Godwin JD, Dietrich PA, et al: Swyer-James syndrome: CT findings in eight patients. AJR Am J Roentgenol 158:1211-1215, 1992.

862. Margolin HN, Rosenberg LS, Felson B, et al: Idiopathic unilateral hyperlucent lung: A roentgenologic syndrome. Am J Roentgenol Radium Ther Nucl Med 82:63-75, 1959.

863. Davison A, Heard B, McAllister W, et al: Steroid-responsive relapsing cryptogenic organizing pneumonitis. Thorax 37:785, 1982.

864. Cordier JF: Cryptogenic organizing pneumonitis. Bronchiolitis obliterans organizing pneumonia. Clin Chest Med 14:677-692, 1993.

865. Akira M, Yamamoto S, Sakatani M: Bronchiolitis obliterans organizing pneumonia manifesting as multiple large nodules or masses. AJR Am J Roentgenol 170:291-295, 1998.

866. Spiteri MA, Klenerman P, Sheppard MN, et al: Seasonal cryptogenic organising pneumonia with biochemical cholestasis: A new clinical entity. Lancet 340:281-284, 1992.

867. Chandler PW, Shin MS, Friedman SE, et al: Radiographic manifestations of bronchiolitis obliterans with organizing pneumonia vs usual interstitial pneumonia. AJR Am J Roentgenol 147:899-906, 1986.

868. Müller NL, Guerry-Force ML, Staples CA, et al: Differential diagnosis of bronchiolitis obliterans with organizing pneumonia and usual interstitial pneumonia: Clinical, functional, and radiologic findings. Radiology 162:151-156, 1987.

869. Cordier JF, Loire R, Brune J: Idiopathic bronchiolitis obliterans organizing pneumonia. Definition of characteristic clinical profiles in a series of 16 patients. Chest 96:999-1004, 1989.

870. Nishimura K, Itoh H: High-resolution computed tomographic features of bronchiolitis obliterans organizing pneumonia. Chest 102:26S-31S, 1992.

871. Bouchardy LM, Kuhlman JE, Ball WC Jr, et al: CT findings in bronchiolitis obliterans organizing pneumonia (BOOP) with radiographic, clinical, and histologic correlation. J Comput Assist Tomogr 17:352-357, 1993.

872. King TE Jr, Mortenson RL: Cryptogenic organizing pneumonitis. The North American experience. Chest 102:8S-13S, 1992.

873. Epler GR: Bronchiolitis obliterans organizing pneumonia. Arch Intern Med 161:158-164, 2001.

874. Cordier JF: Organising pneumonia. Thorax 55:318-328, 2000.

875. Guerry-Force ML, Müller NL, Wright JL, et al: A comparison of bronchiolitis obliterans with organizing pneumonia, usual interstitial pneumonia, and small airways disease. Am Rev Respir Dis 135:705-712, 1987.

876. Nizami IY, Kissner DG, Visscher DW, et al: Idiopathic bronchiolitis obliterans with organizing pneumonia. An acute and life-threatening syndrome. Chest 108:271-277, 1995.

877. Cohen AJ, King TE Jr, Downey GP: Rapidly progressive bronchiolitis obliterans with organizing pneumonia. Am J Respir Crit Care Med 149:1670-1675, 1994.

878. Lohr RH, Boland BJ, Douglas WW, et al: Organizing pneumonia. Features and prognosis of cryptogenic, secondary, and focal variants. Arch Intern Med 157:1323-1329, 1997.

879. Cosio MG, Hale KA, Niewoehner DE: Morphologic and morphometric effects of prolonged cigarette smoking on the small airways. Am Rev Respir Dis 122:265-221, 1980.

880. Wright JL, Lawson LM, Paré PD, et al: Morphology of peripheral airways in current smokers and ex-smokers. Am Rev Respir Dis 127:474-477, 1983.

881. Fraig M, Shreesha U, Savici D, et al: Respiratory bronchiolitis: A clinicopathologic study in current smokers, ex-smokers, and never-smokers. Am J Surg Pathol 26:647-653, 2002.

882. King TE Jr: Respiratory bronchiolitis–associated interstitial lung disease. Clin Chest Med 14:693-6.98, 1993.

883. Moon J, du Bois RM, Colby TV, et al: Clinical significance of respiratory bronchiolitis on open lung biopsy and its relationship to smoking related interstitial lung disease. Thorax 54:1009-1014, 1999.

884. Remy-Jardin M, Remy J, Gosselin B, et al: Lung parenchymal changes secondary to cigarette smoking: Pathologic-CT correlations. Radiology 186:643-651, 1993.

885. Park JS, Brown KK, Tuder RM, et al: Respiratory bronchiolitis–associated interstitial lung disease: Radiologic features with clinical and pathologic correlation. J Comput Assist Tomogr 26:13-20, 2002.

886. Yousem SA, Colby TV, Carrington CB: Follicular bronchitis/bronchiolitis. Hum Pathol 16:700-706, 1985.

887. Fortoul TI, Cano-Valle F, Oliva E, et al: Follicular bronchiolitis in association with connective tissue diseases. Lung 163:305-314, 1985.

888. Howling SJ, Hansell DM, Wells AU, et al: Follicular bronchiolitis: Thin-section CT and histologic findings. Radiology 212:637-642, 1999.

889. Iwata M, Colby TV, Kitaichi M: Diffuse panbronchiolitis: Diagnosis and distinction from various pulmonary diseases with centrilobular interstitial foam cell accumulations. Hum Pathol 25:357-363, 1994.

890. Krishnan P, Thachil R, Gillego V: Diffuse panbronchiolitis: A treatable sinobronchial disease in need of recognition in the United States. Chest 121:659-661, 2002.

891. Homma H, Yamanaka A, Tanimoto S, et al: Diffuse panbronchiolitis. A disease of the transitional zone of the lung. Chest 83:63-69, 1983.

892. Hoiby N: Diffuse panbronchiolitis and cystic fibrosis: East meets West. Thorax 49:531-532, 1994.

893. Sugiyama Y, Saitoh K, Kano S, et al: An autopsy case of diffuse panbronchiolitis accompanying rheumatoid arthritis. Respir Med 90:175-177, 1996.

894. Ono K, Shimamoto Y, Matsuzaki M, et al: Diffuse panbronchiolitis as a pulmonary complication in patients with adult T-cell leukemia. Am J Hematol 30:86-90, 1989.

895. Randhawa P, Hoagland MH, Yousem SA: Diffuse panbronchiolitis in North America. Report of three cases and review of the literature. Am J Surg Pathol 15:43-47, 1991.

896. Maeda M, Saiki S, Yamanaka A: Serial section analysis of the lesions in diffuse panbronchiolitis. Acta Pathol Jpn 37:693-704, 1987.

897. Nakata K, Tanimoto H: [Diffuse panbronchiolitis (authors' transl).] Rinsho Hoshasen 26:1133-1142, 1981.

898. Akira M, Kitatani F, Lee YS, et al: Diffuse panbronchiolitis: Evaluation with high-resolution CT. Radiology 168:433-438, 1988.

899. Keicho N, Kudoh S: Diffuse panbronchiolitis: Role of macrolides in therapy. Am J Respir Med 1:119-131, 2002.

PULMONARY DISEASE CAUSED BY INHALED INORGANIC DUST

Pneumoconiosis can be defined as "a condition characterized by permanent deposition of substantial amounts of particulate matter in the lungs, usually of occupational or environmental origin, and by the tissue reaction to its presence."[1] This reaction usually takes one of two histologic forms:

1. Fibrosis, which can be focal and nodular (as in silicosis) or diffuse (as in asbestosis); it often results in radiologic abnormalities and may lead to significant lung impairment.
2. Aggregates of particle-laden macrophages with minimal or no accompanying fibrosis. This reaction is typically seen with inert dust such as iron, tin, and barium; though sometimes causing radiologic abnormalities, it is associated with minimal, if any, functional or clinical consequences.

Although the death rate from pneumoconiosis has been declining gradually in the United States over the past 35 years,[2] the condition remains an important cause of morbidity and mortality: during the 29-year period from 1968 to 1996, there were more than 113,000 pneumoconiosis deaths among U.S. residents.[2]

The possibility of dust-related disease should be considered in almost any patient who presents with virtually any kind of pulmonary problem. Identification of a work-related cause of

disease is important both for the affected individual and for those who work under similar conditions: removal of the worker from exposure could modulate disease progression, identification of other affected workers could be facilitated, and preventive measures in the workplace could be initiated or improved. Unfortunately, establishment of a relationship between an inhaled dust and pulmonary disease is not always straightforward, for several reasons:

1. A particular job can be associated with multiple dust exposures, in which case it can be difficult to attribute pathologic changes to one specific substance. For example, in shale miners, progressive massive fibrosis sometimes develops similar to that seen in coal miners; their lungs have been shown to contain dust composed of a combination of kaolinite, mica, and silica,[3] each of which by itself can cause pulmonary disease.
2. Exposure to any given dust can be seen in a number of occupations.
3. Some particulates cause disease in more than one site and of several types[4]; for example, asbestos dust can cause interstitial pulmonary fibrosis, obstructive airway disease, pleural fibrosis, and pulmonary carcinoma.
4. Significant dust exposure can occur in para-occupational settings[5] (e.g., we have seen a laundry worker in whom chronic berylliosis developed after washing the uniforms of workers from a copper

recycling plant) or in nonoccupational (environmental) settings (e.g., silicosis has been reported in the inhabitants of a Himalayan village who experienced frequent dust storms[6]).

5. Some new substances that are introduced into the workplace are found to cause lung disease, and there is an inevitable delay in the recognition of their toxicity.[7]

The reaction of the lung to inhaled inorganic dust depends on several factors. The effects of particle size and shape, the rate and pattern of breathing, the distribution and concentration of inhaled particles, and pulmonary clearance are considered in Chapter 1 (see page 50). There is no doubt that different workers exposed to identical amounts of dust can have profoundly different reactions and severity of disease. This variability in disease expression may be related to a number of factors, including differences in lung structure,[8] genetic susceptibility,[9] efficiency of dust clearance,[10] exposure to other noxious agents (such as tobacco smoke), and the presence of other disease (such as rheumatoid disease).

INTERNATIONAL CLASSIFICATION OF RADIOGRAPHS OF THE PNEUMOCONIOSES

The chest radiograph is an important tool for detecting the effects of particle deposition in the lungs and assessing the progression of ensuing disease.[11] For it to be useful in epidemiologic studies, however, it is essential that an acceptable classification of the extent of involvement be followed and a standard nomenclature be used. The most widely used schema is the International Labour Office (ILO) 1980 International Classification of Radiographs of the Pneumoconioses.[12]

The object of this classification is to codify the radiographic changes associated with the pneumoconioses in a simple and reproducible manner such that international comparability of pneumoconiosis statistics has some validity. Standard reference radiographs have been selected to illustrate the 1980 classification; these radiographs can be purchased from the ILO office. Because the schema uses radiographic descriptors that are somewhat different from those generally used throughout this book, a short glossary of terms follows.

Small Rounded Opacities. These opacities are well-circumscribed nodules ranging in diameter from barely visible to up to 10 mm. The qualifiers *p*, *q*, and *r* subdivide the predominant opacities into three diameter ranges—*p*, up to 1.5 mm; *q*, 1.5 to 3.0 mm; and *r*, 3 to 10 mm.

Small Irregular Opacities. This term is used to describe a pattern that elsewhere in this book has been designated *linear* or *reticular*—in other words, a netlike pattern. Although the nature of these opacities is such that establishment of quantitative dimensions is considerably more difficult than with rounded opacities, three categories have been created—*s*, width up to 1.5 mm; *t*, width exceeding 1.5 mm and up to 3.0 mm; and *u*, width exceeding 3 mm and up to 10 mm.

To record shape and size, two letters must be used. If the reader of the radiograph thinks that all or virtually all opacities are one shape and size, this is noted by recording the symbol twice, separated by an oblique stroke (e.g., *q/q*). If another shape or size is appreciated, this is recorded as the second letter (e.g., *q/t*). The designation *q/t* means that the predominant small opacity is round and of size *q*, but in addi-

tion there are a significant number of small irregular opacities of size *t*. In this way, any combination of small opacities can be recorded.

Profusion. This term refers to the number of small opacities per unit area or zone of lung. There are four basic categories: category 0, small opacities absent or less profuse than in category 1; category 1, small opacities definitely present but few in number (normal lung markings are usually visible); category 2, numerous small opacities (normal lung markings are generally partly obscured); and category 3, very numerous small opacities (normal lung markings are usually totally obscured). These categories can be further subdivided by using a 12-point scale to describe a continuum of changes from complete normality to the most advanced category or grade:[13]

0/−	0/0	0/1
1/0	1/1	1/2
2/1	2/2	2/3
3/2	3/3	3/+

When using this scale, the radiograph is first classified into one of the four categories—0, 1, 2, or 3. If the category above or below is considered a serious alternative during the process, it is recorded (e.g., a radiograph in which profusion is considered to be category 2 but for which category 1 was seriously considered would be graded 2/1). If no alternative is considered (i.e., the profusion was definitely category 2), it would be classified 2/2.

A subdivision is also possible within categories 0 and 3. If the absence of small opacities is particularly obvious, profusion should be recorded as 0/−. Such a category might be seen in a healthy nonsmoking adolescent. A radiograph that shows profusion markedly higher than that classifiable as 3/3 would be recorded as 3/+. The ILO standard films are the final arbitrators of opacity profusion and take precedence over any application of a verbal description of profusion. A film is placed in category 1 if it resembles the ILO film of the same category and opacity type. Thus, this reading should always be done side by side with the ILO standard films.

Large Opacities. This term is reserved for opacities that are greater than 10 mm in diameter. Three categories are recognized: category A, an opacity having a greatest diameter exceeding 1 cm up to and including 5 cm or several opacities each greater than 1 cm, the sum of whose diameters does not exceed 5 cm; category B, one or more opacities larger or more numerous than those in category A whose combined area does not exceed the equivalent of the area of the right upper lung zone; and category C, one or more opacities whose combined area exceeds the equivalent of the area of the right upper lung zone.

Extent. Each lung is divided into three zones—upper, middle and lower—by horizontal lines one third and two thirds of the vertical distance between the apex of the lung and the dome of the diaphragm.

Radiographic Interpretation. To limit observer error in the radiographic diagnosis of pneumoconiosis and in the determination of its extent, the National Institute of Occupational Safety and Health (NIOSH) has established an examination for physicians who wish to be certified as competent interpreters of chest radiographs in pneumoconiosis programs; the examination is preceded by a weekend course administered by the American College of Radiologists. Attendance at the course establishes the physician as an *A reader*; success at the examination results in the more favorable designation *B reader*. Maintenance of competence is ensured by a mandatory recertification examination every 4 years.

There is little doubt that expert readings are superior to nonexpert readings in the detection of disease[14] and avoidance of "over-reading."[15] However, use of the radiograph as a definitive tool for the diagnosis of pneumoconiosis in any given individual is limited by a significant prevalence of small opacities sufficient for "diagnosis" in nonexposed working populations,[16] as well as a certain degree of inter- and intrareader variability.[17] When assessing radiographic progression of simple pneumoconiosis in individual workers, all films should be viewed together in known temporal order.[11] Side-by-side reading has been shown to lead to substantially lower observer variability and error than independent reading.

SILICA

Silica is a ubiquitous and abundant mineral composed of regularly arranged molecules of silicon dioxide (SiO_2). It exists in three forms: (1) *crystalline*, which occurs primarily as quartz, tridymite, or cristobalite; (2) *microcrystalline*, or minute crystals of quartz bonded together by amorphous silica, exemplified by flint and chert; and (3) *amorphous*, which is noncrystalline and consists of kieselguhr (composed of the skeletal remains of diatoms) and several vitreous forms (derived by heating and rapid cooling of the crystalline types). Pure (free) silica (composed predominantly of silicon dioxide) must be distinguished from other substances in which silicon dioxide is combined with an appreciable proportion of various cations ("combined" silica); such "silicates" include asbestos, talc, and mica and are associated with different forms of disease.

Epidemiology

Exposure to a concentration of silica high enough to result in radiologic and pathologic manifestations of silicosis can occur in many occupations[18]; the most common that have been reported in the United States are mining, quarrying, construction, and manufacturing (including foundry and concrete product workers).[2,19] Because of the ubiquity of silica in the earth's crust, miners and quarry workers of such metals as gold, tin, iron, copper, nickel, silver, tungsten, and uranium have a significant risk. The mining of other minerals recognized as causes of pneumoconiosis, such as coal, can be accompanied by silica exposure, which can explain, at least in part, the lung disease of some of these individuals. Sandblasting is a particularly hazardous job because of the potentially large amount of particles that may be produced in a relatively small space. The use of potter's clay and powdered flint (in the ceramics industry), diatomaceous earth (in the manufacturing of paints, varnishes, and insecticides), and ochre, granite, bentonite, enamel, and silica flour is also potentially hazardous.

Although mortality from silicosis is declining in the United States,[2] the disease continues to be an important one: it has been estimated that as many as 3 million workers in 238,000 processing plants are potentially exposed to silica dust.[20] Moreover, respirable levels of silica remain above accepted norms in many industries.[2] When environmental controls are inadequate, silicosis accounts for significant morbidity and mortality, especially in "developing" countries.[21,22] Most individuals in whom the disease develops are men; however, women may also be affected, particularly in the pottery industry[23] and sometimes in association with unusual nonoccupational exposure.[24,25]

Pathogenesis

Two fundamental histologic reactions to inhaled silica can occur: (1) a *silicotic nodule*, which is characterized by dense, often concentric lamellae of collagen and which when multiple and confluent results in a lesion termed *conglomerate silicosis* or *progressive massive fibrosis* (PMF), and (2) *silicoproteinosis*, which typically occurs in individuals exposed to high concentrations of silica. Most studies examining the pathogenesis of silicosis have focused on the first reaction because it is by far the more common.[26]

The interaction of silica with pulmonary macrophages is a key factor in the development of a silicotic nodule. Direct activation of complement in alveolar surfactant induces alveolar macrophages to aggregate around silica particles.[27] After ingestion of these particles, macrophage activation results in the release of a number of substances that promote fibrosis. Two of the most important of these substances are the profibrotic and proinflammatory cytokines tumor necrosis factor-α (TNF-α) and interleukin-1 (IL-1).[28,29] There is evidence that specific genetic polymorphisms related to these two cytokines are associated with both the prevalence and severity of disease,[30,31] which possibly explains some of the individual variation in susceptibility to the effects of inhalation of the dust. Macrophage-derived lymphokines induce lymphocyte aggregation locally and in regional thoracic lymph nodes, from where lymphocytes emigrate to the lung.[32] These cells are predominantly of the CD4+, T_H1 type and facilitate additional lymphocyte and macrophage aggregation within the lung. Macrophages may also contribute to tissue damage by the release of oxidants, which by injuring epithelial cells facilitate exposure of interstitial fibroblasts to the products of other inflammatory cells.[33]

Polymorphonuclear leukocytes also accumulate in the lungs of silica-exposed individuals; they are a source of reactive oxidants and proteolytic enzymes that can contribute to tissue damage[34] if not neutralized by the protease and elastase inhibitors present in bronchoalveolar fluid.[35]

Fas ligand is a membrane-bound and shed protein belonging to the TNF receptor family. Although it is the counterreceptor for the apoptosis-promoting Fas molecule expressed by a wide variety of lymphoid and nonlymphoid tissues, it also has proinflammatory effects.[36] In a murine model of silicosis, antibody to this molecule blocks induction of disease, suggesting that the proinflammatory effects of Fas ligand are of critical importance in pathogenesis.[36]

Crystalline silica is itself cytotoxic. Freshly fractured silica contributes to the formation of a number of bioreactive radicals that can induce both inflammation and fibrosis.[26,37,38] It is possible that adsorption of nonsilica particulates onto the surface of silica diminishes its toxicity[26]; this may explain why the dust burden associated with the development of silicosis is higher when there has been mixed dust exposure than when exposure has been to relatively pure silica alone.

The reasons for the development of PMF in some individuals and not in others are unclear. The complication has been associated with a higher lung dust burden,[39] a history of tuberculosis,[40] a background of increased profusion of small opacities,[41] and genetic[42] and certain environmental (e.g., smoking) influences[43]; however, the precise mechanisms by which these factors might be involved is unclear.

Exposure to a large amount of silica over a relatively short period may result in the production of abundant intra-alveolar lipoproteinaceous material similar to that seen in alveolar proteinosis[44]; typically, there is minimal associated fibrosis. The pathogenesis of this reaction is unclear. Experimentally, instillation of silica into the lungs is followed by type I alveolar cell injury and type II cell hyperplasia and hypertrophy,[45] thus suggesting that an increase in surfactant-producing cells might be a factor. It has also been hypothesized that silica may disturb the ability of macrophages to clear normally produced surfactant from the alveolar air spaces.[46] The reason for the lack of fibrosis in acute silicoproteinosis is likewise unclear; however, it has been shown that coating silica particles with alveolar lining material results in significantly less cytotoxicity for ingesting macrophages.[47]

Pathologic Characteristics

Grossly, silicotic nodules range from 1 to 10 mm in diameter and are typically more numerous in the upper lobes and parahilar regions than elsewhere (see Color Fig. 16–1).[48] Cut sections show the nodules to be more or less well defined, to be spherical or irregularly shaped, and to be firm to hard in texture. Coalescence of nodules results in larger masses that can occupy virtually an entire lobe (PMF) (see Color Fig. 16–2). Such masses are usually associated with emphysema in the adjacent lung and may be cavitated as a result of ischemia, tuberculosis, or infection by anaerobic organisms.[49]

Microscopically, the earliest lesions are characteristically located in the peribronchiolar, interlobular septal, and pleural interstitial tissue. Initially, they consist predominantly of macrophages and scattered reticulin fibers. As the lesions enlarge, the central portions become hypocellular and composed of mature collagen, sometimes arranged in more or less concentric lamellae; a peripheral zone of macrophages and lesser numbers of plasma cells and lymphocytes surrounds this central portion (see Color Fig. 16–3). A variable number of birefringent silicate crystals 1 to 3 μm in length can usually be identified by polarization microscopy in the cellular areas. The larger lesions of PMF are also composed of hyalinized collagen admixed with variable numbers of pigmented macrophages; however, the concentric lamellar appearance of the collagen seen in silicotic nodules is frequently not evident.

In silicoproteinosis, well-defined fibrous nodules are typically absent. Instead, the alveolar air spaces are more or less diffusely filled with somewhat granular periodic acid–Schiff–positive proteinaceous material identical to that seen in idiopathic alveolar proteinosis. Macrophages are present in increased number, and alveolar type II cells show a variable degree of hyperplasia and hypertrophy. Ultrastructurally, the intra-alveolar material contains macrophages and desquamated type II cells as well as membranous material resembling that seen in the normal alveolar lining layer.[44]

Radiologic Manifestations

The classic radiographic pattern of silicosis consists of multiple nodular opacities ranging from 1 to 10 mm in diameter

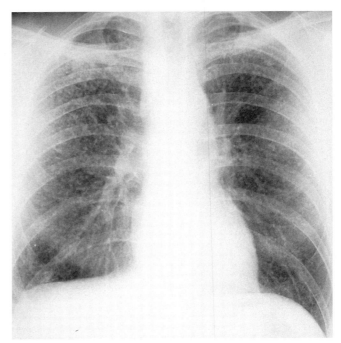

FIGURE 16–1

Silicosis. A posteroanterior chest radiograph demonstrates numerous well-defined small nodules mainly in the upper and middle lung zones. The nodules measure 1.5 to 3 mm in diameter (International Labour Office [ILO] q size nodules), and the profusion is 2/3 (slightly greater than the ILO standard radiograph for profusion 2/2 but considerably less than the standard for profusion 3/3). Early conglomeration is present near the apices. *(From Fraser RS, Müller NL, Colman NC, Paré PD: Fraser and Paré's Diagnosis of Diseases of the Chest, 4th ed. Philadelphia, WB Saunders, 1999.)*

(Fig. 16–1). The nodules are usually well circumscribed and of uniform density. Although profusion can be fairly even throughout both lungs, there is commonly a considerable upper lobe predominance. The nodules tend to involve mainly the posterior portion of the lungs.[50] Calcification is evident on radiographs in 10% to 20% of cases.

The radiographic pattern of small round opacities is commonly referred to as *simple* silicosis, in contrast to *complicated* silicosis (PMF). PMF is characterized by large opacities (conglomerate shadows) usually in the upper lobes. By definition, the opacities measure more than 1 cm in diameter; in practice, they are often larger than this and may exceed the volume of an upper lobe in aggregate (Fig. 16–2). The shadow margins may be irregular and ill defined or smooth[51] and create an interface that parallels the lateral chest wall (see Fig. 16–2). The opacities commonly develop in the midzone or periphery of the lung; with time, they tend to migrate toward the hilum, with emphysematous lung left between the fibrotic tissue and the pleural surface. Though usually bilateral, unilateral opacities may occur and can be confused with carcinoma. Cavitation develops occasionally. The more extensive the conglomerate fibrosis, the less apparent the nodularity in the remainder of the lungs. There is seldom any radiographic evidence of pleural abnormality.

Hilar lymph node enlargement is common and frequently associated with calcification[52]; in a series of 1905 workers, calcification was identified in 4.7%.[53] The calcification may

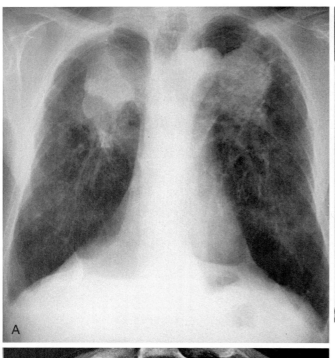

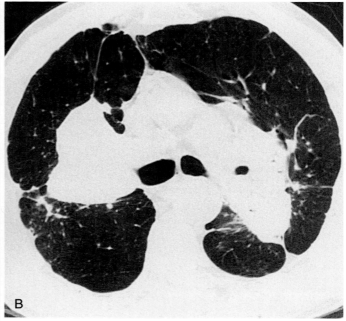

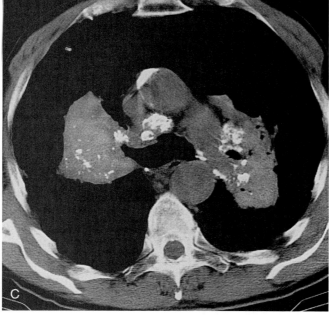

FIGURE 16–2

Silicosis with conglomeration. A posteroanterior chest radiograph (**A**) demonstrates large opacities in the upper lung zones associated with marked retraction of the hila superiorly. Several nodular opacities can be seen, mainly in the midlung zones. HRCT (**B**) demonstrates conglomerate masses and extensive emphysema. Soft tissue windows (**C**) reveal calcification within the lung parenchyma and within the mediastinal and hilar lymph nodes. The patient was a 70-year-old man with long-standing silicosis related to hard rock mining. *(From Fraser RS, Müller NL, Colman NC, Paré PD: Fraser and Paré's Diagnosis of Diseases of the Chest, 4th ed. Philadelphia, WB Saunders, 1999.)*

involve mainly the periphery of the nodes, a finding referred to as *eggshell calcification*. Though occasionally seen in other conditions,[53] this pattern is almost pathognomonic of silica-induced disease; its occurrence in coal and metal miners has been attributed to concomitant exposure to silica.[52] Hilar lymph node enlargement may also be seen in silica-exposed individuals in the absence of pulmonary involvement.

As indicated previously, there are several variants of classic silicosis. Accelerated silicosis has radiographic features similar to those of the classic form except that they develop within 5 to 10 years of exposure. Silicoproteinosis is characterized by bilateral parenchymal consolidation, similar to alveolar proteinosis, that progresses rapidly over a period of months or 1

or 2 years.[54,55] Caplan's syndrome consists of the presence of necrobiotic nodules (rheumatoid nodules), usually superimposed on a background of simple silicosis or coal workers' pneumoconiosis (CWP). It is seen more commonly in CWP than in silicosis. The necrobiotic nodules can be distinguished from those of silicosis by their tendency to occur in crops; they measure 0.5 to 5 cm in diameter and may cavitate.

Radiographic progression of silicosis after removal from the site of exposure has been well established. In a study of 1902 workers who had no radiographic evidence of PMF a maximum of 4 years before leaving the occupation, this complication subsequently developed in 172 on follow-up examination.[56] Despite the development of conglomerate lesions,

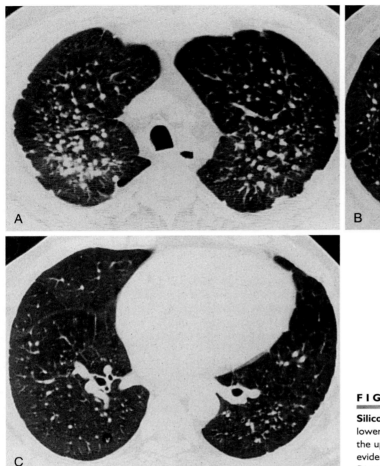

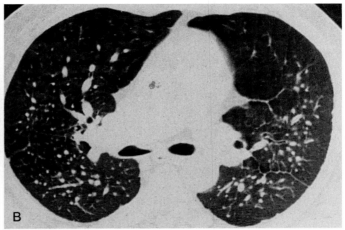

FIGURE 16–3

Silicosis—HRCT findings. HRCT scans from upper (**A**), mid (**B**), and lower (**C**) lung zones demonstrate well-defined nodules mainly involving the upper zones. Pseudoplaques related to subpleural nodules are also evident. *(From Fraser RS, Müller NL, Colman NC, Paré PD: Fraser and Paré's Diagnosis of Diseases of the Chest, 4th ed. Philadelphia, WB Saunders, 1999.)*

there was no progression or regression of the grades of simple pneumoconiosis.

The characteristic CT abnormalities are similar to those on the radiograph:[50,57,58] sharply defined small nodules that may be diffuse throughout the lungs but are frequently most numerous in the upper lung zones (Fig. 16–3). In patients who have relatively mild disease, the nodules may be seen only in the posterior aspect of the upper lobes.[50,59] Nodules adjacent to the visceral pleura may appear as rounded or triangular areas of attenuation, which when confluent may simulate pleural plaques (*pseudoplaques*) (see Fig. 16–3). Confluent nodules (PMF) usually have irregular margins and may contain foci of calcification (see Fig. 16–2); surrounding emphysema is usually present.[57,60,61] Hilar or mediastinal lymph node enlargement is apparent in approximately 40% of patients.[59]

Distinction of small nodules from vessels is easier on CT performed with 5- to 10-mm collimation than on HRCT.[62] However, HRCT allows better assessment of fine parenchymal detail and emphysema. It also allows detection of nodules in patients who have normal radiographic and thick-section CT findings[57] and is particularly helpful in the assessment of nodules smaller than 1.5 mm in diameter.[58] In an investigation of 49 silica-exposed patients, 13 (41%) of 32 who had normal radiographs had evidence of silicosis on CT[57]; in 3 of these patients (9%), the abnormality was visible only on HRCT.

Clinical Manifestations

Many patients who have silicosis are asymptomatic at the time of diagnosis. Dyspnea develops and worsens as the radiographic changes progress[63]; such progression may be evident even after withdrawal from dust exposure in the workplace.[41] With continued destruction of lung tissue, pulmonary hypertension develops and results in cor pulmonale and, eventually, right-sided heart failure. The major determinant of cor pulmonale appears to be the severity of the associated emphysema, the extent of fibrosis being of lesser importance.[64] Although crackles and wheezes are common on auscultation in patients who have advanced disease,[65] in our experience asymptomatic patients usually have no adventitial sounds.

Pulmonary Function Tests

Lung function may be normal in the early stage of disease, and exercise testing is not more sensitive than routine testing in demonstrating early impairment.[66] However, higher degrees of profusion of simple silicosis may be associated with significant loss of lung function.[67] When dyspnea is present, impairment may be restrictive, obstructive, or a combination of both.[67,68] Diffusing capacity may be decreased[69]; the combination of this finding with hyperinflation and a decrease in flow rates constitutes a functional pattern identical to that seen in emphysema. Although arterial oxygen saturation may be normal at rest, exercise gives rise to hypoxemia, especially in patients who have PMF. Advanced disease may be associated with hypercapnia.

Prognosis and Natural History

As might be expected, symptomatic patients with silicosis have a poorer prognosis than asymptomatic ones; in fact, asymptomatic patients who have simple nodular silicosis have a life expectancy similar to that of the general population.[70]

Silicosis is associated with a number of other diseases that can affect the prognosis. It is well established as a predisposing factor for both tuberculosis and nontuberculous mycobacterial infection.[71,72] The risk is increased in patients who have simple disease, but it is particularly marked for those who have PMF.[72,73] There is evidence that concomitant HIV infection increases the risk in a multiplicative fashion.[74]

A second serious complication of silicosis is pulmonary carcinoma. In 1996, silica was recognized by the International Agency for Research on Cancer (IARC) as a group 1 occupational carcinogen.[75] The strength of the association is much greater for workers who have silicosis than for silica-exposed workers alone,[76] thus leaving the putative association between cancer and exposure in the absence of silicosis a controversial one.[77] Excess risk has been reported in workers without apparent exposure to other occupational carcinogens, such as stone cutters,[78] and is independent of cigarette smoking.[76]

The association of both silicosis and silica exposure with progressive systemic sclerosis is well described[79]; limited data suggest that there might be a similar association with rheumatoid arthritis and systemic lupus erythematosus.[80] Regardless of whether established connective tissue disease is present, serologic abnormalities are common in silicosis and include the presence of rheumatoid factor, antinuclear antibodies, immune complexes, and a polyclonal increase in γ-globulin.[81]

There is substantial evidence showing that the dusty environment of silica-exposed workers contributes to the development of chronic airflow obstruction and emphysema. Although it is likely that tobacco smoke is synergistic with the effects of dust, functionally important airway disease can be seen in heavily exposed nonsmoking workers.[82] For example, a significant excess of emphysema as determined by HRCT and pulmonary dysfunction was found in one study of workers who had silicosis, as well as in dust-exposed workers who did not have the disease, after controlling for both age and smoking history.[83] In another investigation, the risk for significant emphysema was 3.5 times greater in miners heavily exposed to dust than in miners who had lighter dust exposure.[84]

COAL AND CARBON

Dust composed predominantly of carbon is inhaled and retained in the lungs of many individuals, particularly those who smoke or live in an urban or industrial environment (a condition often called *anthracosis*). Microscopically, such material is easily recognized as dense black particles, mostly 1 to 2 μm in size, within macrophages adjacent to terminal or proximal respiratory bronchioles and in the pleura. Though predominantly composed of carbon, the particles also contain traces of other substances such as silica and iron.

Nevertheless, associated fibrosis is invariably minimal or absent, and it is generally believed that the presence of such particles is of no pathologic or functional significance.

Such innocuous anthracosis is caused by the inhalation of relatively small amounts of dust. It is clear, however, that the inhalation of large amounts of carbon, either as coal dust or as substances derived from coal or petroleum products, can be associated with significant pulmonary disease. Not surprisingly, disease occurs almost exclusively in the workplace, where the concentration of these materials is much greater than in nonoccupational settings. The most important occupation in terms of the number of individuals affected is coal mining, the resulting disease appropriately being called *coal workers' pneumoconiosis*. Workers in other occupations, such as the production or use of graphite[85] and carbon black,[86] are affected less often. Both acute and chronic pulmonary disease has occasionally been attributed to the inhalation of fly ash (the solid residue that remains after the combustion of coal)[87,88]; however, this association has been disputed.[89]

The pathologic, radiologic, and clinical findings in workers exposed to large amounts of carbon, in whatever form, are similar; however, the vast majority of such individuals are involved in coal mining, and both the literature and the discussion that follows reflect this fact.

Epidemiology

Coal is a sedimentary rock formed by the action of pressure, temperature, and chemical reactions on vegetable material. The percentage of pure carbon varies with the type, brown coal and lignite containing the least and anthracite the most.[90] The degree of exposure to carbon dust thus depends to some extent on the type of coal being mined, a feature that may explain part of the variability in the incidence of CWP from colliery to colliery. Perhaps more important in this regard are local geologic variations[91]; some coal seams are very thick (up to 100 ft), whereas others are much thinner and separated by seams of siliceous rock. Mining in the latter situation can result in significant exposure to silica and other substances in addition to coal, a circumstance that explains the occurrence of silicosis in some coal workers.[92]

Specific tasks within the coal mine also influence the probability that disease will develop and the form that it takes. For example, because the majority of dust is produced at the coal face, operators of cutting and loading machines are exposed to the highest concentration of pure coal dust,[90] whereas surface coal miners drilling through quartz[92] are more likely to come in contact with silica.

The prevalence of CWP has fallen progressively over the past 35 years in the United States.[2,93] The reasons include a fall in dust levels, a decrease in the number of workers employed in mines, and withdrawal of affected miners from the workforce.[94] Despite this decrease, many chest physicians will encounter patients who have CWP: with current environmental standards, it is estimated that category 2 or greater disease will develop in 2% to 12% of American coal miners after a 40-year working life and that PMF will develop in approximately 1% to 7%.[95,96] In 1996, more than 230,000 people received benefits under the Federal Black Lung Act, and there were an estimated 11,000 discharges with a diagnosis of CWP from short-stay nonfederal hospitals.[2]

Pathogenesis

The precise pathogenetic factors involved in the development of simple CWP and complicating PMF are unclear, and several agents or processes, either alone or in combination, may be responsible. One of the most important determinants is the quantity of inhaled dust; both the prevalence of disease and the risk of its progression are related to cumulative dust exposure.[97] In addition, PMF is found at autopsy almost exclusively in workers who have a large amount of dust in their lungs.[98]

Understanding of the cellular and molecular basis of the pulmonary response to inhaled and retained coal dust is complicated by difficulty in distinguishing primary effects from their secondary consequences.[99] As with silicosis, activation of alveolar macrophages and injury to epithelial cells are associated with the production of a number of proinflammatory and profibrotic mediators that contribute to both the initiation and progression of disease. Important among these are TNF-α, IL-1 and IL-8, fibronectin, and transforming growth factor-β (TGF-β).[99-102] Disease is also associated with the production of oxidants derived from neutrophils and activated alveolar macrophages. In addition, oxidants are produced by mechanisms related to the intrinsic properties of the dust itself[33,99]; in fact, variations in oxidant production by different types of coal have been associated with different propensities to disease.[103]

Since Caplan reported the association of CWP and rheumatoid arthritis,[104] it has been noted that pneumoconiotic workers have a high prevalence of a number of serologic abnormalities, including elevated levels of rheumatoid factor and antinuclear antibody.[105] Although one group has described an association between the presence of rheumatoid factor and rapid disease progression,[106] the precise role of antibodies in the pathogenesis of the disease is uncertain.

Pathologic Characteristics

The two morphologic findings characteristic of CWP are the coal macule and PMF.[107] The former is characterized by deposits of anthracotic pigment unassociated with fibrosis, a finding sometimes referred to as *simple* pneumoconiosis. PMF is defined as a focus of fibrosis and pigment deposition larger than 1 cm in diameter and is sometimes designated *complicated* pneumoconiosis. In addition, smaller foci of fibrous tissue (so-called nodular lesions) can be found in many cases, either with or without features of PMF.

Grossly, coal macules are stellate or round, nonpalpable foci that are black and range in size from 1 to 5 mm (Fig. 16–4).

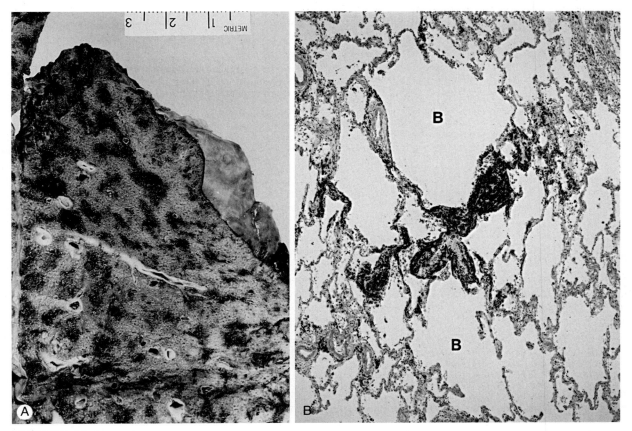

FIGURE 16–4

Coal workers' pneumoconiosis. A magnified view (**A**) of the superior segment of a lower lobe shows multiple foci of dense black pigmentation in the pleura and the lung parenchyma; the latter are irregular in shape and fairly evenly spaced. A section (**B**) shows numerous macrophages containing abundant anthracotic pigment situated in the interstitial tissue adjacent to respiratory bronchioles (**B**). No fibrosis is evident. The bronchioles are mildly dilated. *(From Fraser RS, Müller NL, Colman NC, Paré PD: Fraser and Paré's Diagnosis of Diseases of the Chest, 4th ed. Philadelphia, WB Saunders, 1999.)*

They are distributed fairly uniformly throughout the lung parenchyma, although they tend to be more numerous at the apex than at the base. Microscopically, a macule consists of numerous pigment-laden macrophages in the interstitial tissue adjacent to respiratory bronchioles (see Fig. 16–4); reticulin fibers can be identified between the macrophages, but mature collagen is minimal or absent. Aggregates of pigment-laden macrophages can also be seen in adjacent alveolar air spaces, especially in lung tissue from active miners. Bronchioles within the macules are frequently distended, a finding often designated focal emphysema.

Palpable gray or black nodules smaller than 1 cm in diameter can also be found in the lungs of many coal workers. Although these nodules are described separately, they blend imperceptibly with the macule on the one hand and with PMF on the other,[108] and it is likely that they represent part of a spectrum of changes rather than pathogenetically distinct lesions. The nodules have a variable histologic composition, some consisting of a haphazard mixture of pigment-laden macrophages, free dust, and reticulin and collagen fibers (see Color Fig. 16–4) and others possessing a relatively discrete central zone of pigment-free collagen surrounded by pigment-laden macrophages resembling small silicotic nodules.

Grossly, the lesions of PMF are firm or somewhat rubbery in consistency and either round or irregular in shape. They may be unilateral or bilateral and develop most often in the posterior segment of an upper lobe or the superior segment of a lower lobe, a localization that has been hypothesized to be related to poor lymphatic drainage.[109] Adjacent emphysema is common. Cut sections may reveal a necrotic center containing black fluid that can be washed away to leave a cavity. In most cases, the pathogenesis of the necrosis is ischemia; occasionally, it is caused by tuberculous infection. The microscopic features of PMF are similar to those of the smaller palpable nodules already described: bundles of haphazardly arranged, sometimes hyalinized bands of collagen are interspersed with numerous pigment-laden macrophages and abundant free pigment. Foci of degenerated and frankly necrotic tissue, cholesterol clefts, and mononuclear inflammatory cells are often present.

Radiologic Manifestations

The radiographic pattern of simple CWP is typically one of small (1- to 5-mm-diameter) round nodules.[110,111] These tend to be less well defined and are often smaller (typically p rather than q opacities) than those of silicosis.[112] Despite these observations, it is generally agreed that the radiographic manifestations of CWP cannot be distinguished from those of silicosis with any degree of confidence. Calcification of the nodules can be seen radiographically in 10% to 20% of older coal miners, particularly anthracite workers.[113,114]

Complicated CWP (PMF) is characterized by lesions that range from 1 cm in diameter to the volume of a whole lobe. Though most commonly restricted to the upper half of the lungs, they may occur in the lower lung zones (Fig. 16–5). They are usually observed on a background of simple pneumoconiosis but have been found to develop in miners whose initial chest radiographs 4 to 5 years earlier were considered to be within normal limits.[115] The complication is said to occur in about 30% of patients who have diffuse bilateral opacities.[116,117]

PMF typically starts near the periphery of the lung and is manifested as a mass that has a well-defined lateral border that parallels the rib cage and projects 1 to 3 cm from it.[113] The medial margin of the mass is often ill defined in contrast to its sharp lateral border. The masses tend to be thicker in one dimension than the other; that is, they tend to produce a broad face on a posteroanterior radiograph and a thin shape on a lateral radiograph, frequently paralleling the major fissure.[113] Cavitation occurs only occasionally; it may develop after exposure to coal dust has ceased and, in contrast to simple pneumoconiosis, may progress in the absence of further exposure.[116,118]

As with the conglomerate shadows of silicosis, PMF usually originates in the lung periphery and gradually migrates toward the hilum such that a zone of emphysematous lung is left between it and the chest wall. Particularly when unilateral, a large mass may simulate pulmonary carcinoma closely. Because PMF is occasionally unassociated with radiographic evidence of nodularity,[113] the correct diagnosis may not be suspected in the absence of an appropriate occupational history. The smooth, sharply defined lateral border and the somewhat flattened configuration characteristic of these lesions are useful clues in differentiation from pulmonary carcinoma, whose borders tend to be less well defined and whose configuration is typically spherical.

As discussed previously, Caplan's syndrome consists of the presence of necrobiotic nodules associated with rheumatoid arthritis, usually superimposed on a background of pneumoconiosis (most often silicosis or CWP).[104] The nodules are more regular in contour and more peripherally located than the masses of PMF (Fig. 16–6). They range in size from 0.5 to 5 cm in diameter and are seen most often in workers who have subcutaneous rheumatoid nodules and whose chest radiographs are classified as category 0 or early simple pneumoconiosis.

The CT findings of CWP are similar to those of silicosis and consist of small nodules that may be seen diffusely throughout both lungs but are most numerous in the upper lung zone.[58,119,120] In patients who have mild disease, the nodules may involve only the upper zone and show a posterior predominance.[119] They have a principally centrilobular distribution (Fig. 16–7).[119,121] Subpleural nodules are seen in approximately 80% of patients who have other parenchymal nodules. Confluence of such nodules may result in linear areas of increased attenuation a few millimeters wide (pseudoplaques).[121] Calcification of nodules can be identified in approximately 30% of patients. Hilar or mediastinal lymph node enlargement is seen in about 30% of cases; most enlarged nodes are calcified.[119]

Large opacities (PMF) usually have irregular borders on HRCT and are associated with distortion of the surrounding lung architecture and emphysema.[119,121] Less commonly, they have regular borders and are unassociated with emphysema.[119] They are seen most commonly in the upper lung zone. Though frequently bilateral, they may be unilateral (most commonly on the right).[119]

Clinical Manifestations

Symptoms of cough, sputum production, and dyspnea are more common in miners who have early CWP than in miners

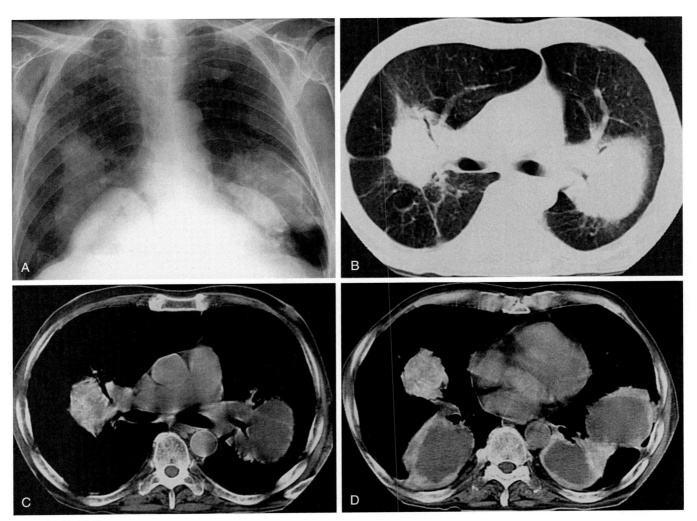

FIGURE 16–5

Coal workers' pneumoconiosis. An anteroposterior chest radiograph (**A**) shows large opacities in the middle and lower lung zones. A 10-mm-collimation CT scan at the level of the right upper lobe bronchus (**B**) demonstrates bilateral perihilar conglomerate masses. Irregular linear opacities and distortion of lung architecture indicative of fibrosis and emphysema are also evident. Soft tissue windows (**C** and **D**) demonstrate that three of the conglomerate masses have large central areas of decreased attenuation suggestive of necrosis. The patient was a 65-year-old man with a 30-year history of exposure to coal dust. *(Courtesy of Dr. Martine Remy-Jardin, Centre Hospitalier Regional et Universitaire de Lille, Lille, France.)*

who have similar smoking and dust exposure histories but no radiographic evidence of disease.[122] These symptoms are even more frequent and severe in workers who have PMF; such workers also suffer from attacks of purulent bronchitis. Copious amounts of black sputum (melanoptysis) may be produced when an ischemic lesion of PMF liquefies and ruptures into a bronchus. With progression of disease, dyspnea worsens and cor pulmonale with right-sided heart failure may ensue.

There is little doubt that coal dust inhalation is related to the development of emphysema and chronic airflow obstruction.[123] Emphysema has been shown to be present more often and to be more severe in patients who have CWP (smokers and nonsmokers alike) than in those who do not[124]; its severity correlates with the degree of dust exposure[125] and is additive to the effects of cigarette smoking.[126] These changes are undoubtedly responsible for many of the alterations in lung function described in workers who have CWP.

Pulmonary Function Tests

The results of early studies in workers who had simple CWP suggested that there was little attributable functional change[127]; however, this finding was probably due to the impact of the "healthy worker effect." Later studies have revealed a correlation between the extent of dust exposure and decline in FEV_1, both in workers who have simple CWP[128] and in miners who do not.[129] Small decrements in diffusing capacity have been noted in smoking and nonsmoking dust-exposed miners, both in those who have simple CWP and in those whose radiographs are normal.[69]

PMF is frequently associated with physiologic evidence of airway obstruction, reduced diffusing capacity, abnormal blood gases, and pulmonary hypertension.[118,130] In one study in which pathology and function were correlated, these changes in lung function were attributed not only to PMF and emphysema but also to small-airway disease and interstitial fibrosis.[131]

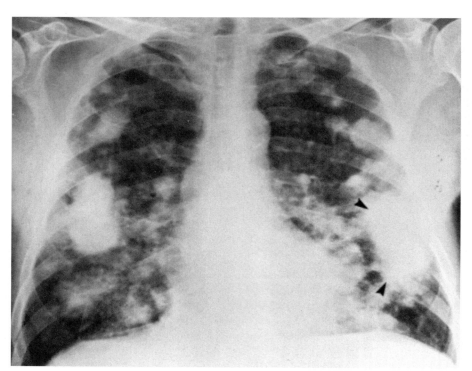

FIGURE 16–6

Caplan's syndrome. A posteroanterior radiograph reveals a multitude of fairly well circumscribed nodules ranging in diameter from 1 to 5 cm and scattered randomly throughout both lungs. No cavitation or calcification is apparent. This patient was a 56-year-old man who had been a coal miner for many years and in recent years had developed arthralgia, which proved to be due to rheumatoid arthritis. Aspiration of the mass in the left lung (*arrowheads*) yielded black fluid. (*From Fraser RS, Müller NL, Colman NC, Paré PD: Fraser and Paré's Diagnosis of Diseases of the Chest, 4th ed. Philadelphia, WB Saunders, 1999.*)

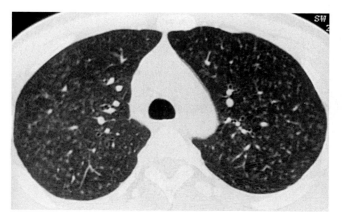

FIGURE 16–7

Coal workers' pneumoconiosis. An HRCT scan in a coal worker shows poorly defined small nodular opacities in the upper lobes. The nodules have a predominantly centrilobular distribution. (*Case courtesy of Dr. Juan Jimenez, Hospital General de Asturias, Oviedo, Spain.*)

Prognosis and Natural History

Mortality from CWP has fallen progressively over the past 35 years in the United States.[2,93] As might be expected, workers with PMF have relatively increased mortality rates[132]; for example, in one investigation, miners in whom PMF developed when young had a third the survival rate of those who did not have CWP after a 22-year period of observation.[133] In contrast to patients who have silicosis, coal workers who have simple pneumoconiosis seldom show progression of disease if removed from the dust-ridden environment.[134]

ASBESTOS

Asbestos is the general term given to a group of fibrous minerals composed of combinations of silicic acid with magnesium, calcium, sodium, and iron. The word is derived from the Greek meaning *inextinguishable*[135] and reflects the resistance of the substance to heat and acid, as well as its strength, durability, and flexibility.

Mineralogically, asbestos can be divided into two major groups: the serpentines, of which the only member of commercial importance is chrysotile, and the amphiboles, which include amosite, crocidolite, anthophyllite, tremolite, and actinolite. Chrysotile fibers are typically curved, whereas the amphiboles are straight. These physical properties, as well as chemical differences, are responsible for the varying uses of asbestos and for their ability to cause disease. Chrysotile, amosite, and tremolite cause the vast majority of pleuropulmonary disease.

Guidelines for diagnosis and initial management of nonmalignant asbestos pleuropulmonary disease have been published.[135a]

Epidemiology

The enormous increase in the use of asbestos in the first three quarters of the 20th century resulted in a dramatic increase in the number of individuals exposed to the mineral. Although concern regarding its toxicity has led to a decline in its use (from a peak of 6.0 million to less than 2.5 million metric tons),[136] it has been estimated that in the United States 8 to 9 million people have had occupational exposure to asbestos and that such exposure will eventually result in 300,000 deaths.[137,138]

Three major sources of asbestos dust are recognized:

1. The primary occupations of asbestos mining and its processing in mills. Exposure in these settings is

predominantly to one fiber type; however, contamination by other fiber types may be present even with commercially "pure" preparations.[139] Though previously an important setting for asbestos-related disease, workers in these occupations currently account for only a small minority of individuals in whom asbestosis develops.[2]

2. Numerous secondary occupations involving the use of asbestos in industrial and commercial products. The most important uses are in the construction and automotive industries (in which asbestos is extensively incorporated in cement piping, tile, molding, paneling, and brake lining), in shipbuilding and repair, and in insulation.[2] Although the risk of exposure applies during the manufacturing process, it is even greater during repair and demolition.

3. Contaminated air inhaled by individuals not directly involved in asbestos-related occupations.[140] That such exposure is common in the general population is indicated by the frequency with which asbestos bodies are found in the lungs in routine autopsies; for example, in a study of individuals who had lived in New York City, 60% had these structures.[141] Despite the lack of evidence that such environmental exposure is a risk for the development of pleuropulmonary disease,[142] it is well established that individuals who live in the vicinity of a mine, mill, or factory where asbestos dust pollution has been heavy have an increased incidence of pleural plaques and mesothelioma.[143] These abnormalities can also occur in persons whose only exposure is the repeated handling of clothes of asbestos workers.[144] Similar environmental exposure and ensuing disease may be seen in specific geographic regions. For example, a high incidence of pleural plaques and mesothelioma has been reported from the Metsovo area of northwest Greece[145] and from isolated villages in Turkey,[146] two places where the soil, which contains tremolite, is used as a whitewash for buildings. It is important to remember that a history of environmental or para-occupational exposure to asbestos may not be readily apparent from the initial inquiry because the exposure may have occurred many years before the recognition of disease, may have been of short duration, or may have been completely unknown to the patient.

Pathogenesis

The pathogenesis of asbestos-related pleuropulmonary disease is complex and incompletely understood.[26] Fiber dose, dimension, and chemical composition may all influence fibrogenicity and carcinogenicity, with longer, thinner, more durable fibers being the most important.[147] Factors related to the host, including pulmonary clearance and immunologic status and exposure to other noxious substances such as cigarette smoke, are also important in determining the nature and severity of the reaction to inhaled fibers. The pathogenesis of asbestosis has been studied the most and is considered in the remainder of this section.

Data concerning the relationship between pulmonary fiber burden and asbestosis are somewhat contradictory and confusing.[26] Although there is a clear relationship with high fiber concentration for amphibole fibers,[148] the situation for chrysotile is less obvious. Fibers of chrysotile are relatively short lived, their half-life being months as opposed to decades for amphiboles. This difference may account for the predominance of amphiboles in lung specimens from workers whose exposure was predominantly to chrysotile, especially when such exposure has been remote. However, the results of both animal and human studies,[149,150] as well as recognition of the adverse effects of cigarette smoking (which increases fiber retention), support the hypothesis that chrysotile fibers are closely associated with disease.

Although the majority of inhaled asbestos fibers are removed by mucociliary clearance, some enter the interstitium within macrophages, by direct penetration across the epithelium, or by organization of intraluminal exudate after epithelial injury.[151,152] Activated macrophages accumulate at the bifurcation of transitional airways and in the interstitium, where they produce cytokines, chemokines, and growth factors that promote inflammation and fibrosis.[153] These products include TNF-α, TGF-β, IL-1, IL-8, and platelet-derived growth factor. The first of these substances may be particularly important since the results of experiments in a TNF-α receptor knockout mouse model of asbestosis show absence of lung damage.[154]

Abundant evidence has shown that free radicals, especially reactive oxygen and nitrogen species,[155] also have an important role in the pathogenesis of asbestosis.[154] Asbestos fibers can induce the formation of reactive oxygen species both directly and indirectly by the activation of inflammatory cells recruited to the site of tissue deposition.[154] These products increase epithelial cell adhesion and uptake of fibers of dust induced by cigarette smoke.[154] They also promote epithelial cell apoptosis, thereby impairing repair.

Asbestosis does not develop in everyone exposed to heavy concentrations of asbestos, which raises the possibility that intrinsic host factors are important in the pathogenesis of the disease. Such hypothesized factors include the efficiency of alveolar and tracheobronchial clearance,[156] underlying lung structure,[150] and immune status. The last has been studied most thoroughly. Circulating rheumatoid factor and antinuclear antibody have been found in 25% to 30% of asbestos workers who have radiographic evidence of asbestosis[157]; however, there is little evidence that B-cell hyperactivity is directly involved in disease pathogenesis.[158] A variety of abnormalities of cell-mediated immunity have also been documented in asbestos-exposed individuals, including delayed skin hypersensitivity,[159] an alteration in the ratio of helper to suppressor T lymphocytes in BAL fluid,[160] and a reduction in natural killer cell activity.[161] As with abnormalities related to antibodies, however, the precise contribution of any of these factors to the development of asbestosis is unknown.

Pathologic Characteristics

Pleural Abnormalities

Parietal Pleural Plaques. These are the most common form of asbestos-related pleuropulmonary disease, the incidence in some series of consecutive routine autopsies ranging from about 5 to 10 per 100 cases.[162] Grossly, they consist of well-defined, pearly-white foci of firm fibrous tissue, usually 2 to 5 mm thick and up to 10 cm in diameter.[163] They may have a smooth surface or show fine or coarse nodularity and can be round, elliptical, or irregularly shaped (Fig. 16–8). Histologic examination typically shows them to consist of dense, almost acellular collagen; occasionally, small aggregates of chronic inflammatory cells are evident at the periphery. Characteristically, plaques are located on the parietal pleura adjacent to the ribs and on the domes of the diaphragm. They are generally absent from the apices, costophrenic angles, and anterior chest wall and are almost always bilateral. The pathogenesis is unclear.

Focal Visceral Pleural Fibrosis. Relatively discrete foci of visceral pleural fibrosis morphologically distinct from pleural plaques are common in association with asbestos exposure. They consist of round or elliptical areas of fibrous tissue 1 to 2 mm thick that often appear to radiate from a central focus. Unless the abnormality is associated with round atelectasis (see later) or located in a fissure, it is unlikely to be detected on chest radiographs.

Diffuse Pleural Fibrosis. In contrast to the relatively discrete foci of visceral and parietal pleural fibrosis described earlier, some patients show more diffuse pleural thickening that may be progressive and associated with clinical and functional abnormalities.[164] The fibrosis usually involves both the parietal and visceral pleural layers and is accompanied by interpleural adhesions. It is not clear whether this form of disease represents an extension of one or both of the other two forms of pleural fibrosis or is a pathogenetically separate process. In a study of seven patients who had diffuse pleural fibrosis, one or more episodes of pleural effusion were identified, suggesting that organization of the effusion might have been responsible for the chronic changes.[164]

Pleural Effusion. Disease in some individuals with a history of asbestos exposure is manifested as pleural effusion. Histologic examination of biopsy specimens from these individuals shows fibrosis, nonspecific chronic inflammation, and an organizing fibrinous exudate. As with other forms of asbestos-related pleural disease, the pathogenesis of the effusion is unclear. It has been suggested that interaction between asbestos fibers and pleural tissue results in the release of non–complement-related chemotactic factors that cause the effusion.[165]

Mesothelioma. There is a strong association between asbestos exposure and the development of mesothelioma. The pathologic features and pathogenesis of this tumor are discussed on page 835.

Pulmonary Abnormalities

Asbestosis. Asbestosis can be defined as more or less diffuse parenchymal interstitial fibrosis secondary to the inhalation of asbestos fibers. Grossly, the fibrosis is most prominent in the subpleural regions of the lower lobes and varies from a slightly coarse appearance of the parenchyma to obvious honeycomb change (Fig. 16–9).[166] Fibrosis of adjacent visceral

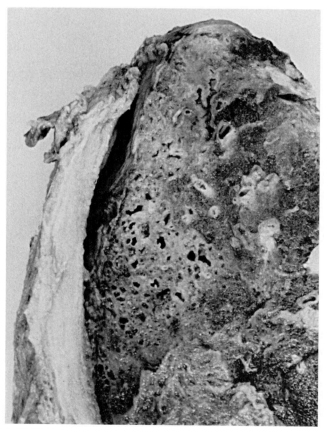

FIGURE 16–9

Diffuse pleural fibrosis and asbestosis. A parasagittal slice through the midportion of a lower lobe shows marked pleural thickening and parenchymal interstitial fibrosis. The pleural lesion consists of fibrous tissue, which extends over most of the costal surface. The pulmonary fibrosis is most evident in the subpleural region and has a honeycomb appearance. *(From Müller NL, Fraser RS, Colman NC, Paré PD: Radiologic Diagnosis of Diseases of the Chest. Philadelphia, WB Saunders, 2001.)*

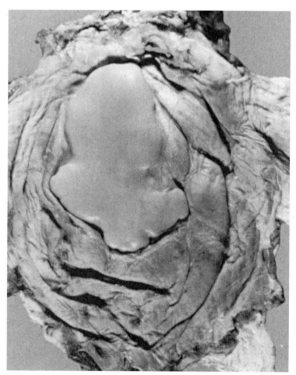

FIGURE 16–8

Parietal pleural plaque. An autopsy specimen of a hemidiaphragm shows a smooth, well-circumscribed focus of fibrosis on the tendinous portion. *(From Müller NL, Fraser RS, Colman NC, Paré PD: Radiologic Diagnosis of Diseases of the Chest. Philadelphia, WB Saunders, 2001.)*

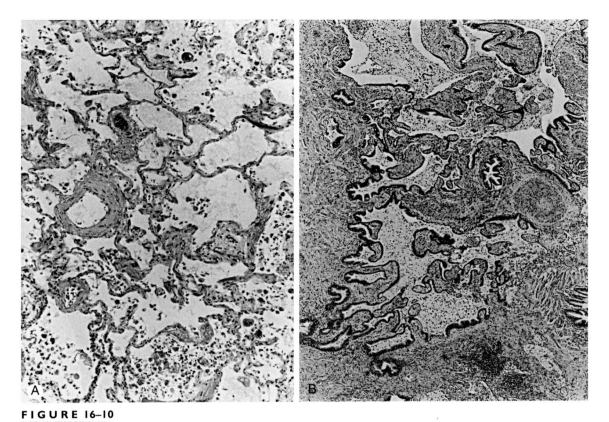

FIGURE 16–10

Asbestosis. Sections show mild (**A**) and severe (**B**) interstitial fibrosis. In **A,** collagen is present in the walls of several transitional airways and alveolar septa. In **B,** there is marked distortion of the lung architecture associated with the presence of broad bands of fibrous tissue and cystic spaces focally lined by metaplastic bronchiolar epithelium (corresponding to honeycomb lung). *(From Müller NL, Fraser RS, Colman NC, Paré PD: Radiologic Diagnosis of Diseases of the Chest. Philadelphia, WB Saunders, 2001.)*

pleura is common and often accompanied by parietal pleural adhesions. As might be expected from the gross description, the microscopic appearance varies from a slight increase in interstitial collagen to complete obliteration of normal lung architecture and the formation of thick fibrous bands and cystic spaces (Fig. 16–10). Asbestos bodies are usually easily identified in tissue sections and may be present in great numbers; in fact, according to most authorities,[166] their presence is required for the histologic diagnosis. Nonetheless, they may be very scarce or apparently absent in some individuals.[167]

The earliest histologic change in asbestosis is thought by some investigators to consist of fibrosis in the walls of respiratory bronchioles.[166] According to this view, the process begins in the most proximal of such airways and extends to involve the terminal bronchioles, the more distal respiratory bronchioles, and the adjacent alveolar interstitium; as the disease progresses, greater portions of lung parenchyma are affected in a centrifugal fashion. Others hypothesize that the peribronchiolar fibrosis seen in association with asbestos exposure (see Color Fig. 16–5) represents a process pathogenetically distinct from pulmonary parenchymal fibrosis.[168] Several observations support this view. For example, peribronchiolar fibrosis has been identified in patients with a history of exposure to mineral dust other than asbestos, thus implying that this pathologic change may be a nonspecific

reaction to dust inhalation rather than a specific manifestation of asbestos toxicity. Experimental studies in sheep have also demonstrated evidence for two distinct pulmonary reactions, one related to small airways and the other to the parenchymal interstitium.[169] Whatever its relationship to interstitial fibrosis, the peribronchiolar fibrosis is likely to be related to the airflow obstruction that is observed in both patients and experimental animals.[169]

The Asbestos Body. The asbestos body is seen commonly in tissue sections in association with asbestos pleuropulmonary disease and consists of a core composed of a transparent asbestos fiber (usually amosite or crocidolite[170]) surrounded by a variably thick coat of iron and protein (see Color Fig. 16–5). Most bodies measure between 2 and 5 μm in width and 20 to 50 μm in length. The shape is quite variable and depends on the length of the asbestos core, the amount and pattern of deposition of the protein-iron coat, and whether the body is whole or fragmented. In tissue sections, they are usually seen within interstitial fibrous tissue or air spaces; they are rarely identified in pleural plaques. Their presence in sputum as well as BAL and transthoracic needle aspiration specimens from individuals with occupational exposure has been well documented.[171-173]

The absolute number of asbestos bodies identified in tissue sections or digested lung samples is a gross underestimation of the total number of uncoated asbestos *fibers*, as determined by electron microscopic examination of tissue samples[174]; thus, the ratio of uncoated to coated fibers in lung digests ranges from approximately 7:1 to 5000:1 in different series.[175] Since it is likely that it is the uncoated form of asbestos that exerts pathologic effects and since there are qualitative as well as quantitative differences between fibers and bodies, these distinctions are important in understanding pathogenesis.

The number of asbestos bodies and fibers per gram of digested lung tissue is roughly proportional to both the presence and severity of disease and the degree of occupational exposure. Thus, individuals who have well-documented high exposure generally have 20 to 100 times the number of fibers in the lung as those not exposed. Individuals who have asbestosis or mesothelioma also usually have a much greater fiber burden than do asbestos-exposed individuals who do not have these complications.[176]

Round Atelectasis. Pathologically, round atelectasis consists of a more or less spherical focus of collapsed parenchyma in the periphery of the lung. Although the abnormality is not related solely to asbestos, the majority of cases are associated with it.[177] Grossly, the atelectatic lung is poorly defined and appears to blend imperceptibly with adjacent normal lung parenchyma.[178] The overlying pleura is invariably fibrotic and shows one or more invaginations 1 mm to 3 cm in length into the adjacent lung.

Radiologic Manifestations

Radiologic manifestations of asbestos-related disease are much more common in the pleura than in the parenchyma.[179,180] CT, in particular HRCT, has higher sensitivity than chest radiography in the detection of abnormalities in both sites.[181-183] For example, in a prospective study of 100 asbestos-exposed workers, pleural abnormalities were evident on the chest radiograph in 53 and on HRCT in 93[183]; parenchymal abnormalities consistent with asbestosis were present on radiograph in 35 and on HRCT in 73.

Pleural Manifestations

Four types of radiologic abnormality occur in the pleura: (1) focal plaque formation, (2) calcification, (3) diffuse thickening, and (4) effusion. Each may occur alone or in combination with the others. The latency period for the development of these abnormalities ranges from approximately 15 to 30 years for plaques, 20 to 40 years for calcified plaques, 10 to 40 years for diffuse thickening, and 5 to 20 years for benign effusion.[112] It has been estimated that there may be 1.3 million people in the United States who have radiographically detectable asbestos-related pleural disease.[137]

Focal Pleural Plaques

Radiographically, pleural plaques are usually more prominent in the lower half of the thorax and tend to follow the ribs when seen en face.[184,185] They may be smooth or nodular and can measure as much as 1 cm thick, although they are generally thinner (Fig. 16–11). They are seen most commonly on the domes of the diaphragm, on the posterolateral aspect of the chest wall between the 7th and 10th ribs, and on the lateral portion of the chest wall between the 6th and 9th ribs.[179] They may be bilateral and symmetrical, bilateral and asymmetrical, or less commonly, unilateral.[186,187]

Although detection of plaques radiographically is highly specific for a history of asbestos exposure, its sensitivity is relatively poor. Depending on the criteria for diagnosis, the frequency with which plaques are recognized on the chest

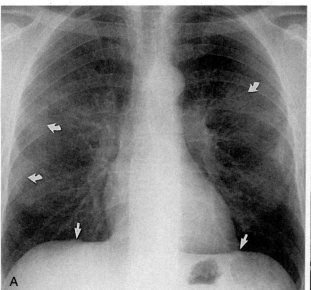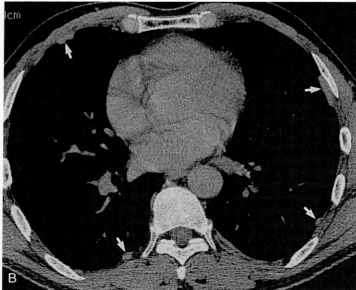

FIGURE 16–11

Pleural plaques. A posteroanterior chest radiograph (**A**) shows multiple pleural-based opacities along the chest wall and diaphragm. Several are viewed tangentially (*straight arrows*), whereas others are ill defined because they are viewed en face *(curved arrows)*, indicative of their origin in the posterolateral or anterolateral aspect of the chest wall. HRCT (**B**) confirms the presence of bilateral plaques *(arrows)*. The patient was a 51-year-old shipyard worker. *(From Müller NL, Fraser RS, Colman NC, Paré PD: Radiologic Diagnosis of Diseases of the Chest. Philadelphia, WB Saunders, 2001.)*

radiograph ranges from 8% to 40% of patients in whom they are demonstrable at autopsy.[162] In one study, the combination of bilateral posterolateral plaques at least 5 mm thick or bilateral calcified diaphragmatic plaques was shown to have a 100% positive predictive value for the diagnosis of autopsy-proven asbestos-related pleural disease[188]; however, these criteria allowed detection of only 12% of plaques. Use of less strict criteria resulted in a considerable number of false-positive diagnoses.

The greatest problem in the radiographic diagnosis of pleural plaques (as well as diffuse pleural thickening) lies in distinguishing them from normal companion shadows of the chest wall—not shadows that are associated with the first three ribs (because this area is rarely involved in asbestos-related pleural disease), but muscle and fat shadows that can be identified in 75% of normal posteroanterior radiographs along the inferior convexity of the thorax. In fact, it may be impossible to differentiate pleural plaques from companion shadows on the radiograph.

HRCT has greater sensitivity than conventional CT or chest radiography does for the detection of these abnormalities.[181,183,189] With this technique, plaques can be identified as circumscribed areas of pleural thickening separated from the underlying ribs and extrapleural soft tissues by a thin layer of fat (see Fig. 16–11). In a study of 30 patients in whom conventional and oblique radiographs revealed pleural shadows of uncertain origin, CT showed that they were the result of subpleural fat accumulation in 14 (47%)[189]; of the remaining 16 patients, 10 had definite pleural plaques, 4 had no evidence of either plaques or fat, and 2 had shadows that could not be attributed with certainty to either plaques or fat.

Calcified Pleural Plaques

Although noncalcified pleural plaques are the most common radiographic manifestation of asbestos-related disease, they are more striking when calcified (Fig. 16–12), a finding that is seen in about 15% of patients.[112] Calcified plaques vary from small linear or circular shadows to shadows that completely encircle the lower portion of a lung.[190] When calcification is minimal, a radiograph overexposed at maximal inspiration facilitates visibility. Although the abnormality may be seen at any location, it is most common in relation to the diaphragm.[191]

Diffuse Pleural Thickening

In contrast to a pleural plaque, diffuse thickening is manifested as a generalized, more or less uniform increase in pleural width. Although the term is not defined precisely in the 1980 ILO classification, the abnormality is generally considered to be present when there is a smooth, uninterrupted pleural density extending over at least a fourth of the chest wall with or without obliteration of the costophrenic angle.[192] Diffuse thickening is diagnosed on CT when a continuous area of pleural thickening greater than 3 mm extends for more than 8 cm craniocaudally and 5 cm around the perimeter of the hemithorax.[193]

On HRCT, the margin between an area of diffuse pleural thickening and the adjacent lung is frequently irregular as a result of parenchymal fibrosis, in contrast to the usually sharply circumscribed margins of pleural plaques.[194] The abnormality is generally associated with contralateral pleural abnormalities, either diffuse pleural thickening or plaques.[195] Although calcification may be present, it is seldom extensive.[195,196] Diffuse thickening rarely involves the mediastinal

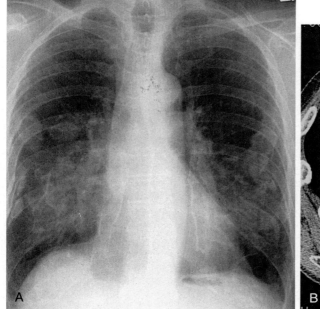
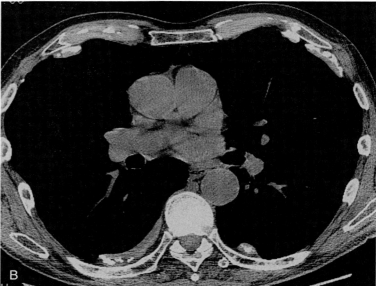

FIGURE 16–12

Calcified pleural plaques. A posteroanterior chest radiograph (**A**) in an 82-year-old man demonstrates numerous calcified pleural plaques. An HRCT scan (**B**) shows the plaques to be located along the posteromedial and anterolateral aspects of the chest wall and the right hemidiaphragm. The patient had worked for many years in a shipyard. *(From Müller NL, Fraser RS, Colman NC, Paré PD: Radiologic Diagnosis of Diseases of the Chest. Philadelphia, WB Saunders, 2001.)*

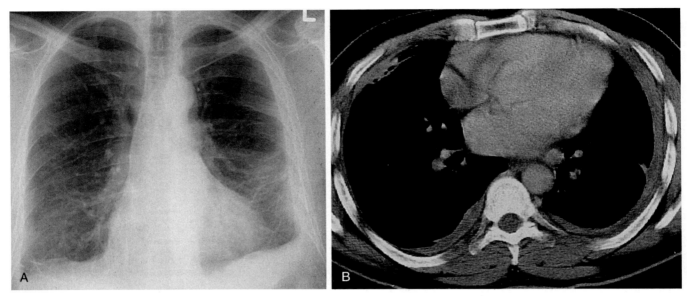

FIGURE 16–13

Diffuse asbestos-related pleural thickening. A posteroanterior chest radiograph (**A**) demonstrates diffuse bilateral pleural thickening as well as blunting of the costophrenic sulci. Curvilinear opacities extending to the thickened pleura are present in the left lung. An HRCT scan (**B**) confirms the presence of pleural thickening. The inner margin of the pleura is irregular because of areas of fibrosis or atelectasis in the adjacent lung. Despite the extensive pleural thickening in the paravertebral portion of the pleura and lateral aspect of the chest wall, there is no evidence of involvement of the mediastinal pleura. The patient was a 47-year-old cement worker with progressive shortness of breath. *(From Müller NL, Fraser RS, Colman NC, Paré PD: Radiologic Diagnosis of Diseases of the Chest. Philadelphia, WB Saunders, 2001.)*

pleura (although it frequently affects the parietal pleura abutting the paravertebral gutters) (Fig. 16–13).[195,197] The absence of mediastinal pleural involvement can be assessed readily on CT scan and is often helpful in distinguishing benign from malignant pleural thickening; in a study of 19 patients, only 1 of 8 with fibrothorax had thickening of the mediastinal pleura, as compared with 8 of 11 with mesothelioma.[195]

Pleural Effusion

The presence of asbestos-associated pleural effusion is often not appreciated.[198,199] The most comprehensive report of its prevalence and incidence was a study of 1135 exposed workers and 717 control subjects in whom benign asbestos effusion was defined by (1) a history of exposure to asbestos; (2) confirmation of the presence of effusion by radiography, thoracentesis, or both; (3) absence of other non-neoplastic disease that could have caused the effusion; and (4) absence of malignant tumor within 3 years.[199] According to these criteria, 34 benign effusions (3%) were identified in the exposed workers versus none in the control subjects. The likelihood of the presence of effusion was dose related. The latency period was shorter than for other asbestos-related disorders, effusion being the most common abnormality detected during the first 20 years after exposure. Most effusions were small, 28% recurred, and 66% were unassociated with symptoms.[199]

Pulmonary Manifestations

Asbestosis

Asbestosis is typically manifested on the chest radiograph by the presence of small, irregular linear opacities (Fig. 16–14).

The development of these abnormalities may be divided into three stages: (1) an early stage of fine reticulation evident predominantly in the lower lung zone and associated with a ground-glass appearance; (2) a stage in which irregular small opacities become more marked and prominent interstitial reticulation is created; during this stage, the combination of parenchymal and pleural abnormalities leads to partial obscuration of the heart border (the so-called shaggy heart sign) and the diaphragm; and (3) a late stage in which reticulation becomes visible in the middle and upper lung zones and the cardiac and diaphragmatic contours become more obscured.[195]

Although the radiographic findings of asbestosis are not specific, the diagnosis should be suspected when irregular linear opacities are associated with pleural plaques or diffuse pleural thickening. In approximately 20% of patients who have radiographic findings of asbestosis, however, there is no radiographic evidence of asbestos pleural disease.[200] Radiographs fail to show any parenchymal abnormalities in 10% to 20% of patients who have pathologically proven asbestosis.[201,202]

As with other conditions, CT, particularly HRCT, allows detection of parenchymal abnormalities not evident on the chest radiograph.[181-183] In a prospective study of 100 asbestos-exposed workers, HRCT findings suggestive of asbestosis were present in 43 of 45 (96%) who satisfied the clinical criteria for asbestosis versus 35 (78%) who had radiographic abnormalities.[183] In a review of the HRCT findings and pulmonary function tests in 169 asbestos-exposed workers who had normal chest radiographs (ILO profusion score <1/0), CT abnormalities consistent with asbestosis were found in 57; these patients had significantly lower VC and DCO values than the workers who had normal CT scans.[182]

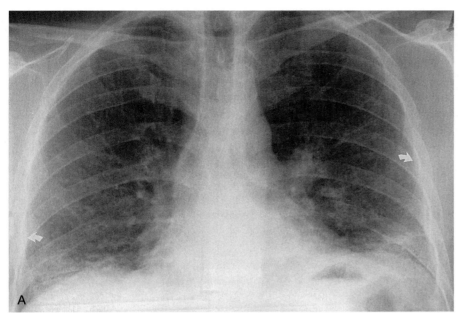

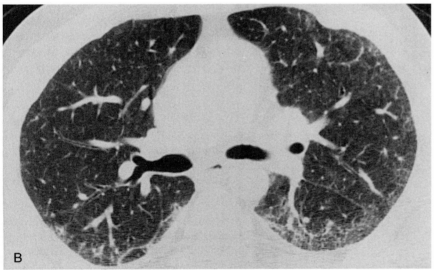

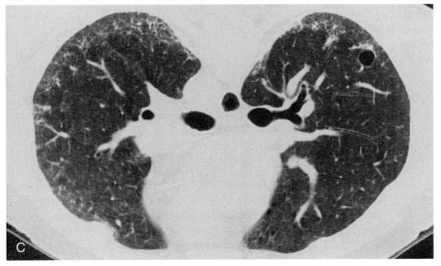

FIGURE 16–14

Asbestosis. A posteroanterior chest radiograph (**A**) in a 54-year-old shipyard worker demonstrates irregular linear opacities in the lower lung zones. Note the associated low lung volumes and bilateral pleural plaques (*arrows*). HRCT scans in the supine (**B**) and prone (**C**) positions demonstrate irregular linear opacities involving predominantly the subpleural regions. The opacities represent both intralobular lines and thickening of interlobular septa. Localized subpleural areas of ground-glass attenuation are also evident. *(From Müller NL, Fraser RS, Colman NC, Paré PD: Radiologic Diagnosis of Diseases of the Chest. Philadelphia, WB Saunders, 2001.)*

The most common HRCT manifestations of asbestosis are intralobular linear opacities; irregular thickening of the interlobular septa; subpleural curvilinear opacities; subpleural small rounded or branching opacities; and parenchymal bands (see Fig. 16–14).[181,182,203] Small, round (dotlike), and branching subpleural opacities are thought to be the earliest manifestation of disease.[203] Typically, they are visible a few millimeters from the pleural surface in a centrilobular location. HRCT-pathologic correlation has shown them to be related to peribronchiolar fibrosis.[203] Subpleural curvilinear opacities are areas of increased attenuation of variable length located within 1 cm of the pleura and parallel to the inner chest wall.[204] Most measure 5 to 10 cm in length. They are seen most commonly in early disease, although they may reflect honeycombing; they may also represent atelectasis adjacent to pleural plaques.[196,203,205]

Parenchymal bands are linear opacities measuring 2 to 5 cm in length that course through the lung and usually abut an area of pleural thickening.[183] Pathologic correlation has shown them to correspond to foci of peribronchovascular or interlobular septal fibrosis associated with distortion of the parenchymal architecture.[205] The bands are more common in asbestosis than in other causes of pulmonary fibrosis; for example, in one study they were present in 79% of patients who had asbestosis as compared with 11% of patients who had idiopathic pulmonary fibrosis.[206]

As in other causes of interstitial pulmonary fibrosis, architectural distortion of secondary lobules and irregular thickening of interlobular septa are seen commonly in asbestosis. With progression of fibrosis, irregular linear opacities and honeycombing predominate.[207,208] At all stages, the abnormalities involve predominantly the subpleural regions of the lower lung zones.[183,205,208]

Because the abnormalities in patients who have mild asbestosis are often limited to the posterior aspects of the lower lung zones, it is recommended that CT scans in these patients be obtained in the supine and prone positions or only in the prone position.[183,207,209] Scans with the patient prone are important to distinguish the normal increased opacity in the dependent lung regions from mild fibrosis. It has been shown that taking a small number of prone images at selected levels in the lower lung zones has high sensitivity for the detection of asbestos-related pulmonary and pleural abnormalities.[209] This procedure, combined with low–radiation dose scans, may become a cost-effective method of screening for asbestosis in high-risk populations.[209,210]

It is important to remember, however, that the HRCT findings of early asbestosis are neither sensitive nor specific.[112,207,211] The condition can be diagnosed with reasonable confidence in the appropriate clinical setting only if the parenchymal abnormalities are bilateral, present at multiple levels, and associated with pleural plaques or diffuse pleural thickening.[112,207] Asbestos-related pleural disease can be seen in 95% to 100% of patients who have evidence of asbestosis on HRCT.[181,183,207]

Round Atelectasis

The characteristic radiologic manifestation of round atelectasis is a rounded or oval, pleural-based opacity associated with loss of volume and curving of adjacent pulmonary vessels and bronchi (the comet tail sign).[212,213] The opacity typically abuts an area of pleural thickening or a pleural effusion. The comet tail sign is easier to identify on CT scan than on radiographs (Fig. 16–15). The abnormality may occur anywhere in the lungs, but it is most common in the posterior aspect of the lower lobes.[214,215] It may be unilateral or bilateral and may measure 2 to 7 cm in diameter. Significant enhancement may occur with administration of intravenous contrast material.[216]

Most cases of round atelectasis are associated with asbestos exposure; however, some have been described in association with other causes of pleural thickening or effusion.[177,215] The lesion may develop and progress over a few months or several years. In a series of 74 patients, it occurred on a background of benign asbestos effusion in 9 and slowly increasing pleural thickening in 13; in the remaining 52 patients, it was a new finding, with earlier radiographs showing only plaques or being normal.[177]

Clinical Manifestations

Most patients who have asbestos-related pleuropulmonary disease are asymptomatic. Pleuritic chest pain may accompany the development of benign asbestos effusion[217]; such effusions are generally less than 500 mL in volume, are often serosanguineous, and may persist from 2 weeks to 6 months. They are recurrent in 15% to 30% of cases. Breathlessness can be the result of interstitial fibrosis, chronic airflow obstruction, or diffuse pleural fibrosis.[218,219] When related to asbestosis, it is generally progressive, even in the absence of continued dust exposure. In patients who have asbestosis, shortness of breath seldom occurs sooner than 20 to 30 years after initial exposure.[220] Signs and symptoms of cor pulmonale develop in some patients. Prolonged asbestos exposure can also cause cough, which may be dry or productive of mucopurulent sputum; it can develop in the absence of physiologic or radiologic evidence of asbestosis.[221]

Physical examination may reveal asymmetry of chest wall motion in patients who have unilateral diffuse pleural fibrosis. Pleural effusion is suggested by the finding of dullness and decreased air entry over the affected lung. Crackles are evident in about 65% of workers who have asbestosis, and clubbing in about 30% to 40%; the presence of clubbing has been associated with a lower diffusing capacity, higher mortality rate, and greater likelihood of disease progression.[222]

Pulmonary Function Tests

Patients with asbestosis may have a restrictive derangement, a mixed restrictive/obstructive derangement, or airflow obstruction alone. When restriction is present, VC, residual volume, TLC, and diffusing capacity are decreased, but good ventilatory function is maintained.[223] Many patients, however, show some degree of airway obstruction as a result of asbestos-induced bronchiolar fibrosis.[223] In addition, emphysema is evident on CT scans in about 50% of workers who have early asbestosis, a figure double that of those who do not.[83] In fact, many workers with significant asbestosis have normal or increased TLC as a result of the presence of associated airflow obstruction.[224] Pulmonary compliance is characteristically greatly reduced and may be an early marker of interstitial fibrosis when the chest radiograph is normal.[225] Hypoxemia may be observed on exercise, but PCO_2 is usually normal or low.

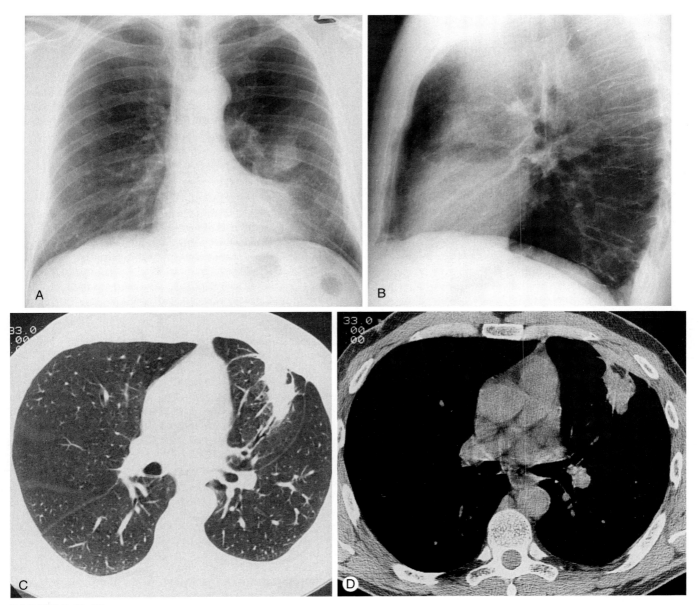

FIGURE 16–15

Round atelectasis. A 54-year-old man with a long-standing history of exposure to asbestos was referred for evaluation of a suspected left lung mass. Posteroanterior (**A**) and lateral (**B**) chest radiographs demonstrate evidence of left pleural thickening and a 3-cm mass in the left lung. The margins of the mass are poorly defined, indicating that it is pleural based. An HRCT scan (**C**) demonstrates an oval soft tissue mass in the lingula associated with loss of volume and anterior displacement of the major fissure. Vessels and bronchi can be seen curving into and sweeping around the area of atelectasis. Soft tissue windows (**D**) demonstrate that the area of atelectasis abuts a focal area of pleural thickening. The size of the mass was stable over a 3-year follow-up period. *(From Müller NL, Fraser RS, Colman NC, Paré PD: Radiologic Diagnosis of Diseases of the Chest. Philadelphia, WB Saunders, 2001.)*

Asbestos-related pleural disease can also cause restrictive lung function.[226] The loss of VC is much more marked in patients who have diffuse pleural thickening than in those who have only plaques.[227]

OTHER SILICATES

A number of fibrous and crystalline silicates other than asbestos can cause pulmonary disease. The most important in terms of numbers of exposed individuals are talc, mica, and kaolin. Additional, less commonly encountered substances include fuller's earth, zeolites (erionite), nepheline,[228] wollastonite,[229] and taconite.[230]

Talc

Talc is a hydrated magnesium silicate that is used in the manufacture of such diverse products as leather, rubber, paper, textiles, ceramic tile, and roofing material. It is also used as an additive in paint, food, many pharmaceuticals, insecticides, and herbicides. Individuals in any of these occupational settings may be exposed to potentially harmful levels of dust. Others at risk include workers involved in talc mining and milling,[231] individuals who work with soapstone,[232] and workers exposed to commercial talcum powder.[233] Pulmonary disease related to talc can also occur in nonoccupational settings, including (1) systemic microembolization of talc after the intravenous injection of oral medications (see page 571), (2) obsessional inhalation of commercial talcum powder,[234] and (3) pleurodesis (which can provoke pulmonary edema).

Because other elements such as iron and nickel are usually incorporated in the talc crystal and because the substance is often found in association with other minerals such as quartz and asbestos, the composition of commercially available talc can differ considerably from region to region and industry to industry.[235] As a result, the pattern of pulmonary disease associated with its inhalation is highly variable. In fact, the ability of talc in pure form to induce fibrosis has been questioned[236]; nonetheless, it is likely that true inhalational talcosis can occur, as evidenced by reports of disease caused by exposure to uncontaminated dust.[235,237]

Pathologic findings include pleural fibrosis (sometimes with calcification and plaque formation identical to that seen in asbestos-related pleural disease), foci of nodular or stellate parenchymal fibrosis, more or less diffuse interstitial fibrosis, non-necrotizing granulomatous inflammation, and accumulation of peribronchiolar and perivascular macrophages.[235,237] Both peribronchiolar and perivascular macrophages and multinucleated giant cells can typically be seen to contain irregularly shaped birefringent plates or needle-like crystals representing talc.

The principal radiologic abnormality consists of pleural plaques similar to those of asbestos-related disease. They may be massive and extend over much of the surface of both lungs.[238,239] Parenchymal involvement is said to be similar to that in asbestosis,[240] the radiographic pattern being one of general haziness, nodulation, and reticulation, with sparing of the apices and costophrenic sulci.[238]

Symptoms are similar to those of other pneumoconioses and include dyspnea and productive cough. Diminished breath sounds, bibasilar crackles, limited chest expansion, and clubbing may be found on physical examination.[241] The level of serum angiotensin-converting enzyme is elevated in some patients.[242]

A restrictive pulmonary function impairment with low diffusing capacity has been reported in patients who have parenchymal lung disease.[241] Restriction has also been described in patients who have apparently isolated pleural disease[243]; however, this report antedates the use of HRCT to exclude parenchymal disease that was unappreciated on the radiograph.

Mica

Micas are complex aluminum silicates, of which three forms are commercially available: (1) muscovite, which is used in the production of windows for stoves and furnaces and is encountered by workers involved in the mining and use of slate (e.g., in roofing, highway construction, and tiling)[244]; (2) phlogopite, which is used in the electrical industry; and (3) vermiculite, whose uses relate primarily to its fire resistance, insulation, and ion-exchange properties.

Similar to talc, micas are often associated with other minerals, particularly tremolite asbestos,[245] and whether they cause disease by themselves has been questioned.[246] However, pulmonary fibrosis has resulted from the inhalation of pure mica alone,[247,248] and it seems reasonable to conclude that the risk of development of pulmonary disease from its inhalation is real, albeit slight. Radiographic and clinical manifestations are indistinguishable from those associated with asbestos or talc.

Kaolin

The term *kaolin* (china clay) refers to a group of clays, of which kaolinite, a hydrated aluminum silicate, is the most important member. This substance is used industrially as a filler in plastics, rubber, paints, and adhesives; as a coating for paper; as an absorbent; and in the making of firebricks.[249] Water is generally used in quarrying or strip mining to minimize the risk of dust exposure; however, subsequent drying, bagging, and transportation can result in exposure to high concentrations of aerosolized dust. Although it seems likely that kaolinite alone can cause pulmonary disease,[249] it is probable that some cases are complicated by the inhalation of other particulates such as silica.

The incidence of significant chest disease in reported series varies from zero[250] to 25%.[251] The presence and severity of abnormalities are related to the number of years of exposure.[252] In a radiographic study of workers from England, 75% were judged to have radiographs of category 0, 20% of category 1, and 5% of categories 2 and 3; 19 workers (1%) were considered to have PMF.[251]

Pathologic findings consist of microscopic, peribronchiolar macules containing pigment-laden macrophages and interspersed reticulin fibers, as well as larger macrophage aggregates that measure up to 12 cm in diameter. Despite their size, the latter may contain only small amounts of collagen. When present, fibrosis appears to correlate with the quartz content.[253]

The radiographic pattern varies. In some cases, there may be no more than a general increase in lung markings. With prolonged and severe exposure, a diffuse nodular and miliary mottling is present; when it develops, the appearance of PMF is identical to that seen in silicosis and CWP.[254] Clnical findings are nonspecific.

Fuller's Earth

Fuller's earth is an aluminum silicate used in the refining of oils, as a filtering agent, as a filler in cosmetics and other products, and in the bonding of molding sands in foundry work. Prolonged exposure can result in the accumulation of dust-containing macrophages, usually with little fibrosis or inflammatory cellular reaction.[255] Radiographic changes are evident mainly in the upper lobes and consist of a prominence of bronchovascular markings and, rarely, PMF.[256]

Zeolites (Erionite)

Zeolites are a group of over 30 naturally occurring minerals composed of hydrated aluminum silicates that are found in deposits of volcanic ash and are widely used as absorbents and for filtration.[257] The richest deposits are in Turkey and the western United States. Most zeolites are not considered toxic; however, erionite has been reported to be associated with pleural plaques, mesothelioma, pulmonary carcinoma, and interstitial fibrosis.[257,258]

INERT RADIOPAQUE DUST

Iron

Workers in many occupations are exposed to dust containing iron, usually in the form of iron oxide (Fe_2O_3). The majority are electric arc or oxyacetylene torch workers, who are exposed to fumes derived from melted and boiled iron emitted during the welding process. Other individuals at risk include those involved in the mining and processing of iron ore and metallic pigments such as ocher, workers in iron and steel rolling mills, foundry workers, boiler scalers, and workers exposed to magnetite.

When inhaled in sufficient quantity in relatively pure form, iron oxide causes *siderosis*, a condition generally believed to be unassociated with fibrosis or functional impairment. This belief is supported by experimental studies in animals in which various inhaled iron compounds did not cause a fibrotic reaction and by the presence of healthy workers exposed to high concentrations of iron dust over a period of many years.[259] However, it is important to realize that workers in occupations associated with iron dust or fume production are frequently exposed to other noxious materials, including asbestos and silica. Such exposure may result in the clinical, radiologic, and pathologic features characteristic of mixed dust pneumoconiosis (siderosilicosis).[260]

Pathologically, pulmonary siderosis is characterized by the presence of macrophages filled with iron oxide, situated predominantly in the peribronchovascular interstitium.[261] Fibrosis is typically absent or minimal. In mixed dust disease, the appearance is similar to that of silicosis and is characterized by solitary or coalescent fibrous nodules, the latter occasionally being large enough to be designated PMF. Unlike in pure silicosis, the nodules are usually rather poorly defined and have stellate borders. Aggregates of iron oxide and other substances, such as carbon and various silicates, can usually be found in the fibrous tissue, either free or within macrophages.

The radiographic pattern in pure siderosis is reticulonodular and widely disseminated. In an evaluation of 661 British electric arc welders, 7% showed small rounded opacities of 0/1 category or higher, there being a clear association between prevalence and years of exposure[262]; only 10 workers had changes greater than 2/2. Opacities have been shown experimentally to correlate with localized aggregates of Fe_2O_3-laden macrophages and are caused by the density of the Fe_2O_3 itself.[263] Individual shadows appear to be of lesser density than the nodules of silicosis. In contrast to the majority of cases of pneumoconiosis, the radiographic abnormalities can disappear partly or completely when patients are removed from dust exposure.[264] In siderosilicosis, the pattern depends somewhat on the concentration of free silica in the inhaled dust: when it is relatively low, the appearance is similar to that of pure siderosis or CWP; when it is high, the pattern is identical to that of silicosis.

Patients who have siderosis are asymptomatic. However, those who have siderosilicosis may complain of cough and dyspnea. Even in the absence of radiographic abnormality, arc welders[265] and foundry workers[264] have been found to have a higher incidence of bronchitis than control subjects. Although some investigators have found the results of pulmonary function tests of welders to be within normal limits,[261] others have identified airflow obstruction, even in nonsmokers.[266]

Iron and Silver

Inhalation of large amounts of iron oxide and silver can produce an unusual pneumoconiosis termed *argyrosiderosis*. This condition results from the use of jeweler's rouge (which is composed in part of iron oxide) as a polishing agent in the finishing of silver products. When it is applied with a buffer, small particles of Fe_2O_3 are generated that may be inhaled. Pathologic examination shows the presence of iron-laden macrophages in a distribution similar to that of pure siderosis; in addition, silver can be identified in the alveolar walls and the walls of small arteries and veins, particularly in the internal elastic laminae.[267] The radiographic manifestation consists of a finely stippled pattern, in contrast to the reticulonodular pattern of siderosis. Patients are typically asymptomatic.

Tin

Pneumoconiosis caused by the inhalation of tin (*stannosis*) occurs predominantly in individuals employed in the handling of ore after it has been mined, especially in industries in which tin oxide fumes have been created. Pathologically, the findings simulate the macule of CWP. Although the condition causes no clinical or functional derangement,[268] the high density of tin (atomic number 50) results in a dramatic radiographic appearance consisting of multiple tiny shadows of high density, about 1 mm in diameter, distributed evenly throughout the lungs[268]; larger, somewhat less numerous nodules are seen occasionally. Linear opacities may be present in the paramediastinal zone, in the vicinity of the costophrenic angles.

Barium

Barium and its salts, particularly barium sulfate, are used as coloring or weighting agents, as fillers in numerous products, and in the manufacturing of glass. Exposure during any of these uses, as well as in mining of the ore itself, can cause pulmonary disease (*barytosis*). The chest radiograph shows a variable number of discrete, high-density shadows (the atomic number of barium is 56) that create an awesome appearance.[269] The lesions may develop after a relatively brief exposure and characteristically regress after removal of the patient from the dust-filled environment. Some patients complain of chronic productive cough and/or asthma-like symptoms[270]; however, many are asymptomatic.

Antimony

Antimony is procured mainly from the mineral stibnite and is handled either as unrefined ore or as a fine white powder.[271]

It is used in cosmetics; in the manufacture of batteries, pewter, printing type, and electrodes; in the compounding of rubber; in textiles, paints, and plastics as a flame retardant; and in ceramics as an opacifier. Both direct pathologic[271] and experimental[272] evidence show that accumulation of the mineral is accompanied by little, if any, fibrosis. The chest radiograph of affected workers reveals minute dense rounded opacities scattered widely throughout both lungs.[272] Lung function is usually normal.

Rare Earth Elements

The rare earth elements include cerium (quantitatively the most important), scandium, yttrium, lanthanum, and 14 other minerals. Although the elements have a wide variety of industrial uses, pneumoconiosis occurs chiefly in individuals working with carbon arc lamps in the graphic arts (such as photoengraving), in printers, or in movie projectionists.[273] Granulomatous inflammation[274] and parenchymal fibrosis[275] have been described in a number of cases; in some, the extent and progression of disease appear to depend on the thorium content of the dust.[276] The typical radiographic appearance consists of diffuse dense punctate opacities,[277] again related to the high atomic number of the inhaled dust, which ranges from 51 to 71. Spirometry may show a restrictive impairment; patients may or may not be symptomatic.

MISCELLANEOUS INORGANIC DUST

Beryllium

Beryllium's properties of low density, high tensile strength, electrical and thermal conductivity, and corrosion resistance have made it an essential material in the manufacture of products for the aerospace, automotive, energy, nuclear, medical, and electronics industries.[278] An estimated 800,000 Americans have been exposed to the substance at some time; disease rates of 2% to 16% have been reported in exposed workers.[279] Sensitization to beryllium[280] does not occur in workers who are exposed to levels less than 0.01 $\mu g/m^3$; however, berylliosis has occurred at exposure levels well below the current Occupational Safety and Health Administration (OSHA) standard of 2.0 $\mu g/m^3$.[281] Disease resulting from nonoccupational and para-occupational exposure (e.g., custodial employees working in a nuclear weapons facility) has been well described.[282]

Berylliosis can occur in acute or chronic forms; however, as a result of improved environmental controls, the acute form is almost never seen today.

Acute Berylliosis

Acute berylliosis has been seen most often after accidental exposure to very high concentrations of dust. It can be manifested as fulminating, often fatal pulmonary edema that develops 1 to 4 weeks after the onset of symptoms. Pathologic findings include bronchitis, bronchiolitis, and diffuse alveolar damage.[283] Sometimes the disease is more insidious, with symptoms of cough, chest pain, dyspnea, anorexia, weakness, and weight loss developing weeks or even months after the initial exposure. Upper airway symptoms may be dominant.[284] Recovery can be complete after withdrawal from exposure.

Chronic Berylliosis

Chronic berylliosis is the result of an immunologic reaction to beryllium particles and is characterized by lymphocyte activation and proliferation, release of various immune cell mediators, and the development of granulomatous inflammation.[278] The pattern of cytokine release from the activated lymphocytes suggests that they are largely of a T_H1 phenotype, producing IL-2 and interferon-γ, the macrophage-activating cytokine that drives the granulomatous reaction.[285] Susceptibility to disease is related to particular HLA-DP alleles that are associated with substitution of a glutamic acid at position 69 in the HLA-DP β-chain,[286] a locus that interacts specifically with beryllium.[287]

The characteristic pathologic abnormality is interstitial pneumonitis,[283] which varies from a more or less diffuse mononuclear cell infiltrate unassociated with granulomatous inflammation to well-formed, discrete, non-necrotizing granulomas indistinguishable from those of sarcoidosis. Interstitial fibrosis is common. In contrast to most other types of dust that cause pneumoconiosis, beryllium is largely removed from the lungs with time and excreted in urine. As a result, quantitative studies show significantly less tissue content of beryllium in chronic than in acute disease.[283]

The most common radiographic pattern consists of bilateral ill-defined nodules, mainly of size p or q, scattered diffusely throughout the lungs, sometimes associated with lymph node enlargement.[112,288] Calcification of the nodules may occur.[289] In a study of 28 patients who had biopsy-proven disease, abnormalities related to beryllium were found in 21 (75%) by HRCT and in 15 (54%) by radiography.[290] The most common findings seen with the former procedure were thickened interlobular septa and small nodular opacities. The nodules were well defined and seen mainly along the bronchovascular bundles or interlobular septa, a distribution similar to that in sarcoidosis.[291,292] Other findings included pleural irregularities—presumably related to coalescence of subpleural nodules—in 7 (25%) patients and hilar or mediastinal lymph node enlargement in 11 (39%). Lymph node enlargement was noted only in patients who had an associated parenchymal abnormality.

In advanced cases, the radiographic pattern may be chiefly reticular and associated with a marked decrease in volume. CT scans in these patients demonstrate a predominantly reticular pattern, frequently associated with honeycombing.[290,293] Conglomeration of nodules may result in the formation of large opacities similar to those seen in silicosis. Spontaneous pneumothorax occurs in slightly more than 10% of cases.[289]

The majority of patients in whom chronic berylliosis develops have been exposed to the dust for more than 2 years. Typically, symptoms begin insidiously 6 to 10 years after exposure has ceased; however, latencies as long as 30 years and as short as 4 months have been reported.[279] Disease can be triggered by specific events, such as pregnancy, surgery, or even performance of the patch test.[294] Symptoms include cough, fatigue, weight loss, increased dyspnea on exertion, and sometimes migratory arthralgia. Crackles may be heard on auscultation, and the liver and spleen may be palpable. Clubbing has been noted in 30% of patients, especially those who have advanced disease.

Hypergammaglobulinemia, hypercalciuria, hypercalcemia, hyperuricemia, abnormal liver function, and polycythemia are not uncommon findings when disease is clinically evident.[279] The serum angiotensin-converting enzyme level may be elevated, although an increase may also be seen in apparently healthy beryllium-exposed workers.[295] Analysis of BAL fluid reveals increased numbers of beryllium-sensitized CD4+ T cells.[296]

Sensitization to beryllium can be demonstrated by patch testing (in which granulomatous inflammation develops as a response to the application of a solution of beryllium sulfate to the skin), by the proliferation of blood lymphocytes on exposure to beryllium,[297] and by beryllium-induced activation and proliferation of lymphocytes obtained by BAL. Since the patch test can itself induce sensitization to beryllium, its use has been relegated to the second tier of diagnostic tools. Because of significant intralaboratory and interlaboratory variation in the results of the blood lymphocyte proliferation test, a worker should be considered sensitized only after two positive tests.[287] Chronic berylliosis does not develop in all sensitized individuals; however, even in the absence of functional, clinical, and radiologic evidence of disease, it can be demonstrated by identifying granulomas on transbronchial biopsy specimens or (according to some authorities[279]) by documenting a proliferative response of lavage fluid lymphocytes to beryllium.

Lung function studies may show restriction, obstruction, or mixed restriction/obstruction.[298] The diffusing capacity may become abnormal only in advanced disease, whereas abnormalities in gas exchange during exercise may be an early finding.

The prognosis of patients who have symptomatic chronic berylliosis is poor,[298] particularly when complicating cor pulmonale is present. Beryllium is a carcinogen that is capable of causing pulmonary carcinoma in animals. The results of large cohort studies support the hypothesis that it is a carcinogen for humans as well,[299] particularly in individuals who have suffered from acute berylliosis.

Aluminum

Individuals can be exposed to the toxic effects of aluminum in a number of situations, including (1) the reduction of alumina to metallic aluminum during smelting,[300] (2) the preparation or use of aluminum powder,[300] (3) aluminum arc welding,[301] (4) the grinding and polishing of aluminum products[302] or the manufacture or use of aluminum-based abrasive grinding tools,[303] and (5) the mining of bauxite.[304] Although each of these situations has been associated with pulmonary disease, the conclusion that aluminum has been the pathogenetic agent is not always definitive since concomitant exposure to other toxic substances may have occurred.[300,303] However, animal studies have revealed a fibrotic response to aluminum alone,[305] thus supporting the notion that the dust can be fibrogenic in humans. It is possible that individual factors such as immune mechanisms are involved in the pathogenesis of disease.[306]

Pathologic findings in the lungs of individuals exposed to aluminum are variable and, as indicated, may be caused in some cases by substances other than aluminum itself. Histologic reactions that have been reported include diffuse interstitial fibrosis,[307] desquamative interstitial pneumonitis,[308] alveolar proteinosis,[302] and diffuse granulomatous inflammation.[306]

Radiographic abnormalities may become apparent after a few months or several years of exposure.[309] Fully developed changes consist of a fine to coarse reticular pattern widely distributed throughout the lungs, sometimes with a nodular component.[309] The fibrosis frequently involves the upper lobes.[303] HRCT findings have been described in a study of six workers, in whom the abnormalities consisted predominantly of small nodular opacities in two and a reticular pattern in four[310]; honeycombing was also present in two patients. In five of the six patients, the abnormalities involved mainly the upper lung zones. Lung volume may be greatly decreased, and the pleura may become thickened; spontaneous pneumothorax is a frequent complication.

Breathlessness is the chief symptom and may be disabling. Chronic airflow obstruction or asthma develops in some individuals.[311] Pulmonary function tests have shown both restrictive and obstructive disease with a reduction in diffusing capacity.[303]

Cobalt and Tungsten Carbide

The term *hard metal* is generally used to refer to an alloy of tungsten, carbon, and cobalt (occasionally with small amounts of other metals[312]). The resulting product is extremely hard and resistant to heat and is used extensively in the drilling and polishing of other metals. Exposure to dust can occur during either manufacture or use of the metal and is well recognized as a cause of interstitial pneumonitis and fibrosis.[313]

The pathogenesis of disease is unclear. Experimental studies in animals suggest that cobalt is the etiologic agent,[312] a hypothesis supported by the finding of disease in diamond polishers,[314] who are exposed to high concentrations of cobalt alone. However, there is evidence that the effects of cobalt are enhanced by the presence of tungsten carbide,[312] and cobalt has not been found in the lung tissue of patients who have interstitial fibrosis and a history of exposure to hard metals in some autopsy studies.[315] Some features of the disease suggest an immunologic pathogenesis, including the lack of correlation of disease with the intensity of exposure, the presence of T cells in the inflammatory infiltrate, and the association between disease and the presence of glutamate-69 in the HLA-DP β-chain (a feature in common with berylliosis).[316]

Pathologic findings are predominantly those of interstitial pneumonitis with a variable degree of fibrosis.[317] Characteristically, numerous macrophages are present in the alveolar air spaces, giving a pattern of desquamative interstitial pneumonitis. In many cases, multinucleated giant cells are also prominent (giant cell interstitial pneumonitis).

The radiographic findings consist of a diffuse micronodular and reticular pattern, sometimes associated with lymph node enlargement; the reticulation may be coarse and in advanced disease may be accompanied by small cystic spaces.[318] In a study of two hard-metal workers, the HRCT findings consisted of bilateral areas of ground-glass attenuation, areas of consolidation, and extensive reticular opacities and traction bronchiectasis indicative of fibrosis[310]; autopsy correlation in one case showed the areas of ground-glass attenuation and consolidation to correspond to aggregates of mononuclear and multinucleated giant cells.

Symptoms include weight loss, dry cough, and dyspnea on exertion; severe respiratory insufficiency sometimes develops and can prove fatal.[319] The identification of multinucleated giant cells in BAL fluid supports the diagnosis.[320] Pulmonary function tests reveal both restrictive and obstructive patterns, and diffusion may be reduced.[321]

Silicon Carbide

Silicon carbide (carborundum) is produced by the fusion of high-grade sand, finely ground carbon (coke), salt, and wood dust at high temperature.[322] The resulting product is extremely hard and used as an abrasive. Some workers in the carborundum industry have been found to have interstitial fibrosis and macrophage accumulation at autopsy, consistent with pneumoconiosis.[323] Radiographic abnormalities include nodular, reticulonodular, or reticular opacities with or without hilar adenopathy[324]; pleural plaques similar to those seen in asbestos-exposed individuals have also been described.[325]

Polyvinyl Chloride

Polyvinyl chloride is produced by polymerization of the gas vinyl chloride under pressure.[326] It is used in the manufacture of plastics, synthetic fibers, and numerous other commercial products. Inhalation of polyvinyl chloride may be associated with the development of interstitial pneumonitis and fibrosis or with the accumulation of interstitial and intra-alveolar macrophages.[327] Epidemiologic studies have shown the presence of radiographic abnormalities consistent with pneumoconiosis in 3% to 20% of workers.[328] Pulmonary function testing may show a restrictive[329] or combined restrictive/obstructive impairment.[330]

Titanium Dioxide

Titanium dioxide is derived from the ore ilmenite and is used chiefly as a pigment in paints, paper, and other products; as a mordant in dyeing; and as an alloy in some hard metals. Histologic examination of the lungs of individuals who have inhaled the substance has shown the accumulation of alveolar and interstitial macrophages but minimal fibrosis.[331] Nonnecrotizing granulomatous inflammation was identified in one patient[332]; because of a positive lymphocyte transformation test on exposure to titanium, the authors considered the possibility of an immunologic reaction similar to that described in workers who have berylliosis. Radiographic changes considered consistent with pneumoconiosis have been reported in some workers involved in pigment production.[332] Restrictive impairment was described in one study.[333]

Volcanic Dust

Volcanic dust can result in liberation of significant quantities of potentially harmful ash into the atmosphere. Asphyxiation resulting from plugging of major airways by mucus and inhaled ash was the cause of death in many individuals who died as a direct result of the eruption of Mount St. Helens in 1980.[334] Patients who survived had a mild increase in the number of acute respiratory complaints such as cough, wheezing, and dyspnea,[335] presumably as a result of acute airway irritation. The long-term consequences, if any, of volcanic ash inhalation are unclear.

Synthetic Mineral Fibers

Synthetic mineral fibers are amorphous silicates derived from slag, rock, or glass. Unlike natural silicates such as asbestos, synthetic fibers break transversely rather than longitudinally when traumatized, thereby resulting in small fragments whose diameter is the same as that of their parents.[336] Because the potential for fibers to cause disease is determined at least in part by a high length-to-diameter ratio,[336] this feature may be important in explaining the relative lack of toxicity of these substances. It is possible that fibers that do cause pulmonary injury are more likely to persist in pulmonary tissue.[337] The major adverse health effect of long-term exposure seems to be functional: a higher prevalence of obstructive lung function is seen in workers than in control populations.[302,338]

Cement Dust

Workers exposed to cement dust have a high prevalence of respiratory tract symptoms.[339] Although some investigators have implicated cement dust as a cause of pneumoconiosis as well,[339,340] others have found few or no radiographic abnormalities.[341]

Zirconium

Zirconium is a heavy metal used as an alloy in the nuclear industry and in the glazing of ceramic tile. Pulmonary disease after exposure seems to be uncommon[342]; however, occasional examples of fibrosis or granulomatous inflammation have been described.[343,344]

Nylon Flock

Flock is finely cut fiber (either natural or synthetic) that is used to give a velvet-like coat to fabric or other material. Nylon flock is widely used in upholstery, clothing, and automobiles. Interstitial lung disease has been described in workers in several nylon flock facilities,[345,346] the overall prevalence being about 4% of exposed workers. Histologic examination of biopsy specimens has shown lymphocytic bronchiolitis and peribronchiolitis, frequently associated with the formation of lymphoid follicles.[346]

Radiographic changes include diffuse reticulonodular opacities and (occasionally) patchy consolidation. HRCT has revealed bilateral areas of ground-glass opacification[345] and is a sensitive diagnostic tool.[7] Symptoms of dry cough and dyspnea have developed with a mean latency of 6 years after initial exposure. Lung function testing shows a restrictive defect with a decrease in diffusing capacity.[346,347] Clinical improvement has been noted with cessation of exposure, and relapse has followed re-exposure to dust.[346]

Dust Exposure in Dental Technicians

Dental technicians are exposed to a variety of inorganic materials during the process of grinding and drilling of dental prostheses, and there are several well-documented cases of lung disease related to inhalation of these substances.[348] Although this form of pneumoconiosis has been attributed to silicon dioxide, it is probable that other agents, such as acrylic resin and cobalt, are implicated as well.[348,349]

REFERENCES

1. Dorland's Illustrated Medical Dictionary. Philadelphia, WB Saunders, 1994.
2. Work-Related Lung Disease Surveillance Report 1999. National Institute for Occupational Safety and Health, Atlanta, GA, 2000.
3. Seaton A, Lamb D, Brown WR, et al: Pneumoconiosis of shale miners. Thorax 36:412-418, 1981.
4. Beckett WS: Occupational respiratory diseases. N Engl J Med 342:406-413, 2000.
5. De Zotti R, Muran A, Zambon F: Two cases of paraoccupational asthma due to toluene diisocyanate (TDI). Occup Environ Med 57:837-839, 2000.
6. Norboo T, Angchuk PT, Yahya M, et al: Silicosis in a Himalayan village population: Role of environmental dust. Thorax 46:341-343, 1991.
7. Kern DG, Kuhn C 3rd, Ely EW, et al: Flock worker's lung: Broadening the spectrum of clinicopathology, narrowing the spectrum of suspected etiologies. Chest 117:251-259, 2000.
8. Pinkerton KE, Plopper CG, Mercer RR, et al: Airway branching patterns influence asbestos fiber location and the extent of tissue injury in the pulmonary parenchyma. Lab Invest 55:688-695, 1986.
9. Richeldi L, Kreiss K, Mroz MM, et al: Interaction of genetic and exposure factors in the prevalence of berylliosis. Am J Ind Med 32:337-340, 1997.
10. Begin R, Masse S, Sebastien P, et al: Asbestos exposure and retention as determinants of airway disease and asbestos alveolitis. Am Rev Respir Dis 134:1176-1181, 1986.
11. Amandus HE, Reger RB, Pendergrass EP, et al: The pneumoconioses: Methods of measuring progression. Chest 63:736-743, 1973.
12. Internal Labour Office: Guidelines for the use of ILO International Classification of Radiographs of Pneumoconioses. Geneva, International Labour Office, 1980, pp 1-48.
13. Liddell FD, Lindars DC: An elaboration of the I.L.O. classification of simple pneumoconiosis. Br J Ind Med 26:89-100, 1969.
14. Albin M, Engholm G, Frostrom K, et al: Chest x ray films from construction workers: International Labour Office (ILO 1980) classification compared with routine readings. Br J Ind Med 49:862-868, 1992.
15. Castellan RM, Sanderson WT, Petersen MR: Prevalence of radiographic appearance of pneumoconiosis in an unexposed blue collar population. Am Rev Respir Dis 131:684-686, 1985.
16. Meyer JD, Islam SS, Ducatman AM, McCunney RJ: Prevalence of small lung opacities in populations unexposed to dusts. A literature analysis. Chest 111:404-410, 1997.
17. Welch LS, Hunting KL, Balmes J, et al: Variability in the classification of radiographs using the 1980 International Labour Organization Classification for Pneumoconioses. Chest 114:1740-1748, 1998.
18. Morgan WK, Seaton A: Occupational Lung Diseases. Philadelphia, WB Saunders, 1995.
19. Rosenman KD, Reilly MJ, Rice C, et al: Silicosis among foundry workers. Implication for the need to revise the OSHA standard. Am J Epidemiol 144:890-900, 1996.
20. International Agency for Research on Cancer: Silica and some silicates. IARC Monogr Eval Carcinog Risks Hum 42, 1986.
21. Murray J, Kielkowski D, Reid P: Occupational disease trends in black South African gold miners. An autopsy-based study. Am J Respir Crit Care Med 153:706-710, 1996.
22. Chen W, Zhuang Z, Attfield MD, et al: Exposure to silica and silicosis among tin miners in China: Exposure-response analyses and risk assessment. Occup Environ Med 58:31-37, 2001.
23. Prowse K, Allen MB, Bradbury SP: Respiratory symptoms and pulmonary impairment in male and female subjects with pottery workers' silicosis. Ann Occup Hyg 33:375-385, 1989.
24. Hirsch M, Bar-Ziv J, Lehmann E, Goldberg GM: Simple siliceous pneumoconiosis of Bedouin females in the Negev desert. Clin Radiol 25:507-510, 1974.
25. Dumontet C, Biron F, Vitrey D, et al: Acute silicosis due to inhalation of a domestic product. Am Rev Respir Dis 143:880-882, 1991.
26. Mossman BT, Churg A: Mechanisms in the pathogenesis of asbestosis and silicosis. Am J Respir Crit Care Med 157:1666-1680, 1998.
27. Warheit DB, Overby LH, George G, Brody AR: Pulmonary macrophages are attracted to inhaled particles through complement activation. Exp Lung Res 14:51-66, 1988.
28. Dubois CM, Bissonnette E, Rola-Pleszczynski M: Asbestos fibers and silica particles stimulate rat alveolar macrophages to release tumor necrosis factor. Autoregulatory role of leukotriene B_4. Am Rev Respir Dis 139:1257-1264, 1989.
29. Mariani TJ, Arikan MC, Pierce RA: Fibroblast tropoelastin and alpha-smooth-muscle actin expression are repressed by particulate-activated macrophage-derived tumor necrosis factor-alpha in experimental silicosis. Am J Respir Cell Mol Biol 21:185-192, 1999.
30. Corbett EL, Mozzato-Chamay N, Butterworth AE, et al: Polymorphisms in the tumor necrosis factor-alpha gene promoter may predispose to severe silicosis in black South African miners. Am J Respir Crit Care Med 165:690-693, 2002.
31. Yucesoy B, Vallyathan V, Landsittel DP, et al: Polymorphisms of the IL-1 gene complex in coal miners with silicosis. Am J Ind Med 39:286-291, 2001.
32. Garn H, Friedetzky A, Kirchner A, et al: Experimental silicosis: A shift to a preferential IFN-gamma–based Th1 response in thoracic lymph nodes. Am J Physiol Lung Cell Mol Physiol 278:L1221-L1230, 2000.
33. Wallaert B, Lassalle P, Fortin F, et al: Superoxide anion generation by alveolar inflammatory cells in simple pneumoconiosis and in progressive massive fibrosis of nonsmoking coal workers. Am Rev Respir Dis 141:129-133, 1990.
34. Gusev VA, Danilovskaja YV, Vatolkina O, et al: Effect of quartz and alumina dust on generation of superoxide radicals and hydrogen peroxide by alveolar macrophages, granulocytes, and monocytes. Br J Ind Med 50:732-735, 1993.
35. Scharfman A, Hayem A, Davril M, et al: Special neutrophil elastase inhibitory activity in BAL fluid from patients with silicosis and asbestosis. Eur Respir J 2:751-757, 1989.
36. Borges VM, Falcao H, Leite-Junior JH, et al: Fas ligand triggers pulmonary silicosis. J Exp Med 194:155-164, 2001.
37. Konecny R, Leonard S, Shi X, et al: Reactivity of free radicals on hydroxylated quartz surface and its implications for pathogenicity; experimental and quantum mechanical study. J Environ Pathol Toxicol Oncol 20(Suppl 1):119-132, 2001.
38. Barrett EG, Johnston C, Oberdorster G, Finkelstein JN: Antioxidant treatment attenuates cytokine and chemokine levels in murine macrophages following silica exposure. Toxicol Appl Pharmacol 158:211-220, 1999.
39. Leibowitz MC, Goldstein B: Some investigations into the nature and cause of massive fibrosis (MF) in the lungs of South African gold, coal, and asbestos mine workers. Am J Ind Med 12:129-143, 1987.
40. Ng TP, Chan SL: Factors associated with massive fibrosis in silicosis. Thorax 46:229-232, 1991.
41. Lee PH, Phoon WH, Ng TP: Radiological progression and its predictive risk factors in silicosis. Occup Environ Med 58:467-471, 2001.
42. Koskinen H, Tiilikainen A, Nordman H: Increased prevalence of HLA-Aw19 and of the phenogroup Aw19,B18 in advanced silicosis. Chest 83:848-852, 1983.
43. Nery LE, Florencio RT, Sandoval PR, et al: Additive effects of exposure to silica dust and smoking on pulmonary epithelial permeability: A radioaerosol study with technetium-99m labelled DTPA. Thorax 48:264-268, 1993.
44. Hoffmann EO, Lamberty J, Pizzolato P, Coover J: The ultrastructure of acute silicosis. Arch Pathol 96:104-107, 1973.
45. Miller BE, Dethloff LA, Gladen BC, Hook GE: Progression of type II cell hypertrophy and hyperplasia during silica-induced pulmonary inflammation. Lab Invest 57:546-554, 1987.
46. Miller BE, Hook GE: Isolation and characterization of hypertrophic type II cells from the lungs of silica-treated rats. Lab Invest 58:565-575, 1988.
47. Emerson RJ, Davis GS: Effect of alveolar lining material–coated silica on rat alveolar macrophages. Environ Health Perspect 51:81-84, 1983.
48. Craighead JE, Kleinerman J, Abraham JL, et al: Diseases associated with exposure to silica and nonfibrous silicate minerals. Silicosis and Silicate Disease Committee. Arch Pathol Lab Med 112:673-720, 1988.
49. del Campo JM, Hitado J, Gea G, et al: Anaerobes: A new aetiology in cavitary pneumoconiosis. Br J Ind Med 39:392-396, 1982.
50. Bergin CJ, Müller NL, Vedal S, Chan-Yeung M: CT in silicosis: Correlation with plain films and pulmonary function tests. AJR Am J Roentgenol 146:477-483, 1986.
51. Greening R, Heslep J: The roentgenology of silicosis. Semin Roentgenol 2:265, 1967.
52. Jacobson G, Felson B, Pendergrass EP, et al: Eggshell calcifications in coal and metal workers. Semin Roentgenol 2:276, 1967.
53. Gross BH, Schneider HJ, Proto AV: Eggshell calcification of lymph nodes: An update. AJR Am J Roentgenol 135:1265-1268, 1980.
54. Dee P, Suratt P, Winn W: The radiographic findings in acute silicosis. Radiology 126:359-363, 1978.
55. Buechner HA, Ansari A: Acute silico-proteinosis. A new pathologic variant of acute silicosis in sandblasters, characterized by histologic features resembling alveolar proteinosis. Dis Chest 55:274-278, 1969.
56. Maclaren WM, Soutar CA: Progressive massive fibrosis and simple pneumoconiosis in ex-miners. Br J Ind Med 42:734-740, 1985.
57. Begin R, Ostiguy G, Fillion R, Colman N: Computed tomography scan in the early detection of silicosis. Am Rev Respir Dis 144:697-705, 1991.
58. Akira M, Higashihara T, Yokoyama K, et al: Radiographic type p pneumoconiosis: High-resolution CT. Radiology 171:117-123, 1989.
59. Grenier P, Chevret S, Beigelman C, et al: Chronic diffuse infiltrative lung disease: Determination of the diagnostic value of clinical data, chest radiography, and CT and Bayesian analysis. Radiology 191:383-390, 1994.
60. Begin R, Bergeron D, Samson L, et al: CT assessment of silicosis in exposed workers. AJR Am J Roentgenol 148:509-514, 1987.
61. Kinsella M, Müller N, Vedal S, et al: Emphysema in silicosis. A comparison of smokers with nonsmokers using pulmonary function testing and computed tomography. Am Rev Respir Dis 141:1497-1500, 1990.
62. Mathieson JR, Mayo JR, Staples CA, Müller NL: Chronic diffuse infiltrative lung disease: Comparison of diagnostic accuracy of CT and chest radiography. Radiology 171:111-116, 1989.

63. Wang XR, Christiani DC: Respiratory symptoms and functional status in workers exposed to silica, asbestos, and coal mine dusts. J Occup Environ Med 42:1076-1084, 2000.
64. Murray J, Reid G, Kielkowski D, de Beer M: Cor pulmonale and silicosis: A necropsy based case-control study. Br J Ind Med 50:544-548, 1993.
65. Munakata M, Homma Y, Matsuzaki M, et al: Rales in silicosis. A correlative study with physiological and radiological abnormalities. Respiration 48:140-144, 1985.
66. Violante B, Brusasco V, Buccheri G: Exercise testing in radiologically-limited, simple pulmonary silicosis. Chest 90:411-415, 1986.
67. Ng TP, Chan SL: Lung function in relation to silicosis and silica exposure in granite workers. Eur Respir J 5:986-991, 1992.
68. Begin R, Ostiguy G, Cantin A, Bergeron D: Lung function in silica-exposed workers. A relationship to disease severity assessed by CT scan. Chest 94:539-545, 1988.
69. Wang X, Yano E, Nonaka K, et al: Respiratory impairments due to dust exposure: A comparative study among workers exposed to silica, asbestos, and coalmine dust. Am J Ind Med 31:495-502, 1997.
70. Infante-Rivard C, Armstrong B, Ernst P, et al: Descriptive study of prognostic factors influencing survival of compensated silicotic patients. Am Rev Respir Dis 144:1070-1074, 1991.
71. Chang KC, Leung CC, Tam CM: Tuberculosis risk factors in a silicotic cohort in Hong Kong. Int J Tuberc Lung Dis 5:177-184, 2001.
72. Corbett EL, Churchyard GJ, Clayton T, et al: Risk factors for pulmonary mycobacterial disease in South African gold miners. A case-control study. Am J Respir Crit Care Med 159:94-99, 1999.
73. Cowie RL: The epidemiology of tuberculosis in gold miners with silicosis. Am J Respir Crit Care Med 150:1460-1462, 1994.
74. Corbett EL, Churchyard GJ, Clayton TC, et al: HIV infection and silicosis: The impact of two potent risk factors on the incidence of mycobacterial disease in South African miners. AIDS 14:2759-2768, 2000.
75. IARC Working Group on the Evaluation of Carcinogenic Risks to Humans: Silica, some silicates, coal dust and para-aramid fibrils. Lyon 15-22 October 1996. IARC Monogr Eval Carcinog Risks Hum 68:1-475, 1997.
76. Smith AH, Lopipero PA, Barroga VR: Meta-analysis of studies of lung cancer among silicotics. Epidemiology 6:617-624, 1995.
77. Checkoway H, Franzblau A: Is silicosis required for silica-associated lung cancer? Am J Ind Med 37:252-259, 2000.
78. Lynge E, Kurppa K, Kristofersen L, et al: Occupational groups potentially exposed to silica dust: A comparative analysis of cancer mortality and incidence based on the Nordic occupational mortality and cancer incidence registers. IARC Sci Publ 7-20, 1990.
79. Beckett W, Abraham J, Becklake M, et al: Adverse effects of crystalline silica exposure. Am J Respir Crit Care Med 155:761-768, 1997.
80. Rosenman KD, Moore-Fuller M, Reilly MJ: Connective tissue disease and silicosis. Am J Ind Med 35:375-381, 1999.
81. Doll NJ, Stankus RP, Hughes J, et al: Immune complexes and autoantibodies in silicosis. J Allergy Clin Immunol 68:281-285, 1981.
82. Oxman AD, Muir DC, Shannon HS, et al: Occupational dust exposure and chronic obstructive pulmonary disease. A systematic overview of the evidence. Am Rev Respir Dis 148:38-48, 1993.
83. Begin R, Filion R, Ostiguy G: Emphysema in silica- and asbestos-exposed workers seeking compensation. A CT scan study. Chest 108:647-655, 1995.
84. Hnizdo E, Sluis-Cremer GK, Abramowitz JA: Emphysema type in relation to silica dust exposure in South African gold miners. Am Rev Respir Dis 143:1241-1247, 1991.
85. Gaensler EA, Cadigan JB, Sasahara AA, et al: Graphite pneumoconiosis of electrotypers. Am J Med 41:864-882, 1966.
86. Miller A, Ramsden F: Carbon pneumoconiosis. Br J Ind Med 18:103, 1961.
87. Shrivastava DK, Kapre SS, Cho K, Cho YJ: Acute lung disease after exposure to fly ash. Chest 106:309-311, 1994.
88. Ghio AJ, Gilbey JG, Roggli VL, et al: Diffuse alveolar damage after exposure to an oil fly ash. Am J Respir Crit Care Med 164:1514-1518, 2001.
89. Borm PJ: Toxicity and occupational health hazards of coal fly ash (CFA). A review of data and comparison to coal mine dust. Ann Occup Hyg 41:659-676, 1997.
90. Green FH, Laqueur WA: Coal workers' pneumoconiosis. Pathol Annu 15:333-410, 1980.
91. Naeye RL, Mahon JK, Dellinger WS: Rank of coal and coal workers pneumoconiosis. Am Rev Respir Dis 103:350-355, 1971.
92. Banks DE, Bauer MA, Castellan RM, Lapp NL: Silicosis in surface coalmine drillers. Thorax 38:275-278, 1983.
93. Goodwin S, Attfield M: Temporal trends in coal workers' pneumoconiosis prevalence. Validating the National Coal Study results. J Occup Environ Med 40:1065-1071, 1998.
94. Lapp NL, Parker JE: Coal workers' pneumoconiosis. Clin Chest Med 13:243-252, 1992.
95. Attfield MD, Morring K: An investigation into the relationship between coal workers' pneumoconiosis and dust exposure in U.S. coal miners. Am Ind Hyg Assoc J 53:486-492, 1992.
96. Attfield MD, Seixas NS: Prevalence of pneumoconiosis and its relationship to dust exposure in a cohort of U.S. bituminous coal miners and ex-miners. Am J Ind Med 27:137-151, 1995.
97. Attfield MD, Morring K: The derivation of estimated dust exposures for U.S. coal miners working before 1970. Am Ind Hyg Assoc J 53:248-255, 1992.

98. Douglas AN, Robertson A, Chapman JS, Ruckley VA: Dust exposure, dust recovered from the lung, and associated pathology in a group of British coalminers. Br J Ind Med 43:795-801, 1986.
99. Schins RP, Borm PJ: Mechanisms and mediators in coal dust induced toxicity: A review. Ann Occup Hyg 43:7-33, 1999.
100. Vanhee D, Gosset P, Marquette CH, et al: Secretion and mRNA expression of TNF alpha and IL-6 in the lungs of pneumoconiosis patients. Am J Respir Crit Care Med 152:298-306, 1995.
101. Vallyathan V, Goins M, Lapp LN, et al: Changes in bronchoalveolar lavage indices associated with radiographic classification in coal miners. Am J Respir Crit Care Med 162:958-965, 2000.
102. Kim KA, Lim Y, Kim JH, et al: Potential biomarker of coal workers' pneumoconiosis. Toxicol Lett 108:297-302, 1999.
103. Huang X, Fournier J, Koenig K, Chen LC: Buffering capacity of coal and its acid-soluble Fe^{2+} content: Possible role in coal workers' pneumoconiosis. Chem Res Toxicol 11:722-729, 1998.
104. Caplan A: Certain unusual radiological appearances in the chest of coal-miners suffering from rheumatoid arthritis. Thorax 8:29, 1953.
105. Lippmann M, Eckert HL, Hahon N, Morgan WK: Circulating antinuclear and rheumatoid factors in coal miners. A prevalence study in Pennsylvania and West Virginia. Ann Intern Med 79:807-811, 1973.
106. Yeh YB, Lai YR: Influence of rheumatoid factor in coalminers' pneumoconiosis in the Fujian Shaowu colliery, south China. Br J Ind Med 47:143-144, 1990.
107. Kleinerman J, Green FH, Harley RA Jr, et al: Pathology standards for coal workers' pneumoconiosis. Arch Pathol Lab Med 103:375, 1979.
108. Davis JM, Chapman J, Collings P, et al: Variations in the histological patterns of the lesions of coal workers' pneumoconiosis in Britain and their relationship to lung dust content. Am Rev Respir Dis 128:118-124, 1983.
109. Goodwin RA, Des Prez RM: Apical localization of pulmonary tuberculosis, chronic pulmonary histoplasmosis, and progressive massive fibrosis of the lung. Chest 83:801-805, 1983.
110. Cockcroft AE, Wagner JC, Seal EM, et al: Irregular opacities in coalworkers' pneumoconiosis—correlation with pulmonary function and pathology. Ann Occup Hyg 26:767-787, 1982.
111. Cockcroft A, Lyons JP, Andersson N, Saunders MJ: Prevalence and relation to underground exposure of radiological irregular opacities in South Wales coal workers with pneumoconiosis. Br J Ind Med 40:169-172, 1983.
112. Kim JS, Lynch DA: Imaging of nonmalignant occupational lung disease. J Thorac Imaging 17:238-260, 2002.
113. Williams JL, Moller GA: Solitary mass in the lungs of coal miners. Am J Roentgenol Radium Ther Nucl Med 117:765-770, 1973.
114. Young RC Jr, Rachal RE, Carr PG, Press HC: Patterns of coal workers' pneumoconiosis in Appalachian former coal miners. J Natl Med Assoc 84:41-48, 1992.
115. Shennan DH, Washington JS, Thomas DJ, et al: Factors predisposing to the development of progressive massive fibrosis in coal miners. Br J Ind Med 38:321-326, 1981.
116. Morgan WK: Respiratory disease in coal miners. JAMA 231:1347-1348, 1975.
117. Davies D: Disability and coal workers' pneumoconiosis. BMJ 2:652-655, 1974.
118. Musk AW, Cotes JE, Bevan C, Campbell MJ: Relationship between type of simple coalworkers' pneumoconiosis and lung function. A nine-year follow-up study of subjects with small rounded opacities. Br J Ind Med 38:313-320, 1981.
119. Remy-Jardin M, Degreef JM, Beuscart R, et al: Coal worker's pneumoconiosis: CT assessment in exposed workers and correlation with radiographic findings. Radiology 177:363-371, 1990.
120. Gevenois PA, Pichot E, Dargent F, et al: Low grade coal worker's pneumoconiosis. Comparison of CT and chest radiography. Acta Radiol 35:351-356, 1994.
121. Remy-Jardin M, Remy J, Farre I, Marquette CH: Computed tomographic evaluation of silicosis and coal workers' pneumoconiosis. Radiol Clin North Am 30:1155-1176, 1992.
122. Rebstock-Bourgkard E, Chau N, Caillier I, et al: [Respiratory symptoms and function of coal miners presenting radiological pulmonary abnormalities.] Rev Epidemiol Sante Publique 42:533-541, 1994.
123. Coggon D, Newman Taylor A: Coal mining and chronic obstructive pulmonary disease: A review of the evidence. Thorax 53:398-407, 1998.
124. Leigh J, Driscoll TR, Cole BD, et al: Quantitative relation between emphysema and lung mineral content in coalworkers. Occup Environ Med 51:400-407, 1994.
125. Leigh J, Outhred KG, McKenzie HI, et al: Quantified pathology of emphysema, pneumoconiosis, and chronic bronchitis in coal workers. Br J Ind Med 40:258-263, 1983.
126. Soutar CA, Hurley JF: Relation between dust exposure and lung function in miners and ex-miners. Br J Ind Med 43:307-320, 1986.
127. Gilson JC, Hugh-Jones P: Lung function in coal worker's pneumoconiosis. Medical Research Council, Special Report 290. London, HMSO, 1955.
128. Bourgkard E, Bernadac P, Chau N, et al: Can the evolution to pneumoconiosis be suspected in coal miners? A longitudinal study. Am J Respir Crit Care Med 158:504-509, 1998.
129. Love RG, Miller BG: Longitudinal study of lung function in coal-miners. Thorax 37:193-197, 1982.
130. Morgan WK, Lapp NL: Respiratory disease in coal miners. Am Rev Respir Dis 113:531-559, 1976.
131. Lyons JP, Campbell H: Relation between progressive massive fibrosis, emphysema, and pulmonary dysfunction in coalworkers' pneumoconiosis. Br J Ind Med 38:125-129, 1981.
132. Sadler RL, Roy TJ: Smoking and mortality from coalworkers' pneumoconiosis. Br J Ind Med 47:141-142, 1990.

133. Miller BG, Jacobsen M: Dust exposure, pneumoconiosis, and mortality of coalminers. Br J Ind Med 42:723-733, 1985.
134. Cochrane AL, Moore F: A 20-year follow-up of men aged 55-64 including coalminers and foundry workers in Staveley, Derbyshire. Br J Ind Med 37:226-229, 1980.
135. Begin R, Dufresne A, Plante F, et al: Asbestos related disorders. Can Respir J 1:167, 1994.
135a. Guidotti TL, Miller A, Christiani D, et al: Diagnosis and initial management of nonmalignant diseases related to asbestos. Am J Respir Crit Care Med 170:691-715, 2004.
136. Wagner GR: Asbestosis and silicosis. Lancet 349:1311-1315, 1997.
137. Rogan WJ, Gladen BC, Ragan NB, Anderson HA: US prevalence of occupational pleural thickening. A look at chest x-rays from the first National Health and Nutrition Examination Survey. Am J Epidemiol 126:893-900, 1987.
138. Landrigan PJ: Commentary: Environmental disease—a preventable epidemic. Am J Public Health 82:941-943, 1992.
139. Craighead JE, Mossman BT: The pathogenesis of asbestos-associated diseases. N Engl J Med 306:1446-1455, 1982.
140. Rogan WJ, Ragan NB, Dinse GE: X-ray evidence of increased asbestos exposure in the US population from NHANES I and NHANES II, 1973-1978. National Health Examination Survey. Cancer Causes Control 11:441-449, 2000.
141. Roberts GH: Asbestos bodies in lungs at necropsy. J Clin Pathol 20:570-573, 1967.
142. Churg A: Lung asbestos content in long-term residents of a chrysotile mining town. Am Rev Respir Dis 134:125-127, 1986.
143. Rey F, Boutin C, Viallat JR, et al: Environmental asbestotic pleural plaques in northeast Corsica: Correlations with airborne and pleural mineralogic analysis. Environ Health Perspect 102(Suppl 5):251-252, 1994.
144. Sider L, Holland EA, Davis TM Jr, Cugell DW: Changes on radiographs of wives of workers exposed to asbestos. Radiology 164:723-726, 1987.
145. Constantopoulos SH, Saratzis NA, Kontogiannis D, et al: Tremolite whitewashing and pleural calcifications. Chest 92:709-712, 1987.
146. Yazicioglu S, Ilcayto R, Balci K, et al: Pleural calcification, pleural mesotheliomas, and bronchial cancers caused by tremolite dust. Thorax 35:564-569, 1980.
147. Donaldson K, Brown RC, Brown GM: Respirable industrial fibres: Mechanisms of pathogenicity. Thorax 48:390, 1993.
148. Becklake MR, Case BW: Fiber burden and asbestos-related lung disease: Determinants of dose-response relationships. Am J Respir Crit Care Med 150:1488-1492, 1994.
149. Begin R, Cantin A, Sebastien P: Chrysotile asbestos exposures can produce an alveolitis with limited fibrosing activity in a subset of high fibre retainer sheep. Eur Respir J 3:81-90, 1990.
150. Becklake MR, Toyota B, Stewart M, et al: Lung structure as a risk factor in adverse pulmonary responses to asbestos exposure. A case-referent study in Quebec chrysotile miners and millers. Am Rev Respir Dis 128:385-388, 1983.
151. Mossman BT, Kessler JB, Ley BW, Craighead JE: Interaction of crocidolite asbestos with hamster respiratory mucosa in organ culture. Lab Invest 36:131-139, 1977.
152. Adamson IY, Bowden DH: Crocidolite-induced pulmonary fibrosis in mice. Cytokinetic and biochemical studies. Am J Pathol 122:261-267, 1986.
153. Robledo R, Mossman B: Cellular and molecular mechanisms of asbestos-induced fibrosis. J Cell Physiol 180:158-166, 1999.
154. Kamp DW, Weitzman SA: The molecular basis of asbestos induced lung injury. Thorax 54:638-652, 1999.
155. Shukla A, Gulumian M, Hei TK, et al: Multiple roles of oxidants in the pathogenesis of asbestos-induced diseases. Free Rad Biol Med 34:1117-1129, 2003.
156. Fasske E: Pathogenesis of pulmonary fibrosis induced by chrysotile asbestos. Longitudinal light and electron microscopic studies on the rat model. Virchows Arch A Pathol Anat Histopathol 408:329-346, 1986.
157. Turner-Warwick M, Parkes WR: Circulating rheumatoid and antinuclear factors in asbestos workers. BMJ 1:886, 1965.
158. deShazo RD, Hendrick DJ, Diem JE, et al: Immunologic aberrations in asbestos cement workers: Dissociation from asbestosis. J Allergy Clin Immunol 72:454-461, 1983.
159. Lange A, Garncarek D, Tomeczko J, et al: Outcome of asbestos exposure (lung fibrosis and antinuclear antibodies) with respect to skin reactivity: An 8-year longitudinal study. Environ Res 41:1-13, 1986.
160. Sprince NL, Oliver LC, McLoud TC, et al: Asbestos exposure and asbestos-related pleural and parenchymal disease. Associations with immune imbalance. Am Rev Respir Dis 143:822-828, 1991.
161. deShazo RD, Morgan J, Bozelka B, Chapman Y: Natural killer cell activity in asbestos workers. Interactive effects of smoking and asbestos exposure. Chest 94:482-485, 1988.
162. Wain SL, Roggli VL, Foster WL Jr: Parietal pleural plaques, asbestos bodies, and neoplasia. A clinical, pathologic, and roentgenographic correlation of 25 consecutive cases. Chest 86:707-713, 1984.
163. Roberts GH: The pathology of parietal pleural plaques. J Clin Pathol 24:348-353, 1971.
164. Miller A, Teirstein AS, Selikoff IJ: Ventilatory failure due to asbestos pleurisy. Am J Med 75:911-919, 1983.
165. Antony VB, Owen CL, Hadley KJ: Pleural mesothelial cells stimulated by asbestos release chemotactic activity for neutrophils in vitro. Am Rev Respir Dis 139:199-206, 1989.
166. Craighead JE, Abraham JL, Churg A, et al: The pathology of asbestos-associated diseases of the lungs and pleural cavities: Diagnostic criteria and proposed grading schema. Report of the Pneumoconiosis Committee of the College of American Pathologists and the National Institute for Occupational Safety and Health. Arch Pathol Lab Med 106:544-596, 1982.
167. Warnock ML, Wolery G: Asbestos bodies or fibers and the diagnosis of asbestosis. Environ Res 44:29-44, 1987.
168. Churg A, Wright JL: Small-airway lesions in patients exposed to nonasbestos mineral dusts. Hum Pathol 14:688-693, 1983.
169. Begin R, Masse S, Bureau MA: Morphologic features and function of the airways in early asbestosis in the sheep model. Am Rev Respir Dis 126:870-876, 1982.
170. Churg AM, Warnock ML: Asbestos and other ferruginous bodies: Their formation and clinical significance. Am J Pathol 102:447-456, 1981.
171. Roggli VL, Greenberg SD, McLarty JW, et al: Comparison of sputum and lung asbestos body counts in former asbestos workers. Am Rev Respir Dis 122:941-945, 1980.
172. De Vuyst P, Dumortier P, Moulin E, et al: Diagnostic value of asbestos bodies in bronchoalveolar lavage fluid. Am Rev Respir Dis 136:1219-1224, 1987.
173. Roggli VL, Johnston WW, Kaminsky DB: Asbestos bodies in fine needle aspirates of the lung. Acta Cytol 28:493-498, 1984.
174. Dodson RF, Williams MG Jr, O'Sullivan MF, et al: A comparison of the ferruginous body and uncoated fiber content in the lungs of former asbestos workers. Am Rev Respir Dis 132:143-147, 1985.
175. Churg A: Fiber counting and analysis in the diagnosis of asbestos-related disease. Hum Pathol 13:381-392, 1982.
176. Roggli VL, Sanders LL: Asbestos content of lung tissue and carcinoma of the lung: A clinicopathologic correlation and mineral fiber analysis of 234 cases. Ann Occup Hyg 44:109-117, 2000.
177. Hillerdal G: Rounded atelectasis. Clinical experience with 74 patients. Chest 95:836-841, 1989.
178. Menzies R, Fraser R: Round atelectasis. Pathologic and pathogenetic features. Am J Surg Pathol 11:674-681, 1987.
179. Fletcher DE, Edge JR: The early radiological changes in pulmonary and pleural asbestosis. Clin Radiol 21:355-365, 1970.
180. Anton HC: Multiple pleural plaques. II. Br J Radiol 41:341-348, 1968.
181. Friedman AC, Fiel SB, Fisher MS, et al: Asbestos-related pleural disease and asbestosis: A comparison of CT and chest radiography. AJR Am J Roentgenol 150:269-275, 1988.
182. Staples CA, Gamsu G, Ray CS, Webb WR: High resolution computed tomography and lung function in asbestos-exposed workers with normal chest radiographs. Am Rev Respir Dis 139:1502-1508, 1989.
183. Aberle DR, Gamsu G, Ray CS, Feuerstein IM: Asbestos-related pleural and parenchymal fibrosis: Detection with high-resolution CT. Radiology 166:729-734, 1988.
184. Sargent EN, Gordonson J, Jacobson G, et al: Bilateral pleural thickening: A manifestation of asbestos dust exposure. AJR Am J Roentgenol 131:579-585, 1978.
185. Sprince NL, Oliver LC, McLoud TC: Asbestos-related disease in plumbers and pipefitters employed in building construction. J Occup Med 27:771-775, 1985.
186. Fisher MS: Asymmetrical changes in asbestos-related disease. J Can Assoc Radiol 36:110-112, 1985.
187. Hu H, Beckett L, Kelsey K, Christiani D: The left-sided predominance of asbestos-related pleural disease. Am Rev Respir Dis 148:981-984, 1993.
188. Hillerdal G, Lindgren A: Pleural plaques: Correlation of autopsy findings to radiographic findings and occupational history. Eur J Respir Dis 61:315-319, 1980.
189. Sargent EN, Boswell WD Jr, Ralls PW, Markovitz A: Subpleural fat pads in patients exposed to asbestos: Distinction from non-calcified pleural plaques. Radiology 152:273-277, 1984.
190. Kleinfeld M: Pleural calcification as a sign of silicatosis. Am J Med Sci 251:215-224, 1966.
191. Solomon A: Radiology of asbestosis. Environ Res 3:320-329, 1970.
192. McLoud TC, Woods BO, Carrington CB, et al: Diffuse pleural thickening in an asbestos-exposed population: Prevalence and causes. AJR Am J Roentgenol 144:9-18, 1985.
193. Lynch DA, Gamsu G, Aberle DR: Conventional and high resolution computed tomography in the diagnosis of asbestos-related diseases. Radiographics 9:523-551, 1989.
194. Hillerdal G, Malmberg P, Hemmingsson A: Asbestos-related lesions of the pleura: Parietal plaques compared to diffuse thickening studied with chest roentgenography, computed tomography, lung function, and gas exchange. Am J Ind Med 18:627-639, 1990.
195. Leung AN, Müller NL, Miller RR: CT in differential diagnosis of diffuse pleural disease. AJR Am J Roentgenol 154:487-492, 1990.
196. Friedman AC, Fiel SB, Radecki PD, Lev-Toaff AS: Computed tomography of benign pleural and pulmonary parenchymal abnormalities related to asbestos exposure. Semin Ultrasound CT MR 11:393-408, 1990.
197. Müller NL: Imaging of the pleura. Radiology 186:297-309, 1993.
198. Gaensler EA, Kaplan AI: Asbestos pleural effusion. Ann Intern Med 74:178-191, 1971.
199. Epler GR, McLoud TC, Gaensler EA: Prevalence and incidence of benign asbestos pleural effusion in a working population. JAMA 247:617-622, 1982.
200. Gefter WB, Conant EF: Issues and controversies in the plain-film diagnosis of asbestos-related disorders in the chest. J Thorac Imaging 3:11-28, 1988.
201. Epler GR, McLoud TC, Gaensler EA, et al: Normal chest roentgenograms in chronic diffuse infiltrative lung disease. N Engl J Med 298:934-939, 1978.
202. Kipen HM, Lilis R, Suzuki Y, et al: Pulmonary fibrosis in asbestos insulation workers with lung cancer: A radiological and histopathological evaluation. Br J Ind Med 44:96-100, 1987.

203. Akira M, Yokoyama K, Yamamoto S, et al: Early asbestosis: Evaluation with high-resolution CT. Radiology 178:409-416, 1991.
204. Yoshimura H, Hatakeyama M, Otsuji H, et al: Pulmonary asbestosis: CT study of subpleural curvilinear shadow. Work in progress. Radiology 158:653-658, 1986.
205. Akira M, Yamamoto S, Yokoyama K, et al: Asbestosis: High-resolution CT-pathologic correlation. Radiology 176:389-394, 1990.
206. al-Jarad N, Strickland B, Pearson MC, et al: High resolution computed tomographic assessment of asbestosis and cryptogenic fibrosing alveolitis: A comparative study. Thorax 47:645-650, 1992.
207. Gamsu G, Salmon CJ, Warnock ML, Blanc PD: CT quantification of interstitial fibrosis in patients with asbestosis: A comparison of two methods. AJR Am J Roentgenol 164:63-68, 1995.
208. Primack SL, Hartman TE, Hansell DM, Müller NL: End-stage lung disease: CT findings in 61 patients. Radiology 189:681-686, 1993.
209. Murray KA, Gamsu G, Webb WR, et al: High-resolution computed tomography sampling for detection of asbestos-related lung disease. Acad Radiol 2:111-115, 1995.
210. Majurin ML, Varpula M, Kurki T, Pakkala L: High-resolution CT of the lung in asbestos-exposed subjects. Comparison of low-dose and high-dose HRCT. Acta Radiol 35:473-477, 1994.
211. Bergin CJ, Castellino RA, Blank N, Moses L: Specificity of high-resolution CT findings in pulmonary asbestosis: Do patients scanned for other indications have similar findings? AJR Am J Roentgenol 163:551-555, 1994.
212. Mintzer RA, Gore RM, Vogelzang RL, Holz S: Rounded atelectasis and its association with asbestos-induced pleural disease. Radiology 139:567-570, 1981.
213. Schneider HJ, Felson B, Gonzalez LL: Rounded atelectasis. AJR Am J Roentgenol 134:225-232, 1980.
214. Lynch DA, Gamsu G, Ray CS, Aberle DR: Asbestos-related focal lung masses: Manifestations on conventional and high-resolution CT scans. Radiology 169:603-607, 1988.
215. Carvalho PM, Carr DH: Computed tomography of folded lung. Clin Radiol 41:86-91, 1990.
216. Taylor PM: Dynamic contrast enhancement of asbestos-related pulmonary pseudotumours. Br J Radiol 61:1070-1072, 1988.
217. Robinson BW, Musk AW: Benign asbestos pleural effusion: Diagnosis and course. Thorax 36:896-900, 1981.
218. Rosenstock L, Barnhart S, Heyer NJ, et al: The relation among pulmonary function, chest roentgenographic abnormalities, and smoking status in an asbestos-exposed cohort. Am Rev Respir Dis 138:272-277, 1988.
219. Hilt B, Lien JT, Lund-Larsen PG: Lung function and respiratory symptoms in subjects with asbestos-related disorders: A cross-sectional study. Am J Ind Med 11:517-528, 1987.
220. Kleinfeld M, Messite J, Shapiro J: Clinical, radiological, and physiological findings in asbestosis. Arch Intern Med 117:813-819, 1966.
221. Enarson DA, Embree V, MacLean L, Grzybowski S: Respiratory health in chrysotile asbestos miners in British Columbia: A longitudinal study. Br J Ind Med 45:459-463, 1988.
222. Coutts II, Gilson JC, Kerr IH, et al: Significance of finger clubbing in asbestosis. Thorax 42:117-119, 1987.
223. Miller A: Pulmonary function in asbestosis and asbestos-related pleural disease. Environ Res 61:1-18, 1993.
224. Kilburn KH: Prevalence and features of advanced asbestosis (ILO profusion scores above 2/2). International Labour Office. Arch Environ Health 55:104-108, 2000.
225. Jodoin G, Gibbs GW, Macklem PT, et al: Early effects of asbestos exposure on lung function. Am Rev Respir Dis 104:525-535, 1971.
226. al Jarad N, Poulakis N, Pearson MC, et al: Assessment of asbestos-induced pleural disease by computed tomography—correlation with chest radiograph and lung function. Respir Med 85:203-208, 1991.
227. Bourbeau J, Ernst P, Chrome J, et al: The relationship between respiratory impairment and asbestos-related pleural abnormality in an active work force. Am Rev Respir Dis 142:837-842, 1990.
228. Olscamp G, Herman SJ, Weisbrod GL: Nepheline rock dust pneumoconiosis. A report of 2 cases. Radiology 142:29-32, 1982.
229. Huuskonen MS, Tossavainen A, Koskinen H, et al: Wollastonite exposure and lung fibrosis. Environ Res 30:291-304, 1983.
230. Gylseth B, Norseth T, Skaug V: Amphibole fibers in a taconite mine and in the lungs of the miners. Am J Ind Med 8:175-184, 1981.
231. Wild P, Leodolter K, Refregier M, et al: A cohort mortality and nested case-control study of French and Austrian talc workers. Occup Environ Med 59:98-105, 2002.
232. Berner A, Gylseth B, Levy F: Talc dust pneumoconiosis. Acta Pathol Microbiol Scand [A] 89:17-21, 1981.
233. Wells IP, Dubbins PA, Whimster WF: Pulmonary disease caused by the inhalation of cosmetic talcum powder. Br J Radiol 52:586-588, 1979.
234. Nam K, Gracey DR: Pulmonary talcosis from cosmetic talcum powder. JAMA 221:492-493, 1972.
235. Gibbs AE, Pooley FD, Griffiths DM, et al: Talc pneumoconiosis: A pathologic and mineralogic study. Hum Pathol 23:1344-1354, 1992.
236. Hildick-Smith GY: The biology of talc. Br J Ind Med 33:217-229, 1976.
237. Vallyathan NV, Craighead JE: Pulmonary pathology in workers exposed to nonasbestiform talc. Hum Pathol 12:28-35, 1981.
238. Wegman DH, Peters JM, Boundy MG, Smith TJ: Evaluation of respiratory effects in miners and millers exposed to talc free of asbestos and silica. Br J Ind Med 39:233-238, 1982.
239. Gamble JF, Fellner W, Dimeo MJ: An epidemiologic study of a group of talc workers. Am Rev Respir Dis 119:741-753, 1979.
240. Seeler AO, Gryboski JS, MacMahon HE: Talc pneumoconiosis. AMA Arch Ind Health 19:392, 1959.
241. Kleinfeld M, Messite J, Shapiro J, et al: Effect of talc dust inhalation on lung function. Arch Environ Health 10:431, 1965.
242. Tukiainen P, Nickels J, Taskinen E, Nyberg M: Pulmonary granulomatous reaction: Talc pneumoconiosis or chronic sarcoidosis? Br J Ind Med 41:84-87, 1984.
243. Gamble J, Greife A, Hancock J: An epidemiological-industrial hygiene study of talc workers. Ann Occup Hyg 26:841-859, 1982.
244. Craighead JE, Emerson RJ, Stanley DE: Slateworker's pneumoconiosis. Hum Pathol 23:1098-1105, 1992.
245. Lockey JE, Brooks SM, Jarabek AM, et al: Pulmonary changes after exposure to vermiculite contaminated with fibrous tremolite. Am Rev Respir Dis 129:952-958, 1984.
246. Davies D, Cotton R: Mica pneumoconiosis. Br J Ind Med 40:22-27, 1983.
247. Landas SK, Schwartz DA: Mica-associated pulmonary interstitial fibrosis. Am Rev Respir Dis 144:718-721, 1991.
248. Zinman C, Richards GA, Murray J, et al: Mica dust as a cause of severe pneumoconiosis. Am J Ind Med 41:139-144, 2002.
249. Lapenas D, Gale P, Kennedy T, et al: Kaolin pneumoconiosis. Radiologic, pathologic, and mineralogic findings. Am Rev Respir Dis 130:282-288, 1984.
250. Edenfield RW: A clinical and roentgenological study of kaolin workers. Arch Environ Health 1:392, 1960.
251. Oldham PD: Pneumoconiosis in Cornish china clay workers. Br J Ind Med 40:131-137, 1983.
252. Altekruse EB, Chaudhary BA, Pearson MG, Morgan WK: Kaolin dust concentrations and pneumoconiosis at a kaolin mine. Thorax 39:436-441, 1984.
253. Wagner JC, Pooley FD, Gibbs A, et al: Inhalation of china stone and china clay dusts: Relationship between the mineralogy of dust retained in the lungs and pathological changes. Thorax 41:190-196, 1986.
254. Bristol LJ: Pneumoconioses caused by asbestos and by other siliceous and non-siliceous dusts. Semin Roentgenol 2:283, 1967.
255. Gibbs AR, Pooley FD: Fuller's earth (montmorillonite) pneumoconiosis. Occup Environ Med 51:644-646, 1994.
256. McNally WD, Trostler IS: Severe pneumoconiosis caused by inhalation of fuller's earth. J Ind Hyg 23:118, 1941.
257. Baris YI, Artvinli M, Sahin AA, et al: Diffuse lung fibrosis due to fibrous zeolite (erionite) exposure. Eur J Respir Dis 70:122-125, 1987.
258. Casey KR, Shigeoka JW, Rom WN, Moatamed F: Zeolite exposure and associated pneumoconiosis. Chest 87:837-840, 1985.
259. Stacy BD, King EJ, Harrison CV, et al: Tissue changes in rats' lungs caused by hydroxides, oxides and phosphates of aluminium and iron. J Pathol Bacteriol 77:417, 1959.
260. Sferlazza SJ, Beckett WS: The respiratory health of welders. Am Rev Respir Dis 143:1134-1148, 1991.
261. Morgan WKC, Kerr HD: Pathologic and physiologic studies of welders' siderosis. Ann Intern Med 58:293, 1963.
262. Attfield MD, Ross DS: Radiological abnormalities in electric-arc welders. Br J Ind Med 35:117-122, 1978.
263. Harding HE, Grout JLA, Davies TAL: The experimental production of x-ray shadows in the lungs by inhalation of industrial dusts: I. Iron oxide. Br J Ind Med 4:223, 1947.
264. Low I, Mitchell C: Respiratory disease in foundry workers. Br J Ind Med 42:101-105, 1985.
265. Antti-Poika M, Hassi J, Pyy L: Respiratory diseases in arc welders. Int Arch Occup Environ Health 40:225-230, 1977.
266. Kilburn KH, Warshaw RH: Pulmonary functional impairment from years of arc welding. Am J Med 87:62-69, 1989.
267. Barrie HJ, Harding HE: Argyro-siderosis of the lungs in silver finishers. Br J Ind Med 4:225, 1947.
268. Robertson AJ, Whitaker PH: Radiological changes in pneumoconiosis due to tin oxide. J Fac Radiol 6:224, 1955.
269. Pendergrass EP, Greening R: Baritosis. Report of a case. Arch Ind Hyg 7:44, 1953.
270. Levi-Valensi P, Drif M, Dat A, Hadjadj G: [Apropos of 57 cases of pulmonary baritosis. (Results of a systematic investigation in a baryta factory)] J Fr Med Chir Thorac 20:443-455, 1966.
271. McCallum RI: Detection of antimony in process workers' lungs by x-radiation. Trans Soc Occup Med 17:134, 1967.
272. Cooper DA, Pendergrass EP, Vorwald AJ, et al: Pneumoconiosis among workers in an antimony industry. Am J Roentgenol Radium Ther Nucl Med 103:496-508, 1968.
273. Porru S, Placidi D, Quarta C, et al: The potential role of rare earths in the pathogenesis of interstitial lung disease: A case report of movie projectionist as investigated by neutron activation analysis. J Trace Elem Med Biol 14:232-236, 2001.
274. Newman LS: Metals that cause sarcoidosis. Semin Respir Infect 13:212-220, 1998.
275. Waring PM, Watling RJ: Rare earth deposits in a deceased movie projectionist. A new case of rare earth pneumoconiosis? Med J Aust 153:726-730, 1990.
276. Cain H, Egner E, Ruska J: [Deposits of rare earth metals in the lungs of man, and in experimental animals (author's transl).] Virchows Arch A Pathol Anat Histol 374:249-261, 1977.
277. Sulotto F, Romano C, Berra A, et al: Rare-earth pneumoconiosis: A new case. Am J Ind Med 9:567-575, 1986.
278. Kolanz ME: Introduction to beryllium: Uses, regulatory history, and disease. Appl Occup Environ Hyg 16:559-567, 2001.

279. Maier LA, Newman LS: Beryllium disease. In Environmental and Occupational Medicine. Philadelphia, Lippincott-Raven, 1998, p 1021.

280. Yoshida T, Shima S, Nagaoka K, et al: A study on the beryllium lymphocyte transformation test and the beryllium levels in working environment. Ind Health 35:374-379, 1997.

281. Eisenbud M: The standard for control of chronic beryllium disease. Appl Occup Environ Hyg 13:25, 1998.

282. Stange AW, Hilmas DE, Furman FJ, Gatliffe TR: Beryllium sensitization and chronic beryllium disease at a former nuclear weapons facility. Appl Occup Environ Hyg 16:405-417, 2001.

283. Freiman DG, Hardy HL: Beryllium disease. The relation of pulmonary pathology to clinical course and prognosis based on a study of 130 cases from the U.S. Beryllium case registry. Hum Pathol 1:25-44, 1970.

284. Beryllium disease. Report of the Section of Nature and Prevalence Committee on Occupational Diseases of the Chest—American College of Chest Physicians. Dis Chest 48:550-558, 1965.

285. Saltini C, Amicosante M: Beryllium disease. Am J Med Sci 321:89-98, 2001.

286. Lombardi G, Germain C, Uren J, et al: HLA-DP allele-specific T cell responses to beryllium account for DP-associated susceptibility to chronic beryllium disease. J Immunol 166:3549-3555, 2001.

287. Deubner DC, Goodman M, Iannuzzi J: Variability, predictive value, and uses of the beryllium blood lymphocyte proliferation test (BLPT): Preliminary analysis of the ongoing workforce survey. Appl Occup Environ Hyg 16:521-526, 2001.

288. Aronchick JM, Rossman MD, Miller WT: Chronic beryllium disease: Diagnosis, radiographic findings, and correlation with pulmonary function tests. Radiology 163:677-682, 1987.

289. Weber AL, Stoeckle JD, Hardy HL: Roentgenologic patterns in long-standing beryllium disease: Report of 8 cases. AJR Am J Roentgenol 93:879, 1965.

290. Newman LS, Buschman DL, Newell JD Jr, Lynch DA: Beryllium disease: Assessment with CT. Radiology 190:835-840, 1994.

291. Brauner MW, Grenier P, Mompoint D, et al: Pulmonary sarcoidosis: Evaluation with high-resolution CT. Radiology 172:467-471, 1989.

292. Müller WJ, Kullnig P, Miller RR: The CT findings of pulmonary sarcoidosis: Analysis of 25 patients. AJR Am J Roentgenol 152:1179-1182, 1989.

293. Harris KM, McConnochie K, Adams H: The computed tomographic appearances in chronic berylliosis. Clin Radiol 47:26-31, 1993.

294. Cotes JE, Gilson JC, McKerrow CB, Oldham PD: A long-term follow-up of workers exposed to beryllium. Br J Ind Med 40:13-21, 1983.

295. Newman LS, Orton R, Kreiss K: Serum angiotensin converting enzyme activity in chronic beryllium disease. Am Rev Respir Dis 146:39-42, 1992.

296. Newman LS, Bobka C, Schumacher B, et al: Compartmentalized immune response reflects clinical severity of beryllium disease. Am J Respir Crit Care Med 150:135-142, 1994.

297. Maier LA: Beryllium health effects in the era of the beryllium lymphocyte proliferation test. Appl Occup Environ Hyg 16:514-520, 2001.

298. Pappas GP, Newman LS: Early pulmonary physiologic abnormalities in beryllium disease. Am Rev Respir Dis 148:661-666, 1993.

299. Ward E, Okun A, Ruder A, et al: A mortality study of workers at seven beryllium processing plants. Am J Ind Med 22:885-904, 1992.

300. Abramson MJ, Wlodarczyk JH, Saunders NA, Hensley MJ: Does aluminum smelting cause lung disease? Am Rev Respir Dis 139:1042-1057, 1989.

301. Vallyathan V, Bergeron WN, Robichaux PA, Craighead JE: Pulmonary fibrosis in an aluminum arc welder. Chest 81:372-374, 1982.

302. Miller RR, Churg AM, Hutcheon M, Lom S: Pulmonary alveolar proteinosis and aluminum dust exposure. Am Rev Respir Dis 130:312-315, 1984.

303. Jederlinic PJ, Abraham JL, Churg A, et al: Pulmonary fibrosis in aluminum oxide workers. Investigation of nine workers, with pathologic examination and microanalysis in three of them. Am Rev Respir Dis 142:1179-1184, 1990.

304. Townsend MC, Sussman NB, Enterline PE, et al: Radiographic abnormalities in relation to total dust exposure at a bauxite refinery and alumina-based chemical products plant. Am Rev Respir Dis 138:90-95, 1988.

305. Gross P, Harley RA Jr, DeTreville RT: Pulmonary reaction to metallic aluminum powders: An experimental study. Arch Environ Health 26:227-236, 1973.

306. De Vuyst P, Dumortier P, Schandene L, et al: Sarcoidlike lung granulomatosis induced by aluminum dusts. Am Rev Respir Dis 135:493-497, 1987.

307. Gilks B, Churg A: Aluminum-induced pulmonary fibrosis: Do fibers play a role? Am Rev Respir Dis 136:176-179, 1987.

308. Herbert A, Sterling G, Abraham J, Corrin B: Desquamative interstitial pneumonia in an aluminum welder. Hum Pathol 13:694-699, 1982.

309. Edling NPG: Aluminium pneumoconiosis: A roentgendiagnostic study of five cases. Acta Radiol 56:170, 1961.

310. Akira M: Uncommon pneumoconioses: CT and pathologic findings. Radiology 197:403-409, 1995.

311. Sorgdrager B, Pal TM, de Looff AJ, et al: Occupational asthma in aluminium potroom workers related to pre-employment eosinophil count. Eur Respir J 8:1520-1524, 1995.

312. Rizzato G, Lo Cicero S, Barberis M, et al: Trace of metal exposure in hard metal lung disease. Chest 90:101-106, 1986.

313. Cugell DW: The hard metal diseases. Clin Chest Med 13:269-279, 1992.

314. Demedts M, Gheysens B, Nagels J, et al: Cobalt lung in diamond polishers. Am Rev Respir Dis 130:130-135, 1984.

315. Ruttner JR, Spycher MA, Stolkin I: Inorganic particulates in pneumoconiotic lungs of hard metal grinders. Br J Ind Med 44:657-660, 1987.

316. Potolicchio I, Mosconi G, Forni A, et al: Susceptibility to hard metal lung disease is strongly associated with the presence of glutamate 69 in HLA-DP beta chain. Eur J Immunol 27:2741-2743, 1997.

317. Cugell DW, Morgan WK, Perkins DG, Rubin A: The respiratory effects of cobalt. Arch Intern Med 150:177-183, 1990.

318. Coates EO Jr, Watson JH: Diffuse interstitial lung disease in tungsten carbide workers. Ann Intern Med 75:709-716, 1971.

319. Forrest ME, Skerker LB, Nemiroff MJ: Hard metal pneumoconiosis: Another cause of diffuse interstitial fibrosis. Radiology 128:609-612, 1978.

320. Kinoshita M, Sueyasu Y, Watanabe H, et al: Giant cell interstitial pneumonia in two hard metal workers: The role of bronchoalveolar lavage in diagnosis. Respirology 4:263-266, 1999.

321. Sprince NL, Chamberlin RI, Hales CA, et al: Respiratory disease in tungsten carbide production workers. Chest 86:549-557, 1984.

322. Funahashi A, Schlueter DP, Pintar K, et al: Pneumoconiosis in workers exposed to silicon carbide. Am Rev Respir Dis 129:635-640, 1984.

323. Masse S, Begin R, Cantin A: Pathology of silicon carbide pneumoconiosis. Mod Pathol 1:104-108, 1988.

324. Marcer G, Bernardi G, Bartolucci GB, et al: Pulmonary impairment in workers exposed to silicon carbide. Br J Ind Med 49:489-493, 1992.

325. Durand P, Begin R, Samson L, et al: Silicon carbide pneumoconiosis: A radiographic assessment. Am J Ind Med 20:37-47, 1991.

326. Cordasco EM, Demeter SL, Kerkay J, et al: Pulmonary manifestations of vinyl and polyvinyl chloride (interstitial lung disease). Newer aspects. Chest 78:828-834, 1980.

327. Antti-Poika M, Nordman H, Nickels J, et al: Lung disease after exposure to polyvinyl chloride dust. Thorax 41:566-567, 1986.

328. Soutar C, Copland L, Thornley P, et al: An epidemiologic study of respiratory disease in workers exposed to polyvinylchloride dust. Chest 80:60, 1981.

329. Soutar CA, Copland LH, Thornley PE, et al: Epidemiological study of respiratory disease in workers exposed to polyvinylchloride dust. Thorax 35:644-652, 1980.

330. Ernst P, De Guire L, Armstrong B, Theriault G: Obstructive and restrictive ventilatory impairment in polyvinylchloride fabrication workers. Am J Ind Med 14:273-279, 1988.

331. Yamadori I, Ohsumi S, Taguchi K: Titanium dioxide deposition and adenocarcinoma of the lung. Acta Pathol Jpn 36:783-790, 1986.

332. Redline S, Barna BP, Tomashefski JF Jr, Abraham JL: Granulomatous disease associated with pulmonary deposition of titanium. Br J Ind Med 43:652-656, 1986.

333. Oleru UG: Respiratory and nonrespiratory morbidity in a titanium oxide paint factory in Nigeria. Am J Ind Med 12:173-180, 1987.

334. Eisele JW, O'Halloran RL, Reay DT, et al: Deaths during the May 18, 1980, eruption of Mount St. Helens. N Engl J Med 305:931-936, 1981.

335. Craighead JE, Adler KB, Butler GB, et al: Health effects of Mount St. Helens volcanic dust. Lab Invest 48:5-12, 1983.

336. Hill JW: Health aspects of man-made mineral fibres. A review. Ann Occup Hyg 20:161-173, 1977.

337. Moore MA, Boymel PM, Maxim LD, Turim J: Categorization and nomenclature of vitreous silicate wools. Regul Toxicol Pharmacol 35:1-13, 2002.

338. Hansen EF, Rasmussen JH, Hardt F, Kamstrup O: Lung function and respiratory health of long-term fiber-exposed stonewool factory workers. Am J Respir Crit Care Med 160:466-472, 1999.

339. Laraqui CH, Laraqui O, Rahhali A, et al: [Prevalence of respiratory problems in workers at two manufacturing centers of ready-made concrete in Morocco.] Int J Tuberc Lung Dis 5:1051-1058, 2001.

340. Albin M, Johansson L, Pooley FD, et al: Mineral fibres, fibrosis, and asbestos bodies in lung tissue from deceased asbestos cement workers. Br J Ind Med 47:767-774, 1990.

341. Abrons HL, Petersen MR, Sanderson WT, et al: Chest radiography in Portland cement workers. J Occup Environ Med 39:1047-1054, 1997.

342. Marcus RL, Turner S, Cherry NM: A study of lung function and chest radiographs in men exposed to zirconium compounds. Occup Med (Lond) 46:109-113, 1996.

343. Bartter T, Irwin RS, Abraham JL, et al: Zirconium compound–induced pulmonary fibrosis. Arch Intern Med 151:1197-1201, 1991.

344. Romeo L, Cazzadori A, Bontempini L, Martini S: Interstitial lung granulomas as a possible consequence of exposure to zirconium dust. Med Lav 85:219-222, 1994.

345. Kern DG, Crausman RS, Durand KT, et al: Flock worker's lung: Chronic interstitial lung disease in the nylon flocking industry. Ann Intern Med 129:261-272, 1998.

346. Eschenbacher WL, Kreiss K, Lougheed MD, et al: Nylon flock–associated interstitial lung disease. Am J Respir Crit Care Med 159:2003-2008, 1999.

347. Washko RM, Day B, Parker JE, et al: Epidemiologic investigation of respiratory morbidity at a nylon flock plant. Am J Ind Med 38:628-638, 2000.

348. Barrett TE, Pietra GG, Maycock RL, et al: Acrylic resin pneumoconiosis: Report of a case in a dental student. Am Rev Respir Dis 139:841-843, 1989.

349. Choudat D, Triem S, Weill B, et al: Respiratory symptoms, lung function, and pneumoconiosis among self employed dental technicians. Br J Ind Med 50:443-449, 1993.

PULMONARY DISEASE CAUSED BY ASPIRATION AND INHALED GASES

ASPIRATION LUNG INJURY

Aspiration of Solid Foreign Bodies

Although aspiration of solid foreign bodies into the tracheo-bronchial tree occurs most often in infants and small children,[1] it is also seen occasionally in older individuals.[2] It can be manifested as acute obstruction of the larynx or trachea, a clinical condition commonly designated *café coronary* because of its frequent occurrence in restaurants and its resemblance to myocardial infarction (see later). In other patients, the condition is more insidious and is often manifested by repeated episodes of pneumonia. In such individuals, the diagnosis is sometimes difficult, particularly when the original episode of aspiration is forgotten.

In children, foreign body aspiration typically occurs in otherwise healthy individuals. By contrast, adults frequently have an underlying condition associated with impairment of airway protection, such as a neurologic disorder, trauma with loss of consciousness, or drug or alcohol abuse.[3] The most commonly implicated aspirated substance is food, usually vegetable.[1,4] Additional relatively frequent foreign bodies, usually seen in adults, are bone and fragments of dental and medical prostheses, such as tracheostomy tube segments (Fig. 17–1).[3,5] Broken fragments of teeth are occasionally aspirated after maxillofacial trauma, particularly in older children,[6] and radiographs of the chest should be obtained as a precautionary measure in all cases in which skull radiographs reveal absence or fracture of teeth after trauma.

Pathologic Characteristics

In the early stages after aspiration, the airway wall in immediate contact with the foreign body shows edema and an acute

inflammatory infiltrate or, if ulcerated, granulation tissue (see Color Fig. 17–1); these reactions contribute directly to airway narrowing. Foreign bodies such as peanuts and other substances high in fatty acid content appear to be associated with an especially severe reaction. Occasionally, the aspirated material becomes incorporated within granulation tissue in the bronchial wall and can appear endoscopically as a fungating "tumor," similar to carcinoma[7]; in such cases, the aspirated substance can usually be identified histologically in material obtained by biopsy.[8] Chronic retention of the aspirated material may result in bronchial wall fibrosis and stenosis, usually accompanied by distal bronchiectasis and obstructive pneumonitis.[9]

Radiologic Manifestations

Although some foreign bodies (such as teeth[4] and coins[5]) are discovered incidentally on routine chest radiographs, in most cases, the radiographic findings reflect the effects of partial or complete airway obstruction. Aspirated foreign bodies can be seen in all lobes, but the most common site is the right lower lobe.[5]

The chest radiograph is helpful in locating the site of foreign body impaction in about 70% of patients[3,5]; in the remainder, it is normal or shows nonspecific air space opacities. In adults, the most common radiographic findings consist of atelectasis and obstructive pneumonitis (Fig. 17–2), with or without visualization of a radiopaque foreign body (see Fig. 17–1).[3,5,10] In most adults, the lung volume distal to an impacted foreign body is decreased; hyperinflation is rare. Other abnormalities include air trapping on expiratory radiographs, abscess formation, and (in long-standing retention) bronchiectasis.[11]

CT is not recommended routinely but can be valuable in selected cases.[12,13] It usually shows the foreign body and its

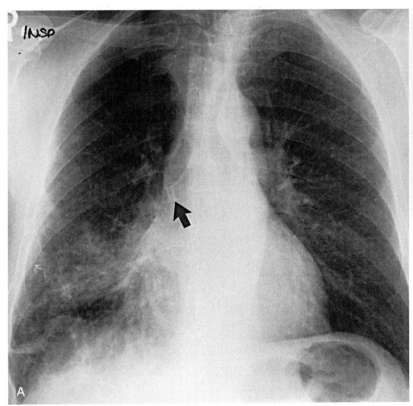

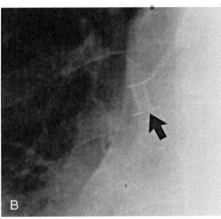

FIGURE 17–1

Aspiration of esophageal speech device. Areas of atelectasis and consolidation in the right middle and lower lobes developed in this 59-year-old man after radical laryngectomy. A chest radiograph (**A**) and magnified view of the right lower portion of the chest (**B**) show an esophageal speech device (*arrows*) in the bronchus intermedius. (*From Müller NL, Fraser RS, Colman NC, Paré PD: Radiologic Diagnosis of Diseases of the Chest. Philadelphia, WB Saunders, 2001.*)

precise location within the bronchial tree, even when the object is radiolucent (Fig. 17–3).[10]

Clinical Manifestations

As might be expected, the most common symptoms of foreign body aspiration are coughing and choking. In children, these symptoms are usually recognized by parents or guardians. Although many adult patients also give a history of choking at the time of aspiration, the physician may require a great deal of persistence to elicit this information when the episode is not recent.[2] In such individuals, an asymptomatic interval may follow aspiration, especially when bronchi are not obstructed; such a latent period can extend to several months or even years, particularly if the aspirated material is bone or inorganic matter.[3] Eventually, disease usually becomes manifested as recurrent pneumonia, chronic cough, or hemoptysis.

The café coronary syndrome occurs in adults and is caused by lodgment of food in the upper airway, with about a third located in a supraglottic position and most of the remainder at the level of the vocal cords (Fig. 17–4).[14] Risk factors include old age, alcohol consumption, use of sedative drugs, institutionalization in a chronic care home, neurologic diseases, mental retardation, and psychiatric disorders. The airway obstruction results in air hunger, cyanosis, and venous distention. As the name suggests, the sudden onset of such a catastrophic episode can lead to a misdiagnosis of myocardial infarction; however, its development during a meal, particularly when associated with an inability to speak, should suggest the true diagnosis.

Aspiration of Gastric Contents or Oropharyngeal Secretions

The term *aspiration pneumonia* is often used to denote pulmonary infection caused by the aspiration of bacteria-laden oropharyngeal secretions. This form of pneumonia is frequently caused by anaerobic organisms in patients who have poor oral hygiene and is commonly associated with abscess formation (see page 248). Though occasionally complicated by such anaerobic bacterial infection, aspiration of oropharyngeal or gastric secretions, with or without admixed food particles, can also cause significant pulmonary disease in the absence of infection. Almost invariably, such aspiration occurs in individuals who have an underlying predisposing condition, such as chronic debilitating disease, oropharyngeal or airway instrumentation (e.g., tube feeding,[15] prolonged mechanical ventilation,[16] endoscopy for upper gastrointestinal hemorrhage,[17] or tracheostomy[18]), loss of consciousness (e.g., from general anesthesia, epileptic seizure, trauma, alcohol, drug overdose, or cerebrovascular accident[19]), cardiopulmonary resuscitation,[20] and swallowing disorders (e.g., esophageal or pharyngeal carcinoma, congenital or acquired tracheoesophageal fistula, and neuromuscular disease). Evidence of aspiration, frequently subclinical, can be demonstrated in many patients who have one of these predisposing conditions.[18,19,21]

In part because of its relatively high prevalence, gastroesophageal reflux may also be an important etiologic factor in pulmonary aspiration. In fact, this process has been implicated in a variety of pulmonary diseases, including asthma, chronic cough (gastroesophageal reflux having been associated

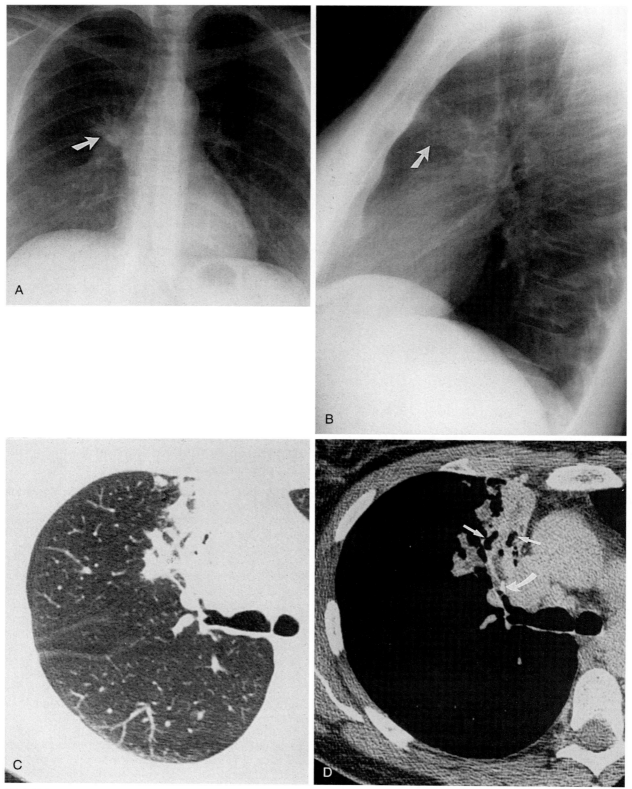

FIGURE 17–2

Obstructive pneumonitis caused by foreign body aspiration. Posteroanterior (**A**) and lateral (**B**) chest radiographs in a 44-year-old woman show localized consolidation and atelectasis involving the anterior segment of the right upper lobe (*arrows*). HRCT scans (**C** and **D**) show evidence of obstructive pneumonitis and bronchiectasis (*straight arrows*) in the same site. The localized area of high attenuation (*curved arrows*) within the bronchial lumen represents an aspirated popcorn kernel. *(From Müller NL, Fraser RS, Colman NC, Paré PD: Radiologic Diagnosis of Diseases of the Chest. Philadelphia, WB Saunders, 2001.)*

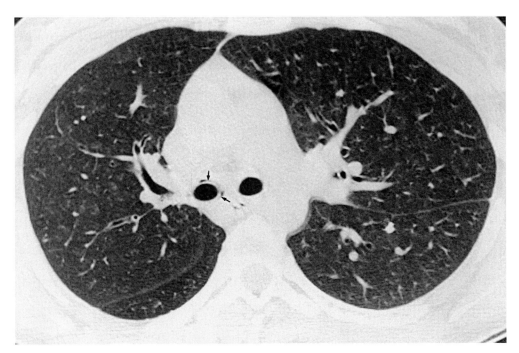

FIGURE 17–3

Foreign body aspiration. A 23-year-old drug addict had a 3-month history of cough productive of increasing amounts of green sputum. An HRCT scan shows tubing within the lumen of the right main bronchus (*arrows*). A small amount of secretions within the bronchial lumen and decreased attenuation, vascularity, and volume of the right lung are evident. (*From Müller NL, Fraser RS, Colman NC, Paré PD: Radiologic Diagnosis of Diseases of the Chest. Philadelphia, WB Saunders, 2001.*)

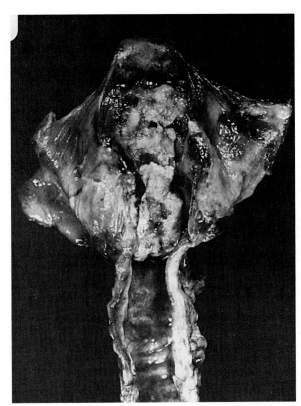

FIGURE 17–4

Acute foreign body aspiration—upper airway obstruction. The specimen consists of the larynx and upper portion of the trachea opened posteriorly. A large fragment of partially masticated meat is completely occluding the laryngeal lumen. The patient was a 58-year-old man who had "passed out" while eating and died (café coronary). (*From Fraser RS, Müller NL, Colman NC, Paré PD: Fraser and Paré's Diagnosis of Diseases of the Chest, 4th ed. Philadelphia, WB Saunders, 1999.*)

in about 20% of patients who have chronic cough[22]), bronchiectasis, recurrent pneumonia, apnea, and diffuse interstitial fibrosis.[23] Evidence supporting these associations is derived from barium studies of the esophagus (particularly those using cineradiography),[24] from scintigraphic investigations involving various foods labeled with radionuclides,[25] and from studies using esophageal pH recordings and manometry.

Pathogenesis

The pathogenesis of pulmonary damage depends on the amount and nature of the aspirated material. The hydrochloric acid in gastric secretions appears to be an important factor; it has been shown that previous neutralization of acid solutions instilled into the trachea reduces the severity of the pulmonary reaction.[26] The results of some experimental studies suggest that pulmonary damage occurs predominantly when the pH of the aspirate is less than 2.5. However, considerable clinical and experimental evidence has indicated that pulmonary damage also occurs when the pH of aspirated fluid is greater than 2.5.[27,28] Perhaps related to this observation is the finding that aspirated acid is unlikely to cause epithelial damage directly; instead, it has been speculated that pulmonary injury is the result of recruitment and activation of neutrophils after acid-induced release of cytokines such as tumor necrosis factor-α and interleukin-8.[29] When aspirated gastric contents include an appreciable quantity of admixed particulates or when the aspirated material is derived from the oropharynx, the pathogenesis of pulmonary damage appears to relate to both a nonspecific reaction to the liquid and a more specific inflammatory response to the various particulates.[30,31]

The risk of aspiration during pregnancy is increased for several reasons, including increased intra-abdominal pressure caused by the enlarged uterus, progesterone-related relaxation of the lower gastroesophageal sphincter, and upper airway intubation and unconsciousness as a result of anesthesia. In addition to the increased risk, the morbidity resulting from aspiration of gastric contents during labor appears to be particularly severe, and mortality is increased.[32]

Pathologic Characteristics

Pathologic changes depend on the nature and quantity of the aspirated material and on the frequency with which bouts of aspiration occur. The histologic reaction to relatively pure gastric liquid of low pH reflects the usually extensive acid-induced epithelial damage. In the airways, bronchitis and bronchiolitis are accompanied by focal ulceration and an intraluminal exudate. In the early stages, the parenchyma shows only air space edema and hemorrhage, followed rapidly by the appearance of necrotic debris, fibrin, and hyaline membranes (an appearance identical to diffuse alveolar damage of other etiologies).

The pathologic appearance differs somewhat when there is admixed particulate material. Edema and hemorrhage are quickly followed by an influx of neutrophils that surround the food particles (Fig. 17–5). Mononuclear phagocytic cells soon appear and develop into foreign body giant cells, typically of highly irregular shape and containing numerous nuclei (Fig. 17–6). Well-organized granulomas often develop around fragments of food or necrotic debris.[33] Although the edema and hemorrhage of the early stage of food aspiration tend to be more or less diffuse throughout the parenchyma, this granulomatous inflammation is often most severe in relation to membranous and respiratory bronchioles; thus, some degree of obliterative bronchiolitis is not uncommon.[34]

The development of secondary bacterial pneumonia or lung abscess in the case of aspirates contaminated by anaerobic or other organisms can alter the typical histologic appearance. In cases of chronic repeated aspiration, there may be extensive fibrosis with evidence of remote, organizing, and acute aspiration.

Radiologic Manifestations

In a patient who has aspirated a large amount of relatively pure gastric secretion at low pH, the chest radiograph typically reveals patchy air space consolidation, similar to the pulmonary edema seen with cardiac failure or early acute respiratory distress syndrome (ARDS).[35] Although discrete air space shadows can be apparent, most opacities are confluent (Fig. 17–7). The distribution is typically bilateral and multicentric but usually favors the perihilar or basal regions. A perihilar distribution has been shown on CT to reflect the presence of predominant consolidation in the posterior segments of the upper lobes or superior segments of the lower lobes.[36] If the patient is lying on the side at the time of aspiration, the changes may be predominantly unilateral.

In uncomplicated cases, the consolidation often worsens for several days and thereafter improves fairly rapidly. Progression of radiographic abnormalities after initial improvement is typically associated with the development of bacterial pneumonia, ARDS, or thromboembolism.[35] The normal size of the heart and the absence of signs of pulmonary venous hypertension differentiate the edema from that of cardiac origin. If the patient survives, resolution is usually relatively rapid; in our experience, it averages about

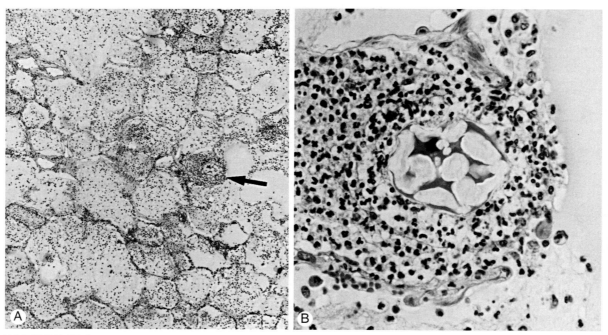

FIGURE 17–5

Acute pneumonia caused by aspiration of gastric contents. A section of lung parenchyma (**A**) shows air spaces consolidated by edema and numerous polymorphonuclear leukocytes, focally aggregated around a small particle of vegetable material (*arrow*) (magnified in **B**). (*From Fraser RS, Müller NL, Colman NC, Paré PD: Fraser and Paré's Diagnosis of Diseases of the Chest, 4th ed. Philadelphia, WB Saunders, 1999.*)

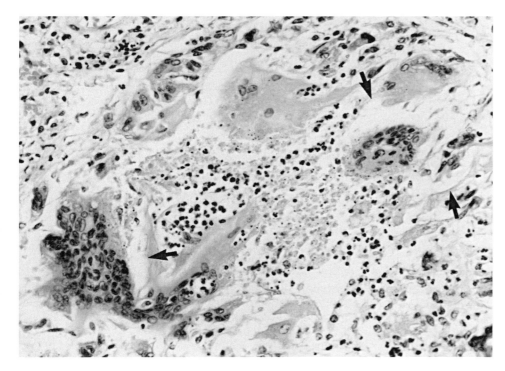

FIGURE 17–6

Foreign body giant cell reaction to aspirated gastric contents. A section through a focus of lower lobe pneumonia shows several multinucleated giant cells surrounding necrotic material and polymorphonuclear leukocytes. Vegetable fragments are partly destroyed and are evident only as clear spaces within and adjacent to the giant cells (*arrows*). *(From Fraser RS, Müller NL, Colman NC, Paré PD: Fraser and Paré's Diagnosis of Diseases of the Chest, 4th ed. Philadelphia, WB Saunders, 1999.)*

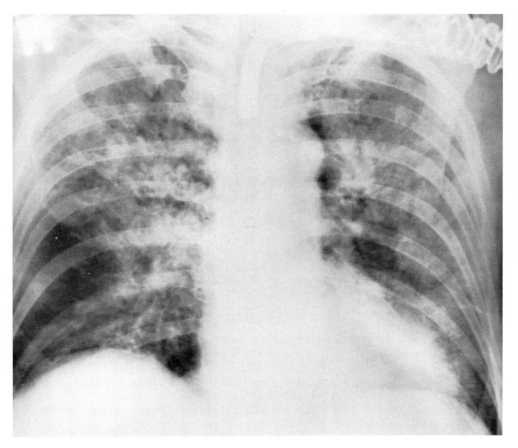

FIGURE 17–7

Acute aspiration pneumonia. While in a supine position after anesthesia, this 68-year-old man aspirated considerable quantities of vomitus. An anteroposterior chest radiograph reveals extensive involvement of both lungs by patchy air space consolidation typical of acute pulmonary edema. Although a few patchy shadows are present in the lower lung zones, the predominant involvement is in the upper zones, a distribution that can be explained, at least partly, by the position of the patient at the time of aspiration. *(From Fraser RS, Müller NL, Colman NC, Paré PD: Fraser and Paré's Diagnosis of Diseases of the Chest, 4th ed. Philadelphia, WB Saunders, 1999.)*

7 to 10 days (about the same as for traumatic fat embolism but much slower than that for edema caused by acute cardiac decompensation).

In patients who have aspirated oropharyngeal secretions or gastric contents containing an appreciable amount of admixed food, the radiographic abnormalities often have a segmental distribution, frequently involving the posterior portions of the upper or lower lobes. The precise localization depends at least partly on the position of the patient at the time of aspiration.[35] Some degree of atelectasis is present in almost all cases, and the picture can be typical of bacterial bronchopneumonia. With repeated aspiration, serial radiography over a period of months or years shows variation in the anatomic distribution of the segments involved, with disease clearing in one segment and appearing in another. A residuum of irregular accentuation of linear markings may remain and represents peribronchial or parenchymal scarring.

Occasionally, the radiographic findings consist of 1- to 5-mm-diameter nodules; HRCT performed in two patients demonstrated the nodules to have a centrilobular distribution.[37] Pathologic correlation has shown the nodules to represent foci of granulomatous inflammation related to vegetable material. Repeated aspiration can also result in diffuse bronchiolitis;[10] HRCT findings consist of centrilobular nodules and branching linear opacities with a tree-in-bud appearance.[10]

Clinical Manifestations

Aspiration of gastric contents of low pH occurs most commonly in patients in a comatose state, often after induction of anesthesia. Intubation does not necessarily protect the lungs because aspirated material situated within the airway above an inflated cuff can flood the lungs when the cuff is deflated; in addition, there is sometimes leakage around an inflated cuff, a complication that has been described even with high-volume, low-pressure endotracheal cuffs.[38]

Respiratory distress may be noted before radiographic abnormalities become evident. In the early stages, diffuse crackles may be heard; once consolidation develops, patchy areas of bronchial breathing may be detected. Hypoxemia may be severe. If the patient survives the stage of acute pulmonary edema, an initially dry cough may supervene and become productive of copious purulent sputum; a variety of aerobic and anaerobic pathogens may be cultured from this material.

The presence of recurrent gastroesophageal reflux or a congenital tracheoesophageal fistula should be considered in a patient who has an unexplained cough or a history of repeated pneumonia without obvious cause. Such patients may also complain of choking, a symptom that is suggestive of esophageal dysfunction. Appropriate investigations include contrast studies, endoscopy, and manometry of the esophagus; prolonged pH monitoring of esophageal secretions and intragastric radioisotope instillation may also be helpful.

As indicated previously, morbidity and mortality depend on the acidity and amount of material aspirated; the death rate of individuals who aspirate a quantity of acidic gastric fluid sufficient for the development of ARDS is as high as 40% to 50%.[29] In our experience, patients who survive a single bout of aspiration do not usually have clinical, physiologic, or radiographic sequelae. However, recovery may be prolonged.[39]

Aspiration of Lipid

Although the term *lipid (lipoid) pneumonia* is sometimes applied to endogenous accumulation of lipid (e.g., in association with airway obstruction or alveolar proteinosis), it is restricted here to exogenous pulmonary disease caused by the aspiration of mineral oil (the most common etiologic agent) or the various vegetable or animal oils present in food.[40]

Etiology and Pathogenesis

Although a variety of cultural[41] and occupational[42] situations predispose to the aspiration of mineral oil, disease is seen most often when the oil is used medically, particularly as a lubricant in infants with feeding difficulties, in older individuals who are constipated, and in patients who have esophageal disease.[43,44] Oil-based nose drops are not used as widely now as formerly; however, cases of lipid pneumonia as a result of nasal medication containing liquid paraffin are still seen occasionally.[45] All these situations are probably associated with repeated subclinical episodes of aspiration that eventually result in sufficient accumulation of lipid to cause radiologic and/or clinical abnormalities.

The pathogenesis of mineral oil–related fibrosis is not well understood. Chemically, the substance is a pure hydrocarbon and is believed to be inert, a feature that may explain the paucity of cough during aspiration. It is possible that altered macrophage function, such as has been hypothesized to occur in silicosis, may be a factor in causing fibrosis. However, it is also likely that other inflammatory or immune mediator cells are involved.[46]

The principal animal oils associated with pneumonia are those in milk or milk products. Aspiration of these substances occurs predominantly in infants and young children during feeding. In contrast to mineral oils, animal fats are hydrolyzed into fatty acids, presumably by lung lipases, and their presence in the lung can cause acute hemorrhagic pneumonitis.

Aspiration of vegetable oils occurs in a variety of circumstances, and there is great variability in their capacity to cause tissue damage. Some oils cause virtually no pulmonary reaction; others cause a tissue reaction similar to that associated with animal oils. It is likely that these oils are aspirated most commonly during eating or in association with vomiting of gastric contents, in which circumstances they are unlikely to be the sole offending agent. As a result, damage to the lung caused by the oil itself is difficult to assess.

Pathologic Characteristics

The degree and quality of tissue reaction to aspirated oil are quite variable and depend on the quantity and frequency of aspiration, the chemical characteristics of the oil itself, and the complicating effects of other substances that may be aspirated at the same time. The reaction to many animal oils and some vegetable oils is an acute bronchopneumonia characterized by edema, intra-alveolar hemorrhage, and a mixed polymorphonuclear and mononuclear infiltrate. By contrast, aspirated mineral oil is associated with minimal, if any, acute inflammatory reaction; instead, there is an intra-alveolar infiltrate of macrophages that rapidly phagocytose the oil. With time, these macrophages become predominantly interstitial in

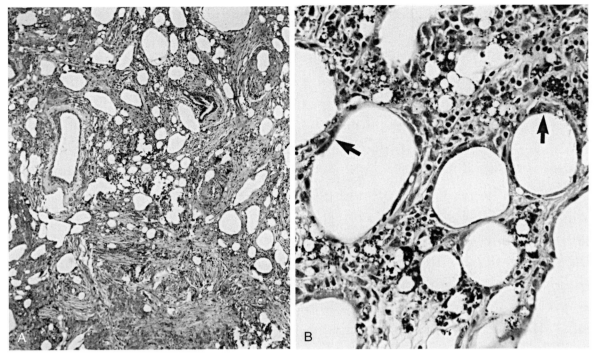

FIGURE 17–8

Mineral oil aspiration. A section from a well-circumscribed parenchymal nodule (**A**) shows fibrous tissue with admixed lymphocytes and numerous clear spaces of variable size and shape. At higher magnification (**B**) many of the clear spaces can be seen to be surrounded by a thin rim of cytoplasm containing multiple, somewhat flattened nuclei (*arrows*). The clear spaces represent foci of mineral oil within multinucleated giant cells. *(From Fraser RS, Müller NL, Colman NC, Paré PD: Fraser and Paré's Diagnosis of Diseases of the Chest, 4th ed. Philadelphia, WB Saunders, 1999.)*

location and decrease in number. The oil droplets are initially small but eventually coalesce to form relatively large round or oval droplets situated within multinucleated giant cells (Fig. 17–8). True granulomas do not develop. Fibrous tissue containing scattered collections of lymphocytes surrounds the giant cells. Grossly, the area of fibrosis can form a fairly well circumscribed, stellate tumor ("paraffinoma") or can be more diffuse and patchy in appearance.

Radiologic Manifestations

The typical appearance of acute lipid aspiration consists of air space consolidation involving mainly the lower lobes.[47] The consolidation can be patchy or confluent and may have a precise segmental distribution (Fig. 17–9). In debilitated patients in a recumbent position, involvement is likely to occur in the superior segment of a lower lobe or the posterior segment of an upper lobe. In the vast majority of cases, CT demonstrates areas of fat attenuation within the consolidated lung.[47] The attenuation may be similar to that of subcutaneous fat (−90 Hounsfield units [HU]) or approach that of water (0 HU).[48] Small pleural effusions are seen on CT in approximately 50% of cases.[47] Most patients demonstrate improvement on follow-up radiographs and CT scans performed weeks or months after the acute episode.[47]

The most common radiographic manifestations of chronic lipoid pneumonia consist of focal or confluent areas of consolidation or a single or multiple masses.[47,48] The consolidated area may be several centimeters in diameter with poorly

defined or sharply defined margins. In 30% to 40% of patients, the appearance is that of a peripheral mass simulating pulmonary carcinoma (Fig. 17–10).[47,48] Less common findings include atelectasis, irregular linear or nodular opacities, and ground-glass opacities.[10,47,48] These abnormalities involve the lower lobes predominantly in approximately 60% of patients but are also frequently seen in the upper lobes or lingula. Calcification or ossification is evident in some cases.[49,50] Areas of fat attenuation (−30 to −90 HU) can be seen on CT in approximately 80% of patients.[44,47,48] Occasionally, multifocal areas of ground-glass attenuation are present in association with interlobular septal thickening, an appearance that resembles the *crazy-paving* pattern seen in alveolar proteinosis.[10] Pleural effusions are uncommon.[47]

Clinical Manifestations

Most patients with mineral oil aspiration are asymptomatic, the abnormality being discovered on a screening chest radiograph. In fact, the diagnosis is sometimes made by histologic examination of transthoracic needle aspiration specimens or tissue removed at thoracotomy after a presumptive diagnosis of pulmonary carcinoma. Some patients complain of chronic, usually nonproductive cough or pleuritic pain. If sufficient oil is aspirated over a long period, diffuse pulmonary fibrosis and cor pulmonale may develop. Clinical findings in cases of animal or vegetable oil aspiration are usually those of acute pneumonia. As indicated, many patients have also aspirated other material in gastric contents at the same time as the lipid,

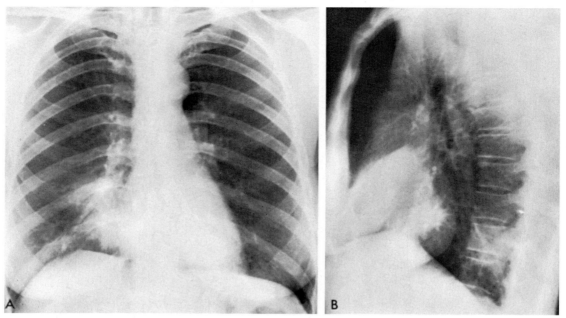

FIGURE 17–9

Lipid pneumonia. Posteroanterior (**A**) and lateral (**B**) radiographs of a 53-year-old symptom-free woman reveal poorly defined shadows of homogeneous density situated in the right middle lobe, the anterior segment of the right lower lobe, and the posterior basal segment of the left lower lobe. *(From Müller NL, Fraser RS, Colman NC, Paré PD: Radiologic Diagnosis of Diseases of the Chest. Philadelphia, WB Saunders, 2001.)*

and the background and course are similar to those outlined in the section on aspiration of gastric secretions.

The diagnosis of mineral oil aspiration should be suspected in any patient with a history of exposure to oily substances, particularly those with an underlying condition predisposing to aspiration. The finding of fat droplets in macrophages in sputum or BAL fluid supports the diagnosis[46]; however, fat can be identified in the sputum of some normal individuals, and its presence is not incontrovertible evidence of pulmonary disease. Quantification of the number of lipid-laden macrophages may be useful.[51] Transthoracic needle aspiration or transbronchial biopsy generally establishes the diagnosis in cases in which the results of lavage are uncertain.

Aspiration of Water (Drowning)

Drowning can be defined as death caused by asphyxia as a result of submersion in liquid (usually water) if the victim dies within 24 hours of the submersion episode. *Near-drowning* is defined as survival for at least 24 hours after a submersion episode and is often considered to apply even if the victim subsequently dies. The term *secondary near-drowning* has been used in patients who die of complications of the initial submersion accident (e.g., superimposed infection). The somewhat incongruous term *dry-drowning* refers to the situation in which death results from asphyxia secondary to laryngeal spasm, with minimal or no aspiration of water into the lungs.[52]

Drowning is an important cause of accidental death, particularly in children; it has been estimated that about 140,000 such deaths occur worldwide each year, about 7000 to 9000 of

which take place in the United States.[53] Of equal or greater importance is the morbidity from anoxic brain damage in patients suffering near-drowning accidents.[52]

Pathogenesis

In experimental animals, the effects of inhaling seawater (which has about three times the tonicity of extracellular fluid) clearly differ from those after the inhalation of fresh water (whose salt content is negligible).[54] The volume of water aspirated is also critical; in experimental animals, the chance of survival is very small if the volume of water inhaled exceeds 10 mL/lb body weight for seawater and 20 mL/lb for fresh water.[55] (These figures correspond to about 1.5 and 3 L, respectively, for a 70-kg human.) Because its tonicity is greater than that of blood, aspirated seawater draws water out of blood into alveoli, and ions of sodium, magnesium, calcium, and chloride pass into the blood. The result is rapid hemoconcentration, hypovolemia, and an increase in the amount of intra-alveolar fluid. This increase leads to V̇/Q̇ imbalance and significant pulmonary venous shunting. There follows a slowing of the pulse, a fall in blood pressure, and death in 4 to 5 minutes from hypoxemia and metabolic acidosis. When fresh water enters the alveoli, the situation is reversed. Because of blood's greater tonicity, inhaled water is rapidly absorbed into the circulation, with resultant hemodilution and hemolysis of red blood cells. The serum potassium level rises and the serum sodium level falls, both potential factors in causing ventricular fibrillation.

These experimentally observed differences between the effects of inhalation of salt and fresh water are not as clear-cut in human near-drowning. In fact, when it has been possible

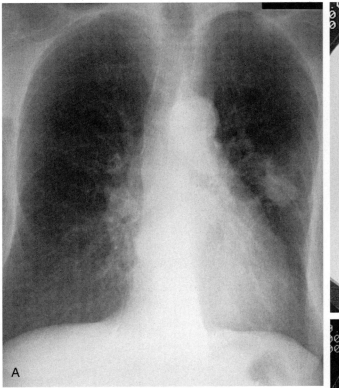

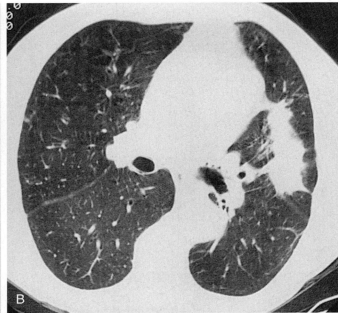

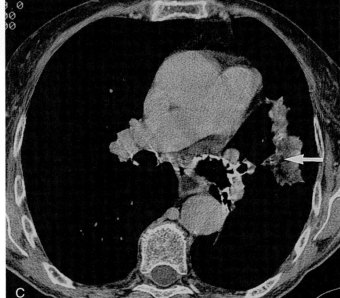

FIGURE 17–10

Mass lesion associated with lipid pneumonia. A chest radiograph (**A**) in an 80-year-old woman shows consolidation in the left upper lobe and lingula. HRCT scans (**B** and **C**) show a focal area of consolidation with surrounding linear opacities and architectural distortion consistent with fibrosis. The presence of localized areas of fat attenuation within the consolidation (*arrow*) permit the diagnosis of lipid pneumonia. *(From Müller NL, Fraser RS, Colman NC, Paré PD: Radiologic Diagnosis of Diseases of the Chest. Philadelphia, WB Saunders, 2001.)*

to carry out appropriate examinations, evidence of significant electrolyte transfer, hemoconcentration, or hemodilution has been found only occasionally.[56,57] Perhaps more importantly, there is little clinical difference between victims of freshwater and saltwater drowning.[58]

Pathologic Characteristics

Pathologic findings consist principally of air space edema. In one study, morphologic evidence of pulmonary parenchymal damage was seen in all victims, whether they survived for a few minutes or for several days[59]; hemorrhagic, desquamative, and exudative reactions developed even in patients who survived only a few minutes. In some cases, the inhaled water contains organisms (e.g., *Aeromonas sobria*[60]) or debris such

as sand, sewage, or other pollutants, all of which can potentially increase pulmonary injury[61]; as a result, deterioration in clinical status may follow initial improvement.

Radiologic Manifestations

The radiographic changes in patients who have experienced near-drowning from freshwater and seawater aspiration are similar.[57] The basic finding is air space consolidation (Fig. 17–11), the severity depending on the amount of water aspirated[62,63]; in the most severe cases, there is almost complete opacification of both lungs. Consolidation is generally bilateral and symmetrical; however, in relatively mild disease, it can be predominantly parahilar and midzonal. An asymmetrical distribution can occur. There may be a delay in the

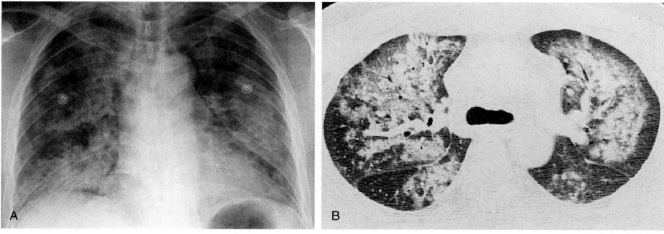

FIGURE 17–11

Near-drowning in seawater. An anteroposterior chest radiograph (**A**) in a 50-year-old man obtained within a few hours of near-drowning in seawater shows extensive, symmetrical bilateral consolidation. An HRCT scan (**B**) shows relative sparing of the peripheral lung, including the dependent regions. The consolidation resolved within 2 days. (*From Müller NL, Fraser RS, Colman NC, Paré PD: Radiologic Diagnosis of Diseases of the Chest. Philadelphia, WB Saunders, 2001.*)

radiographic appearance of edema, sometimes 24 to 48 hours.[63] Sand that is aspirated along with water can be radiopaque as a result of its calcium carbonate content and can cause a *sand bronchogram* on radiographs and CT scans.[64] Pleural effusion occurs in some cases; in one study, it was found to be more likely in saltwater than freshwater drowning[57] and with a longer submersion time.[65]

The air space consolidation generally improves in 3 to 5 days and resolves completely in 7 to 10 days.[62] In some patients, the radiographic changes persist or worsen, usually as a result of superimposed bacterial pneumonia or ARDS.[57]

Clinical Manifestations and Laboratory Findings

Depending on the volume of water aspirated and the duration of submersion, drowning victims may or may not be unconscious when they are first seen by a physician. In more severe cases, respiratory frequency is increased during the initial 24 hours and thereafter returns to normal.[57] Fine inspiratory crackles are common, and wheezing is noted occasionally. Hypoxemia, often severe, is the rule, and metabolic acidosis is frequent (presumably caused by the formation of lactic acid in the hypoxic tissues of a person struggling to survive). Serum electrolyte abnormalities are uncommonly detected in near-drowning victims; nevertheless, hypermagnesemia has been noted in some saltwater victims.[56]

Although respiratory failure is the most important pathogenetic consequence of drowning, other mechanisms play a role in the clinical manifestations in some cases. For example, individuals who have experienced near-drowning after a dive into shallow water may have had head or cervical spine injuries. In addition, a patient who has recovered consciousness and seems to be progressing favorably may, within a few hours, show increasing respiratory distress with progressive breathlessness, cyanosis, and cough. It is probable that the major cause of such deterioration is ARDS or secondary bacterial infection.

Prognosis and Natural History

Among victims of near-drowning, those who are alert on arrival in the emergency room and those who have a normal chest radiograph tend to survive.[66] However, cerebral hypoxia can have important aftereffects in those who live. It has been speculated that the chances of survival are improved when submersion has occurred in cold water, possibly because the hypothermia serves to protect the brain from hypoxic injury[67]; however, the results of some investigations do not support this hypothesis.[68] A clinical staging system in which patients are divided into six groups has been reported to help predict the likelihood of survival.[65]

The long-term effects on pulmonary function are variable. In a study of 10 asymptomatic children examined at a mean interval of 3.3 years after submersion accidents, only mild abnormalities in peripheral airway function were detected[69]; however, 7 of the 10 demonstrated bronchial hyperresponsiveness to inhaled methacholine. Some patients have radiographic evidence of fibrosis (linear opacities) months after recovery.[70]

TOXIC GAS- AND AEROSOL-INDUCED LUNG INJURY

A number of gases and fumes, as well as liquids in a finely dispersed state (aerosols), can cause acute and sometimes chronic damage to the pulmonary airways and parenchyma. Although the concentration of the gas or aerosol and the duration of exposure are the chief factors that determine the clinical manifestations and pulmonary pathology, the effects also depend to some extent on their chemical composition. Some substances—particularly those that are highly soluble, such as sulfur dioxide, ammonia, and chlorine—are so irritating to the mucous membranes of the nose that on exposure, individuals tend to stop breathing and run away, thus reducing the risk of pulmonary damage. By contrast, less soluble gases—

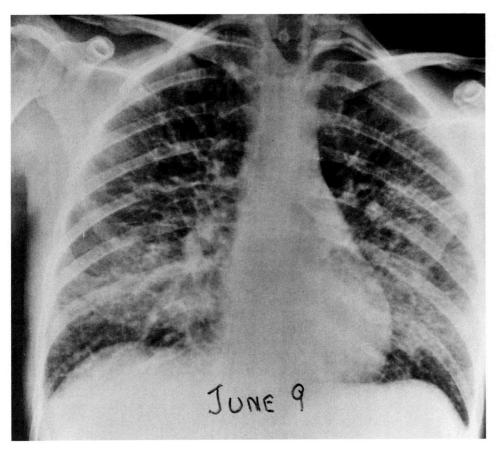

FIGURE 17–12

Acute pulmonary edema caused by the inhalation of mixed fumes. Four days before the radiograph illustrated, this 34-year-old woman had sprayed a lampshade with a plastic substance containing dimethylsulfate and ethylene dichloride (a paint fixative), followed by gold paint. She experienced an abrupt onset of severe dyspnea and nonproductive cough. The radiograph shows diffuse pulmonary edema that is predominantly interstitial in location. Prominent Kerley A and B lines are visible. The heart size is normal. Her recovery was uneventful: a chest radiograph was normal 4 days later. (*Courtesy of Dr. W.G. Brown, Regina Grey Nuns Hospital, Regina, Saskatchewan, Canada.*)

including nitrogen dioxide, ozone, and highly concentrated oxygen—may be inhaled deeply into the lungs before the irritating effect is perceived.

The manifestations of disease that result from inhalation of these toxic substances are variable. In many instances, the underlying abnormality is alveolocapillary damage with resultant permeability pulmonary edema (Fig. 17–12). In others, the chemical injury appears to affect the airways predominantly and results in bronchitis and bronchiolitis, sometimes complicated by atelectasis and bacterial pneumonia. Patients who survive the acute insult may feel relatively well for several weeks and then undergo insidious clinical deterioration with cough, shortness of breath, and fever; this delayed form of disease is reflected pathologically by obliterative bronchiolitis. This complication can also occur in individuals who initially experience diffuse pulmonary edema. Acute exposure to a toxic gas in sufficient concentration may be followed by the development of persistent airway hyperresponsiveness (reactive airways dysfunction syndrome [RADS], see page 652).

In addition to pulmonary disease after a single exposure to a toxic gas, it is probable that repeated exposure to a low concentration of certain gases or aerosols can cause more insidious airway irritation and contribute to the development of chronic bronchitis and COPD. Because of the growth of automobile-based transport and industry throughout the world and the concentration of individuals in large urban centers, atmospheric pollution is probably the most important source of such noxious substances. The health impact of more intense exposure to oxidants such as ozone, sulfur dioxide, and NO_2 in polluted air is graphically demonstrated by the marked increase in hospital visits for respiratory ailments coincident with peaks of atmospheric levels of these gases.[71]

Oxidants

Oxygen, ozone, and nitrogen dioxide have the potential to damage tissue by producing highly reactive metabolic products of oxygen such as hydrogen peroxide, superoxide radical, and hydroxyl radical.[72] Although these oxygen radicals are normally present in small amounts, intracellular production increases markedly under hyperoxic conditions and results in peroxidation of polyunsaturated lipids situated within the cell or on the cell membrane, depolymerization of mucopolysaccharides, protein sulfhydryl oxidation and cross-linking (resulting in enzyme inactivation), and nucleic acid damage. In the lung, the results of such cellular damage include bronchoconstriction, increased mucus secretion, decreased surfactant function, and increased microvascular permeability.[72,73] Additional sources of oxygen radicals are the neutrophils that appear in pulmonary tissue as a result of oxidant-induced tissue damage.

In the presence of hyperoxia, structural abnormalities appear in the lungs of experimental animals within 24 hours. Animals exposed to a low concentration of ozone[74] or to 1 atm of oxygen[75] show similar cellular abnormalities, including vacuolization of ciliated cells, swelling of type I alveolar epithelial cells, and proliferation of type II cells. Pulmonary capillary endothelial cells are also affected,[76] possibly as a result of lipid peroxidation of their cell membranes. Although alveolar macrophages may be somewhat more resistant to oxidizing substances than other cells are, metabolic abnormalities can be found in them after exposure to 100% oxygen for 48 to 72 hours or to NO_2 or ozone after a period of hyperoxia.[77,78] More prolonged exposure results in structural alterations and functional impairment.[79]

Experimental animal studies also demonstrate a remarkable ability of the lung to produce a variety of antioxidant enzymes to prevent damage from cytotoxic oxygen metabolites.[30] The enzymes generally assumed to be responsible for maintaining low levels of oxygen radicals and thus protecting against oxidants include superoxide dismutase (SOD), catalase, glutathione reductase, and glucose-6-phosphate dehydrogenase. Previous exposure to inhaled oxidants, intermittently or in low concentration, exerts a protective effect in some species of animals, an effect that correlates with the production of these antioxidants. Humans have three separate SOD enzymes: manganese (Mn SOD), copper-zinc (CuZn SOD), and extracellular (EC-SOD).[81] Both Mn SOD and CuZn SOD are highly expressed in airway epithelial cells, especially those of small bronchioles. EC-SOD appears to be synthesized by alveolar type II cells and is widely distributed in interstitial tissue.[82]

Oxygen

Studies directed at the assessment of clinical, physiologic, and morphologic alterations in the lungs of patients exposed to high concentrations of oxygen are complicated by the fact that some of the changes observed may be caused by the underlying disease, concurrent drug therapy, or mechanical ventilation. Nevertheless, it is clear from both experimental studies and clinical observations that high concentrations of inhaled oxygen can damage the lung.[83] The most severe form of disease is manifested pathologically as diffuse alveolar damage and clinically as permeability pulmonary edema. Less marked injury may be evident only on function testing.[84]

Although it is difficult to specify the precise level at which oxygen is inevitably toxic, there is ample clinical evidence that humans can tolerate an FIO_2 of 50% for prolonged periods without irreversible pulmonary damage developing.[85] However, the potential deleterious effects of a combination of oxidants should be borne in mind, and unless death from hypoxia appears imminent, higher concentrations of oxygen should be avoided, particularly in patients who have received cytotoxic drugs or radiation therapy.

Ozone

Ozone is clearly a potentially important pulmonary toxin: it constitutes 90% of the measured oxidants in photochemical smog,[86] and in certain urban areas its atmospheric concentration is equal to that known to cause structural and physiologic changes in animals.[74,87,88] In experimental studies, pathologic changes are localized predominantly to small membranous and respiratory bronchioles. Functional abnormalities have included increases in FRC and residual volume and a decrease in DLCO.[89]

Unlike most other toxic gases, ozone has not produced serious acute pulmonary disease in humans. Nevertheless,

several investigators have shown that acute exposure of normal volunteers to low concentrations (0.5 to 0.9 ppm) results in dry cough, chest discomfort, and impaired pulmonary function (manifested as a decrease in bronchial flow rates).[90,91] Considerable variation in these responses is observed among individuals, probably because of differences in airway hyperreactivity, smoking habits, tolerance developed from prolonged exposure, and the degree of exercise performed.[92] The functional derangement that follows ozone exposure is characteristically obstructive.[93,94] However, acute exposure can also cause lung restriction, predominantly by decreasing inspiratory capacity; this effect appears to be mediated by products of arachidonic acid metabolism and is related to stimulation of lung irritant receptors that inhibit full inspiration.[95]

As with oxygen, adaptation to the effects of ozone has been shown in both healthy individuals and patients who have chronic bronchitis.[96,97] It develops within 2 to 5 days of exposure but is relatively short lived, lasting 4 days to 3 weeks after cessation of exposure.

Nitrogen Dioxide

Nitrogen dioxide (NO_2) is a component of photochemical smog that has a biologic effect similar to that of ozone. Animal experiments have shown that short-term exposure to the gas in a concentration lower than 17 ppm can result in injury to bronchopulmonary epithelial and capillary endothelial cells.[98] As with oxygen and ozone, tolerance to such damage develops with repeated exposure. Nonetheless, there is evidence that prolonged exposure can result in pulmonary interstitial fibrosis and emphysema, at least in experimental animals.[99,100]

Experimental studies of the effects of low concentrations of NO_2 in humans have revealed few abnormalities[101]; however, the dangers of exposure to a high concentration are appreciable. This hazard has been recognized for many years in silo fillers and in association with industrial exposure to fuming nitric acid or the use of explosives in mining operations.[102] Silo filler's disease is the most important condition.[103] For 3 to 10 days after a silo has been filled, the fresh silage produces nitric oxide, which on contact with air oxidizes to form NO_2 and its polymer dinitrogen tetroxide. These two gases are heavier than air and are apparent just above the silage as a brownish yellow cloud. Anyone who enters the silo during this period will inhale NO_2 and suffer bronchopulmonary irritation.

After moderate to severe exposure, there is an immediate reaction that consists predominantly of acute bronchiolitis; diffuse alveolar damage has also been documented in some patients.[103] The earliest phase of disease is characterized clinically by the abrupt onset of cough, dyspnea, weakness, and a choking feeling. Pulmonary edema can develop within 4 to 24 hours, but it usually clears without residual lung damage if the patient survives. Symptoms typically abate during the second phase of disease, which lasts 2 to 5 weeks, although weakness may worsen. The chest radiograph is normal. The third phase becomes apparent up to 5 weeks after the initial exposure and is characterized pathologically by obliterative bronchiolitis. Radiographically, there is "miliary nodulation" (reticulonodular pattern), the appearance of which tends to lag somewhat behind the recurrence of symptoms.[104,105] Multiple discrete nodular opacities of varying size are scattered diffusely throughout the lungs (to a point of confluence in more severe cases)[104] or may involve mainly the midlung zones.[105]

The nodules may disappear as the clinical course progresses to a stage of chronic pulmonary insufficiency, although they usually persist for a considerable time after the acute symptoms have subsided. Clinically, this stage is characterized by fever, chills, progressive shortness of breath, cough, and cyanosis. Moist crackles and rhonchi may be heard on auscultation. A neutrophilic leukocytosis develops in most cases, and PaCO$_2$ may be elevated. The patient may die of pulmonary insufficiency or may recover more or less completely during this stage. Some patients have residual chronic obstructive disease or RADS.[106]

Other Gases

Sulfur Dioxide

Sulfur dioxide (SO$_2$) is a highly soluble gas that on contact with moist epithelial surfaces is hydrated and oxidized to form sulfuric acid (H$_2$SO$_4$), which in turn causes mucosal injury. The acid may be partly neutralized—and the damage thereby diminished—by combination with endogenous ammonia in the respiratory tract.[107]

The major source of SO$_2$ is atmospheric pollution, and continuous exposure to low concentrations in an urban environment may play a role in the pathogenesis of COPD. Accidental exposure to a high concentration of the gas can occur in pulp and paper factories, refrigeration plants, and oil-refining and fruit-preserving industries. H$_2$SO$_4$ itself is also used in photographic developing and has been found to cause reversible small-airway obstruction in photographers.[108] It is probable that inhaled SO$_2$ produces the same triphasic course of disease as that caused by NO$_2$[109]; bronchiectasis, obliterative bronchiolitis (Fig. 17–13), and RADS are long-term complications.

Hydrogen Sulfide

Hydrogen sulfide (H$_2$S) produces a characteristic "rotten egg" odor at 0.2 ppm and paralyzes the sense of smell at levels of 150 ppm. Levels of 250 ppm cause irritation of the mucous membranes with resultant keratoconjunctivitis, bronchitis, and pulmonary edema. Higher concentrations affect the central nervous system and can cause rapid death.[110] Like cyanide, sulfide ions act as cytotoxins and selectively bind to cytochrome oxidase within mitochondria and thereby disrupt the electron transport chain. The most common sources of exposure are the petroleum and chemical industries[111] and decaying organic matter such as liquid manure[110] or insufficiently refrigerated fish stored in an unventilated ship's hold.[112]

In a review of 5 years' experience with H$_2$S poisoning in the Alberta oil fields, there were 221 cases of recognized exposure with an overall mortality of 6%[111]; 5% of victims were dead on arrival at the hospital. Acute problems consisted of coma, disequilibrium, and respiratory insufficiency as a result of pulmonary edema; 74% of patients lost consciousness at the accident site. If the patient recovers, respiratory sequelae are uncommon; however, there may be long-term neurologic impairment.[113]

Ammonia

Ammonia is a toxic, highly soluble gas that may play a role along with H$_2$S in causing bronchopulmonary disease on exposure to decaying organic matter. However, it is better known as a cause of lung damage in industry and farming, usually as a result of sudden rupture or leakage of concentrated NH$_3$ from tanks.[114] Vehicular accidents involving tank transportation of the gas can also result in the inhalation of high concentrations by those involved, often with serious consequences. Inhalation of a significant quantity of the gas results in severe acute tracheobronchitis and the production of copious serosanguineous and often purulent secretions. Marked inflammation of the proximal airways can be seen bronchoscopically.[115] Bronchiectasis and obliterative bronchiolitis may develop in survivors.[116]

Chlorine

Exposure to chlorine gas can occur in a variety of occupational, environmental, and household settings.[117] Heavy exposure occurs most often after an industrial accident or when the gas escapes from broken pipes or tank containers; occupational settings at particular risk are the plastic and textile industries, plants for water purification, and pulp mills.[118,119] A less common source of exposure is the use of chlorinated products for swimming pools.[120] The gas can also be generated by mixing bleach (sodium hypochlorite) and cleaning solutions containing phosphoric acid, and a number of cases of pulmonary toxicity have been reported in this situation.[121]

Acute exposure to a high concentration of chlorine results in pulmonary edema, necrosis of airway epithelium, and bronchial inflammation[122]; fever, conjunctivitis, nausea and vomiting, stupor, shock, and hemoptysis may be evident clinically. Cough and influenza-like symptoms, as well as throat and eye irritation, are common consequences of repeated accidental exposure to lower concentrations.[123] Pulmonary function tests show an obstructive pattern, which may return to normal in a few weeks.[124] RADS develops in some patients.[119]

Phosgene

Phosgene is the common name for carbon oxychloride (COCl$_2$), a colorless oxidizing gas that is hydrolyzed to hydrochloric acid and carbon dioxide when inhaled.[125] Necrosis and sloughing of the airway epithelium and interstitial and alveolar edema occur as a result of the action of the acid. Though infamous as a highly poisonous gas used in warfare, it is more important nowadays as an occasional hazard in some industries.[126] Phosgene is also a decomposition product of trichloroethylene, and toxic levels can be generated when welding is performed in an atmosphere containing this substance.[127] As with NO$_2$ inhalation, there is a delay of several hours before the onset of dyspnea. Acute pulmonary edema can cause death, usually within 24 hours of exposure. If the patient survives the acute episode, recovery is usually complete. However, RADS has been described as a long-term complication.

Formaldehyde

Urea formaldehyde resins are used as adhesives in wood products (principally particleboard, fiberboard, and hardwood plywood) and as foam insulation in housing.[128] Occupational exposure occurs in the manufacture of these substances, in carpentry shops, and in those exposed to formalin in pathology

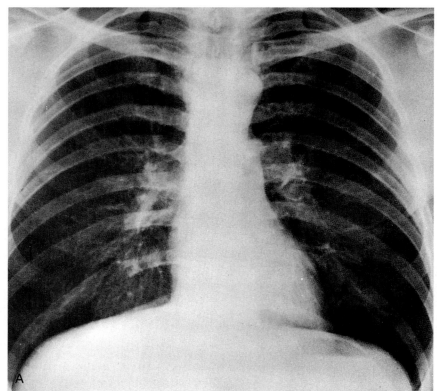

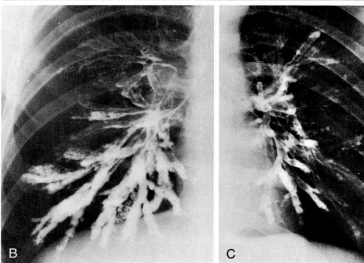

FIGURE 17–13

Obliterative bronchiolitis and bronchiectasis secondary to sulfur dioxide inhalation. Three months before these radiographic studies, this 33-year-old man was exposed to high concentrations of sulfur dioxide fumes rising from a sulfuric acid vat. Acute pulmonary edema was said to have developed immediately after this exposure, but it gradually resolved over a period of days (this acute episode was not documented locally). Three months later, a posteroanterior radiograph (**A**) was essentially normal, although close examination revealed numerous "tram lines" in the central portions of both lungs. The lungs were somewhat overinflated. Bilateral bronchography (**B**) and (**C**) demonstrated severe cylindrical and varicose bronchiectasis of all segmental bronchi of both lungs, the dilated bronchi terminating abruptly in squared or rounded extremities. There was an almost total absence of peripheral filing. These findings are consistent with extensive obliterative bronchiolitis in addition to bronchiectasis. (*From Fraser RS, Müller NL, Colman NC, Paré PD: Fraser and Paré's Diagnosis of Diseases of the Chest, 4th ed. Philadelphia, WB Saunders, 1999.*)

departments and funeral homes.[129-131] Nonoccupational exposure occurs in buildings that contain urea formaldehyde foam insulation.[132] Exposure in any of these settings can cause eye irritation, rhinitis, rash, and upper respiratory symptoms.[133] However, most investigators have found no evidence of either acute or chronic impairment of pulmonary function.[128,130,134]

Metals

Fumes or gaseous forms of several metals, including mercury, zinc (zinc chloride), manganese, cadmium, nickel (nickel carbonyl), and vanadium, can cause acute tracheobronchitis, diffuse lung injury associated with pulmonary edema (ARDS), interstitial pneumonitis and edema, or a syndrome called *metal fume fever*. The latter is a poorly understood systemic reaction clinically characterized by the sudden onset of thirst, a metallic taste in the mouth, substernal tightness, headache, fever, chills, muscle aches, and a neutrophil alveolitis.[135,136] It appears to be related to inhalation of the finely dispersed particles (<1 μm in diameter) that develop when metals are heated to 93°C or higher. Symptoms usually appear within 12 hours of exposure and subside within 24 hours without complications or sequelae. Repeated exposure can result in increased tolerance, although re-exposure on Mondays after off-duty weekends is usually associated with a more severe episode. Moist crackles and rhonchi may be heard on auscultation, and leukocytosis (20,000/mm³ or more) with neutrophilia can occur. The chest radiograph either is normal or shows increased prominence of bronchovascular markings.

Mercury

Occupational exposure to vaporized mercury occurs most often in a confined space such as a tank or a boiler. Accidental exposure can occur in the home when metallic mercury is allowed to burn on a stove.[137] Symptoms and signs tend to develop 3 to 4 hours after exposure and include gingivostomatitis, crampy abdominal pain, and diarrhea; severe tracheitis, bronchitis, bronchiolitis, and pneumonitis can develop.[138] The condition is particularly serious in infants, in whom the bronchiolitis may be fatal. Pulmonary function tests performed shortly after exposure have shown a combination of obstructive and restrictive disease and a lowered diffusing capacity.[137]

Cadmium

This toxic metal is present in many foods and in tobacco. Acute exposure to a high concentration usually occurs during the heating of cadmium-coated metal with an oxyacetylene torch and may result in metal fume fever or pulmonary edema.[139] Chronic exposure occurs most often in cigarette smokers, the metal being present in the smoke itself. The results of some studies have suggested the possibility of a pathogenetic relationship between cadmium inhalation and emphysema[140,141]; however, the importance of this relationship relative to other components of cigarette smoke is unclear.

Epoxides, Trimellitic Anhydride, and Polymers

Trimellitic anhydride (TMA) is a low-molecular-weight chemical widely used in the manufacture of plastics, epoxy resin coatings, and paints. Four syndromes have been associated with its inhalation:[142] (1) an immediate-type airway response (asthma-rhinitis) mediated by an IgE antibody directed against trimellityl-conjugated human respiratory tract proteins; (2) a syndrome characterized by cough, wheezing, dyspnea, myalgia, and arthralgia that develops 4 to 12 hours after exposure and is related to the induction of IgG antibodies by a TMA hapten-protein complex; (3) an alveolar hemorrhage syndrome associated with high levels of antibodies to trimellityl-conjugated proteins and erythrocytes; and (4) an occupational bronchitis resulting from the direct irritant properties of TMA. The first three syndromes have a latent period between initial exposure and the onset of symptoms. Removal from exposure usually results in rapid disappearance of symptoms and decreased levels of serum antibodies. Hypoxemia, which may be severe, and the restrictive functional defect revert to normal in patients who have alveolar hemorrhage syndrome.[143]

Polymer fume fever (polytetrafluoroethylene poisoning) is caused by the inhalation of fumes that evolve as degradation products when polytetrafluoroethylene (Fluon, Teflon) is heated to high temperatures (above 250° C); the pyrolytic products of this plastic material have not been identified. Symptoms are similar to those of metal fume fever and include tightness in the chest, headache, shivering, fever, aching, weakness, and occasionally, shortness of breath.[144] Pulmonary edema has developed in some patients.[145] In most reported cases, fume inhalation has been associated with cigarette smoking, the high temperatures generated by the burning of the tobacco being sufficient to produce pyrolysis products.

BRONCHOPULMONARY DISEASE ASSOCIATED WITH BURNS

Pulmonary parenchymal disease and tracheobronchial disease are common and important complications of burns and can occur by several mechanisms. Assessment of the relative contribution of each can be extremely difficult in an individual patient.[146]

The inhalation of smoke and the various toxic chemicals that it contains is a particularly important mechanism of tracheobronchial injury, especially when exposure has occurred within a confined space. Smoke consists of gases and a suspension of small particles in hot air. The particles are composed of carbon coated with combustible products such as organic acids and aldehydes. The gaseous fraction has a highly variable composition that depends on the material that is burning[147]; although most constituents are usually unknown, carbon monoxide and carbon dioxide are always present. Another toxic combustion product is cyanide, which is a product of fires involving material such as nylon, asphalt, wool, silk, and polyurethane; high carboxyhemoglobin levels correlate with high cyanide levels in the blood of fire survivors.[148]

Polyvinyl chloride (PVC), a plastic solid widely used as a rubber substitute for covering electric and telephone wires and cables and in many manufactured products,[149] has been implicated as a major cause of bronchopulmonary damage because of the release of hydrogen chloride gas when it burns. PVC degrades and releases hydrochloric acid at temperatures higher than 225° C. The effect of the acid in the gas phase is largely restricted to irritability and chiefly involves the upper respiratory tract; however, hydrochloric acid can condense on soot aerosol and thereby gain access to the lower airway mucosa and lung parenchyma.

Direct trauma as a result of heat can cause severe tissue damage, particularly to the airway mucosa. Although the most frequent situation in which such damage occurs is fire, it can also occur in other settings such as the explosion of a steam tube in a ship's boiler room.[150] In addition to injury caused by heat and by the inhalation of smoke, pulmonary disease can be a result of concurrent shock, sepsis, and renal failure.

The histopathologic findings in patients who die within 48 hours of a fire include pulmonary congestion, edema, intravascular fibrin thrombi, intra-alveolar hemorrhage, and necrosis of tracheal and proximal bronchial epithelium.[151] Although the latter abnormality is probably diffuse in most cases, occasionally it results in the formation of localized endobronchial polyps composed of granulation tissue.[152]

Pulmonary complications occur in 20% to 30% of burn victims admitted to a hospital.[153,154] The incidence correlates with the severity of the burn and with a history of being in an enclosed space. During the first 24 hours, complications result from upper airway edema secondary to direct heat injury or toxic products, usually in patients who have head and neck burns. After a latent period of 12 to 48 hours, symptoms and radiographic evidence of lower respiratory tract involvement may be evident.[155] Pulmonary complications that become evident 2 to 5 days after a burn consist of atelectasis, edema, and pneumonia. The first of these complications may be caused by mucus plugging of large bronchi[156]; the last occurs much more frequently in the presence of inhalation injury.[157] Complications that arise after 5 days include pulmonary thromboembolism and ARDS.

The radiographic findings of acute smoke inhalation include focal opacities (which have been interpreted as atelectasis and usually clear within several days)[158] or more diffuse disease that represents pulmonary edema (Fig. 17–14).[155] Several groups of investigators have shown that patients who have an abnormal radiograph within 48 hours after inhalation injury are more likely to require ventilatory support and have a worse prognosis than those who have normal radiographs.[155,159,160] However, in a study of 29 patients who required ventilatory support after acute smoke inhalation and burns, only 13 had initial radiologic findings consistent with inhalation injury, including interstitial or air space edema and linear atelectasis.[161]

The pattern of deposition and rate of clearance of aerosolized technetium 99m–labeled diethylenetriamine pentaacetic acid (DTPA) has been used as a measure of the degree of acute inhalation injury in patients exposed to smoke; a pattern of inhomogeneous distribution and rapid uptake has been found to correlate with radiographic, lung function, and clinical markers of the severity of lung injury.[162]

Radiographic manifestations of large-airway burns include subglottic edema and indistinctness of the trachea.[159] Late manifestations include tracheal stenosis,[163] bronchiectasis,[164,165] and evidence of obliterative bronchiolitis (increased lung volumes and decreased vascularity in the peripheral lung regions).[164] Corresponding HRCT findings include bronchiectasis and areas of decreased attenuation and perfusion (Fig. 17–15).

A number of controlled studies in which pulmonary function has been assessed in firefighters have failed to show short-term deterioration in function[166-168]; however, their findings support the conclusion that a long-term risk for obstructive pulmonary disease exists in this occupation over and above that caused by cigarette smoking. An analysis of causes of death in 2470 Boston firefighters employed during the period 1915 to 1975 failed to reveal an association between occupation and cause-specific mortality.[169]

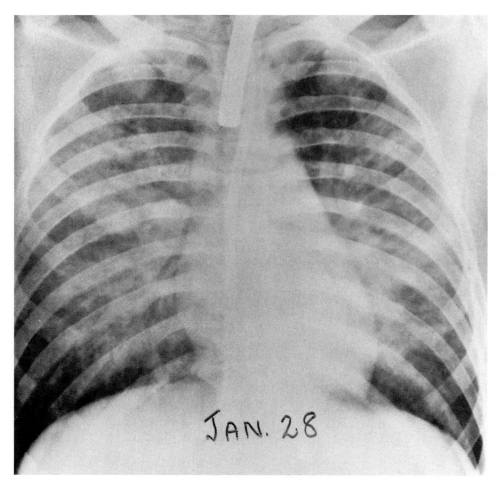

FIGURE 17–14

Acute smoke inhalation. A 30-year-old man was involved in a fire and inhaled large quantities of smoke before being rescued. He was brought to the emergency department in severe respiratory distress, and a tracheostomy was required. An anteroposterior radiograph shows massive consolidation of both lungs in a pattern characteristic of acute pulmonary edema. The patient had an uneventful recovery. *(From Müller NL, Fraser RS, Colman NC, Paré PD: Radiologic Diagnosis of Diseases of the Chest. Philadelphia, WB Saunders, 2001.)*

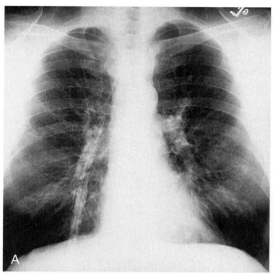

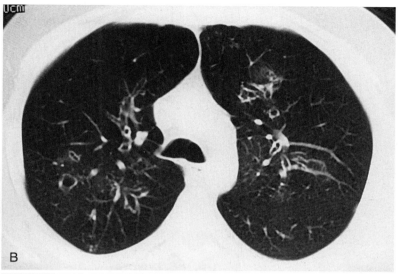

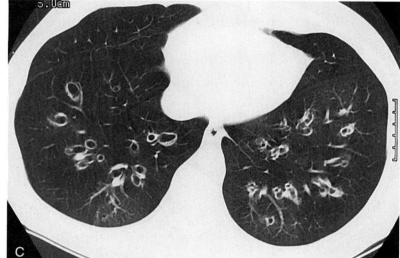

FIGURE 17–15

Bronchiectasis and obliterative bronchiolitis after smoke inhalation. A posteroanterior chest radiograph (**A**) in a 33-year-old man shows increased lung volume, bronchiectasis, and decreased peripheral vascular markings. HRCT scans (**B** and **C**) show extensive bronchiectasis and areas of decreased attenuation and vascularity as a result of obliterative bronchiolitis. The patient had experienced severe smoke inhalation several years earlier. (*Courtesy of Dr. Christopher Griffen, Department of Radiology, Veterans Affairs Hospital, Portland, Oregon.*)

REFERENCES

1. Weissberg D, Schwartz I: Foreign bodies in the tracheobronchial tree. Chest 91:730-733, 1987.
2. Lan RS: Non-asphyxiating tracheobronchial foreign bodies in adults. Eur Respir J 7:510-514, 1994.
3. Chen CH, Lai CL, Tsai TT, et al: Foreign body aspiration into the lower airway in Chinese adults. Chest 112:129-133, 1997.
4. Brown BS, Ma H, Dunbar JS, Macewan DW: Foreign bodies in tracheobronchial tree in childhood. J Can Assoc Radiol 14:158-171, 1963.
5. Limper AH, Prakash UB: Tracheobronchial foreign bodies in adults. Ann Intern Med 112:604-609, 1990.
6. Pochaczevsky R, Leonidas JC, Feldman F, et al: Aspirated and ingested teeth in children. Clin Radiol 24:349-353, 1973.
7. Chopra S, Simmons DH, Cassan SM, et al: Bronchial obstruction by incorporation of aspirated vegetable material in the bronchial wall. Am Rev Respir Dis 112:717-720, 1975.
8. Ristagno RL, Kornstein MJ, Hansen-Flaschen JH: Diagnosis of occult meat aspiration by fiberoptic bronchoscopy. Am J Med 80:154-156, 1986.
9. Tarkka M, Anttila S, Sutinen S: Bronchial stenosis after aspiration of an iron tablet. Chest 93:439-441, 1988.
10. Franquet T, Gimenez A, Roson N, et al: Aspiration diseases: Findings, pitfalls, and differential diagnosis. Radiographics 20:673-685, 2000.
11. Kurklu EU, Williams MA, Le Roux BT: Bronchiectasis consequent upon foreign body retention. Thorax 28:601-602, 1973.
12. Berger PE, Kuhn JP, Kuhns LR: Computed tomography and the occult tracheobronchial foreign body. Radiology 134:133-135, 1980.
13. Kavanagh PV, Mason AC, Müller NL: Thoracic foreign bodies in adults. Clin Radiol 54:353-360, 1999.
14. Mittleman RE, Wetli CV: The fatal cafe coronary. Foreign-body airway obstruction. JAMA 247:1285-1288, 1982.
15. Strauss D, Kastner T, Ashwal S, White J: Tubefeeding and mortality in children with severe disabilities and mental retardation. Pediatrics 99:358-362, 1997.
16. Tolep K, Getch CL, Criner GJ: Swallowing dysfunction in patients receiving prolonged mechanical ventilation. Chest 109:167-172, 1996.
17. Lipper B, Simon D, Cerrone F: Pulmonary aspiration during emergency endoscopy in patients with upper gastrointestinal hemorrhage. Crit Care Med 19:330-333, 1991.
18. Elpern EH, Scott MG, Petro L, Ries MH: Pulmonary aspiration in mechanically ventilated patients with tracheostomies. Chest 105:563-566, 1994.
19. Nakagawa T, Sekizawa K, Arai H, et al: High incidence of pneumonia in elderly patients with basal ganglia infarction. Arch Intern Med 157:321-324, 1997.
20. Lawes EG, Baskett PJ: Pulmonary aspiration during unsuccessful cardiopulmonary resuscitation. Intensive Care Med 13:379-382, 1987.
21. Huxley EJ, Viroslav J, Gray WR, Pierce AK: Pharyngeal aspiration in normal adults and patients with depressed consciousness. Am J Med 64:564-568, 1978.
22. Irwin RS, Curley FJ, French CL: Chronic cough. The spectrum and frequency of causes, key components of the diagnostic evaluation, and outcome of specific therapy. Am Rev Respir Dis 141:640-647, 1990.
23. Barish CF, Wu WC, Castell DO: Respiratory complications of gastroesophageal reflux. Arch Intern Med 145:1882-1888, 1985.
24. Ekberg O, Hilderfors H: Defective closure of the laryngeal vestibule: Frequency of pulmonary complications. AJR Am J Roentgenol 145:1159-1164, 1985.
25. Crausaz FM, Favez G: Aspiration of solid food particles into lungs of patients with gastroesophageal reflux and chronic bronchial disease. Chest 93:376-378, 1988.
26. Chen CT, Toung TJ, Haupt HM, et al: Evaluation of the efficacy of Alka-Seltzer Effervescent in gastric acid neutralization. Anesth Analg 63:325-329, 1984.

27. Schwartz DJ, Wynne JW, Gibbs CP, et al: The pulmonary consequences of aspiration of gastric contents at pH values greater than 2.5. Am Rev Respir Dis 121:119-126, 1980.

28. Bond VK, Stoelting RK, Gupta CD: Pulmonary aspiration syndrome after inhalation of gastric fluid containing antacids. Anesthesiology 51:452-453, 1979.

29. Matthay MA, Rosen GD: Acid aspiration induced lung injury. New insights and therapeutic options. Am J Respir Crit Care Med 154:277-278, 1996.

30. Vidyarthi SC: Diffuse miliary granulomatosis of the lungs due to aspirated vegetable cells. Arch Pathol 83:215-218, 1967.

31. Teabeaut JI: Aspiration of gastric contents: An experimental study. Am J Pathol 28:51, 1952.

32. MacLennan FM: Maternal mortality from Mendelson's syndrome: An explanation? Lancet 1:587-589, 1986.

33. Knoblich R: Pulmonary granulomatosis caused by vegetable particles. So-called lentil pulse pneumonia. Am Rev Respir Dis 99:380-389, 1969.

34. Matsuse T, Oka T, Kida K, Fukuchi Y: Importance of diffuse aspiration bronchiolitis caused by chronic occult aspiration in the elderly. Chest 110:1289-1293, 1996.

35. Landay MJ, Christensen EE, Bynum LJ: Pulmonary manifestations of acute aspiration of gastric contents. AJR Am J Roentgenol 131:587-592, 1978.

36. Müller NL: Aspiration pneumonia. In Siegel B (ed): Chest Disease, 5th series. Test Syllabus. American College of Radiology, 1996, p 378.

37. Marom EM, McAdams HP, Sporn TA, Goodman PC: Lentil aspiration pneumonia: Radiographic and CT findings. J Comput Assist Tomogr 22:598-600, 1998.

38. Macrae W, Wallace P: Aspiration around high-volume, low-pressure endotracheal cuff. Br Med J (Clin Res Ed) 283:1220, 1981.

39. Brandstetter RD, Conetta R, Sander NW, et al: Adult respiratory distress syndrome in adolescents due to aspiration of gastric contents. N Y State J Med 86:513-516, 1986.

40. Genereux GP: Lipids in the lungs: Radiologic-pathologic correlation. J Can Assoc Radiol 21:2-15, 1970.

41. Miller GJ, Ashcroft MT, Beadnell HM, et al: The lipoid pneumonia of blackfat tobacco smokers in Guyana. Q J Med 40:457-470, 1971.

42. Cullen MR, Balmes JR, Robins JM, Smith GJ: Lipoid pneumonia caused by oil mist exposure from a steel rolling tandem mill. Am J Ind Med 2:51-58, 1981.

43. Spickard A 3rd, Hirschmann JV: Exogenous lipoid pneumonia. Arch Intern Med 154:686-692, 1994.

44. Gondouin A, Manzoni P, Ranfaing E, et al: Exogenous lipid pneumonia: A retrospective multicentre study of 44 cases in France. Eur Respir J 9:1463-1469, 1996.

45. Spatafora M, Bellia V, Ferrara G, Genova G: Diagnosis of a case of lipoid pneumonia by bronchoalveolar lavage. Respiration 52:154-156, 1987.

46. Lauque D, Dongay G, Levade T, et al: Bronchoalveolar lavage in liquid paraffin pneumonitis. Chest 98:1149-1155, 1990.

47. Baron SE, Haramati LB, Rivera VT: Radiological and clinical findings in acute and chronic exogenous lipoid pneumonia. J Thorac Imaging 18:217-224, 2003.

48. Lee KS, Müller NL, Hale V, et al: Lipoid pneumonia: CT findings. J Comput Assist Tomogr 19:48-51, 1995.

49. Salm R, Hughes EW: A case of chronic paraffin pneumonitis. Thorax 25:762-768, 1970.

50. Tahon F, Berthezene Y, Hominal S, et al: Exogenous lipoid pneumonia with unusual CT pattern and FDG positron emission tomography scan findings. Eur Radiol 12(Suppl 3):S171-S173, 2002.

51. Gallagher JD, Smith DS, Meranze J, et al: Aspiration during induction of anaesthesia in patients with colon interposition. Can Anaesth Soc J 32:56-59, 1985.

52. Modell JH: Drowning. N Engl J Med 328:253-256, 1993.

53. Weinstein MD, Krieger BP: Near-drowning: Epidemiology, pathophysiology, and initial treatment. J Emerg Med 14:461-467, 1996.

54. Kylstra JA: Survival of submerged mammals. N Engl J Med 272:198-200, 1965.

55. Modell JH, Moya F: Effects of volume of aspirated fluid during chlorinated fresh water drowning. Anesthesiology 27:662-672, 1966.

56. Cohen DS, Matthay MA, Cogan MG, Murray JF: Pulmonary edema associated with salt water near-drowning: New insights. Am Rev Respir Dis 146:794-796, 1992.

57. Hasan S, Avery WG, Fabian C, Sackner MA: Near drowning in humans. A report of 36 patients. Chest 59:191-197, 1971.

58. Bradley M: Near-drowning: CPR is just the beginning. J Respir Dis 2:37, 1981.

59. Fuller RH: The 1962 Wellcome prize essay. Drowning and the postimmersion syndrome. A clinicopathologic study. Mil Med 128:22-36, 1963.

60. Ender PT, Dolan MJ, Dolan D, et al: Near-drowning–associated Aeromonas pneumonia. J Emerg Med 14:737-741, 1996.

61. Noguchi M, Kimula Y, Ogata T: Muddy lung. Am J Clin Pathol 83:240-244, 1985.

62. Hunter TB, Whitehouse WM: Fresh-water near-drowning: Radiological aspects. Radiology 112:51-56, 1974.

63. Putman CE, Tummillo AM, Myerson DA, Myerson PJ: Drowning: Another plunge. Am J Roentgenol Radium Ther Nucl Med 125:543-548, 1975.

64. Dunagan DP, Cox JE, Chang MC, Haponik EF: Sand aspiration with near-drowning. Radiographic and bronchoscopic findings. Am J Respir Crit Care Med 156:292-295, 1997.

65. Szpilman D: Near-drowning and drowning classification: A proposal to stratify mortality based on the analysis of 1,831 cases. Chest 112:660-665, 1997.

66. Modell JH, Graves SA, Ketover A: Clinical course of 91 consecutive near-drowning victims. Chest 70:231-238, 1976.

67. Bolte RG, Black PG, Bowers RS, et al: The use of extracorporeal rewarming in a child submerged for 66 minutes. JAMA 260:377-379, 1988.

68. Suominen PK, Korpela RE, Silfvast TG, Olkkola KT: Does water temperature affect outcome of nearly drowned children. Resuscitation 35:111-115, 1997.

69. Laughlin JJ, Eigen H: Pulmonary function abnormalities in survivors of near drowning. J Pediatr 100:26-30, 1982.

70. Glauser FL, Smith WR: Pulmonary interstitial fibrosis following near-drowning and exposure to short-term high oxygen concentrations. Chest 68:373-375, 1975.

71. Thurston GD, Ito K, Hayes CG, et al: Respiratory hospital admissions and summertime haze air pollution in Toronto, Ontario: Consideration of the role of acid aerosols. Environ Res 65:271-290, 1994.

72. Doelman CJ, Bast A: Oxygen radicals in lung pathology. Free Radic Biol Med 9:381-400, 1990.

73. Putman E, van Golde LM, Haagsman HP: Toxic oxidant species and their impact on the pulmonary surfactant system. Lung 175:75-103, 1997.

74. Boatman ES, Sato S, Frank R: Acute effects of ozone on cat lungs. II. Structural. Am Rev Respir Dis 110:157-169, 1974.

75. Weibel ER: Oxygen effect on lung cells. Arch Intern Med 128:54-56, 1971.

76. Clark JM, Lambertsen CJ: Pulmonary oxygen toxicity: A review. Pharmacol Rev 23:37-133, 1971.

77. Fisher AB, Diamond S, Mellen S, Zubrow A: Effect of 48- and 72-hour oxygen exposure on the rabbit alveolar macrophage. Chest 66(Suppl):4S-7S, 1974.

78. Simons JR, Theodore J, Robin ED: Common oxidant lesion of mitochondrial redox state produced by nitrogen dioxide, ozone, and high oxygen in alveolar macrophages. Chest 66(Suppl):9S-12S, 1974.

79. Huber GL, Mason RJ, LaForce M, et al: Alterations in the lung following the administration of ozone. Arch Intern Med 128:81-87, 1971.

80. Deneke SM, Fanburg BL: Normobaric oxygen toxicity of the lung. N Engl J Med 303:76-86, 1980.

81. Tsan MF: Superoxide dismutase and pulmonary oxygen toxicity. Proc Soc Exp Biol Med 214:107-113, 1997.

82. Su WY, Folz R, Chen JS, et al: Extracellular superoxide dismutase mRNA expressions in the human lung by in situ hybridization. Am J Respir Cell Mol Biol 16:162-170, 1997.

83. Balentine JD: Pathologic effects of exposure to high oxygen tensions. A review. N Engl J Med 275:1038-1040, 1966.

84. Caldwell PR, Lee WL Jr, Schildkraut HS, Archibald ER: Changes in lung volume, diffusing capacity, and blood gases in men breathing oxygen. J Appl Physiol 21:1477-1483, 1966.

85. Jackson RM: Pulmonary oxygen toxicity. Chest 88:900-905, 1985.

86. Cross CE, De Lucia AJ, Reddy AK, et al: Ozone interactions with lung tissue. Biochemical approaches. Am J Med 60:929-935, 1976.

87. Castleman WL, Dungworth DL, Schwartz LW, Tyler WS: Acute respiratory bronchiolitis: An ultrastructural and autoradiographic study of epithelial cell injury and renewal in rhesus monkeys exposed to ozone. Am J Pathol 98:811-840, 1980.

88. Watanabe S, Frank R, Yokoyama E. Acute effects of ozone on lungs of cats. I. Functional. Am Rev Respir Dis 108:1141-1151, 1973.

89. Gross KB, White HJ: Functional and pathologic consequences of a 52-week exposure to 0.5 ppm ozone followed by a clean air recovery period. Lung 165:283-295, 1987.

90. Kagawa J: Respiratory effects of two-hour exposure with intermittent exercise to ozone, sulfur dioxide and nitrogen dioxide alone and in combination in normal subjects. Am Ind Hyg Assoc J 44:14-20, 1983.

91. McDonnell WF, Kehrl HR, Abdul-Salaam S, et al: Respiratory response of humans exposed to low levels of ozone for 6.6 hours. Arch Environ Health 46:145-150, 1991.

92. Frampton MW, Morrow PE, Torres A, et al: Effects of ozone on normal and potentially sensitive human subjects. Part II: Airway inflammation and responsiveness to ozone in nonsmokers and smokers. Res Rep Health Eff Inst 39-72, discussion 81-99, 1997.

93. Kagawa J: Exposure-effect relationship of selected pulmonary function measurements in subjects exposed to ozone. Int Arch Occup Environ Health 53:345-358, 1984.

94. Kerr HD, Kulle TJ, McIlhany ML, Swidersky P: Effects of ozone on pulmonary function in normal subjects. An environmental-chamber study. Am Rev Respir Dis 111:763-773, 1975.

95. Hazucha MJ, Madden M, Pape G, et al: Effects of cyclo-oxygenase inhibition on ozone-induced respiratory inflammation and lung function changes. Eur J Appl Physiol Occup Physiol 73:17-27, 1996.

96. Horvath SM, Gliner JA, Folinsbee LJ: Adaptation to ozone: Duration of effect. Am Rev Respir Dis 123:496-499, 1981.

97. Kulle TJ, Milman JH, Sauder LR, et al: Pulmonary function adaptation to ozone in subjects with chronic bronchitis. Environ Res 34:55-63, 1984.

98. Evans MJ, Stephens RJ, Freeman G: Effects of nitrogen dioxide on cell renewal in the rat lung. Arch Intern Med 128:57-60, 1971.

99. Stephens RJ, Freeman G, Evans MJ: Ultrastructural changes in connective tissue in lungs of rats exposed to NO_2. Arch Intern Med 127:873-883, 1971.

100. Ranga V, Kleinerman J: Lung injury and repair in the blotchy mouse. Effects of nitrogen dioxide inhalation. Am Rev Respir Dis 123:90-97, 1981.

101. Folinsbee LJ, Horvath SM, Bedi JF, Delehunt JC: Effect of 0.62 ppm NO_2 on cardiopulmonary function in young male nonsmokers. Environ Res 15:199-205, 1978.

102. Ramirez J, Dowell AR: Silo-filler's disease: Nitrogen dioxide–induced lung injury. Long-term follow-up and review of the literature. Ann Intern Med 74:569-576, 1971.

103. Douglas WW, Hepper NG, Colby TV: Silo-filler's disease. Mayo Clin Proc 64:291-304, 1989.

104. Cornelius EA, Betlach EH: Silo-filler's disease. Radiology 74:232-238, 1960.

105. Janigan DT, Kilp T, Michael R, McCleave JJ: Bronchiolitis obliterans in a man who used his wood-burning stove to burn synthetic construction materials. CMAJ 156:1171-1173, 1997.

106. Fleming GM, Chester EH, Montenegro HD: Dysfunction of small airways following pulmonary injury due to nitrogen dioxide. Chest 75:720-721, 1979.
107. Larson TV, Frank R, Covert DS, et al: Measurements of respiratory ammonia and the chemical neutralization of inhaled sulfuric acid aerosol in anesthetized dogs. Am Rev Respir Dis 125:502-506, 1982.
108. Kipen HM, Lerman Y: Respiratory abnormalities among photographic developers: A report of three cases. Am J Ind Med 9:341-347, 1986.
109. Woodford DM, Couto RE, Gaensler EA: Obstructive lung disease from acute sulfur dioxide exposure. Respiration 38:238, 1979.
110. Osbern LN, Crapo RO: Dung lung: A report of toxic exposure to liquid manure. Ann Intern Med 95:312-314, 1981.
111. Burnett WW, King EG, Grace M, Hall WF: Hydrogen sulfide poisoning: Review of 5 years' experience. Can Med Assoc J 117:1277-1280, 1977.
112. Glass RI, Ford R, Allegra DT, Markel HL: Deaths from asphyxia among fisherman. JAMA 244:2193-2194, 1980.
113. Snyder JW, Safir EF, Summerville GP, Middleberg RA: Occupational fatality and persistent neurological sequelae after mass exposure to hydrogen sulfide. Am J Emerg Med 13:199-203, 1995.
114. Arwood R, Hammond J, Ward GG: Ammonia inhalation. J Trauma 25:444-447, 1985.
115. Flury KE, Dines DE, Rodarte JR, Rodgers R: Airway obstruction due to inhalation of ammonia. Mayo Clin Proc 58:389-393, 1983.
116. Kass I, Zamel N, Dobry CA, Holzer M: Bronchiectasis following ammonia burns of the respiratory tract. A review of two cases. Chest 62:282-285, 1972.
117. Das R, Blanc PD: Chlorine gas exposure and the lung: A review. Toxicol Ind Health 9:439-455, 1993.
118. Shroff CP, Khade MV, Srinivasan M: Respiratory cytopathology in chlorine gas toxicity: A study in 28 subjects. Diagn Cytopathol 4:28-32, 1988.
119. Bherer L, Cushman R, Courteau JP, et al: Survey of construction workers repeatedly exposed to chlorine over a three to six month period in a pulpmill: II. Follow up of affected workers by questionnaire, spirometry, and assessment of bronchial responsiveness 18 to 24 months after exposure ended. Occup Environ Med 51:225-228, 1994.
120. Martinez TT, Long C: Explosion risk from swimming pool chlorinators and review of chlorine toxicity. J Toxicol Clin Toxicol 33:349-354, 1995.
121. Chlorine gas toxicity from mixture of bleach with other cleaning products—California. MMWR Morb Mortal Wkly Rep 40(36):619-621, 627-629, 1991.
122. Demnati R, Fraser R, Ghezzo H, et al: Time-course of functional and pathological changes after a single high acute inhalation of chlorine in rats. Eur Respir J 11:922-928, 1998.
123. Courteau JP, Cushman R, Bouchard F, et al: Survey of construction workers repeatedly exposed to chlorine over a three to six month period in a pulpmill: I. Exposure and symptomatology. Occup Environ Med 51:219-224, 1994.
124. Hasan FM, Gehshan A, Fuleihan FJ: Resolution of pulmonary dysfunction following acute chlorine exposure. Arch Environ Health 38:76-80, 1983.
125. Lim SC, Yang JY, Jang AS, et al: Acute lung injury after phosgene inhalation. Korean J Intern Med 11:87-92, 1996.
126. Wyatt JP, Allister CA: Occupational phosgene poisoning: A case report and review. J Accid Emerg Med 12:212-213, 1995.
127. Sjogren B, Plato N, Alexandersson R, et al: Pulmonary reactions caused by welding-induced decomposed trichloroethylene. Chest 99:237-238, 1991.
128. Bernstein RS, Stayner LT, Elliott LJ, et al: Inhalation exposure to formaldehyde: An overview of its toxicology, epidemiology, monitoring, and control. Am Ind Hyg Assoc J 45:778-785, 1984.
129. Alexandersson R, Hedenstierna G, Kolmodin-Hedman B: Exposure to formaldehyde: Effects on pulmonary function. Arch Environ Health 37:279-284, 1982.
130. Levine RJ, DalCorso RD, Blunden PB, Battigelli MC: The effects of occupational exposure on the respiratory health of West Virginia morticians. J Occup Med 26:91-98, 1984.
131. Khamgaonkar MB, Fulare MB: Pulmonary effects of formaldehyde exposure—an environmental-epidemiological study. Indian J Chest Dis Allied Sci 33:9-13, 1991.
132. Norman GR, Pengelly LD, Kerigan AT, Goldsmith CH: Respiratory function of children in homes insulated with urea formaldehyde foam insulation. CMAJ 134:1135-1138, 1986.
133. Dally KA, Hanrahan LP, Woodbury MA, Kanarek MS: Formaldehyde exposure in nonoccupational environments. Arch Environ Health 36:277-284, 1981.
134. Nunn AJ, Craigen AA, Darbyshire JH, et al: Six year follow up of lung function in men occupationally exposed to formaldehyde. Br J Ind Med 47:747-752, 1990.
135. Nemery B: Metal toxicity and the respiratory tract. Eur Respir J 3:202-219, 1990.
136. Gordon T, Fine JM: Metal fume fever. Occup Med 8:504-517, 1993.

137. Lien DC, Todoruk DN, Rajani HR, et al: Accidental inhalation of mercury vapour: Respiratory and toxicologic consequences. Can Med Assoc J 129:591-595, 1983.
138. Natelson EA, Blumenthal BJ, Fred HL: Acute mercury vapor poisoning in the home. Chest 59:677-678, 1971.
139. Fuortes L, Leo A, Ellerbeck PG, Friell LA: Acute respiratory fatality associated with exposure to sheet metal and cadmium fumes. J Toxicol Clin Toxicol 29:279-283, 1991.
140. Hirst RN Jr, Perry HM Jr, Cruz MG, Pierce JA: Elevated cadmium concentration in emphysematous lungs. Am Rev Respir Dis 108:30-39, 1973.
141. Snider GL, Hayes JA, Korthy AL, Lewis GP: Centrilobular emphysema experimentally induced by cadmium chloride aerosol. Am Rev Respir Dis 108:40-48, 1973.
142. Zeiss CR, Wolkonsky P, Chacon R, et al: Syndromes in workers exposed to trimellitic anhydride. A longitudinal clinical and immunologic study. Ann Intern Med 98:8-12, 1983.
143. Rice DL, Jenkins DE, Gray JM: Chemical pneumonitis secondary to inhalation of epoxy pipe coating. Arch Environ Health 32:173-178, 1977.
144. Wegman DH, Peters JM: Polymer fume fever and cigarette smoking. Ann Intern Med 81:55-57, 1974.
145. Evans EA: Pulmonary edema after inhalation of fumes from polytetrafluoroethylene (PTFE). J Occup Med 15:599-601, 1973.
146. Demling RH: Smoke inhalation injury. New Horiz 1:422-434, 1993.
147. Done A: The toxic emergency: Where there's smoke, there may be more than fire. Emerg Med 13:111, 1981.
148. Clark CJ, Campbell D, Reid WH: Blood carboxyhaemoglobin and cyanide levels in fire survivors. Lancet 1:1332-1335, 1981.
149. Dyer RF, Esch VH: Polyvinyl chloride toxicity in fires. Hydrogen chloride toxicity in fire fighters. JAMA 235:393-397, 1976.
150. Brinkmann B, Puschel K: Heat injuries to the respiratory system. Virchows Arch A Pathol Anat Histol 379:299-311, 1978.
151. Hasleton PS, McWilliam L, Haboubi NY: The lung parenchyma in burns. Histopathology 7:333-347, 1983.
152. Williams DO, Vanecko RM, Glassroth J: Endobronchial polyposis following smoke inhalation. Chest 84:774-776, 1983.
153. Whitener DR, Whitener LM, Robertson KJ, et al: Pulmonary function measurements in patients with thermal injury and smoke inhalation. Am Rev Respir Dis 122:731-739, 1980.
154. Teixidor HS, Novick G, Rubin E: Pulmonary complications in burn patients. J Can Assoc Radiol 34:264-270, 1983.
155. Teixidor HS, Rubin E, Novick GS, Alonso DR: Smoke inhalation: Radiologic manifestations. Radiology 149:383-387, 1983.
156. Pietak SP, Delahaye DJ: Airway obstruction following smoke inhalation. Can Med Assoc J 115:329-331, 1976.
157. Shirani KZ, Pruitt BA Jr, Mason AD Jr: The influence of inhalation injury and pneumonia on burn mortality. Ann Surg 205:82-87, 1987.
158. Putman CE, Loke J, Matthay RA, Ravin CE: Radiographic manifestations of acute smoke inhalation. AJR Am J Roentgenol 129:865-870, 1977.
159. Lee MJ, O'Connell DJ: The plain chest radiograph after acute smoke inhalation. Clin Radiol 39:33-37, 1988.
160. Darling GE, Keresteci MA, Ibanez D, et al: Pulmonary complications in inhalation injuries with associated cutaneous burn. J Trauma 40:83-89, 1996.
161. Wittram C, Kenny JB: The admission chest radiograph after acute inhalation injury and burns. Br J Radiol 67:751-754, 1994.
162. Lin WY, Kao CH, Wang SJ: Detection of acute inhalation injury in fire victims by means of technetium-99m DTPA radioaerosol inhalation lung scintigraphy. Eur J Nucl Med 24:125-129, 1997.
163. Gaissert HA, Lofgren RH, Grillo HC: Upper airway compromise after inhalation injury. Complex strictures of the larynx and trachea and their management. Ann Surg 218:672-678, 1993.
164. Tasaka S, Kanazawa M, Mori M, et al: Long-term course of bronchiectasis and bronchiolitis obliterans as late complication of smoke inhalation. Respiration 62:40-42, 1995.
165. Slutzker AD, Kinn R, Said SI: Bronchiectasis and progressive respiratory failure following smoke inhalation. Chest 95:1349-1350, 1989.
166. Unger KM, Snow RM, Mestas JM, Miller WC: Smoke inhalation in firemen. Thorax 35:838-842, 1980.
167. Young I, Jackson J, West S: Chronic respiratory disease and respiratory function in a group of fire fighters. Med J Aust 1:654-658, 1980.
168. Sparrow D, Bosse R, Rosner B, Weiss ST: The effect of occupational exposure on pulmonary function: A longitudinal evaluation of fire fighters and nonfire fighters. Am Rev Respir Dis 125:319-322, 1982.
169. Musk AW, Monson RR, Peters JM, Peters RK: Mortality among Boston firefighters, 1915-1975. Br J Ind Med 35:104-108, 1978.

C H A P T E R   E I G H T E E N

PULMONARY DISEASE CAUSED BY DRUGS, POISONS, AND IRRADIATION

DRUGS

Knowledge of adverse drug reactions is important for the pulmonary physician for several reasons. First, they are a significant cause of morbidity and mortality; it has been estimated that as many as 5% of all hospitalizations and about 0.3% of all deaths that occur in the hospital are drug related.[1] Second, drug reactions are surprisingly common; for example, it has been estimated that lung toxicity develops in about 5% of patients receiving amiodarone and that an irritating cough develops in as many as 15% of patients taking angiotensin-converting enzyme (ACE) inhibitors. Finally, early recognition of a potential reaction is important since the ensuing disease can be progressive and fatal, and cessation of drug use may be followed by prompt reversibility of toxicity.[2]

More than 350 agents have been recognized to cause an adverse pulmonary reaction of one kind or another (Table 18–1). Such reactions can imitate virtually any pulmonary syndrome; thus, the *possibility* that an adverse drug response may explain a patient's illness must always be considered and thorough questioning of drug ingestion undertaken. Pulmonary drug reactions can be considered according to the radiologic and clinical patterns of disease that they produce, the main forms being interstitial pneumonia (which may be acute, subacute, or chronic), edema, hemorrhage, airway disease (typically either bronchiolitis or bronchoconstriction), and vascular disease (usually hypertension). Drug-induced

disease involving the pleura (see page 824) and the neuromuscular control of breathing (see page 914) are considered elsewhere in the text, as are specific agents associated with systemic lupus erythematosus (see page 484) and eosinophilia (see page 514).

In most cases, the diagnosis of pulmonary drug-induced disease is suspected because of the insidious onset of dyspnea and cough in a patient receiving a drug (or drugs) recognized as potentially damaging to the lungs. Fever is common, and diffuse crackles are often audible. Drugs that initiate capillary leakage or bronchospasm tend to be associated with a more abrupt clinical manifestation, and physical examination usually reveals profuse crackles or wheezes, respectively. Some patients do not have symptoms, the presence of a reaction being suggested by the appearance of diffuse abnormalities on the chest radiograph or by a significant reduction in diffusing capacity. Pulmonary dysfunction may be barely detectable or may be severe and require mechanical ventilation to maintain life; though generally restrictive in type with a low DLCO, the pattern may be mixed or even predominantly obstructive.

The histologic changes of drug-induced pulmonary disease are usually nonspecific; however, when an abnormality is found in association with a drug known to cause that particular reaction, the diagnosis of toxicity is clearly supported. In some cases, the simultaneous use of multiple drugs can make it difficult to be certain of the specific agent responsible for the pulmonary disease.

TABLE 18–1. Selected Causes of Drug-Induced Lung Disease

Drug	Interstitial Lung Disease	Edema	Hemorrhage	Airways	Pleural	Vascular	Mediastinal Disease	Neuromuscular Disease	Comments
Cytotoxic Antibiotics									
Bleomycin	x	x		x	x		x		See text
Mitomycin	x	x	x			x			See text
Alkylating Agents									
Busulfan	x			x		x			See text
Chlorambucil	x								See text
Cyclophosfamide	x	x		x	x				See text
Melphalan	x			x					See text
Nitrosoureas	x	x			x	x			See text
Vinca alkaloids	x			x					See text
Antimetabolites									
Azathioprine	x		x	x					UAO, hemorrhage, subacute pneumonitis
Cytosine arabinoside		x	x						
Fludarabine	x	x	x						See text
Gemcitabine	x	x		x					
L-Asparaginase						x			Thromboembolic disease
Methotrexate	x	x		x	x				See text
Miscellaneous									
Cyclosporine	x	x	x						
Etoposide	x			x					
Hydroxyurea	x								
Irinotecan	x	x							
Procarbazine	x				x				See text
Taxels	x				x				Acute or subacute
Hormonal Agents									
Estrogens						x			Thromboembolic disease
Nitulamide	x			x					See text
Raloxifene						x			
Tamoxifen						x			
Biologic Response Modifiers									
GM-CSF	x	x				x			See text
Interferon	x			x	x				See text
Interleukin-2	x	x		x	x				See text
TNF		x	x						
Antimicrobial Agents									
Aminoglycosides								x	Respiratory muscle weakness
Amphotericin B		x		x					Acute edema, bronchospasm
Ampicillin	x	x							Subacute, eosinophilia with infiltrates
Cephalosporins Dapsone	x								Eosinophilia with infiltrates
Erythromycin	x	x		x		x			Eosinophilia with infiltrates
Ethambutol	x								Eosinophilia with infiltrates
Isoniazid (INH)	x				x				Lupus reaction, eosinophilia with infiltrates
Maloprim									
Nitrofurantoin	x	x	x	x	x	x			See text
Para-aminosalicylic acid (PAS)	x	x							Eosinophilia with infiltrates

Continued

TABLE 18–1. Selected Causes of Drug-Induced Lung Disease—cont'd

Drug	Interstitial Lung Disease	Edema	Hemorrhage	Airways	Pleural	Vascular	Mediastinal Disease	Neuromuscular Disease	Comments
Antimicrobial Agents—Cont'd									
Penicillin	x			x			x		Eosinophilia with infiltrates
Pyrimethamine									
Streptomycin	x								Eosinophilia with infiltrates
Sulfasalazine	x	x			x	x			
Sulfonamides	x	x		x	x	x	x		
Tetracyclines	x	x		x	x		x		See text
Trimethoprim-sulfamethoxazole	x	x					x		Acute or subacute, eosinophilia with infiltrates, noncardiogenic edema
Antiarrhythmic Drugs									
Amiodarone	x	x	x	x	x				See text
Flecainide	x								
Lidocaine		x							
Quinidine	x		x			x			
Procainamide	x				x			x	Lupus reaction
Sotolol				x					COP
Tocainide	x								
Anticonvulsant Drugs									
Carbamazepine	x	x	x	x	x		x		See text
Diphenylhydantoin	x		x	x	x	x			
Salicylates									
Aspirin	x	x		x		x	x		See text
Mesalamine	x			x	x				
NSAIDs									Bronchospasm, eosinophilia with infiltrates
Diclofenac	x			x					
Diflunisal	x			x					
Tolfenamic acid	x			x					
Antirheumatic Drugs									
Gold salts	x			x					See text
Penicillamine	x		x	x	x				See text
Sympathomimetic Drugs									
Aminorex						x			
(Dex)fenfluramine	x				x	x			Pulmonary hypertension
Methylphenidate	x								Eosinophilia with infiltrates
Tocolytics		x							
Illicit Drugs, Narcotics, and Sedative Drugs									
Bromocarbamide									
Chlordiazepoxide									
Cocaine		x	x	x					See text
Fentanyl				x					Explosive cough
Heroin and other narcotics	x	x		x					See text
Methadone									
Propofol		x		x		x			
Thiopental				x					
Antidepressant and Antipsychotic Drugs									
Amitryptyline	x			x					
Clorimipramine				x					COP

TABLE 18–1. Selected Causes of Drug-Induced Lung Disease—cont'd

Drug	Interstitial Lung Disease	Edema	Hemorrhage	Airways	Pleural	Vascular	Mediastinal Disease	Neuromuscular Disease	Comments
Clozapine	x				x	x			Pulmonary embolism, eosinophilia with infiltrates
Desipramine	x			x					Eosinophilia with infiltrates, bronchospasm
Fluoxetine	x								
Imipramine	x								Eosinophilia with infiltrates
Trimipramine									
Contrast Media									
Lymphangiography		x							See text
Water-soluble contrast media	x	x	x	x					See text
ACE inhibitors	x			x	x				See text
Miscellaneous Drugs									
Abciximab			x						
β-Adrenergic blockers	x			x	x	x			See text
Antilymphocyte globulin	x	x							
Hydralazine	x		x	x					Subacute, COP, lupus reaction
Hydrochlorothiazide	x	x							
Inhaled beclomethasone	x								Eosinophilia with infiltrates
Bromocriptine	x				x				
Clomiphene		x	x		x	x			
Chloroquin	x								Eosinophilia with infiltrates
Colchicine		x							
Curare				x					
Deferoxamine		x				x			
Ergotamine	x			x	x				Subacute pneumonitis, fibrosis; COP
Gefitinib		x			x				See text
Imatinib	x								
IV Immunoglobulins		x		x					Edema, bronchospasm
Injected silicone									
Isotretinoin	x				x	x			Eosinophilia with infiltrates, eosinophilia with effusion
Levodopa					x		x	x	Lupus reaction, lymphadenopathy, respiratory dyskinesia
Methyldopa					x		x		Lupus reaction
Methysergide	x			x		x			Effusion, sclerosing mediastinitis
Naloxone		x							
Propylthiouracil	x	x	x		x	x			
Protamine		x		x					
Retinoic acid	x	x	x		x	x			See text
Sirolimus	x	x							
Statins (HMG-CoA reductase inhibitors)	x			x	x				COP, lupus reaction, eosinophilia with infiltrates
Thiazolidinediones		x							
Valsartan	x			x					Drug-induced antisynthetase syndrome
Zafirlukast						x			Churg-Strauss vasculitis
Zanamivir			x						Bronchospasm

ACE, angiotensin-converting enzyme; COP, cryptogenic organizing pneumonia; GM-CSF, granulocyte-macrophage colony-stimulating factor; HMG-CoA, 3-hydroxy-3-methylglutaryl coenzyme A; NSAIDs, nonsteroidal anti-inflammatory drugs; TNF, tumor necrosis factor; UAO, upper airway obstruction.

Chemotherapeutic and Immunosuppressive Drugs

Bleomycin

Bleomycin is an antibiotic that has significant activity against a variety of cancers, including squamous cell carcinoma of the head and neck, cervix, and esophagus, as well as germ cell tumors and Hodgkin's and non-Hodgkin's lymphomas.[3] The reported incidence of lung toxicity varies from 2% to more than 40%.[3,4] This wide spectrum is related partly to variations in the prevalence of associated risk factors in the populations studied (see later) and partly to the sensitivity of the tests used for diagnosis. Most disease is manifested as subacute to chronic interstitial pneumonia; a minority of patients have an acute illness that appears to have an immunologic pathogenesis and consists of reversible eosinophilic pneumonia.[5] Rarely, the drug causes pulmonary veno-occlusive disease or cryptogenic organizing pneumonia (COP)[6]; the latter can simulate metastatic disease radiologically.

The development of bleomycin-induced pulmonary disease is dose related; however, disease has been reported after the administration of as little as 49 U.[7] Risk is increased in older people,[8] in smokers,[9] and in patients receiving combined cytotoxic drug therapy (particularly with cyclophosphamide),[10] a high concentration of inspired oxygen, or radiation therapy[11]; impaired renal function may also be important.[12]

Bleomycin is concentrated predominantly in lung and skin, where it can cleave DNA by generating oxygen radicals.[6] Theoretically, an imbalance between such oxidants and locally produced antioxidants could lead to epithelial damage and interstitial fibrosis.[13] In support of this hypothesis is the observation that augmentation of bleomycin toxicity is associated with oxygen administration and radiation therapy,[14] both of which are also thought to cause toxicity by production of oxygen radicals. By contrast, both hypoxia and the administration of antioxidants protect against bleomycin toxicity in animal models.[15,16] A complex interaction among macrophages, lymphocytes, fibroblasts, and endothelial and epithelial cells appears to be responsible for both the initiation and maintenance of chronic inflammation and the ensuing fibrosis.[17,18] In animal models, alveolar macrophages are affected early in the course of disease and release a number of chemotactic, proinflammatory, and profibrotic cytokines[19,20] that lead to recruitment and activation of other inflammatory cells and endothelial and epithelial damage. The characteristic pathologic finding in human patients is diffuse alveolar damage.

Radiographic abnormalities usually consist of bibasilar reticular, reticulonodular, or fine nodular opacities, often showing a striking peripheral distribution.[21] With more severe disease, the abnormalities may extend into the middle and upper lung zones or progress to patchy or massive air space consolidation (Fig. 18–1).[22] The abnormalities appear 6 weeks to 3 months after the start of therapy and may be seen before, synchronous with, or after the appearance of clinical symptoms.[23] Occasionally, multiple nodules, sometimes cavitary, are present and simulate metastases.[24]

Findings on HRCT usually consist of bilateral irregular lines of attenuation, ground-glass attenuation, or focal areas of consolidation in a predominantly basal subpleural distribution.[25] Follow-up scans may show complete resolution of the parenchymal abnormalities within 9 months after cessation of therapy.[26]

Symptoms include fever, cough, and dyspnea on exertion[3]; substernal and pleuritic chest pain have also been reported, sometimes of sufficient severity to mimic myocardial infarction or pulmonary thromboembolism.[27] Such symptoms usually develop 4 to 10 weeks after treatment has finished, although toxicity can occur while the drug is being given or shortly after completion of therapy.[28] Crackles may be detected, particularly at the lung bases, but may be absent even in the presence of radiologically evident disease[29]; rhonchi and wheezes are evident occasionally. The tendency for deposition of the drug in the skin can cause hyperpigmentation and swelling of the fingers, palms, and soles of the feet.

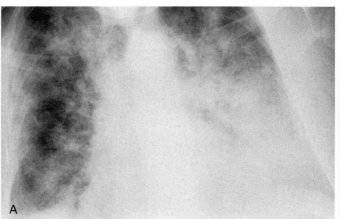
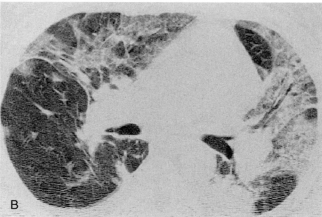

FIGURE 18–1

Bleomycin-induced pulmonary disease. An anteroposterior chest radiograph (**A**) in a 36-year-old man shows extensive bilateral air space consolidation with relative sparing of the right lower lobe. An HRCT scan (**B**) shows bilateral areas of ground-glass attenuation, focal areas of consolidation, and a few linear areas of attenuation. Histologic assessment of a lung biopsy specimen showed diffuse alveolar damage, focal areas of organizing pneumonia, and mild veno-occlusive disease consistent with a drug reaction. *(From Müller NL, Fraser RS, Colman NC, Paré PD: Radiologic Diagnosis of Diseases of the Chest. Philadelphia, WB Saunders, 2001.)*

Assessment of pulmonary function may be helpful. VC and diffusing capacity have been used to monitor patients receiving the drug, and measurement of these pulmonary parameters has been reported by some investigators to detect lung involvement at an early stage when the chest radiograph is still normal. A decrease in TLC has also been found to predict the development of clinically evident toxicity.[30]

The overall mortality rate of bleomycin pulmonary toxicity is about 1% to 2%.[28] Death usually follows a prolonged period of increasing dyspnea.

Mitomycin

Mitomycin is an alkylating antibiotic that is used mainly for the treatment of patients who have gastrointestinal, breast, and cervical malignancies, as well as non–small cell carcinoma of the lung.[31] Clinically evident toxicity has been identified in about 3% to 6% of patients.[32] Although such disease has been described with mitomycin alone,[33] most patients have been treated with other agents, usually the vinca alkaloids. Toxicity is more likely to occur at cumulative doses greater than 20 mg/m^2,[34] although it has been reported after a single course of therapy.[35]

The mechanism by which mitomycin induces pulmonary damage is unclear; however, because it possesses alkylating properties, its mode of action may be similar to that of cyclophosphamide and other alkylating agents. The typical pathologic pattern in patients who die is diffuse alveolar damage.[32]

Radiologic manifestations consist of bilateral reticular opacities that can be diffuse but tend to have a lower lung zone predominance.[25,31] Occasionally, the radiographic and HRCT findings are those of acute respiratory distress syndrome (ARDS), with extensive bilateral areas of consolidation involving mainly the posterior aspects of the lungs. Pleural effusion has been described in many patients and appears to be a more common feature of mitomycin toxicity than are other cytotoxic drug reactions.

Most patients have a clinical picture consistent with interstitial pneumonitis and fibrosis identical to that caused by other cytotoxic agents. Two additional rare but important effects have been described: (1) acute, severe asthma in association with the administration of a vinca alkaloid[36] and (2) noncardiogenic pulmonary edema in the context of hemolytic-uremic syndrome. The latter complication may occur as long as 6 to 12 months after the initiation of therapy and may be precipitated by concomitant blood transfusion or therapy with 5-fluorouracil[37]; the mortality rate exceeds 90%. Diffuse alveolar hemorrhage has also been described in patients who have had mitomycin-induced hemolytic-uremic syndrome.[38]

Busulfan

Busulfan is used in the treatment of myeloproliferative disorders, particularly chronic myelogenous leukemia, and in preparation for autologous or allogeneic bone marrow transplantation in patients who have either hematologic or non-hematologic malignancies.[39] Although clinically recognized pulmonary toxicity occurs in only about 5% of patients,[37] some pathologic studies have found evidence of drug-induced damage in almost 50% of cases.[40] The mechanism of damage

is unknown; however, the primary target appears to be epithelial cells.[4]

Clinically apparent pulmonary toxicity tends to occur only with long-term use, from 8 months to 10 years in several studies (average, 3 to 4 years).[41] Previous use of other cytotoxic drugs or radiation therapy increases the risk.[42] Although toxicity does not appear to be directly dose dependent, pulmonary disease has not developed in any patient receiving a total dose of less than 500 mg in the absence of other potentially toxic influences such as radiation therapy or administration of other chemotherapeutic agents.[41] An acute or subacute pneumonitis (idiopathic pneumonia syndrome) has also been attributed to the use of high-dose, short-course busulfan given as part of a conditioning regimen before autologous bone marrow transplantation.[43]

The pathologic finding most characteristic of busulfan-induced pulmonary disease is the presence of large, cytologically atypical type II pneumocytes (Fig. 18–2).[44] Although similar atypical pneumocytes can be found in pulmonary disease induced by other drugs, the extent and severity of atypia are particularly marked with busulfan. Nonspecific interstitial pneumonitis is also typically present.

The chest radiograph usually shows a bilateral reticular or reticulonodular pattern, which may be diffuse or have a lower lung zone predominance (Fig. 18–3).[4] Less common radiographic and HRCT findings include patchy or widespread air space consolidation. Pleural effusion has been reported occasionally.[45]

The onset of disease is usually insidious. The principal complaints are dry cough, fever, weakness, weight loss, and dyspnea. By removing an inhibitor of tyrosinase, busulfan accelerates the formation of melanin from tyrosine and thus results in hyperpigmentation of the skin; as a consequence, some patients have an appearance resembling that of Addison's disease.[46] Once disease has become evident, lung volumes and diffusing capacity are usually reduced.[47] The mean survival time after the diagnosis of pulmonary fibrosis is 5 months, and the mortality rate is estimated to be greater than 80%.[48] The prognosis may be improved by early detection of disease and cessation of drug therapy.[35]

Cyclophosphamide

The alkylating drug cyclophosphamide is used widely in the treatment of malignancy and autoimmune connective tissue disease. Because it is often combined with other chemotherapeutic agents, it may not be apparent which drug is responsible for pulmonary disease or whether the toxicity is the result of a synergistic effect.[49] Nevertheless, well-documented cases of pulmonary fibrosis have occurred after the use of cyclophosphamide as a single agent.[50] The incidence of pulmonary toxicity is probably less than 1%. The development of interstitial fibrosis has been reported after the administration of as little as 150 mg of the drug,[41] although the risk of serious toxicity appears to be greater with higher doses.[4] Pathologic findings include diffuse alveolar damage and nonspecific interstitial pneumonia.

The chest radiograph usually shows a bilateral basilar reticular pattern, occasionally associated with focal areas of consolidation (Fig. 18–4).[4] In a review of five patients, pleural thickening accompanied the interstitial changes in all.[50]

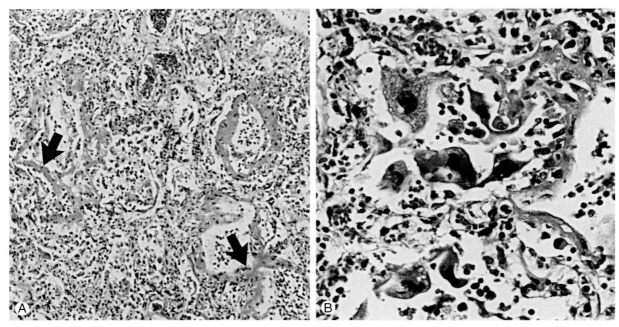

FIGURE 18–2

Busulfan toxicity. A section of lung parenchyma (**A**) obtained at autopsy shows a moderate degree of interstitial thickening by lymphocytes, extensive air space filling by macrophages and other mononuclear inflammatory cells, and several hyaline membranes (*arrows*). A magnified view (**B**) shows type II pneumocytes to be greatly increased in size and to contain hyperchromatic, cytologically atypical nuclei. The patient had been taking busulfan for myelogenous leukemia. *(From Fraser RS, Müller NL, Colman NC, Paré PD: Fraser and Paré's Diagnosis of Diseases of the Chest, 4th ed. Philadelphia, WB Saunders, 1999.)*

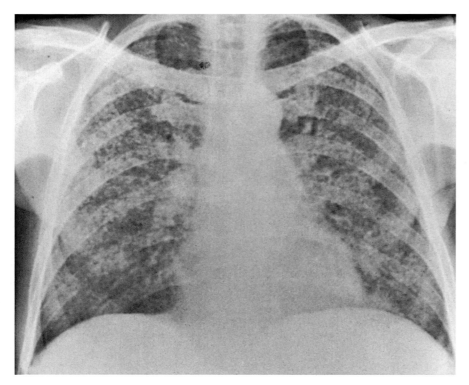

FIGURE 18–3

Busulfan toxicity. A posteroanterior chest radiograph shows a widespread, coarse reticulonodular pattern throughout both lungs without anatomic predominance. The patient was a 61-year-old woman being treated for myelogenous leukemia. *(From Müller NL, Fraser RS, Colman NC, Paré PD: Radiologic Diagnosis of Diseases of the Chest. Philadelphia, WB Saunders, 2001.)*

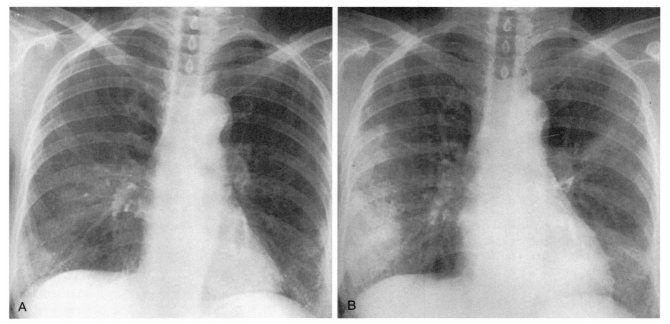

FIGURE 18–4

Cyclophosphamide toxicity. A posteroanterior radiograph (**A**) shows ill-defined opacities in the midportion of the right lung and at both lung bases. The appearance suggests a combination of interstitial and air space abnormalities. Seven months later (**B**), the opacities had become largely air space in character and, on the right side at least, showed considerable peripheral dominance. The patient was a middle-aged woman being treated with cyclophosphamide for lymphoma. *(From Müller NL, Fraser RS, Colman NC, Paré PD: Radiologic Diagnosis of Diseases of the Chest. Philadelphia, WB Saunders, 2001.)*

The onset of pulmonary disease is acute or subacute more often than chronic. The time interval between initiation of therapy and the development of symptoms varies markedly: in some patients, symptoms develop within months,[51] whereas in others, they become apparent after years.[52] Cough and dyspnea are the major complaints; fever occurs in more than 50% of patients. Pulmonary function tests show a restrictive ventilatory defect and reduced diffusing capacity. About 60% of patients recover[53]; cessation of cyclophosphamide therapy can be followed by resolution of the pulmonary disease, especially when it is of early onset.[50]

Nitrosoureas

Nitrosoureas are used chiefly for the treatment of intracranial neoplasms, melanoma, breast and gastrointestinal carcinoma, and lymphoma.[54,55] Their pharmacologic action is similar to that of other alkylating agents and consists of interference with DNA synthesis and impedance of DNA repair.[56] The propensity of the drug to reduce glutathione synthesis, an important antioxidant defense, may lead to oxidant-induced lung injury,[57] particularly when it is combined with other agents such as cyclophosphamide.[58]

Most cases of pulmonary disease have been caused by BCNU (1,3-bis(2-chloroethyl)-1-nitrosourea). Although many of these cases have occurred in patients receiving this drug alone, some have developed in combination with other cytotoxic agents, particularly cyclophosphamide and cisplatin.[59] The rate of drug administration may be important in determining whether toxicity occurs: in a study involving a cyclophosphamide, cisplatin, and BCNU regimen, more rapid

infusion of the BCNU was associated with a syndrome of acute lung injury in 12 of 14 (86%) patients.[60] The incidence of pulmonary toxicity after BCNU therapy as a single agent ranges from 1% to 20% in different series[61]; by contrast, the incidence is as high as 40% to 60% in patients treated with high-dose combination chemotherapy protocols before autologous bone marrow transplantation.[62] An increased risk associated with a total dose of 1 g or more has been well documented.[63] Pathologic findings are similar to those of other forms of cytotoxic pulmonary damage and include nonspecific interstitial pneumonia with alveolar epithelial cell atypia and diffuse alveolar damage.

The chest radiograph becomes abnormal late in the course of pulmonary toxicity, typically after the onset of symptoms.[2] The most frequent manifestation is a bibasilar reticular pattern.[2] Less common findings include focal or patchy bilateral areas of consolidation, upper lobe reticular opacities, and pneumothorax.[64] Findings on HRCT consist of bilateral areas of ground-glass attenuation involving the lower lung zones.[25] Although the early radiographic and CT abnormalities tend to involve mainly the lower lung zones, in a study of six patients who had long-term follow-up (mean, 14 years), upper lobe fibrosis was the predominant finding.[65]

Clinical evidence of pulmonary damage usually appears from 1 month to 1 year after the institution of therapy[66]; however, fibrosis has been first identified as long as 17 years after childhood therapy for brain tumors.[65] Symptoms include dry cough, fatigue, and dyspnea. $DLCO$, PaO_2, and VC are reduced. The course of the disease is usually insidious over a period of months, although it can be rapidly progressive and fatal.[4] Interstitial pneumonia that develops after multidrug therapy before stem cell transplantation is seen a mean of 90 days following drug administration; the response to corticosteroids is good, and most patients survive the complication.[67]

Vinca Alkaloids

The vinca alkaloids vinblastine, vinorelbine, and vindesine are almost invariably used with other drugs, particularly mitomycin, a combination that has been reported to cause both interstitial pneumonia and diffuse alveolar damage.[68,69] Whether the toxicity is caused by the vinca alkaloid, the mitomycin, or the two combined is difficult to determine. However, in a series of 387 patients treated with this regimen, acute dyspnea developed in 25 while being administered the vinca alkaloid[70]; 22 of the 25 (88%) had new focal or diffuse interstitial infiltrates and impairment in gas exchange. Although substantial improvement occurred over a 24-hour period, 15 patients were left with chronic respiratory impairment. Vindesine and vinblastine also appear to be capable of inducing bronchospasm,[71] and vindesine may play a role in the development of progressive interstitial fibrosis when combined with radiation therapy.[72]

Antimetabolic Drugs

Methotrexate

Methotrexate is used in the treatment of malignancy and, in lower doses, in a variety of nonmalignant disorders. It usually causes reversible pulmonary disease, probably as a result of a hypersensitivity reaction (see later)[73]; however, chronic interstitial fibrosis develops in some patients.[74] The latter complication can be difficult to diagnose in patients in whom the condition being treated is itself associated with interstitial fibrosis (e.g., rheumatoid disease). There is evidence that the incidence of methotrexate-induced lung injury is substantial. For example, it has been estimated that the incidence of disease in patients receiving low-dose methotrexate for rheumatoid arthritis is about 2% to 5%[75]; in addition, transient symptoms developed in 20% of patients treated with methotrexate for trophoblastic tumors in one study.[76]

As indicated, there is evidence that a hypersensitivity reaction is the underlying pathogenetic mechanism in many cases.[77] However, the failure of some patients to experience recurrent pneumonitis after rechallenge with the drug argues against the likelihood that a hypersensitivity reaction is the sole mechanism.[1] Both the dose and duration of therapy, as well as the presence of underlying lung disease, increase the risk for toxicity.[78] In a case-control study of 29 patients who were receiving low-dose methotrexate for rheumatoid arthritis, significant risk factors for the development of pulmonary injury included previous use of disease-modifying antirheumatic drugs and hypoalbuminemia[79]; older age, diabetes, and rheumatoid pleuropulmonary disease before the institution of methotrexate were also predictive of the complication.

Interstitial pneumonitis and fibrosis, sometimes associated with granuloma formation resembling extrinsic allergic alveolitis, are the most frequent histologic abnormalities.[80] Diffuse alveolar damage has been seen occasionally, sometimes in patients who have received the drug intrathecally.[81]

Radiographic changes are fairly characteristic and should suggest the diagnosis in the proper clinical setting. Initially, there is a basal or diffuse reticular or ground-glass pattern, followed by rapid progression to patchy air space consolidation that in time reverts to an interstitial pattern and then complete resolution.[82] Multiple nodules and hilar lymph node enlargement may also be seen.[83] The most common HRCT findings consist of bilateral areas of ground-glass attenuation with or without associated intralobular linear opacities.[84] Less frequent findings include centrilobular nodular opacities or areas of consolidation.[85]

The duration of maintenance methotrexate therapy before symptoms and signs of toxicity become clinically apparent ranges from days to several years.[37] In most cases, the onset is acute to subacute and is characterized by fever, cough, dyspnea, and headache[86]; pleuritic pain is unusual.[76] Tachypnea, crackles, and cyanosis are common findings on physical examination.[87] Digital clubbing has also been described, and skin eruptions have been noted in about 15% of cases.[83] A moderate blood eosinophilia occurs in about 40% to 65% of cases. Pulmonary function tests show a restrictive pattern. A very low PaO_2 may be apparent.[88] Monitoring of lung function has not been found to permit early detection of lung injury before the onset of clinical symptoms.[89]

When considering the diagnosis, it should be remembered that low-dose methotrexate therapy predisposes to infection by a variety of opportunistic organisms.[90,91] Because no pathognomonic clinical, radiologic, or laboratory features allow such infections to be distinguished from methotrexate-induced pulmonary injury, a thorough search for potential organisms must be made when drug toxicity is suspected, in some cases including biopsy, BAL, or both.

The overall mortality rate is estimated to be 1% to 10%.[35] Most patients receiving low-dose maintenance therapy experience rapid clearing of symptoms and radiographic abnormalities after withdrawal of the medication.[88] Cases have been reported in which clearing has occurred despite continuation or reinstitution of therapy[83]; however, fatalities have also been reported with rechallenge.[92]

Cytosine Arabinoside

Cytosine arabinoside is an antimetabolite that is used for the treatment of acute leukemia. Pulmonary toxicity has been reported in 15% to 30% of patients who have received the drug intravenously in high dose.[93] Older age appears to be a risk factor.[94] Although diffuse alveolar damage is seen histologically in some cases, an appearance resembling cardiogenic pulmonary edema has been described more commonly.[95] It is possible that the latter reaction is mediated by cytokine release induced by infusion of the drug or by proteolytic enzymes released by tumor lysis.[2,96]

Radiographic manifestations consist of bilateral irregular linear opacities, air space consolidation, or more commonly, both interstitial and air space patterns.[97] Clinical findings are those of noncardiogenic pulmonary edema and fever developing 1 day to 5 weeks after therapy. The prognosis cited in published reports varies widely; for example, in a series of 13 patients, 9 died,[95] whereas in another study of 31 patients, fatality ensued in only 3.[97]

Gemcitabine

Gemcitabine is a cytidine analogue that has activity against several neoplasms, including non–small cell pulmonary carcinoma.[98] It is similar in structure and metabolism to cytosine arabinoside[99]; like the latter, it has been associated with the development of noncardiogenic pulmonary edema.[100]

Azathioprine

Azathioprine (Imuran) is the nitroimidazole derivative of 6-mercaptopurine; it interferes with purine base synthesis and therefore RNA and DNA synthesis.[101] It has been used to suppress rejection in patients who have received organ transplants and as an immunosuppressive agent in a variety of other disorders. In view of its widespread use and the relatively few reports of associated complications, it must be considered an uncommon cause of pulmonary toxicity. Nonetheless, azathioprine has been associated with interstitial pneumonitis and fibrosis,[102] diffuse alveolar damage,[103] and diffuse alveolar hemorrhage.[104] Although some patients die of respiratory insufficiency, others recover, possibly because of the relatively low drug dose, treatment with corticosteroids, or early recognition of toxicity.[102]

Fludarabine

Fludarabine is a nucleotide analogue used in the treatment of refractory chronic lymphocytic leukemia. Both interstitial pneumonia and diffuse alveolar damage have been associated with its use.[105] The clinical course is characterized by cough, dyspnea, and fever usually occurring within days of a treatment course. Exclusion of opportunistic infection is important because *Pneumocystis jiroveci* (*carinii*) and other pathogens are much more frequent causes of this clinical picture.[106]

Biologic Response Modifiers

Interleukin-2

Interleukin-2, with or without autologous lymphokine-activated killer cell infusion, has been used in the treatment of a variety of malignancies, including melanoma and renal cell carcinoma.[107] The toxicity associated with these agents is prominent and includes a syndrome of cardiorespiratory failure with hypotension and peripheral and pulmonary edema.[108] Chest radiographic manifestations range from mild interstitial to extensive air space edema.[2] The mechanism of pulmonary edema is generally considered to be increased capillary permeability; however, small increases in pulmonary capillary wedge pressure and a decrease in blood oncotic pressure have also been implicated.[109]

Granulocyte-Macrophage Colony-Stimulating Factor

Use of the hematopoietic growth factor granulocyte-macrophage colony-stimulating factor (GM-CSF) has been associated with a variety of pulmonary complications, including acute eosinophilic pneumonia,[110] dyspnea (caused by accumulation of aggregated neutrophils in the pulmonary vasculature), a capillary leak syndrome with pleural and pericardial effusions, thromboembolism (possibly related to the development of thrombosis at the catheter tip as a result of local accumulation of granulocytes that damage the vascular endothelium), and ARDS.[111] The last-named condition is the most common clinical manifestation and may be related to neutrophil activation by GM-CSF[112]; enhancement of toxicity by other chemotherapeutic agents may be a factor in some cases.

Interferons

Interferons have been used for a wide variety of malignant and nonmalignant disorders. A number of pulmonary reactions have been reported, including the precipitation of severe bronchospasm in asthmatic patients,[113] the development of a sarcoidosis-like disorder with granulomatous inflammation,[114] and interstitial pneumonia.[115]

Hormonal Agents

Tamoxifen

The administration of tamoxifen, an antiestrogen widely used in the treatment of breast carcinoma, has been associated with the development of thrombotic events in about 1% to 4% of patients.[116] Similar figures have been reported for other antiestrogens.[117] Although many patients have had other risk factors for venous thrombosis and pulmonary thromboembolism, it is likely that tamoxifen itself is associated with an increased risk for the complications.[118]

Nilutamide

Nilutamide, a synthetic antiandrogen used in the treatment of prostatic carcinoma, has been associated with the development of interstitial pneumonitis and fibrosis.[119] Recovery has occurred after drug withdrawal or dose reduction and with corticosteroid therapy.

Antimicrobial Drugs

Nitrofurantoin

Although almost 1000 cases of pulmonary toxicity caused by nitrofurantoin have been reported, overall, pulmonary reactions are rare.[120] The higher incidence in women and the elderly is probably a reflection of the patient population receiving the medication.[121] Disease is most commonly manifested within hours to days after the onset of treatment, a reaction that almost certainly represents hypersensitivity. A more insidious form of disease that becomes evident after weeks to years of continuous therapy probably represents direct tissue damage from oxidants.[122] Histologic examination of the lungs shows interstitial pneumonitis and fibrosis in most patients[123]; some have a pattern of desquamative interstitial pneumonitis or COP.[124,125]

The radiographic manifestations of acute disease consist of a diffuse reticular pattern with some basilar predominance; septal lines may be present (Fig. 18–5).[25] The pattern

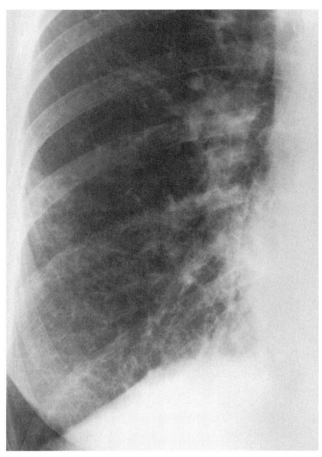

FIGURE 18–5

Nitrofurantoin toxicity. A view of the right lung from a posteroanterior chest radiograph shows a reticular pattern involving predominantly the lower lung zones. A few septal lines and a small right pleural effusion are evident. The patient was a 58-year-old woman with progressive shortness of breath. The findings resolved within a few days after discontinuation of nitrofurantoin therapy. *(From Müller NL, Fraser RS, Colman NC, Paré PD: Radiologic Diagnosis of Diseases of the Chest. Philadelphia, WB Saunders, 2001.)*

occur in 10% to 20%.[131] Symptoms tend to develop more rapidly in patients who have received the drug previously. The chronic form of disease is characterized by dry cough and gradually increasing shortness of breath on exertion that develops after months to years of therapy.[127] Crackles may be heard at the lung bases; pleural effusion and clubbing develop in a minority of patients. A peripheral blood eosinophilia of 5% or more is present in almost 85% of patients who have acute disease and in 40% of those with the chronic form[121]; pleural fluid eosinophilia has also been reported.[132] Diffusing capacity and PaO2 may be very low, particularly in the acute form.

The prognosis is excellent in the acute variety, with all evidence of disease usually disappearing within 4 to 8 weeks.[133] Although complete clearing has been reported after cessation of therapy in patients who have chronic disease, 10% of affected individuals die.[123]

Sulfasalazine

Pulmonary toxicity from sulfasalazine probably represents a hypersensitivity reaction; in most patients, findings consist of acute, transitory radiographic opacities accompanied by peripheral blood eosinophilia, and in some individuals, drug challenge after cessation of therapy has elicited a positive reaction.[134,135] Most biopsy specimens have revealed interstitial pneumonitis and fibrosis or organizing pneumonia (COP)[136]; a histologic appearance resembling eosinophilic pneumonia or extrinsic allergic alveolitis has been documented occasionally.[137]

The radiographic manifestations typically consist of bilateral areas of consolidation that are commonly peripheral in distribution.[138] They involve predominantly the upper lobes, although lower lobe or diffuse abnormalities occur in a small number of cases.[139] The clinical manifestations vary little among patients and consist of dry cough, progressive dyspnea, and fever, often associated with a rash and blood eosinophilia[140]; these findings become manifest 1 to 6 months after initiation of treatment. Both restrictive and obstructive patterns have been found on pulmonary function testing.[141] Follow-up studies after cessation of drug use generally reveal complete resolution.

Tetracycline and Minocycline

Both tetracycline and minocycline have been reported to cause lung disease that usually resembles simple pulmonary eosinophilia.[142,143] Rechallenge with minocycline in several patients has implicated a hypersensitivity reaction in the pathogenesis.[144] However, a CD8-predominant lymphocytosis with an expansion of CD4+ lymphocytes has also been found in BAL fluid, thus suggesting a role for cell-mediated immunity.[144]

The radiographic findings resemble those of simple pulmonary eosinophilia and usually consist of bilateral apical and predominantly subpleural areas of consolidation.[145] Less common findings include unilateral consolidation or a fine bilateral reticular pattern.

Patients usually have dyspnea, fever, and dry cough; chest pain, fatigue, rash, and hemoptysis occur occasionally.[146] Crackles can be appreciated on auscultation of the chest. Hepatitis, pleural effusion, and peripheral lymphadenopathy

resembles interstitial pulmonary edema; the rapid clearing that occurs when use of the drug is withdrawn suggests that edema plays a considerable role in production of the opacities.[126] Pleural effusions are relatively common and may be an isolated finding.[127]

The radiographic manifestations of the chronic form consist of a bilateral reticular pattern, usually involving mainly the lower lung zones. HRCT findings include ground-glass opacities and predominantly subpleural or diffuse reticulation.[128,129] Although the reticulation may be widespread and associated with architectural distortion, it may resolve after withdrawal of the drug. A pattern of predominantly subpleural or peribronchial consolidation resembling COP (bronchiolitis obliterans with organizing pneumonia [BOOP]) may also be seen (Fig. 18–6).[130] Pleural effusions are uncommon.[2]

Clinical manifestations in the acute form of the disease include fever, dyspnea, and a nonproductive cough; about 25% of patients complain of chest pain. A rash and arthralgia

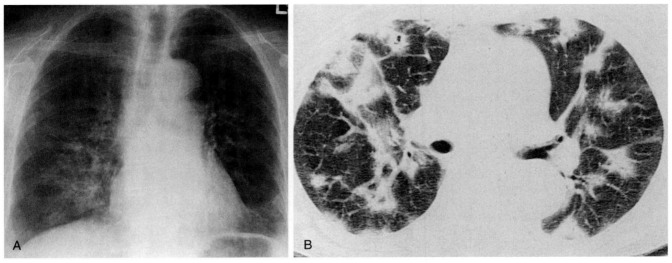

FIGURE 18–6

Chronic nitrofurantoin toxicity. A posteroanterior chest radiograph (**A**) shows a coarse reticular pattern and patchy areas of consolidation involving predominantly the middle and lower lung zones. An HRCT scan (**B**) shows a peribronchial distribution of the areas of consolidation and a few irregular linear opacities. The patient was an 81-year-old woman with progressive shortness of breath. She had been taking nitrofurantoin for 2 years. A transbronchial biopsy specimen showed cryptogenic organizing pneumonia. *(From Müller NL, Fraser RS, Colman NC, Paré PD: Radiologic Diagnosis of Diseases of the Chest. Philadelphia, WB Saunders, 2001.)*

may be seen. The peripheral and BAL eosinophil counts are typically elevated.[147] Hypoxemia is usual and may be severe. Lung function studies have revealed both obstructive and restrictive patterns. The pulmonary opacities resolve with discontinuation of the drug; corticosteroids appear to accelerate improvement when administered in severe disease.[146]

Antiarrhythmic Drugs

Amiodarone

Amiodarone hydrochloride is an iodinated benzofuran derivative used in the treatment of cardiac arrhythmias. Given the vagaries of the clinical findings, different diagnostic criteria, and difficulty distinguishing toxicity from congestive heart failure, thromboembolism, or infection, the precise incidence of pulmonary toxicity is uncertain; however, it has been suggested that with current patterns of use, the complication develops in about 5% of treated patients, 5% to 10% of whom die as a consequence.[148]

The pathogenesis of pulmonary injury is uncertain, but it seems likely that both direct and indirect mechanisms are involved.[149] Amiodarone causes inhibition of phospholipid degradation within the lysosomes of target cells, thereby resulting in an increase in their phospholipid content and a foamy appearance on histologic examination.[150] Although these abnormalities correlate well with tissue levels of the drug and its metabolites and such levels are toxic to lung cells in vitro,[151] foamy macrophages can be found in tissue that shows no evidence of damage histologically; thus, it appears likely that the lipid accumulation represents a marker of amiodarone administration rather than an essential step in the pathogenesis of disease. In fact, there is evidence that an inflammatory or immune response is responsible for the

tissue damage, at least in some patients.[152] For example, the cell composition in BAL fluid is similar to that seen in extrinsic allergic alveolitis, and both pulmonary and blood immune cells are activated in response to the drug.[153]

Most patients have received 400 mg/day or more of amiodarone before the appearance of pulmonary disease; however, problems have occurred with maintenance doses of less than 400 mg/day in some patients.[86] Lung damage generally has its onset months after the initiation of therapy.[154] The preferential concentration of the drug in the lung and its very long half-life probably explain the slow resolution of toxicity after discontinuation of the agent.

Light microscopic examination of the lung typically reveals chronic inflammation and fibrosis of the alveolar septa, hyperplasia of type II pneumocytes, and an increase in macrophages in alveolar air spaces (Fig. 18–7).[155] The macrophages and pneumocytes have coarsely vacuolated cytoplasm that can be seen ultrastructurally to contain numerous, often enlarged lysosomal inclusions composed of thin osmiophilic lamellae surrounded by amorphous electron-dense material (see Fig. 18–7). The inclusion-bearing macrophages can be identified in BAL specimens[156]; however, as indicated previously, such macrophages can also be seen in patients without evidence of disease,[155] and their presence is not diagnostic of drug-related tissue damage. Additional histologic patterns reported to occur in some patients include diffuse alveolar damage and organizing pneumonia (COP).[155]

The chest radiograph usually shows a diffuse bilateral reticular pattern or bilateral areas of consolidation (Fig. 18–8).[2] The latter may be peripheral in distribution and may involve the upper lobes predominantly, similar to chronic eosinophilic pneumonia.[157] Less common manifestations include focal consolidation and nodular opacities.[64]

Because amiodarone contains about 37% iodine by weight, it has a high attenuation value on CT; as a result, this

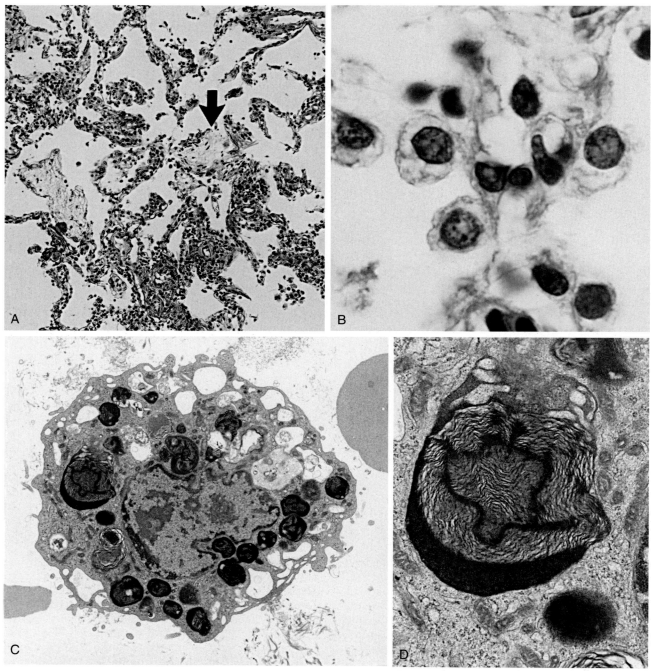

FIGURE 18–7

Amiodarone toxicity—interstitial pneumonitis. A section of lung parenchyma (**A**) shows a moderate degree of interstitial fibrosis and lymphocytic infiltration; focal fibroblastic tissue is also present (*arrow*). A magnified view of one alveolar wall (**B**) shows several type II pneumocytes with coarsely vacuolated cytoplasm. Ultrastructural examination of an alveolar macrophage (**C**) reveals the cytoplasm to contain numerous phagosomes, many of which contain densely osmiophilic material. A magnified view of one phagosome (**D**) shows a laminated inclusion surrounded by a crescent-shaped zone of amorphous electron-dense material. The patient was a 63-year-old man who had been taking amiodarone daily for several months. (*From Fraser RS, Müller NL, Colman NC, Paré PD: Fraser and Paré's Diagnosis of Diseases of the Chest, 4th ed. Philadelphia, WB Saunders, 1999.*)

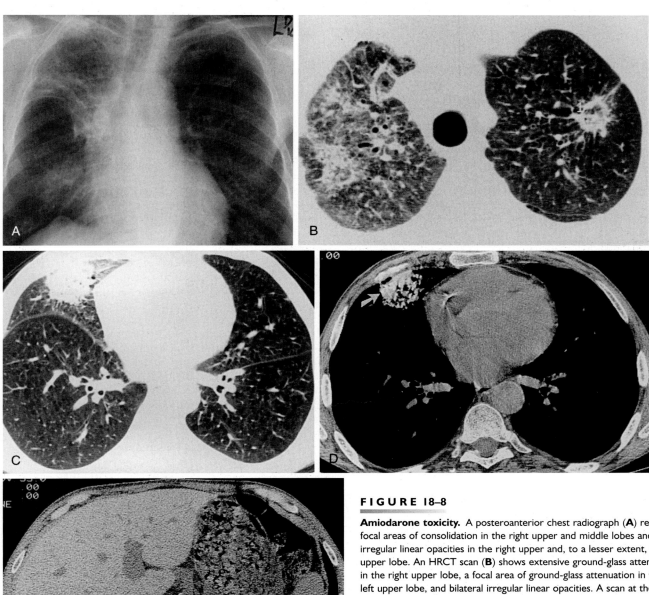

FIGURE 18–8

Amiodarone toxicity. A posteroanterior chest radiograph (**A**) reveals focal areas of consolidation in the right upper and middle lobes and irregular linear opacities in the right upper and, to a lesser extent, the left upper lobe. An HRCT scan (**B**) shows extensive ground-glass attenuation in the right upper lobe, a focal area of ground-glass attenuation in the left upper lobe, and bilateral irregular linear opacities. A scan at the level of the inferior pulmonary veins (**C**) reveals a focal area of consolidation in the right middle lobe. A scan at the same level as that in **C** and photographed with soft tissue windows (**D**) demonstrates that the consolidation in the right middle lobe (*arrow*) has an attenuation greater than that of the chest wall and cardiac muscle. A scan through the upper part of the abdomen (**E**) reveals high attenuation of the liver. The patient was a 61-year-old man. *(From Fraser RS, Müller NL, Colman NC, Paré PD: Fraser and Paré's Diagnosis of Diseases of the Chest, 4th ed. Philadelphia, WB Saunders, 1999.)*

procedure allows confident recognition of drug deposition within pulmonary and other tissues (see Fig. 18–8).[158] High-attenuation (82 to 175 Hounsfield units [HU]) pulmonary abnormalities are seen in approximately 70% of patients who have symptoms of pulmonary toxicity.[159] The appearance of the parenchymal abnormalities is variable and may consist of bilateral areas of consolidation (frequently wedge shaped and pleural based), a reticular pattern, linear atelectasis, or (less commonly) focal round areas of consolidation.[159] Pleural effusions are seen in about 50% of cases.[159] Visceral pleural

thickening may be evident.[160] Distinction of amiodarone pneumonitis from congestive heart failure may be facilitated by the documentation of increased uptake on gallium 67 radionuclide lung scans.[161]

The most common clinical findings are the insidious onset of dyspnea on exertion, dry cough, weight loss, weakness, and (occasionally) fever.[162] About a third of patients have a more acute onset of disease, which may be confused clinically with infection, pulmonary edema, or thromboembolism.[148] Physical findings in both forms of disease are inconsistent and nonspecific. Manifestations of extrapulmonary toxicity are not uncommon and include blue-gray skin discoloration, rash (such as photodermatitis), thyroid dysfunction (both hypothyroidism and hyperthyroidism), corneal microdeposits, gastrointestinal symptoms, neurotoxicity (manifested by muscle weakness, peripheral neuropathy, or extrapyramidal symptoms), hepatic dysfunction, and bradycardia.[163]

Pulmonary function tests show restrictive impairment and a reduction in gas transfer.[164] Although an isolated reduction in diffusing capacity is a sensitive finding in diagnosis, it lacks specificity.[165] However, normal lung function provides reasonable assurance of the absence of toxicity. The diagnosis remains one of exclusion and requires careful correlation of the results of history taking, physical examination, functional and radiologic investigation, and in some cases, BAL and biopsy. The finding of high attenuation of the parenchymal abnormalities on HRCT is particularly useful in this regard.[159]

The response to withdrawal of the drug in early disease appears to be excellent. The long half-life of the drug creates considerable difficulty in assessing the value of corticosteroid therapy in the absence of a controlled clinical trial comparing this therapy with drug withdrawal.[166] Nonetheless, relapse of disease after steroid withdrawal has been reported in patients who had improvement after its institution, suggesting that it has a beneficial effect.[167] There is evidence that patients who are taking amiodarone or have had previous pulmonary toxicity from the drug and who undergo cardiothoracic surgery are at increased risk for the development of postoperative ARDS.[168]

Analgesic Drugs

Acetylsalicylic Acid

Acetylsalicylic acid (aspirin) is well known to provoke asthma attacks in susceptible individuals (see page 650). It can also cause acute pulmonary edema, particularly in middle-aged and elderly people who become habituated as a result of ingesting large doses to alleviate pain. Serum salicylate levels in these individuals are usually 30 mg/mm^3 or more; however, there is no clear dose relationship because edema does not develop in many patients with similar blood levels.[169] Cigarette smoking has been identified as a risk factor in some studies.[170]

The edema results from an increase in capillary permeability.[171] Chest radiographs reveal the typical diffuse air space pattern of pulmonary edema.[169] Patients are dyspneic, lethargic, and confused; they tend to have proteinuria, perhaps because of increased capillary permeability in the systemic circulation. A history of long-term acetylsalicylic acid ingestion, usually in large quantities, is typical.[172] Because the pulmonary edema responds well to measures that decrease serum salicylate levels, the prognosis is good.[170]

Antirheumatic Drugs

Penicillamine

Penicillamine is a derivative of penicillin that can chelate a variety of metals. It is used to treat lead poisoning, Wilson's disease, cystinuria, and several connective tissue diseases, particularly rheumatoid disease. A variety of complications associated with this use can affect the lungs, including lupus-like[173] and myasthenia-like[174] disease, as well as alveolitis, obliterative bronchiolitis, and diffuse alveolar hemorrhage (the latter in association with acute glomerulonephritis).[175-177] Because most published cases of penicillamine-associated bronchiolitis have occurred in patients who have had rheumatoid arthritis, however, it is possible that some such cases, if not all, have been a manifestation of the underlying disease rather than the drug. The risk of toxicity is not dose related.[141] The mechanism of acute reversible pulmonary disease, usually accompanied by eosinophilia,[178] is probably a type I immunologic reaction, whereas limited pathologic findings suggest that the pulmonary hemorrhage is type III.[177]

Pathologic abnormalities vary with the type of disease. Biopsy specimens from some patients have shown nonspecific interstitial pneumonia.[179] Histologic findings in patients who have pulmonary-renal syndrome are those of diffuse alveolar hemorrhage with minimal or no vasculitis. The appearance of bronchiolitis is identical to that seen in rheumatoid disease.

Radiographic manifestations consist of a reticular or reticulonodular pattern (with or without limited air space opacities), overinflation unaccompanied by parenchymal abnormality (associated with obliterative bronchiolitis), and diffuse air space consolidation (typically seen in patients who have diffuse alveolar hemorrhage).[141,180] In patients with obliterative bronchiolitis, HRCT findings consist of areas of decreased attenuation and perfusion (mosaic attenuation) and bronchial dilation.[176]

Patients with interstitial pneumonia or obliterative bronchiolitis usually present with cough and dyspnea that develop insidiously over a period of weeks to months; however, the onset of dyspnea is typically abrupt in patients who have pulmonary hemorrhage.[141] In patients with bronchiolitis, pulmonary function tests reveal evidence of obstruction, sometimes when the chest radiograph is normal. The prognosis for patients with interstitial pneumonitis is excellent, the clinical and radiographic abnormalities characteristically resolving rapidly after withdrawal of medication and initiation of steroid therapy.[178] By contrast, death is common in patients who have pulmonary-renal syndrome or obliterative bronchiolitis.[141]

Gold

Pulmonary toxicity is uncommon after gold therapy, having been estimated to occur in less than 1% of patients. The risk does not appear to be dose related. The mechanism of pulmonary damage is thought to be a hypersensitivity reaction[181]; however, there is also evidence of a cell-mediated immune reaction.[141] A strong association between toxicity and the presence of certain major histocompatibility antigens has been reported.[182]

Histologic examination usually reveals nonspecific interstitial pneumonia.[183] Gold can be identified within the lysosomes of macrophages and pulmonary capillary endothelial cells[184]; however, as with amiodarone, it has not been established whether this finding simply represents a marker of drug administration or is related to the pathogenesis of disease. The chest radiograph has been described as showing diffuse interstitial and patchy air space opacities.[185]

Clinical manifestations usually develop acutely or subacutely, thereby aiding in the differentiation from interstitial fibrosis associated with rheumatoid disease, the onset of which is insidious.[186] Patients are often febrile and complain of progressive shortness of breath on exertion and a dry cough; almost half have associated dermatitis.[141] Physical examination may reveal crackles. About a third of patients have peripheral eosinophilia.[181] A restrictive pattern and hypoxemia are found on physiologic assessment.[187] The response to cessation of therapy is usually good.

Sympathomimetic Drugs

The tocolytic sympathomimetics terbutaline, ritodrine, and isoxsuprine, used in the treatment of preterm labor, have been implicated in the development of permeability pulmonary edema.[188] The differential diagnosis includes other disorders of pregnancy such as amniotic fluid embolism, cardiomyopathy of pregnancy, and fluid overload. The chest radiograph reveals classic signs of air space edema. Symptoms and clinical findings develop within 2 to 3 days of the initiation of therapy and can be associated with extreme hypoxemia. The prognosis is excellent after discontinuation of the drug and initiation of supportive measures.[189]

The association of fenfluramine, phentermine, and related agents with the development of pulmonary hypertension is discussed in Chapter 13 (see page 591).

Illicit Drugs

Narcotic and Sedative Drugs

Opiates and related drugs are well-known causes of pulmonary edema.[190] The complication has also been reported as a result of an overdose of other narcotics and benzodiazepines. A high protein content of the edema fluid has been well documented in affected patients,[191] indicating that the development of edema is related to increased capillary permeability. Although the mechanism by which capillary leakage occurs has not been elucidated, it is probable that the hypoxemia and acidosis that accompany severe respiratory center depression cause endothelial damage. It is also possible that the edema has a neurogenic origin; opiate receptors can be identified near the medullary respiratory center,[192] and the application of drugs in this area has produced edema in dogs. Such a mechanism could explain the paradoxical development of edema after administration of the opiate antagonist naloxone.[193]

The pathologic and radiologic manifestations are indistinguishable from those of edema of other etiologies. The appearance of the edema may be delayed after admission to the hospital, sometimes for as long as 6 to 10 hours[194]; resolution characteristically occurs in as brief a time as 24 to 48 hours. The typical patient is stuporous or comatose and has frothy, pink fluid oozing from the nostrils and mouth. Constricted pupils and respiratory depression are usually evident; however, a depressed level of consciousness is not always present.[195] Hypoxemia is severe and accompanied by a mixed acidosis.[196]

A number of other pulmonary abnormalities can be seen in opiate addicts.[197] Bronchiectasis has been identified in some

individuals with a history of drug-induced pulmonary edema; it is probably explained by recurrent infection and aspiration.[198] Unilateral or bilateral pneumothorax, hemothorax, hemopneumothorax, and pyopneumothorax have been reported as complications of attempted venous access in the neck. Septic emboli, sometimes associated with right ventricular endocarditis, can also be seen.

Cocaine

When smoked, the crystalline precipitate of freebase cocaine ("crack") reaches the cerebral circulation within 6 to 8 seconds and causes virtually instantaneous euphoria. This property, along with its ease of administration and wide availability, has made crack cocaine the most frequently abused controlled substance in the United States.[199] Use of the drug has been associated with a variety of pulmonary complications, including edema, hemorrhage, airway thermal injury (sometimes complicated by tracheal stenosis or the reactive airways dysfunction syndrome), asthma, COP, pneumothorax, pneumomediastinum, and pneumopericardium.[200,201] The combination of widespread abuse and variable manifestations of disease necessitates that inquiry concerning cocaine use be a routine part of history taking.

The radiographic manifestations of pulmonary edema consist of bilateral, symmetrical, and predominantly perihilar interstitial or air space opacities.[202] These abnormalities generally resolve within 24 to 72 hours, regardless of treatment. Pulmonary hemorrhage may result in transient focal or diffuse bilateral air space consolidation.[203] Less commonly, there are fleeting areas of consolidation (resulting in a Löffler's syndrome–like appearance) or a pattern of organizing pneumonia.[199] Barotrauma related to cocaine abuse may result in pneumomediastinum, pneumothorax, or (rarely) hemopneumothorax or pneumopericardium.[204,205]

Symptoms are common within minutes to hours of inhaling crack cocaine; more than 40% of users report intercurrent cough, production of black sputum, pleuritic or nonpleuritic chest pain, shortness of breath, exacerbation of asthma, or hemoptysis.[199] Although the cause of the chest pain is usually unclear despite investigation, myocardial ischemia or infarction, pneumothorax, and pneumomediastinum must be excluded. A persistent reduction in diffusing capacity with otherwise normal pulmonary function has been described in long-term cocaine users,[200] but the precise pathogenesis of this finding is not known.

Marijuana

Habitual marijuana use is associated with the development of acute and chronic bronchitis similar to that seen in tobacco smokers[206]; its effects are probably additive to and independent of those of tobacco in this respect.[207] Reports of wheezing, breathlessness, and chest tightness are also more common in chronic users of marijuana than in individuals who do not smoke tobacco.[208] Chronic, heavy use has no consistent effect on nonspecific airway reactivity[209]; the drug's bronchodilator effects become blunted with repeated use. The common contamination of marijuana with *Aspergillus* species has been implicated in the development of both allergic bronchopulmonary aspergillosis in marijuana users who are asthmatic and opportunistic *Aspergillus* infection in those who are immunocompromised.[195] A reduction in diffusing capacity has also been attributed to long-term marijuana use.[210]

Antidepressant and Antipsychotic Drugs

Antidepressant and antipsychotic agents have been associated with a variety of pulmonary abnormalities, the most common of which is ARDS.[211] In an investigation of 82 patients admitted to an intensive care unit with tricyclic antidepressant overdose, 32 (39%) had radiographic abnormalities, 9 of which were consistent with ARDS.[212] Although aspiration was documented by the finding of charcoal used in nasogastric lavage before intubation in the tracheal aspirates of 18 of 72 patients, there was no correlation between this observation and the radiographic findings of edema. The drugs have also been associated with the development of idiopathic pulmonary fibrosis; for example, in a retrospective review in which the lifetime drug use of patients in whom the disease had developed was compared with that of a control group, the odds ratio associated with a history of imipramine use was 4.8.[213]

Contrast Media

Water-soluble contrast media have occasionally been reported to cause permeability pulmonary edema.[214] Acute reactions to ionic contrast media injected intravenously occur in 5% to 15% of patients.[215] They are usually mild; life-threatening reactions occur in only 0.05% to 0.1% of injections, with a mortality rate of about 1 in 75,000. Manifestations of minor reactions include nausea, vomiting, urticaria, and diaphoresis; more severe disease is associated with faintness, severe vomiting, laryngeal edema, and bronchospasm. The most severe reactions are characterized by pulmonary edema, shock, convulsions, and cardiorespiratory arrest. The risk for such anaphylactoid reactions is increased in patients who have allergies, asthma, or previous reactions to the contrast medium.[215]

Embolization of the ethiodized oil used for lymphangiography can result in a "subacute" form of ARDS that possesses clinical features resembling those of fat embolism and may have a similar pathogenesis (see page 573).

Angiotensin-Converting Enzyme Inhibitors

Persistent nonproductive cough is a common side effect of ACE inhibitor therapy[216]; a reasonable estimate of its overall occurrence is probably about 10%. Most investigators have reported a higher prevalence in women than men. The pathogenesis of the cough is unclear. It does not appear to be the result of inhibition of the renin-angiotensin system because treatment with angiotensin receptor blockers and renin inhibitors has not caused the symptom.[217,218] More likely, it is related to stimulation of vagal afferents of the cough reflex in the airway mucosa by bradykinin or tachykinins, whose accumulation is favored by ACE inhibition.

Cough is often very troublesome. Usually, it begins several months after starting the drug; occasionally, it starts as early as the first dose or as late as 1 year after initiation of therapy.[219] It diminishes significantly within 3 days and disappears entirely within 10 days of drug cessation.[220]

Although ACE inhibitors have also occasionally been associated with the development of asthma,[221] administration of these agents to patients who have established asthma has not been found to result in deterioration of lung function or change in clinical status.[222] Additional rare complications of ACE inhibitors include angioedema (occasionally associated with upper airway obstruction[223]) and peripheral eosinophilia.[224]

Miscellaneous Drugs

Hydrochlorothiazide has rarely been implicated as a cause of permeability pulmonary edema.[225] Clinical symptoms and signs of edema develop 20 to 60 minutes after ingestion of the drug. Complete recovery typically occurs after cessation of therapy. The reaction is probably a hypersensitivity phenomenon.

β-Adrenergic blocking agents (β-blockers) can produce a systemic lupus erythematosus–like syndrome and can also precipitate acute bronchospasm. Propranolol and other β-blockers have also been implicated as the cause of a hypersensitivity pneumonitis characterized by lymphocytic alveolitis on BAL.[226,227] Acute pulmonary edema and bronchospasm have been reported to accompany the use of β-blocker eye drops in the treatment of glaucoma.[60,228]

ARDS has been reported in patients in whom talc was instilled intrapleurally for the treatment of a malignant effusion[229]; in an investigation of 120 patients so treated, arterial oxygen desaturation developed in 7%, and 3 patients required mechanical ventilation.[230] Fever, increasing dyspnea, and finally ARDS develop over a 72-hour period after the injection. Fear of the complication has led some authorities to advocate against its use as a sclerosing agent in patients requiring pleurodesis.[231]

Though most strongly associated with pleural disease, ergotamine and its derivatives bromocriptine and mesulergine have been reported to cause pulmonary fibrosis.[232] Clinical and radiographic improvement after drug withdrawal suggests that this relationship is real.[233]

The vitamin A derivative all-*trans*-retinoic acid has been used for the treatment of patients who have acute promyelocytic leukemia.[234] The retinoic acid syndrome, which consists of fever, weight gain, respiratory distress, interstitial pulmonary infiltrates, thromboembolic events, pleural and pericardial effusion, episodic hypotension, and acute renal failure, develops in some patients.

Both of the tyrosine kinase inhibitors gefitinib (Iressa) and imatinib (Gleevec) have been associated with pulmonary toxicity. The former, which is used as salvage therapy in non–small cell lung carcinoma, has been found to result in diffuse ground-glass changes on CT scan in about 1% of patients.[235] The pathologic findings are those of diffuse alveolar damage. Imatinib has caused interstitial pneumonitis in some patients.[236]

POISONS

Poison-induced pulmonary toxicity almost always occurs as a result of accidental exposure or suicidal intent. The great majority of toxic substances are inhaled as noxious gases or soluble aerosols, usually in an occupational setting or from environmental pollution in the vicinity of production sites or vehicular accidents during transport. A few poisons reach the lungs after absorption through the skin or gastrointestinal tract or directly by intravenous injection.

Insecticides and Herbicides

Organophosphates

The most important examples of this group are parathion and malathion. Poisoning with these agents occurs most commonly in agricultural workers during or shortly after the spraying of crops and less often in industrial workers during manufacture and transport; it can also occur accidentally in children and intentionally in suicide attempts.[237] The chemicals exert their effects by inhibiting acetylcholinesterase at nerve endings. Symptoms and signs are thus attributable mainly to the accumulation of acetylcholine at cholinergic synapses, which results in an initial stimulation and later inhibition of synaptic transmission. Important signs and symptoms include miosis, diaphoresis, increased salivation, bronchorrhea, bronchoconstriction, bradycardia, hyperperistalsis, and coma. Muscular fasciculations, particularly of the diaphragm, can be seen and may be followed by fatigue and eventual paralysis. Depending on the route and the amount of poison taken, the time interval between exposure and the onset of symptoms ranges from 5 minutes (after a massive dose) to 24 hours.

Radiographic findings consist of interstitial or air space pulmonary edema, usually associated with cardiomegaly.[238] In patients who survive, these abnormalities clear within 2 to 4 days. Death can result from central nervous system depression or diaphragmatic paralysis; the effects of the latter are compounded by bronchoconstriction, hypersecretion of airway mucus, and pulmonary edema.[239]

Paraquat

Poisoning with this herbicide usually follows its ingestion, either by mistake or for suicidal purposes; occasionally, it results from absorption of the poison through the skin[240] or from inhalation.[241] Poisoning after absorption tends to be less acute and less severe than that after ingestion, presumably because of a smaller dosage; however, even small amounts may be fatal. Pulmonary damage may also occur as a result of prolonged absorption of low concentrations, as has been described in vineyard sprayers.[242] The pathogenesis of pulmonary injury is complex and probably includes a combination of peroxidation of cell lipid membranes, DNA injury, nitric oxide synthesis, mitochondrial and cytoskeleton damage, and oxygen radical production.[243-245] Pathologic features are those of diffuse alveolar damage.

Radiographic findings include extensive bilateral areas of consolidation (in about 60% of patients), pneumomediastinum with or without pneumothorax (in 40%), and cardiomegaly associated with widening of the superior mediastinum (in 20%).[246] Consolidation may be seen at initial evaluation or may develop over a period of several days in patients whose radiographs were previously normal or had a ground-glass opacity. The most common HRCT findings consist of diffuse bilateral areas of ground-glass attenuation.[247]

Associated areas of parenchymal consolidation involving mainly the lower lung zones are present in 40% of cases.

Vomiting, abdominal pain, and burning of the mouth and throat ensue shortly after ingestion. Death may occur within hours to a few days from pulmonary edema and renal and hepatic failure[248]; however, some patients have a brief period of apparent recovery before respiratory failure develops 5 to 10 days after admission.[249] Overall, about 30% to 55% of affected individuals die, and serious suicide attempts are almost always successful. Once there is clinical or radiographic evidence of pulmonary involvement, death is especially common.[246] Patients who survive may manifest residual pulmonary dysfunction, although it may improve with time.[250]

Miscellaneous Insecticides and Herbicides

The possibility that carbamate insecticides might be a cause of asthma was suggested by a report from Saskatchewan in which the prevalence of the disease in farmers exposed to these agents was greater than that of farmers not so exposed.[251] Other insecticide aerosols can also trigger symptoms, a fall in lung function and an increase in airway hyperresponsiveness in patients who have asthma.[252]

Propoxur (Baygon), a member of the carbamylester family, has an acetylcholinesterase-binding capacity similar to that of the organophosphates. Pulmonary edema, coma, bronchorrhea, and miosis have been described in patients who have used it in suicide attempts.[253]

Thallium, a drug formerly used as a rodenticide and insecticide, is now used industrially in the production of optic lenses, low-temperature thermometers, semiconductors, pigments, and scintillation counters. Although it has been more commonly associated with central nervous system and gastrointestinal toxicity, ARDS has also been reported.[254]

Spanish Toxic Oil Syndrome

In the summer of 1981, a pneumonic-paralytic-eosinophilic syndrome occurred in Spain in epidemic form.[255] The results of epidemiologic studies indicated that the agent responsible was denatured rapeseed oil contaminated with esters of PAP (3-N-[phenylamino]-1,2-propanediol). More than 300 patients died in the first year of the epidemic, many as a result of restrictive lung disease.[256] Clinically, the syndrome often began as an acute respiratory illness characterized by cough, fever, dyspnea, and hypoxemia. Radiography showed lung opacities described as "atypical pneumonia" and pleural effusions. Half the patients recovered from this acute illness without apparent sequelae. In the remainder, pulmonary hypertension and/or chronic systemic disease that included severe myalgia, eosinophilia, and scleroderma-like skin lesions developed.[257] Although most patients eventually improved, many had persistent symptoms, including dyspnea and cough. Abnormalities in lung func-tion (including reduced VC and diffusing capacity) were common.[258]

Hydrocarbons

It has been estimated that 5% of all poisonings in children result from the ingestion of petroleum products,[259] the most common of which is kerosene.[260] Cases of pulmonary disease have also been reported after the accidental aspiration of petroleum in performers demonstrating the art of fire-eating.[261] It is unclear whether pulmonary disease follows absorption of the hydrocarbon from the intestinal tract with subsequent transport to the pulmonary capillaries or whether it follows emesis and aspiration of vomitus with direct alveolocapillary damage.[262]

The chest radiograph is usually abnormal within an hour of the ingestion of kerosene[263]; however, changes have been found to appear somewhat later after the ingestion of furniture polish.[264] The severity of the pulmonary abnormality varies with the amount ingested.

The typical radiographic pattern is one of patchy bilateral air space consolidation involving predominantly the basal portions of the lung.[263] Pneumatoceles, often large, may develop.[265]

Vomiting follows shortly after ingestion and in many cases is probably associated with aspiration. Symptoms are usually mild; however, the greater the amount of hydrocarbon ingested, the greater the severity of the clinical findings and the extent of radiographic abnormalities. In the absence of witnesses to ingestion, the diagnosis may be suspected from the odor of the offending agent on the patient's breath. The prognosis is good; in a survey of 950 children younger than 5 years who were suspected of having ingested products containing hydrocarbons, only 2 died, and progressive pulmonary disease developed in 5.[259]

IRRADIATION

Within the therapeutic range of doses usually administered, the pulmonary parenchyma can be assumed to react to ionizing radiation in virtually all patients. Many variables affect this reaction and its resulting clinical and radiologic manifestations, including the volume of lung tissue irradiated, the radiation dose administered, the time over which it is given, and the nature of the radiation.[266,267] Pulmonary tissue is usually damaged by radiation aimed directly at the lungs; however, it can also be injured when the beam is directed elsewhere in the thorax, such as at the mediastinum or chest wall.

The incidence of pulmonary disease secondary to radiotherapy varies considerably in reported series. In a review of 18 studies involving 5534 patients reported before 1992, symptomatic pneumonitis developed in 7% of patients (range, 1% to 34%) after radiation therapy for carcinoma of the lung or breast, mesothelioma, or Hodgkin's lymphoma[268]; radiologic changes developed in 43% of patients (range, 13% to 100%). In another analysis of 24 series that included 1911 patients who had undergone combined modality therapy for pulmonary carcinoma (in which the total radiation dose ranged from 25 to 63 Gy, with a median dose of 50 Gy [1 Gy = 100 rad]), symptomatic radiation pneumonitis occurred in approximately 8% of patients.[269] The risk was greater with a higher total radiation dose, daily radiation fractions greater than 2.67 Gy, and the use of once-daily as opposed to twice-daily irradiation. Symptomatic radiation pneumonitis occurred in 6% of patients who received a total radiation dose lower than 45 Gy, in 9% who received doses between 45 and 54 Gy, and in 12% who had a total dose of 55 Gy or greater.

Though most often caused by external beam radiation, radiation injury to the lungs can also follow the inhalation of β-emitting radionuclides or (rarely) internal selective radiotherapy of the liver when radioactive microspheres injected into the hepatic artery enter the pulmonary circulation through arterioportal shunts.[270,271] In addition, focal injury to the airways can occur after brachytherapy for palliation of obstructing pulmonary carcinoma.[272]

Pathogenesis

Radiologic Factors

Volume of Lung Irradiated. The likelihood of clinical symptoms and radiologic evidence of pulmonary injury is proportional to the volume of lung irradiated.[266] In fact, this variable is one of the most important factors associated with lung damage; for example, it has been estimated that a total dose of 30 Gy delivered in fractions to 25% of TLC may not produce any symptoms, whereas radiation delivered in the same manner to the entire volume of both lungs would probably prove fatal.[273] Recognition of this potential problem led to the development of tangential ports to deliver radiotherapy, thereby limiting the amount of radiation given to normal structures. This modification has been associated with a considerable reduction in morbidity; for example, the prevalence of symptomatic radiation pneumonitis after treatment of breast carcinoma decreased from about 60% to less than 10% with the use of tangential ports.[274]

Dose. As might be expected, the dose of radiation administered is also important in determining the presence and severity of pneumonitis. Radiologic evidence of pneumonitis seldom occurs with doses less than 30 Gy,[266] is variably present with doses between 30 and 40 Gy, and is almost always present with doses greater than 40 Gy.[266] It is important to remember, however, that there is considerable individual variability in the pulmonary response, and it is impossible to predict in which patient radiologic changes or symptoms will develop.[266,274]

Time and Dose Factor. Because fractionation permits time for repair of sublethal damage between fractions, the effect of radiation on the lung is related less to the total dose than to the rate at which it is delivered.[270] This variable biologic effect of equivalent doses of radiation is related to the total dose absorbed, the number of fractions, and the time elapsed between the first and last treatments.[275] The severity of the radiation effect increases with increased dose per fraction or when the same dose is given over a shorter period.[266]

Previous or Concurrent Therapy. The risk for radiation pneumonitis is increased in patients who have had previous pulmonary irradiation or previous or concurrent chemotherapy[266,274] and in those in whom corticosteroid therapy has been withdrawn.[276] For example, in a study of 328 patients who had breast carcinoma and who received radiotherapy and chemotherapy, symptomatic radiation pneumonitis developed in 11 (3%) as compared with only 6 of 1296 (0.5%) patients who received radiotherapy alone.[277] The risk for pneumonitis is increased when radiation and chemotherapy are administered simultaneously. The term "radiation recall" refers to the development of pneumonitis in a previously irradiated site after the administration of chemotherapeutic agents; it can occur within hours to days of drug administration and can be seen from a few days up to 15 years after radiotherapy.[278,279]

Cellular and Molecular Factors

The molecular basis of radiation-induced pulmonary disease is complex and not completely understood.[280] It is believed that x-rays or gamma rays exert their effects by colliding with and exciting electrons, which in turn generate ion pairs and a variety of free radicals. The latter cause breakage of covalent bonds in both small and large molecules; such damage can be repaired in some instances but may be irreversible, particularly in the presence of oxygen. The resulting molecular changes can lead to significant biochemical, structural, and functional abnormalities in DNA, as well as a variety of non-DNA macromolecules contained in the cell cytoplasm, organelles, and membranes. Damage to the latter group can result in several immediate effects, such as impaired cell membrane integrity and transport of intracellular material; if sufficiently severe, these effects can lead directly to cell death. Such injury may be the mechanism of capillary endothelial and type I epithelial cell damage in early radiation pneumonitis, as reflected by an increase in capillary permeability and the accumulation of intra-alveolar fluid. Increased transudation of fluid and serum proteins into the alveoli may also occur secondary to the increased alveolar surface tension as a consequence of injury to type II pneumocytes and surfactant loss.

Injury to DNA can take several forms, including breaks that are incorrectly repaired, abnormal cross-links, and chromosomal rearrangements. Cells containing such DNA can remain viable and apparently unharmed until they divide, at which time the progeny may die or show functional disturbances. These effects are most evident in capillary endothelial, bronchial epithelial, and alveolar type II cells. The cytologic atypia of type II pneumocytes in radiation pneumonitis presumably reflects this genetic damage.

The precise pathogenesis of the delayed pulmonary fibrosis that occurs after irradiation is unclear. However, there is experimental evidence that it may be the result of endothelial damage (which causes an alteration in the normal endothelial-fibroblast interaction[281]) or cytokine production and release by pulmonary macrophages.[282] It is possible that the involvement of lung tissue outside the radiation field in acute radiation pneumonitis may be the result of a delayed hypersensitivity reaction in response to a radiation-damaged antigen.[282,283]

Pathologic Characteristics

The histologic reaction in acute radiation pneumonitis is that of diffuse alveolar damage (Fig. 18–9) and consists of an exudate of proteinaceous material in the alveolar air spaces associated with hyaline membranes in the alveolar ducts and respiratory bronchioles.[284] The parenchymal interstitium is thickened by congested capillaries, edema, and, with time, fibroblasts and loose connective tissue; an inflammatory

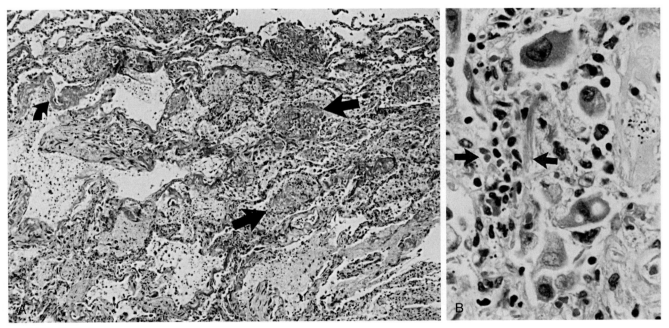

FIGURE 18–9

Acute radiation pneumonitis. A section of lung parenchyma (**A**) from the upper lobe of a patient treated 3 months before death with radiotherapy for breast carcinoma reveals extensive air space filling by a proteinaceous exudate (*straight arrows*), mild interstitial thickening, and focal hyaline membrane formation (*curved arrow*). A magnified view (**B**) shows a mononuclear inflammatory infiltrate in the alveolar septal interstitium (*between arrows*) and several irregularly shaped type II pneumocytes that have hyperchromatic and cytologically atypical nuclei. (*From Fraser RS, Müller NL, Colman NC, Paré PD: Fraser and Paré's Diagnosis of Diseases of the Chest, 4th ed. Philadelphia, WB Saunders, 1999.*)

cellular infiltrate is usually minimal. Type II cells are hyperplastic and often have large nuclei that are sometimes bizarre in shape (see Fig. 18–9).

The fibrotic stage is characterized by fibrosis of the parenchymal air spaces and interstitium (see Color Fig. 18–1) that may be so severe that the underlying architecture is difficult to identify; an increased number plus fragmentation of elastic fibers is common. Although airways can appear unaffected, bronchiolitis obliterans and (occasionally) endobronchial fibrosis are present. Vessels often show intimal thickening as a result of proliferation of myofibroblasts and deposition of connective tissue[285]; focal medial hyalinization and intimal foam cells may also be seen.

Radiologic Manifestations

Radiographic evidence of acute radiation pneumonitis usually becomes evident about 8 weeks after completion of radiotherapy with doses of 40 Gy and about 1 week earlier for every additional 10-Gy increment.[266] Abnormalities are generally most marked 3 to 4 months after completion of radiotherapy; they are rarely seen immediately after its completion and occasionally within 1 to 4 weeks.

The radiographic manifestations may be subtle, consisting of hazy ground-glass opacities with slight indistinctness of the pulmonary vessels, or more marked, consisting of patchy or homogeneous air space consolidation (Fig. 18–10).[274,286] Air bronchograms are commonly present. The abnormalities usually have sharp boundaries, corresponding to the radiation

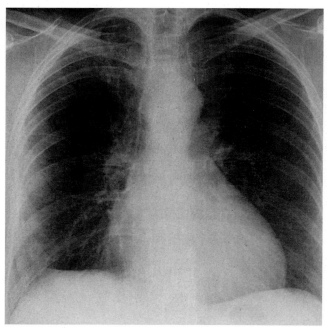

FIGURE 18–10

Acute radiation pneumonitis. A posteroanterior chest radiograph shows areas of consolidation with poorly defined margins in the axillary portion of the right lung. The patient was a 54-year-old woman who had undergone radiotherapy for carcinoma of the right breast 6 weeks previously. *(Courtesy of Dr. Jackie Morgan-Parkes, British Columbia Cancer Agency, Vancouver.)*

portals, and cross normal anatomic structures without segmental or lobar distribution. Typically, there is considerable loss of volume, presumably as a result of a surfactant deficit and adhesive atelectasis. Occasionally, mild abnormalities are seen beyond the radiation ports (Fig. 18–11). In a few patients, areas of consolidation initially limited to the radiation field spread to involve both lungs[287]; lung biopsy performed in some of these patients has shown organizing pneumonia (COP). The complication generally occurs 6 weeks to 10 months after radiation therapy and frequently relapses.[288]

Evidence of acute radiation pneumonitis is seen more commonly and up to 8 weeks earlier on CT scans than on radiographs.[289] The findings consist of homogeneous areas of ground-glass attenuation or patchy or diffuse consolidation involving the radiated portions of the lungs; well-defined borders conforming to the shape of the radiation portals are usually present (Fig. 18–12).[289,290] In a few cases, areas of consolidation within the radiated lung are patchy in distribution and do not conform to the shape of the radiation portal; occasionally, they extend beyond the radiation portals. Other characteristic findings include air bronchograms, loss of volume, and extension across normal anatomic boundaries.

The late or chronic stage of radiation damage is characterized by evidence of fibrosis (Fig. 18–13). Typically, this stage starts after 3 to 4 months, develops gradually, and becomes stable 9 to 12 months after completion of radiotherapy.[266] The affected lung shows severe loss of volume with obliteration of all normal architectural markings. Dense fibrotic strands frequently extend from the hilum to the periphery. Occasionally, the radiographic findings are subtle and consist only of mild elevation of one or both hila, retraction of pulmonary vessels, or pleural thickening.[266] The CT findings consist of dense consolidation or linear strands conforming to the radiation portals and associated with volume loss, architectural distortion, and bronchial dilation (traction bronchiectasis) (Fig. 18–14).[266,286]

Pleural effusions are seldom seen on the chest radiograph during acute radiation pneumonitis,[291] although small effusions are commonly detected on CT.[266] Other pleural complications include spontaneous pneumothorax (in patients with pulmonary carcinoma and thin-walled cavities)[292] and bronchopleural fistula (related to necrosis of a postlobectomy or pneumonectomy stump).[286] Some degree of pleural thickening, occasionally extensive, develops in most patients who have radiation-induced pulmonary fibrosis.[293]

Clinical Manifestations

Many patients who have radiographic evidence of radiation damage remain symptom free. When symptoms do develop, they usually appear between 2 and 3 months after the completion of therapy; occasionally, they arise as late as 6 months and rarely during the first month. Discontinuation of corticosteroids in patients receiving combined steroid therapy and radiotherapy can precipitate severe symptoms.[276] Symptoms generally have an insidious onset and consist of nonproductive cough, weakness, and shortness of breath on exertion.

Acute radiation pneumonitis may persist for 1 month and can resolve completely or progress to fibrosis. The latter develops in most patients who receive therapeutic doses of

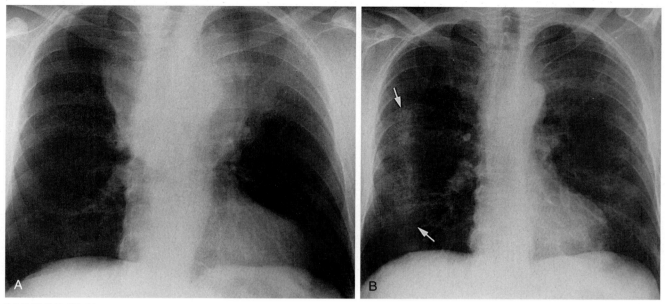

FIGURE 18–11

Acute radiation pneumonitis. A posteroanterior chest radiograph (**A**) before radiotherapy for Hodgkin's lymphoma demonstrates widening of the mediastinum. A chest radiograph 5 weeks later (**B**) shows consolidation in the right lung (*arrows*). The consolidation resolved slowly over the following months. The diagnosis of radiation pneumonitis outside the radiation ports was made clinically. *(Courtesy of Dr. Jackie Morgan-Parkes, British Columbia Cancer Agency, Vancouver.)*

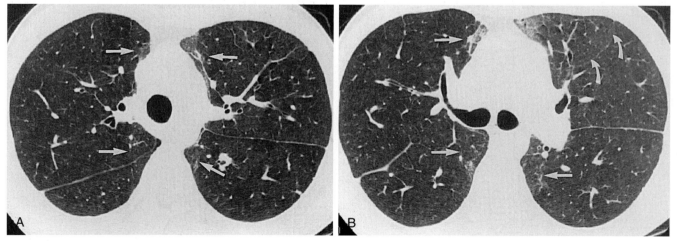

FIGURE 18–12

Acute radiation pneumonitis. HRCT scans (**A** and **B**) demonstrate areas of ground-glass attenuation (*straight arrows*) in the paramediastinal regions of both lungs. Focal extension of radiation pneumonitis outside the radiation portal (*curved arrows*) is evident in the anterior aspect of the left upper lobe. The patient was a 37-year-old man who had completed a course of radiotherapy for Hodgkin's lymphoma 2 months previously. *(From Fraser RS, Müller NL, Colman NC, Paré PD: Fraser and Paré's Diagnosis of Diseases of the Chest, 4th ed. Philadelphia, WB Saunders, 1999.)*

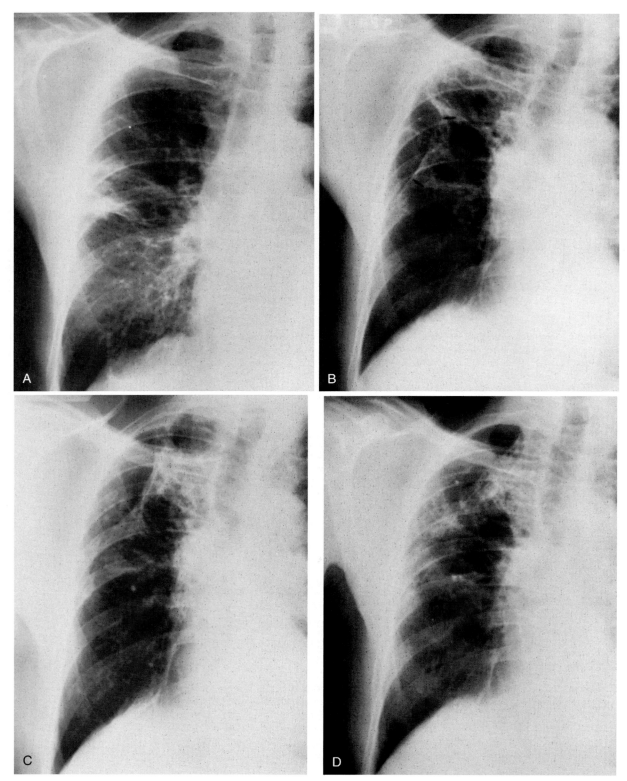

FIGURE 18–13

Progressive cicatrization atelectasis after radiation pneumonitis manifested by migration of a bulla. Several months after completion of a course of radiotherapy to the right hemithorax for inoperable pulmonary carcinoma, a radiograph (**A**) of this 66-year-old man reveals some loss of volume of the right lung and a few patchy opacities in the axillary portion of the right upper lobe. Almost 1.5 years later (**B**), the loss of volume is more severe, and a well-circumscribed cystic space has developed in the axillary portion of the right lung (*arrows*) that proved to be a bulla. Three months later (**C**), the bulla has enlarged somewhat and has migrated superiorly in response to progressive fibrosis of the right upper lobe. An additional 3 months later (**D**), the bulla occupies the apical zone of the right hemithorax. *(From Fraser RS, Müller NL, Colman NC, Paré PD: Fraser and Paré's Diagnosis of Diseases of the Chest, 4th ed. Philadelphia, WB Saunders, 1999.)*

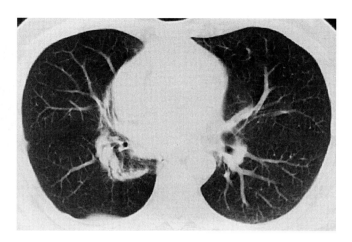

FIGURE 18–14

Radiation fibrosis. A 7-mm-collimation spiral CT scan demonstrates a sharply marginated area of ground-glass attenuation associated with linear opacities and air bronchograms. Focal pleural thickening is also evident. This 47-year-old man had undergone thymectomy and radiotherapy for invasive thymoma 4 years previously. *(From Fraser RS, Müller NL, Colman NC, Paré PD: Fraser and Paré's Diagnosis of Diseases of the Chest, 4th ed. Philadelphia, WB Saunders, 1999.)*

radiation and may be seen in patients who have had no radiographic evidence of acute radiation pneumonitis.[266] With the onset of fibrosis, symptoms of the acute pneumonitis abate gradually. In a few patients, fibrosis develops insidiously without an acute phase being recognized.

Complications of brachytherapy include mucosal fibrosis with bronchostenosis, localized radiation pneumonitis, bronchoesophageal fistula, and hemoptysis.[272,294] The latter has been reported to be fatal in 5% to 10% of cases.[272,295]

REFERENCES

1. Rosenow EC 3rd: Drug-induced pulmonary disease. Dis Mon 40:253-310, 1994.
2. Aronchick JM, Gefter WB: Drug-induced pulmonary disorders. Semin Roentgenol 30:18-34, 1995.
3. Jules-Elysee K, White DA: Bleomycin-induced pulmonary toxicity. Clin Chest Med 11:1-20, 1990.
4. Cooper JA Jr, White DA, Matthay RA: Drug-induced pulmonary disease. Part 1: Cytotoxic drugs. Am Rev Respir Dis 133:321-340, 1986.
5. Yousem SA, Lifson JD, Colby TV: Chemotherapy-induced eosinophilic pneumonia. Relation to bleomycin. Chest 88:103-106, 1985.
6. Sleijfer S: Bleomycin-induced pneumonitis. Chest 120:617-624, 2001.
7. Blum RH, Carter SK, Agre K: A clinical review of bleomycin—a new antineoplastic agent. Cancer 31:903-914, 1973.
8. Snyder LS, Hertz MI: Cytotoxic drug–induced lung injury. Semin Respir Infect 3:217-228, 1988.
9. Waid-Jones MI, Coursin DB: Perioperative considerations for patients treated with bleomycin. Chest 99:993-999, 1991.
10. Ngan HY, Liang RH, Lam WK, et al: Pulmonary toxicity in patients with non-Hodgkin's lymphoma treated with bleomycin-containing combination chemotherapy. Cancer Chemother Pharmacol 32:407-409, 1993.
11. Hirsch A, Vander Els N, Straus DJ, et al: Effect of ABVD chemotherapy with and without mantle or mediastinal irradiation on pulmonary function and symptoms in early-stage Hodgkin's disease. J Clin Oncol 14:1297-1305, 1996.
12. O'Sullivan JM, Huddart RA, Norman AR, et al: Predicting the risk of bleomycin lung toxicity in patients with germ-cell tumours. Ann Oncol 14:91-96, 2003.
13. Cantin AM, Hubbard RC, Crystal RG: Glutathione deficiency in the epithelial lining fluid of the lower respiratory tract in idiopathic pulmonary fibrosis. Am Rev Respir Dis 139:370-372, 1989.
14. Ingrassia TS 3rd, Ryu JH, Trastek VF, et al: Oxygen-exacerbated bleomycin pulmonary toxicity. Mayo Clin Proc 66:173-178, 1991.
15. Berend N: Protective effect of hypoxia on bleomycin lung toxicity in the rat. Am Rev Respir Dis 130:307-308, 1984.
16. Hagiwara SI, Ishii Y, Kitamura S: Aerosolized administration of N-acetylcysteine attenuates lung fibrosis induced by bleomycin in mice. Am J Respir Crit Care Med 162:225-231, 2000.
17. Howell DC, Goldsack NR, Marshall RP, et al: Direct thrombin inhibition reduces lung collagen, accumulation, and connective tissue growth factor mRNA levels in bleomycin-induced pulmonary fibrosis. Am J Pathol 159:1383-1395, 2001.
18. Marshall RP, Gohlke P, Chambers RC, et al: Angiotensin II and the fibroproliferative response to acute lung injury. Am J Physiol Lung Cell Mol Physiol 286:L156-L164, 2004.
19. Takahashi F, Takahashi K, Okazaki T, et al: Role of osteopontin in the pathogenesis of bleomycin-induced pulmonary fibrosis. Am J Respir Cell Mol Biol 24:264-271, 2001.
20. Sato N, Suzuki Y, Nishio K, et al: Roles of ICAM-1 for abnormal leukocyte recruitment in the microcirculation of bleomycin-induced fibrotic lung injury. Am J Respir Crit Care Med 161:1681-1688, 2000.
21. Balikian JP, Jochelson MS, Bauer KA, et al: Pulmonary complications of chemotherapy regimens containing bleomycin. AJR Am J Roentgenol 139:455-461, 1982.
22. Iacovino JR, Leitner J, Abbas AK, et al: Fatal pulmonary reaction from low doses of bleomycin. An idiosyncratic tissue response. JAMA 235:1253-1255, 1976.
23. Samuels ML, Johnson DE, Holoye PY, et al: Large-dose bleomycin therapy and pulmonary toxicity. A possible role of prior radiotherapy. JAMA 235:1117-1120, 1976.
24. McCrea ES, Diaconis JN, Wade JC, et al: Bleomycin toxicity simulating metastatic nodules to the lungs. Cancer 48:1096-1100, 1981.
25. Padley SP, Adler B, Hansell DM, et al: High-resolution computed tomography of drug-induced lung disease. Clin Radiol 46:232-236, 1992.
26. Bellamy EA, Husband JE, Blaquiere RM, et al: Bleomycin-related lung damage: CT evidence. Radiology 156:155-158, 1985.
27. White DA, Schwartzberg LS, Kris MG, et al: Acute chest pain syndrome during bleomycin infusions. Cancer 59:1582-1585, 1987.
28. White DA, Stover DE: Severe bleomycin-induced pneumonitis. Clinical features and response to corticosteroids. Chest 86:723-728, 1984.
29. Van Barneveld PW, Sleijfer DT, van der Mark TW, et al: Natural course of bleomycin-induced pneumonitis. A follow-up study. Am Rev Respir Dis 135:48-51, 1987.
30. Wolkowicz J, Sturgeon J, Rawji M, et al: Bleomycin-induced pulmonary function abnormalities. Chest 101:97-101, 1992.
31. Castro M, Veeder MH, Mailliard JA, et al: A prospective study of pulmonary function in patients receiving mitomycin. Chest 109:939-944, 1996.
32. Buzdar AU, Legha SS, Luna MA, et al: Pulmonary toxicity of mitomycin. Cancer 45:236-244, 1980.
33. Orwoll ES, Kiessling PJ, Patterson JR: Interstitial pneumonia from mitomycin. Ann Intern Med 89:352-355, 1978.
34. Linette DC, McGee KH, McFarland JA: Mitomycin-induced pulmonary toxicity: Case report and review of the literature. Ann Pharmacother 26:481-484, 1992.
35. Twohig KJ, Matthay RA: Pulmonary effects of cytotoxic agents other than bleomycin. Clin Chest Med 11:31-54, 1990.
36. Thomas P, Pradal M, Le Caer H, et al: [Acute bronchospasm due to periwinkle alkaloid and mitomycin association.] Rev Mal Respir 10:268-270, 1993.
37. Rosenow EC 3rd, Limper AH: Drug-induced pulmonary disease. Semin Respir Infect 10:86-95, 1995.
38. Torra R, Poch E, Torras A, et al: Pulmonary hemorrhage as a clinical manifestation of hemolytic-uremic syndrome associated with mitomycin C therapy. Chemotherapy 39:453-456, 1993.
39. Lund MB, Kongerud J, Brinch L, et al: Decreased lung function in one year survivors of allogeneic bone marrow transplantation conditioned with high-dose busulphan and cyclophosphamide. Eur Respir J 8:1269-1274, 1995.
40. Heard BE, Cooke RA: Busulphan lung. Thorax 23:187-193, 1968.
41. Ginsberg SJ, Comis RL: The pulmonary toxicity of antineoplastic agents. Semin Oncol 9:34-51, 1982.
42. Soble AR, Perry H: Fatal radiation pneumonia following subclinical busulfan injury. AJR Am J Roentgenol 128:15-18, 1977.
43. Bilgrami SF, Metersky ML, McNally D, et al: Idiopathic pneumonia syndrome following myeloablative chemotherapy and autologous transplantation. Ann Pharmacother 35:196-201, 2001.
44. Burns WA, McFarland W, Matthews MJ: Busulfan-induced pulmonary disease. Report of a case and review of the literature. Am Rev Respir Dis 101:408-413, 1970.
45. Smalley RV, Wall RL: Two cases of busulfan toxicity. Ann Intern Med 64:154-164, 1966.
46. Harrold BP: Syndrome resembling Addison's disease following prolonged treatment with busulphan. BMJ 5485:463-464, 1966.
47. Littler WA, Ogilvie C: Lung function in patients receiving busulphan. BMJ 4:530-532, 1970.
48. Rosenow EC 3rd, Myers JL, Swensen SJ, et al: Drug-induced pulmonary disease. An update. Chest 102:239-250, 1992.
49. Mileshkin L, Prince HM, Rischin D, et al: Severe interstitial pneumonitis following high-dose cyclophosphamide, thiotepa and docetaxel: Two case reports and a review of the literature. Bone Marrow Transplant 27:559-563, 2001.
50. Malik SW, Myers JL, DeRemee RA, et al: Lung toxicity associated with cyclophosphamide use. Two distinct patterns. Am J Respir Crit Care Med 154:1851-1856, 1996.
51. Spector JI, Zimbler H, Ross JS: Early-onset cyclophosphamide-induced interstitial pneumonitis. JAMA 242:2852-2854, 1979.

52. Alvarado CS, Boat TF, Newman AJ: Late-onset pulmonary fibrosis and chest deformity in two children treated with cyclophosphamide. J Pediatr 92:443-446, 1978.
53. Batist G, Andrews JL Jr: Pulmonary toxicity of antineoplastic drugs. JAMA 246:1449-1453, 1981.
54. Cherniack RM, Abrams J, Kalica AR: NHLBI Workshop summary. Pulmonary disease associated with breast cancer therapy. Am J Respir Crit Care Med 150:1169-1173, 1994.
55. Rubio C, Hill ME, Milan S, et al: Idiopathic pneumonia syndrome after high-dose chemotherapy for relapsed Hodgkin's disease. Br J Cancer 75:1044-1048, 1997.
56. Wu M, Kelley MR, Hansen WK, et al: Reduction of BCNU toxicity to lung cells by high-level expression of O(6)-methylguanine-DNA methyltransferase. Am J Physiol Lung Cell Mol Physiol 280:L755-L761, 2001.
57. Abushamaa AM, Sporn TA, Folz RJ: Oxidative stress and inflammation contribute to lung toxicity after a common breast cancer chemotherapy regimen. Am J Physiol Lung Cell Mol Physiol 283:L336-L345, 2002.
58. Todd NW, Peters WP, Ost AH, et al: Pulmonary drug toxicity in patients with primary breast cancer treated with high-dose combination chemotherapy and autologous bone marrow transplantation. Am Rev Respir Dis 147:1264-1270, 1993.
59. Wong R, Rondon G, Saliba RM, et al: Idiopathic pneumonia syndrome after high-dose chemotherapy and autologous hematopoietic stem cell transplantation for high-risk breast cancer. Bone Marrow Transplant 31:1157-1163, 2003.
60. Jones RB, Matthes S, Shpall EJ, et al: Acute lung injury following treatment with high-dose cyclophosphamide, cisplatin, and carmustine: Pharmacodynamic evaluation of carmustine. J Natl Cancer Inst 85:640-647, 1993.
61. Durant JR, Norgard MJ, Murad TM, et al: Pulmonary toxicity associated with bis-chloroethylnitrosourea (BCNU). Ann Intern Med 90:191-194, 1979.
62. Cao TM, Negrin RS, Stockerl-Goldstein KE, et al: Pulmonary toxicity syndrome in breast cancer patients undergoing BCNU-containing high-dose chemotherapy and autologous hematopoietic cell transplantation. Biol Blood Marrow Transplant 6:387-394, 2000.
63. Melato M, Tuveri G: Pulmonary fibrosis following low-dose 1,3-bis(2-chloroethyl)-1-nitrosourea (BCNU) therapy. Cancer 45:1311-1314, 1980.
64. Holoye PY, Jenkins DE, Greenberg SD: Pulmonary toxicity in long-term administration of BCNU. Cancer Treat Rep 60:1691-1694, 1976.
65. O'Driscoll BR, Hasleton PS, Taylor PM, et al: Active lung fibrosis up to 17 years after chemotherapy with carmustine (BCNU) in childhood. N Engl J Med 323:378-382, 1990.
66. Demeter SL, Ahmad M, Tomashefski JF: Drug-induced pulmonary disease. Part I. Patterns of response. Cleve Clin Q 46:89-99, 1979.
67. Alessandrino EP, Bernasconi P, Colombo A, et al: Pulmonary toxicity following carmustine-based preparative regimens and autologous peripheral blood progenitor cell transplantation in hematological malignancies. Bone Marrow Transplant 25:309-313, 2000.
68. Rao SX, Ramaswamy G, Levin M, et al: Fatal acute respiratory failure after vinblastine-mitomycin therapy in lung carcinoma. Arch Intern Med 145:1905-1907, 1985.
69. Konits PH, Aisner J, Sutherland JC, et al: Possible pulmonary toxicity secondary to vinblastine. Cancer 50:2771-2774, 1982.
70. Rivera MP, Kris MG, Gralla RJ, et al: Syndrome of acute dyspnea related to combined mitomycin plus vinca alkaloid chemotherapy. Am J Clin Oncol 18:245-250, 1995.
71. Luedke D, McLaughlin TT, Daughaday C, et al: Mitomycin C and vindesine associated pulmonary toxicity with variable clinical expression. Cancer 55:542-545, 1985.
72. Figueredo AT, Jones G, Kay MJ, et al: Kaposi's sarcoma of the lung—remission followed by fatal pneumonitis after vinblastine and thoracic irradiation. Acta Oncol 34:532-533, 1995.
73. Fuhrman C, Parrot A, Wislez M, et al: Spectrum of CD4 to CD8 T-cell ratios in lymphocytic alveolitis associated with methotrexate-induced pneumonitis. Am J Respir Crit Care Med 164:1186-1191, 2001.
74. Bedrossian CW, Miller WC, Luna MA: Methotrexate-induced diffuse interstitial pulmonary fibrosis. South Med J 72:313-318, 1979.
75. Salaffi F, Manganelli P, Carotti M, et al: Methotrexate-induced pneumonitis in patients with rheumatoid arthritis and psoriatic arthritis: Report of five cases and review of the literature. Clin Rheumatol 16:296-304, 1997.
76. Gillespie AM, Lorigan PC, Radstone CR, et al: Pulmonary function in patients with trophoblastic disease treated with low-dose methotrexate. Br J Cancer 76:1382-1386, 1997.
77. Schnabel A, Richter C, Bauerfeind S, et al: Bronchoalveolar lavage cell profile in methotrexate induced pneumonitis. Thorax 52:377-379, 1997.
78. Golden MR, Katz RS, Balk RA, et al: The relationship of preexisting lung disease to the development of methotrexate pneumonitis in patients with rheumatoid arthritis. J Rheumatol 22:1043-1047, 1995.
79. Alarcon GS, Kremer JM, Macaluso M, et al: Risk factors for methotrexate-induced lung injury in patients with rheumatoid arthritis. A multicenter, case-control study. Methotrexate-Lung Study Group. Ann Intern Med 127:356-364, 1997.
80. Leduc D, De Vuyst P, Lheureux P, et al: Pneumonitis complicating low-dose methotrexate therapy for rheumatoid arthritis. Discrepancies between lung biopsy and bronchoalveolar lavage findings. Chest 104:1620-1623, 1993.
81. Bernstein ML, Sobel DB, Wimmer RS: Noncardiogenic pulmonary edema following injection of methotrexate into the cerebrospinal fluid. Cancer 50:866-868, 1982.
82. Everts CS, Westcott JL, Bragg DG: Methotrexate therapy and pulmonary disease. Radiology 107:539-543, 1973.
83. Sostman HD, Matthay RA, Putman CE, et al: Methotrexate-induced pneumonitis. Medicine (Baltimore) 55:371-388, 1976.

84. Arakawa H, Yamasaki M, Kurihara Y, et al: Methotrexate-induced pulmonary injury: Serial CT findings. J Thorac Imaging 18:231-236, 2003.
85. Akira M, Ishikawa H, Yamamoto S: Drug-induced pneumonitis: Thin-section CT findings in 60 patients. Radiology 224:852-860, 2002.
86. Imokawa S, Colby TV, Leslie KO, et al: Methotrexate pneumonitis: Review of the literature and histopathological findings in nine patients. Eur Respir J 15:373-381, 2000.
87. Barrera P, Laan RF, van Riel PL, et al: Methotrexate-related pulmonary complications in rheumatoid arthritis. Ann Rheum Dis 53:434-439, 1994.
88. St Clair EW, Rice JR, Snyderman R: Pneumonitis complicating low-dose methotrexate therapy in rheumatoid arthritis. Arch Intern Med 145:2035-2038, 1985.
89. Cottin V, Tebib J, Massonnet B, et al: Pulmonary function in patients receiving long-term low-dose methotrexate. Chest 109:933-938, 1996.
90. Kuitert LM, Harrison AC: Pneumocystis carinii pneumonia as a complication of methotrexate treatment of asthma. Thorax 46:936-937, 1991.
91. Law KF, Aranda CP, Smith RL, et al: Pulmonary cryptococcosis mimicking methotrexate pneumonitis. J Rheumatol 20:872-873, 1993.
92. Kremer JM, Alarcon GS, Weinblatt ME, et al: Clinical, laboratory, radiographic, and histopathologic features of methotrexate-associated lung injury in patients with rheumatoid arthritis: A multicenter study with literature review. Arthritis Rheum 40:1829-1837, 1997.
93. Shearer P, Katz J, Bozeman P, et al: Pulmonary insufficiency complicating therapy with high dose cytosine arabinoside in five pediatric patients with relapsed acute myelogenous leukemia. Cancer 74:1953-1958, 1994.
94. Kumar M, Saleh A, Rao PV, et al: Toxicity associated with high-dose cytosine arabinoside and total body irradiation as conditioning for allogeneic bone marrow transplantation. Bone Marrow Transplant 19:1061-1064, 1997.
95. Andersson BS, Luna MA, Yee C, et al: Fatal pulmonary failure complicating high-dose cytosine arabinoside therapy in acute leukemia. Cancer 65:1079-1084, 1990.
96. Chiche D, Pico JL, Bernaudin JF, et al: Pulmonary edema and shock after high-dose aracytosine-C for lymphoma; possible role of TNF-alpha and PAF. Eur Cytokine Netw 4:147-151, 1993.
97. Tham RT, Peters WG, de Bruine FT, et al: Pulmonary complications of cytosine-arabinoside therapy: Radiographic findings. AJR Am J Roentgenol 149:23-27, 1987.
98. Hui YF, Reitz J: Gemcitabine: A cytidine analogue active against solid tumors. Am J Health Syst Pharm 54:162-170, quiz 197-198, 1997.
99. Pavlakis N, Bell DR, Millward MJ, et al: Fatal pulmonary toxicity resulting from treatment with gemcitabine. Cancer 80:286-291, 1997.
100. Marruchella A, Fiorenzano G, Merizzi A, et al: Diffuse alveolar damage in a patient treated with gemcitabine. Eur Respir J 11:504-506, 1998.
101. Saway PA, Heck LW, Bonner JR, et al: Azathioprine hypersensitivity. Case report and review of the literature. Am J Med 84:960-964, 1988.
102. Bedrossian CW, Sussman J, Conklin RH, et al: Azathioprine-associated interstitial pneumonitis. Am J Clin Pathol 82:148-154, 1984.
103. Weisenburger DD: Interstitial pneumonitis associated with azathioprine therapy. Am J Clin Pathol 69:181-185, 1978.
104. Stetter M, Schmidl M, Krapf R: Azathioprine hypersensitivity mimicking Goodpasture's syndrome. Am J Kidney Dis 23:874-877, 1994.
105. Helman DL Jr, Byrd JC, Ales NC, et al: Fludarabine-related pulmonary toxicity: A distinct clinical entity in chronic lymphoproliferative syndromes. Chest 122:785-790, 2002.
106. Byrd JC, Hargis JB, Kester KE, et al: Opportunistic pulmonary infections with fludarabine in previously treated patients with low-grade lymphoid malignancies: A role for Pneumocystis carinii pneumonia prophylaxis. Am J Hematol 49:135-142, 1995.
107. Vogelzang PJ, Bloom SM, Mier JW, et al: Chest roentgenographic abnormalities in IL-2 recipients. Incidence and correlation with clinical parameters. Chest 101:746-752, 1992.
108. Briasoulis E, Pavlidis N: Noncardiogenic pulmonary edema: An unusual and serious complication of anticancer therapy. Oncologist 6:153-161, 2001.
109. Berthiaume Y, Boiteau P, Fick G, et al: Pulmonary edema during IL-2 therapy: Combined effect of increased permeability and hydrostatic pressure. Am J Respir Crit Care Med 152:329-335, 1995.
110. Seebach J, Speich R, Fehr J, et al: GM-CSF–induced acute eosinophilic pneumonia. Br J Haematol 90:963-965, 1995.
111. Kreisman H, Wolkove N: Pulmonary toxicity of antineoplastic therapy. Semin Oncol 19:508-520, 1992.
112. Azoulay E, Attalah H, Harf A, et al: Granulocyte colony-stimulating factor or neutrophil-induced pulmonary toxicity: Myth or reality? Systematic review of clinical case reports and experimental data. Chest 120:1695-1701, 2001.
113. Bini EJ, Weinshel EH: Severe exacerbation of asthma: A new side effect of interferon-alpha in patients with asthma and chronic hepatitis C. Mayo Clin Proc 74:367-370, 1999.
114. Rubinowitz AN, Naidich DP, Alinsonorin C: Interferon-induced sarcoidosis. J Comput Assist Tomogr 27:279-283, 2003.
115. Kumar KS, Russo MW, Borczuk AC, et al: Significant pulmonary toxicity associated with interferon and ribavirin therapy for hepatitis C. Am J Gastroenterol 97:2432-2440, 2002.
116. Cutuli B, Petit JC, Fricker JP, et al: [Thromboembolic accidents in postmenopausal patients with adjuvant treatment by tamoxifen. Frequency, risk factors and prevention possibilities.] Bull Cancer 82:51-56, 1995.
117. Cummings SR, Eckert S, Krueger KA, et al: The effect of raloxifene on risk of breast cancer in postmenopausal women: Results from the MORE randomized trial. Multiple Outcomes of Raloxifene Evaluation. JAMA 281:2189-2197, 1999.

118. Meier CR, Jick H: Tamoxifen and risk of idiopathic venous thromboembolism. Br J Clin Pharmacol 45:608-612, 1998.
119. Seigneur J, Trechot PF, Hubert J, et al: Pulmonary complications of hormone treatment in prostate carcinoma. Chest 93:1106, 1988.
120. Jick SS, Jick H, Walker AM, et al: Hospitalizations for pulmonary reactions following nitrofurantoin use. Chest 96:512-515, 1989.
121. Holmberg L, Boman G, Bottiger LE, et al: Adverse reactions to nitrofurantoin. Analysis of 921 reports. Am J Med 69:733-738, 1980.
122. Suntres ZE, Shek PN: Nitrofurantoin-induced pulmonary toxicity. In vivo evidence for oxidative stress–mediated mechanisms. Biochem Pharmacol 43:1127-1135, 1992.
123. Simonian SJ, Kroeker EJ, Boyd DP: Chronic interstitial pneumonitis with fibrosis after long-term therapy with nitrofurantoin. Ann Thorac Surg 24:284-288, 1977.
124. Bone RC, Wolfe J, Sobonya RE, et al: Desquamative interstitial pneumonia following long-term nitrofurantoin therapy. Am J Med 60:697-701, 1976.
125. Cameron RJ, Kolbe J, Wilsher ML, et al: Bronchiolitis obliterans organising pneumonia associated with the use of nitrofurantoin. Thorax 55:249-251, 2000.
126. Ngan H, Millard RJ, Lant AF, et al: Nitrofurantoin lung. Br J Radiol 44:21-23, 1971.
127. Holmberg L, Boman G: Pulmonary reactions to nitrofurantoin. 447 cases reported to the Swedish Adverse Drug Reaction Committee 1966-1976. Eur J Respir Dis 62:180-189, 1981.
128. Cleverley JR, Screaton NJ, Hiorns MP, et al: Drug-induced lung disease: High-resolution CT and histological findings. Clin Radiol 57:292-299, 2002.
129. Sheehan RE, Wells AU, Milne DG, et al: Nitrofurantoin-induced lung disease: Two cases demonstrating resolution of apparently irreversible CT abnormalities. J Comput Assist Tomogr 24:259-261, 2000.
130. Ellis SJ, Cleverley JR, Müller NL: Drug-induced lung disease: High-resolution CT findings. AJR Am J Roentgenol 175:1019-1024, 2000.
131. Lee NK, Slavin JD Jr, Spencer RP: Ventilation-perfusion lung imaging in nitrofurantoin-related pulmonary reaction. Clin Nucl Med 17:94-96, 1992.
132. Geller M, Flaherty DK, Dickie HA, et al: Lymphopenia in acute nitrofurantoin pleuropulmonary reactions. J Allergy Clin Immunol 59:445-448, 1977.
133. Taskinen E, Tukiainen P, Sovijarvi AR: Nitrofurantoin-induced alterations in pulmonary tissue. A report on five patients with acute or subacute reactions. Acta Pathol Microbiol Scand [A] 85:713-720, 1977.
134. Parry SD, Barbatzas C, Peel ET, et al: Sulphasalazine and lung toxicity. Eur Respir J 19:756-764, 2002.
135. Hamadeh MA, Atkinson J, Smith LJ: Sulfasalazine-induced pulmonary disease. Chest 101:1033-1037, 1992.
136. Gabazza EC, Taguchi O, Yamakami T, et al: Pulmonary infiltrates and skin pigmentation associated with sulfasalazine. Am J Gastroenterol 87:1654-1657, 1992.
137. Kolbe J, Caughey D, Rainer S: Sulphasalazine-induced sub-acute hyper-sensitivity pneumonitis. Respir Med 88:149-152, 1994.
138. Rossi SE, Erasmus JJ, McAdams HP, et al: Pulmonary drug toxicity: Radiologic and pathologic manifestations. Radiographics 20:1245-1259, 2000.
139. Camus P, Piard F, Ashcroft T, et al: The lung in inflammatory bowel disease. Medicine (Baltimore) 72:151-183, 1993.
140. Yaffe BH, Korelitz BI: Sulfasalazine pneumonia. Am J Gastroenterol 78:493-494, 1983.
141. Cooper JA Jr, White DA, Matthay RA: Drug-induced pulmonary disease. Part 2: Noncytotoxic drugs. Am Rev Respir Dis 133:488-505, 1986.
142. Ho D, Tashkin DP, Bein ME, et al: Pulmonary infiltrates with eosinophilia associated with tetracycline. Chest 76:33-36, 1979.
143. Oddo M, Liaudet L, Lepori M, et al: Relapsing acute respiratory failure induced by minocycline. Chest 123:2146-2148, 2003.
144. Guillon JM, Joly P, Autran B, et al: Minocycline-induced cell-mediated hypersensitivity pneumonitis. Ann Intern Med 117:476-481, 1992.
145. Dykhuizen RS, Zaidi AM, Godden DJ, et al: Minocycline and pulmonary eosinophilia. BMJ 310:1520-1521, 1995.
146. Sitbon O, Bidel N, Dussopt C, et al: Minocycline pneumonitis and eosinophilia. A report on eight patients. Arch Intern Med 154:1633-1640, 1994.
147. Dussopt C, Mornex JF, Cordier JF, et al: [Acute eosinophilic lung after a course of minocycline.] Rev Mal Respir 11:67-70, 1994.
148. Martin WJ 2nd, Rosenow EC 3rd: Amiodarone pulmonary toxicity. Recognition and pathogenesis (part I). Chest 93:1067-1075, 1988.
149. Baritussio A, Marzini S, Agostini M, et al: Amiodarone inhibits lung degradation of SP-A and perturbs the distribution of lysosomal enzymes. Am J Physiol Lung Cell Mol Physiol 281:L1189-L1199, 2001.
150. Dean PJ, Groshart KD, Porterfield JG, et al: Amiodarone-associated pulmonary toxicity. A clinical and pathologic study of eleven cases. Am J Clin Pathol 87:7-13, 1987.
151. Martin WJ 2nd, Rosenow EC 3rd: Amiodarone pulmonary toxicity. Recognition and pathogenesis (part 2). Chest 93:1242-1248, 1988.
152. Akoun GM, Cadranel JL, Blanchette G, et al: Bronchoalveolar lavage cell data in amiodarone-associated pneumonitis. Evaluation in 22 patients. Chest 99:1177-1182, 1991.
153. Akoun GM, Gauthier-Rahman S, Liote HA, et al: Leukocyte migration inhibition in amiodarone-associated pneumonitis. Chest 94:1050-1053, 1988.
154. Raeder EA, Podrid PJ, Lown B: Side effects and complications of amiodarone therapy. Am Heart J 109:975-983, 1985.
155. Myers JL, Kennedy JI, Plumb VJ: Amiodarone lung: Pathologic findings in clinically toxic patients. Hum Pathol 18:349-354, 1987.
156. Liu FL, Cohen RD, Downar E, et al: Amiodarone pulmonary toxicity: Functional and ultrastructural evaluation. Thorax 41:100-105, 1986.
157. Gefter WB, Epstein DM, Pietra GG, et al: Lung disease caused by amiodarone, a new antiarrhythmic agent. Radiology 147:339-344, 1983.
158. Siniakowicz RM, Narula D, Suster B, et al: Diagnosis of amiodarone pulmonary toxicity with high-resolution computerized tomographic scan. J Cardiovasc Electrophysiol 12:431-436, 2001.
159. Kuhlman JE, Teigen C, Ren H, et al: Amiodarone pulmonary toxicity: CT findings in symptomatic patients. Radiology 177:121-125, 1990.
160. Ren H, Kuhlman JE, Hruban RH, et al: CT-pathology correlation of amiodarone lung. J Comput Assist Tomogr 14:760-765, 1990.
161. Zhu YY, Botvinick E, Dae M, et al: Gallium lung scintigraphy in amiodarone pulmonary toxicity. Chest 93:1126-1131, 1988.
162. Kennedy JI, Myers JL, Plumb VJ, et al: Amiodarone pulmonary toxicity. Clinical, radiologic, and pathologic correlations. Arch Intern Med 147:50-55, 1987.
163. Marchlinski FE, Gansler TS, Waxman HL, et al: Amiodarone pulmonary toxicity. Ann Intern Med 97:839-845, 1982.
164. Cazzadori A, Braggio P, Barbieri E, et al: Amiodarone-induced pulmonary toxicity. Respiration 49:157-160, 1986.
165. Gleadhill IC, Wise RA, Schonfeld SA, et al: Serial lung function testing in patients treated with amiodarone: A prospective study. Am J Med 86:4-10, 1989.
166. Adams GD, Kehoe R, Lesch M, et al: Amiodarone-induced pneumonitis. Assessment of risk factors and possible risk reduction. Chest 93:254-263, 1988.
167. Chendrasekhar A, Barke RA, Druck P: Recurrent amiodarone pulmonary toxicity. South Med J 89:85-86, 1996.
168. Ashrafian H, Davey P: Is amiodarone an underrecognized cause of acute respiratory failure in the ICU? Chest 120:275-282, 2001.
169. Walters JS, Woodring JH, Stelling CB, et al: Salicylate-induced pulmonary edema. Radiology 146:289-293, 1983.
170. Heffner JE, Sahn SA: Salicylate-induced pulmonary edema. Clinical features and prognosis. Ann Intern Med 95:405-409, 1981.
171. Bowers RE, Brigham KL, Owen PJ: Salicylate pulmonary edema: The mechanism in sheep and review of the clinical literature. Am Rev Respir Dis 115:261-268, 1977.
172. Andersen R, Refstad S: Adult respiratory distress syndrome precipitated by massive salicylate poisoning. Intensive Care Med 4:211-213, 1978.
173. Gould DM, Daves ML: A review of roentgen findings in systemic lupus erythematosus (SLE). Am J Med Sci 235:596-610, 1958.
174. Adelman HM, Winters PR, Mahan CS, et al: D-Penicillamine–induced myasthenia gravis: Diagnosis obscured by coexisting chronic obstructive pulmonary disease. Am J Med Sci 309:191-193, 1995.
175. Eastmond CJ: Diffuse alveolitis as complication of penicillamine treatment for rheumatoid arthritis. BMJ 1:1506, 1976.
176. Padley SP, Adler BD, Hansell DM, et al: Bronchiolitis obliterans: High resolution CT findings and correlation with pulmonary function tests. Clin Radiol 47:236-240, 1993.
177. Derk CT, Jimenez SA: Goodpasture-like syndrome induced by D-penicillamine in a patient with systemic sclerosis: Report and review of the literature. J Rheumatol 30:1616-1620, 2003.
178. Davies D, Jones JK: Pulmonary eosinophilia caused by penicillamine. Thorax 35:957-958, 1980.
179. Camus P, Degat OR, Justrabo E, et al: D-Penicillamine–induced severe pneumonitis. Chest 81:376-378, 1982.
180. Zitnik RJ, Cooper JA Jr: Pulmonary disease due to antirheumatic agents. Clin Chest Med 11:139-150, 1990.
181. Morley TF, Komansky HJ, Adelizzi RA, et al: Pulmonary gold toxicity. Eur J Respir Dis 65:627-632, 1984.
182. Partanen J, van Assendelft AH, Koskimies S, et al: Patients with rheumatoid arthritis and gold-induced pneumonitis express two high-risk major histocompatibility complex patterns. Chest 92:277-281, 1987.
183. Winterbauer RH, Wilske KR, Wheelis RF: Diffuse pulmonary injury associated with gold treatment. N Engl J Med 294:919-921, 1976.
184. Nickels J, van Assendelft AH, Tukiainen P: Diffuse pulmonary injury associated with gold treatment. Acta Pathol Microbiol Immunol Scand [A] 91:265-267, 1983.
185. Evans RB, Ettensohn DB, Fawaz-Estrup F, et al: Gold lung: Recent developments in pathogenesis, diagnosis, and therapy. Semin Arthritis Rheum 16:196-205, 1987.
186. Blancas R, Moreno JL, Martin F, et al: Alveolar-interstitial pneumopathy after gold-salts compounds administration, requiring mechanical ventilation. Intensive Care Med 24:1110-1112, 1998.
187. James DW, Whimster WF, Hamilton EB: Gold lung. BMJ 1:1523-1534, 1978.
188. Bader AM, Boudier E, Martinez C, et al: Etiology and prevention of pulmonary complications following beta-mimetic mediated tocolysis. Eur J Obstet Gynecol Reprod Biol 80:133-137, 1998.
189. Nimrod C, Rambihar V, Fallen E, et al: Pulmonary edema associated with isoxsuprine therapy. Am J Obstet Gynecol 148:625-629, 1984.
190. Sporer KA, Dorn E: Heroin-related noncardiogenic pulmonary edema: A case series. Chest 120:1628-1632, 2001.
191. Katz S, Aberman A, Frand UI, et al: Heroin pulmonary edema. Evidence for increased pulmonary capillary permeability. Am Rev Respir Dis 106:472-474, 1972.
192. Snyder SH: Opiate receptors in the brain. N Engl J Med 296:266-271, 1977.
193. Taff RH: Pulmonary edema following naloxone administration in a patient without heart disease. Anesthesiology 59:576-577, 1983.
194. Saba GP 2nd, James AE Jr, Johnson BA, et al: Pulmonary complications of narcotic abuse. Am J Roentgenol Radium Ther Nucl Med 122:733-739, 1974.
195. Heffner JE, Harley RA, Schabel SI: Pulmonary reactions from illicit substance abuse. Clin Chest Med 11:151-162, 1990.
196. Schaaf JT, Spivack ML, Rath GS, et al: Pulmonary edema and adult respiratory distress syndrome following methadone abuse. Am Rev Respir Dis 107:1047-1051, 1973.

197. McCarroll KA, Roszler MH: Lung disorders due to drug abuse. J Thorac Imaging 6:30-35, 1991.

198. Banner AS, Rodriguez J, Sunderrajan EV, et al: Bronchiectasis: A cause of pulmonary symptoms in heroin addicts. Respiration 37:232-237, 1979.

199. Haim DY, Lippmann ML, Goldberg SK, et al: The pulmonary complications of crack cocaine. A comprehensive review. Chest 107:233-240, 1995.

200. Tashkin DP, Khalsa ME, Gorelick D, et al: Pulmonary status of habitual cocaine smokers. Am Rev Respir Dis 145:92-100, 1992.

201. Brody SL, Slovis CM, Wrenn KD: Cocaine-related medical problems: Consecutive series of 233 patients. Am J Med 88:325-331, 1990.

202. Hoffman CK, Goodman PC: Pulmonary edema in cocaine smokers. Radiology 172:463-465, 1989.

203. Murray RJ, Albin RJ, Mergner W, et al: Diffuse alveolar hemorrhage temporally related to cocaine smoking. Chest 93:427-429, 1988.

204. Eurman DW, Potash HI, Eyler WR, et al: Chest pain and dyspnea related to "crack" cocaine smoking: Value of chest radiography. Radiology 172:459-462, 1989.

205. Leitman BS, Greengart A, Wasser HJ: Pneumomediastinum and pneumopericardium after cocaine abuse. AJR Am J Roentgenol 151:614, 1988.

206. Gong H Jr, Fligiel S, Tashkin DP, et al: Tracheobronchial changes in habitual, heavy smokers of marijuana with and without tobacco. Am Rev Respir Dis 136:142-149, 1987.

207. Taylor DR, Hall W: Respiratory health effects of cannabis: Position statement of the Thoracic Society of Australia and New Zealand. Intern Med J 33:310-313, 2003.

208. Taylor DR, Poulton R, Moffitt TE, et al: The respiratory effects of cannabis dependence in young adults. Addiction 95:1669-1677, 2000.

209. Tashkin DP, Simmons MS, Chang P, et al: Effects of smoked substance abuse on nonspecific airway hyperresponsiveness. Am Rev Respir Dis 147:97-103, 1993.

210. Tilles DS, Goldenheim PD, Johnson DC, et al: Marijuana smoking as cause of reduction in single-breath carbon monoxide diffusing capacity. Am J Med 80:601-606, 1986.

211. Varnell RM, Godwin JD, Richardson ML, et al: Adult respiratory distress syndrome from overdose of tricyclic antidepressants. Radiology 170:667-670, 1989.

212. Roy TM, Ossorio MA, Cipolla LM, et al: Pulmonary complications after tricyclic antidepressant overdose. Chest 96:852-856, 1989.

213. Hubbard R, Venn A, Smith C, et al: Exposure to commonly prescribed drugs and the etiology of cryptogenic fibrosing alveolitis: A case-control study. Am J Respir Crit Care Med 157:743-747, 1998.

214. Morcos SK: Review article: Effects of radiographic contrast media on the lung. Br J Radiol 76:290-295, 2003.

215. Bush WH, Swanson DP: Acute reactions to intravascular contrast media: Types, risk factors, recognition, and specific treatment. AJR Am J Roentgenol 157:1153-1161, 1991.

216. Visser LE, Stricker BH, van der Velden J, et al: Angiotensin converting enzyme inhibitor associated cough: A population-based case-control study. J Clin Epidemiol 48:851-857, 1995.

217. Lacourciere Y, Brunner H, Irwin R, et al: Effects of modulators of the renin-angiotensin-aldosterone system on cough. Losartan Cough Study Group. J Hypertens 12:1387-1393, 1994.

218. Semple PF: Putative mechanisms of cough after treatment with angiotensin converting enzyme inhibitors. J Hypertens Suppl 13(Suppl 3):S17-S21, 1995.

219. Olsen CG: Delay of diagnosis and empiric treatment of angiotensin-converting enzyme inhibitor–induced cough in office practice. Arch Fam Med 4:525-528, 1995.

220. Yesil S, Yesil M, Bayata S, et al: ACE inhibitors and cough. Angiology 45:805-808, 1994.

221. Lunde H, Hedner T, Samuelsson O, et al: Dyspnoea, asthma, and bronchospasm in relation to treatment with angiotensin converting enzyme inhibitors. BMJ 308:18-21, 1994.

222. Kaufman J, Schmitt S, Barnard J, et al: Angiotensin-converting enzyme inhibitors in patients with bronchial responsiveness and asthma. Chest 101:922-925, 1992.

223. Jain M, Armstrong L, Hall J: Predisposition to and late onset of upper airway obstruction following angiotensin-converting enzyme inhibitor therapy. Chest 102:871-874, 1992.

224. Watanabe K, Nishimura K, Shiode M, et al: Captopril, an angiotensin-converting enzyme inhibitor, induced pulmonary infiltration with eosinophilia. Intern Med 35:142-145, 1996.

225. Fine SR, Lodha A, Zoneraich S, et al: Hydrochlorothiazide-induced acute pulmonary edema. Ann Pharmacother 29:701-703, 1995.

226. Akoun GM, Milleron BJ, Mayaud CM, et al: Provocation test coupled with bronchoalveolar lavage in diagnosis of propranolol-induced hypersensitivity pneumonitis. Am Rev Respir Dis 139:247-249, 1989.

227. Lombard JN, Bonnotte B, Maynadie M, et al: Celiprolol pneumonitis. Eur Respir J 6:588-591, 1993.

228. Diggory P, Heyworth P, Chau G, et al: Unsuspected bronchospasm in association with topical timolol—a common problem in elderly people: Can we easily identify those affected and do cardioselective agents lead to improvement? Age Ageing 23:17-21, 1994.

229. Brant A, Eaton T: Serious complications with talc slurry pleurodesis. Respirology 6:181-185, 2001.

230. Bondoc AY, Bach PB, Sklarin NT, et al: Arterial desaturation syndrome following pleurodesis with talc slurry: Incidence, clinical features, and outcome. Cancer Invest 21:848-954, 2003.

231. Light RW: Talc should not be used for pleurodesis. Am J Respir Crit Care Med 162:2024-2026, 2000.

232. McElvaney NG, Wilcox PG, Churg A, et al: Pleuropulmonary disease during bromocriptine treatment of Parkinson's disease. Arch Intern Med 148:2231-2236, 1988.

233. Melmed S, Braunstein GD: Bromocriptine and pleuropulmonary disease. Arch Intern Med 149:258-259, 1989.

234. Tallman MS, Andersen JW, Schiffer CA, et al: Clinical description of 44 patients with acute promyelocytic leukemia who developed the retinoic acid syndrome. Blood 95:90-95, 2000.

235. Cohen MH, Williams GA, Sridhara R, et al: United States Food and Drug Administration Drug approval summary: Gefitinib (ZD1839; Iressa) tablets. Clin Cancer Res 10:1212-1218, 2004.

236. Rosado MF, Donna E, Ahn YS: Challenging problems in advanced malignancy: Case 3. Imatinib mesylate–induced interstitial pneumonitis. J Clin Oncol 21:3171-3173, 2003.

237. Bardin PG, van Eeden SF, Joubert JR: Intensive care management of acute organophosphate poisoning. A 7-year experience in the western Cape. S Afr Med J 72:593-597, 1987.

238. Li C, Miller WT, Jiang J: Pulmonary edema due to ingestion of organophosphate insecticide. AJR Am J Roentgenol 152:265-266, 1989.

239. Betrosian A, Balla M, Kafiri G, et al: Multiple systems organ failure from organophosphate poisoning. J Toxicol Clin Toxicol 33:257-260, 1995.

240. Wesseling C, Hogstedt C, Picado A, et al: Unintentional fatal paraquat poisonings among agricultural workers in Costa Rica: Report of 15 cases. Am J Ind Med 32:433-441, 1997.

241. George M, Hedworth-Whitty RB: Non-fatal lung disease due to inhalation of nebulised paraquat. BMJ 280:902, 1980.

242. Levin PJ, Klaff LJ, Rose AG, et al: Pulmonary effects of contact exposure to paraquat: A clinical and experimental study. Thorax 34:150-160, 1979.

243. Dusinska M, Kovacikova Z, Vallova B, et al: Responses of alveolar macrophages and epithelial type II cells to oxidative DNA damage caused by paraquat. Carcinogenesis 19:809-812, 1998.

244. Giulivi C, Lavagno CC, Lucesoli F, et al: Lung damage in paraquat poisoning and hyperbaric oxygen exposure: Superoxide-mediated inhibition of phospholipase A_2. Free Radic Biol Med 18:203-213, 1995.

245. Costantini P, Petronilli V, Colonna R, et al: On the effects of paraquat on isolated mitochondria. Evidence that paraquat causes opening of the cyclosporin A–sensitive permeability transition pore synergistically with nitric oxide. Toxicology 99:77-88, 1995.

246. Im JG, Lee KS, Han MC, et al: Paraquat poisoning: Findings on chest radiography and CT in 42 patients. AJR Am J Roentgenol 157:697-701, 1991.

247. Lee SH, Lee KS, Ahn JM, et al: Paraquat poisoning of the lung: Thin-section CT findings. Radiology 195:271-274, 1995.

248. Higenbottam T, Crome P, Parkinson C, et al: Further clinical observations on the pulmonary effects of paraquat ingestion. Thorax 34:161-165, 1979.

249. Fairshter RD, Wilson AF: Paraquat poisoning: Manifestations and therapy. Am J Med 59:751-753, 1975.

250. Lin JL, Liu L, Leu ML: Recovery of respiratory function in survivors with paraquat intoxication. Arch Environ Health 50:432-439, 1995.

251. Senthilselvan A, McDuffie HH, Dosman JA: Association of asthma with use of pesticides. Results of a cross-sectional survey of farmers. Am Rev Respir Dis 146:884-887, 1992.

252. Salome CM, Marks GB, Savides P, et al: The effect of insecticide aerosols on lung function, airway responsiveness and symptoms in asthmatic subjects. Eur Respir J 16:38-43, 2000.

253. Salisbury BG, Tate CF Jr, Davies JE: Baygon-induced pulmonary edema. Chest 65:455-457, 1974.

254. Roby DS, Fein AM, Bennett RH, et al: Cardiopulmonary effects of acute thallium poisoning. Chest 85:236-240, 1984.

255. Rigau-Perez JG, Perez-Alvarez L, Duenas-Castro S, et al: Epidemiologic investigation of an oil-associated pneumonic paralytic eosinophilic syndrome in Spain. Am J Epidemiol 119:250-260, 1984.

256. Alonso-Ruiz A, Calabozo M, Perez-Ruiz F, et al: Toxic oil syndrome. A long-term follow-up of a cohort of 332 patients. Medicine (Baltimore) 72:285-295, 1993.

257. Kilbourne EM, Posada de la Paz M, Abaitua Borda I, et al: Toxic oil syndrome: A current clinical and epidemiologic summary, including comparisons with the eosinophilia-myalgia syndrome. J Am Coll Cardiol 18:711-717, 1991.

258. Martin Escribano P, Diaz de Atauri MJ, Gomez Sanchez MA: Persistence of respiratory abnormalities four years after the onset of toxic oil syndrome. Chest 100:336-339, 1991.

259. Anas N, Namasonthi V, Ginsburg CM: Criteria for hospitalizing children who have ingested products containing hydrocarbons. JAMA 246:840-843, 1981.

260. Singh H, Chugh JC, Shembesh AH, et al: Management of accidental kerosene ingestion. Ann Trop Paediatr 12:105-109, 1992.

261. Brander PE, Taskinen E, Stenius-Aarniala B: Fire-eater's lung. Eur Respir J 5:112-114, 1992.

262. Scharf SM, Heimer D, Goldstein J: Pathologic and physiologic effects of aspiration of hydrocarbons in the rat. Am Rev Respir Dis 124:625-629, 1981.

263. Bruenner S, Rovsing H, Wulf H: Roentgenographic changes in the lungs of children with kerosene poisoning. Am Rev Respir Dis 89:250-254, 1964.

264. Jimenez JP, Lester RG: Pulmonary complications following furniture polish ingestion. A report of 21 cases. Am J Roentgenol Radium Ther Nucl Med 98:323-333, 1966.

265. Harris VJ, Brown R: Pneumatoceles as a complication of chemical pneumonia after hydrocarbon ingestion. Am J Roentgenol Radium Ther Nucl Med 125:531-537, 1975.

266. Libshitz HI: Radiation changes in the lung. Semin Roentgenol 28:303-320, 1993.
267. Park KJ, Chung JY, Chun MS, et al: Radiation-induced lung disease and the impact of radiation methods on imaging features. Radiographics 20:83-98, 2000.
268. Movsas B, Raffin TA, Epstein AH, et al: Pulmonary radiation injury. Chest 111:1061-1076, 1997.
269. Roach M 3rd, Gandara DR, Yuo HS, et al: Radiation pneumonitis following combined modality therapy for lung cancer: Analysis of prognostic factors. J Clin Oncol 13:2606-2612, 1995.
270. Gross NJ: Pulmonary effects of radiation therapy. Ann Intern Med 86:81-92, 1977.
271. Lin M: Radiation pneumonitis caused by yttrium-90 microspheres: Radiologic findings. AJR Am J Roentgenol 162:1300-1302, 1994.
272. Gustafson G, Vicini F, Freedman L, et al: High dose rate endobronchial brachytherapy in the management of primary and recurrent bronchogenic malignancies. Cancer 75:2345-2350, 1995.
273. Rubin P, Casarett G: Clinical Radiation Pathology, vol 1. Philadelphia, WB Saunders, 1968.
274. Davis SD, Yankelevitz DF, Henschke CI: Radiation effects on the lung: Clinical features, pathology, and imaging findings. AJR Am J Roentgenol 159:1157-1164, 1992.
275. Wara WM, Phillips TL, Margolis LW, et al: Radiation pneumonitis: A new approach to the derivation of time-dose factors. Cancer 32:547-552, 1973.
276. Pezner RD, Bertrand M, Cecchi GR, et al: Steroid-withdrawal radiation pneumonitis in cancer patients. Chest 85:816-817, 1984.
277. Lingos TI, Recht A, Vicini F, et al: Radiation pneumonitis in breast cancer patients treated with conservative surgery and radiation therapy. Int J Radiat Oncol Biol Phys 21:355-360, 1991.
278. Burdon J, Bell R, Sullivan J, et al: Adriamycin-induced recall phenomenon 15 years after radiotherapy. JAMA 239:931, 1978.
279. Soh LT, Koo WH, Ang PT: Case report: Delayed radiation pneumonitis induced by chemotherapy. Clin Radiol 52:720-723, 1997.
280. Gross NJ: The pathogenesis of radiation-induced lung damage. Lung 159:115-125, 1981.
281. Adamson IY, Bowden DH: Endothelial injury and repair in radiation-induced pulmonary fibrosis. Am J Pathol 112:224-230, 1983.
282. Morgan GW, Breit SN: Radiation and the lung: A reevaluation of the mechanisms mediating pulmonary injury. Int J Radiat Oncol Biol Phys 31:361-369, 1995.
283. Gibson PG, Bryant DH, Morgan GW, et al: Radiation-induced lung injury: A hypersensitivity pneumonitis? Ann Intern Med 109:288-291, 1988.
284. Fajardo LF, Berthrong M: Radiation injury in surgical pathology. Part I. Am J Surg Pathol 2:159-199, 1978.
285. Wilkinson MJ, Maclennan KA: Vascular changes in irradiated lungs: A morphometric study. J Pathol 158:229-232, 1989.
286. Logan PM: Thoracic manifestations of external beam radiotherapy. AJR Am J Roentgenol 171:569-577, 1998.
287. Crestani B, Valeyre D, Roden S, et al: Bronchiolitis obliterans organizing pneumonia syndrome primed by radiation therapy to the breast. The Groupe d'Etudes et de Recherche sur les Maladies Orphelines Pulmonaires (GERM"O"P). Am J Respir Crit Care Med 158:1929-1935, 1998.
288. Takigawa N, Segawa Y, Saeki T, et al: Bronchiolitis obliterans organizing pneumonia syndrome in breast-conserving therapy for early breast cancer: Radiation-induced lung toxicity. Int J Radiat Oncol Biol Phys 48:751-755, 2000.
289. Ikezoe J, Takashima S, Morimoto S, et al: CT appearance of acute radiation-induced injury in the lung. AJR Am J Roentgenol 150:765-770, 1988.
290. Ikezoe J, Morimoto S, Takashima S, et al: Acute radiation-induced pulmonary injury: Computed tomography evaluation. Semin Ultrasound CT MR 11:409-416, 1990.
291. Whitcomb ME, Schwarz MI: Pleural effusion complicating intensive mediastinal radiation therapy. Am Rev Respir Dis 103:100-107, 1971.
292. Mesurolle B, Qanadli SD, Merad M, et al: Unusual radiologic findings in the thorax after radiation therapy. Radiographics 20:67-81, 2000.
293. Bell J, McGivern D, Bullimore J, et al: Diagnostic imaging of post-irradiation changes in the chest. Clin Radiol 39:109-119, 1988.
294. Khanavkar B, Stern P, Alberti W, et al: Complications associated with brachytherapy alone or with laser in lung cancer. Chest 99:1062-1065, 1991.
295. Speiser BL, Spratling L: Radiation bronchitis and stenosis secondary to high dose rate endobronchial irradiation. Int J Radiat Oncol Biol Phys 25:589-597, 1993.

TRAUMATIC CHEST INJURY

Trauma to the thorax can result in a wide variety of effects on the chest wall, diaphragm, mediastinum, trachea, and lungs.[1,2] The results may be direct (e.g., fractures of the ribs, spine, or shoulder girdles; diaphragmatic hernia; esophageal rupture; and pulmonary contusion or laceration) or indirect (e.g., air embolism resulting from the escape of air into the pulmonary veins subsequent to parenchymal laceration). Because the manifestations of such trauma are dissimilar in different sites, each is considered separately. As might be anticipated, however, a great deal of overlap occurs. The effects of penetrating and nonpenetrating trauma may be different and require separate consideration.

Although the diagnosis of most traumatic abnormalities of the thorax can be established with reasonable confidence by conventional radiography, in some cases significant abnormalities, such as fractures of the thoracic spine, pulmonary lacerations, pneumothorax, and hemothorax, may be apparent only on CT scan.[3,4] Certain conditions, such as laceration of the aorta, often require special diagnostic procedures, including CT angiography or aortography, to confirm the injury and establish its extent. In fact, CT is gradually replacing conventional radiography as the initial imaging modality of choice in the evaluation of severe trauma victims in many centers.[5]

EFFECTS OF NONPENETRATING TRAUMA ON THE LUNGS

Pulmonary Contusion

Pulmonary contusion consists of traumatic extravasation of blood into the lung parenchyma unaccompanied by substantial tissue disruption.[6] It is the most common pulmonary complication of chest trauma.[7] The severity of the injury necessary to produce contusion varies from a trivial glancing blow to major trauma resulting from motor vehicle or aircraft accidents.[8]

The radiographic pattern varies from irregular, patchy areas of air space consolidation to diffuse and extensive homogeneous consolidation (Fig. 19–1). As might be expected, the opacities do not conform to lobes or segments.[4,9] Although the major abnormality usually occurs in lung directly deep to the traumatized areas, damage may also be seen, sometimes predominantly, on the opposite side as a result of a contre-coup effect.[10] An increase in the size and loss of definition of the vascular markings extending from the hila indicate the presence of hemorrhage and edema in the peribronchovascular interstitial tissue.[7,9] The time between trauma and detection of the radiographic abnormality is important in diagnosis, particularly in differentiation from fat embolism. In contusion, changes are radiographically apparent soon after

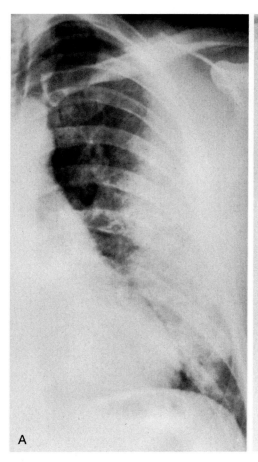
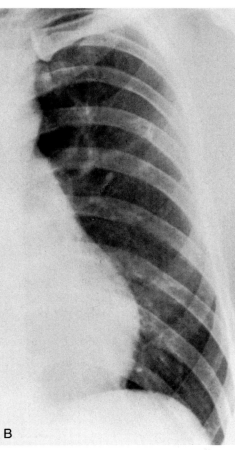

FIGURE 19–1

Pulmonary contusion. Six hours before radiographic examination, this 33-year-old man was involved in a car accident in which he suffered severe trauma to the posterior portion of the left side of his chest. A view of the left hemithorax from an anteroposterior radiograph (**A**) shows homogeneous consolidation of the posterolateral portion of the left lung in a nonsegmental distribution. The margins of the consolidation are defined indistinctly, and there is no air bronchogram. No ribs were fractured. The right lung was clear. Six days later (**B**), complete clearing had occurred. *(From Müller NL, Fraser RS, Colman NC, Paré PD: Radiologic Diagnosis of Diseases of the Chest. Philadelphia, WB Saunders, 2001.)*

trauma (almost invariably within 6 hours),[4,8] whereas in fat embolism, changes usually become evident only 1 to 2 days or more after injury. Resolution of lung contusion typically occurs rapidly, improvement being noted within 24 to 48 hours and complete clearing within 3 to 10 days.[4,11]

CT findings consist of areas of consolidation, which may be patchy or homogeneous.[4,12] Air bronchograms are commonly present.[6] Although contusion is by definition unassociated with radiographic evidence of pulmonary laceration, small lacerations—seen as small round or ovoid air collections with or without an air-fluid level—are commonly evident on CT.[13]

Most patients have no symptoms directly related to the contusion. However, extensive bilateral contusion may lead to respiratory failure and acute respiratory distress syndrome (ARDS).[6,14]

Pulmonary Laceration, Traumatic Pneumatocele, and Hematoma

Uncommonly, closed chest trauma results in the development of radiographically detectable lacerations within the lung that remain air filled (traumatic pneumatocele) or that fill partly or completely with blood (hematoma). The trauma is usually blunt and often severe, as in an automobile accident. Children and young adults are particularly prone to the development of such lacerations, presumably because of the greater flexibility of their thoracic walls.[15]

Radiographically, traumatic pneumatoceles and hematomas are not usually seen until a few hours or several days after trauma, often being initially masked by the surrounding contusion.[16,17] They may be single or multiple, unilocular or multilocular, oval or spherical, and 2 to 14 cm in diameter.[18] In most cases, they are located in the subpleural parenchyma under the point of maximal injury[8]; occasionally, they occur in a remote location as a result of a contrecoup effect. Pneumatoceles are manifested as thin-walled, air-filled spaces with or without air-fluid levels (Fig. 19–2)[19]; they may enlarge rapidly in patients receiving high-pressure mechanical ventilation.[6] Hematomas appear as homogeneous, well-circumscribed masses of soft tissue density (Fig. 19–3).[20] Most lesions resolve over a period of 6 to 11 weeks[21]; however, they may persist for several months and occasionally years (see Fig. 19–3).[13,22] If resolution is not apparent within 6 weeks, the possibility that trauma may have been coincidental with a solitary nodule of other etiology should be considered.[8]

CT is much more sensitive than chest radiography in the detection of pulmonary lacerations.[23,17] The findings consist of one or more round, oval, or multiloculated air collections with or without air-fluid levels.[18,23] Hemorrhage related to a pulmonary laceration may result in an air-fluid level, an air crescent sign, or, when the lacerated region is filled completely with blood, a round or oval soft tissue density.[22,24] Hematomas that persist for several months may have central attenuation slightly greater than that of water and rim enhancement.[22]

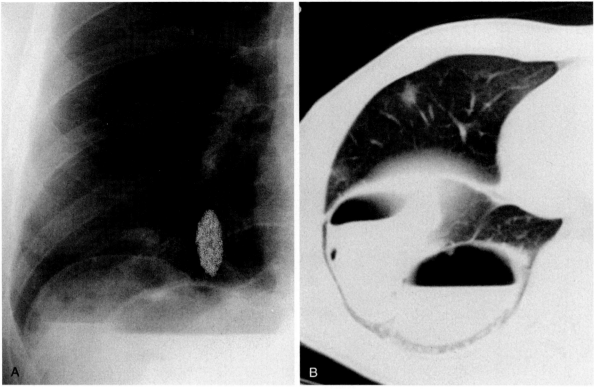

FIGURE 19-2

Traumatic pneumatocele. A view of the right lower portion of the chest from a posteroanterior radiograph (**A**) in a 26-year-old man 2 weeks after a motor vehicle accident reveals thin-walled cystic lesions with air-fluid levels. A CT scan (**B**) essentially confirms the radiographic findings. *(From Müller NL, Fraser RS, Colman NC, Paré PD: Radiologic Diagnosis of Diseases of the Chest. Philadelphia, WB Saunders, 2001.)*

Most patients do not have symptoms related to the pulmonary lesion itself. Hemoptysis occurs rarely and is probably attributable to the emptying of a hematoma.[21]

Fractures of the Trachea and Bronchi

Fractures (rupture, transection) of the tracheobronchial tree as a result of nonpenetrating trauma are usually secondary to blunt injury to the anterior of the chest in a vehicular accident[25]; occasionally, they occur as a result of a fall from height[26] or secondary to overdistention of the cuff of an endotracheal tube.[27] Most fractures associated with blunt trauma follow rapid anteroposterior compression of the chest.[28] This situation may result in a sudden increase in airway pressure causing a "burst" injury; alternatively, the sudden lateral widening of the thorax may pull the lung apart and avulse a bronchus.[28] Although fractures may occur in the absence of thoracic skeletal injury,[7] such injury is often present.

Traumatic tracheobronchial fracture is uncommon; it has been estimated that only about 2% to 3% of patients who die as a result of trauma have the complication.[25] Its rarity probably contributes to the infrequency with which it is recognized early. In one series, 68% of cases were not diagnosed until obstructive pneumonitis had developed in the lung distal to the fracture.[29] Fractures of the bronchi are more frequent than those of the trachea and account for about 80% of injuries.[11,28] They are usually parallel to the cartilage rings and involve the main bronchi 1 to 2 cm distal to the carina.[11,28] The right side is affected more often than the left; associated pulmonary vessels are rarely damaged.[30] Fractures of the intrathoracic trachea are horizontal and generally occur just above the carina.[11,31]

As might be expected, the most common radiographic findings are pneumomediastinum and pneumothorax.[32] Tension pneumothorax occurs in approximately 50% of patients. Certain combinations of findings are highly suggestive of the diagnosis, including (1) a large pneumothorax that does not respond to chest tube drainage (because of free communication between the fractured airway and the pleural space), (2) pneumothorax and pneumomediastinum in the absence of pleural effusion, and (3) mediastinal and deep cervical emphysema in a trauma patient who is not receiving positive pressure ventilation.[33,34]

Displacement of fracture ends can cause bronchial obstruction and atelectasis of an entire lung[35]; it is important to recognize that such atelectasis may be a late development, and the discovery of such a change sometime after an accident should suggest the diagnosis. In about 10% of patients, fracture is unassociated with any radiographically demonstrable abnormality,[11] in which case it is likely that the preservation of peribronchial connective tissue prevents passage of air into the mediastinum or pleura. The consequences of the trauma may not become evident until the patient is evaluated months or even years later and demonstrates atelectasis of a lobe or lung as a result of bronchial stenosis.[36]

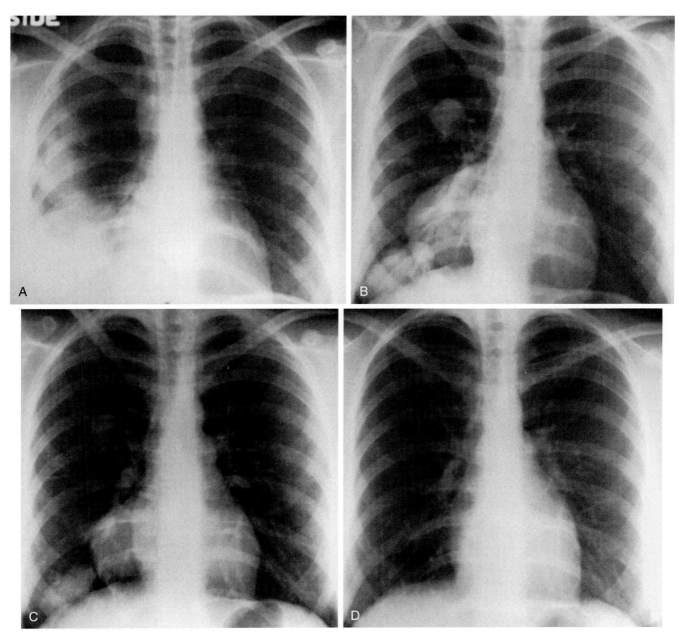

FIGURE 19–3

Multiple unilateral pulmonary hematomas. This 17-year-old girl was involved in a two-car collision in which she sustained fractures of the right scapula and humerus. The day after admission, an anteroposterior radiograph (**A**) showed extensive parenchymal consolidation in the lower two thirds of the right lung in a nonsegmental distribution; the left lung was clear. There was some widening of the superior mediastinum from venous hemorrhage. Two months later (**B**), multiple, sharply circumscribed homogeneous nodules in the right lung ranging from 1 to 6 cm in diameter can be identified. No cavitation was present, and the left lung remained clear. Approximately 1 month later (**C**), the nodules had diminished considerably in size, and several had disappeared altogether. Seven months after the injury, all signs of disease had disappeared, and the chest radiograph (**D**) was normal. *(Courtesy of Dr. John D. Armstrong, Jr., University of Utah College of Medicine, Salt Lake City.)*

Symptoms and signs of tracheobronchial fracture include cyanosis, hemoptysis, and cough. Air is often identifiable in the subcutaneous tissues; it initially involves the neck and upper part of the thorax and later becomes generalized.[37] It may be seen to escape directly from a wound in the neck in cases of tracheal fracture.[25] When fracture is suspected, bronchoscopy should be performed to confirm the diagnosis and locate the site of injury.

EFFECTS OF NONPENETRATING TRAUMA ON THE PLEURA

Hemothorax and pneumothorax are common manifestations of nonpenetrating trauma. Hemothorax occurs in 25% to 50% of patients who have sustained blunt chest trauma.[38] It is usually small and secondary to bleeding from lacerated pulmonary vessels[38]; large accumulations are the result of tears in large pulmonary vessels or systemic arteries or veins.[38]

Pneumothorax occurs in 15% to 40% of patients.[38,39] Most often, it follows alveolar rupture and dissection of gas into the adjacent interstitium and, eventually, the pleural space; occasionally, it is a complication of tracheobronchial fracture or esophageal rupture. It may occur with or without radiographic evidence of rib fracture.[40] When fracture is present, the probable mechanism is laceration of the visceral pleura by rib fragments; in such circumstances, hemothorax may be expected as a concomitant finding. Pneumothorax is detected more commonly on CT than on radiography.[15]

EFFECTS OF NONPENETRATING TRAUMA ON THE MEDIASTINUM

Mediastinal Hemorrhage

Most cases of mediastinal hemorrhage result from trauma, usually of a severe nature, such as that associated with motor vehicle accidents or falls from a height.[41,42] The source of bleeding is often the aorta. Mediastinal blood may also originate in traumatized retropharyngeal soft tissue. In some cases, the trauma is iatrogenic (e.g., occurring after faulty placement of a central venous line[43] or perforation of the superior vena cava[44]).

Radiographically, extensive hemorrhage typically results in uniform, symmetrical widening of the mediastinum (Fig. 19–4). Local accumulation of blood in the form of a

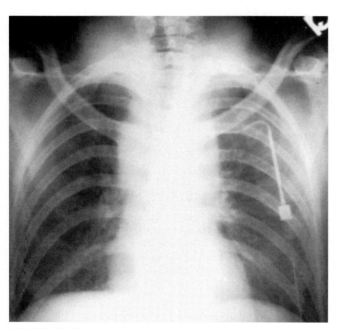

FIGURE 19–4

Traumatic mediastinal hemorrhage. A chest radiograph in anteroposterior projection, supine position, of a young man after severe closed chest trauma reveals moderate widening of the upper half of the mediastinum, roughly symmetrical on both sides. The lungs are unremarkable. *(From Müller NL, Fraser RS, Colman NC, Paré PD: Radiologic Diagnosis of Diseases of the Chest. Philadelphia, WB Saunders, 2001.)*

hematoma is manifested by a homogeneous focal opacity that may project to one or both sides of the mediastinum and may be situated in any compartment. The most important diagnostic consideration in these patients is aortic rupture; however, only about 10% to 20% of patients who have radiographic findings suggestive of mediastinal hemorrhage after trauma have an aortic injury.[3] Further diagnostic procedures, including contrast-enhanced CT, transesophageal ultrasound, and aortography, are required for a definitive diagnosis (see next section).

Symptoms and signs of mediastinal hemorrhage are seldom striking. Suspicion may be aroused when retrosternal pain that radiates to the back develops in a patient who recently suffered chest trauma.

Rupture of the Thoracic Aorta and Its Branches

Patients at risk for aortic injury after blunt trauma include those involved in high-speed motor vehicle accidents in which there is substantial vehicle deformity, pedestrians or cyclists struck by a vehicle, and individuals falling from a height greater than 10 ft (3 m).[45] About 90% of injuries involve the region of the aortic isthmus immediately distal to the left subclavian artery; tears of the ascending aorta, the distal descending aorta, or abdominal aorta are much less common.[3,45]

Laceration is believed to be the result of a shearing force in which the relatively mobile anterior portion of the aortic arch contacts the more fixed posterior arch and descending aorta. It has also been suggested that it may be caused by chest compression pinching the aorta between the anterior and posterior components of the bony thorax.[46] According to this hypothesis, compressive forces depress the anterior thoracic osseous structures, cause them to rotate posteriorly and inferiorly about the posterior rib articulation, and pinch and shear the interposed vascular structures. The aortic injury is almost always a transverse tear that disrupts one or more layers of its wall; the adventitia remains intact in about 60% of cases.[45]

Occasionally, mediastinal hemorrhage after severe chest trauma results from damage to one of the great vessels arising from the aortic arch. Avulsion of the innominate artery from the arch has been stated to be the second most common type of aortic injury in which the patient survives long enough for diagnostic evaluation.[47] The radiographic findings are similar to those of rupture of the aortic isthmus, with the possible exception that the outline of the descending aorta may be preserved. Fractures of the upper thoracic spine may also cause radiographic findings similar to those of aortic rupture.[48]

Radiologic Manifestations

A variety of radiographic signs have been described as being useful in the diagnosis of aortic rupture. Some, particularly mediastinal widening and an abnormal or indistinct contour of the aortic arch, have relatively high sensitivity but low specificity; others, such as rightward deviation of the trachea, downward displacement of the left main bronchus, rightward displacement of a nasogastric tube, and thickening of the right paratracheal stripe, have greater specificity but lower sensitivity.[3,45] In fact, the greatest value of the chest radiograph is in *excluding* traumatic aortic injury, the negative predictive value of a normal erect frontal chest radiograph being approximately 98%.[45,49] The positive predictive value of an abnormal chest radiograph is relatively low; only 10% to 20% of patients who have abnormalities suggestive of mediastinal hemorrhage have an aortic injury.[3,50]

Widening of the Upper Half of the Mediastinum. Plain chest radiographs frequently reveal widening of the superior mediastinum after aortic rupture (Fig. 19–5). Assessment of such widening may be based solely on subjective criteria or on measurement of mediastinal diameter at the level of the aortic arch (>8 cm indicating pathologic widening).[3,51] Using this value as a cutoff, one group found a sensitivity of 36% and a specificity of 81% for aortic rupture on erect anteroposterior chest radiographs and a sensitivity of 67% and specificity of 45% on radiographs performed with the patient supine.[49] (The diagnostic usefulness of widening on supine radiographs is poorer because of the effect of magnification.)

Abnormal Contour of the Aortic Arch. Irregularity or obscuration of the contour of the aortic arch (see Fig. 19–5) is probably the most reliable sign of aortic rupture. In a study of 205 patients who sustained blunt chest trauma and underwent aortography, the sign had a sensitivity of 63% and specificity of 62% on erect radiographs and a sensitivity of 81%

and specificity of 45% on radiographs performed with the patient supine.[49] Other related signs that have been found to be helpful include obscuration of the aortopulmonary window and obscuration of the proximal descending thoracic aorta.[49,52]

Deviation of the Trachea and Left Main Bronchus. As the amount of mediastinal blood increases, the left main bronchus may be deviated anteriorly, inferiorly, and to the right, and the trachea may be displaced to the right. Shift of the left tracheal wall to the right of the T4 spinous process has a specificity of greater than 90% in the detection of traumatic aortic laceration; however, the finding has low sensitivity, being present on erect frontal views of the chest in only 15% of patients in some series.[49] Depression of the left main bronchus greater than 40 degrees below the horizontal in the absence of left lower lobe atelectasis is also suggestive of the diagnosis but, again, is seen in only a few patients.[49]

Deviation of the Nasogastric Tube. Displacement of a nasogastric tube to the right of the T4 spinous process has high specificity in diagnosis. However, the sensitivity is low; in one study the finding was present in only 10% of patients.[49]

Left Apical Cap. A potential space exists between the isthmus of the aorta and the parietal pleura of the left lung.

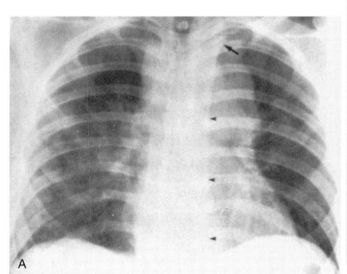
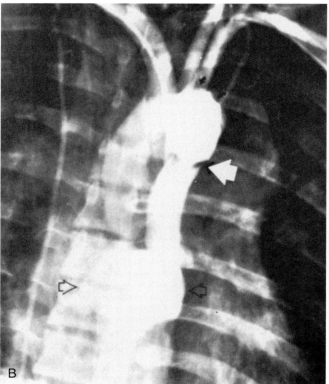

FIGURE 19–5

Traumatic aneurysm and rupture of the thoracic aorta. This 16-year-old boy crashed into a telephone pole in an automobile traveling at 85 mph. Shortly after his arrival in the emergency department, a chest radiograph in anteroposterior projection (**A**) showed marked widening of the upper mediastinum and loss of visualization of the aortic arch. A wide paravertebral opacity (*arrowheads*) extends up to the apex, associated with an extrapleural apical cap (*arrow*). The suspicion of aortic rupture was confirmed by aortography (**B**). The site of primary aortic laceration is indicated by a *thick arrow*, the irregular bulge immediately above (*small arrows*) representing dissection proximally. Several centimeters distally is a large, well-circumscribed collection of contrast medium (*open arrows*) that represents an extra-aortic hematoma from a second rupture. The patient exsanguinated after section of the mediastinal pleura at thoracotomy. *(From Müller NL, Fraser RS, Colman NC, Paré PD: Radiologic Diagnosis of Diseases of the Chest. Philadelphia, WB Saunders, 2001.)*

Provided that the latter is intact, extravasated blood can track cephalad along the course of the left subclavian artery between the parietal pleura and the extrapleural soft tissues and result in a homogeneous opacity over the apex of the left hemithorax and, subsequently, an extrapleural apical cap.[53] By itself, the cap is an unreliable sign of acute aortic rupture.[49,54]

Left Hemothorax. Hemothorax complicating acute aortic rupture is uncommon; in an investigation of patients who had blunt chest trauma, it was present in only 5%.[55] It is almost invariably left sided.

Summary

Many investigators have attempted to assess the relative value of the radiographic signs just described.[49,55,56] The majority opinion, with which we agree, is that the most reliable ones are mediastinal widening and an abnormal outline of the aortic arch. However, no single sign or combination of signs has sufficient sensitivity to avoid the performance of a large number of negative aortographic studies. As a result, the use of additional, noninvasive techniques—primarily CT—is indicated in most patients.

Computed Tomography

CT permits ready distinction of mediastinal widening secondary to hemorrhage from that related to tortuous vessels, fat, or radiographic magnification. Both indirect and direct signs are useful.[57] Mediastinal hematoma abutting the aorta is an indirect sign, whereas irregularity of the wall (Fig. 19–6), the presence of a pseudoaneurysm, an abrupt change in

caliber of the aorta, extravasation of contrast material from the aorta, and the presence of an intraluminal radiolucent filling defect (intimal flap) (Fig. 19–7) constitute direct signs.[41,57,58] In a meta-analysis of the data from 3334 patients published in the literature by 1996 in which the presence of mediastinal hematoma or direct signs of aortic injury were considered to be an indicator for a positive examination, the sensitivity of CT was 99.3%, the specificity was 87.1%, the positive predictive value was 19.9%, and the negative predictive value was 99.9%.[58] The presence of direct signs of aortic injury had a sensitivity of 97%, specificity of 99.8%, positive predictive value of 90.1%, and negative predictive value of 99.9%.

In most studies published before 1996, conventional CT was used for diagnosis. The relatively long time interval between each individual slice and the difference in inspiratory effort between slices often resulted in suboptimal contrast enhancement and interslice artifacts. The shortened scanning time of spiral CT has resulted in greatly improved vascular contrast enhancement (see Figs. 19–6 and 19–7).[59] Rapid scanning of multiple levels during a single breath-hold eliminates interslice artifacts and allows performance of CT angiography with excellent direct visualization of the aortic injury.[60] Assessment of aortic injuries has also improved considerably with the advent of spiral and multidetector CT scanners.[5,61] Because of cardiac motion artifact, ascending aortic injuries may be missed on spiral CT.[62] Some workers have suggested that a normal aorta on spiral CT effectively excludes aortic injury and that aortography is not necessary in this situation, even when mediastinal hematoma is present.[63,64] However, most investigators

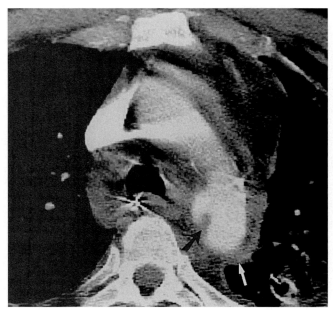

FIGURE 19–6

Traumatic laceration of the aorta on spiral CT. A contrast-enhanced 7-mm-collimation spiral CT scan performed in a 53-year-old man after an automobile accident shows focal irregularity of the proximal descending thoracic aorta (*black arrow*), diagnostic of an aortic laceration. A small amount of blood can be seen adjacent to the aorta (*white arrow*). (*From Müller NL, Fraser RS, Colman NC, Paré PD: Radiologic Diagnosis of Diseases of the Chest. Philadelphia, WB Saunders, 2001.*)

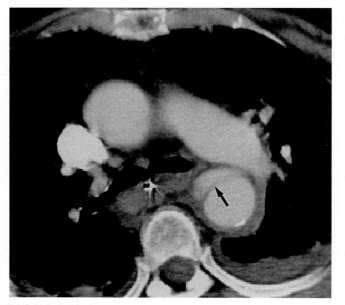

FIGURE 19–7

Traumatic laceration of the aorta with an intimal flap. A contrast-enhanced spiral CT scan shows irregularity of the lateral wall of the aorta and an intimal flap (*arrow*). A small amount of blood is evident around the proximal descending thoracic aorta, and small bilateral pleural effusions are present. (*From Müller NL, Fraser RS, Colman NC, Paré PD: Radiologic Diagnosis of Diseases of the Chest. Philadelphia, WB Saunders, 2001.*)

consider aortography to be mandatory in patients who have periaortic hematoma.[45,65,66]

Based on our review of the literature, we believe that the following recommendations are reasonable in a patient who has suffered blunt chest trauma:

1. Because of the high negative predictive values associated with normal chest radiographs, further investigation is seldom warranted in these patients. However, since it may provide other important diagnostic information, spiral CT of the chest is indicated in patients who are undergoing CT of the abdomen and pelvis after trauma regardless of the chest radiograph findings.[60]
2. Patients who have abnormal chest radiographs and are unstable should proceed directly to aortography or surgery.
3. Patients who are stable and who have suboptimal or abnormal chest radiographs should undergo spiral CT of the chest. Those who have a normal scan need no further evaluation unless serial radiographs show progressive mediastinal widening.[67] Depending on the experience of the radiologist and surgeon, patients who have direct signs of aortic injury on CT scan may undergo transcatheter aortography or proceed directly to surgery. Patients who have a periaortic hematoma evident on CT scan or who have indeterminate or inadequate chest CT scans should undergo emergency aortography.

Aortography

Transfemoral aortography is the definitive imaging modality to diagnose the presence, location, and extent of aortic injury.[51,68] Angiographic findings indicative of aortic injury include an intimal tear, extravasation of contrast material, dissection with an intimal flap, pseudoaneurysm, and pseudocoarctation (see Fig. 19–5).[68] The procedure has a sensitivity of about 95% and a negative predictive value of 99%.[60] The main reasons for false-positive interpretations are the presence of an atypical ductus diverticulum or an ulcerated atherosclerotic plaque.[69] A ductus diverticulum consists of a focal bulge or convexity at the level of the aortic isthmus and has been noted in about 25% of otherwise normal individuals.[69] Reasons for false-negative diagnoses include the presence of a small intimal flap or a small localized rupture through the intima and media.[60,70]

Perforation of the Esophagus

Rupture of the esophagus is a rare but serious complication of closed chest trauma.[71,72] Radiologic manifestations include mediastinal widening secondary to mediastinitis, pneumomediastinum, pleural effusion, pneumothorax, and hydropneumothorax.[24,71] CT scan may show pneumomediastinum not apparent on radiographs.[73] In most cases, the site of rupture can be identified precisely—though sometimes with considerable difficulty—only by radiologic evidence of extravasation of ingested contrast material in the mediastinum or pleural space.[24] The area of greatest esophageal thickening on CT often represents the level of perforation[71]; in most cases, however, the perforation itself is obscured by edema or hemorrhage and is not seen on CT scan.[71]

Rupture of the Thoracic Duct

Thoracic duct injury from blunt trauma is rare[74] and thought to be secondary to hyperextension of the thoracic spine.[75] The site of injury is shown best by lymphangiography.[76] The anatomic course of the thoracic duct and the site of damage determine the side on which the chylothorax develops. As it enters the thorax, the duct lies slightly to the right of the midline, so rupture in its lower third—an unusual site in crush injuries—leads to right-sided chylothorax. The duct crosses the midline to the left in the midthorax; consequently, disruption of the duct above this point tends to produce left-sided chylothorax.

Several days to weeks may elapse between the time of trauma and the development of radiographically demonstrable pleural fluid,[77] a time lag that should suggest the diagnosis. It has been postulated that the delay occurs because the extravasated chyle is initially confined to the mediastinal space and ruptures into the pleural space only when the accumulation has acquired sufficient pressure.[77]

EFFECTS OF NONPENETRATING TRAUMA ON THE CHEST WALL AND DIAPHRAGM

Rupture of the Diaphragm

Diaphragmatic rupture is diagnosed in 1% to 4% of patients admitted to the hospital with blunt trauma and in about 5% of those who subsequently undergo laparotomy or thoracotomy.[7,78] In a review of 1000 diaphragmatic injuries in 980 patients reported by 1995, 75% of ruptures were the result of blunt trauma and 25% followed penetrating injury.[78] Several mechanisms have been postulated for development of rupture of the diaphragm following blunt trauma, including a sudden increase in intrathoracic or intra-abdominal pressure against a fixed diaphragm, shearing stress on a stretched diaphragm, and avulsion of the diaphragm from its points of attachment[78]; the first of these mechanisms is the most commonly accepted.[79,80]

The complication is discovered more commonly on the left, a localization ascribed to a variety of causes, including the buffer action of the liver, the greater strength of the right hemidiaphragm (experimental studies in cadavers having shown a relative weakness of the left hemidiaphragm), and underdiagnosis of right-sided injuries.[78] Although ruptures may occur in any area, most develop through the posterolateral surface along the embryonic fusion lines.[7]

Radiologic Manifestations

The radiographic findings are related to the mechanism of injury (blunt or penetrating), the site of injury (left or right), the presence of herniated viscera, and the presence of concomitant pleural or pulmonary injury.[78,81] Depending on these factors, a preoperative diagnosis based on the radiographic findings in various studies has been made in 4% to 63% of cases.[78,82,83] The likelihood of diagnosis is higher in patients who have left-sided perforation and blunt rather than perforating injury.[84,85]

Diagnostic signs include visualization of herniated stomach or bowel in the chest and cephalad extension of an intragastric tube above the level of the diaphragm (Fig. 19–8).[78,84] Suggestive findings include irregularity of the diaphragmatic contour, inability to visualize the diaphragm, a persistent basilar opacity (which may mimic atelectasis or a supradiaphragmatic mass), an elevated hemidiaphragm in the absence of atelectasis, and a contralateral shift of the mediastinum in the absence of a large pleural effusion or pneumothorax.

The stomach and the colon are the viscera that most commonly herniate into the thorax after rupture of the left hemidiaphragm. The diagnosis can be confirmed by contrast-enhanced studies of these two organs or by CT or MR imaging.[38,86,87] The diagnostic finding is the presence of a focal constriction (*collar sign*) in the stomach or afferent and efferent loop of bowel where they traverse the orifice of the diaphragmatic rupture. This finding is sometimes seen on plain chest radiographs but is visualized more readily on contrast-enhanced stomach or colon studies or on CT scans.[87] When strangulation occurs, unilateral pleural effusion may be present.[88]

After rupture of the right hemidiaphragm, a portion of the liver may herniate through the rent and create a mushroom-like mass within the right hemithorax, with the herniated liver being constricted by the tear. In such circumstances, the diagnosis should be suspected by the high position of the lower border of the liver as indicated by the position of the hepatic flexure.[89] The diagnosis can be confirmed by CT (Fig. 19–9), MR imaging, or ultrasound.[85,87,90]

Several groups have assessed the use of CT in the diagnosis of diaphragmatic rupture.[87,91,92] Characteristic findings include a sharp discontinuity of the diaphragm, intrathoracic visceral herniation, lack of visualization of a hemidiaphragm (*absent diaphragm sign*), and constriction of bowel or stomach at the site of herniation.[87,92]

Focal discontinuity of the diaphragm is seen on CT in 70% to 80% of patients who have a diaphragmatic rupture[87,92]; however, such defects are seen occasionally in healthy people, particularly the elderly, and a diagnosis based solely on this sign should be made with caution.[87,92] A more reliable sign is herniation of omental fat or abdominal viscera, which is seen in 50% to 60% of patients (Fig. 19–10).[87,92] A waistlike narrowing of the stomach, bowel, or liver (see Fig. 19–9) at the site of herniation (collar sign) is seen in 30% to 40%[87,92]; sometimes it is the only CT abnormality.[87]

Clinical Manifestations

Signs and symptoms of diaphragmatic injury can be immediate or delayed. Bleeding from the torn edge of the diaphragm is seldom of sufficient severity to cause hemodynamic compromise. Respiratory distress can be caused by mechanical displacement of lung or by pneumothorax after intrathoracic rupture of an abdominal viscus. An extremely scaphoid anterior abdominal wall (*Gibson's sign*) should make one suspicious of the complication.[93] Strangulation of herniated abdominal viscera may cause nausea and vomiting. However, uncomplicated herniation of abdominal contents may be asymptomatic for years.[94]

As might be expected, patients frequently have other serious injuries, such as rib and pelvic fractures, splenic laceration or rupture, closed head injury, and liver laceration.[81] These abnormalities often obscure the findings related to the diaphragmatic rupture, and the diagnosis is not uncommonly delayed or missed. For example, in a review of 1000 diaphragmatic injuries, the diagnosis was made at the time of admission in 44% of cases and incidentally at thoracotomy, laparotomy, or autopsy in 41%[78]; in the remaining 15%, the diagnosis was delayed 24 hours or more. Failure to make the diagnosis has been associated with a mortality rate of 20% to 35%.[95]

An unusual complication of thoracoabdominal trauma associated with diaphragmatic rupture is thoracic splenosis. Splenosis is the autotransplantation of splenic tissue, most often after splenic rupture. Although it usually affects the peritoneum, omentum, and mesentery, thoracic involvement may occur after combined diaphragmatic and splenic injury.[96,97] The complication is usually identified years after the injury.[97] The splenic nodules may be solitary or multiple and are almost always pleural based and located in the left hemithorax.[97] Radiographic and CT findings include single or multiple pleural-based or paraspinal soft tissue nodules.

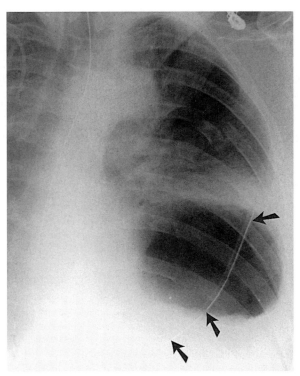

FIGURE 19–8

Traumatic rupture of the left hemidiaphragm. A view of the left side of the chest from an anteroposterior radiograph shows an intrathoracic stomach with cephalad extension of the nasogastric tube (*arrows*). Left rib fractures, areas of atelectasis in the left lung, and a mediastinal shift to the right are visible. (*From Müller NL, Fraser RS, Colman NC, Paré PD: Radiologic Diagnosis of Diseases of the Chest. Philadelphia, WB Saunders, 2001.*)

Fractures of the Ribs

Rib fractures occur in about half of all patients who have major blunt chest trauma.[98,99] Most commonly, they involve the 4th to 10th ribs. Identification of such fractures per se is of limited

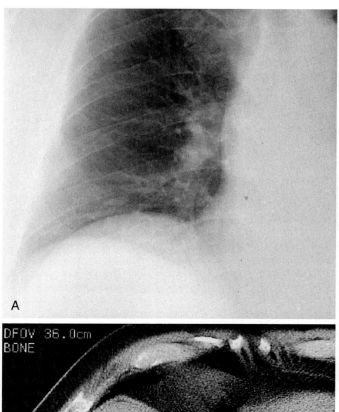

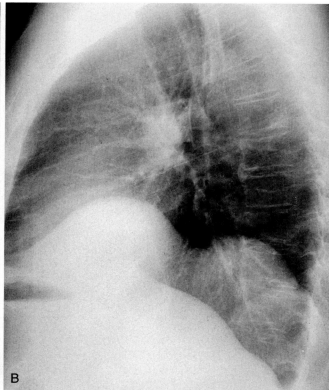

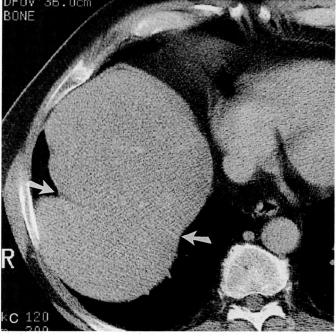

FIGURE 19–9

Traumatic rupture of the right hemidiaphragm. A 53-year-old man was referred for further evaluation of an unusual diaphragmatic contour. Views of the right side of the chest from posteroanterior (**A**) and lateral (**B**) radiographs show apparent elevation of the right hemidiaphragm with a biconvex upper contour. A CT scan (**C**) shows superior herniation of the liver and a focal constriction (*arrows*) characteristic of a traumatic tear. *(From Müller NL, Fraser RS, Colman NC, Paré PD: Radiologic Diagnosis of Diseases of the Chest. Philadelphia, WB Saunders, 2001.)*

clinical significance, the main value of radiography being detection of associated pleural and pulmonary complications.[100] Nonetheless, fractures of certain ribs have specific associations that may be useful in diagnosis. Fractures of the 9th, 10th, or 11th ribs are apt to be associated with splenic or hepatic injury and sometimes with serious intra-abdominal hemorrhage.[93,98] Their presence should prompt investigation with CT of possible associated abdominal organ injury.[20] Because they are relatively protected, fractures of the first, second, and third ribs usually imply severe trauma, often involving the aorta.[101,102]

The diagnosis of fractured ribs may be suggested clinically by the abrupt onset of chest pain after blunt trauma or a severe

bout of coughing. (Cough fractures occur more often in women than men and almost invariably involve the sixth to ninth ribs, most often the seventh, and usually in the posterior axillary line.[103,104]) The pain is accentuated by breathing; in some cases, a sensation of "something snapping" is noted by the patient. Involvement of multiple ribs may result in focal chest wall instability, in which case paradoxical motion of the "flail" chest may be associated with respiratory failure. This complication is usually clinically apparent as paradoxical movement of the chest wall; blood gas analysis is imperative to assess the presence and course of respiratory failure in these cases.

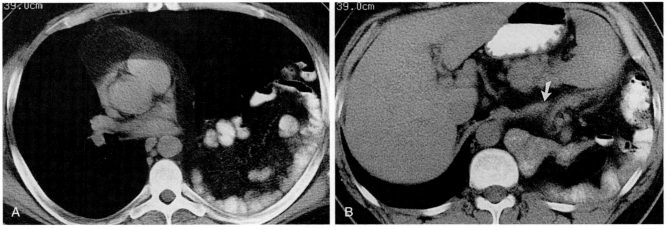

FIGURE 19-10

Traumatic rupture of the left hemidiaphragm. CT scans of the chest (**A**) and upper part of the abdomen (**B**) performed after the oral administration of contrast material show the torn end of the left hemidiaphragm (*arrow*) and intrathoracic herniation of the bowel. The patient was a 28-year-old man with a history of abdominal pain 1 year after trauma sustained during wrestling. (*From Müller NL, Fraser RS, Colman NC, Paré PD: Radiologic Diagnosis of Diseases of the Chest. Philadelphia, WB Saunders, 2001.*)

Fractures of the Spine

Fractures of the thoracic spine account for 15% to 30% of all spine fractures.[20,105] They may result in extraosseous hemorrhage and the development of unilateral or bilateral paraspinal masses or diffuse widening of the mediastinum[106]; in fact, the findings on chest radiographs may mimic those of aortic rupture. About 70% to 90% of fractures are visible on plain radiographs.[3] CT and MR imaging allow detection of otherwise occult fractures and assessment of the relationship between the fracture fragments and the spinal cord. The abnormality is best assessed on multidetector CT scanners using thin sections and multiplanar reconstructions.[5,61] Early recognition is important because of the frequency of associated neurologic deficits: about 60% of patients who have fracture-dislocations of the thoracic spine have complete neurologic deficits, as compared with 30% of patients who have similar injuries to the cervical spine and 2% with injury to the lumbar spine.[3]

Pulmonary Herniation

Protrusion of a portion of lung through an abnormal aperture in the chest wall may be congenital or acquired and may be cervical, thoracic, or (rarely) diaphragmatic in location.[107] The protrusion is covered by parietal and visceral pleura. Congenital hernias occur most frequently in the supraclavicular fossa and less often at the costochondral junction. Traumatic hernias may follow chest trauma or surgery, or chest tube drainage.[107]

The most common location of post-traumatic herniation is the parasternal region just medial to the costochondral junction, where the intercostal musculature is thinnest. The patient usually complains of a bulge appearing during coughing and straining. In most cases, the diagnosis can be made by the observation of a soft crepitant mass that develops under these conditions and disappears during expiration or rest.

Chest radiographs show pulmonary herniation through an obvious defect in the rib cage (Fig. 19–11) or through the supraclavicular fossa.[108] Optimal visualization requires the performance of a Valsalva maneuver or CT.[107]

EFFECTS OF PENETRATING TRAUMA ON THE THORAX

The usual radiographic appearance of the path of a bullet through the lung parenchyma is a poorly defined homogeneous shadow, which, as might be expected, is more or less circular when viewed in the direction in which the bullet passed and longitudinal when viewed in perpendicular projection (Fig. 19–12). The indistinct definition is caused by hemorrhage and edema in the parenchyma surrounding the bullet track; both usually resolve within 3 to 8 days and permit clear visualization of the bullet track, which at that time contains blood and is seen as a soft tissue density that is again circular when seen en face or tubular when seen in profile.[109] The hematoma in the bullet track slowly decreases in size from its periphery.[109] In a few cases, a central radiolucency may be apparent along the bullet's course, indicating communication between the central core of blood and the bronchial tree.[109,110] In such circumstances, a history of hemoptysis can usually be elicited. In most cases, the bullet track resolves completely within a few months. Delay or failure of resolution should suggest the possibility of superimposed infection.[109,111]

Penetrating wounds of the thorax from a knife or bullet may induce traumatic pneumothorax or hemopneumothorax, although the searing effect of a bullet as it passes through the pleura may cauterize the tissues sufficiently to prevent escape of air into the pleural space. In a series of 250 consecutive patients who sustained gunshot wounds involving the thorax, 90% presented with hemothorax or hemopneumothorax, and only 3% presented with pneumothorax alone.[112]

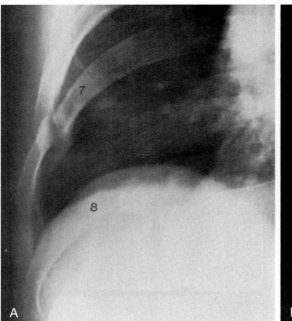
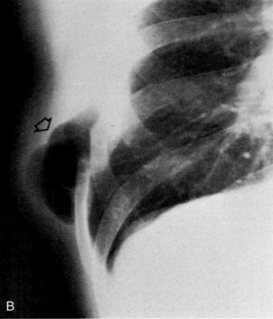

FIGURE 19–11

Hernia of the lung. About 1 year before the radiographs illustrated, this 46-year-old man suffered comminuted fractures of the axillary portions of ribs 6, 7, and 8 on the right in a crush injury to the chest. Healing of the rib fractures had occurred such that there was considerable separation between ribs 7 and 8 (**A**). The patient noted a soft, fluctuant bulge in the axillary region of the chest on coughing and straining. Radiography of the chest in full inspiration during the Valsalva maneuver (**B**) showed herniation of a sizable portion of lung through the defect in the rib cage into the contiguous soft tissues of the axilla (*arrow*). The first radiograph (**A**) was exposed at full expiration and shows no evidence of lung herniation. *(From Müller NL, Fraser RS, Colman NC, Paré PD: Radiologic Diagnosis of Diseases of the Chest. Philadelphia, WB Saunders, 2001.)*

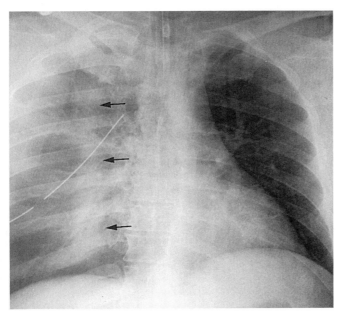

FIGURE 19–12

Bullet track. A 40-year-old man was shot in the back of the neck. The bullet traversed the pleura, lung, diaphragm, and anterior aspect of the liver. An anteroposterior chest radiograph shows the bullet track in the lung (*arrows*), as well as a right hemopneumothorax. *(From Müller NL, Fraser RS, Colman NC, Paré PD: Radiologic Diagnosis of Diseases of the Chest. Philadelphia, WB Saunders, 2001.)*

Penetrating injury to the lungs may be associated with damage to other intrathoracic structures with corresponding radiologic and clinical manifestations. For example, laceration of the esophagus may result in pneumomediastinum, mediastinitis, and/or pleural effusion. The diaphragm can be damaged without evidence of visceral injury and with normal radiographic findings[113]; patients usually complain of abdominal pain, and examination reveals tenderness and rigidity of the abdominal wall. When present, the radiographic abnormalities associated with penetrating diaphragmatic injury are nonspecific and consist of hemothorax, pneumothorax, or apparent elevation of the hemidiaphragm.[85]

COMPLICATIONS OF THORACIC SURGERY

Most complications related to thoracic surgery occur in the immediate postoperative period (up to day 10). Although the radiographic changes observed in the chest wall, pleura, mediastinum, diaphragm, and lungs are in many ways interdependent and should be considered together in interpretation, it is convenient to deal with them separately.

Chest Wall

Thoracotomy. Soft tissue swelling caused by hemorrhage and edema in the vicinity of the incision is common, but it seldom leads to difficulty in radiologic interpretation; in fact, it is often not radiographically apparent. Subcutaneous emphysema is manifested as linear streaks of gas density in the lateral aspect of the chest wall and (frequently) the neck and is almost invariable in the first 2 or 3 postoperative days. It need cause concern only when large in amount, in which case it may be the result of ongoing leak from the surgical anastomosis.

Median Sternotomy. This procedure is the principal surgical approach to the heart and great vessels and to a variety of mediastinal abnormalities. Although the incidence of associated complications is low (<5%), the mortality rate of three of the major complications (sternal dehiscence, mediastinitis, and osteomyelitis) is high.[114,115] Complications usually become evident 1 to 2 weeks postoperatively. Conventional radiography plays a limited role in assessment, and CT is required for adequate evaluation, particularly when mediastinitis is suspected clinically.[116]

Normal postoperative findings that may persist on CT for 2 to 3 weeks after sternotomy include minimal presternal and retrosternal soft tissue thickening by edema fluid and blood, hematoma, a postincisional bone defect, minor sternal irregularities such as slight misalignment, and minimal pericardial thickening.[117] Small localized collections of air may also be seen in the immediate postoperative period and usually resolve within a week.[114,117] Presternal complications, including sinus tracts and abscesses, as well as retrosternal complications such as hematoma, abscess, mediastinitis, pericardial effusion, and empyema, can be diagnosed with CT (Fig. 19–13).[117]

Sternal dehiscence is an uncommon but serious complication of median sternotomy, with an estimated frequency of 1% to 2%.[118] A 2- to 4-mm gap at the sternotomy site (the *midsternal stripe*) can be recognized in 30% to 60% of patients sometime during the postoperative period and is of no diagnostic or prognostic significance.[119] Of much greater importance in establishing sternal separation is migration or reorientation of the sternal wires.[118]

Pleura

After pneumonectomy, fluid gradually fills the empty hemithorax. The rate of accumulation is variable. In most cases, about half to two thirds of the hemithorax fills within the first week; complete filling usually occurs within 2 to 4 months, although it occasionally takes as long as 6 months.[120] Long-term follow-up shows partial or complete resorption of the fluid in many patients.[121] In this situation, there is typically a marked ipsilateral shift of the mediastinum, elevation of the hemidiaphragm, and overinflation of the contralateral lung.

In patients who have not undergone pneumonectomy, little or no fluid is evident during the first 2 or 3 days after thoracotomy because the pleural space is usually effectively drained. After removal of the drainage tube, however, a small amount of fluid often appears, only to disappear quickly during convalescence. Minimal residual pleural thickening may remain, particularly over the lung base.

Accumulation of fluid in larger than expected amounts may result from a variety of causes, including poor positioning of a drainage tube, hemorrhage from an intercostal

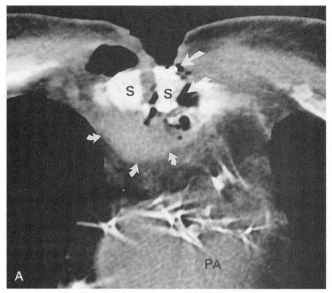

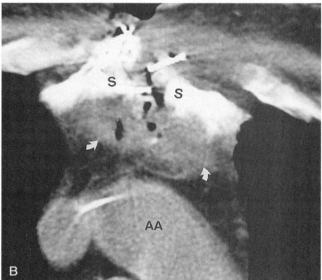

FIGURE 19–13

Retrosternal abscess after sternotomy. A 64-year-old patient had a persistent wound infection 5 weeks after coronary artery bypass surgery. A CT scan at the level of the main pulmonary artery (PA) (**A**) shows a draining sinus (*straight arrows*) communicating with a retrosternal collection (*curved arrows*). The collection extended cephalic to the level of the aortic arch (AA) (**B**). Note the sternal (S) dehiscence and broken sternal wires. The presence of a retrosternal abscess was confirmed at surgery. Cultures grew *Staphylococcus aureus*. (From Müller NL, Fraser RS, Colman NC, Paré PD: Radiologic Diagnosis of Diseases of the Chest. Philadelphia, WB Saunders, 2001.)

vessel, and infection (empyema). In the presence of pleural adhesions, fluid may loculate in areas that are not in communication with the drainage tube, a finding that is particularly common after pleural decortication. In this circumstance, absorption of the fluid may be prolonged, sometimes requiring several weeks. Such local intrapleural collections may be simulated by an extrapleural hematoma secondary to the thoracotomy incision; however, in either event, the finding is not important unless the accumulation is large or infected.

In contrast to the small amount of fluid that often accumulates, gas is seldom visible in the pleural space after removal of the drainage tube, even on radiographs exposed with the patient erect. Postoperative pneumothorax has a variety of causes. Lack of communication with the drainage tube is probably the most common, particularly if the gas is loculated or the tube is positioned incorrectly (e.g., in a major fissure). Other causes include leakage into the pleural space from a "blown" bronchial stump (bronchopleural fistula) or from a bare area of lung after wedge or segmental resection of lung (Fig. 19–14). In the presence of pleural adhesions, a loculated collection of gas may remain for a considerable period; occasionally, it is associated with a collection of fluid in the form of hydropneumothorax.

The incidence of bronchopleural fistula as a complication of pulmonary resection is about 2%[122]; the reported mortality rate ranges from 30% to 70%.[122,123] The complication occurs as a result of necrosis of bronchial stump tissue or dehiscence of sutures. It is most common after right pneumonectomy and occurs rarely after lower lobectomy on either side. Clinical findings include the sudden onset of dyspnea and expectoration of bloody fluid during the first 10 days postoperatively.[123] The chest radiograph may show an unexpected disappearance of fluid as a result of emptying of the pleural space by way of the tracheobronchial tree.[124]

Radiologic evaluation can be facilitated by spiral CT, particularly with the use of thin sections (2-mm collimation).[125]

Esophageal-pleural fistulas may develop after esophagectomy, anterior fusion of the cervical spine, or esophageal dilation. Radiographic findings include mediastinal widening, pleural effusion, pneumothorax, and hydropneumothorax.[126,127] The diagnosis is made readily by demonstration of orally administered contrast material in the pleural space by fluoroscopically guided esophagography or CT.[127,128]

Although rupture of the thoracic duct may be a complication of penetrating or nonpenetrating trauma, the most common cause is iatrogenic; chylothorax is reported as a complication in about 0.2% of patients who have undergone thoracic surgery.[129] As with nonpenetrating duct rupture (see page 799), the anatomic course of the thoracic duct and the site of damage establish on which side the chylothorax develops. The site of injury to the thoracic duct is shown best by lymphangiography.[76]

Mediastinum

The two major radiologic abnormalities that occur in the mediastinum in the postoperative period are enlargement and displacement. The former results from the accumulation of gas or fluid. Pneumomediastinum is a frequent finding after mediastinotomy and should not occasion alarm; however,

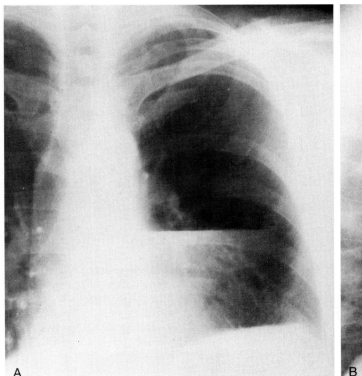
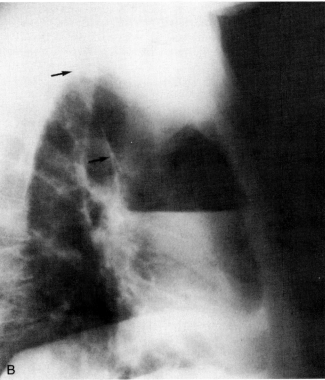

FIGURE 19–14

Loculated hydropneumothorax after lobectomy. Posteroanterior (**A**) and lateral (**B**) radiographs show a large loculated collection of gas and fluid in the anterior portion of the left hemithorax (the upper half of the lower lobe major fissure is indicated by *arrows* in **B**). These films were taken about 2 weeks after left upper lobectomy; the persistence of pneumothorax was caused by an air leak from the lower lobe parenchyma. *(From Müller NL, Fraser RS, Colman NC, Paré PD: Radiologic Diagnosis of Diseases of the Chest. Philadelphia, WB Saunders, 2001.)*

persistence of pneumomediastinum in the absence of other potential causes (such as tracheostomy) should raise suspicion of interstitial pulmonary emphysema associated with some form of pulmonary disease.[130] Venous hemorrhage and edema are also common after mediastinotomy and should not be considered serious unless widening is excessive or progressive. Severe bleeding should be suspected when there is an abrupt increase in the mediastinal width or change in contour after sternotomy.[131] Although the radiographic findings may be helpful in diagnosis, in most cases the diagnosis is based on excessive bloody mediastinal tube drainage.[132] Other causes of mediastinal widening after cardiac surgery include aortic dissection and traumatic venous catheter insertion.[132]

An alteration in the contour of the mediastinum after thoracic surgery may be caused by transposed muscle or by omental or pericardial fat used to obliterate spaces, promote repair and healing, cover a bronchial stump, or reinforce airway and esophageal anastomoses.[133,134] On CT, these "surgical flaps" are visualized as vascularized structures that, depending on their nature, have soft tissue or adipose tissue attenuation.[133,134]

Position of the mediastinum is one of the most important indicators of a pulmonary abnormality during the postoperative period. Displacement may occur toward or away from the side of the thoracotomy. Ipsilateral displacement is an expected finding after lobectomy or pneumonectomy. After lobectomy it is temporary, and the normal midline position is regained as the remainder of the lung undergoes compensatory overinflation. Excessive displacement toward the operated side may be a sign of atelectasis in the ipsilateral lung. In the case of pneumonectomy, ipsilateral mediastinal displacement is progressive and permanent. Mediastinal displacement away from the operated side may occur as a result of atelectasis in the contralateral lung or as a result of an accumulation of excessive fluid or gas in the ipsilateral pleural space.

Within 24 hours of pneumonectomy, the ipsilateral pleural space typically contains air, the mediastinum is shifted slightly to the ipsilateral side, and the hemidiaphragm is elevated slightly (Fig. 19–15).[121] The postpneumonectomy space begins to fill with fluid in a progressive and predictable manner at a rate of about two rib spaces per day. In most cases, there is 80% to 90% obliteration of the space at the end of 2 weeks and complete obliteration by 2 to 4 months. Such obliteration occurs as a result of fluid accumulation, as well as progressive displacement of the mediastinum and elevation of the hemidiaphragm. Mediastinal displacement is an almost invariable finding and constitutes the most reliable indicator of a normal postoperative course. It generally requires 6 to 8 months to reach its maximum. Failure of the mediastinum to shift in the postoperative period almost always indicates an abnormality in the postpneumonectomy space, such as bronchopleural fistula, empyema (Fig. 19–16), or hemorrhage.

The most sensitive indicator of late complications is a return to the midline of a previously shifted mediastinum, particularly the tracheal air column.[121] Such movement usually indicates the presence of recurrent neoplasm, blood, lymph (chylothorax), or pus (empyema) within the postpneumonectomy space. CT can be of great value in documentation of tumor recurrence, either as enlarged mediastinal lymph nodes or as a soft tissue mass projecting into the

near–water density postpneumonectomy space,[135] and in assessment of suspected empyema. Although a shift of the trachea and mediastinal contents back to midline and the sudden appearance of an air-fluid level on the radiograph are helpful clues to the latter complication, they are present in only a few cases.[136] On CT scan, the mediastinal border of the postpneumonectomy space normally has a concave margin[137]; loss of this margin with the development of convex expansion of the postpneumonectomy space has been described as a characteristic finding of empyema.[138]

Rare complications of pneumonectomy include herniation of the heart through a pericardial defect (after radical pneumonectomy in which partial pericardiectomy has been carried out or in which intrapericardial ligation of pulmonary vessels has been performed) and proximal bronchial obstruction resulting from excessive mediastinal shift and rotation (postpneumonectomy syndrome) (Fig. 19–17).[120,139]

Diaphragm

The value of diaphragmatic position in assessment of the postoperative chest radiograph depends largely on the position of the patient at the time of radiography. In the supine position, the normally higher position of the right hemidiaphragm is accentuated, presumably because of the mass of the liver; this finding must not be mistaken for evidence of intrathoracic abnormality. With the patient erect, the usual rules regarding diaphragmatic position pertain.

After pneumonectomy or lobectomy, the ipsilateral hemidiaphragm is almost invariably elevated during the first few days. With pneumonectomy, this elevation persists along with an ipsilateral mediastinal shift despite accumulation of fluid in the pleural space; with lobectomy, elevation and mediastinal displacement disappear over a period of several days or weeks as the remainder of the ipsilateral lung undergoes compensatory overinflation. Marked elevation of a hemidiaphragm can result from injury to the phrenic nerve sustained during surgery. Elevation can also be caused by pulmonary abnormalities such as atelectasis, bronchopneumonia, and thromboembolism. Depression of one hemidiaphragm is an uncommon postoperative abnormality and is invariably caused by a massive pneumothorax or hydrothorax.

Lungs

The radiographic changes in the lungs that can be anticipated after thoracotomy depend on the nature of the surgical procedure. For example, after lobectomy, there is a predictable pattern of reorientation of the remaining lobe or lobes whereby they rotate and hyperinflate to occupy the residual space.[140] The rearrangement of fissures resulting from reorientation of the lobes should not be misinterpreted as evidence of atelectasis. Similarly, the vascular markings become more widely spaced and lung density is reduced (as a result of compensatory overinflation), signs that must not be confused with markings associated with atelectasis or reduced perfusion as a result of thromboembolism.

As might be expected, hematoma formation is common at the site of excision after wedge or segmental pulmonary

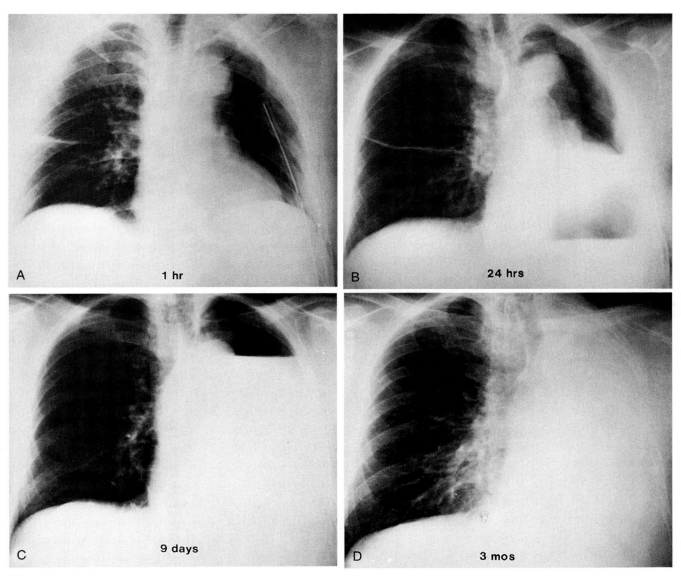

FIGURE 19–15

Postpneumonectomy course—normal. An anteroposterior radiograph obtained in the supine position at the bedside 1 hour after left pneumonectomy (**A**) shows a slight reduction in volume of the left hemithorax. The space is air filled, and the mediastinum is in the midline. After 24 hours, a radiograph in the erect position (**B**) shows moderate elevation of the left hemidiaphragm (as indicated by the gastric air bubble), a moderate shift of the mediastinum to the left, and a prominent air-fluid level in the plane of the third interspace anteriorly. By 9 days (**C**), fluid has filled about two thirds of the cavity of the left hemithorax, but the mediastinum is still displaced to the left (note the curvature of the tracheal air column). By 3 months (**D**), the left hemithorax has become completely airless. Note the persistent shift of the mediastinum to the left and the prominent curve of the air column of the trachea. *(From Müller NL, Fraser RS, Colman NC, Paré PD: Radiologic Diagnosis of Diseases of the Chest. Philadelphia, WB Saunders, 2001.)*

resection. Provided that the physician is aware of the type of surgical procedure carried out, these sometimes ominous-looking yet clinically insignificant opacities should present little difficulty in diagnosis. Apart from such hematomas, any local pulmonary opacity identified in the postoperative period must be regarded as one of the "big four"—atelectasis, pneumonia, infarction, or edema. The manifestations of these complications are no different from those that develop in a nonsurgical setting.

The most common pulmonary complication of surgical procedures is atelectasis, whether the surgery is thoracic or abdominal.[132] The abnormality varies widely in extent, in some cases affecting an entire lobe and in others only lobules. In the latter circumstance, the degree of atelectasis may be insufficient to be appreciated radiographically and is evidenced only by alterations in lung function and gas exchange.[141] The mechanisms by which postoperative atelectasis develops also vary considerably. The most common cause is probably mucus plugging, which occurs chiefly as a result of diminished diaphragmatic excursion (caused by splinting as a result of pain).[141] Disruption of mucociliary clearance has also been documented after major surgery.[142]

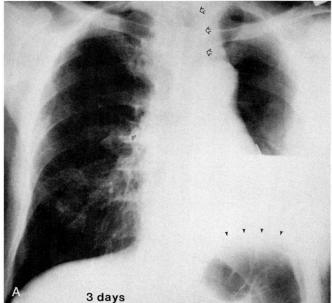

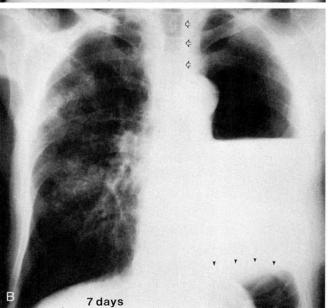

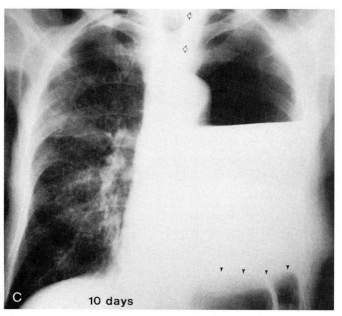

FIGURE 19–16

Postpneumonectomy course complicated by empyema. Three days after left pneumonectomy (**A**), the amount of fluid that has accumulated, the position of the left hemidiaphragm (*arrowheads*), and the shift of the tracheal air column to the left (*open arrows*) are all consistent with a normal postoperative course. At 7 days (**B**), the left hemidiaphragm (*arrowheads*) has undergone some depression, and the tracheal air column (*open arrows*) has returned to the midline. Such a change should suggest empyema, bronchopleural fistula, pleural hemorrhage, or chylothorax. By 10 days (**C**), the left hemidiaphragm (*arrowheads*) has become concave superiorly, and the mediastinum and tracheal air column (*open arrows*) have shifted farther to the right. *(From Müller NL, Fraser RS, Colman NC, Paré PD: Radiologic Diagnosis of Diseases of the Chest. Philadelphia, WB Saunders, 2001.)*

Some degree of atelectasis is present in 60% of patients who have undergone lobectomy.[143] Right upper lobectomy, alone or in combination with middle lobectomy, has been found to have a fivefold greater incidence of severe atelectasis than is noted with other types of resection.[143] Left lower lobe atelectasis, usually seen as a homogeneous opacity behind the heart and often associated with an air bronchogram, is common in patients who have undergone cardiopulmonary bypass during open heart surgical procedures. Right lower lobe atelectasis may also occur in this setting but is less common and less severe.[132,144] Both forms cause little clinical disability and are such a frequent finding after bypass surgery that they can be regarded as an expected part of a satisfactory postoperative appearance.

Pulmonary edema, usually mild, is seen in most patients immediately after cardiac surgery.[131] It may be caused by fluid

overload, left ventricular dysfunction, or increased capillary permeability related to cardiopulmonary bypass.[131] It generally resolves within 24 to 48 hours. Pulmonary edema may occur after lung surgery as a result of fluid overload, congestive heart failure, thromboembolism, or ARDS secondary to aspiration, pneumonia, or sepsis.[145] Occasionally, no cause is apparent. The latter situation is known as postpneumonectomy pulmonary edema and has a high mortality rate (see page 622).[145]

Herniation of lung through the surgical defect is an uncommon complication of thoracotomy, video-assisted thoracoscopic surgery, or chest tube drainage.[107,146] Such hernias may not be detectable on conventional chest radiographs performed at end-inspiration, but they are usually evident on those performed at end-expiration, during cough, or during a Valsalva maneuver or on CT scan (Fig. 19–18). (Lung hernias

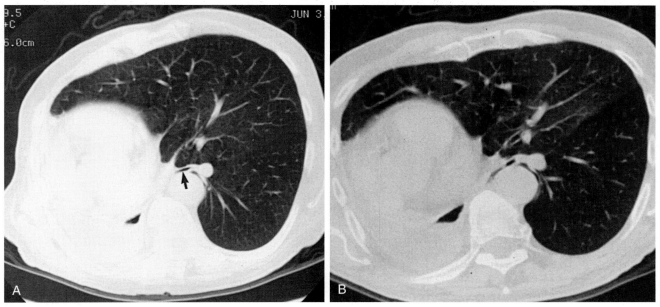

FIGURE 19–17

Postpneumonectomy syndrome. A CT scan performed at end-inspiration (**A**) shows narrowing of the left lower lobe bronchus (*arrow*). An expiratory CT scan (**B**) shows decreased attenuation and vascularity in the left lower lobe as a result of air trapping. *(Case courtesy of Dr. Fred Matzinger, Department of Radiology, The Ottawa Civic Hospital, Ottawa, Canada.)*

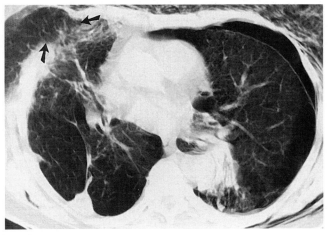

FIGURE 19–18

Lung hernia. A CT scan in a 74-year-old man shows herniation of a portion of the right lung (*arrows*) through a defect in the chest wall. The patient had undergone right thoracotomy and bullectomy several years previously and was being evaluated for recurrent left pneumothorax. Emphysema and scarring in both lungs, left lower lobe atelectasis, left pneumothorax, and subcutaneous emphysema are evident. *(From Müller NL, Fraser RS, Colman NC, Paré PD: Radiologic Diagnosis of Diseases of the Chest. Philadelphia, WB Saunders, 2001.)*

may also be congenital or result from external trauma [see page 802], lifting heavy weights, or playing wind instruments.[107])

Pulmonary torsion is a rare complication of thoracotomy and may involve a lobe or the entire lung.[147] It occurs most commonly after lobectomy but may be seen after wedge resection, pleurectomy, or lung transplantation. Radiologic findings consist of atelectasis, abnormal positioning and orientation of pulmonary vessels and bronchi within the atelectatic lobe, and abnormal position of the hilum in relation to the atelectatic lobe.[147-149] CT shows twisting and narrowing or occlusion of the bronchus, as well as abnormal orientation of the pulmonary vessels and delayed opacification after intravenous administration of contrast material.[138]

COMPLICATIONS OF NONTHORACIC SURGERY

The major thoracic complications of abdominal surgery are atelectasis, pneumonia, thromboembolism, subphrenic abscess, cardiogenic pulmonary edema, and ARDS.[150] The reported incidence of such complications has varied from about 20% to 75%[151]; series associated with the higher figures have undoubtedly included patients who had radiographic abnormalities of little clinical significance.

As discussed previously, atelectasis is the most common complication of surgery and in most patients is related to airway mucus plugging. The process may be complicated by infection[151]; with and without such infection, distinction of atelectasis from pneumonia in the postoperative setting can be difficult because symptoms of cough, sputum production, and fever do not permit accurate differentiation of one from the other. The radiographic and clinical features of acute pneumonia and pulmonary thromboembolism are no different from those observed in other clinical settings. Subphrenic abscess, though uncommon, is almost always a complication of abdominal surgery; its clinical signs (pain in the hypochondrium, limitation of respiratory motion, and fever), timing (10 days after surgery), and radiographic manifestations (pleural effusion and diaphragmatic elevation) do not allow easy distinction from thromboembolism.

COMPLICATIONS OF THERAPEUTIC PROCEDURES

Tracheostomy

Tracheal stenosis, tracheomalacia, and tracheal perforation are well-recognized complications of tracheostomy. The first of these complications is the most common and can occur at the level of the stoma or at the site at which an endotracheal tube impinged on the mucosa. The radiologic and clinical manifestations are discussed in Chapter 15 (see page 628).

Airway and Vascular Stents

Expandable metal or silicone stents have been used in the definitive or (more often) palliative treatment of many intrathoracic diseases.[152] The most common has been carcinoma, usually pulmonary and occasionally esophageal.[153,154] Benign conditions such as relapsing polychondritis,[155] tuberculosis,[156] and airway stenosis following lung transplantation[157] have also been treated in this manner. Stenting of vascular stenoses that have resulted from congenital cardio-

vascular disease,[158] thromboemboli,[159] or lung transplantation[160] has also been performed.

The incidence of complications associated with these stents is low. Such complications include airway perforation,[161] the formation of obstructing granulation tissue or mucous webs,[162] recurrent pneumonia after erosion of an esophageal stent into a bronchus,[163] and recurrent vascular stenosis secondary to intimal fibrosis at the stent site.[164]

Esophageal Procedures

About 75% of cases of esophageal rupture are the result of diagnostic or therapeutic interventions, the most common being associated with esophagoscopy or gastroscopy.[101] The usual sites of perforation are below the cricopharyngeal muscle, at the level of the left main bronchus, and immediately above the gastroesophageal junction. As might be expected, the most common complication is acute mediastinitis, manifested radiographically by mediastinal widening that typically possesses a smooth, sharply defined margin. Other manifestations include pneumomediastinum, left pleural effusion, pneumothorax, hydropneumothorax, and chylothorax (Fig. 19–19).[165]

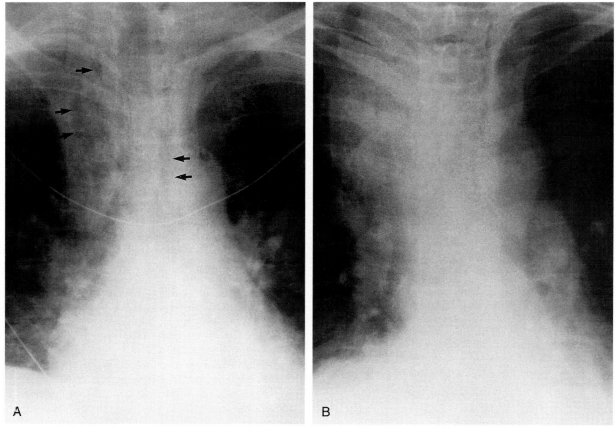

A   B

FIGURE 19–19

Esophageal rupture. A view of the mediastinum from an anteroposterior chest radiograph (**A**) in a 39-year-old woman shows pneumomediastinum (*arrows*) and mild mediastinal widening. A radiograph taken 5 days later (**B**) reveals increased mediastinal widening. Esophageal rupture at the level of the T1 vertebral body, which occurred during attempted endotracheal intubation, was confirmed by Gastrografin swallow. (*From Müller NL, Fraser RS, Colman NC, Paré PD: Radiologic Diagnosis of Diseases of the Chest. Philadelphia, WB Saunders, 2001.*)

Chest Drainage Tubes

Complications of chest drainage tubes are uncommon and are usually readily apparent clinically.[166] They include laceration of an intercostal artery or vein; laceration of the diaphragm, liver, spleen, or stomach; malposition of the tube (such as in the chest wall, abdomen, or interlobar fissure); pulmonary perforation; infection (predominantly empyema); formation of a systemic artery–to–pulmonary artery shunt; and perforation of the right ventricle.[167,168]

Hemorrhage from a lacerated intercostal vessel can be avoided by insertion of the tube in the intercostal space as close as possible to the superior surface of a rib; however, intercostal vessels may be tortuous, especially in the elderly, and even careful insertion carries a risk.[167]

Malposition of the chest tube can occur within the pleural space, in which case the complication is one of inadequate drainage. Such malposition can occur in several ways; for example, a tube inserted anterolaterally and directed posteriorly drains the posterior pleural space but, with the patient lying in a supine position, does not drain a pneumothorax situated anteriorly. The incidence of malposition of a chest tube within a major fissure is probably higher than generally believed.[166,169] Such malposition often cannot be recognized convincingly on a single anteroposterior radiograph; however, when a pneumothorax or hydrothorax is not draining satisfactorily, the abnormal position can be confirmed, if necessary, by lateral radiography. In some cases, suboptimal tube positioning may be unrecognized even when frontal and lateral radiographs are obtained.[170] Although only frontal radiographs are required for assessment of chest tube location in most patients, frontal and lateral radiographs are recommended after every tube insertion for empyema, unless the tube was placed under CT or ultrasound guidance.[171] CT may show unexpected tube malplacement, including an extrapleural location, an intraparenchymal, transdiaphragmatic course, a trans-splenic course, and impingement on the trachea or posterior mediastinum.[172]

Pulmonary perforation is a rare complication of tube insertion.[173] Although it can be suspected on radiographs, it is better depicted on CT, which shows the intraparenchymal location of the tube, as well as the presence of associated laceration and hematoma (Fig. 19–20).[172] Care must be taken, however, when assessing the lung periphery, particularly near the lung apex and diaphragm, where partial volume averaging and indentation of the lung by a chest tube in the pleural space may mimic perforation.[172]

Abdominal Drainage Tubes

Potentially serious complications, including hemothorax, pneumothorax, and empyema, can follow transgression of the pleural space during placement of a drainage catheter into the liver or upper part of the abdomen.[174,175] With this in mind, it is important not to puncture the ninth intercostal space in the midaxillary line because needles inserted through this interspace have been found to traverse the pleura in cadaver studies.[174,175]

Nasogastric Tubes

Because most nasogastric tubes are opaque, any malposition should be readily apparent radiographically. The most

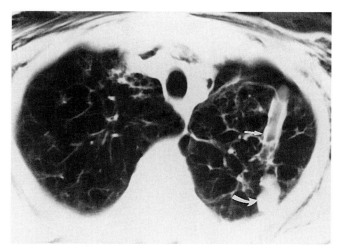

FIGURE 19–20

Intraparenchymal chest tube. A CT scan in a 69-year-old patient shows a left chest tube (*straight arrow*) with its tip in the left upper lobe; a small hematoma (*curved arrow*) is present. Severe emphysema, a small left pneumothorax, pneumomediastinum, and subcutaneous emphysema are evident. (*From Müller NL, Fraser RS, Colman NC, Paré PD: Radiologic Diagnosis of Diseases of the Chest. Philadelphia, WB Saunders, 2001.*)

common findings are coiling within the esophagus and incomplete insertion. Although the function of the tube is not served in both situations, there are usually no serious consequences. Of far greater clinical importance is faulty insertion of the tube into the tracheobronchial tree, a complication that has been reported in about 0.2% to 0.3% of feeding tube placements.[176,177] It is most apt to occur in patients who have impaired mental status or diminished gag, cough, or swallowing reflexes.[178] The malposition is particularly hazardous if the tube is meant for hyperalimentation, in which case fluid injected into the lungs or pleural cavity can lead to pneumonia, abscess, pneumothorax, hydropneumothorax, and empyema.[179,180] In these cases, the tip of the tube sometimes ends up in an unusual location, such as the mediastinum or abdomen (Fig. 19–21).

Endotracheal Tubes

During the first few days after insertion of an endotracheal tube, serious complications are infrequent; they occur more often in association with emergency resuscitation than with more routine interventions.[181] The chief complication is large-airway obstruction resulting from placement of the tube too low in the trachea or in the proximal bronchi. In most instances, the tube enters the right main bronchus, and the balloon cuff occludes the orifice of the left main bronchus and thereby results in atelectasis of the left lung.[181] If the tube is advanced sufficiently into the right main bronchus, occlusion of the right upper lobe bronchus may be the sole result, or both right upper lobe atelectasis and atelectasis of the left lung may be seen. Occasionally, the tube enters the left rather than the right main bronchus and leads to atelectasis of the right lung.

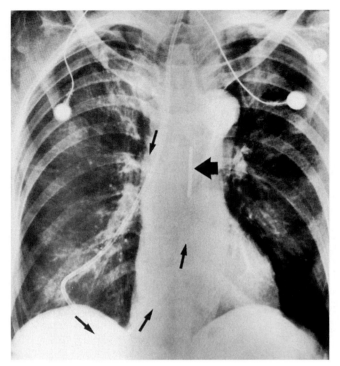

FIGURE 19-21

Faulty insertion of a feeding tube. The circuitous course taken by this feeding tube can be established only partly from this anteroposterior radiograph. It passed into the right lower lobe. As it turned to the left, it presumably penetrated the visceral pleura covering this lobe and then passed superiorly either within the mediastinum or in the pleural space adjacent to the azygoesophageal recess to a point where its tip overlies the region of the tracheal carina (*large arrow*). The patient suffered no ill effects after removal of the tube. (*From Müller NL, Fraser RS, Colman NC, Paré PD: Radiologic Diagnosis of Diseases of the Chest. Philadelphia, WB Saunders, 2001.*)

The rate at which atelectasis occurs depends on the gas content of the lung at the moment of occlusion. Total collapse requires 18 to 24 hours if the parenchyma is air containing, but it may occur in a matter of minutes if the lung contains 100% oxygen (often the case in acute respiratory emergencies). Withdrawal of the tube typically results in rapid re-expansion of the collapsed lung or lobe.

With the head and neck in neutral position, the ideal distance between the tip of the endotracheal tube and the carina is 5 ± 2 cm.[182] Flexion and extension of the neck cause a 2-cm descent and ascent of the tip of the endotracheal tube, respectively; if the position of the neck can be established from the radiograph (through visualization of the mandible), the ideal distance between the tip of the endotracheal tube and the carina should be 3 ± 2 cm with the neck flexed and 7 ± 2 cm with the neck extended. When the carina is not visualized, it is sufficient to establish the relationship of the tip of the endotracheal tube to the fifth, sixth, or seventh thoracic vertebral body.[183]

Malpositioning of an endotracheal tube in the esophagus is uncommon and usually evident clinically. Because the trachea and esophagus are superimposed on anteroposterior radiographs, such malpositioning is seldom apparent radi-

ographically; when present, findings include projection of the tip of the endotracheal tube lateral to the trachea, gaseous distention of the distal part of the esophagus or stomach, and (rarely) deviation of the trachea by an overinflated balloon cuff (Fig. 19–22).[184] Complications that result from prolonged inflation of the cuff of an endotracheal tube, such as tracheal stenosis, are discussed in Chapter 15 (see page 628).

Transtracheal Catheters

The use of long-term indwelling transtracheal catheters to administer oxygen to patients who have COPD was developed in the 1980s to cut the cost and increase the ease of home oxygen care.[185] The catheters may be inserted directly into the trachea through the skin of the neck (percutaneous catheters) or may be implanted through an incision in the suprasternal notch, stitched to the tracheal wall, and tunneled under the skin to exit in the upper part of the abdomen (tunneled catheters).[186]

Complications associated with these catheters include subcutaneous emphysema, localized skin infection or hemorrhage, abnormal tracheal mucus production, breakage of catheter parts into the trachea, and the formation of partly occlusive mucus or mucopurulent plugs around the catheter tip.[185,187] An increase in the size or dislodgment of such a plug may result in tracheal or bronchial obstruction that can compromise airflow significantly.[187,188]

Percutaneous Central Venous Catheters

Insertion of a central venous catheter can be followed by a variety of complications, some of which have serious consequences.[189-191] Some pertain to the procedure itself and relate to abnormalities within or around the catheterized vein; others, perhaps most, arise from incorrect positioning of the catheter tip.

Faulty Insertion. Central venous catheters can be inserted through an arm vein, a subclavian vein (by either an infraclavicular or supraclavicular route), or an external or internal jugular vein. Most faulty placements occur in arm and infraclavicular subclavian approaches. Only about 65% to 75% of catheters reach their proper location after arm vein insertion; the results with external jugular placement are less satisfactory.[192] Supraclavicular subclavian and internal jugular approaches result in a relatively small percentage of improper placements.[193]

Phlebothrombosis. Phlebothrombosis is probably the most common complication of venous catheterization and can be manifested by either sleeve or mural thrombosis.[189] Autopsy studies have shown that circumferential fibrin sleeves develop around indwelling venous catheters 24 hours after insertion in 80% to 100% of cases.[194,195] Although these fibrin sleeves seldom give rise to complications, parts of the thrombus may embolize to the lungs, particularly when the catheter is removed.[189]

Mural thrombosis can lead to partial or complete venous obstruction. In an investigation of 204 patients in the intensive care unit who had internal jugular or subclavian catheters, color Doppler ultrasound examination performed just before or within 24 hours of catheter removal showed thrombosis at the catheter site in 33%.[196] The thrombus was limited (2 to

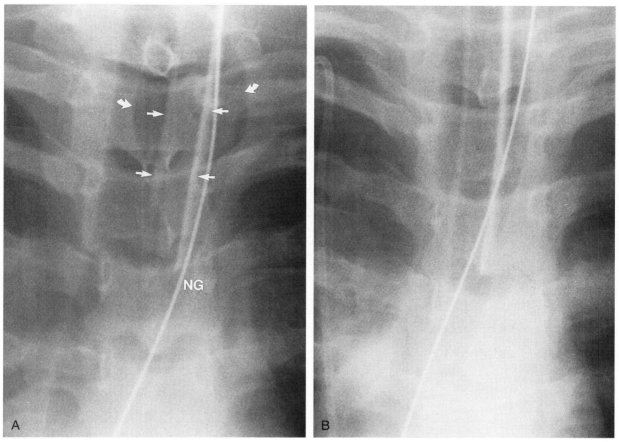

FIGURE 19–22

Esophageal intubation. A view of the thoracic inlet from an anteroposterior chest radiograph (**A**) in a 22-year-old patient after a motor vehicle accident shows an endotracheal tube (*straight arrows*) lying lateral to the trachea and in close proximity to the nasogastric tube (NG); the appearance is consistent with esophageal intubation. Note the inflated cuff of the endotracheal tube (*curved arrows*). A view after reintubation (**B**) shows a normal endotracheal position. *(From Müller NL, Fraser RS, Colman NC, Paré PD: Radiologic Diagnosis of Diseases of the Chest. Philadelphia, WB Saunders, 2001.)*

4 mm) in 8%, large (≥4 mm) in 22%, and occlusive in 3%. The likelihood of such thrombosis is related to the duration that the catheter is left in place.[197]

The radiographic findings are neither sensitive nor specific and include enlargement of the vena cava, pleural effusion, and dilated collateral vessels (including the arch of the azygos vein or left superior intercostal vein).[195] The diagnosis can be confirmed by venography, color flow Doppler ultrasonography, CT, or MR imaging.[196,198,199] All these modalities have limitations, and the technique of choice is influenced by the suspected location of the thrombosis, cost, and local experience.

Complications of thrombosis include loss of central venous access, superior vena cava syndrome, and pulmonary thromboembolism.[200,201] Although most thromboses are sterile, infection may occur, particularly in patients who have long-term indwelling central venous catheters.[190] Other infectious complications related to catheter insertion include mediastinitis, osteomyelitis of the clavicle, and exit site or tunnel infections.[190]

Vascular Perforation. A vein can be perforated at the time of catheter insertion or sometime later[202,203]; later perforation is caused by gradual erosion of a relatively thin-walled intrathoracic vessel, partly as a result of cardiac and respiratory movements affecting the catheter tip.[44] Most perforations occur after the introduction of catheters for pressure measurements and hyperalimentation. Depending on the vein involved, perforation can result in pneumothorax (the most common complication), hemothorax, hydrothorax, mediastinal hemorrhage, a bronchopulmonary-venous fistula, or extrapleural hematoma.[204]

Vascular erosion by central venous catheters usually affects the superior vena cava and is considerably more common with left-sided catheters.[204] It has been postulated that this predisposition is related to the more horizontal orientation of the left brachiocephalic vein than the right vein; as a consequence, the tip of a left-sided catheter inserted an insufficient length tends to abut against the right lateral wall of the superior vena cava within 45 degrees of perpendicular.[204] An early sign of impending perforation of the superior vena cava is a gentle curvature of the distal portion of the catheter with the tip directed toward the right lateral vein wall.[44]

Myocardial Perforation. It is common for the tip of a central venous catheter to reside in one of the right heart chambers; for example, in an investigation of 300 patients, the tip was identified in the right atrium or right ventricle in 40 (13%).[193] This position is potentially hazardous, particularly if the catheter has a firm or sharp tip; perforation of the atrium or ventricle may result in fatal pericardial tamponade (from blood or infused fluid),[205] and irritation of the myocardium may cause arrhythmias.

Catheter Coiling, Knotting, and Breaking. Coiled catheters traumatize the vein and are much more likely to perforate, break, and embolize. They also have a much greater tendency to twist into knots; although these knots can sometimes be manipulated free, this is not always possible, and thoracotomy may be required for removal.[206]

Miscellaneous Complications. Other complications of percutaneous central venous catheter insertion include sepsis, embolization of catheter fragments to the lungs (Fig. 19–23), air embolism (usually asymptomatic), thoracic duct laceration, and damage to the brachial plexus, sympathetic chain, or phrenic, recurrent laryngeal, or 9th to 12th cranial nerves.[207,208]

Pulmonary Arterial Catheters

Complications of flow-directed balloon-tipped (Swan-Ganz) catheters include atrial and ventricular arrhythmias, perforation of the pulmonary artery, perforation of the visceral pleura, pulmonary artery thrombosis with pulmonary infarction, and air embolism.[209] As a group, these events are not rare;

for example, in a prospective study of 528 catheterizations, serious complications were considered to have occurred in 23 (4.4%).[210]

Pulmonary artery occlusion, with or without infarction, is probably the most common pulmonary complication. In a series of 391 patients who had undergone catheterization, evidence of thrombosis/thromboembolism was found in 16 (4%).[211] Although it has been estimated that the pulmonary artery is perforated in only about 0.001% to 0.5% of all cases of catheter insertion,[212] there is evidence that it may be a more common event. In one autopsy review, 4 such cases were identified in a consecutive series of 270 cases (1.5%)[209]; in only 1 case was the perforation suspected clinically.

As might be expected, the usual result of pulmonary artery perforation is hemorrhage, generally into pulmonary parenchyma but occasionally predominantly into the bronchovascular interstitium or pleural space.[213] Shortly after perforation, the chest radiograph may show a localized area of consolidation with hazy margins (Fig. 19–24).[214,215] This finding is replaced within 1 to 3 weeks by a round, well-circumscribed nodule or mass ranging from 2 to 8 cm in diameter that corresponds to the development of an organizing hematoma (false aneurysm). Contrast-enhanced CT shows the latter as an enhancing mass associated with a vessel and sometimes containing a partially thrombosed lumen.[214] The diagnosis can be confirmed by pulmonary angiography.[214]

As might be expected, the primary clinical manifestation is hemoptysis, which can be massive. The mortality rate

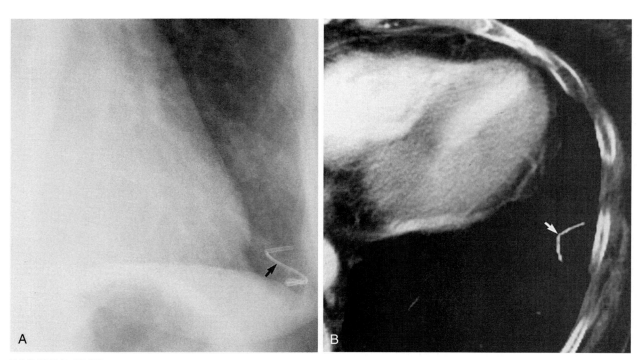

FIGURE 19–23

Embolization of a broken central venous catheter. Views of the left lung from a posteroanterior radiograph (**A**) and a CT scan (**B**) show the broken distal portion of an intravenous catheter (*arrows*) in the left lower lobe. The tip presumably lies within a pulmonary artery. The patient did not have symptoms, and the catheter was left in place; no associated symptoms were observed during a 4-year follow-up period. *(From Müller NL, Fraser RS, Colman NC, Paré PD: Radiologic Diagnosis of Diseases of the Chest. Philadelphia, WB Saunders, 2001.)*

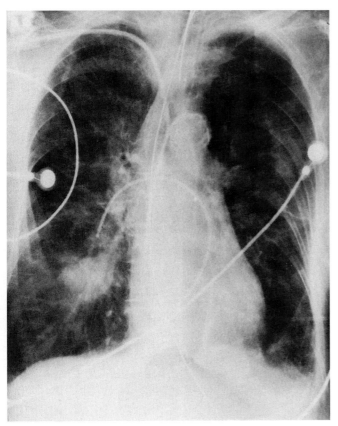

FIGURE 19–24

Pulmonary artery perforation by a Swan-Ganz catheter. A posteroanterior radiograph shows the tip of a Swan-Ganz catheter in the region of the right interlobar artery. Distal to it is a fairly well defined opacity that could be situated in either the middle or lower lobe. Shortly thereafter, this 83-year-old woman coughed up a small amount of blood and died. At autopsy, the right middle lobe showed extensive air space hemorrhage and a defect in a subsegmental pulmonary artery associated with an irregularly shaped intraparenchymal hematoma. *(From Müller NL, Fraser RS, Colman NC, Paré PD: Radiologic Diagnosis of Diseases of the Chest. Philadelphia, WB Saunders, 2001.)*

associated with clinically evident perforation has been estimated to be as high as 45% to 65%.[216] Patients in whom false aneurysms develop can have recurrent life-threatening hemorrhage; the rate of this complication has been estimated to be about 30% to 40% and the mortality rate 40% to 70%.[214,217]

Cardiac Pacemakers

A variety of pleuropulmonary complications are associated with the presence of cardiac pacemakers,[218] including pneumothorax, pleural effusion, and embolism of the distal segment to the pulmonary artery. Venous thrombosis may also lead to partial or complete occlusion of the subclavian and brachiocephalic veins or superior vena cava.[219] Complications associated with automatic implantable cardioverter-defibrillators include hemoptysis as a result of erosion of the ventricular patch into a bronchus and bronchopericardial fistula.[218,220]

REFERENCES

1. Boyd AD, Glassman LR: Trauma to the lung. Chest Surg Clin N Am 7:263-284, 1997.
2. Mayberry JC: Imaging in thoracic trauma: The trauma surgeon's perspective. J Thorac Imaging 15:76-86, 2000.
3. Groskin SA: Selected topics in chest trauma. Semin Ultrasound CT MR 17:119-141, 1996.
4. Zinck SE, Primack SL: Radiographic and CT findings in blunt chest trauma. J Thorac Imaging 15:87-96, 2000.
5. Rivas LA, Fishman JE, Munera F, Bajayo DE: Multislice CT in thoracic trauma. Radiol Clin North Am 41:599-616, 2003.
6. Greene R: Lung alterations in thoracic trauma. J Thorac Imaging 2:1-11, 1987.
7. Shorr RM, Crittenden M, Indeck M, et al: Blunt thoracic trauma. Analysis of 515 patients. Ann Surg 206:200-205, 1987.
8. Errion AR, Houk VN, Kettering DL: Pulmonary hematoma due to blunt, nonpenetrating thoracic trauma. Am Rev Respir Dis 88:384-392, 1963.
9. Stevens E, Templeton AW: Traumatic nonpenetrating lung contusion. Radiology 85:247-252, 1965.
10. Williams J, Stembridge V: Pulmonary contusion secondary to nonpenetrating chest trauma. AJR Am J Roentgenol 91:284, 1964.
11. Wiot JF: The radiologic manifestations of blunt chest trauma. JAMA 231:500-503, 1975.
12. Smejkal R, O'Malley KF, David E, et al: Routine initial computed tomography of the chest in blunt torso trauma. Chest 100:667-669, 1991.
13. Reid JD, Kommareddi S, Lankerani M, Park MC: Chronic expanding hematomas. A clinicopathologic entity. JAMA 244:2441-2442, 1980.
14. Kollmorgen DR, Murray KA, Sullivan JJ, et al: Predictors of mortality in pulmonary contusion. Am J Surg 168:659-663, discussion 663-664, 1994.
15. Wagner RB, Crawford WO Jr, Schimpf PP: Classification of parenchymal injuries of the lung. Radiology 167:77-82, 1988.
16. Hollister M, Stern EJ, Steinberg KP: Type 2 pulmonary laceration: A marker of blunt high-energy injury to the lung. AJR Am J Roentgenol 165:1126, 1995.
17. Athanassiadi K, Gerazounis M, Kalantzi N, et al: Primary traumatic pulmonary pseudocysts: A rare entity. Eur J Cardiothorac Surg 23:43-45, 2003.
18. Kang EY, Müller NL: CT in blunt chest trauma: Pulmonary, tracheobronchial, and diaphragmatic injuries. Semin Ultrasound CT MR 17:114-118, 1996.
19. Santos GH, Mahendra T: Traumatic pulmonary pseudocysts. Ann Thorac Surg 27:359-362, 1979.
20. Collins J: Chest wall trauma. J Thorac Imaging 15:112-119, 2000.
21. Melloni G, Cremona G, Ciriaco P, et al: Diagnosis and treatment of traumatic pulmonary pseudocysts. J Trauma 54:737-743, 2003.
22. Takahashi N, Murakami J, Murayama S, et al: MR evaluation of intrapulmonary hematoma. J Comput Assist Tomogr 19:125-127, 1995.
23. Kuhlman JE, Pozniak MA, Collins J, Knisely BL: Radiographic and CT findings of blunt chest trauma: Aortic injuries and looking beyond them. Radiographics 18:1085-1106 discussion 1107-1108, quiz 1, 1998.
24. Mirvis SE, Templeton P: Imaging in acute thoracic trauma. Semin Roentgenol 27:184-210, 1992.
25. Rossbach MM, Johnson SB, Gomez MA, et al: Management of major tracheobronchial injuries: A 28-year experience. Ann Thorac Surg 65:182-186, 1998.
26. Song JK, Beaty CD: Diagnosis of pulmonary contusions and a bronchial laceration after a fall. AJR Am J Roentgenol 167:1510, 1996.
27. Roxburgh JC: Rupture of the tracheobronchial tree. Thorax 42:681-688, 1987.
28. Barmada H, Gibbons JR: Tracheobronchial injury in blunt and penetrating chest trauma. Chest 106:74-78, 1994.
29. Burke JF: Early diagnosis of traumatic rupture of the bronchus. JAMA 181:682-686, 1962.
30. Collins JP, Ketharanathan V, McConchie I: Rupture of major bronchi resulting from closed chest injuries. Thorax 28:371-375, 1973.
31. Weir IH, Müller NL, Connell DG: CT diagnosis of bronchial rupture. J Comput Assist Tomogr 12:1035-1036, 1988.
32. Unger JM, Schuchmann GG, Grossman JE, Pellett JR: Tears of the trachea and main bronchi caused by blunt trauma: Radiologic findings. AJR Am J Roentgenol 153:1175-1180, 1989.
33. Harvey-Smith W, Bush W, Northrop C: Traumatic bronchial rupture. AJR Am J Roentgenol 134:1189-1193, 1980.
34. Lotz PR, Martel W, Rohwedder JJ, Green RA: Significance of pneumomediastinum in blunt trauma to the thorax. AJR Am J Roentgenol 132:817-819, 1979.
35. Silbiger ML, Kushner LN: Tracheobronchial perforation: Its diagnosis and treatment. Radiology 85:242-246, 1965.
36. Vidinel I: Displacement of the mediastinum. Chest 62:215-216, 1972.
37. Larizadeh R: Rupture of the bronchus. Thorax 21:28-31, 1966.
38. Groskin SA: Selected topics in chest trauma. Radiology 183:605-617, 1992.
39. Ashbaugh DG, Peters GN, Halgrimson CG, et al: Chest trauma. Analysis of 685 patients. Arch Surg 95:546-555, 1967.
40. Robertson HT, Lakshminarayan S, Hudson LD: Lung injury following a 50-metre fall into water. Thorax 33:175-180, 1978.
41. Raptopoulos V, Sheiman RG, Phillips DA, et al: Traumatic aortic tear: Screening with chest CT. Radiology 182:667-673, 1992.
42. Fisher RG, Chasen MH, Lamki N: Diagnosis of injuries of the aorta and brachiocephalic arteries caused by blunt chest trauma: CT vs aortography. AJR Am J Roentgenol 162:1047-1052, 1994.
43. Mitchell SE, Clark RA: Complications of central venous catheterization. AJR Am J Roentgenol 133:467-476, 1979.

44. Tocino IM, Watanabe A: Impending catheter perforation of superior vena cava: Radiographic recognition. AJR Am J Roentgenol 146:487-490, 1986.

45. Patel NH, Stephens KE Jr, Mirvis SE, et al: Imaging of acute thoracic aortic injury due to blunt trauma: A review. Radiology 209:335-348, 1998.

46. Crass JR, Cohen AM, Motta AO, et al: A proposed new mechanism of traumatic aortic rupture: The osseous pinch. Radiology 176:645-649, 1990.

47. Eller JL, Ziter FM Jr: Avulsion of the innominate artery from the aortic arch. An evaluation of roentgenographic findings. Radiology 94:75-78, 1970.

48. Dennis LN, Rogers LF: Superior mediastinal widening from spine fractures mimicking aortic rupture on chest radiographs. AJR Am J Roentgenol 152:27-30, 1989.

49. Mirvis SE, Bidwell JK, Buddemeyer EU, et al: Value of chest radiography in excluding traumatic aortic rupture. Radiology 163:487-493, 1987.

50. Pretre R, Chilcott M: Blunt trauma to the heart and great vessels. N Engl J Med 336:626-632, 1997.

51. Creasy JD, Chiles C, Routh WD, Dyer RB: Overview of traumatic injury of the thoracic aorta. Radiographics 17:27-45, 1997.

52. Heystraten FM, Rosenbusch G, Kingma LM, et al: Chest radiography in acute traumatic rupture of the thoracic aorta. Acta Radiol 29:411-417, 1988.

53. Simeone JF, Minagi H, Putman CE: Traumatic disruption of the thoracic aorta: Significance of the left apical extrapleural cap. Radiology 117:265-268, 1975.

54. Simeone JF, Deren MM, Cagle F: The value of the left apical cap in the diagnosis of aortic rupture: A prospective and retrospective study. Radiology 139:35-37, 1981.

55. Mirvis SE, Bidwell JK, Buddemeyer EU, et al: Imaging diagnosis of traumatic aortic rupture. A review and experience at a major trauma center. Invest Radiol 22:187-196, 1987.

56. Marnocha KE, Maglinte DD: Plain-film criteria for excluding aortic rupture in blunt chest trauma. AJR Am J Roentgenol 144:19-21, 1985.

57. Marotta R, Franchetto AA: The CT appearance of aortic transection. AJR Am J Roentgenol 166:647-651, 1996.

58. Mirvis SE, Shanmuganathan K, Miller BH, et al: Traumatic aortic injury: Diagnosis with contrast-enhanced thoracic CT—five-year experience at a major trauma center. Radiology 200:413-422, 1996.

59. Rigauts H, Marchal G, Baert AL, Hupke R: Initial experience with volume CT scanning. J Comput Assist Tomogr 14:675-682, 1990.

60. Gavant ML, Menke PG, Fabian T, et al: Blunt traumatic aortic rupture: Detection with helical CT of the chest. Radiology 197:125-133, 1995.

61. Lomoschitz FM, Eisenhuber E, Linnau KF, et al: Imaging of chest trauma: Radiological patterns of injury and diagnostic algorithms. Eur J Radiol 48:61-70, 2003.

62. Trerotola SO: Can helical CT replace aortography in thoracic trauma. Radiology 197:13-15, 1995.

63. Gavant ML, Flick P, Menke P, Gold RE: CT aortography of thoracic aortic rupture. AJR Am J Roentgenol 166:955-961, 1996.

64. Zeiger MA, Clark DE, Morton JR: Reappraisal of surgical treatment of traumatic transection of the thoracic aorta. J Cardiovasc Surg (Torino) 31:607-610, 1990.

65. Van Hise ML, Primack SL, Israel RS, Müller NL: CT in blunt chest trauma: Indications and limitations. Radiographics 18:1071-1084, 1998.

66. Dyer DS, Moore EE, Mestek MF, et al: Can chest CT be used to exclude aortic injury? Radiology 213:195-202, 1999.

67. Morgan PW, Goodman LR, Aprahamian C, et al: Evaluation of traumatic aortic injury: Does dynamic contrast-enhanced CT play a role? Radiology 182:661-666, 1992.

68. Hunink MG, Bos JJ: Triage of patients to angiography for detection of aortic rupture after blunt chest trauma: Cost-effectiveness analysis of using CT. AJR Am J Roentgenol 165:27-36, 1995.

69. Morse SS, Glickman MG, Greenwood LH, et al: Traumatic aortic rupture: False-positive aortographic diagnosis due to atypical ductus diverticulum. AJR Am J Roentgenol 150:793-796, 1988.

70. Smith MD, Cassidy JM, Souther S, et al: Transesophageal echocardiography in the diagnosis of traumatic rupture of the aorta. N Engl J Med 332:356-362, 1995.

71. Ketai L, Brandt MM, Schermer C: Nonaortic mediastinal injuries from blunt chest trauma. J Thorac Imaging 15:120-127, 2000.

72. Stanbridge RD: Tracheo-oesophageal fistula and bilateral recurrent laryngeal nerve palsies after blunt chest trauma. Thorax 37:548-549, 1982.

73. Kerns SR, Gay SB: CT of blunt chest trauma. AJR Am J Roentgenol 154:55-60, 1990.

74. Dulchavsky SA, Ledgerwood AM, Lucas CE: Management of chylothorax after blunt chest trauma. J Trauma 28:1400-1401, 1988.

75. Worthington MG, de Groot M, Gunning AJ, von Oppell UO: Isolated thoracic duct injury after penetrating chest trauma. Ann Thorac Surg 60:272-274, 1995.

76. Sachs PB, Zelch MG, Rice TW, et al: Diagnosis and localization of laceration of the thoracic duct: Usefulness of lymphangiography and CT. AJR Am J Roentgenol 157:703-705, 1991.

77. Reynolds J, Davis JT: Injuries of the chest wall, pleura, pericardium, lungs, bronchi and esophagus. Radiol Clin North Am 4:383-401, 1966.

78. Shah R, Sabanathan S, Mearns AJ, Choudhury AK: Traumatic rupture of diaphragm. Ann Thorac Surg 60:1444-1449, 1995.

79. de la Rocha AG, Creel RJ, Mulligan GW, Burns CM: Diaphragmatic rupture due to blunt abdominal trauma. Surg Gynecol Obstet 154:175-180, 1982.

80. Leaman PL: Rupture of the right hemidiaphragm due to blunt trauma. Ann Emerg Med 12:351-357, 1983.

81. Meyers BF, McCabe CJ: Traumatic diaphragmatic hernia. Occult marker of serious injury. Ann Surg 218:783-790, 1993.

82. Miller L, Bennett EV Jr, Root HD, et al: Management of penetrating and blunt diaphragmatic injury. J Trauma 24:403-409, 1984.

83. Beauchamp G, Khalfallah A, Girard R, et al: Blunt diaphragmatic rupture. Am J Surg 148:292-295, 1984.

84. Gelman R, Mirvis SE, Gens D: Diaphragmatic rupture due to blunt trauma: Sensitivity of plain chest radiographs. AJR Am J Roentgenol 156:51-57, 1991.

85. Shackleton KL, Stewart ET, Taylor AJ: Traumatic diaphragmatic injuries: Spectrum of radiographic findings. Radiographics 18:49-59, 1998.

86. Shanmuganathan K, Mirvis SE, White CS, Pomerantz SM: MR imaging evaluation of hemidiaphragms in acute blunt trauma: Experience with 16 patients. AJR Am J Roentgenol 167:397-402, 1996.

87. Worthy SA, Kang EY, Hartman TE, et al: Diaphragmatic rupture: CT findings in 11 patients. Radiology 194:885-888, 1995.

88. Aronchick JM, Epstein DM, Gefter WB, Miller WT: Chronic traumatic diaphragmatic hernia: The significance of pleural effusion. Radiology 168:675-678, 1988.

89. Salomon NW, Zukoski CF: Isolated rupture of the right hemidiaphragm with eventration of the liver. JAMA 241:1929-1930, 1979.

90. Somers JM, Gleeson FV, Flower CD: Rupture of the right hemidiaphragm following blunt trauma: The use of ultrasound in diagnosis. Clin Radiol 42:97-101, 1990.

91. Voeller GR, Reisser JR, Fabian TC, et al:: Blunt diaphragm injuries. A five-year experience. Am Surg 56:28-31, 1990.

92. Murray J, Caoili E, Gruden J: Acute rupture of the diaphragm due to blunt trauma: Diagnostic sensitivity and specificity of CT. AJR Am J Roentgenol 166:1035, 1996.

93. Wilson RF, Murray C, Antonenko DR: Nonpenetrating thoracic injuries. Surg Clin North Am 57:17-36, 1977.

94. Root H, Harmen P: Injury to the diaphragm. In Moore E, Mattox K, Feliciano D (eds): Trauma. Norwalk, CT, Appleton & Lange, 1991.

95. Mansour KA: Trauma to the diaphragm. Chest Surg Clin N Am 7:373-383, 1997.

96. Normand JP, Rioux M, Dumont M, et al: Thoracic splenosis after blunt trauma: Frequency and imaging findings. AJR Am J Roentgenol 161:739-741, 1993.

97. Madjar S, Weissberg D: Thoracic splenosis. Thorax 49:1020-1022, 1994.

98. Tocino I, Miller MH: Computed tomography in blunt chest trauma. J Thorac Imaging 2:45-59, 1987.

99. Dougall AM, Paul ME, Finely RJ, et al: Chest trauma—current morbidity and mortality. J Trauma 17:547-553, 1977.

100. DeLuca SA, Rhea JT, O'Malley TO: Radiographic evaluation of rib fractures. AJR Am J Roentgenol 138:91-92, 1982.

101. Stark P: Radiology of thoracic trauma. Invest Radiol 25:1265-1275, 1990.

102. Albers JE, Rath RK, Glaser RS, Poddar PK: Severity of intrathoracic injuries associated with first rib fractures. Ann Thorac Surg 33:614-618, 1982.

103. Wynn-Williams N, Young RD: Cough fracture of the ribs including one complicated by pneumothorax. Tubercle 40:47-49, 1959.

104. Pearson JE: Cough fracture of the ribs. Br J Tuberc Dis Chest 51:251-254, 1957.

105. Meyer S: Thoracic spine trauma. Semin Roentgenol 27:254-261, 1992.

106. Bolesta MJ, Bohlman HH: Mediastinal widening associated with fractures of the upper thoracic spine. J Bone Joint Surg Am 73:447-450, 1991.

107. Bhalla M, Leitman BS, Forcade C, et al: Lung hernia: Radiographic features. AJR Am J Roentgenol 154:51-53, 1990.

108. Taylor DA, Jacobson HG: Post-traumatic herniation of the lung. Am J Roentgenol Radium Ther Nucl Med 87:896-899, 1962.

109. George PY, Goodman P: Radiographic appearance of bullet tracks in the lung. AJR Am J Roentgenol 159:967-970, 1992.

110. Larose JH: Cavitation of missile tracks in the lung. Radiology 90:995-998, 1968.

111. Spees EK, Strevey TE, Geiger JP, Aronstam EM: Persistent traumatic lung cavities resulting from medium- and high-velocity missiles. Ann Thorac Surg 4:133-142, 1967.

112. Oparah SS, Mandal AK: Penetrating gunshot wounds of the chest in civilian practice: Experience with 250 consecutive cases. Br J Surg 65:45-48, 1978.

113. Sandrasagra FA: Penetrating thoracoabdominal injuries. Br J Surg 64:638-640, 1977.

114. Goodman LR, Kay HR, Teplick SK, Mundth ED: Complications of median sternotomy: Computed tomographic evaluation. AJR Am J Roentgenol 141:225-230, 1983.

115. Carrol CL, Jeffrey RB Jr, Federle MP, Vernacchia FS: CT evaluation of mediastinal infections. J Comput Assist Tomogr 17:449-454, 1987.

116. Li AE, Fishman EK: Evaluation of complications after sternotomy using single- and multidetector CT with three-dimensional volume rendering. AJR Am J Roentgenol 181:1065-1070, 2003.

117. Templeton PA, Fishman EK: CT evaluation of poststernotomy complications. AJR Am J Roentgenol 159:45-50, 1992.

118. Boiselle PM, Mansilla AV: A closer look at the midsternal stripe sign. AJR Am J Roentgenol 178:945-948, 2002.

119. Goodman LR: Postoperative chest radiograph: II. Alterations after major intrathoracic surgery. AJR Am J Roentgenol 134:803-813, 1980.

120. Tsukada G, Stark P: Postpneumonectomy complications. AJR Am J Roentgenol 169:1363-1370, 1997.

121. Hansen R, Kloiber R, Lesperance R: Unpublished data.

122. Asamura H, Naruke T, Tsuchiya R, et al: Bronchopleural fistulas associated with lung cancer operations. Univariate and multivariate analysis of risk factors, management, and outcome. J Thorac Cardiovasc Surg 104:1456-1464, 1992.

123. Hollaus PH, Lax F, el-Nashef BB, et al: Natural history of bronchopleural fistula after pneumonectomy: A review of 96 cases. Ann Thorac Surg 63:1391-1396, discussion 1396-1397, 1997.

124. Leading article: Bronchopleural fistula. BMJ 2:1093-1094, 1976.

125. Westcott JL, Volpe JP: Peripheral bronchopleural fistula: CT evaluation in 20 patients with pneumonia, empyema, or postoperative air leak. Radiology 196:175-181, 1995.

126. Wechsler RJ: CT of esophageal-pleural fistulae. AJR Am J Roentgenol 147:907-909, 1986.
127. Wechsler RJ, Steiner RM, Goodman LR, et al: Iatrogenic esophageal-pleural fistula: Subtlety of diagnosis in the absence of mediastinitis. Radiology 144:239-243, 1982.
128. Heiken JP, Balfe DM, Roper CL: CT evaluation after esophagogastrectomy. AJR Am J Roentgenol 143:555-560, 1984.
129. Cevese PG, Vecchioni R, D'Amico DF, et al: Postoperative chylothorax. Six cases in 2,500 operations, with a survey of the world literature. J Thorac Cardiovasc Surg 69:966-971, 1975.
130. Westcott JL, Cole SR: Interstitial pulmonary emphysema in children and adults: Roentgenographic features. Radiology 111:367-378, 1974.
131. Henry DA, Jolles H, Berberich JJ, Schmelzer V: The post–cardiac surgery chest radiograph: A clinically integrated approach. J Thorac Imaging 4:20-41, 1989.
132. Carter AR, Sostman HD, Curtis AM, Swett HA: Thoracic alterations after cardiac surgery. AJR Am J Roentgenol 140:475-481, 1983.
133. Bhalla M, Wain JC, Shepard JA, McLoud TC: Surgical flaps in the chest: Anatomic considerations, applications, and radiologic appearance. Radiology 192:825-830, 1994.
134. Coppage L, Jolles H, Wornom IL 3rd: Computed tomography findings in patients who have undergone muscle flap and omental transposition procedures in the treatment of poststernotomy mediastinitis. J Thorac Imaging 9:14-22, 1994.
135. Peters JC, Desai KK: CT demonstration of postpneumonectomy tumor recurrence. AJR Am J Roentgenol 141:259-262, 1983.
136. Kerr WF: Late-onset post-pneumonectomy empyema. Thorax 32:149-154, 1977.
137. Heater K, Revzani L, Rubin JM: CT evaluation of empyema in the postpneumonectomy space. AJR Am J Roentgenol 145:39-40, 1985.
138. Kim EA, Lee KS, Shim YM, et al: Radiographic and CT findings in complications following pulmonary resection. Radiographics 22:67-86, 2002.
139. Grillo HC, Shepard JA, Mathisen DJ, Kanarek DJ: Postpneumonectomy syndrome: Diagnosis, management, and results. Ann Thorac Surg 54:638-650, discussion 650-651, 1992.
140. Holbert JM, Chasen MH, Libshitz HI, Mountain CF: The postlobectomy chest: Anatomic considerations. Radiographics 7:889-911, 1987.
141. Hamilton WK: Atelectasis, pneumothorax, and aspiration as postoperative complications. Anesthesiology 22:708-722, 1961.
142. Gamsu G, Singer MM, Vincent HH, et al: Postoperative impairment of mucous transport in the lung. Am Rev Respir Dis 114:673-679, 1976.
143. Korst RJ, Humphrey CB: Complete lobar collapse following pulmonary lobectomy. Its incidence, predisposing factors, and clinical ramifications. Chest 111:1285-1289, 1997.
144. Wilcox P, Baile EM, Hards J, et al: Phrenic nerve function and its relationship to atelectasis after coronary artery bypass surgery. Chest 93:693-698, 1988.
145. van der Werff YD, van der Houwen HK, Heijmans PJ, et al: Postpneumonectomy pulmonary edema. A retrospective analysis of incidence and possible risk factors. Chest 111:1278-1284, 1997.
146. Bousson V, Arrive L, Brauner M: Lung herniation occurring after video-assisted thoracic surgery. AJR Am J Roentgenol 172:1145-1146, 1999.
147. Moser ES Jr, Proto AV: Lung torsion: Case report and literature review. Radiology 162:639-643, 1987.
148. Felson B: Lung torsion: Radiographic findings in nine cases. Radiology 162:631-638, 1987.
149. Collins J, Love R: Pulmonary torsion: Complication of lung transplantation. Clin Pulm Med 3:297, 1996.
150. Kroenke K, Lawrence VA, Theroux JF, et al: Postoperative complications after thoracic and major abdominal surgery in patients with and without obstructive lung disease. Chest 104:1445-1451, 1993.
151. Hall JC, Tarala RA, Hall JL, Mander J: A multivariate analysis of the risk of pulmonary complications after laparotomy. Chest 99:923-927, 1991.
152. Nesbitt JC, Carrasco H: Expandable stents. Chest Surg Clin N Am 6:305-328, 1996.
153. Hauck RW, Lembeck RM, Emslander HP, Schomig A: Implantation of Accuflex and Strecker stents in malignant bronchial stenoses by flexible bronchoscopy. Chest 112:134-144, 1997.
154. Takamori S, Fujita H, Hayashi A, et al: Expandable metallic stents for tracheobronchial stenoses in esophageal cancer. Ann Thorac Surg 62:844-847, 1996.
155. Sacco O, Fregonese B, Oddone M, et al: Severe endobronchial obstruction in a girl with relapsing polychondritis: Treatment with Nd YAG laser and endobronchial silicon stent. Eur Respir J 10:494-496, 1997.
156. Watanabe Y, Murakami S, Oda M, et al: Treatment of bronchial stricture due to endobronchial tuberculosis. World J Surg 21:480-487, 1997.
157. Higgins R, McNeil K, Dennis C, et al: Airway stenoses after lung transplantation: Management with expanding metal stents. J Heart Lung Transplant 13:774-778, 1994.
158. Abdulhamed JM, Alyousef SA, Mullins C: Endovascular stent placement for pulmonary venous obstruction after Mustard operation for transposition of the great arteries. Heart 75:210-212, 1996.
159. Haskal ZJ, Soulen MC, Huettl EA, et al: Life-threatening pulmonary emboli and cor pulmonale: Treatment with percutaneous pulmonary artery stent placement. Radiology 191:473-475, 1994.
160. Clark SC, Levine AJ, Hasan A, et al: Vascular complications of lung transplantation. Ann Thorac Surg 61:1079-1082, 1996.
161. Hramiec JE, Haasler GB: Tracheal wire stent complications in malacia: Implications of position and design. Ann Thorac Surg 63:209-212, discussion 213, 1997.

162. Remacle M, Lawson G, Minet M, et al: Endoscopic treatment of tracheal stenosis using the carbon dioxide laser and the Gianturco stent: Indications and results. Laryngoscope 106:306-312, 1996.
163. Hendra KP, Saukkonen JJ: Erosion of the right mainstem bronchus by an esophageal stent. Chest 110:857-858, 1996.
164. Hijazi ZM, al-Fadley F, Geggel RL, et al: Stent implantation for relief of pulmonary artery stenosis: Immediate and short-term results. Cathet Cardiovasc Diagn 38:16-23, 1996.
165. Nygaard SD, Berger HA, Fick RB: Chylothorax as a complication of oesophageal sclerotherapy. Thorax 47:134-135, 1992.
166. Stark DD, Federle MP, Goodman PC: CT and radiographic assessment of tube thoracostomy. AJR Am J Roentgenol 141:253-258, 1983.
167. Miller KS, Sahn SA: Chest tubes. Indications, technique, management and complications. Chest 91:258-264, 1987.
168. Dalbec DL, Krome RL: Thoracostomy. Emerg Med Clin North Am 4:441-457, 1986.
169. Webb WR, LaBerge JM: Radiographic recognition of chest tube malposition in the major fissure. Chest 85:81-83, 1984.
170. Mirvis SE, Tobin KD, Kostrubiak I, Belzberg H: Thoracic CT in detecting occult disease in critically ill patients. AJR Am J Roentgenol 148:685-689, 1987.
171. Curtin JJ, Goodman LR, Quebbeman EJ, Haasler GB: Thoracostomy tubes after acute chest injury: Relationship between location in a pleural fissure and function. AJR Am J Roentgenol 163:1339-1342, 1994.
172. Cameron EW, Mirvis SE, Shanmuganathan K, et al: Computed tomography of malpositioned thoracostomy drains: A pictorial essay. Clin Radiol 52:187-193, 1997.
173. Daly RC, Mucha P, Pairolero PC, Farnell MB: The risk of percutaneous chest tube thoracostomy for blunt thoracic trauma. Ann Emerg Med 14:865-870, 1985.
174. Neff CC, Mueller PR, Ferrucci JT Jr, et al: Serious complications following transgression of the pleural space in drainage procedures. Radiology 152:335-341, 1984.
175. Nichols DM, Cooperberg PL, Golding RH, Burhenne HJ: The safe intercostal approach? Pleural complications in abdominal interventional radiology. AJR Am J Roentgenol 142:1013-1018, 1984.
176. Hendry PJ, Akyurekli Y, McIntyre R, et al: Bronchopleural complications of nasogastric feeding tubes. Crit Care Med 14:892-894, 1986.
177. Ghahremani GG, Gould RJ: Nasoenteric feeding tubes. Radiographic detection of complications. Dig Dis Sci 31:574-585, 1986.
178. Roubenoff R, Ravich WJ: Pneumothorax due to nasogastric feeding tubes. Report of four cases, review of the literature, and recommendations for prevention. Arch Intern Med 149:184-188, 1989.
179. Miller KS, Tomlinson JR, Sahn SA: Pleuropulmonary complications of enteral tube feedings. Two reports, review of the literature, and recommendations. Chest 88:230-233, 1985.
180. Wiener MD, Garay SM, Leitman BS, et al: Imaging of the intensive care unit patient. Clin Chest Med 12:169-198, 1991.
181. Twigg HL, Buckley CE: Complications of endotracheal intubation. Am J Roentgenol Radium Ther Nucl Med 109:452-454, 1970.
182. Conrardy PA, Goodman LR, Lainge F, Singer MM: Alteration of endotracheal tube position. Flexion and extension of the neck. Crit Care Med 4:7-12, 1976.
183. Goodman LR, Conrardy PA, Laing F, Singer MM: Radiographic evaluation of endotracheal tube position. AJR Am J Roentgenol 127:433-434, 1976.
184. Smith GM, Reed JC, Choplin RH: Radiographic detection of esophageal malpositioning of endotracheal tubes. AJR Am J Roentgenol 154:23-26, 1990.
185. Heimlich HJ, Carr GC: Transtracheal catheter technique for pulmonary rehabilitation. Ann Otol Rhinol Laryngol 94:502-504, 1985.
186. Shneerson J: Transtracheal oxygen delivery. Thorax 47:57-59, 1992.
187. Fletcher EC, Nickeson D, Costarangos-Galarza C: Endotracheal mass resulting from a transtracheal oxygen catheter. Chest 93:438-439, 1988.
188. Borer H, Frey M, Keller R: Ulcerous tracheitis and mucus ball formation: A nearly fatal complication of a transtracheal oxygen catheter. Respiration 63:400-402, 1996.
189. Wechsler RJ, Spirn PW, Conant EF, et al: Thrombosis and infection caused by thoracic venous catheters: Pathogenesis and imaging findings. AJR Am J Roentgenol 160:467-471, 1993.
190. Clarke DE, Raffin TA: Infectious complications of indwelling long-term central venous catheters. Chest 97:966-972, 1990.
191. Kidney DD, Nguyen DT, Deutsch LS: Radiologic evaluation and management of malfunctioning long-term central vein catheters. AJR Am J Roentgenol 171:1251-1257, 1998.
192. Dunbar RD, Mitchell R, Lavine M: Aberrant locations of central venous catheters. Lancet 1:711-715, 1981.
193. Langston CS: The aberrant central venous catheter and its complications. Radiology 100:55-59, 1971.
194. Hoshal VL Jr, Ause RG, Hoskins PA: Fibrin sleeve formation on indwelling subclavian central venous catheters. Arch Surg 102:253-258, 1971.
195. Ahmed N: Thrombosis after central venous cannulation. Med J Aust 1:217-220, 1976.
196. Falk RL, Smith DF: Thrombosis of upper extremity thoracic inlet veins: Diagnosis with duplex Doppler sonography. AJR Am J Roentgenol 149:677-682, 1987.
197. Brismar B, Hardstedt C, Jacobson S: Diagnosis of thrombosis by catheter phlebography after prolonged central venous catheterization. Ann Surg 194:779-783, 1981.
198. Yedlicka JW Jr, Cormier MG, Gray R, Moncada R: Computed tomography of superior vena cava obstruction. J Thorac Imaging 2:72-78, 1987.
199. Hansen ME, Spritzer CE, Sostman HD: Assessing the patency of mediastinal and thoracic inlet veins: Value of MR imaging. AJR Am J Roentgenol 155:1177-1182, 1990.

200. Horattas MC, Wright DJ, Fenton AH, et al: Changing concepts of deep venous thrombosis of the upper extremity—report of a series and review of the literature. Surgery 104:561-567, 1988.

201. Hill SL, Berry RE: Subclavian vein thrombosis: A continuing challenge. Surgery 108:1-9, 1990.

202. Maggs PR, Schwaber JR: Fatal bilateral pneumothoraces complicating subclavian vein catheterization. Chest 71:552-553, 1977.

203. Chute E, Cerra FB: Late development of hydrothorax and hydromediastinum in patients with central venous catheters. Crit Care Med 10:868-869, 1982.

204. Duntley P, Siever J, Korwes ML, et al: Vascular erosion by central venous catheters. Clinical features and outcome. Chest 101:1633-1638, 1992.

205. Hunt R, Hunter TB: Cardiac tamponade and death from perforation of the right atrium by a central venous catheter. AJR Am J Roentgenol 151:1250, 1988.

206. Rossleigh MA: Unusual complication of intravenous catheterisation. Med J Aust 1:236, 1982.

207. McGoon MD, Benedetto PW, Greene BM: Complications of percutaneous central venous catheterization: A report of two cases and review of the literature. Johns Hopkins Med J 145:1-6, 1979.

208. Woodring JH, Fried AM: Nonfatal venous air embolism after contrast-enhanced CT. Radiology 167:405-407, 1988.

209. Fraser RS: Catheter-induced pulmonary artery perforation: Pathologic and pathogenic features. Hum Pathol 18:1246-1251, 1987.

210. Boyd KD, Thomas SJ, Gold J, Boyd AD: A prospective study of complications of pulmonary artery catheterizations in 500 consecutive patients. Chest 84:245-249, 1983.

211. Katz JD, Cronau LH, Barash PG, Mandel SD: Pulmonary artery flow-guided catheters in the perioperative period. Indications and complications. JAMA 237:2832-2834, 1977.

212. Kearney TJ, Shabot MM: Pulmonary artery rupture associated with the Swan-Ganz catheter. Chest 108:1349-1352, 1995.

213. Rosenblum SE, Ratliff NB, Shirey EK, et al: Pulmonary artery dissection induced by a Swan-Ganz catheter. Cleve Clin Q 51:671-675, 1984.

214. Ferretti GR, Thony F, Link KM, et al: False aneurysm of the pulmonary artery induced by a Swan-Ganz catheter: Clinical presentation and radiologic management. AJR Am J Roentgenol 167:941-945, 1996.

215. Dieden JD, Friloux LA 3rd, Renner JW: Pulmonary artery false aneurysms secondary to Swan-Ganz pulmonary artery catheters. AJR Am J Roentgenol 149:901-906, 1987.

216. Urschel JD, Myerowitz PD: Catheter-induced pulmonary artery rupture in the setting of cardiopulmonary bypass. Ann Thorac Surg 56:585-589, 1993.

217. Kirton OC, Varon AJ, Henry RP, Civetta JM: Flow-directed, pulmonary artery catheter–induced pseudoaneurysm: Urgent diagnosis and endovascular obliteration. Crit Care Med 20:1178-1180, 1992.

218. Goodman LR, Almassi GH, Troup PJ, et al: Complications of automatic implantable cardioverter defibrillators: Radiographic, CT, and echocardiographic evaluation. Radiology 170:447-452, 1989.

219. Bejvan SM, Ephron JH, Takasugi JE, et al: Imaging of cardiac pacemakers. AJR Am J Roentgenol 169:1371-1379, 1997.

220. Nolan RL, McAdams HP: Bronchopericardial fistula after placement of an automatic implantable cardioverter defibrillator: Radiographic and CT findings. AJR Am J Roentgenol 172:365-368, 1999.

PLEURAL DISEASE

PLEURAL EFFUSION

Effusion develops when an alteration in hydrostatic and osmotic forces affects the formation of pleural fluid, when lymphatic drainage is impaired, or when mesothelial or capillary endothelial permeability is increased.[1] It may occur by itself or in association with disease of the lung, mediastinum, or chest wall. Radiologic abnormalities reflecting such disease may provide important clues about the etiology of the effusion. For example, when effusion accompanies enlargement of the heart or multiple rib fractures, it is reasonable to conclude that it is the result of cardiac failure or chest wall trauma, respectively. It is important to remember, however, that underlying pulmonary or mediastinal disease is not always detectable on initial radiographs; large effusions may mask parenchymal opacities or mediastinal masses, which may become evident only when fluid has been removed or other imaging procedures render the underlying lung or mediastinal structures visible. In practice, the diagnosis of a specific etiology of an effusion is often difficult, even after thorough radiologic, bacteriologic, biochemical, and pathologic investigation; in some series, it remains undetermined in as many as 25% of cases.[2]

This chapter is concerned with the diagnosis and differential diagnosis of diseases of the pleura. The radiologic signs of pleural disease (see page 144) and analysis of cell number and type in pleural fluid (see page 172) are discussed elsewhere.

Before reviewing the specific causes of pleural effusion—of which there are many (Table 20–1)[2]—the general features of clinical and pulmonary function disturbances, findings on biochemical analysis of pleural fluid, and the means of investigation are summarized briefly.

Clinical Manifestations

Approximately 15% of patients with pleural effusion are asymptomatic.[2] When symptoms are evident, they are usually related either to the space-occupying nature of the fluid or to accompanying pleuritis. Pleural pain that is sharp, localized, and exacerbated by inspiration is a frequent manifestation of pleuritis; however, it often diminishes when effusion develops. In some cases, the pain is not accentuated by breathing and is felt as a dull ache. Since branches of the intercostal nerves innervate the parietal pleura, pleural pain is usually well localized, although it may be referred to the abdomen. When phrenic nerve endings are irritated by inflammation of the diaphragmatic pleura, the pain may be felt in the shoulder. Dry cough may be seen and can become productive if associated with pneumonia.

Dyspnea is a common complaint and may be severe as a result of either compromise of respiratory reserve by the fluid or concomitant pulmonary parenchymal or vascular disease. The mediastinal displacement that occurs in tension

TABLE 20–1. Pleural Effusion—Etiology

Pleuropulmonary Infection

Mycobacterium tuberculosis
Nontuberculous bacteria
Actinomyces and *Nocardia* species
Fungi
Parasites
Viruses, *Mycoplasma*, and Rickettsiae

Pleuropulmonary Malignancy

Pulmonary carcinoma
Metastatic neoplasm to pleura and mediastinal lymph nodes
Lymphoma
Leukemia

Connective Tissue Disease

Systemic lupus erythematosus
Rheumatoid disease
Others

Asbestos

Drugs

See Table 20–2, page 824

Heart Failure

Trauma

Penetrating and nonpenetrating injury
Coronary artery bypass procedures
Pulmonary resection
Esophageal rupture
Intravascular therapeutic or monitoring devices
Abdominal surgery
Subarachnoid-pleural fistula

Metabolic and Endocrine Disease

Myxedema
Diabetes mellitus
Amyloidosis

Skeletal Disease

Neoplasms
Langerhans cell histiocytosis
Spondylitis
Gorham's disease

Liver Disease

Cirrhosis
Biliary tract fistula
Transplantation

Kidney Disease

Dialysis
Urinoma
Nephrotic syndrome
Acute glomerulonephritis
Uremia

Pancreatic Disease

Acute pancreatitis
Chronic pancreatitis with pleuropancreatic fistula

Gynecologic Tumors

Ovary, uterus, fallopian tube
Ovarian hyperstimulation syndrome

TABLE 20–1. Pleural Effusion—Etiology—cont'd

Gastrointestinal Tract

Gastric/duodenal-pleural fistula
Diaphragmatic hernia
Idiopathic inflammatory bowel disease

Miscellaneous Causes

Subphrenic abscess
Lymphatic hypoplasia
Dressler's syndrome
Familial paroxysmal polyserositis
Rupture of silicon gel mammoplasty device
Systemic cholesterol embolization
Extramedullary hematopoiesis

Idiopathic

From Fraser RS, Müller NL, Colman NC, Paré PD: Fraser and Paré's Diagnosis of Diseases of the Chest, 4th ed. Philadelphia, WB Saunders, 1999.

hydrothorax can cause respiratory distress, dysphagia, engorged neck veins, a tender liver, and edema of the lower extremities[3]; thoracentesis is characteristically followed by immediate relief of symptoms and signs.

Physical examination reveals dullness on percussion and a decrease or absence of breath sounds. Although breath sounds are usually absent when the effusion is large, sometimes an area of bronchial breath sounds may be appreciated, especially at the lung-fluid interface. Chest wall edema has been described when the effusion is large and protracted.[4]

Pulmonary Function Tests

In the absence of pulmonary disease, the effects of pleural effusion on pulmonary function reflect the combination of a space-occupying process and a reduction in lung volume as a consequence of relaxation atelectasis. The former results in a reduction in all subdivisions of lung volume, including TLC, FRC, and VC; nonetheless, ventilatory ability may be little impaired when the other lung is normal and there is no pleural pain inhibiting chest wall movement.[5] Depending on the amount of fluid and therefore the degree of ipsilateral pulmonary collapse, diffusing capacity may be moderately diminished, although it often remains within the predicted normal range. Blood gas tensions may also be normal; arterial oxygen saturation is usually unaffected, even with significant atelectasis, because regional perfusion diminishes in response to the reduction in regional ventilation. When hypoxemia is present, the major mechanism appears to be intrapulmonary shunting.[6] Arterial PCO_2 may decrease if unilateral pulmonary collapse results in hyperventilation but otherwise remains unaffected.

The slight but significant increase in PaO_2 and lung volumes and the decrease in $PAO_2 - PaO_2$ that occur in some patients after thoracentesis are insufficient to explain the relief of dyspnea that is commonly experienced. This improvement may result from a reduction in size of the thoracic cage that allows the inspiratory muscles to operate on a more advantageous portion of their length-tension curve.[7] In some patients, thoracentesis results in hypoxemia as a result of the development of re-expansion pulmonary edema (see page 622).[8]

Laboratory Findings

The diagnosis of pleural effusion of uncertain etiology often begins with characterization of the effusion as an exudate or transudate. An *exudative effusion* is usually associated with disease of the pleural surface itself or the adjacent lung, whereas a *transudative effusion* generally results from an alteration in the systemic circulation that influences the movement of fluid into and out of the pleural space. When the distinction between an exudate and a transudate is obvious (e.g., by the identification of pus in the context of empyema or blood in the context of trauma), biochemical, hematologic, and cytologic investigation of the fluid is not necessary. However, when these findings are not clearly present, such investigations are frequently helpful in diagnosis.

Light and colleagues have identified three biochemical characteristics that independently differentiate an exudate from a transudate:[9] (1) a fluid-to-serum protein ratio greater than 0.5, (2) a pleural fluid lactate dehydrogenase (LDH) level greater than 200 IU, and (3) a fluid-to-serum LDH ratio greater than 0.6. Isolated measurement of other chemicals has not been found to be useful.[10,11] However, using the criteria of pleural fluid LDH greater than 45% of the upper limit of the normal serum value, pleural cholesterol greater than 45 mg/dL (1.2 mmol/L), and pleural fluid protein greater than 29 g/L to define an exudate avoids the necessity of obtaining a simultaneous serum sample when performing thoracentesis for diagnosis.[12] The value of biochemical tests for other substances is discussed in the sections in which they are most pertinent.

SPECIFIC CAUSES OF PLEURAL EFFUSION

Infection

Mycobacteria

The incidence of tuberculous pleural effusion depends on the prevalence of tuberculosis in the population studied. Where the disease is common, it may be the most frequent cause of pleural effusion or empyema,[13] whereas in "developed" countries such as the United States, Canada, and parts of Europe, it is infrequent.[14] In regions of high prevalence, tuberculous effusion occurs most often in young people[15]; where it is less prevalent, it is seen more commonly in middle-aged or elderly patients.[16]

Tuberculous pleural effusion is believed to result from rupture of subpleural foci of necrosis into the adjacent pleural space.[17] Although such foci cannot usually be seen on conventional chest radiographs, they have been documented pathologically[18] and on CT scans.[19] T lymphocytes in tuberculous pleural fluid, mostly of the CD4+ type,[20] are specifically sensitized to purified protein derivative (PPD).[21] Such activated lymphocytes, as well as macrophages, produce a variety of cytokines that participate in production and regulation of the local inflammatory process.[22,23]

When associated with acute symptoms and the absence of radiographically evident pulmonary disease, tuberculous effusion is often believed to represent primary infection. Generally, this clinical and radiologic constellation has been seen in children and young adults.[24] By contrast, tuberculous effusion that is associated with an indolent course and with parenchymal lung disease on the chest radiograph has been seen more frequently in older patients and has been thought to be a manifestation of postprimary (reactivation) infection.[14] However, categorization as primary or postprimary disease on the basis of these criteria is not always correct since parenchymal lung disease may be obscured by the effusion, and primary tuberculosis occurring in immunologically naive or debilitated older patients may have an indolent clinical course. Occasionally, tuberculous effusion is chronic and is manifested by loculation of frankly purulent material that is surrounded by a thick layer of calcified fibrous tissue; the bacterial load in such an effusion is high.[25]

Thoracentesis usually yields a serous, lymphocyte-predominant exudate.[26] Although neutrophils may be numerous in early disease and in the setting of chronic loculation, effusions containing more than 50% of these cells are generally of a nontuberculous etiology. The glucose content of pleural fluid may be low; however, this finding can also be seen in nontuberculous bacterial pneumonia, rheumatoid disease, and metastatic carcinoma. In fact, the majority of patients with effusions of tuberculous etiology have pleural fluid glucose levels above 3.3 mmol/L.[17] Identification of adenosine deaminase, a marker of lymphocyte activation, has very high sensitivity and specificity for the diagnosis in patients who have lymphocyte-predominant effusion.[27] Its major value in areas of low tuberculosis prevalence is its very high negative predictive power (99%).[28] Measurement of interferon-γ levels is also useful, the sensitivity and specificity of the test being 99% and 98%, respectively.[29]

A diagnosis of tuberculous pleural effusion should be considered when there is a combination of a positive tuberculin test and a predominantly lymphocytic response in the pleural fluid. However, a negative PPD reaction does not exclude the diagnosis, and the skin test should be repeated in any patient suspected of having the disease. Microscopic examination of pleural biopsy specimens shows granulomas in about 60% to 80% of proven cases. Although this finding is virtually diagnostic, *definitive* diagnosis still requires the identification of organisms in pleural fluid or tissue by acid-fast stain, polymerase chain reaction (PCR), or culture. Culture of biopsy specimens is positive in 55% to 80% of patients, and culture of fluid in 20% to 25%.[30] The sensitivity of PCR has been reported to be as high as 75%[31]; although a positive reaction should generally be considered to confirm the diagnosis,[32] the possibility of a false-positive result must always be kept in mind.[33] Sputum culture is positive in about 50% of patients, sometimes in those who do not have radiographically identifiable lung disease.[34]

The natural history of tuberculous pleuritis and effusion is usually complete absorption of fluid and apparently complete restoration of the patient's health (although some degree of pleural fibrosis may be evident pathologically or radiologically). However, the likelihood of subsequent development of pulmonary tuberculosis is high,[35] and the long-term prognosis is partly determined by recognition of the disease and the initiation of effective therapy.

Bacteria Other Than Mycobacteria

Pleural effusion occurs in about 40% of patients who have acute bacterial pneumonia (parapneumonic effusion).[36] In some cases, the fluid is sterile, the fluid accumulation representing part of the inflammatory reaction to infection in the adjacent lung. In others, organisms spread to the pleura and ultimately the pleural space itself, where they directly influence fluid accumulation. About 25% of patients who have the latter complication will require drainage of the pleural space. Such infection occurs more commonly in men than women[37]; the presence of comorbid conditions such as diabetes, malignancy, or underlying pulmonary disease increases the risk.

Pleural effusion of nontuberculous bacterial origin is characterized by a predominance of polymorphonuclear leukocytes; in a few patients, the fluid is grossly cloudy or frankly purulent (empyema).[38] The initial response to bacteria in the pleural space is an exudative inflammatory reaction consisting of a thin fluid containing few leukocytes.[39] Under the influence of a variety of chemotactic cytokines released by activated mesothelial cells,[40] this response is followed by the accumulation of large numbers of neutrophils and fibrin. At this stage, the pleural surface may be covered by a shaggy white exudate several millimeters thick; if untreated, the empyema may drain spontaneously through the chest wall (empyema necessitans). Organization of the exudate may result in a fibrous pleural "peel" that can measure several centimeters in thickness.

As with bacterial pneumonia, the organisms responsible for empyema vary with the host's state of health. In "developed" countries, about two thirds of cases have been attributed to aerobic bacteria[41]; however, anaerobic organisms, often mixed with aerobic species, have been identified in up to 75% of cases of empyema when microbiology has been performed by research laboratories that specialize in their identification.[42] Among aerobic organisms, *Staphylococcus aureus* and enteric gram-negative bacilli are important pathogens,[43,44] particularly in the post-trauma setting. The same organisms, as well as anaerobic bacteria, are a common cause of empyema in HIV-positive drug abusers.[45] *Streptococcus pneumoniae* is also an important cause in some series.[43] Most cases of *Klebsiella-Enterobacter-Serratia* infection occur in elderly hospitalized patients compromised by major medical or surgical illnesses. Pneumonia caused by *Klebsiella* usually develops in alcoholic, diabetic, or otherwise debilitated patients and is rarely hospital acquired[46]; empyema is a frequent complication. Radiologic features of necrotizing pneumonia, including gangrene or lung abscess, can often be appreciated in affected patients.[47] Other hospital-acquired gram-negative pneumonias that are associated with a high incidence of empyema include those caused by *Escherichia coli* and *Pseudomonas aeruginosa*.[17]

Although most patients with empyema are febrile and have blood neutrophilia, compromised hosts and patients receiving corticosteroid therapy can be afebrile and have a normal white blood cell count.[48] Patients with aerobic bacterial pneumonia and effusion usually have an acute onset of chest pain, fever,

cough, and sputum, whereas symptoms are more indolent in patients with anaerobic infection.[49]

It is important to recognize that parapneumonic effusion encompasses a spectrum of disease that ranges from the incidental to the life-threatening, with each patient requiring an individual diagnostic and therapeutic approach. At one end of this spectrum are patients who have only a small amount of free-flowing fluid (<10 mm on lateral decubitus radiographs); usually, these patients do not require thoracentesis or tube thoracostomy for either diagnosis or therapy. At the other end are patients who have loculated effusion that is associated with a thick pleural peel; these patients often require surgical intervention or fibrinolytic therapy to effect a successful outcome.[50] Between these two extremes, patients may or may not require chest tube drainage or other procedures. In the absence of frank empyema, the finding of a pH higher than 7.20, glucose level greater than 2.2 mmol/L, and LDH level less than 1000 U/L indicates that medical management alone will be sufficient in most patients.[51] It is also reasonable to consider other factors when determining the need for drainage procedures, including the initial response to antibiotic therapy alone, the initial clinical state of the patient (e.g., whether previously healthy or compromised in some manner), the virulence of the organism and its propensity to evolve rapidly in an adverse fashion, the size of effusion, and the presence of loculations.[52]

Uninfected parapneumonic effusions clear spontaneously and do not alter the prognosis of pneumonia. By contrast, pleural effusions that require drainage or thoracotomy are associated with increased morbidity and mortality.[53] The prognosis also varies with the age of the patient, the presence or absence of underlying disease, and the specific organism responsible for the empyema.[54] Failure to drain the empyema adequately has also been associated with an increase in morbidity and mortality.[55,56]

Actinomyces and *Nocardia* Species

Radiographic evidence of pulmonary involvement is an almost invariable accompaniment of pleural disease caused by *Actinomyces* organisms, usually in the form of nonsegmental homogeneous air space consolidation and often accompanied by abscess formation. The pleural disease (typically empyema) may itself extend across the parietal pleura into the chest wall and lead to rib destruction and subcutaneous abscess formation.[57] Although pulmonary nocardiosis is also often associated with empyema, chest wall involvement is less commonly seen.[58]

Fungi

Pleural effusion caused by fungi is uncommon[59]; for example, in a series of 100 patients who had primary pulmonary infection with *Histoplasma capsulatum*, only 2 had the complication.[60] Effusion has been reported to occur in about 20% of symptomatic patients who have primary coccidioidomycosis[61]; the effusion may be associated with erythema nodosum and peripheral blood eosinophilia. In addition, hydropneumothorax can develop when a coccidioidal cavity ruptures into the pleural space, a complication said to occur in 1% to 5% of patients who have chronic cavitary disease.[17] Effusions caused by *Blastomyces dermatitidis* and *Cryptococcus neoformans* are usually associated with acute air space pneumonia[62];

the complication may be more common in patients who have AIDS.[63] Isolation of the fungus or, in the case of cryptococcosis, detection of antigen in pleural fluid[64] is essential for definitive diagnosis. Pleural effusion may also accompany *Pneumocystis jiroveci* pneumonia in patients who are severely immunocompromised (particularly those who have AIDS).[65]

Candida species usually infect the pleural space in association with other organisms that originate in the gastrointestinal tract; the complication typically occurs after aspiration from the oropharynx or spread of organisms directly into the pleural space via an esophagopleural fistula or across the diaphragm from a contiguous intra-abdominal source.[44,66] Pleural invasion by *Aspergillus* species occurs most commonly after thoracoplasty for tuberculosis (typically many years after the procedure and often associated with a bronchopleural fistula),[17] resectional surgery of an aspergilloma,[67] or invasive pulmonary infection. Pleural effusion has also been seen in some patients who have allergic bronchopulmonary aspergillosis.[68]

Viruses, Mycoplasmas, and Rickettsiae

Pleural effusion can be demonstrated in as many as 20% of patients who have pneumonia caused by these organisms, although radiographs in the lateral decubitus position may be required.[69] The effusion is usually small, transient, and unassociated with symptoms; occasionally, it provides material sufficient for diagnosis.[44]

Parasites

Entamoeba histolytica. Pleuropulmonary involvement in amebiasis generally occurs by spread of infection from a hepatic or subphrenic abscess across the diaphragm into the pleural space and lung. It is said to occur in about 5% to 40% of patients who have liver involvement.[70] The effusion is usually serofibrinous in the early stage, when it is sterile and represents an inflammatory reaction to adjacent diaphragmatic disease; when the abscess penetrates the pleural space, it may have an "anchovy paste" appearance as a result of the presence of liquefied liver tissue.[70] In addition to right-sided pleural effusion, radiography commonly reveals elevation and fixation of the right hemidiaphragm and consolidation of the right lower lobe, with or without abscess formation. This combination of findings should suggest the diagnosis, especially in a patient from an area endemic for amebiasis whose liver is enlarged.

Echinococcus granulosus. Pleural effusion is uncommon in hydatid disease. It occurs when a pulmonary cyst ruptures into the pleural space rather than into the lung or airway. Because air is present in most cases, the radiographic appearance is that of a hydropneumothorax. Daughter cysts floating on the surface of the fluid may produce irregularities in the fluid surface that are known as the "water lily" sign or "sign of the camalote." The finding of acid-fast hooklets and scolices in pleural fluid confirms the diagnosis.[44]

Paragonimus westermani. This organism enters the thorax through the diaphragm, during which time effusion may be apparent. The complication may also be seen in patients who have chronic pulmonary paragonimiasis.[71] Pleural lesions containing the parasite have been reported in up to 70% of infected patients[72] and may be bilateral and have associated pneumothorax. Detection of the eggs in pleural fluid is diagnostic.[44]

Immunologic Disease

Pleural effusion associated with systemic lupus erythematosus (SLE) and rheumatoid disease is relatively common and often caused by the connective tissue disease itself. By contrast, in patients who have other connective tissue disorders, such as progressive systemic sclerosis, dermatomyositis, and Sjögren's syndrome, effusion more commonly develops as a result of causes other than the primary disease (e.g., heart failure). To the extent that pleural disease is found in these last-named disorders, it is discussed in Chapter 10.

Systemic Lupus Erythematosus

Clinically evident involvement of the pleura occurs during the course of SLE in up to 70% of patients and is the initial manifestation in about 5%. Patients typically have pleuritic pain accompanied by dyspnea, cough, and fever.[73] Effusions are generally bilateral and small to moderate in size, but they may be unilateral, massive, or both.[74] They are generally serous or serosanguineous. The cell count ranges from several hundred to 15,000/μL; the effusion may be predominantly neutrophilic at the onset of pleuritis but becomes lymphocytic with time. The finding of LE cells in cytology specimens has very high specificity for the diagnosis[75]; by contrast, the finding of antinuclear antibody lacks specificity, even when present in high titer (although the sensitivity of the test is high).[76]

In addition to the effusion, radiographs may show a minimal to moderate degree of enlargement of the cardiopericardial silhouette. This enlargement may be secondary to lupus-induced pericarditis, endocarditis, or myocarditis or to the effects of hypertension, renal disease, or anemia. Silhouette enlargement usually takes place over a period of weeks but may occur with startling abruptness; in the latter situation, effusion is the most likely cause. When enlargement is associated with bilateral pleural effusion, the diagnosis of lupus serositis should be strongly considered, particularly in young women.

Rheumatoid Disease

Pleural effusion is a common thoracic manifestation of rheumatoid disease. For unexplained reasons, it has a distinct male preponderance despite the fact that rheumatoid arthritis occurs more often in women. Middle-aged individuals are usually affected.[77] Patients are frequently asymptomatic, the effusion being found by chance during radiographic examination. In occasional cases, it develops abruptly and is associated with pain, fever, or dyspnea. Although the effusion generally appears sometime after the clinical onset of rheumatoid arthritis and is often associated with episodic exacerbations of arthritis, it may antedate both signs and symptoms of joint disease. It occurs more often in patients who have subcutaneous nodules than in those without and usually develops independently of pulmonary rheumatoid disease.[78] The effusions are generally unilateral, slightly more often on the right side. The only distinctive radiographic characteristic is a tendency to remain relatively unchanged for months or, sometimes, years.

The fluid is typically an exudate, usually turbid and greenish yellow, with a predominance of lymphocytes and a paucity of mesothelial cells. Neutrophils are prominent in some cases. Cytologic examination may reveal the presence of multinucleated giant cells and clumps of amorphous granular material, an appearance caused by rupture of a subpleural necrobiotic nodule into the pleural space.[79] The glucose content is characteristically very low.[80] Rheumatoid factor is frequently present in the effusion,[80] typically when it is also elevated in serum; however, its presence alone is not diagnostic.[81] Measurement of complement components and their activation products may be useful in distinguishing rheumatoid effusion from effusion associated with malignancy or tuberculosis; in the former, levels of SC5b-9 are higher than 2 AU/mL, and the C4d/C4 ratio is higher than in effusions of the latter two.[82] The pH of the fluid is also reduced, usually below 7.20. The combination of low pH, glucose, and complement levels and a high rheumatoid factor level is virtually diagnostic.

Drug-Induced Pleural Effusion

Many drugs have been reported to cause pleural effusion (Table 20–2), and the diagnosis should be considered in any patient who is taking a medication and in whom pleural disease of unknown etiology develops.[83,84] Some medications, such as bromocriptine, methysergide, and dantrolene sodium, appear to affect the pleura almost selectively.[85] Others initiate a lupus-like syndrome that is associated with development of the effusion.[76]

Neoplasia

The most common cause of exudative pleural effusion is malignancy.[17] The most frequent sites of origin are the lung, breast, ovary, and stomach (carcinoma) and the lymph nodes (lymphoma)[86]; in fact, pulmonary carcinoma, breast carcinoma, and lymphoma account for about 75% of all malignant pleural effusions.[87] Most such effusions are unilateral; bilateral involvement is frequently associated with hepatic metastases.[88]

The pathogenesis of pleural effusion in malignancy is varied and includes[17] (1) direct neoplastic invasion of the pleura, which is similar to an inflammatory reaction associated with capillary fluid leak; (2) invasion of the pleuropulmonary lymphatics and bronchopulmonary, hilar, and/or mediastinal lymph nodes, which hinders return of lymphatic fluid to the circulation; (3) bronchial obstruction by carcinoma, which creates an increased negative intrapleural pressure and increased transudation; (4) hypoproteinemia (in debilitated patients), which leads to increased transudation; (5) infection associated with obstructive pneumonitis, which results in a parapneumonic effusion; and (6) a drug reaction, radiation therapy, or deposition of immune complexes related to circulating tumor antigens, which causes increased pleural capillary permeability.[89] It is important to remember that pleural involvement by carcinoma/lymphoma does not necessarily result in effusion, nor does the volume of effusion bear any relation to the extent of pleural tumor involvement.[88]

The diagnosis of carcinoma as the etiology of pleural effusion may be strongly suspected from findings on the chest radiograph, such as a mass or reticular or nodular opacities

TABLE 20–2. Drug Causes of Pleural Effusion

Drug-Induced Lupus Syndrome
β-Adrenoreceptor blocking agents (acebutolol, labetalol, pindolol, propranolol)
Chlorpromazine
Etanercept
Fluvastatin
Hydralazine
Isoniazid
Methyldopa
Olsalazine
Phenytoin and other anticonvulsants
Procainamide
Quinidine
Sulfasalazine

Drugs That Affect the Pleural Space Selectively
Bromocriptine
Dantrolene sodium
Methysergide

Drugs That Affect the Pleural Space Nonselectively
Chemotherapeutic Agents
Bleomycin
Busulfan
Cytosine arabinoside
Melphalan
Methotrexate
Mitomycin C
Biologic Response Modifiers
Granulocyte-macrophage colony-stimulating factor
Infliximab
Interleukin-2
Antibiotics
Itraconazole
Minocycline
Metronidazole
Nitrofurantoin
Praziquantel
Simvastatin
Antiarrhythmia Drugs
Amiodarone
Miscellaneous Drugs
Acyclovir
Clomiphene
Clozapine
Ergotamine and other derivatives
Ethchlorvynol
Gliclazide
Isotretinoin
Minoxidil
Pergolide
Propylthiouracil

characteristic of metastatic carcinoma. In the absence of radiologic abnormalities or symptoms such as hemoptysis or a very large effusion, bronchoscopy is unlikely to be helpful in identifying malignancy as the cause of effusion.[90]

Pleural effusions associated with malignancy are almost invariably exudates[91]; when a malignant effusion is a transudate, the patient almost always has another disorder that explains the findings.[92] Although lymphocytes typically predominate, a significant number of neutrophils are frequently present; eosinophils are uncommon.[93] A minority of effusions are grossly bloody.[88] The great majority have a normal glucose level and a pH above 7.30[94]; those that have a glucose level below 3.3 mmol/L and a pH below 7.30 are more likely to be large, to be positive on cytologic examination, and to be associated with a poor performance status that portends a poor prognosis.[95]

Examination of a small volume of pleural fluid produces positive cytologic findings in about 35% to 85% of patients who have a malignant effusion.[96] As a diagnostic procedure, such examination has higher yield than closed pleural biopsy, although the two procedures are complementary.[97] The distinction between benign and malignant cells can be difficult, and many techniques have been studied in an attempt to identify markers useful for differential diagnosis, including immunohistochemistry, electron microscopy, cytogenetic analysis, flow cytometry, and molecular biologic tests. When an effusion persists and cytologic and other analyses are negative for malignancy, open or thoracoscopic biopsy may be required for diagnosis; when technically feasible, the latter is the procedure of choice.[98]

Pulmonary Carcinoma

Pleural involvement is evident in about 5% to 15% of patients who have pulmonary carcinoma at the time that they first seek medical attention.[94] During the course of the disease, the complication develops in at least 50% of patients who have disseminated carcinoma.[17] Effusion in this setting is almost always associated with radiographically evident pulmonary abnormalities. Documentation of malignant cells in pleural fluid or biopsy specimens of patients who have proven pulmonary carcinoma is generally regarded as evidence of inoperability and is associated with a very poor prognosis[99]; for example, in a series of 96 patients, 54% were dead within 1 month and 84% within 6 months.[94]

Metastatic Nonpulmonary Carcinoma

As indicated previously, the most common extrathoracic primary sites associated with malignant pleural effusion are the breast, ovary, and stomach, with the breast being the most common.[86] A history of such primary tumor is present in most cases; however, about 5% of patients with malignant pleural effusion have an unknown primary at the time of diagnosis.

Effusion in breast carcinoma is generally unilateral and on the same side as the primary tumor, suggesting that tumor spread occurs via the lymphatics.[100,101] Although bilateral malignant effusion is uncommon in association with breast carcinoma, it is still among the major causes of this manifestation of malignancy.[102] As with pulmonary carcinoma, the development of malignant pleural effusion associated with an extrapulmonary primary carries a dismal prognosis, with death usually occurring within a year and often within months.[103]

Lymphoma

About 10% of malignant pleural effusions are the result of lymphoma.[104] The vast majority of patients have had a previous diagnosis of lymphoma, or additional findings in the thorax or elsewhere that suggest it. However, effusion is occasionally the sole radiographic finding at the time of diagnosis, usually in non-Hodgkin's lymphoma. Primary pleural lymphoma (i.e., unassociated with significant nodal or visceral tumor) is rare but has been reported in patients who have chronic pyothorax associated with Epstein-Barr virus–infected cells[105] and in those who have AIDS associated with herpesvirus 8 infection.[106]

Pleural effusion is uncommon in multiple myeloma.[107] In many cases, it is probably caused by direct extension of neoplastic cells from the ribs into the pleura.[108] A high level of the specific paraprotein produced by the tumor cells can sometimes be identified in pleural fluid.[109] Effusion is not uncommon in Waldenström's macroglobulinemia and can occur in the absence of parenchymal disease[110]; atypical lymphocytes and a high level of IgM can be identified in the pleural fluid.

Pleural effusion in lymphoma can be the result of a variety of mechanisms, including impaired lymphatic drainage as a result of mediastinal lymph node or thoracic duct obstruction, pleural or pulmonary infiltration by tumor,[14] venous obstruction, pulmonary infection, or radiation therapy.[107] In non-Hodgkin's lymphoma, direct pleural invasion seems to be the most important factor.[111] However, the relative contribution of the various mechanisms is less clear in Hodgkin's lymphoma.

The cytologic diagnosis of lymphoma in pleural fluid specimens can be difficult, particularly with small lymphocytic tumors. (It should be remembered that cytologically atypical lymphocytes can be present in tuberculous effusions and result in an appearance that has been mistaken for lymphoma.[112]) Immunohistochemical and molecular analysis can help establish the diagnosis.

Leukemia

As a radiographic abnormality, pleural effusion in leukemia is second in frequency only to mediastinal lymph node enlargement and is identified in up to 25% of patients. It is probably caused by leukemic infiltration of the pleura in no more than 5% of cases, the majority being secondary to cardiac failure or infection. It is generally unilateral. Cytochemical and immunocytochemical studies of cells obtained from the fluid may be helpful in diagnosis.[113] Pleural effusion is also a common feature of retinoic acid syndrome.[114]

Thromboembolic Disease

As a radiographic manifestation of clinically evident pulmonary thromboembolism (PTE), pleural effusion is as common as parenchymal consolidation and occurs in about 35% of patients.[115] As might be expected, such effusion is often associated with pulmonary infarction. Sometimes the associated parenchymal opacity is diminutive or hidden by the fluid; in these cases the diagnostic possibilities are confused to such an extent that an embolic episode will be suggested only if there is a high index of suspicion. The amount of pleural fluid is frequently small but may be abundant and is most often unilateral.[116] The effusion usually develops and is resorbed synchronously with the infarct but occasionally appears later and clears sooner.[117]

Transudative effusions occur rarely in association with thromboemboli[118]; it is likely that most, if not all, are caused by clinically unrecognized heart failure. In a patient suspected on clinical grounds of having PTE, a bloody pleural effusion is strong confirmatory evidence of associated infarction.

The radiographic manifestations of PTE and infarction are varied and generally lack both sensitivity and specificity for the diagnosis.[119] However, the combination of diaphragmatic elevation, basal pulmonary opacity of almost any type (but usually homogeneous), and a small pleural effusion constitutes a triad of signs that are highly suggestive of the diagnosis. Patients who have effusions that progress during therapy should be evaluated for recurrent PTE, secondary infection, or pleural hemorrhage secondary to anticoagulation.[14]

Cardiac Failure

One of the most common forms of pleural effusion is that associated with cardiac decompensation. The fluid is usually a transudate; an exudative effusion is relatively rare but has been described after intravenous diuretic therapy close to the time of thoracentesis and in patients in whom previous coronary bypass surgery might have interfered with lymphatic drainage of the pleural space.[120,121] Pulmonary hypertension alone is not associated with the development of pleural effusion[122]; however, an increase in systemic venous pressure secondary to such hypertension could *contribute* to the development of effusion by increasing hydrostatic pressure in the systemic circulation that drains the pleural cavity.

Pleural effusion in congestive heart failure is most often bilateral; for unknown reasons, it is more likely to be right sided than left sided when unilateral.[123] Associated clinical findings and radiographic evidence of cardiac enlargement, with or without pulmonary venous hypertension, make the diagnosis obvious in most cases.

Trauma

Pleural effusion is a common manifestation of penetrating and nonpenetrating trauma and may develop by several mechanisms. Hemothorax may result from laceration of the parietal or visceral pleura by fractured ribs; however, it can also occur in closed chest trauma without evidence of fracture. It commonly complicates traumatic rupture of the aorta, in which case it is almost invariably left sided.

Pleural effusion or hydropneumothorax, again almost always left sided, frequently develops after esophageal perforation, usually as a complication of esophagoscopy or gastroscopy.[124] In these circumstances, identification of ingested material such as milk or food particles in pleural fluid is diagnostic. The level of pleural fluid amylase (derived from the salivary glands) is raised in most patients.[125] In the majority of cases, the site of rupture must be identified precisely (and sometimes with considerable difficulty) by radiologic evidence of extravasation of ingested contrast material. Small exudative effusions sometimes develop after endoscopic sclerotherapy for esophageal varices, presumably as a result of inflammation of the mediastinal parietal pleura.[126]

Pleural effusion is also very common after myocardial revascularization procedures, in which it occurs in up to 90% of patients.[127] The accumulation of fluid in large amounts is uncommon and usually seen in association with internal mammary bypass grafts.[128] Such effusions are generally left sided and resolve spontaneously.[129] Those occurring early in the postoperative period are bloody, whereas those that occur more than 1 month after surgery are exudates with a predominance of lymphocytes.[130]

Malpositioning of central venous and Swan-Ganz catheters[131] can cause vascular perforation, either at the time of insertion or sometime later as a result of gradual erosion of the vessel wall by the catheter tip. Depending on the vessel involved, the result may be mediastinal hemorrhage, hemothorax, pneumothorax, massive hydrothorax, or extrapleural hematoma. In patients receiving hyperalimentation, the infusion of potentially toxic solutions obviously increases the hazard.

Pleural Effusion Related to Abdominal Disease

Several intra-abdominal and pelvic disorders are associated with pleural effusion. The pathogenesis of the fluid accumulation varies with the underlying disease and can be related to secondary effects on cardiac function, changes in plasma oncotic pressure, or the passage of ascitic fluid or secretions from the peritoneal cavity into the pleural space via diaphragmatic lymphatics or stomata.[132,133]

Kidney

Because of transdiaphragmatic fluid flow, peritoneal dialysis is occasionally followed by hydrothorax.[134] Pleural effusion may also develop in patients receiving long-term hemodialysis,[135] the fluid often being serosanguineous as a consequence of the use of heparin during the procedure. Heart failure is the cause of effusion in about half the cases; most of the remainder have been attributed to uremia or infection.[136]

Urinary tract obstruction is occasionally associated with unilateral or bilateral accumulation of urine in the pleural space.[137,138] In most cases, the urine is believed to originate in retroperitoneal collections (urinomas) that develop by extravasation from the obstructed urinary tract. The diagnosis of urinothorax is made by the demonstration of a higher level of creatinine in pleural fluid than in blood.[139] Surgical drainage of the retroperitoneal collection usually results in rapid clearing of the effusion.

Pleural effusion is common in patients who have nephrotic syndrome. Although a number of causes are possible, the principal mechanism is diminution in plasma osmotic pressure.[140] The fluid is usually a transudate. Because of the increased risk of thrombosis in patients who have the syndrome, it is particularly important to exclude thromboembolic disease.[141]

Both the pericardium and the pleura may become inflamed in patients who have uremia, in some cases associated with fluid accumulation. Affected patients sometimes complain of pain; friction rubs are frequently heard on auscultation.[142] The effusion generally clears slowly on long-term hemodialysis.[143]

Pancreas

Acute or chronic pancreatitis is sometimes associated with pleural effusion, often without radiographic evidence of other intrathoracic abnormality. When associated with acute pancreatitis, it is a marker of severe disease and has a relatively poor prognosis.[144] Effusions are predominantly left sided.[145] In the majority of patients, symptoms suggest an acute upper abdominal disorder; however, the clinical features may suggest a primary or parapneumonic effusion.[146]

Chronic pancreatitis is associated with pleural effusion more often than acute disease is.[147] The effusion is frequently recurrent, and symptoms often direct attention to the thorax rather than the abdomen.[147] Duct disruption can lead to the creation of a pancreaticopleural fistula, with or without pseudocyst formation.[148] The fistulous tract can also communicate with the peritoneal cavity (causing ascites),[149] the mediastinum (resulting in bilateral pleural effusions and sometimes pericarditis),[150] and the tracheobronchial tree.[151]

The pleural fluid in both acute and chronic pancreatitis has the characteristics of an exudate; it may be serosanguineous and is occasionally frankly bloody. In acute pancreatitis, the effusion is more likely to be slight or moderate in amount and bloody, whereas in chronic disease it tends to be serous and massive. The amylase content in the pleural fluid is characteristically very high and almost invariably greater than that in serum. A pancreaticopleural fistula is best demonstrated by endoscopic retrograde cholangiopancreatography (ERCP) or CT.[152]

Ovary

The association of an ovarian neoplasm with a nonmalignant pleural effusion is known as the *Meigs-Salmon syndrome.*[153,154] A variety of tumors have been implicated, including fibroma, thecoma, granulosa cell tumor, and (occasionally) adenocarcinoma. It is believed that large tumor size is the most important pathogenetic factor. Although the precise mechanism of fluid formation is unclear, sufficient fluid accumulates to cause ascites and (via transdiaphragmatic flow) pleural effusion.[17] The effusion may be massive; it occurs more frequently on the right but may be left sided or bilateral. Although it is usually a transudate, it may contain blood. Removal of the pelvic tumor is generally followed by disappearance of both the ascites and the effusion.

Pleural effusion is commonly present in patients with the ovarian hyperstimulation syndrome, a postovulatory complication seen in women receiving exogenous gonadotropins for induction of ovulation.[155] The syndrome has two main components: (1) sudden bilateral ovarian enlargement, readily recognized by ultrasound, and (2) a rapid shift of intravascular fluid into the third space. The majority of patients seek medical attention within 2 weeks after receiving human chorionic gonadotropin. Clinical symptoms include abdominal distention and discomfort, nausea, vomiting, and shortness of breath. Radiologic manifestations include unilateral or bilateral pleural effusion and, less commonly, pericardial effusion or hydrostatic pulmonary edema.[155,156]

Liver

A large pleural effusion in a patient who has cirrhosis and no evidence of primary pulmonary or cardiac disease has been termed *hepatic hydrothorax.*[157] The effusion is usually right sided and transudative.[158]

Subphrenic Abscess

Small pleural effusions are often found in association with infection in the subphrenic region.[159] Associated findings include elevation and restriction of movement of the ipsilateral hemidiaphragm and basal linear atelectasis or pneumonitis. This combination of findings should suggest the diagnosis, especially in the postoperative period after laparotomy or gastrointestinal perforation.

Miscellaneous Causes of Pleural Effusion

Asbestos. Disease in some individuals who have a history of asbestos exposure is manifested as pleural effusion (see page 730). The likelihood of the complication is dose related. The latency period is shorter than for other asbestos-related disorders, and it is the most common abnormality during the first 20 years after exposure. Most effusions are small.[160]

Abdominal Surgery. Small exudative effusions are common after abdominal surgery, especially when the upper part of the abdomen is involved.[161] They generally resolve without specific therapy.[162]

Myxedema. Although most pleural effusions in patients with hypothyroidism have cardiovascular, renal, or another cause, they occasionally occur in the absence of an etiology other than myxedema. There are no distinctive radiographic characteristics. The effusions are not inflammatory, and biochemically they are usually borderline between exudates and transudates.[163]

Lymphatic Hypoplasia. Pleural effusion is occasionally associated with hypoplasia of the lymphatic system. In some cases, the clinical findings are those of Milroy's disease (congenital lymphedema)[164]; in others, the effusion is associated with lymphedema of the extremities, yellow nails, and (sometimes) bronchiectasis (*yellow nail syndrome*).[165] The pleural fluid characteristically has a high protein content.

Dressler's Syndrome. The *postpericardiectomy* or *post–myocardial infarction syndrome*, known eponymously as *Dressler's syndrome*, is characterized by chest pain, fever, and pericardial and pleural effusion. When related to myocardial damage, it is most common when the damage is transmural and associated with epicardial involvement.[166] The pathogenesis is unknown but is believed to be the result of an immunologic reaction, presumably to mesothelial cells or other serosal components.[167] Clinical findings of chest pain, fever, pericardial rub, dyspnea, crackles, pleural rub, and leukocytosis occur relatively soon after the myocardial/pericardial injury (on average 20 days)[168]; however, they can recur several years after the initial episode.[169]

Familial Paroxysmal Polyserositis. Familial paroxysmal polyserositis (familial Mediterranean fever, recurrent hereditary polyserositis) is a rare cause of pleural effusion.[170] It occurs predominantly in Sephardic Jews, Arabs, Turks, and Armenians and is transmitted in an autosomal recessive fashion in most affected families.[171] The gene responsible has been mapped to chromosome 16 and designated *MEFV*; it encodes for a protein called *pyrin* (marenostrin), which may be a transcription factor regulating genes involved in the suppression of inflammation.[172] The actual cause of the precipitation of attacks is unknown.

In a large study of 175 Arabs with the disease,[173] the most common manifestation was peritonitis (94%), followed by arthritis (34%) and pleuritis (32%). Most attacks of pleuritis are painful and associated with arthritis or arthralgia, usually involving the large joints. Fever, sometimes as high as 104°F (40°C), persists for 12 to 48 hours. The disorder is characterized by remissions and relapses, the former sometimes lasting for years. Though historically complicated by amyloidosis, this has now been shown to be preventable with colchicine therapy, and apart from the disability associated with the attacks themselves, the long-term prognosis is good.[174]

CHYLOTHORAX

The term *chylothorax* designates the presence of lymphatic fluid in the pleural space.[175] The fluid is characteristically "milky" in appearance; however, not all milky effusions are chylous, and not all chylous effusions are milky.[176] A *chyliform* effusion results from degeneration of malignant and other cells in pleural fluid or from an accumulation of cholesterol (usually associated with tuberculosis, rheumatoid disease, or nephrotic syndrome). Chylous effusions are high in neutral fat and fatty acid but low in cholesterol, whereas chyliform effusions are low in neutral fat and high in cholesterol and lecithin.[176] Simultaneous analysis of fasting samples of serum and pleural fluid by lipoprotein electrophoresis readily distinguishes between the two[177]; as a quick test, high triglyceride values are very likely to be found in chylous effusions, whereas low values are not.[178]

The disorder results from obstruction or disruption of the thoracic duct or one of its major divisions. There are numerous causes of such abnormality (Table 20–3), the most frequent being neoplasia and trauma. Chyle may reflux from an obstructed thoracic duct by two routes—the left posterior intercostal lymphatics to the parietal pleural lymphatics and the left bronchomediastinal trunk to lymphatics of the pulmonary parenchyma and visceral pleura. It then extravasates into the pleural cavity from either the visceral or parietal lymphatics.

Although malignancy is responsible for many cases of chylous effusion, it should be noted that such effusion is an infrequent complication of neoplasia as a whole, even when the thoracic duct is completely occluded. The explanation is probably related to the presence of collateral channels between the thoracic duct and the right posterior intercostal lymphatics and to the opening of preexisting lymphovenous channels.[179] Lymphoma is the most common neoplasm associated with chylothorax, being the cause in about 75% of patients who have malignancy.[180] When associated with cancer, the effusion is often bilateral and usually accompanied by chylous ascites.[181]

Trauma is the second most common cause of chylothorax, most cases being related to surgery and some to penetrating or nonpenetrating thoracic injury.[182] Because the thoracic duct crosses to the left of the spine between the fifth and the seventh thoracic vertebrae, disruption tends to cause right-sided chylothorax when the lower portion is affected and left-sided disease when the upper half is involved. Once the thoracic duct has been disrupted, chyle can leak into the mediastinum and thence into the pleural cavity, either because of damage to the parietal pleura by the initial trauma or because the pleura "breaks down" under the pressure of the mediastinal fluid collection. Because of its anatomic course, the thoracic duct is particularly vulnerable to traumatic injury during

TABLE 20–3. Chylothorax—Etiology

Neoplasia
Metastatic carcinoma
Lymphoma/leukemia
Kaposi's sarcoma

Penetrating or Nonpenetrating Thoracic Injury
Surgery

Congenital Anomalies
Congenital lymphangiectasis
Noonan's syndrome
Jaffe-Campanacci syndrome
Adams-Oliver syndrome
46,XY/46,XX mosaicism
Hennekam's syndrome

Miscellaneous
Pancreatitis
Tuberculous spondylitis or lymphadenitis
Fibrosing mediastinitis
Subclavian vein thrombosis
Sarcoidosis
Severe heart failure
Retrosternal goiter
Behçet's syndrome
Gorham's syndrome
Lymphangioleiomyomatosis
Thoracic aortic aneurysm
Castleman's disease
Cirrhosis
Constrictive pericarditis
Systemic lupus erythematosus
Radiation

surgery on the vertebral column[183] or on the left hemithorax near the hilum.

Lymphangiography has an important role in the investigation of patients who have chylothorax and has been shown to be superior to CT.[183] The clinical features of chylothorax are no different from those of pleural effusion of other etiologies. The prognosis is generally good, with the exception of patients in whom it is caused by neoplasm, in which case it is usually a late manifestation of disease.[184]

PNEUMOTHORAX

The presence of air within the pleural space, or pneumothorax, is one of the more common forms of thoracic disease. It is caused most often by trauma, either accidental or iatrogenic. For example, in a series of 318 cases it was the responsible mechanism in 177 (56%)[185]; the trauma was iatrogenic in 102 cases and noniatrogenic in 75. The pneumothorax can be caused by direct communication of the pleural space with the atmosphere through a chest wall puncture or by disruption of the proximal tracheobronchial tree or the visceral pleura. A variety of investigative and biopsy procedures can be followed by the complication (Table 20–4).[186]

In the absence of a history of trauma, pneumothorax is referred to as spontaneous; in this situation it can be primary (unassociated with clinical or radiographic evidence of significant pulmonary disease) or secondary (in which significant pulmonary disease is present). Pneumothorax can also

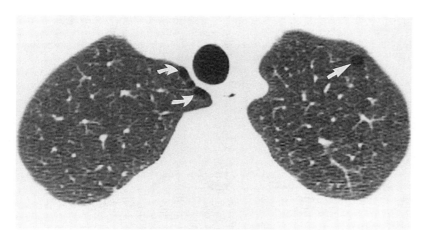

FIGURE 20–1

Localized emphysema in a nonsmoker. An HRCT scan in an 18-year-old man shows small subpleural bullae in the right lung apex (*curved arrows*) and a localized area of emphysema in the left lung apex (*straight arrow*). The patient was a lifelong nonsmoker who had previously undergone chest tube drainage for recurrent right pneumothorax. The emphysema and bullae could not be visualized on the chest radiograph even in retrospect. (*From Müller NL, Fraser RS, Colman NC, Paré PD: Radiologic Diagnosis of Diseases of the Chest. Philadelphia, WB Saunders, 2001.*)

TABLE 20–4. Iatrogenic Causes of Pneumothorax

Biopsy Procedures

Transthoracic needle aspiration
Transbronchial biopsy
Transtracheal biopsy
Colonoscopy
Liver biopsy
Fine-needle aspiration of the breast

Therapeutic Procedures

Thoracentesis
Central venous catheterization
Feeding tube insertion
Positive pressure ventilation
Tracheal intubation
Pacemaker insertion
Electromyographic electrode insertion
Acupuncture
Percutaneous nephrolithotomy
Use of a voice box prosthesis

From Müller NL, Fraser RS, Colman NC, Paré PD: Radiologic Diagnosis of Diseases of the Chest. Philadelphia, WB Saunders, 2001.

occur secondary to pneumomediastinum, air tracking from that location into the pleural space through the mediastinal pleura. In this situation, there is evidence that the most likely sites of rupture are small areas just above the root of the left lung and at the junction with the pericardium.

The primary form of pneumothorax occurs most commonly in men in their twenties or thirties. Although the male-to-female predominance varies in different studies, most investigators have found a ratio of about 4 to 5:1.[187-189] This section is concerned principally with the epidemiology, etiology, pathogenesis, and clinical manifestations of pneumothorax; radiologic signs are discussed on page 157.

Primary Spontaneous Pneumothorax

This form of pneumothorax is believed to be caused by rupture of an air-containing space within or immediately deep to the visceral pleura. These spaces may be either *bullae* (defined as sharply demarcated foci of emphysema >1 cm in diameter) or *blebs* (focal gas-containing spaces situated entirely within the pleura). Though often referred to as blebs, it is likely that most of the air-containing spaces associated with spontaneous pneumothorax are bullae. At surgery or after pathologic examination of resected lung, emphysema is evident in more than 90% of patients[190]; CT scans show focal areas of emphysema in 80% to 90%, even those who are lifelong nonsmokers.[188,189,191] The latter are situated predominantly in the peripheral portion of the apex of the upper lobes and are seen as localized areas of low attenuation measuring 3 mm or more in diameter that may or may not be delineated by thin walls (Fig. 20–1).[188] Bullae are more likely to be identified on radiographs when they cause an irregular outline of the visceral pleura, a finding most easily appreciated in the presence of pneumothorax (Fig. 20–2). Even in the latter situation, however, they are often not visible[192,193]; by contrast, they can be seen on CT in most patients.[187,188,190]

Blebs are believed to be caused by rupture of alveoli adjacent to perivascular or interlobular septal connective tissue, followed by dissection of air through this tissue to the visceral pleura, where it accumulates in the form of a "cyst." Theoretically, alveolar rupture may be the result of check-valve obstruction of a small airway leading to distention of the distal air spaces. Such airway obstruction could have several causes, including recent or remote infection and accumulation of intraluminal mucus. Support for this obstructive hypothesis is provided by the high incidence of cigarette smoking in patients who have spontaneous pneumothorax, tobacco smoke clearly being associated with increased mucus production.[194,195]

The mechanisms underlying the formation of bullae in the apical region of the upper lobes are less clear than those for blebs. Most speculation has centered on the possibility of regional damage to this portion of the lung as a result of either ischemia or the greater distending forces on apical alveoli caused by more negative pleural pressure.[196] In support of both these mechanisms is the observation that primary spontaneous pneumothorax shows a predilection for tall, thin men.[185,197] An intrinsic abnormality of connective tissue resulting in an increased tendency to bulla or bleb formation is probably also important in patients who have Marfan's syndrome or Ehlers-Danlos syndrome.[198,199]

The immediate cause of rupture of a bleb or bulla is often unknown. It is not related to exertional effort because most patients are at rest when the pneumothorax occurs.[200] Localized areas of emphysema distend with a decrease in atmospheric pressure (e.g., with increasing altitude during flight[201]

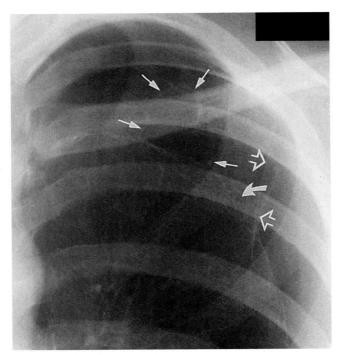

FIGURE 20–2

Bullae in a patient with recurrent pneumothorax. A view of the upper portion of the left side of the chest from a posteroanterior radiograph in a 17-year-old man who had recurrent pneumothorax shows large bullae (*straight arrows*). Irregularity of the margins of the visceral pleura as a result of subpleural bullae (*curved arrow*) and adhesions between the visceral and parietal pleura (*open arrows*) are evident. The patient was a three-pack-per-year smoker. (*From Müller NL, Fraser RS, Colman NC, Paré PD: Radiologic Diagnosis of Diseases of the Chest. Philadelphia, WB Saunders, 2001.*)

and with rapid surfacing after diving[202]), and this mechanism is probably important in some cases.

Secondary Spontaneous Pneumothorax

Numerous conditions have been associated with secondary spontaneous pneumothorax (Table 20–5), the most frequent being COPD. Catamenial pneumothorax—the development of pneumothorax at the time of menstruation—is an uncommon one. It is likely that most cases are related to tissue disruption caused by foci of pleural endometriosis.[203,204] Symptoms of shoulder or chest pain and dyspnea usually appear within 72 hours of the onset of menses and are typically recurrent.[205] The radiologic manifestations are those of pneumothorax, hemothorax, or pleural effusion.[206,207] About 90% of cases occur on the right side, 5% on the left, and 5% bilaterally.[206]

PLEURAL FIBROSIS

As with effusion, pleural fibrosis has numerous etiologies and is the outcome of many primary pleural diseases, as well as a potential complication of virtually every inflammatory condition that affects the lungs. In most cases, the fibrosis is patchy or is localized to a single, relatively small area; in these circumstances, clinical and functional abnormalities are

TABLE 20–5. Secondary Spontaneous Pneumothorax—Etiology

Developmental disease
  Congenital cystic adenomatoid malformation
Connective tissue disease
  Lymphangioleiomyomatosis
  Tuberous sclerosis
  Neurofibromatosis
  Marfan's syndrome
  Ehlers-Danlos syndrome
  Mitral valve prolapse
Infection
  Fungal pneumonia (particularly *Pneumocystis jiroveci* pneumonia in patients who have AIDS)
  Hydatid disease
  Bacterial pneumonia
Neoplasms
  Primary pulmonary carcinoma
  Carcinoid tumor
  Mesothelioma
  Metastatic carcinoma
  Metastatic sarcoma
  Metastatic germ cell tumors
Drugs and toxins
  Chemotherapy for malignancy
  Paraquat poisoning
  Hyperbaric oxygen therapy
  Radiation therapy
  Aerosolized pentamidine therapy in patients with AIDS
Immunologic disease
  Wegener's granulomatosis
  Idiopathic pulmonary hemorrhage
  Idiopathic pulmonary fibrosis
  Langerhans cell histiocytosis
  Sarcoidosis
Obstructive pulmonary disease
  Asthma
  Chronic obstructive pulmonary disease (COPD)
  Cystic fibrosis
Pneumoconiosis
  Silicoproteinosis
  Berylliosis
  Bauxite pneumoconiosis
Vascular disease
  Pulmonary infarction
Metabolic disease
  Pulmonary alveolar proteinosis
Intra-abdominal disease
  Gastropleural fistula
  Colopleural fistula

From Müller NL, Fraser RS, Colman NC, Paré PD: Radiologic Diagnosis of Diseases of the Chest. Philadelphia, WB Saunders, 2001.

absent, and the condition is recognized on a screening radiograph or CT scan during the investigation of other intrathoracic disease or at autopsy. Less commonly, the fibrosis is more or less diffuse in one or both pleural cavities, in which case functional abnormalities may be apparent. Because of this important difference, the two forms are discussed separately.

Local Pleural Fibrosis

Healed Pleuritis

The most common cause of localized pleural fibrosis is organized fibrinous or fibrinopurulent pleuritis secondary to pneumonia. Because pleural effusions of an infectious etiology are almost invariably basal, it is not surprising that this is the anatomic location of most pleural thickening related to this cause. The usual radiographic abnormality is partial obliteration or blunting of the posterior and lateral costophrenic sulci, in some cases associated with line shadows. Thickening of the pleural line may extend for a variable distance up the lateral and posterior thoracic walls and diminish gradually toward the apex; it seldom amounts to more than 1 to 2 mm in width. Obliteration of the costophrenic sulci sometimes has a radiographic appearance difficult to differentiate from that of a small pleural effusion, in which case radiography in the lateral decubitus position, ultrasound, or CT is required for clarification.

Apical Cap

An apical cap is defined radiographically as a curved soft tissue opacity at the apex of one or both hemithoraces (Fig. 20–3).[208] The abnormality is fairly common: in a review of the chest radiographs of 258 patients, a unilateral cap was seen in 11% and bilateral caps in 12%.[209] The prevalence increased with age, being identified in 6% of patients younger than 45 years and 16% of patients older than 45 years. In most cases a specific cause is not identified. Such idiopathic caps usually measure less than 5 mm in height and have a sharply marginated smooth or undulating lower margin (Color Fig. 20–1). Histologic examination shows them to consist of fibrosis of the pleura and underlying parenchymal interstitium and air spaces.

Tuberculosis is probably the most frequently identified cause.[210] In this situation, the cap is often larger than in the idiopathic variety and commonly measures several centimeters in thickness (Fig. 20–4). In some cases the cap is the result of an accumulation of extrapleural fat.[210] Apical caps may also be the result of pleural and subpleural fibrosis after radiation therapy for carcinoma of the breast, lung, or neck.[208,211]

An apical cap may be confused radiologically with the companion shadows of the first and second ribs. Of greater importance from a differential diagnostic point of view is the early stage of an apical pulmonary carcinoma (Pancoast tumor) (Fig. 20–5). Suspicion of neoplasia should be aroused when the apical abnormality is unilateral, when the difference in height between the right and left apical caps is greater than 5 mm, when a focal convexity is present, or when sequential radiographs show progressive enlargement.

Pleural Plaques

Pleural plaques are well-circumscribed foci of dense fibrous tissue located on the parietal pleura (see pages 725 and 728). Because the cause in most cases is asbestos, the prevalence is influenced by the population studied; for example, the prevalence was found to be approximately 4% in an autopsy study of a general urban population[212] and 39% in a population situated in an asbestos-mining region.[213] The latency period between such exposure and the development of radiologically visible plaques is approximately 15 years; for calcified plaques, it is at least 20 years.[214,215]

The earliest radiographic manifestation is a thin line of soft tissue density under a rib in the axillary region, usually the seventh or eighth rib, on one or both sides. The plaques may be difficult to visualize, particularly when viewed en face, and tangential radiographs or CT scans may be necessary. Radiologic-pathologic correlation studies at autopsy have shown that many plaques are missed on chest radiographs.[216] The majority of plaques are bilateral. For unexplained reasons, when unilateral, the left side is more commonly affected.[217,218] Moreover, the width and extent of pleural thickening and the extent of pleural plaque calcification are frequently greater on the left than on the right (Fig. 20–6).[218]

The greatest problem in the recognition of early plaque formation lies in distinguishing plaques from normal companion shadows of the chest wall—not those associated with the first three ribs (because this area is rarely involved in asbestos-related disease), but rather the muscle and fat shadows that can be identified in 75% of normal posteroanterior radiographs along the convexity of the thorax inferiorly. Noncalcified plaques may also be difficult to differentiate from normal diaphragmatic undulations and from focal postinfectious pleural thickening. The accuracy of detection of noncalcified plaques on the chest radiograph is related to their thickness; for example, in an autopsy study no plaques measuring less than 3 mm in thickness were detected radiographically. Overall, the sensitivity of radiography in the detection of pleural plaques ranges from about 30% to 80% and the specificity from 60% to 80%.[212,219,220]

As might be expected, CT is superior in detection (see Fig. 20–6).[221,222] Pleural plaques are identified as circumscribed areas of pleural thickening, usually separated from the underlying rib and extrapleural soft tissues by a thin layer of fat. Most plaques are seen along the posterolateral surface of the parietal pleura in the lower part of the thorax, with sparing of the lung apex and costophrenic angles.

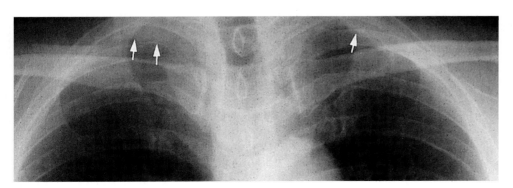

FIGURE 20–3

Apical cap. A view of the upper hemithorax from a posteroanterior chest radiograph in a 72-year-old man shows bilateral apical caps (*arrows*). (*From Müller NL, Fraser RS, Colman NC, Paré PD: Radiologic Diagnosis of Diseases of the Chest. Philadelphia, WB Saunders, 2001.*)

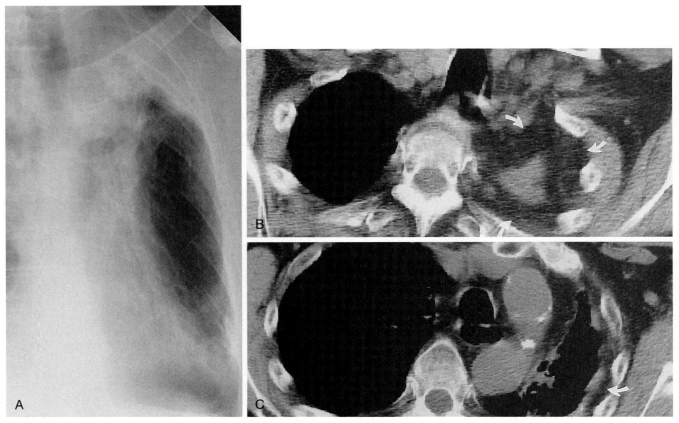

FIGURE 20–4

Apical cap—previous tuberculosis. A view of the left hemithorax from a posteroanterior chest radiograph (**A**) in a 72-year-old man shows marked loss of volume of the left upper lobe with superior retraction of the hilum. A large left apical cap is present. HRCT scans (**B** and **C**) show that most of the apparent pleural thickening is due to the accumulation of extrapleural fat (*arrows*). The patient had been treated for tuberculosis 20 years previously. *(From Müller NL, Fraser RS, Colman NC, Paré PD: Radiologic Diagnosis of Diseases of the Chest. Philadelphia, WB Saunders, 2001.)*

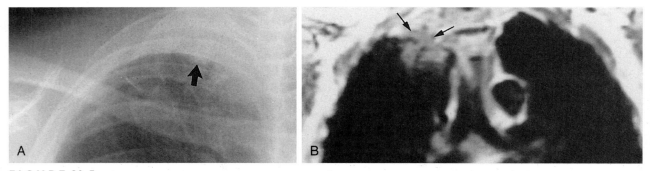

FIGURE 20–5

Pancoast tumor. A view of the right upper hemithorax from a posteroanterior chest radiograph (**A**) in a 44-year-old woman shows a poorly defined right apical opacity with a focal inferior convexity (*arrow*). Localized areas of scarring in the right upper lobe are evident. A cardiac-gated T1-weighted (TR/TE 706/20) spin-echo coronal MR image (**B**) shows tumor in the right lung apex with focal infiltration of the pleura and extrapleural soft tissues (*arrows*). *(From Müller NL, Fraser RS, Colman NC, Paré PD: Radiologic Diagnosis of Diseases of the Chest. Philadelphia, WB Saunders, 2001.)*

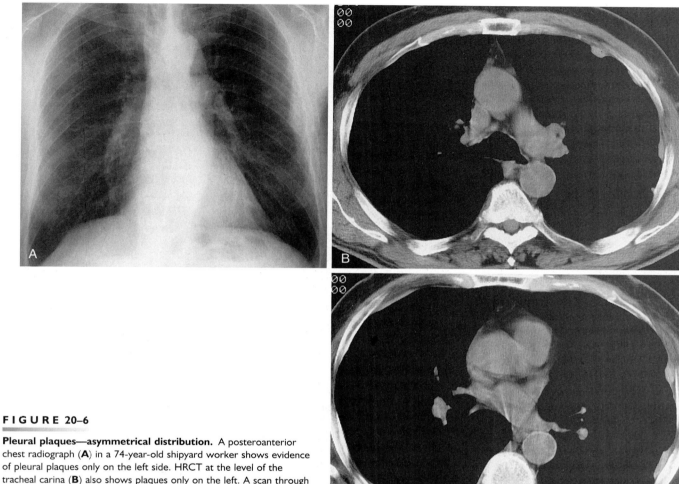

FIGURE 20–6

Pleural plaques—asymmetrical distribution. A posteroanterior chest radiograph (**A**) in a 74-year-old shipyard worker shows evidence of pleural plaques only on the left side. HRCT at the level of the tracheal carina (**B**) also shows plaques only on the left. A scan through the lower lung zones (**C**) reveals prominent plaques on the left side and thin plaques on the right side. *(From Müller NL, Fraser RS, Colman NC, Paré PD: Radiologic Diagnosis of Diseases of the Chest. Philadelphia, WB Saunders, 2001.)*

The frequency of radiologically detectable plaque calcification is variable (Fig. 20–7); some investigators have found calcified and noncalcified plaques in about equal numbers,[223] whereas others have observed calcification in only about 20% of patients.[224] These differences may be related to the variety of asbestos to which the individuals were exposed. Radiologically, calcified plaques vary from small linear or circular shadows usually situated over the diaphragmatic domes to large shadows that completely encircle the lower portion of the lungs. When extensive and viewed en face, they may obscure or be confused with interstitial lung disease.

Diffuse Pleural Fibrosis

Diffuse pleural thickening (fibrothorax) has several causes, including infectious pleuritis (particularly tuberculosis), hemothorax, connective tissue diseases (particularly rheumatoid disease), and asbestos. Radiographically, it is considered to be present when a smooth, uninterrupted pleural opacity is seen extending over at least a fourth of the chest wall with or without obliteration of the costophrenic sulci.[225,226] The

thickness of the pleural "peel" is usually less than 1 cm.[227] The abnormality is diagnosed as diffuse on CT when it extends for more than 8 cm in a craniocaudad direction and 5 cm in a lateral direction and the pleura is more than 3 mm thick.[226] Depending to some extent on the severity and duration of the fibrosis, calcification may or may not be evident (Fig. 20–8).

Fibrothorax seldom affects the mediastinal pleura (Fig. 20–9).[227] (The mediastinal pleura is defined as the pleura that abuts the mediastinum, the posterior extent of which is demarcated by the anterior aspect of the vertebrae; the paravertebral pleura is considered part of the costal pleura.) This observation is useful in the differential diagnosis of malignancy since thickening of the mediastinal pleura on CT is not uncommon in patients who have mesothelioma or metastatic carcinoma.[227]

The distribution and character of the fibrosis may yield clues to its cause. Fibrothorax secondary to tuberculosis, nontuberculous bacterial empyema, and hemorrhagic effusion is most often unilateral, whereas asbestos disease is usually bilateral (manifested either as diffuse pleural thickening or as plaques).[226-228] Extensive calcification is seen most commonly in patients who have had previous tuberculosis, empyema, or

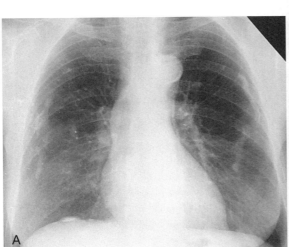
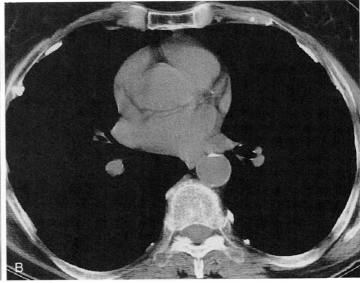

FIGURE 20–7

Calcified asbestos-related pleural plaques. A posteroanterior chest radiograph (**A**) and CT scan (**B**) reveal bilateral discrete calcified plaques involving the costal, diaphragmatic, and paravertebral pleura. The patient was a 79-year-old man who previously had occupational asbestos exposure. (*From Müller NL, Fraser RS, Colman NC, Paré PD: Radiologic Diagnosis of Diseases of the Chest. Philadelphia, WB Saunders, 2001)*

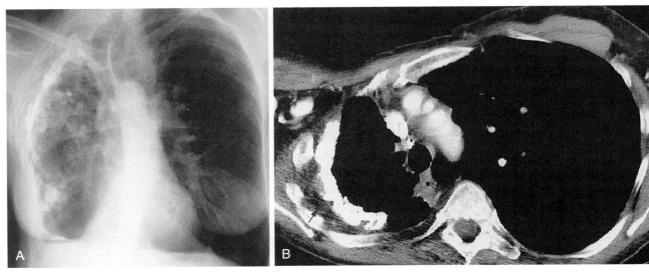

FIGURE 20–8

Calcified fibrothorax. A view of the right side of the chest from a posteroanterior chest radiograph (**A**) shows extensive right pleural calcification associated with loss of volume. Increased thickness of the extrapleural soft tissues is evident. A contrast-enhanced CT scan (**B**) shows marked calcification of the right costal pleura. On this examination, the increased thickness of the extrapleural tissues is related mainly to the accumulation of extrapleural fat (*arrow*). The patient was a 71-year-old woman who previously had tuberculosis. (*From Müller NL, Fraser RS, Colman NC, Paré PD: Radiologic Diagnosis of Diseases of the Chest. Philadelphia, WB Saunders, 2001.)*

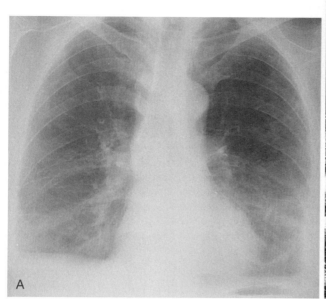
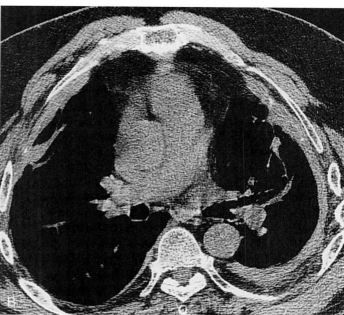

FIGURE 20–9

Diffuse pleural fibrosis. A posteroanterior chest radiograph (**A**) shows extensive bilateral pleural thickening. The blunted costophrenic angles are angulated sharply rather than meniscus shaped, a finding helpful in distinguishing pleural thickening from effusion. Curved bands of increased opacity can be seen to extend from the left lung to the pleural thickening. This feature is seen most commonly with pleural thickening related to asbestos. A CT scan (**B**) shows marked bilateral pleural thickening with small areas of calcification. Although there is marked thickening of the costal and paravertebral pleura, the mediastinal pleura is not affected. The patient was a 53-year-old man who had a history of exposure to asbestos. *(From Müller NL, Fraser RS, Colman NC, Paré PD: Radiologic Diagnosis of Diseases of the Chest. Philadelphia, WB Saunders, 2001.)*

hemothorax and is uncommon in asbestos-related thickening.[229] Assessment of the underlying lungs may also be helpful in determining the etiology. If the lung appears relatively normal, the antecedent abnormality was most likely traumatic hemothorax; by contrast, if there is local scarring and loss of volume, the pleural change was probably the result of remote empyema secondary to *Mycobacterium tuberculosis* or a pyogenic organism.

Diffuse pleural thickening can result in a marked decrease in volume of the affected hemithorax and impaired ventilation of the underlying lung. The degree of ventilation impairment can be gauged, at least roughly, by assessing pulmonary vascularity. If the pulmonary vessels of the affected lung are smaller than those of the opposite side, it can be assumed that the reduction in perfusion has occurred in response to reduced ventilation, presumably as a result of hypoxic vasoconstriction. If the vascularity of the two lungs is roughly symmetrical, it is reasonable to assume that reflex vasoconstriction has not occurred and that ventilation is therefore preserved.

Diffuse pleural fibrosis related to asbestos exposure may cause restrictive impairment in the absence of radiologic evidence of pulmonary disease.[230] The characteristic alteration in lung function consists of a decrease in static lung volumes, reduced diffusing capacity (DLCO), and a normal or increased transfer coefficient (KCO). In a study of 36 patients, serial measurements of lung function over a mean follow-up period of 9 years showed a progressive decrease in FEV_1 and FVC[231]; although there was also a progression in the thickness and extent of fibrothorax on the radiograph, no significant correlation could be found between the change in lung function and the increase in radiographic score.

PLEURAL NEOPLASMS

Mesothelioma

Diffuse mesothelioma is an uncommon but increasingly recognized malignant neoplasm derived from mesothelial cells of the pericardium, peritoneum, or pleura.[232] The neoplasm is important not only because of its dismal prognosis but also because of the potential economic impact of litigation and workers' compensation.[233] Most tumors are associated with a history of asbestos exposure.[232,234]

Overall, the tumor is very uncommon; for example, the incidence in the United States has been estimated to be only about 2 cases per million per year.[235] However, incidence figures vary considerably in different geographic regions, largely reflecting the likelihood of environmental or occupational asbestos exposure. There is evidence that the incidence has been increasing in the recent past, at least in men and in some geographic regions.[236] The incidence also shows a striking sex predominance, a finding largely related to the increased likelihood of occupational asbestos exposure in men; it has been estimated that 85% to 90% of all mesotheliomas occur in men.[237] However, in women who have had occupational asbestos exposure, the incidence rate is similar to that of men.[238]

Etiology

As indicated, the most important cause of mesothelioma is asbestos. However, some patients have had no recognized exposure to the mineral, and other factors are probably important in occasional cases.

Asbestos. Abundant epidemiologic evidence has shown a close association between asbestos exposure and the development of mesothelioma. For example, a history of such exposure is noted in more than 50% of patients in most studies[239,240] and in as many as 80% to 90% in other studies.[241,242] An increased incidence of the tumor has been reported in individuals involved in the mining and production of asbestos, in the numerous secondary occupations associated with its use, and in the demolition of buildings that contain it.[243,244] Some occupations have been associated with an especially high risk, including shipbuilding and spraying of asbestos-based insulation material.[245-247] It should be remembered that occupational asbestos exposure can also occur in uncommon or apparently unlikely occupations; for example, exposure and mesothelioma have been documented in workers involved in the manufacture of cigarette filters,[248] in the production of jewelry,[249] and after the preparation of an asbestos-based cement product in a home basement.[250]

There is good evidence that exposure to asbestos outside the workplace is also potentially hazardous.[251] Such contact can be secondarily related to occupation, as in the home in spouses, children, and siblings of individuals who are directly exposed to asbestos.[252,253] Similarly, an increased incidence of tumors has been documented in individuals who reside near factories or workshops that process or use asbestos, presumably as a result of an increased level of asbestos in the atmosphere.[254,255] Cases of nonoccupational environmental mesothelioma are also related to the presence of tremolite asbestos in the soil in some eastern Mediterranean regions.[256,257]

The risk of mesothelioma's developing varies with the type of asbestos to which an individual is exposed. The majority of evidence indicates that the greatest risk occurs with the amphiboles crocidolite and amosite[258,259]; the risk with anthophyllite appears to be very small.[260] The importance of chrysotile has been the subject of some debate.[261,262] Although the results of most studies suggest that exposure to this substance is indeed associated with increased risk, there is evidence that the risk is much smaller than that of crocidolite and amosite.[263,264]

The variable pathogenicity of the different types of asbestos may be related to their different physicochemical characteristics. Long straight fibers, such as those of the amphiboles, tend to be transported to the periphery of the lung, whereas the irregular curly shape of the chrysotile fiber predisposes to deposition in the more central airways.[265] Thus, amosite and crocidolite tend to accumulate in relatively large numbers in the peripheral portions of the lung close to the pleura. There is also evidence that chrysotile fibers fragment with time and are transported out of the lung via the mucociliary escalator or lymphatics.[265] Amphiboles, on the other hand, are relatively stable; they remain constant in number in an individual who is no longer exposed, and they continue to accumulate over the lifetime of an individual who is continually exposed.

Other Fibrous Minerals. Because the risk for mesothelioma appears to be closely related to the size and shape of inhaled asbestos fibers, attention has been directed to the possibility that other minerals that have the same physical characteristics as asbestos may also be pathogenic. The most clearly implicated of these minerals is erionite, a member of the zeolite group that is found in the soil of central Turkey and the western United States.[266] A variety of artificial fibers, including fiberglass, can also induce cancer when introduced directly into the pleural space of animals[265,267]; however, inhalation of these substances by humans does not appear to be associated with an increased risk for mesothelioma.[268]

Infection. Simian virus 40 (SV40) is a double-stranded DNA organism that normally infects the kidneys of rhesus monkeys.[269] The virus was inadvertently transmitted to many humans in contaminated polio vaccines in the late 1950s and early 1960s. It was subsequently found that the virus has a variety of oncogenic effects in tissue culture and can induce mesothelioma in some experimental animals.[270] Moreover, a number of investigators have found DNA sequences identical to those of the virus in a substantial proportion of human mesotheliomas.[271] An oncoprotein associated with the virus (SV40 large cell antigen [Tag]) has been found to bind and inactivate retinoblastoma family proteins and p53,[272,273] suggesting that the virus may mediate oncogenesis by inactivating tumor suppressor genes. These observations provide evidence of a possible role for SV40 in the pathogenesis of mesothelioma, either by itself or as a cofactor with asbestos. However, not all investigators have been able to demonstrate evidence of the virus or associated oncogene mutations in mesothelioma,[274,275] and further studies are necessary before it can be concluded that SV40 has a pathogenic role in development of the tumor.

Genetic Factors. A familial occurrence of mesothelioma has been documented by several investigators.[276] Although some cases are probably the result of a common source of environmental or occupational asbestos exposure,[255] it is also possible that there is a degree of genetic susceptibility. For example, in an investigation of the first-degree relatives of 196 patients who had pathologically confirmed mesothelioma, a twofold increased risk for the tumor was found in asbestos-exposed men who had two or more relatives with a history of cancer.[277] Mutations of the neurofibromatosis type 2 gene have been noted in a substantial proportion of tumors by some investigators.[278] The tumor suppressor gene *WT1*, which is frequently the site of mutation in Wilms' tumor, can also be identified in many mesotheliomas.[279]

Radiation. The findings of several studies suggest that external radiation is responsible for occasional cases of mesothelioma.[280,281] Experimental evidence suggests that the risk is significantly increased when radiation is combined with asbestos exposure.[282]

Pathologic Characteristics

Mesothelioma typically appears as a plaquelike or lobulated thickening encasing a portion of the lung or, in autopsy specimens, the entire lung (Color Fig. 20–2).[283] Extension of the neoplasm along fissures and into adjacent tissues, such as the chest wall, diaphragm, and pericardium, is not uncommon. Although the tumor may expand in a nodular fashion into the lung, more often it does not extend beneath the pleura.

The tumors can be classified histologically into three forms—epithelial, sarcomatous (mesenchymal or spindle cell), and biphasic (mixed).[284] The first of these forms is the most common and accounts for 60% to 70% of cases in most series; however, the number of mixed tumors increases as more tissue is examined.[285] The epithelial form has a variable appearance, with cells being organized in papillary or tubular structures, acinar clusters, or relatively solid sheets (Fig. 20–10). Individual tumor cells are usually cuboidal or round and possess a moderate amount of eosinophilic cytoplasm. Nuclei are often rather uniform in size and shape, although significant pleomorphism is seen in the less differentiated forms. Nucleoli are characteristically prominent.

The sarcomatous form typically consists of spindle cells arranged haphazardly or in a fascicular or storiform pattern (see Fig. 20–10). Interstitial collagen may be apparent and suggests fibroblastic differentiation; occasionally, this tissue is abundant and leads to the designation "desmoplastic" mesothelioma.[286] Differentiation of the latter form of tumor from a benign fibrous proliferation can be difficult, particularly with small biopsy specimens or when mild cytologic atypia is present. Other forms of mesenchymal differentiation, including cartilage, bone, and fat, are seen occasionally.[287]

As the name implies, mixed tumors consist of a combination of epithelial and mesenchymal patterns; although the proportion of each that is necessary for such classification is arbitrary, a minimum of 10% seems reasonable.

The pathologic diagnosis of mesothelioma is confounded by two major practical problems: (1) distinguishing mesothelial hyperplasia from neoplasia[288] and (2) distinguishing mesothelioma from metastatic carcinoma, especially adenocarcinoma. Each of these differential diagnostic problems is particularly troublesome with the small tissue fragments commonly obtained by closed chest pleural biopsy; however, these problems may also be encountered with material derived from open or thoracoscopic biopsy. These difficulties in pathologic diagnosis are reflected in the results of interobserver variability studies, in which significant disagreement in diagnosis has been documented in 5% to 15% of cases.[289,290]

Reactive mesothelial cells after pleural injury can have a variety of morphologic patterns, including simple or complex papillary projections and aggregates of cells of variable thickness covering the pleural surface; occasionally, mitotic figures, cytologic atypia, and entrapment of mesothelial cell clusters in underlying fibrous tissue can be seen.[288] Although histologic criteria have been proposed to aid in the distinction between such benign proliferations and mesothelioma,[291] in some cases it may be impossible to be definitive. In fact, it is possible that some cases represent examples of dysplastic mesothelium analogous to the preinvasive neoplastic process that occurs in epithelia throughout the body.[292] A variety of ancillary pathologic procedures have been investigated in an attempt to distinguish reactive from neoplastic mesothelium.[293-295] However, none has sufficient specificity to have been accepted as a definitive test.

The second major problem in the pathologic diagnosis of mesothelioma lies in distinguishing it from metastatic carcinoma. This difficulty is predominantly related to the fact that epithelial forms of mesothelioma histologically resemble adenocarcinoma. In addition, some carcinomas, particularly those of the lung, can spread along the pleura in a fashion grossly identical to that of mesothelioma.[296] As with the distinction between hyperplasia and neoplasia, a variety of ancillary techniques have been used to aid in the solution of this problem, including histochemistry,[297] immunohistochemistry (particularly for the presence of "anticarcinoma" antibodies such as CEA and "antimesothelial" antibodies such as calretinin),[298] electron microscopy,[299] and biochemical analysis.

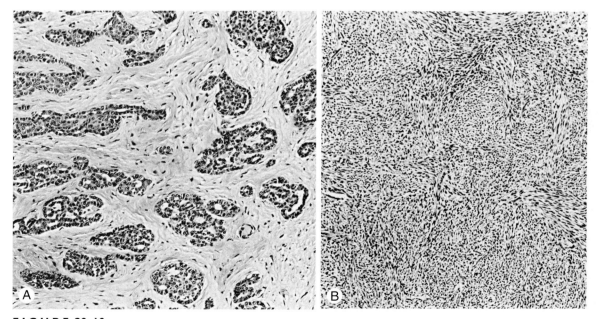

FIGURE 20–10

Diffuse mesothelioma—epithelial and sarcomatous types. A section of an epithelial tumor (**A**) reveals small nests of cells with round or elongated slitlike spaces separated by a fibroblastic stroma. A section of another tumor (**B**) reveals fascicles of spindle-shaped cells arranged in an interdigitating pattern; a storiform appearance is present focally. *(From Müller NL, Fraser RS, Colman NC, Paré PD: Radiologic Diagnosis of Diseases of the Chest. Philadelphia, WB Saunders, 2001.)*

Radiologic Manifestations

The most frequent radiographic manifestation of malignant mesothelioma is unilateral sheetlike or lobulated pleural thickening encasing the entire lung (Fig. 20–11).[300,301] Additional relatively common findings include volume loss of the ipsilateral hemithorax and extension of tumor into a fissure. Less commonly, the tumor is manifested as multiple pleural-based masses. Unilateral effusion is identified at initial evaluation in 30% to 80% of cases and often obscures the underlying neoplasm. In advanced tumors, chest wall invasion may be manifested by a periosteal reaction along the ribs, rib erosion, or rib destruction.[301] Occasionally, hematogenous metastases to the lung are seen as lung nodules or masses.[302]

CT is superior to conventional radiography in determining the presence and extent of tumor in the pleura and in assessing invasion of the mediastinum, chest wall, and upper part of the abdomen.[300,303,304] Again, the most common findings

consist of pleural thickening and effusion. In a review of 70 patients, the thickening was nodular in 72% and uniform in 28%.[305] Less common findings included loss of volume of the ipsilateral hemithorax, a contralateral shift of the mediastinum, lymph node enlargement, and chest wall invasion. Calcification within a mesothelioma is seen in approximately 10% of cases and usually represents engulfment of calcified plaques.[306] With respect to the differential diagnosis, it should be remembered that diffuse sheetlike or nodular pleural thickening identical to that of mesothelioma may be seen on CT with metastatic carcinoma or lymphoma but rarely with benign processes.[226,227]

Findings suggestive of chest wall invasion include obscuration of fat planes, infiltration of intercostal muscles, periosteal reaction, and bone destruction. Features of mediastinal invasion include obliteration of fat planes, nodular pericardial thickening, and direct soft tissue extension. The sensitivity of CT in assessing such invasion is very good; in a study of 34 patients who underwent potentially curative surgery, the

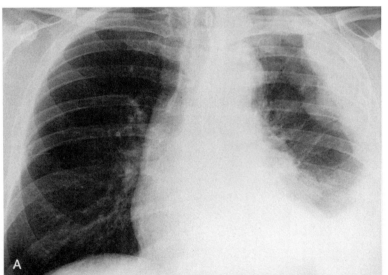

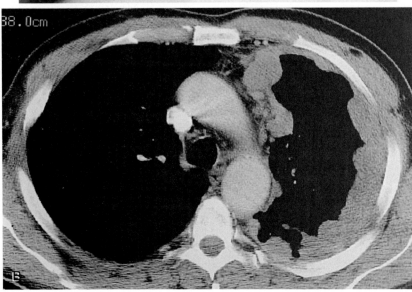

FIGURE 20–11

Mesothelioma. A posteroanterior chest radiograph (**A**) in a 70-year-old man shows marked lobulated left pleural thickening encasing the entire lung. A contrast-enhanced CT scan (**B**) shows a nodular pleural rind. *(From Müller NL, Fraser RS, Colman NC, Paré PD: Radiologic Diagnosis of Diseases of the Chest. Philadelphia, WB Saunders, 2001.)*

sensitivity was 93% for excluding chest wall involvement, 94% for excluding transdiaphragmatic extension, and 100% for excluding mediastinal involvement.[307] The most helpful findings in assessing resectability were preservation of normal extrapleural fat for excluding chest wall invasion, a clear fat plane between the inferior diaphragmatic surface and the adjacent abdominal organs for excluding transdiaphragmatic extension, and preservation of normal mediastinal fat for exclusion of mediastinal invasion.

MR imaging is comparable or slightly superior to CT in assessment of tumor morphology and extent.[307,308] Mesothelioma has slightly greater signal intensity than the intercostal muscles on T1-weighted imaging but considerably greater signal intensity on proton-density and T2-weighted images. In one study, all six mesotheliomas had a hyperintense signal relative to intercostal muscle on proton-density and T2-weighted images, whereas 14 of 16 benign causes of pleural thickening, including all pleural plaques and cases of fibrothorax, were isointense or hypointense.[308] The procedure is comparable to CT in predicting tumor resectability. Preliminary results suggest that positron emission tomography (PET) imaging with 2-(^{18}F)-fluoro-2-deoxy-D-glucose (FDG) may also be helpful in assessment. In an investigation of 28 patients, uptake of FDG was significantly higher in the 24 who had biopsy-proven malignant disease (22 with mesothelioma, 2 with metastatic adenocarcinoma) than in the 4 who had benign disease (2 with pleuritis, 1 with angiolipoma, and 1 with asbestos-related pleural fibrosis).[309]

Clinical Manifestations

The most common clinical manifestations consist of vague chest or shoulder ache or true pleuritic pain[242,310]; however, a substantial number (a third of patients in some series[242]) have pleural effusion unassociated with pain. As the disease progresses, shortness of breath and a dry, sometimes hacking cough can develop; fatigue and weight loss are common. Physical examination may reveal clubbing, and retraction of the thorax and dullness on percussion are common. Occasionally, the neoplasm invades the chest wall along a needle track used for previous thoracentesis or thoracoscopy; in this circumstance, a localized tumor may be palpated in relation to the puncture site, a finding highly suggestive of the diagnosis.

Cardiac abnormalities are common, usually as a result of direct spread of tumor into the pericardial space. In a series of 64 patients, electrocardiographic abnormalities were present in 55 (86%) and consisted of arrhythmia (60%) and conduction abnormalities (37%).[311] Echocardiography revealed pericardial effusion in 13 patients.

An occupational history of asbestos exposure should suggest the diagnosis, particularly in a patient who has an unexplained unilateral pleural effusion. Such history will usually be evident on routine questioning because the majority of tumors occur in individuals who have jobs that are clearly associated with asbestos and the period of exposure is generally long. However, as discussed previously, some patients have only minimal exposure or have worked in occupations not clearly linked to asbestos, so careful questioning may be necessary to elicit evidence of an asbestos association. Compounding this difficulty is the latent period between exposure and the development of clinically evident disease, which is not infrequently 40 years or longer.[310,312]

Laboratory Findings

As indicated, pleural effusion is present in the majority of patients who have mesothelioma and is often considerable in amount; it may be either straw colored or serosanguineous, in roughly equal numbers. Cytologic examination of the fluid can be helpful in diagnosis.[313] However, as with histologic diagnosis, difficulty may be encountered in distinguishing reactive from neoplastic mesothelial cells and mesothelioma from metastatic adenocarcinoma. A variety of ancillary procedures have been investigated in an attempt to overcome these difficulties, and some observers have reported a high degree of accuracy with cytologic diagnosis.[314,315] Nonetheless, the overall sensitivity is probably low,[316] and examination of tissue specimens obtained by closed chest needle biopsy or thoracoscopic biopsy is often necessary for definitive diagnosis.[317]

Measurement of the pleural fluid content of a variety of substances, including CEA,[318] surfactant protein-A (SP-A),[318] hyaluronic acid,[319] α_1-acid glycoprotein, and phosphohexose isomerase,[320] has been performed in an attempt to distinguish between reactive and neoplastic processes and between mesothelioma and metastatic carcinoma. As with such investigations in tissue, however, none is sufficiently specific by itself to yield a definitive diagnosis.

Prognosis and Natural History

The course of untreated mesothelioma is characterized by progressive spread of tumor over the pleural surface until the entire lung is encased. Concomitant spread to the opposite pleural and pericardial spaces and across the diaphragm into the peritoneum is not infrequent. Although microscopic lymphangitic spread or hematogenous metastases are not uncommonly seen in the lung at autopsy, they are uncommonly identified during life.[321] Similarly, metastases outside the thorax are common at autopsy but are infrequently detected clinically[302]; they are most common in tumors that have a sarcomatous morphology.[322] Mediastinal lymph node metastases are often discovered during staging when the tumor is initially identified.[323]

The prognosis is extremely poor: most patients die within the first year of the onset of symptoms, and "long-term" survival is rare.[324,325] For example, in two series of 281 patients, only 7 (2.5%) lived more than 5 years.[326,327] As with most other cancers, the prognosis is related to the extent of local or distant tumor spread[328,329]; several staging systems have been described.[323] The prognosis is better in patients who have tumors with an epithelial rather than a sarcomatous morphology,[329,330] an effect that seems to be independent of stage. Some investigators have also found evidence for longer survival in younger patients independent of stage and histologic type.[330]

It is possible that surgery—either pleurectomy/decortication in cases of minimal disease or extrapleural pneumonectomy (en bloc excision of parietal pleura, lung, pericardium, diaphragm, and attached tumor) in more extensive tumor[331]—followed by irradiation and chemotherapy may offer some benefit in selected patients.[323] For example, in a series of 120 patients who underwent these procedures, overall survival rates were 45% at 2 years and 27% at 5 years.[332] Unfortunately, it is not clear to what extent this relatively good survival is related to patient selection.

Solitary Fibrous Tumor

Solitary fibrous tumor (local, fibrous, or benign mesothelioma; subpleural, submesothelial, or pleural fibroma) is an uncommon mesenchymal neoplasm that can occur in many sites throughout the body but is most often identified in the pleura. Approximately 600 cases had been documented by 2000[333]; an additional 101 were reported from the files of the Armed Forces Institute of Pathology (AFIP) in 2003.[334] It occurs slightly more often in women than men.[334] Although it can be seen at any age,[335] the mean age at diagnosis is 55 years.[334] The cause is unknown in most cases; however, occasional tumors have developed after radiation therapy to the chest wall.[336,337] There is no association with cigarette smoking or asbestos exposure.[338,339] Most investigators believe that the tumor originates from the pleural connective tissue.[339,340]

Pathologic Characteristics

About 65% to 80% of tumors arise in the visceral pleura.[338,339] Most project into the pleural space and compress the adjacent lung to a variable degree. Occasionally, tumors that arise in the medial pleura extend into the mediastinum,[341] and those in a fissure extend into the pulmonary parenchyma.[339] Most are spherical or oval and well circumscribed; many are attached to the pleura by a short vascular pedicle. They can grow to a huge size, some occupying more than half a hemithorax.[334] Cut sections often show a lobulated or whorled appearance reminiscent of a leiomyoma (Color Fig. 20–3). Histologically, the tumor consists of haphazardly arranged or interlacing fascicles of spindle cells (Fig. 20–12), occasionally with a storiform or palisade pattern resembling other soft tissue tumors.[342] Between the cells is a variable amount of collagen, in some regions virtually undetectable and in others so abundant that the spindle cells themselves may be almost inapparent. Blood vessels are prominent in some tumors, a feature that has been associated with significant enhancement on CT.[343] Immunohistochemical studies typically show a negative reaction for cytokeratin and a positive one for CD34, in contrast to the sarcomatous form of diffuse malignant mesothelioma, in which the keratin reaction is often positive and CD34 negative.[344]

Radiologic Manifestations

Radiographically, solitary fibrous tumors are sharply defined, smooth, or lobulated masses of homogeneous density ranging in diameter from 1 cm to the size of a hemithorax.[334,345,346] They may be located in an interlobar fissure or adjacent to the diaphragm, mediastinum, or chest wall.[334] Small lesions (<4 cm) typically have tapering margins and form obtuse angles with the chest wall or mediastinum, important findings in establishing the extrapulmonary nature of a thoracic mass (Fig. 20–13). When a tumor is large, however, its site of origin is frequently difficult or impossible to determine. Calcification or effusion is evident occasionally,[339] the latter more commonly in malignant than benign tumors.[345]

A finding of considerable diagnostic value is a change in position of the tumor with respiration, needling, or a modification in body position.[346,347] If the tumor originates in the visceral pleura, movement is detected by relating its position to contiguous ribs or mediastinal structures; if its origin is in the parietal pleura, movement may be related to the presence of a pedicle. Occasionally the pedicle becomes twisted and results in detachment of the tumor from the pleura and the formation of a free intrapleural body.[348]

Similar findings have been described with CT.[349-351] Helpful signs in determining the extrapulmonary nature of the lesion include the presence of tapering margins and displacement of adjacent lung parenchyma (see Fig. 20–13).[351] Heterogeneous

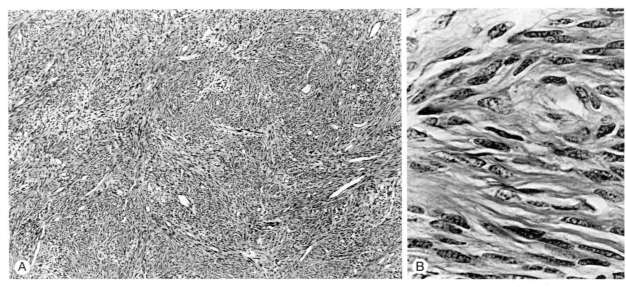

FIGURE 20-12

Solitary fibrous tumor of the pleura. A section of a well-circumscribed tumor attached to the visceral pleura (**A**) shows interlacing fascicles of spindle cells with little intercellular collagen. A magnified view (**B**) demonstrates mild nuclear pleomorphism. *(From Müller NL, Fraser RS, Colman NC, Paré PD: Radiologic Diagnosis of Diseases of the Chest. Philadelphia, WB Saunders, 2001.)*

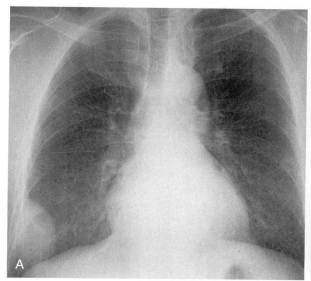
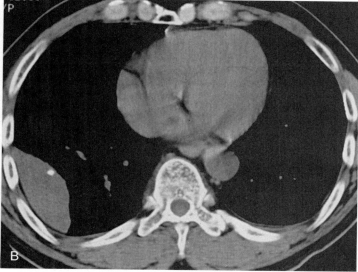

FIGURE 20–13

Solitary tumor of the pleura. A posteroanterior chest radiograph (**A**) in a 62-year-old man shows a well-defined pleural-based tumor in the lower right hemithorax. The cephalic border of the tumor tapers smoothly and forms an obtuse angle with the chest wall. A CT scan without intravenous contrast (**B**) shows a smoothly marginated pleural-based soft tissue lesion with a focal area of calcification. *(From Müller NL, Fraser RS, Colman NC, Paré PD: Radiologic Diagnosis of Diseases of the Chest. Philadelphia, WB Saunders, 2001.)*

attenuation as a result of localized areas of low attenuation or foci of calcification are seen before the administration of intravenous contrast in approximately 60% of benign tumors and virtually 100% of malignant ones.[334] After the administration of contrast, approximately 80% of benign tumors exhibit heterogeneous attenuation.[334] In a series of 78 patients, pleural effusion was present in 21 of 61 (34%) with benign tumors and 8 of 17 (47%) with malignant ones.[334]

MR imaging is superior to CT in determining the tissue characteristics of these tumors. With this technique, benign variants usually have low signal intensity on T1- and T2-weighted images, consistent with the presence of fibrous tissue.[352,353] These characteristics allow distinction from pulmonary carcinoma, which usually has increased signal intensity on T2-weighted images. Although the low signal intensity is not pathognomonic for fibrous tumor, it allows a presumptive diagnosis and may obviate the need for transthoracic needle biopsy. Fibrous tumors also show a marked increase in signal intensity after the intravenous injection of gadolinium.[345,354]

Clinical Manifestations

Most patients are asymptomatic[339]; cough, chest pain, and dyspnea occur occasionally,[338] especially in association with larger tumors.[355] One particularly common finding is hypertrophic osteoarthropathy,[338] an association that is much stronger than with pulmonary carcinoma; in fact, its presence in a patient who has a large intrathoracic mass should suggest the diagnosis. Surgical removal of the tumor relieves the symptoms of arthropathy in most cases.[356] Symptomatic hypoglycemia (Doege-Potter syndrome) has been documented in about 5% of patients[355,357]; it is more common in malignant than in benign tumors and three times more frequent in women than men.[339]

Prognosis and Natural History

The majority of solitary fibrous tumors behave in a benign fashion, with intrathoracic growth resulting in compression but not invasion of contiguous structures. Most tumors grow slowly. Surgical excision usually results in complete cure, particularly when the tumor possesses a well-defined pedicle; however, there can be local recurrence if the initial surgery is inadequate. Patients who have unresectable primary or recurrent disease usually die within 2 years as a result of extensive intrathoracic disease[338]; extrathoracic metastases are rare.

Prediction of an aggressive or benign behavior of these neoplasms can be difficult. As indicated, the radiologic features associated with an increased risk for aggressive behavior include pleural effusion and chest wall invasion.[339] Although most tumors that behave in malignant fashion have significant cellular pleomorphism and a high mitotic rate,[358] these features do not necessarily imply a bad prognosis; in one review, almost half the patients judged to have a malignant neoplasm by light microscopic criteria were considered clinically cured.[339] Moreover, occasional tumors that have a bland histologic appearance recur.

Lipoma

Lipomas related to the pleura are seen on the chest radiograph as soft tissue masses that have well-defined margins where they abut the lung and poorly defined margins where they abut the chest wall. When small, they often have tapering margins and form obtuse angles with the chest wall.[126,359] CT allows a specific diagnosis by showing uniform attenuation similar to that of subcutaneous fat (Fig. 20–14). A few linear strands of soft tissue attenuation may be seen related to their fibrous stroma[359]; however, when the lesion has a

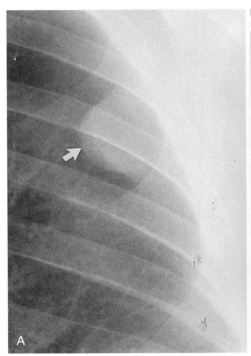

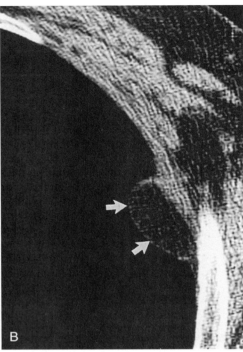

FIGURE 20–14

Pleural lipoma. A view of the upper portion of the left side of the chest from a posteroanterior radiograph (**A**) shows a homogeneous opacity (*arrow*) with smooth margins, a sharply defined medial edge, and an ill-defined lateral border characteristic of a pleural-based lesion. A view from an HRCT scan (**B**) shows characteristic homogeneous fat attenuation (*arrows*). (*From Müller NL, Fraser RS, Colman NC, Paré PD: Radiologic Diagnosis of Diseases of the Chest. Philadelphia, WB Saunders, 2001.*)

heterogeneous appearance with attenuation values greater than −50 Hounsfield units, liposarcoma should be suspected.[226]

REFERENCES

1. Zocchi L: Physiology and pathophysiology of pleural fluid turnover. Eur Respir J 20:1545-1558, 2002.
2. Marel M, Stastny B, Melinova L, et al: Diagnosis of pleural effusions. Experience with clinical studies, 1986 to 1990. Chest 107:1598-1603, 1995.
3. DeSouza R, Lipsett N, Spagnolo SV: Mediastinal compression due to tension hydrothorax. Chest 72:782-783, 1977.
4. Naschitz JE, Yeshurun D: Unilateral chest wall edema in carcinomatous pleurisy. Respiration 47:73-77, 1985.
5. Gilmartin JJ, Wright AJ, Gibson GJ: Effects of pneumothorax or pleural effusion on pulmonary function. Thorax 40:60-65, 1985.
6. Agusti AG, Cardus J, Roca J, et al: Ventilation-perfusion mismatch in patients with pleural effusion: Effects of thoracentesis. Am J Respir Crit Care Med 156:1205-1209, 1997.
7. Wang JS, Tseng CH: Changes in pulmonary mechanics and gas exchange after thoracentesis on patients with inversion of a hemidiaphragm secondary to large pleural effusion. Chest 107:1610-1614, 1995.
8. Brandstetter RD, Cohen RP: Hypoxemia after thoracentesis. A predictable and treatable condition. JAMA 242:1060-1061, 1979.
9. Light RW, Macgregor MI, Luchsinger PC, Ball WC Jr: Pleural effusions: The diagnostic separation of transudates and exudates. Ann Intern Med 77:507-513, 1972.
10. Burgess LJ, Maritz FJ, Taljaard JJ: Comparative analysis of the biochemical parameters used to distinguish between pleural transudates and exudates. Chest 107:1604-1609, 1995.
11. Rubins JB, Colice GL: Evaluating pleural effusions. How should you go about finding the cause? Postgrad Med 105:39-42, 45-48, 1999.
12. Heffner JE, Brown LK, Barbieri CA: Diagnostic value of tests that discriminate between exudative and transudative pleural effusions. Primary Study Investigators. Chest 111:970-980, 1997.
13. Liam CK, Lim KH, Wong CM: Causes of pleural exudates in a region with a high incidence of tuberculosis. Respirology 5:33-38, 2000.
14. Sahn SA: The pleura. Am Rev Respir Dis 138:184, 1988.
15. Batungwanayo J, Taelman H, Allen S, et al: Pleural effusion, tuberculosis and HIV-1 infection in Kigali, Rwanda. AIDS 7:73-79, 1993.
16. Seibert AF, Haynes J Jr, Middleton R, Bass JB Jr: Tuberculous pleural effusion. Twenty-year experience. Chest 99:883-886, 1991.
17. Light RW: Pleural Diseases. Philadelphia, Lea & Febiger, 1983.
18. Stead W, Eichenholz A, Stauss H: Operative and pathologic findings in twenty-four patients with syndrome of idiopathic pleurisy with effusion, presumably tuberculous. Am Rev Respir Dis 71:473, 1955.
19. Hulnick DH, Naidich DP, McCauley DI: Pleural tuberculosis evaluated by computed tomography. Radiology 149:759-765, 1983.
20. Gambon-Deza F, Pacheco Carracedo M, Cerda Mota T, Montes Santiago J: Lymphocyte populations during tuberculosis infection: V beta repertoires. Infect Immun 63:1235-1240, 1995.
21. Lorgat F, Keraan MM, Ress SR: Cellular immunity in tuberculous pleural effusions: Evidence of spontaneous lymphocyte proliferation and antigen-specific accelerated responses to purified protein derivative (PPD). Clin Exp Immunol 90:215-218, 1992.
22. Barnes PF, Lu S, Abrams JS, et al: Cytokine production at the site of disease in human tuberculosis. Infect Immun 61:3482-3489, 1993.
23. Park JS, Kim YS, Jee YK, et al: Interleukin-8 production in tuberculous pleurisy: Role of mesothelial cells stimulated by cytokine network involving tumour necrosis factor-alpha and interleukin-1 beta. Scand J Immunol 57:463-469, 2003.
24. Antoniskis D, Amin K, Barnes PF: Pleuritis as a manifestation of reactivation tuberculosis. Am J Med 89:447-450, 1990.
25. Sahn SA, Iseman MD: Tuberculous empyema. Semin Respir Infect 14:82-87, 1999.
26. Valdes L, Alvarez D, San Jose E, et al: Tuberculous pleurisy: A study of 254 patients. Arch Intern Med 158:2017-2021, 1998.
27. Lee YC, Rogers JT, Rodriguez RM, et al: Adenosine deaminase levels in nontuberculous lymphocytic pleural effusions. Chest 120:356-361, 2001.
28. Jimenez Castro D, Diaz Nuevo G, Perez-Rodriguez E, Light RW: Diagnostic value of adenosine deaminase in nontuberculous lymphocytic pleural effusions. Eur Respir J 21:220-224, 2003.
29. Villena V, Lopez-Encuentra A, Echave-Sustaeta J, et al: Interferon-gamma in 388 immunocompromised and immunocompetent patients for diagnosing pleural tuberculosis. Eur Respir J 9:2635-2639, 1996.
30. Kirsch CM, Kroe DM, Azzi RL, et al: The optimal number of pleural biopsy specimens for a diagnosis of tuberculous pleurisy. Chest 112:702-706, 1997.
31. Villegas MV, Labrada LA, Saravia NG: Evaluation of polymerase chain reaction, adenosine deaminase, and interferon-gamma in pleural fluid for the differential diagnosis of pleural tuberculosis. Chest 118:1355-1364, 2000.
32. Querol JM, Minguez J, Garcia-Sanchez E, et al: Rapid diagnosis of pleural tuberculosis by polymerase chain reaction. Am J Respir Crit Care Med 152:1977-1981, 1995.
33. de Wit D, Maartens G, Steyn L: A comparative study of the polymerase chain reaction and conventional procedures for the diagnosis of tuberculous pleural effusion. Tuber Lung Dis 73:262-267, 1992.
34. Conde MB, Loivos AC, Rezende VM, et al: Yield of sputum induction in the diagnosis of pleural tuberculosis. Am J Respir Crit Care Med 167:723-725, 2003.
35. Roper W, Waring J: Primary serofibrinous pleural effusion in military personnel. Am Rev Respir Dis 71:616, 1955.
36. Light RW, Girard WM, Jenkinson SG, George RB: Parapneumonic effusions. Am J Med 69:507-512, 1980.
37. Strange C, Sahn SA: The definitions and epidemiology of pleural space infection. Semin Respir Infect 14:3-8, 1999.
38. LeMense GP, Strange C, Sahn SA: Empyema thoracis. Therapeutic management and outcome. Chest 107:1532-1537, 1995.

39. Light RW: A new classification of parapneumonic effusions and empyema. Chest 108:299-301, 1995.
40. Antony VB, Mohammed KA: Pathophysiology of pleural space infections. Semin Respir Infect 14:9-17, 1999.
41. Alfageme I, Munoz F, Pena N, Umbria S: Empyema of the thorax in adults. Etiology, microbiologic findings, and management. Chest 103:839-843, 1993.
42. Bartlett JG: Bacterial infections of the pleural space. Semin Respir Infect 3:308-321, 1988.
43. Brook I, Frazier EH: Aerobic and anaerobic microbiology of empyema. A retrospective review in two military hospitals. Chest 103:1502-1507, 1993.
44. Everts RJ, Reller LB: Pleural space infections: Microbiology and antimicrobial therapy. Semin Respir Infect 14:18-30, 1999.
45. Borge J, Michavila I, Mendez J, et al: Thoracic empyema in HIV-infected patients. Chest 113:732, 1998.
46. Chen KY, Hsueh PR, Liaw YS, et al: A 10-year experience with bacteriology of acute thoracic empyema: Emphasis on *Klebsiella pneumoniae* in patients with diabetes mellitus. Chest 117:1685-1689, 2000.
47. Moon WK, Im JG, Yeon KM, Han MC: Complications of *Klebsiella* pneumonia: CT evaluation. J Comput Assist Tomogr 19:176-181, 1995.
48. Sahn SA, Lakshminarayan S, Char DC: "Silent" empyema in patients receiving corticosteroids. Am Rev Respir Dis 107:873-876, 1973.
49. Light RW: Pleural diseases. Dis Mon 38:261-331, 1992.
50. Colice GL, Curtis A, Deslauriers J, et al: Medical and surgical treatment of parapneumonic effusions: An evidence-based guideline. Chest 118:1158-1171, 2000.
51. Ferrer J, Roldan J: Clinical management of the patient with pleural effusion. Eur J Radiol 34:76-86, 2000.
52. Heffner JE: Indications for draining a parapneumonic effusion: An evidence-based approach. Semin Respir Infect 14:48-58, 1999.
53. Jess P, Brynitz S, Friis Moller A: Mortality in thoracic empyema. Scand J Thorac Cardiovasc Surg 18:85-87, 1984.
54. Pothula V, Krellenstein DJ: Early aggressive surgical management of parapneumonic empyemas. Chest 105:832-836, 1994.
55. Cham CW, Haq SM, Rahamim J: Empyema thoracis: A problem with late referral? Thorax 48:925-927, 1993.
56. Ashbaugh DG: Empyema thoracis. Factors influencing morbidity and mortality. Chest 99:1162-1165, 1991.
57. Murray J, Finegold S, Foman S, et al: The changing spectrum of nocardiosis. A review and presentation of nine cases. Am Rev Respir Dis 83:315, 1961.
58. Neu HC, Silva M, Hazen E, Rosenheim SH: Necrotizing nocardial pneumonitis. Ann Intern Med 66:274-284, 1967.
59. Lambert RS, George RB: Fungal diseases of the pleura: Clinical manifestations, diagnosis, and treatment. Semin Respir Infect 3:343-351, 1988.
60. Curry F, Wier J: Histoplasmosis: A review of one hundred consecutively hospitalized patients. Am Rev Tuberc 77:749, 1958.
61. Takamura M, Stark P: Diagnostic case study. Coccidioidomycosis: Pleural involvement. Semin Respir Infect 16:280-285, 2001.
62. Failla PJ, Cerise FP, Karam GH, Summer WR: Blastomycosis: Pulmonary and pleural manifestations. South Med J 88:405-410, 1995.
63. Mauri M, Fernandez Sola A, Capdevila JA, et al: [Pleural cryptococcosis in patients with human immunodeficiency virus infection.] Med Clin (Barc) 106:380-382, 1996.
64. Fukuchi M, Mizushima Y, Hori T, Kobayashi M: Cryptococcal pleural effusion in a patient with chronic renal failure receiving long-term corticosteroid therapy for rheumatoid arthritis. Intern Med 37:534-537, 1998.
65. Horowitz ML, Schiff M, Samuels J, et al: *Pneumocystis carinii* pleural effusion. Pathogenesis and pleural fluid analysis. Am Rev Respir Dis 148:232-234, 1993.
66. Ko SC, Chen KY, Hsueh PR, et al: Fungal empyema thoracis: An emerging clinical entity. Chest 117:1672-1678, 2000.
67. Meredith HC, Cogan BM, McLaulin B: Pleural aspergillosis. AJR Am J Roentgenol 130:164-166, 1978.
68. Light RW: Useful tests on the pleural fluid in the management of patients with pleural effusions. Curr Opin Pulm Med 5:245-249, 1999.
69. Fine NL, Smith LR, Sheedy PF: Frequency of pleural effusions in mycoplasma and viral pneumonias. N Engl J Med 283:790-793, 1970.
70. Shamsuzzaman SM, Hashiguchi Y: Thoracic amebiasis. Clin Chest Med 23:479-492, 2002.
71. Uchida K, Sekiguchi S, Doi Y, Yamazaki H: Pulmonary paragonimiasis with pleural effusion containing *Paragonimus* ova: Sonographical appearance of pleural effusion. Intern Med 34:1178-1180, 1995.
72. Nakamura-Uchiyama F, Mukae H, Nawa Y: Paragonimiasis: A Japanese perspective. Clin Chest Med 23:409-420, 2002.
73. Good JT Jr, King TE, Antony VB, Sahn SA: Lupus pleuritis. Clinical features and pleural fluid characteristics with special reference to pleural fluid antinuclear antibodies. Chest 84:714-718, 1983.
74. Bouros D, Panagou P, Papandreou L, et al: Massive bilateral pleural effusion as the only first presentation of systemic lupus erythematosus. Respiration 59:173-175, 1992.
75. Orens JB, Martinez FJ, Lynch JP 3rd: Pleuropulmonary manifestations of systemic lupus erythematosus. Rheum Dis Clin North Am 20:159-193, 1994.
76. Wang DY: Diagnosis and management of lupus pleuritis. Curr Opin Pulm Med 8:312-316, 2002.
77. Wiedemann HP, Matthay RA: Pulmonary manifestations of the collagen vascular diseases. Clin Chest Med 10:677-722, 1989.
78. Campbell GD, Ferrington E: Rheumatoid pleuritis with effusion. Dis Chest 53:521-527, 1968.
79. Naylor B: The pathognomonic cytologic picture of rheumatoid pleuritis. The 1989 Maurice Goldblatt Cytology award lecture. Acta Cytol 34:465-473, 1990.
80. Lillington GA, Carr DT, Mayne JG: Rheumatoid pleurisy with effusion. Arch Intern Med 128:764-768, 1971.
81. Levine H, Szanto M, Grieble HG, et al: Rheumatoid factor in nonrheumatoid pleural effusions. Ann Intern Med 69:487-492, 1968.
82. Salomaa ER, Viander M, Saaresranta T, Terho EO: Complement components and their activation products in pleural fluid. Chest 114:723-730, 1998.
83. Antony VB: Drug-induced pleural disease. Clin Chest Med 19:331-340, 1998.
84. Morelock SY, Sahn SA: Drugs and the pleura. Chest 116:212-221, 1999.
85. Jurivich DA: Iatrogenic pleural effusions. South Med J 81:1417-1420, 1988.
86. Sahn SA: Malignancy metastatic to the pleura. Clin Chest Med 19:351-361, 1998.
87. Vargas FS, Teixeira LR: Pleural malignancies. Curr Opin Pulm Med 2:335-340, 1996.
88. Meyer PC: Metastatic carcinoma of the pleura. Thorax 21:437-443, 1966.
89. Andrews BS, Arora NS, Shadforth MF, et al: The role of immune complexes in the pathogenesis of pleural effusions. Am Rev Respir Dis 124:115-120, 1981.
90. Poe RH, Levy PC, Israel RH, et al: Use of fiberoptic bronchoscopy in the diagnosis of bronchogenic carcinoma. A study in patients with idiopathic pleural effusions. Chest 105:1663-1667, 1994.
91. Assi Z, Caruso JL, Herndon J, Patz EF Jr: Cytologically proved malignant pleural effusions: Distribution of transudates and exudates. Chest 113:1302-1304, 1998.
92. Ashchi M, Golish J, Eng P, O'Donovan P: Transudative malignant pleural effusions: Prevalence and mechanisms. South Med J 91:23-26, 1998.
93. Kuhn M, Fitting JW, Leuenberger P: Probability of malignancy in pleural fluid eosinophilia. Chest 96:992-994, 1989.
94. Chernow B, Sahn SA: Carcinomatous involvement of the pleura: An analysis of 96 patients. Am J Med 63:695-702, 1977.
95. Burrows CM, Mathews WC, Colt HG: Predicting survival in patients with recurrent symptomatic malignant pleural effusions: An assessment of the prognostic values of physiologic, morphologic, and quality of life measures of extent of disease. Chest 117:73-78, 2000.
96. Sallach SM, Sallach JA, Vasquez E, et al: Volume of pleural fluid required for diagnosis of pleural malignancy. Chest 122:1913-1917, 2002.
97. Hsu C: Cytologic detection of malignancy in pleural effusion: A review of 5,255 samples from 3,811 patients. Diagn Cytopathol 3:8-12, 1987.
98. Kendall SW, Bryan AJ, Large SR, Wells FC: Pleural effusions: Is thoracoscopy a reliable investigation? A retrospective review. Respir Med 86:437-440, 1992.
99. Sawabata N, Matsumura A, Motohiro A, et al: Malignant minor pleural effusion detected on thoracotomy for patients with non–small cell lung cancer: Is tumor resection beneficial for prognosis? Ann Thorac Surg 73:412-415, 2002.
100. Banerjee AK, Willetts I, Robertson JF, Blamey RW: Pleural effusion in breast cancer: A review of the Nottingham experience. Eur J Surg Oncol 20:33-36, 1994.
101. Thomas JM, Redding WH, Sloane JP: The spread of breast cancer: Importance of the intrathoracic lymphatic route and its relevance to treatment. Br J Cancer 40:540-547, 1979.
102. Blackman NS, Rabin CB: Bilateral pleural effusion; its significance in association with a heart of normal size. J Mt Sinai Hosp N Y 24:45-53, 1957.
103. Dieterich M, Goodman SN, Rojas-Corona RR, et al: Multivariate analysis of prognostic features in malignant pleural effusions from breast cancer patients. Acta Cytol 38:945-952, 1994.
104. Sahn SA: State of the art. The pleura. Am Rev Respir Dis 138:184-234, 1988.
105. Ibuka T, Fukayama M, Hayashi Y, et al: Pyothorax-associated pleural lymphoma. A case evolving from T-cell–rich lymphoid infiltration to overt B-cell lymphoma in association with Epstein-Barr virus. Cancer 73:738-744, 1994.
106. Gaidano G, Pastore C, Gloghini A, et al: Human herpesvirus type-8 (HHV-8) in haematopoietic neoplasia. Leuk Lymphoma 24:257-266, 1997.
107. Rodriguez-Garcia JL, Fraile G, Moreno MA, et al: Recurrent massive pleural effusion as a late complication of radiotherapy in Hodgkin's disease. Chest 100:1165-1166, 1991.
108. Kapadia SB: Cytological diagnosis of malignant pleural effusion in myeloma. Arch Pathol Lab Med 101:534-535, 1977.
109. Shoenfeld Y, Pick AI, Weinberger A, et al: Pleural effusion—presenting sign in multiple myeloma. Respiration 36:160-164, 1978.
110. Teo SK, Lee SK: Recurrent pleural effusion in Waldenström's macroglobulinaemia. BMJ 2:607-608, 1978.
111. Celikoglu F, Teirstein AS, Krellenstein DJ, Strauchen JA: Pleural effusion in non-Hodgkin's lymphoma. Chest 101:1357-1360, 1992.
112. Spieler P: The cytologic diagnosis of tuberculosis in pleural effusions. Acta Cytol 23:374-379, 1979.
113. Janckila AJ, Yam LT, Li CY: Immunocytochemical diagnosis of acute leukemia with pleural involvement. Acta Cytol 29:67-72, 1985.
114. Jung JI, Choi JE, Hahn ST, et al: Radiologic features of all-*trans*-retinoic acid syndrome. AJR Am J Roentgenol 178:475-480, 2002.
115. Worsley DF, Alavi A, Aronchick JM, et al: Chest radiographic findings in patients with acute pulmonary embolism: Observations from the PIOPED Study. Radiology 189:133-136, 1993.
116. Bynum LJ, Wilson JE 3rd: Radiographic features of pleural effusions in pulmonary embolism. Am Rev Respir Dis 117:829-834, 1978.
117. Figley M, Gerdes A, Ricketts H: Radiographic aspects of pulmonary embolism. Semin Roentgenol 2:389, 1967.
118. Romero Candeira S, Hernandez Blasco L, Soler MJ, et al: Biochemical and cytologic characteristics of pleural effusions secondary to pulmonary embolism. Chest 121:465-469, 2002.

119. Shah AA, Davis SD, Gamsu G, Intriere L: Parenchymal and pleural findings in patients with and patients without acute pulmonary embolism detected at spiral CT. Radiology 211:147-153, 1999.

120. Eid AA, Keddissi JI, Samaha M, et al: Exudative effusions in congestive heart failure. Chest 122:1518-1523, 2002.

121. Gotsman I, Fridlender Z, Meirovitz A, et al: The evaluation of pleural effusions in patients with heart failure. Am J Med 111:375-378, 2001.

122. Wiener-Kronish JP, Matthay MA: Pleural effusions associated with hydrostatic and increased permeability pulmonary edema. Chest 93:852-858, 1988.

123. Logue R, Rogers JJ, Gay BJ, et al: Subtle roentgenographic signs of left heart failure. Am Heart J 65:464, 1963.

124. Traumatic perforation of oesophagus. BMJ 1:524, 1972.

125. Abbott OA, Mansour KA, Logan WD Jr, et al: Atraumatic so-called "spontaneous" rupture of the esophagus. A review of 47 personal cases with comments on a new method of surgical therapy. J Thorac Cardiovasc Surg 59:67-83, 1970.

126. Edling JE, Bacon BR: Pleuropulmonary complications of endoscopic variceal sclerotherapy. Chest 99:1252-1257, 1991.

127. Peng MJ, Vargas FS, Cukier A, et al: Postoperative pleural changes after coronary revascularization. Comparison between saphenous vein and internal mammary artery grafting. Chest 101:327-330, 1992.

128. Light RW, Rogers JT, Cheng D, Rodriguez RM: Large pleural effusions occurring after coronary artery bypass grafting. Cardiovascular Surgery Associates, PC. Ann Intern Med 130:891-896, 1999.

129. Light RW, Rogers JT, Moyers JP, et al: Prevalence and clinical course of pleural effusions at 30 days after coronary artery and cardiac surgery. Am J Respir Crit Care Med 166:1567-1571, 2002.

130. Sadikot RT, Rogers JT, Cheng DS, et al: Pleural fluid characteristics of patients with symptomatic pleural effusion after coronary artery bypass graft surgery. Arch Intern Med 160:2665-2668, 2000.

131. Hart U, Ward DR, Gillilian R, Brawley RK: Fatal pulmonary hemorrhage complicating Swan-Ganz catheterization. Surgery 91:24-27, 1982.

132. Johnston RF, Loo RV: Hepatic hydrothorax studies to determine the source of the fluid and report of thirteen cases. Ann Intern Med 61:385-401, 1964.

133. Alberts WM, Salem AJ, Solomon DA, Boyce G: Hepatic hydrothorax. Cause and management. Arch Intern Med 151:2383-2388, 1991.

134. Rudnick MR, Coyle JF, Beck LH, McCurdy DK: Acute massive hydrothorax complicating peritoneal dialysis, report of 2 cases and a review of the literature. Clin Nephrol 12:38-44, 1979.

135. Galen MA, Steinberg SM, Lowrie EG, et al: Hemorrhagic pleural effusion in patients undergoing chronic hemodialysis. Ann Intern Med 82:359-361, 1975.

136. Jarratt MJ, Sahn SA: Pleural effusions in hospitalized patients receiving long-term hemodialysis. Chest 108:470-474, 1995.

137. Shanes JG, Senior RM, Stark DD, Baron RL: Pleural effusion associated with urinary tract obstruction. Thorax 37:160, 1982.

138. Nusser RA, Culhane RH: Recurrent transudative effusion with an abdominal mass. Urinothorax. Chest 90:263-264, 1986.

139. Miller KS, Wooten S, Sahn SA: Urinothorax: A cause of low pH transudative pleural effusions. Am J Med 85:448-449, 1988.

140. Eid AA, Keddissi JI, Kinasewitz GT: Hypoalbuminemia as a cause of pleural effusions. Chest 115:1066-1069, 1999.

141. Llach F, Arieff AI, Massry SG: Renal vein thrombosis and nephrotic syndrome. A prospective study of 36 adult patients. Ann Intern Med 83:8-14, 1975.

142. Nidus BD, Matalon R, Cantacuzino D, Eisinger RP: Uremic pleuritis—a clinicopathological entity. N Engl J Med 281:255-256, 1969.

143. Yoshii C, Morita S, Tokunaga M, et al: Bilateral massive pleural effusions caused by uremic pleuritis. Intern Med 40:646-649, 2001.

144. Gumaste V, Singh V, Dave P: Significance of pleural effusion in patients with acute pancreatitis. Am J Gastroenterol 87:871-874, 1992.

145. Kaye MD: Pleuropulmonary complications of pancreatitis. Thorax 23:297-306, 1968.

146. Falk A, Gustafsson L, Gamklou R: Silent pancreatitis. Report of 4 cases of acute pancreatitis with atypical symptomatology. Acta Chir Scand 150:341-342, 1984.

147. Uchiyama T, Suzuki T, Adachi A, et al: Pancreatic pleural effusion: Case report and review of 113 cases in Japan. Am J Gastroenterol 87:387-391, 1992.

148. Williams SG, Bhupalan A, Zureikat N, et al: Pleural effusions associated with pancreaticopleural fistula. Thorax 48:867-868, 1993.

149. Gertsch P, Marquis J, Diserens H, Mosimann R: Chronic pancreatic pleural effusions and ascites. Int Surg 69:145-147, 1984.

150. Zeilender S, Turner MA, Glauser FL: Mediastinal pseudocyst associated with chronic pleural effusions. Chest 97:1014-1016, 1990.

151. Cooper CB, Bardsley PA, Rao SS, Collins MC: Pleural effusions and pancreaticopleural fistulae associated with asymptomatic pancreatic disease. Br J Dis Chest 82:315-320, 1988.

152. McCarthy S, Pellegrini CA, Moss AA, Way LW: Pleuropancreatic fistula: Endoscopic retrograde cholangiopancreatography and computed tomography. AJR Am J Roentgenol 142:1151-1154, 1984.

153. Salmon V: Benign pelvic tumors associated with ascites and pleural effusion. J Mt Sinai Hosp 1:169, 1934.

154. Meigs J: Fibroma of the ovary with ascites and hydrothorax. With a report of seven cases. Am J Obstet Gynecol 33:249, 1937.

155. Pride S, James C, Yuen B: The ovarian hyperstimulation syndrome. Semin Reprod Endocrinol 8:247, 1990.

156. Abramov Y, Elchalal U, Schenker JG: Pulmonary manifestations of severe ovarian hyperstimulation syndrome: A multicenter study. Fertil Steril 71:645-651, 1999.

157. Lazaridis KN, Frank JW, Krowka MJ, Kamath PS: Hepatic hydrothorax: Pathogenesis, diagnosis, and management. Am J Med 107:262-267, 1999.

158. Assouad J, Barthes Fle P, Shaker W, et al: Recurrent pleural effusion complicating liver cirrhosis. Ann Thorac Surg 75:986-989, 2003.

159. Miller WT, Talman EA: Subphrenic abscess. Am J Roentgenol Radium Ther Nucl Med 101:961-969, 1967.

160. Epler GR, McLoud TC, Gaensler EA: Prevalence and incidence of benign asbestos pleural effusion in a working population. JAMA 247:617-622, 1982.

161. Light RW, George RB: Incidence and significance of pleural effusion after abdominal surgery. Chest 69:621-625, 1976.

162. Nielsen PH, Jepsen SB, Olsen AD: Postoperative pleural effusion following upper abdominal surgery. Chest 96:1133-1135, 1989.

163. Gottehrer A, Roa J, Stanford GG, et al: Hypothyroidism and pleural effusions. Chest 98:1130-1132, 1990.

164. Hurwitz PA, Pinals DJ: Pleural effusion in chronic hereditary lymphedema (Nonne, Milroy, Meige's disease). Report of two cases. Radiology 82:246-248, 1964.

165. Morandi U, Golinelli M, Brandi L, et al: "Yellow nail syndrome" associated with chronic recurrent pericardial and pleural effusions. Eur J Cardiothorac Surg 9:42-44, 1995.

166. Wen J, Baughman K: The Dressler syndrome. Johns Hopkins Med J 148:179, 1981.

167. Kim S, Sahn SA: Postcardiac injury syndrome. An immunologic pleural fluid analysis. Chest 109:570-572, 1996.

168. Stelzner TJ, King TE Jr, Antony VB, Sahn SA: The pleuropulmonary manifestations of the postcardiac injury syndrome. Chest 84:383-387, 1983.

169. Domby WR, Whitcomb ME: Pleural effusion as a manifestation of Dressler's syndrome in the distant post-infarction period. Am Heart J 96:243-245, 1978.

170. Lidar M, Pras M, Langevitz P, Livneh A: Thoracic and lung involvement in familial Mediterranean fever (FMF). Clin Chest Med 23:505-511, 2002.

171. Yuval Y, Hemo-Zisser M, Zemer D, et al: Dominant inheritance in two families with familial Mediterranean fever (FMF). Am J Med Genet 57:455-457, 1995.

172. Babior BM, Matzner Y: The familial Mediterranean fever gene—cloned at last. N Engl J Med 337:1548-1549, 1997.

173. Barakat MH, Karnik AM, Majeed HW, et al: Familial Mediterranean fever (recurrent hereditary polyserositis) in Arabs—a study of 175 patients and review of the literature. Q J Med 60:837-847, 1986.

174. Drenth JP, van der Meer JW: Hereditary periodic fever. N Engl J Med 345:1748-1757, 2001.

175. Miller JI Jr: Diagnosis and management of chylothorax. Chest Surg Clin N Am 6:139-148, 1996.

176. Latner A: Cantarow and Trumper Clinical Biochemistry. Philadelphia, WB Saunders, 1975.

177. Staats BA, Ellefson RD, Budahn LL, et al: The lipoprotein profile of chylous and nonchylous pleural effusions. Mayo Clin Proc 55:700-704, 1980.

178. Chinnock B: Chylothorax: Case report and review of the literature. J Emerg Med 24:259, 2002.

179. Schulman A, Fataar S, Dalrymple R, Tidbury I: The lymphographic anatomy of chylothorax. Br J Radiol 51:420-427, 1978.

180. Ampil FL, Burton GV, Hardjasudarma M, Stogner SW: Chylous effusion complicating chronic lymphocytic leukemia. Leuk Lymphoma 10:507-510, 1993.

181. Quinonez A, Halabe J, Avelar F, et al: Chylothorax due to metastatic prostatic carcinoma. Br J Urol 63:325-327, 1989.

182. Haniuda M, Nishimura H, Kobayashi O, et al: Management of chylothorax after pulmonary resection. J Am Coll Surg 180:537-540, 1995.

183. Fine PG, Bubela C: Chylothorax following celiac plexus block. Anesthesiology 63:454-456, 1985.

184. Mares DC, Mathur PN: Medical thoracoscopic talc pleurodesis for chylothorax due to lymphoma: A case series. Chest 114:731-735, 1998.

185. Melton LJ 3rd, Hepper NG, Offord KP: Influence of height on the risk of spontaneous pneumothorax. Mayo Clin Proc 56:678-682, 1981.

186. Despars JA, Sassoon CS, Light RW: Significance of iatrogenic pneumothoraces. Chest 105:1147-1150, 1994.

187. Lesur O, Delorme N, Fromaget JM, et al: Computed tomography in the etiologic assessment of idiopathic spontaneous pneumothorax. Chest 98:341-347, 1990.

188. Bense L, Lewander R, Eklund G, et al: Nonsmoking, non–alpha 1-antitrypsin deficiency–induced emphysema in nonsmokers with healed spontaneous pneumothorax, identified by computed tomography of the lungs. Chest 103:433-438, 1993.

189. Andrivet P, Djedaini K, Teboul JL, et al: Spontaneous pneumothorax. Comparison of thoracic drainage vs immediate or delayed needle aspiration. Chest 108:335-339, 1995.

190. Jordan KG, Kwong JS, Flint J, Müller NL: Surgically treated pneumothorax. Radiologic and pathologic findings. Chest 111:280-285, 1997.

191. Mitlehner W, Friedrich M, Dissmann W: Value of computer tomography in the detection of bullae and blebs in patients with primary spontaneous pneumothorax. Respiration 59:221-227, 1992.

192. Inouye WY, Berggren RB, Johnson J: Spontaneous pneumothorax: Treatment and mortality. Dis Chest 51:67-73, 1967.

193. Ruckley CV, McCormack RJ: The management of spontaneous pneumothorax. Thorax 21:139-144, 1966.

194. Bense L, Eklund G, Wiman LG: Smoking and the increased risk of contracting spontaneous pneumothorax. Chest 92:1009-1012, 1987.

195. Jansveld CA, Dijkman JH: Primary spontaneous pneumothorax and smoking. BMJ 4:559-560, 1975.

196. Spontaneous pneumothorax and apical lung disease. BMJ 4:573, 1971.

197. Peters RM, Peters BA, Benirschke SK, Friedman PJ: Chest dimensions in young adults with spontaneous pneumothorax. Ann Thorac Surg 25:193-196, 1978.
198. Hall JR, Pyeritz RE, Dudgeon DL, Haller JA Jr: Pneumothorax in the Marfan syndrome: Prevalence and therapy. Ann Thorac Surg 37:500-504, 1984.
199. Smit J, Alberts C, Balk AG: Pneumothorax in the Ehlers-Danlos syndrome: Consequence or coincidence? Scand J Respir Dis 59:239-242, 1978.
200. Bense L, Wiman LG, Hedenstierna G: Onset of symptoms in spontaneous pneumothorax: Correlations to physical activity. Eur J Respir Dis 71:181-186, 1987.
201. Dermksian G, Lamb LE: Spontaneous pneumothorax in apparently healthy flying personnel. Ann Intern Med 51:39-51, 1959.
202. Rose DM, Jarczyk PA: Spontaneous pneumoperitoneum after scuba diving. JAMA 239:223, 1978.
203. Schoenfeld A, Ziv E, Zeelel Y, Ovadia J: Catamenial pneumothorax—a literature review and report of an unusual case. Obstet Gynecol Surv 41:20-24, 1986.
204. Carter EJ, Ettensohn DB: Catamenial pneumothorax. Chest 98:713-716, 1990.
205. Karpel JP, Appel D, Merav A: Pulmonary endometriosis. Lung 163:151-159, 1985.
206. Shiraishi T: Catamenial pneumothorax: Report of a case and review of the Japanese and non-Japanese literature. Thorac Cardiovasc Surg 39:304-307, 1991.
207. Van Schil PE, Vercauteren SR, Vermeire PA, et al: Catamenial pneumothorax caused by thoracic endometriosis. Ann Thorac Surg 62:585-586, 1996.
208. McLoud TC, Isler RJ, Novelline RA, et al: The apical cap. AJR Am J Roentgenol 137:299-306, 1981.
209. Renner RR, Markarian B, Pernice NJ, Heitzman ER: The apical cap. Radiology 110:569-573, 1974.
210. Im JG, Webb WR, Han MC, Park JH: Apical opacity associated with pulmonary tuberculosis: High-resolution CT findings. Radiology 178:727-731, 1991.
211. Fennessy JJ: Irradiation damage to the lung. J Thorac Imaging 2:68-79, 1987.
212. Hourihane D, Lessof L, Richardson P: Hyaline and calcified pleural plaques as an index of exposure to asbestos: A study of radiological and pathological features of 100 cases with a consideration of epidemiology. BMJ 1:1069, 1966.
213. Meurman L: Asbestos bodies and pleural plaques in a Finnish series of autopsy cases. Acta Pathol Microbiol Scand Suppl 181:1, 1966.
214. Schwartz DA: New developments in asbestos-induced pleural disease. Chest 99:191-198, 1991.
215. Fletcher DE, Edge JR: The early radiological changes in pulmonary and pleural asbestosis. Clin Radiol 21:355-365, 1970.
216. Svenes KB, Borgersen A, Haaversen O, Holten K: Parietal pleural plaques: A comparison between autopsy and x-ray findings. Eur J Respir Dis 69:10-15, 1986.
217. Withers BF, Ducatman AM, Yang WN: Roentgenographic evidence for predominant left-sided location of unilateral pleural plaques. Chest 95:1262-1264, 1989.
218. Hu H, Beckett L, Kelsey K, Christiani D: The left-sided predominance of asbestos-related pleural disease. Am Rev Respir Dis 148:981-984, 1993.
219. Hillerdal G, Lindgren A: Pleural plaques: Correlation of autopsy findings to radiographic findings and occupational history. Eur J Respir Dis 61:315-319, 1980.
220. Wain SL, Roggli VL, Foster WL Jr: Parietal pleural plaques, asbestos bodies, and neoplasia. A clinical, pathologic, and roentgenographic correlation of 25 consecutive cases. Chest 86:707-713, 1984.
221. Friedman AC, Fiel SB, Fisher MS, et al: Asbestos-related pleural disease and asbestosis: A comparison of CT and chest radiography. AJR Am J Roentgenol 150:269-275, 1988.
222. Staples CA, Gamsu G, Ray CS, Webb WR: High resolution computed tomography and lung function in asbestos-exposed workers with normal chest radiographs. Am Rev Respir Dis 139:1502-1508, 1989.
223. Anton HC: Multiple pleural plaques. II. Br J Radiol 41:341-348, 1968.
224. Freundlich I, Greening R: Asbestosis and associated medical problems. Radiology 89:224, 1967.
225. McLoud TC, Woods BO, Carrington CB, et al: Diffuse pleural thickening in an asbestos-exposed population: Prevalence and causes. AJR Am J Roentgenol 144:9-18, 1985.
226. Müller NL: Imaging of the pleura. Radiology 186:297-309, 1993.
227. Leung AN, Müller NL, Miller RR: CT in differential diagnosis of diffuse pleural disease. AJR Am J Roentgenol 154:487-492, 1990.
228. Lynch DA, Gamsu G, Aberle DR: Conventional and high resolution computed tomography in the diagnosis of asbestos-related diseases. Radiographics 9:523-551, 1989.
229. Friedman AC, Fiel SB, Radecki PD, Lev-Toaff AS: Computed tomography of benign pleural and pulmonary parenchymal abnormalities related to asbestos exposure. Semin Ultrasound CT MR 11:393-408, 1990.
230. Schwartz DA, Fuortes LJ, Galvin JR, et al: Asbestos-induced pleural fibrosis and impaired lung function. Am Rev Respir Dis 141:321-326, 1990.
231. Yates DH, Browne K, Stidolph PN, Neville E: Asbestos-related bilateral diffuse pleural thickening: Natural history of radiographic and lung function abnormalities. Am J Respir Crit Care Med 153:301-306, 1996.
232. Parker C, Neville E: Lung cancer: Management of malignant mesothelioma. Thorax 58:809-813, 2003.
233. Hoogsteden HC, Langerak AW, van der Kwast TH, et al: Malignant pleural mesothelioma. Crit Rev Oncol Hematol 25:97-126, 1997.
234. McDonald JC, McDonald AD: The epidemiology of mesothelioma in historical context. Eur Respir J 9:1932-1942, 1996.
235. Spirtas R, Beebe GW, Connelly RR, et al: Recent trends in mesothelioma incidence in the United States. Am J Ind Med 9:397-407, 1986.
236. Karjalainen A, Pukkala E, Mattson K, et al: Trends in mesothelioma incidence and occupational mesotheliomas in Finland in 1960-1995. Scand J Work Environ Health 23:266-270, 1997.

237. Driscoll TR, Baker GJ, Daniels S, et al: Clinical aspects of malignant mesothelioma in Australia. Aust N Z J Med 23:19-25, 1993.
238. Rosler JA, Woitowitz HJ, Lange HJ, et al: Mortality rates in a female cohort following asbestos exposure in Germany. J Occup Med 36:889-893, 1994.
239. Edge JR, Choudhury SL: Malignant mesothelioma of the pleura in Barrow-in-Furness. Thorax 33:26-30, 1978.
240. Hasan FM, Nash G, Kazemi H: The significance of asbestos exposure in the diagnosis of mesothelioma: A 28-year experience from a major urban hospital. Am Rev Respir Dis 115:761-768, 1977.
241. Spirtas R, Heineman EF, Bernstein L, et al: Malignant mesothelioma: Attributable risk of asbestos exposure. Occup Environ Med 51:804-811, 1994.
242. Yates DH, Corrin B, Stidolph PN, Browne K: Malignant mesothelioma in south east England: Clinicopathological experience of 272 cases. Thorax 52:507-512, 1997.
243. Huncharek M: Changing risk groups for malignant mesothelioma. Cancer 69:2704-2711, 1992.
244. Teschke K, Morgan MS, Checkoway H, et al: Mesothelioma surveillance to locate sources of exposure to asbestos. Can J Public Health 88:163-168, 1997.
245. Dorward AJ, Stack BH: Diffuse malignant pleural mesothelioma in Glasgow. Br J Dis Chest 75:397-402, 1981.
246. Sheers G, Coles RM: Mesothelioma risks in a naval dockyard. Arch Environ Health 35:276-282, 1980.
247. Oksa P, Pukkala E, Karjalainen A, et al: Cancer incidence and mortality among Finnish asbestos sprayers and in asbestosis and silicosis patients. Am J Ind Med 31:693-698, 1997.
248. Talcott JA, Thurber WA, Kantor AF, et al: Asbestos-associated diseases in a cohort of cigarette-filter workers. N Engl J Med 321:1220-1223, 1989.
249. Driscoll RJ, Mulligan WJ, Schultz D, Candelaria A: Malignant mesothelioma. A cluster in a native American pueblo. N Engl J Med 318:1437-1438, 1988.
250. Otte KE, Sigsgaard TI, Kjaerulff J: Malignant mesothelioma: Clustering in a family producing asbestos cement in their home. Br J Ind Med 47:10-13, 1990.
251. Howel D, Arblaster L, Swinburne L, et al: Routes of asbestos exposure and the development of mesothelioma in an English region. Occup Environ Med 54:403-409, 1997.
252. Magnani C, Terracini B, Ivaldi C, et al: A cohort study on mortality among wives of workers in the asbestos cement industry in Casale Monferrato, Italy. Br J Ind Med 50:779-784, 1993.
253. Dodson RF, O'Sullivan M, Brooks DR, Hammar SP: Quantitative analysis of asbestos burden in women with mesothelioma. Am J Ind Med 43:188-195, 2003.
254. Begin R, Gauthier JJ, Desmeules M, Ostiguy G: Work-related mesothelioma in Quebec, 1967-1990. Am J Ind Med 22:531-542, 1992.
255. Ascoli V, Carnovale-Scalzo C, Nardi F, et al: A one-generation cluster of malignant mesothelioma within a family reveals exposure to asbestos-contaminated jute bags in Naples, Italy. Eur J Epidemiol 18:171-174, 2003.
256. Constantopoulos SH, Malamou-Mitsi VD, Goudevenos JA, et al: High incidence of malignant pleural mesothelioma in neighbouring villages of Northwestern Greece. Respiration 51:266-271, 1987.
257. Metintas S, Metintas M, Ucgun I, Oner U: Malignant mesothelioma due to environmental exposure to asbestos: Follow-up of a Turkish cohort living in a rural area. Chest 122:2224-2229, 2002.
258. Sluis-Cremer GK, Liddell FD, Logan WP, Bezuidenhout BN: The mortality of amphibole miners in South Africa, 1946-80. Br J Ind Med 49:566-575, 1992.
259. Nicholson WJ, Raffn E: Recent data on cancer due to asbestos in the U.S.A. and Denmark. Med Lav 86:393-410, 1995.
260. Karjalainen A, Meurman LO, Pukkala E: Four cases of mesothelioma among Finnish anthophyllite miners. Occup Environ Med 51:212-215, 1994.
261. Stayner LT, Dankovic DA, Lemen RA: Occupational exposure to chrysotile asbestos and cancer risk: A review of the amphibole hypothesis. Am J Public Health 86:179-186, 1996.
262. Smith AH, Wright CC: Chrysotile asbestos is the main cause of pleural mesothelioma. Am J Ind Med 30:252-266, 1996.
263. Dufresne A, Harrigan M, Masse S, Begin R: Fibers in lung tissues of mesothelioma cases among miners and millers of the township of Asbestos, Quebec. Am J Ind Med 27:581-592, 1995.
264. Elmes P: Mesotheliomas and chrysotile. Ann Occup Hyg 38:547-553, 415, 1994.
265. Craighead JE: Current pathogenetic concepts of diffuse malignant mesothelioma. Hum Pathol 18:544-557, 1987.
266. Selcuk ZT, Coplu L, Emri S, et al: Malignant pleural mesothelioma due to environmental mineral fiber exposure in Turkey. Analysis of 135 cases. Chest 102:790-796, 1992.
267. Infante PF, Schuman LD, Dement J, Huff J: Fibrous glass and cancer. Am J Ind Med 26:559-584, 1994.
268. De Vuyst P, Dumortier P, Swaen GM, et al: Respiratory health effects of man-made vitreous (mineral) fibres. Eur Respir J 8:2149-2173, 1995.
269. Stenton SC: Asbestos, simian virus 40 and malignant mesothelioma. Thorax 52(Suppl 3):S52-S57, 1997.
270. Cicala C, Pompetti F, Carbone M: SV40 induces mesotheliomas in hamsters. Am J Pathol 142:1524-1533, 1993.
271. Vilchez RA, Kozinetz CA, Arrington AS, et al: Simian virus 40 in human cancers. Am J Med 114:675-684, 2003.
272. De Luca A, Baldi A, Esposito V, et al: The retinoblastoma gene family pRb/p105, p107, pRb2/p130 and simian virus-40 large T-antigen in human mesotheliomas. Nat Med 3:913-916, 1997.
273. Carbone M, Rizzo P, Grimley PM, et al: Simian virus-40 large-T antigen binds p53 in human mesotheliomas. Nat Med 3:908-912, 1997.

274. Mor O, Yaron P, Huszar M, et al: Absence of p53 mutations in malignant mesotheliomas. Am J Respir Cell Mol Biol 16:9-13, 1997.

275. Mayall F, Barratt K, Shanks J: The detection of simian virus 40 in mesotheliomas from New Zealand and England using real time FRET probe PCR protocols. J Clin Pathol 56:728-730, 2003.

276. Dawson A, Gibbs A, Browne K, et al: Familial mesothelioma. Details of 17 cases with histopathologic findings and mineral analysis. Cancer 70:1183-1187, 1992.

277. Heineman EF, Bernstein L, Stark AD, Spirtas R: Mesothelioma, asbestos, and reported history of cancer in first-degree relatives. Cancer 77:549-554, 1996.

278. Sekido Y, Pass HI, Bader S, et al: Neurofibromatosis type 2 (NF2) gene is somatically mutated in mesothelioma but not in lung cancer. Cancer Res 55:1227-1231, 1995.

279. Upham JW, Garlepp MJ, Musk AW, Robinson BW: Malignant mesothelioma: New insights into tumour biology and immunology as a basis for new treatment approaches. Thorax 50:887-893, 1995.

280. Cavazza A, Travis LB, Travis WD, et al: Post-irradiation malignant mesothelioma. Cancer 77:1379-1385, 1996.

281. Shannon VR, Nesbitt JC, Libshitz HI: Malignant pleural mesothelioma after radiation therapy for breast cancer. A report of two additional patients. Cancer 76:437-441, 1995.

282. Warren S, Brown CE, Chute RN, Federman M: Mesothelioma relative to asbestos, radiation, and methylcholanthrene. Arch Pathol Lab Med 105:305-312, 1981.

283. Whitaker D, Shilkin KB: Diagnosis of pleural malignant mesothelioma in life—a practical approach. J Pathol 143:147-175, 1984.

284. Attanoos RL, Gibbs AR: Pathology of malignant mesothelioma. Histopathology 30:403-418, 1997.

285. Johansson L, Linden CJ: Aspects of histopathologic subtype as a prognostic factor in 85 pleural mesotheliomas. Chest 109:109-114, 1996.

286. Wilson GE, Hasleton PS, Chatterjee AK: Desmoplastic malignant mesothelioma: A review of 17 cases. J Clin Pathol 45:295-298, 1992.

287. Yousem SA, Hochholzer L: Malignant mesotheliomas with osseous and cartilaginous differentiation. Arch Pathol Lab Med 111:62-66, 1987.

288. McCaughey WT, Al-Jabi M: Differentiation of serosal hyperplasia and neoplasia in biopsies. Pathol Annu 21(Pt 1):271-293, 1986.

289. Andrion A, Magnani C, Betta PG, et al: Malignant mesothelioma of the pleura: Interobserver variability. J Clin Pathol 48:856-860, 1995.

290. Skov BG, Lauritzen AF, Hirsch F, Nielsen HW: The histopathological diagnosis of malignant mesothelioma v. pulmonary adenocarcinoma: Reproducibility of the histopathological diagnosis. Histopathology 24:553-557, 1994.

291. Tuder RM: Malignant disease of the pleura: A histopathological study with special emphasis on diagnostic criteria and differentiation from reactive mesothelium. Histopathology 10:851-865, 1986.

292. Whitaker D, Henderson DW, Shilkin KB: The concept of mesothelioma in situ: Implications for diagnosis and histogenesis. Semin Diagn Pathol 9:151-161, 1992.

293. Cagle PT, Brown RW, Lebovitz RM: P53 immunostaining in the differentiation of reactive processes from malignancy in pleural biopsy specimens. Hum Pathol 25:443-448, 1994.

294. Frierson HF Jr, Mills SE, Legier JF: Flow cytometric analysis of ploidy in immunohistochemically confirmed examples of malignant epithelial mesothelioma. Am J Clin Pathol 90:240-243, 1988.

295. Bogers J, Jacobs W, Segers K, et al: Stereological evaluation of malignant mesothelioma versus benign pleural hyperplasia. Pathol Res Pract 192:10-14, 1996.

296. Koss M, Travis W, Moran C, Hochholzer L: Pseudomesotheliomatous adenocarcinoma: A reappraisal. Semin Diagn Pathol 9:117-123, 1992.

297. Citas ES, Corson JM, Pinkus GS: The distinction of adenocarcinoma from malignant mesothelioma in cell blocks of effusions: The role of routine mucin histochemistry and immunohistochemical assessment of carcinoembryonic antigen, keratin proteins, epithelial membrane antigen, and milk fat globule–derived antigen. Hum Pathol 18:67-74, 1987.

298. Ordonez NG: The immunohistochemical diagnosis of mesothelioma: A comparative study of epithelioid mesothelioma and lung adenocarcinoma. Am J Surg Pathol 27:1031-1051, 2003.

299. Coleman M, Henderson DW, Mukherjee TM: The ultrastructural pathology of malignant pleural mesothelioma. Pathol Annu 24(Pt 1):303-353, 1989.

300. Alexander E, Clark RA, Colley DP, Mitchell SE: CT of malignant pleural mesothelioma. AJR Am J Roentgenol 137:287-291, 1981.

301. Miller BH, Rosado-de-Christenson ML, Mason AC, et al: From the archives of the AFIP: Malignant pleural mesothelioma: Radiologic-pathologic correlation. Radiographics 16:613-644, 1996.

302. Krumhaar D, Lange S, Hartmann C, Anhuth D: Follow-up study of 100 malignant pleural mesotheliomas. Thorac Cardiovasc Surg 33:272-275, 1985.

303. Rabinowitz JG, Efremidis SC, Cohen B, et al: A comparative study of mesothelioma and asbestosis using computed tomography and conventional chest radiography. Radiology 144:453-460, 1982.

304. Rusch VW, Godwin JD, Shuman WP: The role of computed tomography scanning in the initial assessment and the follow-up of malignant pleural mesothelioma. J Thorac Cardiovasc Surg 96:171-177, 1988.

305. Ng CS, Munden RF, Libshitz HI: Malignant pleural mesothelioma: The spectrum of manifestations on CT in 70 cases. Clin Radiol 54:415-421, 1999.

306. Kawashima A, Libshitz HI: Malignant pleural mesothelioma: CT manifestations in 50 cases. AJR Am J Roentgenol 155:965-969, 1990.

307. Patz EF Jr, Shaffer K, Piwnica-Worms DR, et al: Malignant pleural mesothelioma: Value of CT and MR imaging in predicting resectability. AJR Am J Roentgenol 159:961-966, 1992.

308. Falaschi F, Battolla L, Mascalchi M, et al: Usefulness of MR signal intensity in distinguishing benign from malignant pleural disease. AJR Am J Roentgenol 166:963-968, 1996.

309. Benard F, Sterman D, Smith RJ, et al: Metabolic imaging of malignant pleural mesothelioma with fluorodeoxyglucose positron emission tomography. Chest 114:713-722, 1998.

310. Tammilehto L, Maasilta P, Kostiainen S, et al: Diagnosis and prognostic factors in malignant pleural mesothelioma: A retrospective analysis of sixty-five patients. Respiration 59:129-135, 1992.

311. Wadler S, Chahinian P, Slater W, et al: Cardiac abnormalities in patients with diffuse malignant pleural mesothelioma. Cancer 58:2744-2750, 1986.

312. Mowe G, Gylseth B, Hartveit F, Skaug V: Occupational asbestos exposure, lung-fiber concentration and latency time in malignant mesothelioma. Scand J Work Environ Health 10:293-298, 1984.

313. Leong AS, Stevens MW, Mukherjee TM: Malignant mesothelioma: Cytologic diagnosis with histologic, immunohistochemical, and ultrastructural correlation. Semin Diagn Pathol 9:141-150, 1992.

314. DiBonito L, Falconieri G, Colautti I, et al: Cytopathology of malignant mesothelioma: A study of its patterns and histological bases. Diagn Cytopathol 9:25-31, 1993.

315. Stevens MW, Leong AS, Fazzalari NL, et al: Cytopathology of malignant mesothelioma: A stepwise logistic regression analysis. Diagn Cytopathol 8:333-341, 1992.

316. Renshaw AA, Dean BR, Antman KH, et al: The role of cytologic evaluation of pleural fluid in the diagnosis of malignant mesothelioma. Chest 111:106-109, 1997.

317. Boutin C, Rey F: Thoracoscopy in pleural malignant mesothelioma: A prospective study of 188 consecutive patients. Part 1: Diagnosis. Cancer 72:389-393, 1993.

318. Shijubo N, Honda Y, Fujishima T, et al: Lung surfactant protein-A and carcinoembryonic antigen in pleural effusions due to lung adenocarcinoma and malignant mesothelioma. Eur Respir J 8:403-406, 1995.

319. Nurminen M, Dejmek A, Martensson G, et al: Clinical utility of liquid-chromatographic analysis of effusions for hyaluronate content. Clin Chem 40:777-780, 1994.

320. Martinez-Vea A, Gatell JM, Segura F, et al: Diagnostic value of tumoral markers in serous effusions: Carcinoembryonic antigen, alpha1-acidglycoprotein, alpha-fetoprotein, phosphohexose isomerase, and beta 2-microglobulin. Cancer 50:1783-1788, 1982.

321. Ohishi N, Oka T, Fukuhara T, et al: Extensive pulmonary metastases in malignant pleural mesothelioma. A rare clinical and radiographic presentation. Chest 110:296-298, 1996.

322. Law MR, Hodson ME, Heard BE: Malignant mesothelioma of the pleura: Relation between histological type and clinical behaviour. Thorax 37:810-815, 1982.

323. Rusch VW, Venkatraman E: The importance of surgical staging in the treatment of malignant mesothelioma. J Thorac Cardiovasc Surg 111:815-825, discussion 825-826, 1996.

324. De Pangher Manzini V, Brollo A, Franceschi S, et al: Prognostic factors of malignant mesothelioma of the pleura. Cancer 72:410-417, 1993.

325. Marinaccio A, Nesti M: Analysis of survival of mesothelioma cases in the Italian register (ReNaM). Eur J Cancer 39:1290-1295, 2003.

326. Brenner J, Sordillo PP, Magill GB, Golbey RB: Malignant mesothelioma of the pleura: Review of 123 patients. Cancer 49:2431-2435, 1982.

327. Chailleux E, Dabouis G, Pioche D, et al: Prognostic factors in diffuse malignant pleural mesothelioma. A study of 167 patients. Chest 93:159-162, 1988.

328. Tammilehto L, Kivisaari L, Salminen US, et al: Evaluation of the clinical TNM staging system for malignant pleural mesothelioma: An assessment in 88 patients. Lung Cancer 12:25-34, 1995.

329. Baas P: Predictive and prognostic factors in malignant pleural mesothelioma. Curr Opin Oncol 15:127-130, 2003.

330. Van Gelder T, Damhuis RA, Hoogsteden HC: Prognostic factors and survival in malignant pleural mesothelioma. Eur Respir J 7:1035-1038, 1994.

331. Sugarbaker DJ, Mentzer SJ, Strauss G: Extrapleural pneumonectomy in the treatment of malignant pleural mesothelioma. Ann Thorac Surg 54:941-946, 1992.

332. Sugarbaker DJ, Garcia JP, Richards WG, et al: Extrapleural pneumonectomy in the multimodality therapy of malignant pleural mesothelioma. Results in 120 consecutive patients. Ann Surg 224:288-294, discussion 294-296, 1996.

333. Cardillo G, Facciolo F, Cavazzana AO, et al: Localized (solitary) fibrous tumors of the pleura: An analysis of 55 patients. Ann Thorac Surg 70:1808-1812, 2000.

334. Rosado-de-Christenson ML, Abbott GF, McAdams HP, et al: From the archives of the AFIP: Localized fibrous tumor of the pleura. Radiographics 23:759-783, 2003.

335. Coffin CM, Dehner LP: Mesothelial and related neoplasms in children and adolescents: A clinicopathologic and immunohistochemical analysis of eight cases. Pediatr Pathol 12:333-347, 1992.

336. Bilbey JH, Müller NL, Miller RR, Nelems B: Localized fibrous mesothelioma of pleura following external ionizing radiation therapy. Chest 94:1291-1292, 1988.

337. Hill JK, Heitmiller RF 2nd, Askin FB, Kuhlman JE: Localized benign pleural mesothelioma arising in a radiation field. Clin Imaging 21:189-194, 1997.

338. Briselli M, Mark EJ, Dickersin GR: Solitary fibrous tumors of the pleura: Eight new cases and review of 360 cases in the literature. Cancer 47:2678-2689, 1981.

339. England DM, Hochholzer L, McCarthy MJ: Localized benign and malignant fibrous tumors of the pleura. A clinicopathologic review of 223 cases. Am J Surg Pathol 13:640-658, 1989.

340. el-Naggar AK, Ro JY, Ayala AG, et al: Localized fibrous tumor of the serosal cavities. Immunohistochemical, electron-microscopic, and flow-cytometric DNA study. Am J Clin Pathol 92:561-565, 1989.

341. Witkin GB, Rosai J: Solitary fibrous tumor of the mediastinum. A report of 14 cases. Am J Surg Pathol 13:547-557, 1989.
342. Moran CA, Suster S, Koss MN: The spectrum of histologic growth patterns in benign and malignant fibrous tumors of the pleura. Semin Diagn Pathol 9:169-180, 1992.
343. Lee KS, Im JG, Choe KO, et al: CT findings in benign fibrous mesothelioma of the pleura: Pathologic correlation in nine patients. AJR Am J Roentgenol 158:983-986, 1992.
344. Flint A, Weiss SW: CD-34 and keratin expression distinguishes solitary fibrous tumor (fibrous mesothelioma) of pleura from desmoplastic mesothelioma. Hum Pathol 26:428-431, 1995.
345. Ferretti GR, Chiles C, Choplin RH, Coulomb M: Localized benign fibrous tumors of the pleura. AJR Am J Roentgenol 169:683-686, 1997.
346. Desser TS, Stark P: Pictorial essay: Solitary fibrous tumor of the pleura. J Thorac Imaging 13:27-35, 1998.
347. Soulen MC, Greco-Hunt VT, Templeton P: Cases from A3CR2. Migratory chest mass. Invest Radiol 25:209-211, 1990.
348. Mengeot PM, Gailly C: Spontaneous detachment of benign mesothelioma into the pleural space and removal during pleuroscopy. Eur J Respir Dis 68:141-145, 1986.
349. Dedrick CG, McLoud TC, Shepard JA, Shipley RT: Computed tomography of localized pleural mesothelioma. AJR Am J Roentgenol 144:275-280, 1985.
350. Mendelson DS, Meary E, Buy JN, et al: Localized fibrous pleural mesothelioma: CT findings. Clin Imaging 15:105-108, 1991.
351. Saifuddin A, Da Costa P, Chalmers AG, et al: Primary malignant localized fibrous tumours of the pleura: Clinical, radiological and pathological features. Clin Radiol 45:13-17, 1992.
352. Harris GN, Rozenshtein A, Schiff MJ: Benign fibrous mesothelioma of the pleura: MR imaging findings. AJR Am J Roentgenol 165:1143-1144, 1995.
353. Ferretti GR, Chiles C, Cox JE, et al: Localized benign fibrous tumors of the pleura: MR appearance. J Comput Assist Tomogr 21:115-120, 1997.
354. Padovani B, Mouroux J, Raffaelli C, et al: Benign fibrous mesothelioma of the pleura: MR study and pathologic correlation. Eur Radiol 6:425-428, 1996.
355. Kniznik DO, Roncoroni AJ, Rosenberg M, et al: Giant fibrous pleural mesothelioma associated with myocardial restriction and hypoglycemia. Respiration 37:346-351, 1979.
356. Okike N, Bernatz PE, Woolner LB: Localized mesothelioma of the pleura: Benign and malignant variants. J Thorac Cardiovasc Surg 75:363-372, 1978.
357. Mandal AK, Rozer MA, Salem FA, Oparah SS: Localized benign mesothelioma of the pleura associated with a hypoglycemic episode. Arch Intern Med 143:1608-1610, 1983.
358. Hanau CA, Miettinen M: Solitary fibrous tumor: Histological and immunohistochemical spectrum of benign and malignant variants presenting at different sites. Hum Pathol 26:440-449, 1995.
359. Buxton RC, Tan CS, Khine NM, et al: Atypical transmural thoracic lipoma: CT diagnosis. J Comput Assist Tomogr 12:196-198, 1988.

MEDIASTINAL DISEASE

MEDIASTINITIS

Infections of the mediastinum can be acute or chronic. Acute infections are usually caused by bacteria and sometimes progress to abscess formation; they are often associated with signs and symptoms (especially retrosternal pain and fever), and many are fulminating and lethal. By contrast, chronic disease is most often the result of tuberculous or fungal infection; even though such infections are characteristically insidious in onset and unassociated with clinical manifestations, some patients have symptoms or signs related to obstruction or compression of one or more mediastinal structures. Although most cases of chronic mediastinitis are infectious in origin, some are of unknown cause and are characterized by the accumulation of dense fibrous tissue (fibrosing mediastinitis).

Acute Mediastinitis

Acute infection of the mediastinum is uncommon. Most cases are associated with esophageal perforation or with esophageal or cardiac surgery.[1-3] A less common cause is direct extension of infection from adjacent tissues such as the retropharyngeal space, bones and sternoclavicular or costochondral joints, mediastinal lymph nodes, lungs, or pleural space.[1,3,4]

Over 75% of cases of esophageal rupture follow diagnostic and therapeutic endoscopic procedures,[5] most commonly esophagoscopy and balloon dilation.[6] Perforation may also occur in association with necrotic esophageal carcinoma, radiation esophagitis, or penetrating or blunt trauma. Spontaneous perforation following a sudden rise in intra-esophageal pressure (Boerhaave's syndrome) occurs most frequently after an episode of severe vomiting[7] but can also develop during labor, a severe asthmatic attack, or strenuous exercise. The usual site of rupture is the lower 8 cm, often adjacent to the gastroesophageal junction. Although the usual etiology of mediastinitis in all these situations is infection, gastric acid introduced into the mediastinum can also damage the mediastinal soft tissue.[8]

Postoperative mediastinitis occurs in approximately 0.5% to 1% of patients who have undergone median sternotomy for cardiac surgery.[9,10] The risk is increased in patients who are immunocompromised or obese or who have diabetes.

Radiologic Manifestations

The main radiographic manifestation of acute mediastinitis is widening of the mediastinum, usually more evident superiorly; typically, the abnormal region possesses a smooth, sharply defined margin (Fig. 21–1). Air may be visible within the mediastinum, as well as in the soft tissues of the neck.[11] Pneumothorax or hydropneumothorax may also be evident. Distal esophageal perforation usually results in left-sided hydrothorax or hydropneumothorax, whereas midesophageal perforation tends to cause pleural changes on the right.[12] The diagnosis can be readily confirmed by demonstrating extravasation of ingested contrast material into the mediastinum or pleural space under fluoroscopy.[13]

CT can be helpful both in diagnosis and in guiding percutaneous aspiration and drainage of mediastinal abscesses.[3] Manifestations include esophageal thickening, obliteration of the normal fat planes, periesophageal areas of soft tissue or fluid attenuation, single or multiple abscesses, and extraluminal gas and/or contrast material (Fig. 21–2).[14] However, because the first three of these manifestations are often present after surgery, it may be difficult to distinguish normal postoperative findings from those of early mediastinitis.

Clinical Manifestations

The principal symptom is retrosternal pain, often severe and abrupt in onset; radiation to the neck may occur. Chills and high fever are common, and the effects of obstruction of the superior vena cava (SVC) may be seen. Physical examination of a patient who has a perforated esophagus commonly reveals subcutaneous emphysema in the soft tissues of the neck or a loud crunching or clicking sound synchronous with the heartbeat on auscultation over the apex of the heart (Hamman's sign). Though suggestive of pneumomediastinum, the latter

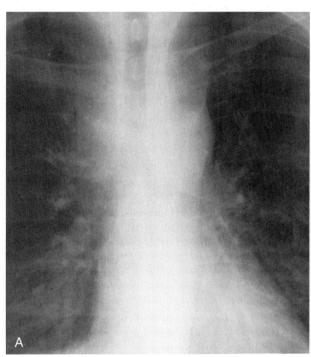

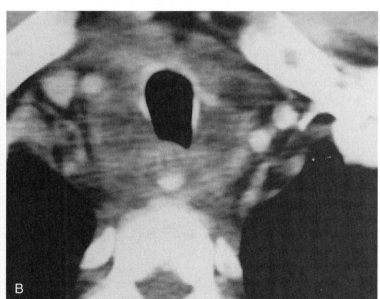

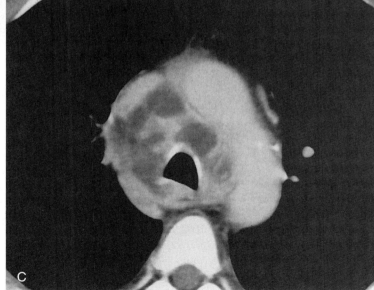

FIGURE 21–1

Acute mediastinitis secondary to retropharyngeal abscess.
A 47-year-old man presented with acute dysphagia and high fever. Clinical examination demonstrated a retropharyngeal abscess. A close-up view from a posteroanterior chest radiograph (**A**) demonstrates smooth widening of the upper mediastinum. An intravenous contrast-enhanced CT scan at the level of the thoracic inlet (**B**) demonstrates inhomogeneous areas of attenuation surrounding the trachea. A scan at the level of the aortic arch (**C**) shows localized areas of low attenuation consistent with abscess formation anterior and lateral to the trachea. *(From Fraser RS, Müller NL, Colman NC, Paré PD: Fraser and Paré's Diagnosis of Diseases of the Chest, 4th ed. Philadelphia, WB Saunders, 1999.)*

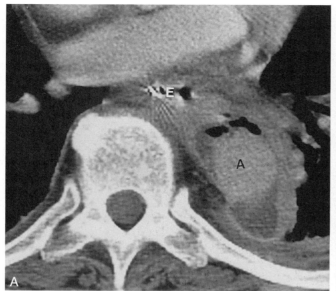
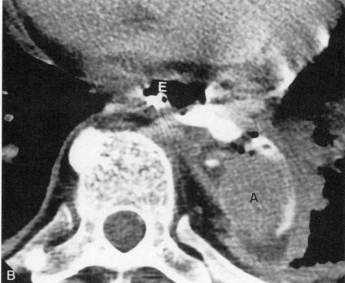

FIGURE 21–2

Carcinoma of the esophagus with perforation. A CT scan obtained after the intravenous administration of contrast (**A**) demonstrates a nasogastric tube within the esophagus (E), increased soft tissue between the esophagus and the aorta (A), and localized collections of gas and fluid consistent with abscess formation. Also noted is a small left pleural effusion. A CT scan obtained after oral administration of contrast (**B**) demonstrates extravasation of contrast, confirming the presence of esophageal perforation and communication with the periaortic fluid and air collections. *(From Fraser RS, Müller NL, Colman NC, Paré PD: Fraser and Paré's Diagnosis of Diseases of the Chest, 4th ed. Philadelphia, WB Saunders, 1999.)*

sign is not pathognomonic since it is heard in some patients who have pneumothorax and occasionally in patients who have moderate elevation of the left hemidiaphragm associated with gaseous distention of the fundus of the stomach or the splenic flexure of the colon.

When treatment is not instituted promptly, acute mediastinitis can progress to abscess formation, which in turn can rupture into the lung, a bronchus, or the pleural cavity. The presence of such fistulas can usually be confirmed by contrast radiographic or CT examination. Acute mediastinitis is a serious disease; for example, in a series of 16 patients who had the complication after esophageal rupture, 6 (38%) died, all of polymicrobial sepsis.[15]

Fibrosing Mediastinitis

Fibrosing mediastinitis is a rare condition characterized by chronic inflammation and fibrosis of mediastinal soft tissues. The process is often progressive and can occur either focally or more or less diffusely throughout the mediastinum. It can cause compression and sometimes obliteration of vessels, airways, and the esophagus and result in a variety of functional and radiologic manifestations and, occasionally, death.

Etiology and Pathogenesis

A consideration of the etiology and pathogenesis of fibrosing mediastinitis is complicated to some extent by the fact that the disease has been reported to have two distinct pathologic manifestations: (1) more or less diffuse involvement of mediastinal tissues by inflammatory cells and fibrous tissue and (2)

a relatively localized granulomatous inflammatory mass ("pseudotumor") centered on one or several lymph nodes. Because it is not always clear in published articles which cases represent the localized form of mediastinal granulomatous inflammation and which the diffuse fibrosing type, statements about the relative importance of specific organisms in the etiology of fibrosing mediastinitis are sometimes difficult to interpret. However, it is clear that infection is an important cause, particularly in relatively localized disease. The most frequently implicated organism is *Histoplasma capsulatum*[16]; in geographic regions in which histoplasmosis is not endemic, *Mycobacterium tuberculosis* is more important.[17] The pathogenesis of progressive mediastinal fibrosis in patients who have infection is not clear. It has been hypothesized that it is related to spillage of necrotic material from affected lymph nodes, followed by either infection of the mediastinum or a hypersensitivity reaction.[18,19]

A second group of cases has no cultural and little or no histologic evidence of an infectious origin.[20] Although some of these cases may represent the end stage of chronic infection in which the organism is not identifiable, in others the etiology and pathogenesis are undoubtedly noninfectious. Evidence for such an origin derives from the occasional patient in whom a similar fibrotic process can be identified elsewhere, including the retroperitoneal space (retroperitoneal fibrosis), the orbit ("pseudotumor of the orbit"), the thyroid ("Riedel's struma"), and the cecum ("ligneous perityphlitis").[21] The etiology and pathogenesis of this abnormality are probably varied, and there is evidence for both genetic and immunologic components.[21,22] Methysergide, a drug used for the alleviation of headache, has also clearly been associated with its development.[23]

Pathologic Characteristics

The fibrosis tends to affect the upper half of the mediastinum, predominantly anterior to the trachea and around the hilum, but it can extend from the brachiocephalic veins to the base of a lung.[20] Compression of vessels (especially the SVC and pulmonary veins), airways, and (occasionally) the esophagus may be apparent (Fig. 21–3). The histologic appearance varies with the underlying cause. In some cases—particularly those in which an infectious organism is identified—there is necrotizing granulomatous inflammation; in others, the granulomatous component is minimal or absent, the abnormal tissue being composed predominantly of mature fibrous tissue containing a mononuclear inflammatory cell infiltrate (see Fig. 21–3).

Secondary effects on the lung are common. Parenchymal interstitial fibrosis and pneumonitis, intra-alveolar aggregates of hemosiderin-laden macrophages, and vascular changes consistent with pulmonary hypertension may be seen in lobes in which the draining veins are affected.[24,25] Venous or arterial thrombi (or both) in various stages of organization, with or without associated parenchymal infarcts, are seen occasionally.

Radiologic Manifestations

As indicated previously, fibrosing mediastinitis can be manifested as a focal mass or as diffuse widening.[26,27] Focal lesions involve the right paratracheal region most commonly (Fig. 21–4); less often, the left paratracheal, subcarinal, or posterior mediastinal regions are affected. Because the majority of the masses are the result of histoplasmosis or tuberculosis, areas of calcification may be evident, particularly on CT scan. In a minority of patients, pulmonary parenchymal disease or bronchopulmonary lymph node enlargement suggests a pulmonary origin for the mediastinal disease. The diffuse form typically results in widening of the mediastinum, most commonly involving its upper portion; the mediastinal outline may be smooth or lobulated. Calcification is rare.[26]

In some cases of either focal or diffuse disease, the mediastinal silhouette is normal, and the radiographic manifestations result from narrowing of the trachea, major bronchi, or esophagus or obstruction of pulmonary veins or arteries. A variety of findings can be associated with these processes.[26,27] For example, involvement of the SVC frequently results in a prominent aortic nipple as a result of a dilated left superior intercostal vein. Obstruction or narrowing of a pulmonary artery may result in localized areas of decreased opacification and vascularity, volume loss, or thrombosis. We have seen one patient with a combination of total occlusion of the left interlobar artery and compression of multiple pulmonary veins leading to interstitial pulmonary edema in all regions except the left lower lobe (Fig. 21–5). CT allows excellent evaluation of the extent of mediastinal soft tissue infiltration and

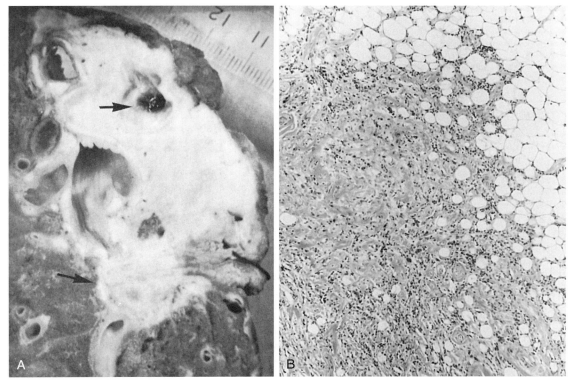

FIGURE 21–3

Fibrosing mediastinitis. A poorly delimited mass of fibrous tissue (**A**) can be seen in the hilar region and adjacent mediastinal tissue in this pneumonectomy specimen. A pulmonary artery (*upper arrow*) and vein (*lower arrow*) are partly or completely obstructed. A section from another "tumor" in the upper mediastinum (**B**) shows it to be composed of fibrous tissue containing scattered lymphocytes. The "tumor" appears to invade the mediastinal adipose tissue. *(From Fraser RS, Müller NL, Colman NC, Paré PD: Fraser and Paré's Diagnosis of Diseases of the Chest, 4th ed. Philadelphia, WB Saunders, 1999.)*

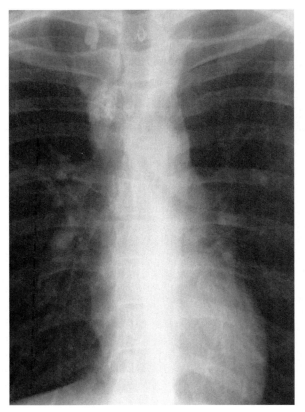

FIGURE 21-4

Fibrosing mediastinitis related to histoplasmosis. A close-up view of the chest from a posteroanterior radiograph demonstrates enlarged and calcified right paratracheal lymph nodes. The patient had superior vena cava syncrome. (*Courtesy of Dr. Robert Tarver, Indiana University Medical Center, Indianapolis.*)

assessment of calcification (Fig. 21–6), narrowing of the tracheobronchial tree, and, with the use of intravenous contrast, involvement of the pulmonary arteries, veins, and SVC.[26,27]

In the appropriate clinical context, the presence of a localized mediastinal soft tissue mass with calcification is virtually diagnostic of the disease and obviates the need for tissue sampling.[26] However, if the mass is not calcified or if there is clinical or radiologic evidence of disease progression, biopsy may be required to exclude a neoplasm.[26] Esophageal involvement is best demonstrated by contrast esophagography.[28]

Clinical Manifestations

Symptoms and signs of fibrosing mediastinitis are quite variable and depend on the extent of the fibrosis and the particular structures within the mediastinum that are affected.[16] Involvement of the SVC is probably the most common cause of clinical abnormalities and results in the typical manifestations of the SVC syndrome, including giddiness, tinnitus, headache, epistaxis, cyanosis, and puffiness of the face, neck, and arms. The severity of these symptoms can lessen with time as collateral venous channels develop. Additional findings may be seen with involvement of the pulmonary veins (signs of pulmonary venous hypertension and edema), pulmonary arteries (pulmonary hypertension with recurrent, sometimes

copious hemoptysis), thoracic duct (chylothorax), and the recurrent laryngeal nerve (hoarseness).[20]

Definitive diagnosis usually requires histologic examination of tissue removed at mediastinoscopy or thoracotomy. The prognosis is generally good, particularly in patients whose initial complaints can be relieved surgically.[16,17]

PNEUMOMEDIASTINUM

Pneumomediastinum (mediastinal emphysema) connotes the presence of gas in the mediastinal space. The gas can originate from five sites: the lung, the mediastinal airways (most often after trauma), the esophagus (usually in association with episodes of severe vomiting and occasionally after trauma or perforation of an esophageal neoplasm or during labor, a severe asthma attack, or strenuous exercise),[7] the neck (gas passing along deep fascial planes after trauma to the neck or after surgical or dental procedures),[29] and (rarely) the abdominal cavity.[30]

Etiology and Pathogenesis

The pulmonary parenchyma is the most common source of gas. The initial event is probably a sudden increase in alveolar pressure resulting in rupture of alveoli adjacent to airways or pulmonary arteries or veins; gas then passes into the perivascular or peribronchial interstitium and tracks through the interstitial tissue to the hilum and mediastinum.[31-33]

In most patients, the development of pneumomediastinum can be clearly related to an incident that results in a sudden rise in alveolar pressure or to a disease process in which such an incident is likely to occur. Such incidents or diseases include acute bronchiolitis, as may be seen with aspiration and viral infection (which predisposes to alveolar rupture as a result of check-valve bronchiolar obstruction and a local increase in air space pressure)[34]; deep respiratory maneuvers, such as those that occur during strenuous exercise or forced vital capacity breaths[35,36]; Valsalva maneuvers, such as those that occur during parturition or weight-lifting[37]; asthma (particularly in children)[38]; vomiting from any cause; artificial ventilation (particularly in patients who have obstructive pulmonary disease and in those being maintained on positive end-expiratory pressure)[39]; closed chest trauma; and a sudden drop in atmospheric pressure, such as occurs during the rapid ascent of a scuba diver or pilot.

When sufficient gas accumulates in the pneumomediastinum, pressure can build up and impede blood flow, particularly in low-pressure veins. This occurs only when gas is prevented from passing into the neck, a situation particularly likely to occur in neonates. More frequently, air escapes from the mediastinum by way of the fascial planes of the great vessels into the neck and anterior chest wall, thereby producing subcutaneous emphysema. Gas can also pass via the peribronchovascular interstitial tissue to the visceral pleura, which may rupture and lead to pneumothorax. This complication can also result directly from rupture of the mediastinal pleura when sufficient gas accumulates at this site.

Radiologic Manifestations

The radiographic manifestations consist of radiolucent streaks or focal bubble-like or larger collections of gas outlining the

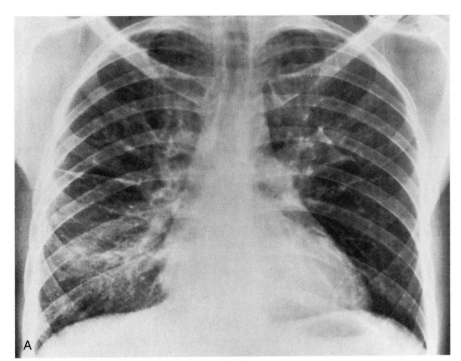

A

B

FIGURE 21-5

Fibrosing mediastinitis with encasement of pulmonary arteries and veins. A posteroanterior radiograph (**A**) reveals interstitial edema throughout the right lung and left upper zone. Septal lines are present in the right costophrenic angle. A striking disparity in density of the lower half of the two lungs is observed, the left being radiolucent and oligemic. A pulmonary arteriogram (**B**) shows almost complete occlusion of the left interlobar artery with virtually no perfusion of the left lower lobe and lingula. Although there appears to be good opacification of the arteries of the right lung, the truncus anterior and interlobar arteries show concentric narrowing medial to the hilum. The venous phase of the angiogram is not available, but it is almost certain that the pulmonary veins were affected in the same manner, which resulted in venous hypertension and the interstitial edema apparent on the plain radiograph. The cause of the fibrosis was *Histoplasma capsulatum* infection. *(Courtesy of Dr. M.J. Palayew, Jewish General Hospital, Montreal.)*

mediastinal structures.[40] In posteroanterior projection, the mediastinal pleura is seen to be displaced laterally, which creates a longitudinal line shadow parallel to the heart border and separated from the heart by gas. This shadow is usually more evident on the left side (Fig. 21–7). Occasionally, pneumomediastinum is more readily identified on the lateral radiograph as lucent streaks that outline the ascending aorta, aortic arch, and pulmonary arteries.[40]

In some cases, gas from a pneumomediastinum extends between the parietal pleura and the diaphragm or between the parietal pleura and the extrapleural tissues at the lung apex.[40]

Although such extrapleural gas can resemble pneumothorax, it does not shift on radiographs exposed with the patient in different body positions. Furthermore, the pleural line in this situation is not smooth, as in pneumothorax, but tends to be irregular as a result of tethering of the parietal pleural by overlying fascia.[40] This tethering is best detected on CT scan.[40]

When gas becomes interposed between the heart and diaphragm, the central portion of the diaphragm can be identified in continuity with the lateral portions, a finding known as the *continuous diaphragm sign* (Fig. 21–8).[41] In theory, gas within the pericardial sac should also permit visualization

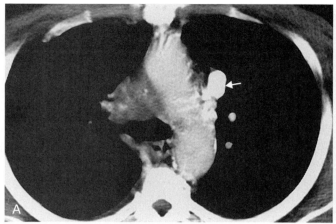
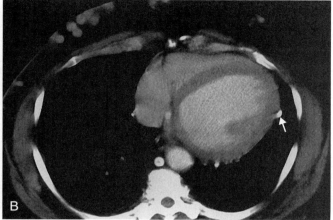

FIGURE 21–6

Fibrosing mediastinitis related to histoplasmosis. A contrast-enhanced CT scan at the level of the aortic arch (**A**) demonstrates complete obstruction of the superior vena cava and collateral venous circulation through the left superior intercostal vein (*arrow*). Note the foci of calcification within the right paratracheal mass consistent with previous histoplasmosis. Calcified mediastinal lymph nodes were present at several levels. A CT scan at a more caudal level (**B**) shows extensive collateral circulation through the left pericardiophrenic vein (*arrow*), azygos vein, and chest wall veins. (*Courtesy of Dr. Robert Tarver, Indiana University Medical Center, Indianapolis.*)

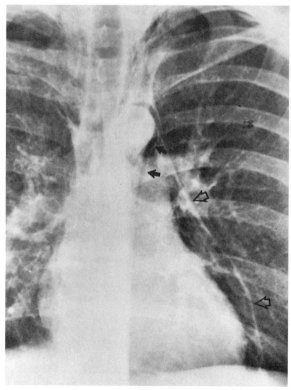

FIGURE 21–7

Spontaneous pneumomediastinum. A view of the chest in posteroanterior projection reveals a long linear opacity roughly paralleling the left heart border (*open arrows*) that represents the laterally displaced mediastinal pleura. Considerable gas is present around the aortic arch and proximal descending thoracic aorta (*solid arrows*). The patient was a 20-year-old man who had an abrupt onset of severe retrosternal pain. (*From Fraser RS, Müller NL, Colman NC, Paré PD: Fraser and Paré's Diagnosis of Diseases of the Chest, 4th ed. Philadelphia, WB Saunders, 1999.*)

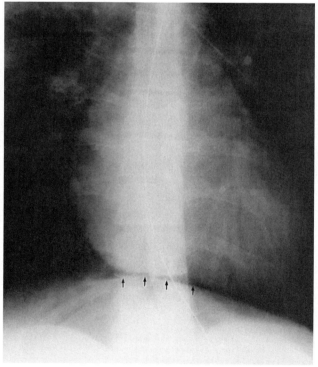

FIGURE 21–8

Pneumomediastinum—continuous diaphragm sign. An anteroposterior chest radiograph in a 58-year-old woman demonstrates pneumomediastinum outlining the central portion of the diaphragm (*arrows*), a finding known as the "continuous diaphragm sign." (*From Fraser RS, Müller NL, Colman NC, Paré PD: Fraser and Paré's Diagnosis of Diseases of the Chest, 4th ed. Philadelphia, WB Saunders, 1999.*)

of the central portion of the diaphragm; however, pneu-mopericardium is almost always associated with pericardial fluid, thus leading to obliteration of the central portion of the diaphragm, at least on radiographs exposed with the patient in the erect position.[41] When it is not certain whether a collection of gas is within the pericardial sac or the medi-astinal space, differentiation is readily established by demon-strating a change in position of the gas in the pericardial sac on radiographs exposed with the patient in different body positions.[42]

Sometimes, gas within the interstitial tissue of the lung ("interstitial emphysema") can be detected radiographically. Such gas should not be apparent in the interstitium of other-wise normal lung because of the lack of contrast; thus, its identification requires the presence of disease in contiguous parenchyma, a finding seen most often in patients who have acute respiratory distress syndrome. The radiographic findings include focal lucent areas that result in a mottled or stippled appearance of the parenchyma, lucent bands, perivas-cular lucencies, and subpleural and parenchymal cysts.[43] Although these findings are often difficult to identify on radi-ographs, they can be readily seen on CT scan.[44] With the latter,

air may also be seen to extend along the peribronchovascular interstitium into the mediastinum (Fig. 21–9).

Clinical Manifestations

Symptoms and signs depend largely on the amount of air in the mediastinal space and on the presence or absence of associated infection. There may be a history of an abrupt onset of retrosternal pain radiating to the shoulders and down both arms, usually preceded by an event that resulted in an excessive increase in intrathoracic pressure, such as a spasm of coughing, sneezing, or vomiting. The pain is usually aggravated by respiration; dyspnea may be severe. Physical examination generally reveals the presence of air in the sub-cutaneous tissues of the neck or over the thoracic wall. Hamman's sign (a crunching or clicking noise synchronous with the heartbeat) may be detected on auscultation over the apex of the heart. Patients in whom air does not freely escape from the mediastinum into the neck may have engorged neck veins, a rapid thready pulse, and significant systemic hypotension.

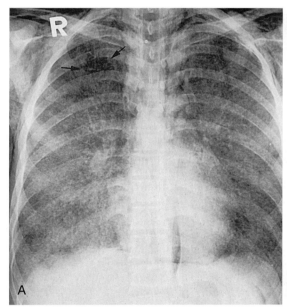

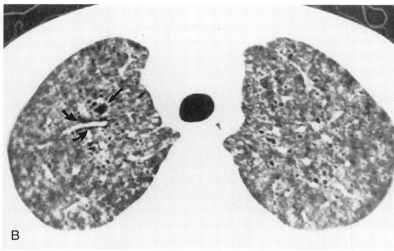

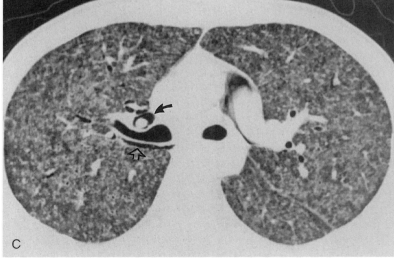

FIGURE 21–9

Interstitial emphysema and pneumomediastinum in miliary tuberculosis. An anteroposterior chest radiograph (**A**) in a 21-year-old man demonstrates focal lucencies in the right upper lobe (*arrows*), pneumomediastinum, and subcutaneous emphysema. An HRCT scan in the region of the apical segment of the right upper lobe (**B**) shows focal lucency (*straight arrow*) and perivascular dissection of gas (*curved arrows*). A scan at the level of the right upper lobe bronchus (**C**) demonstrates peribronchial (*open arrow*) and perivascular gas (*curved arrow*) and pneumomediastinum. (*Courtesy of Dr. Kun-Il Kim, Pusan National University Hospital, Pusan, South Korea.*)

MEDIASTINAL HEMORRHAGE

As might be expected, most cases of mediastinal hemorrhage result from trauma, usually of a severe nature such as that associated with an automobile accident or vigorous cardiopulmonary resuscitation.[45,46] Less common causes include perforation of a vein by faulty insertion of a central venous line and migration of a central venous catheter, rupture of an aortic aneurysm, and spontaneous hemorrhage in patients who have mediastinal tumors or a coagulopathy or who are undergoing chronic hemodialysis.[5,34,47]

Radiologically, hemorrhage typically results in uniform, symmetrical widening of the mediastinum.[48] Local accumulation of blood in the form of hematoma is manifested as a homogeneous mass that can project to one or both sides of the mediastinum and may be situated in any compartment (Fig. 21–10).[48] Hemorrhage caused by nontraumatic rupture of the aorta often results in obscuration or a convex appearance of the aortopulmonary window and displacement of the left paraspinal interface.[34] When mediastinal hemorrhage is due to a ruptured aorta, the blood may also extend into the pleural space, usually the left only but sometimes the right as well.[46] CT is superior to plain radiography in demonstrating both the presence of mediastinal hemorrhage and the underlying cause.

The majority of cases of mediastinal hemorrhage are probably unrecognized, the amount of bleeding being insufficient to produce symptoms and signs. Retrosternal pain radiating into the back develops in some patients. Hemorrhage related to a coagulation disorder may be suspected if local symptoms are associated with evidence of bleeding elsewhere, such as into the skin or retropharyngeal space. Hemorrhage related to a dissecting aneurysm may be associated with decreased pulsation in the arteries of the extremities.

MEDIASTINAL MASSES

A wide variety of lesions can be manifested as a localized tumor in the mediastinum.[49,50] Because many of these lesions arise in a specific tissue or structure that is situated in a particular site within the mediastinum, it is logical to classify them on the basis of their anatomic location. The scheme used in this text considers these lesions to occur in three sites, as defined by radiographic criteria: (1) the *anterior mediastinum*, when a tumor is situated predominantly in the region in front of a line drawn along the anterior border of the trachea and the posterior border of the heart (Fig. 21–11); (2) the *middle-posterior mediastinum*, when it is located predominantly between this line and the anterior aspect of the vertebral bodies; and (3) the *paravertebral region*, when a tumor is situated predominantly in the potential space adjacent to a vertebral body.

Overlap is bound to occur in such a classification; for example, aortic aneurysms may be situated in any of the three compartments, as may certain neoplasms such as leiomyoma and neurofibroma. Nevertheless, separation into these three groups is helpful in suggesting the diagnosis of many tumors, particularly if this information is combined with knowledge of the patients' clinical manifestations and the CT characteristics of the mass. In fact, a diagnosis can be made with a high degree of confidence in some cases on the basis of this information alone (e.g., an anterior mediastinal mass in a patient who has myasthenia gravis is almost certainly a thymoma). Despite this relatively high degree of diagnostic accuracy, tissue confirmation is necessary in most cases and is available in the majority after surgical excision of the tumor. Needle aspiration biopsy is often helpful when this is not possible.[51]

Most mediastinal abnormalities are initially suspected after chest radiography; the need for further investigation

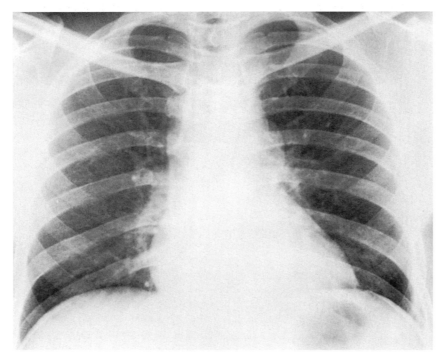

FIGURE 21–10

Spontaneous mediastinal hemorrhage. A 35-year-old hemophiliac was admitted to the hospital with evidence of recent extrathoracic hemorrhage. He had no symptoms referable to the thorax. A posteroanterior radiograph demonstrates bilateral widening of the mediastinum by a process whose lateral margins are somewhat lobulated. Involvement appears to be chiefly of the midmediastinal compartment. (A lateral radiograph was not helpful in localizing the abnormality.) The lesion resolved completely in 10 days without residua and was assumed to represent spontaneous hemorrhage. *(From Fraser RS, Müller NL, Colman NC, Paré PD: Fraser and Paré's Diagnosis of Diseases of the Chest, 4th ed. Philadelphia, WB Saunders, 1999.)*

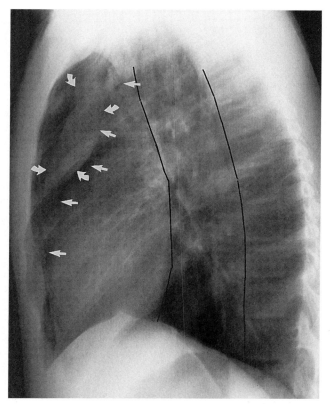

FIGURE 21–11

Mediastinal compartments. The presence of pneumomediastinum in this patient allows identification of the anterior border of the heart, ascending aorta, and brachiocephalic vessels (*straight arrows*). The anatomic anterior mediastinum is composed of the tissue anterior to these structures and includes the thymus (*curved arrows*), adipose tissue, and lymph nodes. However, the anterior margins of the ascending aorta and brachiocephalic vessels are normally difficult to visualize. Furthermore, anterior mediastinal masses often project over the heart. Therefore, on the lateral chest radiograph a mass can be considered to probably lie in the anterior mediastinum if it is situated predominantly in the region in front of a line drawn along the anterior border of the trachea and the posterior border of the heart. A mass probably lies in the middle or posterior mediastinum if it is situated between this line and a line drawn along the anterior aspect of the vertebral bodies. Extrapulmonary masses located posterior to this line lie outside the mediastinum and should therefore be considered paravertebral in location. (*From Fraser RS, Müller NL, Colman NC, Paré PD: Fraser and Paré's Diagnosis of Diseases of the Chest, 4th ed. Philadelphia, WB Saunders, 1999.*)

and the optimal imaging modality or other test by which it should be conducted are largely dictated by the tentative diagnosis made on this examination. CT and MR imaging allow visualization of the exact location of the lesions and, in some cases, identification of the structures from which they arise; one or both of these techniques are indicated in almost all cases. Because of their anatomic precision, it is preferable to describe the exact location of a lesion in relation to the adjacent mediastinal structures with both of these techniques rather than limiting the description to a particular mediastinal compartment.

The wide variety of tissues within the mediastinum is reflected in the many forms of neoplastic, developmental, and inflammatory masses that are seen.[52] In one representative

review,[53] the frequency of tumors (excluding metastatic pulmonary carcinoma) was as follows: neurogenic neoplasms, 19%; lymphoma, 16%; bronchial and pericardial cysts, 14%; germ cell tumors, 13%; thymoma, 12%; and thyroid tumors, 6%; a variety of miscellaneous tumors accounted for the remainder.

Masses Situated Predominantly in the Anterior Mediastinum

The anterior mediastinum is the site of the majority of clinically important primary mediastinal masses, including thymoma and a variety of other thymic abnormalities, lymphoma, germ cell tumors, and hyperplastic and neoplastic abnormalities of thyroid and ectopic parathyroid tissue. Abnormalities involving the ascending aorta can also mimic an anterior mediastinal mass.

Thymic Tumors

Thymic Hyperplasia

True thymic hyperplasia, as opposed to the lymphoid hyperplasia that is associated with myasthenia gravis (see next section), can be defined as an increase in size of the thymus gland asso-ciated with a more or less normal gross architecture and histologic appearance.[54,55] The pathogenesis is variable. Most commonly, it appears to be a rebound phenomenon secondary to atrophy caused by chemotherapy for malignancy (usually lymphoma or a germ cell tumor) or by hypercortisolism.[56,57] Occasionally, a history of hyperthyroidism,[58] a "stressful" event such as sepsis or a massive burn,[59,60] or other disease is present. Analysis of excised hyperplastic tissue has shown no immunochemical, structural, or functional differences from normal thymic tissue.[61]

Thymic hyperplasia is seldom apparent on the chest radiograph in adults.[62] On CT, the most helpful measurement for determining an increase in the size of the thymus is its thickness (Fig. 21–12)[63]: the maximal normal thickness in individuals younger than 20 years is 1.8 cm; in those older than 20, it is 1.3 cm. Measurements greater than these are consistent with hyperplasia. In patients who have lymphoma, rebound thymic hyperplasia must be distinguished from residual or recurrent tumor.[64] Although such distinction cannot be achieved reliably with CT or MR imaging, it may be possible with gallium scintigraphy,[65] gallium uptake being seen in residual tumor but not in fibrotic or necrotic tissue. However, although increased uptake is relatively common in children who have rebound thymic hyperplasia,[65] it is rare in adults.[66]

Most patients are children or young adults.[54,55] Symptoms are usually absent, although respiratory distress and dysphagia can occur. The diagnosis should be suspected in those with a history of previous chemotherapy; in the absence of such a history, excision of the enlarged thymus is almost certainly required for diagnosis.

Thymic Lymphoid Hyperplasia

In approximately two thirds of individuals who have myasthenia gravis, the thymic cortex is the site of multiple well-defined lymphoid follicles, many containing germinal centers. Because of this finding and because the weight of the thymus

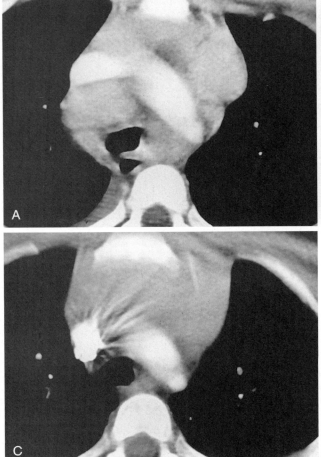

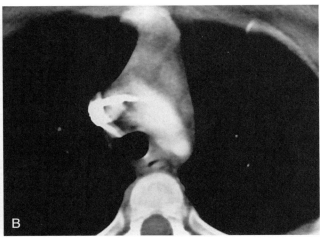

FIGURE 21–12

Thymic "rebound"—hyperplasia. A contrast-enhanced CT scan in a 9-year-old child (**A**) demonstrates extensive mediastinal lymphadenopathy (proven to be due to Hodgkin's lymphoma). The patient underwent successful treatment. A CT scan performed 6 months later (**B**) shows a small residual thymus. A scan performed 1 year after the initial scan (**C**) demonstrates a significant increase in thymic size representing "rebound" hyperplasia. There was no evidence of tumor recurrence. *(Courtesy of Dr. Ella Kazerooni, Department of Radiology, University of Michigan Hospital, Ann Arbor.)*

in these cases is usually within normal limits, it has been suggested that the terms *lymphoid* or *follicular* hyperplasia be used to describe the abnormality.[67] The large number of cases of myasthenia gravis and thymic lymphoid hyperplasia, as well as the favorable response to thymectomy in many patients who have the abnormality, suggests a pathogenetic association between the two conditions[68]; however, the details of this relationship remain unclear.

Thymic lymphoid hyperplasia seldom leads to radiographically apparent abnormalities.[62,69] CT may demonstrate a normal-appearing thymus, a diffusely enlarged thymus, or less commonly, a focal mass.[70]

Thymolipoma

Thymolipomas are uncommon anterior mediastinal tumors that consist of an admixture of fat and histologically normal thymic lymphoepithelial tissue.[71] The precise nature of the tumor is uncertain.[72] It has been thought to represent no more than a lipoma occurring within the thymus gland; however, because the thymic tissue itself appears to be increased in amount,[73] this hypothesis appears unlikely. It has also been suggested that the tumor begins as true thymic hyperplasia (i.e., an increase in the amount of normal thymic tissue) that subsequently regresses and is replaced by adipose tissue.[73] Grossly, thymolipomas are typically yellow, soft, and roughly

bilobed in shape, somewhat resembling the normal thymus gland. They are often large and can grow to huge proportions.[71]

The characteristic radiographic appearance consists of an anterior mediastinal mass that droops into the lower part of the chest (Fig. 21–13)[49,74]; extension into one or both hemithoraces may be seen. The tumor typically conforms to adjacent structures and may mimic cardiomegaly or elevation of one or both hemidiaphragms. When small, it is round or oval, similar to other mediastinal masses. CT scans characteristically show predominant fat attenuation or equivalent fat and soft tissue attenuation. The soft tissue may appear as linear whorls intermixed with fat or, less commonly, as small rounded opacities embedded within it. MR imaging demonstrates high signal intensity on T1-weighted spin-echo images as a result of fat and areas of intermediate signal intensity related to soft tissue.[74]

Thymolipomas characteristically cause few or no symptoms even when large; thus, the lesion is usually discovered on a screening radiograph. Their behavior is typically benign.

Thymic Cysts

Thymic cysts account for about 1% to 2% of all tumors in the anterior compartment.[75] Many are probably derived from remnants of the fetal thymopharyngeal duct. Occasional cysts have been reported after thoracic surgery or chemotherapy

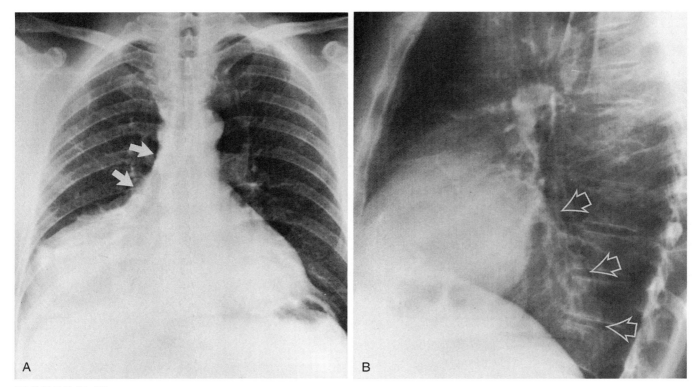

FIGURE 21-13

Thymolipoma. Posteroanterior (**A**) and lateral (**B**) radiographs demonstrate a large mass situated in the lower half of the right hemithorax. The obtuse angle that the mass creates with the mediastinum (*arrows* in **A**) indicates its origin from that structure. In lateral projection, note that the mass extends to almost the entire anteroposterior depth of the thorax and is obscuring most of the right hemidiaphragm (the posterior margin of the mass is indicated by *open arrows* in **B**). The anterior mediastinum looks "empty." *(Courtesy of Dr. R. Hedvigi, Montreal Chest Institute.)*

for a malignant neoplasm, thus suggesting a relationship to trauma or drug-related involution.[76,77] An association with HIV infection has also been documented in some cases.[78]

Pathologically, the cysts are unilocular or multilocular and can contain straw-colored fluid or, if hemorrhage has occurred, brown gelatinous or friable material. Histologically, the cyst wall is lined by squamous, transitional, or simple cuboidal or columnar epithelium; ulceration associated with underlying fibrosis and chronic inflammation is fairly common. Thymic tissue can be identified focally in the cyst wall. An important point in the pathologic differential diagnosis is the observation that some neoplasms, including thymoma, Hodgkin's lymphoma, and germ cell tumors,[79,80] can show prominent cystic change, with only a relatively small amount of neoplastic tissue; consequently, thorough sampling of every "thymic cyst" must be carried out to exclude the possibility of neoplasia.

The appearance on the chest radiograph consists of a smoothly marginated anterior mediastinal mass.[49,81] When large, the cyst may obscure the margins of adjacent structures and simulate cardiomegaly (Fig. 21–14). On CT, cysts typically have water density and thin walls. Occasionally, soft tissue septa or ringlike calcifications are seen within the cyst, or foci of linear calcification in the cyst wall are observed, presumably as a result of previous hemorrhage.[81] The cysts have low signal intensity on T1-weighted MR images and high signal intensity on T2-weighted images.[82]

Most patients are asymptomatic. Provided that a neoplastic cyst has been excluded, the prognosis is excellent.

Thymoma

Thymomas are best defined simply as neoplasms of thymic epithelium.[83,84] They are the most common primary neoplasm to occur in the anterior mediastinum and overall account for approximately 20% of all primary mediastinal tumors.[85] Most are discovered in adults between 40 and 50 years of age. The etiology and pathogenesis are unknown in the vast majority of cases.

The tumors have a complex histologic appearance, which has resulted in a variety of classification schemes that have engendered considerable debate among pathologists about their validity and usefulness.[86-88] Traditionally, the term "thymoma" has been used to refer to tumors that are composed of rather uniform epithelial cells and that have a variable amount of admixed lymphocytes; though cytologically bland, such tumors can behave in either a benign or a malignant fashion. Tumors composed of cells that have significant cytologic atypia, a high mitotic rate, and necrosis are often clinically much more aggressive and have been categorized separately as *thymic carcinoma*.[89] A more recent classification scheme proposed by the World Health Organization (WHO) considers the latter tumors to be part of the spectrum of thymoma.[90] According to this scheme (Table 21–1), thymomas

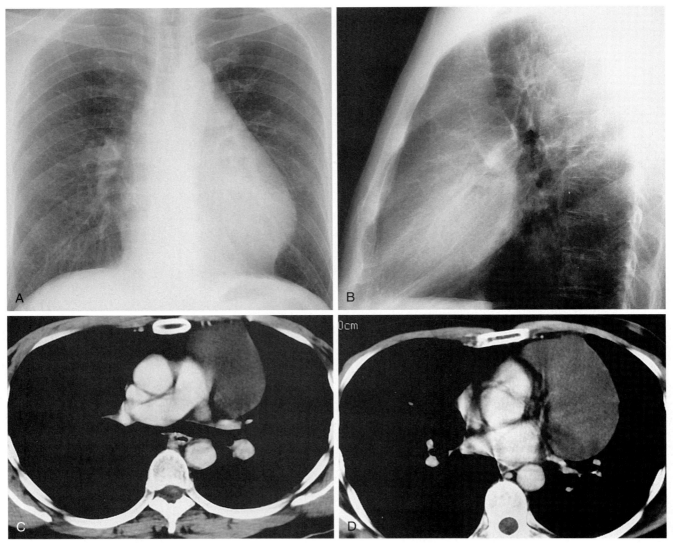

FIGURE 21–14

Thymic cyst. A posteroanterior chest radiograph (**A**) in a 53-year-old man shows an unusual contour of the mediastinum and apparent cardiomegaly. A lateral radiograph (**B**) shows a poorly defined increased opacity in the anterior mediastinum and normal heart size. Contrast-enhanced CT scans (**C** and **D**) demonstrate a thin-walled, fluid-filled cyst. The presence of a thymic cyst was confirmed surgically. *(From Fraser RS, Müller NL, Colman NC, Paré PD: Fraser and Paré's Diagnosis of Diseases of the Chest, 4th ed. Philadelphia, WB Saunders, 1999.)*

are separated into three major categories—A, B, and C—on the basis of the degree of cytologic atypia, the shape of the neoplastic epithelial cells, and the proportion of admixed lymphocytes.

Pathologic Characteristics. Grossly, most type A and B thymomas are well encapsulated and round or slightly lobulated. They are usually between 5 and 15 cm in diameter,[91] although they tend to be somewhat smaller in individuals who have myasthenia gravis, presumably because of the presence of symptoms at an earlier stage. Sections often reveal the tumors to be subdivided into numerous lobules by variably thick fibrous bands (see Color Fig. 21–1). One or more cysts are not infrequent and are sometimes large and comprise most of the tumor volume (see Color Fig. 21–2)[79]; foci of fibrosis, calcification, and hemorrhage may also be seen. Apparent infiltration of the pleura, lung, and (less commonly) the pericardium, chest wall, diaphragm, or mediastinal vessels occurs in 30% to 50% of cases[92]; however, since the tumor can be adherent to

these structures without actually invading them,[91] such infiltration must be clearly confirmed histologically.

As suggested by the existence of multiple classifications, there is considerable variability in the histologic appearance of thymomas. The epithelial cells can have a polygonal to a distinctly spindled shape, and the associated lymphocytic infiltrate can be absent or can be so marked that it almost completely obscures the presence of the epithelial cells. Such variability was perhaps most simply reflected in one of the earliest and most widely used histologic classifications, which divided the tumors into predominantly lymphocytic, mixed lymphoepithelial, and predominantly epithelial (the latter often being further subdivided into polygonal and spindle cell variants) (see Color Fig. 21–3).[91,93]

A second, somewhat more complicated classification based on epithelial cell morphology and possible functional characteristics was subsequently proposed:[94] tumors were divided into cortical, medullary, and mixed forms, the first in turn being subdivided into "predominantly" cortical (organoid) and "pure" cortical types. Because of morphologic, immuno-histochemical, and functional differences between the cortical and medullary regions of a normal thymus,[94,95] such a classi-fication has some theoretical merit. Perhaps more impor-tantly, there is evidence that the histologic types defined in this classification are associated with different biologic behavior and prognosis.[96,97] This concept of histologic types has become the basis of the categories defined in the WHO classification.[90]

Radiologic Manifestations. Most type A and B thymomas are situated near the junction of the heart and great vessels. Radiographically, they are round or oval, and their margins are usually smooth or lobulated (Fig. 21–15).[49,98] They can protrude to one or both sides of the mediastinum and can displace the heart and great vessels posteriorly. In some cases, calcification is apparent at the periphery of the lesion or

throughout its substance.[98] Occasionally, a tumor simulates cardiac enlargement or is located in an unusual site, such as the cardiophrenic angle or middle-posterior mediastinum.[81,98] The radiographic appearance of invasive and noninvasive tumors is usually indistinguishable.

On CT, the majority of thymomas are manifested as round or oval soft tissue masses that have sharply demarcated margins. Typically, they are located in the region of the thymus anterior to the aortic root and main pulmonary artery and project to one side of the mediastinum (see Fig. 21–15).[49,98] Most tumors have homogeneous attenuation and show homogeneous enhancement with contrast; less commonly and usually in large tumors, the presence of hemorrhage, necrosis, or cyst formation leads to focal areas of low attenu-ation.[99] Foci of calcification may be seen in the capsule or throughout the tumor.[81,98] Areas of low attenuation, multifo-cal calcification, and irregular margins are seen more

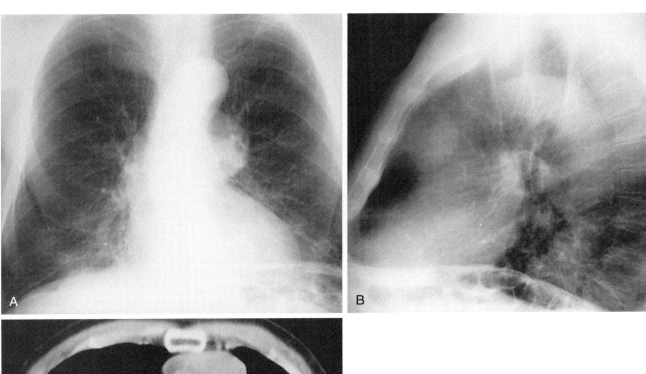

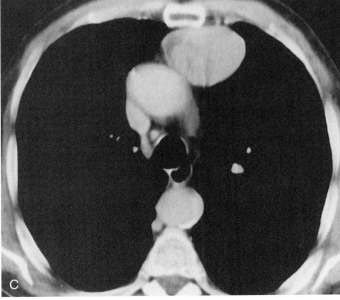

FIGURE 21–15

Thymoma. Posteroanterior (**A**) and lateral (**B**) chest radiographs in a 75-year-old man demonstrate an anterior mediastinal mass. A contrast-enhanced CT scan (**C**) shows a smoothly marginated mass with heterogeneous enhancement. *(From Fraser RS, Müller NL, Colman NC, Paré PD: Fraser and Paré's Diagnosis of Diseases of the Chest, 4th ed. Philadelphia, WB Saunders, 1999.)*

TABLE 21–1. Thymoma—World Health Organization Histologic Classification

Type	Description
A	A tumor composed of a population of neoplastic thymic epithelial cells having a spindle/oval shape, lacking nuclear atypia, and accompanied by few or no non-neoplastic lymphocytes
AB	A tumor in which foci having the features of type A thymoma are admixed with foci rich in lymphocytes
B1	A tumor that resembles the normal functional thymus in that it combines large expanses that have an appearance practically indistinguishable from normal thymic cortex with areas resembling thymic medulla
B2	A tumor in which the neoplastic epithelial component appears as scattered plump cells with vesicular nuclei and distinct nucleoli among a heavy population of lymphocytes
B3	A type of thymoma predominantly composed of epithelial cells that have a round or polygonal shape and exhibit no or mild atypia. They are admixed with a minor component of lymphocytes
C	A thymic tumor exhibiting clear-cut cytologic atypia and a set of cytoarchitectural features no longer specific to the thymus, but rather analogous to those seen in carcinomas of other organs

TABLE 21–2. Staging of Thymoma

Stage I
Macroscopically completely encapsulated and microscopically no capsular invasion

Stage II
Macroscopic invasion into surrounding fatty tissue or mediastinal pleura or microscopic invasion into the capsule

Stage III
Macroscopic invasion into the neighboring organ (i.e., pericardium, great vessels, or lung)

Stage IV
a. Pleural or pericardial dissemination b. Lymphogenous or hematogenous metastasis

From Masaoka A, Monden Y, Nakahara K, et al. Follow-up study of thymomas with special reference to their clinical stages. Cancer 48:2485, 1981.

commonly in invasive than noninvasive thymomas[99]; however, CT does not allow reliable distinction of invasive from noninvasive tumors. Although preservation of fat planes between the tumor and adjacent structures is most suggestive of a noninvasive tumor, limited invasion cannot be excluded. Similarly, although obliteration of the fat planes is suggestive of invasion (Fig. 21–16), such obliteration may be seen with noninvasive tumors.[100]

Thymomas have intermediate signal intensity (equal to that of skeletal muscle) on T1-weighted MR images and increased signal intensity (approaching that of fat) on T2-weighted images (see Fig. 21–16).[98,101] The capsule has low signal intensity. Cystic regions and areas of hemorrhage have low signal intensity on T1-weighted images and high signal intensity on T2-weighted images. Inhomogeneous areas of signal intensity on T2-weighted images are seen more commonly in invasive than in noninvasive tumors.[101] It has been suggested that MR imaging is superior to CT in distinguishing invasive from noninvasive thymomas and in assessing tumor recurrence.[102]

CT or MR imaging is also indicated in the investigation of patients who have myasthenia gravis.[102] In an investigation of 45 such patients, 26 had normal CT findings, 7 had a diffusely enlarged thymus, and 12 had a focal mass.[70] Pathologic assessment demonstrated that 16 of 26 patients who had normal findings had normal thymic tissue, and 10 had lymphoid hyperplasia; all 7 patients who had a diffusely enlarged thymus had lymphoid hyperplasia. Five of 12 patients who had a focal mass at CT had lymphoid hyperplasia, and 7 had thymoma.

Clinical Manifestations. About 50% of patients are asymptomatic when the tumor is discovered[103]; the remainder have symptoms related to local compression or invasion of thoracic structures or to systemic paraneoplastic disease. Symptoms of thoracic disease are seen in about a third of patients, the most frequent being chest pain, shortness of breath, dysphagia, and cough[91]; hoarseness, evidence of pericarditis, and SVC syndrome can also be seen.[104,105]

Myasthenia gravis is by far the most common paraneoplastic disease associated with thymoma. Approximately 10% to 15% of patients with myasthenia have the tumor,[91] and about 35% to 40% of all patients with type A or B thymoma have myasthenia.[91,97] The tumor is sometimes occult.[106] A variety of hematologic abnormalities are associated with thymoma.[107-109] Red blood cell aplasia (hypoplasia) is the most common[110]; of all patients who have this disorder, approximately 10% to 15% have a thymoma.[111] Many autoimmune connective tissue diseases, such as polymyositis and lupus erythematosus, have also been associated with thymoma. Although some of these conditions probably represent true paraneoplastic complications of the tumor, the development of the connective tissue disease some years after thymectomy suggests that absence of the thymus itself may be the pathogenetic link in some cases.[112]

Prognosis and Natural History. Most type A and B thymomas are slow-growing encapsulated neoplasms whose excision results in cure; however, some are locally aggressive tumors that are unresectable or recur after apparent complete excision. Recurrence or local invasion at the time of initial diagnosis occurs most commonly in the anterior mediastinal soft tissue, pericardium, or pleura; occasionally, a tumor extends into the lung parenchyma or large mediastinal vessels. The most common sites of metastasis are the lung, pleura, thoracic skeleton, and mediastinal, supraclavicular, or cervical lymph nodes. Extrathoracic metastases are very uncommon and should raise the possibility that the tumor is type C (thymic carcinoma).[91,113]

Numerous investigations have been carried out in an attempt to identify criteria that can accurately assess the likelihood of tumor recurrence or metastasis. Though histologic type and stage are to some extent correlated, there is evidence that both are useful in this regard. Several staging schemes have been proposed, the most widely used being that of Masaoka and colleagues (Table 21–2).[114]

There is little question that the best criterion of malignancy or benignancy (apart from metastasis) is the presence or absence of local invasion, a finding that is usually established by the surgeon at the time of thoracotomy. The percentage of thymomas that are reported to show such invasion varies

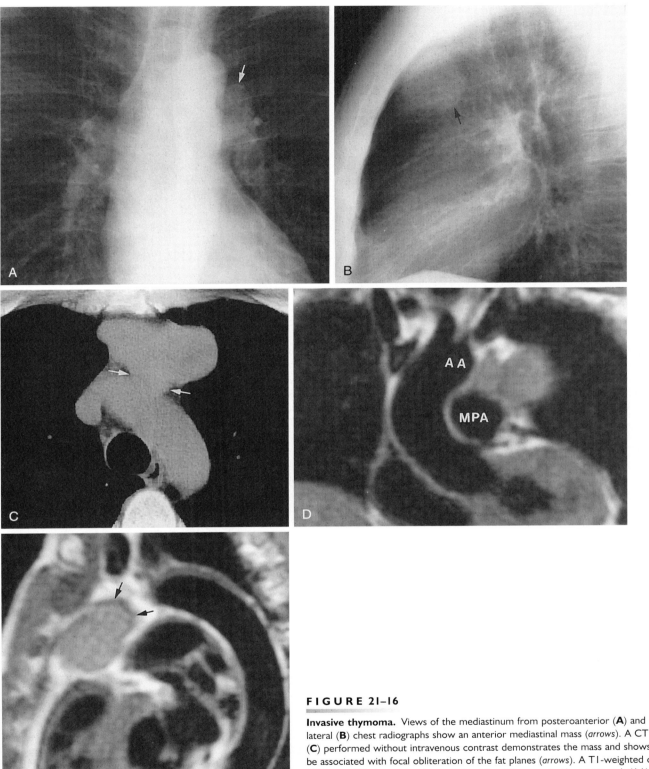

FIGURE 21–16

Invasive thymoma. Views of the mediastinum from posteroanterior (**A**) and lateral (**B**) chest radiographs show an anterior mediastinal mass (*arrows*). A CT scan (**C**) performed without intravenous contrast demonstrates the mass and shows it to be associated with focal obliteration of the fat planes (*arrows*). A T1-weighted coronal MR image (**D**) shows the close relationship of the mass to the aortic arch (AA) and main pulmonary artery (MPA). A sagittal T1-weighted MR image (**E**) shows low–signal intensity capsule (*arrows*) and high–signal intensity mediastinal fat. *(From Fraser RS, Müller NL, Colman NC, Paré PD: Fraser and Paré's Diagnosis of Diseases of the Chest, 4th ed. Philadelphia, WB Saunders, 1999.)*

widely in different series, ranging from about 5% to 50%. Recurrence is not uncommon in individuals who have such grossly invasive tumors because complete resection is usually impossible; however, because many tumors are slow growing, residual disease may be associated with prolonged survival.[115] Recurrence may be seen many years after thymectomy,[116] so long-term follow-up is necessary before a patient can be considered to be cured. Microscopic invasion into fat, pleura, or pericardium adjacent to the thymic tumor is also associated with an increased likelihood of recurrence, even if the tumor appears to have been completely excised.[117] In an investigation of 273 patients, the 20-year survival rates were 89%, 91%, 49%, 0%, and 0% for patients who had stage I, II, III, IVa, and IVb, respectively.[118]

As indicated previously, there is evidence that tumor behavior is also associated with histologic type: several groups of investigators have shown that the probability of tumor recurrence is relatively high and the prognosis relatively poor with type B versus types A and AB.[96,97] For example, in the investigation cited previously, 20-year survival rates were 100%, 87%, 91%, 59%, and 36% for types A, AB, B1, B2, and B3, respectively.[118] Because the likelihood of local invasion is also associated with the histologic type, its usefulness in predicting behavior can be questioned[119]; nevertheless, multivariate analysis in some studies has shown it to be independent of stage in predicting long-term survival.[120]

Investigations of other parameters that theoretically might help predict biologic behavior, such as nuclear DNA content (by flow cytometry),[121,122] cell proliferative activity (as manifested by argyrophilic nucleolar organizer region counts or MIB-1 immunoreactivity),[123,124] and oncogene expression,[125] have yielded variable and overall unhelpful results.

Thymic Carcinoma (Type C Thymoma)

As discussed in the previous section, some thymomas that have histologic features suggestive of a benign neoplasm invade adjacent mediastinal tissues and lung and occasionally metastasize. Although this behavior indicates that such tumors are malignant and hence might be called carcinomas, the term *carcinoma* is usually reserved for neoplasms that possess the traditional histologic and cytologic features of malignancy, such as nuclear atypia, significant mitotic activity, and necrosis.[126] In the WHO classification, these neoplasms are termed type C thymomas.

Pathologically, the tumors are usually large (5 to 15 cm in diameter) and are often found to invade adjacent structures at the time of diagnosis (see Color Fig. 21–4).[127] A variety of histologic patterns have been reported, the most common being squamous cell carcinoma. Distinction between primary thymic and metastatic carcinoma can be difficult on histologic examination alone and relies in part on the lack of a neoplasm in another site, particularly the lung. Some investigators have found CD5—a molecule associated with T-cell growth—to be present in many thymic carcinomas but not in extrathymic carcinomas.[128]

Radiologically, thymic carcinomas are usually manifested as large anterior mediastinal masses that have irregular or poorly defined margins (Fig. 21–17).[49,129] On CT, the tumors can have homogenous soft tissue attenuation or heterogeneous attenuation as a result of necrosis; foci of calcification

are present in approximately 10% of cases.[129,130] The majority of tumors have irregular margins and show evidence of extension outside the thymus with focal or diffuse obliteration of the adjacent fat planes. Although local pleural infiltration and associated effusion are common, distal pleural implants are seldom seen. Mediastinal lymph node enlargement (almost always reactive) is present in about 40% of cases.[129,130]

Clinically, most patients are symptomatic at the time of diagnosis, the most common complaints being chest pain and cough; systemic findings such as fever, weight loss, fatigue, and night sweats are also common.[127] The presence of a paraneoplastic syndrome is very uncommon.[131] As might be expected, the prognosis is poor, with progressive intrathoracic growth and extrathoracic metastases developing in the majority of patients.[132,133] The overall survival rate at 5 years is about 30% to 35%.[127,134]

Thymic Neuroendocrine Neoplasms

The term *thymic neuroendocrine neoplasm* encompasses several tumors, each of which has histologic, immunohistochemical, and occasionally clinical features of neuroendocrine function.[135] They are believed to be derived from neuroendocrine cells present in the normal thymus. The most common histologic subtype is carcinoid tumor; as with their pulmonary counterparts, these neoplasms may be well differentiated (typical carcinoid tumor) or may have histologic features suggestive of a more aggressive nature (atypical carcinoid).[136,137] Occasional tumors are classified as small cell carcinoma or large cell neuroendocrine carcinoma.[138,139] From a practical point of view, metastasis from pulmonary carcinoma must be carefully excluded before a tumor that has one of the last two appearances can be considered primary in the mediastinum.

The chest radiograph can be normal, a feature that is particularly likely in patients who have corticotropin-producing carcinoid tumors.[140] Nonsecreting tumors or tumors associated with multiple endocrine neoplasia (MEN) syndromes more commonly appear as large anterior mediastinal masses.[141] On CT, the tumors range from 1 to 25 cm in diameter and have homogeneous or heterogeneous attenuation as a result of necrosis or calcification.[49] Evidence of invasion of adjacent structures and metastases to the regional lymph nodes or lungs is not uncommon.[141]

Many mediastinal carcinoid tumors produce no symptoms and are discovered on screening chest radiography. Signs and symptoms caused by compression or invasion of mediastinal structures may be present and include chest or shoulder pain, dyspnea, cough, and SVC syndrome.[138] About 5% of patients have MEN syndrome[142]; almost all affected patients are male, and the majority have MEN type I (pituitary adenoma, parathyroid adenoma, and pancreatic islet cell tumor). Clinical findings of paraneoplastic disease are present in about a third of patients[135]; Cushing's syndrome is by far the most common.[136]

Complete excision of typical thymic carcinoid tumors is associated with a good prognosis, even in the few patients in whom regional lymph node metastases are present.[138] By contrast, death occurs in many patients who have atypical tumors, particularly if extension outside the thymus is detected at initial evaluation[138]; the overall 5-year survival rate has been reported to be about 65%.[136]

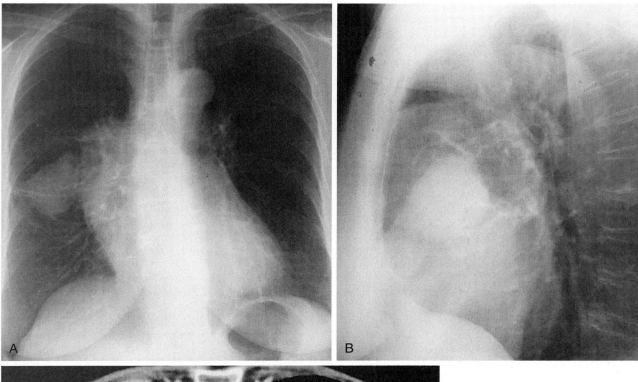

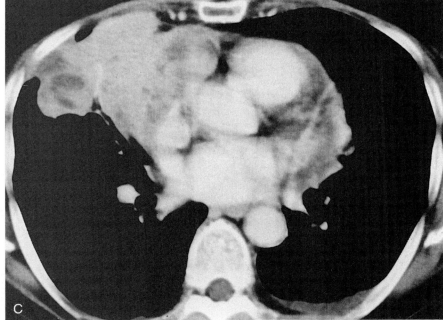

FIGURE 21-17

Thymic carcinoma. Posteroanterior (**A**) and lateral (**B**) chest radiographs in a 69-year-old woman show a large, lobulated anterior mediastinal mass. A soft tissue component projecting into the right midlung zone is evident. A contrast-enhanced CT scan (**C**) also demonstrates a lobulated anterior mediastinal mass with inhomogeneous attenuation and obliteration of the adjacent fat planes. The mass can be seen extending into the right middle lobe. At surgery it was shown to be a thymic carcinoma with pericardial, pleural, and right middle lobe involvement. (*From Fraser RS, Müller NL, Colman NC, Paré PD: Fraser and Paré's Diagnosis of Diseases of the Chest, 4th ed. Philadelphia, WB Saunders, 1999.*)

Germ Cell Neoplasms

The vast majority of mediastinal germ cell tumors are located in the anterior compartment.[143,144] The most common form is mature teratoma, which represented about 45% to 75% of tumors in three reviews.[143,145,146] The most common malignant tumor is seminoma.[143,147] Additional histologic varieties include embryonal carcinoma, malignant teratoma, choriocarcinoma, and endodermal sinus tumor[148,149]; many tumors have a mixed histologic appearance. Most tumors become evident in early adulthood.[147,150] For unexplained reasons,

benign lesions appear to be more common in women and malignant ones in men.[143,147,151]

Mediastinal germ cell tumors are generally thought to arise from cells whose journey along the urogenital ridge to the primitive gonad is interrupted in the mediastinum during fetal development.[150] Sometimes, clinical or pathologic examination of a testicle reveals either viable tumor or focal scarring consistent with regressed tumor,[152] findings indicating that the mediastinal neoplasm represents a metastasis. Although careful clinical examination must be performed in every case of mediastinal germ cell tumor to exclude this possibility, the relatively large number of negative pathologic examinations at autopsy and biopsy and the usual lack of emergence of a gonadal primary tumor during prolonged clinical follow-up indicate that it is a rare event.[153,154]

A relationship between mediastinal germ cell neoplasms and Klinefelter's syndrome has been documented in about 5% of patients.[155] The reason for the association is unclear; possible explanations include the abnormal androgen and gonadotropin secretion that is characteristic of the syndrome or the intrinsically abnormal germ cell tissue in patients who have Klinefelter's syndrome. Hematologic malignancies, most commonly nonlymphocytic leukemia, have also been associated with mediastinal germ cell neoplasms, particularly teratomas.[156] Some of the leukemias have developed after the institution of chemotherapy or radiotherapy, thus raising the possibility of therapeutically induced neoplasia; in most, however, the teratoma and hematologic malignancy have been recognized synchronously or within a short time after the induction of therapy, suggesting a common pathogenesis. The basis of this relationship is unclear.[156]

Although pathologic diagnosis of a mediastinal germ cell tumor can be made with small tissue samples, such as those obtained by transthoracic needle aspiration,[157] because of the tumor's varied histologic appearance, such diagnosis is sometimes difficult. Although this problem is relatively unimportant with respect to specific typing of germ cell tumors, advances in chemotherapy make the distinction from metastatic carcinoma of considerable significance. Because such distinction is sometimes difficult on histologic examination, it is reasonable that the possibility of a primary germ cell neoplasm be considered in any young patient who has an anterior mediastinal mass and in whom a diagnosis of metastatic carcinoma is made in the absence of an extramediastinal primary focus.[158] In this situation, review of pathologic material and testing for the presence of serum and tissue tumor markers, such as α-fetoprotein, β-human chorionic gonadotropin, and CD30, may result in a change in diagnosis.

As a group, nonseminomatous malignant germ cell tumors are typically seen on radiographs as large anterior mediastinal masses that may have smooth, lobulated, or irregular margins.[159,160] On CT, they usually have heterogeneous attenuation and contain large areas of low attenuation.[159,160] Focal areas of calcification may be seen. The fat planes between the tumor and adjacent structures are usually obliterated, and pleural and pericardial effusions are common. CT may also demonstrate pulmonary metastases, irregular interfaces between the tumor and the lung as a result of direct pulmonary extension, extension into the chest wall, and mediastinal lymph node enlargement.[49,160]

Although the prognosis of malignant nonseminomatous germ cell tumors has improved markedly with some chemotherapeutic regimens,[161] it is worse than that associated with their testicular counterparts, and approximately 50% to 70% of patients die of local or metastatic disease.[151,162] A staging system that may aid in predicting prognosis has been proposed.[150]

Teratoma

A teratoma can be defined as a neoplasm that consists of one or more types of tissue, usually derived from more than one germ cell layer, at least some of which are not native to the area

in which the tumor arises. In the mediastinum, the majority of such lesions are cystic and benign (see Color Fig. 21–5); solid neoplasms are usually malignant. The tumors can be divided into three histologic types: mature teratoma, immature teratoma, and teratoma with malignant transformation. *Mature teratomas* are by far the most common form. Most are large (average diameter, 8 to 10 cm) and multicystic.[163] Histologically, ectodermal elements predominate, particularly epidermis and skin appendages; a relatively high incidence of pancreatic tissue has been documented.[164] *Immature teratomas* consist of the same adult tissues as the mature variety but in addition contain foci of primitive, less well organized tissue resembling that seen in a developing fetus. *Teratomas with malignant transformation* contain a frankly malignant neoplasm in addition to the fetal or well-differentiated adult tissues that are found in the immature and mature varieties. The most common malignancy is sarcoma, usually angiosarcoma or rhabdomyosarcoma,[165] followed by adenocarcinoma.[166]

The majority of mediastinal teratomas are seen on radiographs as a localized mass in the anterior compartment close to the origin of the major vessels from the heart (Fig. 21–18).[49,160] Occasionally, they are seen in the middle/posterior mediastinum.[167] Calcification is evident in 20% of cases.[167]

On CT, mature teratomas can have smooth or lobulated margins and typically contain one or more cystic areas.[160,167] Areas of fat attenuation are evident in approximately 65% of cases and foci of calcification in 40% (Fig. 21–19).[167] Although soft tissue attenuation is present in all mature cystic teratomas, it is the dominant component (occupying more than 50% of the total volume of the mass) in less than 5%.[167] The combination of fat, fluid, and soft tissue allows confident diagnosis in the majority of cases.[159] Similar findings have been described on MR imaging.[167] Complications of teratoma that may be evident on either radiographs or CT include atelectasis and obstructive pneumonitis (as a result of airway

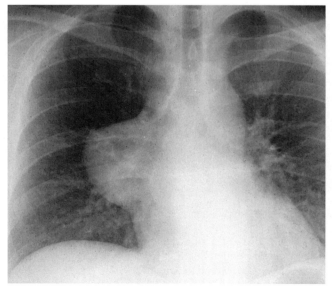

FIGURE 21–18

Mature teratoma. A view of a posteroanterior chest radiograph in a 36-year-old man shows a smoothly marginated mediastinal mass. *(From Fraser RS, Müller NL, Colman NC, Paré PD: Fraser and Paré's Diagnosis of Diseases of the Chest, 4th ed. Philadelphia, WB Saunders, 1999.)*

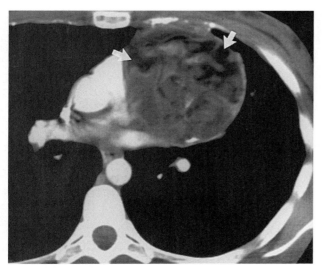

FIGURE 21–19

Mature teratoma. A view of an intravenous contrast–enhanced CT scan in a 29-year-old woman shows a heterogeneous anterior mediastinal mass that contains areas of fat attenuation (*arrows*). *(From Müller NL, Fraser RS, Colman NC, Paré PD: Radiologic Diagnosis of Diseases of the Chest. Philadelphia, WB Saunders, 2001.)*

compression), pneumonitis (after rupture into the lung), and effusion (secondary to rupture into the pleural space or pericardium).[167,168]

Mature teratomas do not usually produce symptoms and are discovered on a screening chest radiograph. Those that grow to large size can cause shortness of breath, cough, and a sensation of pressure or pain in the retrosternal area. Large lesions, particularly the malignant forms, may also obstruct the SVC. Occasionally, a cystic tumor ruptures and spills its contents into the mediastinum or pleural cavity, thereby resulting in mediastinitis, empyema, or fistula formation with a mediastinal vessel, airway, or esophagus.[169,170] The pathogenesis of cyst rupture may be related to infection or erosion by locally produced pancreatic enzymes.

Mature teratomas are benign tumors; provided that they are completely excised, cure is the rule. Thorough pathologic sampling, however, must be carried out to ensure that small foci of immature tissue, other germ cell tumors, or carcinoma or sarcoma is not present. Immature teratomas that develop in adults and teratomas with malignant transformation are usually aggressive and cause death within a few months of diagnosis as a result of local spread and/or metastases.[146,150]

Seminoma

Seminoma is the most frequent mediastinal germ cell neoplasm after teratoma and is the most common form of histologically pure malignant tumor.[171] The tumor occurs almost exclusively in men; most patients are in their twenties or thirties. The majority are solid; occasionally, there is prominent multilocular cystic change.[80] Histologically, the tumor is composed of nests of clear cells separated by a variably thick fibrovascular stroma that contains numerous lymphocytes and (often) loosely formed, non-necrotizing granulomas.

Radiographically, seminomas usually appear as large masses that project into one or both sides of the anterior

mediastinum.[160] They typically have homogeneous attenuation on CT and enhance only slightly after the intravenous administration of contrast material. Occasionally, a few localized areas of low attenuation or ringlike and stippled foci of calcification are seen.[160,172] Evidence of invasion of adjacent structures is seldom apparent.[49,172]

Approximately 20% to 30% of patients are asymptomatic at the time of initial diagnosis. Symptoms generally derive from pressure on or invasion of mediastinal vessels or the major airways and include chest pain and shortness of breath.[171] SVC obstruction develops in about 10% of patients. Pure seminomas are radiosensitive, and the overall 5-year survival rate is in the range of 60% to 80%.[146]

Primary Mediastinal Lymphoma

Lymphoma is one of the most common causes of mediastinal abnormality (see page 388); it has been estimated that it accounts for about 20% of all mediastinal neoplasms in adults and 50% in children.[173] Most often, such involvement occurs in association with clinical or radiologic evidence of extrathoracic lymphoma; in about 5% of cases, the mediastinum is the sole site of abnormality,[174] in which case differentiation from other mediastinal abnormalities can be difficult on the basis of radiologic findings alone. The most common causes of such primary disease are Hodgkin's lymphoma, diffuse large cell lymphoma, and lymphoblastic lymphoma. Many of these tumors appear to originate in the thymus.

Thyroid Tumors

Although extension of thyroid tissue into the thorax is seen in only a small percentage of patients subjected to thyroidectomy, such tissue nevertheless constitutes a significant percentage of anterior mediastinal masses. The most frequent pathologic finding is multinodular goiter, a condition that occurs most commonly in women in their forties[175]; occasionally, the abnormality is thyroiditis or thyroid carcinoma.[176,177]

Seventy-five percent to 80% of mediastinal thyroid tumors arise from a lower pole or the isthmus and extend into the anterior or middle mediastinum. Most of the remainder arise from the posterior aspect of either thyroid lobe and extend into the posterior aspect of the mediastinum behind the trachea, innominate or brachiocephalic vein, and innominate or subclavian arteries[178]; in the last-mentioned location, they are situated almost exclusively on the right. Radiographically, the appearance is that of a sharply defined, smooth or lobulated mass that causes displacement and narrowing of the trachea (Fig. 21–20).[179] Anterior and middle mediastinal goiters displace the trachea posteriorly and laterally, whereas those in the posterior mediastinum displace it anteriorly.

Characteristic features on CT include continuity with the cervical thyroid and focal calcification (Fig. 21–21).[180] The attenuation value of the intrathoracic thyroid is often greater than 100 Hounsfield units before the administration of contrast material; because the gland concentrates iodine, it enhances intensely and for a prolonged period (more than 2 minutes) after intravenous injection. Focal nonenhancing areas of low attenuation as a result of hemorrhage or cyst formation are common.[179] Distinction between thyroid carcinoma and a goiter can be made on CT when there is evidence

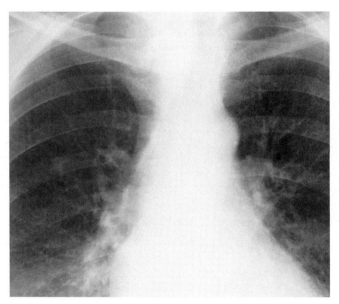

FIGURE 21–20

Retrosternal multinodular goiter. A view from a posteroanterior chest radiograph in a 64-year-old woman demonstrates extrinsic compression and smooth displacement of the trachea by a soft tissue mass extending from the lower part of the neck into the thoracic inlet. *(From Fraser RS, Müller NL, Colman NC, Paré PD: Fraser and Paré's Diagnosis of Diseases of the Chest, 4th ed. Philadelphia, WB Saunders, 1999.)*

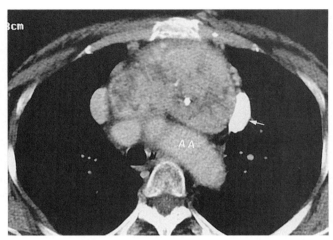

FIGURE 21–21

Multinodular goiter. A CT scan performed during intravenous administration of contrast demonstrates a large anterior mediastinal mass that has inhomogeneous attenuation and contains small foci of calcification. The mass lies anterior to the aortic arch (AA) and innominate artery and is displacing the left brachiocephalic vein *(arrow)*. The patient was a 67-year-old woman with long-standing multinodular goiter. *(From Fraser RS, Müller NL, Colman NC, Paré PD: Fraser and Paré's Diagnosis of Diseases of the Chest, 4th ed. Philadelphia, WB Saunders, 1999.)*

of spread into the adjacent tissue or lymph node enlargement.[181,182] In many cases, however, the borders of a carcinoma are well defined.[181] Localized areas of low attenuation and foci of calcification can be seen in both benign and malignant masses.

Although MR imaging can also demonstrate the extent of intrathoracic thyroid tissue and its relationship to adjacent structures,[183] because of its low sensitivity in the detection of calcification and its high cost, it has a limited role, if any, in assessment. The vast majority of intrathoracic goiters show evidence of function on radionuclide imaging.[184]

Many patients who have an intrathoracic goiter are asymptomatic,[175] the abnormality being discovered on a screening chest radiograph. Symptoms include respiratory distress (which can be worsened by certain movements of the neck) and hoarseness. Posterior mediastinal goiters can cause dysphagia, whereas those in the anterior and middle compartment can cause SVC syndrome as a result of obstruction of brachiocephalic vessels.[145] Physical examination usually reveals evidence of a goiter in the neck; inspiratory and expiratory stridor may be apparent.

Soft Tissue Tumors and Tumor-like Conditions

Although most specific types of soft tissue tumor are rare in the mediastinum, overall they account for about 5% of all masses in this site. They include benign and malignant neoplasms of fat, fibrous tissue, smooth and striated muscle, blood and lymphatic vessels, bone, and neural tissue.[185] In addition, several developmental and acquired abnormalities composed predominantly of mesenchymal tissue (such as hemangioma and lipomatosis) can be manifested as mediastinal masses. Each of these abnormalities can occur in any mediastinal compartment; however, tumors of neural tissue are most common in the paravertebral region (see page 888), whereas most of the others are most frequently located anteriorly.

Lipoma

Extrathymic lipoma is probably the most common non-neurogenic mesenchymal tumor that occurs in the mediastinum; in a series of 396 mediastinal neoplasms, it constituted 2.3% of the total.[186] Certain radiographic findings aid in diagnosis. Because the density of fat is lower than that of other soft tissues, the radiographic density of lipomas is often—albeit not always—less than that of other mediastinal masses. This is particularly true if the mass happens to be surrounded by mediastinal tissue of unit density (Fig. 21–22).[187] In some patients the mass has an hourglass configuration, with part of the lesion being in either the neck or the chest wall.[188,189] CT is usually diagnostic, the characteristic finding consisting of a mass that has homogeneous fat attenuation.[190] The presence of heterogeneous attenuation with soft tissue components should raise the possibility of a liposarcoma. Perhaps because of their pliability, mediastinal lipomas do not usually cause symptoms, even when massive.[186] Surgical excision is curative in virtually all cases.

Lipomatosis

Lipomatosis is a non-neoplastic abnormality of mediastinal adipose tissue characterized by excessive accumulation of fat in its normal locations. It is seen most commonly in conditions associated with hypercortisolism, such as Cushing's syndrome, ectopic adrenocorticotropic hormone syndrome, and long-term corticosteroid therapy.[191] The abnormality has also

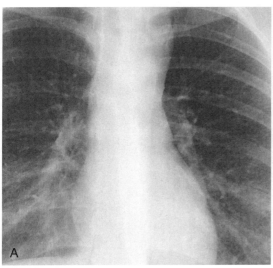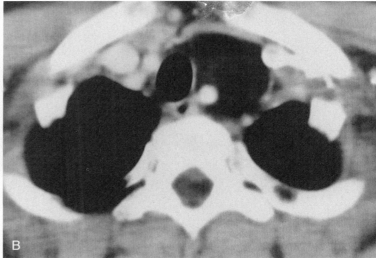

FIGURE 21–22

Mediastinal lipoma. A posteroanterior chest radiograph (**A**) in a 23-year-old asymptomatic woman shows widening of the left upper mediastinum. Note that the abnormality has lower opacity than the aortic arch, the contour of which is not obscured by the mass. A CT scan performed during intravenous administration of contrast (**B**) shows a smoothly marginated mass with homogeneous fat density in the thoracic inlet. *(From Fraser RS, Müller NL, Colman NC, Paré PD: Fraser and Paré's Diagnosis of Diseases of the Chest, 4th ed. Philadelphia, WB Saunders, 1999.)*

been described in obese individuals not receiving corticosteroid therapy.[192] Typically, patients do not have symptoms from the fat deposits.

Radiologically, mediastinal widening tends to be smooth and symmetrical, although the margins can be lobulated if the accumulation is large (Fig. 21–23). The widening usually extends from the thoracic inlet to the hila bilaterally; occasionally, the accumulation is predominantly paraspinal and symmetrical.[193] Increasing size of the pleuropericardial fat pads may be evident on serial radiographs.[194] In cases in which conventional radiographs are inconclusive, CT is invariably diagnostic.[191]

Hemangioma

Hemangiomas are uncommon mediastinal tumors.[195,196] The majority, if not all, probably represent developmental malformation rather than true neoplasm. They can be an isolated abnormality or can occur as part of a multifocal hemangiomatous malformation affecting several organs (Osler-Weber-Rendu syndrome).[197] Pathologically, they are often encapsulated or well circumscribed and can be composed of thin-walled or thick-walled vessels of large, small, or mixed size.

Radiographically, hemangiomas tend to be smooth in outline but are sometimes lobulated. Most are located in the upper portion of the anterior mediastinum.[198] Phleboliths can be identified in approximately 10% of cases and can be considered a virtually diagnostic sign.[198] Findings highly suggestive of the diagnosis on CT include the presence of phleboliths, predominantly central enhancement, and prolonged enhancement after intravenous contrast.[133,198]

Most tumors are discovered in young individuals.[199] Many patients are symptomatic at initial evaluation, the chief complaints being chest pain and dyspnea. The prognosis is good, even for tumors that are incompletely excised.[196]

Lymphangioma

Mediastinal lymphangiomas have two clinicopathologic forms: (1) a variety that extends from the neck into the mediastinum and usually occurs in infants (cystic hygroma) and (2) a more or less well circumscribed variety that is usually discovered in adults and is located in the lower anterior (occasionally middle posterior) mediastinum remote from the neck.[200] As with hemangiomas, they probably represent developmental anomalies rather than true neoplasms. Pathologically, the lesions consist of thin-walled, usually multilocular cysts containing numerous thin-walled vascular spaces lined by endothelial cells.

The radiographic findings are nonspecific and consist of a sharply defined, smoothly marginated mediastinal mass that frequently displaces adjacent mediastinal structures.[201] In an investigation of 19 adult patients, 7 tumors (37%) were located in the anterior mediastinum, 5 (26%) in the middle mediastinum, 3 (16%) in the posterior mediastinum, 3 (16%) in the thoracic inlet, and 1 in the lung.[202] The most common CT appearance consists of a smoothly marginated cystic mass with homogeneous water density that can either displace or surround adjacent vessels (Fig. 21–24).[203] Multiple loculations can be seen in approximately a third of cases. Hemorrhage results in an increase in size of the mass and an increase in attenuation values.[203]

Because of their soft consistency, lymphangiomas seldom cause symptoms, even when large.

Tumors Situated in the Anterior Cardiophrenic Angle

Although masses in the vicinity of the cardiophrenic angle on either side originate in the middle mediastinum, they project into the anterior compartment and are thus discussed at this

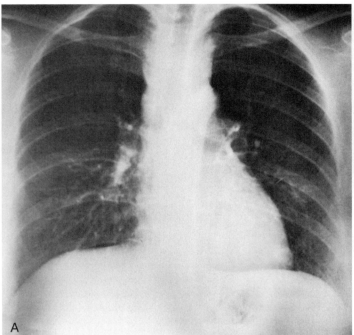
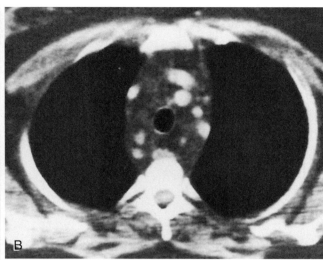

FIGURE 21–23

Mediastinal lipomatosis. A posteroanterior radiograph (**A**) reveals widening of the upper mediastinum to an equal extent on both sides. The contour is smooth. No other abnormalities are apparent other than thickening of the bronchial walls consistent with chronic bronchitis. A CT scan at the level of the left brachiocephalic vein (**B**) demonstrates wide separation of vessels as a result of an accumulation of a large amount of fat. This 58-year-old woman was not receiving any therapy, nor did she have any underlying condition to which the lipomatosis could be attributed; she was simply obese. The widened mediastinum returned to normal after a 40-lb weight loss. *(From Fraser RS, Müller NL, Colman NC, Paré PD: Fraser and Paré's Diagnosis of Diseases of the Chest, 4th ed. Philadelphia, WB Saunders, 1999.)*

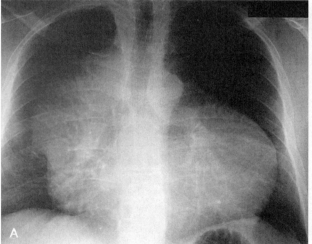
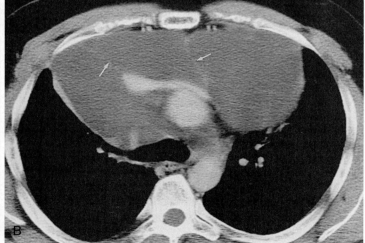

FIGURE 21–24

Lymphangioma. A posteroanterior chest radiograph (**A**) in a 37-year-old man shows diffuse mediastinal widening. A contrast-enhanced CT scan (**B**) demonstrates a predominantly anterior mediastinal cystic mass. The mass has homogeneous water attenuation and contains a few soft tissue septations (*arrows*). *(From Fraser RS, Müller NL, Colman NC, Paré PD: Fraser and Paré's Diagnosis of Diseases of the Chest, 4th ed. Philadelphia, WB Saunders, 1999.)*

point. The differential diagnosis of such masses is extensive and includes lesions arising in the lung parenchyma, in the visceral or parietal pleura, in the pericardium or contiguous myocardium, and in or beneath the diaphragm. Even though lesions arising in any of these structures usually produce similar radiographic findings, specific diagnoses can often be made on CT.[159,181] Only three are considered at this point—pleuropericardial fat, mesothelial cysts, and enlargement of diaphragmatic lymph nodes. Although hernia through the foramina of Morgagni appears radiographically as a homogeneous shadow generally indistinguishable from a large pleuropericardial fat pad, for convenience these lesions are discussed in Chapter 22 (see page 900).

Pleuropericardial Fat

Accumulations of fat that normally occupy the cardiophrenic angles can attain considerable size. Although such pleuropericardial fat pads are always bilateral, they may be asymmetrical. They can enlarge substantially over time as a result of either obesity or hyperadrenocorticism (e.g., Cushing's syndrome); hence, they can cause a potentially confusing radiographic opacity. The diagnosis can be made readily with CT or MR imaging.[204] Affected patients are typically obese.

Mesothelial (Pericardial) Cysts

The vast majority of mesothelial cysts are congenital and result from aberrations in formation of the coelomic cavities. Although they may be seen anywhere in the mediastinum (see Color Fig. 21–6), they are particularly common in the vicinity of the heart. They are spherical or oval, thin walled, and often translucent; most are unilocular and contain clear or straw-colored fluid.[143] Histologically, the cyst wall is composed of a thin layer of fibrous tissue lined by a single layer of flattened or cuboidal cells resembling mesothelial cells.

Radiographically, the majority of mesothelial cysts are located in the cardiophrenic angles, most commonly on the right side (Fig. 21–25).[205,206] Typically, they are smooth and round or oval. Most are between 3 and 8 cm in diameter. The benign cystic nature of these masses can usually be confirmed by CT, MR imaging, or echocardiography.[206,207] The characteristic CT appearance consists of a water-density, smooth, round, or oval cystic lesion abutting the pericardium. Occasional cysts have soft tissue attenuation, presumably as a result of the presence of viscous material[208]; such lesions cannot be reliably distinguished from a neoplasm. Cysts typically have low echogenicity and increased through-transmission on echocardiography.

Symptoms are almost invariably absent, most cysts being discovered on a screening chest radiograph. Occasionally, a large cyst gives rise to a sensation of retrosternal pressure or dyspnea.[209]

Enlargement of Diaphragmatic Lymph Nodes

The superior diaphragmatic lymph nodes are distributed in three clusters: anterior (prepericardiac), middle (lateral pericardiac), and posterior.[210,211] They can be affected by tumors arising above the diaphragm—most commonly lymphoma and less commonly carcinoma of the breast and lung—or by tumors arising below the diaphragm, particularly carcinoma of the colon and ovary.[212]

Normally, the nodes are not visible on chest radiographs because of their small size and their investment with fat and other connective tissue adjacent to the pleura. When enlarged, they displace the pleura laterally and produce a smooth or lobulated mass projecting out of the cardiophrenic angle, an appearance that can simulate pleuropericardial fat pads. Although such enlargement may be apparent on conventional radiographs, CT is a superior method of assessment.[211,213]

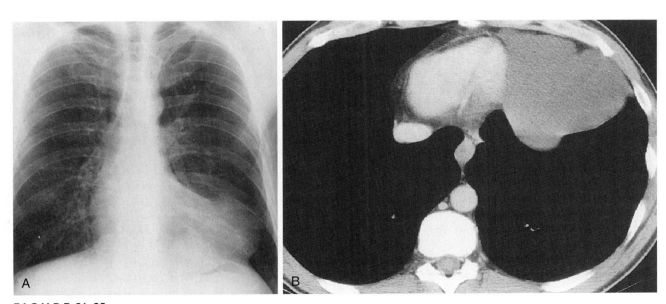

FIGURE 21–25

Mesothelial cyst. A posteroanterior chest radiograph (**A**) in a 46-year-old man demonstrates smoothly marginated increased opacity in the left cardiophrenic angle. A contrast-enhanced CT scan (**B**) demonstrates a water-density cyst. *(From Fraser RS, Müller NL, Colman NC, Paré PD: Fraser and Paré's Diagnosis of Diseases of the Chest, 4th ed. Philadelphia, WB Saunders, 1999.)*

Masses Situated Predominantly in the Middle-Posterior Mediastinum

The most common abnormalities of this region are lymph node enlargement and aortic aneurysms[50]; tracheal carcinoma, esophageal lesions, and congenital cysts are less frequent, and most other lesions are rare.

Lymph Node Enlargement

Lymph node enlargement is the most common abnormality of the middle-posterior mediastinum. It is caused most often by lymphoma, metastatic carcinoma, sarcoidosis, and infection (either directly by organisms such as *H. capsulatum* and *M. tuberculosis* or as a hyperplastic reaction to the presence of organisms within the lungs). Most of these and other less common conditions are discussed elsewhere in this book; only giant lymph node hyperplasia (Castleman's disease) and granulomatous lymphadenitis are considered here.

The clinicopathologic effects of enlarged lymph nodes in the middle-posterior mediastinum are usually minimal or absent altogether. However, because of their intimate association with the airways and vessels that course through this region, stenosis or obstruction may ensue and result in signs and symptoms, sometimes associated with life-threatening consequences.

Giant Lymph Node Hyperplasia (Castleman's Disease)

Giant lymph node hyperplasia (Castleman's disease) is an uncommon lymphoproliferative disorder that has several clinicopathologic variants.[214] The *hyaline vascular type* is the more common and is characterized histologically by enlarged lymph nodes that contain numerous germinal centers interspersed in a population of mononuclear cells (predominantly lymphocytes) and prominent capillaries (Fig. 21–26); some of the capillaries have thickened, hyalinized walls and extend into the germinal centers themselves. This form of disease is usually unassociated with symptoms and is manifested as a mass in the mediastinum or hilum on the chest radiograph. The second variant, the *plasma cell type*, is characterized histologically by the presence of numerous plasma cells between the germinal centers and relatively few capillaries. Patients usually have systemic manifestations of disease, most often nonspecific findings such as fever, anemia, weight loss, and hypergammaglobulinemia.

In many patients, the lesions of both these histologic forms appear to be confined predominantly or entirely to the mediastinum. Such disease tends to occur in young adults and is associated with a good prognosis after surgical excision; systemic manifestations associated with the plasma cell variant usually resolve, and there is typically no tendency to recurrence or the development of new disease. Other patients, however, have multifocal disease that tends to affect superficial lymph node groups with or without involvement of the mediastinum. Such "multicentric Castleman's disease" often affects persons older than those who have isolated Castleman's disease and is frequently associated with evidence of systemic disease such as hepatosplenomegaly, anemia, hypergammaglobulinemia, rash, and renal and central nervous system abnormalities.[215,216] The condition appears to represent an unusual histologic reaction to a number of agents rather than a specific entity[207]; for example, some patients are HIV positive or have Kaposi's sarcoma, in which case evidence of infection by herpesvirus 8 is not uncommon.[217] The prognosis of

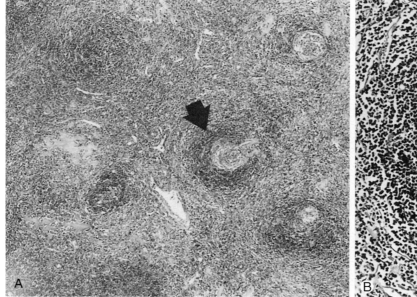
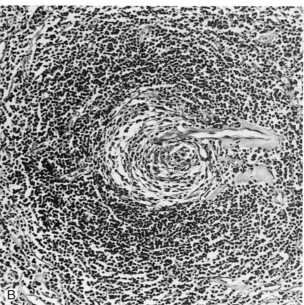

FIGURE 21–26

Giant lymph node hyperplasia (Castleman's disease). A section from a large mediastinal mass (**A**) reveals an infiltrate of lymphoid cells admixed with numerous vessels and several germinal centers (*arrow*). A magnified view of one germinal center (**B**) shows a small vessel with a thickened wall extending into its midportion. (*From Fraser RS, Müller NL, Colman NC, Paré PD: Fraser and Paré's Diagnosis of Diseases of the Chest, 4th ed. Philadelphia, WB Saunders, 1999.*)

the multicentric variant of giant lymph node hyperplasia is distinctly poorer than that of the solitary form; in many patients, there is progression of the lymphoid proliferation, the development of serious infectious complications, or evolution to frank lymphoma.

The radiographic appearance of the localized form of disease is that of a solitary, smooth or lobulated mass situated most commonly in the left or right hilum or middle-posterior mediastinum (Fig. 21–27).[218] In multicentric disease, the lymphadenopathy often involves multiple mediastinal compartments.[219] Multicentric disease can be associated with pulmonary parenchymal involvement.[219] The enlarged nodes typically show marked homogeneous enhancement after the intravenous administration of contrast; such enhancement is less marked in the plasma cell type than in the hyaline vascular type of disease. Focal calcification can be seen.

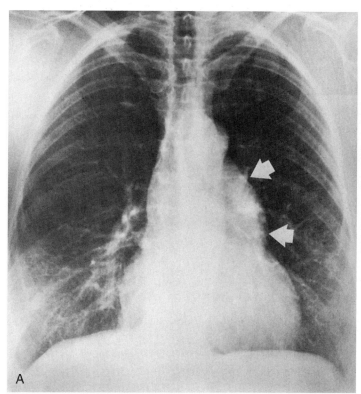

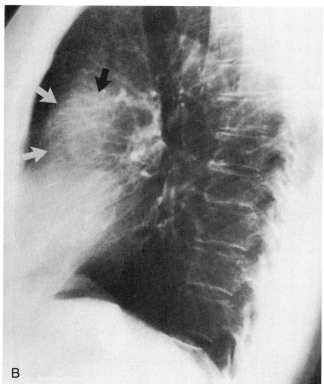

FIGURE 21–27

Giant lymph node hyperplasia (Castleman's disease). Posteroanterior (**A**) and lateral (**B**) radiographs reveal a well-defined opacity protruding to the left from the region of the main pulmonary artery (*arrows* in **A**). In the lateral projection, an ill-defined opacity can be identified in the anterior mediastinum (*arrows*). A CT scan at the level of the main pulmonary artery (**C**) reveals a well-defined, homogeneous mass (*arrows*) contiguous with the left side of the mediastinum and protruding into the left hemithorax. The patient was a 63-year-old woman who had no symptoms referable to her chest. (*From Fraser RS, Müller NL, Colman NC, Paré PD: Fraser and Paré's Diagnosis of Diseases of the Chest, 4th ed. Philadelphia, WB Saunders, 1999.*)

Granulomatous Lymphadenitis

The term *granulomatous lymphadenitis* refers mainly to chronic disease attributable to infection, such as tuberculosis or histoplasmosis, or to sarcoidosis. In both forms, paratracheal and tracheobronchial lymph node enlargement may be the predominant finding. In infectious disease, node enlargement tends to be predominantly unilateral, whereas in sarcoidosis, it tends to be bilateral and symmetrical; in contrast to lymphoma, the latter is almost invariably associated with bronchopulmonary node enlargement.

The presence of granulomatous inflammation of the middle-posterior mediastinal lymph nodes does not by itself result in untoward effects in most cases. Occasionally, infection spreads outside the nodal capsule into adjacent tissue; in some cases, such spread results in localized or diffuse acute mediastinitis or in fibrosing mediastinitis (see page 850). Involvement of the posterior mediastinal lymph nodes can also be associated with local effects on the esophagus, including traction diverticula and esophagobronchial fistula.

Tumors and Cysts

Primary Tracheal Neoplasms

Carcinoma that arises in the trachea or main bronchi just distal to the carina may extend outward into the paratracheal space and cause widening of the mediastinum to either or both sides. An irregular, shaggy mass is also usually evident within the tracheal air column on standard radiographs or CT scans (Fig. 21–28).

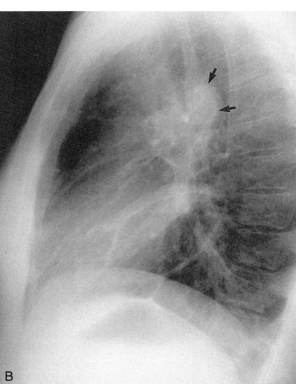

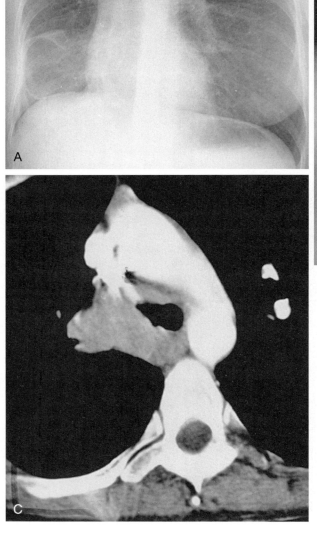

FIGURE 21–28

Middle/posterior mediastinal mass—adenoid cystic carcinoma.
Posteroanterior (**A**) and lateral (**B**) chest radiographs from a 27-year-old man demonstrate a mass posterior to the lower part of the trachea (*arrows*) associated with thickening of the posterior wall of the distal portion of the trachea and right bronchus. Foci of atelectasis in the right middle and lower lobes are also evident. A contrast-enhanced CT scan (**C**) demonstrates circumferential tumor at the level of the tracheal carina. *(From Fraser RS, Müller NL, Colman NC, Paré PD: Fraser and Paré's Diagnosis of Diseases of the Chest, 4th ed. Philadelphia, WB Saunders, 1999.)*

Symptoms include cough, hemoptysis, and (sometimes) severe dyspnea and wheezing; stridor may be apparent.

Paraganglioma

Paragangliomas (chemodectomas) arise from small macroscopic or microscopic collections of neuroendocrine cells (paraganglia) in intimate association with the autonomic nervous system. In the thorax, they generally occur in one of two locations:[220] (1) the perivascular adventitial tissue bounded by the aorta superiorly, the pulmonary artery inferiorly, and the ligamentum arteriosum and right pulmonary artery on each side (aorticopulmonary paragangliomas)[221] and (2) in association with the segmental ganglia of the sympathetic chain in the paravertebral region adjacent to the posterior aspects of the ribs (paravertebral paragangliomas; see page 889). The mean age at the time of diagnosis of tumors in the former site is about 45 to 50 years, and there is a slight female preponderance.[222] They can be manifested grossly as discrete, encapsulated nodules or as poorly circumscribed growths that encompass adjacent vascular structures.[223] Histologic features consist of nests of clear cells separated by a prominent fibrovascular stroma. The cells have minimal cytologic atypia and show evidence of neuroendocrine differentiation.

The radiographic features of aorticopulmonary paragangliomas are those of a mass in the mediastinum in close relation to the base of the heart and aortic arch.[222] Some tumors are located in the subcarinal region or extend into the paratracheal soft tissue (Fig. 21–29). CT demonstrates a soft tissue mass that can have homogeneous attenuation or can contain large central areas of low attenuation as a result of necrosis.[224,225] The mass usually shows marked enhancement after the intravenous administration of contrast.[226] Scintigraphy is the imaging modality of choice to confirm the diagnosis.[227] The vast majority of tumors show abnormal uptake on [131]I- or ^{123}I-metaiodobenzylguanidine (MIBG) or ^{111}In-octreotide scintigraphy.[228,229] The main role of contrast-enhanced CT or MR imaging is in providing detailed assessment of the extent of tumor and its relationship to adjacent structures before surgical resection.[226]

Clinically, most aorticopulmonary paragangliomas do not induce symptoms and are discovered on a screening chest radiograph; sometimes, they compress or invade local structures and cause cough, hoarseness, dysphagia, or the SVC syndrome. Some patients, invariably young women, have a gastric stromal neoplasm and pulmonary chondromas (Carney's triad; see page 397). The prognosis is guarded. Because of their location and vascularity, operative mortality is significant. Moreover, complete excision frequently cannot be achieved, and the local recurrence rate is high.[221] Nonetheless, the growth rate may be slow, and survival for years after partial excision is possible.

Bronchogenic Cyst

Although congenital mediastinal bronchogenic cysts can occur anywhere in the mediastinum, the majority are located in the paratracheal or subcarinal region (see page 194).[50,230] They are usually discovered in childhood or early adult life but can be seen as an incidental finding at autopsy in elderly persons. They may grow very large without inducing symptoms.

Esophageal Cyst

Esophageal cysts (esophageal duplication cysts) have been hypothesized to result from either abnormal budding of the foregut or failure of complete vacuolation of the originally solid esophagus to produce a hollow tube.[231] The cysts are lined by nonkeratinizing squamous or ciliated columnar epithelium. A double layer of smooth muscle in their walls and a lack of cartilage are necessary findings to exclude a diagnosis of bronchogenic cyst; however, distinction between the two may be difficult, and the relatively noncommittal term *simple cyst* is sometimes the best designation.

The cysts are usually located within or adjacent to the wall of the esophagus. The CT findings consist of a round mass of homogeneous water density or soft tissue density that does not enhance after the intravenous administration of contrast (Fig. 21–30).[232] On MR studies, the cysts can have low or high signal intensity on T1-weighted images but characteristically have very high signal intensity on T2-weighted images.[233] Transesophageal ultrasonography has been used successfully for diagnosis.[234]

Most patients are asymptomatic, the abnormality sometimes being discovered incidentally at an advanced age. Occasionally, esophageal compression is manifested by dysphagia and airway impingement by chronic cough.[231,235]

Vascular Abnormalities

Dilation of the Main Pulmonary Artery

Dilation of the main pulmonary artery may be of sufficient degree to suggest a mediastinal mass. The great majority of cases are associated with either pulmonary arterial hypertension or a left-to-right shunt. On the posteroanterior chest

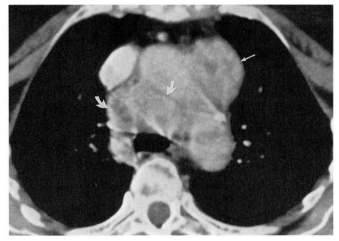

FIGURE 21–29

Aorticopulmonary paraganglioma. A contrast-enhanced CT scan demonstrates an inhomogeneous soft tissue mass involving the aortopulmonary window (*straight arrow*) and paratracheal region (*curved arrows*). The patient was a 68-year-old woman. (*From Fraser RS, Müller NL, Colman NC, Paré PD: Fraser and Paré's Diagnosis of Diseases of the Chest, 4th ed. Philadelphia, WB Saunders, 1999.*)

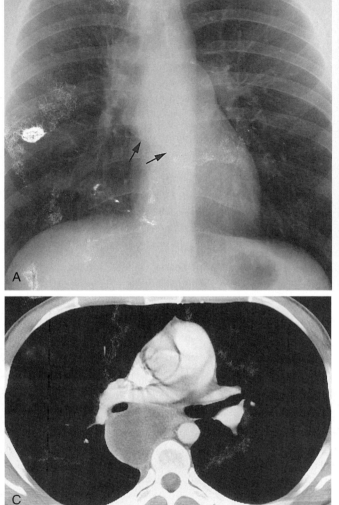

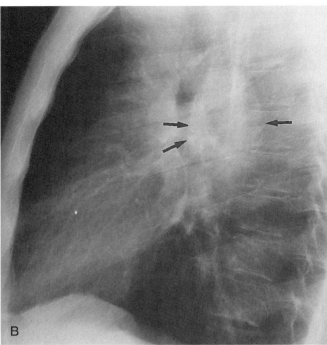

FIGURE 21–30

Esophageal cyst. A posteroanterior chest radiograph (**A**) from a 22-year-old man shows a subcarinal mass displacing the azygoesophageal recess interface (*arrows*). A lateral radiograph (**B**) shows the mass posterior to the bronchus intermedius (*arrows*). A CT scan obtained after the intravenous administration of contrast (**C**) demonstrates a nonenhancing cystic mass adjacent to the esophagus. (*From Fraser RS, Müller NL, Colman NC, Paré PD: Fraser and Paré's Diagnosis of Diseases of the Chest, 4th ed. Philadelphia, WB Saunders, 1999.*)

radiograph, the abnormality is seen as a focal convexity caudal to the aortic arch and cephalic to the left main bronchus (Fig. 21–31). It is usually accompanied by dilation of the pulmonary trunk and enlargement of the right ventricle, findings that are most readily apparent on the lateral radiograph.

The dilation is usually unassociated with symptoms or evidence of hemodynamic abnormality on radiologic examination or during cardiac catheterization. Physical examination of a patient who has a severe degree of dilation may reveal a widely split second heart sound that varies little with respiration.[236]

Dilation of the Superior and Inferior Vena Cava

The great majority of cases of dilation of the SVC are the result of raised central venous pressure, most commonly from cardiac decompensation. The radiographic appearance is distinctive and consists of a smooth, well-defined widening of the right side of the mediastinum (Fig. 21–32). The azygos vein is almost always dilated as well; in fact, such dilation is a more dependable sign of systemic venous hypertension because the diameter of the vein in the right tracheobronchial angle can be precisely measured. (The azygos vein can be considered to be dilated if its diameter is greater than 10 mm when the patient is in the erect position or 15 mm when the patient is recumbent.)

Superior Vena Cava Syndrome

SVC syndrome is caused by obstruction to blood flow as a result of external compression, intraluminal thrombosis, or neoplastic infiltration; not infrequently, a combination of all three processes is involved.[237] Most patients have underlying malignancy[238,239]; pulmonary carcinoma is the cause in 80% to 85%, and lymphoma and metastatic carcinoma of nonpulmonary origin in 5% to 10%. Of the pulmonary carcinomas, small cell is the most frequent histologic type.[240] Although precise figures are not available, it is possible that the most

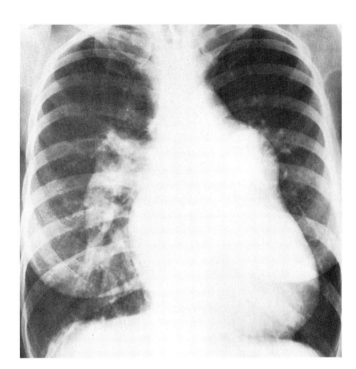

FIGURE 21–31

Dilation of the main pulmonary artery. A posteroanterior chest radiograph shows dilation of the hilar and peripheral pulmonary arteries, indicative of pulmonary pleonemia. The main pulmonary artery is greatly dilated, creating a smooth protuberance of the left border of the cardiovascular silhouette. The patient was known to have a patent ductus arteriosus. (*From Fraser RS, Müller NL, Colman NC, Paré PD: Fraser and Paré's Diagnosis of Diseases of the Chest, 4th ed. Philadelphia, WB Saunders, 1999.*)

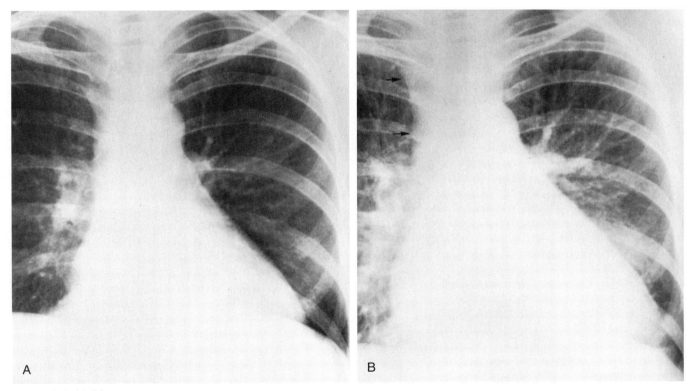

A   B

FIGURE 21–32

Dilation of the superior vena cava. During a remission, the chest radiograph (**A**) of a 35-year-old woman with systemic lupus erythematosus revealed no significant abnormalities. On the occasion of an exacerbation several months later (at which time she had clinical evidence of cardiac decompensation), a chest radiograph (**B**) demonstrated moderate cardiac enlargement (caused predominantly by pericardial effusion) and generalized interstitial pulmonary edema. Note the widening of the superior mediastinum secondary to dilation of the superior vena cava (*arrows*). (*From Fraser RS, Müller NL, Colman NC, Paré PD: Fraser and Paré's Diagnosis of Diseases of the Chest, 4th ed. Philadelphia, WB Saunders, 1999.*)

common benign mechanism causing the syndrome is the insertion of intravenous devices such as cardiac pacemakers and Hickman catheters.[241,242] The pathogenesis of the obstruction in these cases is presumably thrombosis and (after thrombus organization) fibrosis. The most common non-iatrogenic underlying benign disorder is probably fibrosing mediastinitis.[243]

In most cases, the chest radiograph shows a mass widening the mediastinum on the right; a prominent azygos vein may also be evident (Fig. 21–33). In patients in whom vena cava thrombosis develops as a result of indwelling central venous catheters, radiographs commonly show lateral displacement of the catheter.[244] The diagnosis can be confirmed by CT, MR imaging, or venography.[239,245,246] With CT, it is based on decreased or absent opacification of the SVC and the presence of opacification of collateral veins after the intravenous administration of contrast. Both findings need to be present to make a definitive diagnosis because opacification of collateral vessels is seen in about 5% of patients who do not have SVC obstruction.[247]

SVC syndrome is characterized clinically by edema of the face, neck, upper extremities, and thorax, often associated with prominent, dilated chest wall veins. The most common symptoms are dyspnea and a feeling of fullness in the head. In an investigation of patients in whom the syndrome was caused by metastatic pulmonary carcinoma, symptoms were present in about 30% for 1 week or less before diagnosis and in 50% for over 2 weeks.[248] The concept that SVC syndrome represents a medical emergency is no longer generally accepted.[238]

Dilation of the Azygos and Hemiazygos Veins

The most common cause of dilation of these veins is elevated central venous pressure secondary to cardiac decompensation; other causes of elevated right-sided pressure, such as tricuspid stenosis, acute pericardial tamponade, or constrictive pericarditis, are less frequent. The typical radiographic manifestation is a round or oval shadow in the right tracheobronchial angle (see Fig. 21–33) that measures more than 10 mm in diameter on radiographs exposed with the patient in the erect position or more than 15 mm in the supine position. A dilated vein can be differentiated from an enlarged azygos lymph node fairly easily by comparing the diameters of the shadow on radiographs exposed in the erect and supine

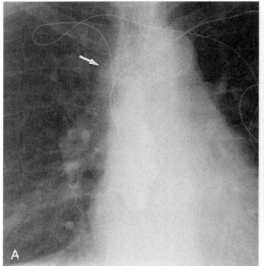

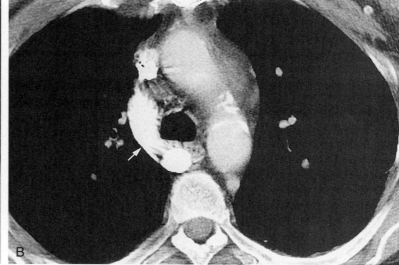

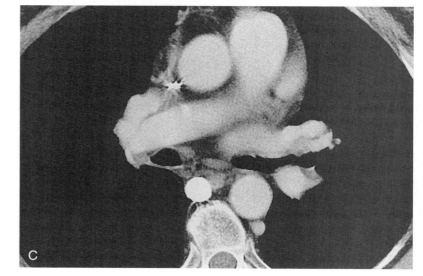

FIGURE 21–33

Superior vena cava syndrome. A 53-year-old woman previously underwent surgery for mitral valve disease. Superior vena cava (SVC) syndrome developed several years after insertion of a cardiac pacemaker and sequential atrial ventricular leads. A close-up view of the chest from a posteroanterior radiograph (**A**) shows dilation of the azygos vein (*arrow*). A contrast-enhanced CT scan (**B**) demonstrates intravenous contrast within the SVC and azygos vein (*arrow*). A CT scan at a more caudal level shows complete obstruction of the SVC with collateral flow through the azygos vein. (The metallic density seen within the SVC in **C** represents the two pacemaker wires.) (*From Fraser RS, Müller NL, Colman NC, Paré PD: Fraser and Paré's Diagnosis of Diseases of the Chest, 4th ed. Philadelphia, WB Saunders, 1999.*)

positions: when the shadow is the vein, there is a noticeable difference in size. Dilation of the posterior portions of the azygos or hemiazygos vein may result in widening and irregularity of the paraspinal line on the right or left side, respectively.[249] The normal anatomy of the azygos and hemiazygos veins and their abnormalities are well visualized by both CT and MR imaging.[250,251]

The symptoms and signs of azygos and hemiazygos vein dilation depend entirely on the cause. Azygos continuation of the inferior vena cava (IVC) is often associated with a congenital cardiac malformation,[252,253] with errors in abdominal situs,[254] or with asplenia or polysplenia.[255] Most patients are asymptomatic; however, some have symptoms or signs attributable to the associated heart disease.

Dilation of the Left Superior Intercostal Vein

Dilation of the left superior intercostal vein has the same causes as those associated with dilation of the azygos vein, although visibility of this vein radiographically is not nearly as frequent as that of the azygos. The normal left superior intercostal vein originates from a confluence of the second, third, and fourth left intercostal veins. As it passes anteriorly from the spine it relates intimately to some portion of the aortic arch and in this location is seen end-on as the "aortic nipple," a local protuberance in the contour of the arch that is identifiable in about 10% of normal individuals.[256] On posteroanterior chest radiographs taken with the patient in an erect position, the maximum normal diameter of the aortic nipple is 4.5 mm.[257] A diameter larger than 4.5 mm is a useful sign of a vascular abnormality, the most common of which are azygos continuation of the IVC, hypoplasia of the left innominate vein, cardiac decompensation, portal hypertension,

Budd-Chiari syndrome, obstruction of the SVC or IVC (Fig. 21–34), and congenital absence of the azygos vein.[257]

Aneurysms of the Thoracic Aorta

The normal diameter of the thoracic aorta is 3.7 ± 0.3 cm at its root, 3.3 ± 0.6 cm in the ascending portion, and 2.4 ± 0.3 cm in the descending portion.[258] An aneurysm is considered to be present when the diameter at any site is 5 cm or more. They can be classified according to the composition of their wall, their location, or their shape. Pathologically, the wall of a true aneurysm is composed of intima, media, and adventitia, whereas that of a false aneurysm (pseudoaneurysm) is composed of fibrous tissue, thrombus, or both.

Most true thoracic aortic aneurysms are the result of atherosclerosis and occur in the descending portion.[259] They are usually fusiform, start immediately distal to the takeoff of the left subclavian artery, and often extend into the abdomen.[260] Such aneurysms are typically seen in elderly persons and are more common in men. Aneurysms of the ascending aorta are less common and can be the result of atherosclerosis, cystic medial degeneration ("cystic medial necrosis"), or rarely, infection (mycotic aneurysm). Cystic medial degeneration is the most common pathologic finding and can be idiopathic or associated with a connective tissue disorder such as Marfan's syndrome or Ehlers-Danlos syndrome.[261] Mycotic aneurysms can occur anywhere; predisposing conditions include bacterial endocarditis, drug abuse, and immunosuppression.[261] False aneurysms are most often the result of blunt trauma; occasionally, they follow penetrating trauma or iatrogenic injury. Typically, they are eccentric or saccular in shape and are located in the proximal descending thoracic aorta just beyond the origin of the left subclavian artery.[262,263]

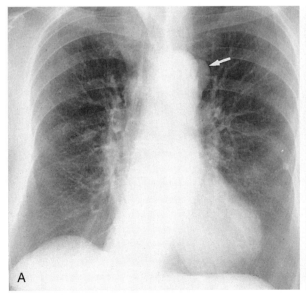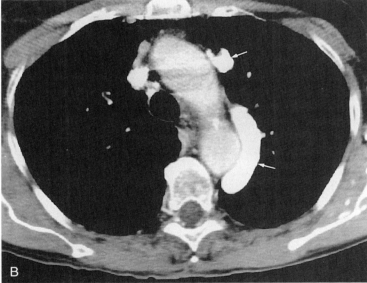

FIGURE 21–34

Enlarged left superior intercostal vein. A posteroanterior chest radiograph (**A**) demonstrates a prominent aortic nipple (*arrow*). (Incidental note is made of a calcified granuloma in the left lung.) A contrast-enhanced CT scan (**B**) demonstrates a dilated left superior intercostal vein (*arrows*) as a result of collateral blood flow from the left brachiocephalic vein into the hemiazygos and azygos veins. Also note collateral blood flow in the left axilla. The patient was a 77-year-old woman who had long-standing superior vena cava obstruction related to fibrosing mediastinitis (presumed to be due to histoplasmosis). Note the calcified paratracheal lymph nodes. (*From Fraser RS, Müller NL, Colman NC, Paré PD: Fraser and Paré's Diagnosis of Diseases of the Chest, 4th ed. Philadelphia, WB Saunders, 1999.*)

On the chest radiograph, aneurysms of the ascending aorta and proximal aortic arch usually project anteriorly and to the right (Fig. 21–35), whereas those of the distal arch and descending aorta project posteriorly and to the left (Fig. 21–36). In fact, aortic aneurysms should be considered in the differential diagnosis for any abnormal opacity that is contiguous with any part of the aorta. Calcification of the aneurysm wall is relatively common.

The diagnosis can be confirmed by CT, MR imaging, transesophageal echocardiography, or angiography.[264-266] Contrast-enhanced CT is currently the most commonly used technique (Fig. 21–37). It allows accurate assessment of the presence and extent of the aneurysm, its relationship to adjacent structures, and the presence of complications such as compression of the trachea, bronchi, pulmonary arteries or veins, or SVC.[261] Foci of intimal calcification are seen on CT scans in approximately 75% of cases. Mural thrombus is also frequently evident, particularly in patients who have large aneurysms (see Fig. 21–37).

Many patients are asymptomatic. When present, clinical manifestations depend on the size and location of the aneurysm. Symptoms caused by aneurysms of the transverse arch are particularly notable and result from compression of the SVC, recurrent laryngeal nerve, or tracheobronchial tree. They include a brassy cough, hemoptysis, and hoarseness. Aneurysms of the descending aorta may cause bone erosion leading to severe pain; they can also cause dysphagia as a result of esophageal compression.

Aortic Dissection

Aortic dissection occurs when blood collects in the media and divides it into two distinct layers. In the majority of patients, the primary event is an intimal tear.[267,268] Because it is under high pressure, the blood cleaves a channel in the media, which results in the formation of a false lumen for blood flow, in addition to the true aortic lumen. Such dissection can proceed proximally into the perivalvular region and lead to aortic insufficiency or into the pericardial sac and cause tamponade[269,270] and can proceed distally to occlude the branches of the aortic arch.[269] The most widely accepted classification is the Stanford classification system, which designates dissections involving the ascending aorta as type A, regardless of the distal extension of the dissection, and all other dissections as type B. Depending on the series, about 55% to 90% of cases are type A.[271,272]

Aortic dissection is seen most commonly in patients who have systemic arterial hypertension or Marfan's syndrome; less common causes include Ehlers-Danlos syndrome, aortitis, and vascular catheterization.[269,273] In many cases, cystic medial degeneration is evident in the aortic wall. Because most patients are older, atherosclerosis is often present; however, it is more likely to be a coincidental finding than a significant contributing factor in the dissection.

The most common radiographic manifestations are widening of the superior mediastinum and aorta (Fig. 21–38), a double contour of the aortic arch, an increase in size of the aorta or change in its configuration on serial chest radi-

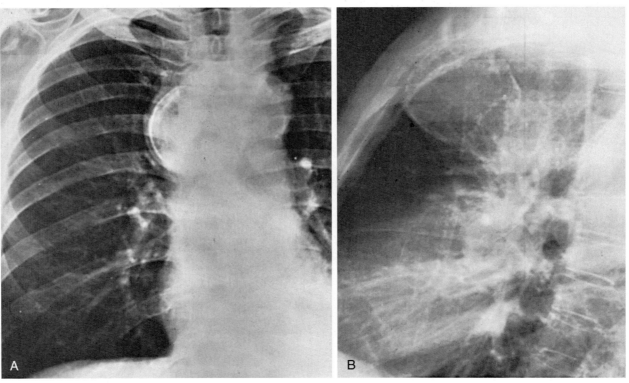

FIGURE 21–35

Saccular aneurysm of the ascending thoracic aorta. Posteroanterior (**A**) and lateral (**B**) radiographs from a 52-year-old asymptomatic man reveal a well-circumscribed mass projecting anteriorly and to the right. Its wall is densely calcified. *(From Fraser RS, Müller NL, Colman NC, Paré PD: Fraser and Paré's Diagnosis of Diseases of the Chest, 4th ed. Philadelphia, WB Saunders, 1999.)*

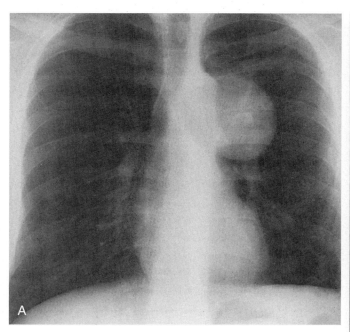

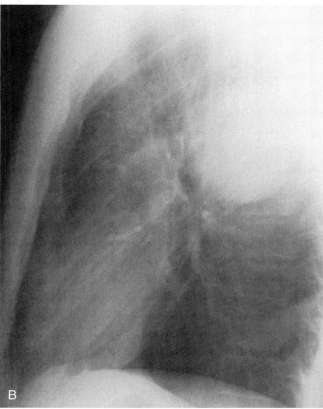

FIGURE 21–36

Mycotic aneurysm of the proximal descending thoracic aorta. Posteroanterior (**A**) and lateral (**B**) radiographs from a 22-year-old man demonstrate a well-circumscribed mass abutting the aorta and projecting posteriorly and to the left. *(From Fraser RS, Müller NL, Colman NC, Paré PD: Fraser and Paré's Diagnosis of Diseases of the Chest, 4th ed. Philadelphia, WB Saunders, 1999.)*

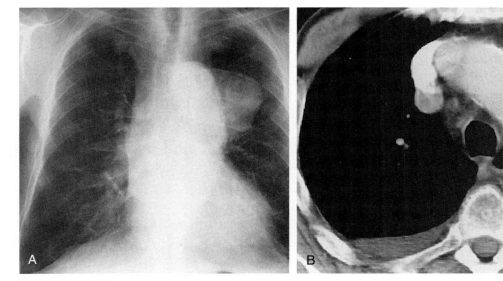

FIGURE 21–37

Aneurysm of the aorta. A posteroanterior chest radiograph (**A**) from an 87-year-old man demonstrates a homogeneous soft tissue opacity abutting the proximal descending thoracic aorta. A contrast-enhanced CT scan (**B**) shows a focal saccular aneurysm involving the proximal descending thoracic aorta and containing a large mural thrombus. Small bilateral pleural effusions are also evident. *(From Fraser RS, Müller NL, Colman NC, Paré PD: Fraser and Paré's Diagnosis of Diseases of the Chest, 4th ed. Philadelphia, WB Saunders, 1999.)*

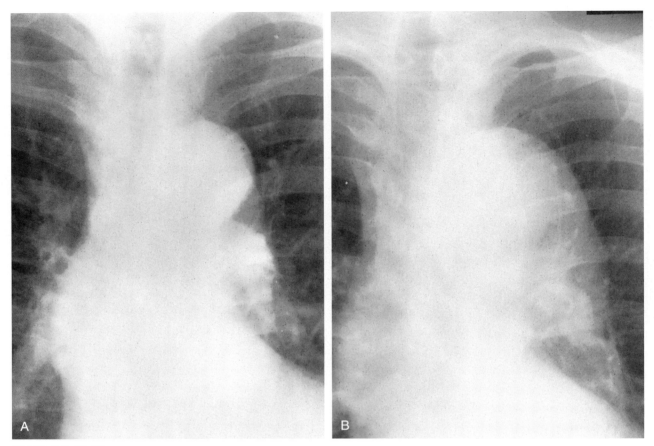

FIGURE 21–38

Dissection of the descending thoracic aorta. A close-up view of the upper mediastinum from a posteroanterior radiograph (**A**) in an elderly man reveals marked elongation of the thoracic aorta consistent with atherosclerosis. Approximately 1 year later, shortly after the abrupt onset of severe pain in the back, a repeat radiograph (**B**) reveals marked widening of the mediastinum in the region of the aorta that possesses a configuration consistent with acute dissection. *(From Fraser RS, Müller NL, Colman NC, Paré PD: Fraser and Paré's Diagnosis of Diseases of the Chest, 4th ed. Philadelphia, WB Saunders, 1999.)*

ographs, and displacement of a calcified plaque by 10 mm or more.[260,270] Enlargement of the aorta is a nonspecific finding seen in many patients who have systemic arterial hypertension or atherosclerosis. However, acute enlargement on serial chest radiographs should raise suspicion of dissection.[274] A normal configuration of the aorta does not exclude the diagnosis because it is seen in approximately 25% of patients who have acute dissection. Displacement of intimal calcification is also not a reliable diagnostic finding:[270,274] the lateral border of the visualized aorta may not be at the same level as that of the calcified plaque, thus mimicking displacement of the calcification; in addition, other tissue such as fat or a neoplasm can simulate the appearance of aortic wall thickening.[270] Because of the equivocal significance of these findings, the plain chest radiograph is of limited value in the diagnosis of aortic dissection.[275]

CT is a rapid and relatively noninvasive method for diagnosis. Moreover, the reported sensitivity of spiral CT after the intravenous administration of contrast for detecting acute aortic dissection is 93% to 98%.[272,276] Characteristic CT findings consist of a linear filling defect (intimal flap) and the presence of a false lumen (Fig. 21–39). The true lumen and the false lumen have differential enhancement on CT scans,

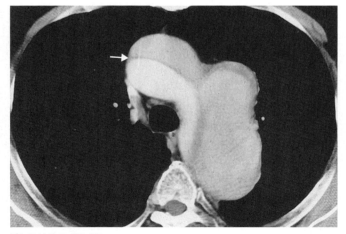

FIGURE 21–39

Aortic dissection. A contrast-enhanced CT scan at the level of the aortic arch from a 57-year-old man demonstrates marked enhancement of the true aortic lumen and poor enhancement of the false lumen of the dissection. Note the presence of a linear filling defect (intimal flap) (*arrow*) separating the true from the false lumen. *(From Fraser RS, Müller NL, Colman NC, Paré PD: Fraser and Paré's Diagnosis of Diseases of the Chest, 4th ed. Philadelphia, WB Saunders, 1999.)*

the former showing greater enhancement than the latter. Another sign of dissection is increased attenuation of the thrombosed false lumen or the aortic wall.[270,274] Such increased attenuation is present in the acute phase and decreases gradually as the hematoma resolves.

MR imaging is comparable or slightly superior to CT in evaluation (Fig. 21–40).[272] The diagnosis can usually be made by using a conventional spin-echo MR technique with electrocardiographic gating and T1 weighting; however, slow flow of blood within the false lumen may mimic intramural thrombus on spin-echo imaging.[265] The distinction can be made readily by using gradient-echo imaging, cine phase-contrast imaging, or gadolinium-enhanced MR angiography.[265] Transthoracic echocardiography is also a rapid and

noninvasive method for assessment of the ascending aorta, but it does not provide adequate visualization of the aortic arch and descending aorta. Better assessment of these portions of the vessel can be obtained with transesophageal echocardiography.[272]

Typically, the onset of dissection is sudden and associated with severe pain, which may be described as tearing or ripping and often radiates to the throat, jaw, back, or abdomen as the dissection extends from its point of origin.[277] Nausea and vomiting, sweating, and faintness are other manifestations in some individuals. Most patients have a history of hypertension. Physical examination may reveal evidence of acute peripheral arterial occlusion, aortic insufficiency, or bruits over the affected portion of aorta.

FIGURE 21–40

Dissection of the ascending aorta in a patient with a right aortic arch. A posteroanterior radiograph (**A**) reveals evidence of a former right thoracotomy that had been performed many years previously for repair of a coarctation and aortic valvotomy. The trachea is markedly deviated to the left by a right-sided aortic arch. The width of the aorta at the point of maximal tracheal displacement is obviously greater than normal. A T1-weighted MR image in transverse section (**B**) at the level of the right pulmonary artery (RPA) shows a markedly dilated ascending aorta (*open arrows*). Situated within it is a curvilinear shadow (*arrows*) representing an intimal flap; the smaller area to the left of the flap represents the true lumen, and the larger area to the right, the false lumen. Note that the descending aorta (A) at this level is still on the right side. A coronal reconstruction (**C**) again reveals the markedly dilated ascending aorta (*arrows*) containing the intimal flap (*arrowheads*); again, the true lumen is on the left and the false lumen is on the right. The patient was a 27-year-old woman who had Turner's syndrome. (*From Fraser RS, Müller NL, Colman NC, Paré PD: Fraser and Paré's Diagnosis of Diseases of the Chest, 4th ed. Philadelphia, WB Saunders, 1999.*)

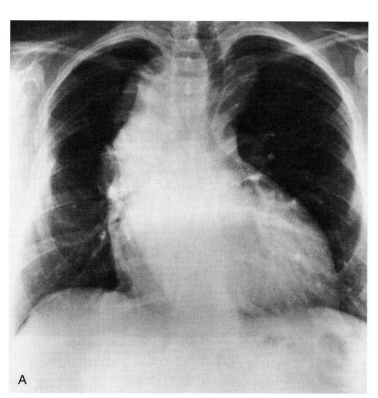

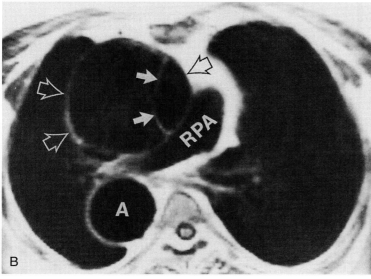

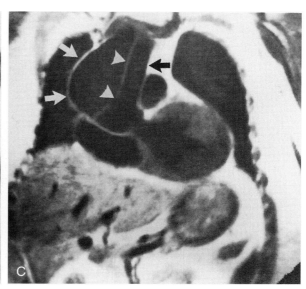

As might be expected, untreated aortic dissection is often rapidly fatal, particularly if it involves the ascending aorta; in fact, the death rate in this situation is about 1% per hour for the first 48 hours. With prompt treatment, survival rates are about 80% to 90% at 30 days and 60% to 70% at 5 years.[269,278]

Penetrating Aortic Ulcer

The term *penetrating aortic ulcer* has been used to refer to ulceration of an atheromatous plaque through the intima into the media of the aortic wall.[279,280] Such lesions usually occur in elderly patients who have hypertension and severe atherosclerosis. They can be single or multiple and typically involve the aortic arch and descending thoracic aorta. They are identified on CT and MR as an outpouching extending beyond the contour of the normal lumen, similar to a peptic ulcer.[281] These ulcers can become quite large and may be associated with a variable amount of intramural hematoma. They are often associated with thickening of the aortic wall, which enhances after the intravenous administration of contrast.[282] Associated aneurysm formation or rupture occurs occasionally.[283]

Buckling and Aneurysm of the Innominate Artery

Both of these abnormalities are manifested radiographically as a smooth, well-defined opacity in the right superior paramediastinal area that extends upward from the aortic arch (Fig. 21–41). Buckling is a relatively common condition that occurs in about 15% of patients who have hypertension or atherosclerosis, or both.[284] Aneurysms are much less common.

The innominate artery is about 5 cm long and is firmly fixed proximally at its origin from the aorta and distally by the subclavian and carotid arteries. When the thoracic aorta elongates and dilates as a result of atherosclerosis, the arch moves cephalad and carries with it the origin of the innominate artery. Because of its fixation superiorly, the latter buckles to

the right.[285] Occasionally, the buckling occurs posteriorly and laterally, in which case the vessel becomes almost completely surrounded by lung parenchyma and simulates a nodule.[286]

Aneurysms of the innominate artery can cause pain, cough, dyspnea, hoarseness, dysphagia, Horner's syndrome, and clubbing of the fingers of the right hand. A pulsatile mass may be evident at the base of the neck. Buckling occurs most often in middle-aged or older obese women who have clinical evidence of atherosclerosis and hypertension. It seldom causes symptoms.

Congenital Anomalies of the Aorta

Although most congenital malformations of the aortic arch become evident during the first year of life,[287] occasional cases are not recognized until adulthood.[288,289] A congenital aortic vascular ring results from persistence of the two aortic arches or persistence of the right aortic arch and the left ductus arteriosus; in a minority of patients, the right subclavian artery, also of anomalous origin, arises from the descending aorta.[290] A radiographic diagnosis can be made by the demonstration of a double aortic arch and a vessel posterior to the esophagus. On the frontal view, the trachea is midline; on the lateral radiograph, the trachea is displaced posteriorly by the larger anterior arch. A specific diagnosis can be made with CT or MR imaging.[291,292] Symptoms result from compression of the trachea or esophagus and include symptoms caused by recurrent respiratory infections, shortness of breath, and dysphagia.

Other congenital anomalies of the aorta that result in abnormalities in mediastinal contour include (1) pseudocoarctation of the aorta, in which a left paramediastinal "mass" is visible just above the aortic arch as a result of elongation and buckling of the aorta[293]; (2) a cervical aortic arch, in which the aortic arch extends into the soft tissues of the neck before turning downward on itself to become the

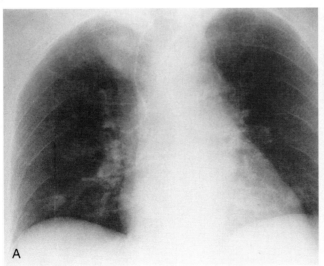
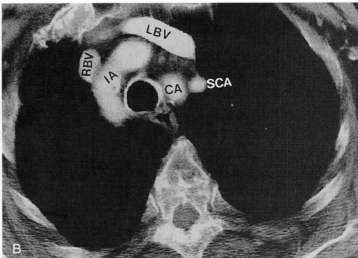

FIGURE 21–41

Buckling of the innominate artery. An anteroposterior chest radiograph (**A**) from an 86-year-old woman shows a focal opacity in the right superior paramediastinal area. A contrast-enhanced CT scan (**B**) shows that the opacity is the result of buckling of the innominate artery (IA). Contrast is also present in the left brachiocephalic vein (LBV), right brachiocephalic vein (RBV), left carotid artery (CA), and left subclavian artery (SCA). *(From Fraser RS, Müller NL, Colman NC, Paré PD: Fraser and Paré's Diagnosis of Diseases of the Chest, 4th ed. Philadelphia, WB Saunders, 1999.)*

descending aorta[294]; (3) aortic diverticula[295]; and (by far the most common) (4) a right aortic arch (Fig. 21–42).[296] The last-named anomaly is present in about 0.1% to 0.2% of the general population.[297] In approximately 70% of cases there is also an aberrant left subclavian artery. Occasionally, the abnormal arch compresses the trachea sufficiently to result in a clinical picture that can be confused with asthma.[298]

In approximately 0.5% of the population, a normal left aortic arch is associated with an aberrant right subclavian artery.[297] Occasionally, this vessel is visualized as a soft tissue opacity that typically has an oblique course from left to right and extends cephalad from the aortic arch.[299] The proximal portion of the aberrant artery is frequently dilated, a finding known as the diverticulum of Kommerell.[297] The diagnosis can be readily confirmed with contrast-enhanced CT (Fig. 21–43) or MR imaging.

Diseases of the Esophagus

Carcinoma

Although barium examination and esophagoscopy are the two definitive procedures in the diagnosis of primary carcinoma of the esophagus, conventional radiographs of the chest can provide clues to its presence (Fig. 21–44).[300,301] The most fre-

quent abnormalities include an abnormal azygoesophageal recess interface, a widened mediastinum, a posterior tracheal indentation or mass, and tracheal deviation.

CT manifestations include esophageal wall thickening, proximal dilation, obscuration of the periesophageal fat planes, and periesophageal lymph node enlargement.[300,302] Although wall thickening is the earliest manifestation, it is by no means diagnostic, other causes including reflux and monilial esophagitis, varices, and postirradiation scarring.[303] CT is also helpful in identifying advanced local disease and the presence of metastases to the lungs, liver, and intra-abdominal lymph nodes. However, it has limited value in the detection of early periesophageal tumor extension.[304] Several investigators have shown that endoscopic ultrasound examination is superior to CT in the detection of such local tumor spread.[305,306] Preliminary results suggest that positron emission tomography using 2-[18F]-fluoro-2-deoxy-D-glucose (FDG) is comparable to CT in demonstrating the extent of esophageal carcinoma and involvement of periesophageal nodes and is superior to it in detecting distant metastases.[307]

Diverticula

Diverticula can occur at several places in the esophagus. Zenker's diverticulum originates between the transverse

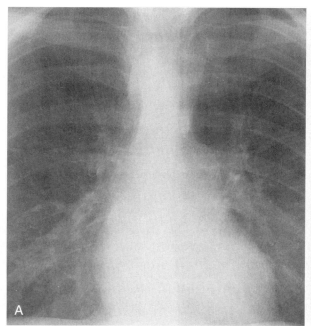
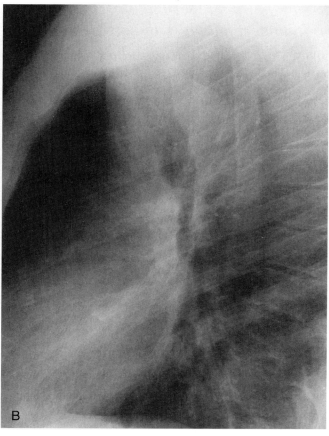

FIGURE 21–42

Right aortic arch. Close-up views of posteroanterior (**A**) and lateral (**B**) chest radiographs from a 33-year-old man demonstrate a right aortic arch causing smooth deviation of the trachea anteriorly and to the left. The patient was asymptomatic. (From Fraser RS, Müller NL, Colman NC, Paré PD: Fraser and Paré's Diagnosis of Diseases of the Chest, 4th ed. Philadelphia, WB Saunders, 1999.)

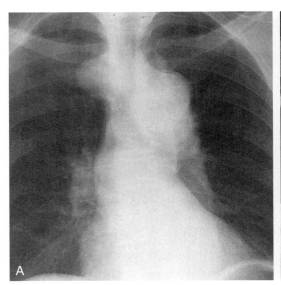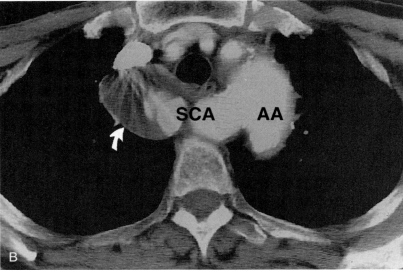

FIGURE 21–43

Diverticulum of Kommerell. A close-up view of a posteroanterior chest radiograph (**A**) from a 74-year-old woman shows a soft tissue opacity in the superior mediastinum. A contrast-enhanced CT scan (**B**) demonstrates the upper aspect of the aortic arch (AA) and the aberrant right subclavian artery (SCA). The latter is ectatic (diverticulum of Kommerell) and contains thrombus (*curved arrow*). *(From Fraser RS, Müller NL, Colman NC, Paré PD: Fraser and Paré's Diagnosis of Diseases of the Chest, 4th ed. Philadelphia, WB Saunders, 1999.)*

and oblique fibers of the inferior pharyngeal constrictor muscle. It may become large enough to be identified in the superior mediastinum on plain radiographs, in which case it frequently contains an air-fluid level. If large, it can compress the esophagus. Barium studies not only clearly outline the sac but also reveal the degree of anterior displacement of the proximal portion of the esophagus. The diagnosis can also be readily made with CT. Symptoms include dysphagia, chronic cough as a result of aspiration, and recurrent pneumonia.

Diverticula arising from the lower third of the esophagus are almost always congenital in origin and are manifested as round, cystlike structures to the right of the midline just above the diaphragm. An air-fluid level is usually present. Barium studies are again diagnostic.[308] Diverticula that develop in the midthoracic region are usually the result of cicatricial contraction from healed infected lymph nodes (traction diverticula); they are seldom, if ever visible on plain radiographs.

Megaesophagus

Esophageal dilation has many causes, including stenosis secondary to reflux esophagitis or fibrosing mediastinitis, progressive systemic sclerosis (PSS), carcinoma, and achalasia. Among these etiologies, achalasia causes the most severe generalized dilation. The dilated esophagus is usually radiographically apparent as a shadow projecting to the right side of the mediastinum. Because it is behind the heart, it does not cause a silhouette sign with that structure. The trachea may be displaced anteriorly. Depending on the underlying cause, an air-fluid level may be observed in the dilated esophagus, most frequently in achalasia and seldom in PSS.

Although a barium study is the diagnostic procedure of choice, CT also enables diagnosis, even in patients in whom the condition is not suspected.[309,310] On conventional chest radiographs, an air-containing esophagus may be identified in some patients who have PSS and, in the appropriate clinical context, is suggestive of the diagnosis. Air in the esophagus can also be seen postoperatively and in patients who use esophageal speech after laryngectomy.[311,312]

Symptoms of achalasia include dysphagia, pain on swallowing, and chronic cough; recurrent pneumonia may result from aspiration. Stridor is observed occasionally.[313]

Tracheoesophageal and Bronchoesophageal Fistulas

Fistulas between the esophagus and the airways can be congenital or acquired. Although the former is identified most often in neonates, it may not be recognized until adolescence or adulthood. In most cases of delayed recognition, there is a long history of cough, often with expectoration of food; occasionally, associated bronchiectasis is present (see page 198).

The most common cause of an acquired fistula between the esophagus and the respiratory tract is carcinoma of the esophagus.[314] In some instances, it represents direct extension of tumor from the esophagus to an airway; in others, it is associated with radiation therapy. This complication is not rare; in a series of 474 patients it occurred in 25 (approximately 5%).[315] As might be expected, once a fistula has developed, the prognosis is extremely poor, most patients dying within weeks to months. Acquired nonmalignant tracheoesophageal fistulas can be caused by cuffed tracheal tubes, surgical trauma, blunt injuries, and foreign bodies.[316]

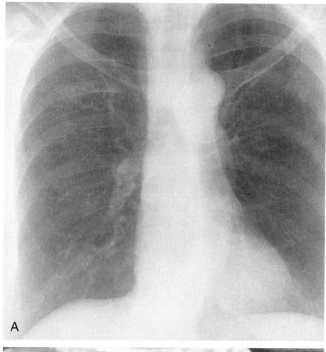

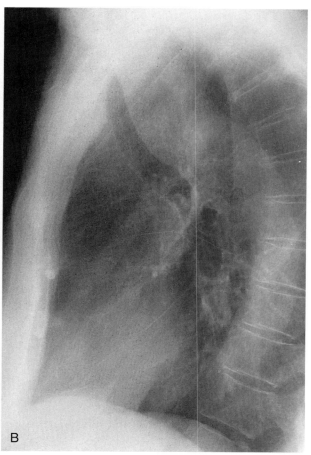

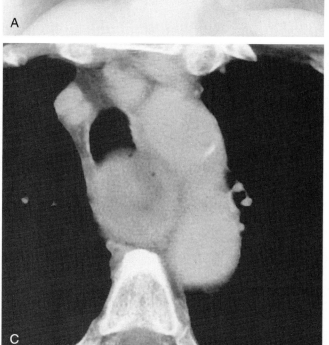

FIGURE 21–44

Esophageal carcinoma. A posteroanterior chest radiograph (**A**) from a 77-year-old woman demonstrates a poorly defined opacity in the left upper mediastinum. A lateral view (**B**) shows increased opacity in the retrotracheal region and anterior displacement of the trachea. A CT scan (**C**) demonstrates marked inhomogeneous thickening of the esophageal wall. The patient was unable to tolerate any oral contrast. (*From Fraser RS, Müller NL, Colman NC, Paré PD: Fraser and Paré's Diagnosis of Diseases of the Chest, 4th ed. Philadelphia, WB Saunders, 1999.*)

Esophageal Varices

These ectatic veins occasionally result in abnormalities on the chest radiograph. In a review of 352 patients who had portal hypertension, abnormalities were evident in 17 (5%) and included middle-posterior mediastinal or paravertebral opacities, a soft tissue opacity adjacent to the descending thoracic aorta, and obscuration of the aorta.[317] The diagnosis can be made readily by CT.[318] Although the varices do not in themselves occasion respiratory symptoms, complicating hematemesis may be confused with hemoptysis. In addition, transient pleural effusions and mediastinal opacities have been identified on radiographs after endoscopic injection sclerotherapy.[319]

Masses Situated Predominantly in the Paravertebral Region

The paravertebral region is in a sense a potential space because it normally contains only a small amount of connective tissue, blood vessels, the sympathetic nerve chains, and peripheral nerves. However, neoplasms that originate in the last two structures, as well as abnormalities related to the spinal canal, can expand to be manifested as masses in this region. Although herniation of abdominal contents through a posterior diaphragmatic defect and infectious, traumatic, or neoplastic diseases of the thoracic spine can also be manifested as a paravertebral mass, for convenience these conditions are discussed elsewhere (see pages 900 and 907).

Tumors and Tumor-like Conditions of Neural Tissue

Neoplasms of neural tissue account for about 20% of all primary "mediastinal" neoplasms in adults and as many as 35% in children[85,320]; they are by far the most common type in the paravertebral compartment. From a histogenetic point of view, there are two basic types: those arising from the peripheral nerves and those originating from sympathetic ganglia, the latter including paragangliomas and ganglioneuromas.

Tumors Arising from Peripheral Nerves

Most neural tumors that arise in the thorax originate in an intercostal nerve in the paravertebral region. Neoplasms arising from other nerves, including the vagus and phrenic nerves and small unnamed branches, are rare.[321] Some

tumors, particularly malignant ones, are associated with neurofibromatosis.[322]

Several histologic forms can be seen, including neurilemoma (schwannoma), neurofibroma (both plexiform and nonplexiform types), and neurogenic sarcoma (malignant schwannoma); neurilemoma is the most common. The majority of neurilemomas and neurofibromas are encapsulated, more or less spherical masses that expand into the paravertebral space; some tumors extend through a spinal foramen and grow in a dumbbell fashion in both the spinal canal and paravertebral region.[323] Although malignant tumors can show invasion of contiguous structures at the time of diagnosis, they can also be encapsulated.

In most cases, neurilemomas and neurofibromas are manifested radiographically as sharply defined round, smooth or lobulated paraspinal masses (Fig. 21–45).[50] They typically span only one or two posterior rib interspaces but can become quite large. In approximately 50% of cases, they are associated

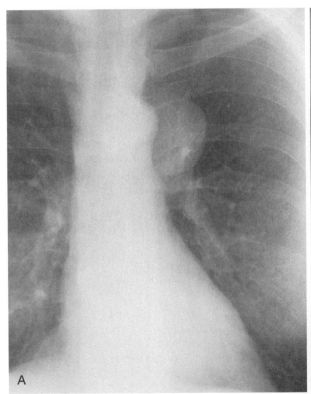

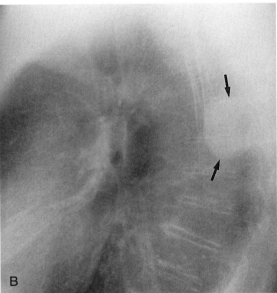

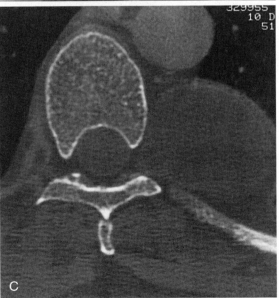

FIGURE 21–45

Neurilemoma. Close-up views from posteroanterior (**A**) and lateral (**B**) chest radiographs show a left paraspinal mass (*arrows*). On thin-section CT scan (**C**), the mass has lower attenuation than the paraspinal muscles. The patient was a 58-year-old asymptomatic man.

with bony abnormalities such as expansion of the neural foramina, erosion of the vertebral bodies, and erosion or deformity of the ribs. On CT scans, both forms of tumor can have homogeneous or heterogeneous attenuation; in most cases, attenuation is slightly lower than that of chest wall muscle (see Fig. 21–45).[50,324] Tumors usually show heterogeneous enhancement after the intravenous administration of contrast medium, a feature related to the presence of lipid within myelin and to areas of hypocellularity, cystic degeneration, or hemorrhage. Punctate foci of calcification are seen in 10% of cases.[324] On MR imaging, schwannomas and neurofibromas have low to intermediate signal intensity on T1-weighted images and focal areas with intermediate to high signal intensity on T2-weighted images (Fig. 21–46).[325] The procedure is particularly helpful in determining the nerve of origin for tumors in the thoracic inlet.[326]

Neurogenic sarcomas are usually manifested radiographically as round masses larger than 5 cm in diameter.[50,327] CT typically demonstrates areas of low attenuation related to hemorrhage and necrosis.[328] The tumors may have either well-defined smooth margins or poorly defined margins because of infiltration of the chest wall or adjacent mediastinal structures. Calcification is evident in some cases.

Most tumors are discovered in young adults. The majority do not cause symptoms and are discovered on a screening chest radiograph.[145] In some patients, compression of intercostal nerves gives rise to pain.[85] As might be expected, signs and symptoms are more frequent in patients who have malignant tumors.[320] The majority of tumors are benign, only about 5% to 25% having pathologic or clinical features of malignancy.[85,322,329] Provided that complete surgical excision can be achieved, the prognosis associated with the former group is excellent. By contrast, malignant neoplasms are typically aggressive and not uncommonly associated with hematogenous metastases, usually to the lungs.[50]

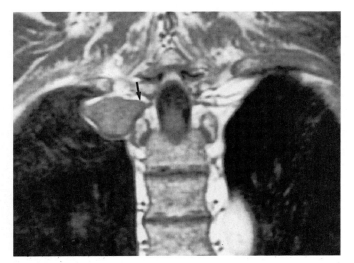

FIGURE 21–46

Neurofibroma. A coronal MR image obtained by using a T1-weighted spin-echo technique (TR/TE 800/15) demonstrates a paraspinal tumor. The mass has heterogeneous signal intensity and can be seen to originate from a nerve root (arrow). *(From Fraser RS, Müller NL, Colman NC, Paré PD: Fraser and Paré's Diagnosis of Diseases of the Chest, 4th ed. Philadelphia, WB Saunders, 1999.)*

Tumors Arising from Sympathetic Ganglia

Ganglioneuroma, Ganglioneuroblastoma, and Neuroblastoma. These three tumors have somewhat overlapping histologic features. Ganglioneuromas are composed of an admixture of mature Schwann cells, collagen, and ganglion cells, whereas neuroblastomas consist of primitive-appearing cells, usually with scanty cytoplasm and pleomorphic, hyperchromatic nuclei. Ganglioneuroblastomas show features of both tumors in varying degrees. Because of this histologic continuum, distinction between the neoplasms is sometimes difficult.[330]

The radiographic appearance consists of sharply defined oblong masses located along the anterolateral surface of the thoracic spine.[50] The tumors can usually be distinguished from other neurogenic tumors by their vertical orientation and elongated, tapering appearance. Calcification occurs in approximately 25% of cases.[331] The ribs or vertebrae are eroded in some cases, just as often by benign as by malignant forms; such erosion can be striking in neuroblastoma but tends to be more subtle in ganglioneuroma.[332] The tumors can exhibit homogeneous or heterogeneous attenuation on CT.[50] MR imaging usually demonstrates homogeneous, intermediate signal intensity on both T1- and T2-weighted images.[50,333]

Neuroblastomas and ganglioneuroblastomas occur most commonly in infants and children, whereas ganglioneuromas tend to occur in adolescents and young adults.[330] Many patients are asymptomatic, but some have chest wall pain. Ganglioneuromas are benign neoplasms that may grow very slowly over a period of many years, and complete excision typically results in cure. By contrast, neuroblastomas are aggressive tumors; although there is evidence that the course may be more prolonged in adults than in children, recurrence and metastases are common even in these patients, in whom the 5-year survival rate may be no more than 30%.[334] The prognosis of patients who have ganglioneuroblastoma is considerably better; in a review of 55 patients monitored for 2 to 23 years, the 5-year actuarial survival rate was approximately 90%.[330]

Paraganglioma. As discussed previously (see page 875), intrathoracic paragangliomas occur either in the middle mediastinum in relation to the aortopulmonary paraganglia or in the paravertebral region in relation to the aorticosympathetic paraganglia. As with tumors arising in the former location, those in the paravertebral region are uncommon.[335] The average age at the time of diagnosis is about 30 to 40 years, and there is a male-to-female preponderance of about 2:1. The pathologic features are similar to those of aorticopulmonary tumors.[223]

Radiographically, most tumors are sharply defined round or oval masses indistinguishable from other neurogenic neoplasms. Most are located in the midthoracic region adjacent to the fifth, sixth, or seventh rib; there is a right-sided predominance of 2:1.[336] CT demonstrates a soft tissue mass that can have homogeneous attenuation or can contain large central areas of low attenuation as a result of necrosis; marked enhancement after the intravenous administration of contrast is typical.[225] Approximately 90% of tumors show abnormal uptake on [131]I- or ^{123}I-MIBG scintigraphy.[228] Preliminary results suggest that ^{111}In-octreotide scintigraphy may be superior to MIBG scintigraphy.[337]

About 50% of patients are asymptomatic or complain of chest pain.[336] The remainder have signs and symptoms related to excess catecholamine production, including headache, sweating, tachycardia, palpitations, dyspnea, and nausea.

Hypertension is present in most patients, as are increased levels of plasma and urinary catecholamines.[338] The prognosis is better than that in those who have aorticopulmonary tumors, complete surgical excision and cure being possible in many cases.[223,356] In a few patients, local invasion precludes complete excision, in which situation the neoplasm usually recurs, though sometimes after a prolonged interval. Many patients have adrenal or other extrathoracic paraganglionic tumors that can occur either synchronously or metachronously.[336]

Meningocele and Meningomyelocele

Meningocele and meningomyelocele are rare anomalies that consist of herniation of the leptomeninges through an intervertebral foramen; a meningocele contains cerebrospinal fluid only, whereas a meningomyelocele also contains neural tissue. The abnormalities occur slightly more often on the right side than on the left and can be situated anywhere between the thoracic inlet and the diaphragm. Approximately 75% of patients

are between the ages of 30 and 60 years at diagnosis[339]; many have neurofibromatosis.[340]

On conventional radiographs, the lesions do not have any specific features that distinguish them from neurogenic neoplasms. However, the diagnosis can usually be made readily with CT or MR imaging, both of which demonstrate continuity between the cerebrospinal fluid in the thecal sac and the meningocele (Fig. 21–47).[50] Kyphoscoliosis is frequent.[339] Enlargement of the intervertebral foramen is present in the vast majority of cases. An association with vertebral and rib anomalies is fairly frequent and should suggest the diagnosis.[143,341]

Cysts

Gastroenteric (Neurenteric) Cyst

Gastroenteric cysts are lined in whole or in part by gastric and/or small intestinal epithelium; when such a cyst is associated with anomalies of the spinal column (such as spina bifida

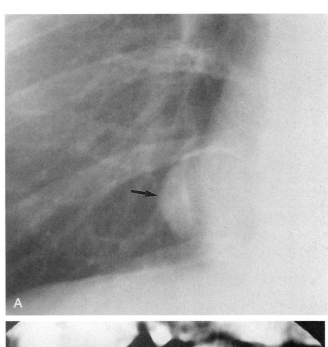

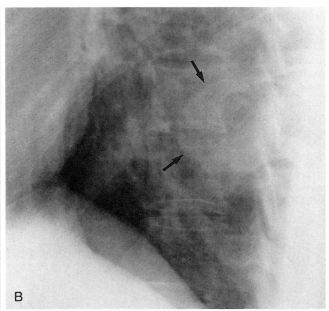

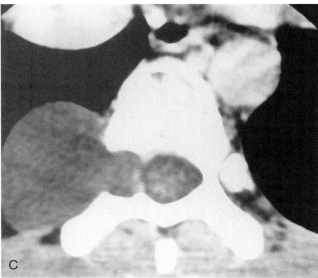

FIGURE 21–47

Meningocele. Close-up views from posteroanterior (**A**) and lateral (**B**) chest radiographs show a paraspinal opacity (*arrows*) at the level of T10. A CT scan (**C**) demonstrates characteristic fluid attenuation of the meningocele, which communicates with the thecal sac. The patient was a 29-year-old man. *(From Fraser RS, Müller NL, Colman NC, Paré PD: Fraser and Paré's Diagnosis of Diseases of the Chest, 4th ed. Philadelphia, WB Saunders, 1999.)*

and hemivertebrae), the designation *neurenteric* is usually applied. It has been hypothesized that the cysts result from incomplete separation of endoderm from the notochord during early fetal life or that they are the result of herniation of a portion of the gut anlage into a gap in the notochord ("split notochord" syndrome).[230,342]

The radiographic appearance is that of a sharply defined round or lobulated opacity of homogeneous density.[50] Because of their fluid content, the cysts tend to mold themselves to surrounding structures. They are often connected by a stalk to the meninges and commonly also to a portion of the gastrointestinal tract.[343] If attachment is to the esophagus, communication is rare; however, if it is to the gastrointestinal tract, there is usually communication that permits gas to enter the cyst. Approximately 50% of cases are associated with incomplete closure of the neural tube (spinal dysraphism) or with butterfly vertebrae or hemivertebrae.[50] MR imaging is required to exclude intraspinal extension.[50]

Neurenteric cysts typically produce symptoms and therefore manifest themselves in neonates. They can grow very large and cause compression atelectasis, thereby leading to respiratory distress. Gastric epithelium can be functional and associated with peptic ulceration and perforation.[344]

Hydatid Cyst

Mediastinal echinococcosis is most common in the paravertebral region; in a review of 80 cases, cysts were identified at this site in 65%, in the anterior mediastinum in 36%, and in the posterior or middle mediastinum in only 9%.[345] Cysts situated in the paravertebral region tend to erode ribs and vertebrae and compress the spinal cord. CT is helpful in determining the presence of the cysts and in demonstrating their relationship to adjacent structures.[346]

Extramedullary Hematopoiesis

Extramedullary hematopoiesis occurs as a compensatory phenomenon in various diseases characterized by inadequate production or excessive destruction of blood cells. The most common underlying conditions are congenital hemolytic anemia (usually hereditary spherocytosis) and thalassemia.[347,348] The most frequent sites are the liver and spleen; however, foci can occur in many other organs and tissues, including the paravertebral areas of the thorax.[347] It has been postulated that lesions develop at this site either by extension of hyperplastic marrow from adjacent bone or lymph nodes or by "primary" growth from embryonic rests of hematopoietic tissue.[349] In one study, CT showed that the bone in the region in which the mass had developed was usually wider and thinner than elsewhere,[350] supporting the hypothesis that extrusion of marrow occurs through thinned rib trabeculae. Foci of extramedullary hematopoiesis can be solitary or multiple and appear grossly as soft, reddish nodules that resemble hematomas. Histologically, all marrow elements can be identified, usually with erythroid hyperplasia.[351]

The characteristic radiographic finding is one or several smooth but often lobulated masses situated in the paravertebral regions in the lower portion of the chest (Fig. 21–48).[352]

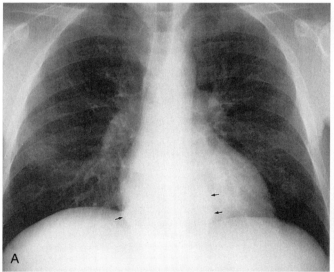
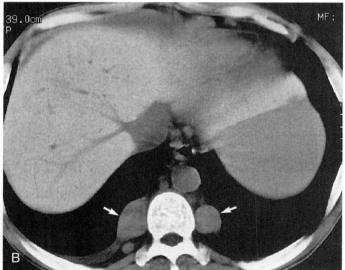
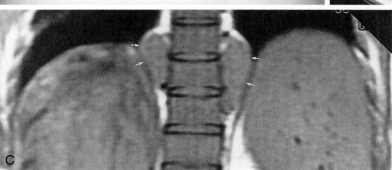

FIGURE 21–48

Extramedullary hematopoiesis. A posteroanterior chest radiograph (**A**) from a 39-year-old man shows displacement of the paraspinal interfaces (*arrows*). A CT scan obtained without intravenous contrast (**B**) reveals paraspinal soft tissue masses (*arrows*). Note the increased attenuation of the liver as a result of hemosiderosis. A coronal T1-weighted MR image (**C**) better demonstrates the extent of the extramedullary hematopoiesis (*arrows*). The patient had thalassemia intermedia. (*From Fraser RS, Müller NL, Colman NC, Paré PD: Fraser and Paré's Diagnosis of Diseases of the Chest, 4th ed. Philadelphia, WB Saunders, 1999.*)

Less commonly, masses occur at multiple levels or involve the entire paravertebral region. On CT scans, the masses usually have homogeneous soft tissue density[352]; occasionally, a large fatty component is present.[353] Other features include widening of the ribs as a result of expansion of the medullary cavity, a lacy appearance of the vertebrae, and absence of bony erosion. Radionuclide bone marrow scans may or may not show uptake within the mass.[354,355]

The masses seldom induce symptoms; however, hemothorax has been documented and paraplegia has been reported to develop as a result of spinal cord compression.[347,356]

REFERENCES

1. Carrol CL, Jeffrey RB Jr, Federle MP, et al: CT evaluation of mediastinal infections. J Comput Assist Tomogr 11:449-454, 1987.
2. El Oakley RM, Wright JE: Postoperative mediastinitis: Classification and management. Ann Thorac Surg 61:1030-1036, 1996.
3. Breatnach E, Nath PH, Delany DJ: The role of computed tomography in acute and subacute mediastinitis. Clin Radiol 37:139-145, 1986.
4. Levine TM, Wurster CF, Krespi YP: Mediastinitis occurring as a complication of odontogenic infections. Laryngoscope 96:747-750, 1986.
5. Tocino IM, Miller MH: Mediastinal trauma and other acute mediastinal conditions. J Thorac Imaging 2:79-100, 1987.
6. LaBerge JM, Kerlan RK Jr, Pogany AC, et al: Esophageal rupture: Complication of balloon dilatation. Radiology 157:56, 1985.
7. Rogers LF, Puig AW, Dooley BN, et al: Diagnostic considerations in mediastinal emphysema: A pathophysiologic-roentgenologic approach to Boerhaave's syndrome and spontaneous pneumomediastinum. Am J Roentgenol Radium Ther Nucl Med 115:495-511, 1972.
8. Jenkins IR, Raymond R: Boerhaave's syndrome complicated by a large bronchopleural fistula. Chest 105:964-965, 1994.
9. Loop FD, Lytle BW, Cosgrove DM, et al: J. Maxwell Chamberlain memorial paper. Sternal wound complications after isolated coronary artery bypass grafting: Early and late mortality, morbidity, and cost of care. Ann Thorac Surg 49:179-186, discussion 186-187, 1990.
10. Ivert T, Lindblom D, Sahni J, et al: Management of deep sternal wound infection after cardiac surgery—Hanuman syndrome. Scand J Thorac Cardiovasc Surg 25:111-117, 1991.
11. Appleton DS, Sandrasagra FA, Flower CD: Perforated oesophagus: Review of twenty-eight consecutive cases. Clin Radiol 30:493-497, 1979.
12. Han SY, McElvein RB, Aldrete JS, et al: Perforation of the esophagus: Correlation of site and cause with plain film findings. AJR Am J Roentgenol 145:537-540, 1985.
13. Christoforidis A, Nelson SW: Spontaneous rupture of esophagus with emphasis on the roentgenologic diagnosis. Am J Roentgenol Radium Ther Nucl Med 78:574-580, 1957.
14. White CS, Templeton PA, Attar S: Esophageal perforation: CT findings. AJR Am J Roentgenol 160:767-770, 1993.
15. Goldstein LA, Thompson WR: Esophageal perforations: A 15 year experience. Am J Surg 143:495-503, 1982.
16. Mathisen DJ, Grillo HC: Clinical manifestation of mediastinal fibrosis and histoplasmosis. Ann Thorac Surg 54:1053-1057, discussion 1057-1058, 1992.
17. Mole TM, Glover J, Sheppard MN: Sclerosing mediastinitis: A report on 18 cases. Thorax 50:280-283, 1995.
18. Dines DE, Payne WS, Bernatz PE, et al: Mediastinal granuloma and fibrosing mediastinitis. Chest 75:320-324, 1979.
19. Loyd JE, Tillman BF, Atkinson JB, et al: Mediastinal fibrosis complicating histoplasmosis. Medicine (Baltimore) 67:295-310, 1988.
20. Schowengerdt CG, Suyemoto R, Main FB: Granulomatous and fibrous mediastinitis A review and analysis of 180 cases. J Thorac Cardiovasc Surg 57:365-379, 1969.
21. Comings DE, Skubi KB, Van Eyes J, et al: Familial multifocal fibrosclerosis. Findings suggesting that retroperitoneal fibrosis, mediastinal fibrosis, sclerosing cholangitis, Riedel's thyroiditis, and pseudotumor of the orbit may be different manifestations of a single disease. Ann Intern Med 66:884-892, 1967.
22. Dozois RR, Bernatz PE, Woolner LB, et al: Sclerosing mediastinitis involving major bronchi. Mayo Clin Proc 43:557-569, 1968.
23. Graham JR, Suby HI, LeCompte PR, et al: Fibrotic disorders associated with methysergide therapy for headache. N Engl J Med 274:359-368, 1966.
24. Katzenstein AL, Mazur MT: Pulmonary infarct: An unusual manifestation of fibrosing mediastinitis. Chest 77:521-524, 1980.
25. Sobrinho-Simoes MA, Vaz Saleiro J, Wagenvoort CA: Mediastinal and hilar fibrosis. Histopathology 5:53-60, 1981.
26. Sherrick AD, Brown LR, Harms GF, et al: The radiographic findings of fibrosing mediastinitis. Chest 106:484-489, 1994.
27. Rossi SE, McAdams HP, Rosado-de-Christenson ML, et al: Fibrosing mediastinitis. Radiographics 21:737-757, 2001.
28. Ramakantan R, Shah P: Dysphagia due to mediastinal fibrosis in advanced pulmonary tuberculosis. AJR Am J Roentgenol 154:61-63, 1990.
29. Sandler CM, Libshitz HI, Marks G: Pneumoperitoneum, pneumomediastinum and pneumopericardium following dental extraction. Radiology 115:539-540, 1975.
30. Cyrlak D, Milne EN, Imray TJ: Pneumomediastinum: A diagnostic problem. Crit Rev Diagn Imaging 23:75-117, 1984.
31. Rouby JJ, Lherm T, Martin de Lassale E, et al: Histologic aspects of pulmonary barotrauma in critically ill patients with acute respiratory failure. Intensive Care Med 19:383-389, 1993.
32. Caldwell EJ, Powell RD Jr, Mullooly JP: Interstitial emphysema: A study of physiologic factors involved in experimental induction of the lesion. Am Rev Respir Dis 102:516-525, 1970.
33. Jamadar DA, Kazerooni EA, Hirschl RB: Pneumomediastinum: Elucidation of the anatomic pathway by liquid ventilation. J Comput Assist Tomogr 20:309-311, 1996.
34. Fultz PJ, Melville D, Ekanej A, et al: Nontraumatic rupture of the thoracic aorta: Chest radiographic features of an often unrecognized condition. AJR Am J Roentgenol 171:351-357, 1998.
35. Morgan EJ, Henderson DA: Pneumomediastinum as a complication of athletic competition. Thorax 36:155-156, 1981.
36. Varkey B, Kory RC: Mediastinal and subcutaneous emphysema following pulmonary function tests. Am Rev Respir Dis 108:1393-1396, 1973.
37. Karson EM, Saltzman D, Davis MR: Pneumomediastinum in pregnancy: Two case reports and a review of the literature, pathophysiology, and management. Obstet Gynecol 64:39S-43S, 1984.
38. Dattwyler RJ, Goldman MA, Bloch KJ: Pneumomediastinum as a complication of asthma in teenage and young adult patients. J Allergy Clin Immunol 63:412-416, 1979.
39. Rohlfing BM, Webb WR, Schlobohm RM: Ventilator-related extra-alveolar air in adults. Radiology 121:25-31, 1976.
40. Bejvan SM, Godwin JD: Pneumomediastinum: Old signs and new signs. AJR Am J Roentgenol 166:1041-1048, 1996.
41. Levin B: The continuous diaphragm sign. A newly-recognized sign of pneumomediastinum. Clin Radiol 24:337-338, 1973.
42. Felson B: The mediastinum. Semin Roentgenol 4:40, 1969.
43. Unger JM, England DM, Bogust GA: Interstitial emphysema in adults: Recognition and prognostic implications. J Thorac Imaging 4:86-94, 1989.
44. Satoh K, Kobayashi T, Kawase Y, et al: CT appearance of interstitial pulmonary emphysema. J Thorac Imaging 11:153-154, 1996.
45. Creasy JD, Chiles C, Routh WD, et al: Overview of traumatic injury of the thoracic aorta. Radiographics 17:27-45, 1997.
46. Gavant ML, Menke PG, Fabian T, et al: Blunt traumatic aortic rupture: Detection with helical CT of the chest. Radiology 197:125-133, 1995.
47. Gomelsky A, Barry MJ, Wagner RB: Spontaneous mediastinal hemorrhage: A case report with a review of the literature. Md Med J 46:83-87, 1997.
48. Woodring JH, Loh FK, Kryscio RJ: Mediastinal hemorrhage: An evaluation of radiographic manifestations. Radiology 151:15-21, 1984.
49. Strollo DC, Rosado de Christenson ML, Jett JR: Primary mediastinal tumors. Part 1: Tumors of the anterior mediastinum. Chest 112:511-522, 1997.
50. Strollo DC, Rosado-de-Christenson ML, Jett JR: Primary mediastinal tumors: Part II. Tumors of the middle and posterior mediastinum. Chest 112:1344-1357, 1997.
51. Powers CN, Silverman JF, Geisinger KR, et al: Fine-needle aspiration biopsy of the mediastinum. A multi-institutional analysis. Am J Clin Pathol 105:168-173, 1996.
52. Marchevsky A: The mediastinum. Pathology (Phila) 3:339-348, 1996.
53. Ingels GW, Campbell DC Jr, Giampetro AM, et al: Malignant schwannomas of the mediastinum. Report of two cases and review of the literature. Cancer 27:1190-1201, 1971.
54. Linegar AG, Odell JA, Fennell WM, et al: Massive thymic hyperplasia. Ann Thorac Surg 55:1197-1201, 1993.
55. Langer CJ, Keller SM, Erner SM: Thymic hyperplasia with hemorrhage simulating recurrent Hodgkin disease after chemotherapy-induced complete remission. Cancer 70:2082-2086, 1992.
56. Kissin CM, Husband JE, Nicholas D, et al: Benign thymic enlargement in adults after chemotherapy: CT demonstration. Radiology 163:67-70, 1987.
57. Tabarin A, Catargi B, Chanson P, et al: Pseudo-tumours of the thymus after correction of hypercortisolism in patients with ectopic ACTH syndrome: A report of five cases. Clin Endocrinol (Oxf) 42:207-213, 1995.
58. Bergman TA, Mariash CN, Oppenheimer JH: Anterior mediastinal mass in a patient with Graves' disease. J Clin Endocrinol Metab 55:587-588, 1982.
59. Williams DJ: True thymic hyperplasia: An unrecognised cause of cardiac murmur? Thymus 12:135-137, 1988.
60. Gelfand DW, Goldman AS, Law EJ, et al: Thymic hyperplasia in children recovering from thermal burns. J Trauma 12:813-817, 1972.
61. Rice HE, Flake AW, Hori T, et al: Massive thymic hyperplasia: Characterization of a rare mediastinal mass. J Pediatr Surg 29:1561-1564, 1994.
62. Freundlich IM, McGavran MH: Abnormalities of the thymus. J Thorac Imaging 11:58-65, 1996.
63. Baron RL, Lee JK, Sagel SS, et al: Computed tomography of the normal thymus. Radiology 142:121-125, 1982.
64. Suzuki K, Kurokawa K, Suzuki T, et al: Anterior mediastinal metastasis of testicular germ cell tumor: Relation to benign thymic hyperplasia. Eur Urol 32:371-374, 1997.
65. Front D, Ben-Haim S, Israel O, et al: Lymphoma: Predictive value of Ga-67 scintigraphy after treatment. Radiology 182:359-363, 1992.
66. Small EJ, Venook AP, Damon LE: Gallium-avid thymic hyperplasia in an adult after chemotherapy for Hodgkin disease. Cancer 72:905-908, 1993.
67. Levine GD, Rosai J: Thymic hyperplasia and neoplasia: A review of current concepts. Hum Pathol 9:495-515, 1978.

68. Clark RE, Marbarger JP, West PN, et al: Thymectomy for myasthenia gravis in the young adult. Long-term results. J Thorac Cardiovasc Surg 80:696-701, 1980.
69. Mizuno T, Hashimoto T, Masaoka A, et al: Thymic follicular hyperplasia manifested as an anterior mediastinal mass. Surg Today 27:275-277, 1997.
70. Nicolaou S, Müller NL, Li DK, et al: Thymus in myasthenia gravis: Comparison of CT and pathologic findings and clinical outcome after thymectomy. Radiology 201:471-474, 1996.
71. Moran CA, Rosado-de-Christenson M, Suster S: Thymolipoma: Clinicopathologic review of 33 cases. Mod Pathol 8:741-744, 1995.
72. Le Marc'hadour F, Pinel N, Pasquier B, et al: Thymolipoma in association with myasthenia gravis. Am J Surg Pathol 15:802-809, 1991.
73. Rosai J, Levine G: Atlas of Tumor Pathology: Tumors of the Thymus. Washington, DC, Armed Forces Institute of Pathology, 1976.
74. Rosado-de-Christenson ML, Pugatch RD, Moran CA, et al: Thymolipoma: Analysis of 27 cases. Radiology 193:121-126, 1994.
75. McCafferty MH, Bahnson HT: Thymic cyst extending into the pericardium: A case report and review of thymic cysts. Ann Thorac Surg 33:503-506, 1982.
76. Jaramillo D, Perez-Atayde A, Griscom NT: Apparent association between thymic cysts and prior thoracotomy. Radiology 172:207-209, 1989.
77. Borgna-Pignatti C, Andreis IB, Rugolotto S, et al: Thymic cyst appearing after treatment of mediastinal non-Hodgkin lymphoma. Med Pediatr Oncol 22:70-72, 1994.
78. Avila NA, Mueller BU, Carrasquillo JA, et al: Multilocular thymic cysts: Imaging features in children with human immunodeficiency virus infection. Radiology 201:130-134, 1996.
79. Suster S, Rosai J: Cystic thymomas. A clinicopathologic study of ten cases. Cancer 69:92-97, 1992.
80. Moran CA, Suster S: Mediastinal seminomas with prominent cystic changes. A clinicopathologic study of 10 cases. Am J Surg Pathol 19:1047-1053, 1995.
81. Brown LR, Aughenbaugh GL: Masses of the anterior mediastinum: CT and MR imaging. AJR Am J Roentgenol 157:1171-1180, 1991.
82. Molina PL, Siegel MJ, Glazer HS: Thymic masses on MR imaging. AJR Am J Roentgenol 155:495-500, 1990.
83. Johnson SB, Eng TY, Giaccone G, et al: Thymoma: Update for the new millennium. Oncologist 6:239-246, 2001.
84. Muller-Hermelink HK, Marx A: Thymoma. Curr Opin Oncol 12:426-433, 2000.
85. Hoffman OA, Gillespie DJ, Aughenbaugh GL, et al: Primary mediastinal neoplasms (other than thymoma). Mayo Clin Proc 68:880-891, 1993.
86. Harris NL, Muller-Hermelink HK: Thymoma classification. A siren's song of simplicity. Am J Clin Pathol 112:299-303, 1999.
87. Kornstein MJ: Thymoma classification: My opinion. Am J Clin Pathol 112:304-307, 1999.
88. Suster S, Moran CA: Thymoma classification. The ride of the Valkyries? Am J Clin Pathol 112:308-310, 1999.
89. Chung DA: Thymic carcinoma—analysis of nineteen clinicopathological studies. Thorac Cardiovasc Surg 48:114-119, 2000.
90. Rosai J, Sobin L: Histologic typing of tumours of the thymus. In International Histologic Classification of Tumours, ed 2. New York, Springer, 1999.
91. Lewis JE, Wick MR, Scheithauer BW, et al: Thymoma. A clinicopathologic review. Cancer 60:2727-2743, 1987.
92. Maggi G, Casadio C, Cavallo A, et al: Thymoma: Results of 241 operated cases. Ann Thorac Surg 51:152-156, 1991.
93. Salyer WR, Eggleston JC: Thymoma: A clinical and pathological study of 65 cases. Cancer 37:229-249, 1976.
94. Marino M, Muller-Hermelink HK: Thymoma and thymic carcinoma. Relation of thymoma epithelial cells to the cortical and medullary differentiation of thymus. Virchows Arch A Pathol Anat Histopathol 407:119-149, 1985.
95. Lee D, Wright DH: Immunohistochemical study of 22 cases of thymoma. J Clin Pathol 41:1297-1304, 1988.
96. Ho FC, Fu KH, Lam SY, et al: Evaluation of a histogenetic classification for thymic epithelial tumours. Histopathology 25:21-29, 1994.
97. Pan CC, Wu HP, Yang CF, et al: The clinicopathological correlation of epithelial subtyping in thymoma: A study of 112 consecutive cases. Hum Pathol 25:893-899, 1994.
98. Rosado-de-Christenson ML, Galobardes J, Moran CA: Thymoma: Radiologic-pathologic correlation. Radiographics 12:151-168, 1992.
99. Tomiyama N, Müller NL, Ellis SJ, et al: Invasive and noninvasive thymoma: Distinctive CT features. J Comput Assist Tomogr 25:388-393, 2001.
100. Chen JL, Weisbrod GL, Herman SJ: Computed tomography and pathologic correlations of thymic lesions. J Thorac Imaging 3:61-65, 1988
101. Sakai F, Sone S, Kiyono K, et al: MR imaging of thymoma: Radiologic-pathologic correlation. AJR Am J Roentgenol 158:751-756, 1992.
102. Pirronti T, Rinaldi P, Batocchi AP, et al: Thymic lesions and myasthenia gravis. Diagnosis based on mediastinal imaging and pathological findings. Acta Radiol 43:380-384, 2002.
103. Schmidt-Wolf IG, Rockstroh JK, Schuller H, et al: Malignant thymoma: Current status of classification and multimodality treatment. Ann Hematol 82:69-76, 2003.
104. Shishido M, Yano K, Ichiki H, et al: Pericarditis as the initial manifestation of malignant thymoma. Disappearance of pericardial effusion with corticosteroid therapy. Chest 106:313-314, 1994.
105. Dib HR, Friedman B, Khouli HI, et al: Malignant thymoma. A complicated triad of SVC syndrome, cardiac tamponade, and DIC. Chest 105:941-942, 1994.
106. Puglisi F, Finato N, Mariuzzi L, et al: Microscopic thymoma and myasthenia gravis. J Clin Pathol 48:682-683, 1995.
107. De Giacomo T, Rendina EA, Venuta F, et al: Pancytopenia associated with thymoma resolving after thymectomy and immunosuppressive therapy. Case report. Scand J Thorac Cardiovasc Surg 29:149-151, 1995.
108. Postiglione K, Ferris R, Jaffe JP, et al: Immune mediated agranulocytosis and anemia associated with thymoma. Am J Hematol 49:336-340, 1995.
109. Lishner M, Ravid M, Shapira J, et al: Delta-T-lymphocytosis in a patient with thymoma. Cancer 74:2924-2929, 1994.
110. Masaoka A, Hashimoto T, Shibata K, et al: Thymomas associated with pure red cell aplasia. Histologic and follow-up studies. Cancer 64:1872-1878, 1989.
111. Wong KF, Chau KF, Chan JK, et al: Pure red cell aplasia associated with thymic lymphoid hyperplasia and secondary erythropoietin resistance. Am J Clin Pathol 103:346-347, 1995.
112. Mevorach D, Perrot S, Buchanan NM, et al: Appearance of systemic lupus erythematosus after thymectomy: Four case reports and review of the literature. Lupus 4:33-37, 1995.
113. Nickels J, Franssila K: Thymoma metastasizing to extrathoracic sites. A case report. Acta Pathol Microbiol Scand [A] 84:331-334, 1976.
114. Masaoka A, Monden Y, Nakahara K, et al: Follow-up study of thymomas with special reference to their clinical stages. Cancer 48:2485-492, 1981.
115. Park HS, Shin DM, Lee JS, et al: Thymoma. A retrospective study of 87 cases. Cancer 73:2491-2498, 1994.
116. Gotti G, Paladini P, Haid MM, et al: Late recurrence of thymoma and myasthenia gravis. Scand J Thorac Cardiovasc Surg 29:37-38, 1995.
117. Wilkins EW Jr, Grillo HC, Scannell JG, et al: J. Maxwell Chamberlain Memorial Paper. Role of staging in prognosis and management of thymoma. Ann Thorac Surg 51:888-892, 1991.
118. Okumura M, Ohta M, Tateyama H, et al: The World Health Organization histologic classification system reflects the oncologic behavior of thymoma: A clinical study of 273 patients. Cancer 94:624-632, 2002.
119. Moran C, Suster S: Current status of the histologic classification of thymoma. Int J Surg Path 3:67, 1995.
120. Blumberg D, Port JL, Weksler B, et al: Thymoma: A multivariate analysis of factors predicting survival. Ann Thorac Surg 60:908-913, discussion 914, 1995.
121. Kuo TT, Lo SK: DNA flow cytometric study of thymic epithelial tumors with evaluation of its usefulness in the pathologic classification. Hum Pathol 24:746-749, 1993.
122. Pollack A, el-Naggar AK, Cox JD, et al: Thymoma. The prognostic significance of flow cytometric DNA analysis. Cancer 69:1702-1709, 1992.
123. Pich A, Chiarle R, Chiusa L, et al: Argyrophilic nucleolar organizer region counts predict survival in thymoma. Cancer 74:1568-1574, 1994.
124. Yang W-I, Elfird J, Quintanilla-Martinez L, et al: Cell kinetic study of thymic epithelial tumors using PCNA (PC 10) and Ki-67 antibodies. Hum Pathol 27:70, 1996.
125. Gilhus NE, Jones M, Turley H, et al: Oncogene proteins and proliferation antigens in thymomas: Increased expression of epidermal growth factor receptor and Ki67 antigen. J Clin Pathol 48:447-455, 1995.
126. Suster S, Moran CA: Thymic carcinoma: Spectrum of differentiation and histologic types. Pathology 30:111-122, 1998.
127. Wick MR, Scheithauer BW, Weiland LH, et al: Primary thymic carcinomas. Am J Surg Pathol 6:613-630, 1982.
128. Dorfman DM, Shahsafaei A, Chan JK: Thymic carcinomas, but not thymomas and carcinomas of other sites, show CD5 immunoreactivity. Am J Surg Pathol 21:936-940, 1997.
129. Tomiyama N, Johkoh T, Mihara N, et al: Using the World Health Organization Classification of thymic epithelial neoplasms to describe CT findings. AJR Am J Roentgenol 179:881-886, 2002.
130. Do YS, Im JG, Lee BH, et al: CT findings in malignant tumors of thymic epithelium. J Comput Assist Tomogr 19:192-197, 1995.
131. Sungur A, Ruacan S, Gungen Y, et al: Myasthenia gravis and primary squamous cell carcinoma of the thymus. Arch Pathol Lab Med 117:937-938, 1993.
132. Suster S, Rosai J: Thymic carcinoma. A clinicopathologic study of 60 cases. Cancer 67:1025-1032, 1991.
133. Cheung YC, Ng SH, Wan YL, et al: Dynamic CT features of mediastinal hemangioma: More information for evaluation. Clin Imaging 24:276-278, 2000.
134. Hsu CP, Chen CY, Chen CL, et al: Thymic carcinoma. Ten years' experience in twenty patients. J Thorac Cardiovasc Surg 107:615-620, 1994.
135. Wick MR, Rosai J: Neuroendocrine neoplasms of the mediastinum. Semin Diagn Pathol 8:35-51, 1991.
136. Viebahn R, Hiddemann W, Klinke F, et al: Thymus carcinoid. Pathol Res Pract 180:445-451, 1985.
137. Valli M, Fabris GA, Dewar A, et al: Atypical carcinoid tumour of the thymus: A study of eight cases. Histopathology 24:371-375, 1994.
138. Rosai J, Levine G, Weber WR, et al: Carcinoid tumors and oat cell carcinomas of the thymus. Pathol Annu 11:201-226, 1976.
139. Chetty R, Batitang S, Govender D: Large cell neuroendocrine carcinoma of the thymus. Histopathology 31:274-276, 1997.
140. Felson B, Castleman B, Levinsohn EM, et al: Radiologic-Pathologic Correlation Conference: SUNY Upstate Medical Center. Cushing syndrome associated with mediastinal mass. AJR Am J Roentgenol 138:815-819, 1982.
141. Wang DY, Chang DB, Kuo SH, et al: Carcinoid tumours of the thymus. Thorax 49:357-360, 1994.
142. Zeiger MA, Swartz SE, MacGillivray DC, et al: Thymic carcinoid in association with MEN syndromes. Am Surg 58:430-434, 1992.
143. Wychulis AR, Payne WS, Clagett OT, et al: Surgical treatment of mediastinal tumors: A 40 year experience. J Thorac Cardiovasc Surg 62:379-392, 1971.

144. Nichols CR: Mediastinal germ cell tumors. Semin Thorac Cardiovasc Surg 4:45-50, 1992.
145. Benjamin SP, McCormack LJ, Effler DB, et al: Primary tumors of the mediastinum. Chest 62:297-303, 1972.
146. Dulmet EM, Macchiarini P, Suc B, et al: Germ cell tumors of the mediastinum. A 30-year experience. Cancer 72:1894-1901, 1993.
147. Knapp RH, Hurt RD, Payne WS, et al: Malignant germ cell tumors of the mediastinum. J Thorac Cardiovasc Surg 89:82-89, 1985.
148. Truong LD, Harris L, Mattioli C, et al: Endodermal sinus tumor of the mediastinum. A report of seven cases and review of the literature. Cancer 58:730-739, 1986.
149. Moran CA, Suster S: Primary mediastinal choriocarcinomas: A clinicopathologic and immunohistochemical study of eight cases. Am J Surg Pathol 21:1007-1012, 1997.
150. Moran CA, Suster S: Primary germ cell tumors of the mediastinum: I. Analysis of 322 cases with special emphasis on teratomatous lesions and a proposal for histopathologic classification and clinical staging. Cancer 80:681-690, 1997.
151. Moran CA, Suster S, Koss MN: Primary germ cell tumors of the mediastinum: III. Yolk sac tumor, embryonal carcinoma, choriocarcinoma, and combined non-teratomatous germ cell tumors of the mediastinum—a clinicopathologic and immunohistochemical study of 64 cases. Cancer 80:699-707, 1997.
152. Aliotta PJ, Castillo J, Englander LS, et al: Primary mediastinal germ cell tumors. Histologic patterns of treatment failures at autopsy. Cancer 62:982-984, 1988.
153. Luna MA, Valenzuela-Tamariz J: Germ-cell tumors of the mediastinum, post-mortem findings. Am J Clin Pathol 65:450-454, 1976.
154. Daugaard G, Rorth M, von der Maase H, et al: Management of extragonadal germ-cell tumors and the significance of bilateral testicular biopsies. Ann Oncol 3:283-289, 1992.
155. Lachman MF, Kim K, Koo BC: Mediastinal teratoma associated with Klinefelter's syndrome. Arch Pathol Lab Med 110:1067-1071, 1986.
156. deMent SH: Association between mediastinal germ cell tumors and hematologic malignancies: An update. Hum Pathol 21:699-703, 1990.
157. Motoyama T, Yamamoto O, Iwamoto H, et al: Fine needle aspiration cytology of primary mediastinal germ cell tumors. Acta Cytol 39:725-732, 1995.
158. Greco FA, Vaughn WK, Hainsworth JD: Advanced poorly differentiated carcinoma of unknown primary site: Recognition of a treatable syndrome. Ann Intern Med 104:547-553, 1986.
159. Ahn IM, Lee KS, Goo JM, et al: Predicting the histology of anterior mediastinal masses: Comparison of chest radiography and CT. J Thorac Imaging 11:265-271, 1996.
160. Rosado-de-Christenson ML, Templeton PA, Moran CA: From the archives of the AFIP Mediastinal germ cell tumors: Radiologic and pathologic correlation. Radiographics 12:1013-1030, 1992.
161. Childs WJ, Goldstraw P, Nicholls JE, et al: Primary malignant mediastinal germ cell tumours: Improved prognosis with platinum-based chemotherapy and surgery. Br J Cancer 67:1098-1101, 1993.
162. Gerl A, Clemm C, Lamerz R, et al: Cisplatin-based chemotherapy of primary extragonadal germ cell tumors. A single institution experience. Cancer 77:526-532, 1996.
163. Pachter MR, Lattes R: "Germinal" tumors of the mediastinum: A clinicopathologic study. Dis Chest 45:301, 1964.
164. Dunn PJ: Pancreatic endocrine tissue in benign mediastinal teratoma. J Clin Pathol 37:1105-1109, 1984.
165. Caballero C, Gomez S, Matias-Guiu X, et al: Rhabdomyosarcomas developing in association with mediastinal germ cell tumours. Virchows Arch A Pathol Anat Histopathol 420:539-543, 1992.
166. Morinaga S, Nomori H, Kobayashi R, et al: Well-differentiated adenocarcinoma arising from mature cystic teratoma of the mediastinum (teratoma with malignant transformation). Report of a surgical case. Am J Clin Pathol 101:531-534, 1994.
167. Moeller KH, Rosado-de-Christenson ML, Templeton PA: Mediastinal mature teratoma: Imaging features. AJR Am J Roentgenol 169:985-990, 1997.
168. Sasaka K, Kurihara Y, Nakajima Y, et al: Spontaneous rupture: A complication of benign mature teratomas of the mediastinum. AJR Am J Roentgenol 170:323-328, 1998.
169. Cobb CJ, Wynn J, Cobb SR, et al: Cytologic findings in an effusion caused by rupture of a benign cystic teratoma of the mediastinum into a serous cavity. Acta Cytol 29:1015-1020, 1985.
170. Southgate J, Slade PR: Teratodermoid cyst of the mediastinum with pancreatic enzyme secretion. Thorax 37:476-477, 1982.
171. Moran CA, Suster S, Przygodzki RM, et al: Primary germ cell tumors of the mediastinum: II. Mediastinal seminomas—a clinicopathologic and immunohistochemical study of 120 cases. Cancer 80:691-698, 1997.
172. Lee KS, Im JG, Han CH, et al: Malignant primary germ cell tumors of the mediastinum: CT features. AJR Am J Roentgenol 153:947-951, 1989.
173. Waldron JA Jr, Dohring EJ, Farber LR: Primary large cell lymphomas of the mediastinum: An analysis of 20 cases. Semin Diagn Pathol 2:281-295, 1985.
174. Levitt LJ, Aisenberg AC, Harris NL, et al: Primary non-Hodgkin's lymphoma of the mediastinum. Cancer 50:2486-2492, 1982.
175. Katlic MR, Wang CA, Grillo HC: Substernal goiter. Ann Thorac Surg 39:391-399, 1985.
176. Irwin RS, Pratter MR, Hamolsky MW: Chronic persistent cough: An uncommon presenting complaint of thyroiditis. Chest 81:386-388, 1982.
177. Ward MJ, Davies D: Riedel's thyroiditis with invasion of the lungs. Thorax 36:956-957, 1981.
178. Fragomeni LS, Ceratti de Azambuja P: Intrathoracic goitre in the posterior mediastinum. Thorax 35:638-629, 1980.
179. Bashist B, Ellis K, Gold RP: Computed tomography of intrathoracic goiters. AJR Am J Roentgenol 140:455-460, 1983.
180. Glazer GM, Axel L, Moss AA: CT diagnosis of mediastinal thyroid. AJR Am J Roentgenol 138:495-498, 1982.
181. Tecce PM, Fishman EK, Kuhlman JE: CT evaluation of the anterior mediastinum: Spectrum of disease. Radiographics 14:973-990, 1994.
182. Takashima S, Morimoto S, Ikezoe J, et al: CT evaluation of anaplastic thyroid carcinoma. AJR Am J Roentgenol 154:1079-1085, 1990.
183. Noma S, Nishimura K, Togashi K, et al: Thyroid gland: MR imaging. Radiology 164:495-499, 1987.
184. Park HM, Tarver RD, Siddiqui AR, et al: Efficacy of thyroid scintigraphy in the diagnosis of intrathoracic goiter. AJR Am J Roentgenol 148:527-529, 1987.
185. Swanson PE: Soft tissue neoplasma of the mediastinum. Semin Diagn Pathol 8:14-34, 1991.
186. Pachter MR, Lattes R: Mesenchymal tumors of the mediastinum. I. Tumors of fibrous tissue, adipose tissue, smooth muscle, and striated muscle. Cancer 16:74-94, 1963.
187. Wilson ES: Radiolucent mediastinal lipoma. Radiology 118:44, 1976.
188. Hodge J, Aponte G, McLaughin E: Primary mediastinal tumors. J Thorac Surg 37:730-744, 1959.
189. Lyons HA, Calvy GL, Sammons BP: The diagnosis and classification of mediastinal masses. 1. A study of 782 cases. Ann Intern Med 51:897-932, 1959.
190. Mendez G Jr, Isikoff MB, Isikoff SK, et al: Fatty tumors of the thorax demonstrated by CT. AJR Am J Roentgenol 133:207-212, 1979.
191. Nguyen KQ, Hoeffel C, Le LH, et al: Mediastinal lipomatosis. South Med J 91:1169-1172, 1998.
192. Lee WJ, Fattal G: Mediastinal lipomatosis in simple obesity. Chest 70:308-309, 1976.
193. Streiter ML, Schneider HJ, Proto AV: Steroid-induced thoracic lipomatosis: Paraspinal involvement. AJR Am J Roentgenol 139:679-681, 1982.
194. van de Putte LB, Wagenaar JP, San KH: Paracardiac lipomatosis in exogenous Cushing's syndrome. Thorax 28:653-656, 1973.
195. Cohen AJ, Sbaschnig RJ, Hochholzer L, et al: Mediastinal hemangiomas. Ann Thorac Surg 43:656-659, 1987.
196. Moran CA, Suster S: Mediastinal hemangiomas: A study of 18 cases with emphasis on the spectrum of morphological features. Hum Pathol 26:416-421, 1995.
197. Kings GL: Multifocal haemangiomatous malformation: A case report. Thorax 30:485-488, 1975.
198. McAdams HP, Rosado-de-Christenson ML, Moran CA: Mediastinal hemangioma: Radiographic and CT features in 14 patients. Radiology 193:399-402, 1994.
199. Pachter M, Lattes R: Mesenchymal tumors of the mediastinum: II. Tumors of blood vascular origin. Cancer 16:95, 1963.
200. Topcu S, Soysal O, Balkan E, et al: Mediastinal cystic lymphangioma: Report of two cases. Thorac Cardiovasc Surg 45:209-210, 1997.
201. Pannell TL, Jolles H: Adult cystic mediastinal lymphangioma simulating a thymic cyst. J Thorac Imaging 7:86-89, 1991.
202. Shaffer K, Rosado-de-Christenson ML, Patz EF Jr, et al: Thoracic lymphangioma in adults: CT and MR imaging features. AJR Am J Roentgenol 162:283-289, 1994.
203. Miyake H, Shiga M, Takaki H, et al: Mediastinal lymphangiomas in adults: CT findings. J Thorac Imaging 11:83-85, 1996.
204. Glazer HS, Wick MR, Anderson DJ, et al: CT of fatty thoracic masses. AJR Am J Roentgenol 159:1181-1187, 1992.
205. Stoller JK, Shaw C, Matthay RA: Enlarging, atypically located pericardial cyst. Recent experience and literature review. Chest 89:402-406, 1986.
206. Wang ZJ, Reddy GP, Gotway MB, et al: CT and MR imaging of pericardial disease. Radiographics 23(Spec No):S167-S180, 2003.
207. Patel J, Park C, Michaels J, et al: Pericardial cyst: Case reports and a literature review. Echocardiography 21:269-272, 2004.
208. Brunner DR, Whitley NO: A pericardial cyst with high CT numbers. AJR Am J Roentgenol 142:279-280, 1984.
209. Daniel RA Jr, Diveley WL, Edwards WH, et al: Mediastinal tumors. Ann Surg 151:783-795, 1960.
210. Aronberg DJ, Peterson RR, Glazer HS, et al: Superior diaphragmatic lymph nodes: CT assessment. J Comput Assist Tomogr 10:937-941, 1986.
211. Schwartz EE, Wechsler RJ: Diaphragmatic and paradiaphragmatic tumors and pseudotumors. J Thorac Imaging 4:19-28, 1989.
212. Vock P, Hodler J: Cardiophrenic angle adenopathy: Update on causes and significance. Radiology 159:395-399, 1986.
213. Sussman SK, Halvorsen RA Jr, Silverman PM, et al: Paracardiac adenopathy: CT evaluation. AJR Am J Roentgenol 149:29-34, 1987.
214. Keller AR, Hochholzer L, Castleman B: Hyaline-vascular and plasma-cell types of giant lymph node hyperplasia of the mediastinum and other locations. Cancer 29:670-683, 1972.
215. Frizzera G: Castleman's disease: More questions than answers. Hum Pathol 16:202-205, 1985.
216. Weisenburger DD, Nathwani BN, Winberg CD, et al: Multicentric angiofollicular lymph node hyperplasia: A clinicopathologic study of 16 cases. Hum Pathol 16:162-172, 1985.
217. Oksenhendler E, Duarte M, Soulier J, et al: Multicentric Castleman's disease in HIV infection: A clinical and pathological study of 20 patients. AIDS 10:61-67, 1996.
218. McAdams HP, Rosado-de-Christenson M, Fishback NF, et al: Castleman disease of the thorax: Radiologic features with clinical and histopathologic correlation. Radiology 209:221-218, 1998.

219. Johkoh T, Müller NL, Ichikado K, et al: Intrathoracic multicentric Castleman disease: CT findings in 12 patients. Radiology 209:477-481, 1998.

220. Glenner G, Grimley P: Atlas of Tumor Pathology: Second Series, Fascicle 9. Tumors of the Extra-Adrenal Paraganglion System (Including Chemoreceptors). Washington, DC, Armed Forces Institute of Pathology, 1974.

221. Lamy AL, Fradet GJ, Luoma A, et al: Anterior and middle mediastinum paraganglioma: Complete resection is the treatment of choice. Ann Thorac Surg 57:249-252, 1994.

222. Lack EE, Stillinger RA, Colvin DB, et al: Aortico-pulmonary paraganglioma: Report of a case with ultrastructural study and review of the literature. Cancer 43:269-278, 1979.

223. Moran CA, Suster S, Fishback N, et al: Mediastinal paragangliomas. A clinicopathologic and immunohistochemical study of 16 cases. Cancer 72:2358-2364, 1993.

224. Ros PR, Rosado-de-Christenson ML, Buetow PC, et al: The Radiological Society of North America 83rd Scientific Assembly and Annual Meeting. Image Interpretation session: 1997. Radiographics 18:195, 1998.

225. Drucker EA, McLoud TC, Dedrick CG, et al: Mediastinal paraganglioma: Radiologic evaluation of an unusual vascular tumor. AJR Am J Roentgenol 148:521-522, 1987.

226. Hamilton BH, Francis IR, Gross BH, et al: Intrapericardial paragangliomas (pheochromocytomas): Imaging features. AJR Am J Roentgenol 168:109-113, 1997.

227. Bomanji J, Conry BG, Britton KE, et al: Imaging neural crest tumours with ^{123}I-metaiodobenzylguanidine and x-ray computed tomography: A comparative study. Clin Radiol 39:502-506, 1988.

228. van Gils AP, Falke TH, van Erkel AR, et al: MR imaging and MIBG scintigraphy of pheochromocytomas and extraadrenal functioning paragangliomas. Radiographics 11:37-57, 1991.

229. van Gelder T, Verhoeven GT, de Jong P, et al: Dopamine-producing paraganglioma not visualized by iodine-123-MIBG scintigraphy. J Nucl Med 36:620-622, 1995.

230. Salyer DC, Salyer WR, Eggleston JC: Benign developmental cysts of the mediastinum. Arch Pathol Lab Med 101:136-139, 1977.

231. Snyder ME, Luck SR, Hernandez R, et al: Diagnostic dilemmas of mediastinal cysts. J Pediatr Surg 20:810-815, 1985.

232. Rappaport DC, Herman SJ, Weisbrod GL: Congenital bronchopulmonary diseases in adults: CT findings. AJR Am J Roentgenol 162:1295-1299, 1994.

233. Murayama S, Murakami J, Watanabe H, et al: Signal intensity characteristics of mediastinal cystic masses on T1-weighted MRI. J Comput Assist Tomogr 19:188-191, 1995.

234. Endo S, Sohara Y, Yamaguchi T, et al: The effectiveness of transesophageal ultrasonography in preoperatively diagnosing an esophageal cyst in a 75-year-old woman: Report of a case. Surg Today 24:356-359, 1994.

235. Bowton DL, Katz PO: Esophageal cyst as a cause of chronic cough. Chest 86:150-152, 1984.

236. Kumar S, Murthy K, Brandfonbrenner M: Possible mechanisms of wide splitting of second sound in idiopathic dilatation of the pulmonary artery. Chest 68:739, 1975.

237. Escalante CP: Causes and management of superior vena cava syndrome. Oncology (Huntingt) 7:61-68, discussion 71-72, 75-77, 1993.

238. Schraufnagel DE, Hill R, Leech JA, et al: Superior vena caval obstruction. Is it a medical emergency? Am J Med 70:1169-1174, 1981.

239. Davies PF, Shevland JE: Superior vena caval obstruction: An analysis of seventy-six cases, with comments on the safety of venography. Angiology 36:354-357, 1985.

240. Chan RH, Dar AR, Yu E, et al: Superior vena cava obstruction in small-cell lung cancer. Int J Radiat Oncol Biol Phys 38:513-520, 1997.

241. Kastner RJ, Fisher WG, Blacky AR, et al: Pacemaker-induced superior vena cava syndrome with successful treatment by balloon venoplasty. Am J Cardiol 77:789-790, 1996.

242. Richmond G, Handwerger S, Schoenfeld N, et al: Superior vena cava syndrome: A complication of Hickman catheter insertion in patients with the acquired immunodeficiency syndrome. N Y State J Med 92:65-66, 1992.

243. Doty DB: Bypass of superior vena cava: Six years' experience with spiral vein graft for obstruction of superior vena cava due to benign and malignant disease. J Thorac Cardiovasc Surg 83:326-338, 1982.

244. Brown G, Husband JE: Mediastinal widening—a valuable radiographic sign of superior vena cava thrombosis. Clin Radiol 47:415-420, 1993.

245. Gosselin MV, Rubin GD: Altered intravascular contrast material flow dynamics: Clues for refining thoracic CT diagnosis. AJR Am J Roentgenol 169:1597-1603, 1997.

246. Weinreb JC, Mootz A, Cohen JM: MRI evaluation of mediastinal and thoracic inlet venous obstruction. AJR Am J Roentgenol 146:679-684, 1986.

247. Kim HJ, Kim HS, Chung SH: CT diagnosis of superior vena cava syndrome: Importance of collateral vessels. AJR Am J Roentgenol 161:539-542, 1993.

248. Gauden SJ: Superior vena cava syndrome induced by bronchogenic carcinoma: Is this an oncological emergency? Australas Radiol 37:363-366, 1993.

249. Floyd GD, Nelson WP: Developmental interruption of the inferior vena cava with azygos and hemiazygos substitution. Unusual radiographic features. Radiology 119:55-57, 1976.

250. Lawler LP, Corl FM, Fishman EK: Multi-detector row and volume-rendered CT of the normal and accessory flow pathways of the thoracic systemic and pulmonary veins. Radiographics 22(Spec No):S45-S60, 2002.

251. White CS, Baffa JM, Haney PJ, et al: MR imaging of congenital anomalies of the thoracic veins. Radiographics 17:595-608, 1997.

252. Petersen RW: Infrahepatic interruption of the inferior vena cava with azygos continuation (persistent right cardinal vein). Radiology 84:304-307, 1965.

253. Milledge RD: Absence of the inferior vena cava. Radiology 85:860-865, 1965.

254. Pacofsky KB, Wolfel DA: Azygos continuation of the inferior vena cava. Am J Roentgenol Radium Ther Nucl Med 113:362-365, 1971.

255. Berdon WE, Baker DH: Plain film findings in azygos continuation of the inferior vena cava. Am J Roentgenol Radium Ther Nucl Med 104:452-457, 1968.

256. Ball JB Jr, Proto AV: The variable appearance of the left superior intercostal vein. Radiology 144:445-452, 1982.

257. Friedman AC, Chambers E, Sprayregen S: The normal and abnormal left superior intercostal vein. AJR Am J Roentgenol 131:599-602, 1978.

258. Guthaner DF, Wexler L, Harell G: CT demonstration of cardiac structures. AJR Am J Roentgenol 133:75-81, 1979.

259. Hirose Y, Hamada S, Takamiya M, et al: Aortic aneurysms: Growth rates measured with CT. Radiology 185:249-252, 1992.

260. Chen JT: Plain radiographic evaluation of the aorta. J Thorac Imaging 5:1-17, 1990.

261. Posniak HV, Olson MC, Demos TC, et al: CT of thoracic aortic aneurysms. Radiographics 10:839-855, 1990.

262. Mirvis SE, Shanmuganathan K, Miller BH, et al: Traumatic aortic injury: Diagnosis with contrast-enhanced thoracic CT—five-year experience at a major trauma center. Radiology 200:413-422, 1996.

263. Gavant ML, Flick P, Menke P, et al: CT aortography of thoracic aortic rupture. AJR Am J Roentgenol 166:955-961, 1996.

264. Hartnell GG: Imaging of aortic aneurysms and dissection: CT and MRI. J Thorac Imaging 16:35-46, 2001.

265. Ho VB, Prince MR: Thoracic MR aortography: Imaging techniques and strategies. Radiographics 18:287-309, 1998.

266. Kamp O, van Rossum AC, Torenbeek R: Transesophageal echocardiography and magnetic resonance imaging for the assessment of saccular aneurysm of the transverse thoracic aorta. Int J Cardiol 33:330-333, 1991.

267. Wilson SK, Hutchins GM: Aortic dissecting aneurysms: Causative factors in 204 subjects. Arch Pathol Lab Med 106:175-180, 1982.

268. Roberts WC: Aortic dissection: Anatomy, consequences, and causes. Am Heart J 101:195-214, 1981.

269. DeBakey ME, McCollum CH, Crawford ES, et al: Dissection and dissecting aneurysms of the aorta: Twenty-year follow-up of five hundred twenty-seven patients treated surgically. Surgery 92:1118-1134, 1982.

270. Petasnick JP: Radiologic evaluation of aortic dissection. Radiology 180:297-305, 1991.

271. Wolff KA, Herold CJ, Tempany CM, et al: Aortic dissection: Atypical patterns seen at MR imaging. Radiology 181:489-495, 1991.

272. Nienaber CA, von Kodolitsch Y, Nicolas V, et al: The diagnosis of thoracic aortic dissection by noninvasive imaging procedures. N Engl J Med 328:1-9, 1993.

273. Sakamoto I, Hayashi K, Matsunaga N, et al: Aortic dissection caused by angiographic procedures. Radiology 191:467-471, 1994.

274. Fisher ER, Stern EJ, Godwin JD 2nd, et al: Acute aortic dissection: Typical and atypical imaging features. Radiographics 14:1263-1271, discussion 1271-1274, 1994.

275. Luker GD, Glazer HS, Eagar G, et al: Aortic dissection: Effect of prospective chest radiographic diagnosis on delay to definitive diagnosis. Radiology 193:813-819, 1994.

276. Moore AG, Eagle KA, Bruckman D, et al: Choice of computed tomography, transesophageal echocardiography, magnetic resonance imaging, and aortography in acute aortic dissection: International Registry of Acute Aortic Dissection (IRAD). Am J Cardiol 89:1235-1238, 2002.

277. Eagle KA, DeSanctis RW: Aortic dissection. Curr Probl Cardiol 14:225-278, 1989.

278. Crawford ES, Svensson LG, Coselli JS, et al: Aortic dissection and dissecting aortic aneurysms. Ann Surg 208:254-273, 1988.

279. Coady MA, Rizzo JA, Hammond GL, et al: Penetrating ulcer of the thoracic aorta: What is it? How do we recognize it? How do we manage it? J Vasc Surg 27:1006-1015, discussion 1015-1016, 1998.

280. Nienaber CA, von Kodolitsch Y, Petersen B, et al: Intramural hemorrhage of the thoracic aorta. Diagnostic and therapeutic implications. Circulation 92:1465-1472, 1995.

281. Castaner E, Andreu M, Gallardo X, et al: CT in nontraumatic acute thoracic aortic disease: Typical and atypical features and complications. Radiographics 23(Spec No):S93-S110, 2003.

282. Kazerooni EA, Bree RL, Williams DM: Penetrating atherosclerotic ulcers of the descending thoracic aorta: Evaluation with CT and distinction from aortic dissection. Radiology 183:759-765, 1992.

283. Quint LE, Williams DM, Francis IR, et al: Ulcerlike lesions of the aorta: Imaging features and natural history. Radiology 218:719-723, 2001.

284. Green RA: Enlargement of the innominate and subclavian arteries simulating mediastinal neoplasm. Am Rev Tuberc 79:790-798, 1959.

285. Schneider HJ, Felson B: Buckling of the innominate artery simulating aneurysm and tumor. Am J Roentgenol Radium Ther Nucl Med 85:1106-1110, 1961.

286. Tamaki M, Tanabe M, Kamiuchi H, et al: Buckling of the distal innominate artery simulating a nodular lung mass. Chest 83:829-830, 1983.

287. Hallman GL, Cooley DA: Congenital aortic vascular ring. Surgical considerations. Arch Surg 88:666-674, 1964.

288. Lam CR, Kabbani S, Arciniegas E: Symptomatic anomalies of the aortic arch. Surg Gynecol Obstet 147:673-681, 1978.

289. Idbeis B, Levinsky L, Srinivasan V, et al: Vascular rings: Management and a proposed nomenclature. Ann Thorac Surg 31:255-258, 1981.

290. Engelman RM, Madayag M: Aberrant right subclavian artery aneurysm: A rare cause of a superior mediastinal tumor. Chest 62:45-47, 1972.

291. van Son JA, Julsrud PR, Hagler DJ, et al: Imaging strategies for vascular rings. Ann Thorac Surg 57:604-610, 1994.

292. VanDyke CW, White RD: Congenital abnormalities of the thoracic aorta presenting in the adult. J Thorac Imaging 9:230-245, 1994.

293. Gaupp EJ, Fagan CJ, Davis M, et al: Pseudocoarctation of the aorta. J Comput Assist Tomogr 5:571-573, 1981.

294. Kennard DR, Spigos DG, Tan WS: Cervical aortic arch: CT correlation with conventional radiologic studies. AJR Am J Roentgenol 141:295-297, 1983.

295. Salomonowitz E, Edwards JE, Hunter DW, et al: The three types of aortic diverticula. AJR Am J Roentgenol 142:673-679, 1984.

296. Shuford WH, Sybers RG, Edwards FK: The three types of right aortic arch. Am J Roentgenol Radium Ther Nucl Med 109:67-74, 1970.

297. Raymond GS, Miller RM, Müller NL, et al: Congenital thoracic lesions that mimic neoplastic disease on chest radiographs of adults. AJR Am J Roentgenol 168:763-769, 1997.

298. Bevelaqua F, Schicchi JS, Haas F, et al: Aortic arch anomaly presenting as exercise-induced asthma. Am Rev Respir Dis 140:805-808, 1989.

299. Branscom JJ, Austin JH: Aberrant right subclavian artery. Findings seen on plain chest roentgenograms. Am J Roentgenol Radium Ther Nucl Med 119:539-542, 1973.

300. Wolfman NT, Scharling ES, Chen MY: Esophageal squamous carcinoma. Radiol Clin North Am 32:1183-1201, 1994.

301. Levine MS: Esophageal cancer. Radiologic diagnosis. Radiol Clin North Am 35:265-279, 1997.

302. Rankin S, Mason R: Staging of oesophageal carcinoma. Clin Radiol 46:373-377, 1992.

303. Reinig JW, Stanley JH, Schabel SI: CT evaluation of thickened esophageal walls. AJR Am J Roentgenol 140:931-934, 1983.

304. Maerz LL, Deveney CW, Lopez RR, et al: Role of computed tomographic scans in the staging of esophageal and proximal gastric malignancies. Am J Surg 165:558-560, 1993.

305. Vilgrain V, Mompoint D, Palazzo L, et al: Staging of esophageal carcinoma: Comparison of results with endoscopic sonography and CT. AJR Am J Roentgenol 155:277-281, 1990.

306. Botet JF, Lightdale CJ, Zauber AG, et al: Preoperative staging of esophageal cancer: Comparison of endoscopic US and dynamic CT. Radiology 181:419-425, 1991.

307. Kato H, Kuwano H, Nakajima M, et al: Comparison between positron emission tomography and computed tomography in the use of the assessment of esophageal carcinoma. Cancer 94:921-928, 2002.

308. Jalundhwala JM, Shah RC: Epiphrenic esophageal diverticulum. Chest 57:97-99, 1970.

309. Tishler JM, Shin MS, Stanley RJ, et al: CT of the thorax in patients with achalasia. Dig Dis Sci 28:692-697, 1983.

310. Rabushka LS, Fishman EK, Kuhlman JE: CT evaluation of achalasia. J Comput Assist Tomogr 15:434-439, 1991.

311. Blomquist G, Mahoney P: Noncollapsing air-filled esophagus in diseased and postoperative chests. Acta Radiol 55:32, 1961.

312. Schabel SI, Stanley JH: Air esophagram after laryngectomy. AJR Am J Roentgenol 136:19-21, 1981.

313. McLean RD, Stewart CJ, Whyte DG: Acute thoracic inlet obstruction in achalasia of the oesophagus. Thorax 31:456-459, 1976.

314. Little AG, Ferguson MK, DeMeester TR, et al: Esophageal carcinoma with respiratory tract fistula. Cancer 53:1322-1328, 1984.

315. Fitzgerald RH Jr, Bartles DM, Parker EF: Tracheoesophageal fistulas secondary to carcinoma of the esophagus. J Thorac Cardiovasc Surg 82:194-197, 1981.

316. Hjelms E, Jensen H, Lindewald H: Non-malignant oesophago-bronchial fistula. Eur J Respir Dis 63:351-355, 1982.

317. Ishikawa T, Saeki M, Tsukune Y, et al: Detection of paraesophageal varices by plain films. AJR Am J Roentgenol 144:701-704, 1985.

318. Wachsberg RH, Yaghmai V, Javors BR, et al: Cardiophrenic varices in portal hypertension: Evaluation with CT. Radiology 195:553-556, 1995.

319. Saks BJ, Kilby AE, Dietrich PA, et al: Pleural and mediastinal changes following endoscopic injection sclerotherapy of esophageal varices. Radiology 149:639-642, 1983.

320. Azarow KS, Pearl RH, Zurcher R, et al: Primary mediastinal masses. A comparison of adult and pediatric populations. J Thorac Cardiovasc Surg 106:67-72, 1993.

321. Dabir RR, Piccione W Jr, Kittle CF: Intrathoracic tumors of the vagus nerve. Ann Thorac Surg 50:494-497, 1990.

322. Gale AW, Jelihovsky T, Grant AF, et al: Neurogenic tumors of the mediastinum. Ann Thorac Surg 17:434-443, 1974.

323. Heltzer JM, Krasna MJ, Aldrich F, et al: Thoracoscopic excision of a posterior mediastinal "dumbbell" tumor using a combined approach. Ann Thorac Surg 60:431-433, 1995.

324. Ko SF, Lee TY, Lin JW, et al: Thoracic neurilemomas: An analysis of computed tomography findings in 36 patients. J Thorac Imaging 13:21-26, 1998.

325. Sakai F, Sone S, Kiyono K, et al: Intrathoracic neurogenic tumors: MR-pathologic correlation. AJR Am J Roentgenol 159:279-283, 1992.

326. Sakai F, Sone S, Kiyono K, et al: Magnetic resonance imaging of neurogenic tumors of the thoracic inlet: Determination of the parent nerve. J Thorac Imaging 11:272-278, 1996.

327. Ducatman BS, Scheithauer BW, Piepgras DG, et al: Malignant peripheral nerve sheath tumors. A clinicopathologic study of 120 cases. Cancer 57:2006-2021, 1986.

328. Coleman BG, Arger PH, Dalinka MK, et al: CT of sarcomatous degeneration in neurofibromatosis. AJR Am J Roentgenol 140:383-387, 1983.

329. Harjula A, Mattila S, Luosto R, et al: Mediastinal neurogenic tumours. Early and late results of surgical treatment. Scand J Thorac Cardiovasc Surg 20:115-118, 1986.

330. Adam A, Hochholzer L: Ganglioneuroblastoma of the posterior mediastinum: A clinicopathologic review of 80 cases. Cancer 47:373-381, 1981.

331. Schweisguth O, Mathey J, Renault P, et al: Intrathoracic neurogenic tumors in infants and children; a study of forty cases. Ann Surg 150:29-41, 1959.

332. Bar-Ziv J, Nogrady MB: Mediastinal neuroblastoma and ganglioneuroma. The differentiation between primary and secondary involvement on the chest roentgenogram. Am J Roentgenol Radium Ther Nucl Med 125:380-390, 1975.

333. Wang YM, Li YW, Sheih CP, et al: Magnetic resonance imaging of neuroblastoma, ganglioneuroblastoma, and ganglioneuroma. Zhonghua Min Guo Xiao Er Ke Yi Xue Hui Za Zhi 36:420-424, 1995.

334. Franks LM, Bollen A, Seeger RC, et al: Neuroblastoma in adults and adolescents: An indolent course with poor survival. Cancer 79:2028-2035, 1997.

335. Odze R, Begin LR: Malignant paraganglioma of the posterior mediastinum. A case report and review of the literature. Cancer 65:564-569, 1990.

336. Gallivan MV, Chun B, Rowden G, et al: Intrathoracic paravertebral malignant paraganglioma. Arch Pathol Lab Med 104:46-51, 1980.

337. Kwekkeboom DJ, van Urk H, Pauw BK, et al: Octreotide scintigraphy for the detection of paragangliomas. J Nucl Med 34:873-878, 1993.

338. Ogawa J, Inoue H, Koide S, et al: Functioning paraganglioma in the posterior mediastinum. Ann Thorac Surg 33:507-510, 1982.

339. Miles J, Pennybacker J, Sheldon P: Intrathoracic meningocele. Its development and association with neurofibromatosis. J Neurol Neurosurg Psychiatry 32:99-110, 1969.

340. Glazer HS, Siegel MJ, Sagel SS: Low-attenuation mediastinal masses on CT. AJR Am J Roentgenol 152:1173-1177, 1989.

341. Cabooter M, Bogaerts Y, Javaheri S, et al: Intrathoracic meningocele. Eur J Respir Dis 63:347-350, 1982.

342. Bajpai M, Mathur M: Duplications of the alimentary tract: Clues to the missing links. J Pediatr Surg 29:1361-1365, 1994.

343. Ochsner JL, Ochsner SF: Congenital cysts of the mediastinum: 20-year experience with 42 cases. Ann Surg 163:909-920, 1966.

344. Kirwan WO, Walbaum PR, McCormack RJ: Cystic intrathoracic derivatives of the foregut and their complications. Thorax 28:424-428, 1973.

345. Rakower J, Milwidsky H: Primary mediastinal echinococcosis. Am J Med 29:73-83, 1960.

346. von Sinner WN, Linjawi T, al watban JA: Mediastinal hydatid disease: Report of three cases. Can Assoc Radiol J 41:79-82, 1990.

347. Verani R, Olson J, Moake JL: Intrathoracic extramedullary hematopoiesis: Report of a case in a patient with sickle-cell disease–beta-thalassemia. Am J Clin Pathol 73:133-137, 1980.

348. Papavasiliou CG: Tumor simulating intrathoracic extramedullary hemopoiesis: Clinical and roentgenologic considerations. Am J Roentgenol Radium Ther Nucl Med 93:695-702, 1965.

349. Da Costa JL, Loh YS, Hanam E: Extramedullary hemopoiesis with multiple tumor-simulating mediastinal masses in hemoglobin E–thalassemia disease. Chest 65:210-212, 1974.

350. Long JA Jr, Doppman JL, Nienhuis AW: Computed tomographic studies of thoracic extramedullary hematopoiesis. J Comput Assist Tomogr 4:67-70, 1980.

351. Moran CA, Suster S, Fishback N, et al: Extramedullary hematopoiesis presenting as posterior mediastinal mass: A study of four cases. Mod Pathol 8:249-251, 1995.

352. Gumbs RV, Higginbotham-Ford EA, Teal JS, et al: Thoracic extramedullary hematopoiesis in sickle-cell disease. AJR Am J Roentgenol 149:889-893, 1987.

353. Joy G, Logan PM: Residents' corner. Answer to case of the month #55. Intrathoracic extramedullary hematopoiesis secondary to idiopathic myelofibrosis. Can Assoc Radiol J 49:200-202, 1998.

354. Coates GG, Eisenberg B, Dail DH: Tc-99m sulfur colloid demonstration of diffuse pulmonary interstitial extramedullary hematopoiesis in a patient with myelofibrosis. A case report and review of the literature. Clin Nucl Med 19:1079-1084, 1994.

355. Harnsberger HR, Datz FL, Knochel JQ, et al: Failure to detect extramedullary hematopoiesis during bone-marrow imaging with indium-111 or technetium-99m sulfur colloid. J Nucl Med 23:589-591, 1982.

356. Smith PR, Manjoney DL, Teitcher JB, et al: Massive hemothorax due to intrathoracic extramedullary hematopoiesis in a patient with thalassemia intermedia. Chest 94:658-660, 1988.

DISEASE OF THE DIAPHRAGM AND CHEST WALL

THE DIAPHRAGM

Abnormalities of Diaphragmatic Position or Motion

Unilateral Diaphragmatic Paralysis

Paralysis of a hemidiaphragm usually results from interruption of transmission of nerve impulses through the phrenic nerve and is associated with many causes. The most common is invasion of the nerve by a neoplasm, usually of pulmonary origin. The second most frequent category is paralysis of unknown etiology; in these idiopathic cases, the paralysis is almost invariably right sided.

Unilateral diaphragmatic paralysis can also occur as a complication of radical neck or thoracic surgery, especially coronary artery bypass surgery.[1] The mechanism by which the hemidiaphragm is paralyzed has not been definitely determined in the latter circumstance; however, there is evidence that it may be the result of cold topical cardioplegia. During cardiopulmonary bypass and aortocoronary bypass grafting, ice slush cooled to subfreezing temperatures by the addition of salt is sometimes packed into the pericardial cavity. The left phrenic nerve runs within the posterior pericardium on the left side; thus, temporary cold-induced injury can theoretically occur.[2,3]

Radiologically, a paralyzed hemidiaphragm appears elevated and has an accentuated dome configuration in both posteroanterior and lateral projections. Since the peripheral points of attachment of the diaphragm are fixed, the costophrenic and costovertebral sulci tend to be deepened, narrowed, and sharpened (Fig. 22–1). If the paralysis is left sided, the stomach and splenic flexure of the colon relate to the inferior surface of the hemidiaphragm and usually contain more gas than normal. Invasion or compression of the phrenic nerve by abnormalities such as pulmonary carcinoma or calcified lymph nodes can be clarified by CT if necessary.[4]

The most reliable radiologic maneuver for detecting hemidiaphragmatic paralysis is the sniff test performed while visualizing the diaphragm with fluoroscopy. Normally, both hemidiaphragms descend sharply during a sniff; with unilateral diaphragmatic paralysis there is paradoxical upward motion of the affected side. Although significant paradoxical motion provides strong evidence of diaphragmatic paralysis, sniffing can cause paradoxical motion of one hemidiaphragm in some normal individuals, and for it to be considered pathologic, it should consist of a reverse excursion of at least 2 cm.[5] False-negative results can occur if the patient uses the abdominal musculature to elevate the diaphragm during the expiratory phase of breathing.[6] Normal and abnormal diaphragmatic motion and hemidiaphragmatic paralysis can also be assessed with ultrasound and MR imaging.[7,8,9,10]

Patients with a paralyzed hemidiaphragm do not usually have symptoms; however, some complain of dyspnea on effort or (rarely) orthopnea.[11] The severity of either symptom relates to the rapidity of development of the paralysis and to the presence or absence of underlying pulmonary disease.

Bilateral Diaphragmatic Paralysis

The most common cause of bilateral diaphragmatic paralysis is spinal cord injury. Neuritis, diabetes mellitus, and congenital central nervous system or spinal cord anomalies are seen occasionally.

The radiographic appearance consists of elevated hemidiaphragms in both posteroanterior and lateral projections.[6] Linear atelectasis may be present at the lung bases. Paradoxical upward motion of both hemidiaphragms during an inspiratory effort or sniff is usually observed on fluoroscopic examination, although recruitment of abdominal expiratory muscles

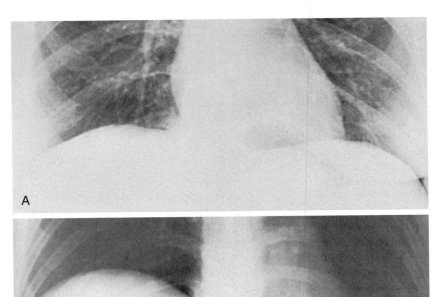

FIGURE 22-1

Paralysis of the right hemidiaphragm. A 33-year-old woman was admitted to the hospital for repair of a lacerated finger tendon. A view of the lower half of the thorax from a preoperative radiograph (**A**) reveals a normal position of both hemidiaphragms. After anesthesia was established by brachial plexus block, the patient complained of mild dyspnea, and a radiograph of the chest (**B**) revealed marked elevation of the right hemidiaphragm in a contour typical of diaphragmatic paralysis. (*From Müller NL, Fraser RS, Colman NC, Paré PD: Radiologic Diagnosis of Diseases of the Chest. Philadelphia, WB Saunders, 2001.*)

can result in a false-negative test.[12,13] Some patients actively expire to a lung volume below true FRC and then use the elastic recoil forces of the abdominothoracic structures to assist the next inspiration passively; sudden downward motion of the diaphragm coincident with abdominal muscle relaxation may be misinterpreted as diaphragmatic contraction when one views it fluoroscopically. Despite these potential pitfalls, fluoroscopy can be effectively used to evaluate the condition.[14] The characteristic findings consist of cephalad movement of the paralyzed diaphragm during inspiration, accompanied by outward chest wall and inward abdominal wall motion, a phenomenon known as the "thoracoabdominal paradox."[14]

Diaphragmatic motion can also be monitored by ultrasonography.[15,16] In fact, the ability of ultrasound to assess diaphragmatic thickness and changing thickness with respiration makes it possibly superior to fluoroscopy.[8,17]

Patients with bilateral diaphragmatic paralysis have profound respiratory symptoms and functional derangement.[12] Ventilatory failure and hypercapnia eventually develop in most; some have evidence of cor pulmonale and right ventricular failure. Breathlessness on exertion and orthopnea are characteristic.

Eventration

Eventration is a congenital anomaly consisting of failure of muscular development of part or all of one or both hemidiaphragms.[18] When marked diaphragmatic elevation can be attributed to a specific cause (e.g., interruption of the phrenic nerve by invasive neoplasm or surgical section), it is clearly possible to use specific terminology in describing the situation; sometimes, however, there is no way of knowing whether the elevation is caused by congenital absence of muscle or by phrenic nerve paralysis (Fig. 22–2).[19,20]

Pathologically, a totally eventrated hemidiaphragm consists of a thin membranous sheet attached peripherally to normal muscle at points of origin from the rib cage. It occurs almost exclusively on the left side. Partial eventration is more common than the total form and is usually present in the anteromedial portion of the right hemidiaphragm; it occurs with equal frequency in men and women, rarely on the left and occasionally in the central portion of either cupola.[21]

The radiologic signs of complete eventration are identical to those described for diaphragmatic paralysis. In patients with only partial failure of muscular development of one hemidiaphragm, the affected hemidiaphragm shows a smaller than normal inspiratory excursion. On fluoroscopy or real-time ultrasound, it may have an initial inspiratory lag or small paradoxical motion; however, later in inspiration it has downward motion.[22]

A confident diagnosis of partial eventration can be established by CT, ultrasonography, or MR imaging.[23] The main value of these procedures is in distinguishing the abnormality from a focal bulge on the diaphragmatic contour caused by a

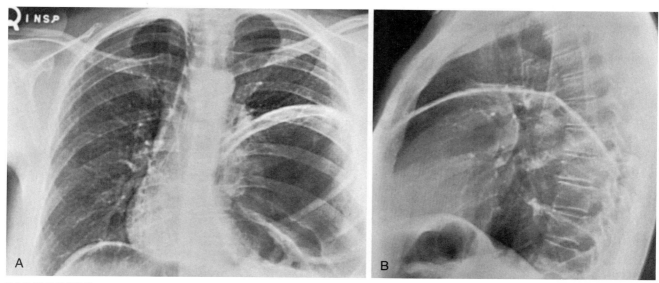

FIGURE 22–2

Paralysis or eventration of the left hemidiaphragm associated with severe colonic dilatation. Posteroanterior (**A**) and lateral (**B**) radiographs reveal a remarkable degree of elevation of the left hemidiaphragm. Severely dilated loops of colon are situated beneath this hemidiaphragm and to a lesser extent beneath the right one. The mediastinum is displaced considerably into the right hemithorax. *(From Müller NL, Fraser RS, Colman NC, Paré PD: Radiologic Diagnosis of Diseases of the Chest. Philadelphia, WB Saunders, 2001.)*

tumor or hernia. In eventration, the diaphragm, though thin, can be seen as a continuous layer above the elevated abdominal viscera and retroperitoneal or omental fat. On fluoroscopy and real-time ultrasound, the area of eventration can be seen to move downward with the normal portions of the hemidiaphragm, although it may have a slight lag in its inspiratory excursion.[22]

Characteristically, eventration is unassociated with symptoms and is discovered on a screening chest radiograph. However, symptoms may be present in obese patients as a result of raised intra-abdominal pressure. Although these symptoms are usually related to the gastrointestinal tract, respiratory embarrassment has been attributed to the anomaly.[24]

Restriction of Diaphragmatic Motion

A great variety of diseases of the lungs, pleura, abdominal organs, and the diaphragm itself may lead to restriction of diaphragmatic motion. In some, the limitation in motion is imposed by the character of the disease itself—for example, the severe pulmonary overinflation and air trapping that characterize diffuse emphysema or asthma prevent normal ascent of the diaphragm during expiration. In other diseases, local irritation causes "splinting" of a hemidiaphragm that is manifested not only by reduced excursion but also by elevation; such splinting can be caused by acute lower lobe pneumonia or infarction, acute pleuritis, rib fractures, and intra-abdominal processes such as subphrenic abscess, acute cholecystitis, and peritonitis.

Although other skeletal muscle groups react to irritation or injury by spasm, the diaphragm appears to react by relaxation; this is the only way of explaining the elevation that characteristically accompanies local inflammation. The mechanism by which the diaphragm is splinted in the postoperative period is thought to be neural inhibition,[25,26] possibly caused by

stimulation of diaphragmatic or splanchnic afferents. Diaphragmatic dysfunction is maximal 8 hours after upper abdominal surgery, with function improving over the subsequent 2 to 7 days.[25]

Diaphragmatic Hernias

Herniation of abdominal or retroperitoneal organs or tissues into the thorax may occur through congenital or acquired weak areas in the diaphragm or through rents resulting from trauma (see page 799). The most frequent nontraumatic form occurs through the esophageal hiatus; hernias through the pleuroperitoneal hiatus (Bochdalek's hernia) or the parasternal hiatus (Morgagni's hernia) are seen less commonly.

Hernia through the Esophageal Hiatus

Although a congenital weakness of the esophageal hiatus may be partly responsible for the development of hiatus hernia, there is little doubt that acquired factors play a significant role, the most important being obesity and pregnancy. The prevalence increases with age; the abnormality is evident on CT in approximately 5% of individuals younger than 40 years, 30% of those between 40 and 59, and 65% of those between 60 and 79.[27] Most patients do not have symptoms, the abnormality being discovered on a chest radiograph or CT performed for unrelated complaints.

The chest radiograph typically shows a retrocardiac mass, usually containing air or an air-fluid level (Fig. 22–3). Definitive diagnosis sometimes requires barium study of the esophagogastric junction or the use of CT.[27,28] In cases in which most of the stomach has herniated through the hiatus, the stomach may undergo volvulus, resulting in the presence of a large mass containing a double air-fluid level; incarceration of such

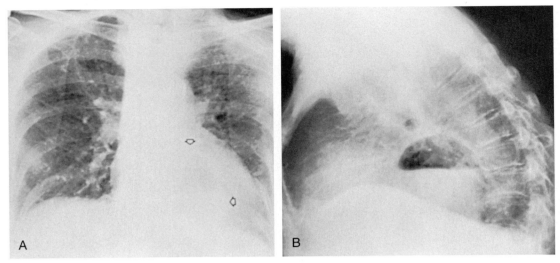

FIGURE 22–3

Large hiatus hernia. Posteroanterior (**A**) and lateral (**B**) radiographs of the chest of an 87-year-old woman reveal a large soft tissue mass containing a prominent air-fluid level occupying the posteroinferior portion of the mediastinum (*arrows* in **A**). The patient had no symptoms referable to this hernia. *(From Müller NL, Fraser RS, Colman NC, Paré PD: Radiologic Diagnosis of Diseases of the Chest. Philadelphia, WB Saunders, 2001.)*

hernial contents is common, and strangulation may occur.[29] The development of acute upper gastrointestinal tract symptoms in a patient who has a herniated stomach should immediately raise suspicion of this complication because it is life-threatening and necessitates immediate surgical intervention.[30]

Although the stomach is the most common hernial content, other structures, such as a portion of the transverse colon, omentum, or liver, can also be seen.[31] In addition, ascitic fluid can extend from the peritoneal cavity into the posterior mediastinum through the esophageal hiatus, an occurrence that can be demonstrated to excellent advantage with CT.[32]

Hernia through the Foramen of Bochdalek

In infants, herniation through a persistent embryonic pleuroperitoneal hiatus is both the most common and the most serious form of diaphragmatic hernia. Its incidence is approximately 1 in 2200 live births.[22,33] Most (75% to 90%) occur on the left side.[34] When large, the hernias are associated with high mortality; even after successful surgical correction, mortality is about 30% as a result of hypoplasia of the underlying lung and pulmonary arterial hypertension (see page 189).[34]

The size of the defect varies widely. When large, as with complete or nearly complete absence of a hemidiaphragm, almost the entire abdominal contents, including the stomach, may be in the left hemithorax, thereby interfering with normal lung development and resulting in hypoplasia.[35,36] Most large hernias have no peritoneal sac, so communication between the pleural and the peritoneal cavities is wide open. When the defect is small, a sac lined by pleura and containing retroperitoneal fat, a portion of the spleen or kidney,[37] or omentum may be the only discernible abnormality.[38]

In adults, small Bochdalek's hernias are much more common than in infants; in fact, small Bochdalek hernias are

seen on CT in about 5% to 10% of adults.[27,39] Their incidence increases with age, suggesting that they are acquired; they are rare in patients younger than 40 but are seen in approximately 5% of patients between 40 and 49 years of age, 15% of patients between 50 and 69 years of age, and 35% of older patients.[27] Unlike the infantile form, hernias seen in adults are almost always unassociated with symptoms.

On the chest radiograph, Bochdalek's hernia can be manifested as a focal bulge in the hemidiaphragm or as a mass adjacent to the posteromedial aspect of either hemidiaphragm (Fig. 22–4). Although the diagnosis can often be suspected on the radiograph by the typical location and by the lower than soft tissue density of the mass because of its fat content, the appearance can mimic that of pulmonary, mediastinal, or paravertebral masses.[40] The diagnosis is readily made on CT.[40-42]

Hernia through the Foramen of Morgagni

Morgagni's (retrosternal or parasternal) hernia is uncommon. The left foramen relates to the heart; as a result, most herniations are seen on the right side.[43] Although the defects are developmental in origin, hernias are more common in adults than children and are often associated with obesity or other situations involving increased intra-abdominal pressure or trauma[22,44]; in fact, affected patients are usually overweight, middle-aged women. In contrast to Bochdalek's hernias, a peritoneal sac is present in most cases. The content of the hernial sac is usually omentum and sometimes liver or bowel. Cases have been reported in which the defect has extended into the pericardial sac, thereby allowing displacement of abdominal contents into this site.[45]

Radiologically, the typical appearance is that of a smooth, well-defined opacity in the right cardiophrenic angle (Fig. 22–5). In most patients, the shadow is of homogeneous density. Occasionally, it is inhomogeneous as a result of either

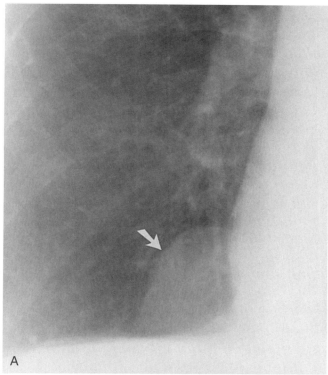

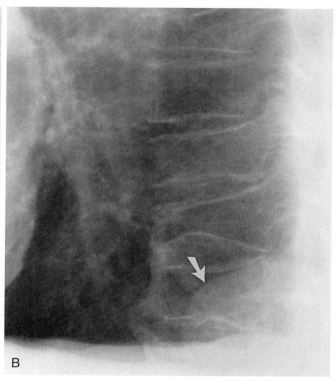

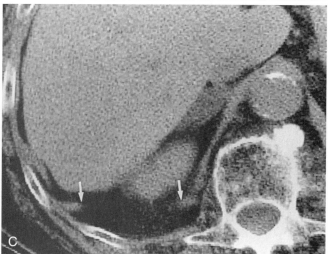

FIGURE 22–4

Bochdalek's hernia. Views of posteroanterior (**A**) and lateral
(**B**) radiographs in a 78-year-old woman demonstrate a large mass adjacent
to the posteromedial aspect of the right hemidiaphragm (*arrows*). The
mass has lower opacity than the heart and soft tissues of the abdomen,
consistent with fat. A view of the right hemidiaphragm from a CT scan
(**C**) demonstrates a focal defect (*arrows*) in the posterior aspect of the right
hemidiaphragm with herniation of omental fat. The patient had no symptoms
related to the hernia. *(From Müller NL, Fraser RS, Colman NC, Paré PD:
Radiologic Diagnosis of Diseases of the Chest. Philadelphia, WB Saunders,
2001.)*

an air-containing loop of bowel or the predominantly fatty
nature of the hernial contents. In the latter situation, the
hernia is likely to contain omentum, and CT or barium enema
reveals the transverse colon to be situated high in the abdomen
with a peak situated anteriorly and superiorly, a finding that
is virtually diagnostic. In the rare case in which the hernia penetrates into the pericardial sac, loops of air-containing bowel
may be identified anterior to the cardiac shadow.[45] The diagnosis of Morgagni's hernia can be readily made on CT or MR
imaging.[22,40,46]

Most hernias do not give rise to symptoms. The few
patients who have symptoms complain of epigastric or lower
sternal pressure and discomfort and sometimes cardiorespiratory and gastrointestinal symptoms.[47]

Neoplasms of the Diaphragm

Primary Neoplasms

Primary neoplasms of the diaphragm are uncommon.[48,49]
Most develop from the tendinous or anterior muscular
portion. The most common benign form is lipoma[50,51]; neural
tumors, leiomyoma, hemangioma, and other soft tissue
tumors are seen rarely.[52,53,54] Fat pads and herniations of
omental fat are common in the region of the diaphragm; thus,
a diagnosis of lipoma requires demonstration of a true
capsule.[55] Fibrosarcoma is the most common malignant
neoplasm[55,56]; many other soft tissue tumor types have
been reported rarely. Various non-neoplastic abnormalities

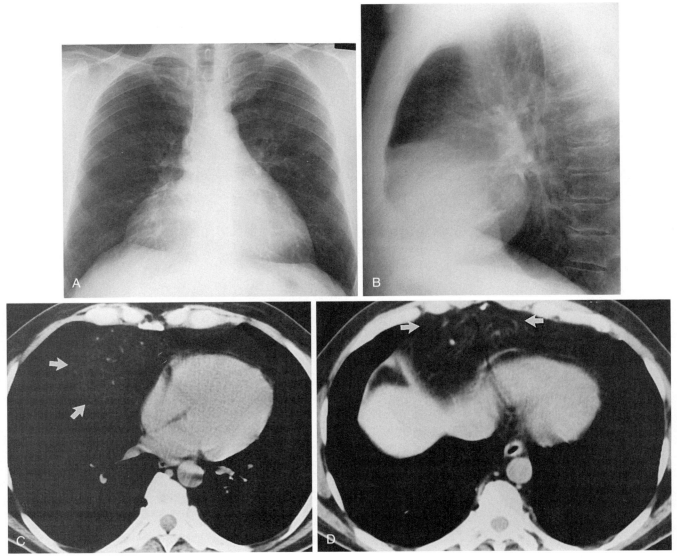

FIGURE 22–5

Morgagni's hernia. Posteroanterior (**A**) and lateral (**B**) chest radiographs demonstrate a mass in the right costophrenic sulcus. The mass has a density lower than that of soft tissue, consistent with fat. CT scans (**C** and **D**) demonstrate herniation of omental fat (*arrows*) through the right lower parasternal region (*arrows*). The patient was a 49-year-old man. (*From Müller NL, Fraser RS, Colman NC, Paré PD: Radiologic Diagnosis of Diseases of the Chest. Philadelphia, WB Saunders, 2001.*)

that form localized tumors, such as lymphangioma and endometrioma,[48] are also found occasionally.

Most diaphragmatic tumors are manifested radiologically as smooth or lobulated soft tissue masses protruding into the inferior portion of the lung (Fig. 22–6). In many cases, malignant tumors involve much of one hemidiaphragm and thus simulate diaphragmatic elevation; associated pleural effusion is common. The presence of an intradiaphragmatic mass can be established most easily by CT.[22,55,57] When the tumor is large, it may not be possible to determine whether it originates in the diaphragm, pleura, lungs, or liver.[55] Variations in diaphragmatic thickness on CT occasionally mimic an intradiaphragmatic mass or a tumor in an adjacent organ.[58] The distinction can be made readily by careful analysis of sequential images and on multiplanar reformations.

As might be expected, benign neoplasms typically occasion no symptoms; by contrast, the majority of patients who have primary malignant neoplasms complain of epigastric or lower chest pain, cough, dyspnea, and gastrointestinal discomfort.[48,49]

Secondary Neoplasms

Secondary neoplastic involvement of the diaphragm occurs most frequently by direct extension of neoplasm from the basal pleura in cases of pulmonary carcinoma or mesothelioma; however, any neoplasm that metastasizes to the pleura or that involves the basal lung, liver, or subphrenic peritoneum can spread into the diaphragm. Ovarian carcinoma is particularly likely to be the cause when the initial site of involvement

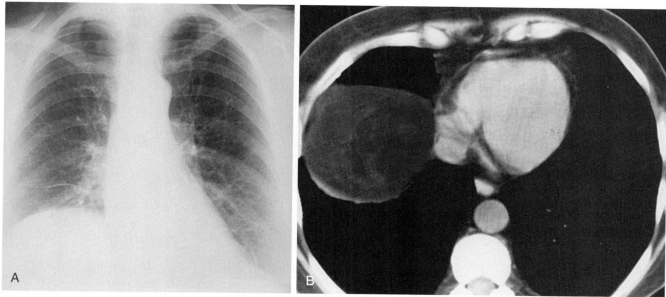

FIGURE 22–6

Lipoma of the diaphragm. A posteroanterior chest radiograph (**A**) in a 62-year-old woman demonstrates apparent elevation of the right hemidiaphragm. A CT scan (**B**) demonstrates a large, round mass in the right lower hemithorax. The mass contains fat and a few blood vessels. *(From Müller NL, Fraser RS, Colman NC, Paré PD: Radiologic Diagnosis of Diseases of the Chest. Philadelphia, WB Saunders, 2001.)*

is the peritoneum.[59] Discrete diaphragmatic metastases derived from either lymphatic or hematogenous spread are rare. The radiographic features and clinical manifestations are usually related to the presence of neoplasm in contiguous structures or elsewhere rather than in the diaphragm itself.

Miscellaneous Abnormalities of the Diaphragm

An accessory diaphragm is a rare anomaly in which the right hemithorax is partitioned into two compartments by a musculotendinous membrane resembling a diaphragm.[60] The accessory leaf is usually situated within the oblique fissure and separates the lower lobe from the remainder of the right lung. Radiologically, it may be mistaken for a somewhat thickened major fissure.

Diaphragmatic defects too small to allow passage of a hernial sac may explain the pleural effusions that develop in patients who have conditions such as Meigs' syndrome or cirrhosis and ascites.[61,62] Such defects may be congenital or acquired and can be demonstrated either directly at autopsy or surgery or indirectly by the development of pneumothorax after the intraperitoneal administration of gas.[62] Similar small defects have been postulated as the entry sites for tissue or air in some cases of pleural endometriosis and catamenial pneumothorax.[63,64]

Intradiaphragmatic cysts are rare and usually represent extralobar sequestration. In most cases, the cyst receives its blood supply from the abdominal aorta or one of its branches and characteristically drains by way of the systemic veins.[65] The anomaly is seen in the left hemidiaphragm in 90% of cases and is usually associated with diaphragmatic eventration.[66]

THE CHEST WALL

Abnormalities of the Pectoral Girdle and Adjacent Structures

A variety of congenital anomalies affect the bones and muscles of the chest wall. The most common anomaly involving the clavicle is *cleidocranial dysostosis*, a syndrome characterized by incomplete ossification associated with defective development of the pubic bones, vertebral column, and long bones. *Sprengel's deformity* is characterized by failure of the scapula to descend normally so that its superior angle lies on a plane higher than the neck of the first rib. It is frequently associated with fusion of two or more cervical vertebrae and results in a short, wide neck with considerably limited movement (the Klippel-Feil deformity).[67] *Poland's syndrome* consists of hypoplasia or aplasia of the pectoralis major muscle and ipsilateral syndactyly[68]; rarely, the hypoplasia-aplasia is bilateral.[68a] Unilateral absence of the pectoralis muscles results in unilateral hyperlucency on the chest radiograph, not to be confused with Swyer-James syndrome (Fig. 22–7).

A pulmonary hernia occurs when the lung protrudes beyond the confines of the thoracic cage. It is an uncommon abnormality, with only approximately 300 cases having been reported by 1996.[69] Approximately 20% are congenital and the remainder acquired. The hernias can be classified according to their location; intercostal hernias are the most common (approximately two thirds of cases), followed by cervical (approximately a third) and diaphragmatic (about 1%).[69,70] The majority of acquired hernias develop after penetrating injury, blunt trauma associated with multiple rib fractures, thoracotomy, or chest tube insertion (see pages 802 and 808).[69,70] Most patients are asymptomatic. Occasionally, a painless bulge

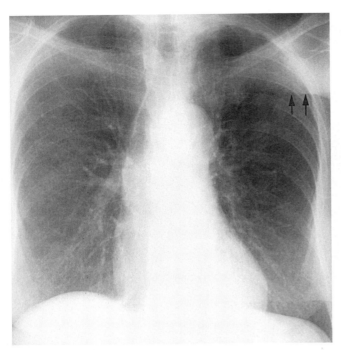

FIGURE 22-7

Congenital absence of the pectoralis muscle. A posteroanterior radiograph demonstrates increased radiolucency of the left hemithorax. The course of the left anterior axillary fold (*arrows*) is horizontal as a result of absence of the left pectoralis muscle. Note that the breast shadows are symmetrical. The patient was a 67-year-old woman. *(From Müller NL, Fraser RS, Colman NC, Paré PD: Radiologic Diagnosis of Diseases of the Chest. Philadelphia, WB Saunders, 2001.)*

can be palpated during cough. Radiographic manifestations include a well-circumscribed lucency extending beyond the rib cage or an air collection in the tissues overlying the chest wall.[69,70] Unless the hernia is tangential to the x-ray beam, it may not be apparent on the radiograph. The diagnosis can be readily made on CT (Fig. 22–8).[70,71]

Abnormalities of the Ribs

Cervical Rib

An anomalous accessory rib in the cervical region is a relatively common finding that is seen in about 0.5% of the general population.[72] It usually arises from the seventh cervical vertebra. Both the anomaly and the symptoms that derive therefrom are said to be more common in women in a ratio of approximately 2.5:1.[72] In about 90% of cases, the ribs do not cause symptoms; however, when they compress the cervical spinal cord,[73] the subclavian vessels, or the brachial plexus (thoracic outlet syndrome), symptoms can be present and are sometimes disabling.[74,75]

Rib Notching and Erosion

Notching of ribs is most frequent on the inferior aspect and has many causes (Table 22–1).[76] By far the most common is coarctation of the aorta, which typically produces notching several centimeters lateral to the costovertebral junction on

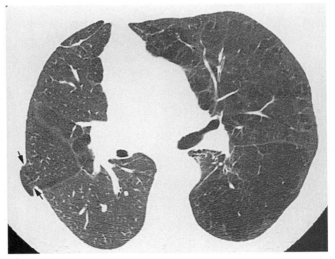

FIGURE 22-8

Lung hernia. An HRCT scan demonstrates a focal defect in right chest wall (*arrows*) associated with a lung hernia. The patient was a 64-year-old woman who had undergone right lung transplantation for emphysema. *(From Müller NL, Fraser RS, Colman NC, Paré PD: Radiologic Diagnosis of Diseases of the Chest. Philadelphia, WB Saunders, 2001.)*

TABLE 22–1. Causes of Inferior Rib Notching

Arterial
Aortic obstruction
Coarctation of the aortic arch
Thrombosis of the abdominal aorta
Subclavian artery obstruction
Blalock-Taussig operation
Takayasu's arteritis
Widened arterial pulse pressure
Decreased pulmonary blood flow
Tetralogy of Fallot
Pulmonary atresia (pseudotruncus)
Ebstein's malformation
Pulmonary valve stenosis
Unilateral absence of the pulmonary artery
Pulmonary emphysema
Venous
Superior vena cava obstruction
Arteriovenous
Pulmonary arteriovenous fistula
Intercostal arteriovenous fistula
Neurogenic
Intercostal neurogenic tumor
Osseous
Hyperparathyroidism
Idiopathic

ribs 3 to 9 (Fig. 22–9). The notches result from erosion of bone by dilated intercostal arteries taking part in collateral arterial flow. These arteries may become extremely tortuous and may even extend to and erode the superior aspects of contiguous ribs. Rib notching secondary to coarctation of the aorta is seldom seen in patients before the age of 6 or 7 years and is not usually well developed until the early teens.[77]

Notching or erosion of the superior aspects of the ribs is considerably less common than that of the inferior aspect; however, it may be present more often than generally recognized because its more subtle radiographic appearance

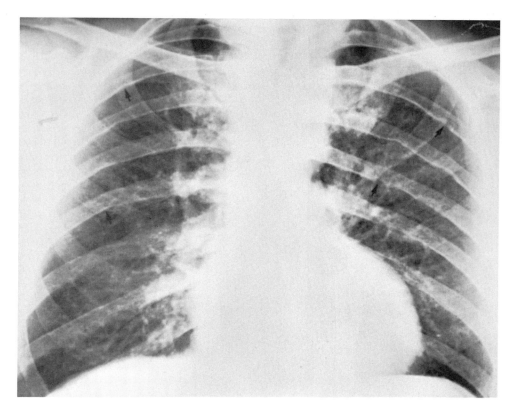

FIGURE 22–9

Rib notching—coarctation of the aorta. A posteroanterior radiograph demonstrates numerous defects in the inferior surfaces of ribs 4 to 8 bilaterally (several are indicated by *arrows*). The configuration of vascular shadows in the region of the aortic arch is strongly suggestive of coarctation. *(From Müller NL, Fraser RS, Colman NC, Paré PD: Radiologic Diagnosis of Diseases of the Chest. Philadelphia, WB Saunders, 2001.)*

TABLE 22–2. Causes of Superior Rib Notching

Disturbance of osteoblastic activity (decreased or deficient bone formation)
    Connective tissue diseases (rheumatoid arthritis, progressive systemic sclerosis, lupus erythematosus, Sjögren's syndrome)
    Localized pressure (rib retractors, chest tubes, multiple hereditary exostoses, neurofibromatosis, thoracic neuroblastoma, coarctation of the aorta)
    Osteogenesis imperfecta
    Marfan's syndrome
    Radiation damage
Disturbance of osteoclastic activity (increased bone resorption)
    Hyperparathyroidism
    Hypervitaminosis D
Idiopathic

hinders its appreciation. The causes of superior marginal rib defects can be classified into three groups:[78] (1) those associated with a disturbance in osteoblastic activity (decreased or deficient bone formation); (2) those associated with a disturbance in osteoclastic activity (increased bone resorption); and (3) idiopathic (Table 22–2). The radiographic appearance typically consists of shallow indentations ranging from 1 to 4 cm in length on ribs 3 to 9 posterolaterally.

Osteomyelitis

Primary infection of the ribs is rare and may be difficult to appreciate radiologically until bone destruction is advanced. More commonly, osteomyelitis is secondary to infectious processes in the lung (usually the result of *Mycobacterium tuberculosis*, *Actinomyces israelii*, or *Nocardia asteroides*) or to empyema (empyema necessitatis).

Costochondral Osteochondritis

Costochondral osteochondritis (Tietze's syndrome) is clinically characterized by painful, nonsuppurative swelling of one or more costochondral or sternochondral joints.[79] It is usually seen in adolescents and young adults. The etiology and pathogenesis are unknown but have been speculated to be related to infection or an immunologic disorder.[80] Weeks or months may elapse before the swelling and pain disappear, and slight chest wall deformity may persist.

Although the majority of patients undoubtedly manifest no radiologic changes, hypertrophy and excess calcification of costal cartilage can be identified in some.[81] The second ribs are the most commonly involved. Affected ribs may show evidence of periosteal reaction and increased size and density anteriorly. Enlargement and alteration of the trabecular pattern of the anterior portion of the first ribs can also occur and may lead to an extremely dense appearance of the bone. CT is helpful in distinguishing the abnormality from more serious disease: the most common abnormalities are enlargement of costal cartilage at the site of the complaint and ventral angulation of the involved costal cartilage.[82] Costochondral osteochondritis can result in increased uptake of 2-[^{18}F]-fluoro-2-deoxy-D-glucose (FDG) and mimic a lung nodule on positron emission tomography.[83]

Abnormalities of the Sternum

Pectus Excavatum

Pectus excavatum ("funnel chest") is a common deformity that consists of depression of the sternum so that the ribs on

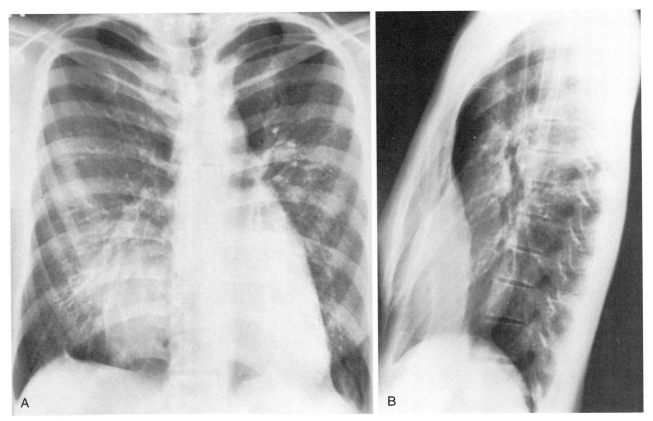

FIGURE 22-10

Pectus excavatum. Posteroanterior (**A**) and lateral (**B**) radiographs of the chest reveal a fairly large opacity projected over the lower portion of the right hemithorax contiguous with the shadow of the thoracic spine. The pulmonary arteries to the right lower lobe are displaced laterally and the heart is displaced to the left. The deformity of the sternum can be readily identified in lateral projection and is of sufficient degree to displace the heart posteriorly so that the contour of the left ventricle is projected over the thoracic vertebral bodies. The patient was a young woman who had no symptoms. *(From Müller NL, Fraser RS, Colman NC, Paré PD: Radiologic Diagnosis of Diseases of the Chest. Philadelphia, WB Saunders, 2001.)*

each side protrude anteriorly more than the sternum itself. It is believed to result from a genetically determined abnormality of the sternum and related portions of the diaphragm; the condition can occur either sporadically or with a dominant pattern of inheritance.[84,85] The prevalence in the general population has been estimated to range from about 0.1% to 0.4%.[84] The vast majority of patients are asymptomatic.

The radiographic manifestations are easily recognized (Fig. 22–10). In posteroanterior projection, the heart is displaced to the left and rotated. The parasternal soft tissues of the anterior chest wall, which are seen in profile rather than straight on, are apparent as increased density over the inferomedial portion of the right hemithorax and should not be mistaken for disease of the right middle lobe, even though the right heart border is obscured. The degree of sternal depression is easily seen on a lateral radiograph. Possibly as a result of upward compression deformity of the heart and great vessels, the abnormality is occasionally associated with an unusual mediastinal configuration that can simulate a mediastinal mass[86]; in such cases, the true nature of the configuration can usually be readily clarified by CT.

Infection

Infection of the sternum and its articulations is seen most frequently after median sternotomy for heart surgery. It has been reported in 0.5% to 5% of patients undergoing sternotomy.[87,88] Occasionally, evidence of sternal osteomyelitis or a retrosternal abscess is apparent on the lateral radiograph[89,90]; however, CT is the imaging method of choice for the assessment of patients suspected of having the complication.[88,90] Findings include irregularity of the bony sternotomy margins, periosteal new bone formation, bony sclerosis, and peristernal soft tissue masses that may contain areas of low attenuation as a result of abscess formation.[88,90,91] Bone scintigraphy or the sequential use of bone scintigraphy and gallium 67 scintigraphy can also be helpful in evaluating these patients.

Abnormalities of the Thoracic Spine

Kyphoscoliosis

Abnormalities in curvature of the thoracic spine may be predominantly lateral (scoliosis), predominantly posterior (kyphosis), or a combination of the two (kyphoscoliosis).

Although such abnormalities are common, particularly scoliosis, deformity of a degree sufficient to cause symptoms and signs of cardiac or pulmonary disease is rare.

Causes of the abnormal curvature can be considered in three groups: (1) congenital, including anomalies of the thoracic spine such as hemivertebrae and various hereditary disorders in which spinal deformity constitutes only a part of the clinical picture (e.g., neurofibromatosis, Friedreich's ataxia, Ehlers-Danlos syndrome, and Marfan's syndrome); (2) paralytic, including poliomyelitis, muscular dystrophy, and cerebral palsy; and (3) idiopathic. Patients in the last group constitute approximately 80% of those who have severe kyphoscoliosis; this variety has a female sex preponderance of 4:1.

In the great majority of cases, the scoliosis is convex to the right. The severity is best determined by the Cobb method:[92] lines are drawn parallel to the upper border of the highest and the lower border of the lowest vertebral bodies of the curvature as seen on an anteroposterior radiograph of the spine, and the angle is measured at the intersection of lines drawn perpendicular to these lines. The angle can also be measured simply by drawing lines parallel to the upper and lower borders of the vertebral bodies encompassing the curvature and calculating the angle at the intersection.

Disability from kyphoscoliosis is related to the angle of scoliosis and to age.[93] It has been suggested that it is the combination of the kyphotic and scoliotic defects that determines the severity of symptoms and the likelihood of ventilatory failure's developing,[94] with lesser degrees of scoliosis causing more severe impairment in the presence of severe kyphosis and vice versa. In general, ventilatory failure will develop in adults whose scoliotic angle is 100 degrees or more.

The major pathophysiologic effect of severe kyphoscoliosis is restrictive lung disease resulting in alveolar hypoventilation, hypoxic vasoconstriction, and eventually, pulmonary arterial hypertension and cor pulmonale. Symptoms and signs of cardiopulmonary disease do not usually appear until the fourth or fifth decade, at which time the course may be rapidly downhill and characterized by repeated episodes of ventilatory and right heart failure, often precipitated by pulmonary infection.

Tests of pulmonary function characteristically reveal a decrease in VC and TLC and normal or increased values of residual volume.[95] Restriction is the result of decreased compliance of both the lung and the chest wall.[96] The decrease in chest wall compliance may be profound and correlates significantly with the angle of scoliosis.[97] The mechanism by which lung compliance is reduced is unclear, but it could be related to microatelectasis or to an increase in the surface tension resulting from failure of the lung to inflate because of the chest wall restriction (or both). Expiratory flow rates are usually reduced only in proportion to the reduction in VC, and direct measurement of airway resistance reveals normal values in the majority.[98] However, some patients have airway obstruction in addition to lung restriction, which has been shown to be related to bronchial torsion and compression of central airways.[99]

In advanced disease, the presence of both hypoxemia and hypercapnia is a common finding that can be attributed to alveolar hypoventilation secondary to shallow respiration and ventilation-perfusion ($\dot{V}/\dot{Q}$) imbalance.[100] Patients can be particularly susceptible to ventilatory depression and oxygen desaturation during sleep.[101]

Ankylosing Spondylitis

Ankylosing spondylitis is an immunologic disorder that develops in approximately 1 in 2000 persons in the general population. It is strongly associated with the histocompatibility antigen HLA-B27:[102,103] the disease will develop in about 20% of HLA-B27–positive individuals, and approximately 90% of patients who have ankylosing spondylitis have the antigen.[103] Although the disease has been reported to occur four to eight times more frequently in males than in females, the distribution of HLA-B27–positive individuals is equal in the two sexes.[104] The discrepancy in sex incidence is related to the fact that the disease in women tends to be milder and is therefore diagnosed less often.[104] The onset of symptoms is early, usually in the third decade of life.

In addition to the characteristic changes in the thoracic skeleton, approximately 1% to 2% of patients have evidence of pleuropulmonary disease on chest radiographs.[105,106] The most common finding is upper lobe fibrobullous disease.[107-109] The bullae can be secondarily infected and associated with significant hemoptysis[110]; usually, this complication is related to the formation of a fungus ball and, occasionally, to nontuberculous mycobacterial infection. HRCT frequently demonstrates parenchymal abnormalities in patients who have normal radiographs, and it is abnormal in the majority of patients with a longer than 5 year history of ankylosing spondylitis.[111-113] The most common findings are localized areas of decreased attenuation and vascularity, air trapping, bronchial wall thickening, apical emphysema with bulla formation, irregular linear opacities and parenchymal bands predominantly in the apical lung regions, and apical pleural thickening.

The clinical picture is characterized by intermittent or continuous low back pain, sometimes associated with constitutional symptoms such as fatigue, weight loss, anorexia, and low-grade fever. The pain can be distinguished from that of a mechanical or nonspecific type by its insidious onset, its duration (usually more than 3 months before the patient seeks medical help), its association with morning stiffness, and its improvement with exercise.[114]

Infectious Spondylitis

Pyogenic or tuberculous spondylitis can result in destruction of the vertebral body and intervertebral disk and the development of a paraspinal mass on the chest radiograph. The mass is often fusiform and has its maximal diameter at the point of major bone destruction. Tuberculous spondylitis shows a predilection for the lower thoracic and upper lumbar spine.[115,116] CT demonstrates bone destruction and associated soft tissue masses that usually contain areas of low attenuation and show rim enhancement after the intravenous administration of contrast medium.[116] Foci of calcification are frequently present within the masses.[116] MR imaging is superior to CT in demonstrating early vertebral osteomyelitis and disk space infection[117-119]; however, CT is superior in the demonstration of calcification.

Neoplasms and Non-neoplastic Tumors of the Chest Wall

Neoplasms of Soft Tissue

Primary neoplasms of the soft tissues of the chest wall are rare. In adults, the most common benign lesion is lipoma; other benign tumors include neurogenic neoplasms of the intercostal nerves, fibromas and angiofibromas of the intercostal muscles, and desmoid tumors (fibromatosis).[120] The most common primary malignant neoplasms are fibrosarcoma, malignant fibrohistiocytoma, and peripheral neuroectodermal tumor; however, virtually any form of mesenchymal tumor can be seen.[121] Lymphoma and plasmacytoma are almost always secondary to adjacent skeletal or pleural disease; however, chest wall involvement is rarely the initial manifestation of Hodgkin's disease, in which case it probably represents direct spread from internal mammary lymph nodes.[122]

Lipoma. The point of origin of a lipoma in the chest wall establishes its mode of expression: when it originates adjacent to the parietal pleura, it causes a soft tissue mass that indents the lung and possesses a contour characteristic of its extrapulmonary origin; when it arises outside the rib cage, it is manifested as a soft tissue mass that may be visualized radiographically if viewed in profile or, if of sufficient size, even en face. Most lipomas that arise between the ribs have a dumbbell or hourglass configuration, part projecting inside and part outside the thoracic cage (Fig. 22–11).

As a result of the specificity of CT in identifying fat-containing structures, this technique is especially valuable in the diagnosis of these tumors.[123,124] The characteristic appearance consists of a well-defined mass that has homogeneous fat attenuation. Foci of calcification may be present in areas of fat necrosis.[124,125] The diagnosis can also be made on MRI, which shows signal intensities characteristic of fat on all pulse sequences.[125,126]

Neurogenic Tumors. Neurogenic tumors may involve the thoracic spine roots, the paraspinal ganglions of the sympathetic chain, the intercostal nerves along the thoracic cage, or the peripheral nerves on the chest wall. Plexiform neurofibromas, seen in patients who have neurofibromatosis, can involve the chest wall extensively.[124] Tumors arising from the intercostal nerves can result in rib erosion, notching, and sclerosis (Fig. 22–12).[124] On CT, they are usually visualized as well-circumscribed cylindrical masses. They may have homogeneous or heterogeneous attenuation that may be lower than or equal to that of chest wall muscle.[127,128] On MR imaging, they generally have low to intermediate signal intensity on T1-weighted images and inhomogeneously high signal intensity on T2-weighted images.[124,129]

Peripheral Primitive Neuroectodermal Tumor. This tumor is part of a group of clinically aggressive neoplasms characterized histologically by the presence of small round cells that have immunohistochemical and ultrastructural evidence of neural differentiation.[130] An abnormality in chromosome 22 is characteristically present.[131] Most tumors are seen in children, adolescents, or young adults. Chest wall pain is the usual initial symptom. Radiologic findings include a unilateral chest wall mass, rib destruction, pleural thickening or effusion, and evidence of extension into the adjacent lung.[132] The prognosis is poor.

Neoplasms and Non-neoplastic Tumors of Bone

Primary bone tumors arise most commonly in a rib and less often in the vertebrae, clavicles, and sternum.[133,134] Both CT

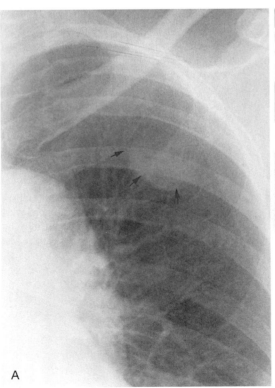

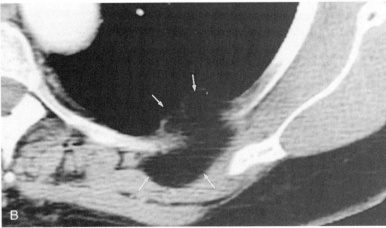

FIGURE 22–11

Chest wall lipoma. A view of the upper left side of the chest from a posteroanterior chest radiograph (**A**) shows a soft tissue opacity (*arrows*) projecting over the left posterior fifth rib. It has well-defined lower margins and poorly defined upper margins, thus suggesting that it abuts the lung and the chest wall. A CT scan (**B**) demonstrates that the mass (*arrows*) has homogeneous fat attenuation and an hourglass configuration. The findings are diagnostic of a lipoma, presumably originating from extrapleural fat. The patient was a 22-year-old woman with chest wall pain. (*From Müller NL, Fraser RS, Colman NC, Paré PD: Radiologic Diagnosis of Diseases of the Chest. Philadelphia, WB Saunders, 2001.*)

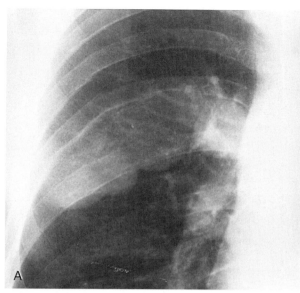
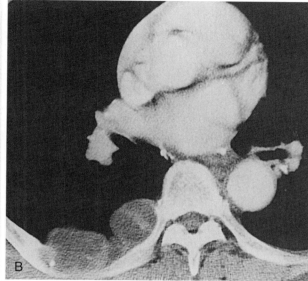

FIGURE 22–12

Intercostal neurilemoma. A close-up view of the right side of the chest from an anteroposterior radiograph (**A**) in a 69-year-old man demonstrates a soft tissue tumor adjacent and parallel to the right seventh rib. Also note notching and sclerosis of the undersurface of the rib and widening of the interspace between the seventh and the eighth ribs. A contrast-enhanced CT scan (**B**) shows the tumor to have nonhomogeneous attenuation and to contain cystic areas. Note the erosion of the posterior seventh rib. *(Case courtesy of Dr. Eun-Young Kang, Department of Radiology, Korea University Guro Hospital, Seoul, South Korea.)*

and MR imaging are helpful in characterizing a tumor and in assessing its extent.[135] The former is superior to MR imaging in demonstrating the foci of calcification seen in chondrosarcomas and osteosarcomas[90,124,126]; however, because of its greater ability to distinguish tumor from normal soft tissue, MR imaging is the modality of choice for assessment of the extent of chest wall tumors and their relationship to adjacent structures.[90,126,135]

The most frequent benign tumor of the thoracic skeleton is osteochondroma.[136] The most common non-neoplastic abnormality is fibrous dysplasia. The latter is usually monostotic and unassociated with symptoms; rarely, multiple lesions are sufficient to result in progressive restrictive lung disease, pulmonary hypertension, and cor pulmonale.[137] Involvement of the rib cage by Paget's disease produces a typical radiographic appearance similar to that in any other bone.

Metastatic carcinoma is by far the most common form of malignancy to affect the bones. It originates most frequently in the breast, thyroid, or lung.[138] Hodgkin's lymphoma can involve the sternum and parasternal chest wall as a result of contiguous spread from retrosternal lymph nodes.[139] The most frequent primary malignant neoplasm of the thoracic skeleton is chondrosarcoma.[140] Radiographically, the tumor usually appears as a mass on the lateral chest wall; sometimes, it arises in the posterior aspect of a rib, in which case it may appear as a paravertebral mass.[141] The tumors are usually large and have indistinct margins and soft tissue involvement.[136] Foci of calcification may be seen within the cartilaginous matrix. As indicated, these foci are best seen on CT.

Multiple myeloma and, occasionally, solitary plasmacytoma are the most frequent malignant lymphoid neoplasms, followed by Hodgkin's and non-Hodgkin's lymphoma.[133,142] In

older patients, particularly men, the association of a destructive lesion of one or more ribs with a soft tissue mass that protrudes into the thorax and indents the lung is highly suggestive of myeloma. However, a similar appearance can be seen in association with a primary pulmonary carcinoma that invades the chest wall and with other primary or metastatic chest wall neoplasms. Advanced myelomatosis of the rib cage may be associated with expansion of bone. Pathologic fractures, particularly of the sternum, may result in severe deformity of the chest wall.

The clinical manifestations of these tumors are varied. A pathologic fracture often causes a patient to seek medical advice; however, some patients have chest pain unassociated with fracture. Tumors of the vertebrae may compress the cord and result in neurologic signs and symptoms.[143]

REFERENCES

1. Wilcox P, Baile EM, Hards J, et al: Phrenic nerve function and its relationship to atelectasis after coronary artery bypass surgery. Chest 93:693-698, 1988.
2. Benjamin JJ, Cascade PN, Rubenfire M, et al: Left lower lobe atelectasis and consolidation following cardiac surgery: The effect of topical cooling on the phrenic nerve. Radiology 142:11-14, 1982.
3. Rousou JA, Parker T, Engelman RM, et al: Phrenic nerve paresis associated with the use of iced slush and the cooling jacket for topical hypothermia. J Thorac Cardiovasc Surg 89:921-925, 1985.
4. Shin MS, Ho KJ: Computed tomographic evaluation of the pathologic lesion for the idiopathic diaphragmatic paralysis. J Comput Tomogr 6:257-259, 1982.
5. Arborelius M Jr, Lilja B, Senyk J: Regional and total lung function studies in patients with hemidiaphragmatic paralysis. Respiration 32:253-264, 1975.
6. Alexander C: Diaphragm movements and the diagnosis of diaphragmatic paralysis. Clin Radiol 17:79-83, 1966.
7. Houston JG, Fleet M, Cowan MD, et al: Comparison of ultrasound with fluoroscopy in the assessment of suspected hemidiaphragmatic movement abnormality. Clin Radiol 50:95-98, 1995.
8. Gottesman E, McCool FD: Ultrasound evaluation of the paralyzed diaphragm. Am J Respir Crit Care Med 155:1570-1574, 1997.

9. Taylor AM, Jhooti P, Keegan J, et al: Magnetic resonance navigator echo diaphragm monitoring in patients with suspected diaphragm paralysis. J Magn Reson Imaging 9:69-74, 1999.

10. Iwasawa T, Kagei S, Gotoh T, et al: Magnetic resonance analysis of abnormal diaphragmatic motion in patients with emphysema. Eur Respir J 19:225-231, 2002.

11. Ridyard JB, Stewart RM: Regional lung function in unilateral diaphragmatic paralysis. Thorax 31:438-442, 1976.

12. Davis J, Goldman M, Loh L, et al: Diaphragm function and alveolar hypoventilation. Q J Med 45:87-100, 1976.

13. Loh L, Goldman M, Davis JN: The assessment of diaphragm function. Medicine (Baltimore) 56:165-169, 1977.

14. Ch'en IY Armstrong JD 2nd: Value of fluoroscopy in patients with suspected bilateral hemidiaphragmatic paralysis. AJR Am J Roentgenol 160:29-31, 1993.

15. Ambler R, Gruenewald S, John E: Ultrasound monitoring of diaphragm activity in bilateral diaphragmatic paralysis. Arch Dis Child 60:170-172, 1985.

16. Diament MJ, Boechat MI, Kangarloo H: Real-time sector ultrasound in the evaluation of suspected abnormalities of diaphragmatic motion. J Clin Ultrasound 13:539-543, 1985.

17. Ueki J, De Bruin PF, Pride NB: In vivo assessment of diaphragm contraction by ultrasound in normal subjects. Thorax 50:1157-1161, 1995.

18. Prasad R, Nath J, Mukerji PK: Eventration of diaphragm. J Indian Med Assoc 84:187-189, 1986.

19. Tamas A, Dunbar J: Eventration of the diaphragm. J Can Assoc Radiol 8:1, 1957.

20. Paris F, Blasco E, Canto A, et al: Diaphragmatic eventration in infants. Thorax 28:66-72, 1973.

21. Tarver RD, Godwin JD, Putman CE: Symposium on Nonpulmonary Aspects in Chest Radiology. The diaphragm. Radiol Clin North Am 22:615-631, 1984.

22. Tarver RD, Conces DJ Jr, Cory DA, et al: Imaging the diaphragm and its disorders. J Thorac Imaging 4:1-18, 1989.

23. Yamashita K, Minemori K, Matsuda H, et al: MR imaging in the diagnosis of partial eventration of the diaphragm. Chest 104:328, 1993.

24. Symbas PN, Hatcher CR Jr, Waldo W: Diaphragmatic eventration in infancy and childhood. Ann Thorac Surg 24:113-119, 1977.

25. Ford GT, Whitelaw WA, Rosenal TW, et al: Diaphragm function after upper abdominal surgery in humans. Am Rev Respir Dis 127:431-436, 1983.

26. Road JD, Burgess KR, Whitelaw WA, et al: Diaphragm function and respiratory response after upper abdominal surgery in dogs. J Appl Physiol 57:576-582, 1984.

27. Caskey CI, Zerhouni EA, Fishman EK, et al: Aging of the diaphragm: A CT study. Radiology 171:385-389, 1989.

28. Bogaert J, Weemaes K, Verschakelen JA, et al: Spiral CT findings in a postoperative intrathoracic gastric herniation: A case report. Eur Radiol 5:192, 1995.

29. Pearson S: Strangulated diaphragmatic hernia; report of four cases. AMA Arch Surg 66:155-166, 1953.

30. Menuck L: Plain film findings of gastric volvulus herniating into the chest. AJR Am J Roentgenol 126:1169-1174, 1976.

31. Poe RH, Schowengerdt CG: Two cases of atraumatic herniation of the liver. Am Rev Respir Dis 105:959-963, 1972.

32. Godwin JD, MacGregor JM: Extension of ascites into the chest with hiatal hernia: Visualization on CT. AJR Am J Roentgenol 148:31-32, 1987.

33. Naeye RL, Shochat SJ, Whitman V, et al: Unsuspected pulmonary vascular abnormalities associated with diaphragmatic hernia. Pediatrics 58:902-906, 1976.

34. Mallik K, Rodgers BM, McGahren ED: Congenital diaphragmatic hernia: Experience in a single institution from 1978 through 1994. Ann Thorac Surg 60:1331-1335, discussion 1335-1336, 1995.

35. Vanamo K: A 45-year perspective of congenital diaphragmatic hernia. Br J Surg 83:1758-1762, 1996.

36. Muraskas JK, Husain A, Myers TF, et al: An association of pulmonary hypoplasia with unilateral agenesis of the diaphragm. J Pediatr Surg 28:999-1002, 1993.

37. Lundius B: Intrathoracic kidney. Am J Roentgenol Radium Ther Nucl Med 125:678-681, 1975.

38. Leroux BT: Supraphrenic herniation of perinephric fat. Thorax 20:376-381, 1965.

39. Gale ME: Bochdalek hernia: Prevalence and CT characteristics. Radiology 156:449-452, 1985.

40. Raymond GS, Miller RM, Müller NL, et al: Congenital thoracic lesions that mimic neoplastic disease on chest radiographs of adults. AJR Am J Roentgenol 168:763-769, 1997.

41. Yamana D, Ohba S: Three-dimensional image of Bochdalek diaphragmatic hernia; a case report. Radiat Med 12:39-41, 1994.

42. Van Hise ML, Primack SL, Israel RS, et al: CT in blunt chest trauma: Indications and limitations. Radiographics 18:1071-1084, 1998.

43. Comer TP, Clagett OT: Surgical treatment of hernia of the foramen of Morgagni. J Thorac Cardiovasc Surg 52:461-468, 1966.

44. Paris F, Tarazona V, Casillas M, et al: Hernia of Morgagni. Thorax 28:631-636, 1973.

45. Wallace DB: Intrapericardial diaphragmatic hernia. Radiology 122:596, 1977.

46. Graham NJ, Müller NL: The diaphragm. Can Assoc Radiol J 43:250-257, 1992.

47. Boyd DP, Wooldridge BF: Diaphragmatic hernia through the foramen of Morgagni. Surg Gynecol Obstet 104:727-732, 1957.

48. Anderson LS, Forrest JV: Tumors of the diaphragm. Am J Roentgenol Radium Ther Nucl Med 119:259-265, 1973.

49. Olafsson G, Rausing A, Holen O: Primary tumors of the diaphragm. Chest 59:568-570, 1971.

50. Ferguson DD, Westcott JL: Lipoma of the diaphragm. Report of a case. Radiology 118:527-528, 1976.

51. Tihansky DP, Lopez GM: Bilateral lipomas of the diaphragm. N Y State J Med 88:151-152, 1988.

52. McHenry CR, Pickleman J, Winters G, et al: Diaphragmatic neurilemoma. J Surg Oncol 37:198-200, 1988.

53. Ohsaki Y, Morimoto H, Osanai S, et al: Extensively calcified hemangioma of the diaphragm with increased ^{99m}Tc-hydroxymethylene diphosphonate uptake. Intern Med 39:576-578, 2000.

54. Soysal O, Libshitz HI: Diaphragmatic desmoid tumor. AJR Am J Roentgenol 166:1496-1497, 1996.

55. Schwartz EE, Wechsler RJ: Diaphragmatic and paradiaphragmatic tumors and pseudotumors. J Thorac Imaging 4:19-28, 1989.

56. Sbokos CG, Salama FD, Powell V, et al: Primary fibrosarcoma of the diaphragm. Br J Dis Chest 71:49-52, 1977.

57. Müller NL: CT features of cystic teratoma of the diaphragm. J Comput Assist Tomogr 10:325-326, 1986.

58. Federle MP, Mark AS, Guillaumin ES: CT of subpulmonic pleural effusions and atelectasis: Criteria for differentiation from subphrenic fluid. AJR Am J Roentgenol 146:685-689, 1986.

59. Kapnick SJ, Griffiths CT, Finkler NJ: Occult pleural involvement in stage III ovarian carcinoma: Role of diaphragm resection. Gynecol Oncol 39:135, 1990.

60. Becmeur F, Horta P, Donato L, et al: Accessory diaphragm—review of 31 cases in the literature. Eur J Pediatr Surg 5:43-47, 1995.

61. Lieberman FL, Hidemura R, Peters RL, et al: Pathogenesis and treatment of hydrothorax complicating cirrhosis with ascites. Ann Intern Med 64:341-351, 1966.

62. Lieberman FL, Peters RL: Cirrhotic hydrothorax. Further evidence that an acquired diaphragmatic defect is at fault. Arch Intern Med 125:114-117, 1970.

63. Müller NL, Nelems B: Postcoital catamenial pneumothorax. Report of a case not associated with endometriosis and successfully treated with tubal ligation. Am Rev Respir Dis 134:803-804, 1986.

64. Shiraishi T: Catamenial pneumothorax: Report of a case and review of the Japanese and non-Japanese literature. Thorac Cardiovasc Surg 39:304-307, 1991.

65. Ranniger K, Valvassori GE: Angiographic diagnosis of intralobar pulmonary sequestration. Am J Roentgenol Radium Ther Nucl Med 92:540-546, 1964.

66. Wier JA: Congenital anomalies of the lung. Ann Intern Med 52:330-348, 1960.

67. Greenspan A, Cohen J, Szabo RM: Klippel-Feil syndrome. An unusual association with Sprengel deformity, omovertebral bone, and other skeletal, hematologic, and respiratory disorders. A case report. Bull Hosp Jt Dis Orthop Inst 51:54-62, 1991.

68. Pearl M, Chow TF, Friedman E: Poland's syndrome. Radiology 101:619-623, 1971.

68a. Karnak I, Tanyel FC, Tuncbilek E, et al: Bilateral Poland anomaly. Am J Med Genet 75:505-507, 1998.

69. Moncada R, Vade A, Gimenez C, et al: Congenital and acquired lung hernias. J Thorac Imaging 11:75-82, 1996.

70. Bhalla M, Leitman BS, Forcade C, et al: Lung hernia: Radiographic features. AJR Am J Roentgenol 154:51-53, 1990.

71. Tamburro F, Grassi R, Romano S, et al: Acquired spontaneous intercostal hernia of the lung diagnosed on helical CT. AJR Am J Roentgenol 174:876-877, 2000.

72. Fisher M: Eve's rib [letter]. Radiology 140:841, 1981.

73. Rock JP, Spickler EM: Anomalous rib presenting as cervical myelopathy: A previously unreported variant of Klippel-Feil syndrome. Case report. J Neurosurg 75:465-467, 1991.

74. Novak CB, Mackinnon SE: Thoracic outlet syndrome. Orthop Clin North Am 27:747-762, 1996.

75. Mackinnon SE, Patterson GA, Novak CB: Thoracic outlet syndrome: A current overview. Semin Thorac Cardiovasc Surg 8:176-182, 1996.

76. Boone ML, Swenson BE, Felson B: Rib notching: Its many causes. Am J Roentgenol Radium Ther Nucl Med 91:1075-1088, 1964.

77. Ferris RA, LoPresti JM: Rib notching due to coarctation of the aorta: Report of a case initially observed at less than one year of age. Br J Radiol 47:357-359, 1974.

78. Sargent EN, Turner AF, Jacobson G: Superior marginal rib defects. An etiologic classification. Am J Roentgenol Radium Ther Nucl Med 106:491-505, 1969.

79. Aeschlimann A, Kahn MF: Tietze's syndrome: A critical review. Clin Exp Rheumatol 8:407-412, 1990.

80. Gill GV: Epidemic of Tietze's syndrome. BMJ 2:499, 1977.

81. Skorneck AB: Roentgen aspects of Tietze's syndrome. Painful hypertrophy of costal cartilage and bone—osteochondritis? Am J Roentgenol Radium Ther Nucl Med 83:748-755, 1960.

82. Edelstein G, Levitt RG, Slaker DP, et al: Computed tomography of Tietze syndrome. J Comput Assist Tomogr 8:20-23, 1984.

83. Lin EC: Costochondritis mimicking a pulmonary nodule on FDG positron emission tomographic imaging. Clin Nucl Med 27:591-592, 2002.

84. Guller B, Hable K: Cardiac findings in pectus excavatum in children: Review and differential diagnosis. Chest 66:165-171, 1974.

85. Leung AK, Hoo JJ: Familial congenital funnel chest. Am J Med Genet 26:887-890, 1987.

86. Soteropoulos GC, Cigtay OS, Schellinger D: Pectus excavatum deformities simulating mediastinal masses. J Comput Assist Tomogr 3:596-600, 1979.

87. Goodman LR, Kay HR, Teplick SK, et al: Complications of median sternotomy: Computed tomographic evaluation. AJR Am J Roentgenol 141:225-230, 1983.

88. Templeton PA, Fishman EK: CT evaluation of poststernotomy complications. AJR Am J Roentgenol 159:45-50, 1992.

89. Biesecker GL, Aaron BL, Mullen JT: Primary sternal osteomyelitis. Chest 63:236-238, 1973.

90. Franquet T, Gimenez A, Alegret X, et al: Imaging findings of sternal abnormalities. Eur Radiol 7:492-497, 1997.

91. Kay HR, Goodman LR, Teplick SK, et al: Use of computed tomography to assess mediastinal complications after median sternotomy. Ann Thorac Surg 36:706-714, 1983.

92. James J: Scoliosis. Baltimore, Williams & Wilkins, 1968.
93. Bjure J, Grimby G, Kasalicky J, et al: Respiratory impairment and airway closure in patients with untreated idiopathic scoliosis. Thorax 25:451-456, 1970.
94. Bergofsky EH, Turino GM, Fishman AP: Cardiorespiratory failure in kyphoscoliosis. Medicine (Baltimore) 38:263-317, 1959.
95. Weber B, Smith JP, Briscoe WA, et al: Pulmonary function in asymptomatic adolescents with idiopathic scoliosis. Am Rev Respir Dis 111:389-397, 1975.
96. Conti G, Rocco M, Antonelli M, et al: Respiratory system mechanics in the early phase of acute respiratory failure due to severe kyphoscoliosis. Intensive Care Med 23:539-544, 1997.
97. Kafer ER: Idiopathic scoliosis. Mechanical properties of the respiratory system and the ventilatory response to carbon dioxide. J Clin Invest 55:1153-1163, 1975.
98. Bates D, Macklem P, Christie R: Respiratory Function in Disease: An Introduction to the Integrated Study of the Lung, ed 2. Philadelphia, WB Saunders, 1971.
99. Al-Kattan K, Simonds A, Chung KF, et al: Kyphoscoliosis and bronchial torsion. Chest 111:1134-1137, 1997.
100. Kafer ER: Respiratory function in paralytic scoliosis. Am Rev Respir Dis 110:450-457, 1974.
101. McNicholas WT: Impact of sleep in respiratory failure. Eur Respir J 10:920-933, 1997.
102. Brewerton DA, Hart FD, Nicholls A, et al: Ankylosing spondylitis and HL-A 27. Lancet 1:904-907, 1973.
103. Schlosstein L, Terasaki PI, Bluestone R, et al: High association of an HL-A antigen, W27, with ankylosing spondylitis. N Engl J Med 288:704-706, 1973.
104. Calin A, Fries JF: Striking prevalence of ankylosing spondylitis in "healthy" w27 positive males and females. N Engl J Med 293:835-859, 1975.
105. Rosenow E, Strimlan CV, Muhm JR, et al: Pleuropulmonary manifestations of ankylosing spondylitis. Mayo Clin Proc 52:641-649, 1977.
106. Luthra HS: Extra-articular manifestations of ankylosing spondylitis. Mayo Clin Proc 52:655-656, 1977.
107. Jessamine AG: Upper lung lobe fibrosis in ankylosing spondylitis. Can Med Assoc J 98:25-29, 1968.
108. Campbell AH, Macdonald CB: Upper lobe fibrosis associated with ankylosing spondylitis. Br J Dis Chest 59:90-101, 1965.
109. Ferdoutsis M, Bouros D, Meletis G, et al: Diffuse interstitial lung disease as an early manifestation of ankylosing spondylitis. Respiration 62:286-289, 1995.
110. Strobel ES, Fritschka E: Case report and review of the literature. Fatal pulmonary complication in ankylosing spondylitis. Clin Rheumatol 16:617-622, 1997.
111. Casserly IP, Fenlon HM, Breatnach E, et al: Lung findings on high-resolution computed tomography in idiopathic ankylosing spondylitis—correlation with clinical findings, pulmonary function testing and plain radiography. Br J Rheumatol 36:677-682, 1997.
112. Senocak O, Manisali M, Ozaksoy D, et al: Lung parenchyma changes in ankylosing spondylitis: Demonstration with high resolution CT and correlation with disease duration. Eur J Radiol 45:117-122, 2003.
113. Kiris A, Ozgocmen S, Kocakoc E, et al: Lung findings on high resolution CT in early ankylosing spondylitis. Eur J Radiol 47:71-76, 2003.
114. Calin A, Porta J, Fries JF, et al: Clinical history as a screening test for ankylosing spondylitis. JAMA 237:2613-2614, 1977.
115. Weaver P, Lifeso RM: The radiological diagnosis of tuberculosis of the adult spine. Skeletal Radiol 12:178-186, 1984.
116. Coppola J, Müller NL, Connell DG: Computed tomography of musculoskeletal tuberculosis. Can Assoc Radiol J 38:199-203, 1987.
117. de Roos A, van Persijn van Meerten EL, Bloem JL, et al: MRI of tuberculous spondylitis. AJR Am J Roentgenol 147:79-82, 1986.
118. Modic MT, Feiglin DH, Piraino DW, et al: Vertebral osteomyelitis: Assessment using MR. Radiology 157:157-166, 1985.
119. Smith AS, Weinstein MA, Mizushima A, et al: MR imaging characteristics of tuberculous spondylitis vs vertebral osteomyelitis. AJR Am J Roentgenol 153:399-405, 1989.
120. Rami-Porta R, Bravo-Bravo JL, Aroca-Gonzalez MJ, et al: Tumours and pseudotumours of the chest wall. Scand J Thorac Cardiovasc Surg 19:97-103, 1985.
121. Jain SK, Afzal M, Mathew M, et al: Malignant mesenchymoma of the chest wall in an adult. Thorax 48:407-408, 1993.
122. Meis JM, Butler JJ, Osborne BM: Hodgkin's disease involving the breast and chest wall. Cancer 57:1859-1865, 1986.
123. Castillo M, Shirkhoda A: Computed tomography of diaphragmatic lipoma. J Comput Tomogr 9:167-170, 1985.
124. Kuhlman JE, Bouchardy L, Fishman EK, et al: CT and MR imaging evaluation of chest wall disorders. Radiographics 14:571-595, 1994.
125. Sulzer MA, Goei R, Bollen EC, et al: Lipoma of the external thoracic wall. Eur Respir J 7:207-209, 1994.
126. Fortier M, Mayo JR, Swensen SJ, et al: MR imaging of chest wall lesions. Radiographics 14:597-606, 1994.
127. Cohen LM, Schwartz AM, Rockoff SD: Benign schwannomas: Pathologic basis for CT inhomogeneities. AJR Am J Roentgenol 147:141-143, 1986.
128. Ko SF, Lee TY, Lin JW, et al: Thoracic neurilemomas: An analysis of computed tomography findings in 36 patients. J Thorac Imaging 13:21-26, 1998.
129. Sakai F, Sone S, Kiyono K, et al: Intrathoracic neurogenic tumors: MR-pathologic correlation. AJR Am J Roentgenol 159:279-283, 1992.
130. Contesso G, Llombart-Bosch A, Terrier P, et al: Does malignant small round cell tumor of the thoracopulmonary region (Askin tumor) constitute a clinicopathologic entity? An analysis of 30 cases with immunohistochemical and electron-microscopic support treated at the Institute Gustave Roussy. Cancer 69:1012-1020, 1992.
131. Ambros IM, Ambros PF, Strehl S, et al: MIC2 is a specific marker for Ewing's sarcoma and peripheral primitive neuroectodermal tumors. Evidence for a common histogenesis of Ewing's sarcoma and peripheral primitive neuroectodermal tumors from MIC2 expression and specific chromosome aberration. Cancer 67:1886-1893, 1991.
132. Winer-Muram HT, Kauffman WM, Gronemeyer SA, et al: Primitive neuroectodermal tumors of the chest wall (Askin tumors): CT and MR findings. AJR Am J Roentgenol 161:265-268, 1993.
133. Ochsner A Jr, Lucas GL, McFarland GB Jr: Tumors of the thoracic skeleton. Review of 134 cases. J Thorac Cardiovasc Surg 52:311-321, 1966.
134. Pairolero PC, Arnold PG: Chest wall tumors. Experience with 100 consecutive patients. J Thorac Cardiovasc Surg 90:367-372, 1985.
135. Tateishi U, Gladish GW, Kusumoto M, et al: Chest wall tumors: Radiologic findings and pathologic correlation: Part 2. Malignant tumors. Radiographics 23:1491-1508, 2003.
136. Meyer CA, White CS: Cartilaginous disorders of the chest. Radiographics 18:1109-1123, quiz 1241-1242, 1998.
137. King RM, Payne WS, Olafsson S, et al: Surgical palliation of respiratory insufficiency secondary to massive exuberant polyostotic fibrous dysplasia of the ribs. Ann Thorac Surg 39:185-187, 1985.
138. Urovitz EP, Fornasier VL, Czitrom AA: Sternal metastases and associated pathological fractures. Thorax 32:444-448, 1977.
139. Goldman JM: Parasternal chest wall involvement in Hodgkin's disease. Chest 59:133-137, 1971.
140. Marcove RC, Huvos AG: Cartilaginous tumors of the ribs. Cancer 27:794-801, 1971.
141. Ishida T, Kuwada Y, Motoi N, et al: Dedifferentiated chondrosarcoma of the rib with a malignant mesenchymomatous component: An autopsy case report. Pathol Int 47:397-403, 1997.
142. Eygelaar A, Homan Van Der Heide: Diagnosis and treatment of primary malignant costal and sternal tumors. Dis Chest 52:683-687, 1967.
143. Morisaki Y, Takagi K, Ishii Y, et al: Periosteal chondroma developing in a rib at the side of a chest wall wound from a previous thoracotomy: Report of a case. Surg Today 26:57-59, 1996.

CHAPTER TWENTY-THREE

RESPIRATORY DISEASE ASSOCIATED WITH A NORMAL RADIOGRAPH

Significant pulmonary and pleural disease, sometimes of life-threatening severity, can be present with a normal chest radiograph. In some cases this is a significant, positive diagnostic feature that excludes diseases in which respiratory symptoms and signs are commonly associated with radiographic abnormalities.

In addition to cases in which the radiograph is undoubtedly normal, a radiographic pattern may be encountered that is judged to be at the outer range of normal but not unequivocally abnormal. An example is elevation of one or both hemidiaphragms beyond the normal range; although a high diaphragm is often a reflection of suboptimal inspiration, it can be an important indication of decreased lung volume. In such cases, comparison with previous radiographs may establish whether there has been a change in the radiographic pattern; alternatively, a subsequent radiograph may resolve the problem by showing progression or regression.

PULMONARY PARENCHYMAL, AIRWAY, AND VASCULAR DISEASE ASSOCIATED WITH A NORMAL RADIOGRAPH

Disease of the Pulmonary Parenchyma

Localized Disease

Localized acute air space disease such as that caused by bacterial infection or alveolar hemorrhage characteristically produces radiographic shadows at a very early stage. By contrast, acute local disease affecting predominantly the pulmonary interstitium (e.g., viral or mycoplasmal pneumonia) can cause symptoms that precede radiographic signs by 48 hours or longer. Localized abnormalities of the pulmonary vascular system, particularly acute thromboembolism, may likewise show no radiographic signs on the chest film.[2]

Chronic pulmonary disease may also be present and "active" for months or even years before it becomes radiographically visible. It has been estimated, for example, that a focus of tuberculosis does not become radiologically detectable until 2 or 3 months after initial infection.[3] Similarly, most pulmonary carcinomas are present for years before they become visible; studies of the growth rate of such tumors and back-extrapolation of the doubling time indicate that they are invisible for two thirds to three quarters of their existence.[4]

Solitary uncalcified lesions smaller than 6 mm in diameter are rarely identified and then usually only in retrospect when the lesion has grown and is detected on subsequent radiographs. A solitary nodule 8 to 10 mm in diameter has an approximately 50% chance of being detected.[1] Larger nodules—sometimes as big as 4 cm in diameter—may also be overlooked, particularly if they are situated over the convexity of the lung or in the paramediastinal area, where the rib cage, large vessels, and mediastinal contents tend to obscure them.

Generalized Disease

In contrast to localized pulmonary tuberculosis, in which symptoms and signs may not appear for many weeks *after* the chest radiograph has become abnormal, clinical manifestations such as fever, general malaise, and headaches may develop some weeks *before* the detection of radiologic abnormality in miliary tuberculosis; in some instances, the pulmonary lesions are not recognized before death.[5] Despite this, multiple micronodular opacities measuring no more than 1 or 2 mm in diameter are usually appreciated, presumably because of the effect of superimposition.

A variety of conditions, including sarcoidosis,[6] idiopathic pulmonary fibrosis,[7] and extrinsic allergic alveolitis,[8] may have radiographically invisible interstitial disease, even in the presence of symptoms and disturbances of pulmonary function. In systemic lupus erythematosus, the presence and extent of parenchymal abnormalities are frequently underestimated on the chest radiograph.[9] Significant pulmonary vascular disease, such as primary pulmonary hypertension and thromboembolism, may also be present without radiographic manifestations.

Disease of the Airways

Many patients with diseases of the conducting airways have normal chest radiographs. In fact, in simple chronic bronchitis, this is the rule rather than the exception. Although the majority of patients who experience acute asthma attacks show evidence of pulmonary overinflation on pulmonary function testing,[10] radiographic evidence of its presence is seldom convincing except in children and adolescents who have early-onset asthma. About 10% of patients with bronchiectasis fail to show evidence of the disease on standard chest radiographs.[11] Patients with emphysema, particularly advanced disease, have distinctly abnormal radiographs; however, patients with mild to moderate disease may have completely normal radiographs.[12]

Patients who have endobronchial or endotracheal tumors that only partly obstruct an airway can have normal chest radiographs, at least when films are exposed at full inspiration. (A radiograph exposed after full expiration may reveal air trapping distal to the partial obstruction.) When the obstruction is in the trachea or a major bronchus, dyspnea and generalized wheezing may suggest a diagnosis of asthma. Lesions arising within the trachea or compressing it from outside should be suspected when wheezing (sometimes relieved by a change in position) is more pronounced during inspiration than expiration or is accompanied by hemoptysis, or when the patient's symptoms fail to respond to the usual therapy for asthma.

Pulmonary Arteriovenous Shunts

Arteriovenous shunts may be acquired or congenital. The latter are characteristic of Rendu-Osler-Weber disease and may be found in patients who have Fanconi's syndrome[13] or polysplenia syndrome associated with multiple cardiac anomalies[14]; although the larger malformations are usually detectable radiographically, small ones may not be evident.

The intrapulmonary form of shunting that occurs in patients who have cirrhosis can also develop in the presence of a normal chest radiograph.[15] Intrapulmonary right-to-left shunting in such patients can be demonstrated by contrast echocardiography.[16] Normally, when ultrasound contrast material (which contains microbubbles) is injected into the peripheral circulation, it is removed during the first pass through the pulmonary circulation, and no echogenic material reaches the left side of the heart; in patients who have intrapulmonary or extrapulmonary right-to-left shunt, bubbles reach the left side of the heart and can be detected ultrasonographically. Quantitative perfusion scintigraphy using radioactively labeled macroaggregated albumin has been used to detect pulmonary arteriovenous communications that are too small to be detected angiographically.[17]

The hypoxemia observed in patients who have cirrhosis may be more severe in the erect than the recumbent position (orthodeoxia),[18] a phenomenon that is attributable to the increased blood flow through the lung bases, where most shunts are found. When orthodeoxia is severe, the patient may complain of increased dyspnea when in the erect position (platypnea).[19]

PLEURAL DISEASE ASSOCIATED WITH A NORMAL RADIOGRAPH

The chest radiograph may be normal in cases of acute pleuritis. However, pleurisy without an effusion ("dry pleurisy") is often associated with diaphragmatic elevation and a reduction in diaphragmatic excursion. Effusions with a volume as large as 500 mL may not be visible on standard posteroanterior chest radiographs exposed with the patient in the erect position.[20] However, films exposed with the patient in the lateral decubitus position can reveal effusions of 100 mL or less.[21] Asbestos-associated pleural plaques may also be invisible on standard radiographs.[22]

ALVEOLAR HYPOVENTILATION

The term *alveolar hypoventilation* is used to designate a deficiency in ventilation that is sufficient to raise the arterial carbon dioxide level ($PaCO_2$) to greater than 45 mm Hg. The diagnosis cannot be made by clinical examination or by measurement of minute ventilation. In patients breathing room air, alveolar hypoventilation is necessarily accompanied by a degree of alveolar hypoxia and therefore arterial hypoxemia. Although regional underventilation can contribute to ventilation-perfusion mismatch and arterial hypoxemia without causing hypercapnia, the term *hypoventilation* should be reserved for a generalized decrease in ventilation that is characterized by the presence of hypercapnia.

Respiratory failure associated with hypercapnia occurs in two broad groups of disorders: those of pulmonary origin (Table 23–1) and those of nonpulmonary origin (Table 23–2). The latter are dealt with more extensively in this chapter because they are frequently associated with a normal chest radiograph.

Disorders of the mechanisms that drive the chest bellows may result in either acute or chronic ventilatory failure. For purposes of clarity, these disorders are considered in two groups: those that result from defective ventilatory control and those caused by an inadequate respiratory pump (see Table 23–2). Included in disorders of ventilatory control are disorders of cerebral and brainstem respiratory center function and abnormalities of the efferent outputs from the upper motor neurons that drive the respiratory muscles, as well as abnormalities of the afferent inputs into the central nervous system from peripheral receptors. Disorders of the respiratory pump include abnormalities of the anterior horn cells, the myoneural junction, the respiratory muscles, the phrenic and intercostal nerves that innervate these muscles, and the chest wall.

Chest radiographs are normal in the majority of patients in whom hypoventilation results from central nervous system

TABLE 23–1. Pulmonary Causes of Ventilatory Failure with Hypercapnia

Upper Airway Obstruction

Acute

Infection (pharyngitis, tonsillitis, epiglottitis, laryngotracheitis)
Edema (irritant gases, angioneurotic edema)
Retropharyngeal hemorrhage (trauma, postoperative, hemophilia, acute leukemia)
Foreign bodies

Chronic

Postintubation stenosis (fibrosis, granulation tissue)
Neoplasm (squamous cell carcinoma, adenoid cystic carcinoma)
Vocal cord paralysis
Hypertrophied tonsils and adenoids
Macroglossia
Micrognathia
Obstructive sleep apnea

Lower Airway Obstruction

Acute

Infection (acute bronchiolitis)
Edema (pulmonary venous hypertension, capillary leakage)
Bronchospasm (asthma, anaphylactoid reactions)

Chronic

Chronic obstructive pulmonary disease
Bronchiolitis
Extensive idiopathic bronchiectasis
Cystic fibrosis
Familial dysautonomia

From Fraser RS, Müller NL, Colman NC, Paré PD: Fraser and Paré's Diagnosis of Diseases of the Chest, 4th ed. Philadelphia, WB Saunders, 1999.

or neuromuscular disease. In instances in which the hypoventilation is caused by respiratory muscle weakness or paralysis, the diaphragm is often elevated. Prolonged hypoventilation may be complicated by atelectasis and pneumonia.[23]

Disorders of Ventilatory Control

Central control of ventilation resides in two anatomically and functionally separate systems that subserve voluntary and automatic breathing (see page 79).[24,25] A variety of abnormalities affecting either system can result in hypoventilation.

Disorders of the Central Nervous System

Cerebral Dysfunction. Many disorders that affect cerebral function are associated with respiratory depression, especially during sleep.[26] Narcotic, analgesic, and sedative agents in prescribed amounts frequently produce hypoventilation and respiratory failure in patients who have underlying chronic pulmonary disease; however, this occurs only rarely in individuals who have normal lungs. In individuals with normal lungs, drug-induced hypoventilation usually occurs after suicide attempts (in adults) or accidental ingestion (in children). Drugs that have been associated with respiratory depression include the narcotics,[27] barbiturates,[28] phenothiazines and benzodiazepines,[29] tricyclic antidepressants,[30] diphenhydramine,[31] and meprobamate.[32]

TABLE 23–2. Nonpulmonary Causes of Ventilatory Failure with Hypercapnia

Disorders of Ventilatory Control

Cerebral Dysfunction

Infection (encephalitis), trauma, vascular accident
Status epilepticus
Narcotic and sedative overdose
Respiratory dyskinesia

Respiratory Center Dysfunction

Impaired Brainstem Controller

Primary alveolar hypoventilation (Ondine's curse)
Obesity-hypoventilation syndrome
Myxedema
Metabolic alkalosis (compensatory)
Sudden infant death syndrome
Parkinson's syndrome
Tetanus

Ablation of Afferent and Efferent Spinal Pathways

Bilateral high cervical cordotomy
Cervical spinal cord trauma
Transverse myelitis
Multiple sclerosis
Parkinson's disease

Peripheral Receptor Dysfunction

Carotid body destruction (bilateral carotid endarterectomy and carotid body resection for asthma)
Bilateral damage to afferent nerves (Arnold-Chiari syndrome with syringomyelia)
Familial dysautonomia
Diabetic neuropathy
Tetanus

Disorders of the Respiratory Pump

Neuromuscular Disease

Anterior Horn Cells

Poliomyelitis
Amyotrophic lateral sclerosis

Peripheral Nerves

Guillain-Barré syndrome
Acute intermittent porphyria
Toxic dinoflagellate poisoning
Neurotoxic shellfish poisoning (*Ptychodiscus brevis*)
Paralytic shellfish poisoning (*Protogonyaulyx cantenella* and *tamarensis*)
Ciguatera fish poisoning (*Gambierdiscus toxicus*)
Puffer fish poisoning (tetrodotoxin)

Myoneural Junction

Myasthenia gravis
Myasthenia-like syndromes (medications, particularly antibiotics, and neoplasms)
Clostridium botulinum poisoning

Respiratory Muscles

Muscular dystrophies
Acid maltase deficiency
Nemaline myopathy
Polymyositis
Hypokalemia (in treatment of diabetes with insulin, renal tubular acidosis)
Hypophosphatemia
Hypermagnesemia
Idiopathic rhabdomyolysis (myoglobinuria)

Chest Wall Disorders

Flail chest
Kyphoscoliosis
Thoracoplasty

From Fraser RS, Müller NL, Colman NC, Paré PD: Fraser and Paré's Diagnosis of Diseases of the Chest, 4th ed. Philadelphia, WB Saunders, 1999.

Cerebral damage resulting from infection, trauma, or vascular accidents can also cause hypoventilation, usually after an initial period of hyperventilation.

Primary Alveolar Hypoventilation. Alveolar hypoventilation that occurs predominantly as a result of an abnormality in central neurogenic control has been termed *primary alveolar hypoventilation of the nonobese* ("Ondine's curse" or central sleep apnea).[33] Affected individuals have normal or almost normal gas exchange and lung function when they are awake and breathing under voluntary ventilatory control, but they may experience respiratory failure and even death during sleep. The disorder can be caused by a specific congenital or hereditary defect in the respiratory center,[34] or it can be secondary to a variety of diseases that affect the central nervous system.

The characteristic physiologic feature is a decrease in sensitivity of the central nervous system to CO_2 that results in alveolar hypoventilation, especially during sleep. A profound decrease in the ventilatory response to hypoxemia has also been seen in some patients.[35] Typically, patients can voluntarily increase their ventilation and lower their $PaCO_2$ to within the normal range.

Although upper airway obstruction is the pathophysiologic mechanism in the vast majority of patients who have sleep apnea, it is important to identify the occasional individual in whom central neurogenic hypoventilation is the cause, because the management of such patients is very different. The apneic episodes are usually of shorter duration and are associated with less bradycardia in patients with central neurogenic hypoventilation than in those who have obstruction. Patients who have primary alveolar hypoventilation also complain more of insomnia and less of daytime hypersomnolence.[36]

The congenital form of the disease becomes manifest within minutes or hours of birth as cyanosis and respiratory acidosis necessitating prolonged mechanical ventilation.[37] In adults, it often occurs in association with another primary neurologic abnormality, such as infarct or hemorrhage, primary tumor, or Parkinson's disease[38,39]; in about 50% of cases there is no associated neurologic disorder.

Clinical manifestations are variable. Hypoventilation occurs only at night in some patients, and arterial blood gas tensions become normal during waking hours. The hypoventilation persists throughout the day in others; as might be expected, these patients have a poorer prognosis.[40] In some patients, nocturnal oxygen therapy decreases the frequency of apnea and increases nocturnal ventilation, suggesting that hypoxic depression of ventilation may occur.[41] In others, nocturnal oxygen alleviates the hypoxemia but also exacerbates hypercapnia[42]; headache and lethargy can result.

Obesity-Hypoventilation Syndrome. The constellation of cyanosis, polycythemia, and obesity became widely recognized as the "pickwickian syndrome" after its description in 1956 because of the similarity in appearance and behavior of affected patients to the fat boy Joe in the novel *Pickwick Papers* by Charles Dickens.[43] Since then, study of breathing during sleep has allowed separation of affected patients into those in whom the primary problem is obstructive sleep apnea and those in whom the problem appears to be primarily one of ventilatory control, and it is these terms rather than "pickwickian syndrome" that should be used.[44]

Considerable confusion exists in the literature regarding precisely what the term "obesity-hypoventilation syndrome"

means. Morbidly obese patients with obstructive sleep apnea are more likely to have persistent hypoventilation; such patients have been considered to have "sleep apnea/obesity-hypoventilation syndrome."[45] Other patients who have sleep apnea without obesity may experience persistent hypoventilation and have been considered to have "sleep hypoventilation syndrome."

We and others believe that the term "obesity-hypoventilation syndrome" should be reserved for cases in which the patient hypoventilates but does not meet the criteria for a diagnosis of obstructive sleep apnea. In some of these patients, there may be a primary hypothalamic defect that causes both obesity and hypoventilation. Alternatively, affected persons may have a ventilatory response to CO_2 and hypoxemia that is at the low end of the normal range; when challenged by the increased work of breathing associated with obesity, they may hypoventilate in much the same way that so-called blue bloaters hypoventilate when faced with the increased work of breathing associated with COPD.[46]

Chronic Mountain Sickness (Monge's Disease). This unusual cause of chronic hypoventilation occurs in long-time residents of high-altitude regions and is characterized by decreased ventilation associated with polycythemia, headache, dizziness, loss of memory, fatigue, and in the later stages of the disease, dyspnea and peripheral edema.[47] The reason why the abnormality develops in only a small percentage of the population is unknown.[48]

Myxedema. A decrease in the central neurogenic drive to breathe can be a contributing factor in the hypoventilation sometimes observed in patients who have myxedema.[49] An additional factor in some patients is obstructive sleep apnea, which is not uncommon in hypothyroidism,[50] possibly as a result of narrowing of the upper airway by macroglossia secondary to deposition of mucopolysaccharides.[49] Patients who have hypothyroidism also demonstrate significant respiratory muscle weakness, which is ameliorated by thyroid replacement therapy.[51]

Metabolic Alkalosis. Hypoventilation can occur in response to metabolic alkalosis when CO_2 retention and an increase in serum bicarbonate follow repeated episodes of vomiting as a result of either psychological or organic causes.[52] This combination has also been reported after gastric resection and in association with Cushing's syndrome,[53,54] in which case the hypoventilation represents a compensatory mechanism that permits a rise in serum bicarbonate, thereby enabling the acid-base balance to return toward normal.

Parkinson's Syndrome. Hypoventilation and hypoxemia appear to be related to central hypoventilation in some patients who have Parkinson's syndrome.[55] Patients with Parkinson's syndrome may also demonstrate decreased maximal expiratory flow and oscillatory fluctuations in expiratory flow that are believed to be related to tremor involving the upper airway and expiratory muscles.[56]

Tetanus. Tetanus toxin is produced by *Clostridium tetani* and causes blockade of inhibitory synapses in both the cerebral cortex and spinal cord. Ventilatory failure is attributable to prolonged spasm of the respiratory musculature. The disease is seen most often in "developing" countries in which hygiene is poor and there is an increased likelihood of wound contamination by *C. tetani*.[57] It is frequently associated with symptoms and signs of autonomic dysfunction, including hypertension, tachycardia, bradycardia, cardiac arrhythmias, profuse sweating, pyrexia, increased urinary catecholamine excretion, and in some cases, the development of hypotension.[58] Patients who have mild disease experience trismus (inability to open the mouth) and hypertonicity of the chest wall and abdominal muscles; those with moderate and severe disease also have tetanic spasms.

Disorders of the Spinal Cord

Lesions of the cervical and thoracic segments of the spinal cord can interfere with both the afferent and efferent spinal pathways to and from the respiratory center. The diaphragm is innervated by nerve roots from C3 to C5, which join to form the phrenic nerve, whereas the parasternal and lateral external intercostal muscles are innervated by nerve roots from T1 to T12 via the intercostal nerves. Of the accessory muscles, the scalenes are innervated by nerve roots from C4 to C8, whereas the sternocleidomastoid is innervated by cranial nerve XI and the cervical nerve roots C1 and C2. The expiratory muscles consist of the lateral internal intercostal muscles, which derive innervation from T1 to T12 via the intercostal nerves, and the rectus abdominis, external and internal obliques, and transversus abdominis, which are innervated by nerves originating from nerve roots T7 to L1.

Patients who suffer spinal cord injury at the level of C5 or lower have preserved diaphragmatic function but paralyzed intercostal muscles. In this circumstance, diaphragmatic contraction during inspiration results in exaggerated protrusion of the abdomen and in-drawing of the sternum and lower ribs; on expiration, the diaphragm relaxes and ascends, with the abdomen flattening and the lower part of the chest expanding as a result of the elasticity of the rib cage.[59] This pattern, termed *paradoxical chest wall motion*, tends to decrease with time after the development of quadriplegia, presumably because spasticity develops in the denervated intercostal muscles. As a result, pulmonary function tends to improve in the first 6 to 12 months after injury.[60]

Surgical cervical cordotomy for pain relief can interfere with respiratory control and result in sleep-induced apnea and even sudden death.[61] Similar physiologic dysfunction has been described in patients who have multiple sclerosis, presumably as a result of destruction of cervical spinal pathways or midline ventral medullary structures.[62] Unilateral cervical spinal cord injury can result in hemiplegia and unilateral paradoxical chest wall motion that mimics a flail chest.[63]

Disorders of Peripheral Chemoreceptors

Peripheral chemoreceptors situated in the carotid bodies account for virtually all the hypoxic drive in humans. Bilateral carotid endarterectomy,[64] or removal of both carotid bodies (a "therapeutic procedure" that was once used for relief of asthma[65]), can abolish the compensatory hyperventilation that normally occurs during hypoxemia. Bilateral carotid body resection also causes a decreased ventilatory response to exercise.[66] Sleep apnea has been reported as a complication after bilateral excision of carotid body tumors.[67]

Abnormalities in ventilatory control and episodes of apnea caused by abnormalities in peripheral chemoreceptor and mechanoreceptor input to the respiratory center can occur in patients who have autonomic dysfunction.[68] These syndromes represent a heterogeneous group of congenital and acquired

disorders that are usually characterized by orthostatic hypotension, hypohidrosis, a relatively fixed heart rate, and bladder and sexual dysfunction.[69]

A number of investigators have demonstrated depressed ventilatory responses to hypoxia and hypercapnia in diabetic patients, especially those with autonomic neuropathy.[70] Patients who have Arnold-Chiari malformation and syringomyelia in whom the central respiratory failure is presumably caused by destruction of afferent pathways in the ninth cranial nerve have been described.[71]

Disorders of the Respiratory Pump

For descriptive purposes, the respiratory pump includes the anterior horn cells in the spinal cord, the neural connections to respiratory muscles in the phrenic and intercostal nerves, the myoneuronal junctions, and the respiratory muscles themselves.

The respiratory muscles can be divided into three distinct groups with different mechanisms of action: the diaphragm, the intercostal and accessory muscles, and the abdominal muscles.[72] Only dysfunction of the inspiratory muscles causes significant ventilatory impairment. However, the expiratory muscles are important for generation of an effective cough, and an inadequate cough can result in mucus plugging and/or pulmonary infection in patients who have neuromuscular disease.

It is not necessary that respiratory muscle weakness be profound to provoke symptoms and signs. Disability from weakened respiratory muscles can be accentuated or precipitated by an increased load on the respiratory system, such as that occasioned by exercise or concomitant COPD. Like other skeletal muscles, respiratory muscles may become fatigued; in fact, such fatigue is probably the final common pathway causing ventilatory failure in patients who have neuromuscular and chest wall abnormalities.

Disorders of Anterior Horn Cells

Poliomyelitis and amyotrophic lateral sclerosis are the most common disorders of anterior horn cells that lead to respiratory failure. Although respiratory failure secondary to poliomyelitis has been almost eradicated in "developed" countries by immunization, occasional cases are still seen, and affected patients can experience unexpected life-threatening hypoventilation.[73] The disease should be suspected as the cause of acute respiratory failure when symptoms of bulbar palsy are present in an unvaccinated person. Patients who have apparently recovered from polio may be susceptible to the later development of a postpolio syndrome that can be associated with obstructive sleep apnea or hypoventilation, or both.[74]

Amyotrophic lateral sclerosis often results in ventilatory failure, although respiratory muscle involvement is rarely the initial manifestation.[75] Involvement of neurons supplying the abdominal expiratory muscles and the muscles of the upper airway can result in abnormalities in expiratory flow. A characteristic flow-volume curve has been described in which expiratory flow is decreased and residual volume increased, a combination that occurs in patients who have predominant expiratory muscle weakness.[76] Selective paralysis of upper airway and oropharyngeal muscles can also influence maximal expiratory flow.[77]

Disorders of Peripheral Nerves

Guillain-Barré Syndrome. Acute polyneuritis (Guillain-Barré syndrome) is probably the most common neuromuscular disease that causes ventilatory failure. It can be associated with either acute or subacute hypoventilation. The disease shows a striking predilection for patients younger than 25 years; a second, smaller peak incidence occurs between the ages of 45 and 60 years. Characteristic clinical findings include symmetrical ascending paralysis associated with a lack of cellular response in cerebrospinal fluid. Patients sometimes have evidence of autonomic dysfunction, including elevated blood pressure, tachycardia, cardiac arrhythmias, and episodes of pyrexia and hyperhidrosis.[78]

Between 15% and 60% of patients have sufficient respiratory muscle paralysis to require mechanical ventilation.[79,80] These patients experience slow but progressive improvement in respiratory muscle strength, although assisted ventilation may be required for several months. The need for such aid should be assessed by repeated measurements of VC or maximal inspiratory pressure.[81] Serial measurements of phrenic nerve conduction velocity may be a more sensitive method of assessing the severity of the disease and predicting impending ventilatory failure.[82]

Porphyria. The hepatic porphyrias—acute intermittent porphyria, porphyria variegata, and hereditary coproporphyria—are abnormalities in porphyrin metabolism that are inherited in an autosomal dominant fashion. Associated peripheral neuropathy is caused by the toxic effect of the accumulated porphyrin precursors aminolevulinic acid and porphobilinogen.[83] Some patients also manifest symptoms of bulbar involvement and experience difficulty clearing bronchial secretions. The diagnosis is supported when it is learned that other members of the family are afflicted, and confirmation can be obtained by the discovery of porphyrin precursors in urine. Each form of porphyria can be associated with ascending paralysis and respiratory failure. Exacerbations of the disease may require prolonged mechanical ventilation.[84]

Fish and Shellfish Poisoning. Several species of toxic dinoflagellates can cause shellfish and fish poisoning that can involve the respiratory muscles.[85] *Neurotoxic shellfish poisoning* is caused by clams or oysters that have ingested *Ptychodiscus brevis* (*Gymnodinium breve*) and concentrated its toxins (brevetoxins, the classic "red tide" toxins).[86] The syndrome is characterized by nausea, diarrhea, abdominal pain, and neurologic symptoms such as circumoral paresthesia; onset can range from a few minutes to 3 hours after ingestion of the clams or oysters. Paresthesia typically progresses to involve the pharynx, trunk, and extremities. Cerebellar symptoms, vertigo, incoordination, convulsions, bradycardia, and respiratory depression may develop.

Paralytic shellfish poisoning results from the ingestion of mussels, clams, scallops, and oysters that have concentrated saxitoxin, the neurotoxin present in *Protogonyaulux cantenella* and *Protogonyaulux tamarensis*. The symptoms are similar to those associated with the ingestion of brevetoxins.[87] *Ciguatera fish poisoning* results from eating fish contaminated with toxins derived from *Gambierdiscus toxicus*.[88] Although the disease occurs primarily in the tropics, cases in temperate

climates have been reported in people who have eaten fish imported from tropical areas.[89] Paralysis can develop up to 1 week after onset of the illness,[90] and muscle weakness can persist for long periods.[85]

Severe neuromuscular paralysis with rapid ventilatory failure can also occur after the ingestion of *puffer fish*. The neurotoxin responsible, tetrodotoxin, blocks sodium channels in the peripheral nerves. The case fatality rate when ventilatory failure occurs is approximately 50%.[91]

Disorders of the Myoneural Junction

Conditions that cause impaired neuromuscular transmission at the myoneural junction with consequent acute or chronic hypoventilation include myasthenia gravis, myasthenia-like syndromes associated with neoplasms, ingestion of various medications, and infection with or ingestion of toxins from *Clostridium botulinum*.

Myasthenia Gravis. The defect in myasthenia gravis is postsynaptic and related to IgG autoantibodies that attach to and destroy acetylcholine receptors at the motor end plate. Ventilatory failure is a frequent complication.[92] Exacerbations of respiratory muscle weakness and the development of respiratory failure can be precipitated by a variety of events, including surgery and infection. Before the onset of hypoventilation, patients who have myasthenia and myasthenia-like syndromes usually manifest paresthesia, diplopia, dysphagia, ptosis, generalized weakness, and dyspnea. The diagnosis may become evident only after a surgical procedure in which the effects of sedation and muscle relaxants cause a prolonged period of inadequate ventilation postoperatively.[93]

Myasthenia-like syndromes, such as Eaton-Lambert syndrome, occur in association with neoplasia, particularly small cell carcinoma of the lung.[94] The presence of neuronal antinuclear antibodies and the response to plasmapheresis and immunosuppressive therapy are consistent with an autoimmune pathogenesis.[95]

Drugs and Poisons. More than a hundred drugs have been reported to impair muscle function by inhibiting neural drive, causing peripheral neuropathy, blocking neuromuscular junctions, producing myopathy, or precipitating myasthenia gravis.[96] The use of nondepolarizing neuromuscular blocking agents in critically ill ventilated patients can cause prolonged muscle weakness,[97] especially when combined with systemic corticosteroids.[98]

Organophosphate poisoning by the insecticides parathion and malathion results from inhibition of acetylcholinesterase at nerve endings with consequent paralysis of the respiratory muscles.[99] Acetylcholine accumulates at cholinergic synapses and results in an initial stimulation and later inhibition of synaptic transmission.

***Clostridium botulinum* Poisoning.** The neurotoxin of *C. botulinum* causes a presynaptic blockade at the cholinergic neuromuscular junction.[100] The disease can occur after the ingestion of food contaminated with the toxin or as a result of wound infection by the organism. Peripheral muscle weakness and bulbar symptoms secondary to cranial nerve involvement usually appear within 18 to 36 hours after the ingestion of contaminated food. Patients complain of blurred vision, weakness, dizziness, dysphonia, dysphagia, respiratory difficulty, and urinary retention. The pupils are dilated and nonreactive, and there is marked dryness of the mouth and tongue associated with muscle weakness. Ocular findings may be prominent and early features.[101] Ventilatory failure secondary to muscle weakness occurs in 30% to 60% of affected patients and is the primary cause of mortality.[102]

Disorders of Respiratory Muscles

Muscular Dystrophy. The muscular dystrophies are inherited disorders characterized by progressive weakness of skeletal muscle. *Duchenne-type muscular dystrophy* has a sex-linked recessive inheritance pattern and begins in childhood. It is commonly associated with respiratory disease and in fact causes death from ventilatory failure in at least 80% of affected patients.[103] Respiratory involvement typically develops insidiously. *Facioscapulohumeral dystrophy* is a disorder of autosomal dominant inheritance that begins in adolescence.[104] *Myotonic dystrophy*, inherited in autosomal dominant fashion, can begin at any age. Ventilatory failure develops in approximately 10% of patients[105]; the respiratory difficulties relate both to weakness and to an increase in impedance of the respiratory system secondary to the increased tone in the abdominal and chest wall muscles.[106]

Acid Maltase Deficiency. This abnormality has a recessive inheritance pattern and is being recognized with increasing frequency as a cause of neuromuscular ventilatory failure.[107] It is due to a deficiency of the enzyme acid maltase (acid α-glucosidase), which leads to an accumulation of glycogen in the intracellular vacuoles of muscle and other tissues. The condition occurs in three forms, depending on the age at onset: (1) an infantile form, in which patients usually die before the age of 2 years and in which hepatic and splenic enlargement is a prominent finding; (2) a childhood form, characterized by variable muscle and organ involvement and usually by slow progression to respiratory failure; and (3) an adult form, in which specific muscle groups can be involved and the course is even more insidiously progressive.[108] Ventilatory failure is an inevitable development in the majority of patients.[109]

Myopathy in Connective Tissue Disease. Respiratory muscle weakness can occasionally be sufficient to cause acute or chronic hypoventilation in polymyositis and dermatomyositis. Respiratory muscular dysfunction is sometimes not recognized because undue attention is directed to associated bronchiolitis or interstitial pulmonary disease; in such cases, withdrawal of corticosteroid therapy may uncover the underlying muscle weakness. Generalized neuropathic and myopathic processes are known to occur in patients who have systemic lupus erythematosus,[110,111] and either process can involve the diaphragm. In fact, such muscular weakness has been postulated to be the mechanism underlying the "shrinking lung syndrome" sometimes seen in these patients.[112]

Respiratory Muscle Fatigue

Muscle fatigue is defined as the inability of a muscle to generate a predetermined force continuously. For the inspiratory muscles, force is assessed by measuring maximal inspiratory pressure (which gives an overall estimate of inspiratory muscle strength) or maximal transdiaphragmatic pressure (which provides a specific estimate of the force generated by the diaphragm).

Respiratory muscle fatigue can be either central or peripheral. The former is characterized by a diminution in force generation that is greater during voluntary effort than during electrical stimulation. Ultimately, respiratory muscles fatigue when an imbalance exists between their energy demand and the energy supply. Factors that determine the energy demand on a respiratory muscle are the work of breathing and the strength and endurance of the muscle; the strength in turn is affected by the length-tension relationship. As with all skeletal muscles, respiratory muscles display distinct length-tension behavior. There is a specific muscle length at which the overlap between actin and myosin filaments is optimal for the generation of pressure. When contracting at this length, the muscle is most efficient in terms of tension generation for a given consumption of adenosine triphosphate. At lengths shorter or longer than optimal, less tension can be generated despite similar activation and similar levels of fuel consumption. Thus, any factor that acutely alters resting length (such as lung hyperinflation) will have a profound effect on efficiency. Respiratory muscle strength is also decreased in patients who have neuromuscular disease or who are malnourished.

Respiratory muscles will inevitably fatigue when they are forced to continuously generate greater than 40% to 50% of the maximal pressure of which they are capable.[113] Such fatigability is increased in the presence of respiratory acidosis and hypoxemia.[114,115]

Clinical Manifestations

Patients who have respiratory failure secondary to neuromuscular abnormalities complain of anxiety, lethargy, headache, dyspnea, and (sometimes) a feeling of suffocation. When ventilation is severely restricted, confusion, coma, and death can ensue rapidly. Cyanosis may or may not be present, depending on the degree of hypoventilation. It is important to remember that in the presence of a normal hemoglobin concentration, hypoxemia can be detected clinically by a change in color of the nail beds and mucous membranes only when SaO_2 has dropped to 80% or less. Similarly, appreciation of the degree of alveolar ventilation clinically is unreliable except when apnea has occurred,[116] by which time the patient will be severely cyanotic.

Because the diaphragm is the principal muscle of inspiration, evidence of diaphragmatic weakness or paralysis on physical examination is important in identifying a neuromuscular cause for the respiratory failure. When a normal diaphragm contracts, it descends and thereby increases intra-abdominal pressure and causes the abdominal wall to protrude (Fig. 23–1). When one hemidiaphragm is paralyzed or weakened, paradoxical movement may be apparent on physical examination or fluoroscopy (Fig. 23–2). On inspiration, the paralyzed hemidiaphragm moves upward coincident with expansion of the rib cage and descent of the normal hemidiaphragm, a motion that can be appreciated to better advantage during "sniffing" by the patient.

When both hemidiaphragms are paralyzed, as in bilateral phrenic nerve palsy, or when a neuropathic or myopathic disorder causes bilateral diaphragmatic weakness, paradoxical abdominal wall motion is more apparent clinically. With each inspiratory effort of the external intercostal and accessory muscles of respiration, the rib cage expands and causes a

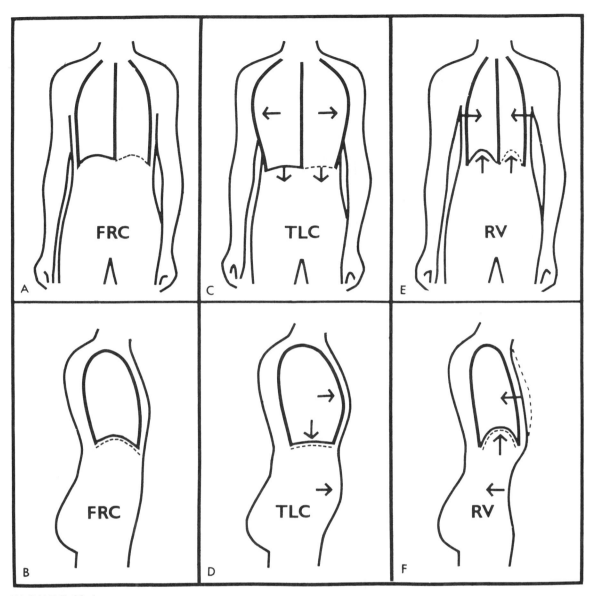

FIGURE 23–1

Schematic depiction of chest cage and diaphragmatic movements throughout the respiratory cycle—normal.
Anteroposterior (**A**) and lateral (**B**) views show the position of the chest wall and diaphragm at resting lung volume (FRC). At full inspiration (**C** and **D**), the diaphragm contracts with resultant expansion of the chest cage, an increase in intra-abdominal pressure, and protrusion of the abdominal wall. At full expiration (**E** and **F**), abdominal muscle contraction causes a rise in intra-abdominal pressure and elevation of the relaxed diaphragm. *(From Fraser RS, Müller NL, Colman NC, Paré PD: Fraser and Paré's Diagnosis of Diseases of the Chest, 4th ed. Philadelphia, WB Saunders, 1999.)*

decrease in intrapleural pressure and "sucking" of the diaphragm into the thorax (Fig. 23–3A to D). In patients who have incipient diaphragmatic fatigue, paradoxical abdominal wall motion can develop during or after a period of increased respiratory muscle activity (e.g., when they are being weaned from ventilatory support).

Recruitment of abdominal expiratory muscles can mask paradoxical breathing and diaphragmatic weakness.[117] During expiration, the abdominal wall muscles may contract and force the flaccid diaphragm into the thoracic cavity; at the onset of inspiration, sudden relaxation of these

muscles causes rapid diaphragmatic descent and apparent outward movement of the abdomen (Fig. 23–3E and F). Recruitment of expiratory abdominal muscles during tidal breathing can be detected by palpation of the anterior abdominal wall. Abdominal muscle contraction can restore an apparently normal pattern of movement to the anterior abdominal wall (Fig. 23–3G to J). This pattern of expiratory muscle recruitment may be responsible for the false-negative findings on fluoroscopic examination in some patients who have bilateral diaphragmatic paralysis or weakness.

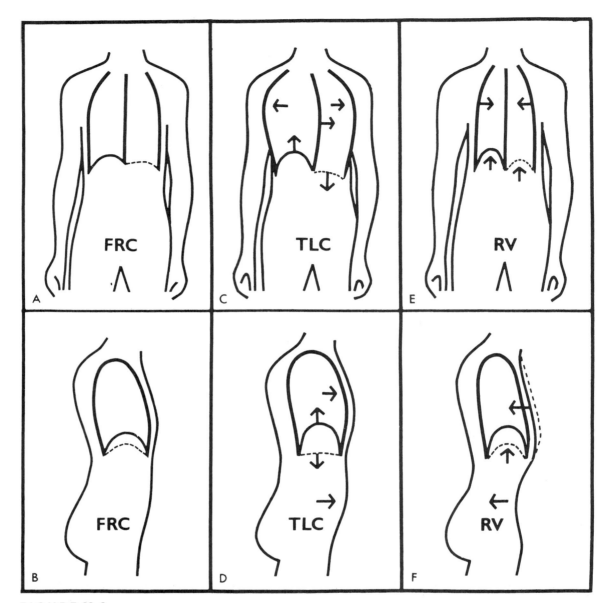

FIGURE 23–2

Schematic depiction of chest cage and diaphragmatic movements throughout the respiratory cycle—right hemidiaphragmatic paralysis. At FRC (**A** and **B**), the right hemidiaphragm is elevated. On full inspiration to TLC (**C** and **D**), the left hemidiaphragm contracts and descends, whereas the right hemidiaphragm passively elevates in response to the more negative intrapleural pressure. On full expiration to RV (**E** and **F**), a rise in intra-abdominal pressure evokes an even greater elevation of the paralyzed right hemidiaphragm. *(From Fraser RS, Müller NL, Colman NC, Paré PD: Fraser and Paré's Diagnosis of Diseases of the Chest, 4th ed. Philadelphia, WB Saunders, 1999.)*

Pulmonary Function Tests

When the lung parenchyma is normal, a decrease in TLC or an increase in residual volume (and thus a decrease in VC) may indicate respiratory muscle weakness.[72] When VC is reduced to 25% or less of predicted, ventilatory failure is either present or imminent.[118] The characteristic expiratory and inspiratory flow-volume curve of patients who have global muscle weakness is an egg-shaped loop; there is a delay in achieving peak expiratory flow, and both maximal expiratory flow and inspiratory flow are reduced.

Abnormalities in arterial blood gas tensions constitute a late finding in patients who have primary neuromuscular disease. In those with severe weakness or complete paralysis of the diaphragm, assumption of the supine posture causes further deterioration in gas exchange. The explanation for this is related to a change in gravitational forces: the weight of the abdominal organs displaces the flaccid diaphragm upward into the thoracic cavity, thus further reducing the effectiveness of the remaining inspiratory muscles.[119] In addition, a further drop in PaO_2 and a rise in $PaCO_2$ often occur during sleep, when the control of breathing is solely automatic.[119]

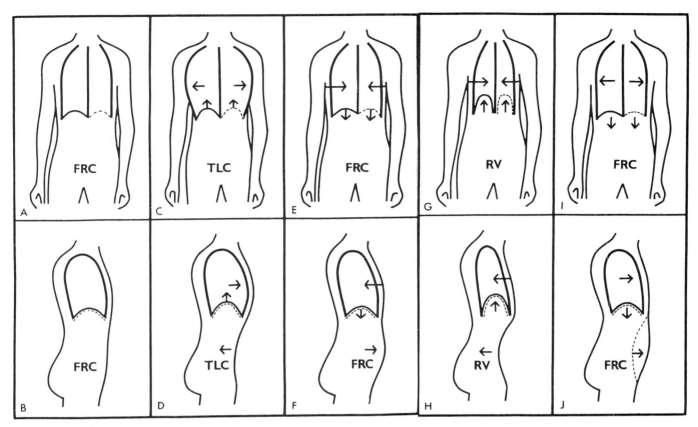

FIGURE 23–3

Schematic depiction of chest cage and diaphragmatic movements throughout the respiratory cycle—bilateral diaphragmatic paralysis. On inspiration to TLC from FRC (**A** to **D**), the increased negative intrapleural pressure "sucks" the diaphragm up and draws the abdominal wall in. On expiration to FRC (**E** and **F**), the diaphragm descends and the abdomen protrudes. With a deeper expiration to RV accompanied by active contraction of the abdominal muscles (**G** and **H**), the diaphragm rises. Subsequently, during the first part of inspiration to FRC (**I** and **J**), abdominal muscle recoil is associated with descent of the flaccid diaphragm, which creates the false impression of active contraction. *(From Fraser RS, Müller NL, Colman NC, Paré PD: Fraser and Paré's Diagnosis of Diseases of the Chest, 4th ed. Philadelphia, WB Saunders, 1999.)*

Measurements of maximal inspiratory and expiratory pressure provide useful indices of respiratory muscle strength. Serial measurement of these pressures is also a practical means of recognizing the development of respiratory muscle weakness or fatigue and documenting recovery of respiratory muscle strength.[120]

Weakness or paralysis of the diaphragm can be detected by measuring transdiaphragmatic pressure. Phrenic nerve function can be measured by recording the diaphragmatic muscle action potential with either esophageal or surface electrodes after transcutaneous stimulation of the phrenic nerve in the neck.[121,122] A positive response in the presence of documented diaphragmatic paralysis indicates that the disorder is myopathic rather than neuropathic.

ALVEOLAR HYPERVENTILATION

Hyperventilation is present when $PaCO_2$ is less than 35 mm Hg. It can result from both pulmonary and extrapulmonary causes.

Pulmonary Disease

Hyperventilation can occur in patients who have asthma, pneumonia, thromboembolism, or diffuse granulomatous or fibrotic interstitial disease. In these circumstances, the hypocapnia is usually associated with hypoxemia. If the hyperventilation is recent in origin, bicarbonate levels remain relatively elevated, as reflected in a lower hydrogen ion concentration (elevated pH). If the overventilation is of longer duration, renal compensation for the lowered $PaCO_2$ results in increased urinary excretion of bicarbonate and a lowered serum bicarbonate level; the hydrogen ion concentration is maintained within normal limits.

Extrapulmonary Disorders

Central Nervous System Abnormalities. These abnormalities include infarct/hemorrhage, trauma, meningitis, and encephalitis. Although the mechanism is not certain, it is possible that metabolites related to inflammation or necrotic tissue cause a rise in hydrogen ion concentration in cerebrospinal fluid that directly stimulates the respiratory center.

Cheyne-Stokes Respiration. This breathing pattern is characterized by a cyclic fluctuation in ventilation in which periods of central apnea or hypopnea alternate with periods of hyperpnea in a gradual crescendo-decrescendo fashion.[123] Tidal volume increases progressively during the phase of hyperpnea and subsequently decreases without change in the respiratory rate. This cyclic form of breathing is caused by instability of the ventilatory control system, in which the circulation time, the sensitivity of the central ventilatory controller, and the damping characteristics of the O_2 and CO_2 stores play important roles.[124] It occurs in patients who have left ventricular failure or impaired cerebrovascular circulation.

Psychogenic Hyperventilation. The *hyperventilation syndrome* is the most common cause of hyperventilation. It has been defined as "a syndrome characterized by a variety of somatic symptoms induced by physiologically inappropriate hyperventilation and usually reproduced in whole or in part by voluntary hyperventilation."[125] The syndrome has been closely related to a psychiatric condition termed *panic disorder* that is characterized by the sudden onset of extreme fear for which there is no known cause.[126]

Psychogenic hyperventilation varies considerably in degree and clinical findings: affected patients range from those who complain of dyspnea at rest and require frequent deep respiratory effort to those who overbreathe to the extent of inducing coma or tetany. Symptoms include giddiness or light-headedness, paresthesias, visual disturbances, and loss of consciousness.[126] The mechanism for these symptoms is probably a combination of cerebral hypoxia secondary to cerebral vasoconstriction and metabolic alkalosis.[127] Dyspnea and palpitations are the most common cardiorespiratory symptoms. The majority of patients describe the shortness of breath as an inability to "get enough air down into the lungs" or an inability to take a satisfying breath.[128]

Although the diagnosis of psychogenic hyperventilation is often made readily on the basis of its characteristic history, in some patients the manifestations closely simulate those of organic disease. Careful monitoring of breathing aids in diagnosis, the characteristic pattern being highly irregular breathing punctuated by deep inspiration.

METHEMOGLOBINEMIA

Methemoglobin is hemoglobin in which the ferrous iron has been oxidized to the ferric form. Blood turns a chocolate-brown color when approximately 15% of hemoglobin is so oxidized; the result is "cyanosis" that is unresponsive to O_2 therapy.[129] Acquired methemoglobinemia can result from exposure to drugs or chemicals[130,131] that increase the rate of hemoglobin oxidation or exhaust the mechanisms that protect hemoglobin against oxidation. Two types of hereditary methemoglobinemia have been described.[132,133]

Patients usually have symptoms and signs related to tissue anoxia, including headache, nausea, dizziness, pounding pulse, and listlessness.[134] In most cases there is a diffuse, persistent, grayish discoloration of the skin; however, this finding may not be obvious. The diagnosis may be suspected when pulse oximetry shows SaO_2 values that are inappropriately low for the measured PaO_2.

CARBON MONOXIDE POISONING

Carbon monoxide (CO) is an odorless, colorless gas that binds in a reversible manner with hemoglobin; it has an affinity for the hemoglobin-binding site that is 200 times greater than that of O_2. It is the most frequent cause of poisoning death in the United States.[135] Acute poisoning most often results from inhalation of motor vehicle exhaust fumes in suicide attempts[136]; less often, it occurs in association with defective heating and cooking systems or the inappropriate use of such systems indoors.[137] A wide variety of additional scenarios have also been associated with unintentional CO poisoning, including house fires, mine explosions, and the use of concrete saws and other devices indoors.[138,139]

Chronic CO exposure occurs in smokers. The blood COHb level in healthy nonsmoking individuals is about 0.5%,[140] whereas it is about 6% in someone who smokes one pack of cigarettes per day.[141] With heavy smoking, the figure may be as high as 20%.[142] The percentage of inspired CO may be increased in heavy traffic because car exhaust contains between 1% and 7% CO[143]; it may also rise in closed breathing circuits during anesthesia or in closed air systems such as in submarines.

The deleterious effects of CO are attributable primarily to tissue hypoxia resulting from the formation of COHb, which reduces the O_2 transport capacity of the blood and causes a shift of the oxyhemoglobin dissociation curve to the left, thus curtailing the amount of O_2 available to tissues. A direct cytotoxic effect of CO may also be responsible for tissue damage.[144] Symptoms of acute poisoning include headache, nausea and vomiting, and decreased manual dexterity. Characteristically, these symptoms develop when carboxyhemoglobin saturation reaches 20%; unconsciousness and convulsions occur at about 50% to 60% and death at about 80%.[145]

CO toxicity can be detected by measuring COHb levels. Pulse oximetry is unreliable in detecting O_2 saturation in CO-exposed patients because it cannot distinguish between COHb and oxyhemoglobin.[146]

REFERENCES

1. Austin JH, Romney BM, Goldsmith LS: Missed bronchogenic carcinoma: Radiographic findings in 27 patients with a potentially resectable lesion evident in retrospect. Radiology 182:115-122, 1992.
2. Worsley DF, Alavi A, Aronchick JM, et al: Chest radiographic findings in patients with acute pulmonary embolism: Observations from the PIOPED Study. Radiology 189:133-136, 1993.
3. Rigler L: Roentgen examination of the chest. Its limitations in the diagnosis of disease. JAMA 142:773, 1950.
4. Steele JD, Buell P: Asymptomatic solitary pulmonary nodules. Host survival, tumor size, and growth rate. J Thorac Cardiovasc Surg 65:140-151, 1973.
5. Kwong JS, Carignan S, Kang EY, et al: Miliary tuberculosis. Diagnostic accuracy of chest radiography. Chest 110:339-342, 1996.
6. Muller NL: Clinical value of high-resolution CT in chronic diffuse lung disease. AJR Am J Roentgenol 157:1163-1170, 1991.
7. Orens JB, Kazerooni EA, Martinez FJ, et al: The sensitivity of high-resolution CT in detecting idiopathic pulmonary fibrosis proved by open lung biopsy. A prospective study. Chest 108:109-115, 1995.
8. Remy-Jardin M, Remy J, Wallaert B, et al: Subacute and chronic bird breeder hypersensitivity pneumonitis: Sequential evaluation with CT and correlation with lung function tests and bronchoalveolar lavage. Radiology 189:111-118, 1993.
9. Bankier AA, Kiener HP, Wiesmayr MN, et al: Discrete lung involvement in systemic lupus erythematosus: CT assessment. Radiology 196:835-840, 1995.
10. Blackie SP, al-Majed S, Staples CA, et al: Changes in total lung capacity during acute spontaneous asthma. Am Rev Respir Dis 142:79-83, 1990.
11. van der Bruggen-Bogaarts BA, van der Bruggen HM, van Waes PF, et al: Screening for bronchiectasis. A comparative study between chest radiography and high-resolution CT. Chest 109:608-611, 1996.

12. Thurlbeck W, Henderson J, Fraser R: Chronic obstructive lung disease. A comparison between clinical, roentgenologic, functional and morphological criteria in chronic bronchitis, emphysema, asthma and bronchiectasis. Medicine (Baltimore) 49:91, 1970.

13. Taxman RM, Halloran MJ, Parker BM: Multiple pulmonary arteriovenous malformations in association with Fanconi's syndrome. Chest 64:118-120, 1973.

14. Papagiannis J, Kanter RJ, Effman EL, et al: Polysplenia with pulmonary arteriovenous malformations. Pediatr Cardiol 14:127-129, 1993.

15. Berthelot P, Walker JG, Sherlock S, et al: Arterial changes in the lungs in cirrhosis of the liver—lung spider nevi. N Engl J Med 274:291-298, 1966.

16. Shub C, Tajik AJ, Seward JB, et al: Detecting intrapulmonary right-to-left shunt with contrast echocardiography. Observations in a patient with diffuse pulmonary arteriovenous fistulas. Mayo Clin Proc 51:81-84, 1976.

17. Vergnon JM, De Bonadona JF, Riffat J, et al: [Technics for the exploration of pulmonary arteriovenous shunts in liver cirrhosis. Apropos of 2 cases.] Rev Mal Respir 3:145-152, 1986.

18. Robin ED, Horn B, Goris ML, et al: Detection, quantitation and pathophysiology of lung "spiders." Trans Assoc Am Physicians 88:202-216, 1975.

19. Kennedy TC, Knudson RJ: Exercise-aggravated hypoxemia and orthodeoxia in cirrhosis. Chest 72:305-309, 1977.

20. Colins JD, Burwell D, Furmanski S, et al: Minimal detectable pleural effusions. A roentgen pathology model. Radiology 105:51-53, 1972.

21. Hessen I: Roentgen examination of pleural fluid: A study of the localization of free effusion, the potentialities of diagnosing minimal quantities of fluid and its existence under physiological conditions. Acta Radiol Suppl 86:1, 1951.

22. Svenes KB, Borgersen A, Haaversen O, et al: Parietal pleural plaques: A comparison between autopsy and x-ray findings. Eur J Respir Dis 69:10-15, 1986.

23. Wathen CG, Capewell SJ, Heath JP, et al: Recurrent lobar pneumonia associated with idiopathic Eaton-Lambert syndrome. Thorax 43:574-575, 1988.

24. Bianchi AL, Denavit-Saubie M, Champagnat J: Central control of breathing in mammals: Neuronal circuitry, membrane properties, and neurotransmitters. Physiol Rev 75:1-45, 1995.

25. Mateika JH, Duffin J: A review of the control of breathing during exercise. Eur J Appl Physiol Occup Physiol 71:1-27, 1995.

26. Guilleminault C, Stoohs R, Quera-Salva MA: Sleep-related obstructive and nonobstructive apneas and neurologic disorders. Neurology 42:53-60, 1992.

27. White JM, Irvine RJ: Mechanisms of fatal opioid overdose. Addiction 94:961-972, 1999.

28. Jay SJ, Johanson WG Jr, Pierce AK: Respiratory complications of overdose with sedative drugs. Am Rev Respir Dis 112:591-598, 1975.

29. Hall SC, Ovassapian A: Apnea after intravenous diazepam therapy. JAMA 238:1052, 1977.

30. Biggs JT, Spiker DG, Petit JM, et al: Tricyclic antidepressant overdose: Incidence of symptoms. JAMA 238:135-138, 1977.

31. Management of unconscious poisoned patients. BMJ 2:647-648, 1969.

32. Maddock RK Jr, Bloomer HA: Meprobamate overdosage. Evaluation of its severity and methods of treatment. JAMA 201:999-1003, 1967.

33. Thalhofer S, Dorow P: Central sleep apnea. Respiration 64:2-9, 1997.

34. Kerbl R, Litscher H, Grubbauer HM, et al: Congenital central hypoventilation syndrome (Ondine's curse syndrome) in two siblings: Delayed diagnosis and successful noninvasive treatment. Eur J Pediatr 155:977-980, 1996.

35. Farmer WC, Glenn WW, Gee JB: Alveolar hypoventilation syndrome. Studies of ventilatory control in patients selected for diaphragm pacing. Am J Med 64:39-49, 1978.

36. Kryger MH: Central apnea. Arch Intern Med 142:1793-1794, 1982.

37. Yasuma F, Nomura H, Sotobata I, et al: Congenital central alveolar hypoventilation (Ondine's curse): A case report and review of the literature. Eur J Pediatr 146:81-83, 1987.

38. Vingerhoets F, Bogousslavsky J: Respiratory dysfunction in stroke. Clin Chest Med 15:729-737, 1994.

39. Valente S, De Rosa M, Culla G, et al: An uncommon case of brainstem tumor with selective involvement of the respiratory centers. Chest 103:1909-1910, 1993.

40. Bradley TD, McNicholas WT, Rutherford R, et al: Clinical and physiologic heterogeneity of the central sleep apnea syndrome. Am Rev Respir Dis 134:217-221, 1986.

41. Raetzo MA, Junod AF, Kryger MH: Effect of aminophylline and relief from hypoxia on central sleep apnoea due to medullary damage. Bull Eur Physiopathol Respir 23:171-175, 1987.

42. Barlow PB, Bartlett D Jr, Hauri P, et al: Idiopathic hypoventilation syndrome: Importance of preventing nocturnal hypoxemia and hypercapnia. Am Rev Respir Dis 121:141-145, 1980.

43. Bickelmann AG, Burwell CS, Robin ED, et al: Extreme obesity associated with alveolar hypoventilation; a pickwickian syndrome. Am J Med 21:811-818, 1956.

44. Bass JB Jr: Pickwickian, obesity-hypoventilation, or Fee-fi-fo-fum syndrome? Am Rev Respir Dis 122:657, 1980.

45. Ahmed Q, Chung-Park M, Tomashefski JF Jr: Cardiopulmonary pathology in patients with sleep apnea/obesity hypoventilation syndrome. Hum Pathol 28:264-269, 1997.

46. Ahmad M, Cressman M, Tomashefski JF: Central alveolar hypoventilation syndromes. Arch Intern Med 140:29-30, 1980.

47. Monge CC, Arregui A, Leon-Velarde F: Pathophysiology and epidemiology of chronic mountain sickness. Int J Sports Med 13(Suppl 1):S79-S81, 1992.

48. Sun SF, Huang SY, Zhang JG, et al: Decreased ventilation and hypoxic ventilatory responsiveness are not reversed by naloxone in Lhasa residents with chronic mountain sickness. Am Rev Respir Dis 142:1294-1300, 1990.

49. Millman RP, Bevilacqua J, Peterson DD, et al: Central sleep apnea in hypothyroidism. Am Rev Respir Dis 127:504-507, 1983.

50. McNamara ME, Southwick SM, Fogel BS: Sleep apnea and hypothyroidism presenting as depression in two patients. J Clin Psychiatry 48:164-165, 1987.

51. Weiner M, Chausow A, Szidon P: Reversible respiratory muscle weakness in hypothyroidism. Br J Dis Chest 80:391-395, 1986.

52. Blank MJ, Lew SQ: Hypoventilation in a dialysis patient with severe metabolic alkalosis: Treatment by hemodialysis. Blood Purif 9:109-113, 1991.

53. Shear L, Brandman IS: Hypoxia and hypercapnia caused by respiratory compensation for metabolic alkalosis. Am Rev Respir Dis 107:836-841, 1973.

54. Tanaka M, Yano T, Ichikawa Y, et al: A case of Cushing's syndrome associated with chronic respiratory failure due to metabolic alkalosis. Intern Med 31:385-390, 1992.

55. Fraser RS, Sproule BJ, Dvorkin J: Hypoventilation, cyanosis and polycythemia in a thin man. Can Med Assoc J 89:1178-1182, 1963.

56. Estenne M, Hubert M, De Troyer A: Respiratory-muscle involvement in Parkinson's disease. N Engl J Med 311:1516-1517, 1984.

57. Abhyankar NY, Bhambure NM, Kasekar SG, et al: Intensive respiratory care service—our eight-year experience. Indian J Chest Dis Allied Sci 34:65-72, 1992.

58. Udwadia FE, Lall A, Udwadia ZF, et al: Tetanus and its complications: Intensive care and management experience in 150 Indian patients. Epidemiol Infect 99:675-684, 1987.

59. Sandor F: Diaphragmatic respiration: A sign of cervical cord lesion in the unconscious patient ("horizontal paradox"). BMJ 5485:465-466, 1966.

60. Loveridge B, Sanii R, Dubo HI: Breathing pattern adjustments during the first year following cervical spinal cord injury. Paraplegia 30:479-488, 1992.

61. Lahuerta J, Lipton S, Wells JC: Percutaneous cervical cordotomy: Results and complications in a recent series of 100 patients. Ann R Coll Surg Engl 67:41-44, 1985.

62. Yamamoto T, Imai T, Yamasaki M: Acute ventilatory failure in multiple sclerosis. J Neurol Sci 89:313-324, 1989.

63. Jaspar N, Kruger M, Ectors P, et al: Unilateral chest wall paradoxical motion mimicking a flail chest in a patient with hemilateral C7 spinal injury. Intensive Care Med 12:396-398, 1986.

64. Wade JG, Larson CP Jr, Hickey RF, et al: Effect of carotid endarterectomy on carotid chemoreceptor and baroreceptor function in man. N Engl J Med 282:823-829, 1970.

65. Lugliani R, Whipp BJ, Seard C, et al: Effect of bilateral carotid-body resection on ventilatory control at rest and during exercise in man. N Engl J Med 285:1105-1111, 1971.

66. Honda Y, Myojo S, Hasegawa S, et al: Decreased exercise hyperpnea in patients with bilateral carotid chemoreceptor resection. J Appl Physiol 46:908-912, 1979.

67. Zikk D, Shanon E, Rapoport Y, et al: Sleep apnea following bilateral excision of carotid body tumors. Laryngoscope 93:1470-1472, 1983.

68. Gozal D, Harper RM: Novel insights into congenital hypoventilation syndrome. Curr Opin Pulm Med 5:335-338, 1999.

69. Hines S, Houston M, Robertson D: The clinical spectrum of autonomic dysfunction. Am J Med 70:1091-1096, 1981.

70. Montserrat JM, Cochrane GM, Wolf C, et al: Ventilatory control in diabetes mellitus. Eur J Respir Dis 67:112-117, 1985.

71. Bullock R, Todd NV, Easton J, et al: Isolated central respiratory failure due to syringomyelia and Arnold-Chiari malformation. BMJ 297:1448-1449, 1988.

72. Derenne JP, Macklem PT, Roussos C: The respiratory muscles: Mechanics, control, and pathophysiology. Am Rev Respir Dis 118:119-133, 1978.

73. Saxton GA Jr, Rayson GE, Moody E, et al: Alveolar-arterial gas tension relationships in acute anterior poliomyelitis. Am J Med 30:871-883, 1961.

74. Hsu AA, Staats BA: "Postpolio" sequelae and sleep-related disordered breathing. Mayo Clin Proc 73:216-224, 1998.

75. Meyrignac C, Poirier J, Degos JD: Amyotrophic lateral sclerosis presenting with respiratory insufficiency as the primary complaint. Clinicopathological study of a case. Eur Neurol 24:115-120, 1985.

76. Kreitzer SM, Saunders NA, Tyler HR, et al: Respiratory muscle function in amyotrophic lateral sclerosis. Am Rev Respir Dis 117:437-447, 1978.

77. Brach BB: Expiratory flow patterns in amyotrophic lateral sclerosis. Chest 75:648-650, 1979.

78. O'Donohue WJ Jr, Baker JP, Bell GM, et al: Respiratory failure in neuromuscular disease. Management in a respiratory intensive care unit. JAMA 235:733-735, 1976.

79. Hu-Sheng W, Qi-Fen Y, Tian-Ci L, et al: The treatment of acute polyradiculoneuritis with respiratory paralysis. Brain Dev 10:147, 1988.

80. Gracey DR, McMichan JC, Divertie MB, et al: Respiratory failure in Guillain-Barré syndrome: A 6-year experience. Mayo Clin Proc 57:742-746, 1982.

81. Chevrolet JC, Deleamont P: Repeated vital capacity measurements as predictive parameters for mechanical ventilation need and weaning success in the Guillain-Barré syndrome. Am Rev Respir Dis 144:814-818, 1991.

82. Gourie-Devi M, Ganapathy GR: Phrenic nerve conduction time in Guillain-Barré syndrome. J Neurol Neurosurg Psychiatry 48:245-249, 1985.

83. Becker DM, Kramer S: The neurological manifestations of porphyria: A review. Medicine (Baltimore) 56:411-423, 1977.

84. Doll SG, Bower AG, Affeldt JE: Acute intermittent porphyria with respiratory paralysis. JAMA 168:1973-1976, 1958.

85. Sakamoto Y, Lockey RF, Krzanowski JJ Jr: Shellfish and fish poisoning related to the toxic dinoflagellates. South Med J 80:866-872, 1987.

86. Ellis S: Brevetoxins: Chemistry and pharmacology of 'red tide' toxins from Ptychodiscus brevis (formerly Gymnodinium breve). Toxicon 23:469-472, 1985.

87. Paralytic shellfish poising. Laboratory for Disease Control, Ottawa, Ontario. Can Dis Wkly Rep 4:21, 1978.

88. Morris JG Jr: Ciguatera fish poisoning. JAMA 244:273-274, 1980.

89. Tatnall FM, Smith HG, Welsby PD, et al: Ciguatera poisoning. BMJ 281:948-949, 1980.
90. Morris JG Jr, Lewin P, Hargrett NT, et al: Clinical features of ciguatera fish poisoning: A study of the disease in the US Virgin Islands. Arch Intern Med 142:1090-1092, 1982.
91. Mills AR, Passmore R: Pelagic paralysis. Lancet 1:161-164, 1988.
92. Zulueta JJ, Fanburg BL: Respiratory dysfunction in myasthenia gravis. Clin Chest Med 15:683-691, 1994.
93. Suxamethonium apnoea. Lancet 1:246-247, 1973.
94. Dropcho EJ, Stanton C, Oh SJ: Neuronal antinuclear antibodies in a patient with Lambert-Eaton myasthenic syndrome and small-cell lung carcinoma. Neurology 39:249-251, 1989.
95. Lang B, Newsom-Davis J, Wray D, et al: Autoimmune aetiology for myasthenic (Eaton-Lambert) syndrome. Lancet 2:224-226, 1981.
96. Aldrich TK, Prezant DJ: Adverse effects of drugs on the respiratory muscles. Clin Chest Med 11:177-189, 1990.
97. Gooch JL: Prolonged paralysis after neuromuscular blockade. J Toxicol Clin Toxicol 33:419-426, 1995.
98. Behbehani NA, Al-Mane F, D'Yachkova Y, et al: Myopathy following mechanical ventilation for acute severe asthma: The role of muscle relaxants and corticosteroids. Chest 115:1627-1631, 1999.
99. Namba T, Nolte CT, Jackrel J, et al: Poisoning due to organophosphate insecticides. Acute and chronic manifestations. Am J Med 50:475-492, 1971.
100. Kao I, Drachman DB, Price DL: Botulinum toxin: Mechanism of presynaptic blockade. Science 193:1256-1258, 1976.
101. Terranova W, Palumbo JN, Breman JG: Ocular findings in botulism type B. JAMA 241:475-477, 1979.
102. Wilcox P, Andolfatto G, Fairbarn MS, et al: Long-term follow-up of symptoms, pulmonary function, respiratory muscle strength, and exercise performance after botulism. Am Rev Respir Dis 139:157-163, 1989.
103. Begin R, Bureau MA, Lupien L, et al: Control of breathing in Duchenne's muscular dystrophy. Am J Med 69:227-234, 1980.
104. Yasukohchi S, Yagi Y, Akabane T, et al: Facioscapulohumeral dystrophy associated with sensorineural hearing loss, tortuosity of retinal arterioles, and an early onset and rapid progression of respiratory failure. Brain Dev 10:319-324, 1988.
105. Gillam PM, Heaf PJ, Kaufman L, et al: Respiration in dystrophia myotonica. Thorax 19:112-120, 1964.
106. Begin R, Bureau MA, Lupien L, et al: Pathogenesis of respiratory insufficiency in myotonic dystrophy: The mechanical factors. Am Rev Respir Dis 125:312-318, 1982.
107. Wokke JH, Ausems MG, van den Boogaard MJ, et al: Genotype-phenotype correlation in adult-onset acid maltase deficiency. Ann Neurol 38:450-454, 1995.
108. Rosenow EC 3rd, Engel AG: Acid maltase deficiency in adults presenting as respiratory failure. Am J Med 64:485-491, 1978.
109. Moufarrej NA, Bertorini TE: Respiratory insufficiency in adult-type acid maltase deficiency. South Med J 86:560-567, 1993.
110. Gibson T, Myers AR: Nervous system involvement in systemic lupus erythematosus. Ann Rheum Dis 35:398-406, 1975.
111. Isenber DA, Snaith ML: Muscle disease in systemic lupus erythematosus: A study of its nature, frequency and cause. J Rheumatol 8:917-924, 1981.
112. Gibson CJ, Edmonds JP, Hughes GR: Diaphragm function and lung involvement in systemic lupus erythematosus. Am J Med 63:926-932, 1977.
113. Roussos C, Fixley M, Gross D, et al: Fatigue of inspiratory muscles and their synergic behavior. J Appl Physiol 46:897-904, 1979.
114. Juan G, Calverley P, Talamo C, et al: Effect of carbon dioxide on diaphragmatic function in human beings. N Engl J Med 310:874-879, 1984.
115. Jardim J, Farkas G, Prefaut C, et al: The failing inspiratory muscles under normoxic and hypoxic conditions. Am Rev Respir Dis 124:274-279, 1981.
116. Mithoefer JC, Bossman OG, Thibeault DW, et al: The clinical estimation of alveolar ventilation. Am Rev Respir Dis 98:868-871, 1968.
117. Grinman S, Whitelaw WA: Pattern of breathing in a case of generalized respiratory muscle weakness. Chest 84:770-772, 1983.
118. Harrison BD, Collins JV, Brown KG, et al: Respiratory failure in neuromuscular diseases. Thorax 26:579-584, 1971.
119. Davis J, Goldman M, Loh L, et al: Diaphragm function and alveolar hypoventilation. Q J Med 45:87-100, 1976.
120. Black LF, Hyatt RE: Maximal static respiratory pressures in generalized neuromuscular disease. Am Rev Respir Dis 103:641-650, 1971.
121. Delhez L: [Manifestations, in normal man, of the electrical response of the diaphragmatic pillars to electric stimulation of the phrenic nerves by single shocks.] Arch Int Physiol Biochim 73:832-839, 1965.
122. Davis JN: Phrenic nerve conduction in man. J Neurol Neurosurg Psychiatry 30:420-426, 1967.
123. Morse SR, Chandrasekhar AJ, Cugell DW: Cheyne-Stokes respiration redefined [editorial]. Chest 66:345-346, 1974.
124. Cherniack NS, Longobardo GS: Cheyne-Stokes breathing. An instability in physiologic control. N Engl J Med 288:952-957, 1973.
125. Lewis RA, Howell JB: Definition of the hyperventilation syndrome. Bull Eur Physiopathol Respir 22:201-205, 1986.
126. Ley R: Panic disorder and agoraphobia: Fear of fear or fear of the symptoms produced by hyperventilation? J Behav Ther Exp Psychiatry 18:305-316, 1987.
127. Nisam M, Albertson TE, Panacek E, et al: Effects of hyperventilation on conjunctival oxygen tension in humans. Crit Care Med 14:12-15, 1986.
128. Bass C, Gardner WN: Respiratory and psychiatric abnormalities in chronic symptomatic hyperventilation. Br Med J (Clin Res Ed) 290:1387-1390, 1985.
129. Harris JC, Rumack BH, Peterson RG, et al: Methemoglobinemia resulting from absorption of nitrates. JAMA 242:2869-2871, 1979.
130. Guertler AT, Pearce WA: A prospective evaluation of benzocaine-associated methemoglobinemia in human beings. Ann Emerg Med 24:626-630, 1994.
131. Kennedy N, Smith CP, McWhinney P: Faulty sausage production causing methaemoglobinaemia. Arch Dis Child 76:367-368, 1997.
132. Vieira LM, Kaplan JC, Kahn A, et al: Four new mutations in the NADH–cytochrome b5 reductase gene from patients with recessive congenital methemoglobinemia type II. Blood 85:2254-2262, 1995.
133. Manabe J, Arya R, Sumimoto H, et al: Two novel mutations in the reduced nicotinamide adenine dinucleotide (NADH)–cytochrome b5 reductase gene of a patient with generalized type, hereditary methemoglobinemia. Blood 88:3208-3215, 1996.
134. Wetherhold J, Linch A, Charsha R: Chemical cyanosis—causes, effects, prevention. Arch Environ Health 1:353, 1960.
135. Hardy KR, Thom SR: Pathophysiology and treatment of carbon monoxide poisoning. J Toxicol Clin Toxicol 32:613-629, 1994.
136. Ostrom M, Thorson J, Eriksson A: Carbon monoxide suicide from car exhausts. Soc Sci Med 42:447-451, 1996.
137. Houck PM, Hampson NB: Epidemic carbon monoxide poisoning following a winter storm. J Emerg Med 15:469-473, 1997.
138. Walker AR: Emergency department management of house fire burns and carbon monoxide poisoning in children. Curr Opin Pediatr 8:239-242, 1996.
139. Hawkes AP, McCammon JB, Hoffman RE: Indoor use of concrete saws and other gas-powered equipment. Analysis of reported carbon monoxide poisoning cases in Colorado. J Occup Environ Med 40:49-54, 1998.
140. Astrup P: Some physiological and pathological effects of moderate carbon monoxide exposure. BMJ 4:447-452, 1972.
141. Goldsmith JR, Landaw SA: Carbon monoxide and human health. Science 162:1352-1359, 1968.
142. Cowie J, Sillett RW, Ball K: Carbon-monoxide absorption by cigarette smokers who change to smoking cigars. Lancet 1:1033-1035, 1973.
143. Carbon monoxide poisoning—a timely warning. N Engl J Med 278:849-850, 1968.
144. Thom SR, Xu YA, Ischiropoulos H: Vascular endothelial cells generate peroxynitrite in response to carbon monoxide exposure. Chem Res Toxicol 10:1023-1031, 1997.
145. Jackson DL, Menges H: Accidental carbon monoxide poisoning. JAMA 243:772-774, 1980.
146. Buckley RG, Aks SE, Eshom JL, et al: The pulse oximetry gap in carbon monoxide intoxication. Ann Emerg Med 24:252-255, 1994.

INDEX

Note: Page numbers followed by f indicate figures; those followed by t indicate tables.

A

Abdomen
  disease of
    in sarcoidosis, 453
    pleural effusion with, 826-827
  surgery of, pleural effusion in, 827
  viscera of, metastases to, 356
Abdominal drainage tubes, complications of, 811
Abscess(es)
  hepatic, in *Entamoeba histolytica* infection, 309
  pulmonary, 226-227, 228f
    cavity wall thickening with, 126, 128f
    in anaerobic bacterial disease, 248, 249f
    in melioidosis, 243
    Klebsiella pneumoniae, 241, 241f
    Legionella pneumophila, 246, 247f
    Staphylococcus aureus, 238, 238f
  retropharyngeal
    acute mediastinitis and, 849f, 850
    upper airway obstruction with, 630, 630f
  retrosternal, 804, 804f
  subphrenic, pleural effusion with, 827
Absent diaphragm sign, 800
Accessory cardiac bronchus, 198, 199f
Acetylsalicylic acid (aspirin)
  asthma and, 650
  drug-induced lung disease and, 778
Acid maltase deficiency, ventilatory failure with, 918
Acid reflux, idiopathic pulmonary fibrosis and, 463
Acid-base status, 48-49
  in chronic obstructive pulmonary disease, 675
  in gastric aspiration, 747, 748, 750
Acidemia, 48
Acidosis, 48
  hypercapnic, in control of breathing, 79
  metabolic, 49
    in control of breathing, 79
  respiratory, 49
Acinetobacter species, 244
Acinus(i), 32
  capillary blood flow in, ventilation matching and, 45-47, 46f
  definition and structure of, 12-13, 23f
  development of, 54-55
  diffusion of gas from, to red blood cells, 44-45
  in emphysema, 666-667, 667f, 669, 672f, 673f
  perfusion of, 39-40
  ventilation of, 28
Acquired immunodeficiency syndrome (AIDS)
  bacillary angiomatosis in, 425
  epidemiology of, 423
  extrapulmonary tuberculosis and, 259
  Kaposi's sarcoma and, 394-396, 396f

Acquired immunodeficiency syndrome (AIDS) *(Continued)*
  lymphocytic interstitial pneumonitis in, 377, 378, 439f, 439-440
  lymphoma in, 438
  Pneumocystis jiroveci pneumonia and, 277, 278, 279, 280, 428-433
  pulmonary hypertension in, 440
  tuberculosis and, 425, 426, 427
    mortality and, 264, 427
Acromegaly, 216
Acrylate glues, liquid, emboli of, 573-574
Actinomyces species, 290-291, 291f, 292f
Actinomycosis, 290-291, 291f, 292f
  pleural effusion with, 822
Acute chest syndrome, in sickle cell disease, 565
Acute lupus pneumonitis, in systemic lupus erythematosus, 482, 482f
Acute respiratory distress syndrome (ARDS)
  acute interstitial pneumonia and, 470, 471
  aspiration pneumonia and, 748, 750
  cardiovascular tests for, 619-620, 621f
  clinical manifestations of, 617-619
  diabetes mellitus and, 216
  incidence of, 615
  microvascular thrombosis in, 543
  pathogenesis of, 615-617
  pathologic characteristics of, 617
  prognosis for, 620-621
  pulmonary function tests for, 619-620
  radiologic characteristics of, 617, 618f-620f
ADAM33 gene, allergy and asthma phenotypes and, 645
Adenocarcinoma
  fetal, well-differentiated, 401
  metastatic, 404, 405f, 406
    vs. mesothelioma, 837
  pathologic and histologic characteristics of, 343-344, 344f
  prognosis for, 365
Adenoid(s), hypertrophy of, airway obstruction with, 631
Adenoid cystic carcinoma, 372, 374f, 375f
  metastatic, 404f
  tracheal, 874f, 874-875
Adenoma, pulmonary, 374, 377
Adenomatoid malformation, congenital, 196, 196f
Adenosine deaminase, tuberculous pleural effusion and, 821
Adenosquamous carcinoma, pathologic and histologic characteristics of, 344
Adenovirus, 300
Adhesins, 236
Adhesion molecules
  in asthma, 645
  in Wegener's granulomatosis, 497

Adiaspiromycosis, 290
Adipose tissue
  embolism of, 565-567, 566f, 566t
    permeability edema and, 623
  in neck, obstructive sleep apnea diagnosis and, 639, 640
  neoplasms of, 399, 908
  pleuropericardial, 871
Adrenergic receptors, in lung muscle, 57
β-Adrenergic blocking drugs
  asthma and, 651
  lung disease and, 780
Adverse drug reactions. *See* Drug-induced lung disease.
Aerosol(s), inhalation of, 754-759
Age
  forced expiratory volume and, smoking and, 661f
  pulmonary carcinoma and, 338, 364
  pulmonary thromboembolic disease and, 543
  tuberculosis and, 250
Agenesis, pulmonary, 189, 190f, 191
AIDS. *See* Acquired immunodeficiency syndrome (AIDS).
Air, unconditioned, isocapnic hyperventilation of, in exercise-induced asthma, 649
Air bronchogram
  in bronchioloalveolar carcinoma, 349, 349f
  in radiation pneumonitis, 784, 787f
  of solitary pulmonary nodules, 349, 349f
Air crescent sign, in aspergillosis, 282, 283f, 286, 287f
Air embolism, 569t, 569-571
  arterial, 569t, 569-570
  clinical manifestations of, 571
  pathogenesis of, 569t, 569-570, 570t
  pathologic characteristics of, 571
  prognosis for, 571
  pulmonary (venous), 570, 570t
  radiologic manifestations of, 571
  systemic (arterial), 569t, 569-570
  venous, 570, 570t
Air excess, lung diseases causing
  general, 131, 131f
  local, 131-132, 132f, 133f
Air pollution
  asthma and, 650-651
  chronic obstructive pulmonary disease and, 662
  pulmonary disease and, 755
Air space(s)
  alveolar, calculi in, in alveolar microlithiasis, 213-214, 214f
  cystic, in diffuse interstitial disease, 115-117, 118f, 118t
  disease of, pulmonary hypertension with, 595